Imaging Atlas of Orthopedic Appliances and Prostheses

Imaging Atlas of Orthopedic Appliances and Prostheses

Editor

Thomas H. Berquist, M.D.
Professor of Diagnostic Radiology
Mayo Medical School
Chair, Department of Diagnostic Radiology
Mayo Clinic Jacksonville
Jacksonville, Florida

Raven Press New York

Raven Press, Ltd., 1185 Avenue of the Americas, New York, New York 10036

Made in the United States of America

Library of Congress Cataloging-in-Publication Data

Berquist, Thomas H. (Thomas Henry), 1945–
Imaging atlas of orthopedic appliances and prostheses/Thomas H. Berquist.
p. cm.
Includes bibliographical references and index.
ISBN 0-7817-0222-4
1. Orthopedic implants—Radiography—Atlases. 2. Orthopedic implants—Complications—Atlases. I. Title.
[DNLM: 1. Musculoskeletal Diseases—diagnosis—atlases. 2. Diagnostic Imaging—atlases. 3. Orthopedic Fixation Devices—atlases. 4. Prosthesis—atlases. WE 17 B532i 1994]
RD755.5.B47 1994
617'.0754—dc20
DNLM/DLC
for Library of Congress 94-20580
CIP

9 8 7 6 5 4 3 2 1

Past publications have been dedicated to my family—without their support my work would be unrewarding and incomplete.

In my career there have been three special people I have had the opportunity to work with and learn from. These individuals have served as role models throughout my career. They have challenged, cajoled, and encouraged me. I am grateful for the impact they have had on my life and career.

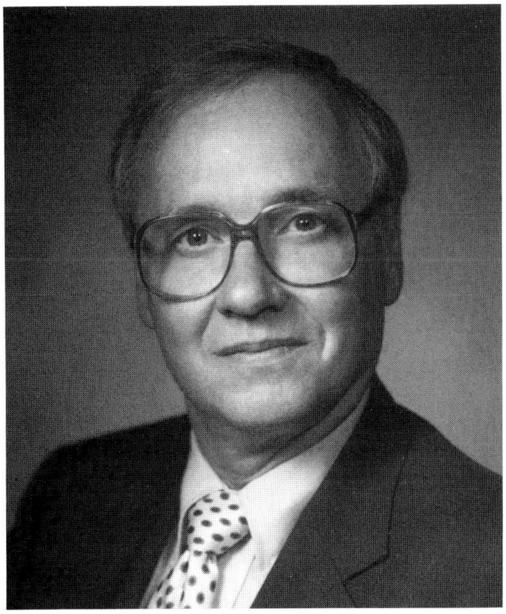

Robert R. Hattery, M. D.

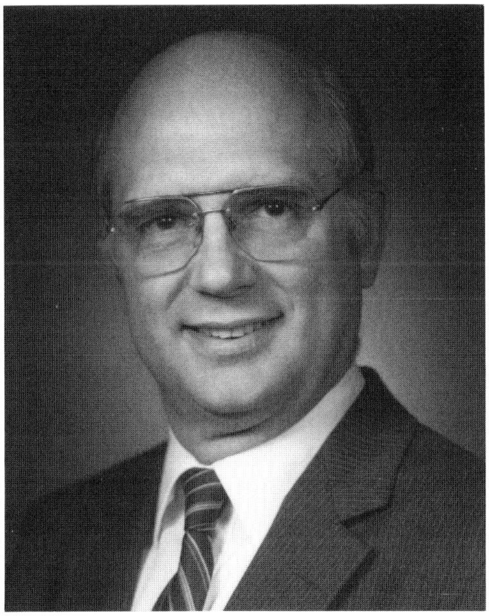

Glen W. Hartman, M.D.

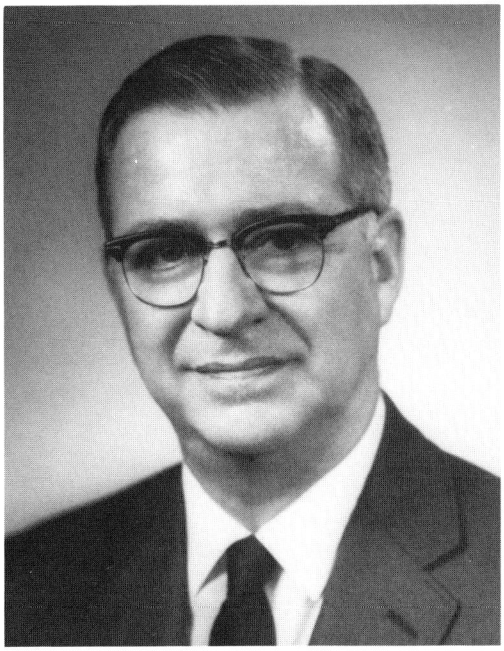

C. Allen Good, M.D.

Contents

Contributing Authors

Claire E. Bender, M.D. *Associate Professor, Mayo Medical School, and Consultant in Diagnostic Radiology, Mayo Clinic, Rochester, Minnesota 55903*

Thomas H. Berquist, M.D. *Professor of Diagnostic Radiology, Mayo Medical School, and Chair, Department of Diagnostic Radiology, Mayo Clinic Jacksonville, Jacksonville, Florida 32224*

Kurt E. Blasser, M.D. *Instructor and Consultant in Orthopedics, Mayo Clinic Jacksonville, Jacksonville, Florida 32224*

Daniel F. Broderick, M.D. *Senior Associate Consultant, Department of Diagnostic Radiology, Mayo Clinic Jacksonville, Jacksonville, Florida 32224*

Mark P. Brodersen, M.D. *Assistant Professor of Orthopedics, Mayo Medical School, and Consultant in Orthopedic Surgery, Mayo Clinic Jacksonville, Jacksonville, Florida 32224*

Bradford L. Currier, M.D. *Assistant Professor of Orthopedics, Mayo Medical School, and Consultant, Department of Orthopedic Surgery, Mayo Clinic, Rochester, Minnesota 55903*

Jon N. Dalton, M.D. *Instructor, Mayo Medical School, and Consultant in Diagnostic Radiology, Mayo Clinic Jacksonville, Jacksonville, Florida 32224*

James K. DeOrio, M.D. *Assistant Professor, Mayo Medical School, and Clinical Assistant Professor, USUHS, and Chair, Department of Orthopedics, Mayo Clinic Jacksonville, Jacksonville, Florida 32224*

Nolan Karstaedt, M.D. *Associate Professor, Mayo Medical School, and Consultant in Diagnostic Radiology, Mayo Clinic Jacksonville, Jacksonville, Florida 32224*

Harold B. Kitaoka, M.D. *Assistant Professor of Orthopedics, Mayo Medical School, and Consultant in Orthopedic Surgery, Mayo Clinic, Rochester, Minnesota 55903*

David G. Lewallen, M.D. *Associate Professor, Mayo Medical School, and Consultant in Orthopedic Surgery, Mayo Clinic, Rochester, Minnesota 55903*

Barbara L. McComb, M.D. *Consultant in Diagnostic Radiology, Mayo Clinic Jacksonville, Jacksonville, Florida 32224*

Mary I. O'Connor, M.D. *Assistant Professor of Orthopedics, Mayo Medical School, Rochester, Minnesota 55903; and Senior Associate Consultant, Mayo Clinic Jacksonville, Jacksonville, Florida 32224*

Jerald H. Pietan, M.D. *Instructor, Mayo Medical School, and Consultant in Diagnostic Radiology, Mayo Clinic Jacksonville, Jacksonville, Florida 32224*

Stephen D. Trigg, M.D. *Instructor, Mayo Medical School, Rochester, Minnesota 55903; and Consultant in Orthopedic Surgery, Mayo Clinic Jacksonville, Jacksonville, Florida 32224*

Preface

I have devoted much of my radiology career to working with orthopedic surgeons and trying to bridge the gap between that group and radiology. One area where this gap seems particularly wide is orthopedic fixation devices and prostheses. These devices continue to evolve, and there are constant modifications made in search of the "perfect implant." Radiologists have difficulty keeping up with these implant changes and the indications, image appearance, and problems associated with them. Simply stated, what does the orthopedic surgeon want to know?

This atlas was developed to answer that question with regard to orthopedic fixation devices and prostheses. Chapter 1 reviews imaging techniques with basic concepts on applications. Chapter 2 reviews general orthopedic devices that can be used in several anatomic regions. Chapters 3–13 are anatomically oriented and deal with specific fixation devices or prostheses used in a given anatomic region. Emphasis is placed on indications, preoperative and postoperative imaging and complications of implants used for trauma, joint replacement, and other common orthopedic procedures. The emphasis is on adult disorders, although pediatric problems are included in several chapters when implants used or procedures performed are common in radiologic practice.

Chapter 14 covers more custom-designed implants used for musculoskeletal neoplasms.

The atlas provides numerous examples of orthopedic fixation devices and prostheses with extensive references for those who wish further information about specific disorders and the surgical approaches to treatment. Because the variations available make it impossible to represent every possible device, we selected representative components used commonly in our practice and primarily in this country. This required borrowing a large number of examples from other authors and institutions to provide a more representative sample. Radiologists and orthopedic surgeons were involved in each chapter, which demonstrates the importance of communication in daily clinical practice.

The atlas will be most useful for radiology staff, residents, and musculoskeletal fellows. Other physicians who deal with orthopedic problems will benefit as well.

Thomas H. Berquist, M.D.

Acknowledgments

Preparation of this atlas was in some ways more difficult than writing an in-depth text because of the number of prostheses and fixation devices available. Representative radiographs and photographs or illustrations of the implants presented in this book could not have been obtained without the assistance of my orthopedic colleagues and representatives from the orthopedic equipment companies. The companies and representatives who provided support are the following:

Jerome T. Glickman, Ed.D. of AcroMed Corporation, Cleveland, Ohio; Michael A. Pentopoulos of Applied Osteo Systems, Inc., Walnut Creek, California; Joe Bend, Associate Distributor of Biomet, Warsaw, Indiana; Nancy June, Administrative Assistant of Danek Group, Inc., Memphis, Tennessee; Rod Kestler, DePuy-Moore and Associates, DePuy, Warsaw, Indiana; Karen Julian, Territory Manager of EBI Medical Products, Parsippany, New Jersey; Jim Rohl, Principle Agent, Bowers and Rohl, Inc., Howmedica, Rutherford, New Jersey; Robert Roche, Sales Representative of Intermedics Orthopedics, Inc., Austin, Texas; Mark DeBiase, Sales Representative of Johnson and Johnson Orthopedics, Raynham, Massachusetts; Bonnie L. Burns, Manager-Advertising of Joint Medical Products, Stamford, Connecticut; Link America-Waldemark Link GMBH and Company, Denville, New Jersey; Scott Johnson, Sales Representative of Linvatec, Largo, Florida; Ron K. Meridith, National Sales Manager of Mitek Surgical Products, Norwood, Massachusetts; Ron Chambers, National Sales Manager of Orthomet, Inc., Minneapolis, Minnesota; Ches E. Adams, Osteonic Distributor, Osteomedics, Inc., Allendale, New Jersey; Protek, A company of Sulzer medica, Berne, Switzerland, distributed by Intermedics Orthopedics, Inc., Austin, Texas; Andy Pettit, Sales Representative of Smith and Nephew Richards, Memphis, Tennessee; Lee Anderson, Spine Sales Specialist of Stuart Medical Inc., Greensburg, Pennsylvania; Distributor for Sofamor, Berck Sur Mer, France of Stuart Specialty, Inc., Spine Division, Greenburg, Pennsylvania; Karen L. McPhail, Marketing Support Manager of Sutter Corporation: Small Joint Orthopedics, San Diego, California; Mark Pickard, Authorized Representative of Wright Medical Technology, Arlington, Tennessee; and Jim Durrett of Zimmer-Wright Association, Zimmer, Warsaw, Indiana, and Sanford, Florida.

The department of photographics at the Mayo Clinic provided the quality radiographic prints for publication. John Hagen provided the excellent medical illustrations that demonstrate classifications and orthopedic procedures.

The manuscript, permissions, and figures were prepared by secretarial support from Cindy Franke, Laura Ulrich, and Rebecca Richmond. I thank them for their diligence and patience throughout this project.

Finally, I wish to thank Craig Percy of Raven Press for his assistance and support with this project.

Imaging Atlas of Orthopedic Appliances and Prostheses,
edited by T.H. Berquist.
Mayo Clinic Foundation © 1995.
Published by Raven Press, Ltd., New York.

CHAPTER 1

Imaging Techniques

Thomas H. Berquist, Jon N. Dalton, Nolan Karstaedt, and Claire E. Bender

Diagnostic imaging techniques are essential for the pre- and postoperative assessment of orthopedic problems. Preoperative imaging plays a significant role in planning the surgical approach and selecting the appropriate fixation device or prostheses. The evaluation of local bone and soft tissue injury and any associated trauma is essential. Multiple imaging techniques, including computed tomography (CT) and magnetic resonance imaging (MRI), may be necessary to support routine radiographic data.

The postoperative evaluation of fixation devices and prostheses can be even more difficult. Correct patient positioning, minimization of the metal artifact, and technical consistency are essential for optimal follow-up evaluations. Routine radiographs remain the primary method of evaluation. However, radionuclide scans, interventional procedures, and other imaging techniques play a significant role in patients with complications that are related to the orthopedic procedures. An understanding of the components, operative methods, and potential complications is essential for the proper selection and evaluation of imaging studies.

This chapter discusses basic concepts and principles of the imaging techniques used to evaluate orthopedic fixation devices and prostheses. More specific data is discussed in the anatomic chapters that follow because imaging approaches vary with anatomy and the types of devices used.

ROUTINE RADIOGRAPHY

Routine radiographs remain the most important screening technique for evaluating orthopedic problems.[1,2] Optimal equipment, consistent patient positioning, and appropriate chronologic labeling of radiographs are required for proper pre- and postoperative evaluations. Chronologic labeling is particularly important when multiple radiographs are performed on the same day (e.g., fracture reduction, operative positioning, and traction changes).[2]

Equipment and Screen-Film Combinations

An orthopedic radiographic suite should include a three-phase generator, a radiographic tube with a small focal spot (0.6 mm), and a four-way floating table. A wall bucky system is also required for standing radiographs and motion studies (i.e., lateral bending and flexion-extension spine views). Typically, a 48-inch target-to-film distance with a 16:1 grid is used for skeletal radiography. A 6-foot target-to-film distance is used for scoliosis and full-length lower-extremity standing views. We use TML film (Eastman Kodak, Rochester, NY) and Lanex fine screens for skeletal radiography.[2]

Fluoroscopic equipment is required in the operating suite and the radiology department. Portable C-arm fluoroscopic equipment is adequate for the operating room to document the placement of devices during surgery. In the radiographic suite, we prefer an overhead fluoroscopic unit (Fig. 1-1) because it offers more flexibility, better geometry, and easier patient access. Fluoroscopic positioning is essential for evaluating specific abnormalities, such as pin tracts, and for ascertaining that the components of a joint prosthesis are optimally positioned for imaging (Fig. 1-2).[2,3,5] The latter is particularly important for knee and shoulder arthroplasties.

Film Labeling

Radiographs must be properly labeled with the patient's name, registration number, date, and side (right

(text continues on page 3)

T. H. Berquist, J. N. Dalton, and N. Karstaedt: Mayo Medical School and Department of Diagnostic Radiology, Mayo Clinic Jacksonville, Jacksonville, Florida 32224.

C. E. Bender: Mayo Medical School and Department of Diagnostic Radiology, Mayo Clinic, Rochester, Minnesota 55903.

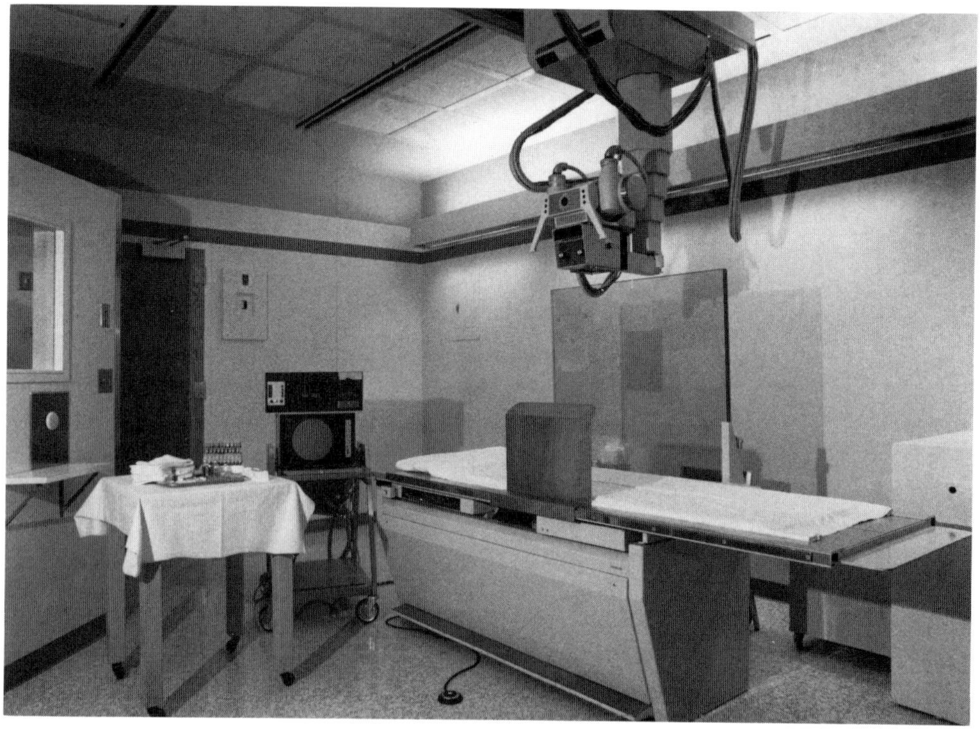

FIG. 1-1. Orthopedic fluoroscopic suite with overhead image tube and floating table top. A movable surgical table is used for interventional materials.

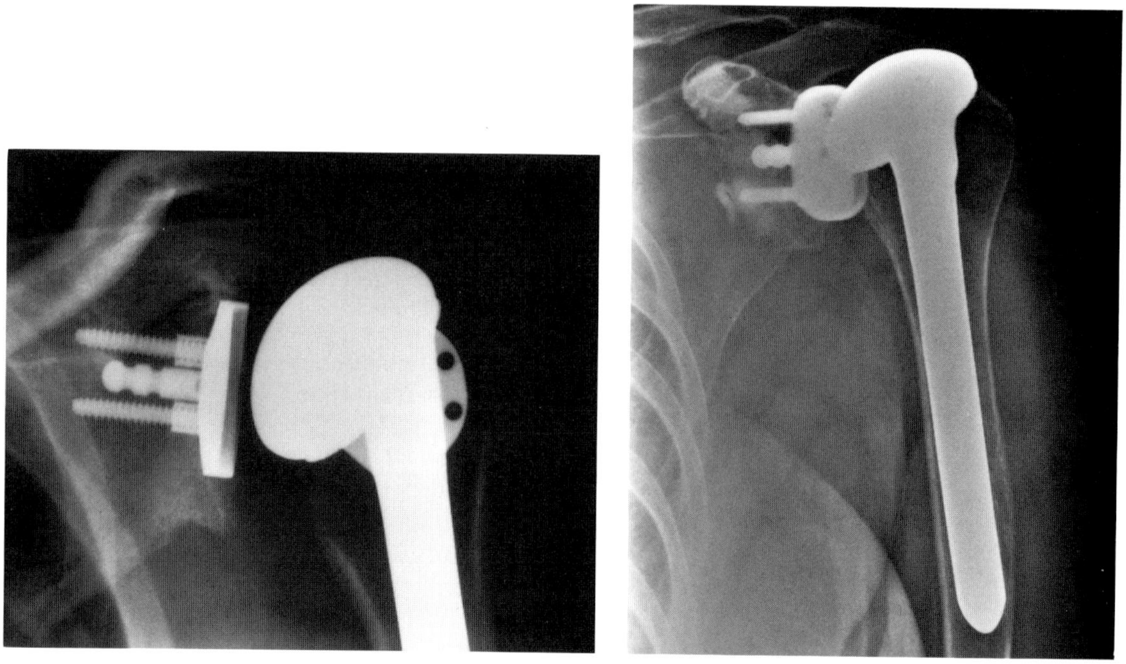

A B

FIG. 1-2. A: Fluoroscopically positioned view of the glenoid component of a left shoulder arthroplasty. The articular portion and fixation peg and screws are in perfect profile. **B:** Routine shoulder radiograph. The glenoid component is not optimally positioned on the film to evaluate the metal-cement or bone-cement interfaces.

or left). Multiple films on the same date are frequently obtained during fracture reduction or traction adjustment or when the components are being positioned for arthroplasty. These films must be numbered chronologically to document the process properly. We also label the films with the technologist's initials as part of our quality control process.[2]

Special radiographic views are discussed in anatomic chapters.

Conventional Tomography

Tomography is still a valuable addition to conventional radiography in certain situations. The detection of subtle abnormalities or the confirmation of suspicious areas on routine radiographs is useful preoperatively. Following surgery, metal artifact may create problems with CT and MRI.[2,4,5] In this setting, conventional tomography may still be an effective tool.

Conventional tomography allows improved detail of a specific body section to be obtained while blurring the structures above and below the selected plane.[2] The film and radiographic tube move in opposite directions during the exposure. Several motion patterns are available, including linear, circular, trispiral, and elliptical. Selection of the type of motion varies with the clinical setting. Complex motion provides the best image quality in skeletal radiography. Thin slices (1.5 to 3 mm) are commonly used. In the postoperative setting, other motion patterns may be sufficient or preferred (Fig. 1-3).[2] Routine radiographs should be reviewed and the type of motion and direction selected to minimize the metal artifact (Fig. 1-4).

CT

The role of CT in evaluating musculoskeletal disorders has expanded. Initially, this technique was primarily used to study musculoskeletal neoplasms.[8] However, CT can also provide valuable information in regard to other orthopedic problem areas, such as preoperative planning in patients with complex trauma or prior to joint reconstruction procedures.[6,7,9–15]

Equipment

The CT scanners use highly collimated x-ray beams, highly efficient detectors, and computer-image reconstruction and display to produce images that have superior contrast but slightly reduced spatial resolution compared with routine radiographs. The CT images are displayed in the axial plane but can be reformatted into coronal, sagittal, and three-dimensional displays.[7,9,11,12,15]

The scanning gantry contains the x-ray source, detection system, and couch for patient positioning. The patient typically lies on the couch and moves through the x-ray source and detectors. Although the gantry may be tilted a few degrees, the orientation of the system allows only axial images in most situations. Extremity positioning changes do allow direct sagittal or coronal images in some cases.[8] In a typical CT scanner, the x-ray tube moves through 360° during a single CT scan slice. The x-ray detectors take several hundred measurements as the tube rotates. In conventional scanners, one slice takes 1 or more seconds. New fast-scan systems use electron-beam CT scanning, allowing images to be obtained in about 50 ms. Dynamic images of the extremities can be obtained in this manner.[8]

The data from the x-ray detectors are processed by a computer that uses an algorithm to manipulate the data and reconstruct an image. The reconstruction time varies from 1 to 60 seconds. The computer divides the scanned area into a matrix of (256×256 or 512×512) small picture elements or pixels. The x-ray attenuation coefficient is determined for each pixel or square by applying the reconstruction algorithm to the data obtained by the detectors. Each square is assigned a CT number that is related to the attenuation coefficient (e.g., the CT number of water is 0).[8]

Because the x-ray beam has a thickness of approximately 3 to 13 mm in most scanners, the attenuation coefficient for each pixel thus represents a volume element or voxel. These factors can introduce an artifact, which is called a partial-volume effect, into the final image. This occurs when two or more structures with different attenuation coefficients are included in the volume scanned. This partial-volume artifact can result in significant errors. For example, a fracture line contained within the plane of the scanned section can be missed because it is averaged in with the rest of the bone in the voxel (Fig. 1-5).[8]

The reconstruction images are displayed on a console that allows the operator to manipulate the window width (i.e., the range of CT numbers in the gray scale) and the window level (i.e., the center of the gray scale) optimally to display either bone or soft tissue detail. In addition, the operator can obtain sagittal, coronal, and three-dimensional reconstructions of the scanned object by using computer reconstruction of the axial data (Fig. 1-6).[8,9,14]

Most CT scanners can also produce digital radiographs of any area of the body by moving the patient through the x-ray beam (gantry) and sampling at intervals from the x-ray detectors. These digital images are of lesser quality but can be useful for the localization of pathologic conditions to be scanned. In addition, accurate measurements can be obtained, which are useful for orthopedic problems, such as leg-length discrepancy.[6,13]

The x-ray dose delivered by CT scanning varies with a

(text continues on page 8)

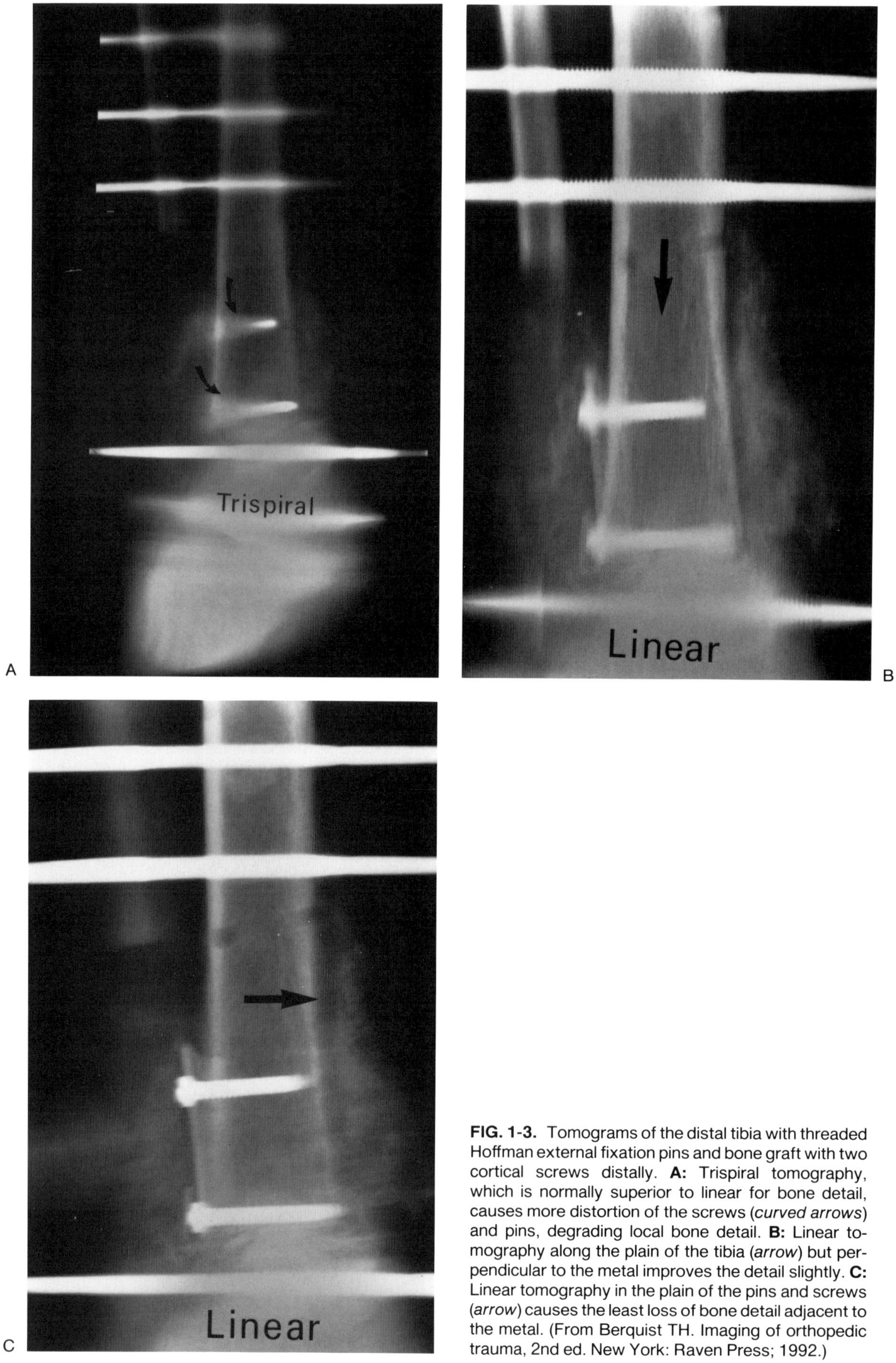

FIG. 1-3. Tomograms of the distal tibia with threaded Hoffman external fixation pins and bone graft with two cortical screws distally. **A:** Trispiral tomography, which is normally superior to linear for bone detail, causes more distortion of the screws (*curved arrows*) and pins, degrading local bone detail. **B:** Linear tomography along the plain of the tibia (*arrow*) but perpendicular to the metal improves the detail slightly. **C:** Linear tomography in the plain of the pins and screws (*arrow*) causes the least loss of bone detail adjacent to the metal. (From Berquist TH. Imaging of orthopedic trauma, 2nd ed. New York: Raven Press; 1992.)

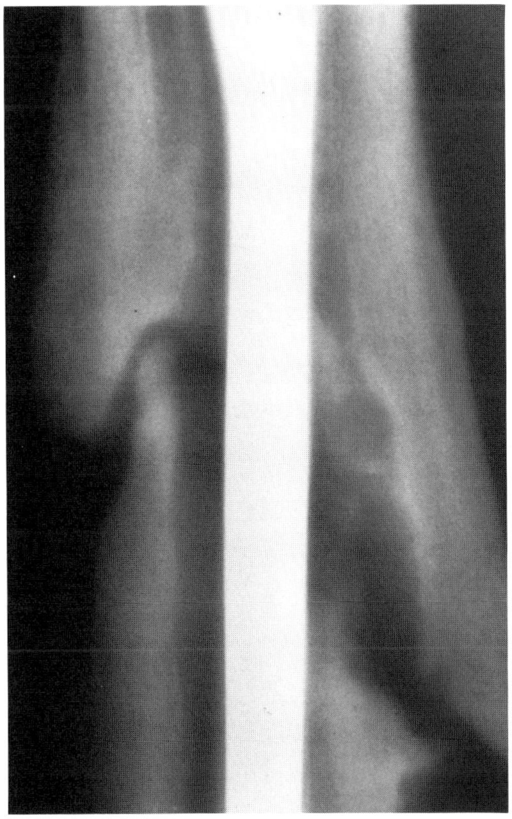

FIG. 1-4. Tomogram of a hypertrophic nonunion with medullary nail in place.

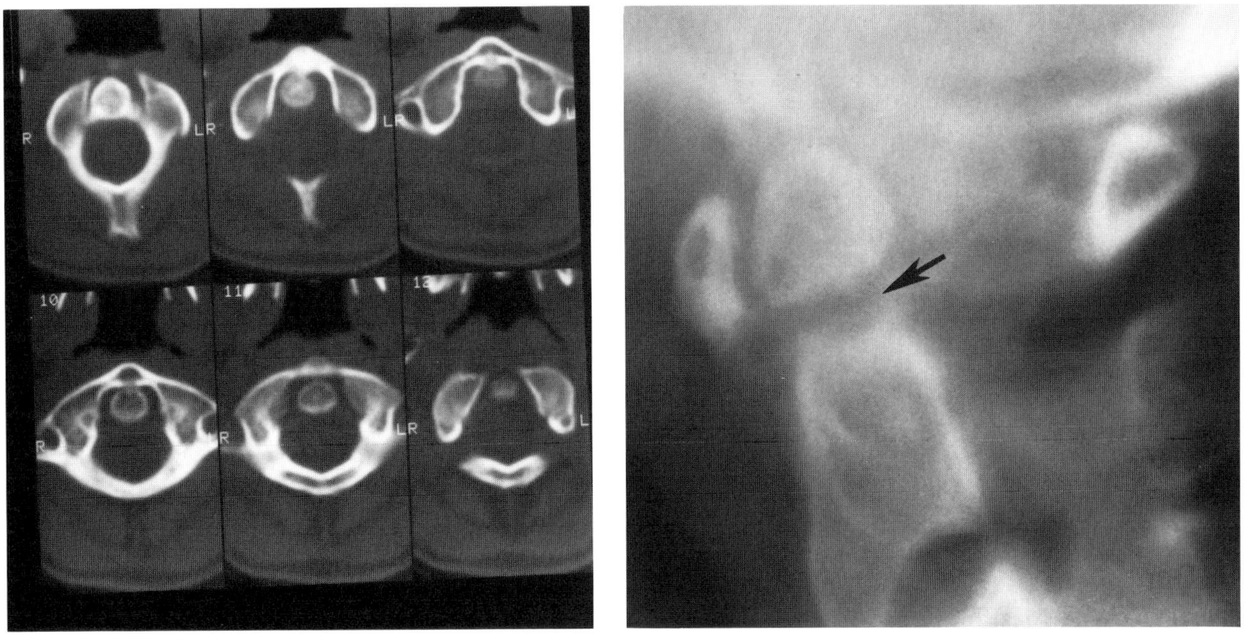

A B

FIG. 1-5. Type II odontoid fracture. The fracture line is in the plane of section on CT **(A)**, and the fracture was overlooked. Lateral tomography **(B)** easily identified the fracture (*arrow*).

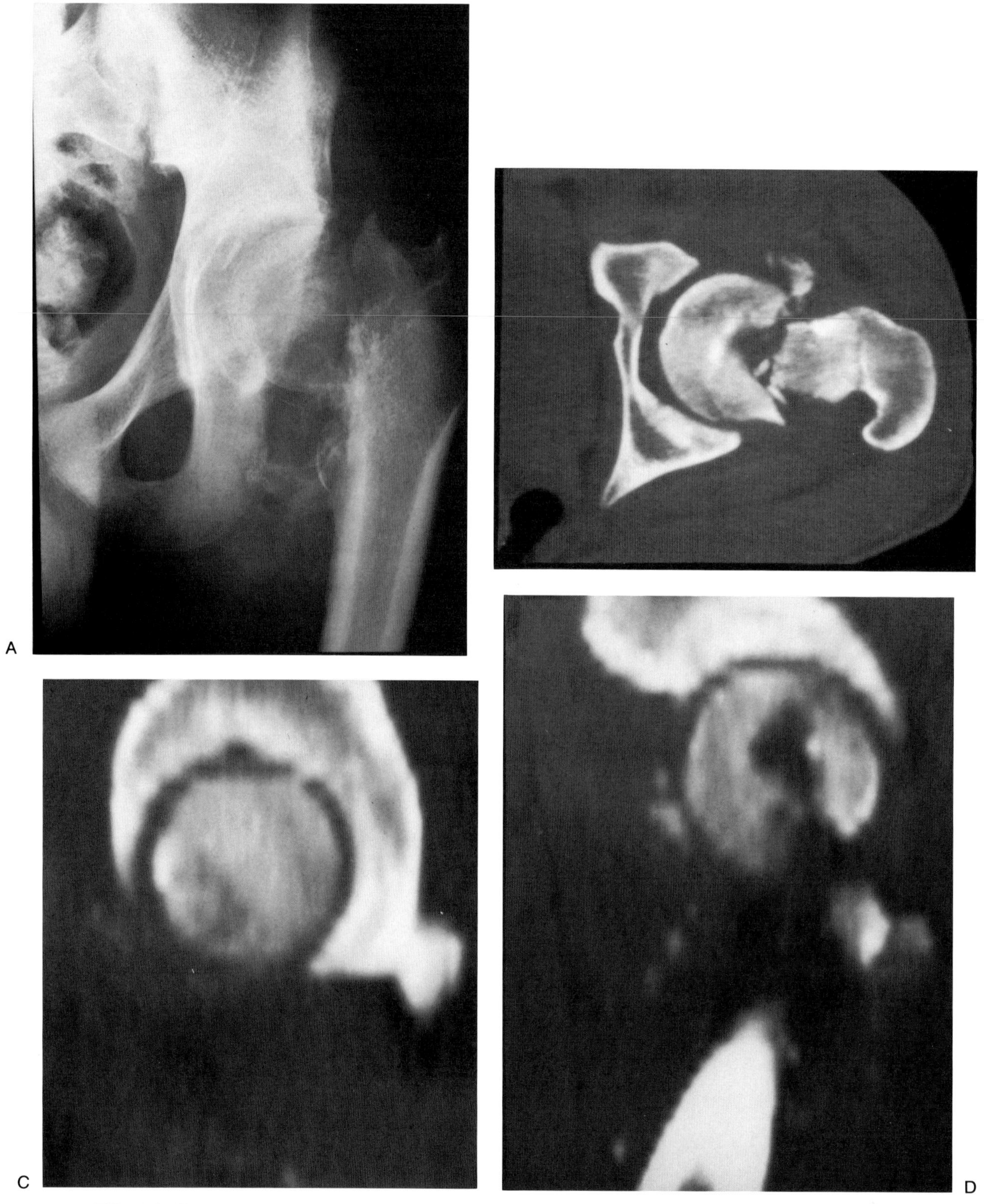

FIG. 1-6. Routine radiograph **(A)** and conventional axial CT image **(B)** of a complex femoral neck and intertrochanteric fracture. Images were reconstructed in the sagittal **(C,D)** and coronal **(E)** planes. Three-dimensional reconstructions **(F,G)** in different degrees of rotation may be useful and more easily interpreted for surgical planning purposes.

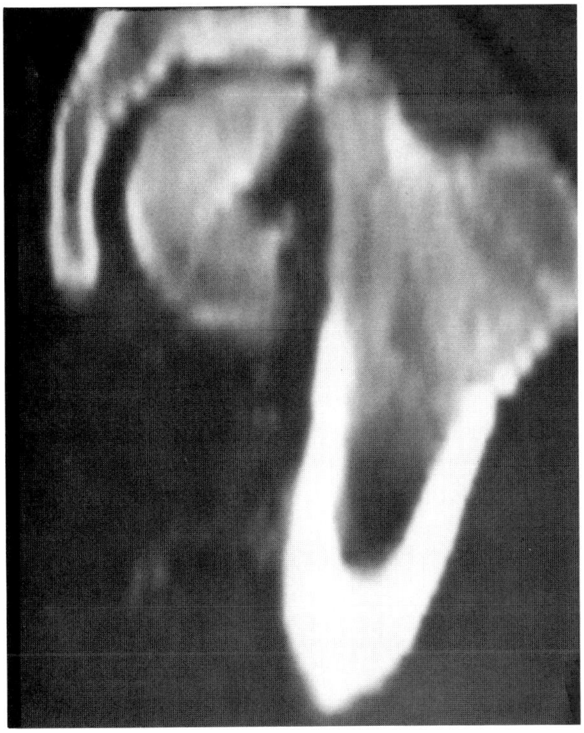

E

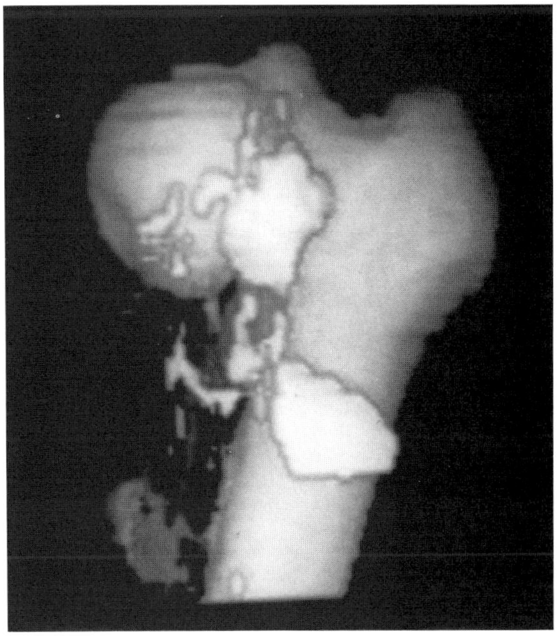

F

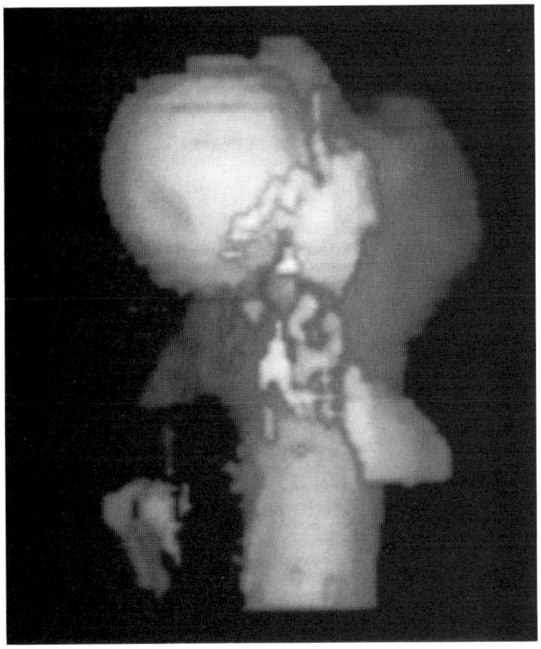

G

FIG. 1-6. *Continued.*

number of factors, some of which are related to the unit (e.g., kVp, MAS, and slice thickness) and some of which are related to the type of examination, such as the number of slices obtained and the degree of overlap of the slices. In general, the dose is greater than that for a single radiograph but less than conventional tomography of the same body part. The CT doses may vary from less than 1 cGy to greater than 10 cGy.[8]

Indications

We find that CT is a valuable technique in both the pre- and postoperative setting. Preoperatively, conventional axial or reconstructed (sagittal, coronal, or three-dimensional) images provide valuable information for planning the surgical approach for the orthopedic surgeon (Fig. 1-6). This information is particularly useful in areas of complex anatomy, such as the shoulder, spine, pelvis, foot, and hand and wrist.[8,9]

It is essential for the radiologist and orthopedic surgeon to communicate regarding the operative options so the CT examination can be performed optimally. Patient positioning, section thickness, and reconstruction needs must be considered prior to the examination. Normally, we use the bone algorithm for bone imaging. If reconstruction is required, thin sections (1.5-mm slices at 1.5-mm intervals or 3-mm slices at 2-mm intervals) are generally best to ensure optimal reconstruction images. In certain cases, 4-mm thick sections at 3-mm intervals are adequate for sagittal and coronal reconstruction. This format can be used to reduce metal artifacts in patients with orthopedic appliances or prosthesis.[7,9,11,12,15]

In the postoperative setting, CT may be less valuable because of the artifact created by metal components, screws, and other devices.[8,12,15] However, even in this setting, valuable information in regard to bone stock, marrow volume, and soft tissue abnormalities can be obtained. This is especially true if the metal is not immediately adjacent to the area of interest (Fig. 1-7). New reconstruction techniques are available to reduce the artifact in postoperative patients.[9,11,15]

MRI

The use of MRI is established for the evaluation of musculoskeletal pathologic conditions. It is frequently used for detection, classification, and staging of musculoskeletal neoplasms prior to therapy planning and soft tissue trauma.[19] It is also useful for evaluating the spinal canal and nerve roots, but MRI is less frequently used prior to other skeletal orthopedic procedures discussed in this atlas (see Chapter 14 for limb salvage techniques). In addition to preoperative studies, it is important to review certain basic principles, indications, and limitations of MRI as they apply to patients with orthopedic prostheses and fixation devices.[16,17–19]

Basic Principles

A complete discussion of the basic principles of MRI is beyond the scope of this chapter. However, certain basic concepts are important to review to understand the indications and limitations of MRI in orthopedic practice. The basic components of an imaging unit include a strong magnet (0.5 to 1.5 T), a radio transmitter, and a radio receiver. To obtain images, additional magnetic gradient coils are required to encode the signal and determine its origin in the object being studied. A computer controls the pulse sequences used to generate the images and reconstructs the data obtained.[19]

Most high-field MRI gantries are more confining than conventional fluoroscopic or CT units (Fig. 1-8). New mid- and low-field units (0.02 to 0.5 T) have shorter, more open gantries, which allow easier patient access. The gantry configuration and the presence of ferromagnetic materials in the patient and in the bulky external fixation devices or traction devices that are on the patient can preclude patients from having the MRI examination (Fig. 1-9).[19,21,23,25,26] Body coils are typically only 53 × 35 cm, which also limits patient size. In addition, most gantry tables do not function properly with patients who weigh greater than 285 pounds.[19]

The patient's clinical status must also be considered. When significant discomfort or inability to maintain necessary positions is a problem, the examination may be difficult to complete. Premedication with Valium™ (Roche, Nutley, NJ) or Demerol™ (Winthrop, New York, NY) may be useful in these cases. Initially, there was concern that severely ill patients requiring cardiac and respiratory monitoring might be difficult, if not impossible, to examine. Remember, ferromagnetic anesthesia equipment cannot be moved into the magnet room or near the gantry without affecting the images. Our experience shows that patients can be successfully monitored with proper equipment. Typical equipment includes a blood pressure cuff with plastic connectors, chest bellows for respiratory evaluation, and an electrocardiogram (ECG) telemetry system. The respiratory rate and ECG are monitored on a Saturn monitor. Generally satisfactory monitoring can be achieved in patients without affecting the image quality.[19]

Magnetic fields may affect certain metallic implants and electrical devices. In most situations, the exact chemical structure of surgically implanted materials cannot be determined.[19,20,22,24,25] Fortunately, early efforts to determine which implants are potentially dangerous to the patient[16–26] or may affect image quality have been successful. Synchronous pacemakers convert to the asynchronous mode when placed in a magnetic field.

(text continues on page 11)

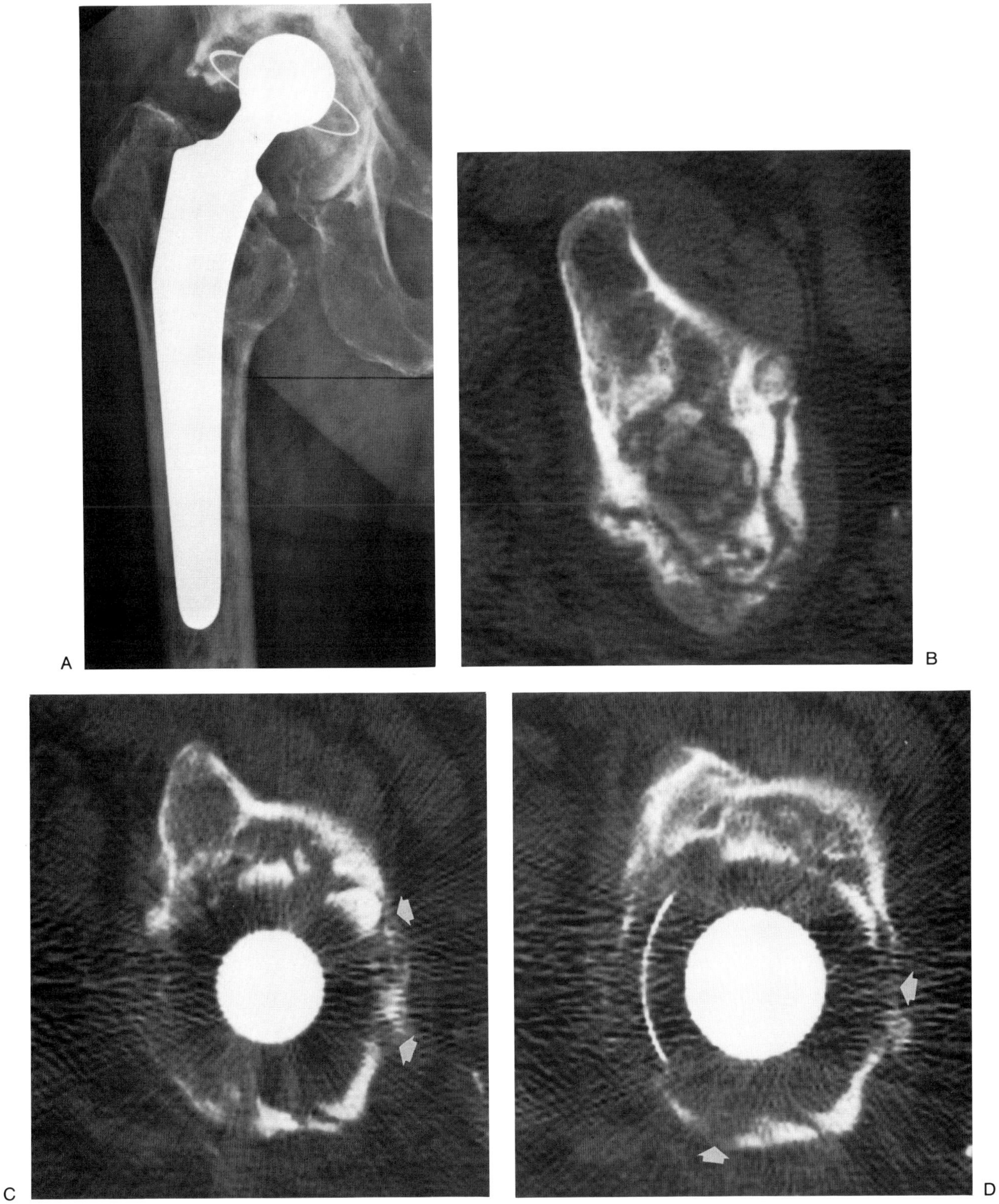

FIG. 1-7. A: Right total hip arthroplasty with loose acetabular component. The CT images through the acetabular region **(B–E)** are degraded to some degree by the metal artifact. However, the lack of adequate bone stock is clearly demonstrated medially and posteriorly (*arrows*) with multiple fractures.

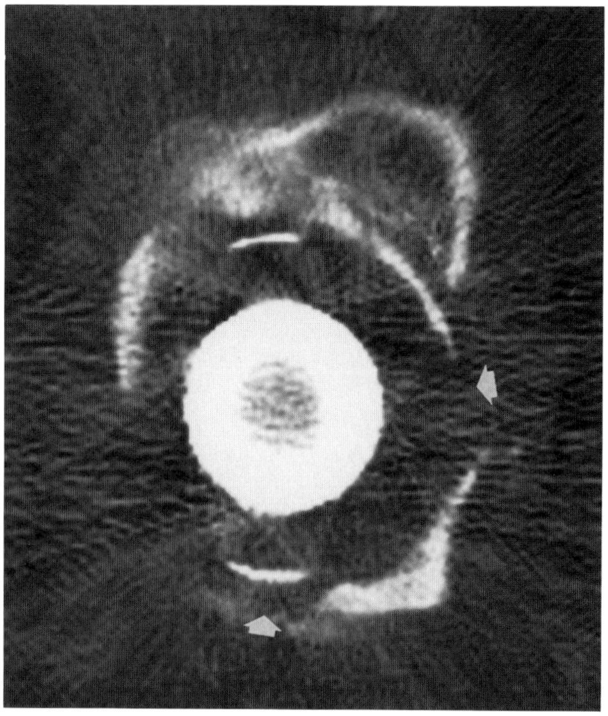

E

FIG. 1-7. *Continued.*

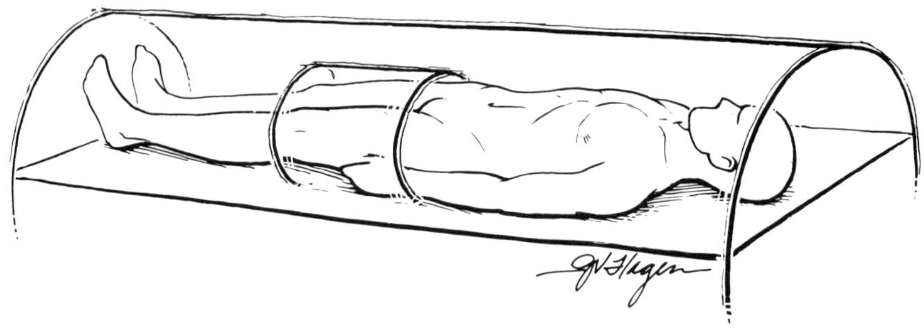

FIG. 1-8. A patient positioned supine in the MRI gantry with a body coil around the thighs. (From Berquist TH. MRI of the musculoskeletal system, 2nd ed. New York: Raven Press, 1990.)

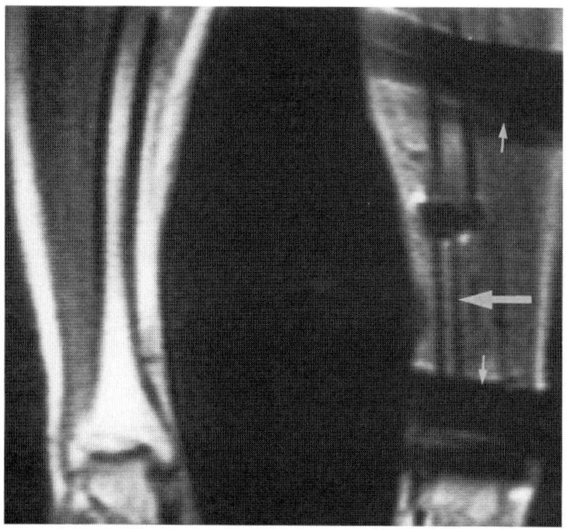

FIG. 1-9. Coronal spin-echo (SE) 500/20 images of the legs with an external fixator (Fischer) on the left. The fibular graft (*large white arrow*) is well seen. The external fixator obscures portions of the anatomy (*small white arrows*).

The pacemaker's power pack may also rotate in the magnetic field. In addition, significant degradation may occur if the power pack is in the region being examined.[21] Numerous heart valves and other metallic materials have been studied and artifacts created are negligible without significant risk to the patient.[21,25]

Most surgical clips at our institution are not ferromagnetic (Fig. 1-10). However, a significant number of aneurysm clips (approximately 75%) are ferromagnetic, and rotation can be demonstrated in a magnetic environment.[20] Therefore, patients with aneurysm clips or pacemakers are currently not examined by MRI.[19]

The manufacturers of most orthopedic appliances (e.g., plates, screws, and joint prostheses) generally use high-grade stainless steel, cobalt/chromium, titanium, or multiphase alloys. These materials are usually not ferromagnetic but may contain small quantities of iron impurities. All orthopedic appliances at our institution have been tested for magnetic properties, including heating. No heating or magnetic response could be detected.[19]

Metallic materials with ferromagnetic impurities can cause significant artifacts on both CT and MRI scans.[19,23] Nonferromagnetic materials cause areas of no signal but less artifact. The degree of artifact is dependent on the size and configuration of the metal (Fig. 1-11). When imaging a hip prosthesis, more artifact is created by the large irregular neck and head region than by the more regular and small femoral portion. There are also significant artifacts created by orthopedic screws, probably related to the configuration of the screw, its increased ferromagnetic impurities, and the fragments from the metal bits used for drilling (Fig. 1-12). Even these small amounts of ferromagnetic material can cause significant artifacts.[18,19] Early experience with metal implants at low and high field strengths (0.15 to 1.5T) shows that artifacts are more significant at higher field strengths (Fig. 1-13).[19]

An evaluation of patients with casts and bulky dressings is also possible with MRI without causing significant problems with image quality. Methyl methacrylate causes an area of no signal (black on MRI scans, Fig. 1-14) but no local artifact to interfere with image quality.

External fixation devices, although bulky, may not be ferromagnetic and can be easily checked with a handheld magnet prior to imaging (Fig. 1-9).

Patient Positioning and Coil Selection

Patient positioning considerations include the body part, the patient's size, and the expected examination time. Typically, the patient is examined with the most closely coupled coil possible to achieve the maximum signal-to-noise ratio and the best spatial resolution.[19] The knees, legs, foot, and ankle can be examined in the circumferential extremity coil or with flat coils (Fig. 1-15). Both are available with high-field magnets and should be used when they fit the clinical setting. With noncircumferential surface coils (flat or incomplete circle), the depth of view is limited. This can result in a loss of uniform signal in structures farther from the coil. As a rule, the depth of view of the flat coils is approximately one half the diameter or width of the coil. A larger head coil may be used when a comparison with the opposite extremity is required. More recently, dual coils have become available for the evaluation of both extremities simultaneously. Patients with casts, external fixators, or bulky dressings can usually not be examined with typical circumferential extremity coils. Head or body coils can be used in this setting.[18,19]

The position and course of the anatomic structures being studied must also be considered. The ability to obtain coronal and sagittal images does not necessarily mean that partial-volume effects are less significant than previously demonstrated with axial CT images. This must be kept in mind when evaluating the extent of disease processes in the coronal and sagittal planes. When possible, image planes should be chosen to fit the structure being studied. This may require off-axis oblique planes to evaluate these anastomotic regions best.[19]

Pulse Sequences and Imaging Parameters

The use of different pulse sequences (inversion recovery, spin-echo, partial saturation, chemical shift, and gradient-echo techniques) and many available echo time (TE) and repetition time (TR) selections at first seem cumbersome. However, current experience indicates that most musculoskeletal pathologic conditions can be evaluated with simple T1- and T2-weighted spin-echo sequences.[19] Short TE and TR spin-echo sequences are T1 weighted and can be performed quickly, providing excellent anatomic detail. Long TE and TR sequences are T2 weighted and are particularly useful for evaluating hemorrhage and other traumatic changes in the muscles, tendons, ligaments, and other soft tissues. More specific information regarding pulse sequences is presented in the anatomic chapters when the imaging evaluation of specific conditions is discussed.

Clinical Applications

The superior soft tissue contrast, multiple image planes, and excellent spatial resolution give MRI many advantages over other techniques in evaluating soft tissue, articular, and even subtle osseous pathologic conditions. Also, MRI is useful in evaluating conditions that may be associated with surgery, such as osteonecrosis and infection. The role of MRI is more limited following internal fixation or joint replacement. More specific applications are discussed in the specific anatomic chapters.

(text continues on page 16)

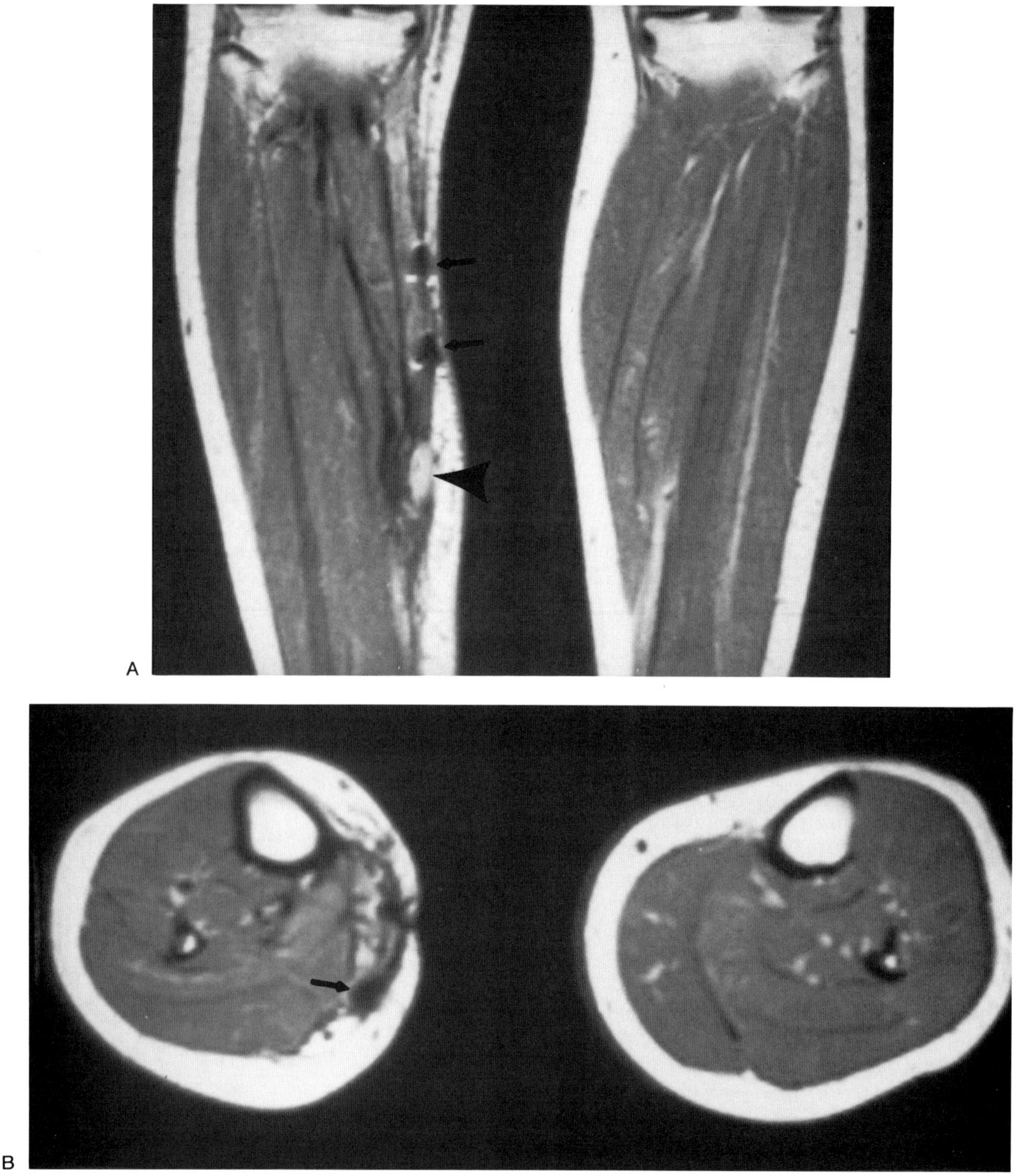

FIG. 1-10. Coronal SE 500/20 **(A)** and axial SE 2,000/30 **(B)** images of the calves after surgery with two surgical clips, which cause local image distortion (*arrows*). Recurrent tumor is visible distally in A (*arrowhead*).

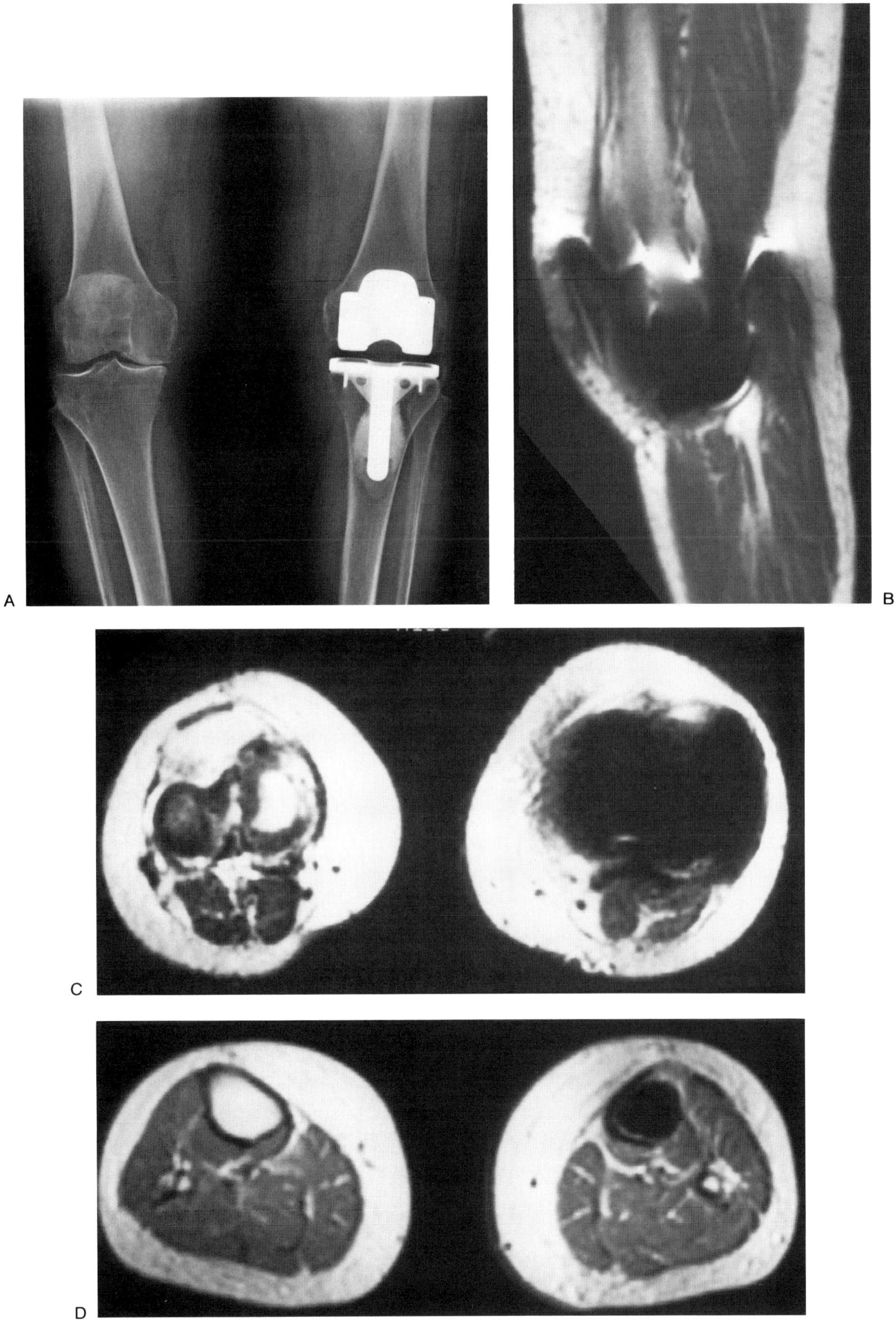

FIG. 1-11. Elderly woman with posterior knee pain and questionable soft tissue mass following total knee arthroplasty. Standing anteroposterior (AP) view **(A)** demonstrating the left knee arthroplasty. Sagittal SE 500/20 image **(B)** and axial SE 2,000/30 images **(C,D)** are degraded to some degree by the metal artifact. However, the soft tissue strictures adjacent to the knee are not affected significantly. No periarticular pathologic condition was identified.

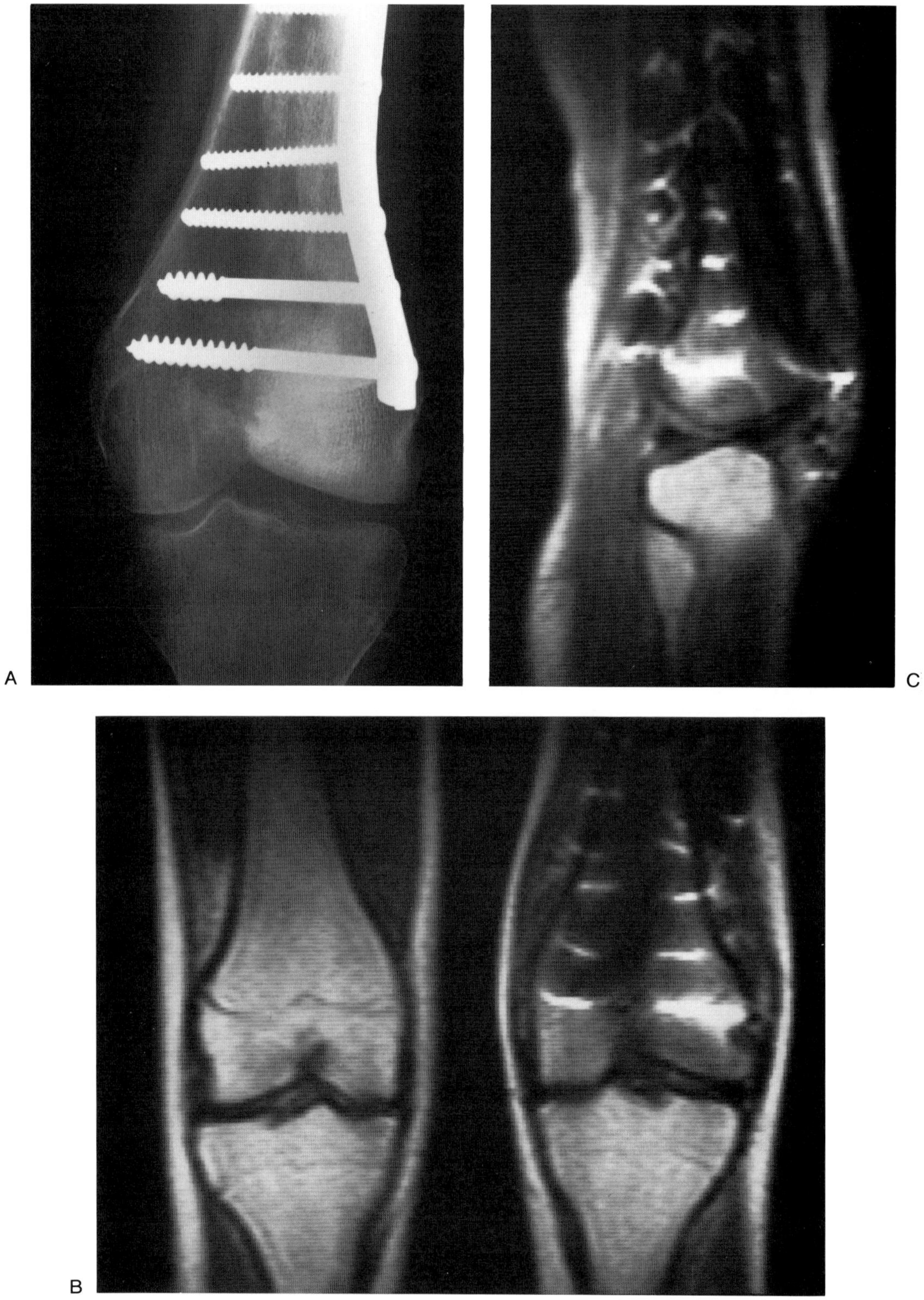

FIG. 1-12. A: An AP radiograph of the distal femur with compression plate and cortical and cancellous screws. The SE 500/20 coronal **(B)** and sagittal **(C)** images at 0.15 T show significant artifacts from the screws.

A 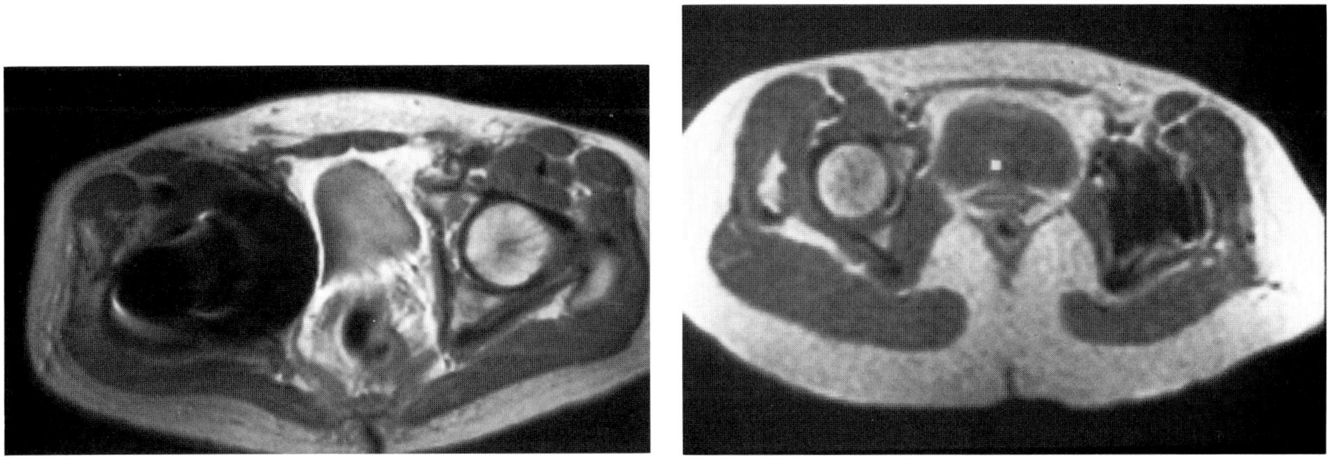 B

FIG. 1-13. Axial SE 500/20 images through the hips in patients with total hip arthroplasty. The artifact in the right hip at 1.5 T **(A)** causes more local image degradation than does the artifact in the left hip at 0.15 T **(B)**.

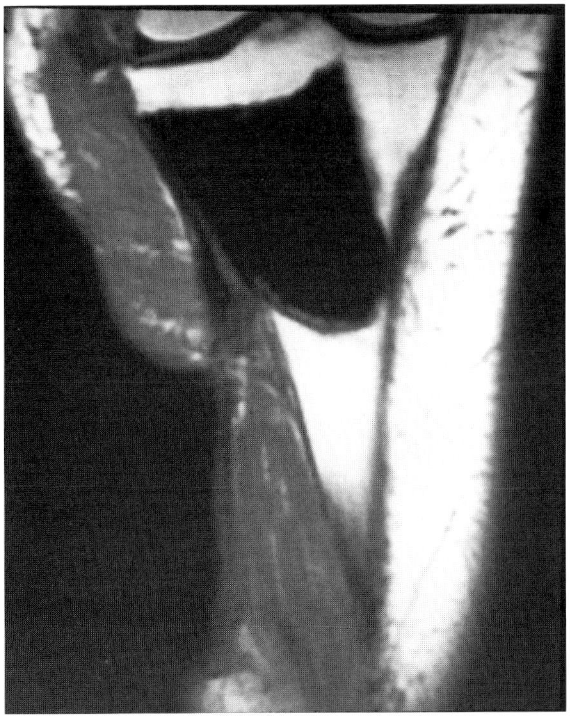

FIG. 1-14. Coronal SE 500/20 image of the knee in a patient with methyl methacrylate after curettage of a benign neoplasm. There is no signal in the region of the methacrylate but no adjacent image distortion.

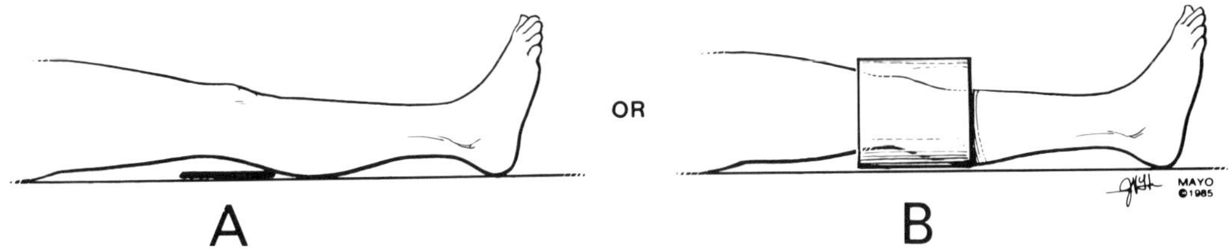

FIG. 1-15. Examination of the knee using a flat coil **(A)** and circumferential extremity coil **(B)**. (From Berquist TH. MRI of the musculoskeletal system, 2nd ed. New York: Raven Press, 1990.)

ULTRASONOGRAPHY

Ultrasonography is not commonly used for the pre- or postoperative evaluation of orthopedic problems discussed in this atlas (i.e., arthropathy, trauma, or prostheses). However, new techniques are evolving that may be useful for evaluating joint prostheses. Ultrasonography is commonly used to investigate the vascular complications related to surgery or trauma.[27,28,30,33,34]

Medical sonography uses frequencies in the range of 2 to 10 MHz.[28,35,36] Unlike CT, the ultrasound transducer can be positioned to allow the visualization of tissue interfaces in many different planes. This flexibility is valuable in demonstrating the continuity or discontinuity of adjacent structures.[28,36]

Doppler ultrasound techniques reflect changes in the frequency of moving structures. The most frequent application is the evaluation of blood flow and vascular patency in patients with arterial or venous (deep venous thrombosis) disease. Both compression and color-flow techniques are commonly used.[29,31,32]

Indications

The inability of sound waves to penetrate bone has limited this technique primarily to soft tissue disorders in orthopedic practice.[28] The most frequent early musculoskeletal application was distinguishing solid from cystic soft tissue masses.[28,31,32] A simple fluid collection, such as an uncomplicated cyst, is represented sonographically as an echo-free area; solid tissue or abscesses with cellular debris provide interfaces for sound reflection and are echogenic. Ultrasonography has also played a role in evaluating soft tissue trauma, joint effusions, arthropathies, and vascular complications related to trauma or orthopedic procedures. Postoperatively, its main role, in addition to vascular studies (Fig. 1-16), is to confirm effusions and assist in joint-space aspirations.[30,33,34]

RADIONUCLIDE IMAGING

Radiopharmaceuticals are used in musculoskeletal imaging (1) to assess pathologic conditions in bone and bone marrow and sites of inflammation or infection and (2) to evaluate painful prosthetic joints. Techniques for specific clinical applications have been developed based on the unique physiology of these radiopharmaceuticals.

RADIOPHARMACEUTICALS

Bone Agents

Technetium-labeled diphosphonate derivatives (Table 1-1), including methylene diphosphonate (MDP) and methylene hydroxydiphosphonate (HDP) are currently the bone agents of choice. Diphosphonates contain organic phosphate-carbon-phosphate bonds that are relatively stable *in vivo*. Both MDP and HDP have rapid blood clearance. Approximately 50% of the radionuclide is cleared by the kidneys and excreted in the urine, providing a high tissue clearance and an improved target-to-background ratio. This allows imaging within 2 to 3 hours following the injection in addition to imaging vascular and blood pool phases for the distribution of the radiotracer.[39,56]

Bone Marrow Agents

Technetium-labeled sulfur colloid (Table 1-1) is the bone marrow imaging agent of choice. These particles average 0.3 to 1.0 mm in size and are phagocytized by reticuloendothelial cells throughout the body after intravenous injection. Larger particles are sequestered by the liver (80% to 85%) and spleen (10% to 15%). Smaller particles reach the bone marrow (1% to 5%) and are phagocytized by resident reticuloendothelial cells. A higher dose, usually two- to threefold that of the dose administered in liver-spleen imaging is used to demonstrate the bone marrow.[56] In Europe, a small technetium-labeled colloid of human serum albumin (nanocolloid) has been studied. A much higher percentage of nanocolloid goes to the bone marrow.[55]

Inflammation and Infection Agents

Indium-111-labeled leukocytes (Table 1-1) is the agent of choice for imaging inflammatory and infectious processes in soft tissue or bone.[45,46,60,73,83] A specimen of the patient's blood is withdrawn, and the leukocytes are separated and labeled with indium-111 oxine. Oxine is a lipophilic ligand capable of chelating metallic ions, such as indium. The formed lipid-soluble complex diffuses through the leukocytic cell membrane. After it becomes intracellular, the indium separates from the oxine and binds to cytoplasmic components. The oxine elutes from the cell and is removed by washing the cells. The labeled leukocytes are injected back into the patient. Activity is seen in the lungs, liver, spleen, and blood pool. The disappearance of labeled leukocytes from the blood has a half-life of about 5 hours. The activity in the blood pool disappears within 18 to 24 hours. Imaging can be performed after this time, typically at 24 hours and, if necessary, 48 hours. Indium-111 has a relatively long physical half-life of 67 hours, enabling delayed imaging.[60,63,67]

Gallium-67 citrate (Table 1-1) is another agent useful in imaging of inflammatory and infectious processes, although it is less specific for infection than indium-111-labeled white blood cells.[38,41,64,65] After intravenous injection, gallium immediately binds to plasma proteins,

TABLE 1-1. *Radiopharmaceuticals for musculoskeletal Imaging*[57,60]

Radiopharmaceutical	Usual dose	Route of administration	Physical half-life (hr)	Time to imaging (hr)	Estimated dose (rads/mCi) Whole body	Gonads	Other	Remarks
Bone								
Technetium-99m diphosphonates	10–20 mCi (370–740 MBq)	IV	6	2–4	0.1	0.01–0.03	Marrow 0.1 Bone 0.02–0.07 Bladder 0.01–0.02	50–60% in bone at 3–4 hr, frequent voiding and forced fluids reduce bladder dose
Bone marrow								
Technetium-99m sulfur colloid	4–6 mCi (148–222 MBq)	IV	6	0.3–2	0.01–0.02	0.01–0.02	Liver 0.2–0.4 Marrow 0.02–0.03 Spleen 0.1–0.4	Localization: liver, 80–90%; spleen, 5–10%; bone marrow, 1–5%
Inflammation and infection								
Indium-111-labeled leukocytes	0.5–1 mCi (18.5–37 MBq)	IV	67	6–24	.4	0.4	Spleen 8.4–18 Liver 1.8–5	
Gallium-67 citrate	2–6 mCi (74–222 MBq)	IV	78	6–72	0.2–0.4	0.3	Kidneys 0.4–0.5 Liver 0.4–0.6 Colon 0.6–0.9	Accumulates in breast milk. Renal excretion first 24 hr. GI excretion after 24 hr
In-111 IgG	2 mCi (74 MBq)	IV	67	4–48				
Prosthesis loosening								
Gallium-67 citrate	1 mCi (37 MBq)	IA	78	1–24				

IV, intravenous; IA, intraarticular.

primarily transferrin. In general, 20% to 30% is excreted by the kidneys within 24 hours. After that time, the intestinal mucosa is the major route of excretion, although some is seen in the liver and biliary tract. Two thirds of the dose is retained in the body in the axial skeleton, liver, spleen, bowel, salivary and lacrimal glands, and external genitalia. It localizes in sites of inflammation and infection as a result of complex mechanisms involving the deposition of transferrin-bound gallium and the migration of lactoferrin-rich leukocytes. Like indium-111, gallium-67 has a relatively long half-life (78 hours), enabling delayed imaging.[64,67] Images are usually obtained at 6 and 24 hours. Delayed imaging may be useful for up to 72 hours.[64,67] Gallium-67 citrate is also useful in tumor imaging, but this topic will not be discussed in this section.[52,59]

Indium-111-labeled nonspecific human immunoglobulin G (In-111 IgG, see Table 1-1) is an investigative agent that has shown promise in the evaluation of inflammatory and infectious processes. Human nonspecific polyclonal IgG is conjugated to bicyclic diethylenetriamine pentaacetic acid (DTPA) and labeled with indium-111 chloride. A dose of 1 mg of IgG labeled with 2 mCi (75 MBq) of indium-111 is administered intravenously. Scintigrams are obtained at 4, 18 to 24, and 42 to 48 hours after the injection.[47,71]

Other Radiolabeled Antibodies

Antibodies labeled with radioiodine, indium-111, and technetium-99m have been under study for some time to evaluate neoplastic, infectious, and inflammatory processes. These agents are investigatory, and a detailed examination of them is beyond the scope of this text. In particular, one that has shown efficacy in inflammation and infection imaging is technetium-99m-labeled nanocolloid.[64]

TECHNIQUES AND SELECTED CLINICAL APPLICATIONS

Bone Imaging

Bone Scan

The patient is injected with 10 to 20 mCi (370 to 740 MBq) of technetium-labeled diphosphonate intravenously, and imaging is performed with a gamma camera 2 to 4 hours later. Whole-body or spot views, patient position, and the number of views depend on the indication of the examination. Routinely, single images require a preset number of counts, usually 500,000 to 1 million (Fig. 1-17).

Selected Clinical Applications
- Evaluation of primary or metastatic bone lesions[56–58,70]
- Evaluation of trauma, such as roentgenographically difficult fractures (Fig. 1-18)[50,69,74,88]
- Evaluation of battered children[54]
- Evaluation of bone pain[39,62,75,85]

Three-Phase Bone Scan

The injection is the same as for a routine bone scan, but imaging is begun immediately after the injection. Blood flow is observed in the first 60 seconds, followed by the blood pool observation 2 to 5 minutes after injection. Delayed images are performed at 2 to 5 hours after injection.

Selected Clinical Applications
- Evaluation of stress fractures[80]
- Differentiation between osteomyelitis and cellulitis[44,48,61,82]
- Determination of infarction or avascular necrosis[51,52]
- Evaluation of reflex sympathetic dystrophy syndrome[53,55]
- Evaluation of frostbite and peripheral vascular disease[66]

Bone Single-Positron Emission CT (SPECT)

This technique is added to the planar bone imaging by the previously described techniques to improve the detection of lesions. Delayed images are acquired on a gamma camera performing SPECT. The computer is used to reconstruct images in multiple planes. This requires extra time to image and process.[40,42,43,68]

Selected Clinical Applications
- Evaluation of low back pain, such as stress-related injuries to the pars interarticularis[49,74,81]

Bone Marrow Imaging

Bone Marrow Scan

The patient is injected with 10 to 15 mCi (370 to 555 MBq) of technetium-labeled sulfur colloid intravenously. Images are obtained with the gamma camera approximately 15 minutes after the injection. A lead shield can be placed over the abdomen to delete counts from the liver and spleen, thus allowing better visualization of the activity in the bone marrow.[56,64]

Selected Clinical Applications
- Define marrow distribution around joint prostheses in the evaluation of the painful prosthetic joint[71,72]
- Identify marrow replacement by a tumor[56]

Inflammation and Infection Imaging

Indium-111-Labeled Leukocyte Scan

A dose of 500 μCi (18.5 MBq) of indium-111-labeled leukocytes is injected intravenously. Imaging with a gamma camera is performed 18 to 24 hours later; 10-minute views of specified areas of interest or of the whole body are obtained (Fig. 1-19).[56,64]

Gallium-67 Citrate Scan

A dose of 5 to 10 mCi (185 to 370 MBq) of gallium-67 citrate is injected intravenously, and images of specified areas of interest or the whole body are obtained 24 to 72 hours after the injection (Fig. 1-20). Bowel cleansing and sequential imaging may help in the interpretation of abdominal activity.[67]

In-111 IgG Scan

A dose of approximately 1 mg of IgG labeled with 2 mCi (75 MBq) of indium-111 is injected intravenously. Imaging is performed with a gamma camera at 4, 18 to 24, and 42 to 48 hours after the injection with a preset time of 10 minutes per view.[71]

Selected Clinical Applications
- Evaluation of osteomyelitis, musculoskeletal sepsis, or abscess with
  - In-111-labeled leukocytes (Fig. 1-19)[73,77,83,84]
  - Gallium-67 citrate (Fig. 1-20)[82,84,86]
  - In-111 IgG[46,71,79,83]
- Evaluation of prosthetic joint infection with
  - In-111-labeled leukocytes[60,65,73,76]
  - Gallium-67 citrate[65]
  - In-111 IgG[71]

Scintigraphic Arthrography

The study involves intraarticular injection of 1 mCi (37 MBq) of gallium-67 citrate, 100 μCi (3.7 MBq) of indium-111 chloride, or 100 μCi (3.7 MBq) indium-111-labeled DTPA. Gallium-67 citrate is preferred because of its widespread availability, low cost, and favorable dosimetry calculations for intraarticular injection. This is generally combined with radiographic iodine contrast arthrography to demonstrate the anatomy better. At the time of contrast arthrography, a localization film with contrast is obtained. With the needle correctly positioned in the joint space, 1 mCi (37 MBq) of gallium-67 citrate is injected and flushed with the remaining contrast material. The contrast arthrogram is completed, and then 10-minute-per-view images are obtained with a gamma camera at 1 hour and 18 to 24 hours postinjec-

(text continues on page 22)

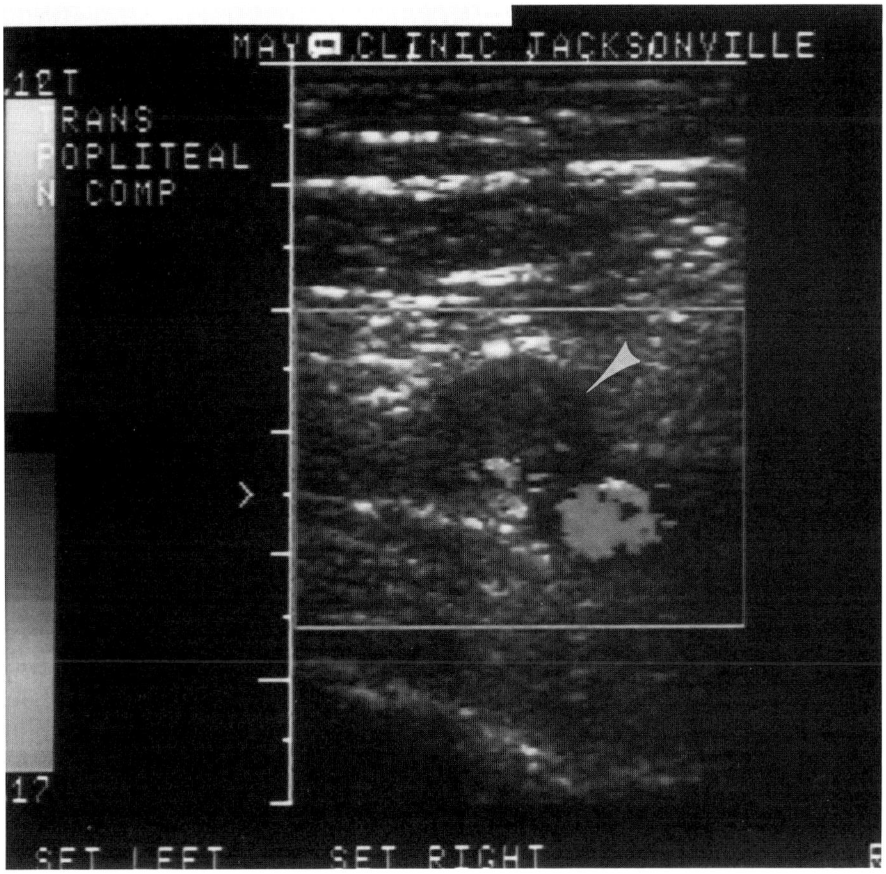

FIG. 1-16. Transverse sonogram of the femoral vein demonstrating thrombosis (*arrow*) in a patient with recent total knee arthroplasty.

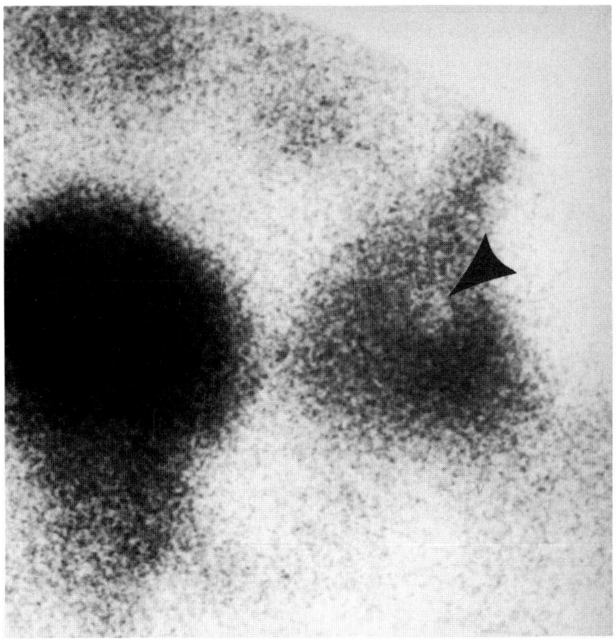

FIG. 1-17. Technetium-99m MDP scan of the pelvis and hips. There is a photopenic area in the left femoral head (*arrow*) caused by early avascular necrosis.

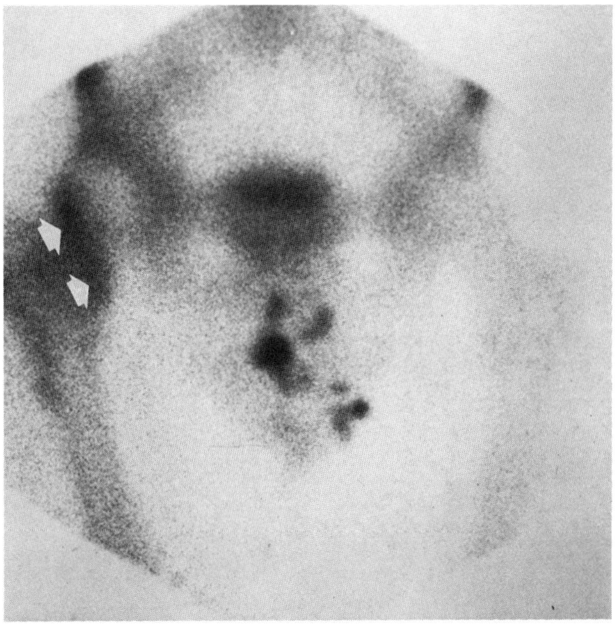

FIG. 1-18. Technetium-99m MDP scan of the pelvis and hips with a linear area of increased uptake (*arrows*) caused by a femoral neck fracture. The femoral head activity is diminished as a result of surgically confirmed avascular necrosis.

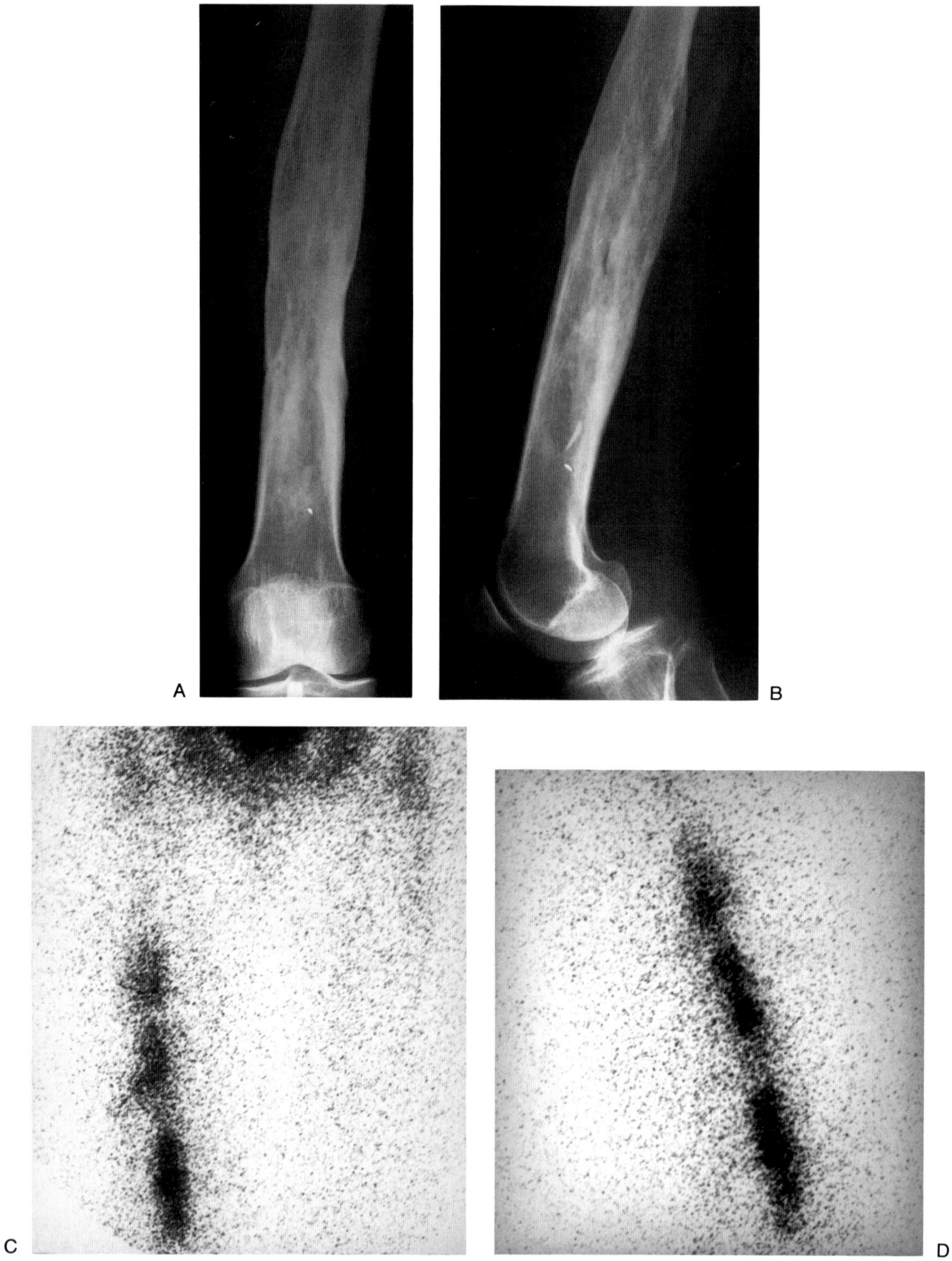

FIG. 1-19. Old fracture of the femur with removal of fixation device. Questionable active infection 6 months later. The AP **(A)** and lateral **(B)** radiographs show the fracture deformity with areas of sclerosis and lucency in the distal femur. The AP **(C)** and lateral **(D)** indium-111-labeled leukocyte images demonstrate extensive marrow uptake as a result of osteomyelitis.

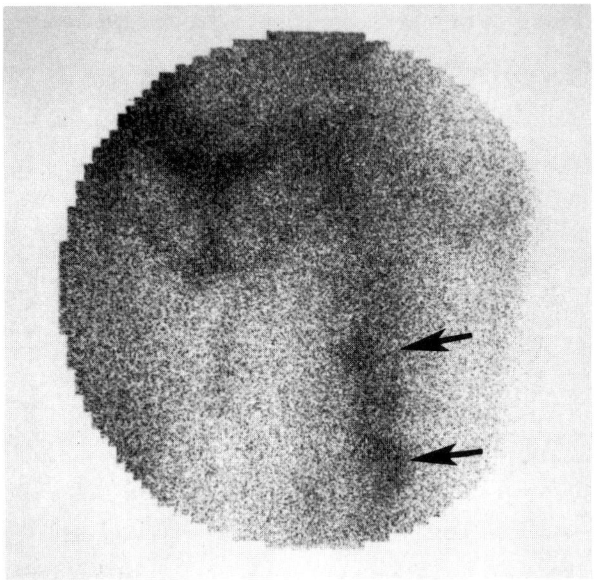

FIG. 1-20. A 48-hour gallium-67 image of the left hip in a patient with hip arthroplasty and questionable infection. There is increased uptake along the distal femoral component (*arrows*) as a result of loosening and infection.

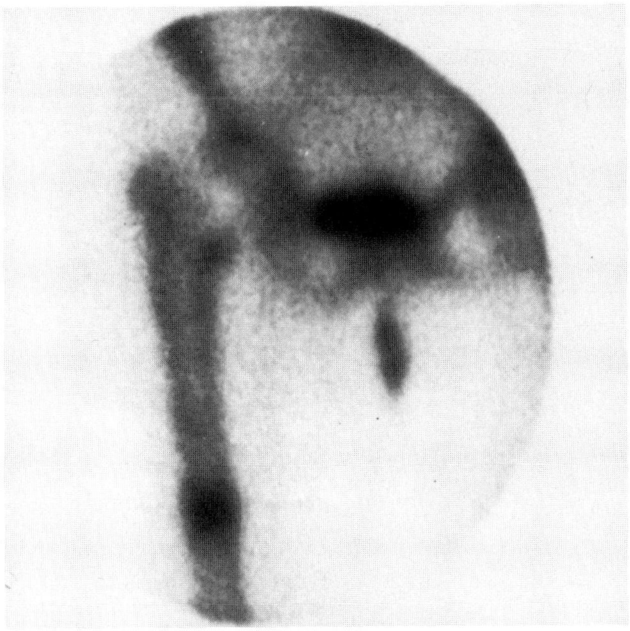

A

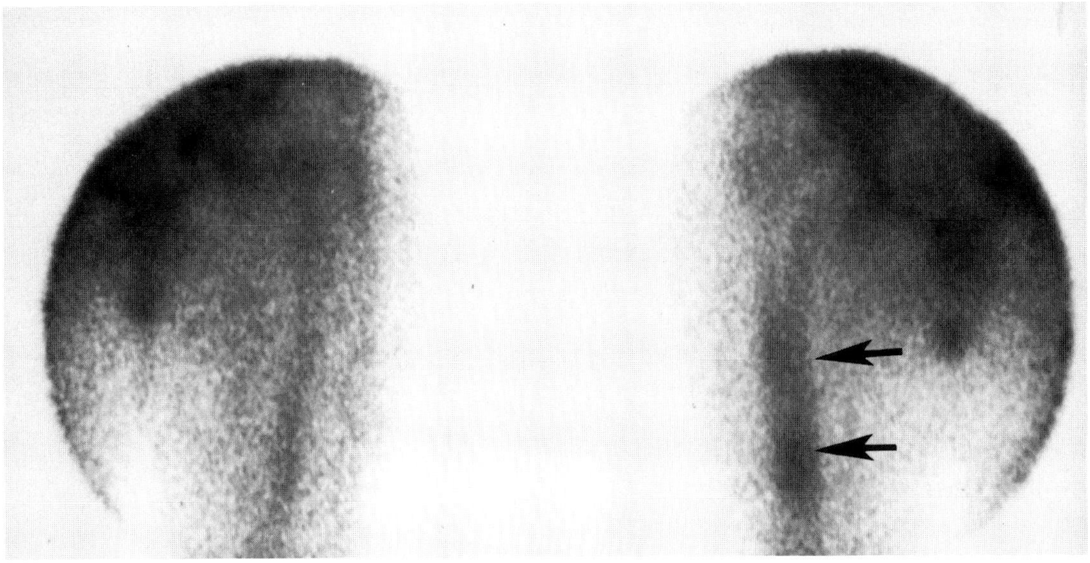

B

FIG. 1-21. Right total hip arthroplasty with suspected infection. **A:** Technetium-99m MDP scan shows uptake around both the femoral and acetabular components (especially at the femoral tip), indicating loosening. **B:** Indium-111-labeled leukocyte scan shows incongruent femoral uptake (*arrows*), indicating infection.

tion. Patients are encouraged to walk or exercise normally prior to delayed imaging.[37,78,89]

Selected Applications
- Evaluation of painful joint prosthesis[63,78,87]
- Detection of dissecting popliteal cysts versus thrombophlebitis[37]

Combined Techniques

Several of the mentioned procedures and other radiographic imaging procedures may be combined to study particular problems to improve the sensitivity and specificity of the detection of pathologic conditions. These techniques are examined in more detail in subsequent anatomic chapter discussions.

Selected Clinical Applications
- Evaluation of the failed hip prosthesis[37,45,63,65,73,76,78,87,89]
  For example: plain films of the affected prosthetic hip are performed to evaluate roentgenographic signs of loosening or infection. If these are questionable or negative, a combined radionuclide study with indium-111-labeled leukocytes and technetium-99m sulfur colloid is performed to detect possible loosening or infection. Identical images from each study are compared to reduced false-positive findings caused by marrow clumping because of previous surgery. If there is an incongruity in the increased indium-111 activity, this supports the diagnosis of an infection (Fig 1-21). If the results are negative or nondiagnostic, fluoroscopic hip aspiration can be performed to increase the sensitivity for finding an infection. This may be combined with a contrast/scintigraphic arthrogram study to evaluate for component loosening.[41]
- Evaluation of suspected osteomyelitis[38,59,82,84,86] For example: Plain films, technetium-99m diphosphonate, and indium-111-labeled leukocytes or gallium-67 citrate scans, and/or MRI findings may be compared to increase the sensitivity and specificity of the detection of osteomyelitis.[41]

INTERVENTIONAL PROCEDURES

Interventional imaging techniques are used preoperatively to localize symptoms and define the anatomy. Postoperatively, these techniques are useful to evaluate potential complications of orthopedic procedures. The techniques used vary with the anatomy and suspected clinical problem. Therefore, specific approaches are discussed in later chapters. However, certain basic concepts are presented here to avoid redundancy in later anatomic chapters.

Arthrography and Diagnostic and/or Therapeutic Injections

The technique of MRI has replaced conventional arthrography in many situations, especially in the knee and shoulder. Conventional arthrography with anesthetic injection may still be useful to assess joint anatomy and capsule size and to clarify the site of symptoms. Arthrography also provides a method for fluid analysis, specifically for the detection of infection.[92–95]

We most commonly perform arthrography or diagnostic injections to define the site of symptoms, check for possible infections, or localize causes of pain following orthopedic procedures.[94] Table 1-2 summarizes the locations and common indications for arthrography and the diagnostic/therapeutic injections in our practice.

Most diagnostic injections are performed with fluoroscopic guidance. The joint or structure to be studied can be optimally positioned to allow direct entry with the needle and minimize the risk of entering vascular or neural structures.[94,108] On occasion, ultrasound guidance may be used.[94]

TABLE 1-2. *Arthrography and diagnostic/therapeutic injections*[92–95]

Location	Indications
Spine	Facet syndrome
	Painful instrumentation (i.e., hooks on rod systems)
	Discograms
Shoulder (Figs. 1-22 and 1-23)	Rotator cuff tears
	Adhesive capsulitis
	Acromioclavicular joint pain
	Subacromial bursitis
	Aspirate calcium deposits
Elbow (Figs. 1-24 to 1-26)	Capsular tears
	Loose bodies
	Bursitis
Hand and wrist (Figs. 1-27 and 1-28)	Ligament tears
	Triangular fibrocartilage tears
	Tendinitis (tendon sheath injections)
	Localize joint symptoms
Pelvis and hips (Fig. 1-29)	Synovial chordromatosis
	PVNS
	Labral tears
	Bursitis
	Snapping iliopsoas tendon
	Sacroiliac pain or instability
	Pubic symphysis pain or instability
Knee (Fig. 1-30)	Evacuate effusion or hemarthrosis
	Proximal tibiofibular joint pain
Foot and ankle (Figs. 1-31 to 1-34)	Ligament tears
	Tendon tears
	Tendinitis
	Localize joint symptoms

PVNS, pigmented villonodular synovitis.

The injection set is devised to accommodate arthrograms, injections, aspirations, and biopsies. An overhead fluoroscopic table (Fig. 1-1) is used for most patients.[91] The procedure tray includes the following items: four sterile drapes, one sterile drape with a central 4-inch hole, six absorbent 6 × 6 gauze sponges, one 5-ml syringe, two 10-ml syringes, one 30-ml syringe, one cup for contrast material, and extension tubing. A needle box is kept in the room. This contains 22- and 18-gauge spinal needles, 1.5-inch 18- to 22-gauge needles, ⅝-inch 25-gauge needles, fine Chiba needles, and biopsy needles. The needle selected varies with the region being studied and the patient's size.[92,93]

Additional items include vials of nonbacteriostatic saline for joint aspiration and irrigation, culture bottles for aerobic and anaerobic bacterial or fungal studies, specimen tubes for synovial fluid analysis, and 1% Xylocaine™ (Astra, Westborough, MA). Celestone™ (Schering, Kenilworth, NJ) and 0.25% Marcaine™ (Sanofi Winthrop, New York, NY) are stocked for diagnostic and therapeutic injections. An additional necessity is an emergency cart in case of contrast medium reactions or other unforeseen emergencies.[92,93]

Specific injection sites and positioning are demonstrated in Figures 1-22 through 1-34. Facet injections and discograms are discussed more completely.

Facet Injections

Injections of the facet joints are most frequently performed in the lumbar spine. This technique is equally useful for preoperative planning and for evaluating symptoms postoperatively.[93,94,96–100]

A brief review of anatomy is essential for understanding this procedure. The anatomic position and alignment of cervical and thoracic facets does not permit easy entry. The lumbar facet joints become more lateral and obliquely oriented as one moves from L-1 inferiorly. The normal facet joint is 2 to 3 mm in width when properly aligned fluoroscopically (Fig. 1-35). Facet joints are true synovial joints surrounded by a fibrous capsule. Innervation (Fig. 1-36) from the posterior rami occurs through the medial branch, which courses through a notch at the base of the transverse process at the inferior margin of the facet joint at that level. A branch from this nerve continues inferiorly to innervate the superior facet joint one level below. Therefore, each posterior ramus innervates two facet joints. This must be taken into consideration when determining the levels for injection.[93,98–100,113]

Indications

Facet injections are performed on patients with suspected facet syndrome.[93,94,100] These patients typically present with low-back pain, which may radiate to the gluteal region or down the leg. Disc protrusion must be excluded. Generally, patients have had MRI examinations, myelograms, or electromyography prior to requesting facet injection. Facet injections in this setting are controversial.[100]

In our practice, we most commonly perform facet injection to localize symptoms prior to lumbar fusion or in postoperative patients with degenerative facet disease following fusion (Fig. 1-37) or laminectomy (Fig. 1-38).[92,94]

Technique

Before performing facet injections, it is important to review the routine radiographs to assess the articulations and determine if they can be entered. In addition, CT scans may be required in certain cases in which severe degeneration or osteophytes may not allow needle entry (Fig. 1-39).

The patient is positioned prone on the fluoroscopic table. Following the sterile preparation of the injection sites, the patient is carefully rotated to allow the proper alignment of the facet to be injected. A slight position change is usually necessary for each facet. Local anesthetic is injected over the entry site. The facet is usually entered with a 22-gauge spinal needle. The capsule can be palpated with the needle tip and its position confirmed with the injection of a small amount of contrast medium. A complete arthrogram is generally not required (Fig. 1-40).[93,97,100] For purely diagnostic purposes, such as preoperatively, we inject approximately 1 ml of Marcaine™. This anesthetic is longer acting than Xylocaine™ and gives the patient more time to reflect on symptomatic improvement. For therapeutic purposes, we inject Marcaine™ with Celestone™ in a 2:1 mixture.[92]

Discography

Discography was first reported in the 1940s and, although useful, has remained somewhat controversial over the years.[104,105] It does, however, play a useful role in the morphologic assessment of the intervertebral disc, and it is complemented by inducing pain that is similar to the patient's symptoms when the level injected is abnormal.[104,106,107,111,118] Combined CT and discography is reported to be particularly useful in evaluating lumbar disorders.[104,111,112,116]

Indications

The indications for discography fall into four general categories: (1) localization of the symptomatic level in degenerative disc disease, (2) localization of symptom-

(text continues on page 37)

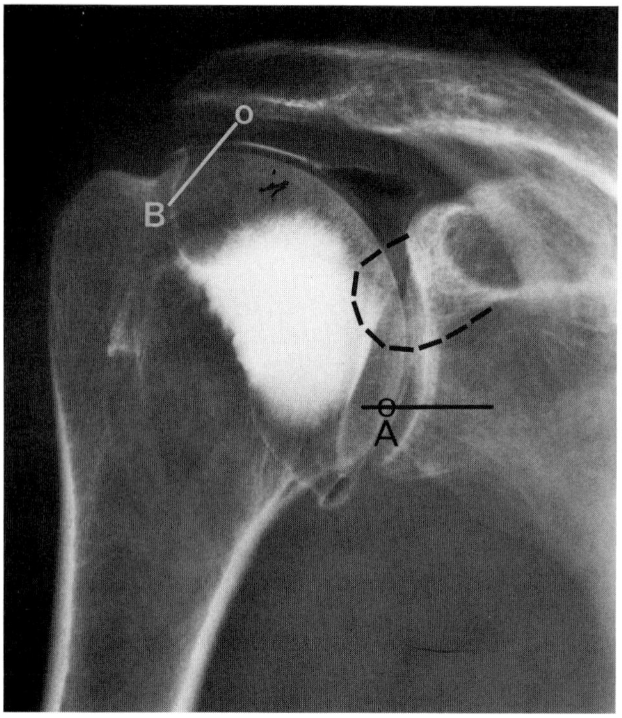

FIG. 1-22. Shoulder injection for arthrography. **A:** Injection sites for the glenohumeral joint. This shoulder demonstrates reduced capsular volume as a result of adhesive capsulitis. The coracoid projects over the joint anteriorly (*broken lines*). Therefore, we typically enter the joint at the junction of the mid and lower third of the glenoid using a direct vertical approach to the medial margin of the humeral head (*o*). **B:** Subacromial bursa injection. The needle enters anteriorly and is angled cephalad until it reaches the undersurface of the acromion. The needle is withdrawn 1 to 2 mm prior to the test injection.

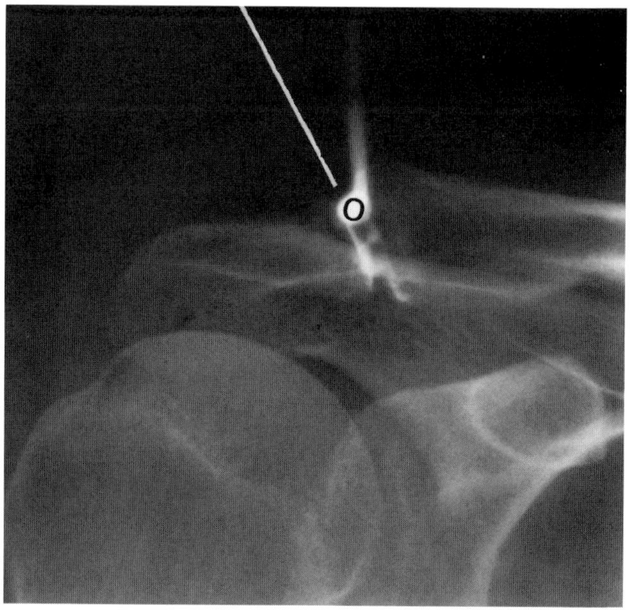

FIG. 1-23. Acromioclavicular joint injection. The joint can be entered anteriorly (*o*) or superiorly (*white line*). The joint has an oblique lateral to medial course, which should be considered when using the superior approach.

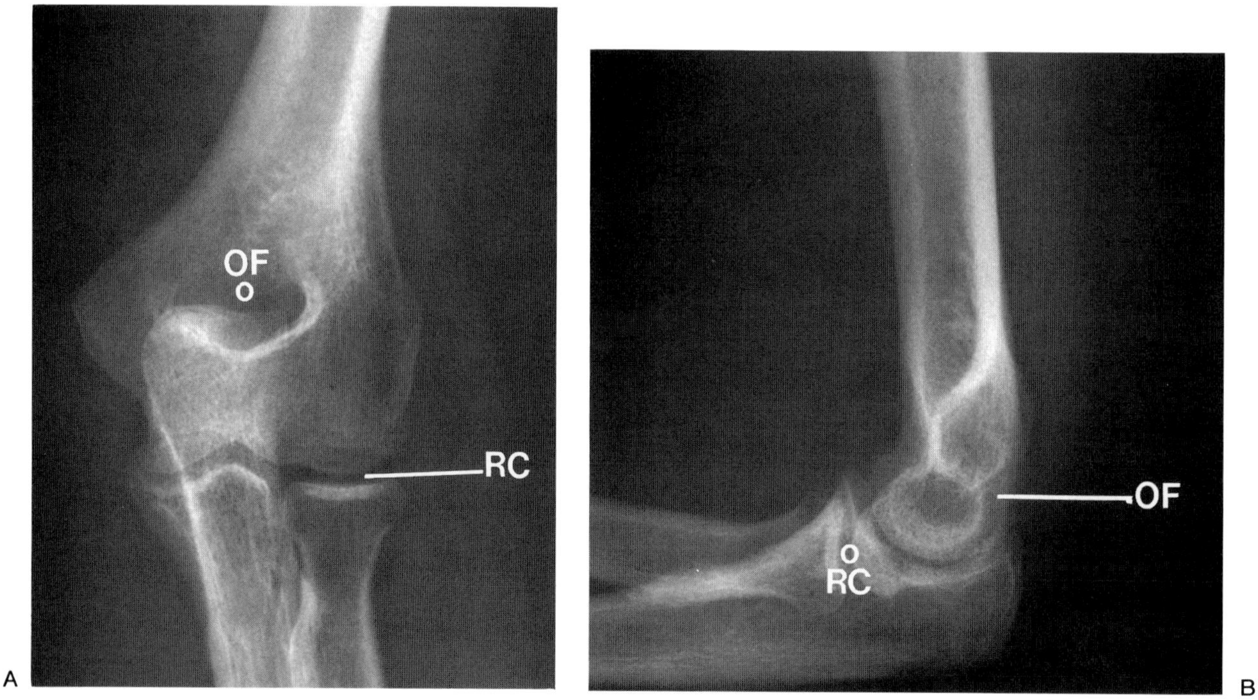

FIG. 1-24. Elbow injection sites on AP **(A)** and lateral **(B)** radiographs. The joint is most easily entered with the elbow flexed 90°. The radiocapitellar joint is approached laterally (*RC*). In certain cases, the posterior approach into the olecranon fossa (*OF*) is selected. The elbow should also be flexed 90° for this approach.

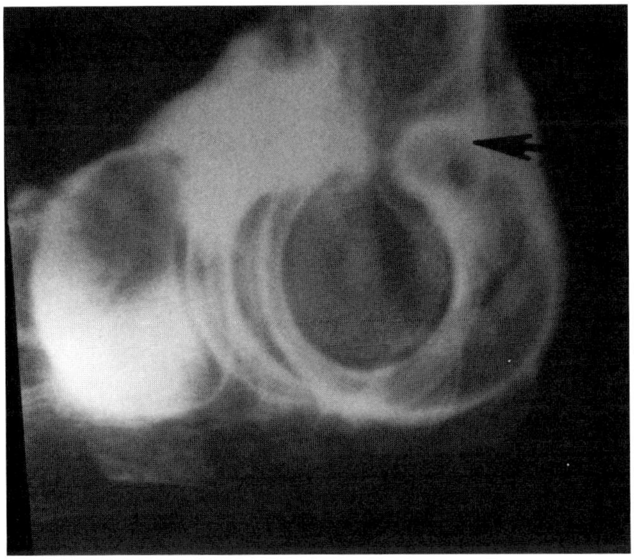

FIG. 1-25. Lateral view of the elbow following contrast injection demonstrates a posterior loose body (*arrow*).

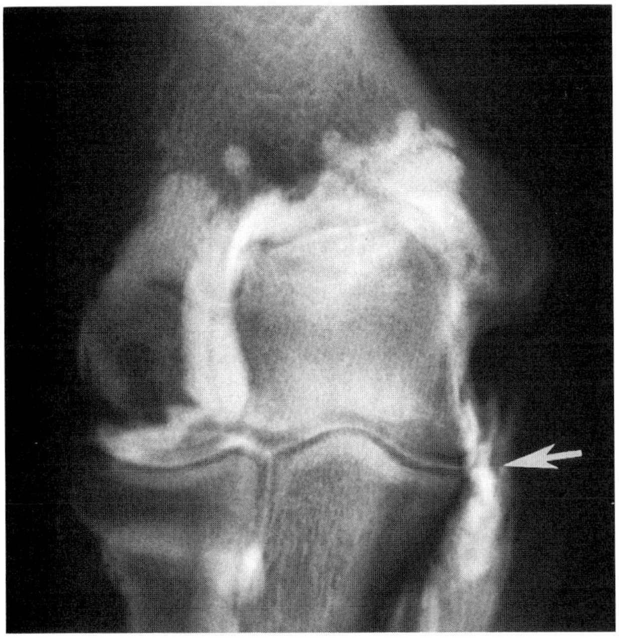

FIG. 1-26. The AP radiograph following contrast injection demonstrates a medial capsular tear (*arrow*).

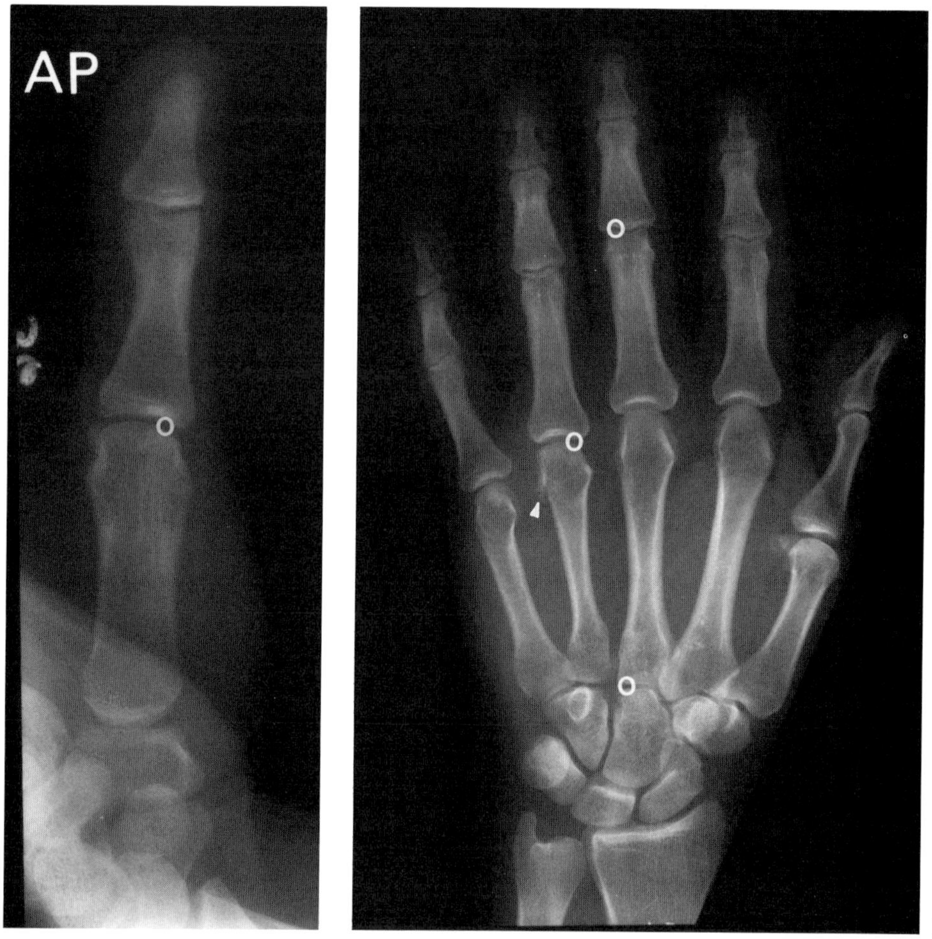

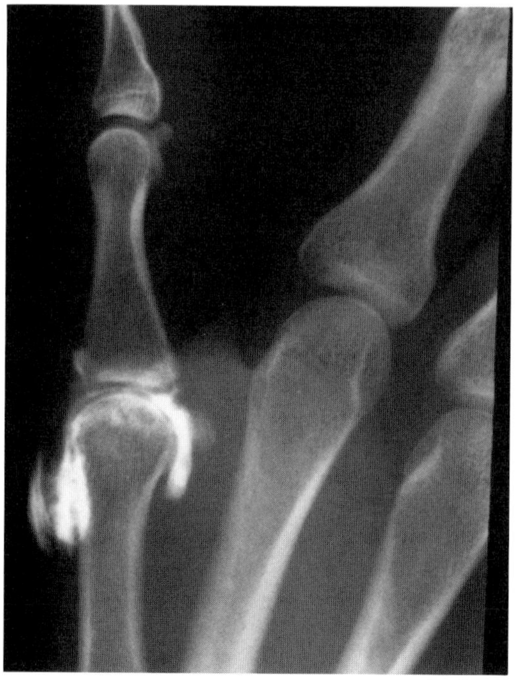

FIG. 1-27. A,B: Injections of the hand are performed using a direct dorsal approach after positioning the hand to optimally visualize the entry site fluoroscopically. Injection sites for the joints of the hand (*o*). The injection is performed either medially or laterally to the overlying extensor tendon, depending on the site of expected pathologic condition. Note the subtle neck fracture in B (*arrow*). **C:** Lateral view of first metacarpophalangeal joint arthrogram. The joint was overdistended with contrast, resulting in dorsal extravasation.

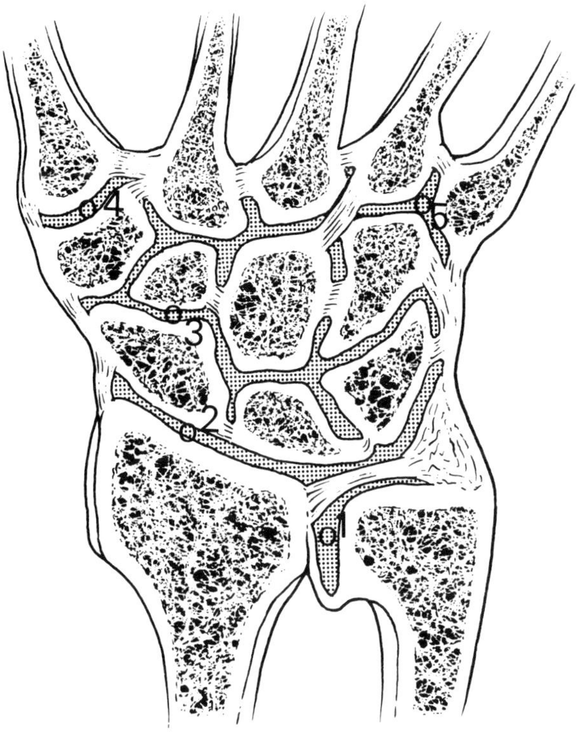

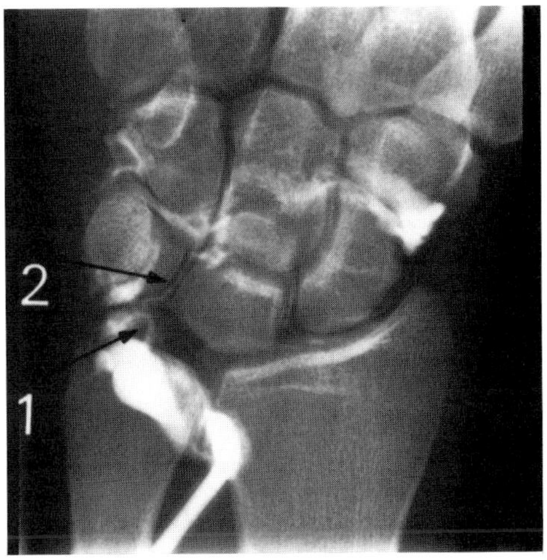

FIG. 1-28. Wrist injections are also performed using a direct dorsal approach. The wrist may have to be deviated in the radial or ulnar position to open the joint optimally. Slight flexion is useful to facilitate entering the radiocarpal joint. **A:** Compartments of the wrist and entry sites (*o*) for injection. *1,* Distal radioulnar joint; *2,* radiocarpal joint; *3,* intercarpal joints; *4,* trapezial-first metacarpal joint; *5,* carpometacarpal joints. **B:** Distal radioulnar joint arthrogram demonstrating flow of contrast through the triangular fibrocartilage (*1*) and lunotriquetral ligament (*2*) into the intercarpal joint. (From Berquist TH. Imaging of orthopedic trauma, 2nd ed. New York: Raven Press, 1992.)

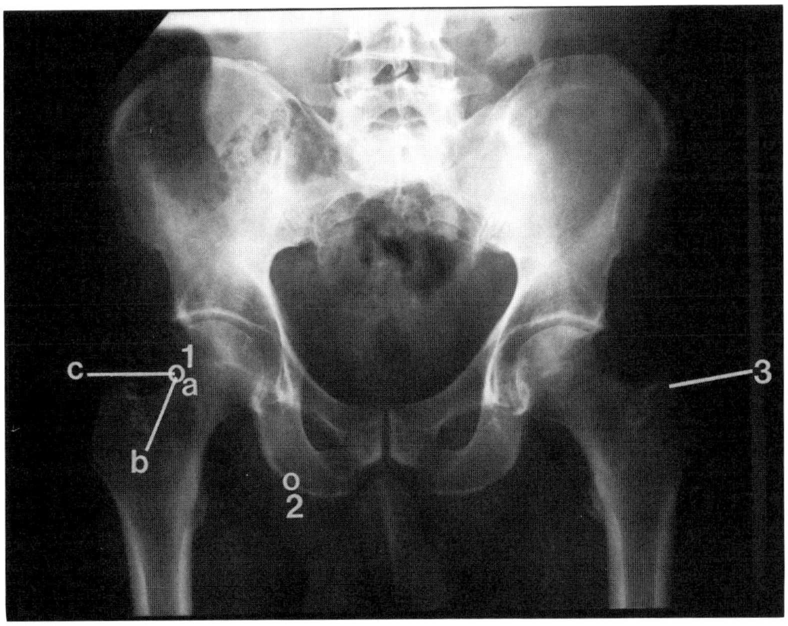

FIG. 1-29. Numerous injections are performed in the pelvis and hips. These include the hip, sacroiliac joint, pubic symphysis, trochanteric bursa, iliopsoas bursa, ischial bursa, and iliopsoas tendon. **A:** An AP view of the pelvis demonstrating injection sites. **1:** The hip may be entered using a direct vertical approach (*a*), slight lateral-to-medial approach (*b*), or a lateral approach (*c*). **2:** The ischial bursa injection is made medial to the sciatic nerve (see Fig. 1-29B). **3:** In the trochanteric bursa, a lateral approach is used. Fluid in the bursa can be localized with ultrasonography or MRI. **B:** Coronal MRI scan demonstrating the position of the nerve roots (*arrows*) and ischial injection site (2–o). (See **B–E** on next page.)

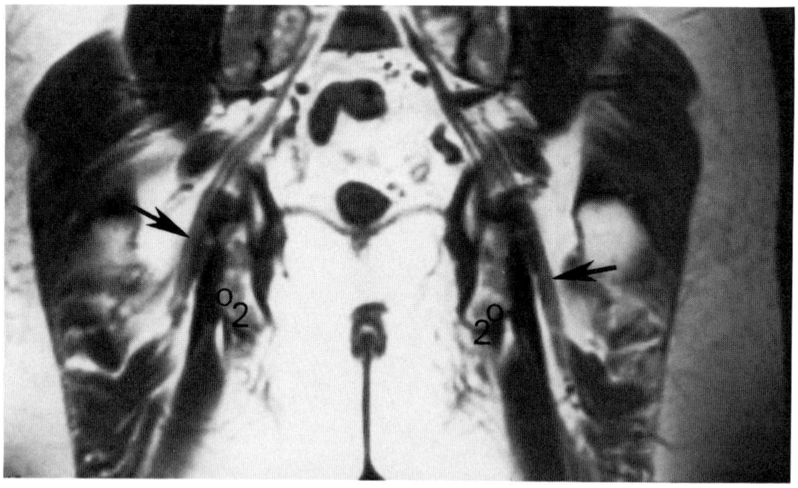

B

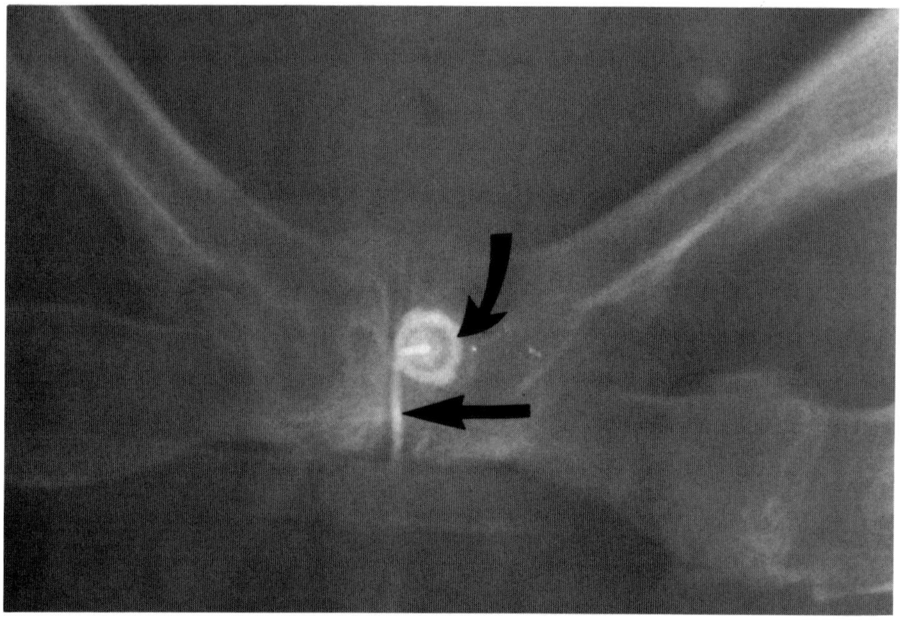

C

FIG. 1-29. *Continued.* **C:** Pubic symphysis. This joint is entered using a vertical approach. Note the needle position (*curved arrow*) and linear appearance of contrast media in the joint (*straight arrow*). **D:** An AP view of the hip with contrast in the iliopsoas muscle and tendon. The hip joint may communicate with the iliopsoas bursa in 20% of patients.[92] Entry of the bursa or tendon (snapping iliopsoas tendon syndrome) may also be accomplished along the path of the tendon, which may be palpable, or by entering near the acetabular rim (*o*). The position of the femoral artery and nerve must be confirmed prior to needle placement. **E:** A CT scan demonstrating the entry of the sacroiliac joint posteriorly with the patient rotated with the involved side down.

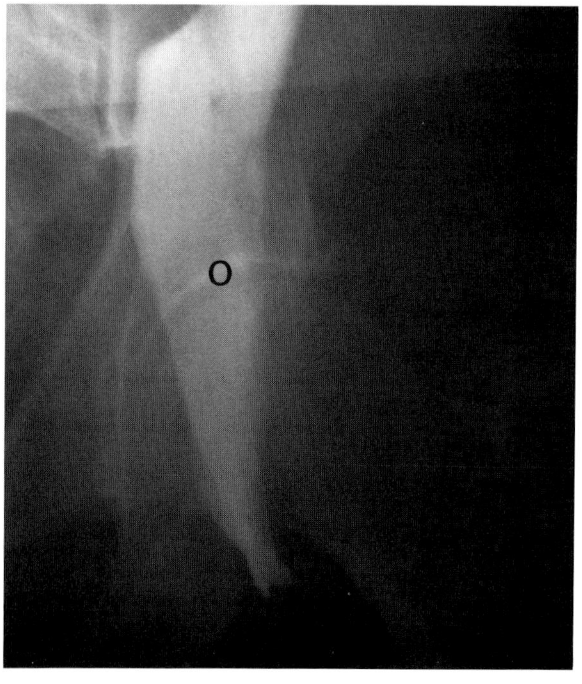

D

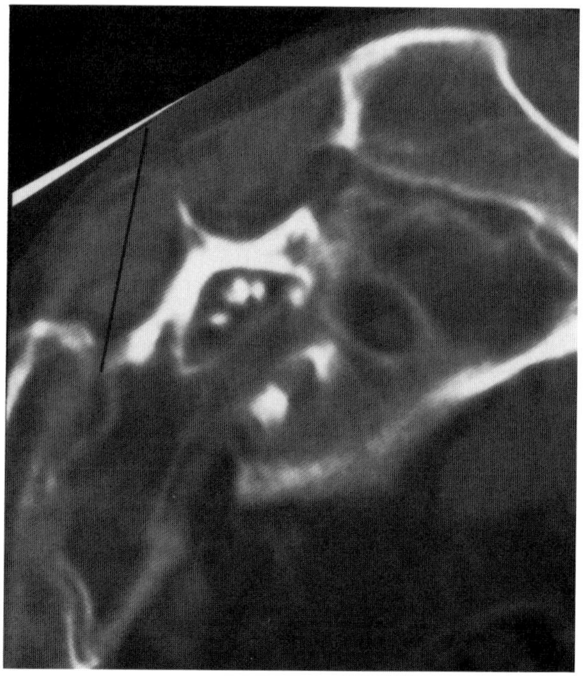

E

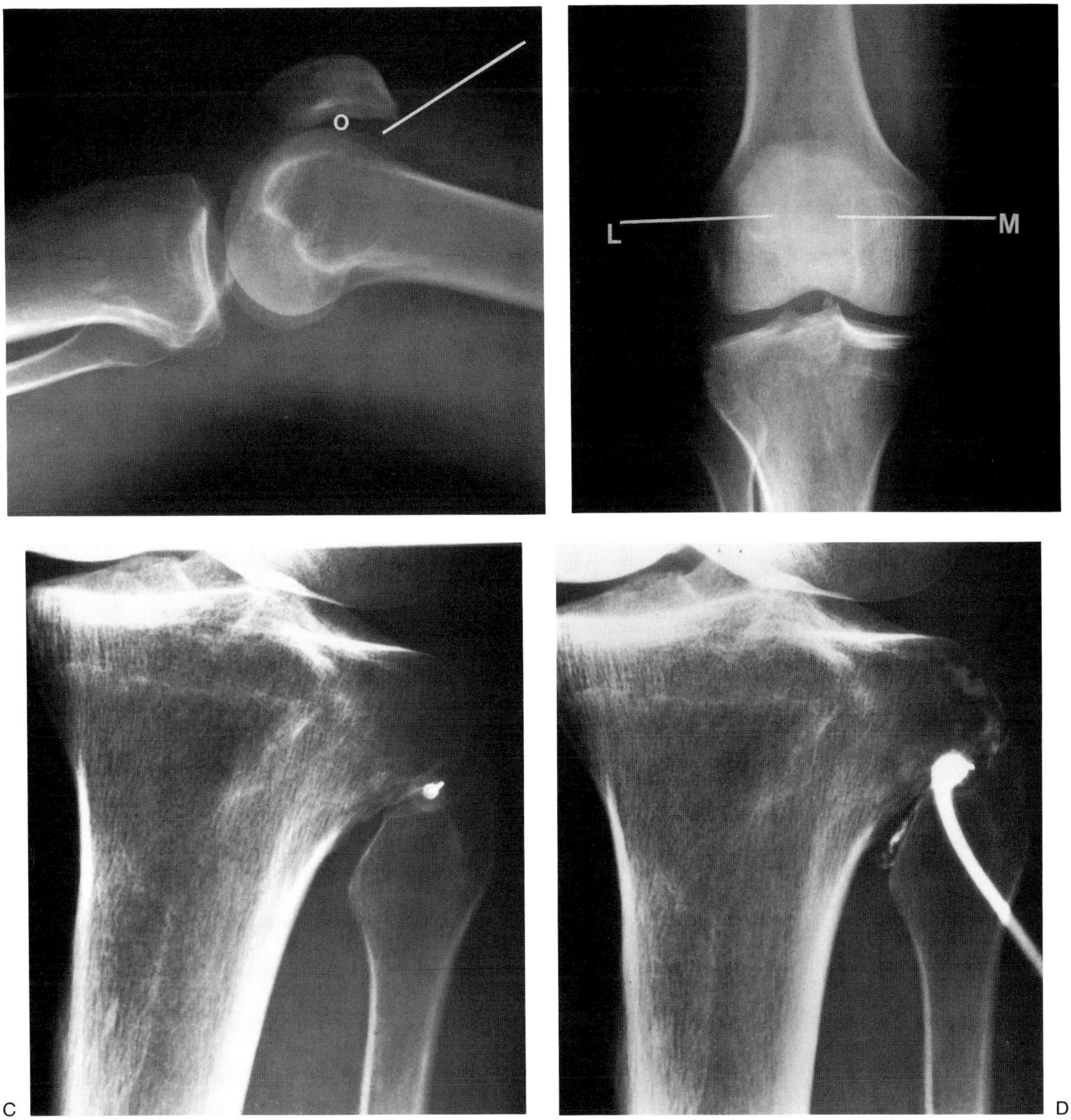

A B C D

FIG. 1-30. Knee injection sites. The knee is usually injected without fluoroscopic guidance. However, in postoperative patients, the joint may be more difficult to enter. Therefore, we prefer to use fluoroscopy in this setting. The knee is most often entered laterally, with the needle inserted below the midpatellar articular surface. Medial and, rarely, superior approaches can also be used. **A:** Lateral view of the knee demonstrating the needle entry site (*o*) beneath the patella. The superior approach (*white line*) is rarely necessary. **B:** The AP view of the knee demonstrating the medial (*m*) and lateral (*l*) approaches to the knee. **C,D:** The knee is rotated medially, and the proximal tibiofibular joint is entered anteriorly to avoid the posterior neurovascular structures. A direct vertical approach with a 1.5-inch 22-gauge needle (C) is easily performed. Contrast injection (D) confirms the needle's position.

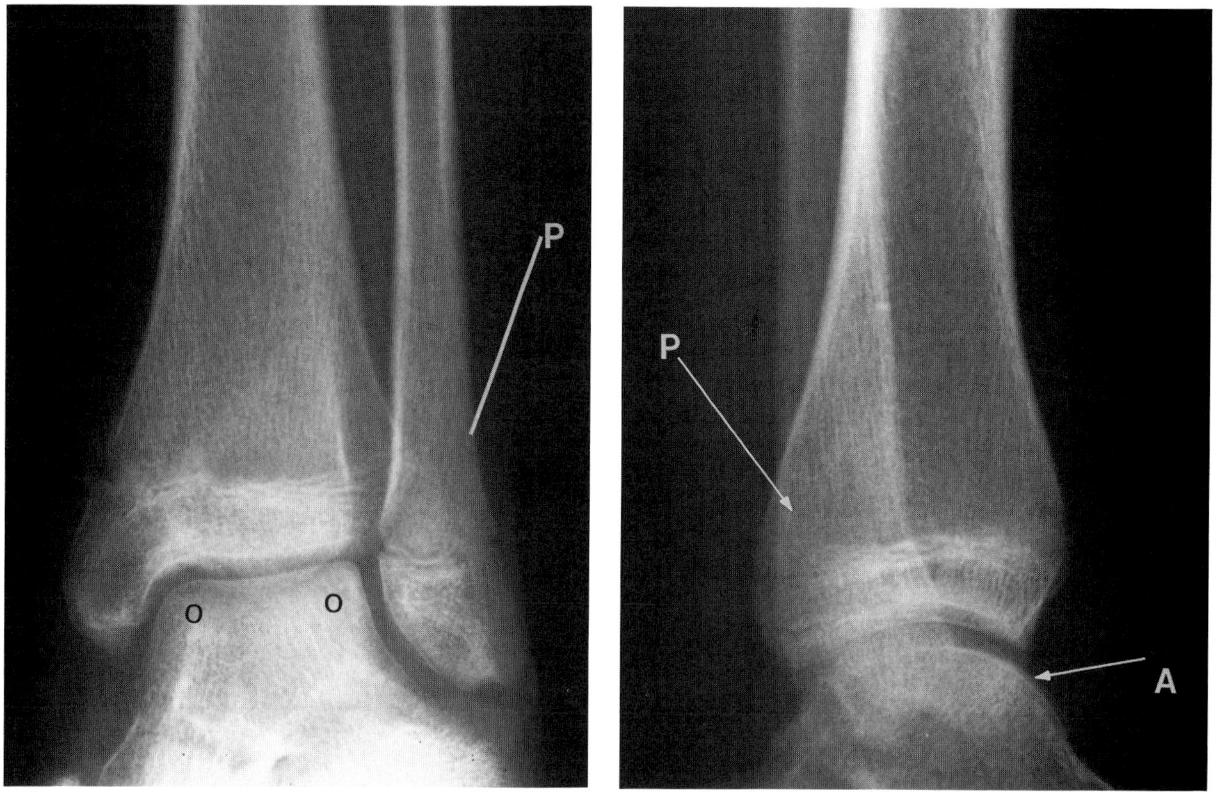

A B

FIG. 1-31. Ankle injections. Injection of the ankle or peroneal tendons is not difficult. The ankle can be entered anteromedially or anterolaterally, depending on the clinical situation. The ankle is turned into the lateral position to check the depth and angle. The tip should be below the anterior tibial lip. The peroneal tendon sheath is most easily accessed above the lateral malleolus in an oblique plane to ensure the entire bevel of the needle tip enters the tendon sheath. **A:** An AP view of the ankle, demonstrating the entry sites for the ankle (*o*) and the approach (*white line*) to the peroneal tendon sheaths. **B:** Lateral view of the ankle, demonstrating ankle (*A*) and peroneal tendon (*P*) approaches.

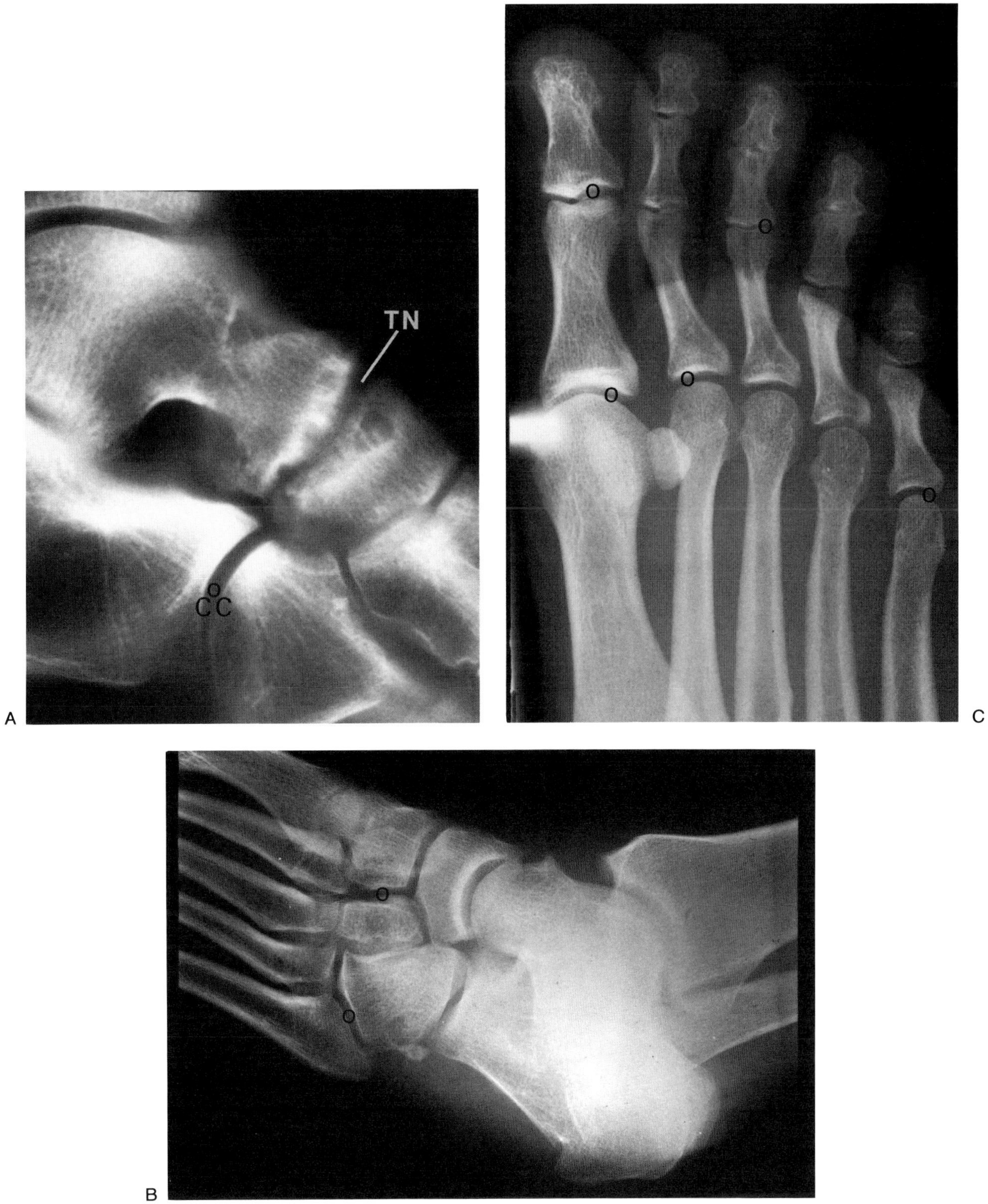

FIG. 1-32. The complex bony anatomy of the foot makes it slightly more difficult to position the patient for selected articular injections. The knee is flexed with the foot on the fluoroscopic table. Rotation of the foot is performed to provide a direct entry site into the desired joints in the mid and hind foot. The foot can be flat on the table for metatarsophalangeal and interphalangeal joint injections. Tendons and pulses are palpated to be sure they are avoided when entering the joints. **A:** Oblique view of the foot allows the calcaneocuboid (*CC*) and talonavicular (*TN*) joints to be more easily entered. Note the advance talonavicular arthrosis. **B:** Oblique position for injection of the lateral tarsometatarsal (*o*) and tarsal joints (lateral-intermediate cuneiform articulation). **C:** Minimal rotation for injection of the metatarsophalangeal and interphalangeal joint (*o*).

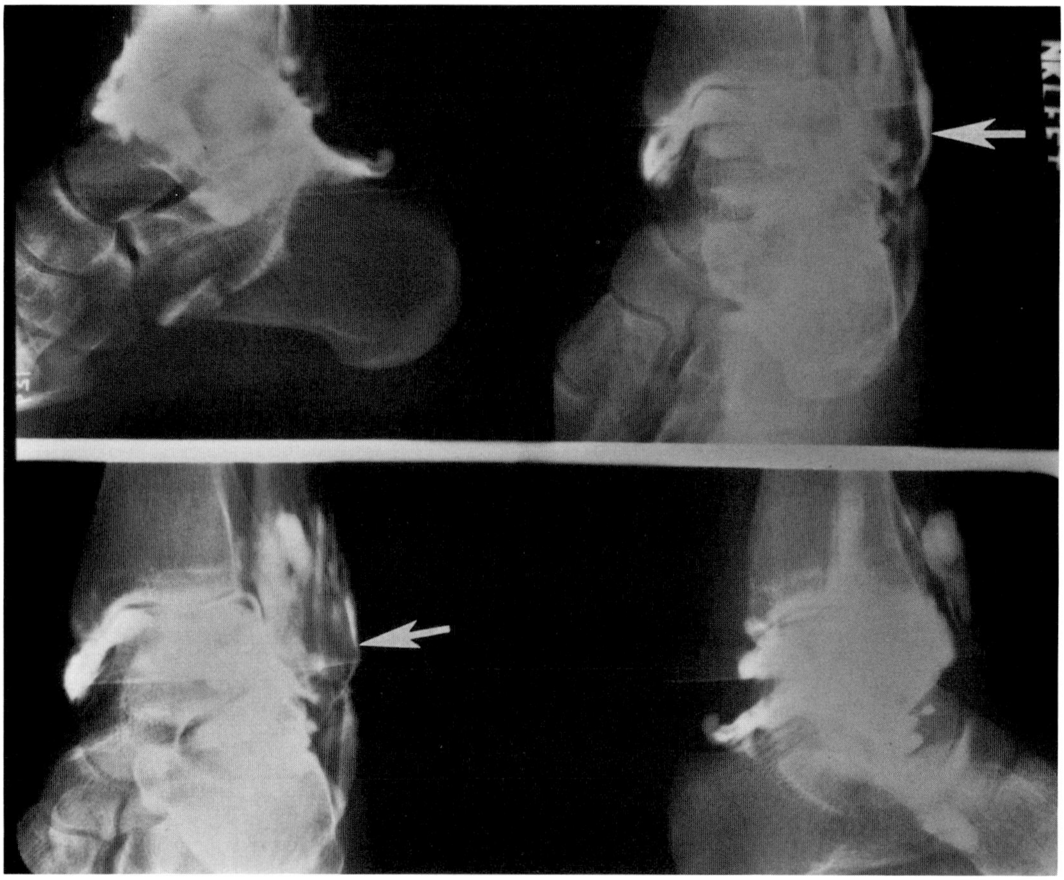

FIG. 1-33. Four-view arthrogram of the left ankle with filling of the peroneal tendon sheaths (*arrows*) caused by calcaneofibular and anterior talofibular ligament tears.

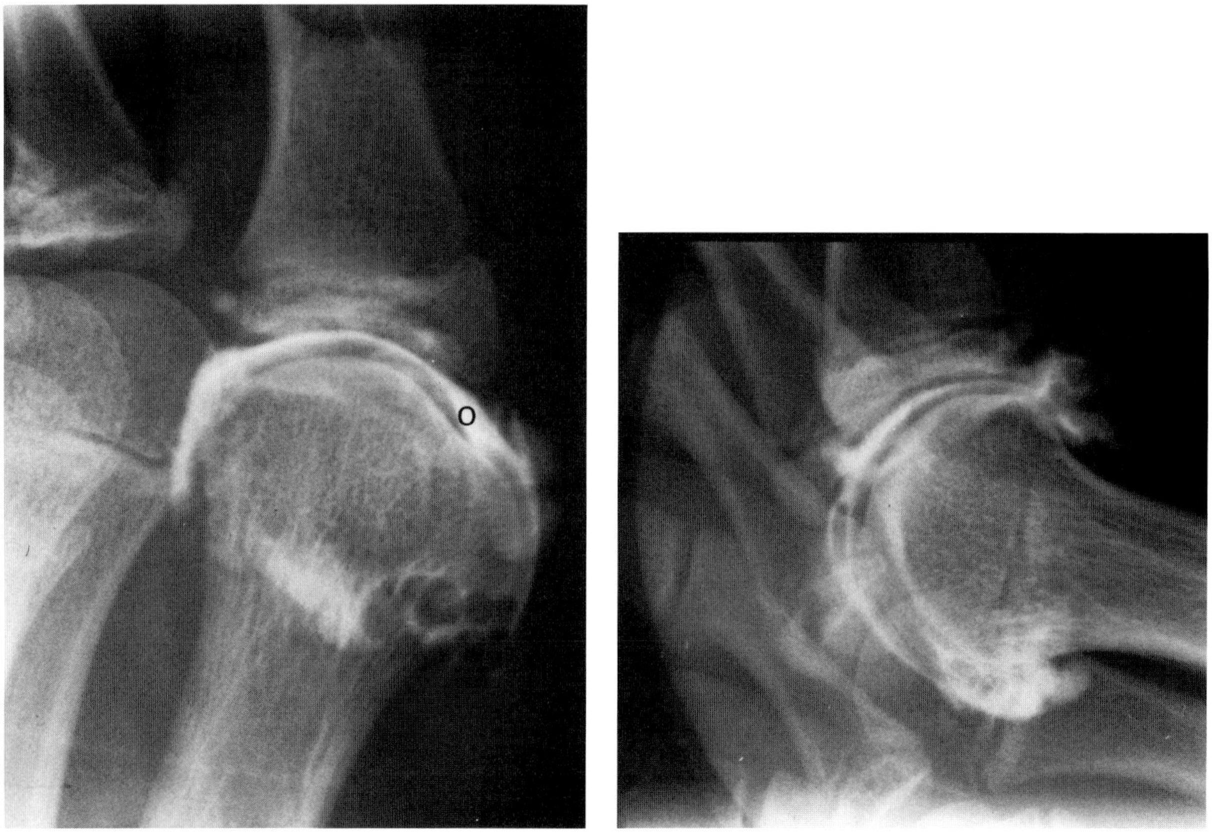

A B

FIG. 1-34. Normal first metatarsophalangeal arthrogram seen on AP **(A)** and lateral **(B)** views. Needle entry site, *o*.

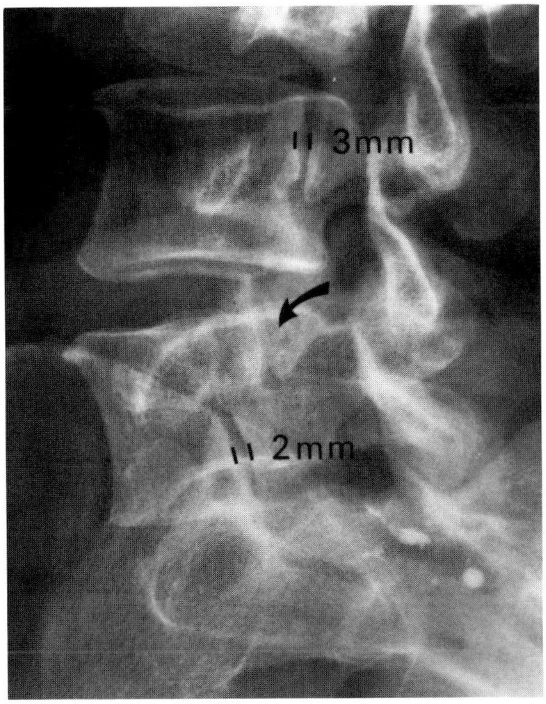

FIG. 1-35. Fluoroscopically positioned oblique view demonstrating normal L-3 to L-4 and L-5 to S-1 facets. The L-4 to L-5 facet (*curved arrow*) is significantly narrowed.

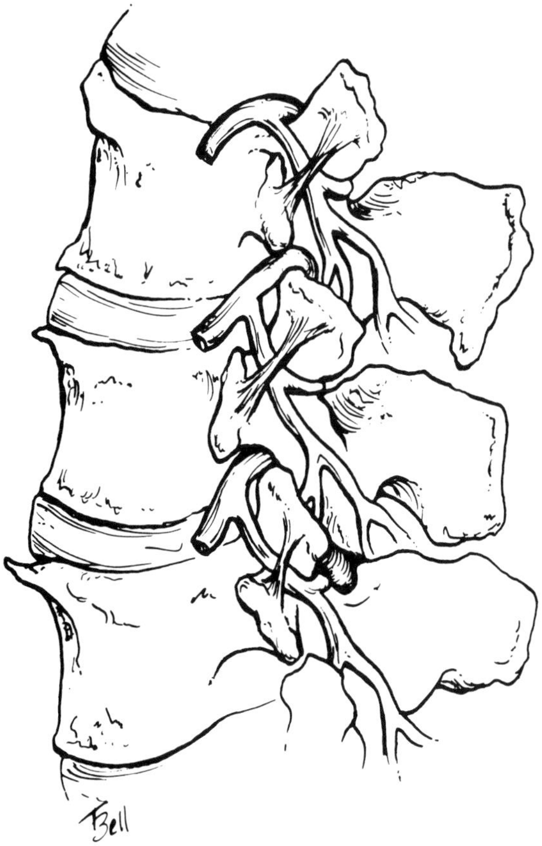

FIG. 1-36. Facet innervation. (From Berquist TH. Imaging of orthopedic trauma and surgery. Philadelphia: WB Saunders, 1986.)

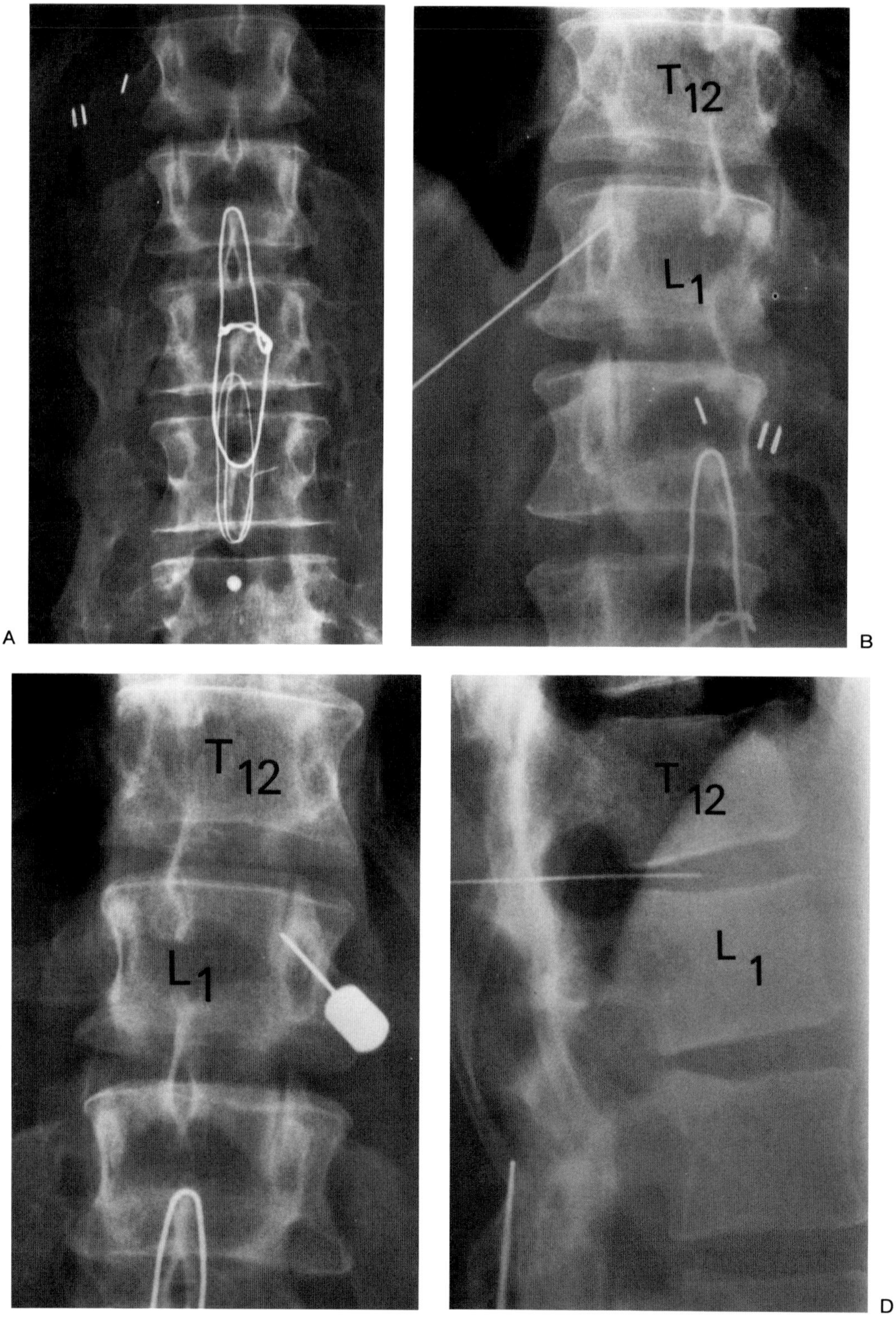

FIG. 1-37. Middle-aged woman with upper lumbar pain after multiple fusions. **A:** An AP radiograph demonstrating solid fusion from L-1 to the sacrum, with posterolateral bone graft and spinous process wiring L-2 to L-4. There are also previous L-4 to L-5 and L-5 to S-1 laminectomies. Bilateral facet injections **(B,C)** and discograms **(D–F)** were performed to localize symptoms prior to considering further surgical therapy. The T-12 to L-1 facets can be entered with the patient supine using a direct vertical approach (B,C). The disc space is entered using a posterolateral approach (D). The discogram shows degeneration on the AP (E) and lateral (F) views.

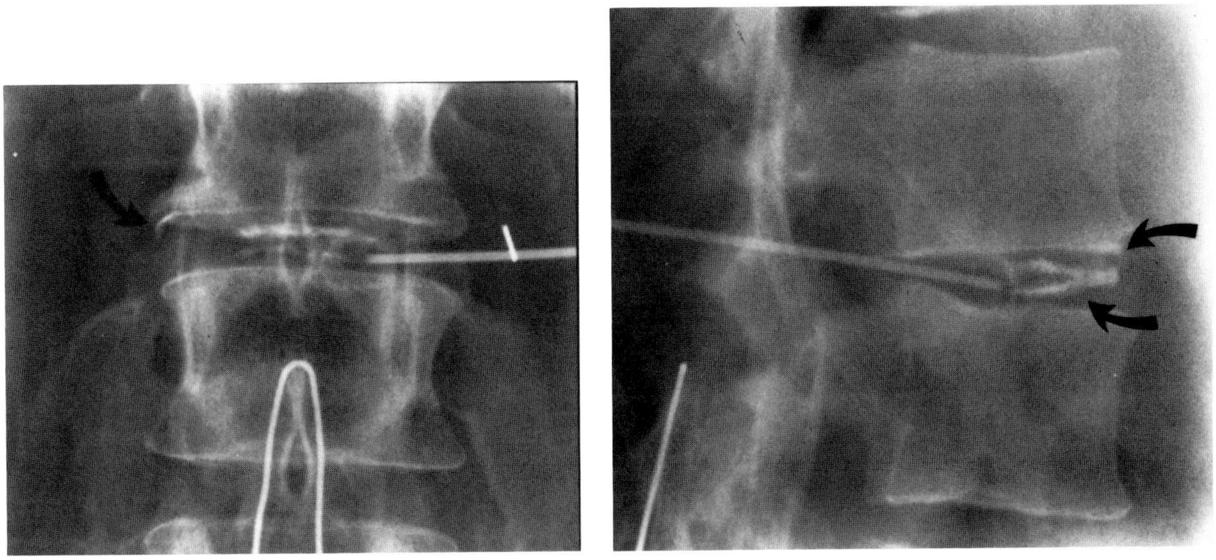

E F

FIG. 1-37. *Continued.*

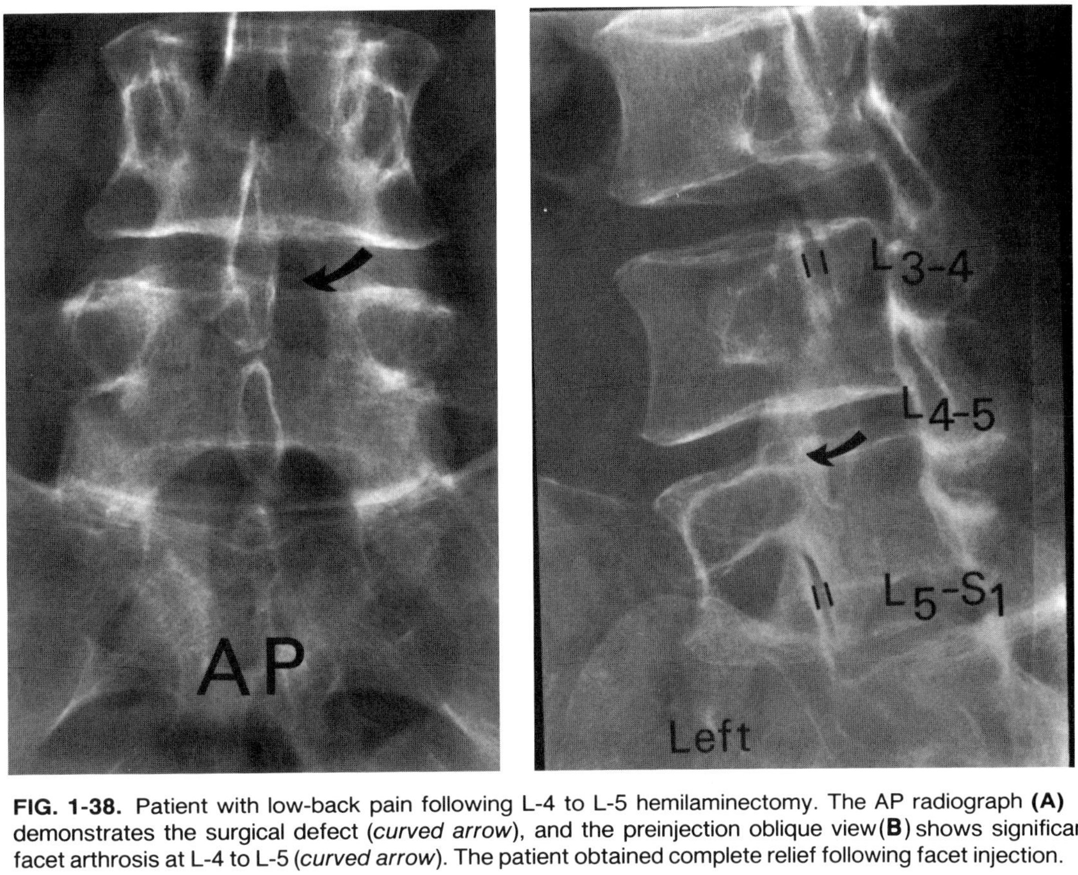

A B

FIG. 1-38. Patient with low-back pain following L-4 to L-5 hemilaminectomy. The AP radiograph **(A)** demonstrates the surgical defect (*curved arrow*), and the preinjection oblique view(**B**) shows significant facet arthrosis at L-4 to L-5 (*curved arrow*). The patient obtained complete relief following facet injection.

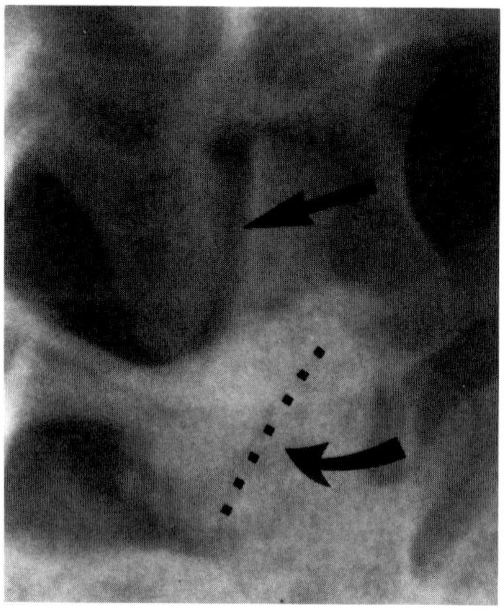

FIG. 1-39. Oblique view demonstrating an open facet joint (*straight arrow*) and ankylosis of the adjacent facet (*dotted line, curved arrow*). This facet would not be possible to inject.

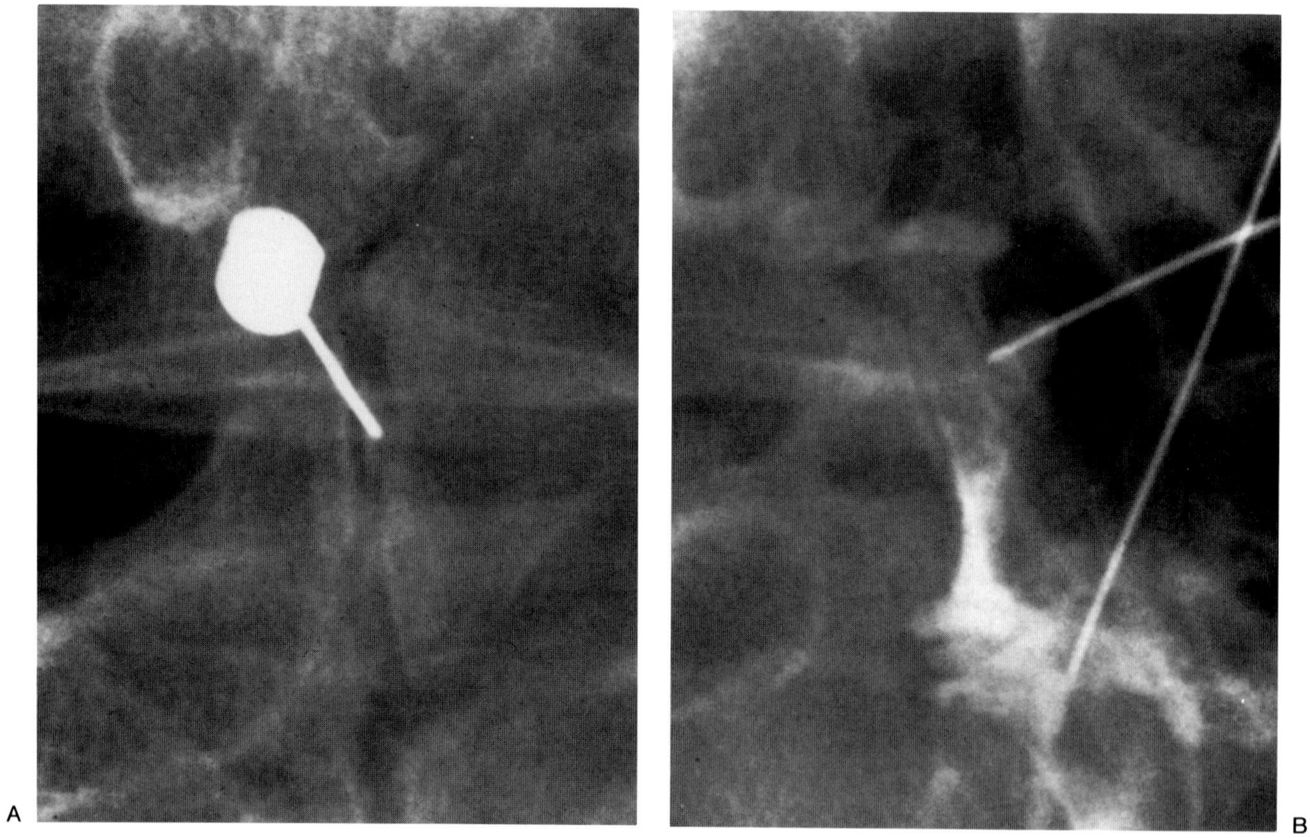

FIG. 1-40. Oblique fluoroscopic view with needle in place **(A)** and after contrast injection **(B)** into two adjacent facet joints.

atic pseudarthrosis, (3) determination of extent for proposed spinal fusion, and (4) use prior to percutaneous discectomy or chemonucleolysis.[104,111] Even these indications remain controversial and vary from institution to institution. Esses et al.[101] indicated that discography had little value in predicting the outcome of spinal surgery.

Technique

The patient is positioned prone on the fluoroscopic table. Following sterile preparation, the patient is positioned to optimize entry into the desired disc space. A posterolateral approach is used at our institution. The transdural approach can also be used in the lumbar region; however, the complications seen with myelography tend to occur using this technique.[104,118] Local anesthetic is injected into the entry site. A 22-gauge spinal needle can be used at most levels. However, the disc at L-5 to S-1 is more difficult to enter. This may require a double-needle technique. The first needle is advanced to the margin of the disc, and a Chiba needle with a slight bend in the distal position is inserted through the first needle and directed into the disc space.[92,104]

The normal lumbar disc will accept 1 to 1.5 ml of contrast medium. A degenerative disc may accept more, and an irregular pattern will be seen fluoroscopically (Fig. 1-41) with extravasation of contrast into the annulus and beyond.[92,104] Distention of the disc space may recreate the patient's symptoms.[92,104]

Subtraction Arthrography

The advent of joint replacement procedures resulted in a new use for the subtraction technique to improve the detection of subtle changes, specifically component loosening.[92,103,117,119]

Subtraction radiography can be performed by using film or digital techniques. Both serve to remove unnecessary information from the image. The result is enhanced specific information, in this case, intraarticular contrast on the images.[90,92]

Indications

Subtraction arthrography is used routinely in patients with joint arthroplasty.[92,110] This technique is most useful with cemented components in which the density of contrast is similar to that of methyl methacrylate impregnated with barium (Fig. 1-42). Subtraction removes the methacrylate and changes the metal density, allowing subtle loosening to be more easily appreciated.[92,117]

Technique

Digital and film subtraction accomplish the same results, but the former requires more expensive equipment. Using either technique, the patient must remain motionless from the time of proper needle placement until the contrast injection is completed. Using the film technique, a second image is taken, and the mask created from the scout is used to create the subtraction image (Fig. 1-42).[92] We do not remove the needle or perform any additional maneuvers that might lead to inadvertent patient motion until the postinjection film has been obtained. Patient motion can cause misregistration (Fig. 1-43), which leads to a poor subtraction and can cause false-positive interpretation.

After the postinjection film has been obtained, the needle can be removed, and additional views, stress views, or postexercise views can be obtained. Regardless of the joint being studied, the result is subtraction in only one position. This technique is most easily accomplished in the hip. We have also used this in other joints, such as the knee. The review of routine films permits the selection of the best position for obtaining subtraction.

Complications of Arthrography and Diagnostic and Therapeutic Injections

Arthrography and diagnostic injections are relatively benign procedures. The main concerns in most anatomic regions are infection or allergy to contrast medium. Infection is rare with careful sterile technique. Freiberger et al.[102] reported 1 infection in 25,000 arthrograms. Painful effusions can occur with intraarticular contrast injections. These usually develop within 12 hours of the injection and may require joint aspiration for relief.[92,95]

An allergy to intraarticular contrast is not as frequent a problem as is that to intravascular contrast. Patients with mild reactions to intravenous contrast in the past can be premedicated with antihistamines. Patients with significant allergies should not be examined, or an alternative, such as air arthrography, may be considered.[92,102]

Injections in certain regions, specifically the spine and in or near nerve roots, may cause some additional problems. Inadvertent nerve block (anesthetic injection along a nerve) may cause numbness or reduced function for several hours. The incidence of disc space infection following discography is slightly higher than that after arthrography (2 in 1,000 versus 1 in 25,000), but this is not a significant risk.[94,104]

Myelography

Positive contrast myelography has been accomplished for many years and provides useful information regard-

(text continues on page 40)

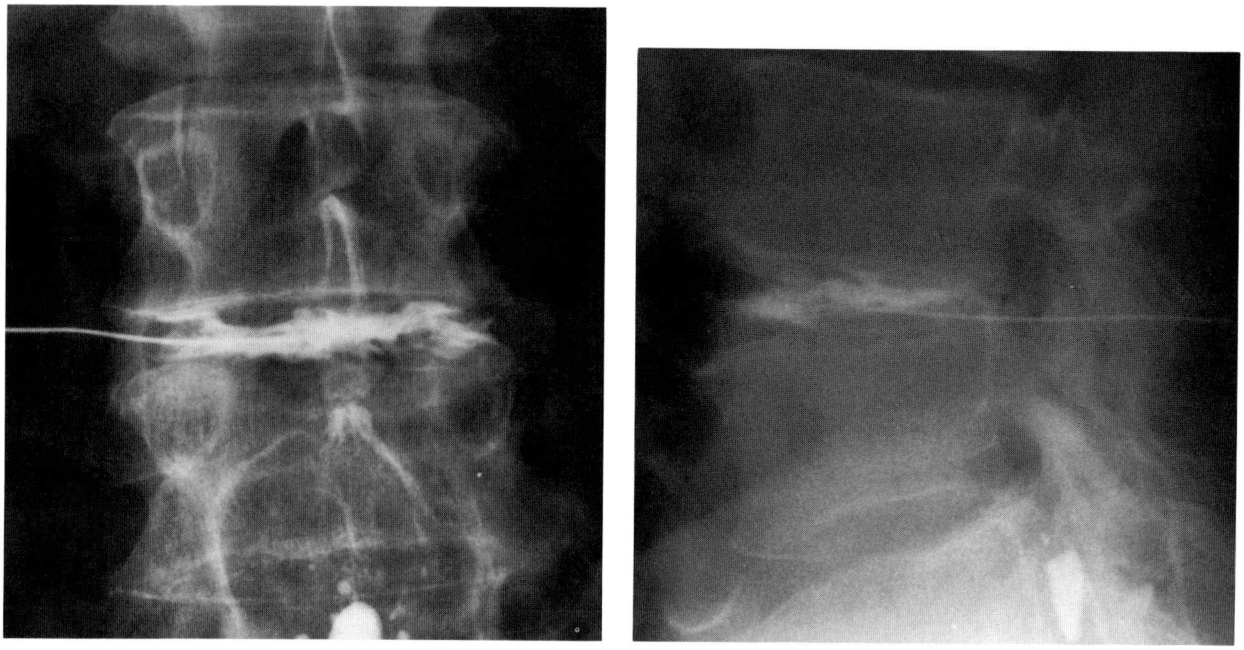

A B

FIG. 1-41. Lumbar discogram in a patient with degenerative disc disease at L-4 to L-5. The AP **(A)** and lateral **(B)** views demonstrate an irregular poorly defined disc.

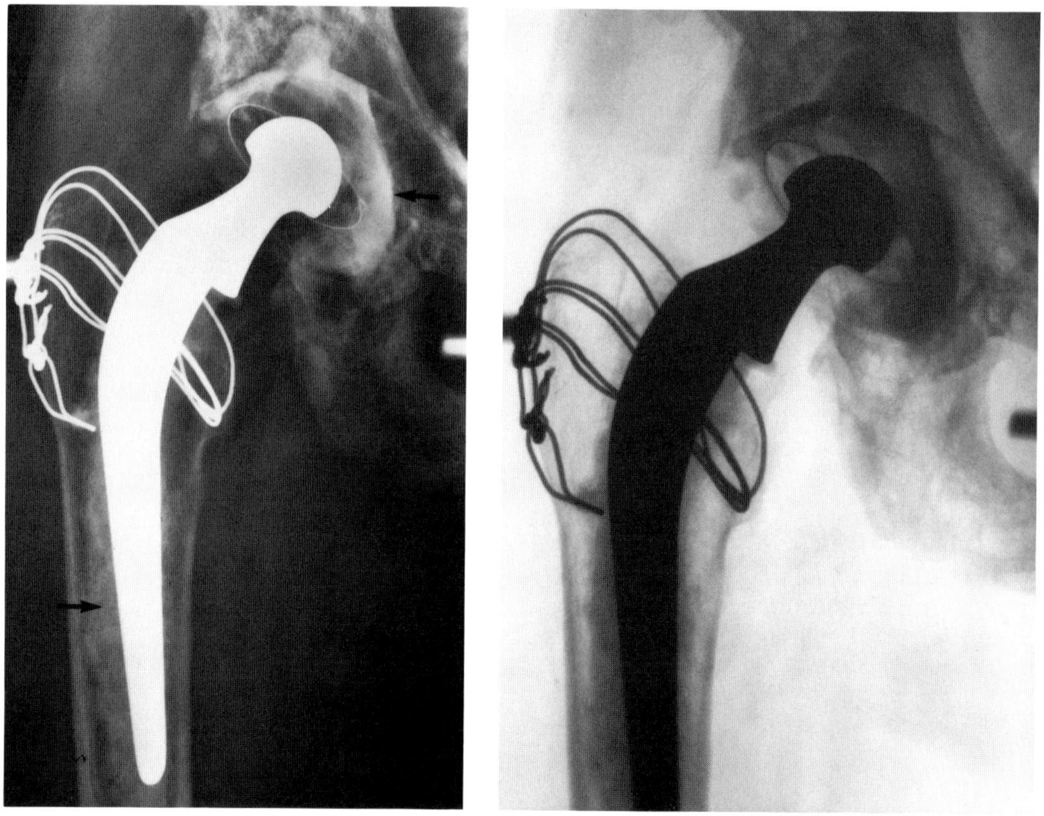

A B

FIG. 1-42. Subtraction arthrogram in a patient with pain caused by component loosening. **A:** Scout film demonstrating a cemented (*arrows*) hip arthroplasty. **B:** Subtraction mask (reverse of scout) used to remove cement and reduce metal interference. **C:** Postarthrogram film demonstrates some extravasation at the cement interface in zone III (*arrow*) of the acetabular component. **D:** Subtraction arthrogram clearly demonstrates contrast in zones I and III (*arrows*) of the acetabular component and along the bone cement interface of the femoral component (*arrow*) due to loosening of both components. (From Berquist TH. Imaging of orthopedic trauma and surgery. Philadelphia: WB Saunders, 1986.)

C

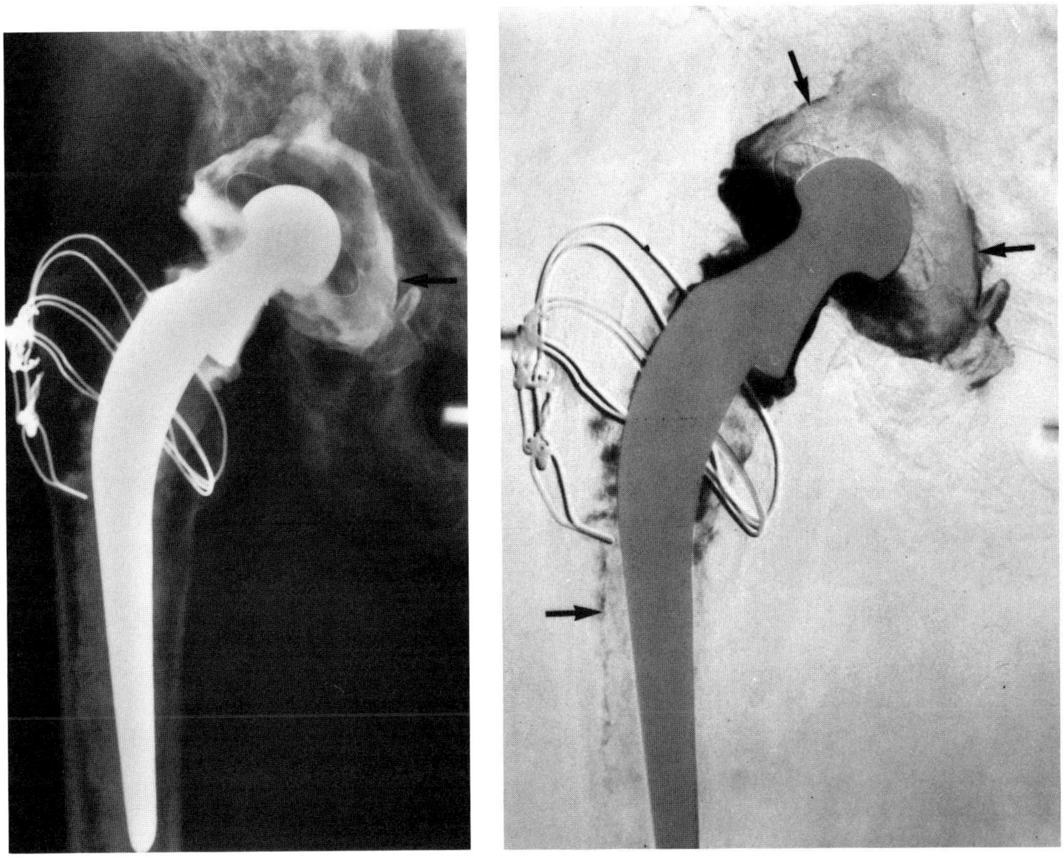

D

FIG. 1-42. *Continued.*

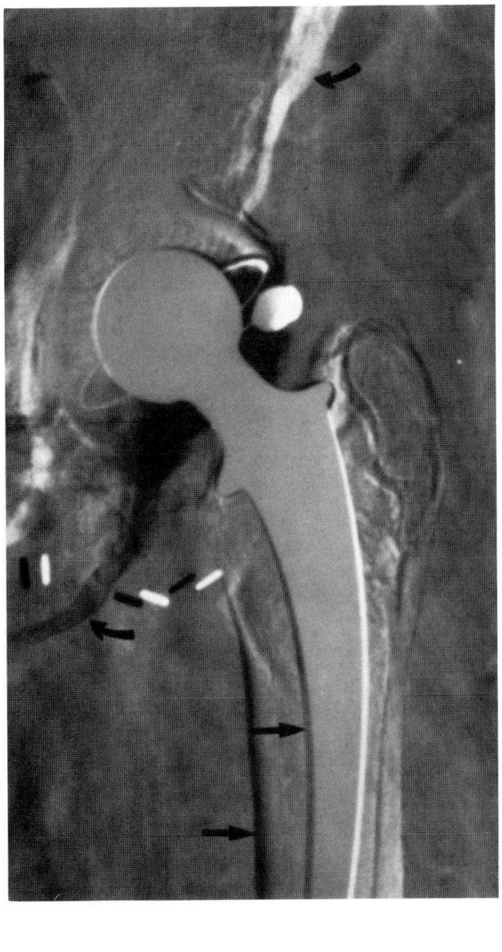

FIG. 1-43. Suboptimal subtraction with misregistration caused by patient motion. This could cause misinterpretation. Note the ischial and femoral cortices (*arrows*) do not cancel out. (From Berquist TH. Imaging of orthopedic trauma and surgery. Philadelphia: WB Saunders, 1986.)

ing the bony spinal canal, spinal cord, and nerve roots.[92,95] In some institutions, its utility has been diminished because of MRI. However, its usefulness following spinal instrumentation and preoperatively, especially in patients with scoliosis, remains strong. An artifact from metal spinal implants reduces the image quality with CT and MRI.[92,93]

Contrast agents for myelography have changed significantly over the years. Pantopaque™ is an oil-based medium that has a long established history in myelography. Amipaque™, a water-soluble agent, followed and was also well accepted. Today, most myelography is performed by using less toxic agents, such as Isovue™ (Squibb). The advantages of the newer agents include thecal absorption (removal no longer necessary), less toxicity, reduced incidence of arachnoiditis, and better delineation of the nerve root sleeves.[92,93]

Myelograms are performed using sterile technique. A table capable of tilting 90° in either direction permits the movement of contrast along the length of the entire spinal canal. We routinely evaluate all segments.[92] The needle is usually inserted into the L-2 to L-3 space. Postoperatively, a C-1 to C-2 disc puncture may be required. The needle puncture is monitored fluoroscopically, and a single-wall midline puncture is performed. Fluid can be obtained for laboratory studies if indicated. Contrast medium (Isovue 200™) is injected under fluoroscopic guidance to ensure proper positioning in the subarachnoid space.[92] Filming is accomplished by tilting the table and moving the contrast through the regions of interest. Posteroanterior, lateral, and oblique views are obtained. The patient is usually turned on the side for lateral views in the thoracic spine. Commonly, CT is performed following conventional filming.[92]

Following myelography with water-soluble agents, the patient's head should be elevated 45° for several hours and hydration maintained. Contrast entering the intracranial region can lead to seizures. The other complication commonly seen, postmyelogram headache, can be reduced by using smaller gauge needles ($8 \leq 22$ gauge).[92]

Vascular Studies

Angiography and venography play a role in the evaluation of orthopedic patients both pre- and postoperatively.[109,114,115]

Angiography is useful in the diagnosis and treatment of vascular injuries following blunt, penetrating, or operative trauma. Vascular injuries include intimal injury, arterial transsection, or thrombosis, pseudoaneurysm, arteriovenous fistula, and venous thrombosis or transsection.[92,114] Vascular trauma may be subtle or result in hemorrhage, pulse deficit, expanding masses, bruits, or signs of distal ischemia.[92,109]

In addition to diagnosis, angiography can be used to treat certain arterial injuries. The introduction of embolic materials can produce temporary or permanent vessel occlusion. These techniques are most useful in pelvic fractures or severe arterial bleeds, which are difficult to manage surgically.[109] The bleeding arteries can be identified and occluded through selective catheterization and injection of embolic materials. Occluding agents include Gelfoam™ (Upjohn, Kalamazoo, MI), Ivalon™ (Ivalon, Inc., San Diego, CA), blood clots, mechanical coils, or detachable balloons.[92,109]

Venography has been replaced by sonography in many situations. However, lower or upper extremity venograms are still useful for the evaluation of suspected venous thrombosis. This technique is most commonly employed in the postoperative setting in regions in which ultrasonography may be less effective.[92]

REFERENCES

Routine Radiography

1. Beabout JW. Radiology of total hip arthroplasty. *Radiol Clin North Am* 1975;13:3–19.
2. Bender CE, Berquist TH, Stears JG, Winkler NT, James EM, Brown ML, Welch TJ, May GR, Forbes GS. Diagnostic techniques. In: Berquist TH, ed. *Imaging of orthopedic trauma.* New York: Raven Press; 1992:1–38.
3. Nguyen VD, London J, Cone RO III. Ring sequestrum: radiographic characteristics of skeletal fixation pin tract osteomyelitis. *Radiology* 1986;158:129–131.
4. Techranzadeh J, Schneider R, Freiberger RH. Radiographic evaluation of painful total hip replacement. *Radiology* 1981;141: 355–362.
5. Weissman BN. The radiology of total joint replacement. *Orthop Clin North Am* 1983;14:171–191.

Computed Tomography

6. Aaron A, Weinstein D, Thickman D, Eilert R. Comparison of orthoroentgenography and computed tomography in measurement of leg length discrepancy. *J Bone Joint Surg* [*Am*] 1992; 74A:897–902.
7. Barmeir E, Dubowitz B, Roffman M. Computed tomography in assessment and planning of computed total hip replacement. *Acta Orthop Scand* 1982;53:597–604.
8. Bender CE, Berquist TH, Stears JG, Winkler NT, James EM, Brown ML, Welch TJ, May GR, Forbes GS. Diagnostic techniques. In: Berquist TH, ed. *Imaging of orthopedic trauma.* New York: Raven Press; 1992:1–37.
9. Fishman EK, Magid D, Robertson DD, Brooker AF, Weiss P, Siegelman SS. Metallic hip implants: CT with multiplanar reconstruction. *Radiology* 1986;160:675–681.
10. Friedman RJ, Hawthorne KB, Genez BM. The use of computerized tomography in the measurement of glenoid version. *J Bone Joint Surg* [*Am*] 1992;74A:1032–1037.
11. Golimbu C, Firoozma H, Rofii M, Engler G, Delman A. CT of thoracic and lumbar spine fractures that have been treated with Harrington instrumentation. *Radiology* 1984;151:731–733.
12. Gross SC, Kowalski JB, Lee SH, Terry B, Honickman SJ. Surgical ligation clip artifact on CT scans. *Radiology* 1985;156:831–832.
13. Helms CA, McCarthy S. CT scanograms for measuring leg length discrepancy. *Radiology* 1984;151:802.
14. Kahlman JE, Fishman EK, Magid D, Scott WW, Brooker AF, Siegelman SS. Fracture non-union: CT assessment with multiplanar reconstruction. *Radiology* 1988;167:483–488.
15. Young SW, Muller HH, Marshall WA. Computed tomography:

beam hardening and environmental density artifact. *Radiology* 1983;148:279–283.

Magnetic Resonance Imaging

16. Augusting N, Gustar K, von Schulthess DM, Bösiger P. MR imaging of large non-ferromagnetic implants at 1.5T. *J Comput Assist Tomogr* 1987;11:678–683.
17. Ballock RT, Hajek PC, Byrne TP, Garten SK. The quality of magnetic resonance imaging affected by the composition of halo arthrosis. *J Bone Joint Surg [Am]* 1989;71A:431–434.
18. Berquist TH. Magnetic resonance imaging: preliminary experience in orthopedic radiology. *Magn Reson Imaging* 1984;2:41–52.
19. Berquist TH. *MRI of the musculoskeletal system.* 2nd ed. New York: Raven Press; 1990.
20. Brown MA, Carden JA, Coleman RE, McKinney R Jr, Spicer LD. Magnetic field effects on surgical ligation clips. *Magn Reson Imaging* 1987;4:443–453.
21. Davis PL, Crooks L, Arakawa M, McRee R, Kaufman L, Margulis AR. Potential hazards of MR imaging: heating and effects of changing magnetic fields on small metallic implants. *AJR Am J Roentgenol* 1981;137:857–860.
22. Lackman RW, Kaufman B, Hans JS, et al. MR imaging in patients with metallic implants. *Radiology* 1985;157:711–714.
23. Mechlin M, Thickman D, Krissel HY, Gefter W, Joseph P. Magnetic resonance imaging of post-operative patients with metallic implants. *AJR Am J Roentgenol* 1984;143:1281–1284.
24. Merritt CRB. Magnetic resonance imaging—a clinical perspective: image quality, safety, and risk management. *Radiographics* 1987;3:1001–1016.
25. Shellock FG. MR imaging of metallic implants and materials: a compilation of the literature. *AJR Am J Roentgenol* 1988; 151: 811–814.
26. Teitelbaum GP, Bradley WG Jr, Klein BD. MR imaging artifacts, ferromagnetism and magnetic torque of intravascular stents and coils. *Radiology* 1988;166:657–664.

Ultrasonography

27. Baratelli M, Cabitza P, Parini L. Ultrasonography in investigation of loose hip prosthesis. *Ital J Orthop Traumatol* 1986;12:77.
28. Bender CE, Berquist TH, Stears JG, Winkler NT, James EM, Brown ML, Welch TJ, May GR, Forbes GS. Diagnostic techniques. In: Berquist TH, ed. *Imaging of orthopedic trauma.* New York: Raven Press; 1992:1–37.
29. Dorfman GS, Froelich JA, Cronan JJ, Urbanek PJ, Herndon JH. Lower extremity venous thrombosis in patients with acute hip fractures: determination of anatomic location and time onset with compression sonography. *AJR Am J Roentgenol* 1990; 154: 851–855.
30. Földes K, Gaal M, Baliut P, Nemeryi K, Kiss C, Bolint GP, Buchanan WW. Ultrasonography after hip arthroplasty. *Skeletal Radiol* 1992;21:297–229.
31. Harcke HT, Grissom LE, Furkelstein MS. Evaluation of the musculoskeletal system with sonography. *AJR Am J Roentgenol* 1988;150:1253–1261.
32. Hermann G, Yeh HC, Lehr-James O. Diagnosis of popliteal cysts: double contrast arthrography and sonography. *AJR Am J Roentgenol* 1981;137:369–372.
33. Komppa GH, Northern JR, Haas DK, Lisecki E, Ghaed N. Ultrasound guidance for needle aspiration of the hip in patients with painful hip prosthesis. *J Clin Ultrasound* 1985;13:433–434.
34. Koski JM, Antilla P, Haalainen M, Isomaki H. Hip joint ultrasonography: correlation with intraarticular effusion and synovitis. *Br J Rheumatol* 1990;29:189–192.
35. Leopold GR. Ultrasonography of superficially located structures. *Radiol Clin North Am* 1980;18:161–173.
36. Winsberg F, Cooperberg PL. *Real-time ultrasonography.* New York: Churchill Livingstone; 1982.

Radionuclide Imaging

37. Abdel-Dayem HM, Brodawala YK, Papolemetriou T. Scintigraphic arthrography: comparison with contrast arthrography and future applications. *Clin Nucl Med* 1982;7:516–522.
38. Amundsen TR, Siegel MJ, Siegel BA. Osteomyelitis and infarction in sickle cell hemoglobinopathies: differentiation by combined technetium and gallium scintigraphy. *Radiology* 1984;153:807–812.
39. Baron NW, Davis LP, Flaherty LE, Muz J, Valdivieso M, Kling GA. Scintigraphic findings in patients with shoulder pain caused by interleukin-2. *AJR Am J Roentgenol* 1990;154:327–330.
40. Bellah RD, Summerville DA, Treves ST, Micheli LJ. Low back pain in adolescent athletes: detection of stress injury to the pars interarticularis with SPECT. *Radiology* 1991;180:509–512.
41. Berquist TH. *Imaging of orthopedic trauma.* 2nd ed. New York: Raven Press; 1992:16–19.
42. Collier BD, Carrera GF, Johnson RP, Isitman AT, Hellman RS, Zielowka JS, Knobel J. Detection of femoral head avascular necrosis in adults by SPECT. *J Nucl Med* 1985;26:979–987.
43. Collier BD, Johnson RP, Carrera GF, Isitman AT, Veluvolu P. Chronic knee pain assessed by SPECT: comparison with other modalities. *Radiology* 1985;157:795–802.
44. Collier BD, Johnson RP, Carrera GF, Meyer GA, Schwab JP, Flatley TS, Isitman AT, Hellman RS, Zielowka AS, Knobel J. Painful spondylolysis or spondylolisthesis studied by radiography and single photon emission computed tomography. *Radiology* 1985;153:207–211.
45. Duszynski DO, Kuhn JF, Afshani E, Riddlesberger MM Jr. Early radionuclide diagnosis of acute osteomyelitis. *Radiology* 1975; 117:337–340.
46. Fink-Bennet DM, Stanisavljevic S, Blake D, Weber K, Weir J, Mayne B. Improved accuracy for detecting an infected hip arthroplasty: sequential technetium-99m sulfur colloid/indium-111 white blood cell imaging. *J Nucl Med* 1988;29:887.
47. Fischman AJ, Rubin RH, Khaw BA, Callahan RJ, Wilkison R, Keech F, Nedelman M, Dragotahes S, Kramer PB, LaMaraglia GM, Lind S, Strauss HW. Detection of acute inflammation with 111-In-labeled nonspecific polyclonal IgG. *Semin Nucl Med* 1988;18:335–344.
48. Gates GF. SPECT imaging of the lumbosacral spine and pelvis. *Clin Nucl Med* 1988;13:907–914.
49. Gilday DL, Paul DJ, Paterson J. Diagnosis of osteomyelitis in children by combined blood pool and bone imaging. *Radiology* 1975;117:331–335.
50. Greaney RB, Gerber FH, Laughlin RL. Distribution and natural history of stress fractures in U.S. Marine recruits. *Radiology* 1983;146:339.
51. Greyson ND, Lotem MM, et al. Radionuclide evaluation of spontaneous femoral osteonecrosis. *Radiology* 1982;142:729–735.
52. Holder LE. Clinical radionuclide bone imaging. *Radiology* 1990;176:607–614.
53. Holder LE, Mackinnon SE. Reflex sympathetic dystrophy in the hands: strict clinical and scintigraphic criteria. *Radiology* 1984;152:517–522.
54. Howard JL, Barron BJ, Smith GG. Bone scintigraphy in the evaluation of extraskeletal injuries from child abuse. *Radiographics* 1990;10:67–81.
55. Intenzo C, Kim S, Millin J, Park C. Scintigraphic patterns of the reflex sympathetic dystrophy syndrome of the lower extremities. *Clin Nucl Med* 1989;14:657–661.
56. Jacobson AF, Stouper PC, Cronin EB, Stomper PC, Kaplan WD. Bone scans with one or two new abnormalities in cancer patients with no known metastases: frequency and serial scintigraphic behavior of benign and malignant lesions. *Radiology* 1990;175: 229–232.
57. Jacobson AF, Stouper PC, Stomper PC, Cronin EB, Kaplan WD. Bone scans with one or two new abnormalities in cancer patients

with known metastases: reliability of interpretation of initial correlative radiographs. *Radiology* 1990;174:503–507.
58. Kagan AR, Steckel RJ. Radiologic contributions to cancer management. *AJR Am J Roentgenol* 1986;147:305–312.
59. Lewin JS, Rosenfield NS, Hoffer PB, Downing D: Acute osteomyelitis in children: combined Tc-99m and Ga-67 imaging. *Radiology* 1986;158:795–804.
60. Magnuson JE, Brown ML, Hauser MF, Berquist TH, Fitzgerald RH Jr, Klee GG. In-111-labeled leukocyte scintigraphy in suspected orthopedic prosthesis infection: comparison with other imaging modalities. *Radiology* 1988;168:235–239.
61. Maurer AH, Chen DCP, Camarge EE, Wong DF, Wagner HN Jr, Alderson PO. Utility of three-phase skeletal scintigraphy in suspected osteomyelitis: concise communication. *J Nucl Med* 1981;22:941–949.
62. Maurice HD, Newman JH, Watt I. Bone scanning of the foot for unexplained pain. *J Bone Joint Surg [Br]* 1987;69B:448–452.
63. Maxon HR, Schneider HJ, Hopson CN, Miller EH, VonStein DE, Kereiakes JG, Cummings DD, McDevitt RM. A comparative study of indium-111 DTPA radionuclide and iothalanate meglumine roentgenographic arthrography in the evaluation of painful total hip arthroplasty. *Clin Orthop* 1989;245:156–159.
64. McAfee JG. Update on radiopharmaceuticals for medical imaging. *Radiology* 1989;171:593–601.
65. McKillop JH, McKay I, Cuthbert GF, Fogelman I, Gray HW, Sturrock RD. Scintigraphic evaluation of the painful prosthetic joint: a comparison of gallium-67 citrate and indium-111 labeled leukocyte imaging. *Clin Radiol* 1984;35:239–241.
66. Mehta RC, Wilson MA. Frostbite injury: prediction of tissue viability with triple-phase bone scanning. *Radiology* 1989;170:511–514.
67. Mettler PA, Guiberteau MJ. *Essentials of nuclear medicine imaging.* 3rd ed. Philadelphia: WB Saunders; 1991.
68. Murray IPC, Dixon J, Kohan L. SPECT for acute knee pain. *Clin Nucl Med* 1990;15:828.
69. Nussbaum AR, Treves ST, Micheli L. Bone stress lesions in ballet dancers: scintigraphic assessment. *AJR Am J Roentgenol* 1988;150:851–855.
70. Orzel JA, Saudaf NW, Richardson ML. Lymphoma of the skeleton: scintigraphic evaluation. *AJR Am J Roentgenol* 1988;150: 1095–1099.
71. Oyen WJG, vanHorn JR, Claessens RAMJ, Slooff TJJH, VanderMeer JWM, Corstens FHM. Diagnosis of bone, joint and joint prosthesis infections with In-111 labeled nonspecific human immunoglobulin G scintigraphy. *Radiology* 1992;182:195–199.
72. Palestro CJ, Kin CK, Swyer AJ, Capozzi JD, Solomon RW, Goldsmith SJ. Total hip arthroplasty: periprosthetic indium-111 labeled leukocyte activity and complementary technetium sulfur colloid imaging in suspected infection. *J Nucl Med* 1990;31: 1950–1955.
73. Palestro CJ, Swyer AJ, Kim CK, Goldsmith SJ. Infected knee prosthesis: diagnosis with In-111 leukocytes, Tc-99m sulfur colloid, and Tc-99m MDP imaging. *Radiology* 1991;179:645–648.
74. Papanicolaou N, Wilkinson RH, Keshavarzian A, Rivett AG, Krause T, Combs RRH, Lavender JP. Bone scintigraphy and radiography in young athletes with low back pain. *AJR Am J Roentgenol* 1985;145:1039–1044.
75. Park WM, Rothschild PA, Kernek CB. Scintigraphic evaluation of extremity pain in children: its efficacy and pitfalls. *AJR Am J Roentgenol* 1985;145:1079–1084.
76. Pring DJ, Henderson RG, et al. Indium-granulocyte scanning in the painful prosthetic joint. *AJR Am J Roentgenol* 1986;146:167–172.
77. Roddie ME, Peters MA, et al. Inflammation: imaging with Tc99m HMPAO-labeled leukocytes. *Radiology* 1988;166:786–772.
78. Rosenthal L, Aldis AJ, Hill OH. Combined radionuclide and radiocontrast arthrography for evaluating hip arthroplasty. *Eur J Nucl Med* 1985;10:531–534.
79. Rubin RH, Fischman AJ, Needleman NM, Wilkinson R, Callahan RJ, Khaw BA, Hansen WP, Kramer PB, Strauss HW. The use of radiolabeled, nonspecific polyclonal human immunoglobulin in the detection of focal inflammation by scintigraphy: comparison with gallium-67 citrate and technetium-99m labeled albumin. *J Nucl Med* 1989;30:385–389.
80. Rupani HD, Holder LE, Espinola DA, Engin SI. Three phase radionuclide bone imaging in sports medicine. *Radiology* 1985;156:187–196.
81. Ryan PJ, Evans PA, Gibson T, Fogelman I. Chronic low back pain: comparison of bone SPECT with radiography and CT. *Radiology* 1992;182:849–854.
82. Schauwecker DS. The scintigraphic diagnosis of osteomyelitis. *AJR Am J Roentgenol* 1992;158:9–18.
83. Schauwecker DS. Osteomyelitis: diagnosis with In-111-labeled leukocytes. *Radiology* 1989;171:141–146.
84. Seabold JE, Nepola JV, Conrad GR, Marsh JL, Montgomery WJ, Brider JA, Kirchner PT. Detection of osteomyelitis at fracture nonunion sites: comparison of two scintigraphic methods. *AJR Am J Roentgenol* 1989;152:1021–1027.
85. Termeulen DC, Majd M. Bone scintigraphy in the evaluation of children with obscure skeletal pain. *Pediatrics* 1987;79:587–592.
86. Tumeh SS, Aliabadi P, Weissman BD, McNeil BJ. Chronic osteomyelitis: bone and gallium scan patterns associated with active disease. *Radiology* 1986;158:685–688.
87. Uri G, Wellman H, Capello W, Robb J, Greenman G. Scintigraphic and x-ray arthrographic diagnosis of femoral prosthesis loosening: concise communication. *J Nucl Med* 1984;25:661–663.
88. Urman M, Ammann W, Sisler J, Lentle BC, Lloyd-Smith R, Loomer R, Fisher C. The role of bone scintigraphy in the evaluation of talar dome fractures. *J Nucl Med* 1991;32:2241–2244.
89. Wellman HN, Schauwecker DS, Capello WN. Evaluation of metallic osseous implants with nuclear medicine. *Semin Nucl Med* 1988;18:126–136.

Interventional Procedures

90. Bassett LW, Loftus AA, Mankouvich NJ. Computer processed subtraction arthrography. *Radiology* 1985;157:821.
91. Bell GR, Modic MT. Radiology of the lumbar spine. In: Simeone FA, Rothman RH, eds. *The spine.* 3rd ed. Philadelphia: WB Saunders; 1992:125–153.
92. Bender CE, Berquist TH, Stears JG, Winkler NT, James EM, Brown ML, Welch TJ, May GR, Forbes GS. Diagnostic techniques. In: Berquist TH, ed. *Imaging of orthopedic trauma.* New York: Raven Press; 1992:1–38.
93. Berquist TH. *Imaging of orthopedic trauma and surgery.* Philadelphia: WB Saunders; 1986.
94. Berquist TH. Diagnostic and therapeutic injections. *Semin Intervent Radiol* 1993; 10(4):326–343.
95. Berquist TH, Bender CE, Maus TP, Williams HJ. Pseudobursae: a useful finding in patients with painful hip arthroplasty. *AJR Am J Roentgenol* 1987;148:103–106.
96. Brodgley CE. The articular facets in relation to low back pain and sciatic radiation. *J Bone Joint Surg* 1941;23:481–496.
97. Carrera GF. Lumbar facet injection in low back pain and sciatica. *Radiology* 1980;137:665–667.
98. Destouset JM, Gilulah A, Murphy WA, Monsees B. Lumbar facet injection. Indication, technique, clinical correlation and preliminary results. *Radiology* 1982;145:321–325.
99. Dory MA. Arthrography of the lumbar facet joints. *Radiology* 1981;140:23–27.
100. El-Koury GY. Facet injection. *Semin Intervent Radiol* 1993; 10(4): 255–261.
101. Esses SJ, Botsford DJ, Kostuik JP. The role of external spine skeletal fixation in assessment of low back disorders. *Spine* 1989;14: 594–601.
102. Freiberger RH, Kaye J. *Arthrography.* New York: Appleton-Century-Crofts; 1979.
103. Garcia-Cumbredo E, Munuera L. Early and late loosening of the acetabular cup after low-friction arthroplasty. *J Bone Joint Surg [Am]* 1992;74A:1119–1128.
104. Guilford WB: Discography. *Semin Intervent Radiol* 1993; 10(4): 291–307.

105. Hirsch C. An attempt to diagnose the level of the disk lesion clinically by disk puncture. *Acta Orthop Scand* 1948;18:132–140.
106. Holt EF Jr. The question of lumbar discography. *J Bone Joint Surg* [*Am*] 1968;50A:720–726.
107. Kikuchi S, McNab I, Moreau P. Localization of the level of symptomatic cervical disk degeneration. *J Bone Joint Surg* [*Br*] 1981;63B:272–277.
108. Kilcoyne RF, Kaplan P. The lateral approach for hip arthrography. *Skeletal Radiol* 1992;21:239–240.
109. Lang EK. Transcatheter embolization of pelvic vessels to control intractable hemorrhage. *Radiology* 1981;140:331–339.
110. Maus TP, Berquist TH, Bender CE, Williams HJ. Arthrographic study of painful hip arthroplasty. Refined criteria. *Radiology* 1987;162:721–727.
111. McCutcheon ME, Thompson WC. CT scanning of lumbar discography. *Spine* 1986;11:257–259.
112. Milette PC, Melanson D. A reappraisal of lumbar discography. *Can Assoc Radiol J* 1982;33:176–182.
113. Pedersen HE, Blinick CFJ, Gardner E. The anatomy of the lumbosacral posterior rami and meningeal branches of the spinal nerves. *J Bone Joint Surg* [*Am*] 1956;38A:377–391.
114. Reid JDS, Redman HC, Wergelt JA, Thol ER, Frances H III. Value of arteriography in detection of arterial injury. *AJR Am J Roentgenol* 1988;151:1035–1039.
115. Slaney G, Ashton F. Arterial injuries and their management. *Postgrad Med* 1971;47:254–269.
116. Vanharanta H, Sachs BL, Spivey MA, Hochschuler SH, Guyer RD, Rashbaum RR, Ohnmeiss DD, Mooney V. A comparison of CT/discography, pain response and radiographic disc height. *Spine* 1988;13:321–324.
117. Weissman BW. The radiology of total joint replacement. *Orthop Clin North Am* 1983;14:171–191.
118. Wilkinson HA. *The failed back syndrome: etiology and therapy.* New York: Harper and Row; 1983.
119. Winkler NT. Roentgenographic subtraction technique. *Radiol Technol* 1968;39:339.

Imaging Atlas of Orthopedic Appliances and Prostheses, edited by T.H. Berquist.
Mayo Clinic Foundation © 1995.
Published by Raven Press, Ltd., New York.

CHAPTER 2

General Orthopedic Fixation Devices

Thomas H. Berquist and Mark P. Brodersen

Fixation devices (Table 2-1) are often poorly understood by radiologists. Fixators may be used for trauma or reconstructive procedures. Selection of the proper device to fit the injury or osteotomy is critical to achieve proper healing and maintain function.[3,5,7,34] This section reviews general fixation devices and describes the selection process, image appearance, and complications related to their use. Devices designed for specific use in certain anatomic regions are discussed more fully in later anatomic chapters.

BASIC PRINCIPLES OF FIXATION

The goals of fracture management and many reconstructive procedures are to restore the normal anatomy and maintain function.[28,41,53] Continued developments in orthopedic hardware have increased the opportunity to achieve better reduction with operative management.[3,4,6,7]

When possible, closed reduction of fractures is used in cases in which alignment with external fixation can be achieved. Most often, casting or an external splint is used. When closed reduction fails or when fractures are better suited to internal fixation (e.g., articular fractures, periarticular fractures, and certain types of long bone fractures), open reduction is selected as the method of treatment.[28,29,40,53]

Prior to demonstrating specific hardware, it is important to review certain basic concepts of internal fixation. Fracture healing is facilitated by proper alignment, preservation of soft tissue support and vascular supply, apposition of the fractured surfaces, and maintenance of the stability of the fractures.[28,41] The principles of internal fixation for fracture treatment are reviewed and disseminated to physicians by the Arbeitsgem einschaft für Osteogynthese fragen (AO) and Association for Study of Internal Fixation (ASIF) group.[39,51]

The object of internal fixation is to improve fracture apposition and maintain stability (prevent motion at the fracture site). There are two basic principles of fixation: compression and splinting. These goals can be achieved in several ways and may be applied separately or in combination.[39]

Interfragment compression increases the contact and stability of the fragments. Uniform compression across the fracture site should be achieved when possible.[53] Adequate compression reduces excess callus formation, which is frequently detected with excess motion at the fracture site. Compression may be static or dynamic.[39,51]

With static compression, the forces act uniformly, and they are constant.[28,39,51] Static compression can be achieved by using several types of fixation devices. External fixation devices (Fig. 2-1) produce axial compression by using threaded pins with external adjustment rods. These devices are most commonly used for arthrodesis, metaphyseal osteotomies, and open lower-extremity fractures.[39] Lag screws are used to create interfragment compression (Fig. 2-2). The term "lag screw" describes its function and does not indicate a specific type of screw. Although the various types of screws are discussed later, it is important to describe their function here. To function as a lag screw, the screw must move freely in the proximal fragment and secure and approximate the distal fragment to the proximal fragment. Therefore, malleolar and cancellous screws that have smooth shafts and distal threads are well suited for this purpose. Cortical screws are threaded over their entire length. Therefore, the proximal cortex must be over-

T. H. Berquist: Mayo Medical School and Department of Diagnostic Radiology, Mayo Clinic Jacksonville, Jacksonville, Florida 32224.

M. P. Brodersen: Mayo Medical School and Department of Orthopedic Surgery, Mayo Clinic Jacksonville, Jacksonville, Florida 32224.

TABLE 2-1. *General fixation devices*

Internal fixation
Screws
Plates
Angled-blade plates
Medullary nails
Wires
Cables
External fixation
Traction devices

drilled (oversized hole) to allow the use of cortical screws as lag screws. When possible, lag screws are inserted perpendicularly to the fracture line (not necessarily perpendicularly to the bone) (Fig. 2-3).[39,51,53] Screw fixation alone provides the needed stability in situations in which the fracture length is two- to threefold the diameter of the bone (Fig. 2-2) or in fractures with a large surface area.[39]

Static compression can also be achieved with short oblique or transverse fractures by using compression or buttress plates. The plates are prestressed by using a tension bending device or placing the screws eccentrically in a compression plate. Either method causes compression of the cortices of the fracture fragment (Fig. 2-4).[39,51,53]

Dynamic compression devices allow muscle forces or body weight to enhance the compressive forces.[39,53] One example of a dynamic compression device is tension-band wiring of the patella (Fig. 2-5).

Compression techniques are best suited to transverse fractures or osteotomies and short oblique fractures. Fractures with comminution or bone loss or fractures susceptible to shortening or instability require additional support with splinting or buttressing.[3,7,40]

Splinting is a less stable method of fixation that typically allows healing to occur by secondary callus formation. It can be accomplished with internal or external devices. External splinting includes cast, cast-pin, and external fixator techniques (Fig. 2-6). Internal splinting can be accomplished with fixation plates or intramedullary nails (Fig. 2-7).[8,40,44] Splinting reduces motion but does not rigidly fix the fracture fragments. Splinting may be accomplished with or without load bearing (Fig. 2-5).

Combination techniques provide both compression and splinting. Examples include compression-screw and side-plate fixation of intratrochanteric fractures (Fig. 2-8), buttress-plate fixation of the upper tibia (Fig. 2-9), and Kirschner-wire (K-wire) tension (and fixation) of olecranon fractures (Fig. 2-10).[39]

INTERNAL FIXATION DEVICES

Screws

Screws may be used alone or with fixation plates. The latter are discussed in the next section. There are two basic screw designs (Fig. 2-11). Cortical screws are threaded along their entire length. Cancellous and malleolar screws are generally partially threaded. Cortical screws are used primarily in the diaphyses, and cancellous screws are used in the metaphyses and epiphyses.[28,39,51,53]

There are numerous types of screws that vary in length, type of point, thread diameter, pitch (thread distance), and head configuration (Figs. 2-12 and 2-13). However, based on their use, two basic types (cancellous and cortical) are commonly used.[28,39,53]

Cortical Screws

Cortical screws are typically threaded over their entire length, and they have a blunt end (Figs. 2-8, 2-9, 2-11, and 2-13). The threads are less prominent (shallower) and more closely spaced than are the cancellous screws. Predrilling and tapping of cortical screws is usually required, although self-tapping screws are available. It is generally thought that tapped screws hold better than do self-tapped ones. Washers or countersinking may be used with thin cortex or thick cortex, respectively, to distribute the force more effectively. In addition, washers protect areas in which the cortex is thin (i.e., metaphysis or osteoporotic bone).[53] Cortical screws should penetrate the opposite cortex by 1 to 2 mm when properly placed, either alone or with a plate (Fig. 2-14).

Cancellous Screws

Cancellous screws have wider threads with more space between threads than do cortical screws (Fig. 2-11). Threads may extend along the length of the screw, but more often, the screws are partially threaded (Figs. 2-9A and 2-11). Partially threaded screws are ideal lag screws because they obtain purchase in the distal fragment but not the proximal fragment. In this setting, the length of the threaded and nonthreaded portions of the screw must be carefully selected prior to insertion. Cancellous screws are most commonly used in metaphyseal or, primarily, cancellous bone.[39,51,53]

Malleolar Screws

At first glance, malleolar screws resemble cancellous screws radiographically (Fig. 2-15). These screws are partially threaded but have close cortical screw threads and a trocar tip; they are self-tapping. The trocar tip (cortical screws are blunt) and finer thread pattern help to differentiate malleolar screws from cortical screws (compare Figs. 2-9A and 2-15).

(text continues on page 54)

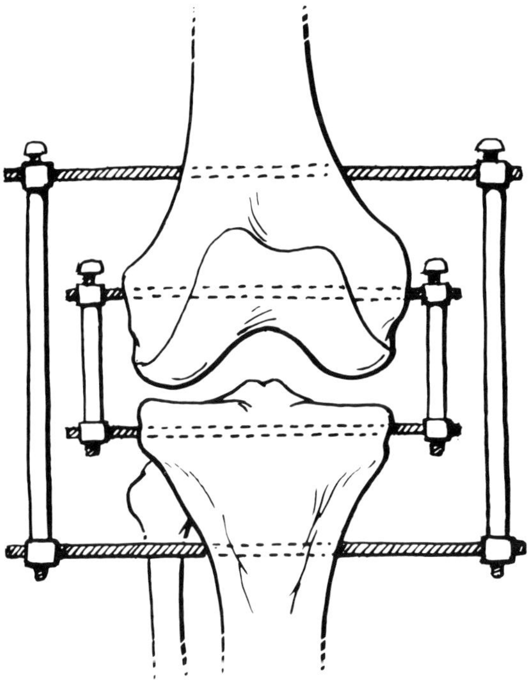

FIG. 2-1. An external fixator used for static compression in knee arthrodesis.

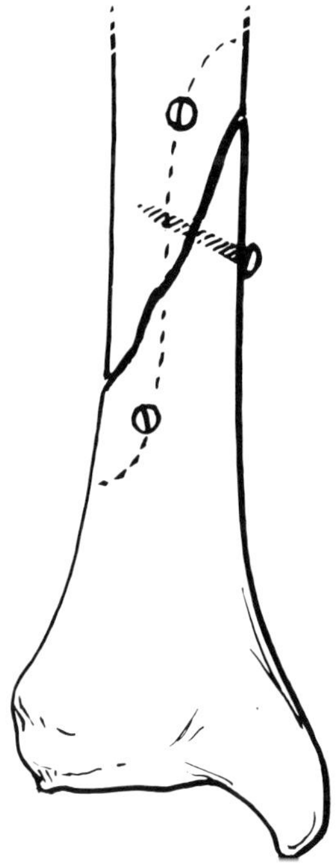

FIG. 2-2. A spiral fracture of the distal tibia fixed with three lag screws. Note the length of the fracture is two- to threefold the diameter of the bone.

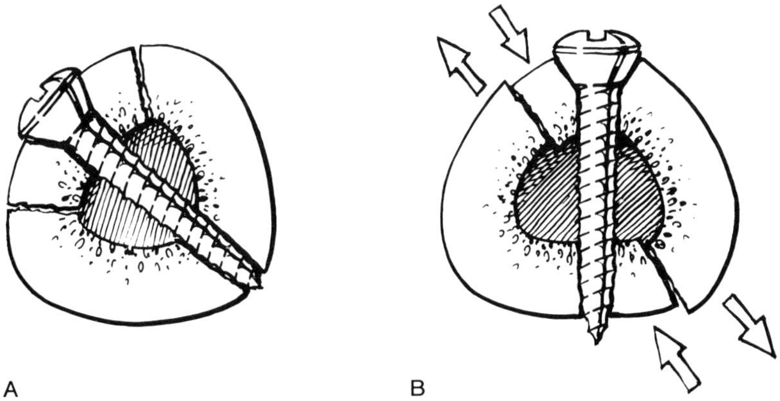

A B

FIG. 2-3. Correct **(A)** and incorrect **(B)** orientation of the lag screw to the fracture line. The screw should be perpendicular to the fracture plane to function optimally.

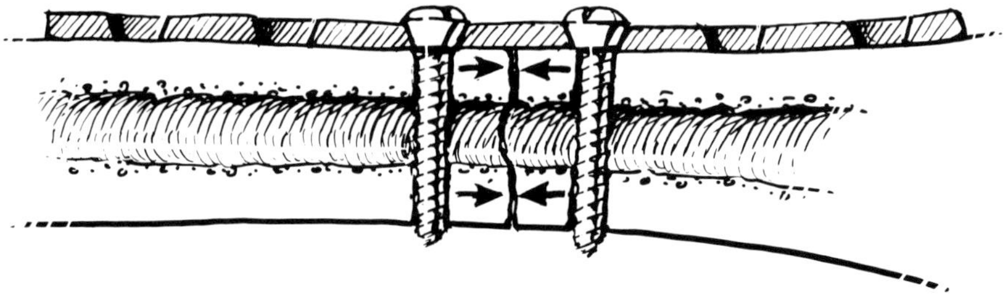

FIG. 2-4. Eccentrically placed screw in a dynamic compression plate, resulting in static interfragment compression. As the large head of the screw rotates into the oval opening, the plate is moved so that compression of the fracture occurs.

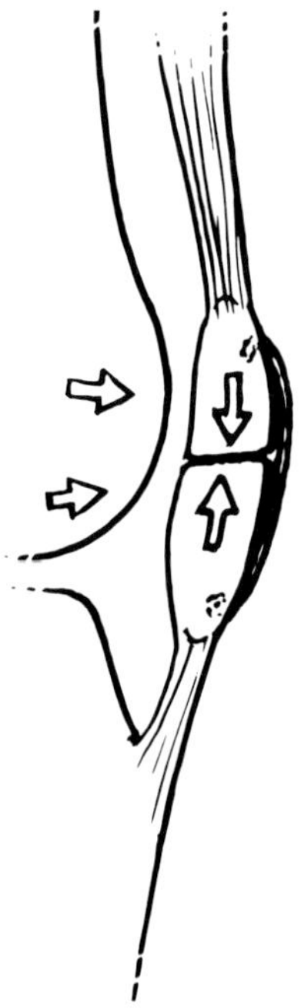

A

FIG. 2-5. Tension-band wiring of a transverse patellar fracture. *A: Arrows* demonstrate the force. Anteroposterior (AP, **B**) and lateral **(C)** views of the knee after "figure-eight" tension-band wiring of a patellar fracture.

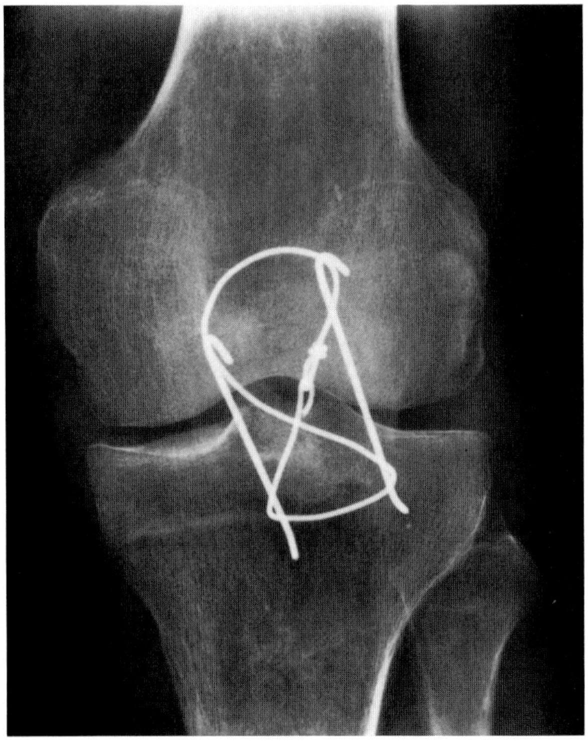

B

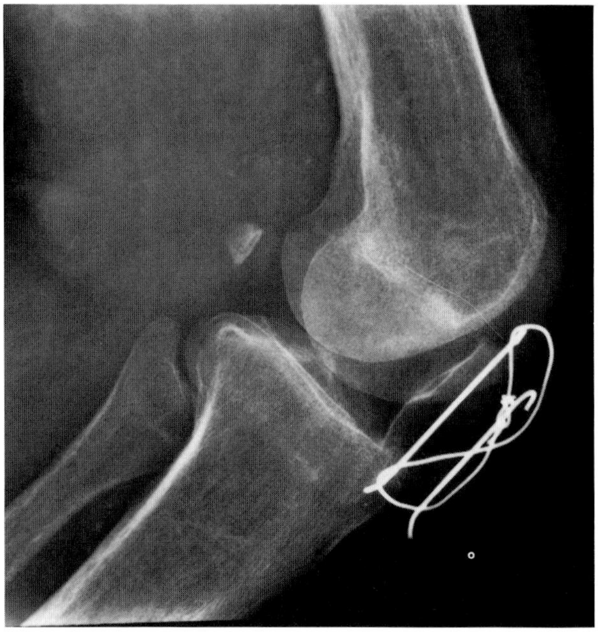

C

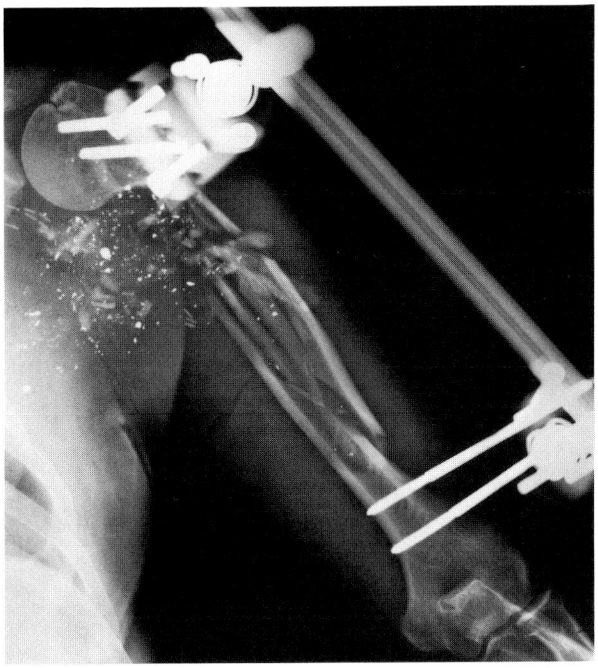

FIG. 2-6. Gunshot injury to the left humerus with severe diaphyseal fragmentation. An external fixator is used to splint the injury.

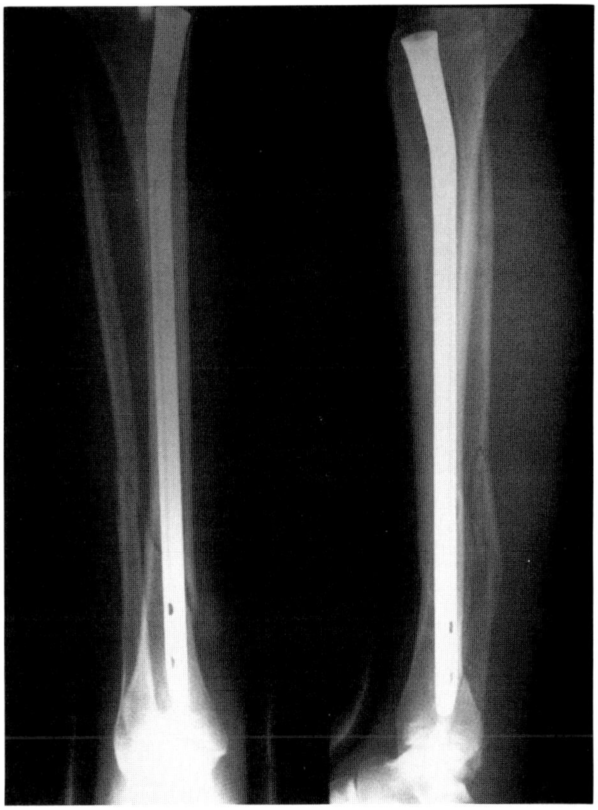

FIG. 2-7. The AP and lateral radiographs of distal third tibial and fibular fractures. The tibial fracture is internally splinted with a medullary nail.

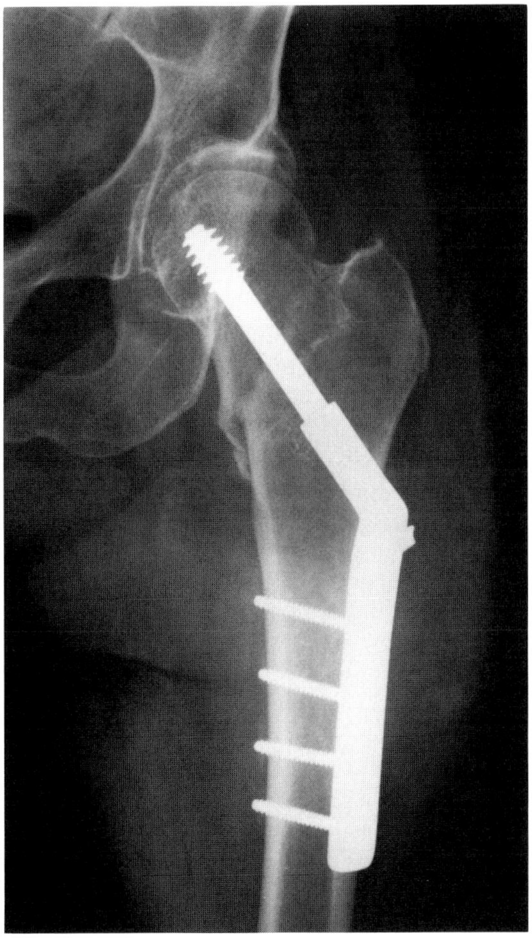

FIG. 2-8. The AP view of the hip after fixation of an intertrochanteric fracture with a dynamic hip screw and 135° angled four-hole plate. There are four cortical screws that properly penetrate both cortices.

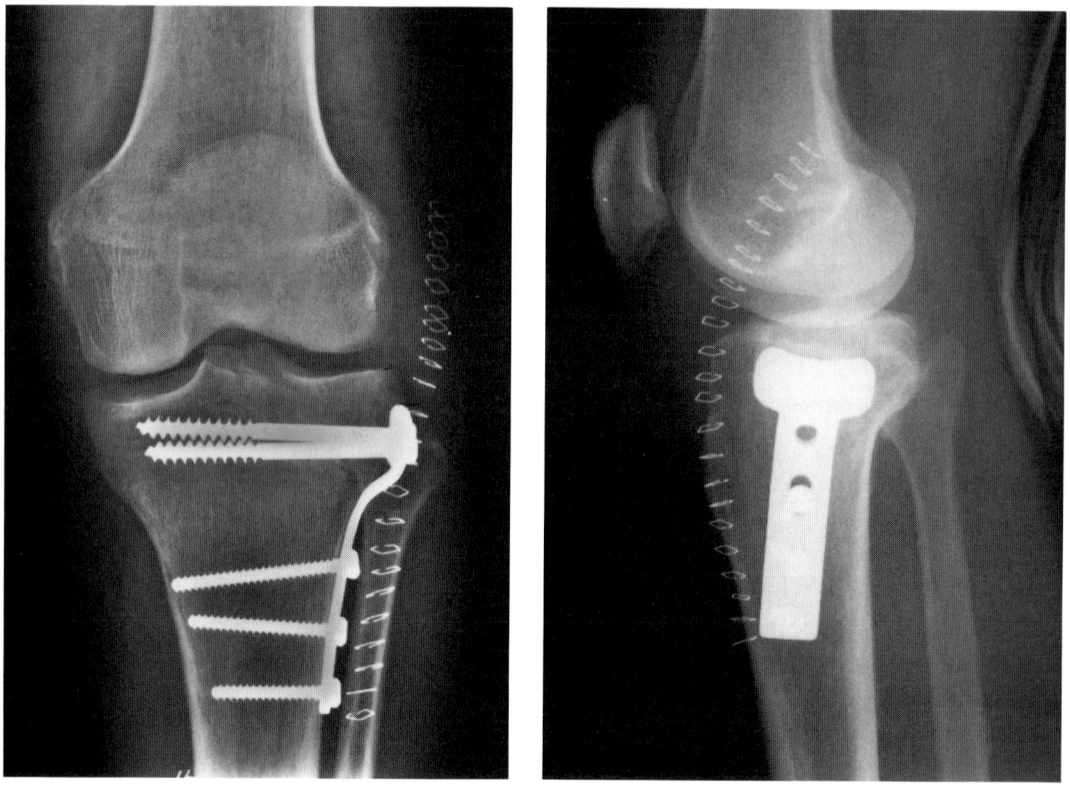

A B

FIG. 2-9. The AP **(A)** and lateral **(B)** views of the knee after internal fixation of a tibial plateau fracture using a "T" buttress plate with two cancellous screws proximally and three cortical screws distally.

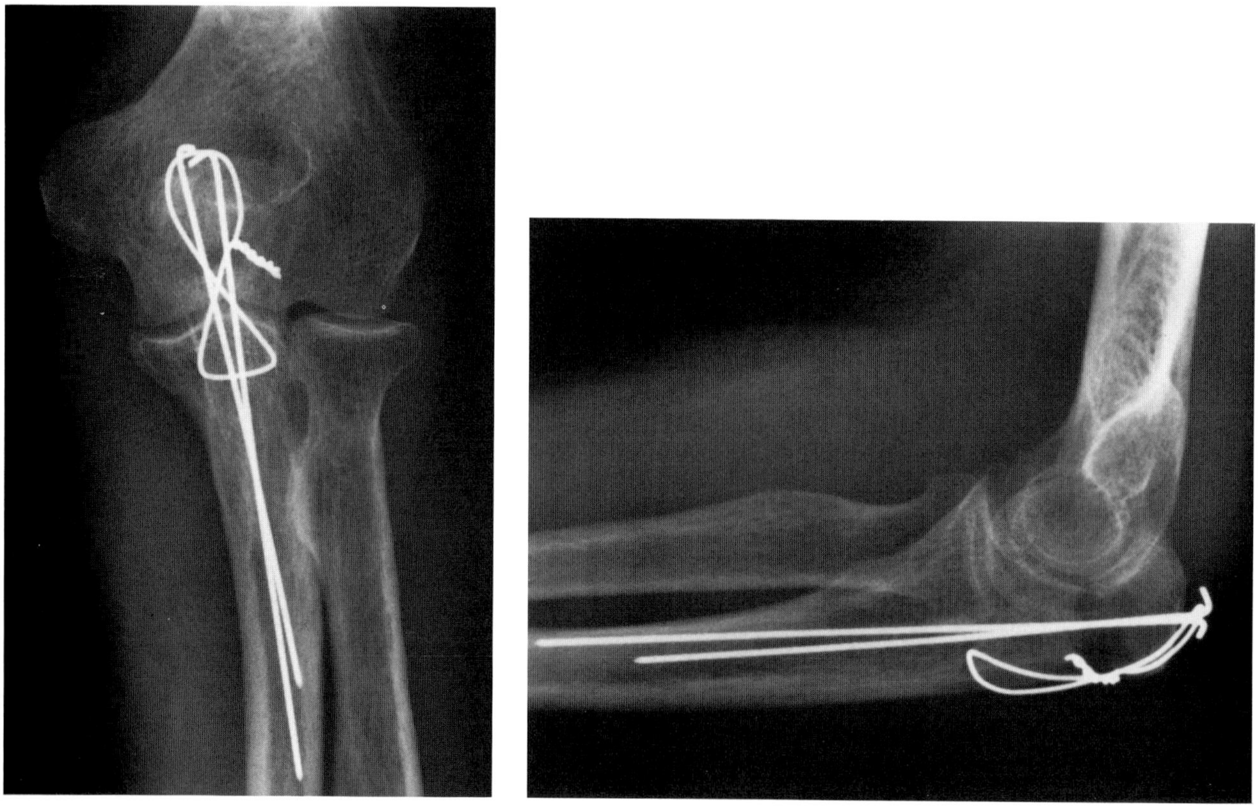

A B

FIG. 2-10. The AP **(A)** and lateral **(B)** views of the elbow, demonstrating an olecranon fracture fixed with two K wires and tension-band wiring technique.

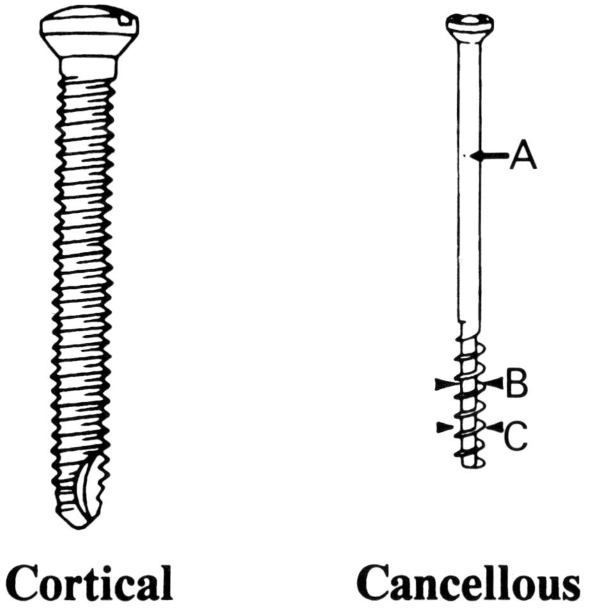

FIG. 2-11. Two basic screw designs: cortical (fully threaded) and cancellous (distal threads). **A:** Shank. **B:** Core diameter. **C:** Thread diameter. (Courtesy of Zimmer, Warsaw, IN.)

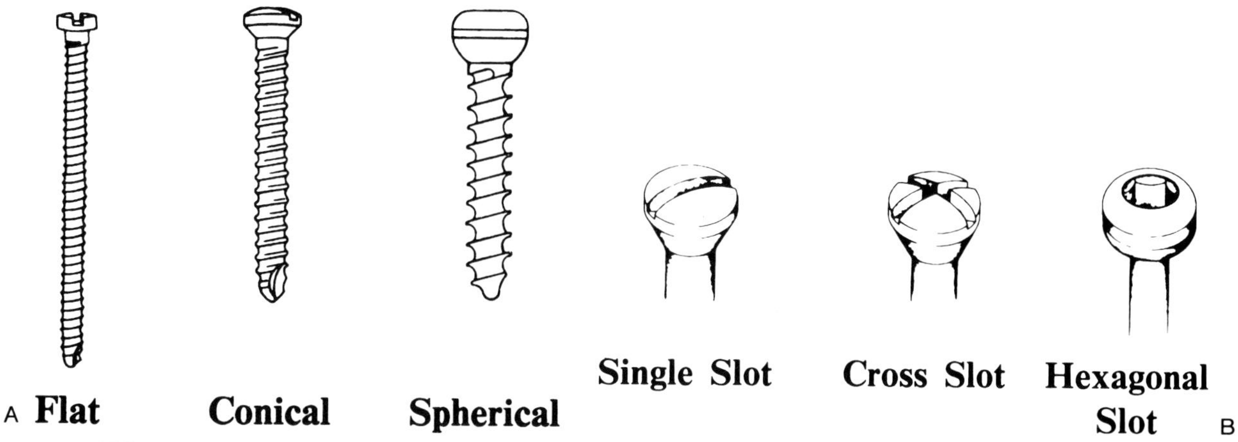

FIG. 2-12. The types of screw head configuration **(A)** and slot **(B)**. (Courtesy of Zimmer, Warsaw, IN.)

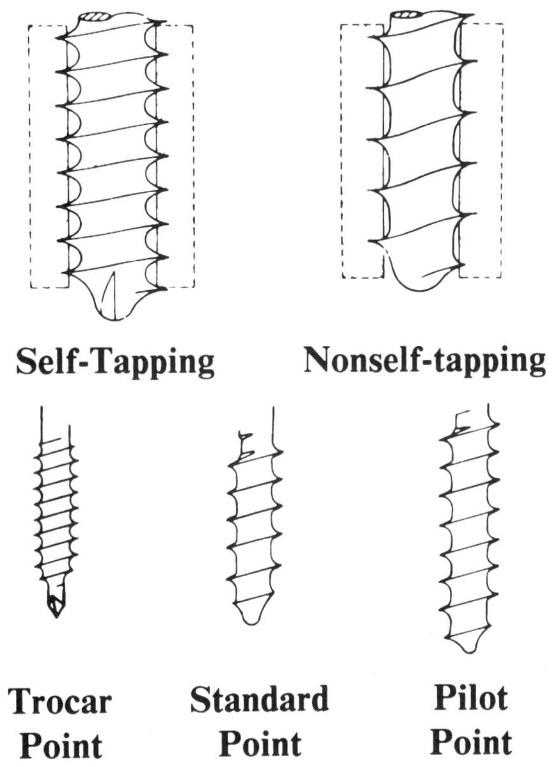

FIG. 2-13. Screw points and self-tapping and nonself-tapping screws. Self-tapping screws (*upper left*) can be inserted after a pilot hole has been drilled. The pilot hole is larger than the core, and the screw must cut its own thread. This can result in breakage, which can pass through cortical bone.[39,51] Nonself-tapping screws (*upper right*) require a pilot hole and tapping (cutting for threads in cortical bone). The threads achieve a deeper cut into adjacent bone with this screw type. The screws are more easily inserted and removed. This type of screw has less advantages in regions in which the cortex is thin (e.g., metaphysis or ilium).[39,51] (Courtesy of Zimmer, Warsaw, IN.)

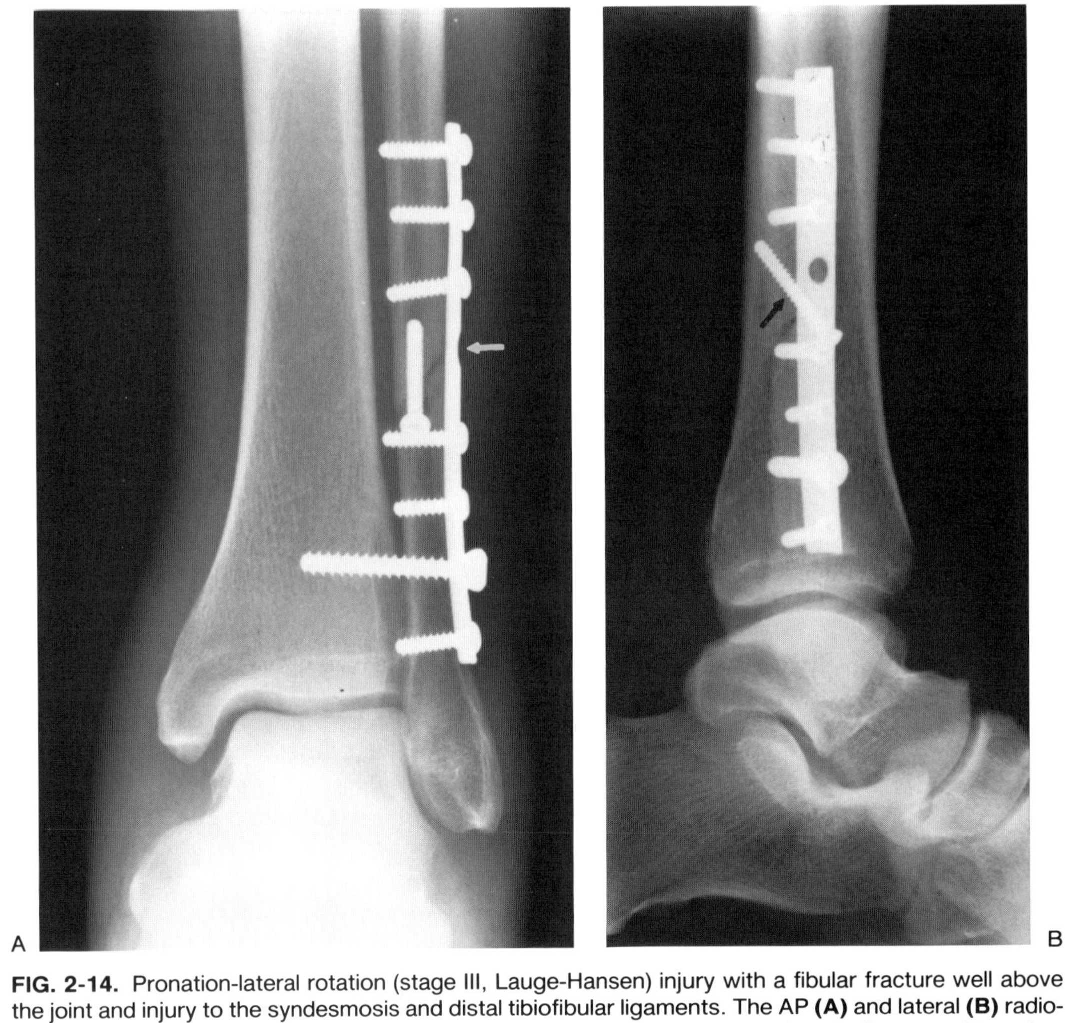

FIG. 2-14. Pronation-lateral rotation (stage III, Lauge-Hansen) injury with a fibular fracture well above the joint and injury to the syndesmosis and distal tibiofibular ligaments. The AP **(A)** and lateral **(B)** radiographs demonstrate internal fixation with an eight-hole semitubular plate and cortical screws. There is a lag screw in the fibula, which is perpendicular to the fracture line. This is best seen on the lateral view (*black arrow*). Obviously, there is no screw in the plate at this level (*white arrow,* AP view). A syndesmosis screw (*second from the bottom*) bridges the tibia and fibula.

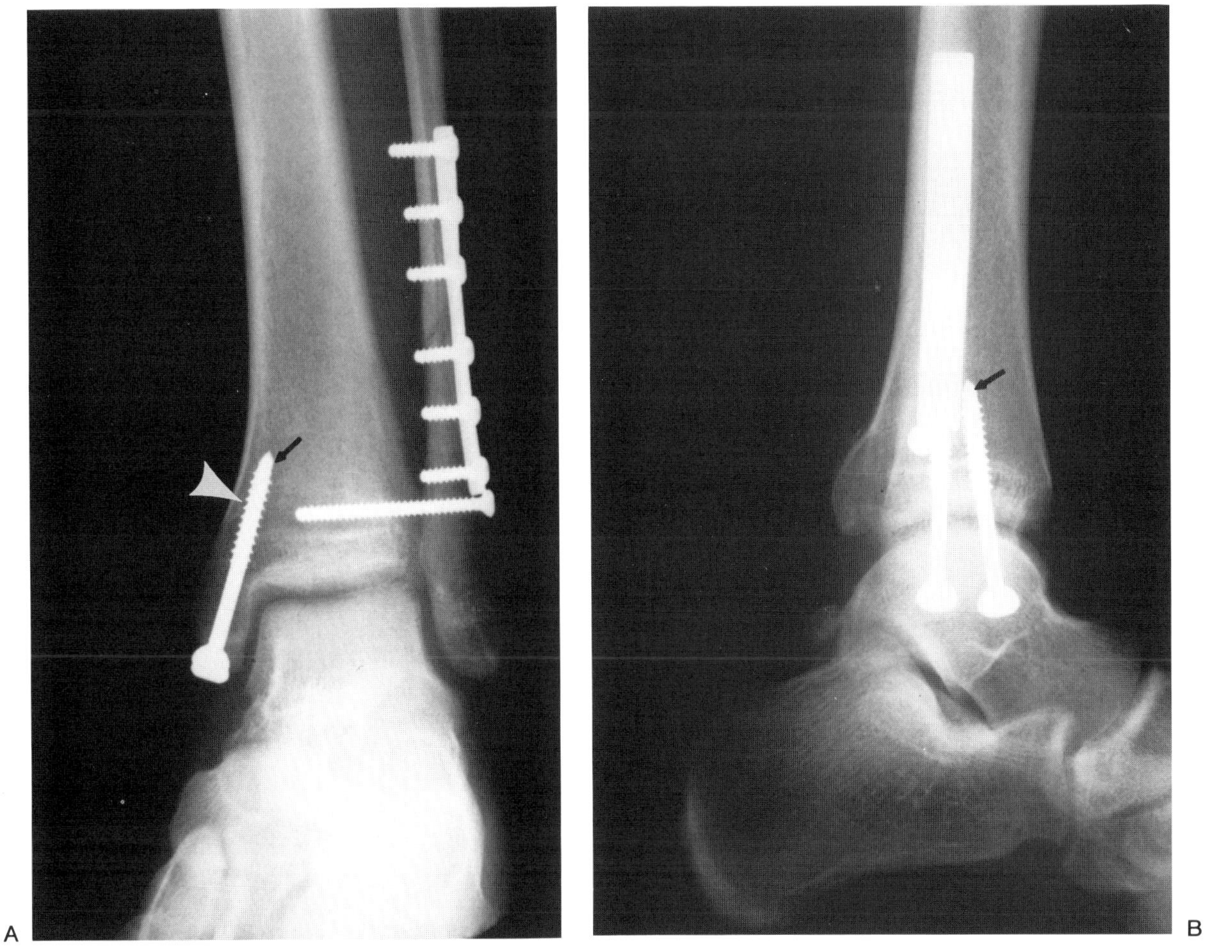

FIG. 2-15. Pronation-lateral rotation stage IV (Lauge-Hansen) injury with cortical screws and semitubular plate fixation of the fibular fracture. There is also a cortical syndesmosis screw below the plate. The medial malleolar fracture is fixed with two malleolar screws. Note the thread pattern (*white arrowhead*) resembles a cortical screw. Also note the trocar point (*black arrow*). See Fig. 2-9A for comparison with typical cancellous screw appearance.

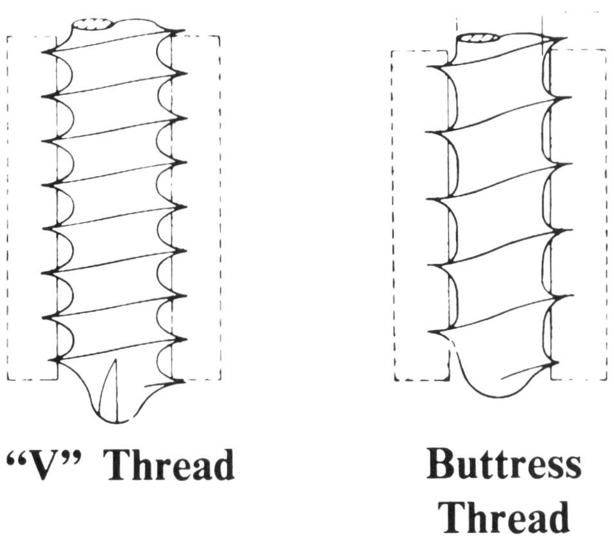

FIG. 2-16. "V" and buttress thread designs for bone screws. (Courtesy of Zimmer, Warsaw, IN.)

Screw Design

Head

The heads on large screws (Fig. 2-12) are typically round with a spheric undersurface to ensure proper contact with plate holes or bone. The spheric head is essential when used with dynamic compression plates (DCP).[39] Hexagonal sockets in the screw heads are used so that the screws can be inserted without pressure. This configuration also facilitates removal of the screws.[40]

Screw Threads

Asymmetric threads are used with bone (Fig. 2-16). The weaker the bone is, the wider the thread spaces are.

Nuts

Nuts can be used to increase the stability in osteopenic bone or to provide additional compression, such as with a tibial bolt for tibial plateau fractures (Fig. 2-17). Methyl methacrylate can also be used with screws to improve their purchase.[39,53]

Washers

Washers are used to enhance the compressive area of a screw and in regions in which the cortex is thin to prevent fractures under the screw. Washers may be flat (Fig. 2-18) or have serrated edges (Fig. 2-19). The latter are used to reattach small avulsed fragments or ligaments to bone. Serrated edges may not be radiopaque, making it difficult to identify these washers radiographically.[39,53]

Special Screw Variations

Specific screw configurations have been developed for certain regions. These are discussed more fully in later anatomic chapters. However, several basic differences are described in this section.

Cannulated Screws

Cannulated screws (Fig. 2-20) are typically used in the juxtaarticular region in which positioning is more critical. The hollow lumen allows the screw to be inserted over a wire guide. Following screw placement, the lumen can be studied with contrast medium to be certain that the joint has not been entered.[38,51] Other categories of screws (discussed subsequently) are also available with cannulation to assist with positioning.

Cannulated screws may have cortical or cancellous threads. Sliding screws are also available (Fig. 2-21) to allow compression at the fracture site.

Interference Screws

Interference screws (Fig. 2-22) are available in several configurations, depending on the function needed and the anatomy. Most are short fully threaded devices with sunken or recessed heads so that the head is not visible radiographically. These screws are used as anchors for bone plugs or bone tendon grafts. These devices are commonly used for cruciate repairs in the knee (Fig. 2-23).[49]

Soft Tissue Anchors

Soft tissue anchors are used to provide a mechanism of anchoring sutures to bone for soft tissue repairs, such to the rotator cuff or shoulder capsule. Several configurations are available. The Mitek anchor system (Mitek Surgical Products, Norwood, MA; Figs. 2-24 and 2-25) uses a suture holder with one, two, or four arcs or barbs. This dcvicc is constructed of nickel-titanium alloy and is fixed to bone in a predrilled hole.

Screw systems are also available. The Revo™ cancellous screw (Linvatec, Largo, FL) is inserted into a small pilot hole. This device was designed specifically for rotator cuff repairs (Fig. 2-26). The Statak™ soft tissue anchor (Zimmer, Warsaw, IN) is also used for shoulder repairs. It is constructed using Tivanium alloy. Both conventional and smaller (Mini-Statak™) sizes are available (Fig. 2-27).

Herbert Screws

The Herbert screw is unique in that it lacks a head and it is threaded on both ends (Fig. 2-28). The end that is introduced into the distal fragment has coarse threads and the proximal end, finer threads. The threads run in the same direction but have different pitch. This configuration allows compression of the fracture fragments. As there is no head, concern about damage to adjacent soft tissues is reduced. The screw is cannulated to allow accurate placement with a K wire. This screw is commonly used for scaphoid fractures of the wrist (Fig. 2-29) and osteochondral fractures.[39,51,53]

Compression Screws

Most dynamic screw systems are designed to be used with a side plate (Fig. 2-21). However, the Universal Compression screw (Howmedica, Rutherford, NJ) is designed as a screw within a screw to allow controlled compression of fracture fragments (Fig. 2-30). The distal threads can be designed for cancellous or cortical bone.

(text continues on page 65)

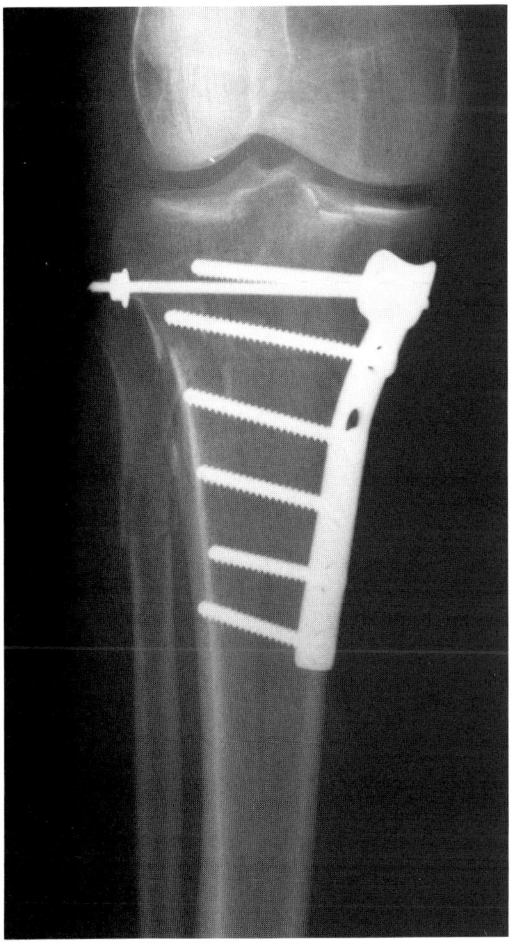

FIG. 2-17. Comminuted tibial plateau fracture. The AP radiograph shows internal fixation with a T-buttress plate and cortical screws. Further compression is achieved using a transtibial bolt and nut.

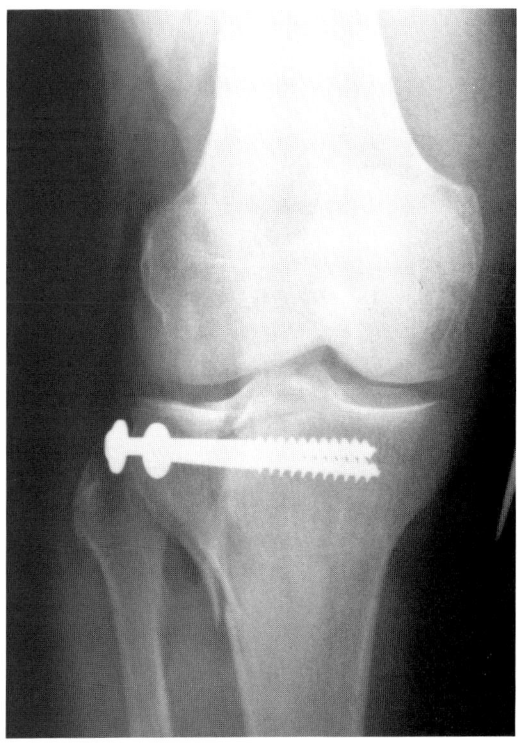

FIG. 2-18. Lateral tibial plateau fracture internally secured using two cancellous screws with washers.

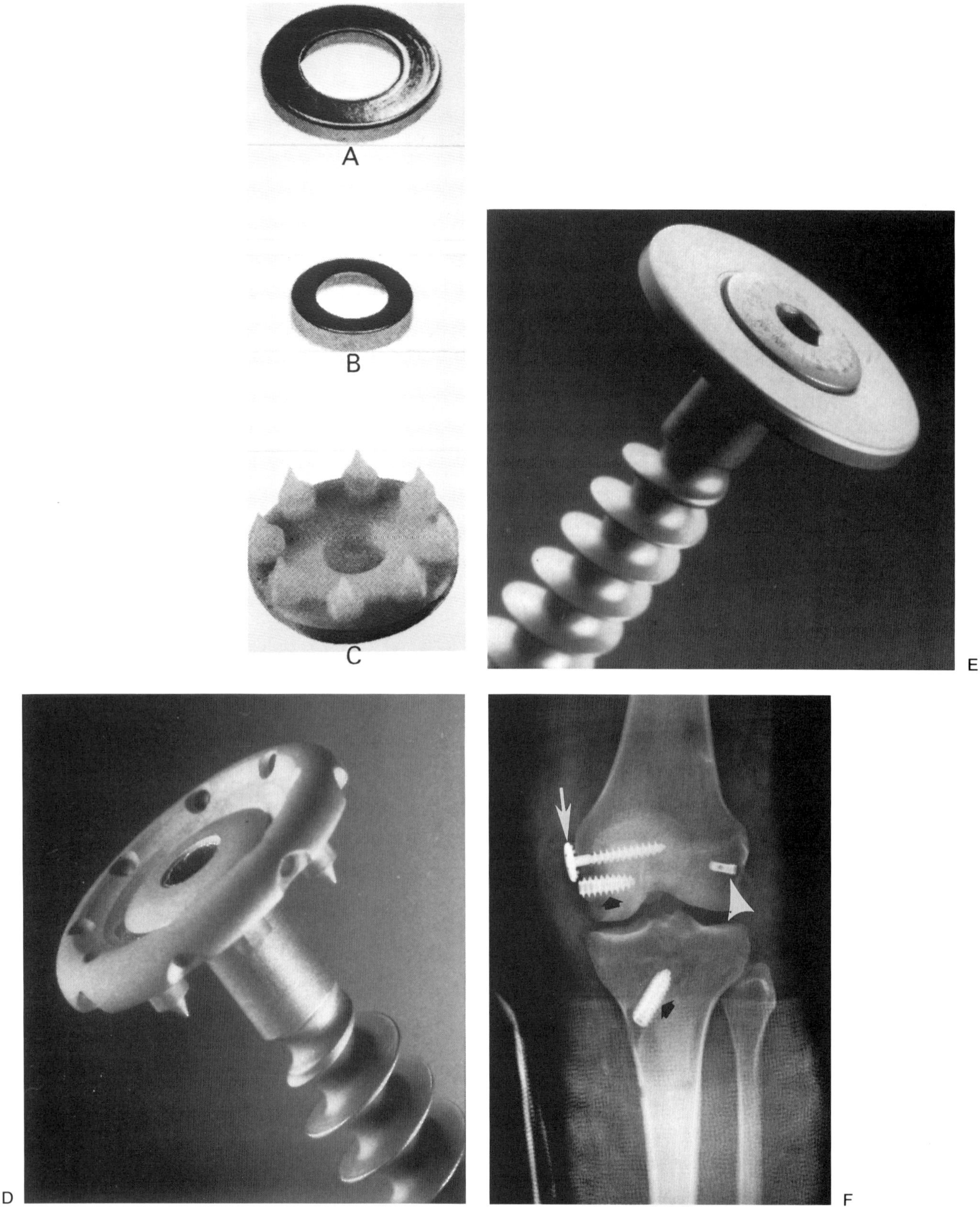

FIG. 2-19. A: Large washer for round-head screw. **B:** Small washer for use with 4-mm cancellous screws. **C:** Spiked washer. (A–C: Courtesy of Zimmer, Warsaw, IN.) Soft tissue anchoring implants. **D:** Spiked washer with screw. **E:** Flat washer with screw. (D,E: Courtesy of Linvatec, Largo, FL.) **F:** Ligament repair left knee with hinged cast in place. The medial collateral ligament has been reattached using a serrated washer (*arrow*) and cancellous screw. There are two interference screws for ligament repair (*black arrows*) and small suture screw [Statak™ (Zimmer) suture attached] laterally (*large white arrowhead*).

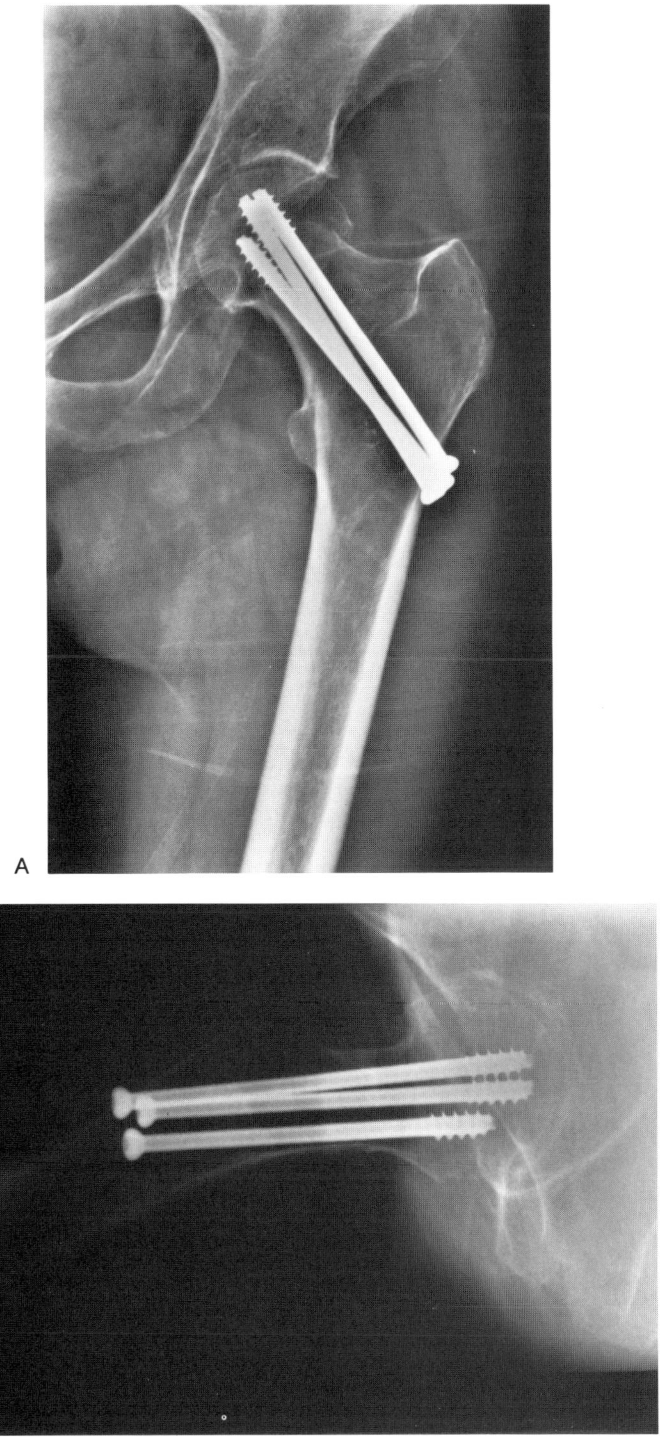

FIG. 2-20. Femoral neck fracture on the left with three cannulated screws for fixation. The central lumen is more easily appreciated on the lateral view **(B)** than the AP view **(A)** as a result of technique.

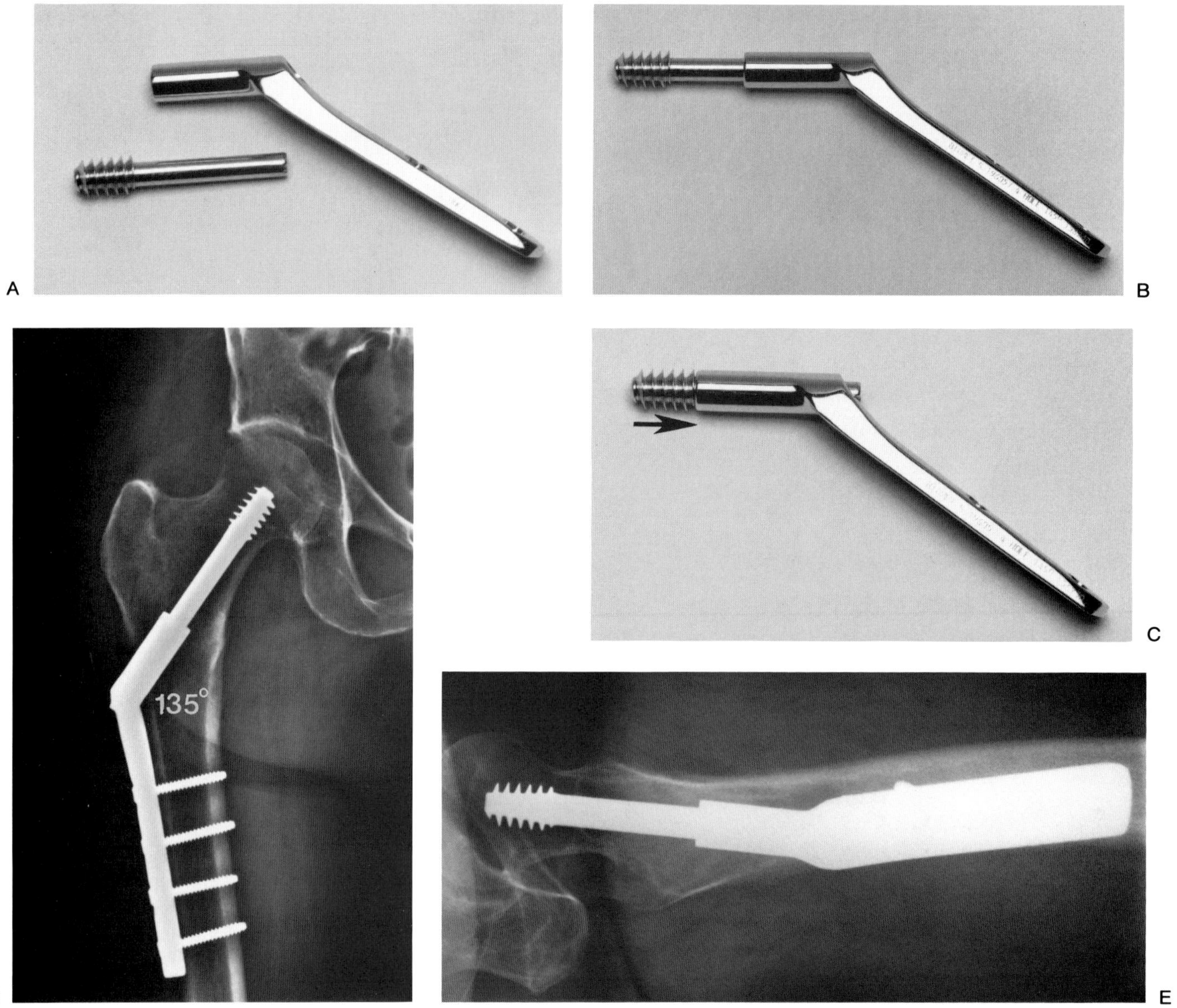

FIG. 2-21. A: Components of the dynamic hip screw (*DHS*) with compression screw and side plate. **B:** With screw in side plate. **C:** Screw can move into the side plate, allowing compression of the fracture fragments. The AP **(D)** and lateral **(E)** views after internal fixation of an intertrochanteric fracture using a dynamic hip screw and 135° four-hole side plate. Note the properly positioned cortical screws, which extend just beyond the far cortex. The most appropriate position for the screw thread of the large hip screw is in the inferior part of the femoral head on the AP and the center of the femoral head on the lateral view.

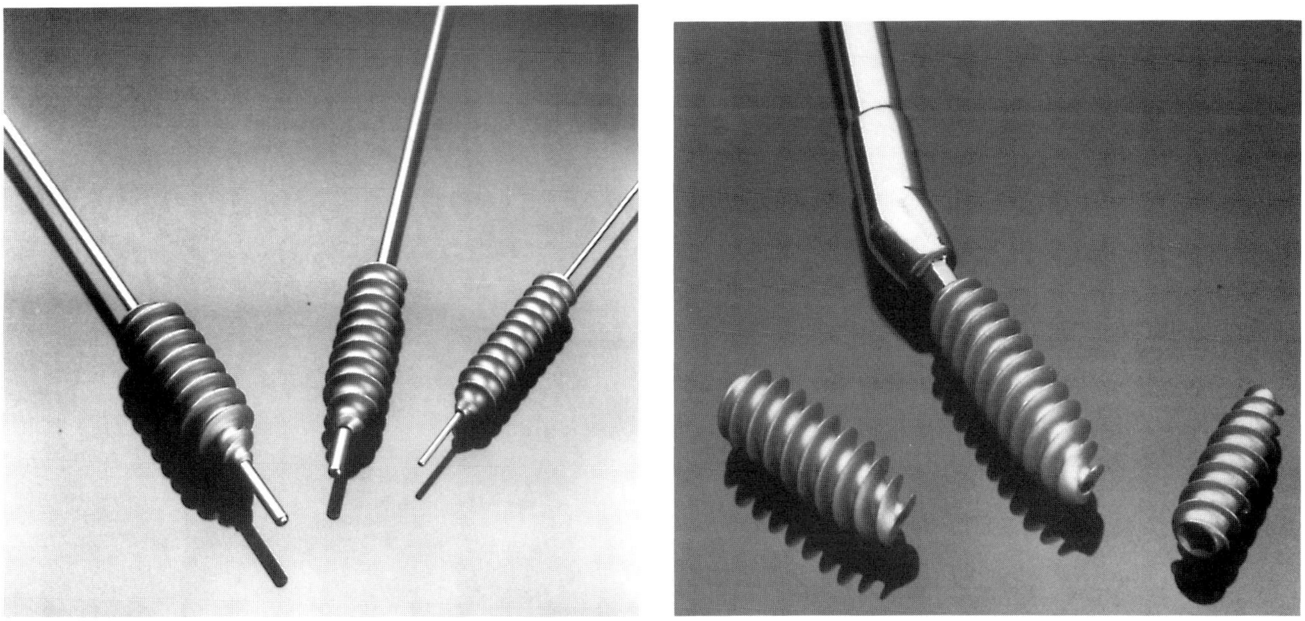

A B

FIG. 2-22. Cannulated interference screws. **A:** Three sizes of cannulated interference screws with guides in place (titanium alloy). Spiral thread design limits divergence with insertion. **B:** Propel™ cannulated interference screws. Double-helix threads permit screw to engage bone evenly on both sides, which reduces divergence with insertion. (Courtesy of Linvatec, Largo, FL.)

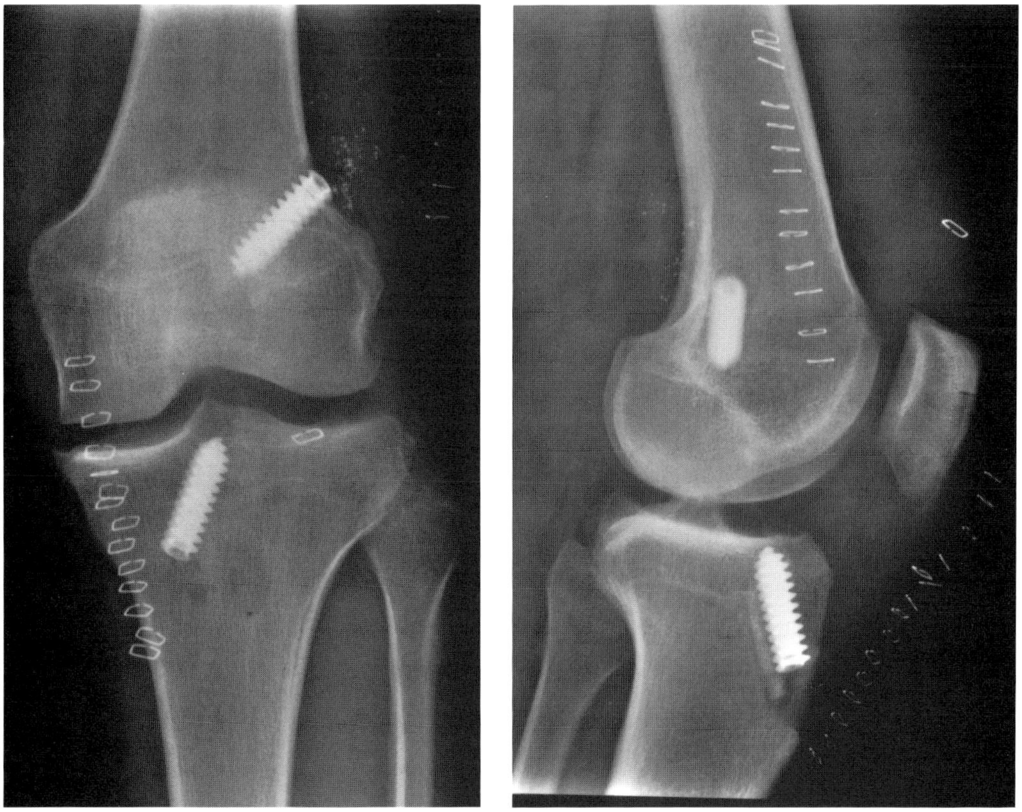

A B

FIG. 2-23. The AP **(A)** and lateral **(B)** views of the knee after anterior cruciate ligament repair. There are two interference screws to secure the ligament graft. The heads on these screws are recessed. This type of screw should not be confused with a fractured screw remnant. Some types of these interference screws are cannulated (see Fig. 2-22).

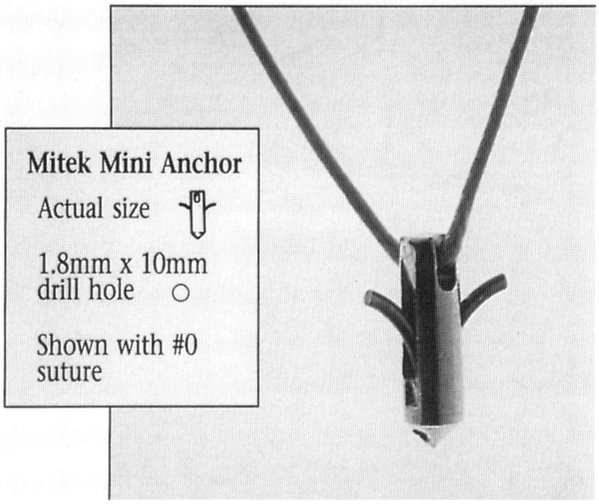

A

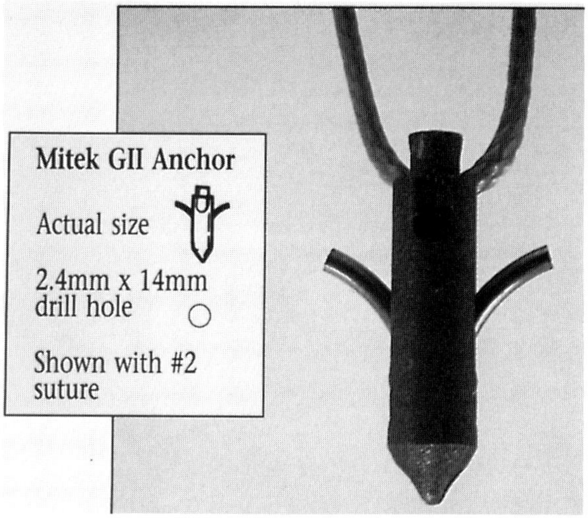

B

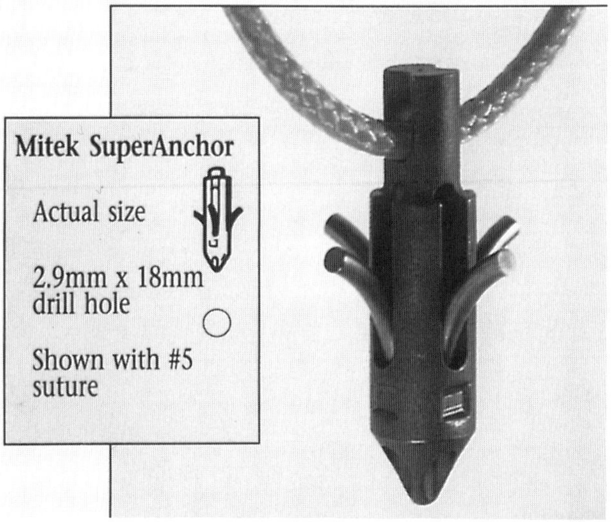

C

FIG. 2-24. Mitek™ soft tissue anchors and sutures with insert, demonstrating actual size. **A:** Minianchor with two barbs or arcs. **B:** GII anchor with suture. **C:** Mitek super anchor with four barbs or arcs. (Courtesy of Mitek Surgical Products, Norwood, MA.)

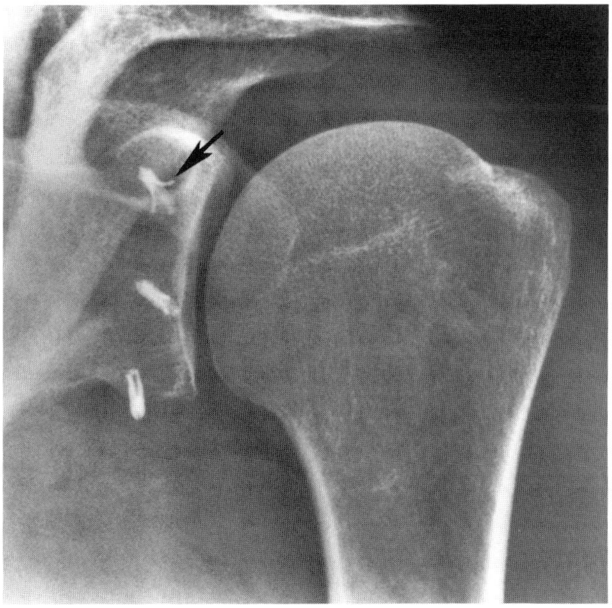

FIG. 2-25. The AP view of the left shoulder with three Mitek™ soft tissue anchors. The two barbs on the upper anchor (*arrow*) are clearly displayed.

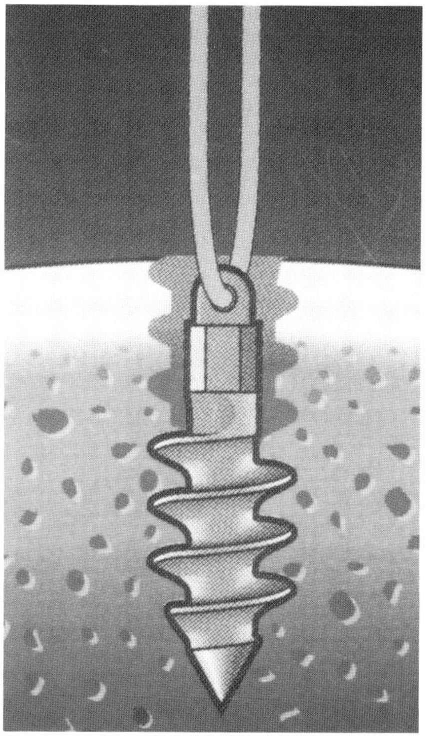

FIG. 2-26. Revo™ cancellous screw and suture in the humeral head. (Courtesy of Linvatec, Largo, FL.)

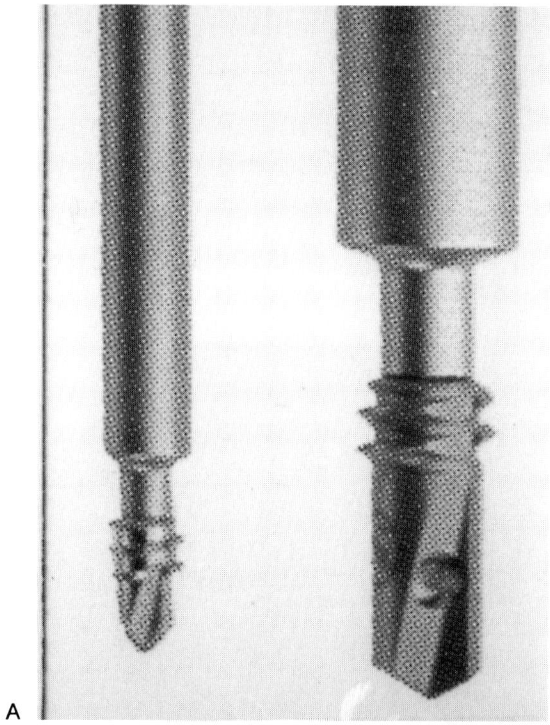

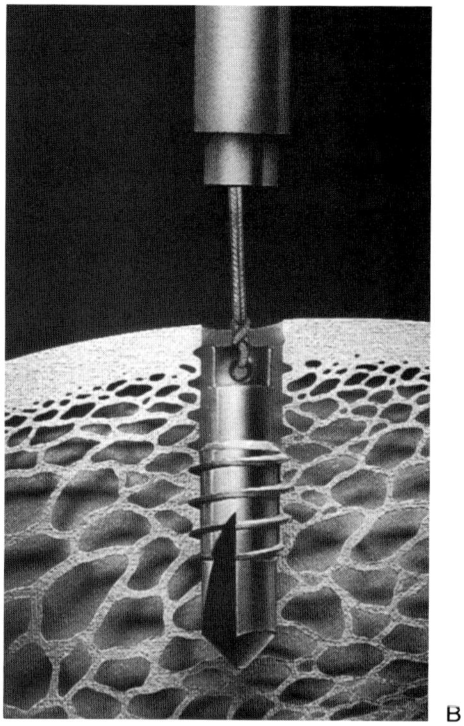

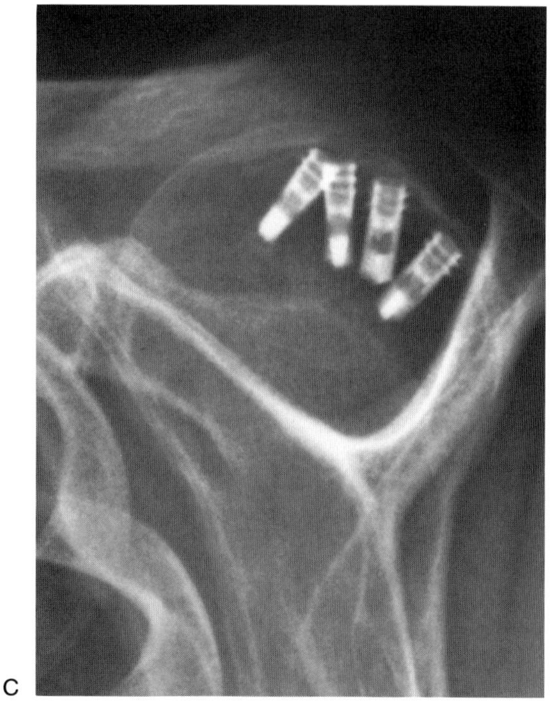

FIG. 2-27. Statak™ soft tissue device. **A:** Statak™(11 mm × 3.8 mm) and Mini-Statak™ (8 mm × 1.9 mm) on 0.25-inch Jacobs Chuck for insertion. **B:** Illustration of Statak™ with suture after insertion. (Courtesy of Zimmer, Warsaw, IN.) **C:** Shoulder outlet view demonstrating four Statak™ devices in the humeral head.

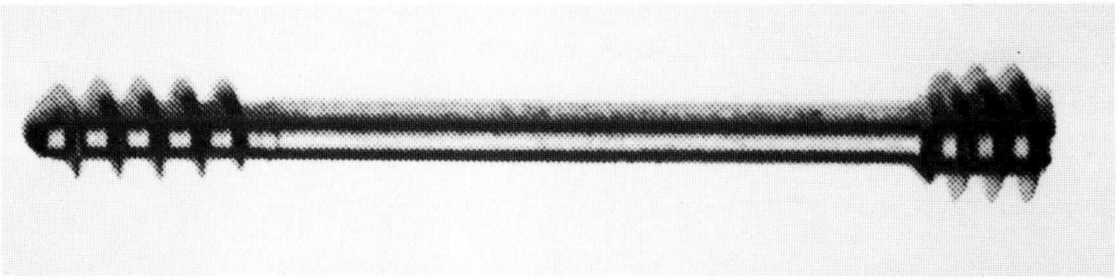

FIG. 2-28. Herbert screw. The screw is threaded at both ends. (Courtesy of Zimmer, Warsaw, IN.)

A

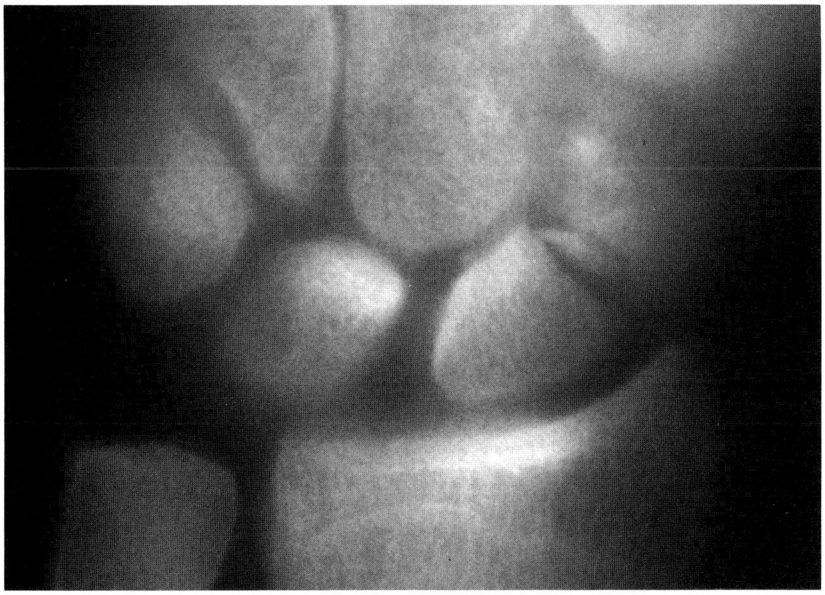

B

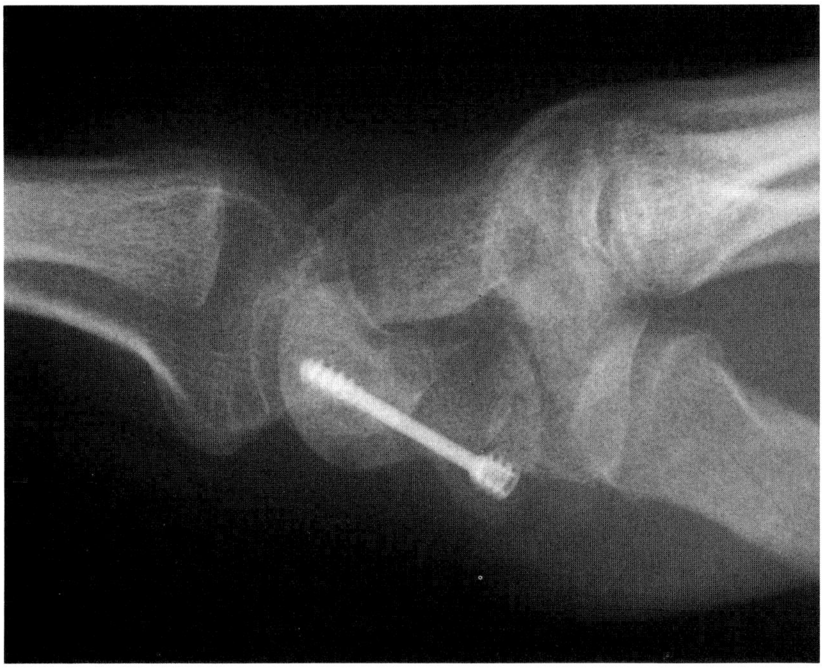

FIG. 2-29. Scaphoid fracture. **A:** Posteroanterior (PA) tomogram of the wrist demonstrates a transverse comminuted scaphoid fracture. **B:** The fracture was internally fixed using a Herbert screw, which is demonstrated on the lateral postoperative radiograph.

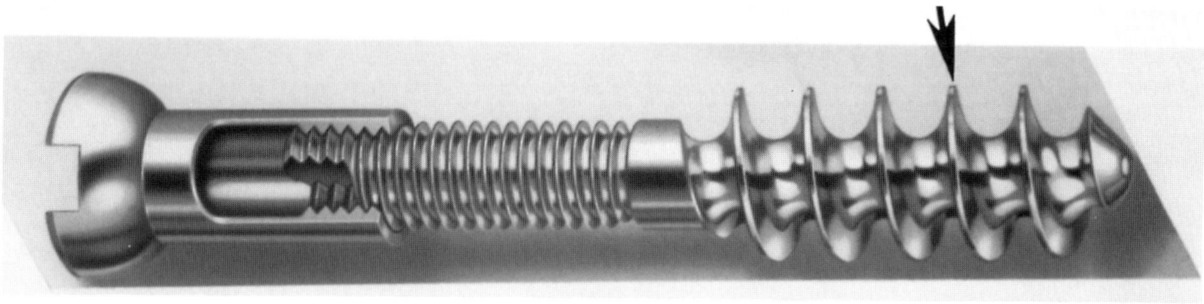

FIG. 2-30. Universal compression screw with cancellous distal threads (*arrow*). (Courtesy of Howmedica, Rutherford, NJ.)

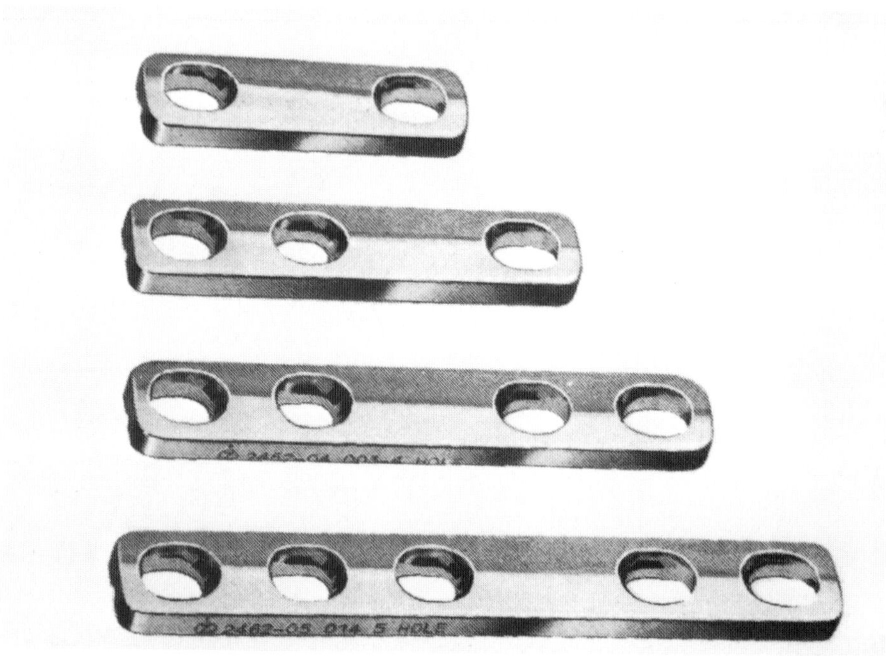

FIG. 2-31. Narrow DCPs with oval holes (two, three, four, and five holes *top to bottom*) in the midline. (Courtesy of Zimmer, Warsaw, IN.)

Plates

Orthopedic plates come in various sizes and shapes with different lengths, numbers, and types of screw holes. Compression plates are used for fractures that can be stabilized with compressive forces. Neutralization plates protect the underlying bone from rotation and axial loading. Buttress plates are generally used in the metaphyseal areas to support fractures that are unstable with compressive or axial loading.[39,53]

There are two basic types of plates: straight and special configuration.[28,39,51] Straight plates are most commonly used in the diaphysis and special plates, in the metaphyseal and epiphyseal regions.[51,53] The plates may function primarily for compression, buttressing, or neutralizing fragments.[53]

Straight Plates

Dynamic Compression Plates (DCP)

The DCP are distinguished by their oval holes. The holes are midline in narrow plates (Fig. 2-31) and offset in broad plates (Fig. 2-32). These plates have several advantages over conventional round-hole plates. Fragment compression can be more readily achieved by positioning or sometimes angling the screw in the oval hole (Fig. 2-3). The ability to angle the screw allows some of the holes to be used for lag screws in the fixation of fractures.[3,49] Drill guides are used to ensure the proper positioning of the screws. Placing screws in the hole eccentrically results in self-compression of the fragments (Fig. 2-3).[36,37] Broad plates are commonly used for the femur and humerus. Narrow plates are used for the tibia, fibula, radius, and ulna.[51,53]

Round-Hole Plates

These plates have round holes and are also available in broad or narrow configurations. These plates may be used for the femur and humerus.

Semitubular Plates

These plates are distinguished by their cross-sectional appearance (Fig. 2-33). Semitubular plates are thin (1 mm) and have less rigidity. The edges dig into the adjacent bone (reduces rotation, Fig. 2-33B), but because of their low rigidity, they are usually used in areas subject to tension forces.

Reconstruction Plates

These plates have scored edges and are designed to be contoured to the bone fragments. Reconstruction plates may be used for the acetabulum, calcaneus (Fig. 2-34), distal humerus, and mandible.[27,28,53]

Small and Miniplates

Smaller plates are designed for use in the smaller bones of the peripheral extremities, specifically the hand and wrist and foot and ankle. Many of these plates are simply smaller versions of the plates described elsewhere in this chapter (Fig. 2-35).

Special Plates

Most special plates are buttress plates designed for the metaphysis or epiphysis of specific anatomic regions. Special plates help prevent articular deformity. Radiographically, these plates are easily identified by their shape.

T and L Plates

T and L plates (Figs. 2-36 and 2-37) may be straight or come with a proximal bend. The latter are chiefly used as buttress plates for the medial tibial plateau and humeral head. The head of either type of T or L plate typically has two holes, which can accommodate 6.5-mm cancellous screws. Proximally, there is an elongated hole (Fig. 2-36) to allow temporary fixation while permitting longitudinal adjustment prior to placing the remaining screws.[28,51] The lateral tibial head plate (Fig. 2-38) has a special proximal design that is better suited to the lateral tibia.[39]

Spoon Plates

This plate is designed for the distal anterior tibia (Fig. 2-39). This plate is specifically shaped for large posterior-fragment comminuted fractures. Current use includes fractures of the distal humerus and tibia, which have not united. There is typically an elongated hole near the midportion of the plate.[39]

Cloverleaf Plates

These plates are commonly used for small-fragment fractures in the distal medial tibia or other metaphyseal regions (Fig. 3-40).

Cobra-Head Plates

These plates are specifically designed for hip fusion (Fig. 2-41).[39]

(text continues on page 74)

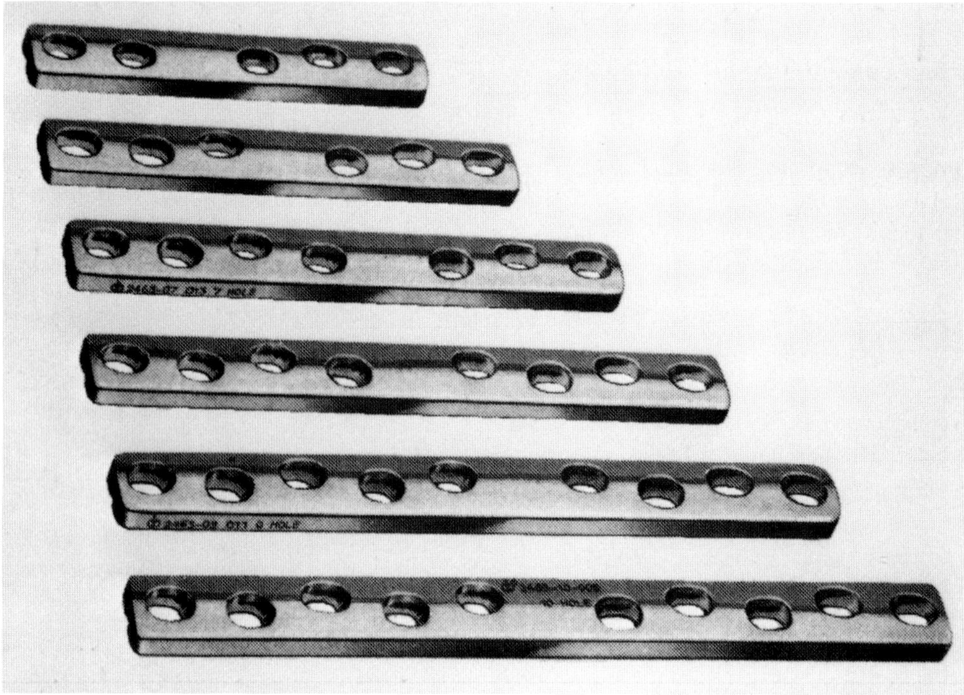

A

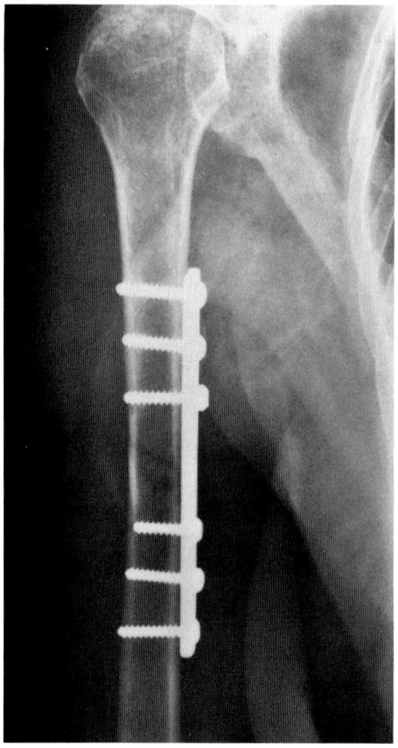

B

FIG. 2-32. A: Broad DCPs with holes (five, six, seven, eight, nine, and ten holes *top to bottom*) offset. (Courtesy of Zimmer, Warsaw, IN.) **B:** Humeral fracture internally fixed with a DCP and six cortical screws. Note the thickness of the plate compared with that of the semitubular plate (Fig. 2-33).

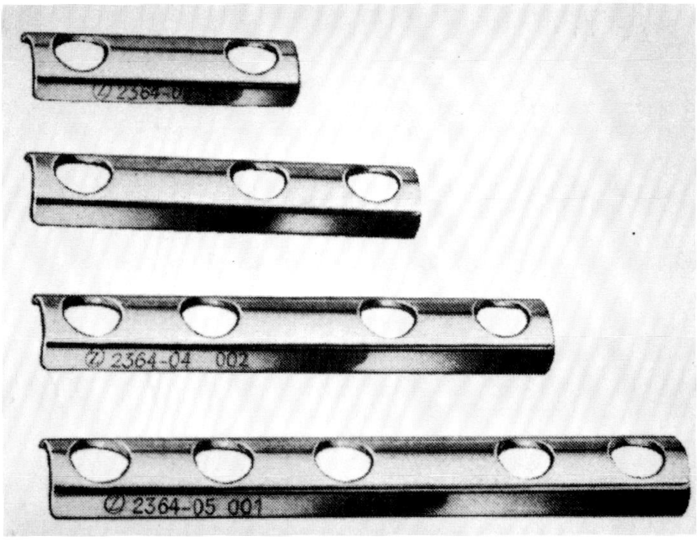

A

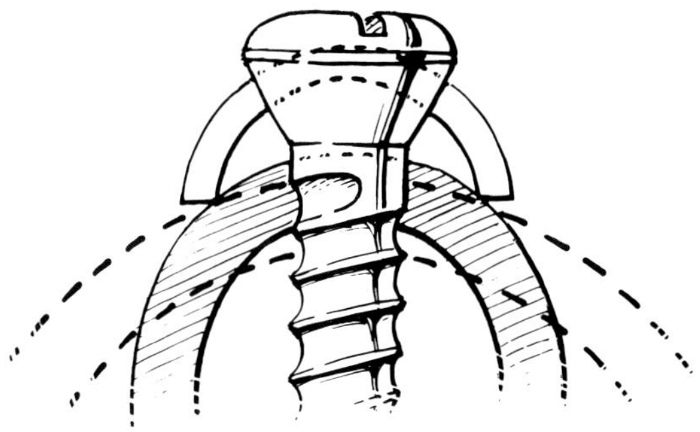

B

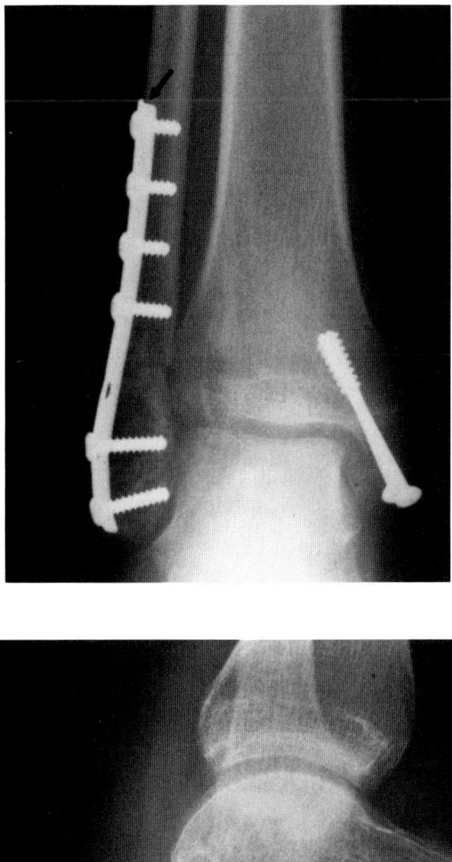

C

FIG. 2-33. A: Semitubular plates (two to five holes). (Courtesy of Zimmer, Warsaw, IN.) **B:** Cross-section of a semitubular plate, demonstrating how the edges cut into the cortex. **C:** The AP view of an ankle with internal fixation of the medial malleolus with two malleolar screws. The fibular fracture is fixed with a preshaped seven-hole semitubular plate and cortical screws. The semitubular plate can be difficult to differentiate from a compression plate. However, it is thinner and, therefore, less opaque, and the curved configuration is easily identified at the ends (*arrow*).

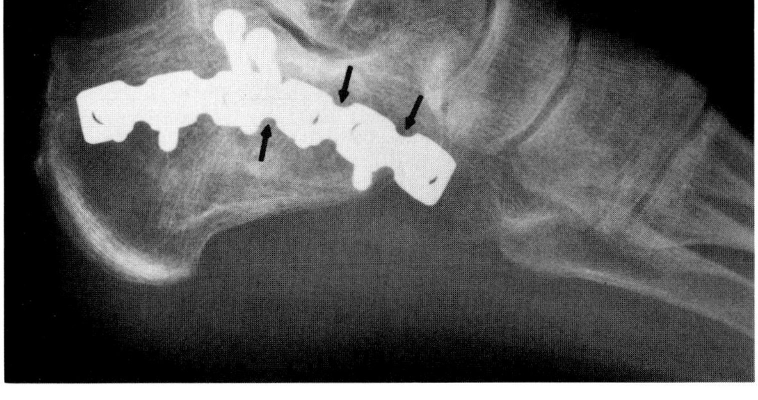

FIG. 2-34. Lateral view of the calcaneus obtained after fracture fixation with a 3.5-mm reconstruction plate. The scalloped edges (*arrows*) allow this plate to be easily identified radiographically. These indentations also allow the plate to be contoured in multiple planes with greater ease. This acts only as a neutralization plate and is not used for compression.

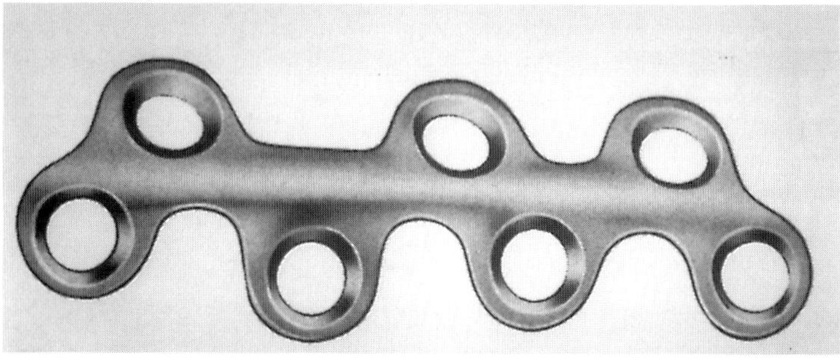
A

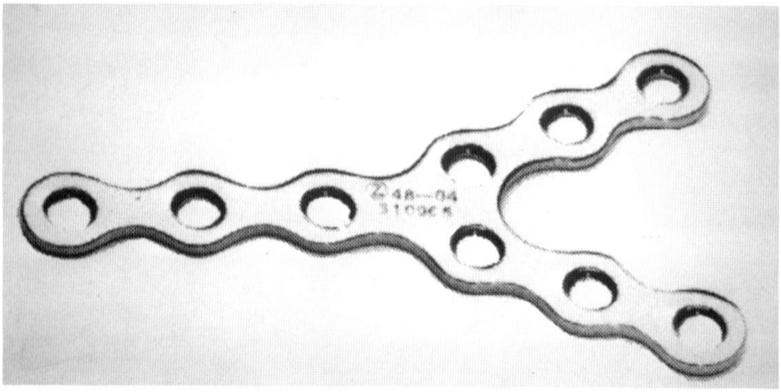
B

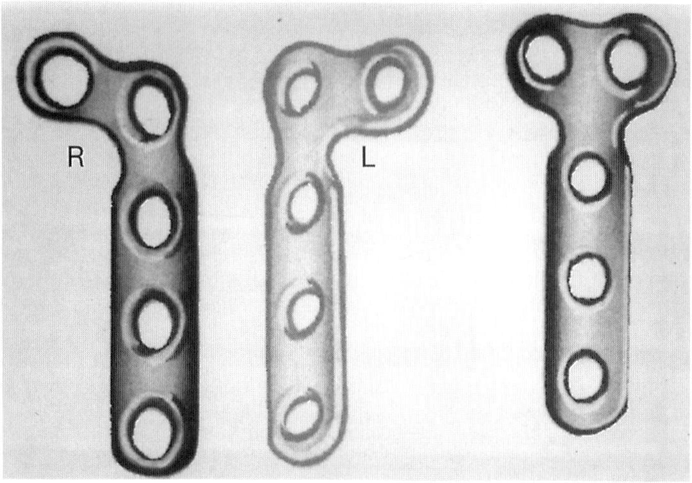

D

FIG. 2-35. Small and miniplates for the peripheral extremities. **A:** Small fragment plate for comminuted small bone fractures. (Courtesy of Zimmer, Warsaw, IN.) **B,C:** Y plate for distal humeral fractures (B). (Courtesy of Zimmer, Warsaw, IN.) The AP view of the elbow, demonstrating Y plate, two K wires, and cancellous screw fixation of a "Y" intercondylar fracture. **D:** Small plates for stabilization with right (*R*), left (*L*), and bilateral end holes. (Courtesy of Zimmer, Warsaw, IN.) **E:** Fracture of the distal humerus with four-hole DCP and small angled plate (*arrow*) for fixation.

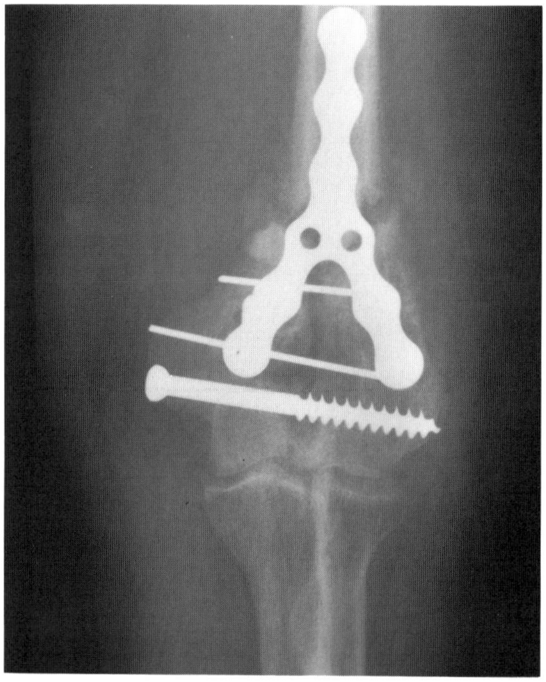
C

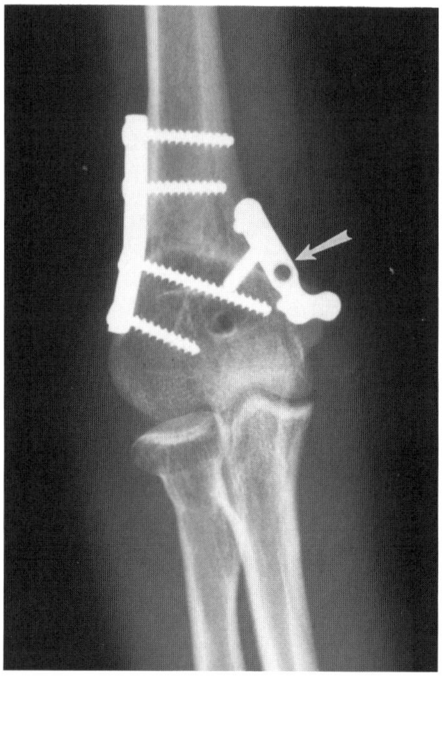
E

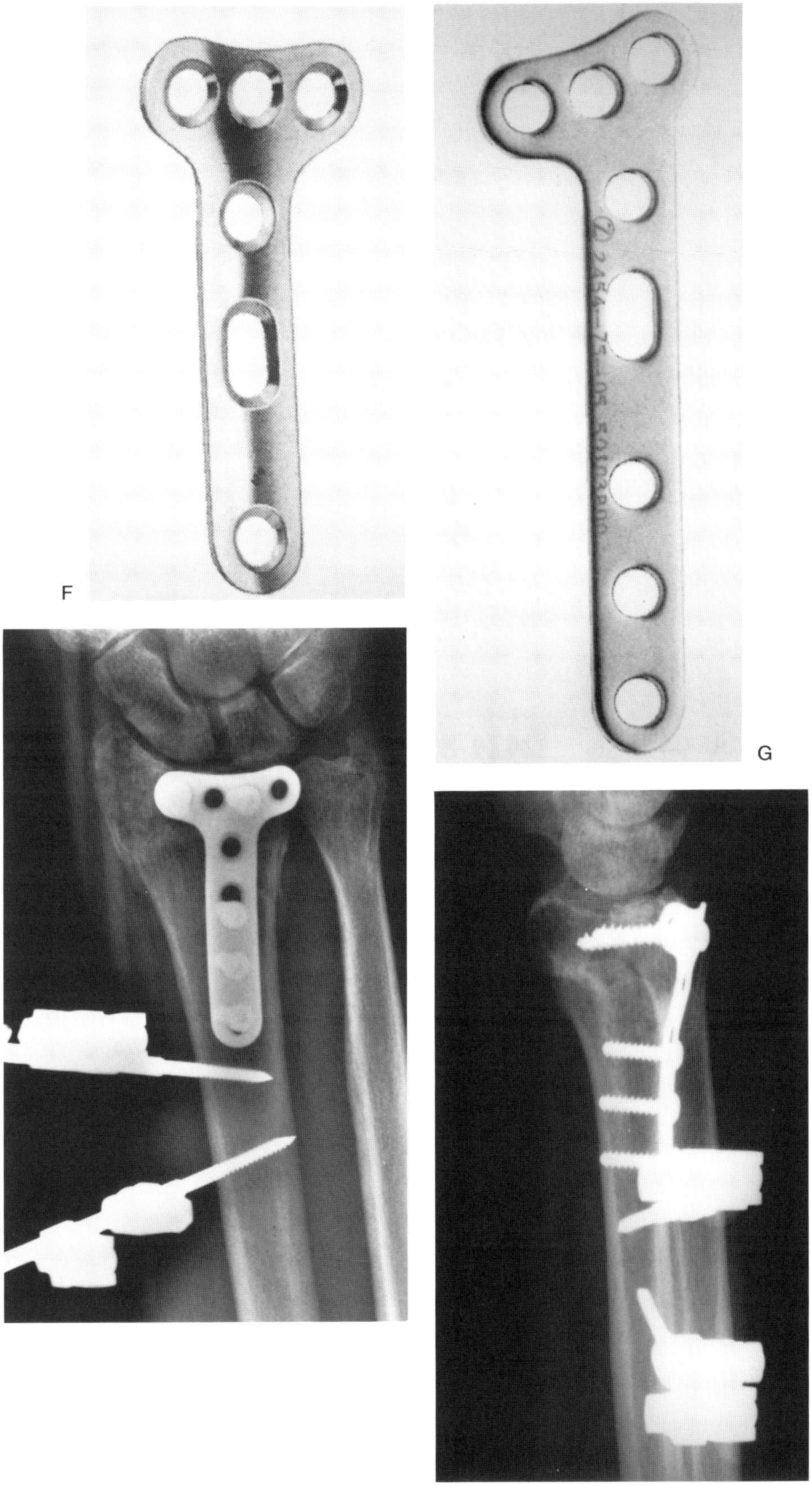

F G H I

FIG. 2-35. *Continued.* **F-I:** Small T plate (F) and oblique T plate (G) for condylar fixation. (Courtesy of Zimmer, Warsaw, IN.) The AP (H) and lateral (I) views of comminuted fracture of the distal radius (Frykman VII) with two external fixation pins and a T plate for fixation.

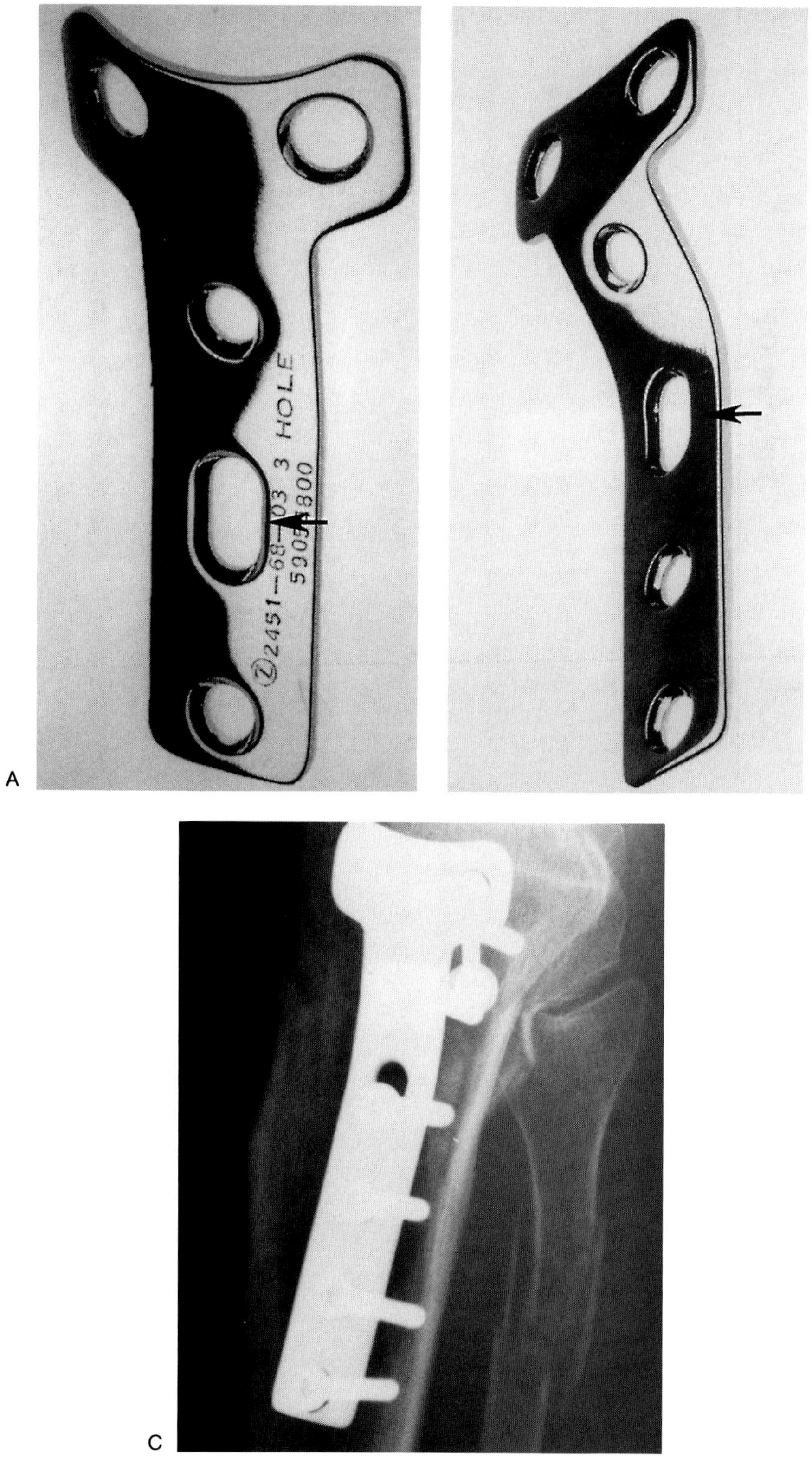

FIG. 2-36. T buttress plates with minimal **(A)** and more obvious curves **(B)**. Note the elongated hole (*arrow*), which allows adjustment after this screw is inserted. (Courtesy of Zimmer, Warsaw, IN.) **C:** Lateral radiograph demonstrating a T buttress plate for fixation of a tibial plateau fracture.

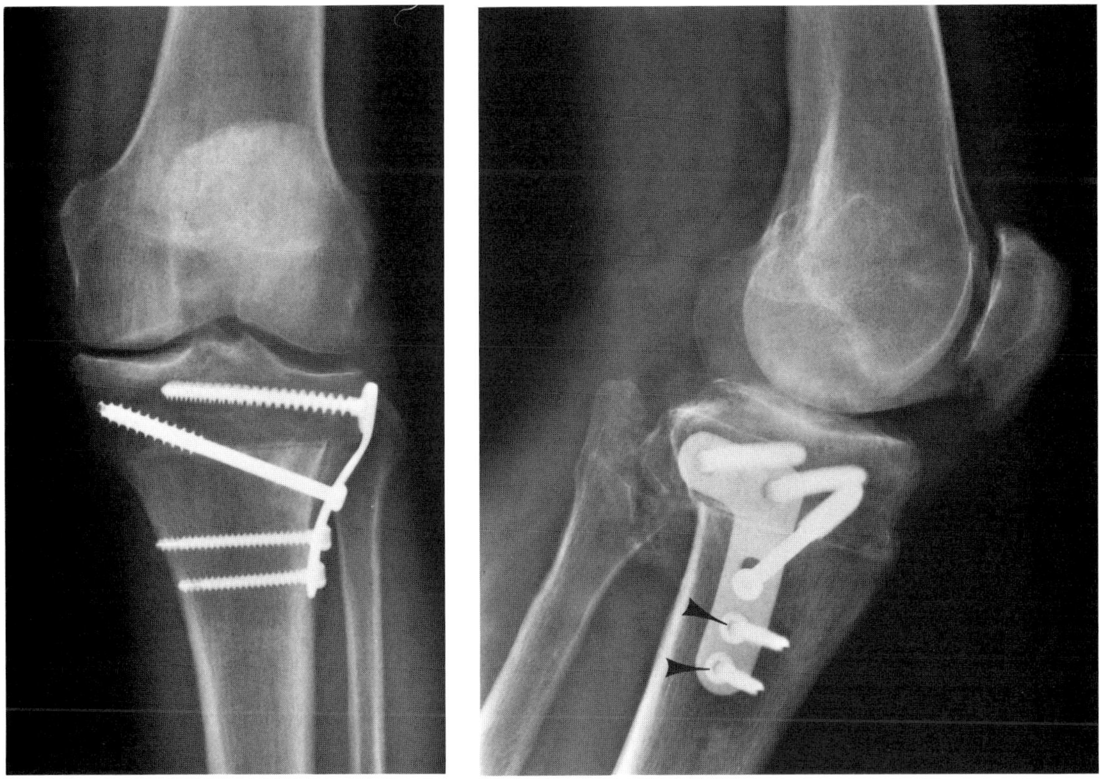

A B

FIG. 2-37. The AP **(A)** and lateral **(B)** radiographs of a tibial osteotomy internally fixed with the L buttress plate. There are two fully threaded cancellous screws superiorly. There is a cannulated obliquely placed lag screw and two distal cortical screws with hexagonal slot heads, which are easily seen radiographically (*arrows*).

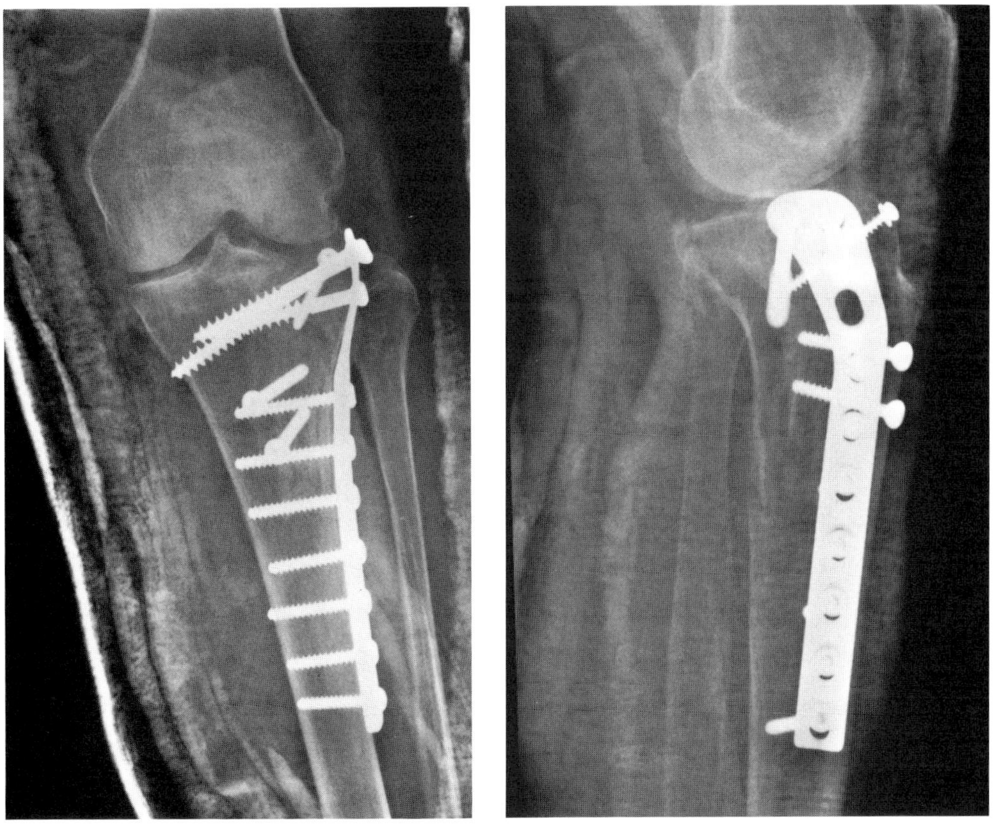

A B

FIG. 2-38. The AP **(A)** and lateral **(B)** radiographs taken following internal fixation of a lateral plateau fracture with a lateral tibial head plate. There are seven cortical screws distally and two cancellous screws proximally. Three separate lag screws.

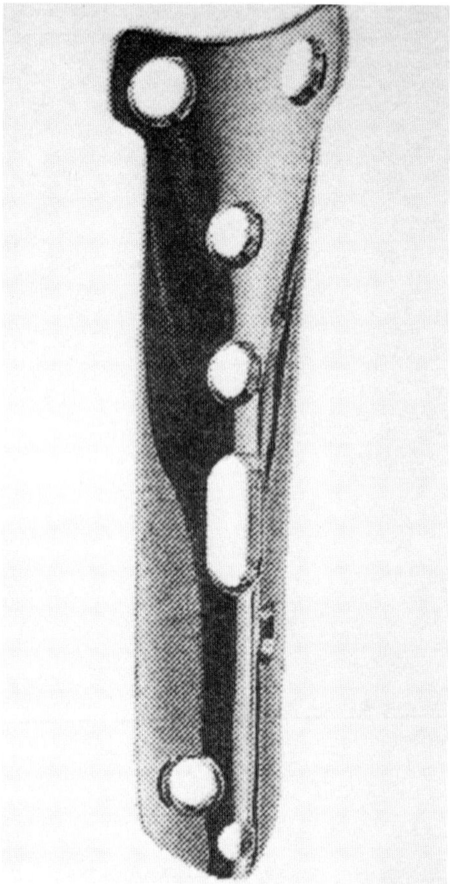

FIG. 2-39. Spoon plate. (Courtesy of DePuy, Warsaw, IN.)

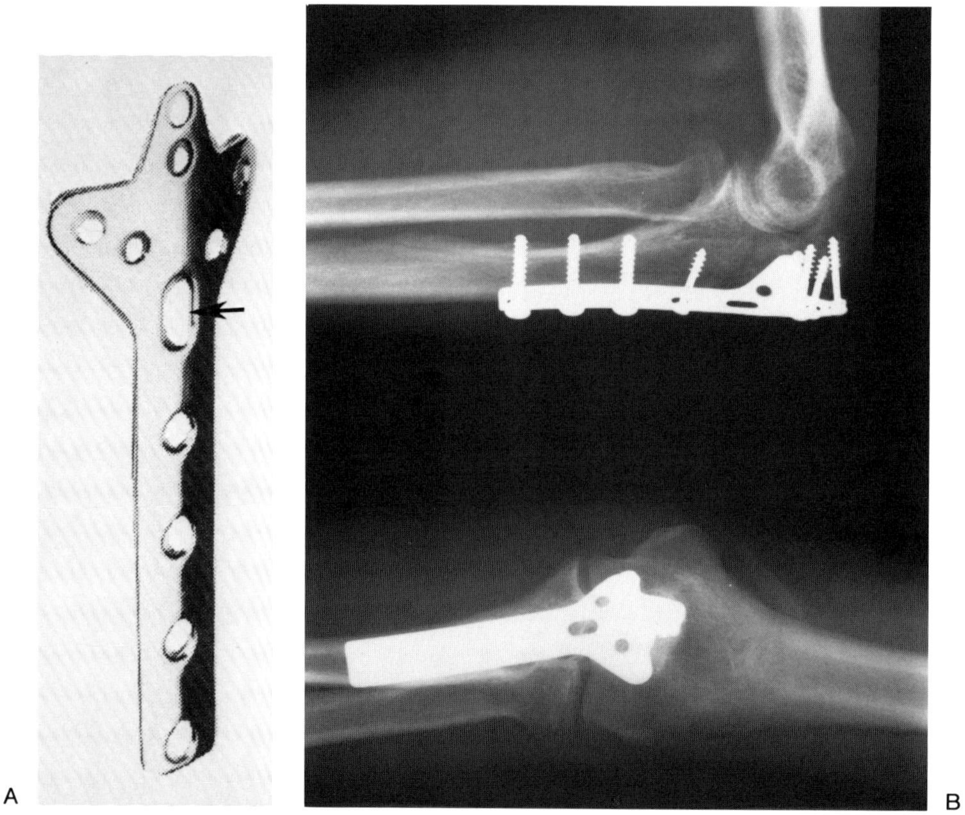

FIG. 2-40. A: Cloverleaf plate. There is an elongated hole (*arrow*) at the base of the cloverleaf. (Courtesy of Zimmer, Warsaw, IN.) **B:** Olecranon fracture internally fixed with a cloverleaf plate and three cortical screws distally. There are five cancellous screws in the proximal plate.

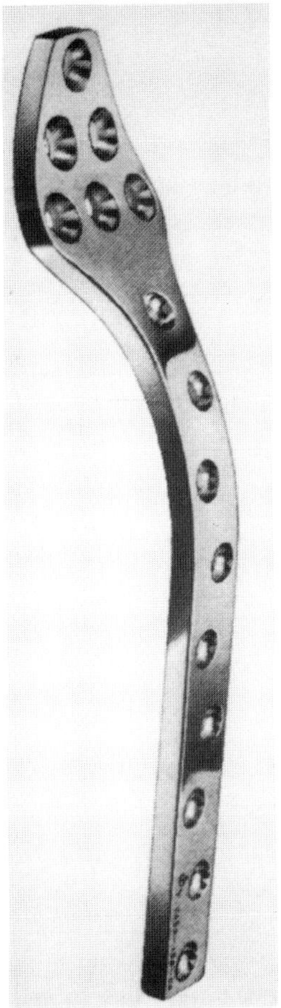

FIG. 2-41. Cobra-head plate designed for hip arthrodesis. (Courtesy of Zimmer, Warsaw, IN.)

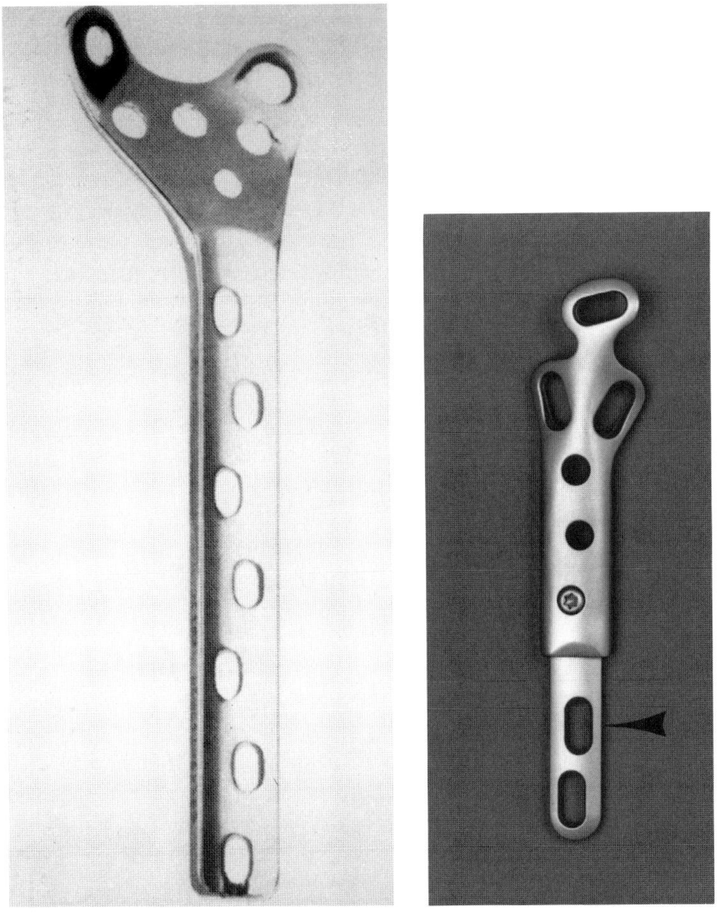

A,B

FIG. 2-42. A: Condylar buttress plate. (Courtesy of Zimmer, Warsaw, IN.) **B:** Alta™ modular distal femoral fracture plate with sliding channel plate (*arrow*), which can be adjusted to different lengths. (Courtesy of Howmedica, Rutherford, NJ.)

Condylar Buttress Plates

These plates come in various lengths, have staggered holes, and are designed for distal femoral fixation (Fig. 2-42).[39]

Lengthening Plates

This plate is used with osteotomies or fractures with severe comminution or bone loss. Lengthening plates are similar to compression plates (Fig. 2-32), except they are longer with no holes in the midportion of the plate. There are holes at the ends, with variable lengths in the midportion and no holes. Union depends on callus formation and preserving as much soft tissue and blood supply to the involved region as possible.[39]

Special plates, as noted earlier, have fairly specific applications. The choice of plate and plate length (Fig. 2-42B) vary with the appearance of the fracture. Therefore, it is essential to demonstrate adequately the fracture fragments and their position preoperatively. Routine radiographs, tomography, and/or computed tomography may be necessary.[7]

The plate should provide an equal number of holes for both main fragments. The type of plate varies with the anatomy. For example, broad plates are used in the femur and humerus, narrow plates in the tibia and forearm, and semitubular plates in the fibula and clavicle.[28,51,53]

Double plates may be used for buttressing metaphyseal fractures (Fig. 2-43). This technique is infrequently used for diaphyseal fractures because bone exposure results in greater devascularization.[3,7]

Angled-Blade Plates

There are four major categories of angled-blade plates.

1. The 130° angled-blade plates. These plates were used primarily for the proximal femur (Fig. 2-44).
2. Condylar plates (Fig. 2-45). These devices are used in the proximal and distal femurs for fracture or osteotomy fixation.[39]
3. Adult osteotomy plates (Fig. 2-45A,B). Osteotomy plates are designed for intertrochanteric osteotomies. They are available with variable angles (90°, 100°, 110°, 120°, and 130°). These plates have four holes with a notch for a tension device.[39]
4. Pediatric angled-blade plate. These plates have a T-shaped cross-section in the blade (Fig. 2-45C) compared with the U-shaped cross-sectional appearance of adult plates (Fig. 2-45D–F).[39]

Angled-blade plates have fixed angles so the blade channel must be properly selected prior to insertion.[28,39,51]

Dynamic Compression Systems

The most commonly used dynamic compression system consists of a plate with an angled sleeve and a large-diameter lag screw (Fig. 2-46).[46,51] These devices are designed in configurations for the upper (Fig. 2-46A) and distal femur (Fig. 2-46B,C). The sliding screw allows weight bearing and muscle forces to compress the fracture fragments. The plate and sleeve are available at different angles and lengths for use in either the proximal or distal femur.[51]

Similar systems are also available with different side plate-sleeve configurations and triphalangeal nails instead of the large cannulated screws (Figs. 2-47 and 2-48).

Intramedullary Fixation

Medullary fixation devices may be solid or hollow (Fig. 2-49). They are available in different configurations for differing diaphyseal regions. Solid devices (the term nail is frequently used) are typically used with unreamed channels.[53] Hollow rods have differing cross-sectional configurations (cloverleaf, triangular, and circular) and blunt tips, which require prereaming of the channel.[8,9] These devices fit the medullary canal more tightly, but interlocking devices are frequently used to prevent rotation and shortening.[35,53] An advantage of the medullary fixation device is the ability to stabilize a fracture without exposing the fracture site. These devices are most commonly used for femoral, tibial, and humeral fractures.[31,39,53]

Radiographic classification is possible with certain devices and more difficult, because of the similarity in appearance, with others. Common systems are reviewed in this section. More specific devices and features are included in later anatomic chapters.

Rush Rod

The Rush rod (Fig. 2-50) is easily identified. The tip is beveled for use in an unreamed channel, and the proximal end is hooked to prevent migration. This rod is typically used in bones with smaller medullary canals. Multiple rods can be used if the medullary canal is larger (humerus).[7,53]

Ender Nail

This device (Fig. 2-49D and Fig. 2-51) is also solid with an oval cross-sectional diameter. Multiple nails are used in most cases. They were designed primarily for femoral fractures. A disadvantage is the lack of ability to prevent rotation of the fragments.[39,53,56]

(text continues on page 82)

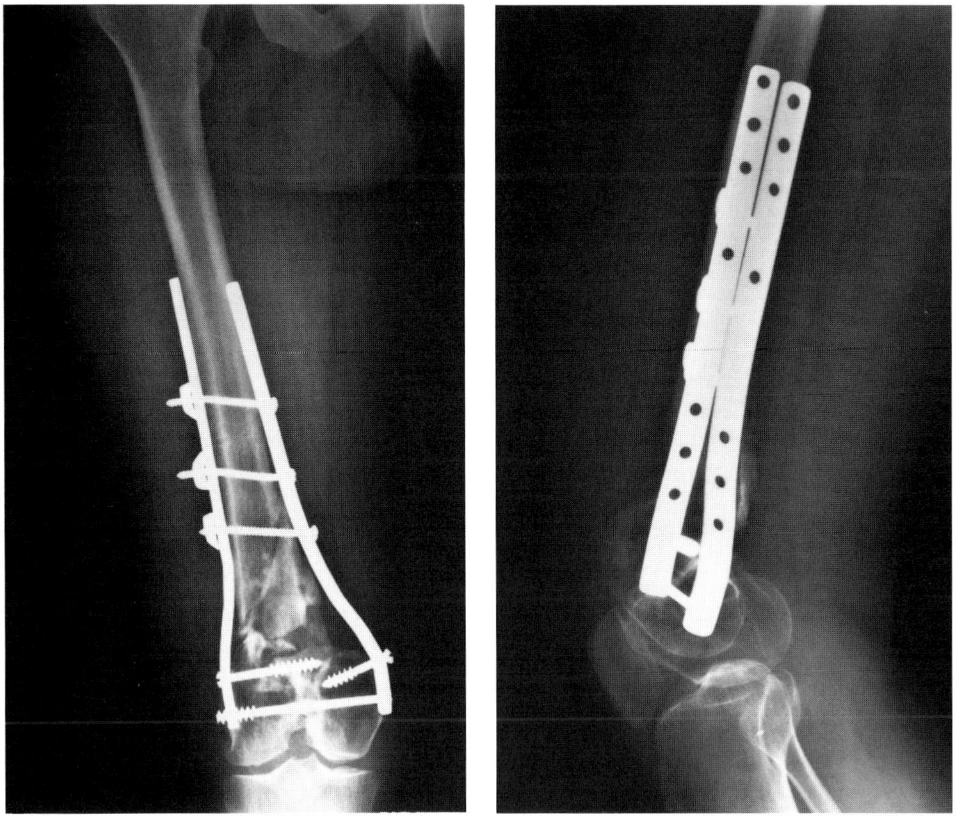

A B

FIG. 2-43. The AP **(A)** and lateral **(B)** radiographs of the right femur, demonstrating double-plate fixation of a comminuted supracondylar fracture. Note the nuts used laterally to fix the plates together.

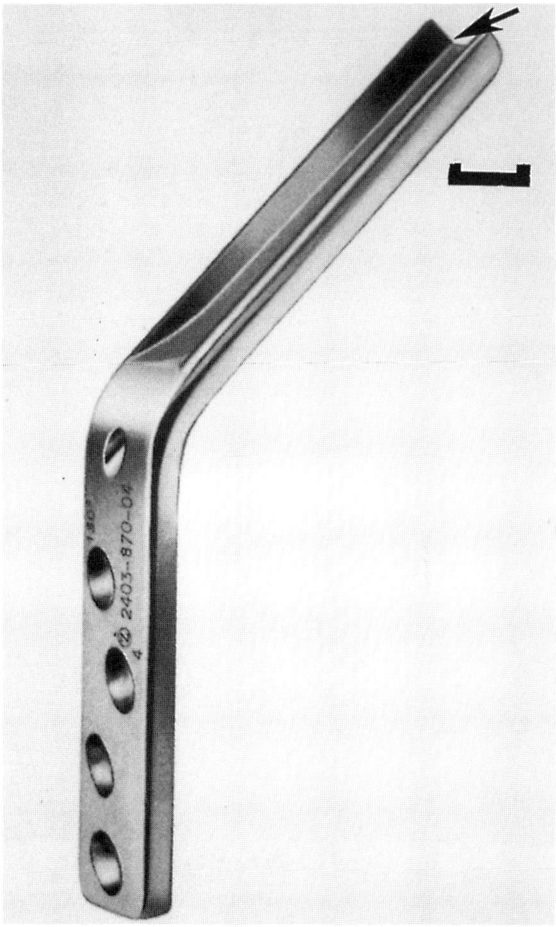

FIG. 2-44. A 130° five-hole angled-blade plate used for fixation of the proximal femur. This blade plate comes with a fixed 130° angle, with lengths varying from 50 to 110 mm. Note the notched or shallow "U" shape (*arrow*) of the femoral neck portion (on the end illustrated below the tip). (Courtesy of Zimmer, Warsaw, IN.)

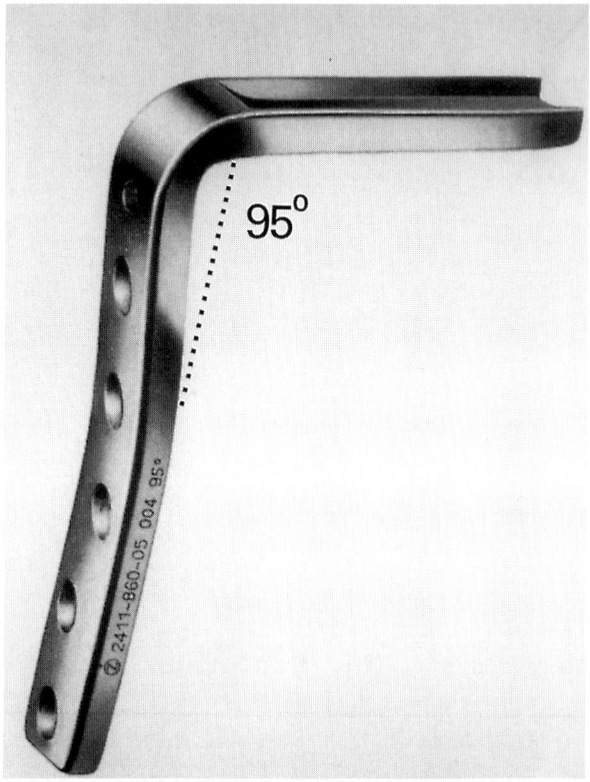

A

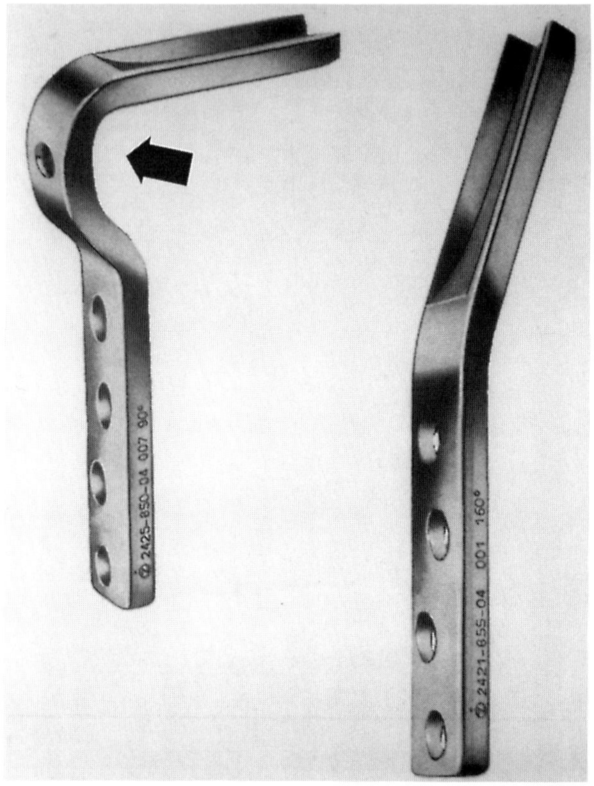

B

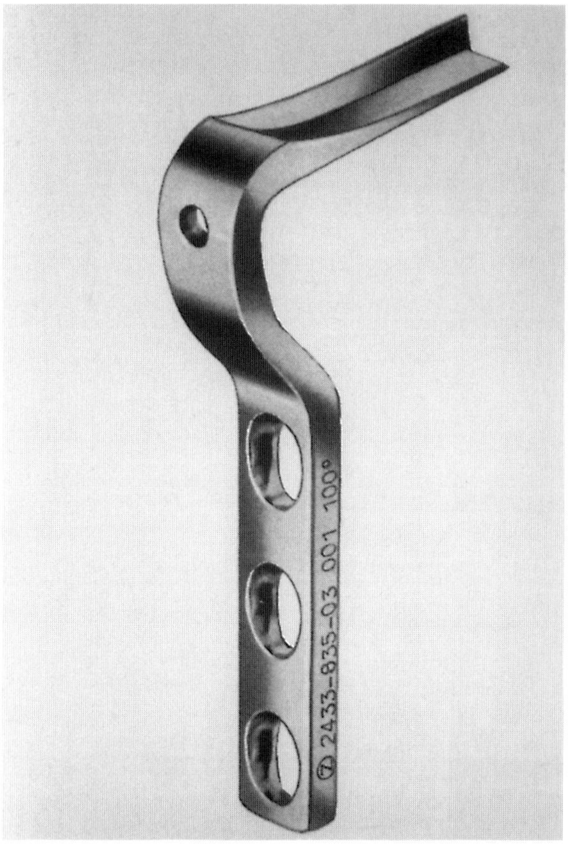

C

FIG. 4-45. Condylar-osteotomy blade plates. **A:** Condylar plate (stainless steel) used for proximal or distal femoral osteotomy or fracture. There is a 95° angle. Plate length varies to allow 5 to 12 holes. **B:** Osteotomy blade plates. The 90° blade plate on the left has a notch (*arrow*). The blade plate on the right is angled 160°. **C:** Pediatric 100° intertrochanteric osteotomy blade plate. (Courtesy of Zimmer, Warsaw, IN.)

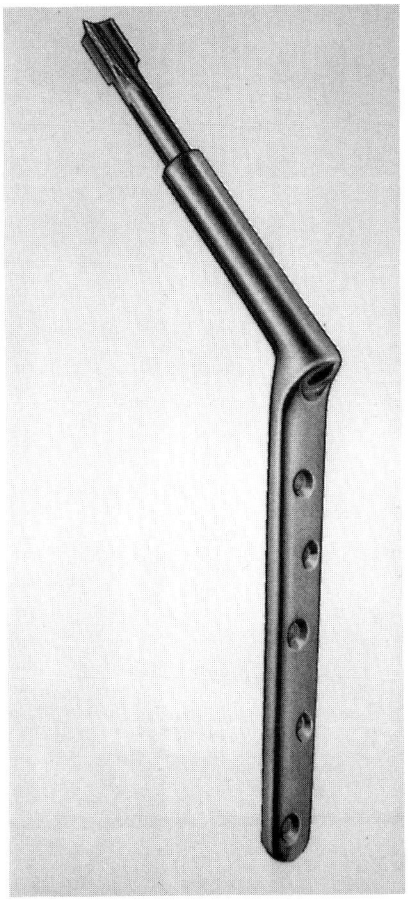

FIG. 2-47. Ken sliding nail for femoral neck and intertrochanteric fractures. (Courtesy of Zimmer, Warsaw, IN.)

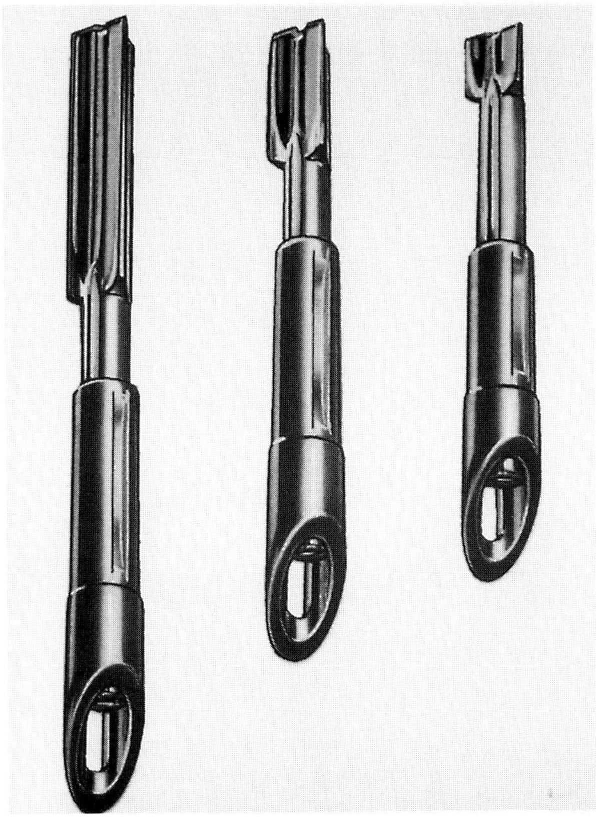

A

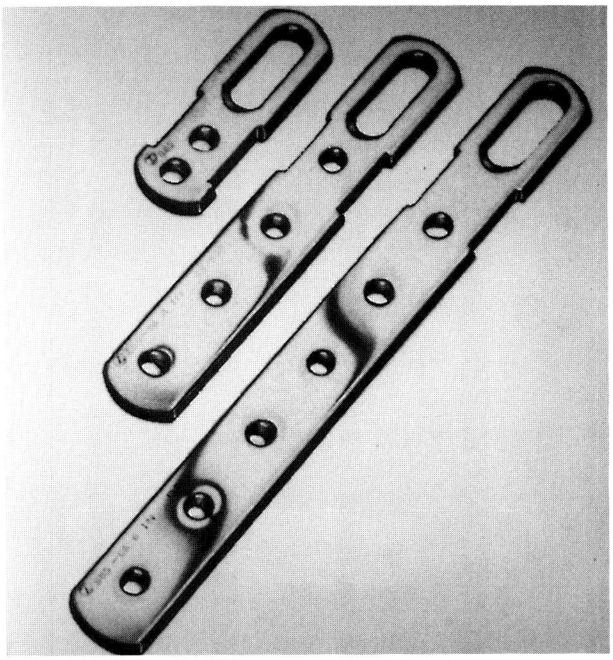

B

FIG. 2-48. Massie sliding nail. **A:** Different lengths and head configuration with nail shaft and sleeve. **B:** Variations in Massie side plate. The proximal oblong hole is for accommodating the tube sleeve assembly. (Courtesy of Zimmer, Warsaw, IN.)

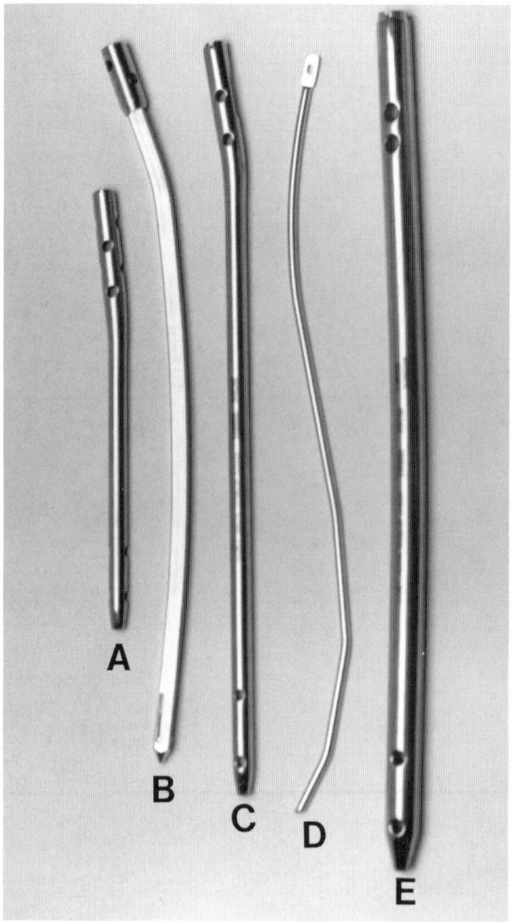

FIG. 2-49. Medullary fixation devices. **A:** Hollow round interlocking humeral rod. **B:** Solid square Hansen-Street nail. **C:** Hollow round interlocking tibial rod. **D:** Ender nail (solid). **E:** Hollow round interlocking femoral rod.

A,B

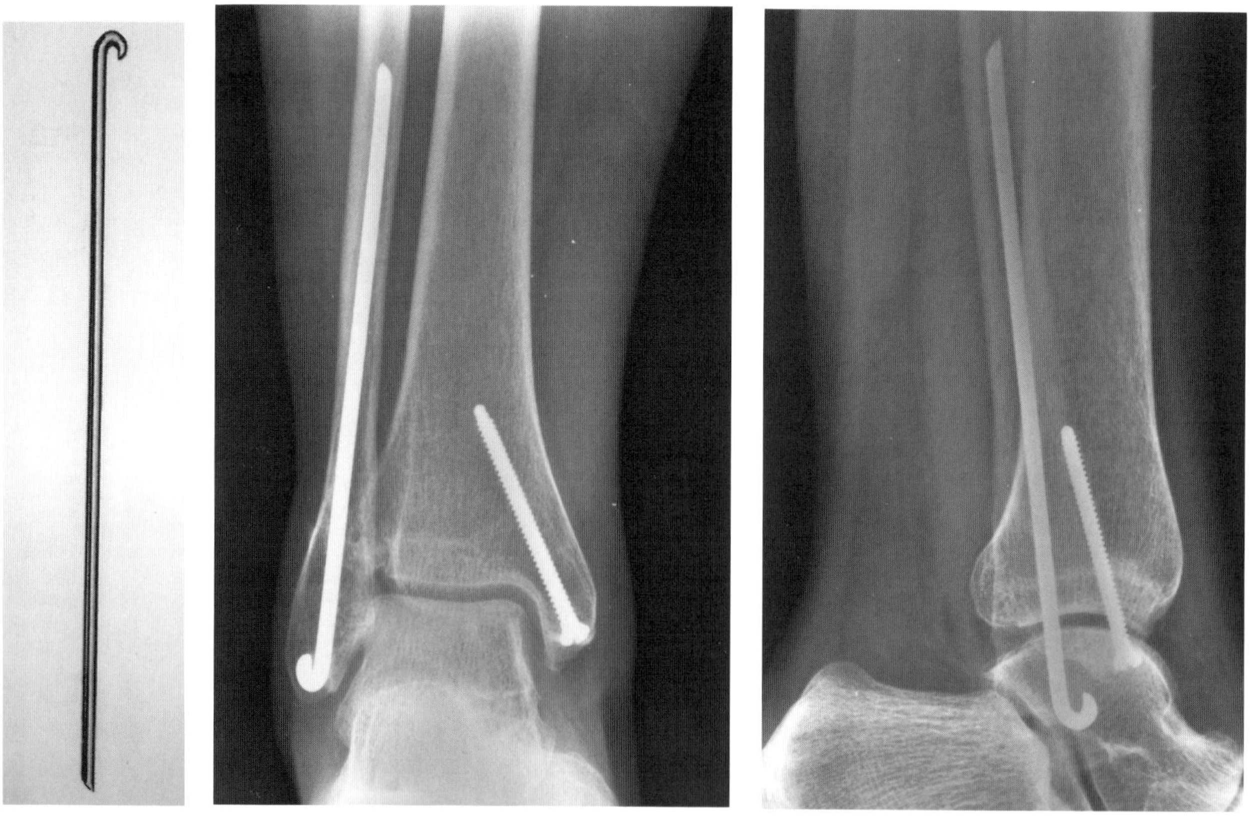

C

FIG. 2-50. A: Rush rod. The AP **(B)** and lateral **(C)** views of the ankle. Healed fibular fracture with Rush rod for fixation. Note the hooked end and beveled tip. There is a cortical screw across the healed medial malleolar fracture.

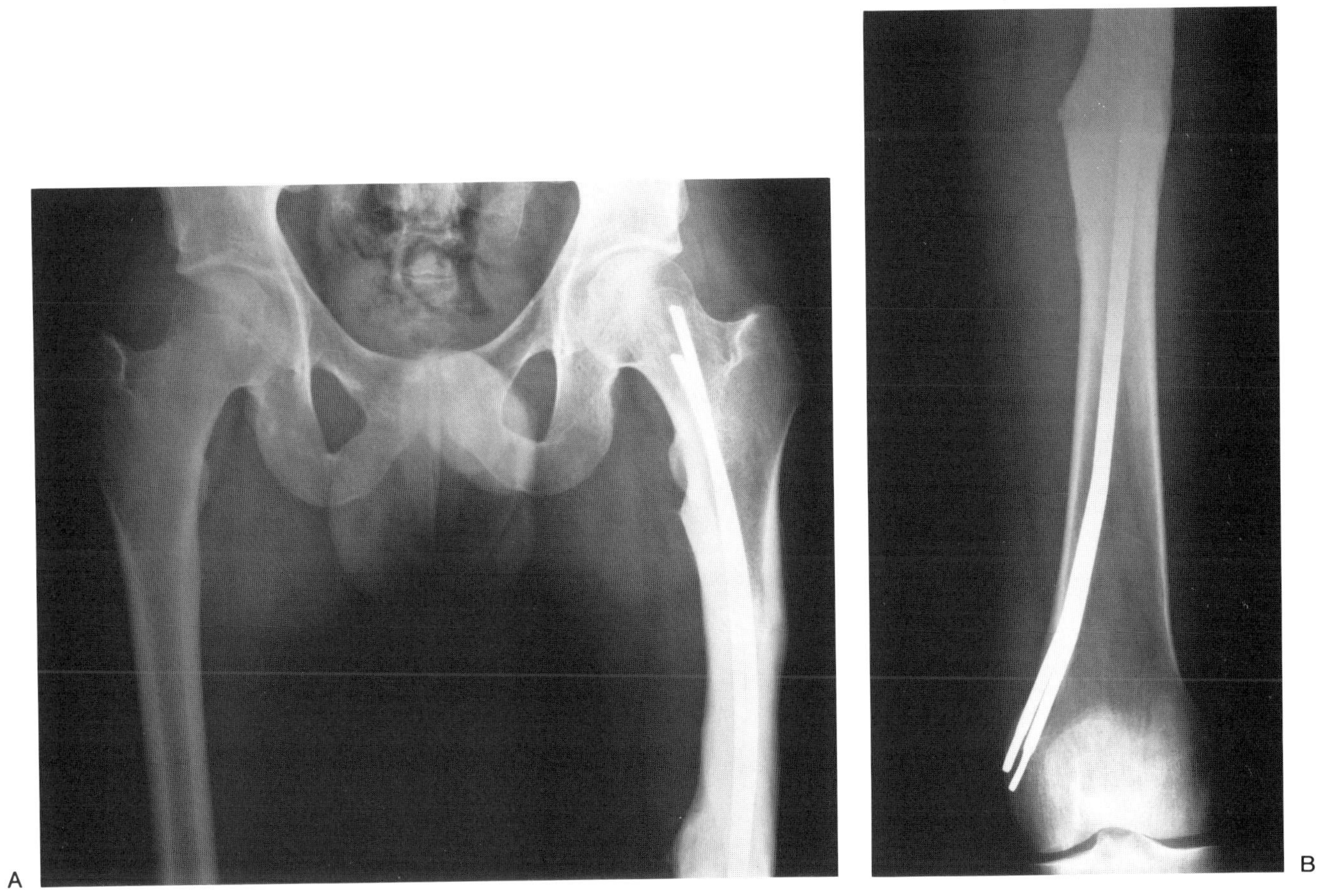

FIG. 2-51. The AP view of the hip and upper femur **(A)** and lower femur **(B)** in a patient with a healed midshaft fracture with two Ender nails for fixation.

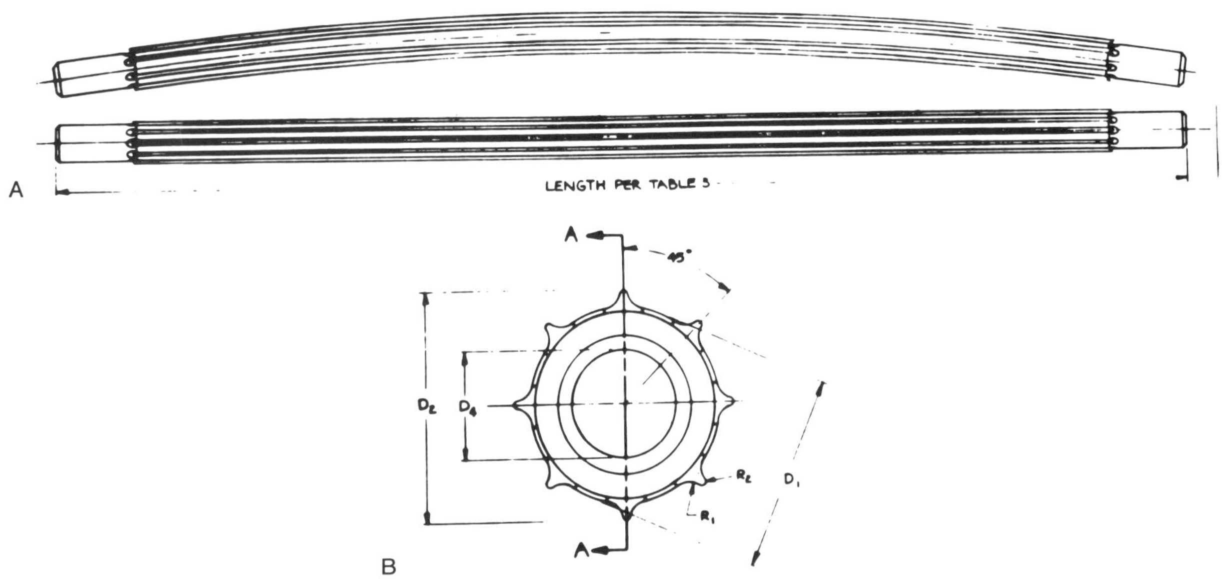

FIG. 2-52. Sampson rod in the AP and lateral views **(A)** and cross-sectional view **(B)**. (From Allen WC, Heiple KG, Burnstein AH. A fluted femoral intramedullary rod. *J Bone Joint Surg [Am]* 1978;60A: 506–515.)

Sampson Rod

This device is a rigid thick-walled fluted rod (Fig. 2-52), which prevents rotation. It is commonly used for knee arthrodesis.

Küntscher Nail

This hollow device has a cloverleaf cross-section with a rounded tip (Fig. 2-53). The configuration provides a press fit in the medullary canal.

Zickel Nail

This is a solid medullary nail with a predrilled proximal opening for placement of a Smith-Peterson triflanged pin (Fig. 2-54). This device is used for subtrochanteric fractures.

Interlocking Medullary Devices

Certain medullary rods or nails are used with pins, screws, or expanding blades to prevent rotation and shortening. Pins and screws may be positioned at one end (dynamic, i.e., allows compression to occur; Fig. 2-55) or both ends (static, i.e., prevents shortening and rotation; Fig. 2-55).

Femoral Interlocking Nails

Proximal screws can be used in the femoral neck and subtrochanteric region. Metaphyseal screws can be positioned distally. Both cortices are engaged distally (Fig. 2-56).

Tibial Interlocking Nail

The nail configuration differs in length, and the proximal end has a curved (Herzog; Fig. 2-55A) end, which distinguishes the tibial interlocking nail from the femoral nail. There are predrilled holes at both ends for either static (both ends) or dynamic (one end) fixation (Fig. 2-55).

Humeral Interlocking Nail

The most commonly used humeral interlocking nail is similar in appearance (Fig. 2-49A) to the tibial nail but smaller in diameter and length. This device is used for humeral fracture fixation and neoplasms (Fig. 2-57).

Expanding humeral nails are also available (Seidel humeral locking nail system, Howmedica, Rutherford, NJ). Proximal interlocking is accomplished with screws. The tip can be expanded with a central screw, which moves proximally, causing the tip to expand, which fixes the nail solidly in the medullary canal (Figs. 2-58 and 2-59).

Interlocking Nails with Distal Flanges

Intramedullary nails may also have distal flanges or blades to provide additional fixation and prevent rotation (Fig. 2-60).[8]

Short Interlocking Nails

Shorter interlocking nail systems are available primarily for intertrochanteric and subtrochanteric femoral fractures (Fig. 2-61).

Pins

There are multiple pin configurations (e.g., Knowles, Hagie, and Steinmann), and both solid and cannulated (hollow) types are available. Pins are also available in smooth and threaded configurations.[39,53] Pins are most often used for fixation of femoral neck fractures. Multiple pins are required. Sliding configurations are also available to allow compression of the fracture fragments.

Pins can also be used with a side plate (Deyerle apparatus, Fig. 2-62). The latter may cause a stress riser, leading to fracture at the lower margin of the plate.

Steinmann Pins

These devices are large wires that may be smooth, threaded, or partially threaded (Fig. 2-63). The tips are pointed. Steinmann pins are used for fracture fixation and with traction systems.

Knowles (Fig. 2-64), Hagie (Fig. 2-65), Guffon, and Deyerle pins (Fig. 2-62) are solid pins used for femoral neck fractures.

Staples

Staples are available with smooth or barbed ends (Fig. 2-66).[14,39] The latter obviously reduces the likelihood of backing out. Special configurations include the stepped osteotomy staple (Coventry, Fig. 2-66C) and the table (Stone) staple (Fig. 2-66 E,F), which has four prongs. The table staple is used for ligament repairs or patellar realignment surgery.[39]

(text continues on page 93)

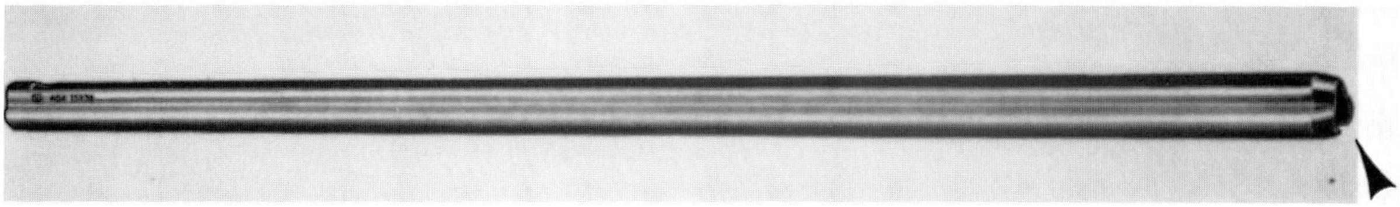

FIG. 2-53. The Küntscher nail. Note the cloverleaf cross-sectional configuration (*arrow*).

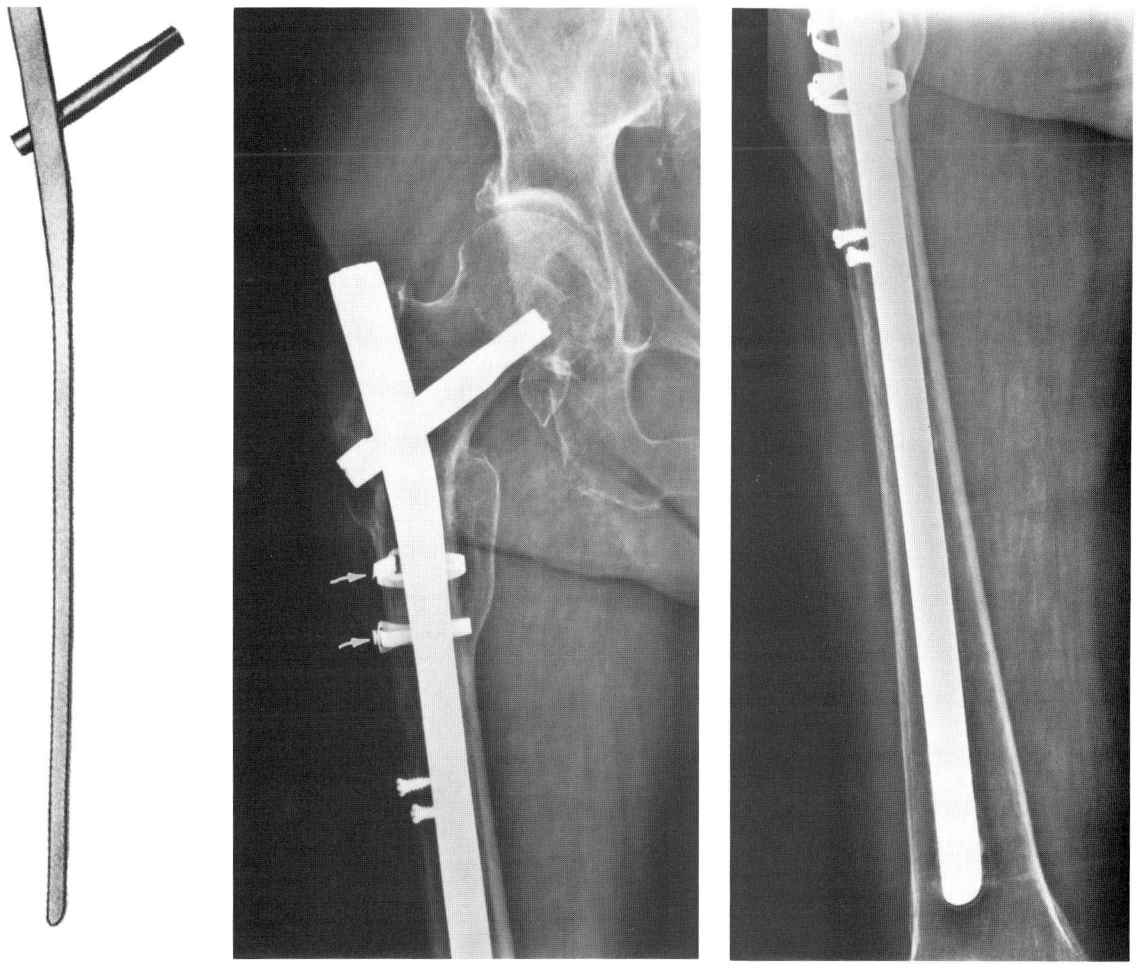

A,B C

FIG. 2-54. Zickel nail. **A:** Zickel nail system. (Courtesy of Howmedica, Rutherford, NJ.) The AP view of the right hip and upper femur **(B)** and lower femur **(C)** in a patient with a healed subtrochanteric fracture treated with a Zickel nail and upper Parham bands (*arrows*).

A 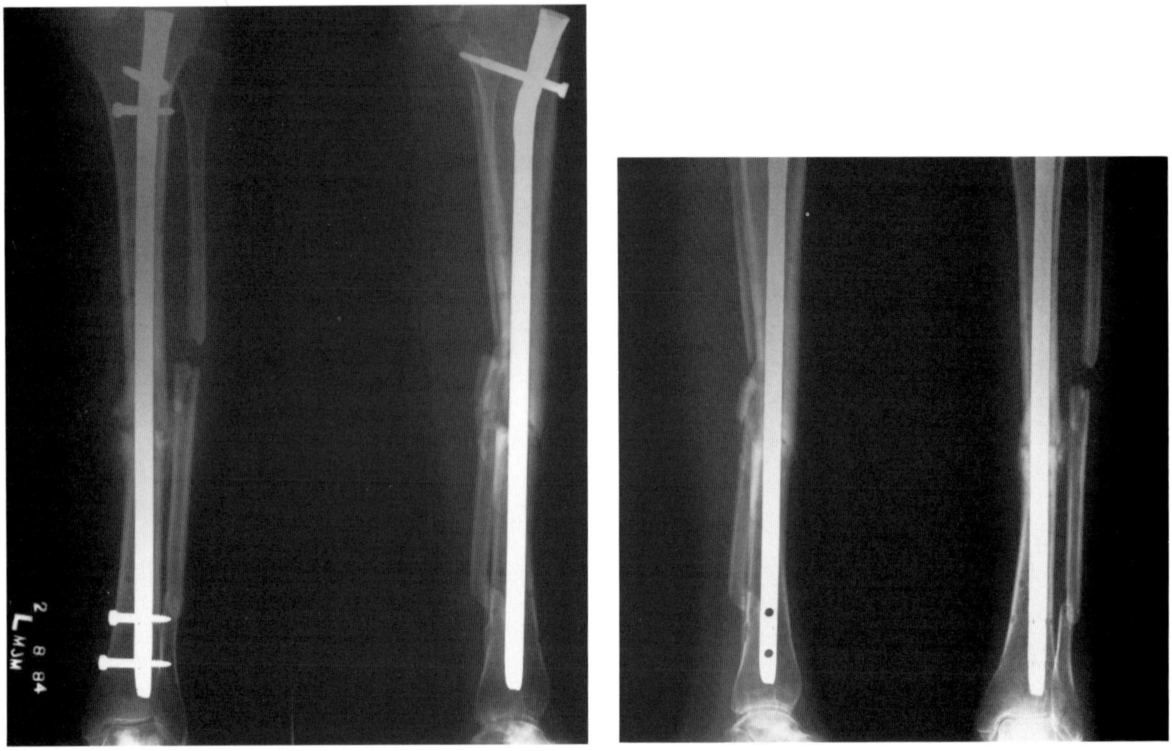 B

FIG. 2-55. Tibial fracture with midfibular fracture treated with Gross and Kempf tibial nail. **A:** The initial AP and lateral views show healing of the tibial fracture with static interlocking (screws used proximally and distally). **B:** The AP and lateral views 4 months later show a healed tibial fracture. The distal screws have been removed, creating a dynamic configuration.

A 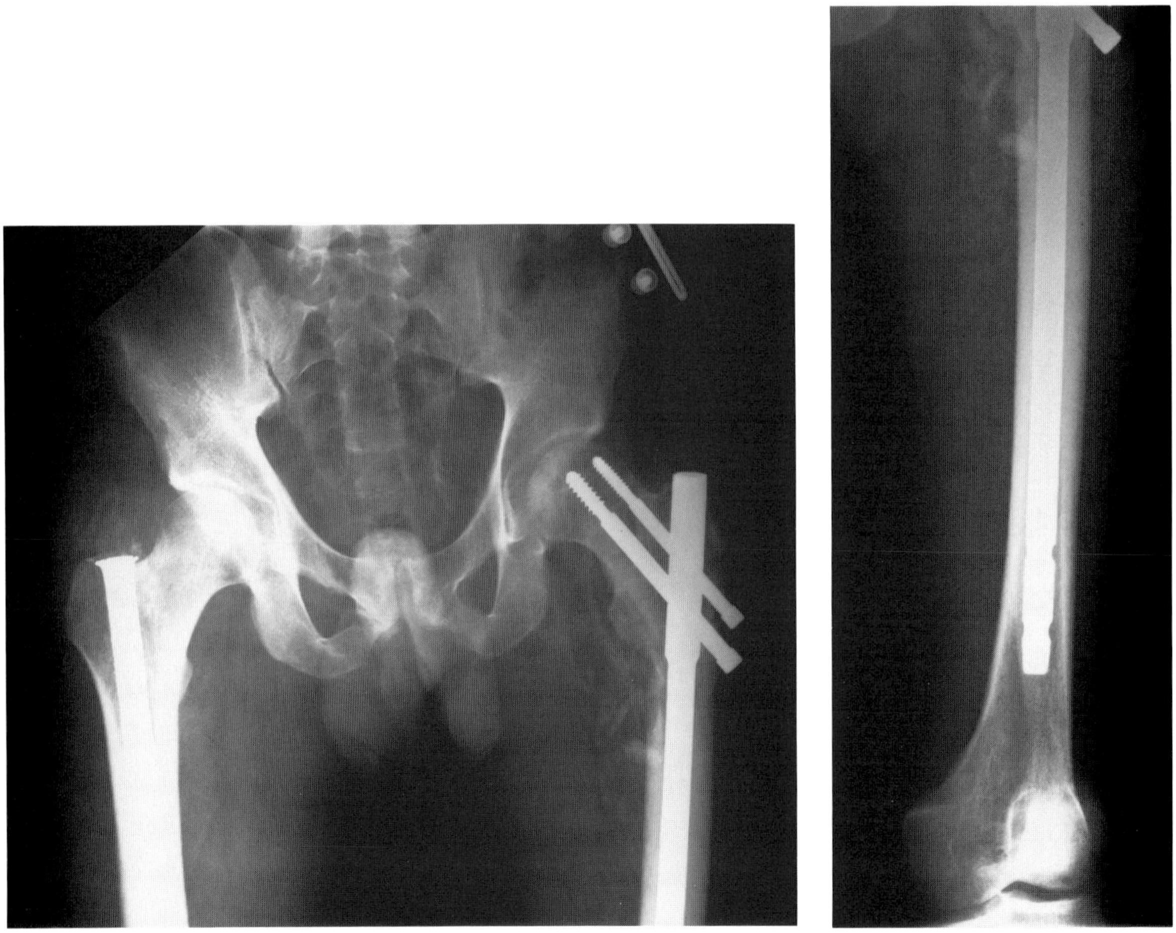 B

FIG. 2-56. The AP views of the pelvis **(A)** and left femur **(B)** demonstrate a Russell-Taylor delta femoral nail with two proximal lag screws and no distal screws for fixation of fractures of the left femoral neck and subtrochanteric region.

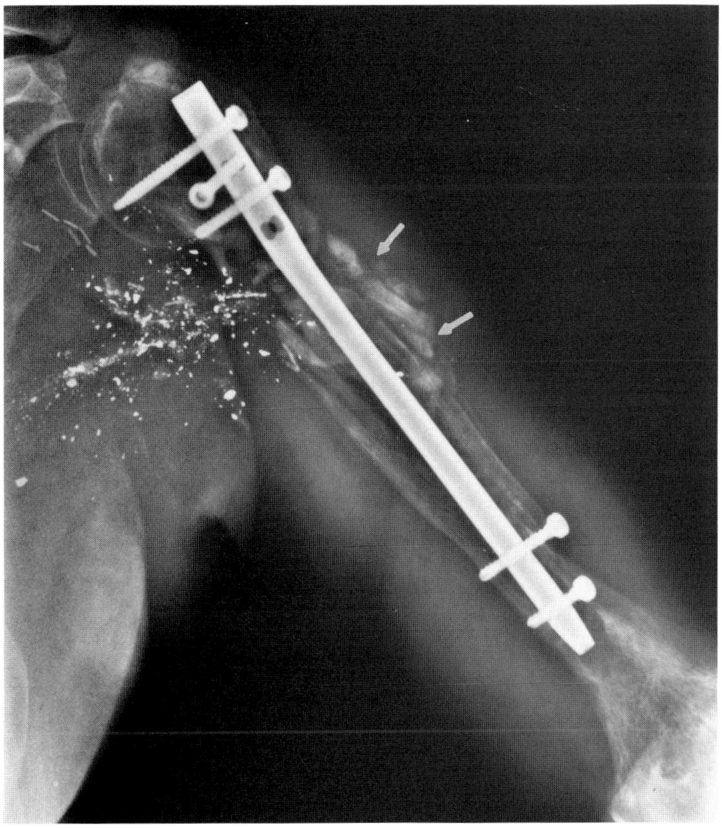

FIG. 2-57. External rotation view of the humerus with a badly comminuted fracture following a gunshot wound. An interlocking medullary nail (9-mm diameter) was positioned with the three proximal and two distal cortical screws. There is bone graft along the midshaft (*arrows*).

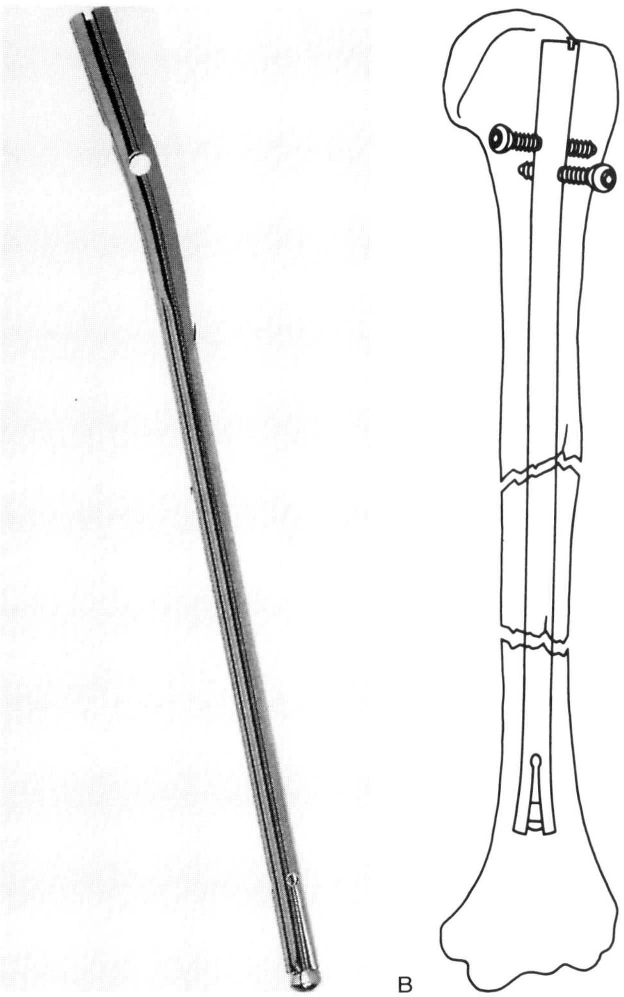

A B

FIG. 2-58. Seidel humeral locking nail system. (Courtesy of Howmedica, Rutherford, NJ.) **A:** Seidel humeral nail. **B:** The Seidel system for fixation of a comminuted mid humeral fracture.

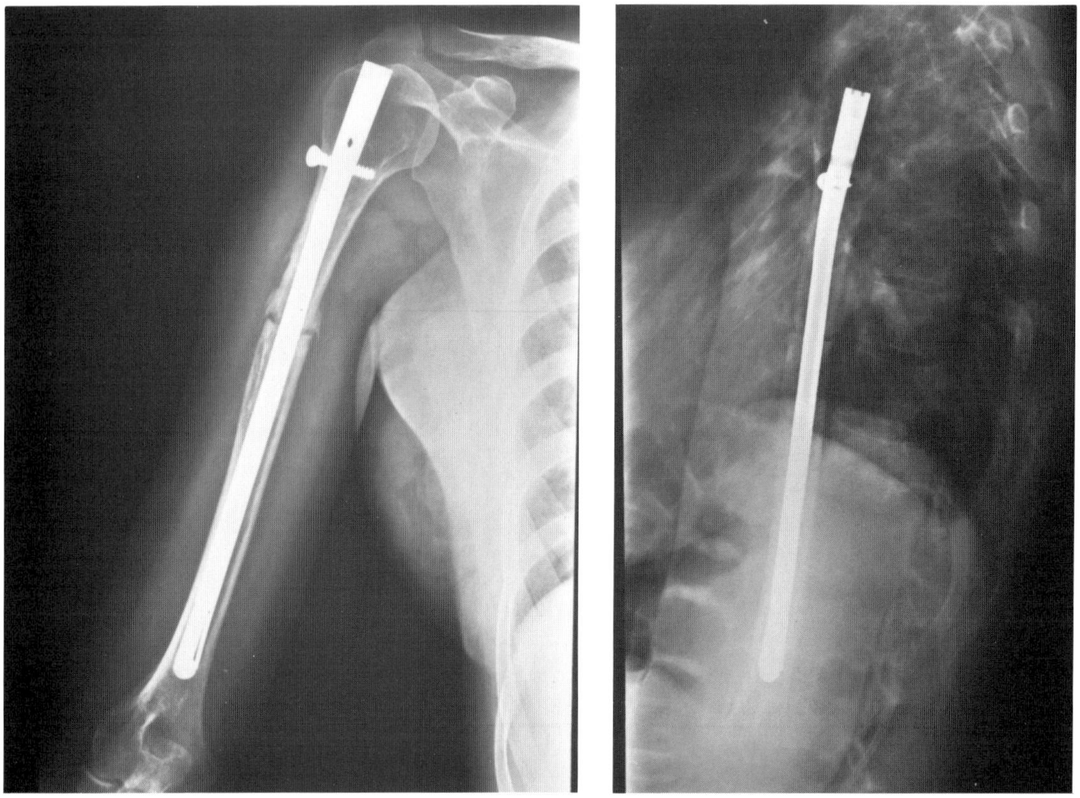

A B

FIG. 2-59. The AP **(A)** and transthoracic **(B)** views of the right humerus, demonstrating internal fixation of a humeral fracture using a Seidel humeral locking nail. Note the expanded tip.

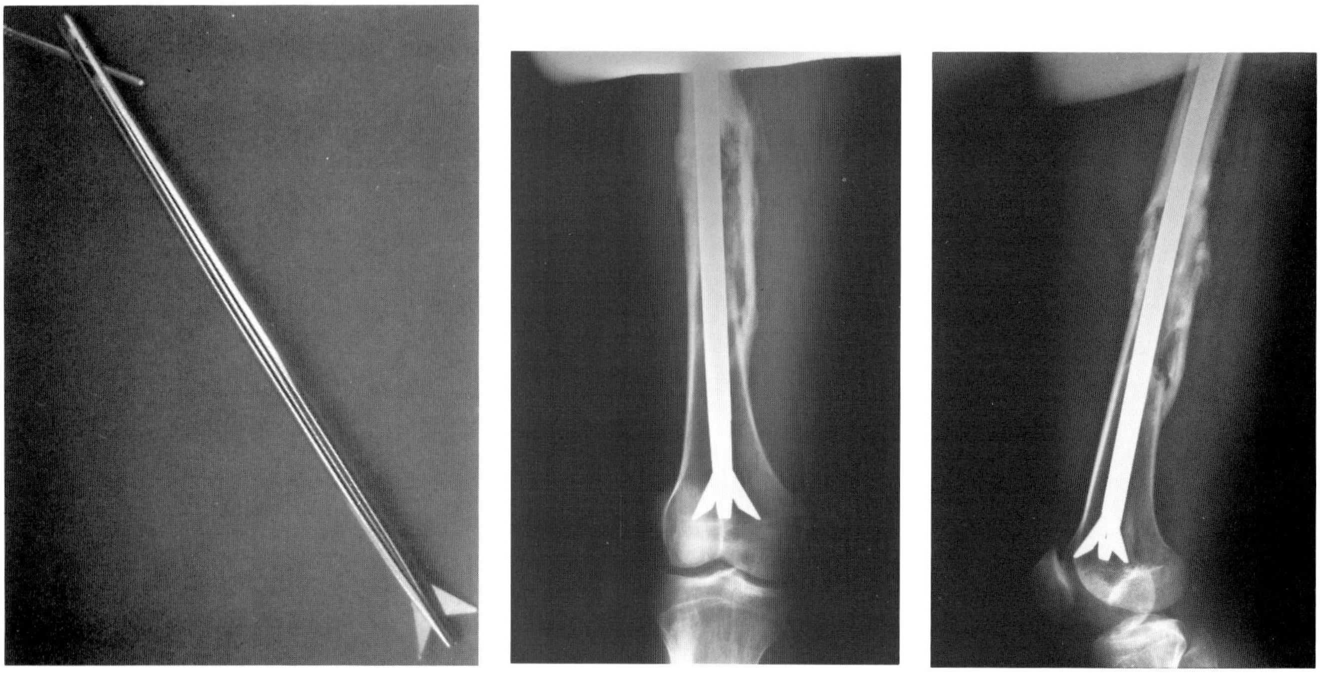

A,B C

FIG. 2-60. A: A Brooker-Wills intramedullary nail with distal flanges. The AP **(B)** and lateral **(C)** views of the distal femur in a patient with a healed midshaft fracture internally fixed with a Brooker-Wills nail.

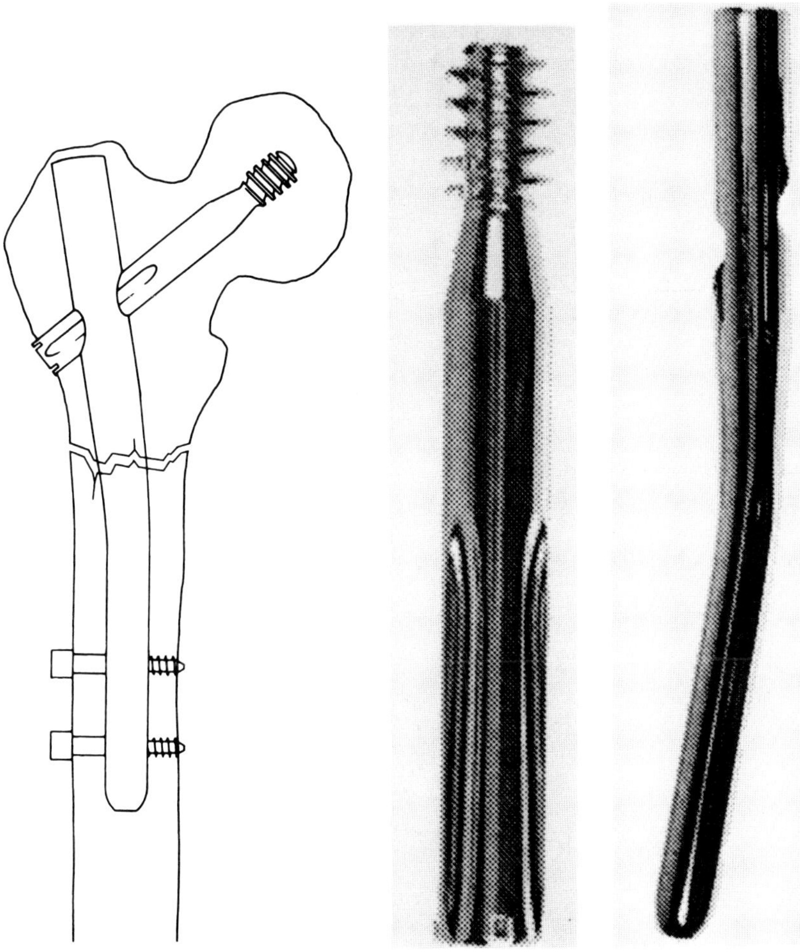

A,B C

FIG. 2-61. A: Gamma™ locking nail system and components. These include the lag screw **(B)** and hollow nail **(C)**. (Courtesy of Howmedica, Rutherford, NJ.) (See **D** and **E** on next page.)

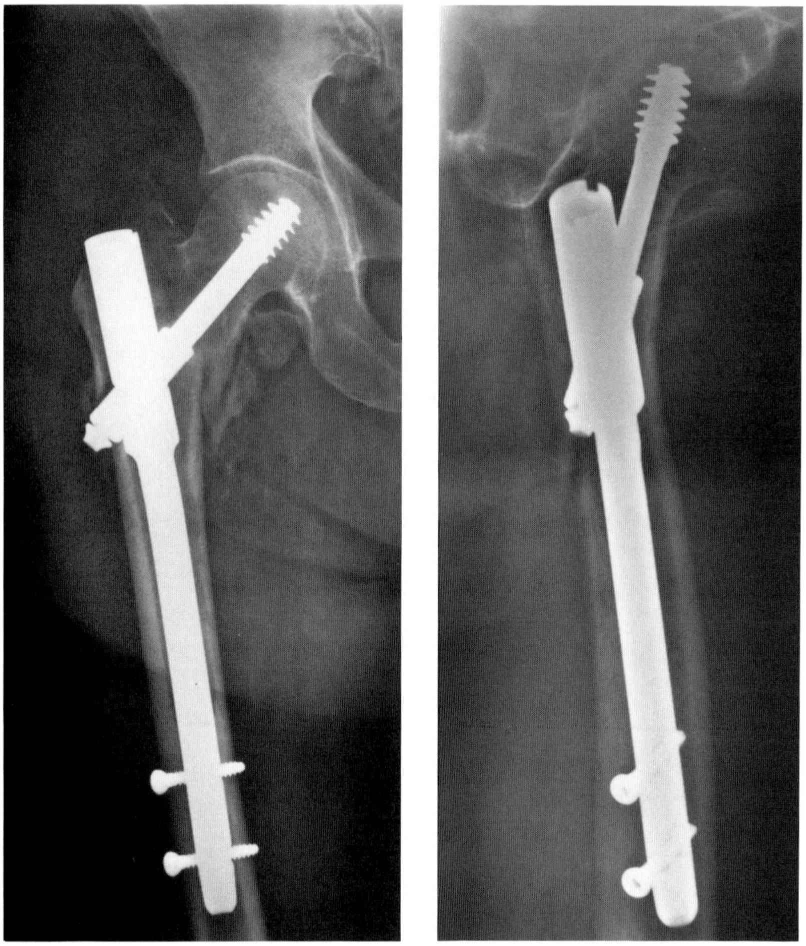

D,E

FIG. 2-61. *Continued.* The AP **(D)** and lateral **(E)** radiograph of a Russell-Taylor short locking nail for fixation of a comminuted trochanteric fracture.

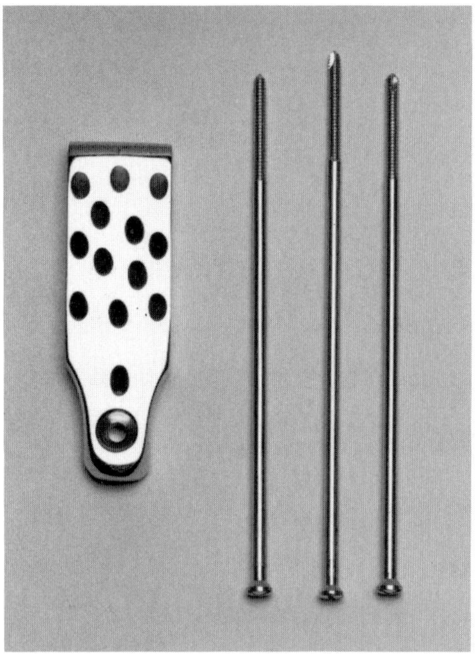

A

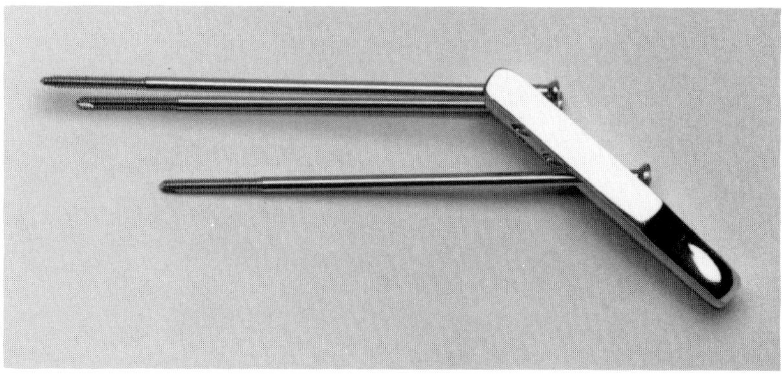

B

FIG. 2-62. Deyerle pins and side plate seen separated **(A)** and in the position used for femoral neck fracture **(B)**.

A,B

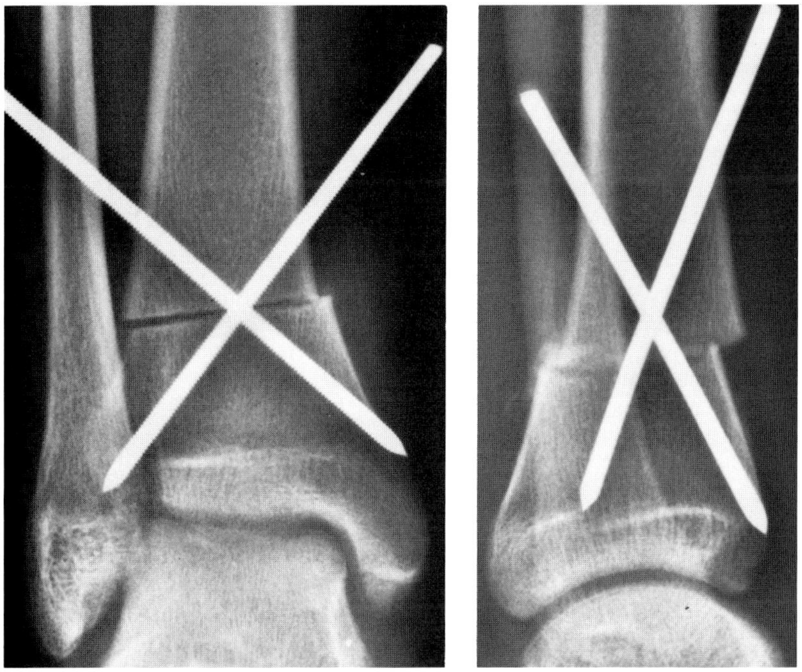

FIG. 2-63. The AP **(A)** and lateral **(B)** radiographs of a distal tibial osteotomy with two threaded Steinmann pins for fixation.

A B C

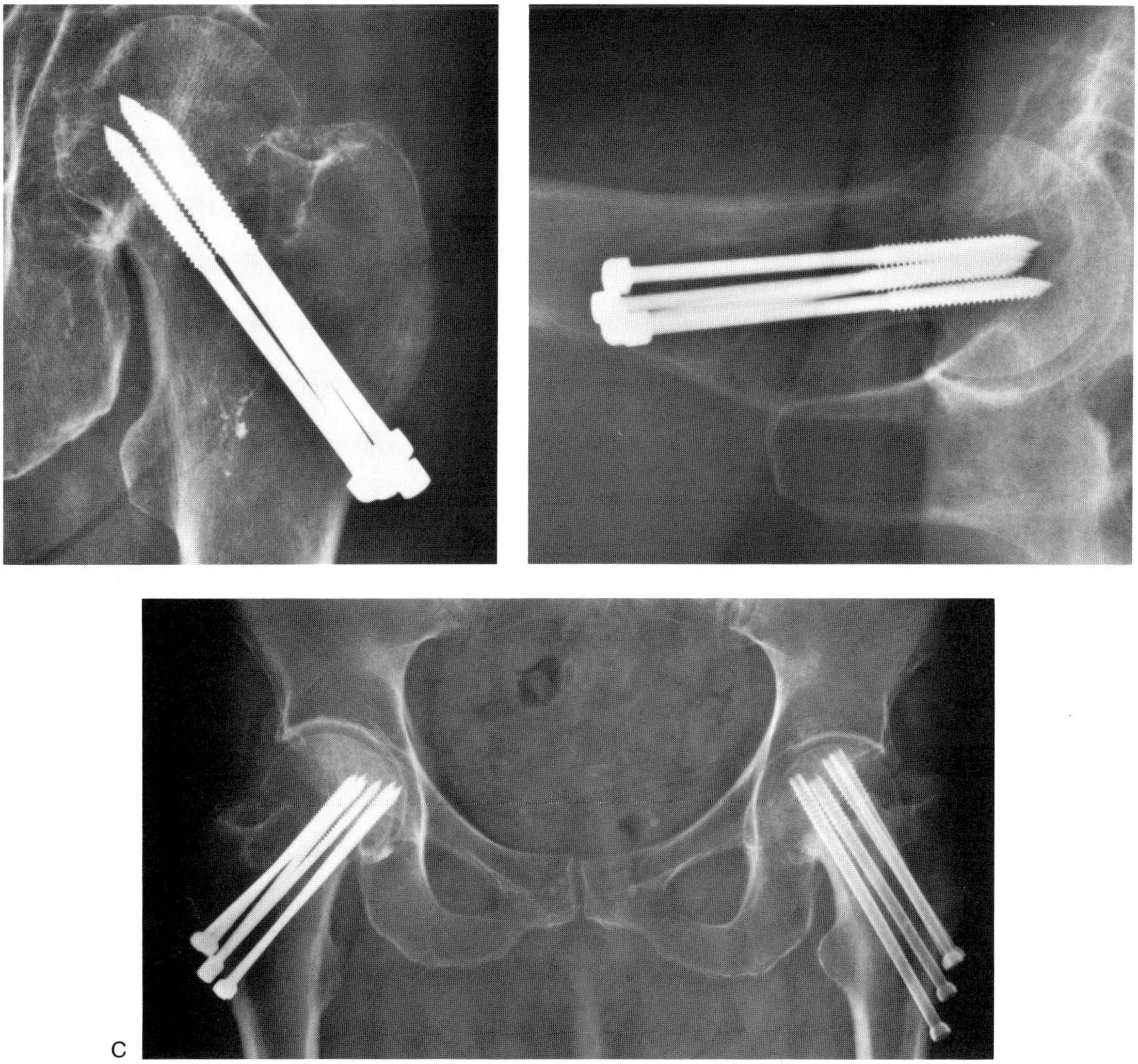

FIG. 2-64. Femoral neck fracture. The AP **(A)** and lateral **(B)** views show fixation with four Knowles pins. **C:** The AP view of the pelvis and hips with bilateral femoral neck fractures. There are Knowles pins for fixation on the right and four Ace cannulated pins on the left.

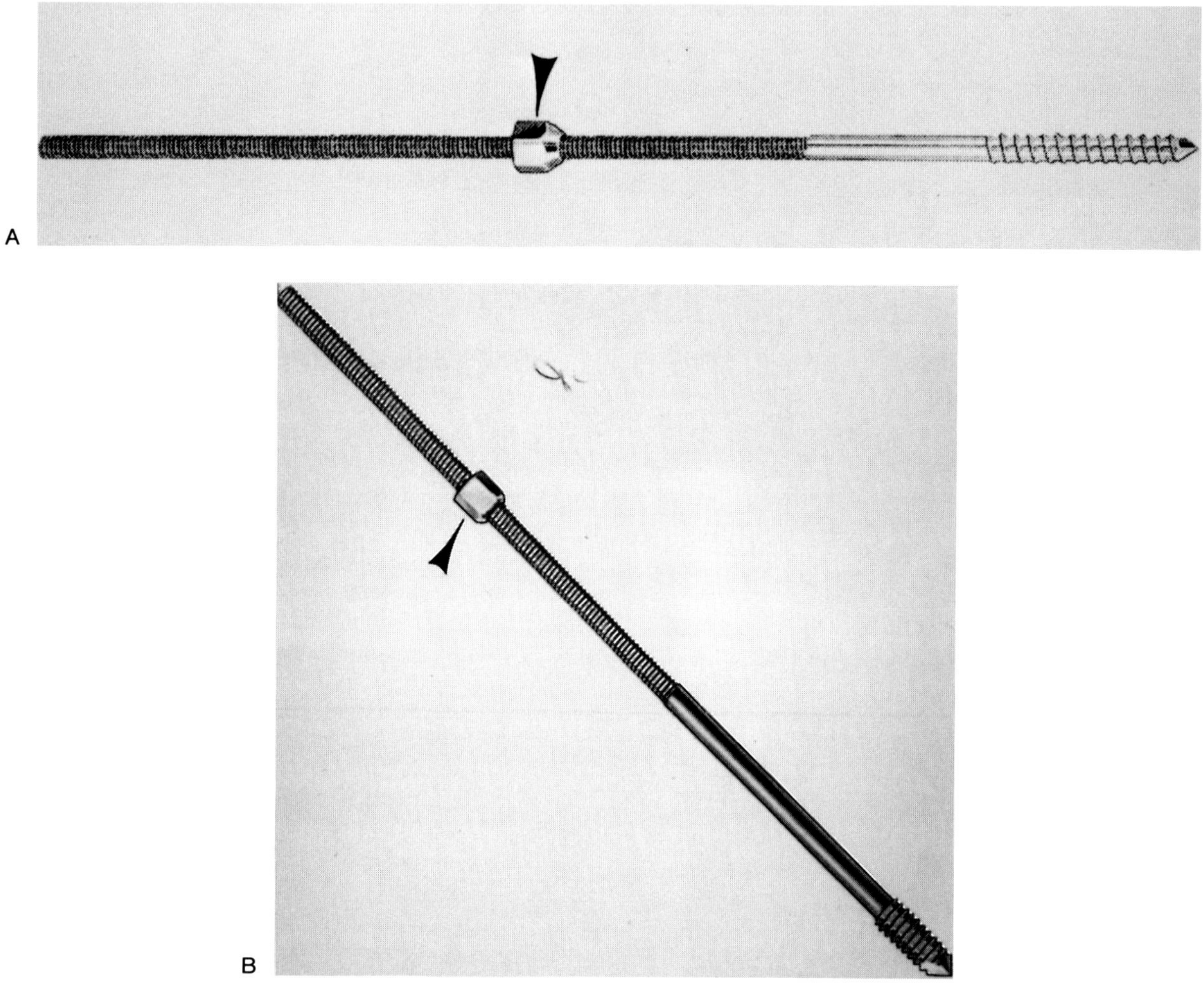

FIG. 2-65. Conventional **(A)** and modified **(B)** Hagie pins configured of stainless steel. The modified pin (B) is threaded for a shorter segment. The hex nuts position (*arrow*) can be varied on the threaded distal portion of the pin.

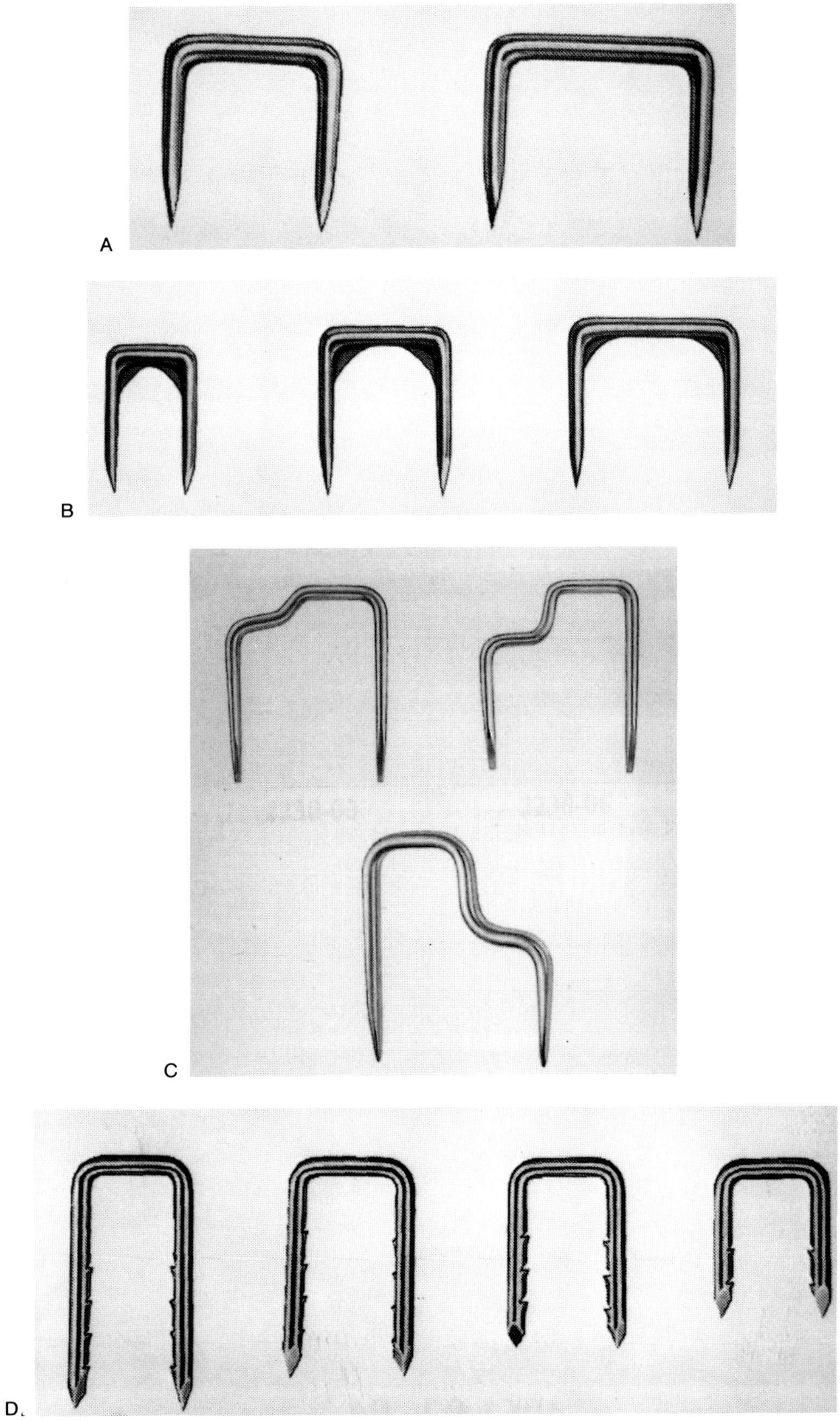

FIG. 2-66. Examples of orthopedic staples. **A:** Fracture staples (cobalt-chromium-molybdenum). **B:** Epiphyseal staples. **C:** Osteotomy staple (Coventry). **D:** Barbed staples (A–D: Courtesy of Zimmer, Warsaw, IN.)

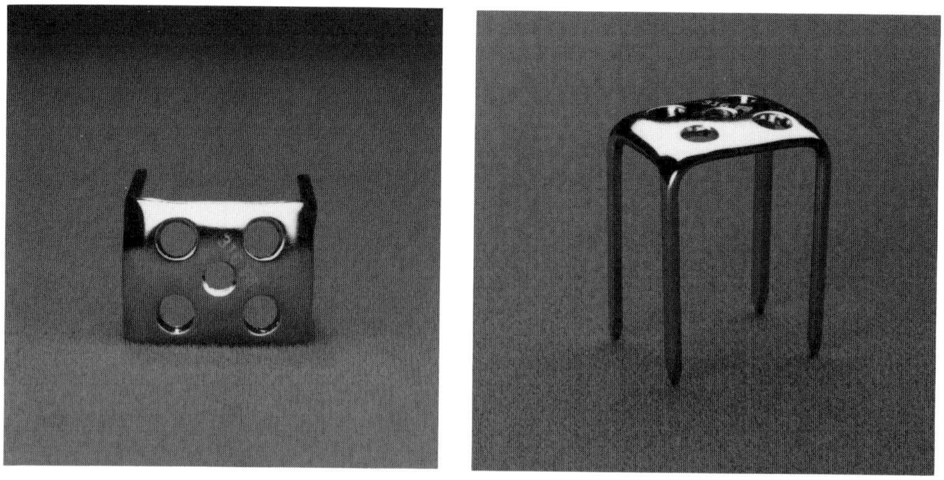

E F

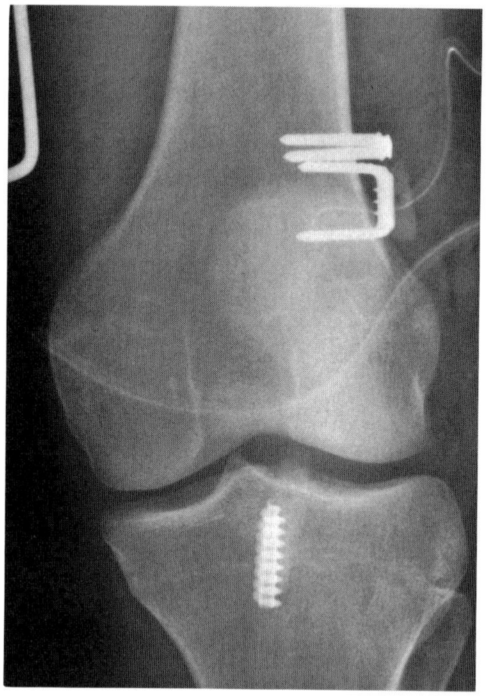

G

FIG. 2-66. *Continued.* Table staple shown on end **(E)** and from the side **(F)**. (Courtesy of Smith and Nephew Richards, Memphis, TN.) **G:** Radiograph after anterior cruciate ligament reconstruction with two barbed staples in the distal lateral femur.

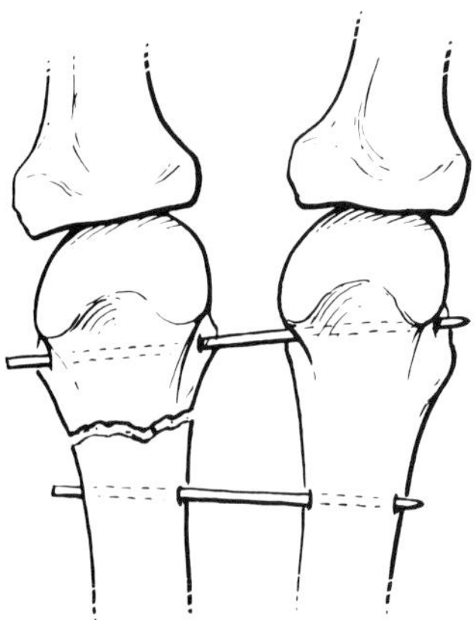

FIG. 2-67. K-wire fixation of the fifth metacarpal. Wires are passed through the adjacent fourth metacarpal to provide stability and prevent rotation of the fragments.

Wires, Cables, and Bands

Wires are used for suture material and tension-band fixation (Figs. 2-5 and 2-10) and K wires, for fracture fixation (generally small fractures, Fig. 2-67) or avulsion fractures.[35,43] Cerclage wire or cable is used for diaphyseal fixation (Fig. 2-68), often in combination with other fixation devices.[16,19,25,34,53]

Wire and K-wire combinations are commonly used for the tension-band technique.[33,39] The parallel K wires (Figs. 2-5 and 2-10) reduce shear and rotational forces.[53]

Dall-Miles cables come in several sizes with compressible fixation clamps (Fig. 2-69) for the support of diaphyseal fractures or bone grafts and with a trochanteric clamp for the reattachment of the greater trochanter after osteotomy (Fig. 2-70). Cables are available in Vitallium alloy or stainless steel. The advantages over conventional wire include increased strength and fewer problems with kinking.

Parham bands are flat strips of metal that are also used to fix cortical bone fragments circumferentially (Fig. 2-54).[32,39]

EXTERNAL FIXATION SYSTEMS

There are many types of external fixation systems designed for specific anatomic regions (Figs. 2-71 to 2-77).[5,9,11,12,15,17,18,29,40,42,47] Their specific functions also vary. For example, fixation devices may be designed to allow the motion of an adjacent joint (Fig. 2-72) or the fixation may be designed to alter the length of the extremity (Wagner external fixator).[10,40,42]

The trend in recent years has been toward simpler unilateral frames (Figs. 2-73 and 2-74).[11,23,24] This approach allows more flexibility for pin insertion and site selection, which reduces the chance for injury to vital structures.[23] Pins and an external frame are ordinarily used. The external frame may be rectangular, pyramidal, or partially circumferential. In some cases, wire under tension may be used to fix small fragments, particularly if the fragment is adjacent to a joint, such as with the Ilizarov device (Fig. 2-75). Full pins may be used that are either smooth or partially threaded (Figs. 2-71D and 2-77C). Figure 2-71D shows two smooth pins with a threaded pin at each end of the construct. Half pins (Figs. 2-75; 2-77A,B; and 2-78) are also used when the direction of the pin might injure neurovascular structures if it continued through the soft tissues on the opposite side of the extremity. Generally, the half pins are larger in diameter than are the full pins.

External fixators should fulfill three major goals. First, they should allow access to the injured area, especially with open fractures. Second, they should be used in situations in which there is no danger of injury to vital structures. Third, the system selected must be able to meet the mechanical demands of the injury.[4,6,24,29,30,38]

External fixation devices have the following advantages:[13]

Three-dimensional stabilization
Limited soft tissue injury or dissection during insertion
Pins used as handles to reduce fragments
Improved wound access for open fractures
Early motion in uninvolved joints

The disadvantages include the following:[1,2,4,54]

Pin tract infection if improper technique is used
Damage to soft tissue or neural structures if improper technique is used
Fixation failure leading to internal fixation procedure

TRACTION

Traction may be applied to the skin or skeleton for brief periods (Fig. 2-79) during fracture reduction or for longer periods (Figs. 2-80 to 2-82) to improve the fragment's position prior to more definitive treatment.

Skeletal traction can be accomplished by using threaded Steinmann pins, smooth pins, or K wires (Fig. 2-82). The latter cause less soft tissue damage but tend to cut through bone.[28] Occasionally, two pins may be used together, depending on the porosity of the bone.

The most common indication for skeletal traction is the femoral fracture (Fig. 2-80). However, traction is also used for certain humeral fractures (Fig. 2-83) and other lower-extremity fractures. Traction pins for lower-extremity fractures are placed in one of the three sites: supracondylar region of the femur, proximal tibia, and calcaneus.[28] The disadvantage of distal femoral traction is quadriceps injury and scarring, which can lead to decreased knee function.[7,28] In addition, passing the pin laterally to medially through the distal femur may injure the neurovascular structures. Calcaneal traction is avoided when possible. The risk of infection in this region carries with it the possibility of a chronic disabling condition.[28] More specific data on traction are provided in the specific anatomic chapters.

COMPLICATIONS

The complications vary with the anatomic region, type of procedure, and fixation device used. More in-depth discussions of complications and imaging techniques are provided in the anatomic chapters that follow. However, certain basic problems and examples are discussed here.

Internal Fixation[7,19–24,46,52,55]
- Screws and plate-screw fixation
  - Loosening and screw pull out (Fig. 2-84)
  - Soft tissue irritation from protruding screws

(text continues on page 106)

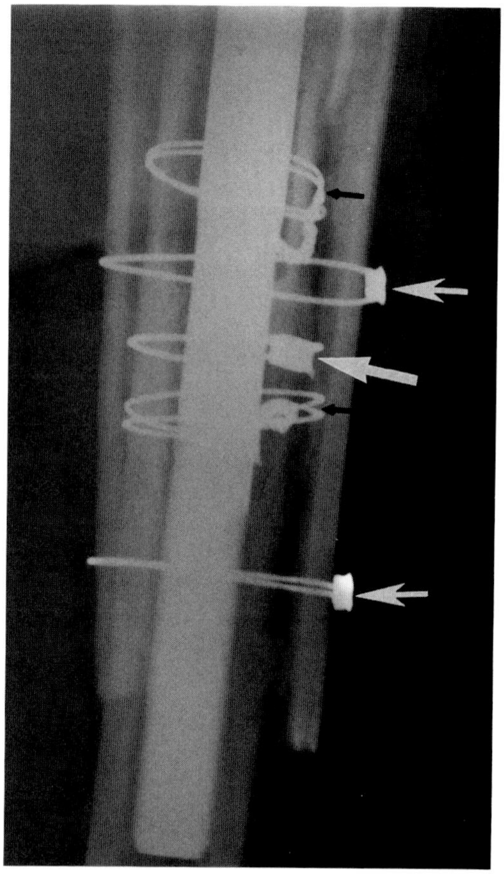

FIG. 2-68. Revision hip arthroplasty with allograft cortical bone grafting. There are double cerclage wires around the native femur (*small black arrows*) and three Dall-Miles cables (*white arrows*) for additional support.

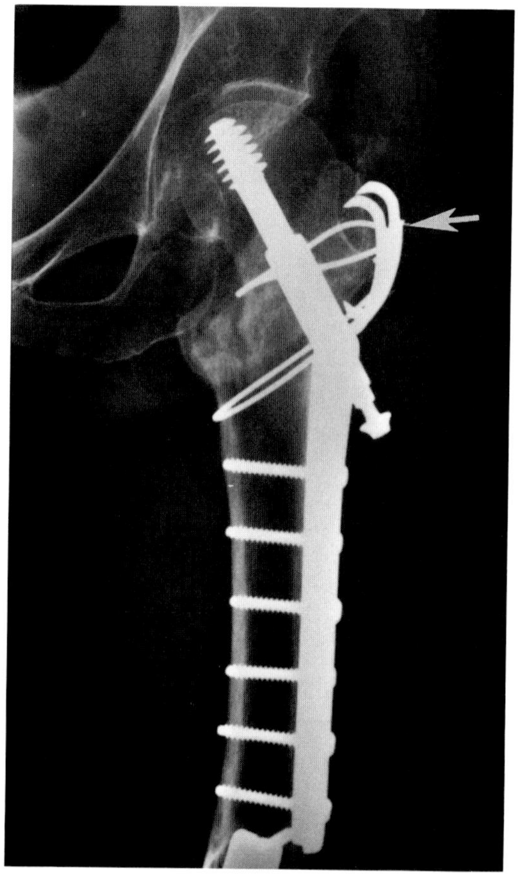

FIG. 2-70. An AP radiograph of the upper femur with an impacted intertrochanteric fracture. The fracture is internally fixed with an Ambi dynamic hip screw and six-hole plate. A Dall-Miles cable system with trochanteric clamp (*arrow*) is placed around the greater trochanter.

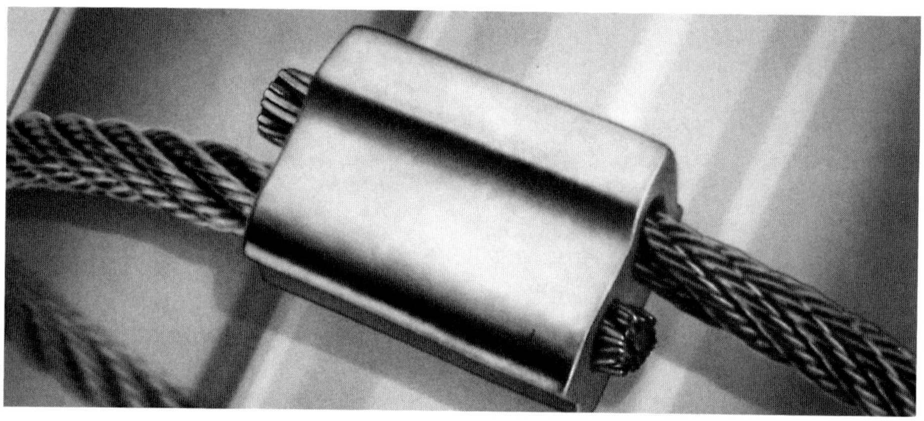

FIG. 2-69. Dall-Miles cable and clamp. (Courtesy of Howmedica, Rutherford, NJ.)

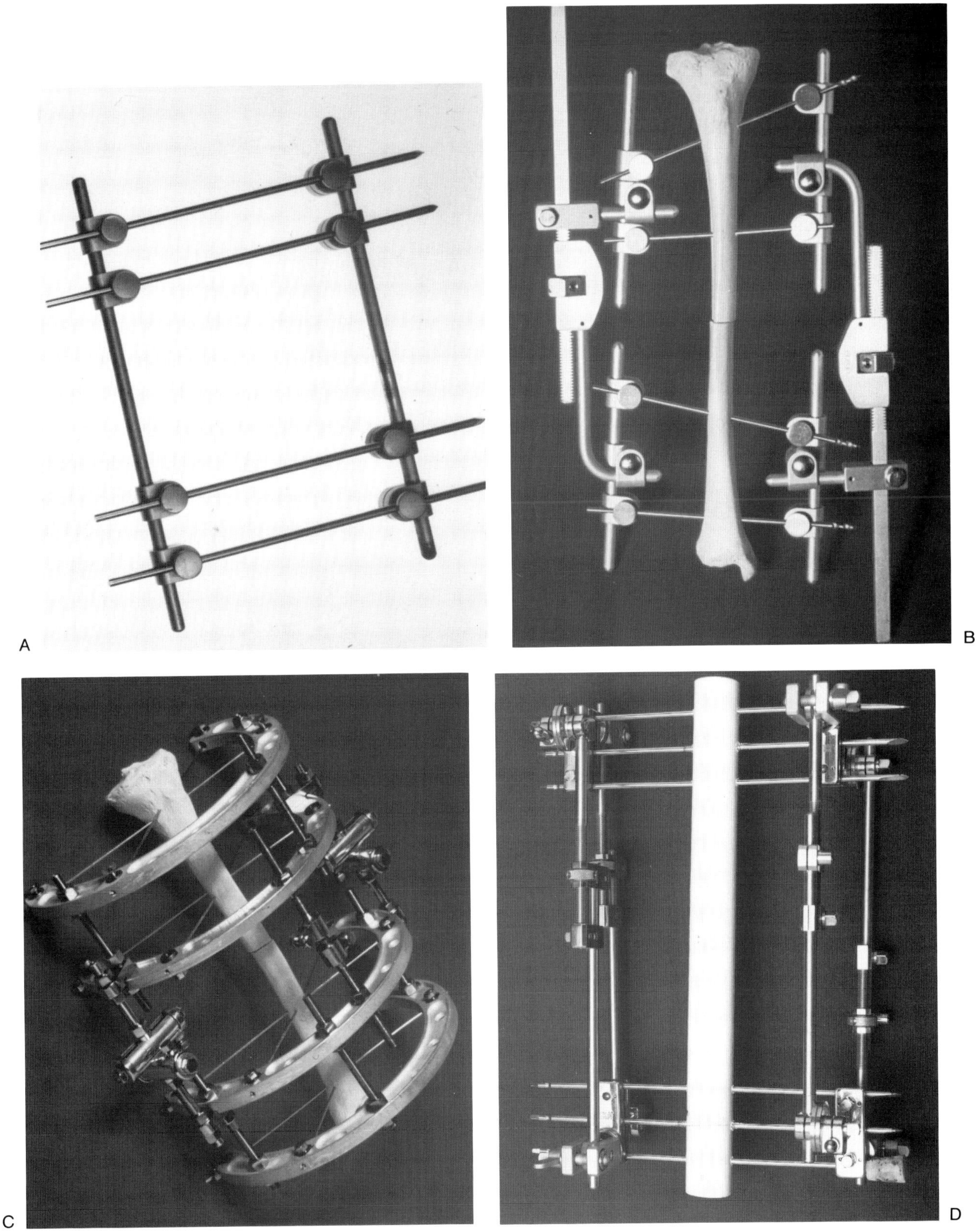

FIG. 2-71. External fixation systems. **A:** Original Roger-Anderson apparatus. **B:** Roger-Anderson apparatus, which allows compression of the fracture surfaces. **C:** Volkov-Oganism device. Hoffman-Vidal quadrangular frame **(D)** and radiograph. (See **E–G** on next page.)

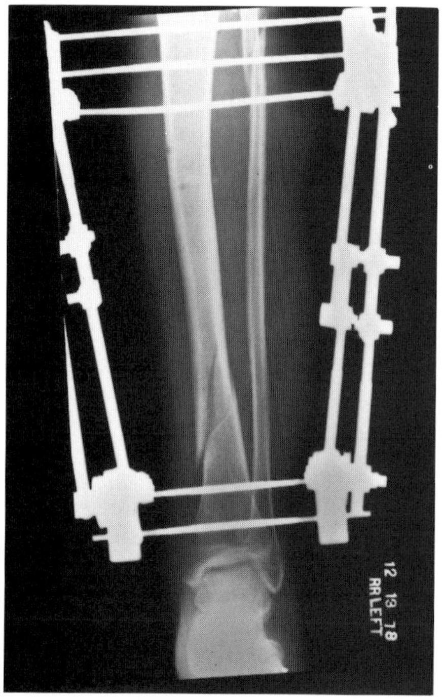

E

FIG. 2-71. (*Continued*). **(E)** of Hoffman-Vidal fixation of distal tibial with upper fibular spiral fractures. **F,G:** Fischer apparatus (F). Radiograph of a refractured femur with Fischer external fixator. (From Berquist, TH. *Imaging of orthopedic trauma,* 2nd ed. New York: Raven Press, 1992.)

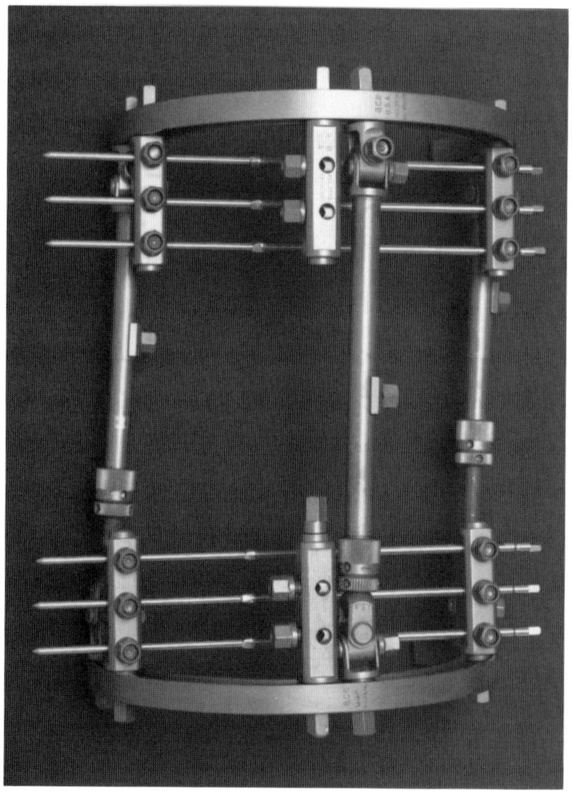

F

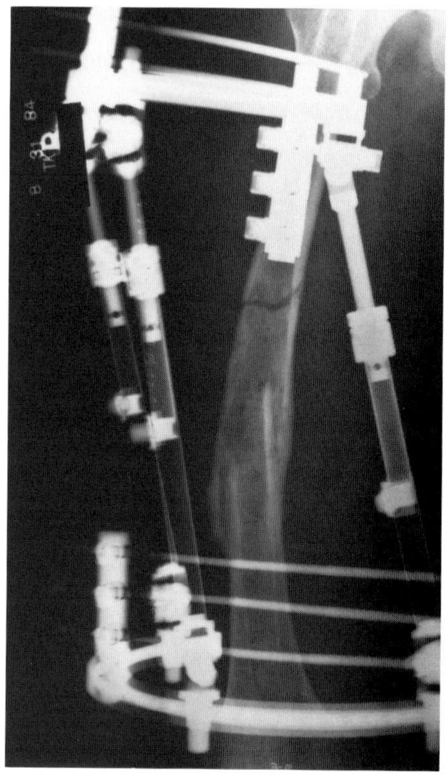

G

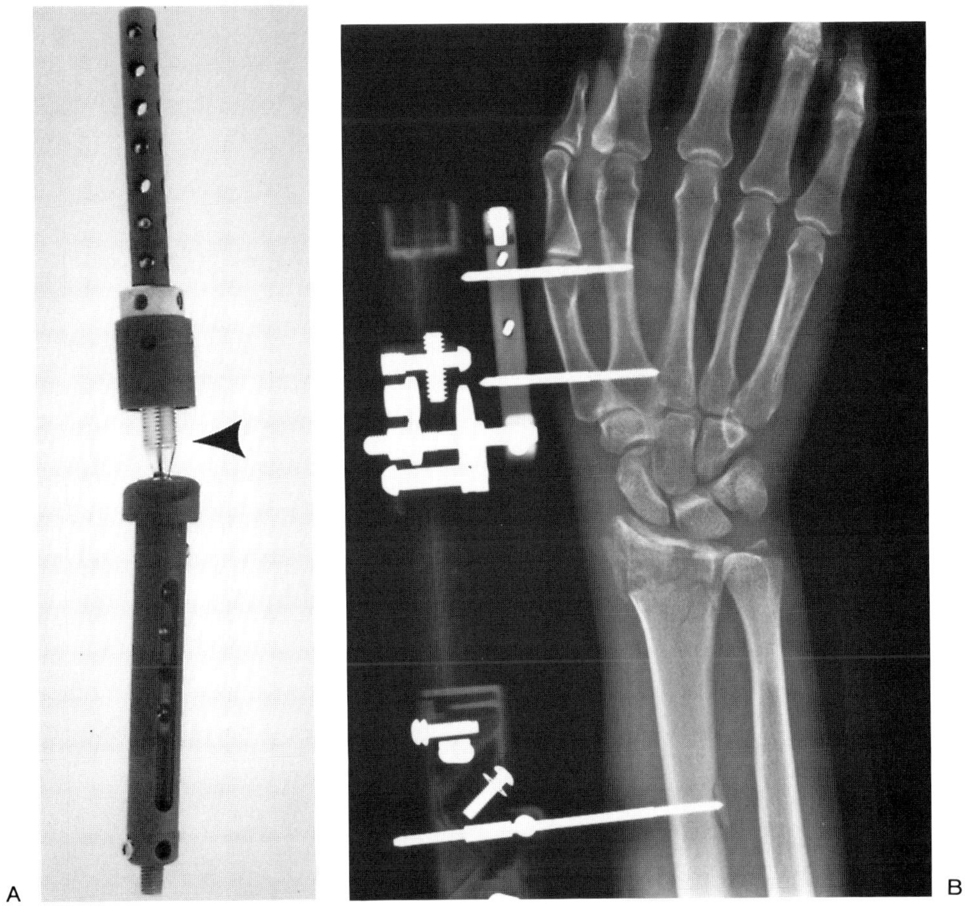

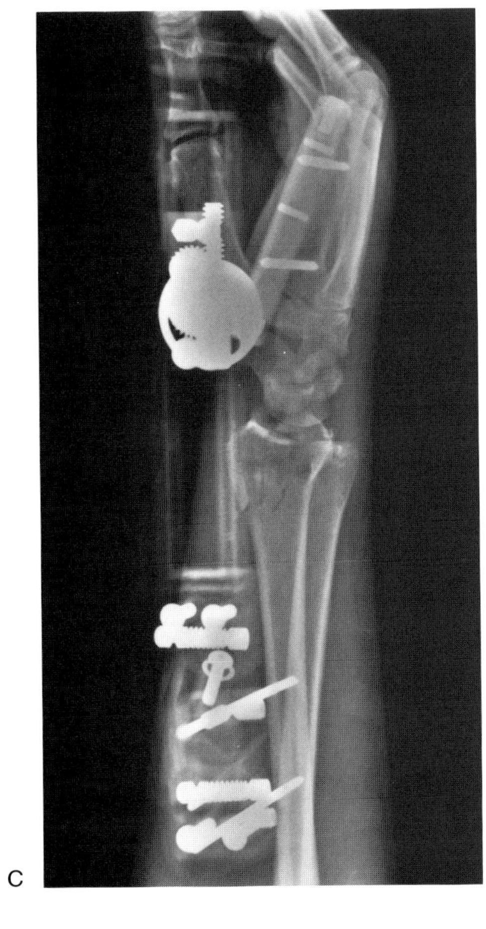

FIG. 2-72. A: Illustration of the Clyburn dynamic Colles fixator system constructed of aluminum and stainless steel. The ball joint (*arrow*) allows motion at this level. (Courtesy of Zimmer, Warsaw, IN.) The PA **(B)** and lateral **(C)** views of the wrist with external fixator for Frykman VIII fracture of the radius and ulnar styloid (Agee Wrist Jack).

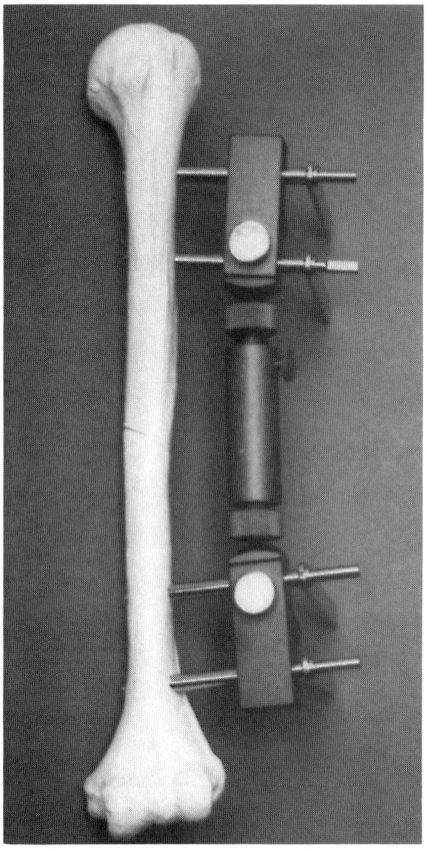

FIG. 2-73. Orthofix™ fixator for humeral fracture. (Courtesy of EBI Medical Systems, Parsippany, NJ.)

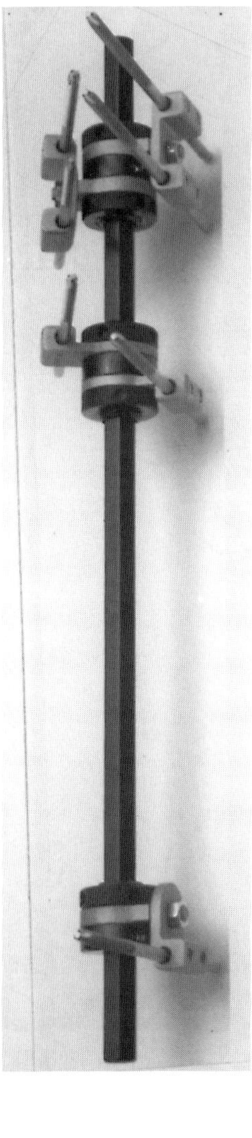

A,B

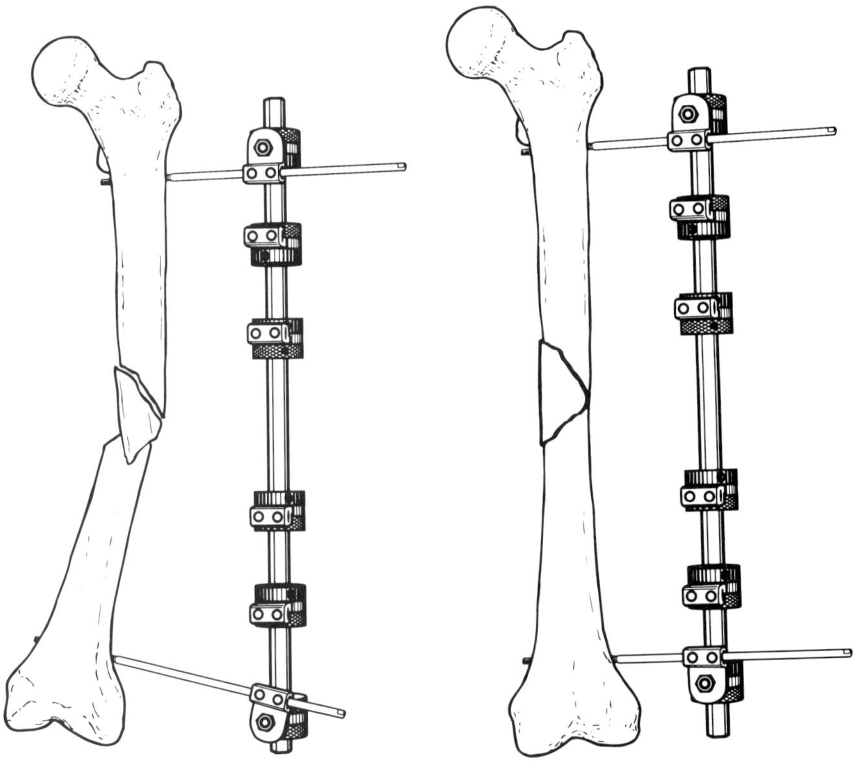

C

FIG. 2-74. Hex-Fix™ fixator system for open or unstable fractures of the femur, tibia, and humerus. **A:** The Hex-fix™ system, which allows multiple pin angles with a single rod system. **B,C:** Illustration of Hex-Fix™ system to reduce a femoral fracture. (Courtesy of Smith and Nephew Richards, Memphis, TN.)

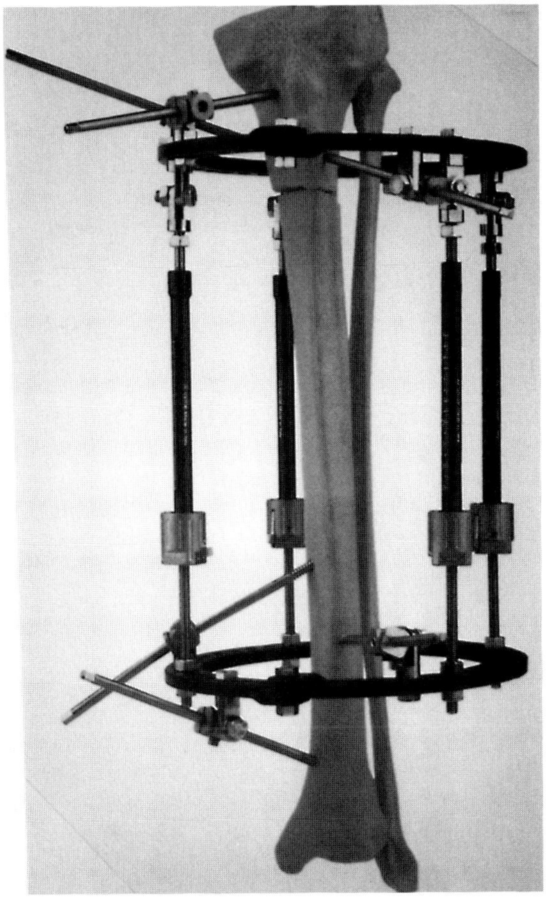

FIG. 2-75. Ilizarov external fixator. (Courtesy of Smith and Nephew Richards, Memphis, TN.)

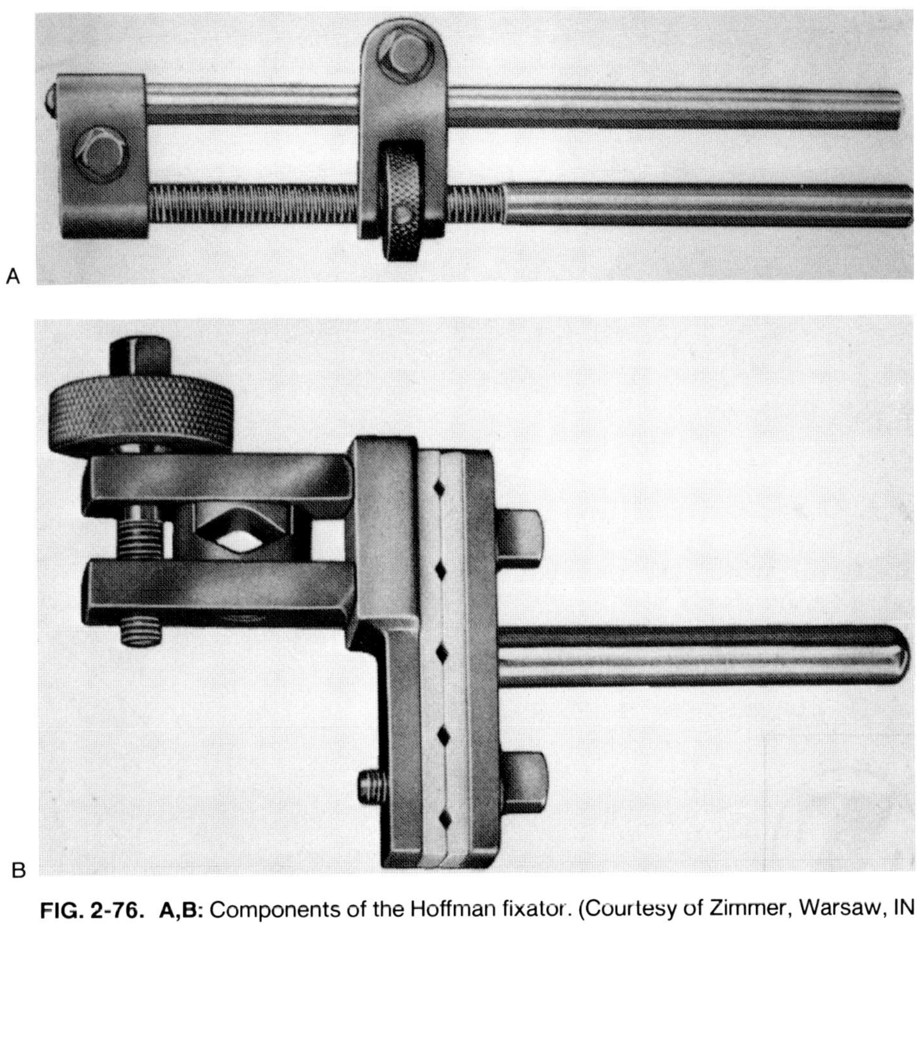

FIG. 2-76. A,B: Components of the Hoffman fixator. (Courtesy of Zimmer, Warsaw, IN.)

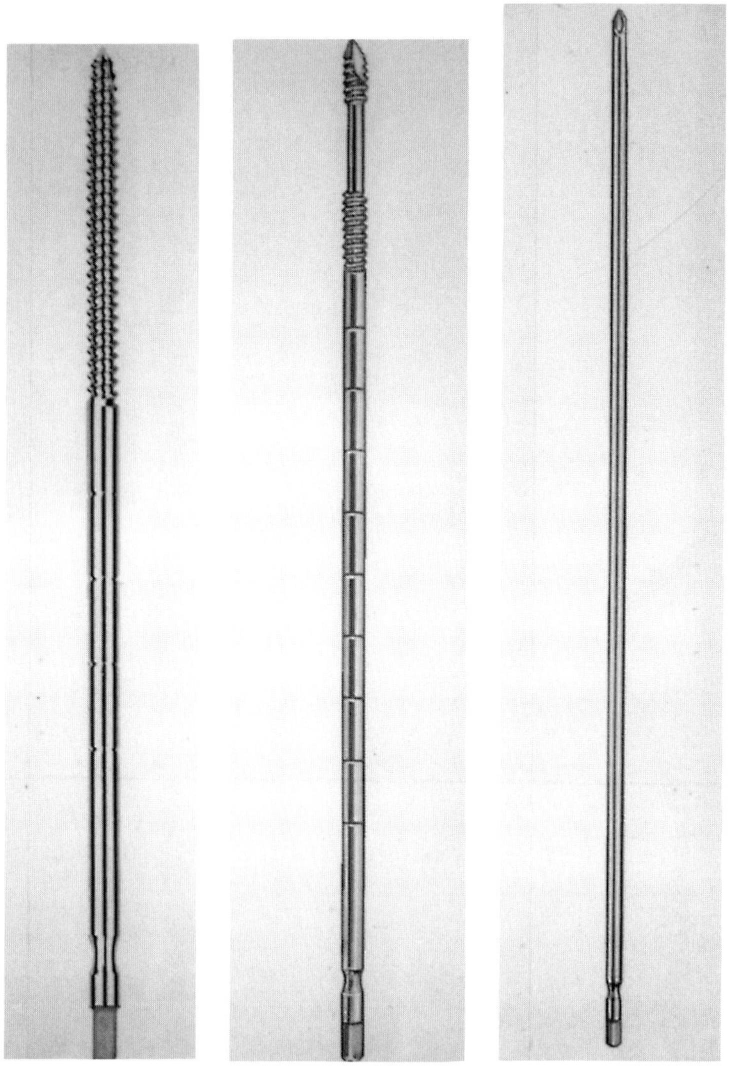

A B C

FIG. 2-77. Fixator pins. **A:** A 4-mm half pin with continuous threads for cancellous bone. **B:** A 4-mm half pin with interrupted threads for cortex of long (diaphyseal) bones. **C:** Unthreaded pin. (Courtesy of Zimmer, Warsaw, IN.)

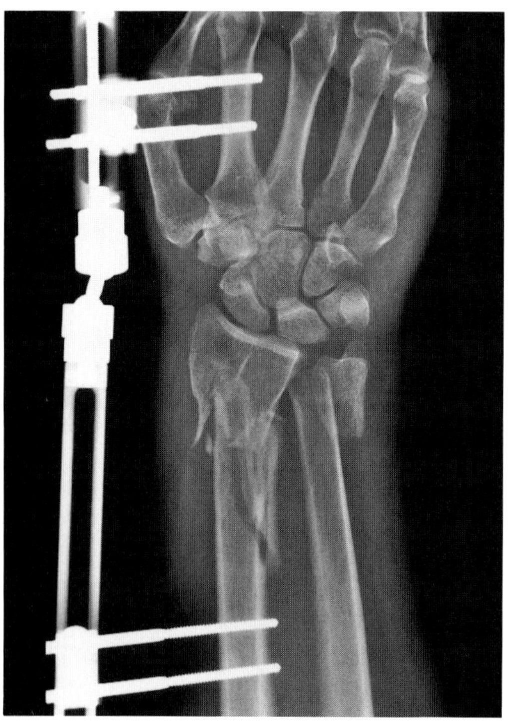

FIG. 2-78. Complex fractures of the distal radius and ulna with unilateral external fixation with fully threaded half pins. The threads pass appropriately through both cortices. There is a ball joint at the wrist to allow some motion.

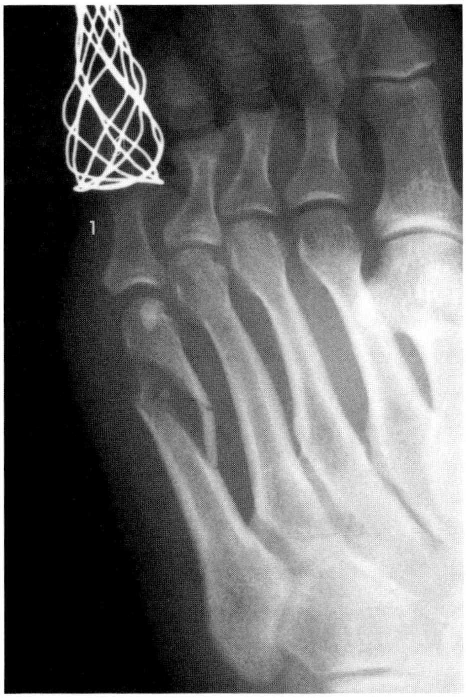

FIG. 2-79. Oblique radiograph of the foot, demonstrating a comminuted fracture of the distal fifth metatarsal. The initial reduction film (*1*) was obtained with finger trap traction on the fifth digit to improve metatarsal length and position of the fracture fragments.

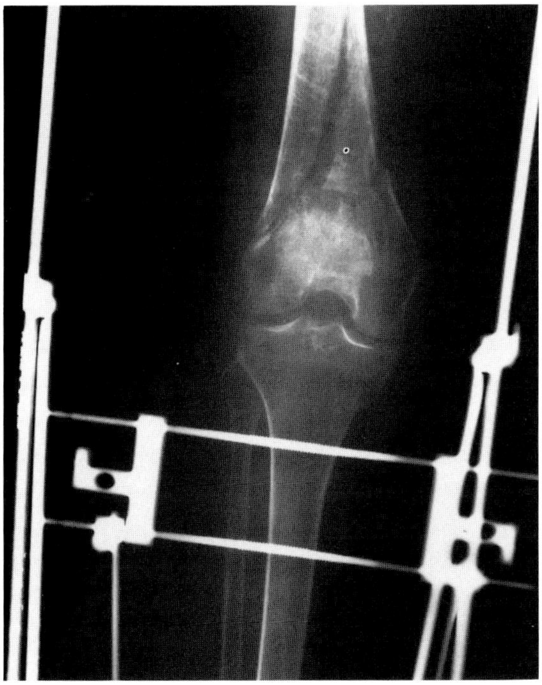

A

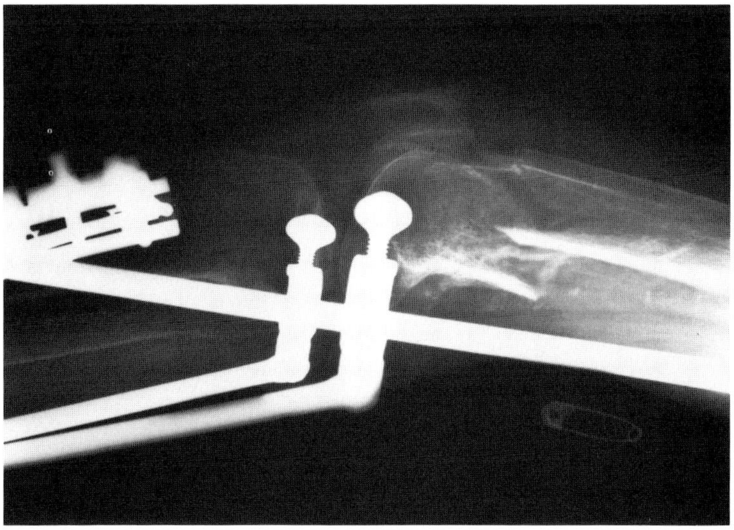

B

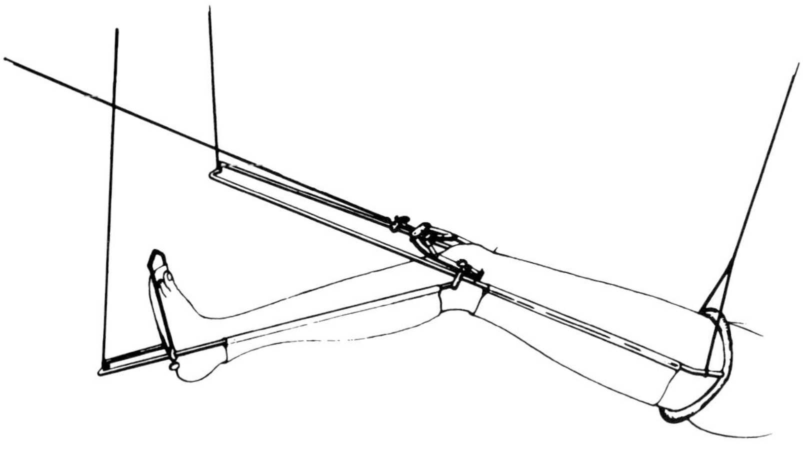

C

FIG. 2-80. The AP **(A)** and lateral **(B)** radiographs of a comminuted fracture of the distal femur. There are two Steinmann pins in the upper tibia with skeletal traction using a Harris splint with Pearson attachment, which is illustrated in **C**. (C: Courtesy of Zimmer, Warsaw, IN.)

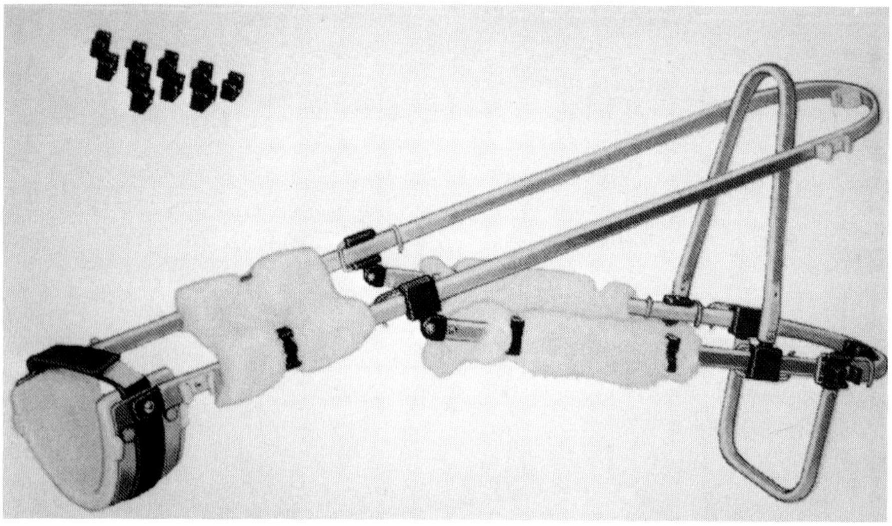

FIG. 2-81. Radiolucent Thomas splint for fractures of the hip, femur, or lower leg. (Courtesy of Zimmer, Warsaw, IN.)

A 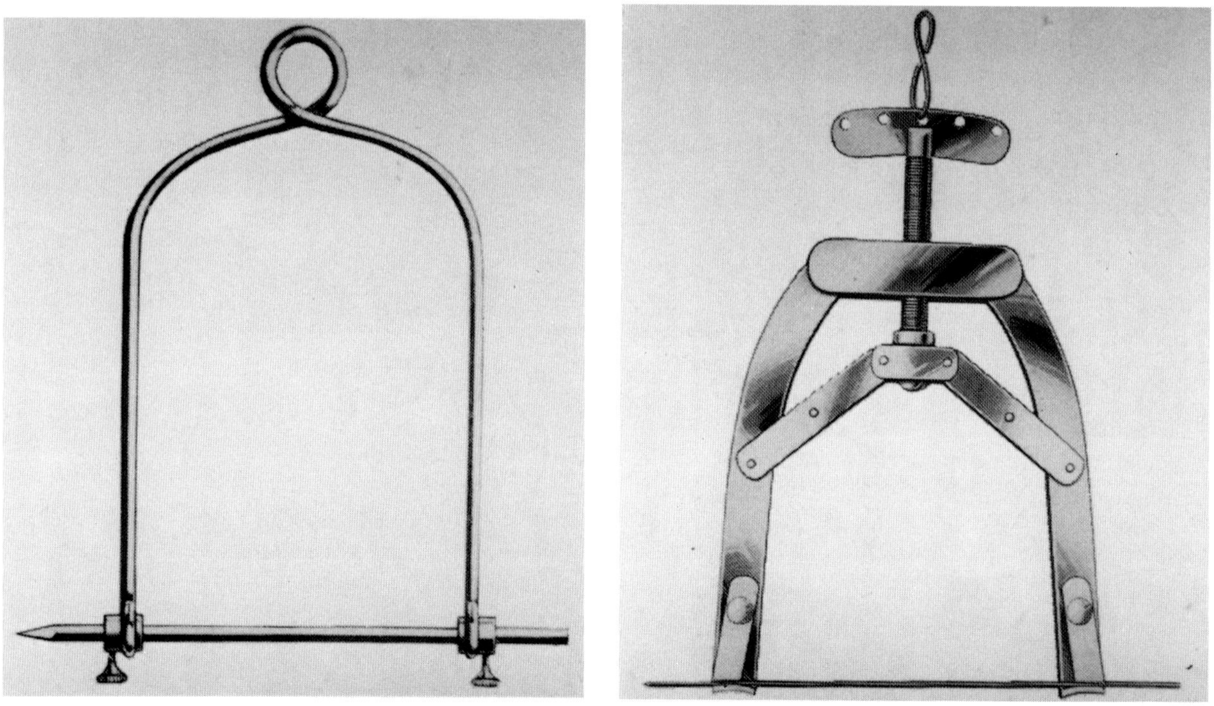 B

FIG. 2-82. A: Böhler-Steinmann pin holder with an unthreaded pin. **B:** K-wire holder with K wire in position. (Courtesy of Zimmer, Warsaw, IN.)

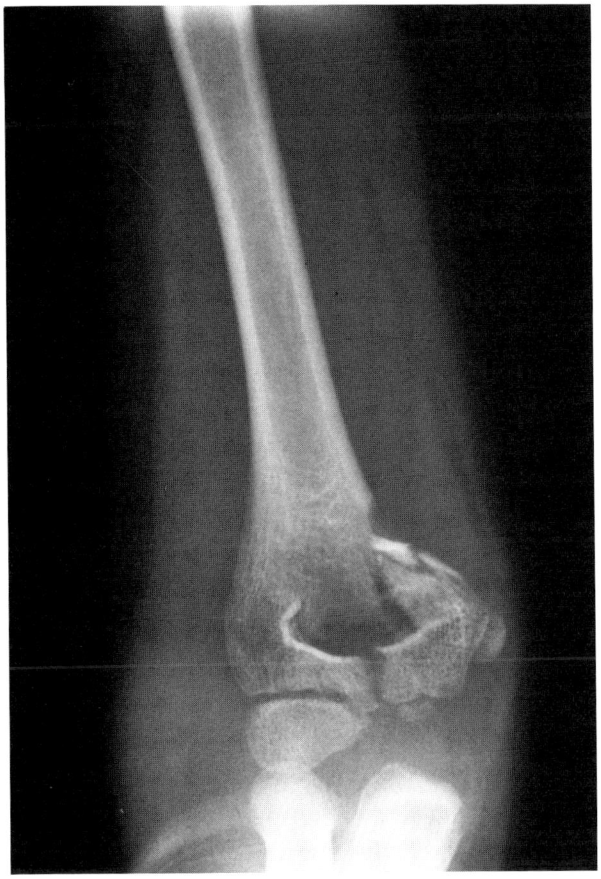

A

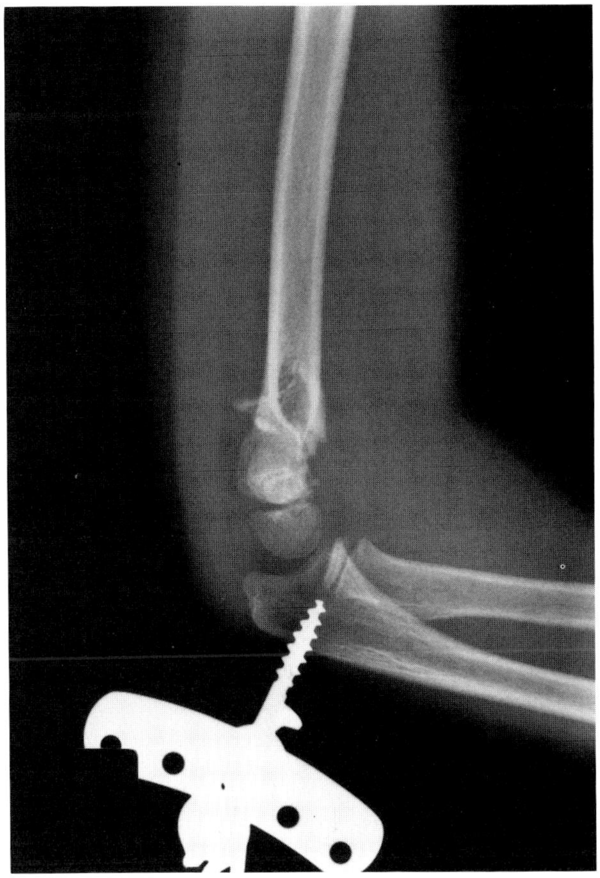

B

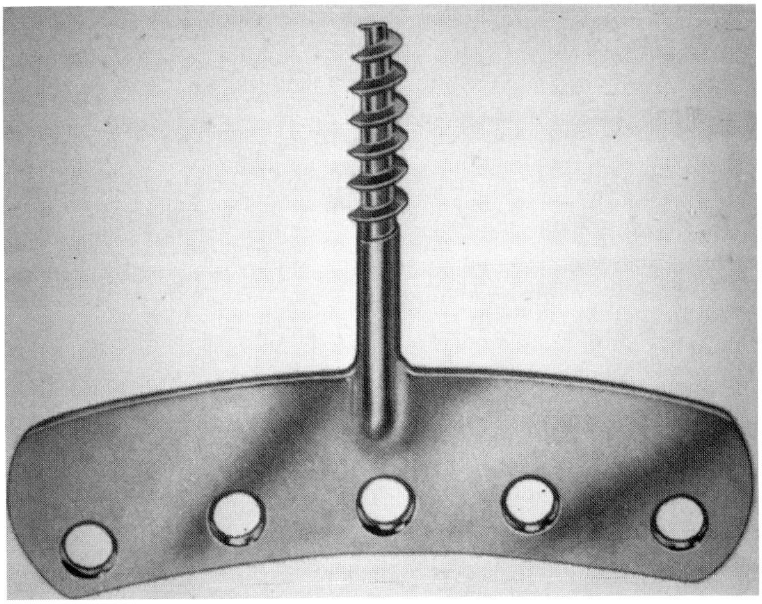

C

FIG. 2-83. The AP **(A)** and lateral **(B)** radiographs of a comminuted supracondylar fracture, which extends through the medial epicondyle. Wing traction screw in place. **C:** Wing traction screw for use in arm-over-body traction for supracondylar fractures of the humerus.

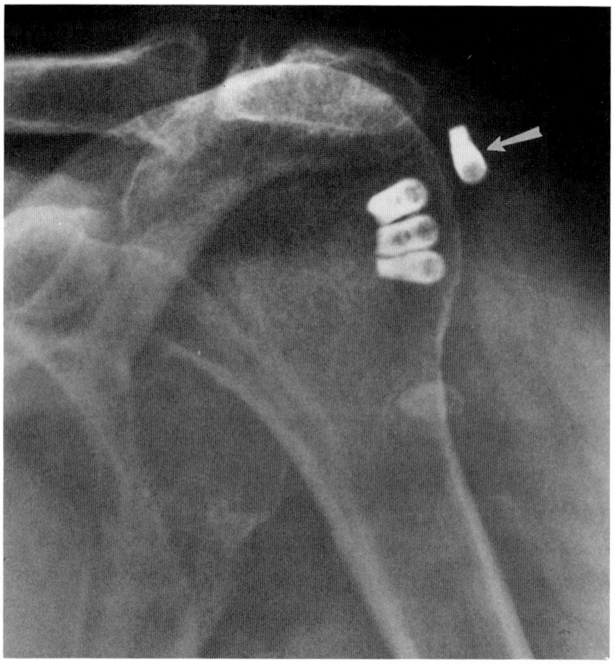

FIG. 2-84. Internal rotation view of the left shoulder after rotator cuff tear repair with suture anchors. One of the anchors (*arrow*) has pulled out.

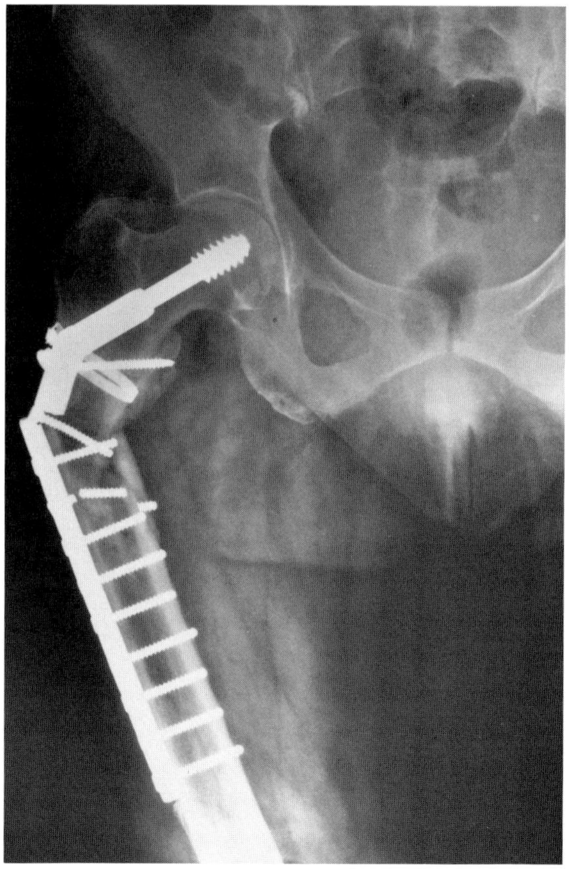

FIG. 2-85. Old subtrochanteric fracture of the right femur with a dynamic hip screw and 12-hole plate. The plate has fractured at one of the upper screw holes, and one of the proximal cortical screws is fractured.

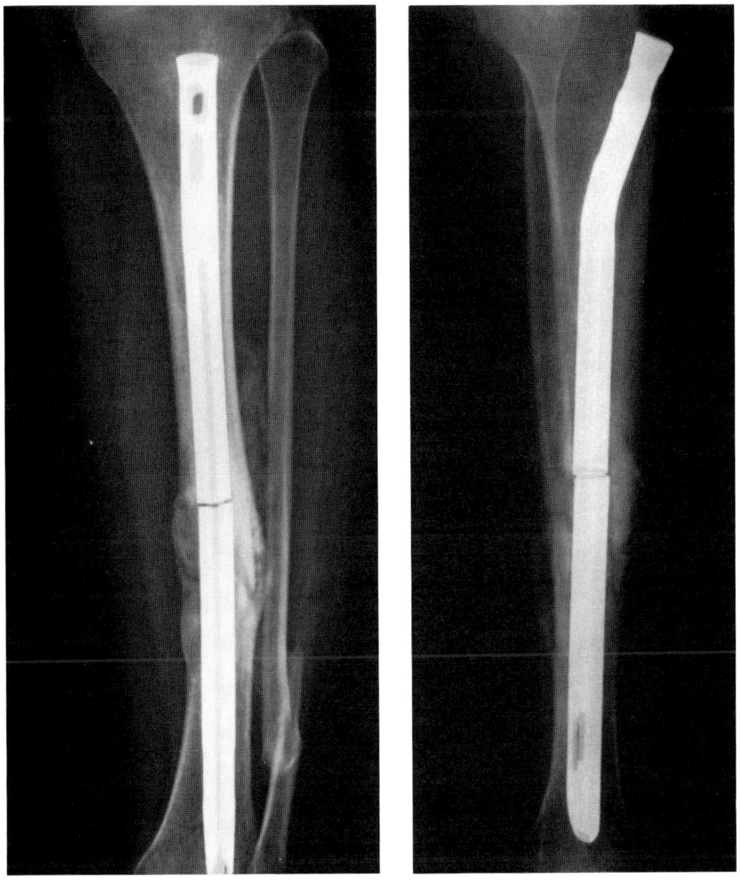

A,B

FIG. 2-86. The AP **(A)** and lateral **(B)** views of the tibia with a medullary nail for fixation. The nail is fractured at the fracture site.

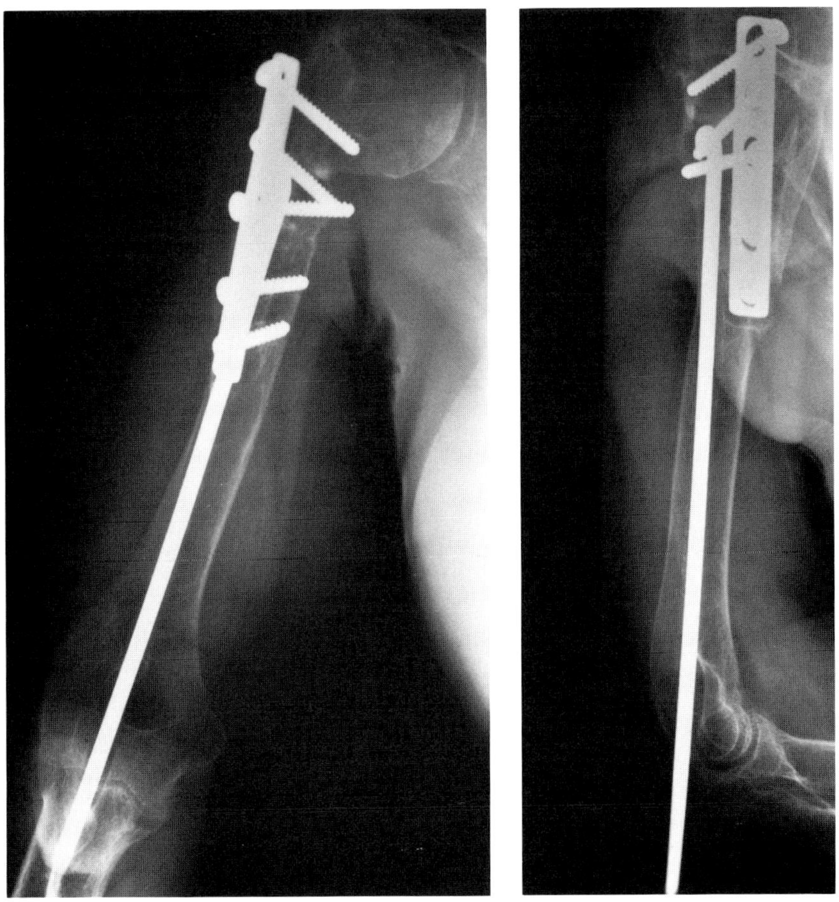

B

FIG. 2-87. Upper humeral fracture with Rush rod and DCP fixation. Follow-up examination in the AP **(A)** and lateral **(B)** views show the rod has migrated through the elbow, the fracture is not united, and the plate and screws are loose.

Stress risers in screw holes, leading to fracture
Instrument failure (Fig. 2-85)
Infection
Delayed union, malunion, or nonunion
Intramedullary nails[7,36,37,51]
Shortening at fracture site
Rotation of fragments
Instrument failure (Fig. 2-86)
Implant migration (Fig. 2-87)
Infection
Traction or External Fixators
Pin tract infection
Pin loosening
Implant removal

Implant removal may be required as a result of failure or persistent symptoms, such as pain related to the implant.[7,50,53] Ideally, implants should be left in place until the fracture or reconstructive procedure has healed. In children, implants are generally removed to avoid stress shielding, to allow complete bone remodeling, and to reduce the risk of infection or metal toxicity.[48] In elderly or osteopenic patients, implants may be left in place. In addition, implants may be left in place in nonweight-bearing bones, such as the upper extremity or upper femoral fractures or in the case of a single cancellous metaphyseal screw.[7,28,53] When multiple devices are in place (i.e., double plates), it may require two procedures to remove the plates separately, approximately 3 to 6 months apart.[28] More detail is provided in the specific anatomic chapters.

REFERENCES

1. Alexander IJ, Kotschi H. Redirecting K-wires and Steinmann pins. *Foot Ankle* 1990;10:243.
2. Aro H, Hein TJ, Chao EYS. Mechanical characteristics of an upper extremity external fixator. *Clin Orthop* 1990;253:240–250.
3. Behrens F. A primer of fixator devices and configurations. *Clin Orthop* 1989;241:5–14.
4. Behrens F. General theory and principles of external fixation. *Clin Orthop* 1989;241:15–23.
5. Behrens F, Kraft EL, Oegema TR Jr. Biochemical changes in articular cartilage after joint immobilization by casting or external fixation. *J Orthop Res* 1989;7:335–343.
6. Behrens F, Searls K. External fixation of the tibia. *J Bone Joint Surg [Br]* 1986;68B:246–254.
7. Berquist TH. *Imaging of orthopedic trauma.* 2nd ed. New York: Raven Press; 1992.
8. Brooker AF, Epps H, Constable D. New tibial interlocking nail system. *J Orthop Trauma* 1987;1:257–259.
9. Carter MD, Gilbert JA, Dahners LE. An evaluation of the bending stiffness of various tibial fixation methods. *Clin Orthop* 1987;224: 289–293.
10. Clyburn TA. Dynamic external fixation for comminuted intra-articular fractures of the distal end of the radius. *J Bone Joint Surg [Am]* 1987;69A:248–254.
11. Cooney WP III, Smith DK. External fixation of the upper extremity. In: *Inst. Course Lectures AAOS (American Academy of Orthopedic Surgeons).* CV Mosby 1987;36:455–469.
12. Cziffer E. The use of the Manuflex disposable mini external fixator. *Orthopedics* 1989;12:163–166.
13. DeCoster T, Alvarez R, Trevino S. External fixation of the foot and ankle. *Foot Ankle* 1986;7:40–48.
14. Duncan KH, Wheeler DK. Staple migration simulating lateral meniscus injury. *Am J Sports Med* 1990;18:211–213.
15. Egan JM, Shearer JR. Behavior of an external fixation frame incorporating an angular separation. A finite element approach. *Clin Orthop* 1987;223:265–274.
16. Fitzgerald JAW, Southgate GW. Cerclage wiring in the management of comminuted fractures of the femoral shaft. *Injury* 1987;18:111–116.
17. Ford LT. Osteotomies. Nomenclature and uses. *Radiol Clin North Am* 1975;13:79–92.
18. Frykman GK, Tooma GS, Boyko K, Henderson R. Comparison of eleven external fixators for treatment of unstable wrist fractures. *J Hand Surg [Am]* 1989;14A:247–254.
19. Fuster S, Palliso F, Combalia A, Sanjuan A, Garcia S. Intrathoracic migration of a Kirschner wire. *Injury* 1990;21:124–126.
20. Garfin SR, Botte MJ, Waters RL, Nickel VL. Complications in the use of the halo fixation device. *J Bone Joint Surg [Am]* 1986;68A: 320–325.
21. Giebel G, Tscherne H, Daiber M. Tibial head osteotomy in the treatment of arthrosis of the knee. *Orthopade* 1985;14:144–153.
22. Glover MG, Convery FR. Migration of fractured greater trochanteric osteotomy wire with resultant sciatica. A report of two cases. *Orthopedics* 1989;12:743–744.
23. Green SA. Ilizarov external fixation technical and anatomic considerations. *Bull Hosp Jt Dis Orthop Inst* 1988;48:28–35.
24. Green SA. Complications of pin and wire external fixation. In: *Clin Orthop* 1983;180:109–116.
25. Habernek H, Walch G, Dengg C. Cerclage for torsional fractures of the tibia. *J Bone Joint Surg [Br]* 1989;71B:311–313.
26. Hammer R. A new device for external fixation. *Acta Orthop Scand* 1988;59:708–711.
27. Hansen ST. Internal fixation of children's fractures of the lower extremity. *Orthop Clin North Am* 1990;21:353–363.
28. Harkness JW, Ramsey WC, Harkness JW. Principles of fractures and dislocations. In: Rockwood CA, Green DP, eds. *Fractures in adults.* 3rd ed. Vol. 1. Philadelphia: JB Lippincott; 1991:1–163.
29. Horne JG, Devane P, Purdie G. A prospective randomized trial of external fixation and plaster cast immobilization in the treatment of distal radial fractures. *J Orthop Trauma* 1990;4:30–34.
30. Howard PW, Stewart HD, Hind RE, Burke FD. External fixation or plaster for severely displaced comminuted Colles' fractures? *J Bone Joint Surg [Br]* 1989;71B:68–73.
31. Johnson KD, Greenberg M. Comminuted femoral shaft fractures. *Orthop Clin North Am* 1987;18:133–147.
32. Jones DG. Bone erosion beneath partridge bands. *J Bone Joint Surg [Br]* 1986;68B:476–477.
33. Jupiter JB, Sheppard JE. Tension wire fixation of avulsion fractures in the hand. *Clin Orthop* 1987;241:113–120.
34. Kanakis TE, Cordey J. Is there mechanical difference between lag screws and double cerclage? *Injury* 1991;22:185–189.
35. Kinast C, Frigg R, Perren SM. Biomechanics of the interlocking nail. A study of the proximal interlock. *Arch Orthop Trauma Surg* 1990;109:197–204.
36. Klaue K, Kowalski M, Perren SM. Internal fixation with self-compressing plate and lag screw: improvements of the plate hole and screw design. 2. In vivo investigations. *J Orthop Trauma* 1991;5: 289–296.
37. Klaue K, Perren SM, Kowalski M. Internal fixation with self-compressing plate and lag screw: improvements of the plate hole and screw design. 1. Mechanical investigation. *J Orthop Trauma* 1991;5:280–288.
38. Moroz TK, Finlay JB, Rorabeck CH, Bourne RB. External skeletal fixation: choosing a system based on biomechanical stability. *J Orthop Trauma* 1989;2:284–296.
39. Müller ME, Allgöwer M, Schneider R, Willenegger H. *Manual of internal fixation: techniques recommended by the AO-ASIF group.* 3rd ed. Berlin: Springer-Verlag; 1991.
40. Murphy CP, D'Ambrosia RD, Dabezies EJ, Acker JH, Shoji H, Chuinard RG. Complex femur fractures: treatment with the Wagner external fixation device or the Grosse-Kempf interlocking nail. *J Trauma* 1988;28:1553–11561.
41. O'Sullivan ME, Chao EYS, Kelly PJ. Current concepts review. The

effects of fixation of fracture healing. *J Bone Joint Surg [Am]* 1989;71A:306–310.

42. Paterson JMH, Waller CS, Catterall A. Lower limb lengthening by a modified Wagner technique. *J Pediatr Orthop* 1989;9:129–133.
43. Polakoff DR, Bucholz RW, Ogden JA. Tension band wiring of displaced tibial tuberosity fractures in adolescents. *Clin Orthop* 1986;209:161–165.
44. Prince H, Worlock P. The small AO external fixator in the treatment of unstable distal forearm fractures. *J Hand Surg [Br]* 1988;13B:294–297.
45. Rezaian SM, Abtahi M. A simple and safe technique for tibial lengthening. *Clin Orthop* 1986;207:216–222.
46. Rommens P, Gielen J, Broos P, Gruwez J. Intrinsic problems with the external fixation device of Hoffmann-Vidal-Adrey: a critical evaluation of 117 patients with complex tibial shaft fractures. *J Trauma* 1989;29:630–638.
47. Rööser B, Bengtson S, Herrlin K, Önnerfält R. External fixation of femoral fractures: experience with 15 cases. *J Orthop Trauma* 1990;4:70–74.
48. Rosson J, Murphy W, Tonge C, Shearer J. Healing of residual screw holes after plate removal. *Injury* 1991;22:383–384.
49. Rostoker G, Robin J, Binet O, Blamoutier J, Paupe J, Lessana-Leibowitch M, Bedouelle J, Sonneck JM, Garrel JB, Millet P. Dermatitis due to orthopaedic implants. *J Bone Joint Surg [Am]* 1987;69A:1408–1412.
50. Schmalzried TP, Grogan TJ, Neumeier DA, Dorey FJ. Metal removal in a pediatric population: benign procedure as necessary evil. *J Pediatr Orthop* 1991;11:72–76.
51. Sequina F, Texhammer R. *AO/ASIF instrumentation manual of use and care.* New York: Springer-Verlag; 1981.
52. Shellock FG, Slimp G. Halo vest for cervical spine fixation during MR imaging. *AJR Am J Roentgenol* 1990;154:631–632.
53. Slone RM, Heare MM, Vander Griend RA, Montgomery WJ. Orthopedic fixation devices. *Radiographics* 1991;11:823–847.
54. Stewart MC, Little RE, Highland TR. Osteomyelitis of the ilium secondary to external pelvic fixation. *J Trauma* 1986;26:284–286.
55. Thompson JD, Talbert CJ, Jackson JP. Late breakage of orthopaedic staple causing peroneal nerve injury. *Am J Sports Med* 1990;18:109–111.
56. Whitelaw GP, Wetzler M, Nelson A, Segal D, Fletcher J, Hadley N, Sawka M. Ender rods versus external fixation in the treatment of open tibial fractures. *Clin Orthop* 1990;253:258–269.

Imaging Atlas of Orthopedic Appliances and Prostheses,
edited by T.H. Berquist.
Mayo Clinic Foundation © 1995.
Published by Raven Press, Ltd., New York.

CHAPTER 3

The Spine

Thomas H. Berquist, Bradford L. Currier, and Daniel F. Broderick

Spinal instrumentation techniques have expanded, but the search for a "perfect" fixation system continues. A system that achieves optimal safety and reliability with low complication rates has not yet been designed. Also, it must be remembered that, except for neoplasms or conditions with short life expectancies, the best fixation system will eventually fail if careful bony fusion is not performed at the time of instrumentation.

Imaging plays a significant role in the pre- and postoperative evaluation of patients requiring orthopedic intervention for spinal disorders. The postoperative imaging to follow the results of the procedure and exclude its direct or indirect complications is particularly difficult.

This section reviews the instrumentation and imaging for common disorders such as scoliosis, spondylolisthesis, and trauma. Neoplasms are discussed in Chapter 14.

SCOLIOSIS

Scoliosis may be idiopathic, congenital, or acquired from any number of neurologic or musculoskeletal abnormalities (Table 3-1).[10,11,28–30,40,51]

Idiopathic scoliosis is classically divided into infantile (≤3 years of age), juvenile (3 years to puberty), and adolescent (puberty and older) categories.[11,29,30,57] Adult scoliosis occurs after skeletal maturity.[24,33]

Infantile scoliosis is more common in male than in female children. A left thoracic curve is most common. Curves less than 30° usually resolve (resolving infantile idiopathic scoliosis). Patients with progressive curves (progressive infantile idiopathic scoliosis) usually have a curve > 70° by age 10 years.[46] With significant curves, cardiorespiratory compromise is not unusual.[33]

Juvenile idiopathic scoliosis is more common in female patients. A right thoracic curve is more common than the left thoracic curve described in infantile scoliosis.[24,34,46] Progression is more common in juvenile scoliosis.[34]

Adolescent idiopathic scoliosis that requires treatment is more common in female patients. A right thoracic curve occurs most frequently.[33,46] Scoliosis is frequently detected during school screening examinations (15% of cases). Curves tend to progress during growth spurts (12 to 14 years).[46,48] A positive family history is common in adolescent idiopathic scoliosis. The family history is positive in 15% to 20% of cases, and if both parents had idiopathic scoliosis, the likelihood that treatment will be necessary is 50-fold that of the normal population. Curves less than 30° at maturity tend not to progress, regardless of the pattern.[42]

Adult scoliosis occurs after skeletal maturity, although some authors include all patients with deformity beyond age 20 years. Adult scoliosis may be detected in young adults or occur in older patients secondary to osteopenia or prior multilevel decompressions for spinal stenosis.[10,30] Except for thoracic curves, many authors did not treat adult scoliosis operatively in the past. More recently, curve progression and pain have been confirmed, resulting in renewed interest in instrumentation.[30]

Congenital scoliosis is commonly caused by vertebral anomalies (Table 3-1). Unilateral segmental bars tend to progress the most rapidly.[33] Multiple hemivertebrae also present a significant problem for the orthopedic surgeon, and the prognosis is less favorable.[42]

Other organ anomalies are not unusual in association with such vertebral changes. In 20% to 25% of patients, associated genitourinary anomalies are found. These are

T. H. Berquist: Mayo Medical School and Department of Diagnostic Radiology, Mayo Clinic Jacksonville, Jacksonville, Florida 32224.

B. L. Currier: Mayo Medical School and Department of Orthopedic Surgery, Mayo Clinic, Rochester, Minnesota 55903.

Daniel F. Broderick: Department of Diagnostic Radiology, Mayo Clinic Jacksonville, Jacksonville, Florida 32224.

TABLE 3-1. *Scoliosis*[20,33,34]

Idiopathic
Infantile
Juvenile
Adolescent
Congenital
Hemivertebrae
Wedge vertebra
Unilateral bar
Bilateral bar (block)
Neuroskeletal development disorders
Myelodysplasia
Diastematomyelia
Meningocele
Extraskeletal developmental disorders
Rib fusion
Myositis ossificans progressiva
Neuromuscular
Syringomyelia
Myopathies
Skeletal dysplasia
Trauma
Metabolic bone diseases
Neoplasms

most often insignificant and include crossed renal ectopia and ureteral duplications.[42] Obstructive uropathy, such as ureteropelvic junction obstruction (5%), may require surgical intervention.[33,42] Lumbar curves are more commonly associated with genitourinary and lower-extremity anomalies and thoracic curves, with cardiac anomalies.[33]

Other common causes of scoliosis are summarized in Table 3-1.[24,33,42]

Imaging

The imaging of patients with scoliosis provides valuable information regarding the extent of deformity, flexibility of the curves, and cause.[5,32,33] Routine radiographs provide essential data for curve classification, measurement, and therapeutic planning.[29] The number of views obtained and positioning (standing, sitting, supine, or bending) vary, depending on the patient's age, clinical status, etiology of the curve, and other factors.[23,34]

Posteroanterior (PA) View

The PA view (Fig. 3-1) should be taken standing with shoes off and include the entire spine or at least T-1 to the iliac crest. The 35 × 120-cm cassettes are used for adults or adolescents and the 35 × 43-cm cassettes, for children. In patients who are unable to stand, we prefer the sitting position.[21,42]

Lateral bending views are included in patients who will require therapy. These views assist in evaluating the flexibility of the curves.[42]

Nonstructural or flexible curves correct when the patient bends laterally to the convex side of the spinal curve. Structural or rigid curves do not correct with lateral bending.[36,37] In addition, the change in the thoracic curve with lateral bending is also a relatively accurate prediction of the correction that can be obtained surgically.[29]

When combined thoracic and lumbar curves are present, the degree of correction of each with lateral bending is important. If lumbar curve correction is equal to or greater than thoracic curve correction with lateral bending, the thoracic curve is fused selectively. When the correction of the lumbar curve is less than the thoracic, both are fused.[29]

Lateral Views

The standing lateral view should include the sacrum (Fig. 3-1).[29] It is important for demonstrating sagittal plane alignment. The appearance of the lumbar lordotic curve and thoracic curve can be assessed. Flexion and extension views can be useful in certain situations, but they are not routinely obtained.[24]

Oblique Views

Oblique views are useful in the postoperative setting or when vertebral anomalies are suspected.[29,42] Cervical, thoracic, and lumbar oblique views are obtained separately using conventional film. We usually only evaluate the involved region.

Special Studies

Additional studies may be required to define spinal abnormalities more clearly. Computed tomography (CT), magnetic resonance imaging (MRI), or myelography may be needed in patients with additional abnormalities, such as diastematomyelia. Associated genitourinary or cardiac anomalies may also need to be evaluated.[5,29,42]

Facet injections and discograms are useful, especially in adults, to confirm symptomatic levels and determine whether surgery is indicated.

Asymmetry in the iliac crest on the standing PA view should raise the question of leg-length discrepancy. Conventional or CT techniques can be used to measure the lower extremities.[5,42]

Measurement Techniques

Measuring the degree of scoliosis and kyphosis and determining the curve patterns are essential in therapeutic planning.[29,36,37,42] The Lippman-Cobb method is most commonly used and has been endorsed by the Scoliosis Research Society.[11,37]

Using the Cobb method (Fig. 3-2), the upper and lower end vertebrae are selected. The vertebrae included in the curve have widened disc spaces on the convex side (Fig. 3-2). The upper vertebra is the most superior segment, the superior end plate of which points maximally to the concavity of the curve. The distal vertebra is the segment in which the inferior end plate points maximally to the concavity of the curve. Lines are drawn along the superior end plate of the upper vertebra and the inferior end plate of the lower vertebra in the curve. In cases in which the end plates are not clearly defined, the lines are drawn along the pedicular margins. With larger curves, the point where the two lines cross forms the angle (Fig. 3-2). With smaller curves, perpendicular lines are drawn to the vertebral lines and the angle formed by these lines is used.[29,42]

Applegren and Willner[3] added an additional measurement to the Cobb method in patients with S-shaped curves. A horizontal line was drawn adjacent to the vertebral lines used to calculate the Cobb angles. The angles formed (Fig. 3-3) were compared. The angles may be equal (symmetric) or unequal (asymmetric). When the lower angle is greater than the upper angle in the curve (Fig. 3-3), brace treatment is not likely to succeed.

The Ferguson technique for the measurement of scoliosis is more difficult to use, especially for larger curves (> 50°).[17,36,37] Using this method, a central point is selected in the apical vertebra by using crossing lines from the vertebral corners (Fig. 3-4). The superior and inferior vertebrae in the curve are marked in the same fashion. Lines drawn through these points determine the angle of the curve. Selecting the proper vertebrae may also be difficult.

The degree of rotation is also important to determine in addition to the spinal curve. This is important for selecting the type and extent of fusion.[34] The degree of vertebral rotation is determined using the spinous process and/or pedicle position on the anteroposterior (AP) radiograph.[30,42] With either method, the degree of rotation is graded 1 to 4+ using the apex vertebra in the curve, which is generally the vertebra that is maximally rotated.

TABLE 3-2. *Scoliosis curve patterns*[34]

Single curves
High thoracic
Thoracic
Thoracolumbar
Lumbar
Double curves
Major thoracic and lumbar
Double major thoracic
Double major thoracic and thoracolumbar
Multiple patterns

TABLE 3-3. *Scoliosis groups based on curve severity*[24]

Group	Angle
I	<20°
II	20–30°
III	31–50°
IV	51–75°
V	76–100°
VI	101–126°
VII	>126°

Figures 3-5 and 3-6 demonstrate these methods. The pedicle method is more accurate.[30,36–38,42]

Vertebral wedging is evaluated by using changes in vertebral height. The vertebral body is divided into six equal segments (Fig. 3-7A). Compression or wedging is graded from 1+ to 4+ (Fig. 3-7B–E) with 1+ equaling a reduction in height of one sixth. When wedging exceeds 4+, the vertebra is greater than 50% wedged.[37]

Vertebral symmetry and the torsobalance line can also be assessed on the standing or sitting AP radiograph (Fig. 3-8). Asymmetry or lateral loss of height is common in scoliosis. The torsobalance line is drawn vertically from C-7 and should fall to the gluteal crease or midsacrum. Radiographically, the line is drawn vertically from the midsacrum (Fig. 3-8) and should pass through the center of T-1. The measurement described in Figure 3-8 is used to follow curve changes postoperatively.[37]

The degree of kyphosis is measured on the lateral radiograph. Lines are drawn from the superior end plate of the upper vertebra and inferior end plate of the lower vertebra. Perpendicular lines are constructed in a fashion similar to the AP measurements to determine the kyphotic angle (Fig. 3-9). Flexion and extension lateral views are used to evaluate rigidity and/or instability.[30,37,42]

The curve patterns (Table 3-2) are determined by the apical vertebra and major (structural) and minor (nonstructural) components defined on the standing AP radiograph.[24,30,42] Curves have also been categorized by the severity of the angles (Table 3-3).[30] King[28] and King et al.[29] described five curve patterns in idiopathic thoracic scoliosis. Type I curves (Fig. 3-10) are S shaped, with both thoracic and lumbar curves crossing the midline. The lumbar curve is more severe. The thoracic curve is more flexible on side-bending radiographs. Type II curve patterns (Fig. 3-11) are similar, except the thoracic curve is greater than the lumbar curve. The type III lumbar curve does not cross the midline (Fig. 3-12). The lumbar curve is centered directly over the sacrum. With type IV curves, there is a long thoracic curve with L-5 centered over the sacrum, and L-4 is tilted into the thoracic curve (Fig. 3-13). Type V curves have a double thoracic pattern (Fig. 3-14). The first thoracic vertebra is tilted into the concavity of the upper curve. The upper curve is a struc-

(text continues on page 116)

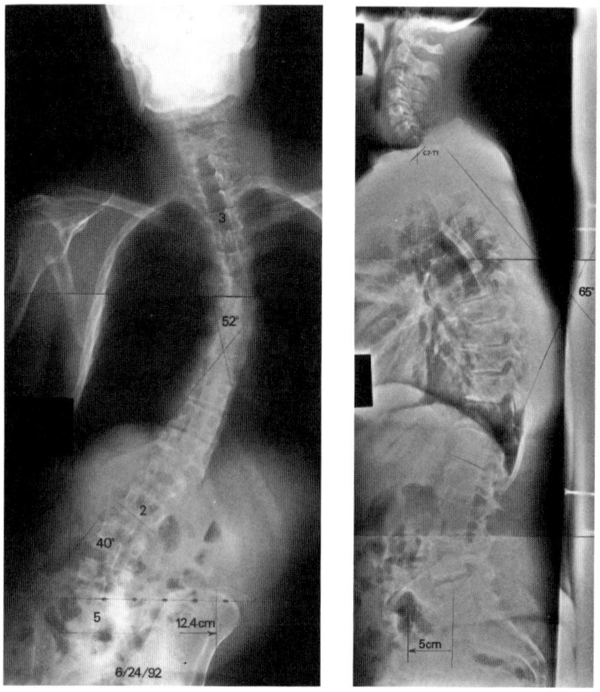

A B

FIG. 3-1. Preoperative PA **(A)** and lateral **(B)** views of the spine with the angles indicated.

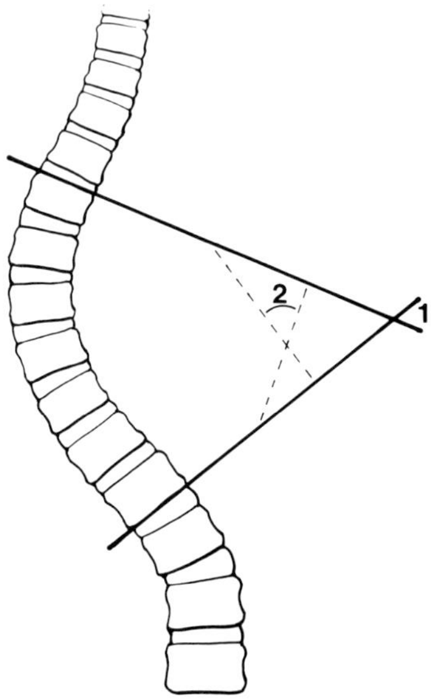

FIG. 3-2. The Lippman-Cobb method for measuring spinal curves. Lines are drawn along the superior body or pedicles of the upper vertebra and along the inferior margin of the lower participating vertebra. The angle formed by these lines in spines with larger curves (*1*) or lines perpendicular to the end vertebra (*2*) define the curves.

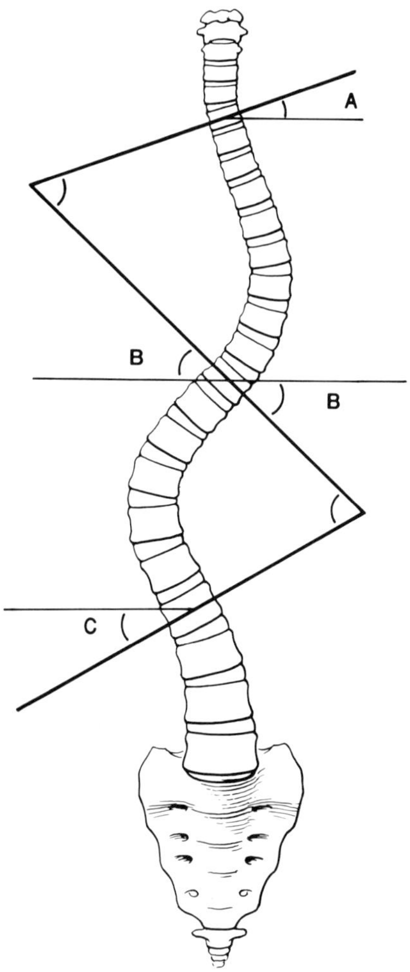

A

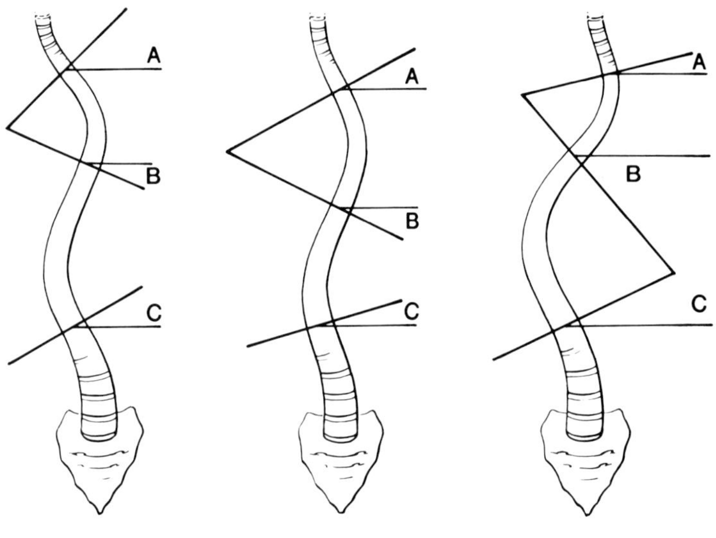

B

FIG. 3-3. A: The Cobb method and end vertebral angle (*EVA*) determination. Angles A and B are compared. When angle B is greater than angle A, brace treatment is not as successful as in symmetric curves or when angle A is greater than angle B. **B:** *Left,* angle A (*upper*) greater than B; *middle,* angle A = B; *right,* angle B > A.[3]

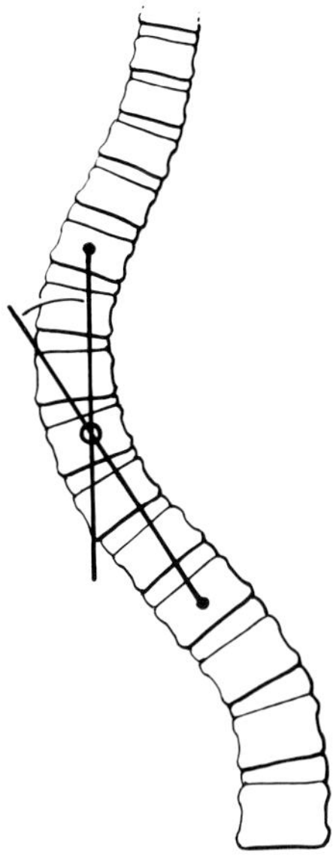

FIG. 3-4. The Ferguson method for measuring spinal curves.

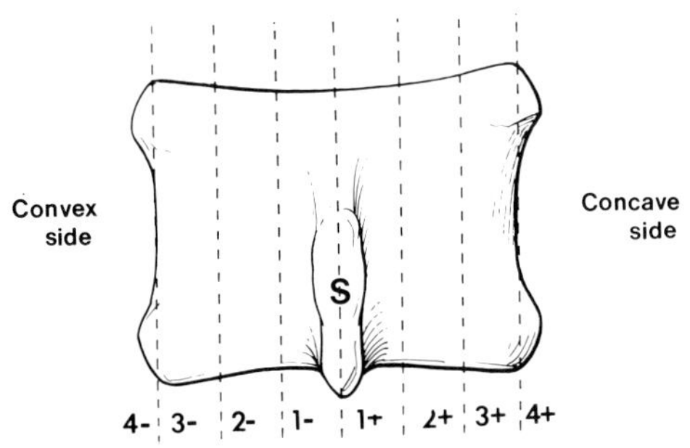

FIG. 3-5. The spinous process technique for measuring vertebral rotation. The vertebral body is divided into six segments (*vertical broken line*). Neutral is used for spinous process (*s*) at the midline and equidistant from lateral vertebral margins. Positive is used for rotation toward the concavity, and negative is used for rotation toward the convexity of the curve.[37]

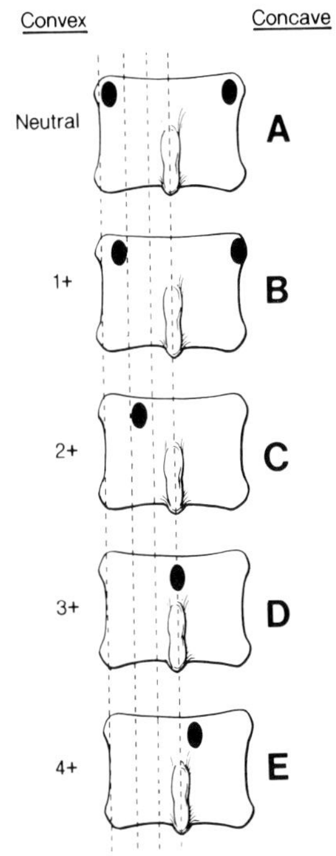

FIG. 3-6. The pedicle technique for grading rotation.[37] **A:** Neutral. **B:** Convex, i.e., moves toward the midline in the first segment and concave, i.e., off the lateral margin. **C:** Convex, moves into segment 2; concave, not readily visible. **D:** Right pedicle moves to midline and left pedicle, not seen. **E:** Right pedicle migrates beyond midline and left pedicle, not seen.

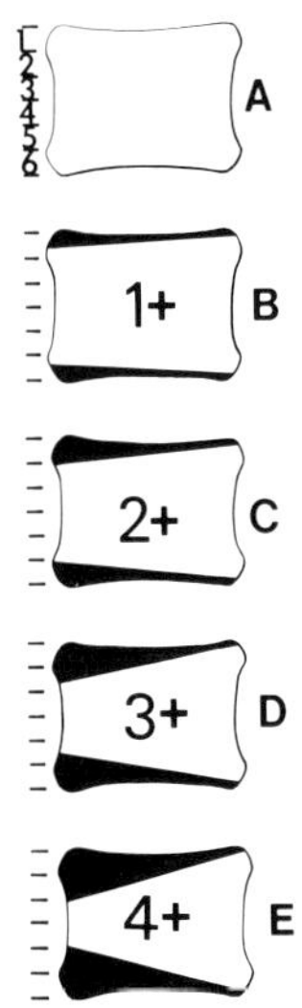

FIG. 3-7. Assessment for vertebral compression. The vertebral body is divided into sixths **(A):** A loss of height can be categorized as 1+ ($\frac{1}{6}$) **(B)** or greater. Lateral wedging of 4+ **(E)** is greater than a one-half reduction in lateral vertebral height.[36,37]

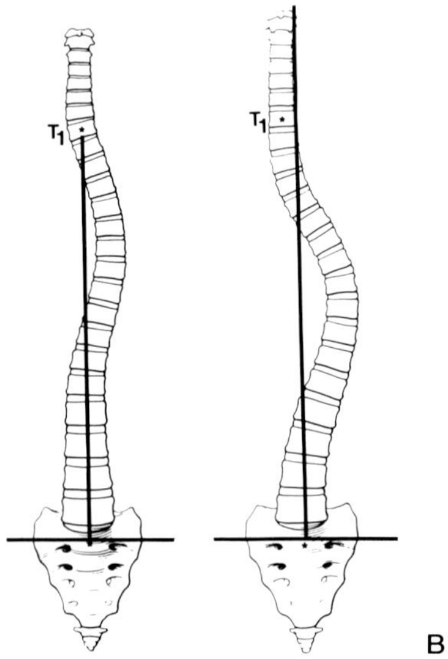

FIG. 3-8. The torso balance line. **A:** The line extending vertically from the midsacrum should pass through the center of T-1. Grade I torso balance passes ≤ 1.5 cm from the midline of T-1; grade II, 1.6 to 3 cm **(B)**; grade III, 3.1 to 5 cm; and grade IV, > 5 cm from the midline of T-1.[37]

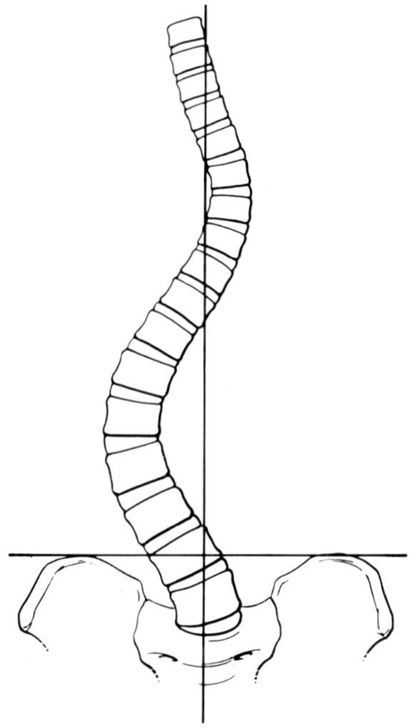

FIG. 3-10. King type I curve pattern. The curve is S shaped, with both thoracic and lumbar curves crossing the midline. The lumbar curve is larger.

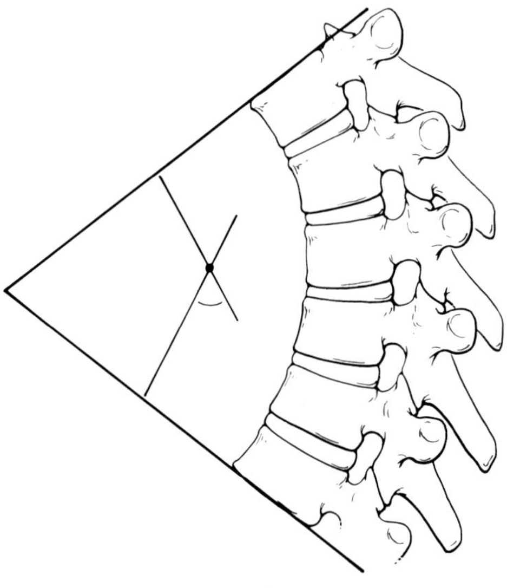

FIG. 3-9. Kyphotic measurement.

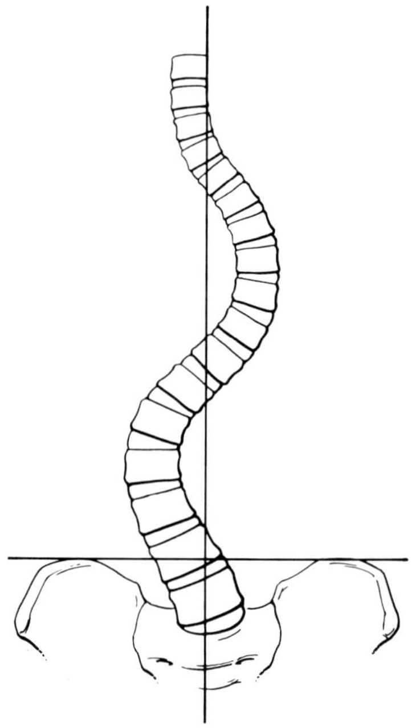

FIG. 3-11. King type II curve pattern. The S-shaped curve has a more severe thoracic component.

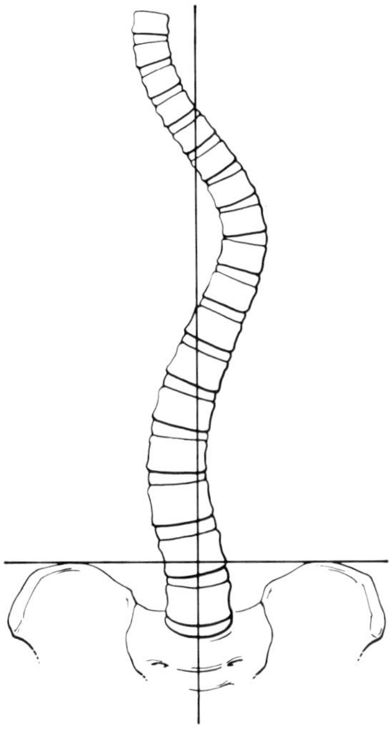

FIG. 3-12. King type III curve pattern. The lumbar curve does not cross the midline and is centered over the sacrum.

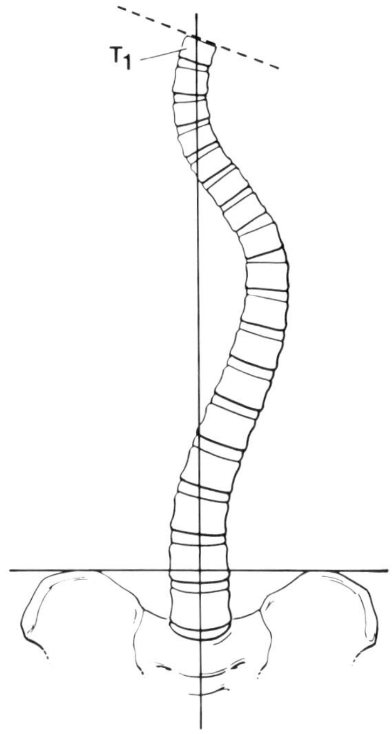

FIG. 3-13. King type IV curve pattern. There is a long thoracic curve with L-5 centered over the sacrum and L-4 tilted to the thoracic curve.

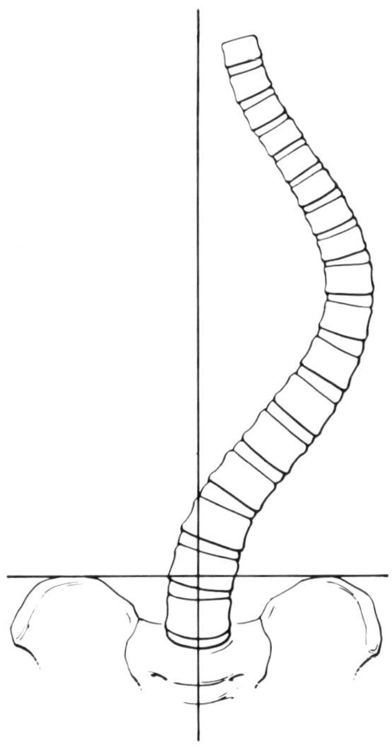

FIG. 3-14. King type V curve pattern. Double-thoracic curve with T-1 tilted into the concavity of the upper curve. The upper curve is a structural curve.

tural curve on side-bending radiographs.[28,29] Using these curve patterns and evaluating vertebral rotation assists in selecting the extent of fusion.[28,29,37]

Instrumentation for Scoliosis

Surgical instrumentation continues to evolve.[1,2,4,43,45,47] The cause, curve configuration and flexibility, and patient status are considered in selecting the most appropriate method of instrumentation.

Harrington instrumentation was introduced in the 1960s and provided adequate results in treatment of idiopathic adolescent scoliosis. Postsurgical recumbency with cast immobilization is required, and less success with other forms of scoliosis led to the development of additional techniques.[2,3,11,20,27]

The Dwyer system of anterior instrumentation evolved in the late 1960s to early 1970s. An anterolateral approach was used, with removal of the discs and interbody fusion. This system was useful in scoliosis but frequently caused an unacceptable loss of lumbar lordosis.[2,7,21]

Others modified the Dwyer system by substituting a compression rod with nuts for the cable used in Dwyer instrumentation (Zielke system).[20] The Dwyer system uses a tension cable on the convex side of the curve. Derotation was achieved more effectively with the Zielke system.[6,20,41]

The Luque system came into use in the 1970s; it consisted of smooth rods with sublaminar wires. This system, although not perfect in every setting, did eliminate the need for postoperative immobilization.[2,38,48]

Cotrel-Dubousset instrumentation for idiopathic scoliosis has been used since 1984.[8] This system achieves rigid fixation by applying bilateral distraction and compression forces. Lumbar lordosis and improvement in thoracic kyphosis are permitted.[8,12,13,24,56]

For purposes of illustration, we review the instrumentation systems as anterior, posterior, or combined.

Anterior Instrumentation

Dwyer Instrumentation (Figs. 3-15 and 3-16)[7,9,22,30]

Indications
- Lumbar and thoracic idiopathic scoliosis
- Neurogenic scoliosis (posterior deficiency)
- Lordotic spinal deformities

Instrumentation
- Flexible titanium cable (Fig. 3-15A) in 30- to 45-cm lengths. Stop on one end with "shoestring tip" for advancing the cable through the collar.
- Screws (Fig. 3-15B). Cancellous screws with cannulated holes for cable transfer.
- Staples (Fig. 3-15C) in 10- to 36-mm widths. Provides additional support and assists in maintaining proper screw position.

Advantages
- Excellent correction of primary curve and limited length of instrumentation

Disadvantages
- Cable breakage
- Kyphotic effect
- Uncertain spontaneous correction of secondary curves[6,8,22,30,51]

Zielke Instrumentation (Figs. 3-17 and 3-18)[25,26,41,46,51]

Zielke modified the Dwyer system by replacing the flexible cable with a solid stainless steel rod passed through slotted screws.[25,51] The device is placed on the convex side of the curve and is most often used for degenerative lumbar scoliosis.

Indications
- Idiopathic and degenerative lumbar and thoracic scoliosis

Instrumentation
- Similar to Dwyer, except for the rod and nuts[25]

Advantages[25]
- Improved derotation capability
- Avoid excessive kyphosis
- Shorter segment instrumentation

Disadvantages
- Technically difficult
- Solid fusion more difficult to obtain if used alone with severe scoliosis[41,46,51]

Texas Scottish Rite Hospital (TSRH) Instrumentation

This is a further modification of the Zielke and Dwyer systems. Screws are inserted into the vertebral body and connected by a single rod. Zielke staples and washers are also generally used.[51] This system is used for shorter-segment fusion than are Harrington rods and other posterior devices (Fig. 3-19).

Posterior Instrumentation

Harrington Instrumentation[11,15,23,51,54,56]

The Harrington system has components for distraction, compression, and sacral purchase. The components are constructed with stainless steel.[22]

Indications
- Thoracic and lumbar scoliosis
- Trauma[56]

(text continues on page 120)

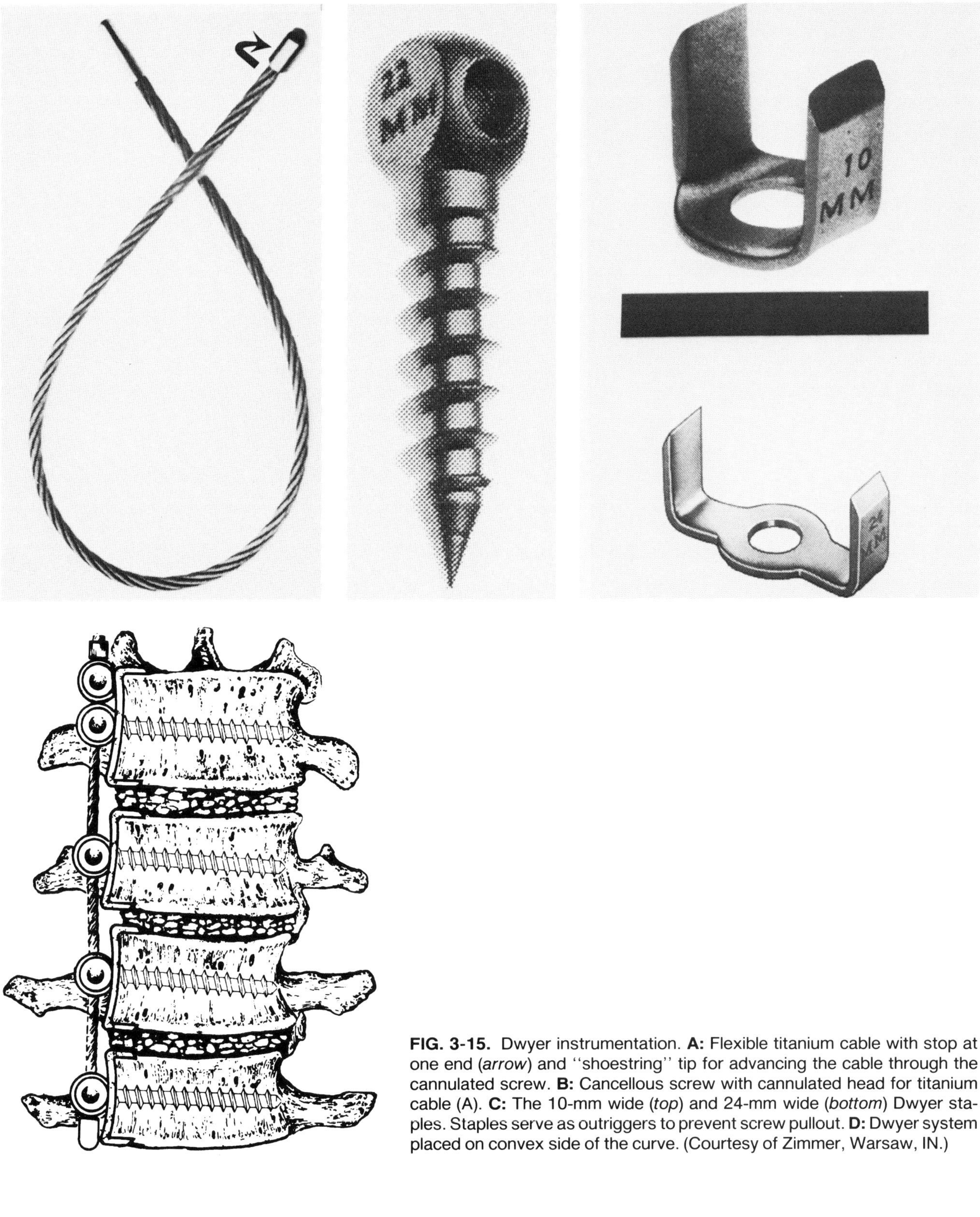

A B,C D

FIG. 3-15. Dwyer instrumentation. **A:** Flexible titanium cable with stop at one end (*arrow*) and "shoestring" tip for advancing the cable through the cannulated screw. **B:** Cancellous screw with cannulated head for titanium cable (A). **C:** The 10-mm wide (*top*) and 24-mm wide (*bottom*) Dwyer staples. Staples serve as outriggers to prevent screw pullout. **D:** Dwyer system placed on convex side of the curve. (Courtesy of Zimmer, Warsaw, IN.)

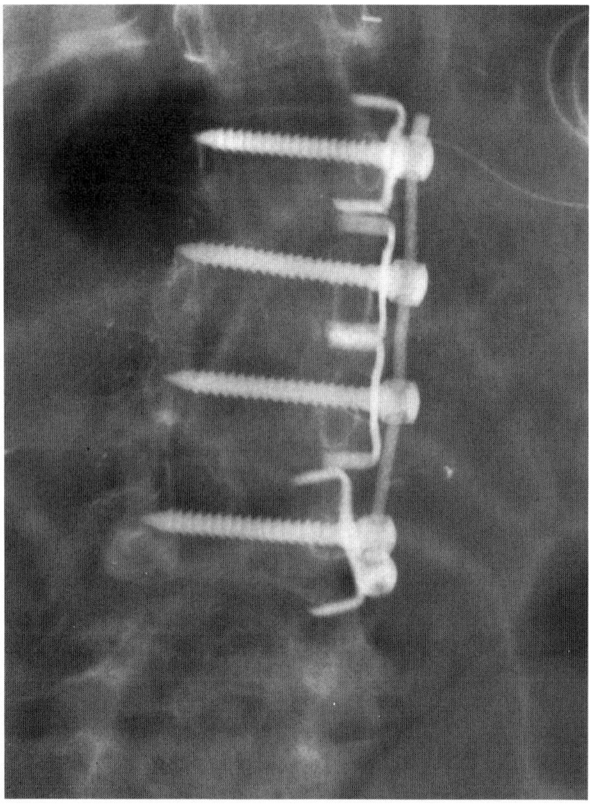

FIG. 3-16. An AP view of the spine with Dwyer instrumentation.

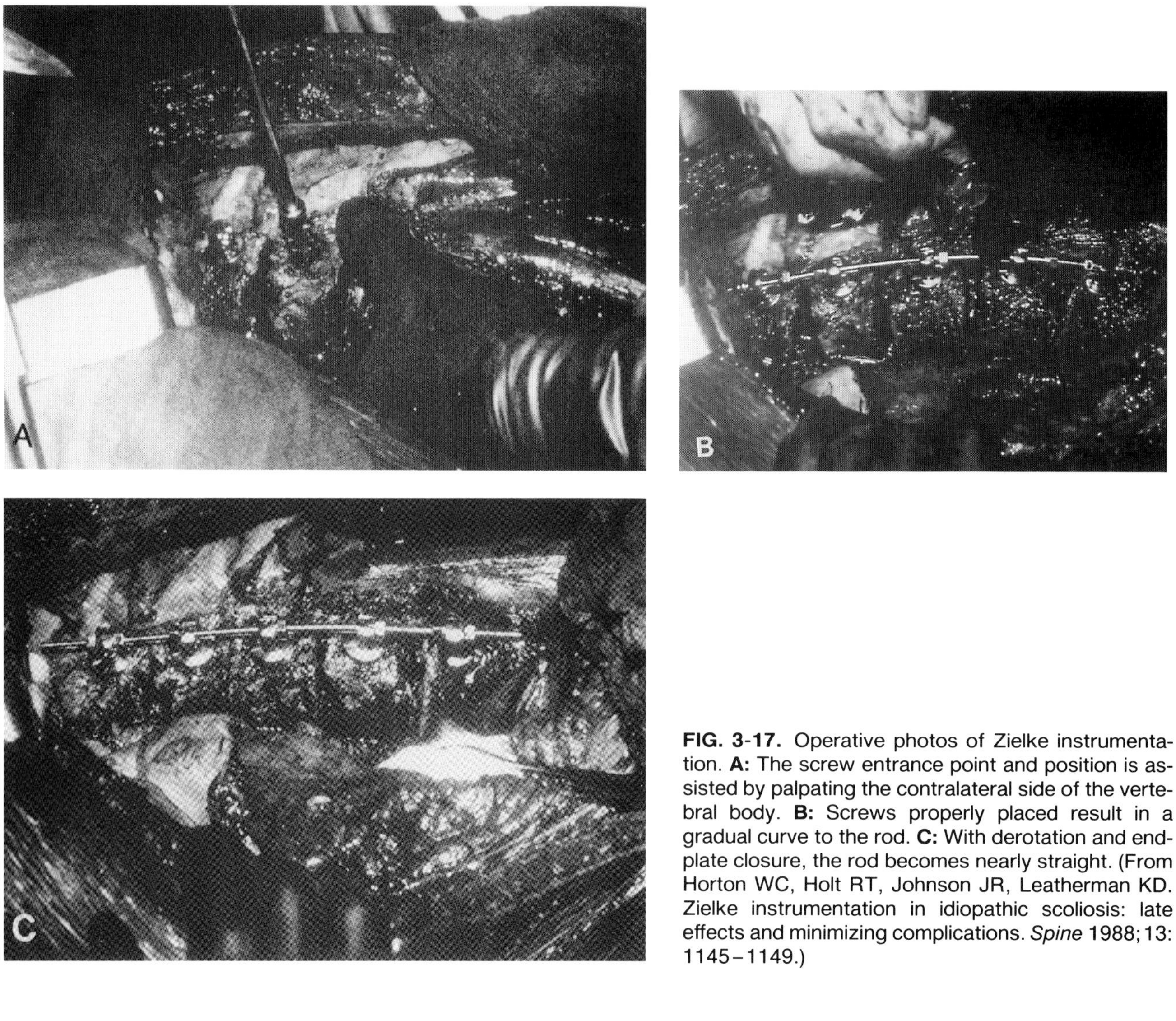

FIG. 3-17. Operative photos of Zielke instrumentation. **A:** The screw entrance point and position is assisted by palpating the contralateral side of the vertebral body. **B:** Screws properly placed result in a gradual curve to the rod. **C:** With derotation and endplate closure, the rod becomes nearly straight. (From Horton WC, Holt RT, Johnson JR, Leatherman KD. Zielke instrumentation in idiopathic scoliosis: late effects and minimizing complications. *Spine* 1988;13: 1145–1149.)

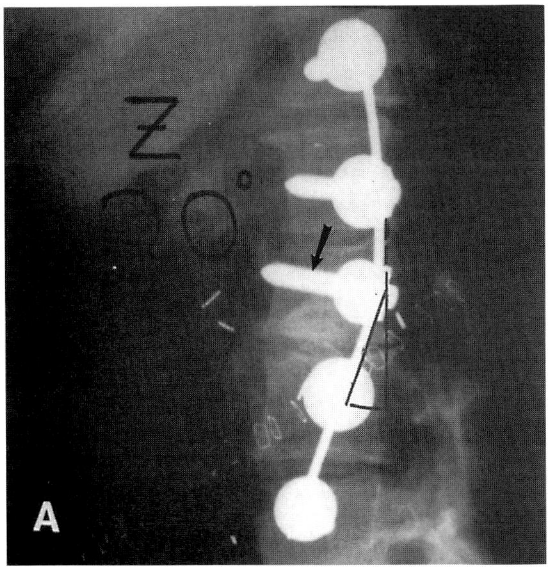

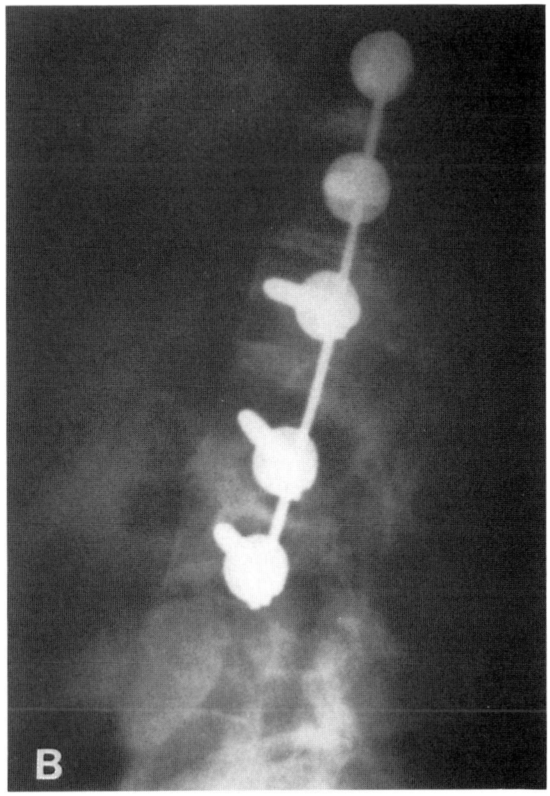

FIG. 3-18. A: Poor screw placement, producing rod angulation. Note the entrance points and direction of the screws. The middle screw (*arrow*) enters more posteriorly and is directed anteriorly. The screw just below it enters more anteriorly and is directed posteriorly. **B:** Better screw placement with no angulation of the rod or abrupt alignment changes in the screws. Any acute angle in the rod (Z angle) may act as a stress riser. Z angles greater than 15° lead to increased instrument failure. (From Horton WC, Holt RT, Johnson JR, Leatherman KD. Zielke instrumentation in idiopathic scoliosis: late effects and minimizing complications. *Spine* 1988; 13:1145–1149.)

A 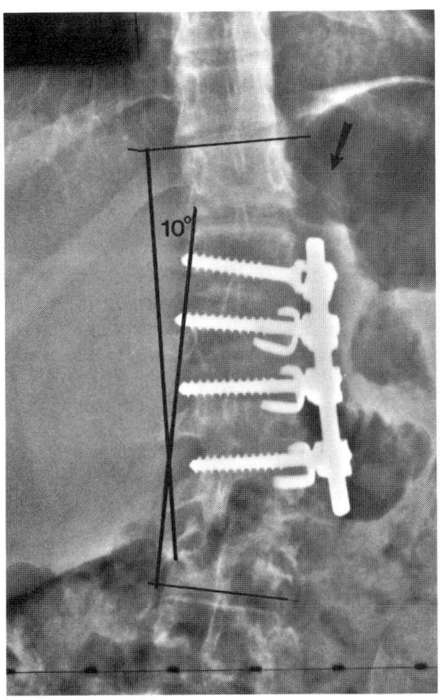

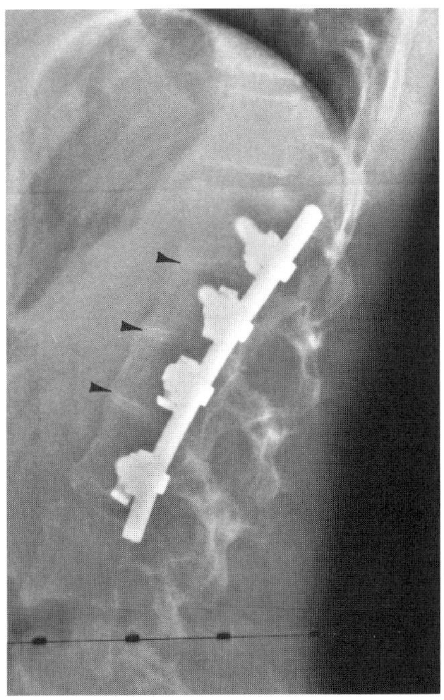 B

FIG. 3-19. The AP **(A)** and lateral **(B)** radiographs following anterior TSRH instrumentation of lumbar scoliosis (six lumbar vertebrae). There are four 6.5-mm cortical TSRH screws in L-1 to L-4, with Zielke staples at L-2 to L-4. A single 0.25-inch stainless steel rod is inserted. The left 12th rib was resected (*arrow*) and used for interbody graft following disc removal (*small arrows*, B) at the L-1 to L-3 interspaces. Postoperatively, the lumbar curve was 10°. Note the pedicles were used for measuring the superior vertebra because of the indistinct end plate on the radiograph (A).

Instrumentation
Rods (Fig. 3-20)
Distraction rods are smooth with collar on one end and notches on the opposite end to allow incremental distraction. The rods are available in 6- to 53.5-cm lengths (Fig. 3-20A).
Shorter collar-end rods are also available (Fig. 3-20B) to prevent rod impingement on bone below inferior hook. Holes below the collar allow wires to be passed around rod and hook to prevent rod rotation and hook displacement. This modification is available in 6- to 40-cm lengths.
Compression rods. Threaded rods are also available in large and smaller diameters (Fig. 3-20C), with hex nuts used for hook positioning and compression.
Hooks (Fig. 3-21)
Hooks are designed differently for purchase, compression, and traction. The hooks are designed in numerous configurations (Fig. 3-21) to be used for the ratchet end, collar end, and threaded Harrington rods. The size of the shoe-and-hook configuration varies with the purpose (i.e., distraction or compression) and the individual patient's laminar anatomy. Figure 3-22 illustrates Harrington-rod fixation in a patient with scoliosis.

Moe System[56]

This system is similar to Harrington instrumentation. However, the rod is square distal to the collar, and the hook holes are square to reduce rotation (Fig. 3-23).

Wisconsin System (Fig. 3-24)[12,27,56,58]

This system is a modification of the Harrington Compression system. Standard Harrington rods are used with Keene™ hooks and bushings. The Keene™ hook has an open back to allow the rod to be pressed into the body of the hook (Fig. 3-24B).

Asher et al.[5] added a modular spinal rod linkage system in conjunction with sublaminar wires to improve torsional stability (Fig. 3-25).

Luque Instrumentation (Figs. 3-26 and 3-27)[1,39,51,56,57]

Unlike the hook-rod systems, the Luque system applies corrective forces at all levels by using two stainless steel rods and sublaminar wires (Fig. 3-26), referred to as segmental spinal instrumentation (SSI).

Indications
Scoliosis
Congenital deformities
Fractures

Instrumentation
Rods are smooth and 4.8 or 6.4 mm in diameter, which can be obtained as straight or L shaped. Rectangular configurations are also available. The rectangular devices are used primarily for short-segment fracture fixation.
Advantages
Corrective forces applied at each vertebral level (Fig. 3-27)
Adaptable to procedure
Eliminates postoperative recumbency and immobilization
Disadvantages
Sublaminar wires may cause neurologic damage. Use of closed-loop wires and H bars with Luque rods or Harrington rods was introduced by Mehdian and Eisenstein[39] to reduce neurologic injury, operating time, and improve pelvic fixation (Fig. 3-28).

Wisconsin Segmental System (Interspinous Segmental Spinal Instrumentation)[16,51,53,56]

This system is a modification of the Luque SSI system. The major difference is the use of segmental spinous process wires with paired buttons to protect the spinous process (Fig. 3-29). This avoids the use of sublaminar wires, avoiding the spinal canal. The spinous processes are wired to Luque or Harrington rods. Luque rods are used on the convex side and Harrington rods, on the concave side.

Cotrel-Dubousset Instrumentation[8,18,34,48–50,55–57]

This system is designed to provide bilateral segmental fixation with distraction and compression forces to preserve lumbar lordosis and increase thoracic kyphosis.[8,18,34] The system provides fixation in the coronal, axial, and sagittal planes.[8,48–50]

Indications[48–50,56]
Idiopathic spinal deformity in children
Adolescent scoliosis
Adult scoliosis
Fractures
Spondylolisthesis
Instrumentation (Figs. 3-30 and 3-31)[48–50]
Rods (Fig. 3-30A) are stainless steel with diamond knurled surface coating to provide more secure hook fixation.
Hooks (Fig. 3-30B-H) are similar to those described earlier, with some variation. Set screws are used to attach the hooks to the rods. Hooks are designed for pedicle (thoracic), transverse process and laminar attachment. Both open and closed body hooks are available.

(text continues on page 128)

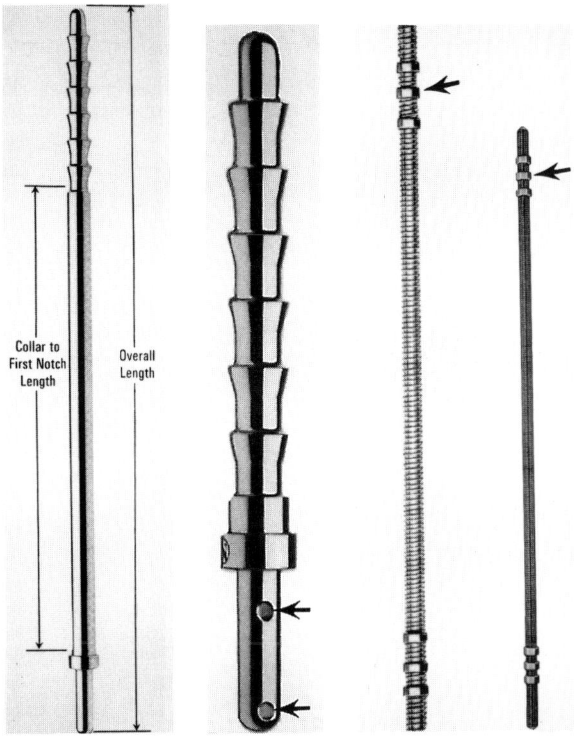

A B,C

FIG. 3-20. A: The Harrington distraction rod with ratchets (*upper end*) to allow incremental distraction, a smooth central portion, and distal collar. **B:** Short collar end rod (compare with Fig. 3-20A) to prevent bone impingement of the inferior hook. There are holes (*arrows*) to allow wire fixation to reduce rotation. **C:** Threaded Harrington compression rods available in large (*left*) and small (*right*) diameters. Hex nuts (*arrows*) are used for hook positioning. (Courtesy of Zimmer, Warsaw, IN.)

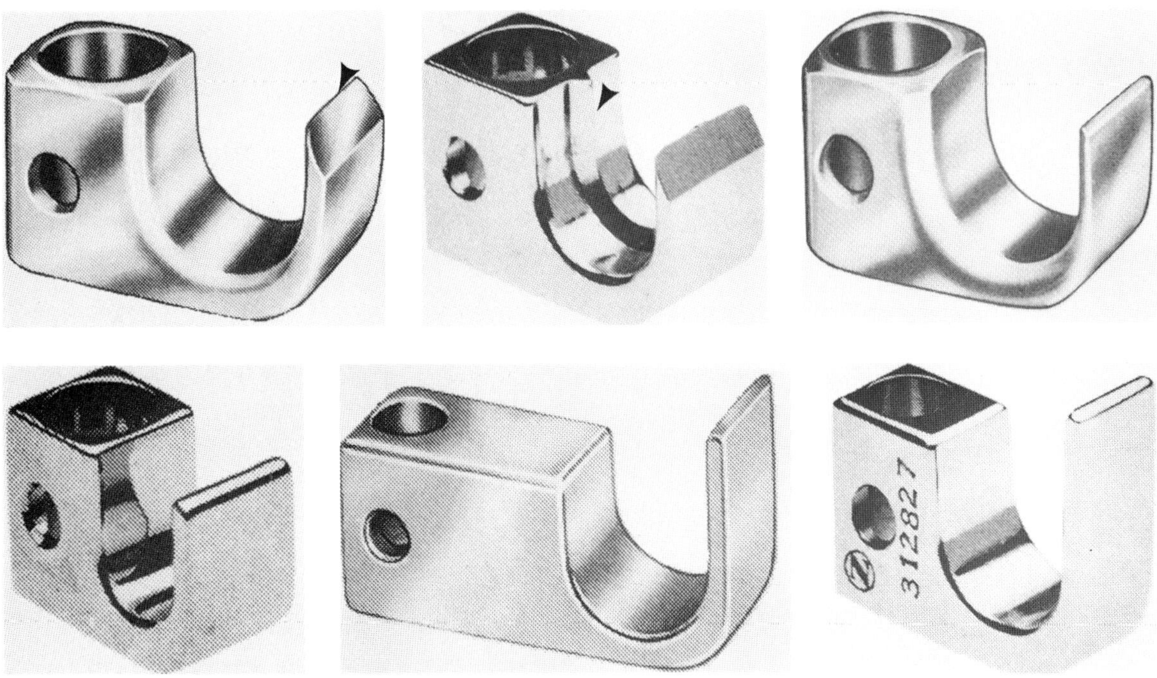

A,B C D,E F

FIG. 3-21. Harrington hooks, selected examples. **A:** Distraction hook with sharp edge (*arrow*) to allow easier engagement. **B:** Distraction hook with central rib (*arrow*) to reduce drift and rotation. **C:** Blunt distraction hook. **D:** Distraction hook with a shorter boot for narrow lamina. **E:** Round collar end hook with an extended shoe and large body. The hook is blunt. **F:** Leatherman hook for patients with increased lumbar lordosis or myelomeningocele with absent posterior elements. (see **G** on next page.)

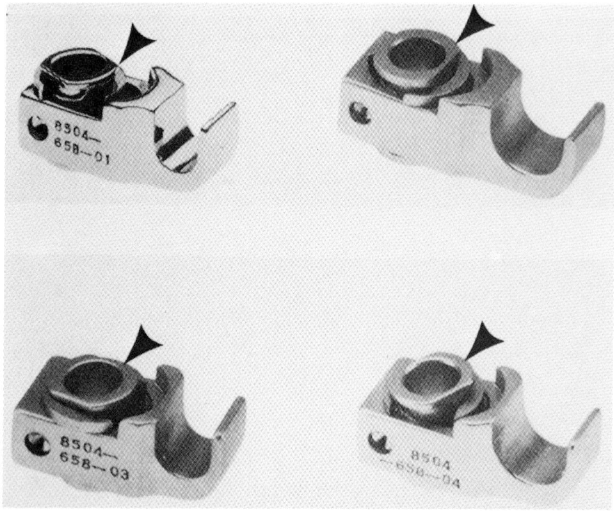

G

FIG. 3-21. *Continued.* **G:** Bobechko hooks with sliding barrels (*arrows*), which allows self-adjustment in the AP plane. Note the different hook sizes. (Courtesy of Zimmer, Warsaw, IN.)

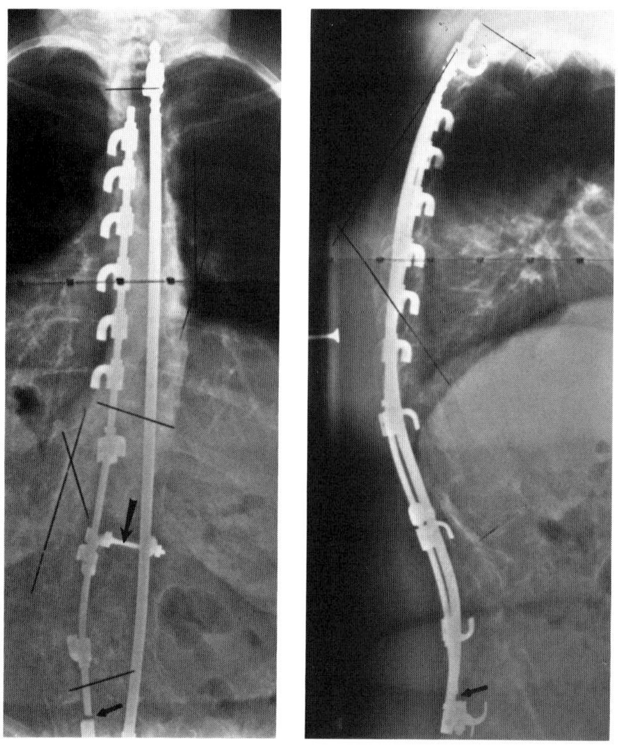

A B

FIG. 3-22. Scoliosis with Harrington instrumentation demonstrated on standing PA **(A)** and lateral **(B)** views. There is a threaded compression rod on the left and a smooth distraction rod on the right. There is a transverse traction assembly (*arrow*) at the thoracolumbar junction. The compression rod is fractured distally (*lower arrows*).

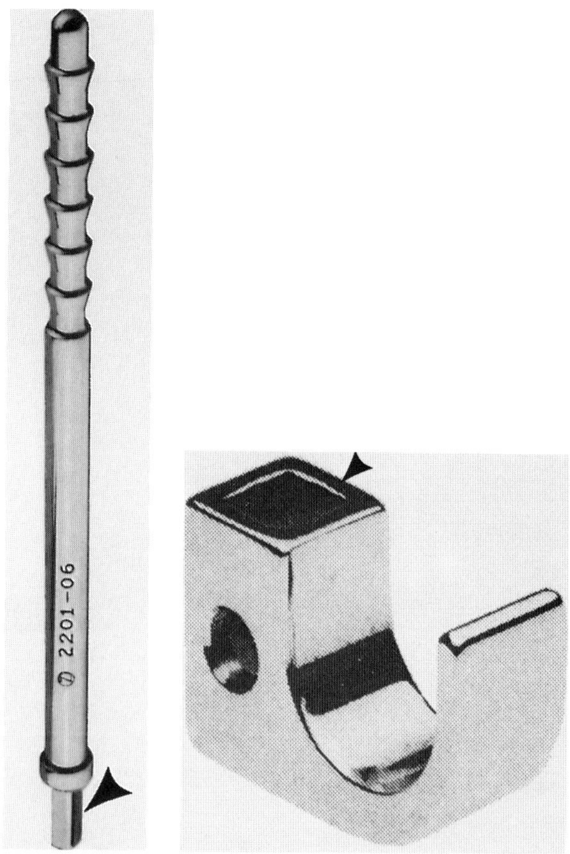

A B

FIG. 3-23. The Moe distraction rod **(A)** with a square end below the collar (*arrow*) and a square entry hole in the hook **(B)**. (Courtesy of Zimmer, Warsaw, IN.)

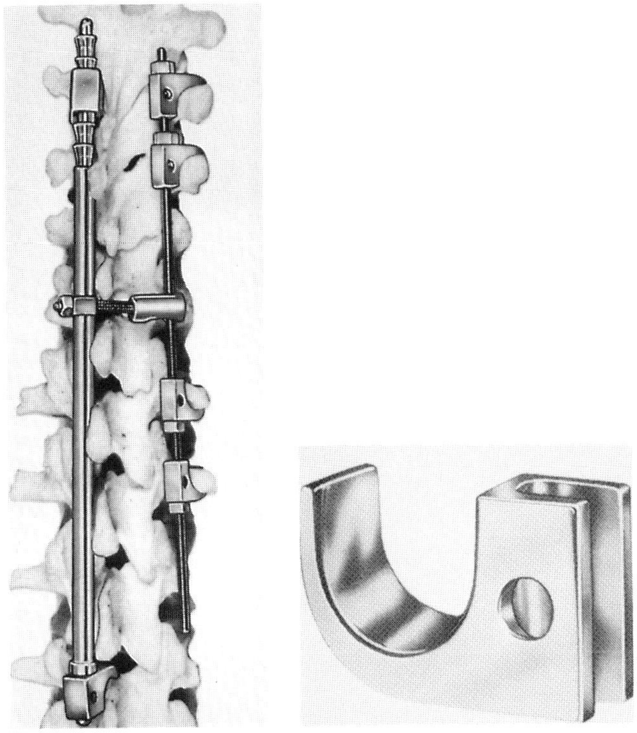

A B

FIG. 3-24. Wisconsin System. (Courtesy of Zimmer, Warsaw, IN.) **A:** Harrington rods with standard hooks and a transverse traction assembly. **B:** Illustration of an open-backed Keene™ hook, which allows the rod to be pressed into the open back of the hook

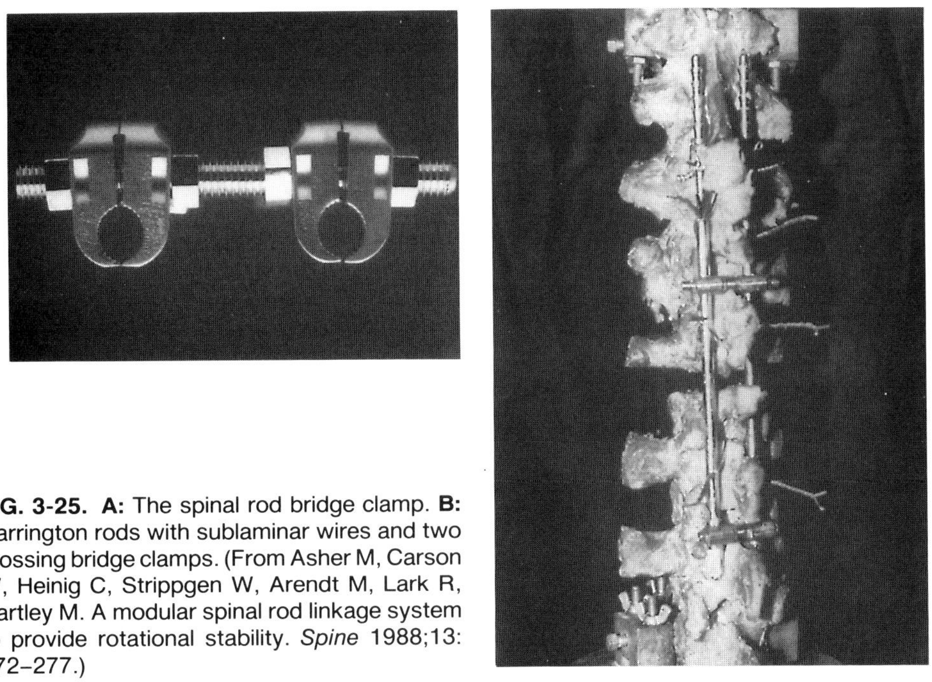

A B

FIG. 3-25. **A:** The spinal rod bridge clamp. **B:** Harrington rods with sublaminar wires and two crossing bridge clamps. (From Asher M, Carson W, Heinig C, Strippgen W, Arendt M, Lark R, Hartley M. A modular spinal rod linkage system to provide rotational stability. *Spine* 1988;13: 272–277.)

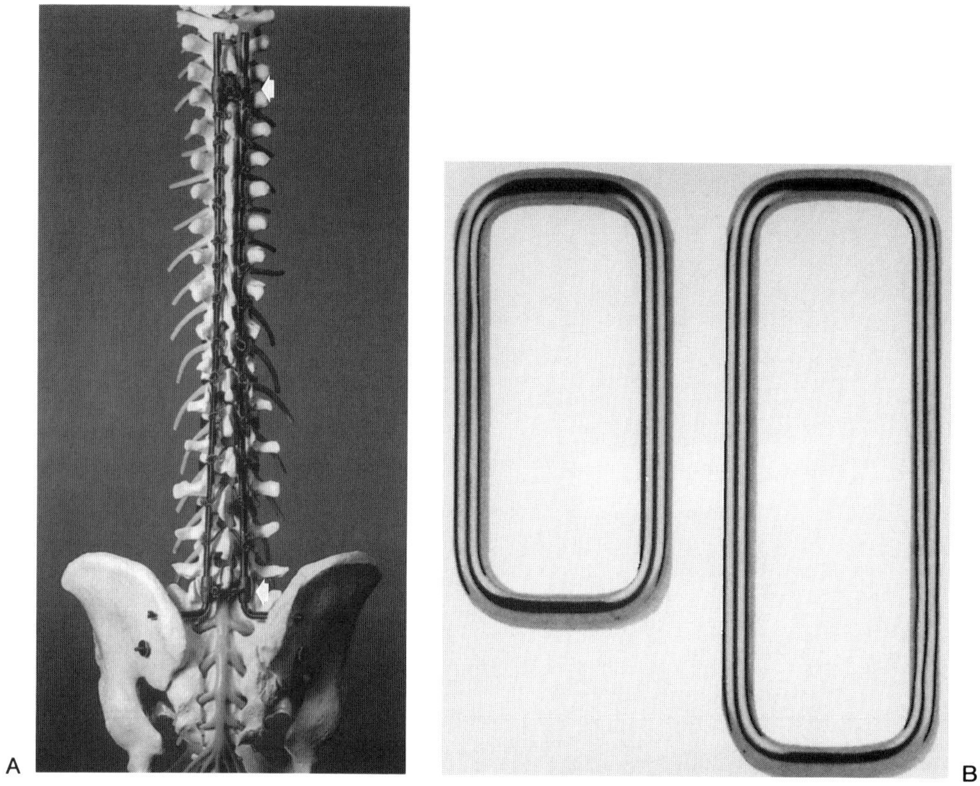

FIG. 3-26. **A:** Luque instrumentation with smooth L-shaped rods, sublaminar wires, and proximal and distal H bars (*arrows*).[38] **B:** Luque rectangles designed for short-segment fixation. (Courtesy of Zimmer, Warsaw, IN.)

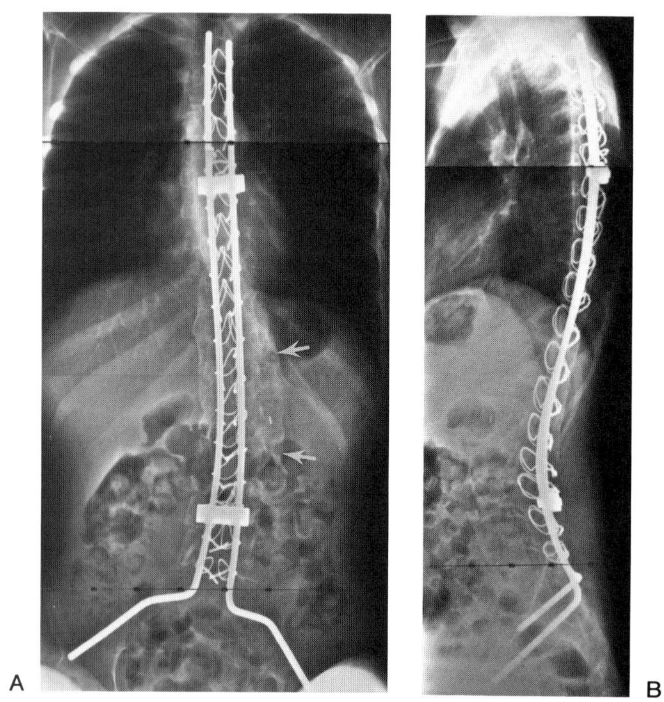

FIG. 3-27. The AP **(A)** and lateral **(B)** standing full-length radiographs with Luque rod and sublaminar wire fixation from T-2 to the sacrum. There are TSRH cross-links proximally at the T-7 level and distally at the L-4 level. The bone graft is also visible (*arrows*).

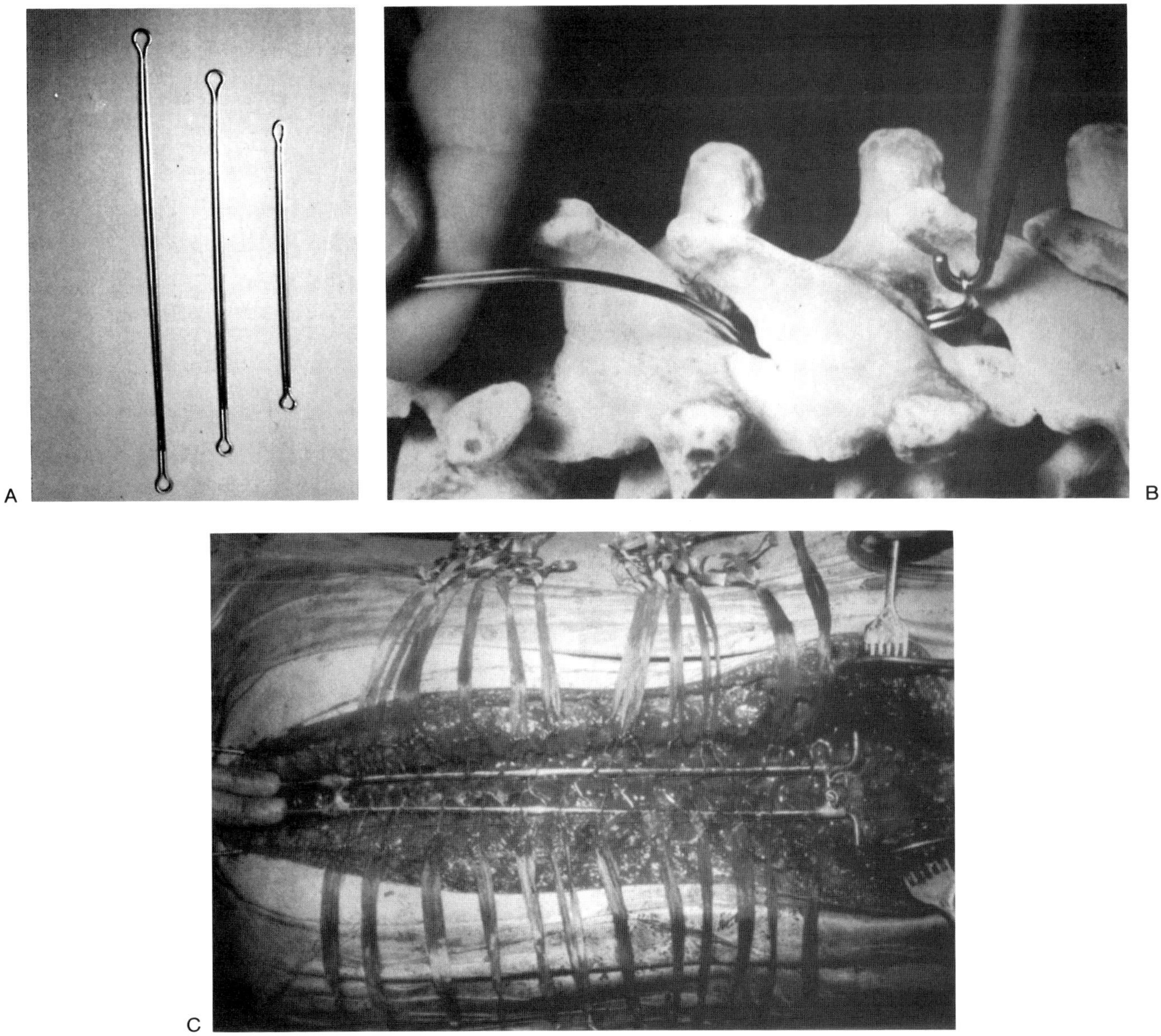

FIG. 3-28. The Mehdian technique uses Luque rods or Harrington rods with closed-loop wires and H bars. **A:** Closed-loop sublaminar wires in 75-, 100-, and 120-mm lengths for the cervical, thoracic, and lumbar spine, respectively. **B:** Sublaminar wire passage with T-handled hook instrument. **C:** Operative photograph after Luque rod sublaminar closed-loop wire and H bar instrumentation. (From Mehdian H. Eisenstein S. Segmental spinal instrumentation using short closed wire loops. *Clin Orthop* 1989; 247:90–96.)

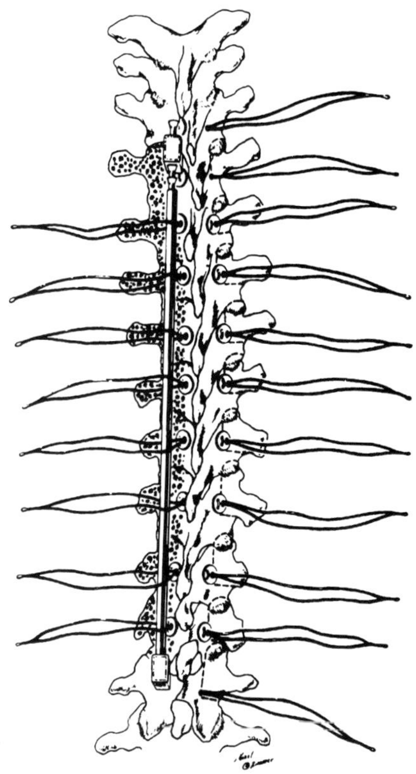

FIG. 3-29. The Wisconsin segmental spinal system (SSI). A paired button-wire implant is passed through the base of the spinous process for fixation to Harrington or Luque rods. This system avoids passage of sublaminar wires. (Courtesy of Zimmer, Warsaw, IN.)

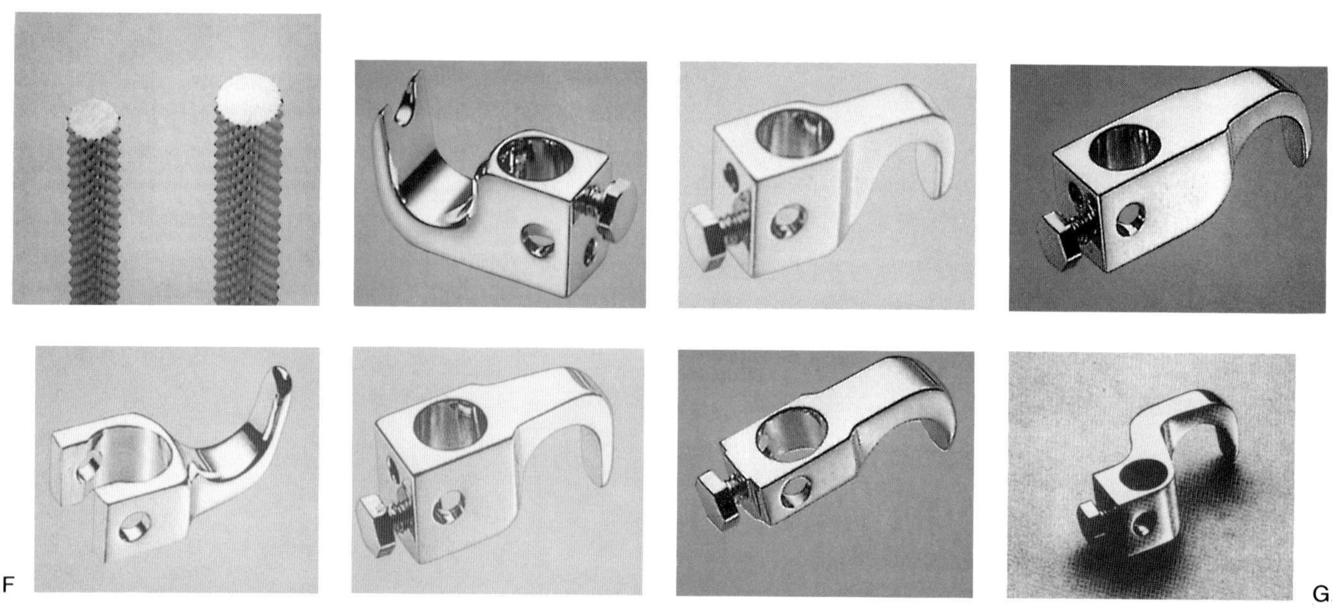

A,B C,D E,F G,H

FIG. 3-30. Cotrel-Dubousset instrumentation (Courtesy of Stuart Specialty, Spine Division, Greensburg, PA.) **A:** Photograph of Cotrel-Dubousset rods with diamond-point surfaces. Rods are available in 5- to 7-mm diameters and lengths from 40 to 600 mm. Various Cotrel-Dubousset hooks are used. **B:** Pedicle hook with closed configuration and set screw. **C:** Thoracic laminar hook with closed configuration. **D:** Supralaminar hook with closed configuration. **E:** Infralaminar hook with open configuration. **F:** Lumbar laminar hook with closed configuration. **G:** Closed transverse process hook. **H:** Closed lumbar laminar hook with left off set. Sacral screws are available in different designs.

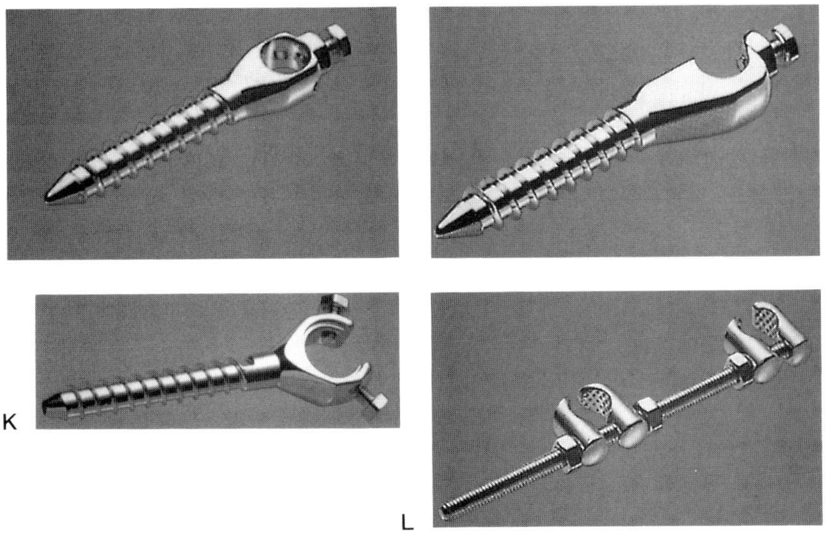

I,J

K

L

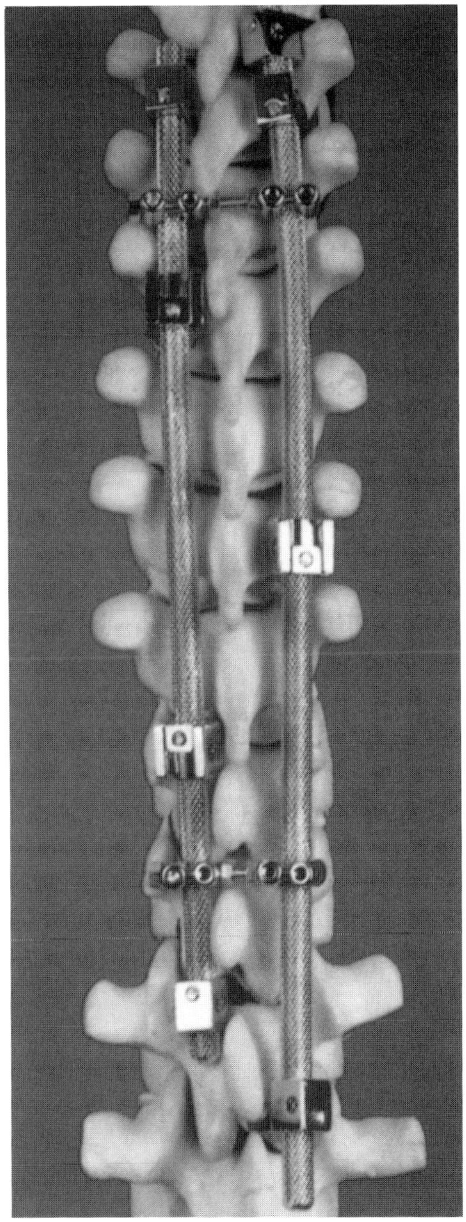

M

FIG. 3-30. *Continued.* **I:** Closed screw. **J:** Lateral open screw. **K:** Posterior open screw. **L:** Transverse traction device. **M:** Cotrel-Dubousset instrumentation on a bone model. There are two transverse connectors.

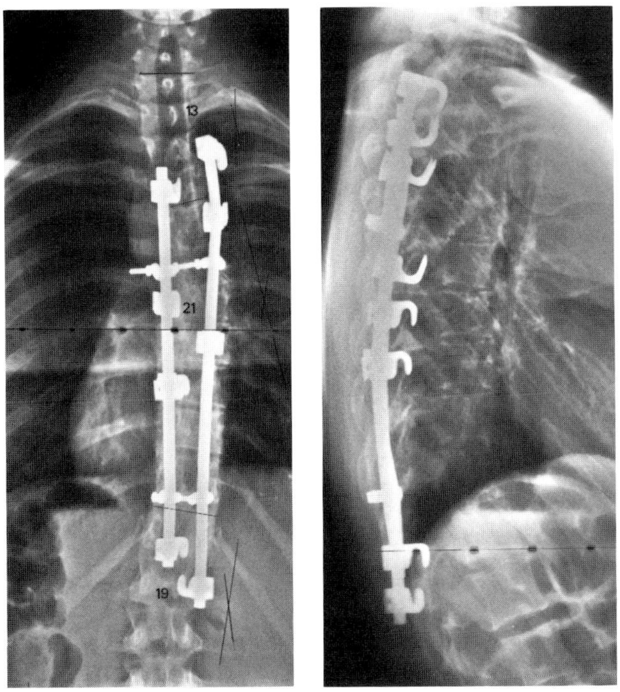

A

B

FIG. 3-31. The AP **(A)** and lateral **(B)** radiographs after Cotrel-Dubousset rod and hook instrumentation. There are transverse stabilizers proximally and distally. The rods appear smooth radiographically.

Transverse traction device. A minimum of two are used to connect rods proximally and distally.
Sacral screws for distal fixation

Advantages
- Improved frontal plane correction
- Improved kyphosis
- Maintain lumbar lordosis
- Postoperative bracing not required in children

Disadvantages
- Rigid fixation may stress shield spine
- Increased instrumentation decreases bone surface for fusion mass

TSRH Instrumentation (Figs. 3-32 and 3-33)[6]

The TSRH system is similar to other rod implants, which use rods and hooks. The TSRH system adds screws and cross plates.

Indications
- Scoliosis
- Trauma
- Spondylolisthesis
- Degenerative disease

The system can be used posteriorly or anteriorly in a configuration similar to Zielke or Dwyer instrumentation.[6,51]

Instrumentation (Fig. 3-32)[6]
- Rods are smooth with hexagonal ends. The hexagonal ends are designed to be used with a small wrench to facilitate rotation. Three different stiffnesses are available (Fig. 3-32A).
- Hooks use the same eyebolt connector. Although there are multiple designs, two basic patterns are used. The central post design allows the hook to be positioned on either side of the rod. The full top hook is positioned in the usual fashion (Fig. 3-32B,C).
- Eyebolts (Fig. 3-32D) are used to attach cross plates and hooks to the rods. They are configured in sizes to match the rod diameters.
- Cross-link plates are available in straight or offset configurations (Fig. 3-32E,F). As with other systems, they are designed to prevent rod migration and increase rigidity of the system.
- Screws are available with open and closed heads (Fig. 3-32 G,H). The eyebolt assembly is used to connect screws to the rods.

ISOLA Spinal System (Figs. 3-34 and 3-35)

This system was designed to simplify the number of implants required and improve sacral fixation. The system is designed for three-dimensional stabilization. Anchor sites include the lamina, pedicles, iliosacral region, and transverse processes.

Indications
- Scoliosis
- Hyperkyphosis
- Spondylolisthesis
- Trauma
- Degenerative disease
- Tumors

Instrumentation (Fig. 3-34)
- Rods are available in several configurations (Fig. 3-34A). Plate-rod combinations, dual-diameter rods, eye rods, and smooth single-diameter rods can be selected.
- Hooks. Top-tightening hooks with variable throat diameters (5.0 to 11.0 mm, Fig. 3-34) are used. Both closed and open hooks (Fig. 3-34C) can be used.
- Screws. Cancellous sacral and partially threaded iliac screws (Fig. 3-34E,F) are used for distal iliosacral fixation.
- Rod connectors are designed to allow fixation in multiple planes (Fig. 3-34G,H).
- Spacer and washers (Fig. 3-34I) are used to position screws and rod connectors properly, increase strength, and provide more space for bone grafts.
- Cross connectors. Transverse rod connectors (Fig. 3-34I) are used to ensure stability.
- Wires. Sublaminar and spinous process wires are used similar to those in Luque and Wisconsin segmental instrumentation.

The ISOLA system (Fig. 3-35) is relatively new but offers three-dimensional stability and multiple anchor sites; minimal external support is required postoperatively.

All new-generation implants (Cotrel-Dubousset, TSRH, and ISOLA) are comparable in terms of indications and components. Selection is based on the surgeon's preference.

Combined Instrumentation

Combined instrumentation may be indicated for rigid thoracic hyperkyphosis, double-thoracic and thoracolumbar curves, and rapidly progressing large thoracic curves.[51,56] Combined anterior and posterior instrumentation may be necessary in these situations (Fig. 3-36).[7,13,31]

Modifications of instrumentation differ slightly and are not truly combined procedures. For example, spinous process or sublaminar wires may be used with Harrington rods.[44] This adds segmental stability and reduces the stress to the lamina by the hooks at the end of the rods. Dual hooks or combined Harrington and Luque

(text continues on page 133)

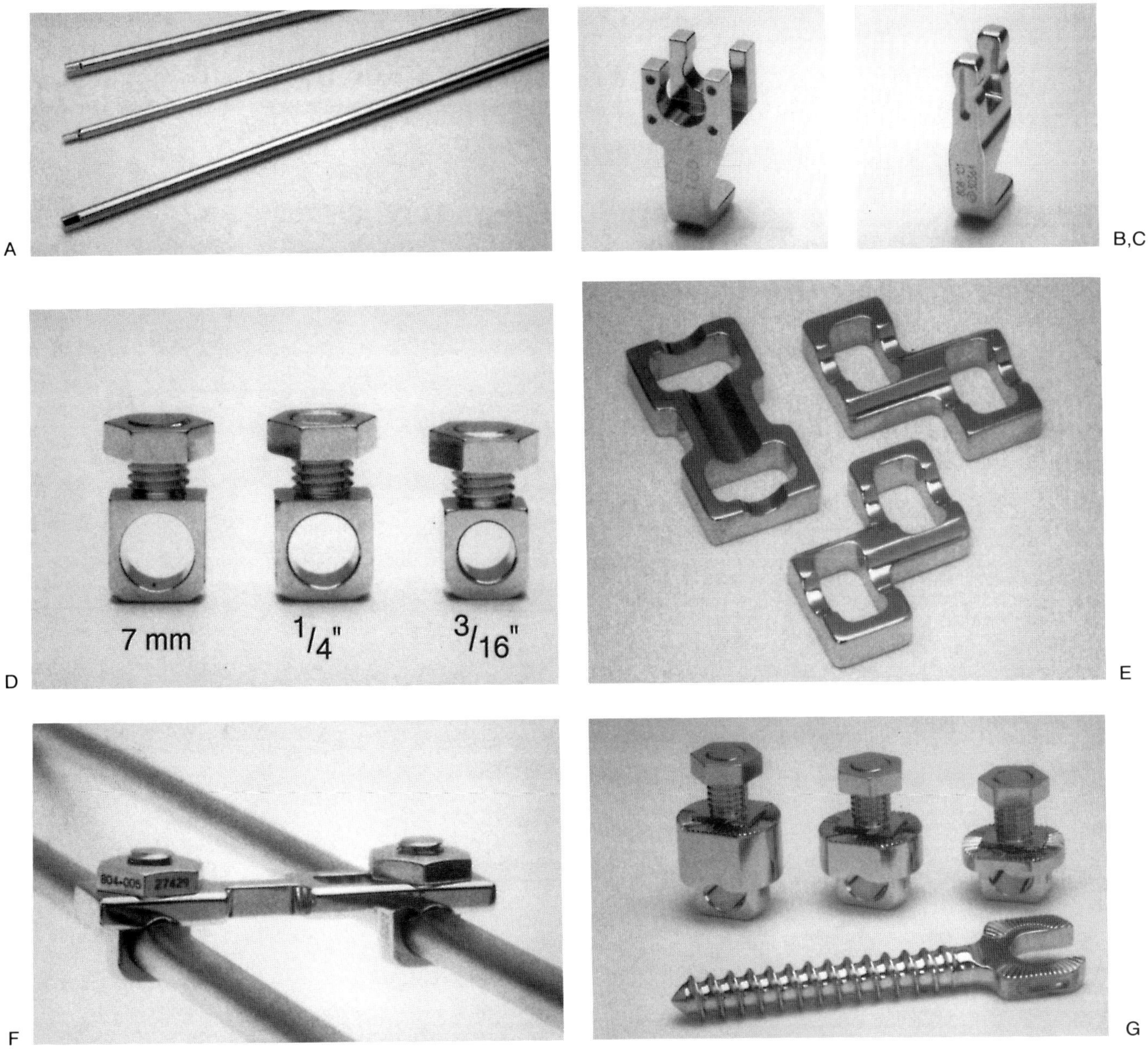

FIG. 3-32. The TSRH instrumentation (Courtesy of Danek Group, Memphis, TN.) **A:** The TSRH smooth rods with hexagonal ends to facilitate rotation during surgery. Full-top **(B)** and central-post **(C)** hooks. The latter can be placed on either side of the rod. **D:** Eyebolt assemblies for three rod sizes. Cross-link plates **(E)** and connected to rods **(F)**. Variably angled eyebolt assemblies with an open screw **(G)** and screws attached to the rod at varying angles **(H)**. (See **H-J** on next page.)

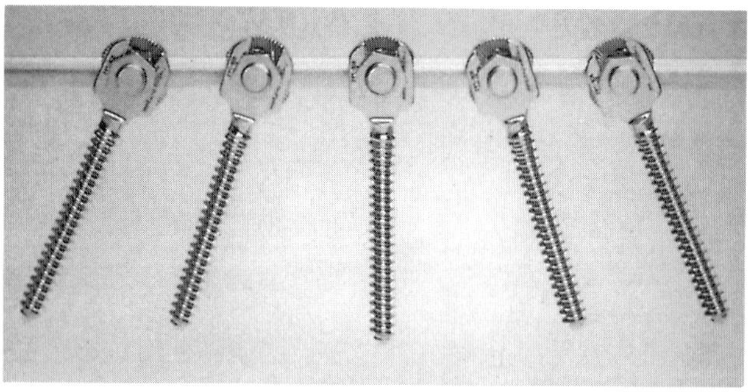

H

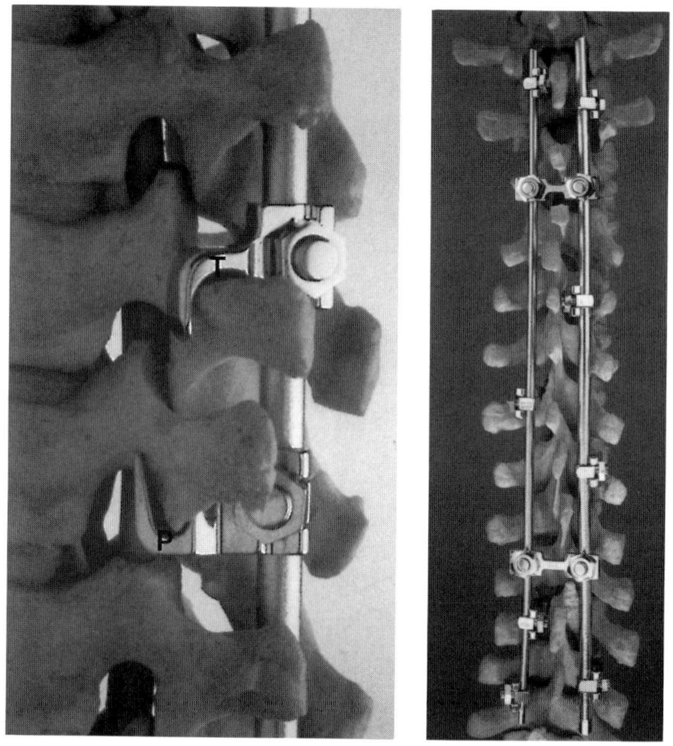

I,J

FIG. 3-32. *Continued.* The TSRH system is shown on a skeletal model. **I:** Rod with two hooks, a caudal facing transverse process hook (*T*) and a cephalad facing pedicle hook (*P*). **J:** the TSRH system with cross links proximally and distally.

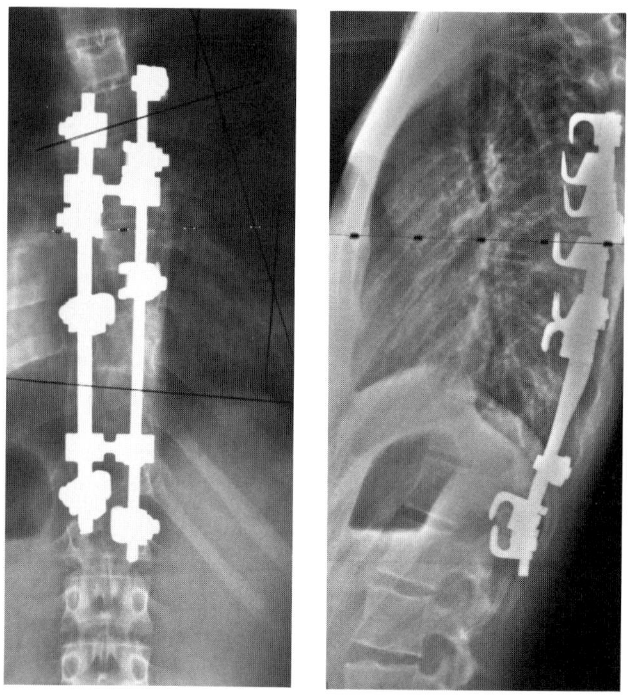

A B

FIG. 3-33. The AP **(A)** and lateral **(B)** radiographs with TSRH instrumentation and proximal and distal cross-links.

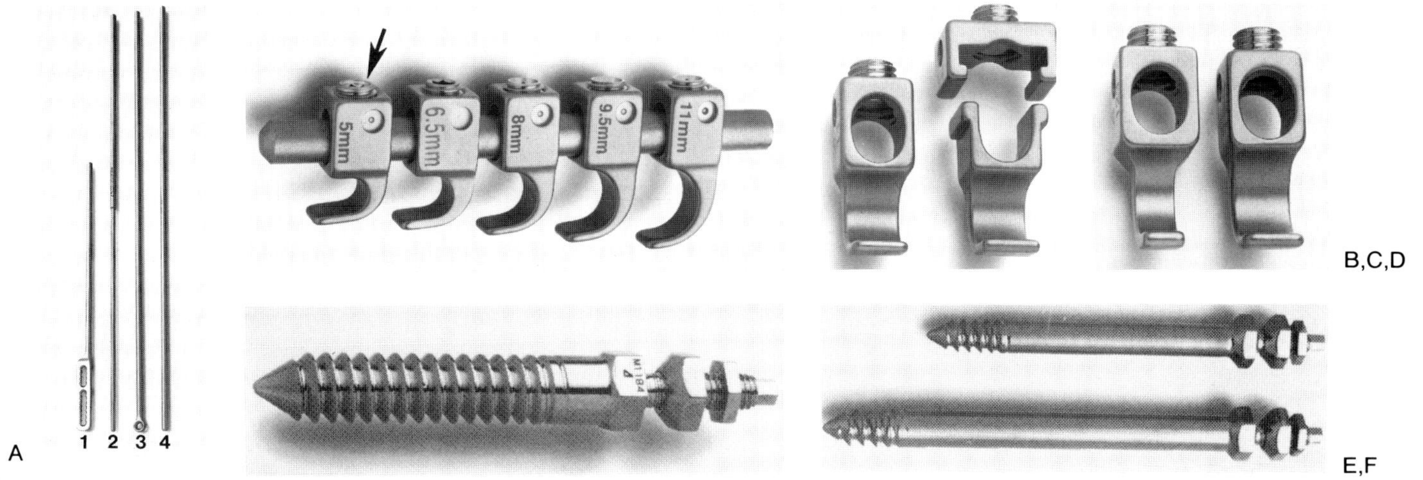

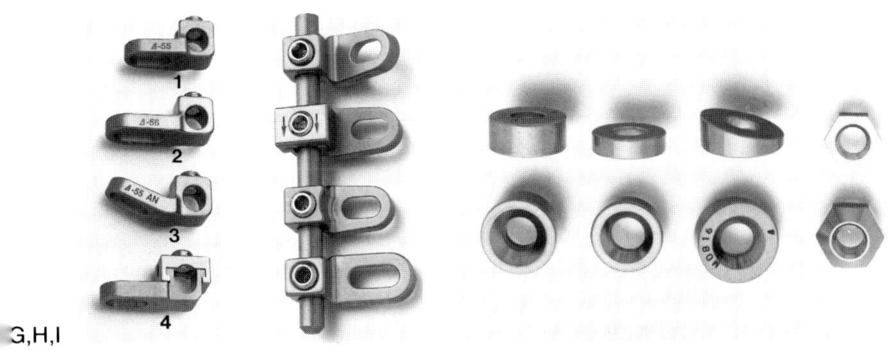

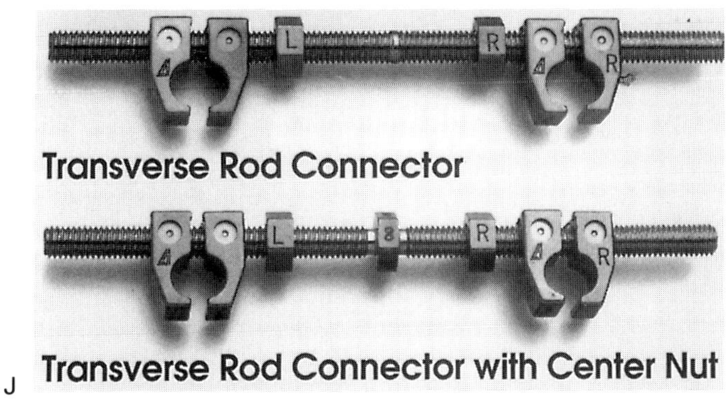

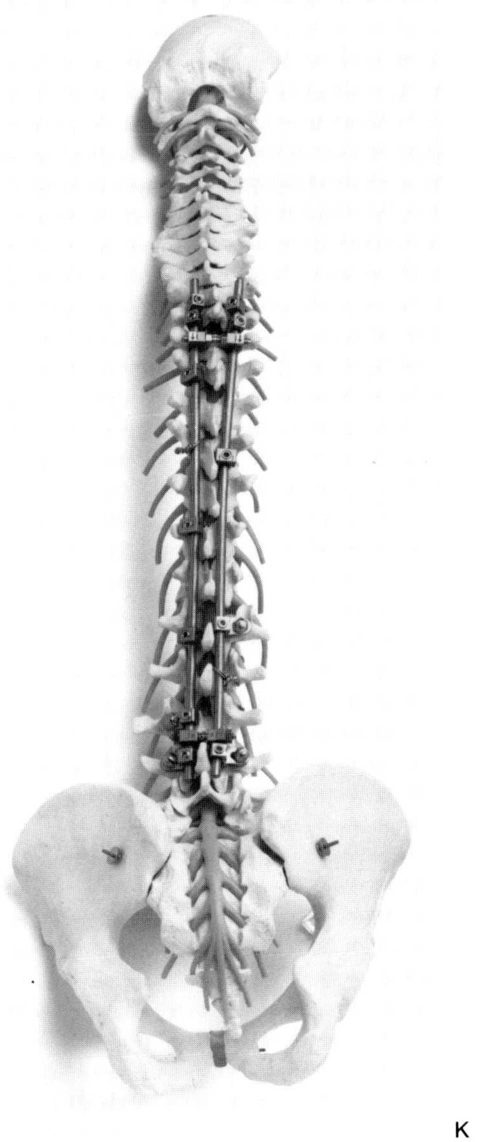

FIG. 3-34. The ISOLA spinal implant system. **A:** Spinal rods (stainless steel and titanium): *1,* plate rod; *2,* dual-diameter rod; *3,* eye rod; and *4,* smooth rod. **B:** The ISOLA hooks with top tightening screw (*arrow*) and throat diameters from 5 to 11 mm. **C:** Closed (*left*) and open (*right*) hook designs. **D:** Narrow and wide blade widths on two closed hooks. **E,F:** Cancellous sacral and partially threaded iliac screws. **G:** Rod connectors with *1,* straight slotted design; *2,* extended straight slotted; *3,* angled; and *4,* open straight slotted design. **H:** Rod connectors attached to a smooth rod. **I:** The ISOLA tapered and flat washers and nuts. **J:** Transverse rod connectors without and with a central nut. **K:** The ISOLA spinal implant system on a skeleton. (Courtesy of AcroMed, Cleveland, OH.)

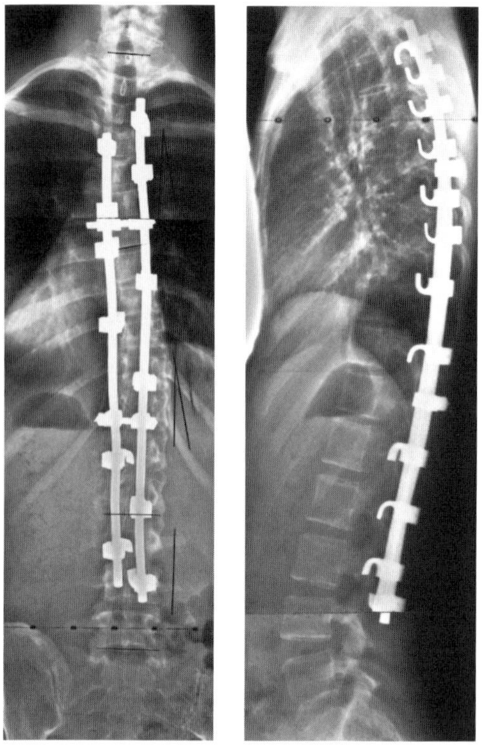

A B

FIG. 3-35. The AP **(A)** and lateral **(B)** standing radiographs demonstrating ISOLA instrumentation with 2 smooth rods, 12 hooks, and 2 transverse rod connectors.

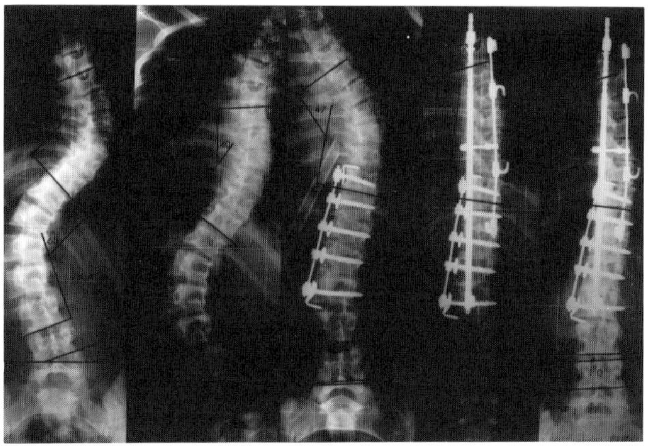

A B C D E

FIG. 3-36. Combined ventral derotational system (VDS) and Harrington instrumentation. The AP radiographs **(A,B)** of a 16-year-old girl with scoliosis and L-4 obliquity. The VDS instrumentation with the Zielke technique **(C)** and after posterior instrumentation with a Harrington distraction rod on the right and threaded compression rod on the left **(D,E)**. (From Korovessis P. Combined VDS and Harrington instrumentation for treatment of idiopathic double major curves. *Spine* 1987;12:244–250.)

TABLE 3-4. *Scoliosis instrumentation complications*[9,11,14,16,19,24,33,35,43,52,55]

Primary
Loss of correction
Rod fracture
Cable rupture
Hook displacement
Screw pull out or fracture
Pseudarthrosis
Increase in secondary curve (untreated)
Neurologic (includes paraplegia)
Infection
Local pain
Secondary
Pneumonia
Pulmonary embolus
Chylothorax
Superior mesenteric artery syndrome
Thrombophlebitis

rod procedures may also be used in certain situations (Fig. 3-37).[32,35,39,57]

Complications

The complications associated with scoliosis instrumentation vary with the type of procedure and the patient's status (e.g., weight, type of curve, and metabolic bone disease). Complications may be related to the procedure (primary) or involve other anatomic regions (secondary). Certain of these complications may be increased with methods requiring immobilization or recumbency (i.e., superior mesenteric artery syndrome and thrombophlebitis; Table 3-4).[9,14,19,24,33,56]

Comparison of pre- and postoperative radiographs is essential to determine the degree of correction and to evaluate a loss of correction should it occur. The AP and lateral standing and side-bending views are used to measure rotation, curve size, and kyphosis. The same vertebra should be selected for measurement on each follow-up examination to ensure accuracy in comparison.[28,29,37,55,56]

Routine radiographs are also generally adequate to evaluate hook, screw, cable, and rod failures (Figs. 3-38 and 3-39). On occasion, fluoroscopic positioning is required to assess the position of the hooks accurately.

It normally takes 6 to 9 months for solid bone graft fusion to occur radiographically. Early recognition of pseudarthrosis or fibrosis union is important to allow early repair and prevent instrument failure.[19,52] Evaluation of bone mass in suspected pseudarthrosis can be difficult. The incidence of pseudarthrosis varies with the type of instrumentation. However, this complication can be seen in 10% to 15% of patients. The metal used for instrumentation interferes with CT and MRI in most cases. The CT images can be improved by reformatting images in the coronal and/or sagittal planes or obtaining more image data.[14,52] Titanium implants cause less artifact on both CT and MRI scans.[52] Radionuclide images can be difficult to interpret in the first year after surgery.[19] Conventional tomography in the AP and lateral views may still be one of the simplest methods of evaluating pseudarthrosis (Fig. 3-40). In difficult cases, diagnostic injection of local anesthetic [1% Xylocaine™ (Astra, Westborough, MA) or 0.25% Marcaine™ (Sanofi Winthrop, New York, NY)] may be helpful. Relief of symptoms localizes the problem. This technique can be used for pseudarthrosis or facet evaluation prior to extending fusion or to confirm the hook site as the source of pain. Fluoroscopic motion studies can be useful in evaluating difficult cases; along with trigger-point symptoms, they assist in selecting injection sites or defining pseudarthrosis (Fig. 3-41). Hook position, as noted previously, can be assessed at this time (Fig. 3-42) because hook-site injections may also provide useful information regarding the patient's symptoms.

LUMBAR FUSIONS (SPONDYLOLISTHESIS AND DEGENERATIVE DISEASE)

Lumbar spine instrumentation may be chosen for the treatment of instability or pain that is due to numerous causes.[65] Spondylolysis and spondylolisthesis are commonly a part of this spectrum of orthopedic problems.

Spondylolysis is a defect in the pars interarticularis. The defect is usually bilateral (74%) and occurs in 5% to 7.2% of the general population.[63,93,96] In patients with low-back pain, the incidence is increased to approximately 10%. The incidence of spondylolysis increases with age and is more common in whites than in blacks. There is also a strong familial tendency.[63,94,102]

Individuals in certain professions, such as football linemen and weight lifters, also demonstrate an increased incidence of spondylolysis. The defect is most commonly noted at the L-5 (67%) and L-4 (10%) levels. Congenital spinous process defects are encountered five- to tenfold more commonly in patients with spondylolysis.[63,94,102]

Many hypotheses have been formulated in an attempt to define the cause of spondylolysis (Table 3-5).[95,97,116–118] The

TABLE 3-5. *Spondylolysis: etiologic hypotheses*[63]

Separate ossification centers
Postnatal fractures
Exaggerated lordosis
Weak supporting structures
Dysplasia
Stress fractures
Pathologic fractures

(text continues on page 138)

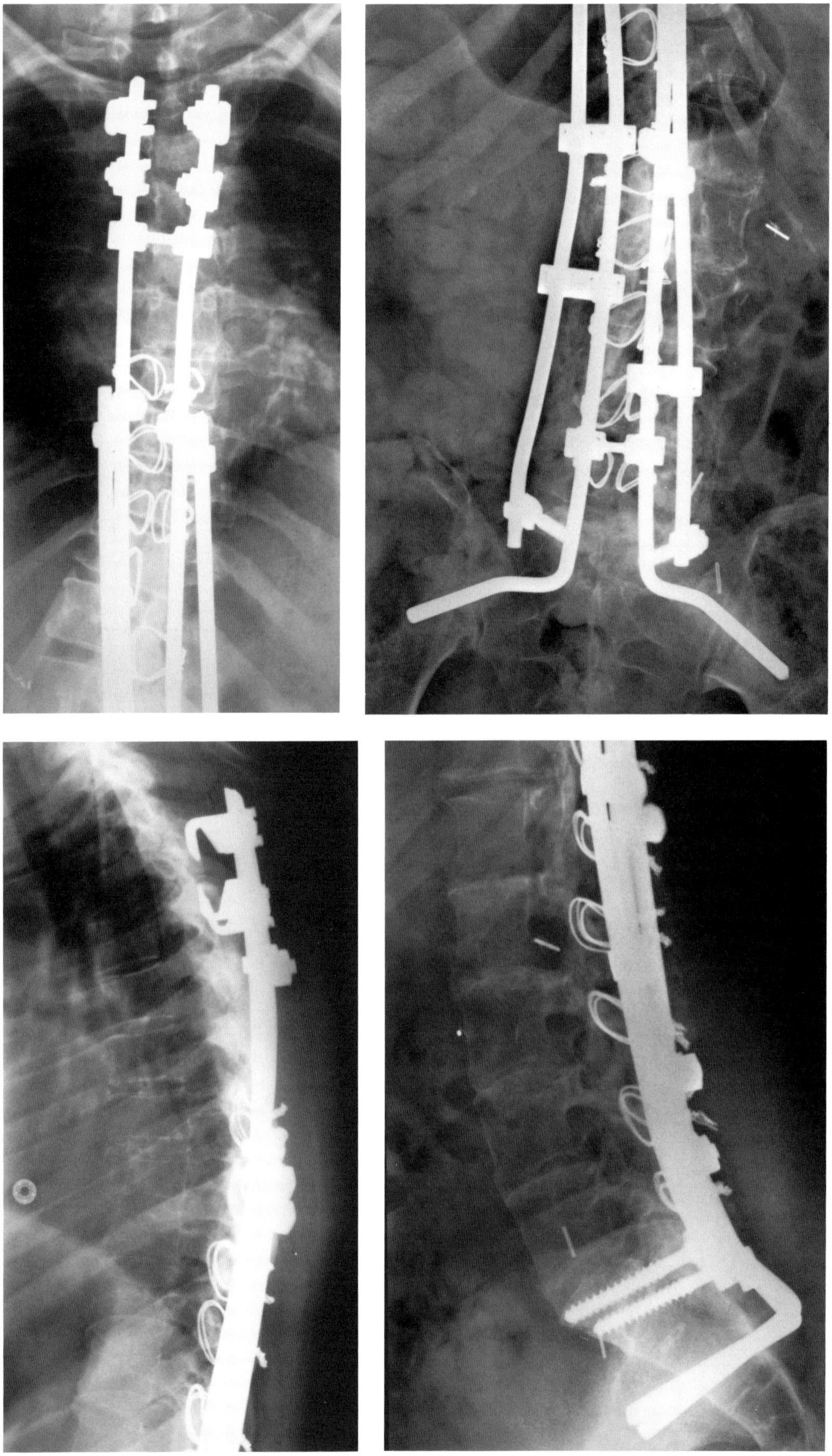

A B C D

FIG. 3-37. The AP (**A, upper**; **B, lower**) and lateral (**C, upper**; **D, lower**) views of the spine with combined Luque rod, TSRH rod, and sublaminar wire instrumentation. There are multiple cross-connectors.

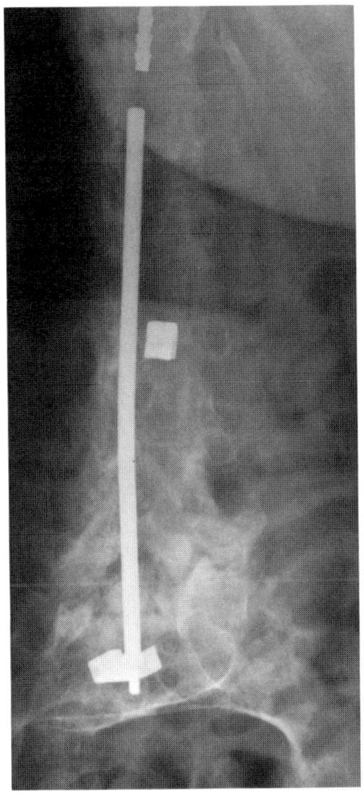

FIG. 3-38. The AP view of the spine, demonstrating fracture of a Harrington distraction rod just below the ratchet end. The hooks are no longer attached.

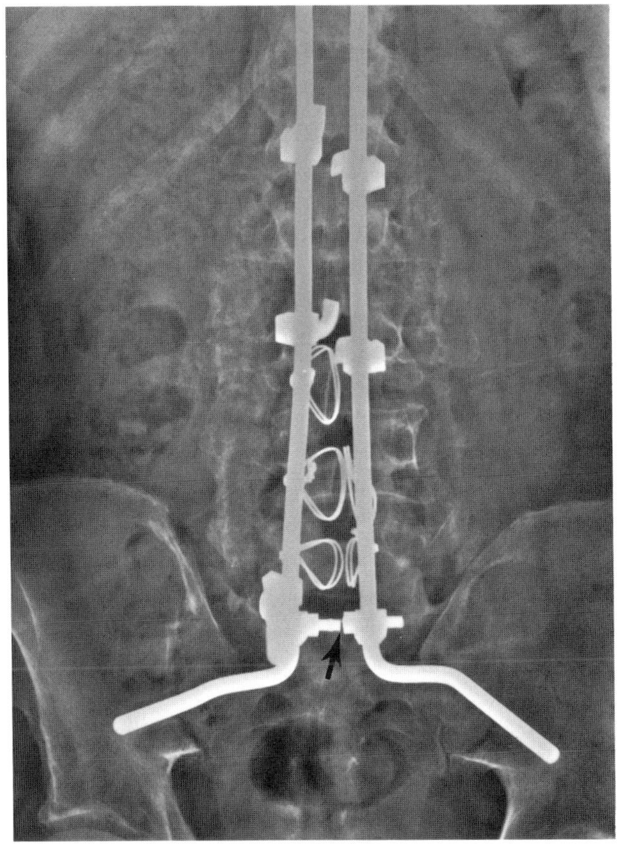

FIG. 3-39. The AP view of the spine after ISOLA rod (with "Galveston" fixation to the ilium) and sublaminar wire and hook instrumentation. The transverse cross-link is fractured (*arrow*).

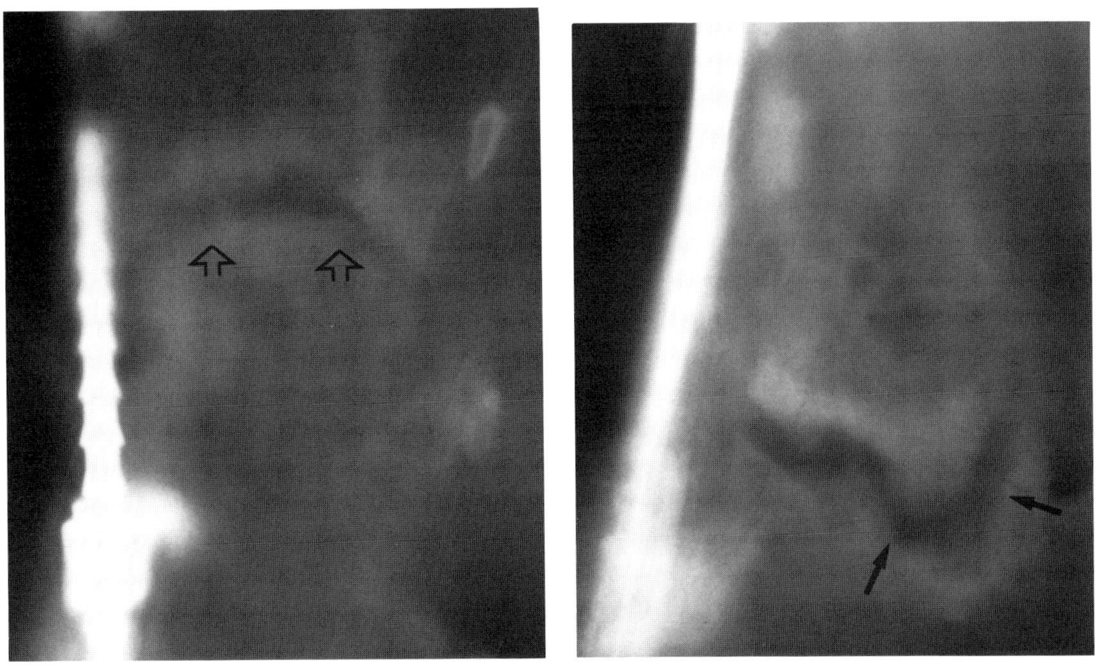

A B

FIG. 3-40. The AP tomograms at the proximal **(A)** and distal **(B)** ends of the Harrington rod, demonstrating fusion failure (pseudarthrosis) (*arrows*).

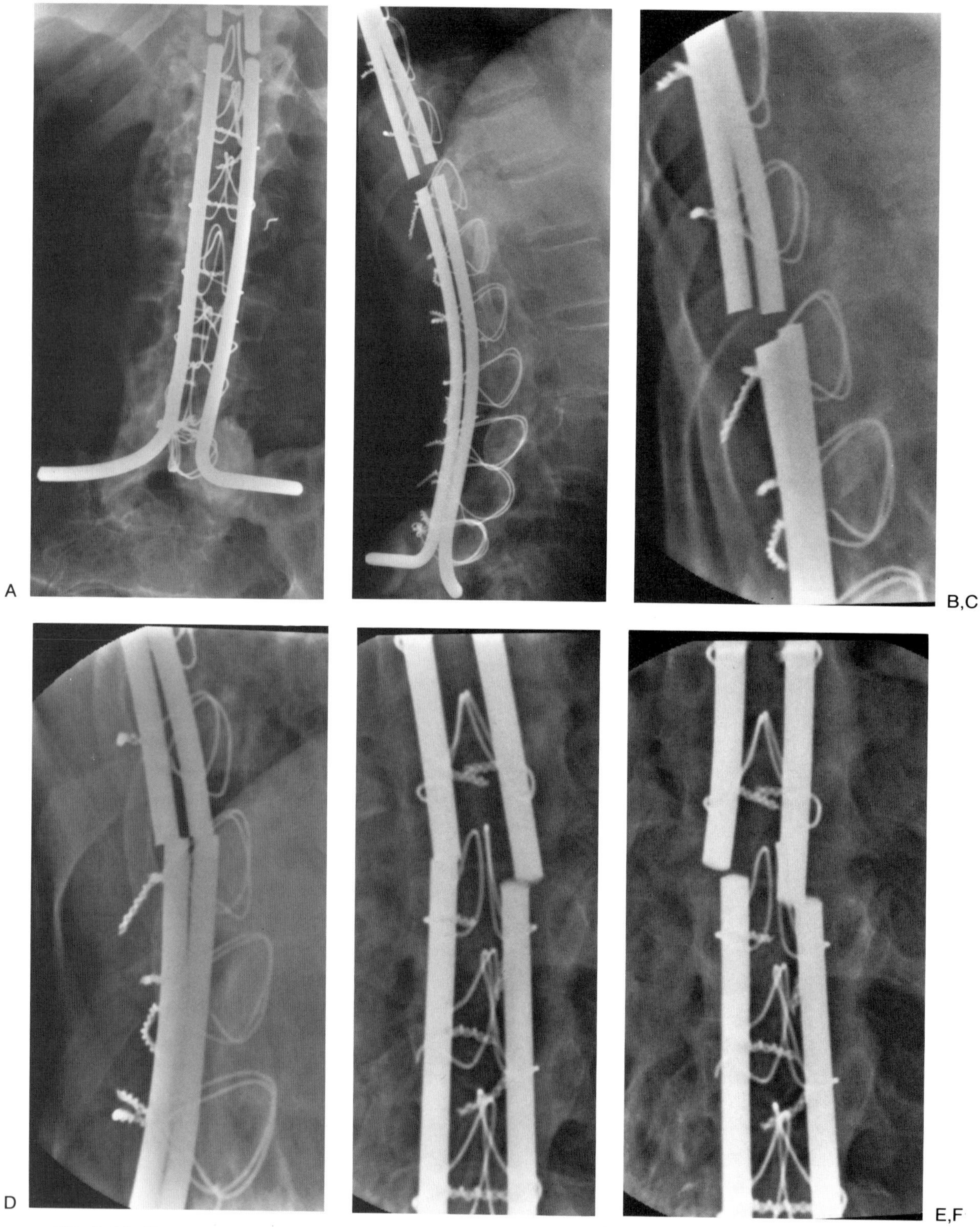

FIG. 3-41. Young male patient with posterior instrumentation for scoliosis using Luque rods and sublaminar wires. The AP **(A)** and lateral **(B)** radiographs show rod fractures at the T-12 level. Fluoroscopic motion studies with flexion **(C)**, extension **(D)**, and lateral bending **(E,F)** show motion of the rods and more clearly define the pseudarthrosis.

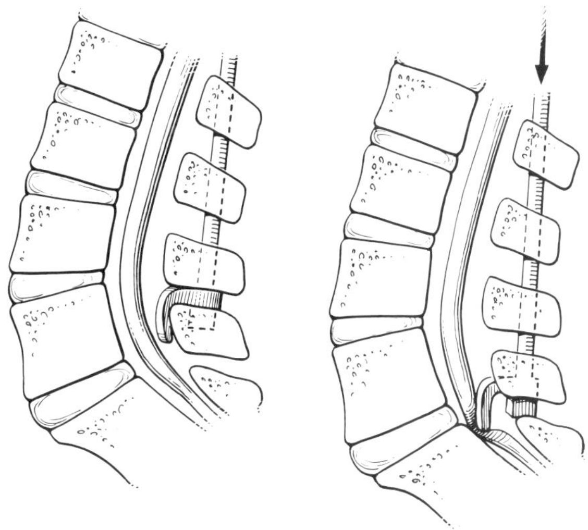

FIG. 3-42. Hook migration, leading to spinal canal compromise. (From Hales DD, Dawson EG, Delamartes R. Late neurological complications of Harrington-rod instrumentation. *J Bone Joint Surg* 1989;71A:1053–1057.)

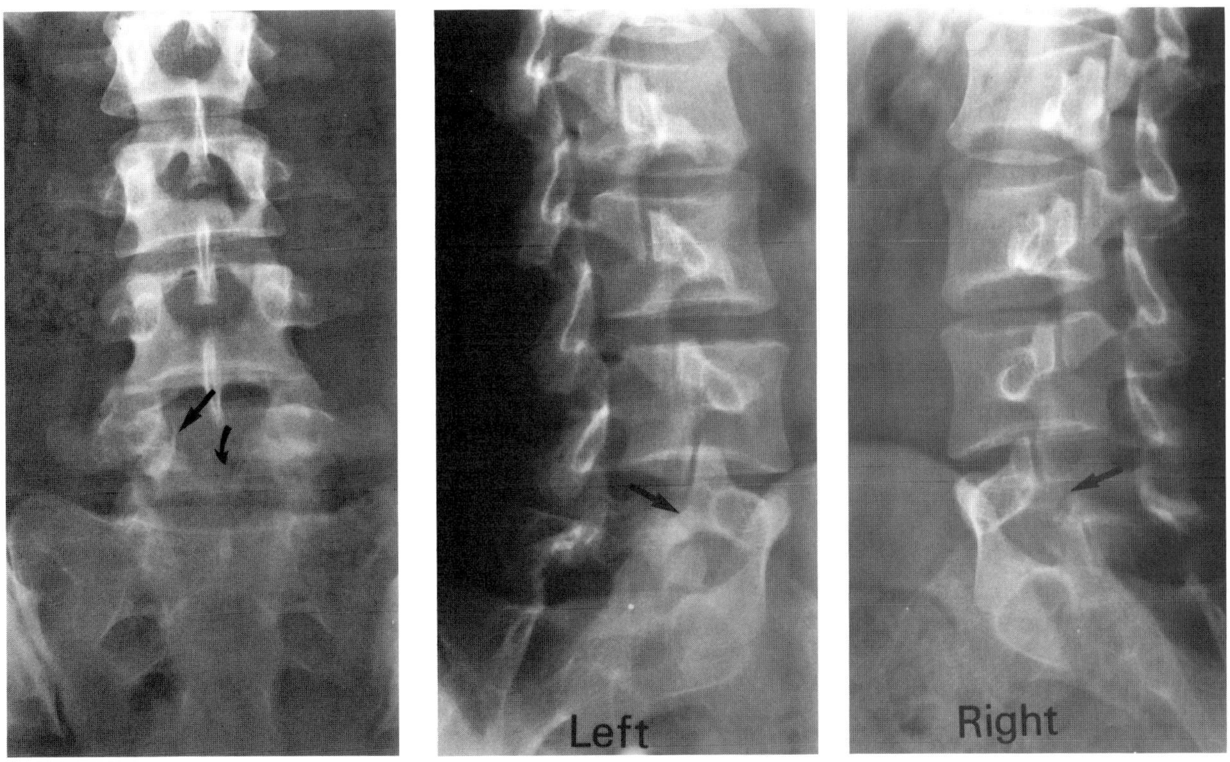

A B,C

FIG. 3-43. A: The AP view of the lumbar spine, demonstrating spina bifida (*curved arrow*) and sclerosis (*straight arrow*) of the right pedicle. Oblique views demonstrate sclerosis and elongation of the pars (*arrow*) on the left **(B)** and a unilateral pars defect (*arrow*) on the right **(C)**. (From Berquist TH. *Imaging of orthopedic trauma.* New York: Raven Press, 1992.)

TABLE 3-6.
Spondylolisthesis: cause[88,118]

Upper sacral dysplasia
Degenerative changes
Pathologic fractures
Previous surgery
Pars defect
Acute fractures
Stress fractures
Elongated pars

suggestion that this may be congenital has been widely disputed and most clearly discussed by Newman and Stone.[97] Evidence against the congenital hypothesis includes the following: (1) the defect has never been found in a fetus or stillborn, (2) the incidence increases with age and is rarely noted in infants prior to walking, and (3) the defect occasionally heals.[88–94,116,118] Others have suggested various acquired causes (Table 3-5).[60,63,93,94,96,102,111] Most authors agree, however, that the defect is due to a combination of (1) a hereditary defect in the cartilage model of the arch and (2) the strain placed on the lower back by upright posture and lumbar lordosis.[63,94,96,102]

Spondylolisthesis is anterior slippage or subluxation of the vertebral body. This is most commonly related to spondylolysis but may also be present without a true interruption of the pars interarticularis.[63,117]

Spondylolisthesis may result from causes other than spondylolysis, such as degenerative facet disease, changes in the facet angles, degenerative disc disease, or previous surgery.[63,75,88] Table 3-6, based on the work of Wiltse, Newman, and MacNab,[88,118] summarizes the possible causes of spondylolisthesis. Degenerative spondylolisthesis usually occurs in patients older than 50 years of age and is fivefold more common in female than in male patients. The location of the level also differs, being more common at the L4-5 level (80%). Multiple levels are involved in 5% of patients, with the degree of slippage rarely exceeding 30%. The incidence of neurologic involvement in degenerative spondylolisthesis is also higher than in spondylolytic spondylolisthesis. Rosenberg[102] noted neurologic complications in 30% of patients in this category.

Preoperative Imaging and Classifications

Radiographic evaluation is usually complete with the AP, lateral, coned-down lateral, and oblique views (Fig. 3-43). Angling the tube 30° to the head on the AP view may also assist in demonstrating the pars defect. Motion views, specifically flexion and extension views, are useful for evaluating stability (Figs. 3-44 and 3-45).[63,76] Findings on the AP view include sclerosis of the opposite pedicle if the lesion is unilateral and foreshortening of the spine in cases of advanced spondylolisthesis.[63,89] The coned lateral view is usually best for the detection of the pars defects and the often associated degenerative disc disease (Fig. 3-46). The degree of subluxation is usually graded according to the systems established by Meyerding or Tillard.[89,93,107,111] Using the Meyerding system, the vertebral body is divided into four equal segments from anterior to posterior, and the degree of slippage is graded I through IV, according to these measurements (Fig. 3-47). The Tillard system is similar but uses a percentage of slippage (Fig. 3-47).[93,111]

The lumbosacral relationship can also be assessed on the lateral cone-down view. This slip angle (Fig. 3-48) is measured using a line along the upper end plate of L-5 and a second perpendicular line to the posterior aspect of the upper sacrum.[61] The upper end plate of L-5 is chosen because the lower end plate is often distorted. A high slip angle indicates a greater risk for instability, progression, and reduced healing potential.[61,118]

Wiltse and Winter,[118] using a sacral-horizontal angle (Fig. 3-49), suggested two-level fusion when this angle exceeds 55°. The angle is measured on a standing lateral radiograph by using a line along the upper end plate of L-5 and a second line that is horizontal. Although the issue was not formally studied, in their experience, patients fused from L4-5 have less back pain than those who undergo an L5-S1 fusion if the sacrohorizontal angle exceeds 55°.

In nonspondylolytic spondylolisthesis, the defect is most commonly at the L-4 to L-5 level, and the degree of associated degenerative change is obvious on the lateral view (Figs. 3-50 and 3-51). The lumbosacral angle is also decreased in these patients compared with that in patients with spondylolytic spondylolisthesis. In normal patients, this angle measures approximately 34°. In patients with nonspondylolytic spondylolisthesis, the angle is about 20°, and if spondylolysis is present, the angle is increased to about 60°. Oblique views are often confirmatory and increase one's confidence in detecting pars defects (Fig. 3-52). The facet joints are also seen to better advantage.[63]

Tomography (Fig. 3-53) or CT (Fig. 3-54) are frequently valuable in studying spondylolysis and other defects in the posterior arch. Although CT may be helpful in selected cases, it can also present a confusing picture. Because of their alignment, the facet joints may be confused with a pars defect. A vacuum sign has been described in the facet joints in patients with degenerative spondylolisthesis. Because CT is used more frequently with newer instrumentation techniques, the decisions regarding pedicle screws can be more accurately assessed.[60,61,63] Conventional myelography or CT studies may be useful in patients with evidence of neurologic involvement.[63]

Subtle cases may also be detected using radionuclide imaging. Specifically, tomographic studies (single-

(text continues on page 144)

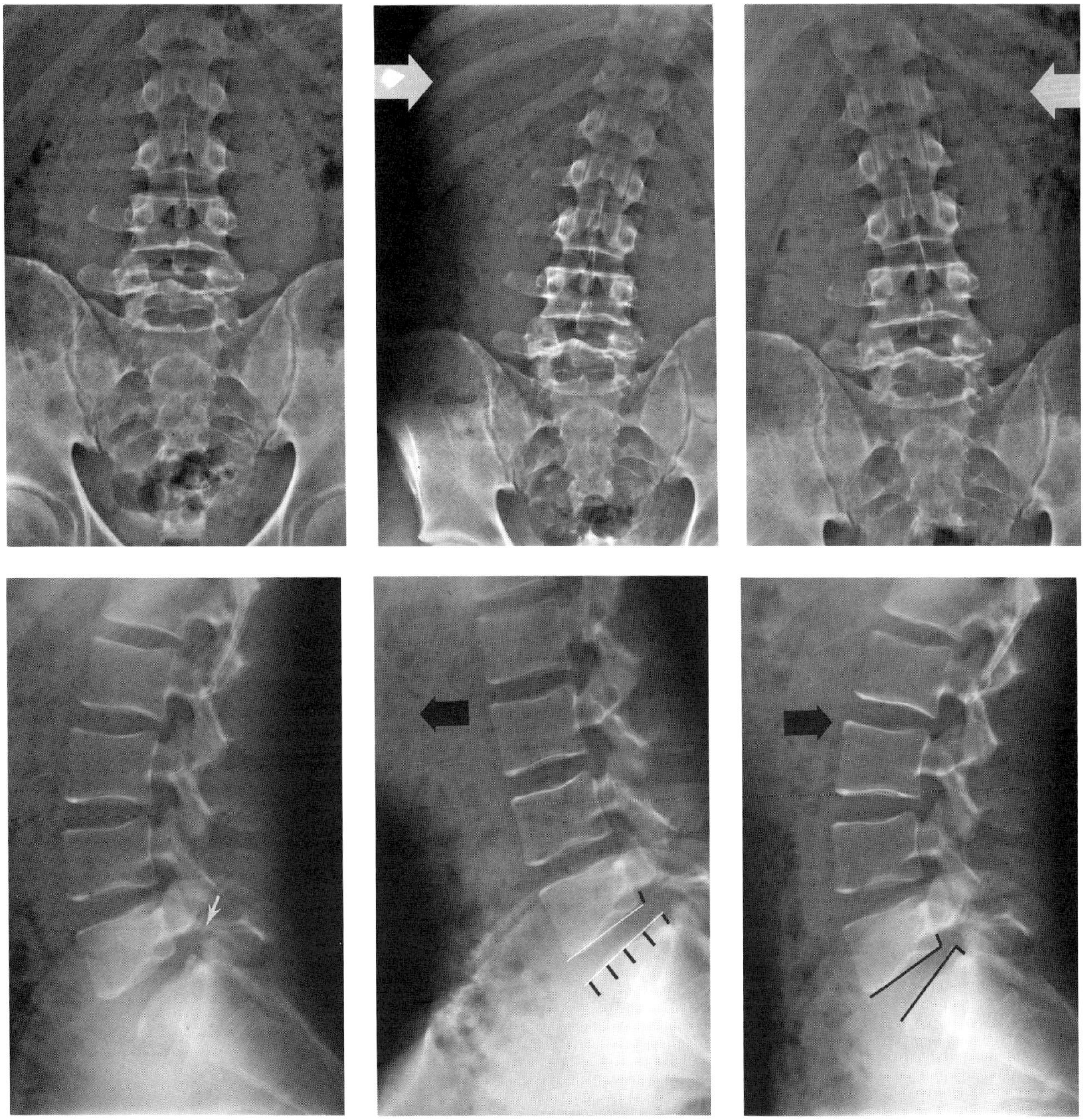

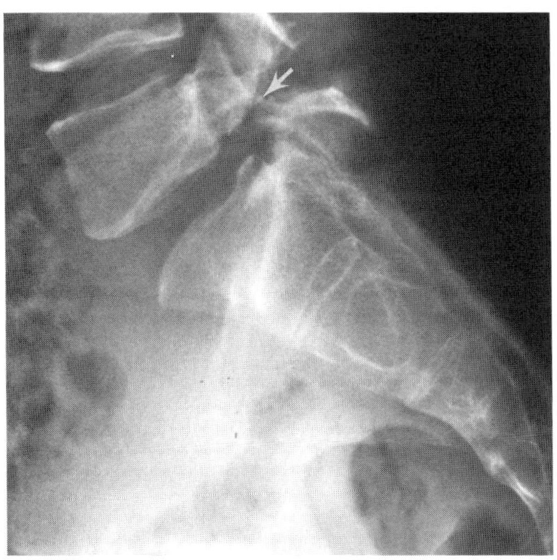

FIG. 3-44. The AP **(A)** and lateral bending **(B,C)** views of the lumbar spine are normal. The lateral views in neutral **(D)**, with flexion **(E)**, and extension **(F)** demonstrate the L-5 pars defect (*arrow*). The degree of subluxation increases, and the posterior disc space widens with flexion (E) and reduces with extension (F). The coned-down lateral view **(G)** is often the most useful for the identification of pars defects (*arrow*) (compare with oblique views, Fig. 3-43).

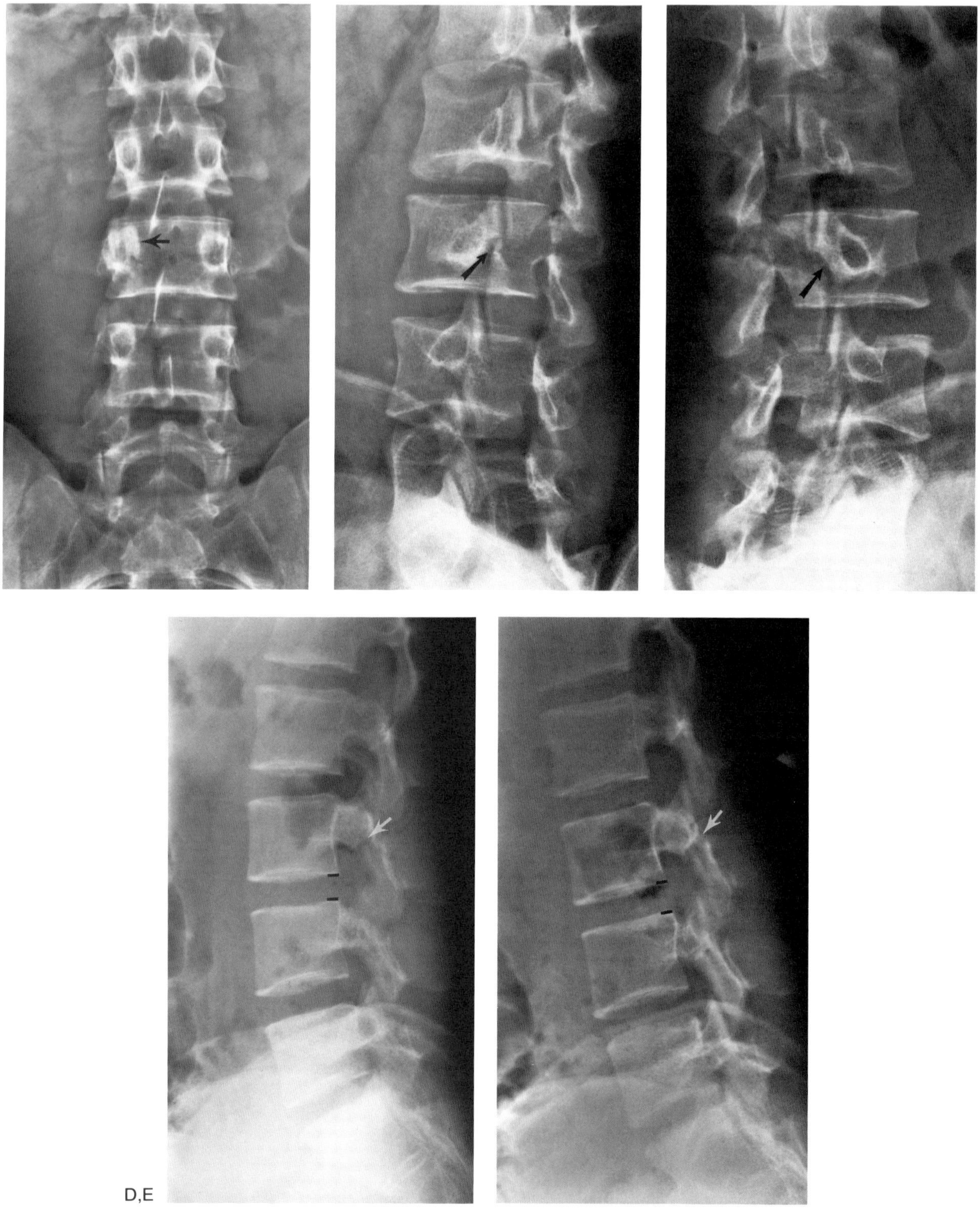

A B,C

D,E

FIG. 3-45. A: The AP view of the lumbar spine in a patient with a L-3 pars defect, demonstrating a sclerotic appearance of the pedicle on the right (*arrow*). **B,C:** Oblique views demonstrate bilateral pars interruptions at L-3 (*arrows*). Neutral lateral **(D)** and flexion views **(E)** show slight widening of the posterior disc space at L-3 with flexion but no subluxation.

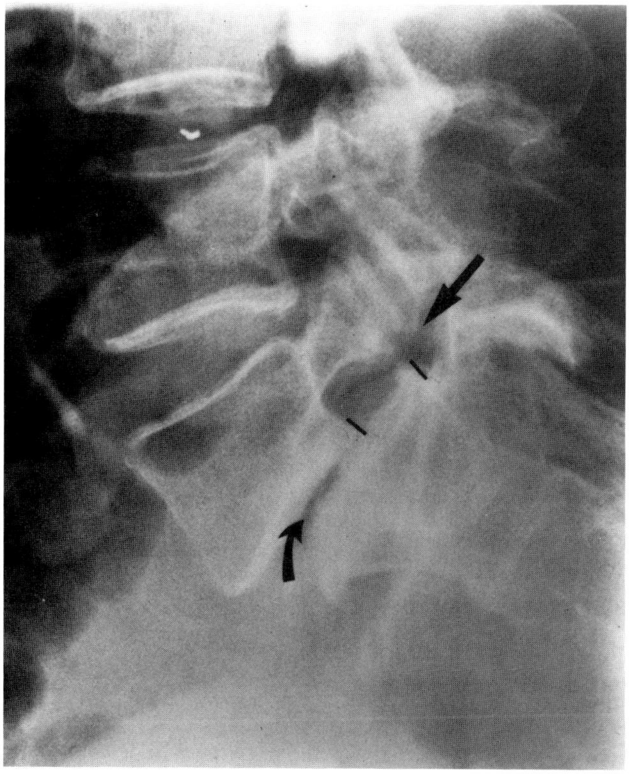

FIG. 3-46. Coned lateral view with bilateral pars defect (*arrow*) and near-grade II subluxation with degenerative disc disease (*curved arrow*).

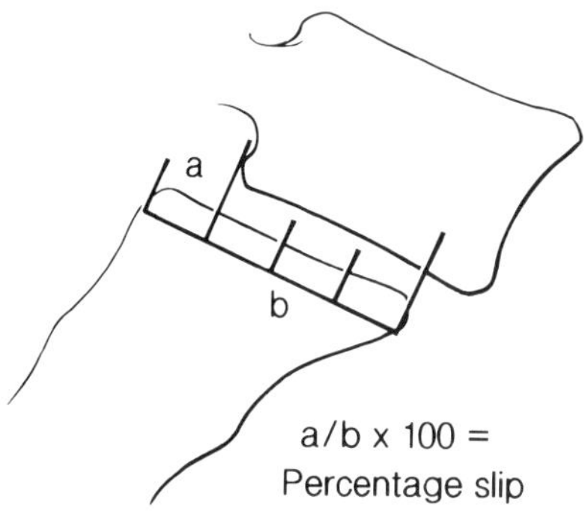

FIG. 3-47. Displacement of L-5 on S-1. Using the Meyerding system, this is grade I or, in the Tillard system, a 25% slip.

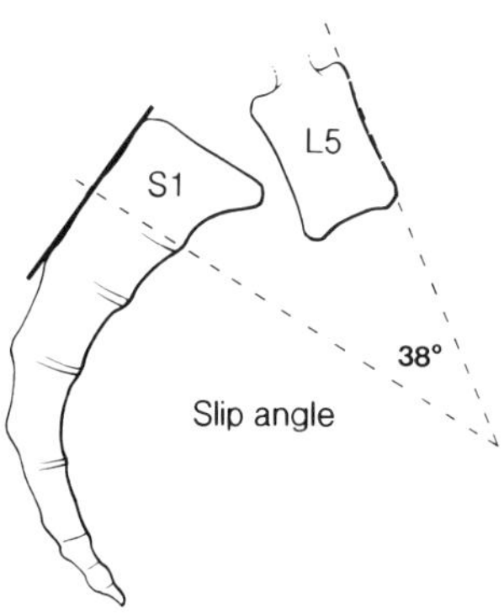

FIG. 3-48. Method for measuring the slip angle. A line is drawn along the upper end plate of L-5, and a second line is drawn perpendicular to the posterior S-1 to S-2 cortical interface.[118]

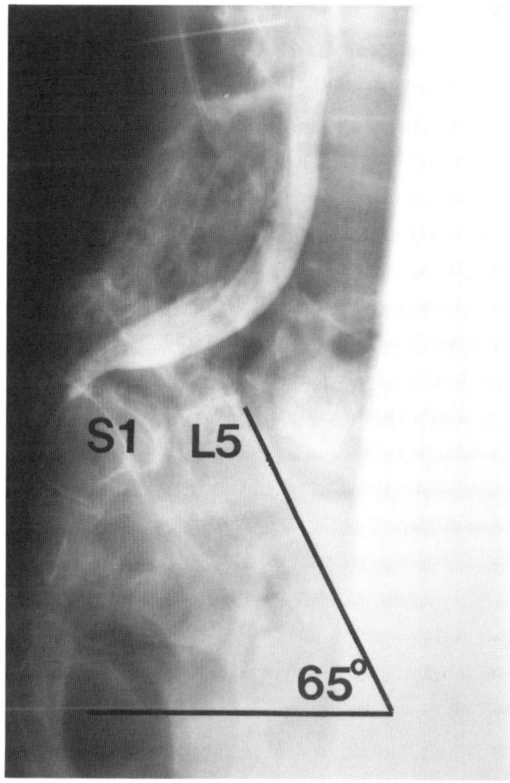

FIG. 3-49. Lateral radiograph of myelogram demonstrating grade IV displacement of L-5 on S-1. The sacrohorizontal angle is formed by a line drawn along the upper end plate of L-5 and a horizontal line. In this case, the angle is 65°, which suggests that two-level fusion should be performed.

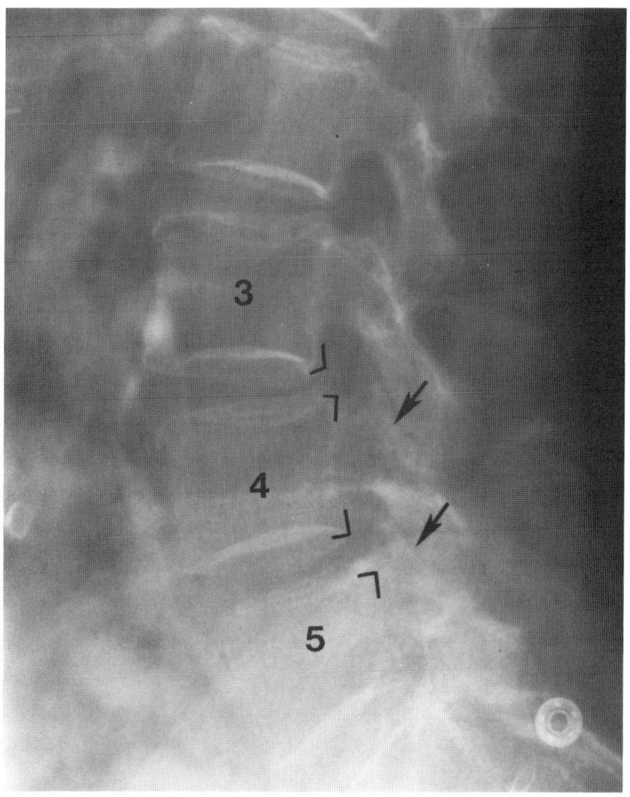

FIG. 3-50. Lateral view of the lumbar spine in a patient with degenerative spondylolisthesis of L-3 on L-4 and L-4 on L-5. Note the changes in the facet joints (*arrows*).

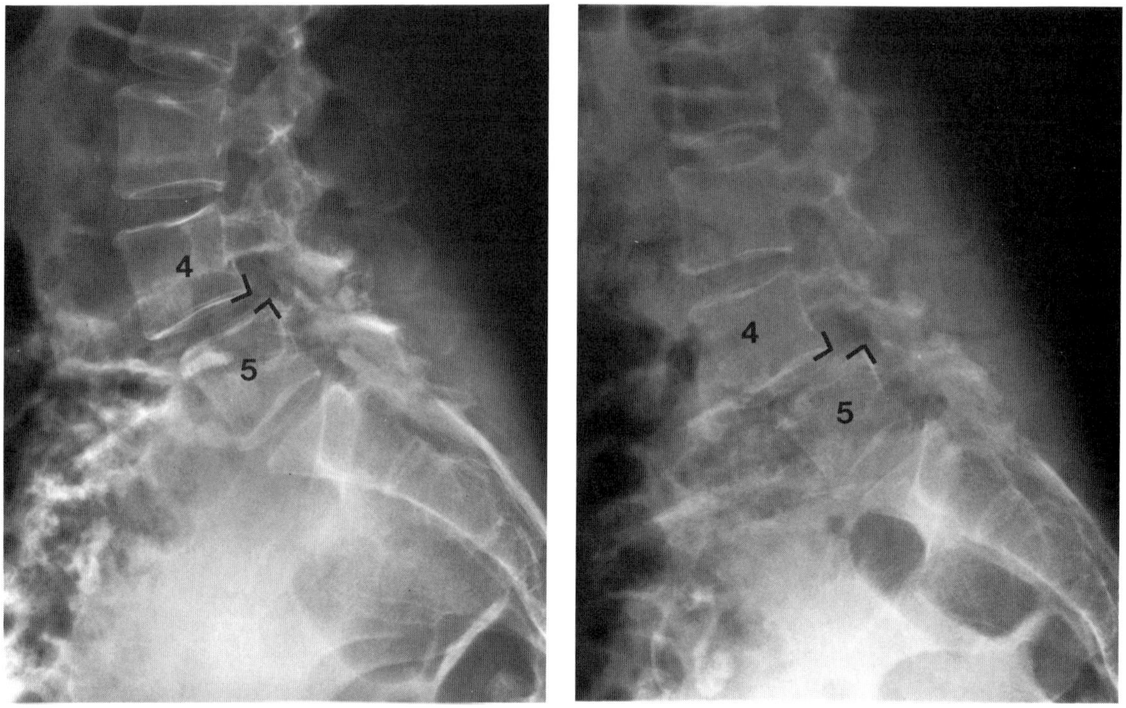

A B

FIG. 3-51. Degenerative subluxation of L-4 on L-5. The findings do not fully reduce with extension **(A)** but increase with flexion **(B)**.

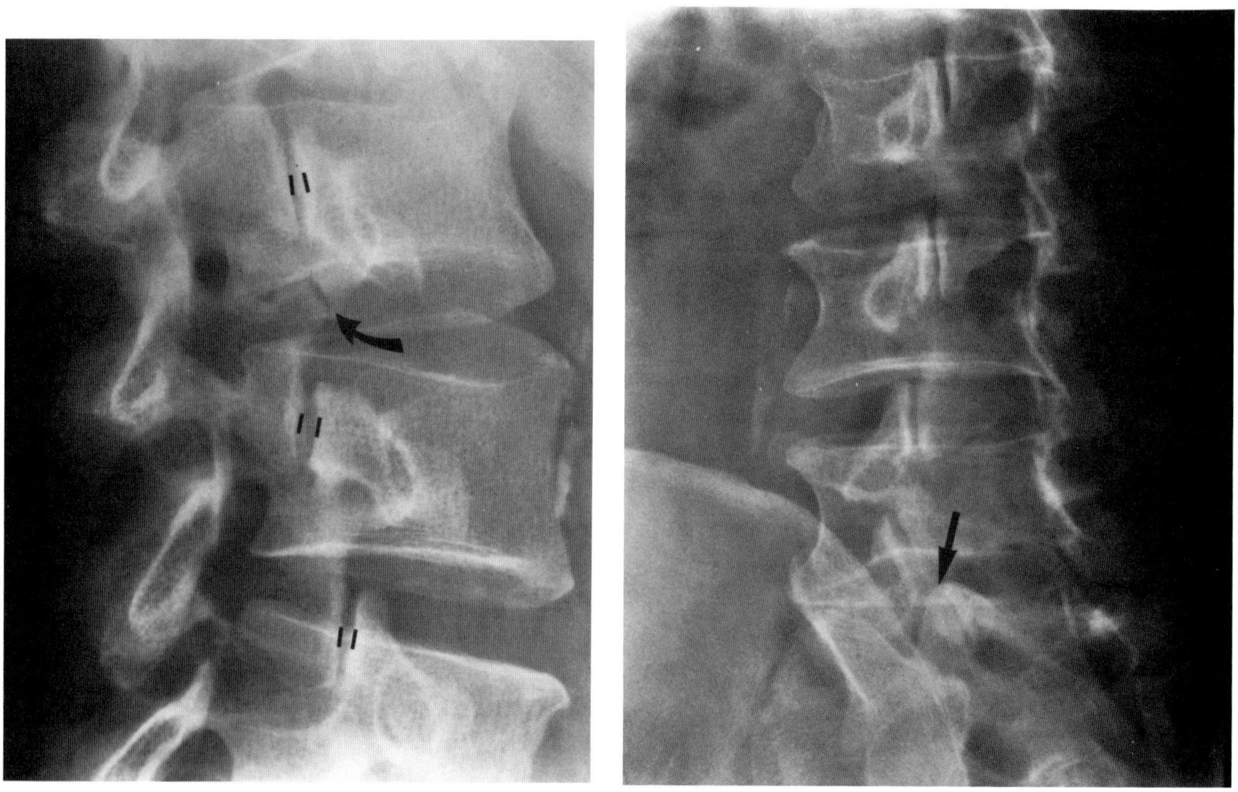

A B

FIG. 3-52. Oblique views of the lumbar spine. **A:** Oblique view demonstrating the facet joints (*vertical lines*) and an acute pars fracture at L-3 (*curved arrow*). **B:** Oblique view demonstrating a typical L-5 pars defect (*arrow*).

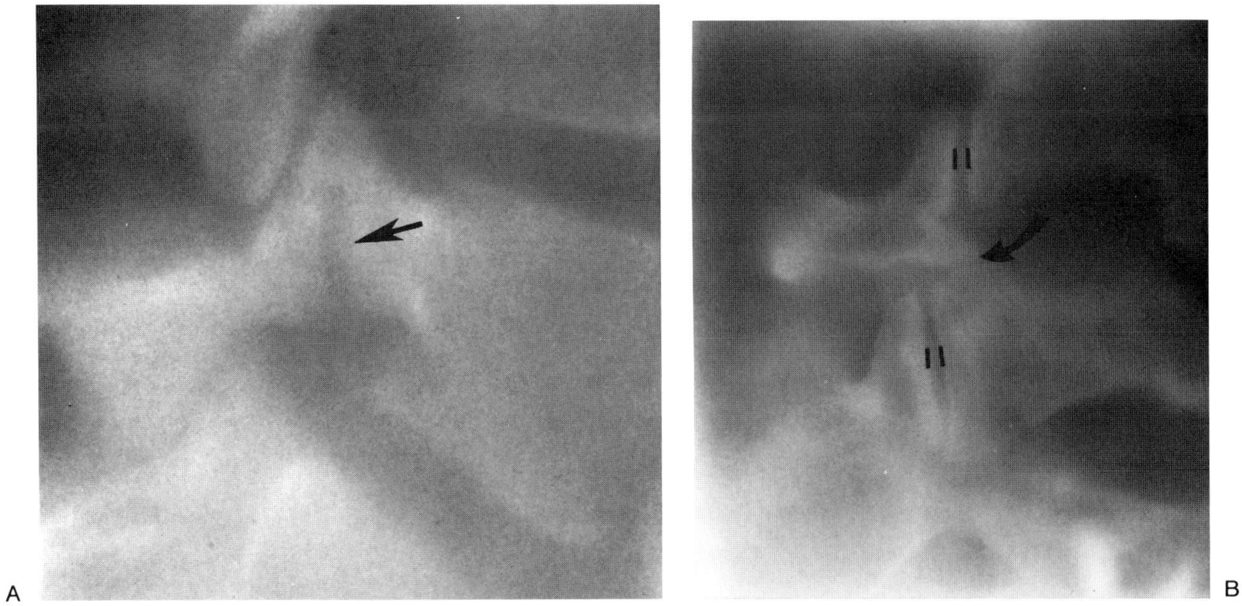

FIG. 3-53. Conventional tomography. **A:** Lateral tomogram demonstrating hockey-stick-shaped L-4 pars defect (*arrow*). **B:** Oblique tomogram demonstrating a pars defect (*curved arrow*).

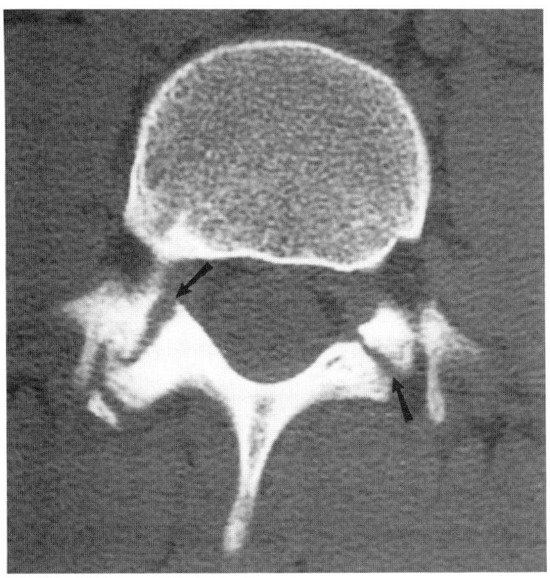

FIG. 3-54. Axial CT image at L-3 demonstrating bilateral pars defect (*arrows*). The facet joints at L-3 to L-4 are nearly straight in the AP plane.

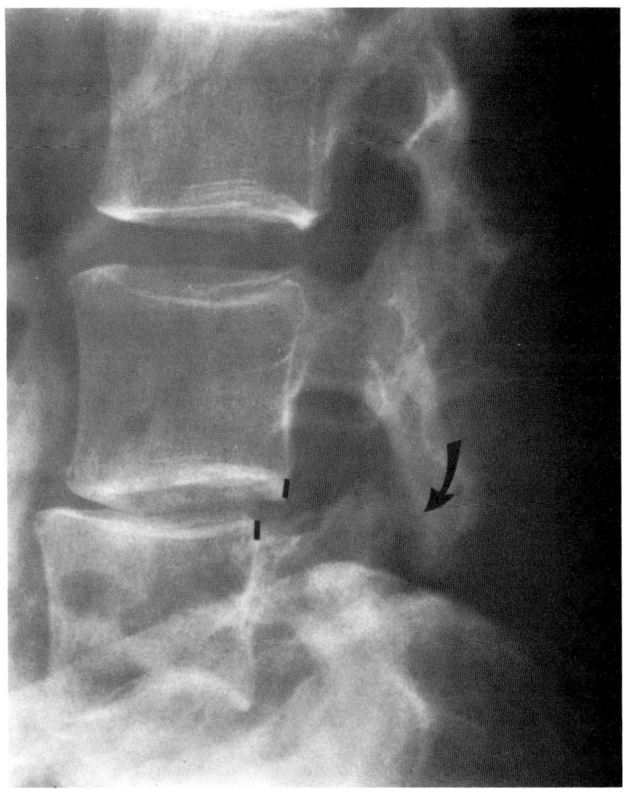

FIG. 3-55. Lateral view of the lumbar spine in a patient with retrolisthesis of L-4 on L-5. Note the L-4 disc space narrowing and widened facet joint (*curved arrow*) as a result of chronic laxity of the ligaments and capsule.

positron emission CT) are useful to identify and clarify the nature (active or chronic) of posterior element abnormalities in the spine.[63,90]

Posterior displacement of the vertebral body may also occur (retrolisthesis, Fig. 3-55).[64] This entity is commonly seen with degenerative disc disease. The incidence in the general population is 4.7%, which is about the same as that of spondylolysis. There is a tendency for retrolisthesis to occur in the upper lumbar region, especially L-2, and in the cervical spine. Most of the features are evident on the lateral view. Degenerative disc changes, abnormal lordosis, narrowing of the intervertebral foramina, prominent spinous processes, and facet joint abnormalities are usually present.[63]

Surgical Instrumentation

Many patients with spondylolysis have symptoms but require only conservative treatment. If symptoms are significant, especially if they are associated with neurologic signs of root irritation or cauda equina claudication, surgical treatment is justified. Spondylolysis of L 5 or grades I and II spondylolisthesis can be managed successfully with posterolateral L5-S1 fusion when low-back pain is the only presenting complaint or with removal of the posterior loose element of L-5 and posterolateral fusion when leg pain is also a problem; in the latter instance, decompression of the involved root (usually the L-5 or S-1 root) may require a rather extensive bony removal on the involved side.[111,117,118]

Grades III and IV spondylolisthesis require more extensive surgical procedures. Posterior decompression combined with L4-S1 lateral mass fusion is the procedure of choice. Attempts to effect reduction of the spondylolisthesis have been associated with a high complication rate but may be indicated in cases with a large slip angle or when the cosmetic deformity is severe.[62,65,66] In severe spondylolisthesis, anterior and posterior procedures may be necessary.[63,74,79,81,82,118]

There are several methods for the reduction or fixation of spondylolisthesis and other causes of lumbar instability. The type of fixation and number of levels fused depends on the degree of subluxation or instability and the type of instrumentation. One-level fixation (above and below) may be adequate for low-grade (grade I or II) displacement. Grade III and IV subluxations require two-level instrumentation.[63,66]

The indications and type of fixation vary with the specific clinical problem. Anterior fusion is used for patients with pseudarthrosis after posterolateral fusion, lumbar scoliosis, and postlaminectomy instability. Posterior fusion is more commonly used for multisegment instability.[82] Combined anterior and posterior instrumentation may be required for scoliosis with degenerative disc disease or postoperative flat back syndrome. Flat back syndrome (loss of lumbar lordosis) may be caused by distraction instrumentation. Knodt rods are an example of a distraction system that may cause this problem. Therefore, this technique is rarely used today.

Posterior Instrumentation

Extensive development of internal fixation implants for the lumbar and lumbosacral regions has occurred over the last decade. This section reviews posterior instrumentation and the evolution of these devices.[65,82,87]

Posterior instrumentation and bone grafting are used to maintain alignment and reduce the incidence of pseudarthrosis seen when bone grafting was used alone.[82] Early techniques included facet joint screws (pseudarthrosis rate, 12% to 55%) and spinous process plates (Fig. 3-56). Spinous process plates were bolted to the spinous processes. The pseudarthrosis rates were reduced to 6% to 15%.

Rod-Laminar Hook Instrumentation

There are several systems available using smooth, threaded, or ratchet-end rods.

Knodt Rod Instrumentation

This system was introduced by Knodt and Larrick in 1964.[82,104] Rods are threaded in opposite directions so that turning causes the cephalad and caudad laminar hooks to distract the lamina to which they have been attached (Fig. 3-57).

Knodt rods are indicated for one- or two-level lumbar fusions. They are used in conjunction with transverse process fusions, especially when laminectomies are performed.[104]

Knodt rods were thought to allow the opening of the intervertebral foramina, resulting in relief of nerve root compression.[86,104] This was accomplished by fusing the spine in flexion with these distraction rods.[86] Therefore, retrolisthesis is improved, but spondylolisthesis may be exaggerated.[104]

Disadvantages of this technique include S-2 nerve root impingement by the lower hooks. Rod removal, as a result of pain, may be required in 7% to 55%.[62,69]

Harrington Rods

The system consists of laminar hooks and rods for compression and distraction (see Scoliosis). The hooks are larger than Knodt rod hooks. The rods are generally bent to conform to the sacral lamina (Figs. 3-58 and 3-59). Square-end rods can be used to avoid rotation.

(text continues on page 147)

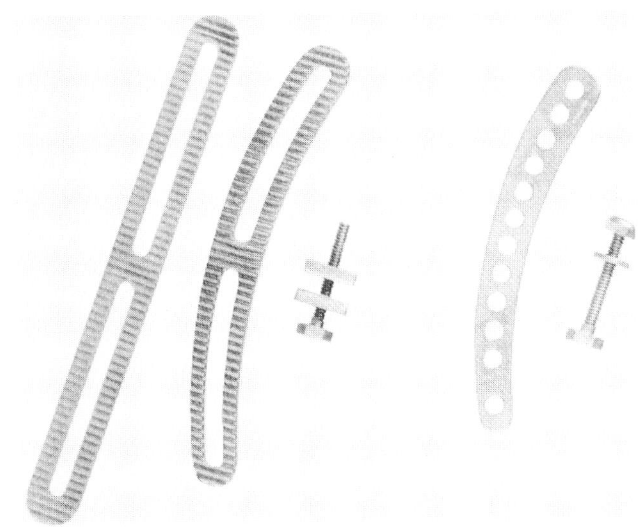

FIG. 3-56. Spinous process plates and bolts. (Courtesy of Howmedica, Rutherford, NJ.)

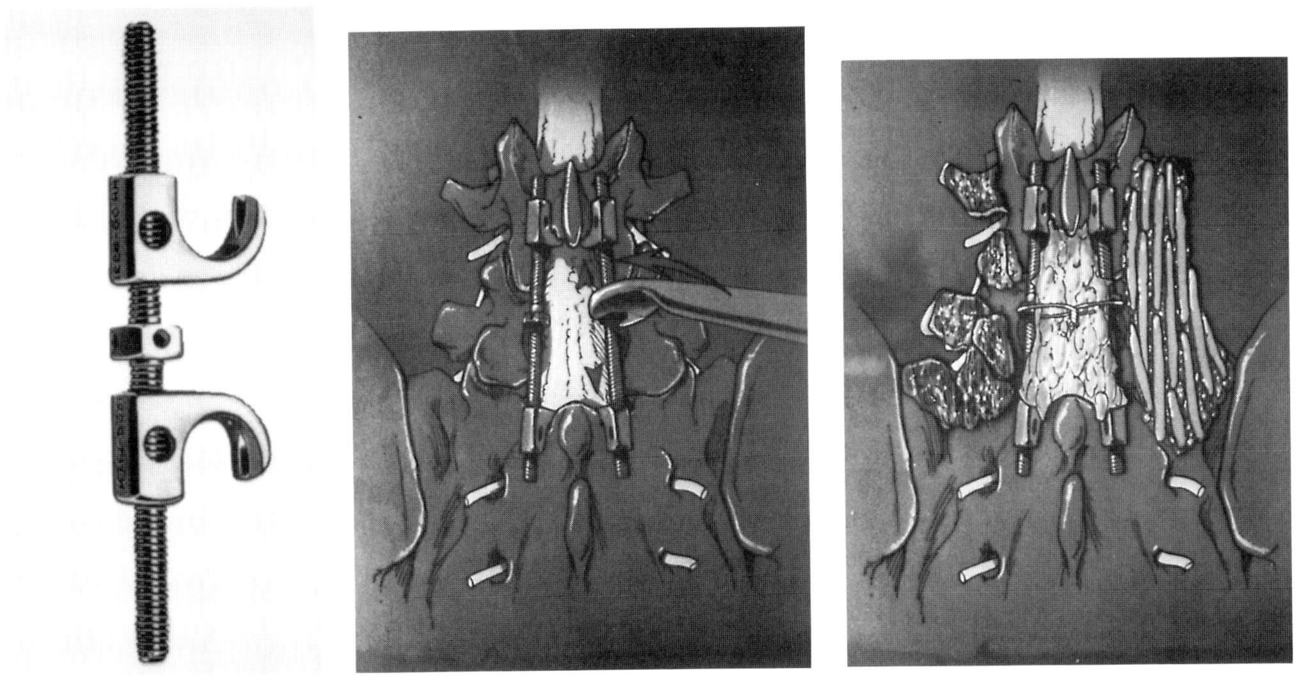

A B,C

FIG. 3-57. A: Knodt rod for lumbar fusion. Knodt rod with distraction hooks and central nut, which when turned, causes the hooks to separate. (Courtesy of Zimmer, Warsaw, IN.) **B:** Tightening the turn buckle to distract the hooks (*arrows*). **C:** Knodt rods, bone graft, and fat centrally to cover the dura. A transverse wire is also used to connect the rods. (B,C: From Selby D. Internal fixation with Knodt's rods. *Clin Orthop* 1986;203:179–184.)

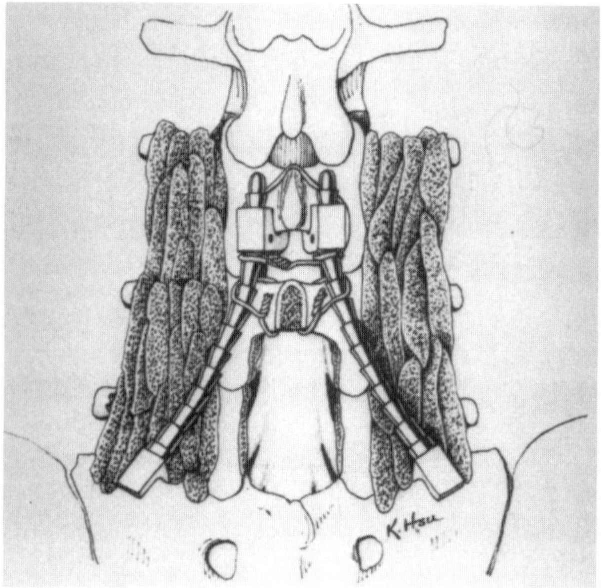

FIG. 3-58. Contoured Harrington distraction rods with upper wire support and posterolateral bone graft from L-3 to the sacrum. (From White AH, Zucherman JF, Hsu K. Lumbosacral fusions with Harrington rods and intersegmental wire. *Clin Orthop* 1986;203:185–190.)

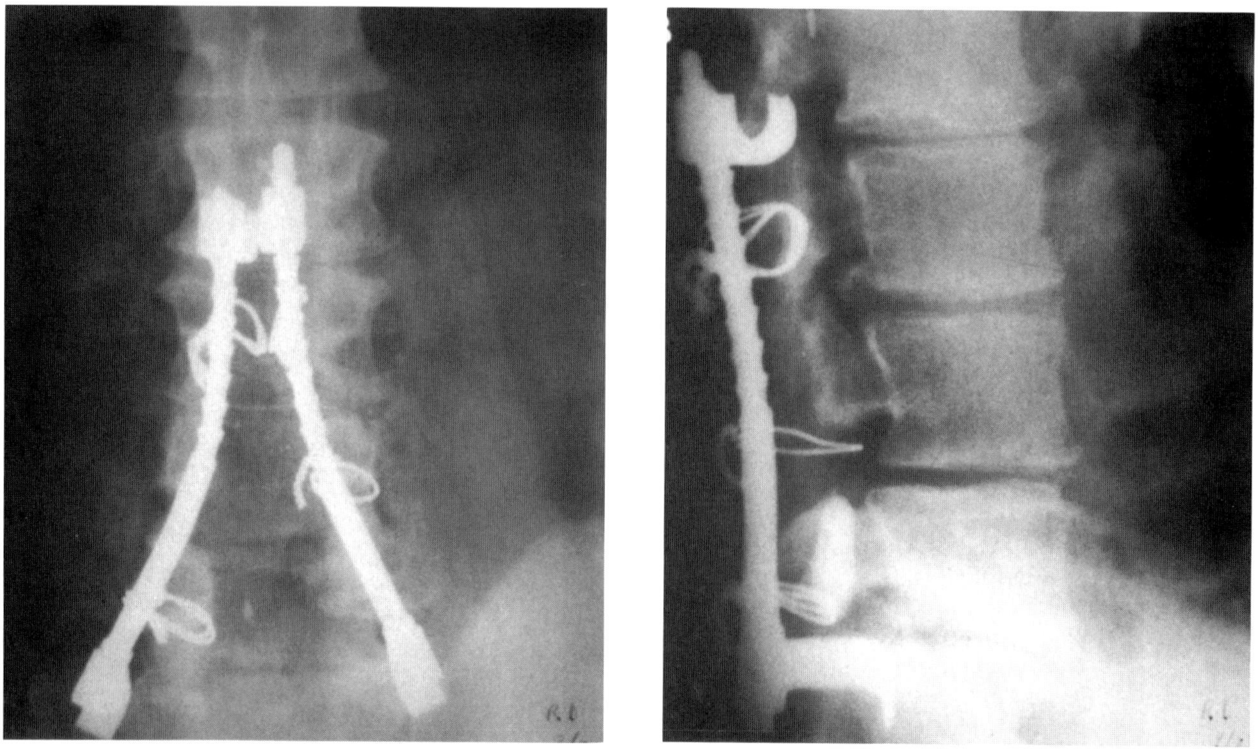

A B

FIG. 3-59. The AP **(A)** and lateral **(B)** radiographs of Harrington distraction rod and wire fixation. (From White AH, Zucherman JF, Hsu K. Lumbosacral fusions with Harrington rods and intersegmental wire. *Clin Orthop* 1986;203:185–190.)

Laminar wires are often used near the upper hooks (Fig. 3-58).[113]

The loss of sacral fixation and flat back syndrome seen with other posterior distraction devices were problems seen with Harrington distraction rods.[82,113]

Harrington compression rods (threaded, see Fig. 3-20C) apply a force opposite to that of distraction rods and can lead to lumbar extension. These implants are not commonly used for lower lumbar degenerative disorders.[82] Although preservation of lumbar lordosis is desirable, the implants may lead to narrowing of the neural foramina and central canal.

Smooth Rods or Rectangles

These devices are used to resist lateral motion and flexion and extension.[82] These systems are most often used for multisegment instability, such as degenerative disease or poststenosis decompression instability. Success rates for fusion are approximately 86% using Luque rods (0.25 inch). The rods are formed to maintain the lumbar lordosis and inserted distally into the ileum above the level of the sciatic notch. This technique was described by Allen and Ferguson.[59] Sublaminar wires are positioned at all levels, except laminectomy sites (Fig. 3-60). Instrumentation is supplemented with posterolateral iliac bone grafts.[79,80]

The risk of cord or dural injury can be reduced by placing wires through the base of the spinous process. Flexible mersilene tapes have also been used instead of wire.[82]

Both Luque (Fig. 3-26B) and Hartshill rectangles (Fig. 3-61A–C) with segmental wires can be used for lumbar fusion.[68]

Pedicle Screw Systems

Both rods and plates are commonly used with pedicle screws today. Plates can be configured in the sagittal plane; rods can be contoured in both planes. The indications and complications are similar; therefore, the selection of the system is usually based on the preference of the surgeon.[70–73,82,91,108–110]

Plate and Screw Systems

Plates and screws, most often transpedicular screws, are commonly used for spinal fusion.

Spinal Process Plates

The combination of spinous process plates and screws or bolts was introduced in the 1940s.[82] Several designs were used.[67,100,115] Wilson and Straub[115] used curved plates (Fig. 3-56), which were bolted to the spinous processes. Cabot et al.[67] designed a plate that crimped onto the dorsal spinous processes in the lumbar spine. The pseudarthrosis rates for these instruments were 15% and 6%, respectively. Other spinous process plates were also designed, but they are not commonly used currently in this country.[67,82,100,115]

Roy-Camille Plates and Pedicle Screws

The Roy-Camille system was one of the first plate and pedicle screw instrumentation methods.[79,103] The plates were configured to match the desired lumbosacral curve, providing good fixation (Fig. 3-62).[103] However, bone resorption under the plates can lead to screw loosening or fracture. Screws may toggle in the upper plate's holes, leading to similar problems.[79,82,103]

Steffee Plate and Pedicle Screws

Steffee et al.[109,110] designed a different plate and screw system in an attempt to address the "toggle" issue described earlier (Fig. 3-63). Using this system, the screw should be perpendicular to the attachment at the plate. This may be difficult to achieve, resulting in screw failure or bending as the nut is tightened.[72,82]

The screws are 5.5 to 7.0 mm in diameter with a dual-nut system to assist in proper positioning with the 16-mm wide notched plates (Fig. 3-64).[71] Modifications have been made in the original plate and screw design (Fig. 3-65).[91,108]

The results have been good thus far. Ninety percent of patients have good to excellent clinical results, and the operating time is short (3 to 4 hours).[69] To date, follow-up has been too short to provide an analysis of long-term results.

AO notched plates are configured with the holes closely spaced. The plates are used with 4.5-mm cortical and 6.5-mm cancellous screws.[73]

Figures 3-66 and 3-67 show radiographs of plate and screw systems.

Trapezoid and Rectangular Plates and Transpedicular Screws

Trapezoid plate and pedicle screws have been developed for spondylolisthesis. The procedure is combined with laminectomy and the removal of as much of the disc between the slipped segments as possible (Fig. 3-68).

The system consists of a trapezoid plate and four cannulated pedicle screws (6.6 mm in diameter and 49 to 52 mm in length). Kirschner wires (K wires) are used for positioning the screws.[77]

(text continues on page 154)

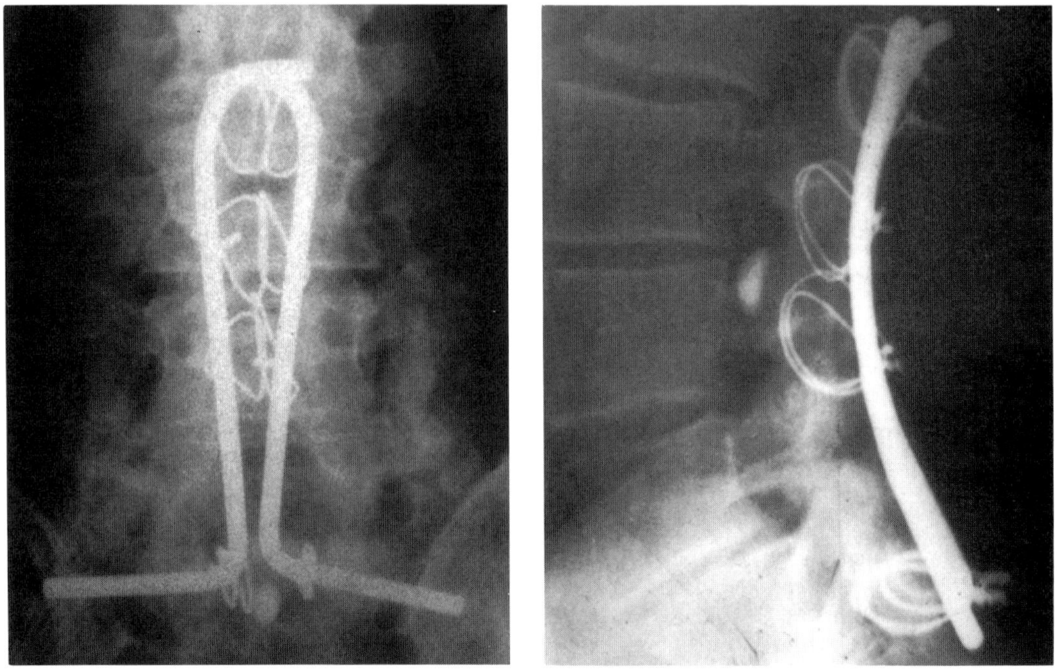

A B

FIG. 3-60. The AP **(A)** and lateral **(B)** Luque rod and sublaminar wire instrumentation from L-2 to the sacrum for degenerative lumbar disease. (From Kostuik JP, Errico TJ, Gleason TF. Luque instrumentation in degenerative conditions of the spine. *Spine* 1990;15:318–321.)

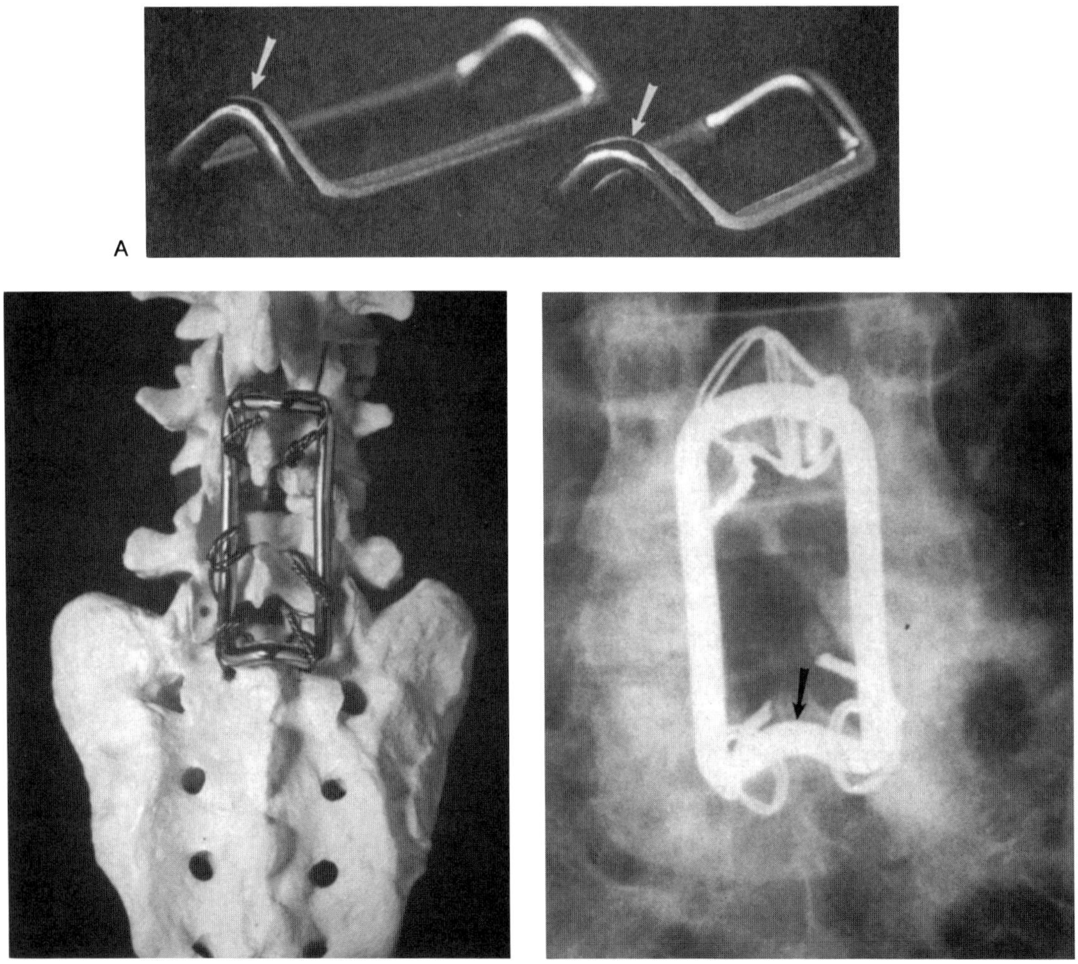

A B C

FIG. 3-61. Hartshill rectangles. **A:** Hartshill rectangles with peaked centers (*arrows*). **B:** Hartshill rectangles with wire fixation. **C:** An AP radiograph of Hartshill rectangle and sublaminar wire fixation. The peaked center (*arrow*) allows differentiation from the Luque rectangle. (From Dove J. Internal fixation of the lumbar spine. The Hartshill rectangle. *Clin Orthop* 1986;203:135–140.)

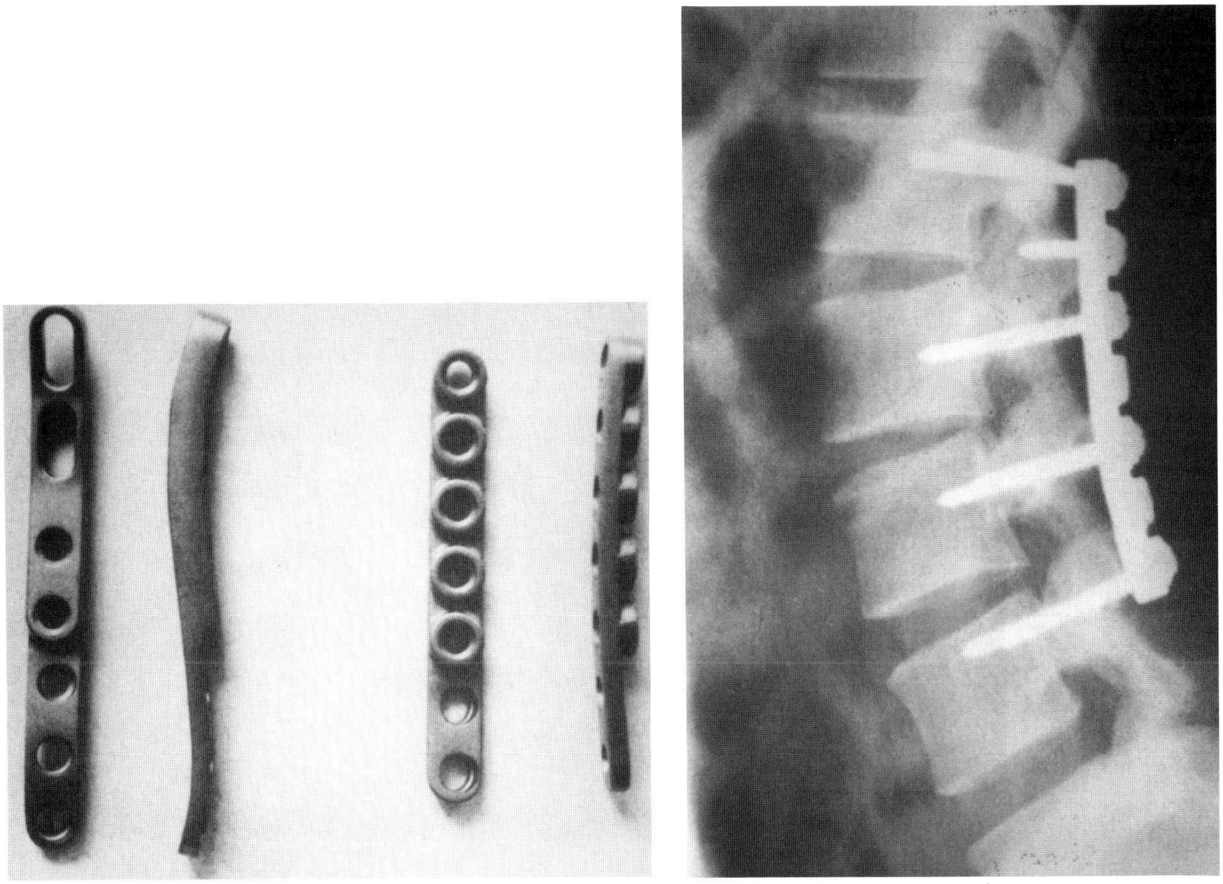

A B

FIG. 3-62. **A:** Roy-Camille plates. *Left:* The AP and lateral views of a plate used for spondylolisthesis from L-4 to S-2. *Right:* The AP and lateral views of the L-4 to S-2 fusion plate. **B:** The raised screw hole can be seen on lateral radiograph. (From Roy-Camille R, Saillant G, Mazel C. Internal fixation of the lumbar spine with pedicle screw plating. *Clin Orthop* 1986;203:7–17.)

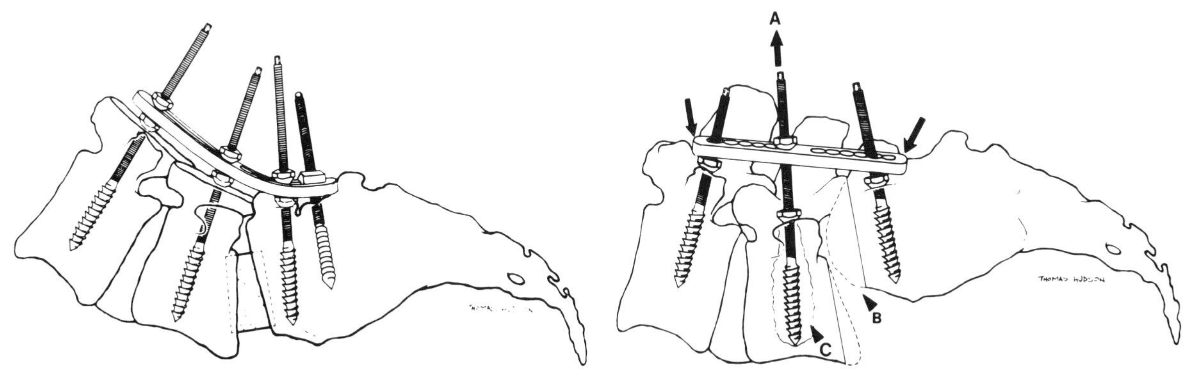

A B

FIG. 3-63. Steffee plate and pedicle screw technique. **A:** Reduction of L-5 to S-1 displacement with a prebent plate and screws in the body above and below. **B:** Reduction of grade IV spondylolisthesis reduced with screw and cement **(C)** in L-5. Bone (B) removed from the lower aspect of L-5 and upper S-1 (*dotted lines*). (From Steffee AD, Sitkowski DJ. Reduction and stabilization of grade IV spondylolisthesis. *Clin Orthop* 1988;227:82–89.)

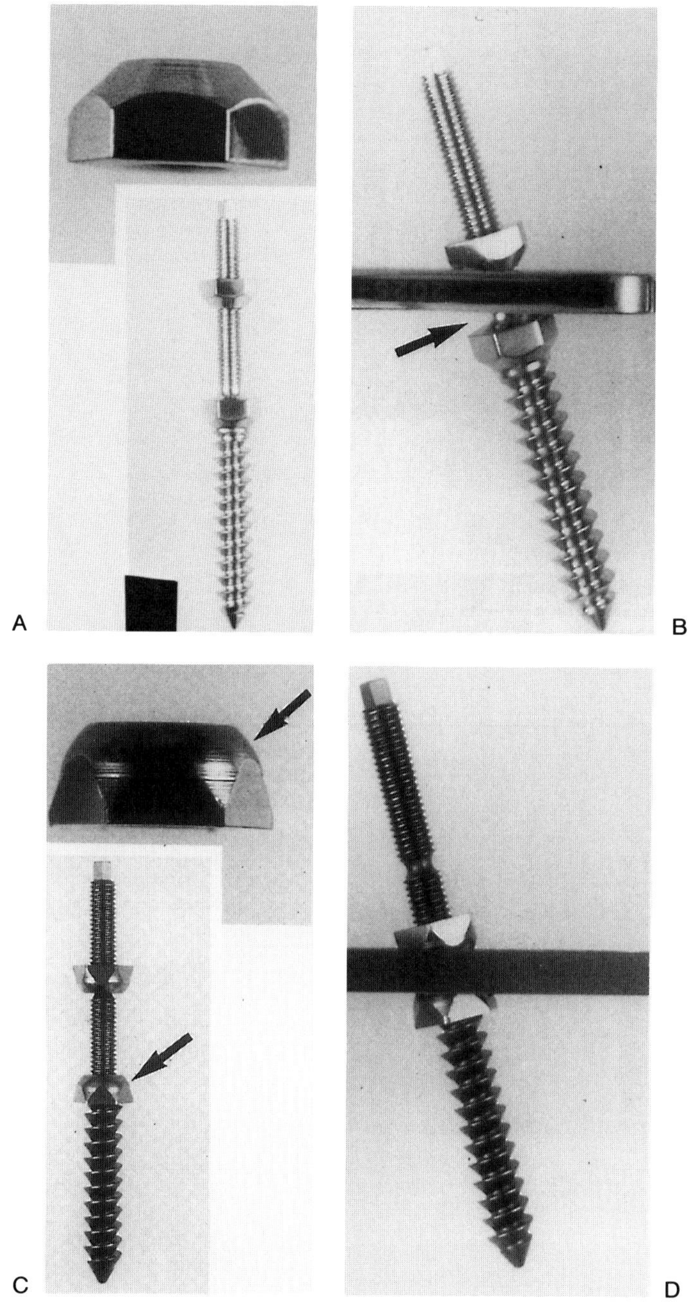

FIG. 3-64. **A:** Original screw and nut configuration. **B:** Lateral appearance of screw in plate. **C:** Modified nut configuration (*arrow*) and improved fit with plate **(D)**. (From Matsuzaki H, Tokuhashi Y, Matsumoto F, Hoshino M, Kiuchi T, Toriyama S. Problems and solutions of pedicle screw plate fixation of lumbar spine. *Spine* 1990;15:1159–1165.)

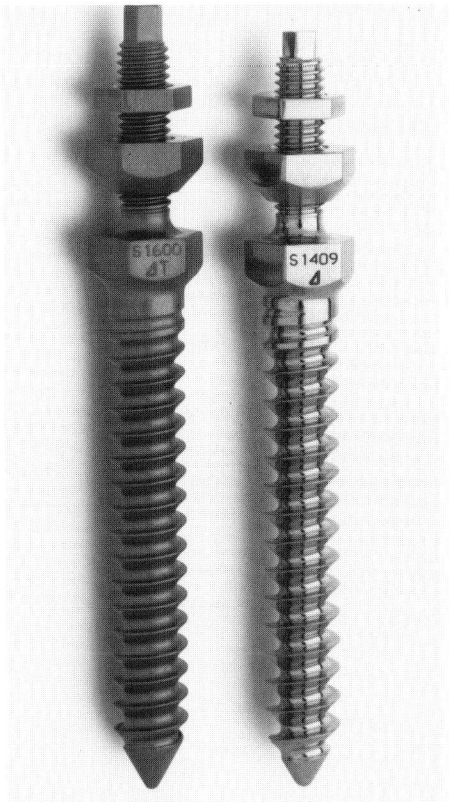

A

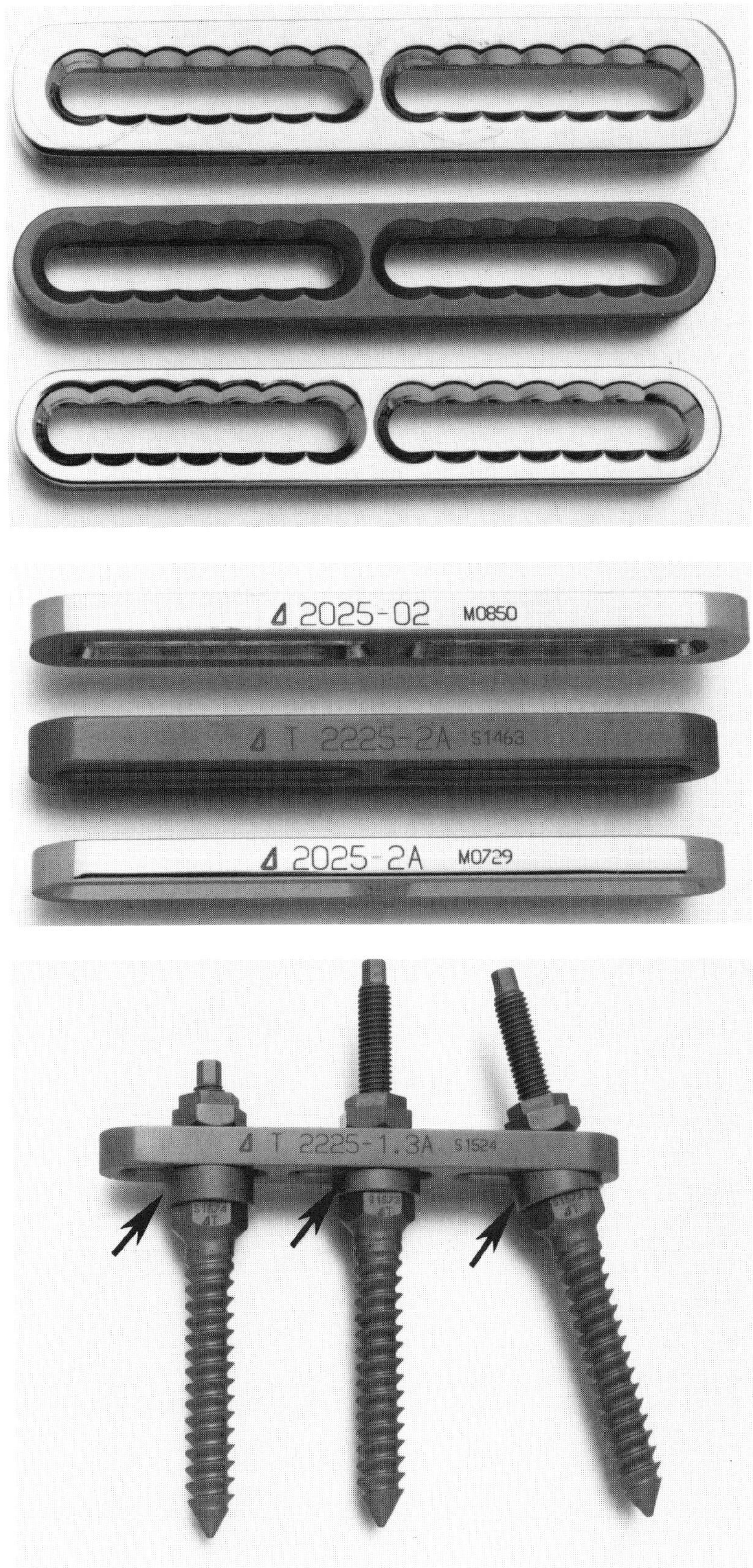

B

C

D

FIG. 3-65. VSP™ implants. **A:** Titanium (*left*) and stainless steel (*right*) screws. Plates seen from the top **(B)** and side **(C)**. **D:** Different washers (*arrows*) assist in screw positioning. (Courtesy of AcroMed, Cleveland, OH.)

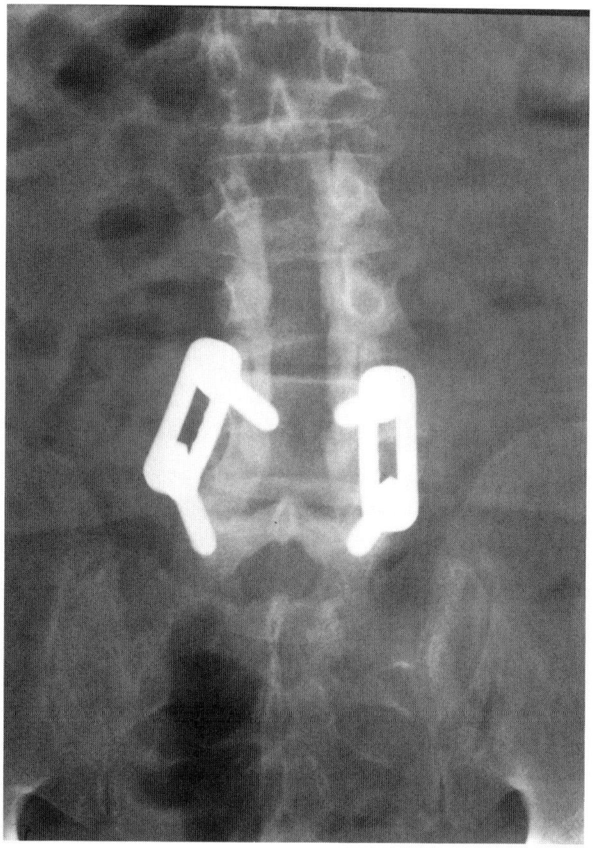

A

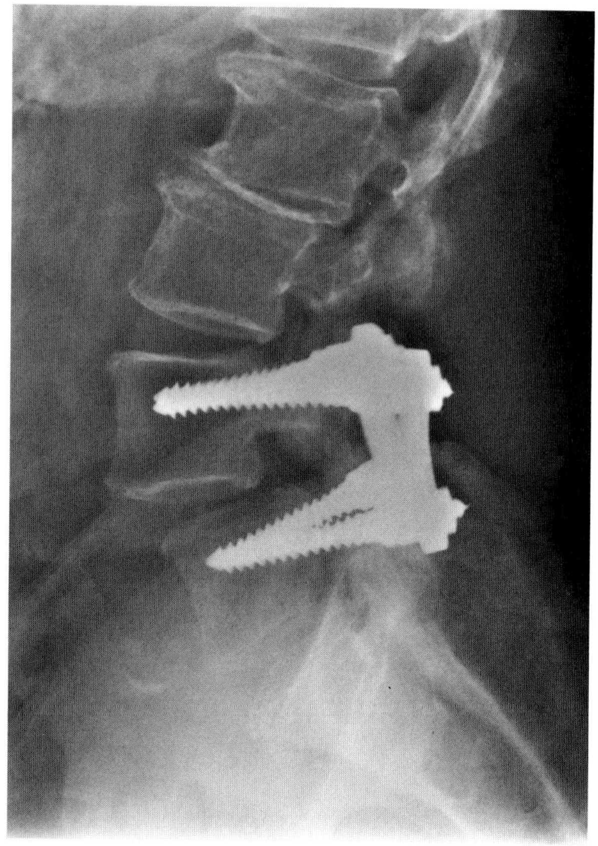

B

FIG. 3-66. The AP **(A)** and lateral **(B)** views of the lumbar spine with laminectomies at L-2 to L-4 and two short Steffee plates and pedicle screws for fixation of the L-4 to L-5 displacement.

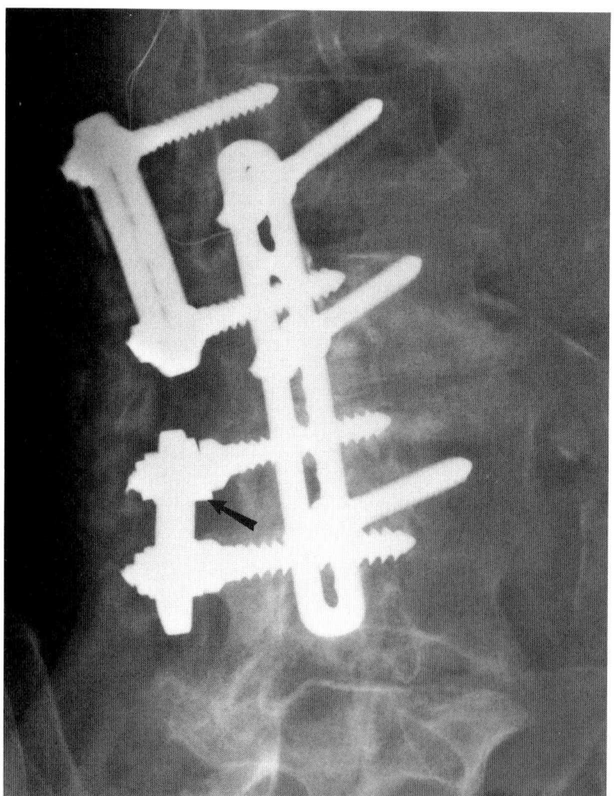

FIG. 3-67. Oblique view of the lumbar spine. There are two short Steffee plates on the left and a long plate with three screws on the right. Note the tapered washer (*arrow*) on the lower left plate.

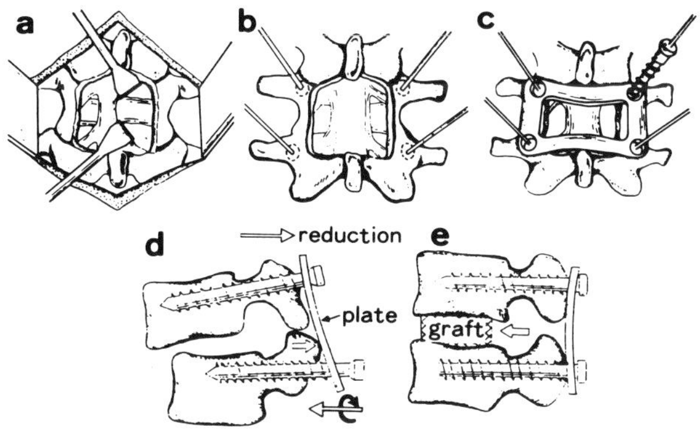

FIG. 3-68. Lumbar trapezoid plate and pedicle screws for instrumentation of spondylolisthesis. **A:** Wide laminectomy. **B:** Screw positioning. **C:** Plate positioned with K wires prior to screw placement. **D:** Leveraged reduction with plate and screws. **E:** Vertebra realigned with bone graft in the disk space. (From Kamioka Y, Yamamoto H. Lumbar trapezoid plate for lumbar spondylolisthesis. *Spine* 1990;15:1198–1203.)

A 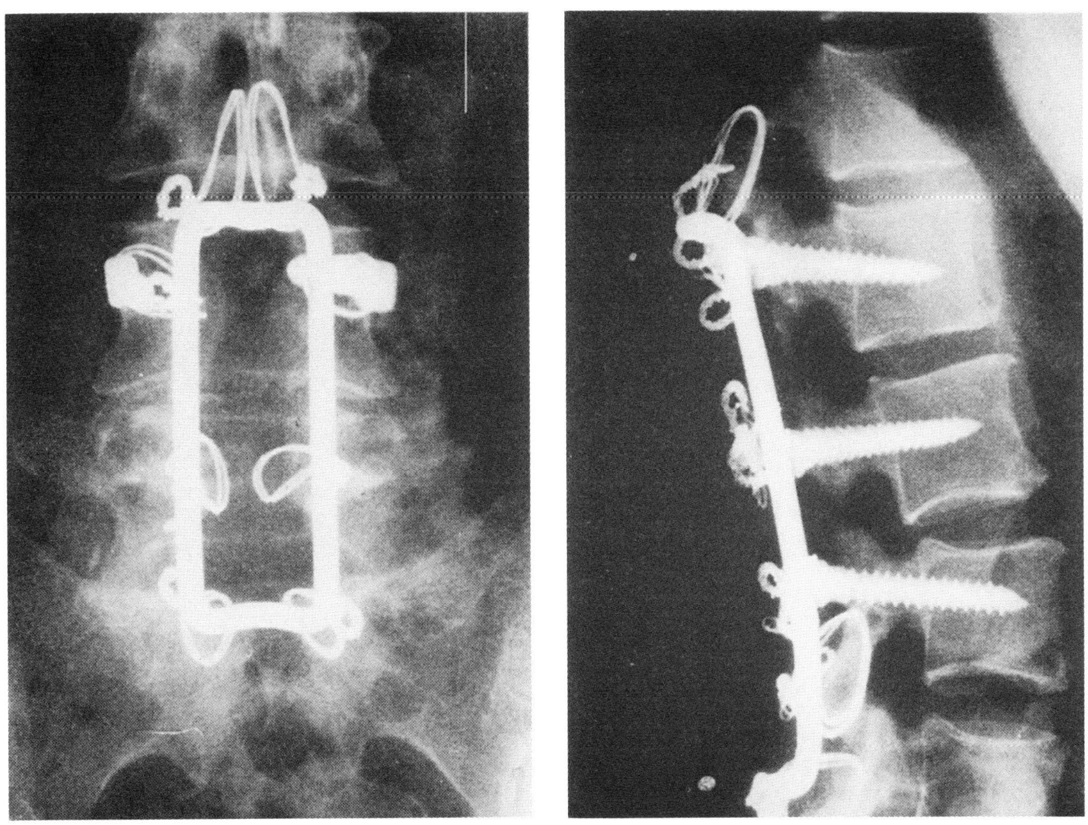 B

FIG. 3-69. The AP **(A)** and lateral **(B)** views of different patients with Hartshill rectangles with sublaminar wires (A) and Dwyer pedicle screws (B). (From Mehdian H, Jaffray D, Eisenstein SM. Dwyer-Hartshill transpedicular fixation for spinal fusion. *J Bone Joint Surg [Br]* 1989;71B:689–691.)

The Dwyer-Hartshill transpedicular technique combines the Hartshill rectangle described earlier with stainless steel Dwyer screws (Fig. 3-69).[92]

Rod and Pedicle Screw Systems

The main advantage of pedicle screw fixators is the long area of purchase provided by the screw, which assists in reduction maneuvers. Also, rods do not interfere with the bone graft bed as much as plate and pedicle screw systems do.[62,74,84,104] Although most early systems were designed for thoracolumbar fracture treatment, lumbar fusions are also possible with rod and pedicle screw instrumentation.[73]

Vermont Spinal Fixator (VSF)

The VSF is a simple system with few components. There are two 0.25-inch smooth rods, which come in lengths that vary by 1 cm and can be used for two to five segments (Fig. 3-70).[85]

Screws have blunt tips for safety and are self-tapping to avoid adjacent tissue injury. The screw has a side gear to adjust flexion and extension prior to inserting the bolt to the screw and rod clamp (Fig. 3-70).[84,85] The screws come in 5-, 6-, and 7-mm diameters, with lengths varying by 5 mm.

The indications are similar to those in other systems. The VSF may be used for trauma, spondylolisthesis, degenerative disease, and pseudarthrosis.[83,85]

This system allows three-dimensional positional adjustment and control and few parts with which to work; rod contouring is not necessary.[83–85]

Wiltse Pedicle Screw Fixation System

The indications for the Wiltse pedicle screw system are similar to those of other pedicle screw systems. The system consists of pedicle screws, saddle clamps, and rods that can be contoured to fit the desired curvature (Fig. 3-71A). An aluminum template rod is used to determine the desired contour for the permanent rod. One or two rods can be used on either side (Fig. 3-71).[72]

AO Spinal Fixator

The AO spinal fixator was originally designed for trauma. However, the indications have expanded to include those listed earlier. The system consists of two 7-mm stainless steel rods (7 to 30 cm in length), 5-mm diameter Schanz screws, and coupling clamps (Fig. 3-72).[70] When additional rotational stabilization is required, a transverse traction device is used to bridge the rods. This gives an appearance similar to the Cotrel-Dubousset system radiographically. The system can be used for compression, distraction, or derotation (Fig. 3-72).[70,71]

Zielke Transpedicular Instrumentation

The Zielke system is primarily used for ventral derotational fixation (Fig. 3-17). The system consists of two 3.2- or 4.0-mm rods, hexagonal nuts, and pedicular screws (Fig. 3-73). The system is less bulky than other systems, which allows generous bone grafting. Zielke instrumentation is usually only adequate for two- or three-level fixation. Cotrel-Dubousset or other pedicle screw-rod systems are often used in more active patients or when more segments require instrumentation.[105]

Rogozinski Spinal Rod System

This system was designed as a rigid spinal fixator to enhance fusion and allow early ambulation as with other systems. Like other rod-pedicle screw systems, it provides the advantages of a shorter length of instrumentation and a lower incidence of pseudarthrosis and flat back syndrome than do hook-rod systems.[101]

This system includes hooks, pedicle screws, rods, and cross bars (Fig. 3-74). Hooks are available in several configurations (neutral, up angle, and down angle) with a slot for the rod. The screws are cannulated to allow wire guidance. The rods have a 0.25-inch diameter and are nonthreaded and flared at one end. Cross bars are attached to the rod-screw assembly.[101] All implants are stainless steel (Fig. 3-74).

Other systems [Dick (AO fixation), Ölerud, and Edwards] are used for similar indications and have similar configurations.[82,99,106] The Cotrel-Dubousset, TSRH, and ISOLA systems described under Scoliosis are also used. These systems are particularly useful for longer-segment fusion revisions (Fig. 3-75).[72] As noted previously, the choice of plate-pedicular screw or rod-pedicular screw systems is heavily dependent on surgical preference (Fig. 3-76).

Imaging Evaluation and Complications of Lumbar Fusion

The evaluation of lumbar instrumentation and potential complications with imaging techniques, although similar in certain aspects, varies with the type of instrumentation and the suspected problem.[63]

A baseline lumbar spine series should be obtained as soon as the patient can tolerate the examination. Routine views should include AP, lateral, and oblique views. Care should be taken to modify centering so that the entire area of interest is included on a single film (Fig. 3-77). When appropriate, standing, lateral bending,

(text continues on page 161)

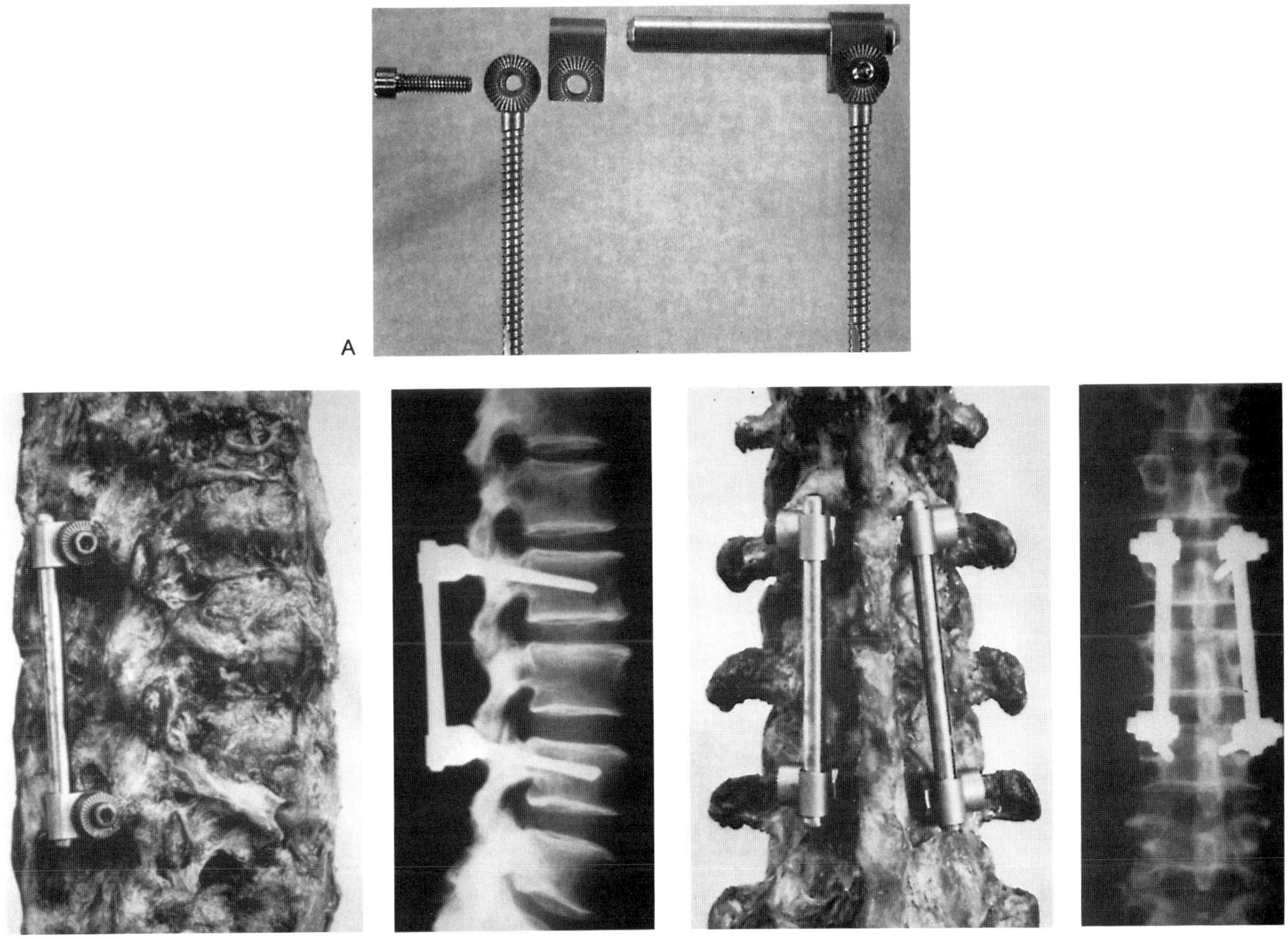

A

B,C

D,E

FIG. 3-70. The VSF. **A:** Components (*left* to *right*): clamp bolt, pedicle screw, articulating clamp, and connecting rod with components attached. Photograph **(B)** and lateral radiograph **(C)** of a cadaver spine with VSF instrumentation from L-2 to L-4. The pedicle screw tips are properly aligned and reach the proper depth. Photograph **(D)** and PA radiograph **(E)** of VSF from L-2 to L-4. (From Krag MH, Beynnon BD, Pope MH, Frymoyer JW, Haurgh LD, Weaver DL. An internal fixator for posterior application to short segments of the thoracic, lumbar, and lumbosacral spine. *Clin Orthop* 1986;203:75–98.)

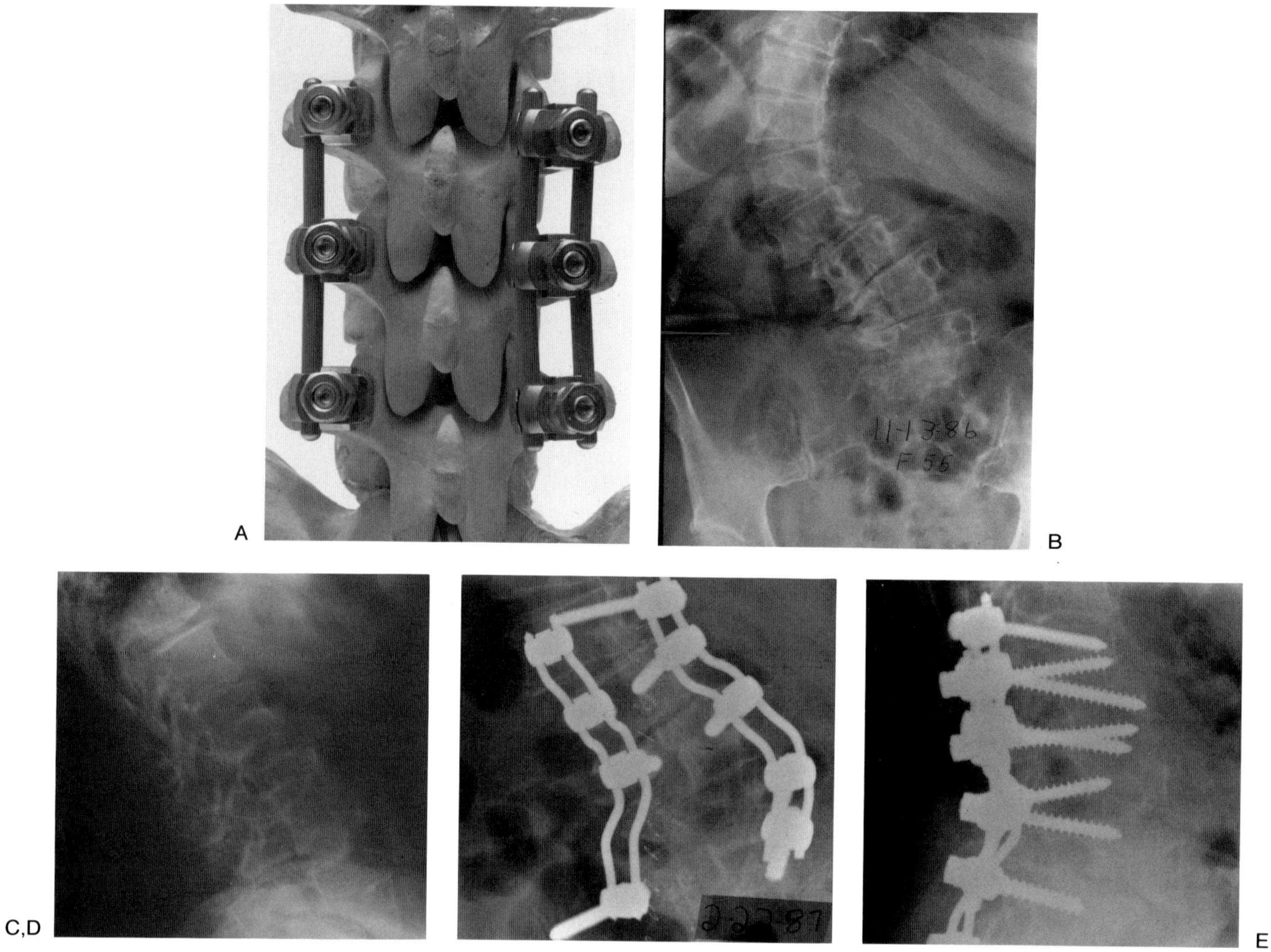

FIG. 3-71. Wiltse pedicle screw fixation system. **A:** The Wiltse system with a single rod on the left and double rods on the right. Preoperative AP **(B)** and lateral **(C)** radiographs of a patient with degenerative scoliosis. Postoperative AP **(D)** and lateral **(E)** radiographs using the double-rod technique right and left. (From Guyer DW, Wiltse LL, Peek RD. The Wiltse pedicle screw fixation system. *Orthopedics* 1988;11: 1455–1460.)

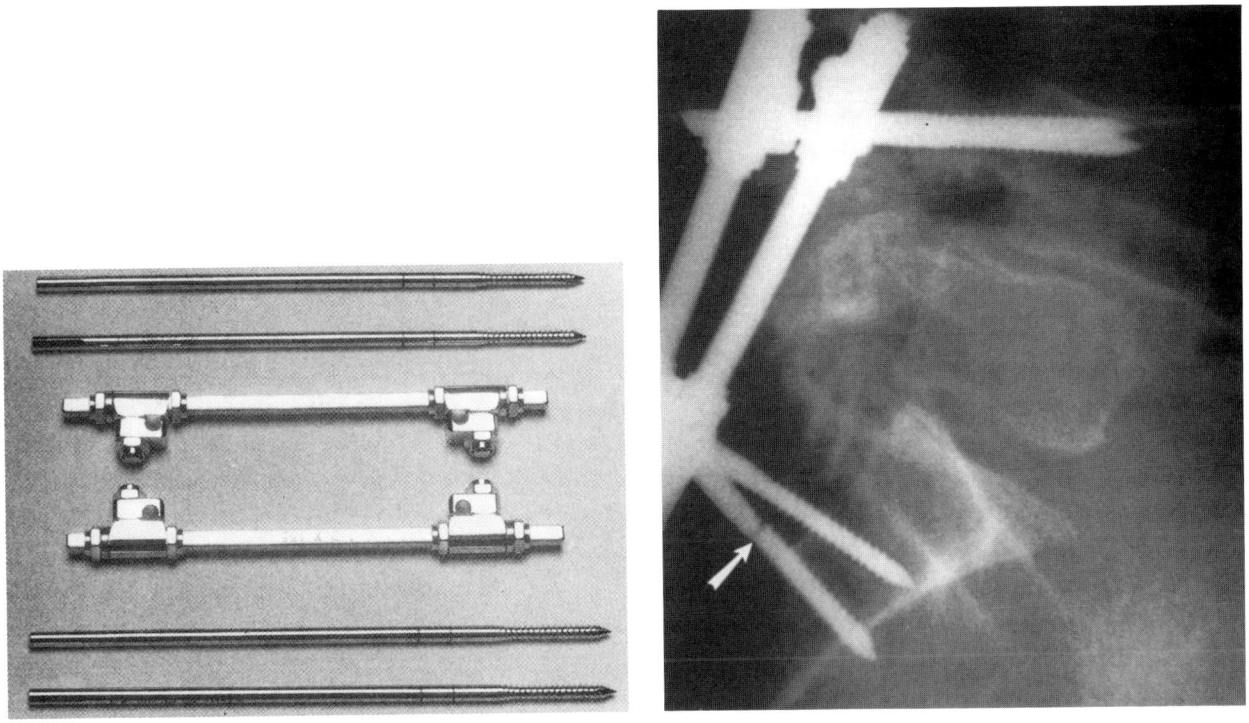

A B

FIG. 3-72. The AO spinal internal fixator. **A:** Components: 5-mm Schanz screws (*top* and *bottom*) and 7-mm flattened stainless steel rods. The coupling devices attached to the rods (*middle*). The Shanz screws provide long lever arms for reduction maneuvers. **B:** Lateral radiographs of an AO fixator for the reduction of L-4 to L-5 displacement. One of the lower screws has fractured (*arrow*). (From Esses SI. The AO spinal internal fixator. *Spine* 1989; 14:373–378.)

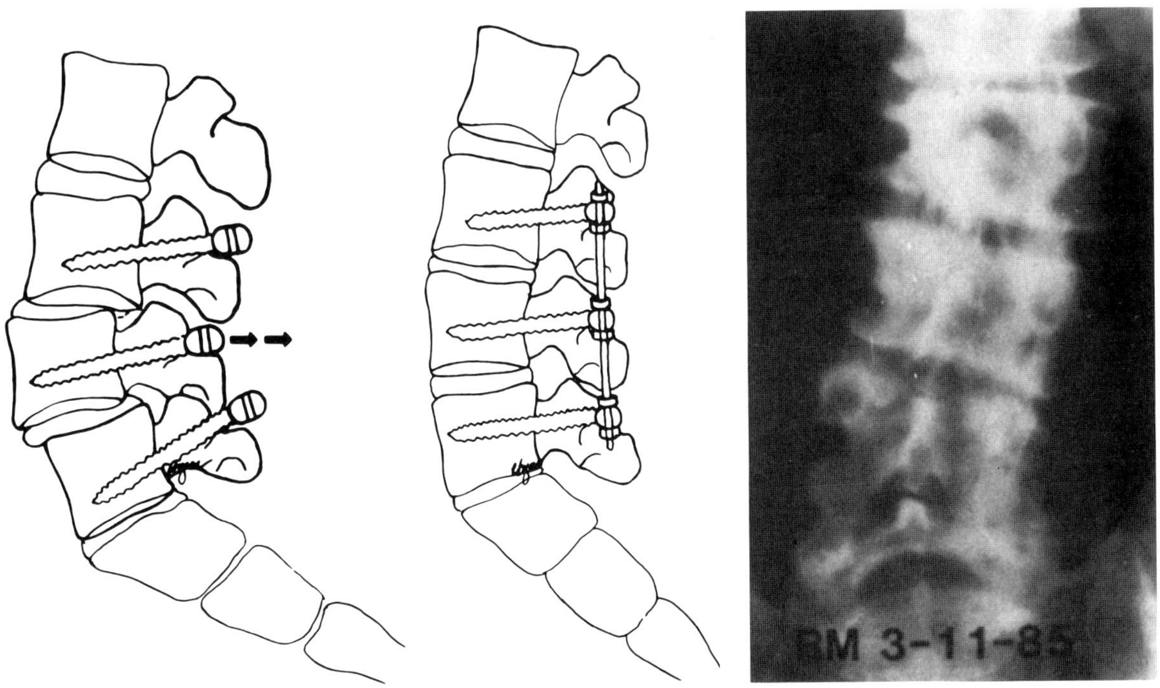

A B,C

FIG. 3-73. Zielke posterior instrumentation. Technique for the reduction of spondylolisthesis, showing pull back of L-4 **(A)** with threaded rod **(B)** to maintain alignment. **C-E:** The AP preoperative radiograph showing degenerative disease with scoliosis. The AP (D) and lateral (E) postoperative radiographs 1 year later showing solid L-2 to L-4 fusion. (See **D** and **E** on next page.) (From Simmons EH, Capicotto WN. Posterior transpedicular Zielke instrumentation of the lumbar spine. *Clin Orthop* 1988; 236:180–191.)

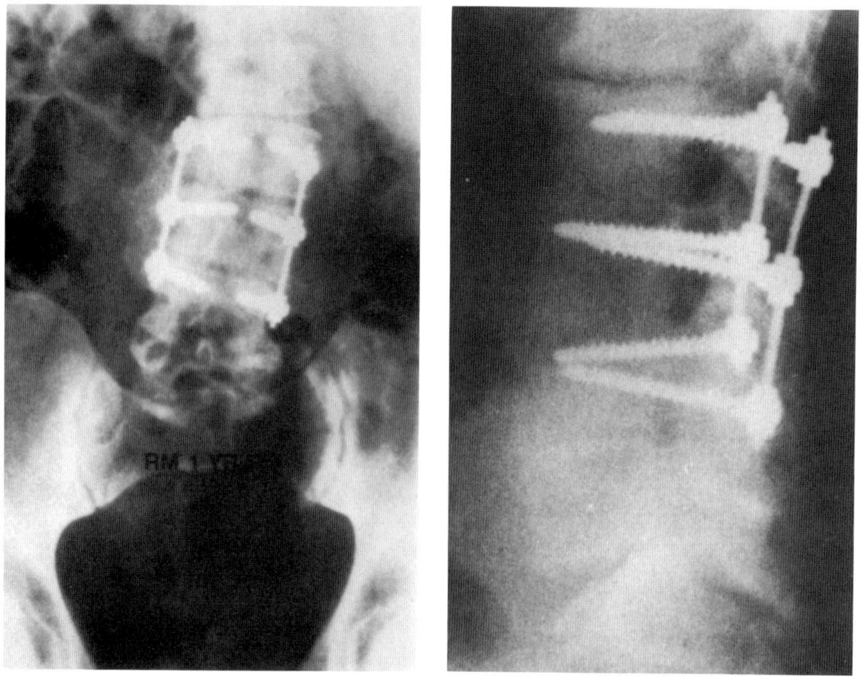

D,E

FIG. 3-73. *Continued.*

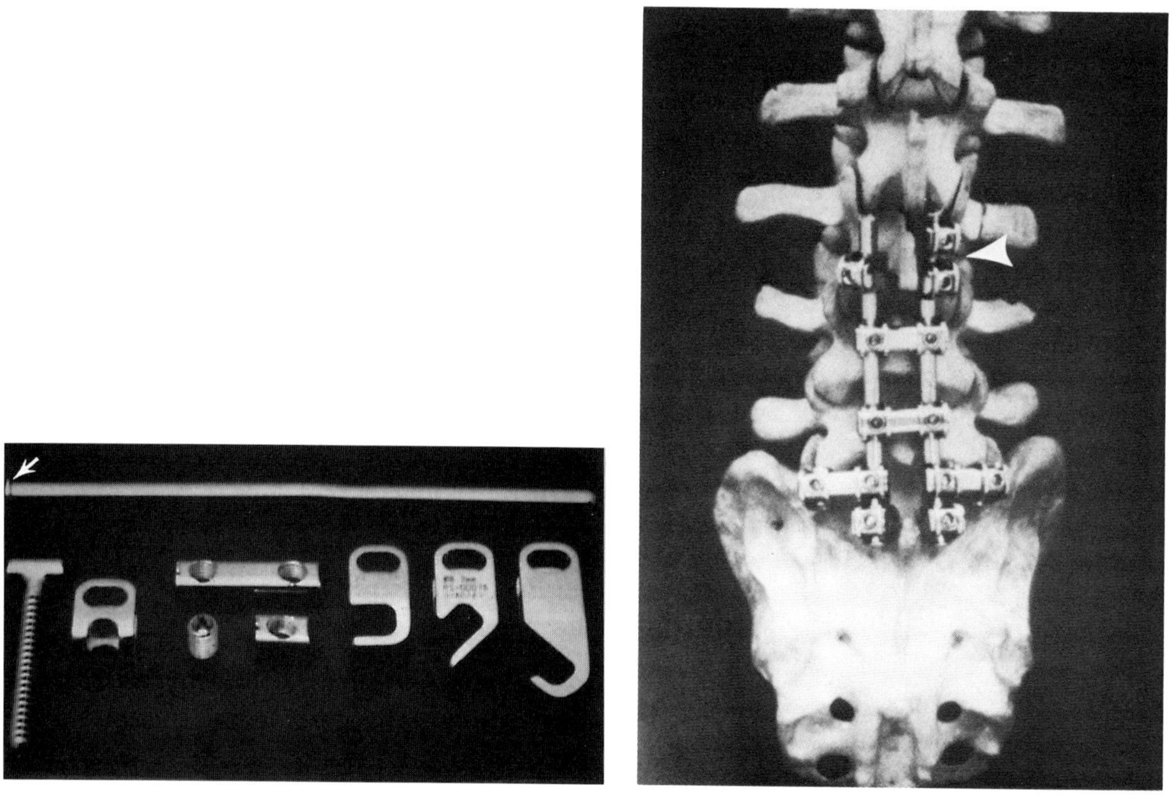

A

B

FIG. 3-74. Rogozinski spinal rod system. **A:** Components. *Top:* Rod with flare (*arrow*) at one end. *Bottom left, right:* Bone screw; coupler, cross-bar with set screw; and neutral, down-angle, and up-angle hooks. **B:** Photograph of system attached to skeleton. The S-1 pedicle hook and screw attachment. Unilateral double (sandwich) hooks at L-3 (*arrow*). (From Rogozinski C, Rognozinski A. The Rogozinski spinal rod system: a new internal fixation of the spine. *Spine* 1992;6:107–120.)

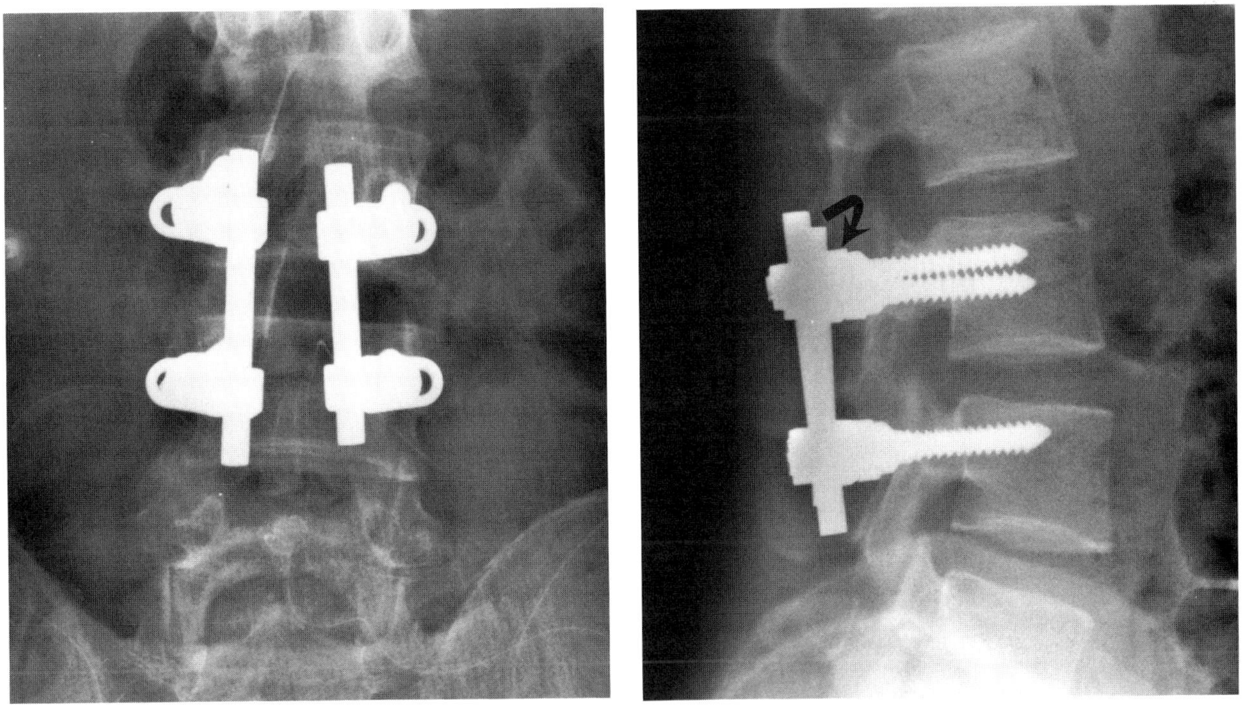

A B

FIG. 3-75. The AP **(A)** and lateral **(B)** radiographs of ISOLA instrumentation at L-3 to L-4 for bilateral pars defects. Note the position of the pedicle screws and tapered washer (*arrow*) on the upper screws (Fig. 3-34).

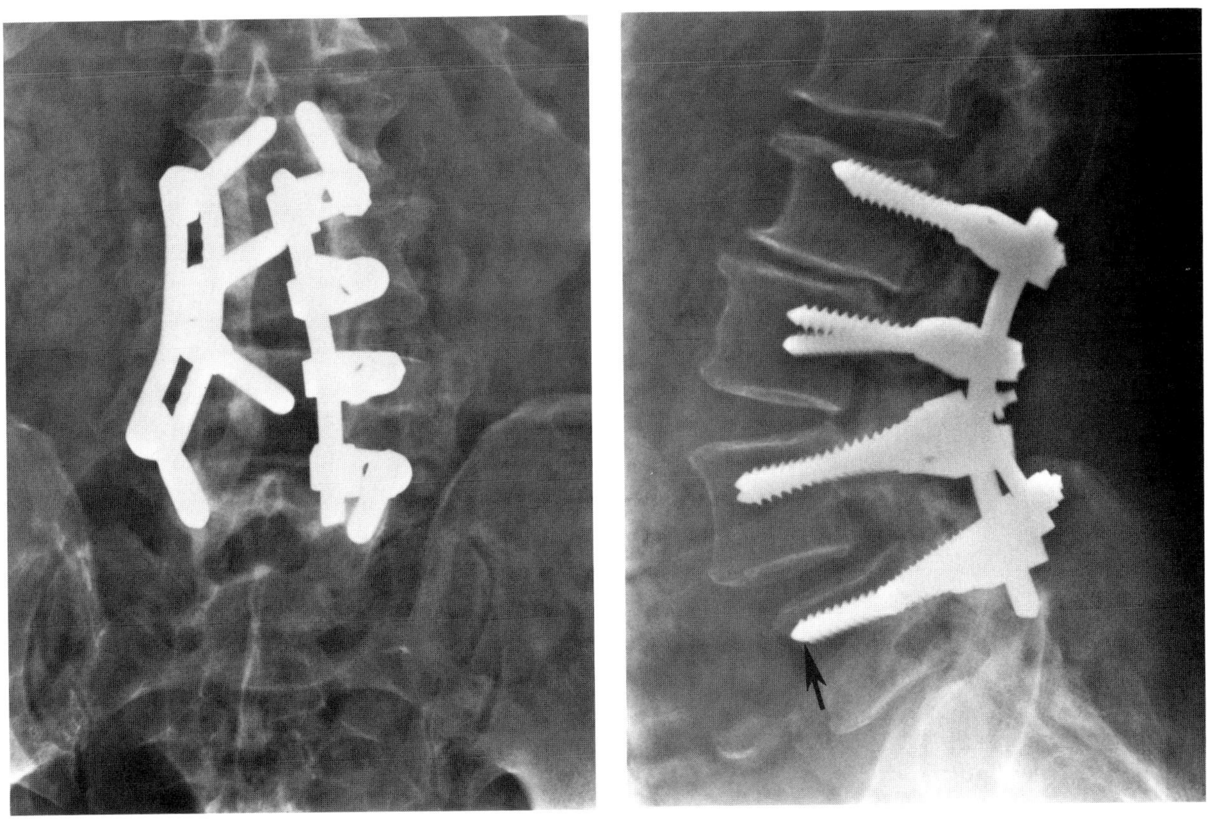

A B

FIG. 3-76. Degenerative disease with wide laminectomies from L-2 to L-5. The AP **(A)** and lateral **(B)** radiographs show degenerative subluxation of L-4 on L-5 and L-2 to L-3 retrolisthesis. Instrumentation with Steffee plate and pedicle screws on the left and ISOLA rod, four-rod connectors, and pedicle screws on the right. One of the pedicle screws in L-5 appears to extend too far anteriorly (*arrow*). Reconstructed CT or fluoroscopic positioning would assist in confirming this.

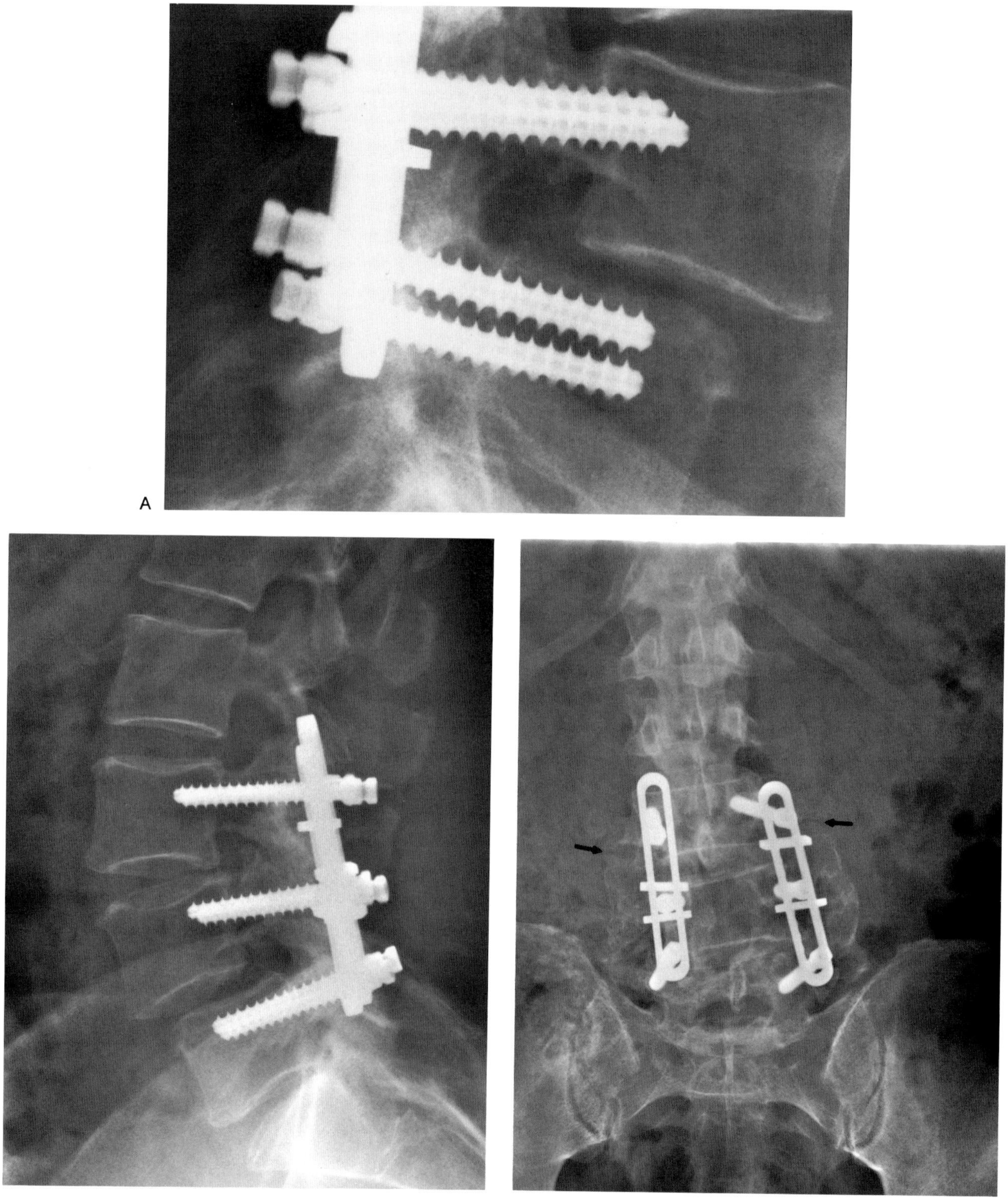

FIG. 3-77. Lateral radiograph after Luque plate and pedicle screw instrumentation at L-3 to L-4. **A:** Improperly coned lateral view does not include the entire operative site or implant. **B:** Lateral view showing the entire operative site and adjacent vertebrae allows proper evaluation. The transpedicular screws penetrate the vertebral body to a greater depth in L-5. The exact position cannot be determined from this view. **C:** The AP view shows the configuration of the Luque slot (compare with Steffee plates, Fig. 3-67). Note the iliac graft has not incorporated into the L-3 transverse processes (*arrows*).

flexion, and extension views should be obtained. Techniques should be performed so they are easily reproduced to ensure accurate comparisons on follow-up studies. Depending on the setting, repeat studies are typically obtained at 3, 6, and 12 months. Measurements made on the lateral view should be compared with those of preoperative examinations and evaluated on follow-up studies.[66] The kyphotic angle is also a useful indication of operative results (Fig. 3-77). Radiographic features, along with cosmetic and symptomatic results and neurologic improvement, are typically used to evaluate the surgical results.[60,66,82]

The disc space angle is formed by lines drawn on the opposing end plates (Fig. 3-78). This angle can be used to evaluate changes in kyphosis or lordosis pre- and postoperatively. The distance from the body cephalad to the tip of the superior articular facet (Fig. 3-78) can be used to evaluate the opening of the foraminal space.[86]

Imaging of complications can be accomplished with routine radiography in some cases. However, additional studies may be required, depending on the clinical setting. Table 3-7 summarizes common complications with common instrumentation techniques.[63,78]

Although many patients respond well to fusion, residual pain and concern regarding pseudarthrosis (Table 3-7) are common indications for more detailed postoperative imaging studies.

The incidence of pseudarthrosis varies with the technique, and it is also predictably higher when longer segments are fused.[98,101] Smokers also have a higher incidence of nonunion. Smokers accounted for up to 79% of nonunions in Rogozinski and Rogozinski's[101] series.

Most implants cause some degree of artifact on CT (Fig. 3-79) or MRI scans. The artifact on MRI scans is less significant with titanium implants than with stainless steel (Fig. 3-80). Also, screws tend to cause more artifacts on MRI scans; therefore, the likelihood of poor image quality is higher with transpedicular screw systems in which the metal surrounds the spinal canal, especially on axial images.[63,91] Conventional tomography is a good choice to assess bone graft incorporation in this setting. Differentiation between pain from pseudarthrosis or pain from other causes may require facet injections (Fig. 3-81B,C) or discograms (Fig. 3-81D,E) in the adjacent segments. This is easily accomplished using fluoroscopic guidance (Fig. 3-81).[63]

TABLE 3-7. *Lumbar instrumentation complications*[70,71,86,87,101,107,112]

Complication	Incidence rates (%)
Pseudarthrosis	5–32
Instrument failure	2–15
Neurologic	3–11
Implant removal	7–54
Removal for pain	3
Iatrogenic flat back syndrome	3
Infection	2.4

TABLE 3-8. *Indications for instrument removal*[84]

Impaired imaging assessment
Increased degenerative disease on adjacent segments
Increased infection risk
Long-term metal toxicity
Implant failure

Neurologic complications may result from improper positioning of transpedicular screws, placement of sublaminar wires, impingement of nerve roots by hooks (which is especially common at the sacral level), and loss of reduction. Screws are usually inserted at the junction of the transverse process and superior articular facet (Fig. 3-82). Preoperative planning with CT (Fig. 3-83) is recommended to reduce this problem.[82,84] The fixation achieved is optimal if the screw depth approaches the anterior cortex. This can be evaluated using lateral and oblique radiographs (Fig. 3-82), but CT is more accurate (Fig. 3-84).[82,107,112,114,119] Complications of pedicle screw placement are demonstrated in Figure 3-85.

Instrument failure (Fig. 3-86) may be associated with pseudarthrosis. Fracture of screws, rods, plates, and hook displacement should all be considered when viewing routine radiographs. Although many of these problems can be easily identified, subtle position changes may not be appreciated unless all films from the time of surgery are available for review. Most cases of hardware failure occur in the first few months after surgery.[75] Longer rods are also more prone to failure than are short-segment rods.[104]

Deep wound infections may be difficult to detect. Significant changes must occur before routine radiographs are abnormal. Thin-section (1 to 3 mm) conventional tomography or CT may demonstrate early bone destruction or sequestra. Combined bone scan imaging with technetium-99m and indium-111-labeled leukocytes may be useful in certain cases and is specific but not sensitive.[63]

Persistent pain and instrument failure may necessitate removal of the fixation devices (Table 3-8).[82]

TRAUMA

Imaging plays a significant role in the detection and classification of spinal injury.[120–124,139] Open or closed techniques are selected for therapy or fixation, based on the clinical and image features of the injury.[126,127]

Acutely injured patients with suspected spinal injury must be immobilized until the extent of the injury is defined and appropriate therapy is instituted. This requires close communication between the examining physician team and the radiologist. A well-organized approach en-

(text continues on page 169)

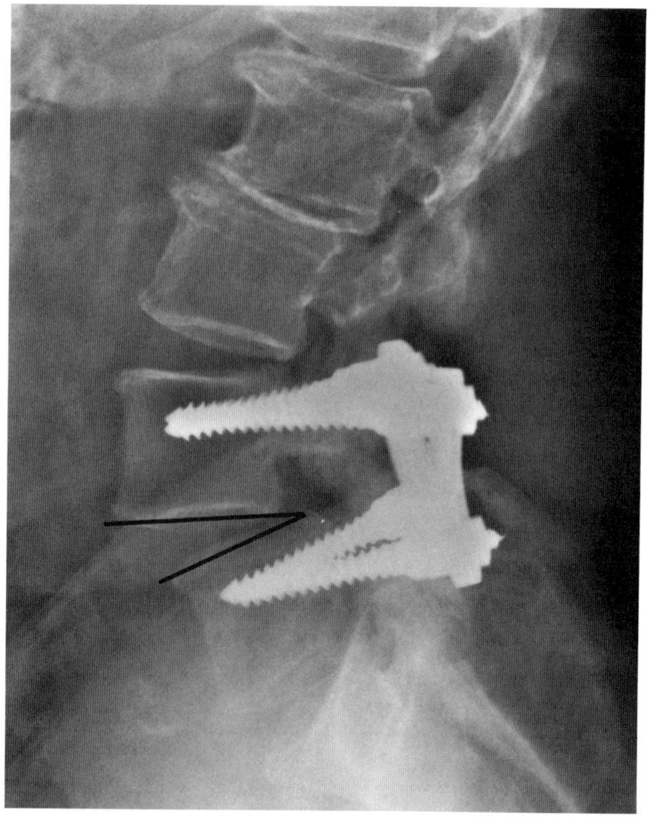

FIG. 3-78. Lateral view after Steffee plate and pedicle screw fixation for L-4 to L-5 displacement. The pedicle screws are in a good position and penetrate to the appropriate depth in the body. The disc space angle (line on end plates) shows an extended configuration (wider anteriorly).

A

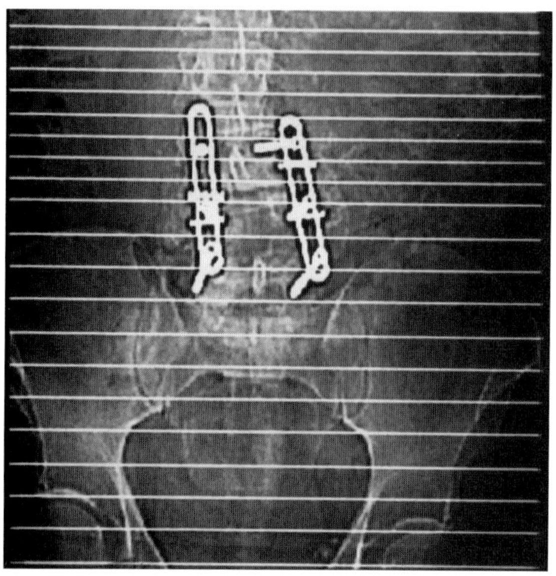

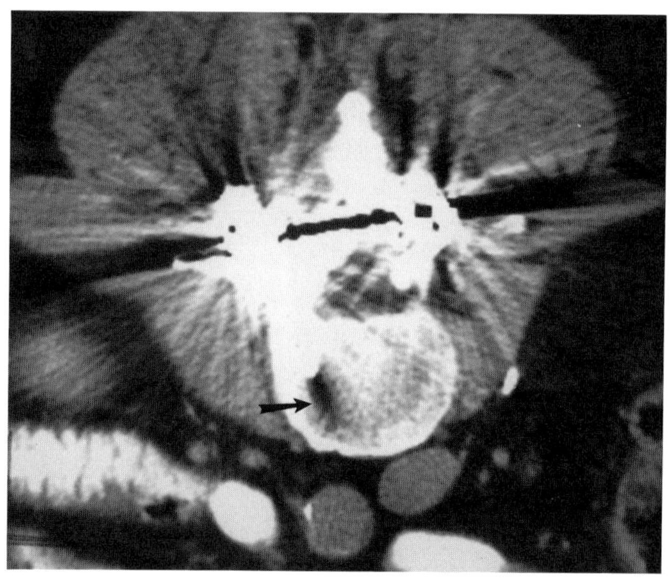

B

FIG. 3-79. The CT scout **(A)** and conventional axial image **(B)** after Luque plate and pedicle screw instrumentation. There is a significant artifact, degrading the detail in the spinal canal and making the exact location of the pedicle screw tip (*arrow*) difficult to identify.

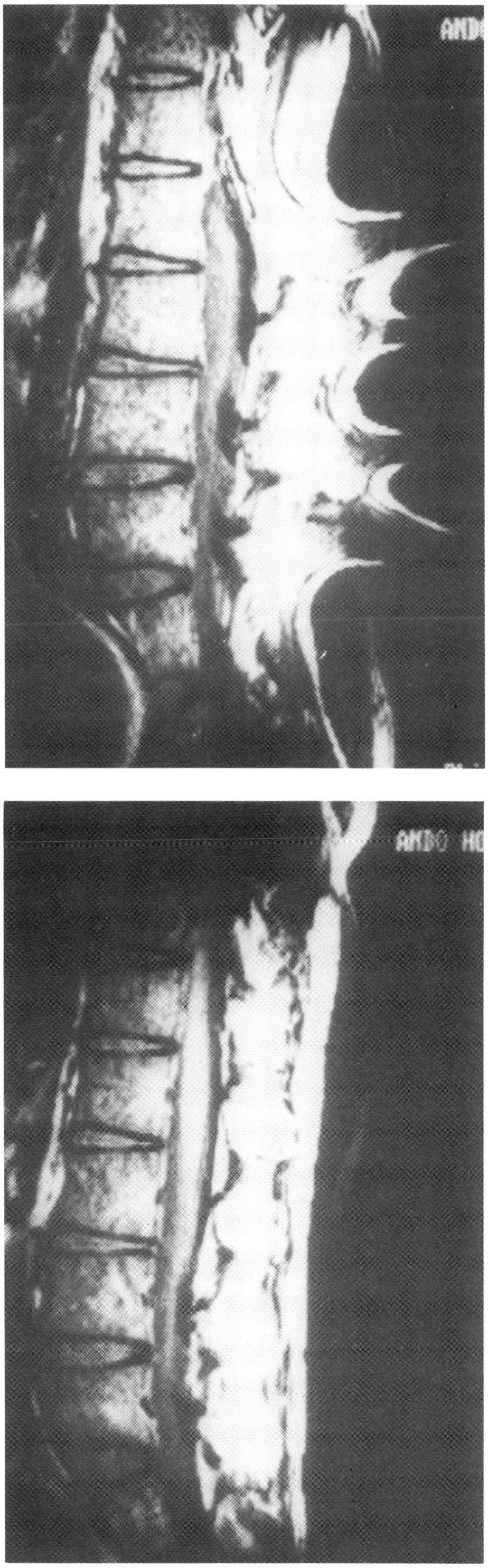

A

B

FIG. 3-80. Sagittal MRI scans with stainless steel **(A)** and titanium **(B)** implants. Note the reduction in artifact in B. (From Matsuzaki H, Tokuhashi Y, Matsumoto F, Hoshino M, Kiuchi T, Toriyama S. Problems and solutions of pedicle screw plate fixation of lumbar spine. *Spine* 1990;15:1159–1165.)

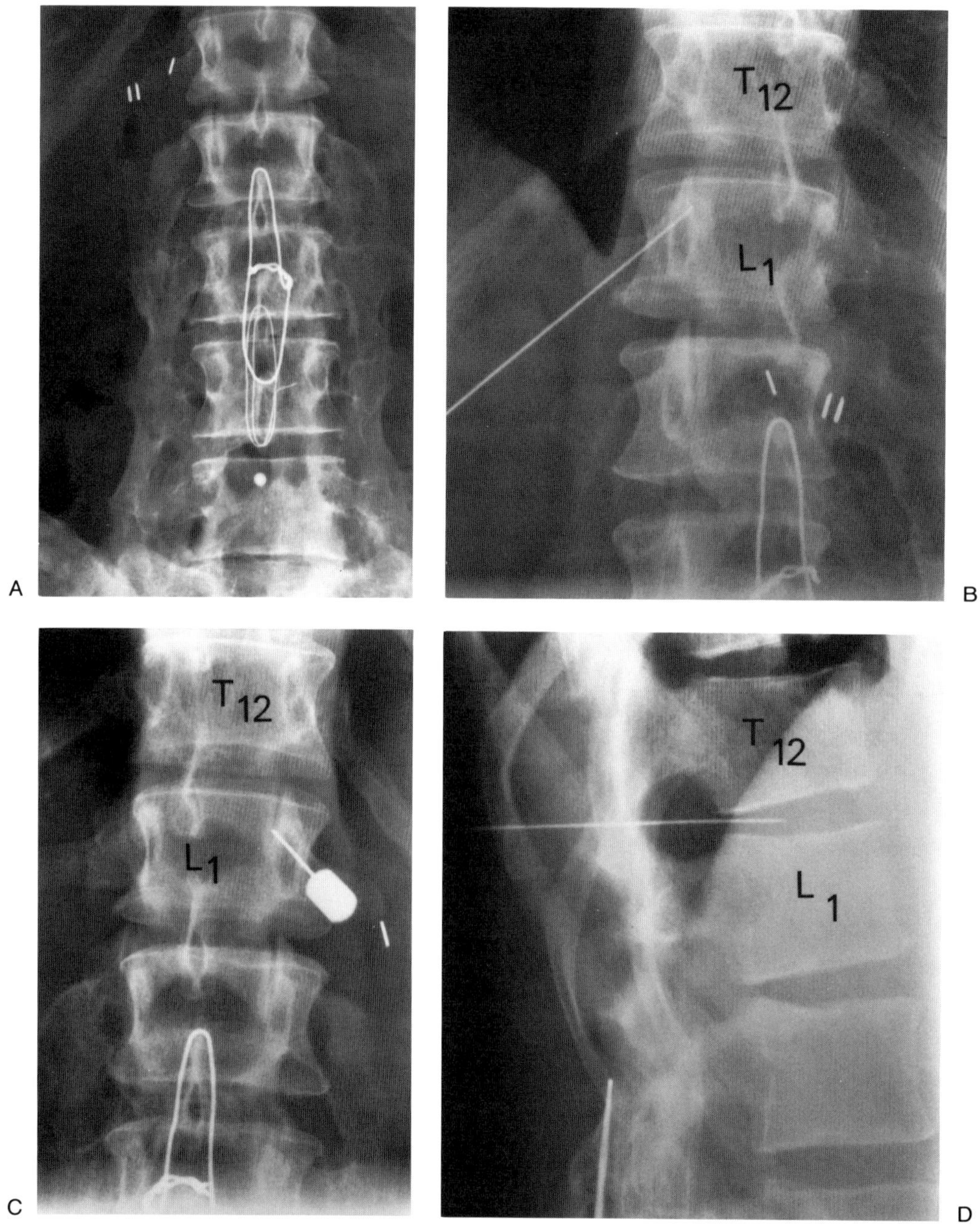

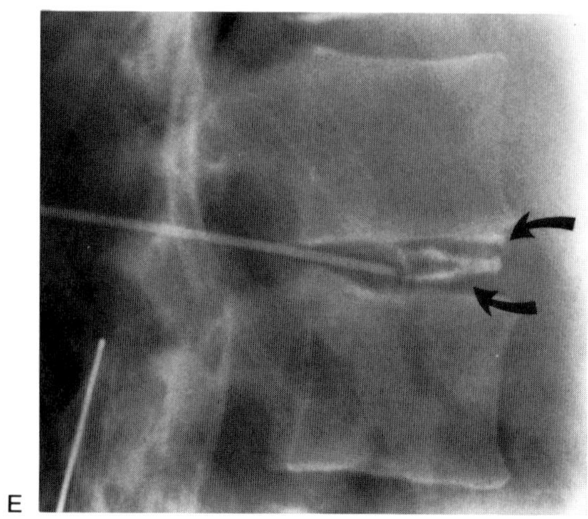

FIG. 3-81. Patient with multiple fusions and midback pain. **A:** The AP radiograph shows bone graft from L-2 to the sacrum, with spinous process wires L-2 to L-4. There were previous hemilaminectomies at L-4 and L-5 on the right. **B,C:** Facet injections, using Xylocaine™ or Marcaine™, can be performed to determine whether this is the site of the symptoms. Fluoroscopic guidance is essential. Discograms can be used to characterize symptoms and evaluate disc anatomy prior to considering further surgery. **D:** Needle in place. **E:** Normal anterior disk (*arrows*) with deformity posteriorly.

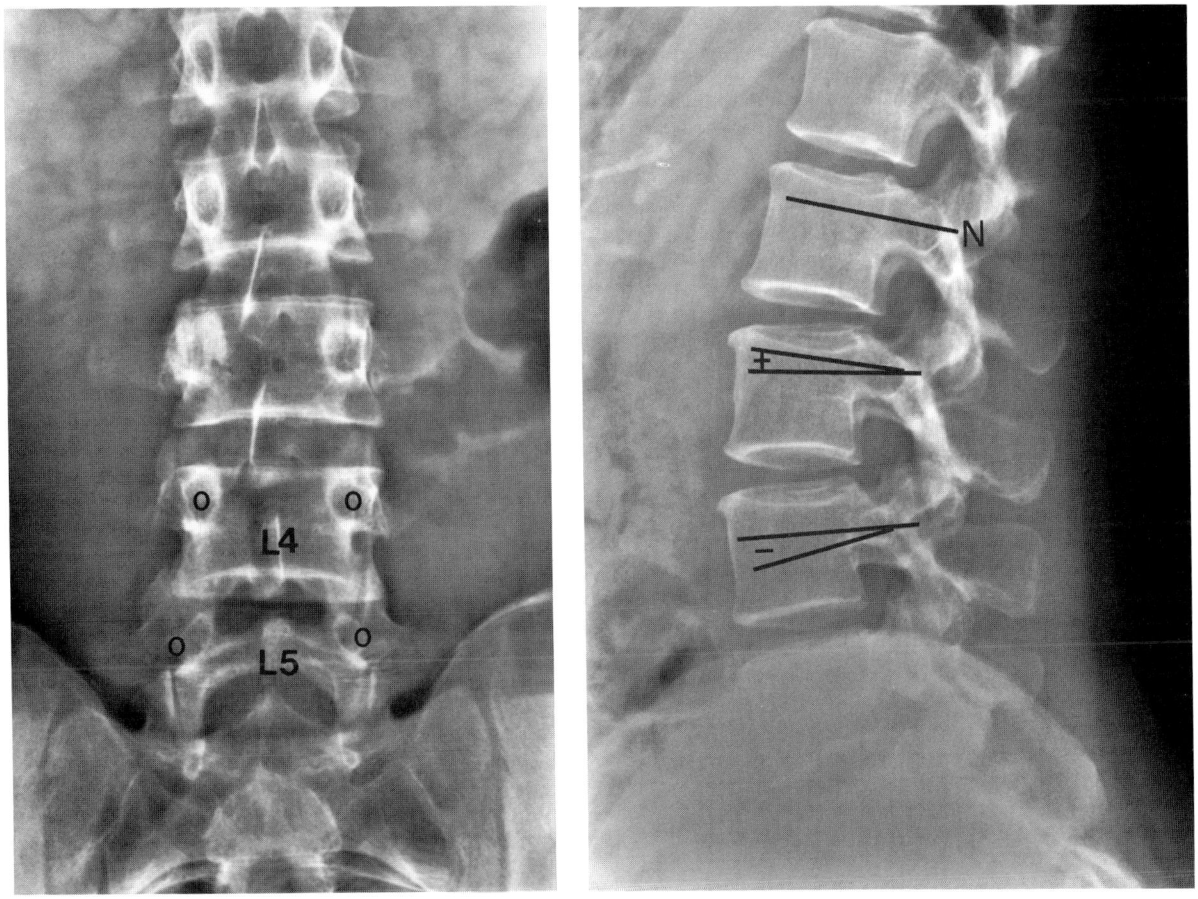

A

B

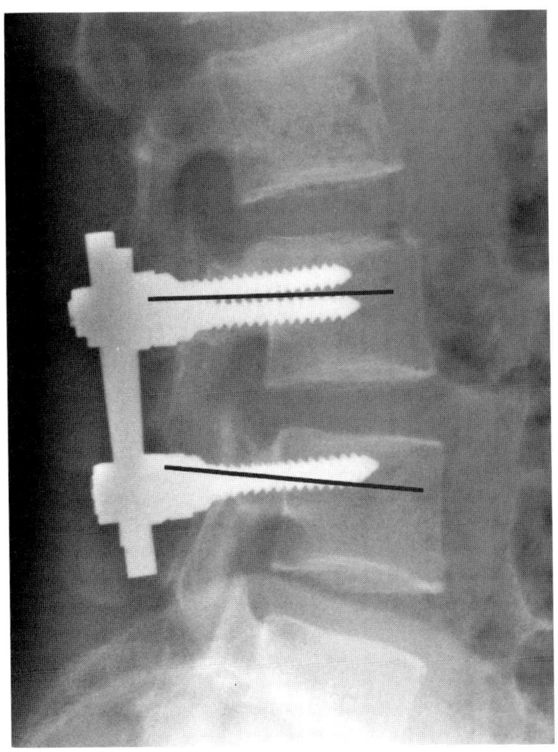

C

FIG. 3-82. Pedicle screw positioning. **A:** An AP radiograph demonstrating entry sites for pedicle screws. Normally, the screw enters at the pedicle near the inferior end of the facet (*o*, at L-4). The screws are usually angled medially 5° to 10° at L-1 and 20° to 25° at L-5 to S-1. Therefore, a slightly more lateral site may be chosen at L-5.[82,91,114] **B:** Lateral view showing normal (*N*), positive (+), and negative (−) sagittal screw angle. A neutral angle is desired, and a positive angle is safe. If the angles are too negative, a nerve root injury is more likely to result. **C:** Lateral view with ISOLA rods and pedicle screws in L-3 and L-4. One screw is slightly positive and one, slightly negative at L-3. Both screws are slightly positive compared with the neutral line in L-4.

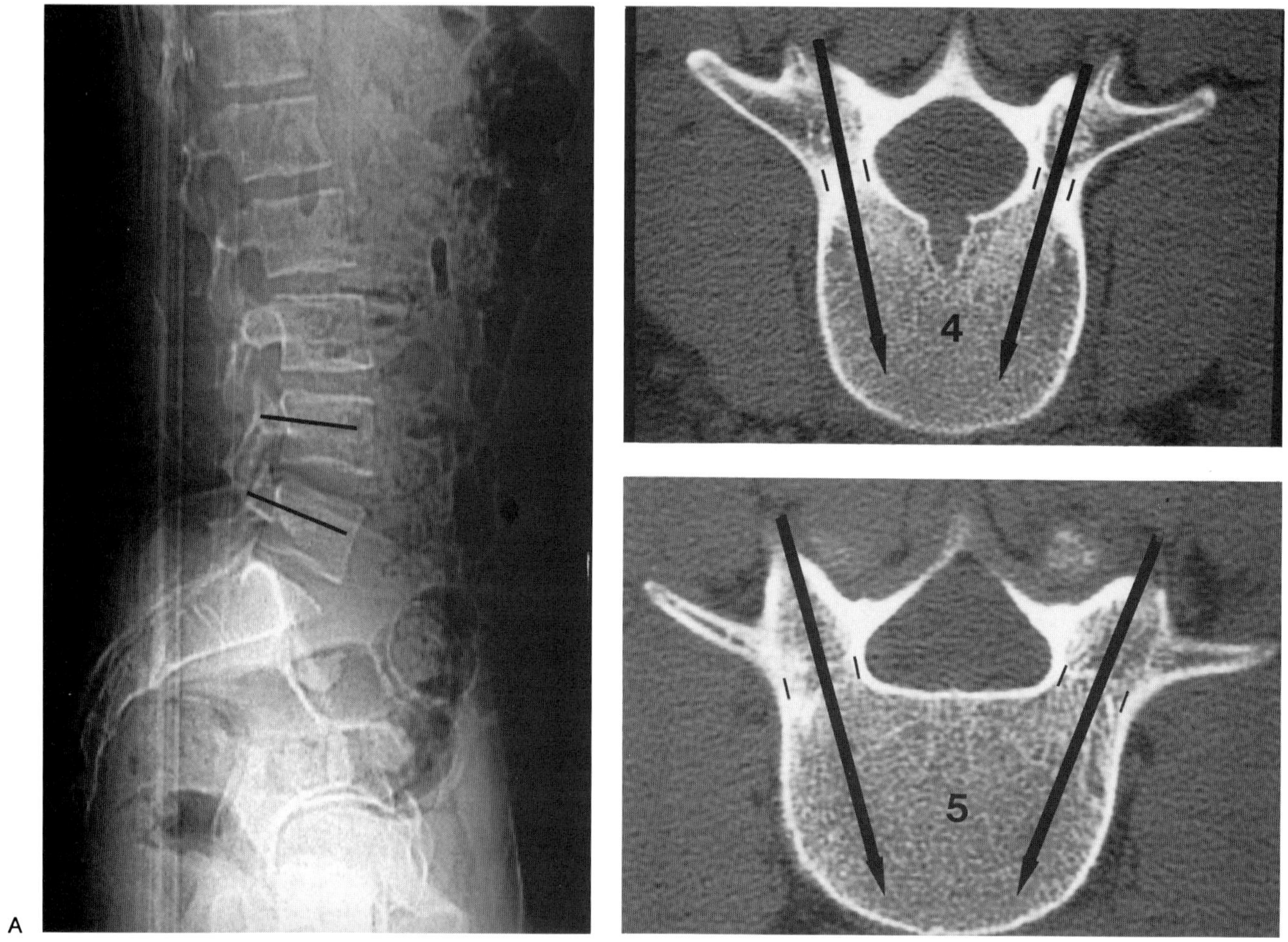

FIG. 3-83. The CT images demonstrating pedicle screw position. **A:** Scout view showing relationships at L-4 and L-5. L-4 **(B)** and L-5 **(C)** showing pedicle width for screw size, angle, and depth. Screws should not be too large in diameter, or pedicle fracture may occur. The depth should approach the anterior cortex, but cortical penetration should be avoided.

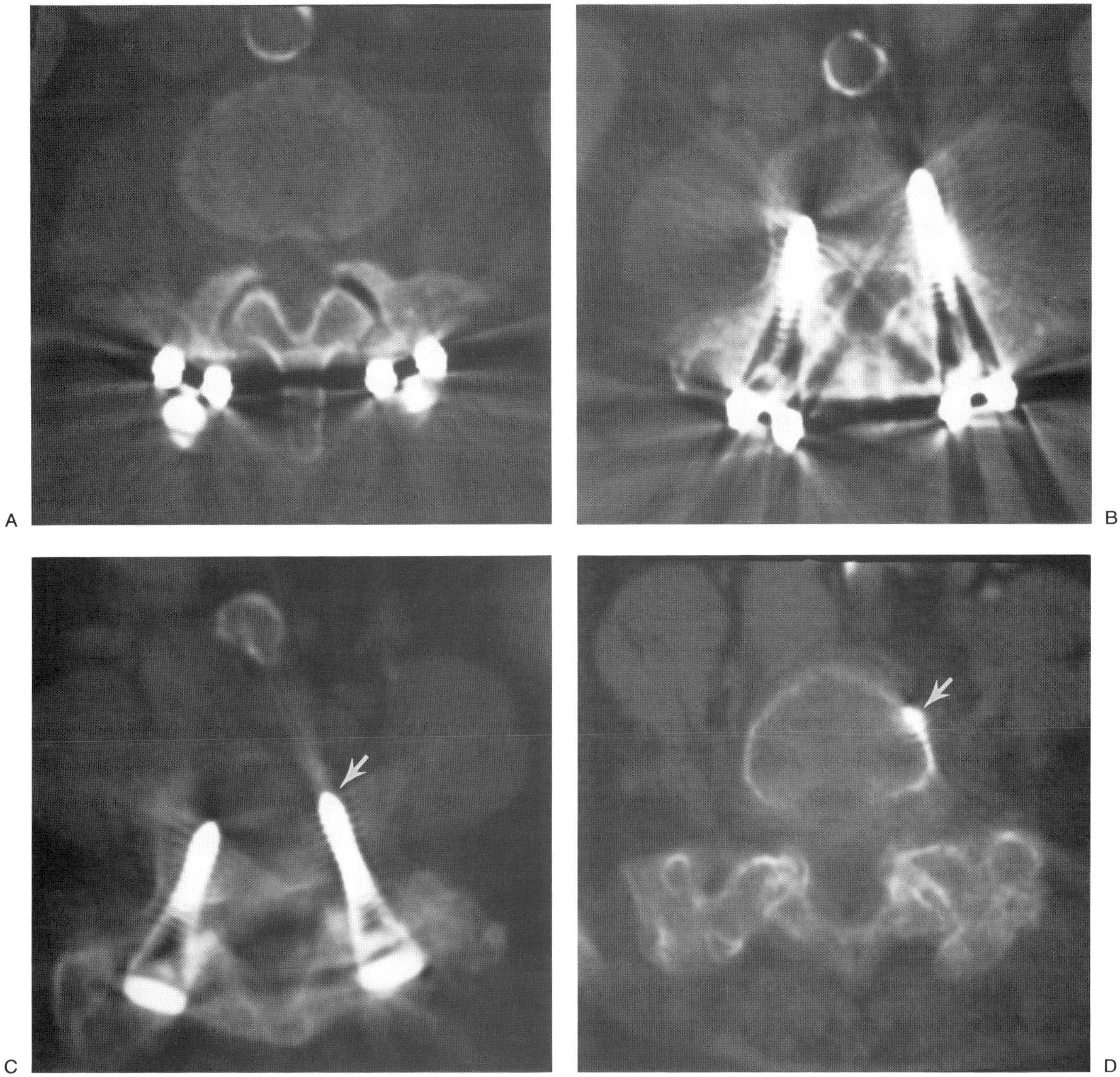

FIG. 3-84. Axial CT images after plate and pedicle screw fixation. **A:** Even at the plate-screw interface, the artifact is not too great to interfere with anatomic detail in the facet joints or spinal canal. **B:** The upper-level screws penetrate to different depths. Pedicles are clearly intact, and the screws do not penetrate the cortex. **C,D:** Screws on the lower level are clearly seen. The right screw is in a normal position. The left screw (*arrow*) is lateral and just penetrates the cortex (D).

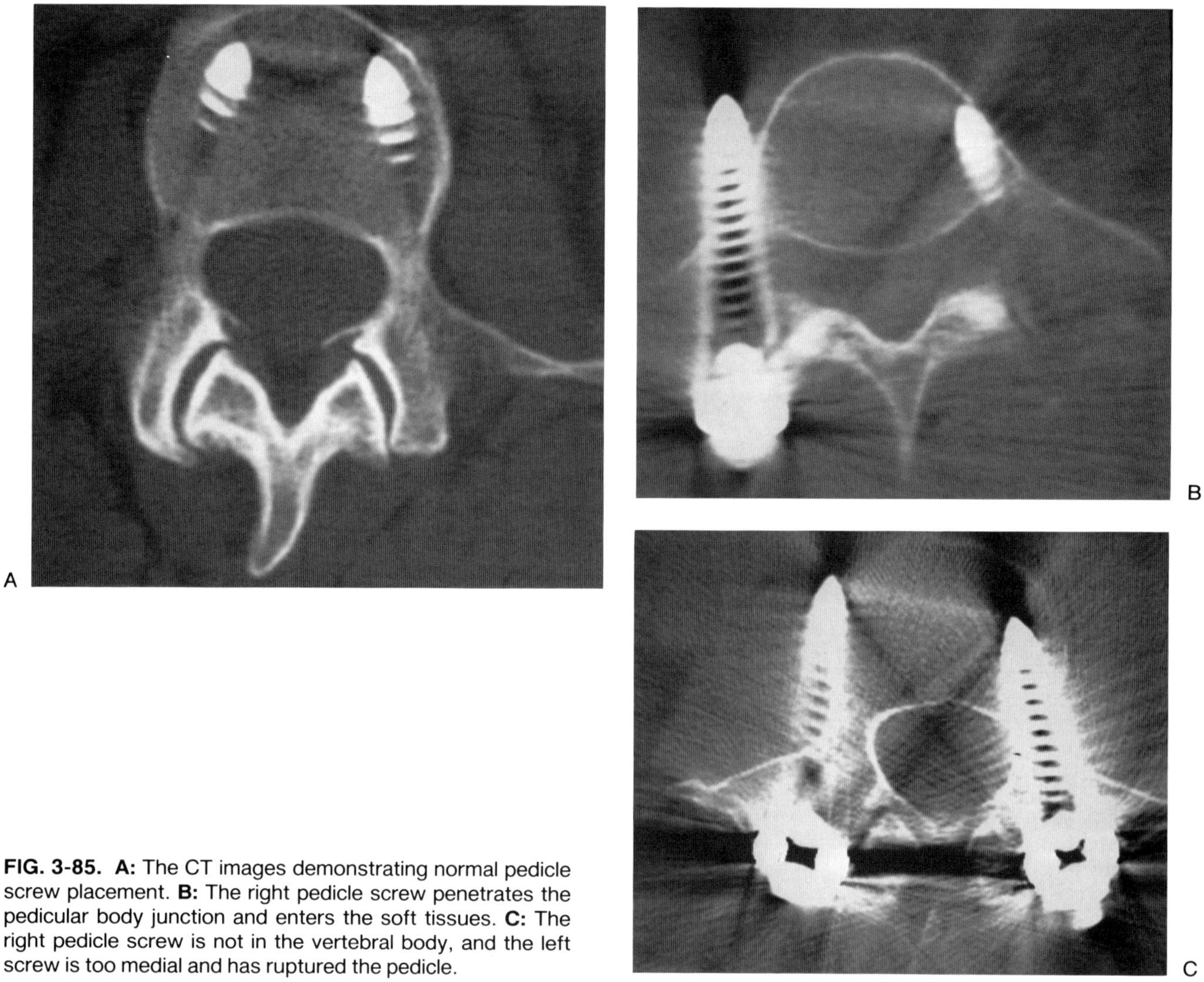

FIG. 3-85. A: The CT images demonstrating normal pedicle screw placement. B: The right pedicle screw penetrates the pedicular body junction and enters the soft tissues. C: The right pedicle screw is not in the vertebral body, and the left screw is too medial and has ruptured the pedicle.

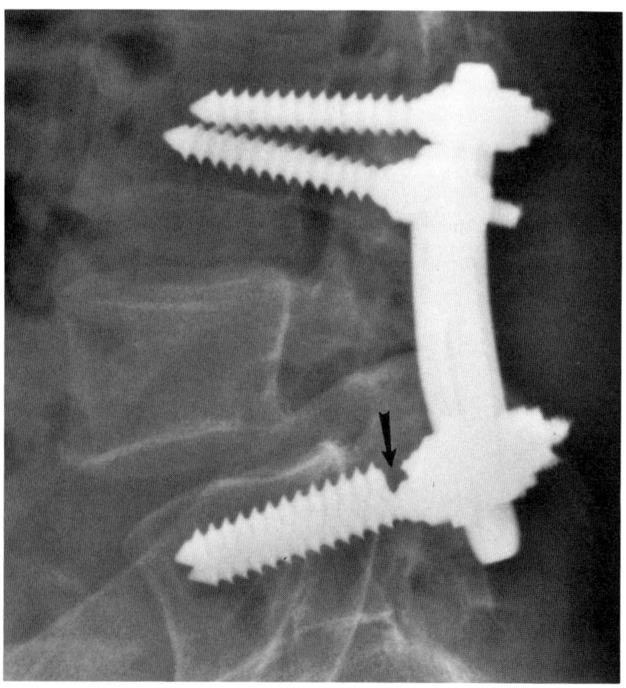

FIG. 3-86. Lateral view of the lumbar spine demonstrating fracture of a pedicle screw (*arrow*).

sures the optimal use of routine films, conventional tomography or CT, or MRI to determine the extent and stability of the injury.[120,122,123,129,131]

Routine radiographs remain the primary screening technique for spinal trauma.[123,124,127,135] The cervical spine trauma series includes AP, lateral, both oblique, and open-mouth AP odontoid views. Special angled views, pillar views, and other techniques may be used, but in most centers, further evaluation is obtained with conventional tomography or CT.[124,128,129,132,135,136] The AP and lateral views are usually adequate for screening the thoracolumbar spine. Areas of suspicion or that require further evaluation are most commonly examined with CT.[124,125,133,136,141,143] Specific techniques are discussed more completely subsequently.

The goals of spinal injury treatment include anatomic reduction, rigid fixation, and neurologic decompression.[130,137,138,140,142]

Cervical Spine Trauma

Approximately 65% of spinal injuries involve the cervical region.[150,154] Trauma to the cervical spine may result in fractures, fracture-dislocation, or isolated soft tissue injuries. The latter may be particularly subtle and can be difficult to detect radiographically.[150,154,165]

A thorough understanding of the mechanisms of injury is critical for selecting imaging techniques and determining the type of therapy. Cervical spine injuries may result from flexion, extension, lateral compression, vertical compression, or shearing forces. Most often the mechanism is not pure. For example, flexion injuries are usually combined with compression forces (flexion-compression injury).[150,153–155]

In our experience, the mechanism of injury can often be determined based on routine radiographic findings (Table 3-9).[150,153] The stability of the lesion can be predicted in many cases, based on features of the lateral radiograph[174] or using the three-column approach described by Denis.[155] The latter is more often applied to thoracolumbar injuries. Features on the lateral view that suggest instability include (1) vertebral subluxation >3.5 mm, (2) relative angular deformity > 11°, (3) increased interspinous distance, (4) narrowed disc space, (5) facet joint widening, and (6) vertebral compression > 25°.[147,150,154,155,173]

Differences in anatomy and biomechanics separate treatment options for the upper (occipital condyles to C-2) and lower cervical spine. Therefore, the discussion of imaging and treatment options is discussed separately.

Upper Cervical Spine (Occipital Condyles to C-2)

Most upper cervical injuries can be detected on AP, lateral, and open-mouth odontoid views (Fig. 3-87).

TABLE 3-9. *Classification and radiographic features of cervical spine injuries*[50,151,153]

Type of injury	Incidence rates (%)[a] in 420 patients
Hyperflexion	46
Distractive hyperflexion	
Hyperflexion sprain (transient dislocation)	
Hyperflexion dislocation	
Locked facets (12% unilateral)[b]	
Spinous process fracture	
Compressive hyperflexion	
Vertebral wedge fracture	
Teardrop fracture	
Fracture dislocation	
Shearing injuries	
Anteriorly displaced odontoid fracture	
Hyperextension	38
Distractive hyperextension	
Hangman's fracture	
Hyperextension sprain	
Anterior inferior vertebral body fracture	
Compressive hyperextension	
Posterior arch fractures	
Hyperextension fracture dislocations	
Shearing injuries	
Posteriorly displaced odontoid fracture	
Axial compression	4
Jefferson's fracture	
Burst fractures	
Hyperrotation injuries	
Rotary fixation of C-1 on C-2	
Anterior and posterior ligament disruptions	
Lateral flexion injuries	
Uncinate process fracture	
Transverse process fracture	
Lateral wedge fracture	
Brachial plexus avulsion	
Indeterminate[a]	10–12

From Berquist,[150] with permission.
[a] 10–12% indeterminate based on radiograph alone (e.g., spinous process fractures or undisplaced odontoid fractures.)
[b] 12% of hyperflexion injuries were due to flexion-rotation with unilateral facet locking.

Careful attention to the prevertebral soft tissues (Fig. 3-88) is useful because prevertebral soft tissue swelling may be the only clue to a subtle fracture.[150,154,165] Further clarification of the injury may require conventional tomography or CT. Although most centers use CT, routine tomography (Fig. 3-89) is still useful for subtle odontoid fractures or occipital condyle fractures in which the fracture line may be located in the slice plane of the CT images.[150] Conventional axial CT images are most useful for vertically oriented fractures or rotary injuries (rotary fixation of C-1 on C-2).[150,161] Thin-section reformatted

(text continues on page 172)

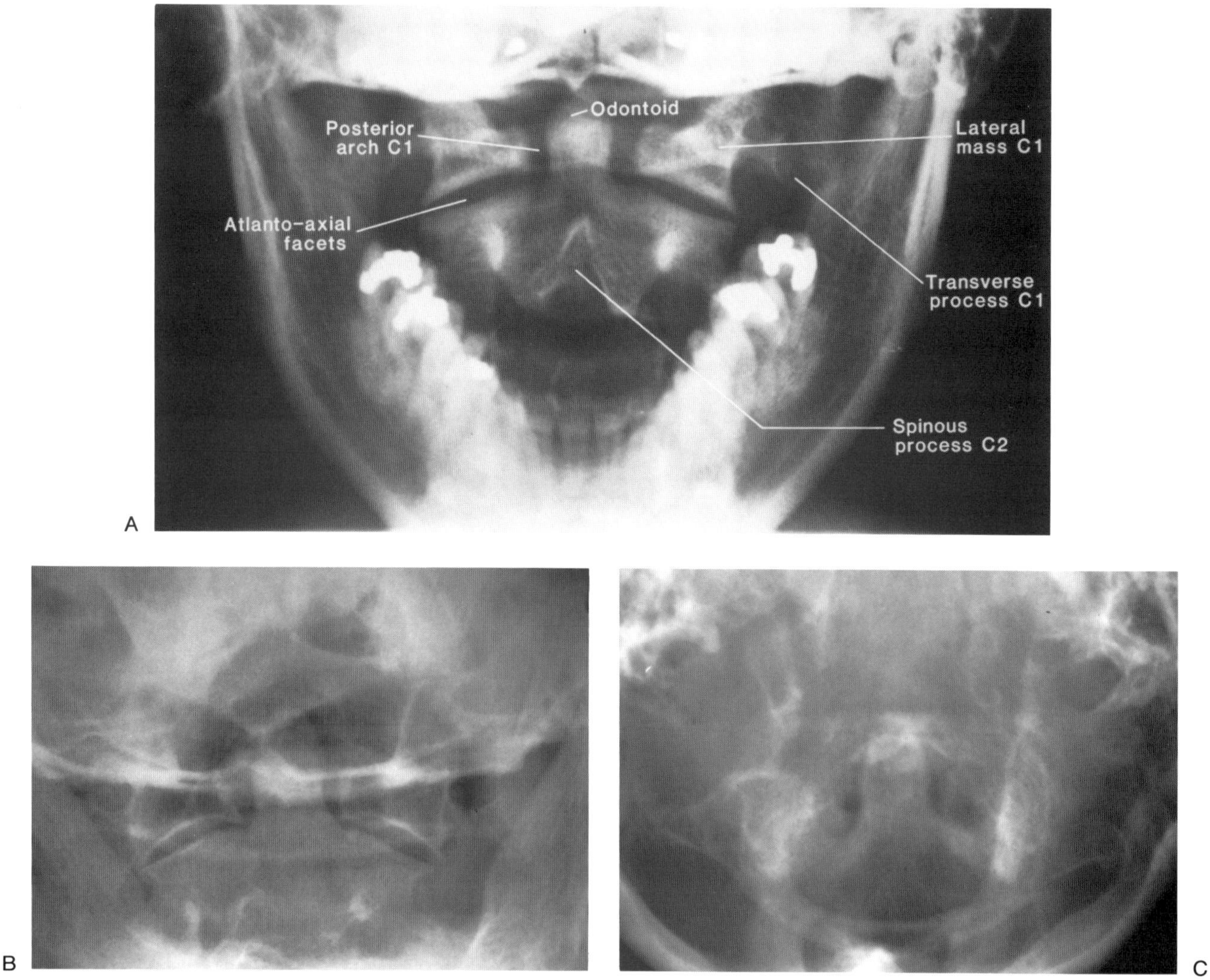

FIG. 3-87. Open mouth odontoid view. **A:** Normal. **B:** Odontoid obscured by overlying bone structures. **C:** Repeat radiograph of B with the tube angled 20° toward the head clearly demonstrates the odontoid.

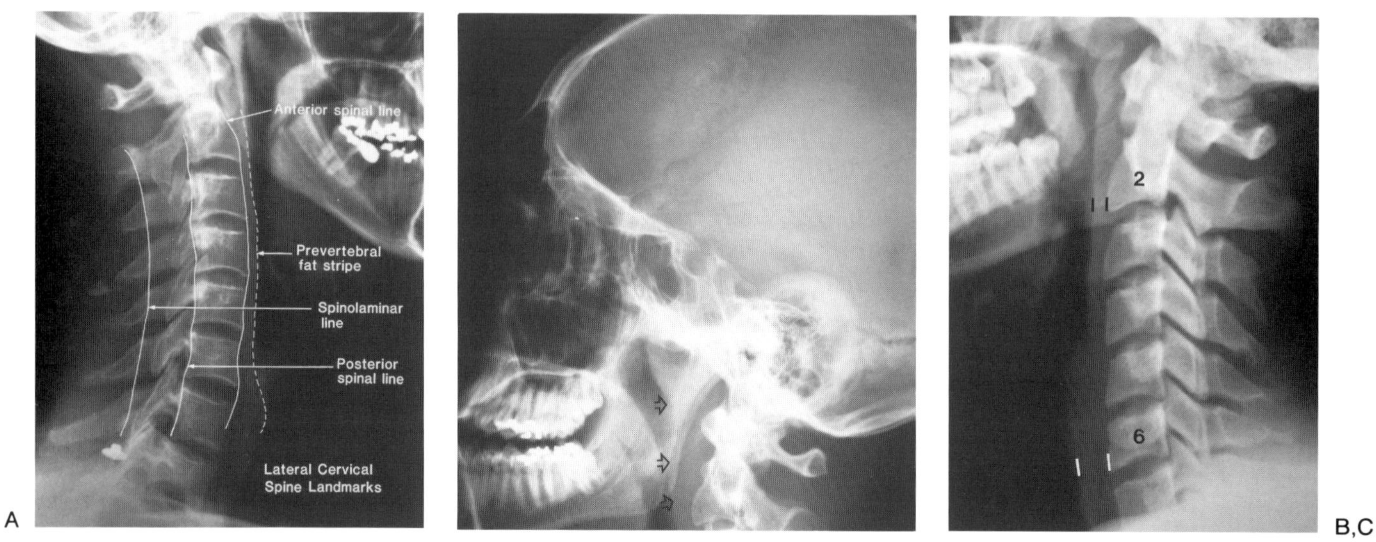

FIG. 3-88. Prevertebral soft tissue evaluation. **A:** Normal lateral view of the cervical spine demonstrating the normal spinolaminal, posterospinal, and anterospinal lines. The prevertebral fat stripe lies just anterior to the vertebral bodies from C-2 to C-6. Anterior displacement or obliteration of this fat stripe is seen with trauma and prevertebral hematoma. (From Berquist TH. *Imaging of orthopedic trauma.* New York: Raven Press, 1992.) **B:** Lateral view of the skull base demonstrating prominent prevertebral soft tissue (*arrows*) as a result of positioning. No injury present. **C:** Normal prevertebral soft tissue (*lines*) at C-2 (normal, 7 mm) and C-6 (normal, approximately one-third vertebral AP diameter).

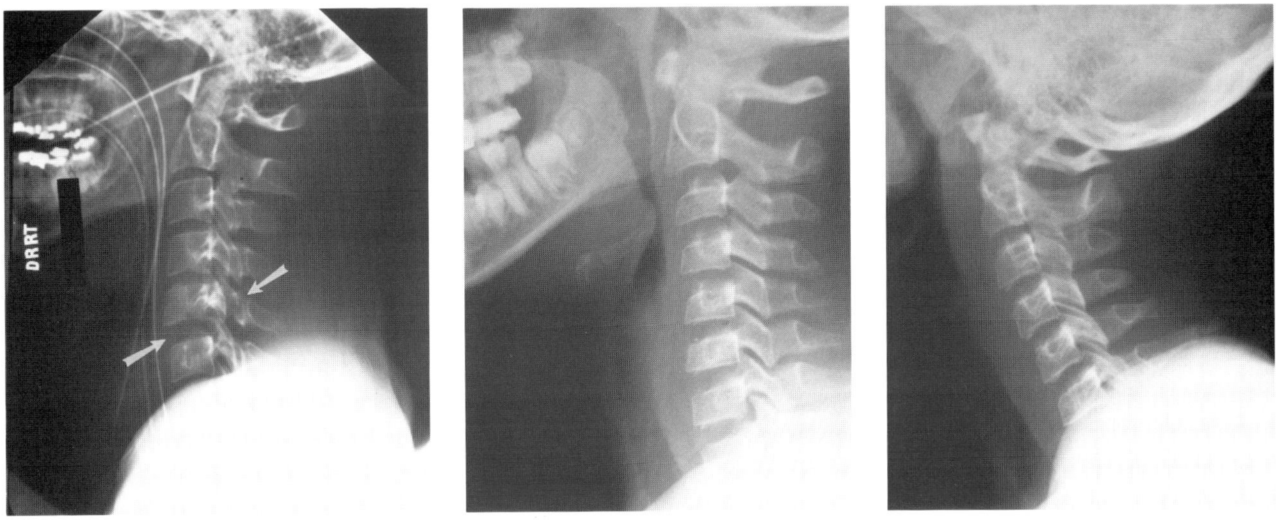

D E,F

FIG. 3-88. *Continued.* **D:** Prevertebral soft tissue measurements are invalid when endotracheal and nasogastric tubes are in position. Hyperextension injury with widened C-5 interspace (*anterior arrow*) and C-5 laminal fracture (*posterior arrow*). Normal lateral view in a child **(E)** and extensive prevertebral swelling **(F)**.

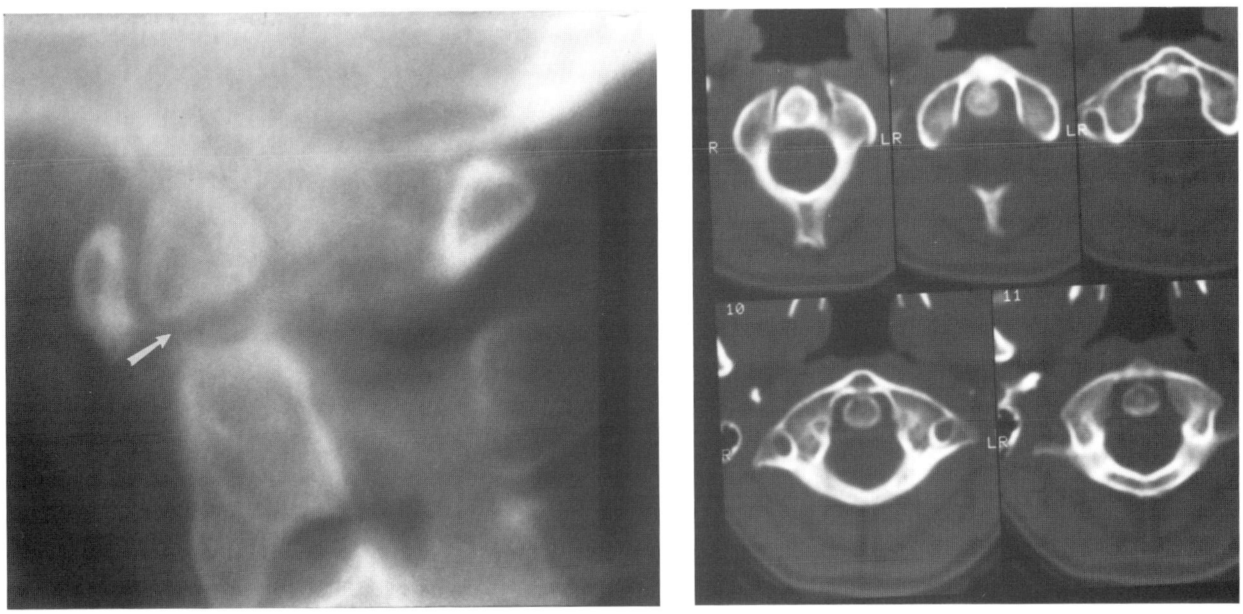

A B

FIG. 3-89. Type II odontoid fracture. **A:** Lateral tomogram demonstrating type II fracture (*arrow*). **B:** Axial CT images did not clearly demonstrate the fracture.

images in the sagittal or coronal plane assist in avoiding these partial-volume effects.[150,171]

Fractures of the upper cervical spine account for 20% to 25% of injuries in adults, but most childhood injuries occur in this location.[178] Table 3-10 lists the types of upper cervical spine fractures and the mechanisms of injury. Combination injuries are not uncommon in the cervical spine. Therefore, a careful evaluation to exclude upper and lower cervical injuries must be made prior to instituting therapy.[150,161]

There are several classifications that radiologists should be familiar with that are used to assist in determining the prognosis and treatment plan for upper cervical spine injuries.

Fielding[157] and Fielding and Hawkins[158] described the classification for rotary subluxation of C-1 on C-2 (Fig. 3-90).

Type I: rotary fixation without anterior subluxation of C-1 on the odontoid (transverse ligament intact)
Type II: rotary fixation with 3 to 5 mm of subluxation
Type III: rotary fixation with > 5 mm of subluxation
Type IV: rotary fixation with posterior subluxation (associated with deficient odontoid)

Types I and II rotary fixations (Fig. 3-91) are the most common and generally follow trauma, upper respiratory infections, or dental procedures.[150,157,158]

The Anderson-D'Alonzo[145] classification is commonly used for odontoid fractures (Fig. 3-92).

Type I: upper odontoid fracture
Type II: base of odontoid
Type III: fracture involving body of C-2 below entry of accessory ligament

TABLE 3-10. *Upper cervical spine fractures*[150,154,161]

Location	Mechanisms of injury
Occipital condyles (rare injury)	Shearing, rotational, or vertical compression
Atlantooccipital dislocation	Shearing, hyperextension
C-1 (~4% of cervical spine injuries)	
Anterior arch	Hyperextension-avulsion
Posterior arch	Hyperextension-compression
Lateral mass	Vertical compression
Transverse process	Lateral compression, avulsion
Jefferson fracture	Vertical compression
C-2 (15–25% of cervical spine injuries)	
Odontoid	Flexion, extension, lateral rotation
Pedicles	Hyperextension
Vertebral body	Hyperextension
Spinous process (rare)	Hyperextension
Lamina	Hyperextension
Facets	Lateral compression, compression rotation

Burke and Harris[152] preferred to use upper (type II) or lower (type III) classifications. Type II fractures are the most common (59% to 67%) and occur above the entry of the accessory ligament, which carries a portion of the blood supply. This may account for the high incidence of nonunion in type II fractures. If displaced, type II fractures frequently require operative fusion.[150,151] Figure 3-93 demonstrates examples of odontoid fractures.

Hangman's fractures were classified by Effendi et al.,[156] which was modified by Levine and Edwards.[170] The fracture classification is based on the relationship of C-2 to C-3 (Fig. 3-94).

Type I: undisplaced C-2 neural arch fracture, with C-2 to C-3 facets intact
Type II: anterior displacement of C-2 on C-3, with facets intact
Type IIA: minimal displacement with severe angulation (distraction injury with C2-3 disc disruption)
Type III: posterior and anterior fragments displaced (facets disrupted)

Most undisplaced fractures heal with collar or halo fixation (Fig. 3-95).[150]

Type III fractures are treated surgically.

Management of Upper Cervical Injuries

Fractures and fracture dislocations of the upper cervical spine and occipital condyles can be managed with external halo fixation or internal fixation procedures. These decisions are based on the type, classification, and stability of the injury.[150,162,169,173]

The goals of upper cervical spine fusion and instrumentation are listed as follows:

Restrict reconstruction to involved segments, as defined by preoperative imaging
Avoid spinal canal invasion with instrumentation
Maintain reduction until bone fusion is solid
Select adequate fixation in the presence of weak or absent posterior elements.[161–163]

Although several techniques have been used, most authors prefer bone grafting, with wire or cable fusion.[162–164,172]

Wire-Cable Techniques. Wires or cables with bone grafts can be used for C-1 to C-2 posterior fusion. Several techniques have been described. The Gallie[159] technique is performed using a single wire (Fig. 3-96) around the posterior arch of C-1 to the spinous process of C-2. A single midline iliac bone graft is used. This technique is referred to as a Gallie fusion.[162,164,172] The single central bone graft has been considered weak and suboptimal by some authors.[162,172]

The Brooks procedure uses sublaminar wires or cables and bone grafts on either side of the midline (Fig. 3-97).[151,162,172] Wires are usually twisted instead of tied

(text continues on page 178)

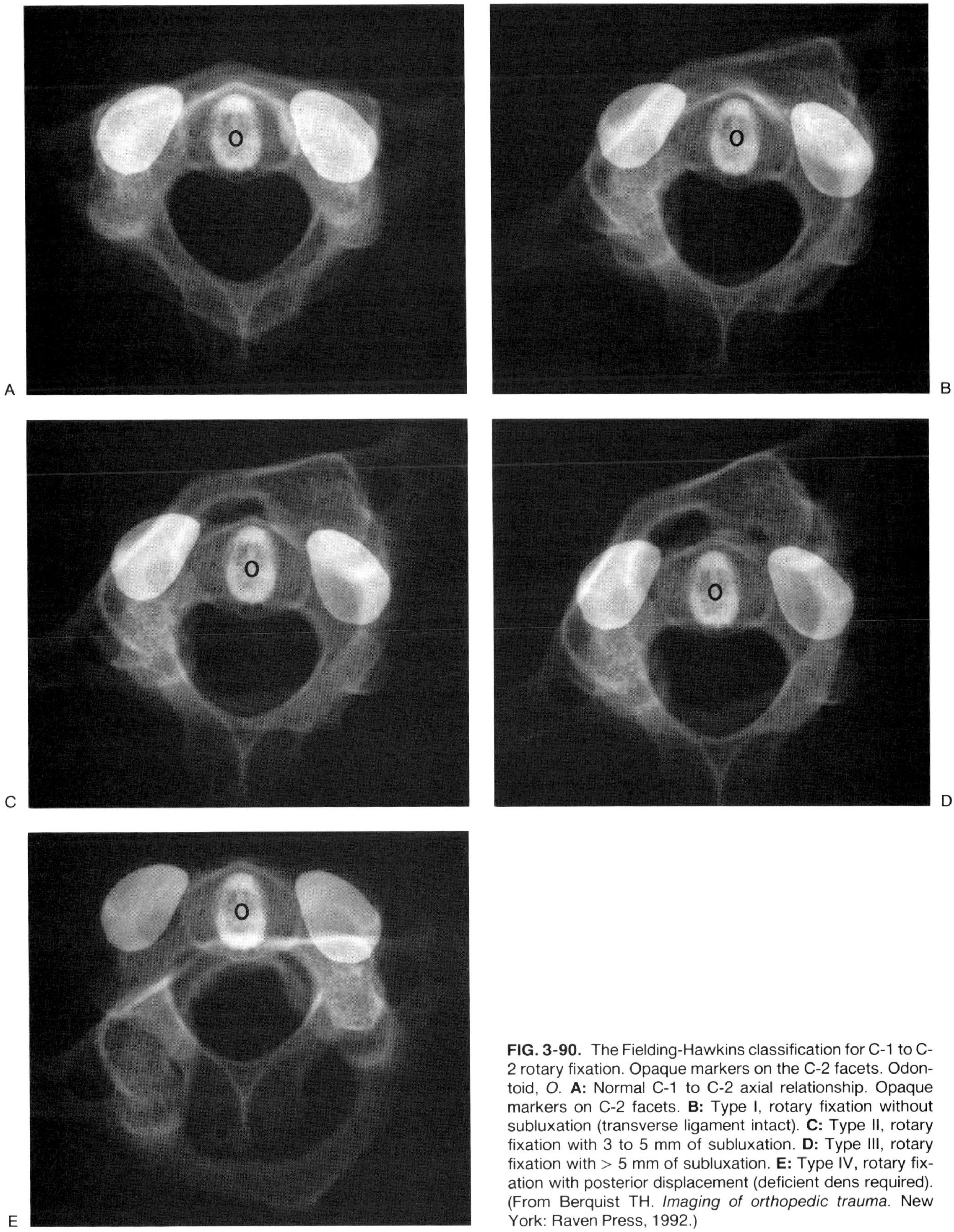

FIG. 3-90. The Fielding-Hawkins classification for C-1 to C-2 rotary fixation. Opaque markers on the C-2 facets. Odontoid, *O.* **A:** Normal C-1 to C-2 axial relationship. Opaque markers on C-2 facets. **B:** Type I, rotary fixation without subluxation (transverse ligament intact). **C:** Type II, rotary fixation with 3 to 5 mm of subluxation. **D:** Type III, rotary fixation with > 5 mm of subluxation. **E:** Type IV, rotary fixation with posterior displacement (deficient dens required). (From Berquist TH. *Imaging of orthopedic trauma.* New York: Raven Press, 1992.)

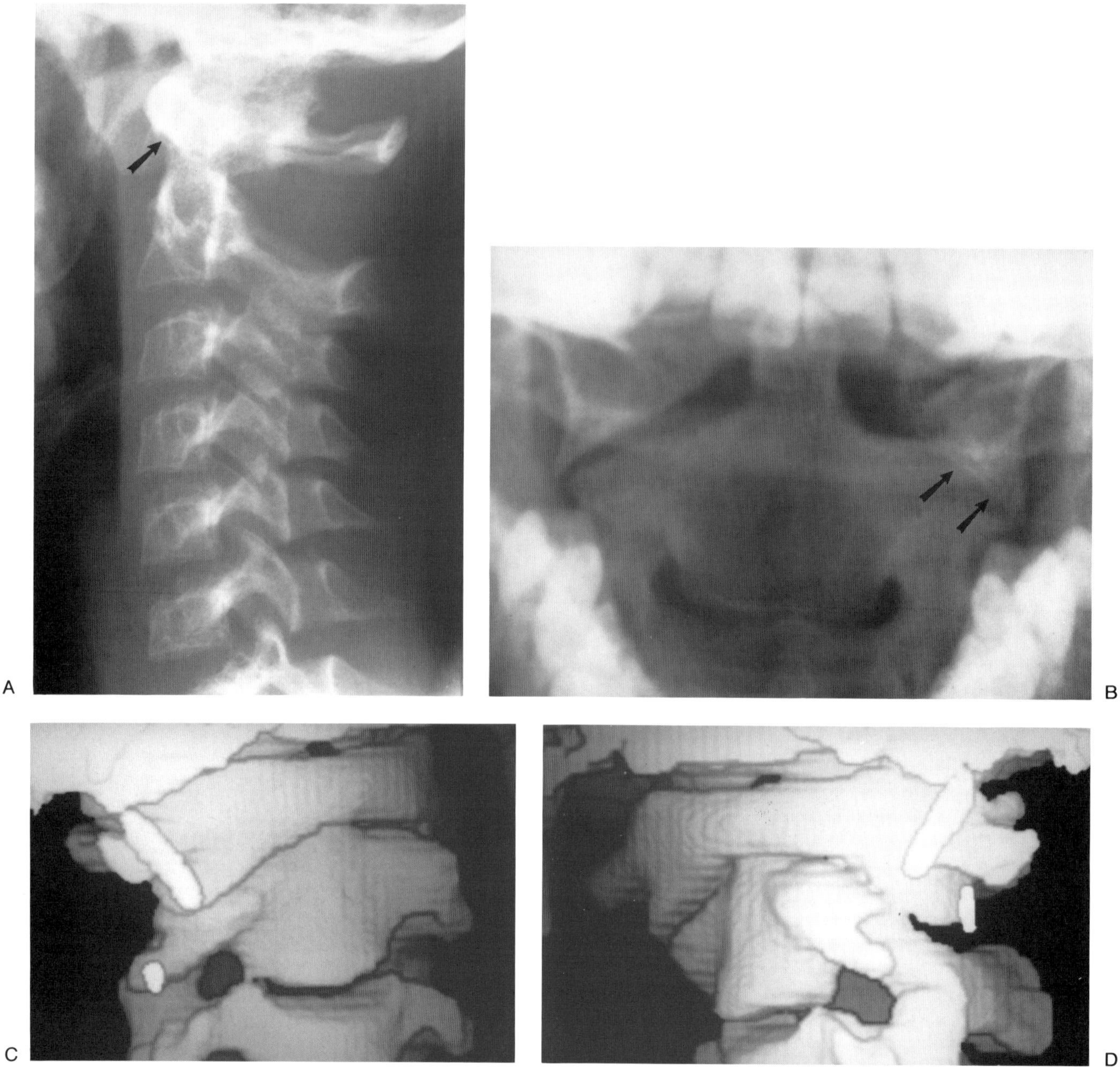

FIG. 3-91. Child with rotary fixation following minor trauma. **A:** Lateral view shows no C-1 to C-2 displacement at the odontoid (*arrow*). **B:** Open-mouth AP odontoid view demonstrates overlap of the C-1 lateral mass on C-2 (*arrows*) on the left. **C,D:** Three-dimensional CT images clearly demonstrate the rotation of C-1 on C-2. Dynamic CT studies may be even more useful in this setting.

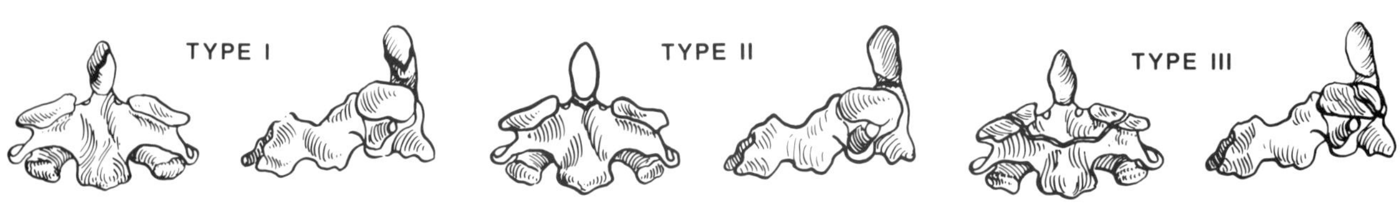

FIG. 3-92. The Anderson-D'Alonzo classification of odontoid fractures. Type I, upper odontoid fracture; Type II, fracture at the odontoid base above the accessory ligament; and Type III, fractures through the body below accessory ligament insertion. (From Berquist TH. Imaging of orthopedic trauma. New York: Raven Press, 1992.)

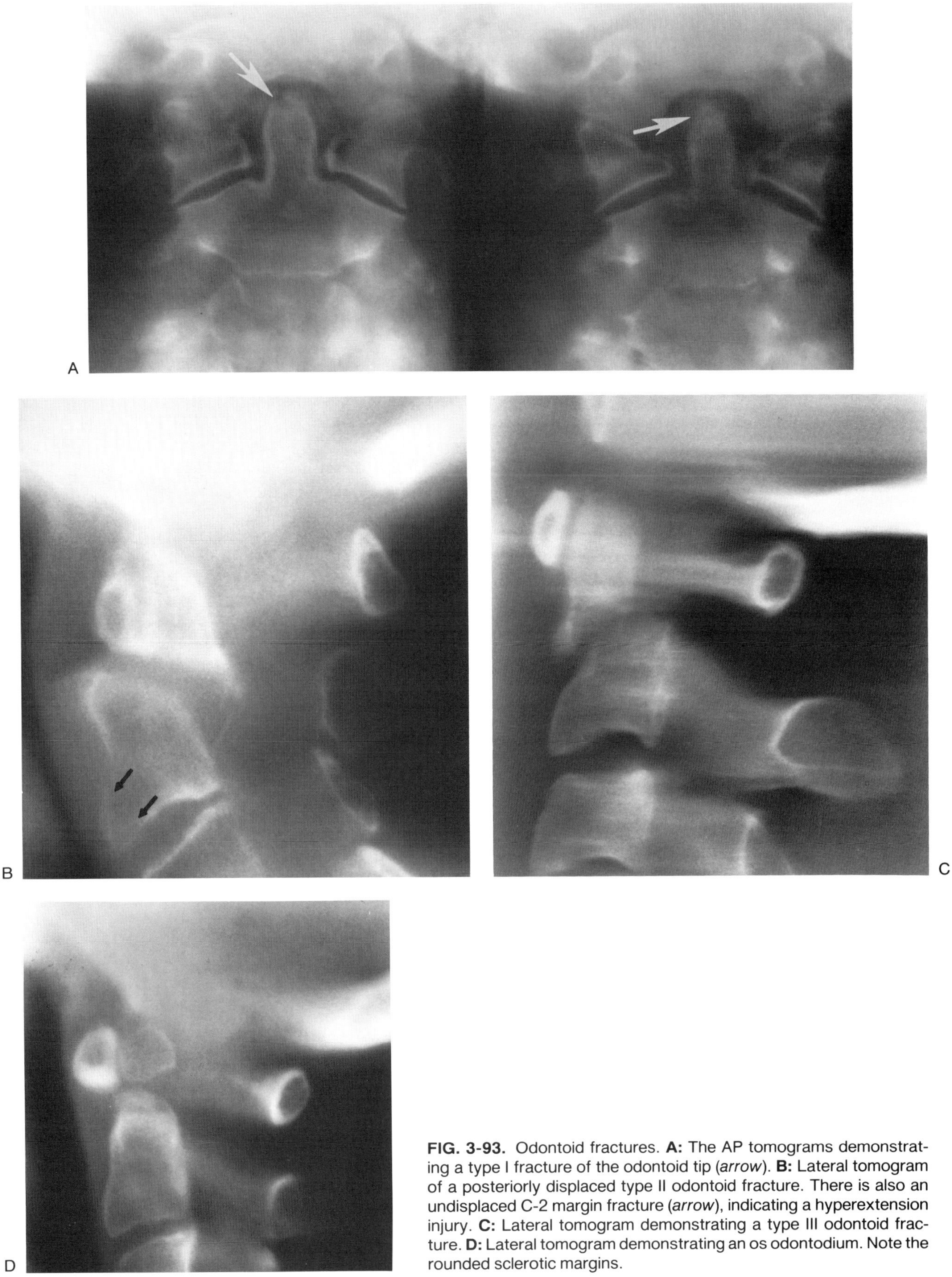

FIG. 3-93. Odontoid fractures. **A:** The AP tomograms demonstrating a type I fracture of the odontoid tip (*arrow*). **B:** Lateral tomogram of a posteriorly displaced type II odontoid fracture. There is also an undisplaced C-2 margin fracture (*arrow*), indicating a hyperextension injury. **C:** Lateral tomogram demonstrating a type III odontoid fracture. **D:** Lateral tomogram demonstrating an os odontodium. Note the rounded sclerotic margins.

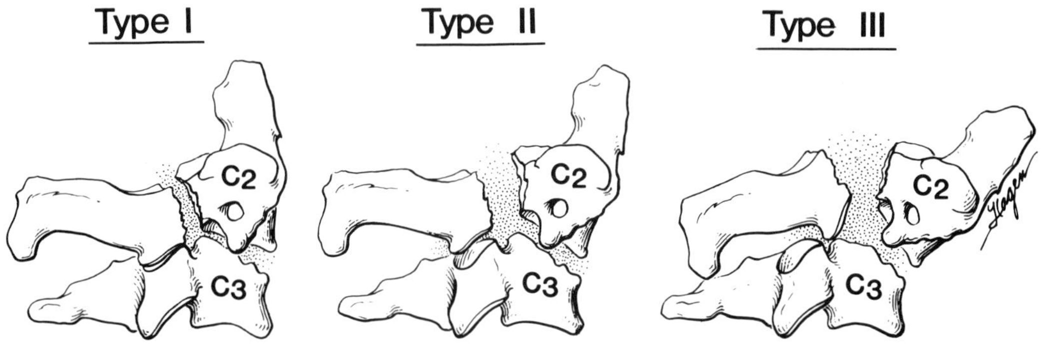

A,B C

FIG. 3-94. Effendi classification for axis ring fractures.[156] **A:** Type I, minimally displaced C-2 neural arch fracture with facet joints intact. **B:** Type II, fracture with C-2 anteriorly displaced on C-3, facets intact. **C:** Type III, posterior and anterior fragments displaced (facets disrupted).

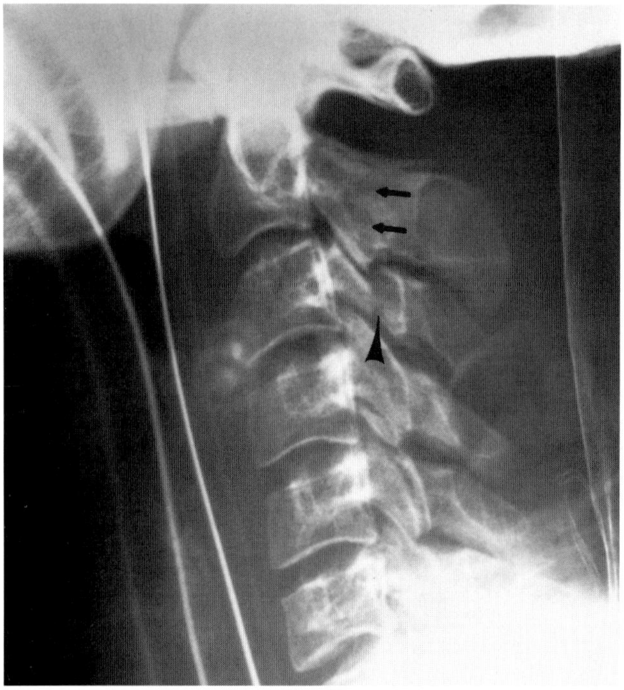

A

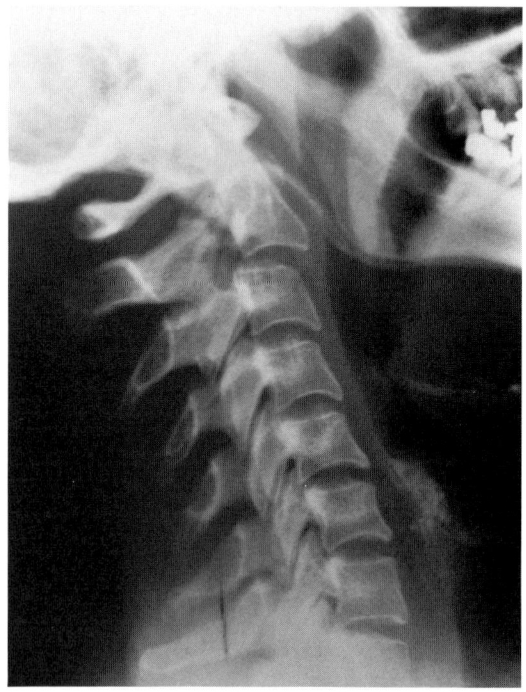

B

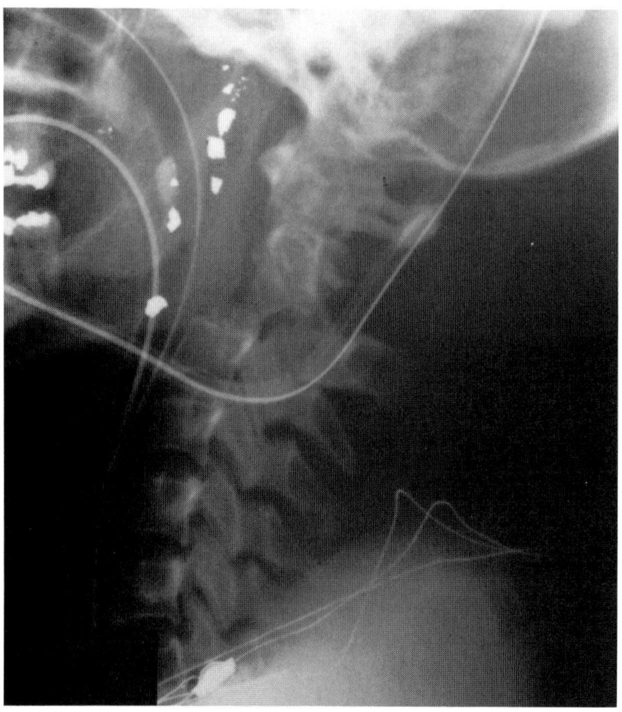

C

FIG. 3-95. Posterior C-2 ring fractures or hangman's fractures. Lateral view of the cervical spine demonstrating an Effendi type I fracture (*arrows*). **A:** There is also a C-3 facet fracture (*lower arrowhead*). Lateral views of the cervical spine demonstrating a slightly displaced type II fracture **(B)** and total posterior dislocation **(C)**.

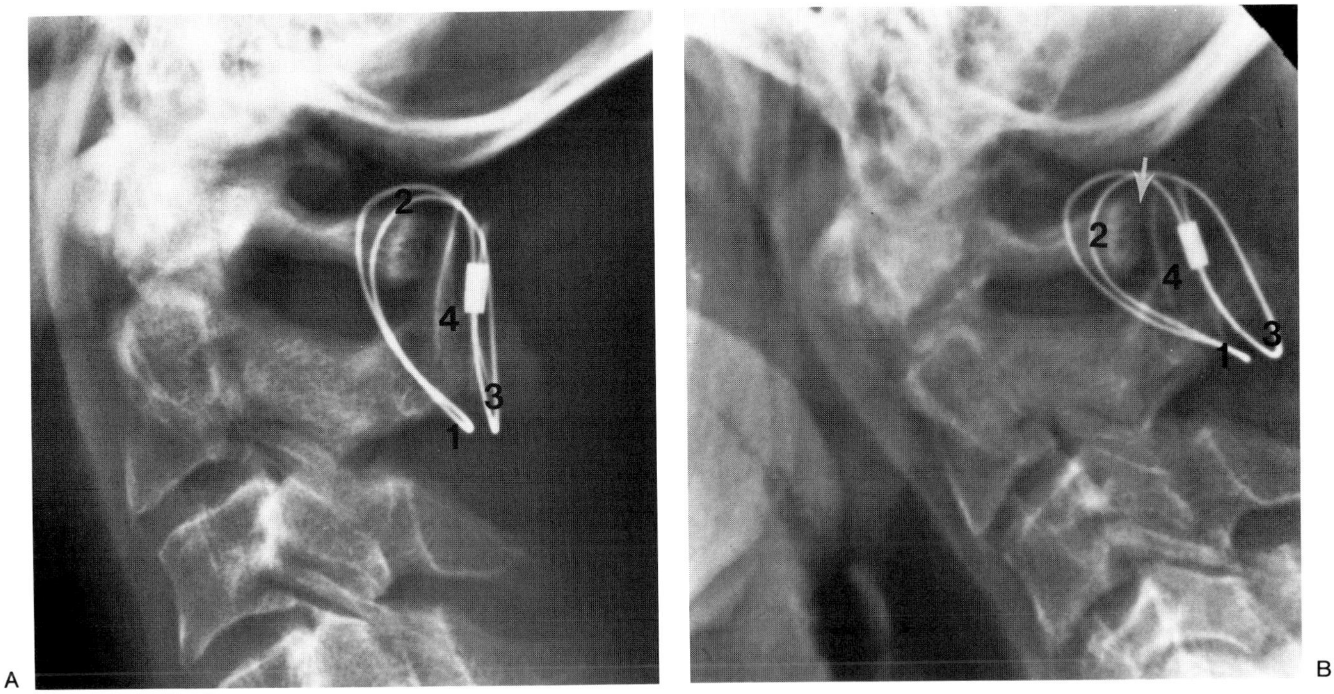

FIG. 3-96. Gallie technique with single cable from the spinous process of C-2 (*1*), around the C-1 arch (*2*), and back over the spinous process (*3*) with a central iliac bone graft (*4*). Neutral **(A)** and flexion **(B)** radiographs show no subluxation. However, the upper end of the graft (*arrow*) changes position, and therefore, union has not occurred.

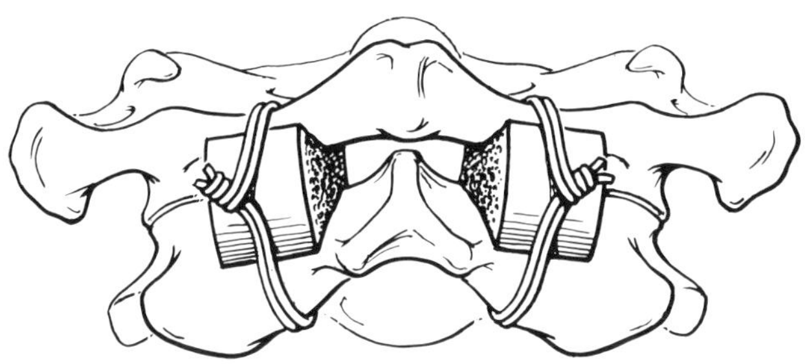

FIG. 3-97. Brooks fusion with paired twisted wires and bone grafts.

to assist in tension adjustment. Cables can be substituted for wires in either setting. These techniques prevent flexion and reduce or retard the anterior subluxation of C-1 on C-2.[172]

Luque Rectangles. Luque rectangles are smooth round rectangular instruments (Fig. 3-26B) that fit the occiput and upper cervical spine (Fig. 3-98). The rectangle is secured to the spine and occipital bone using wire or cables. Bone grafts are also applied to facilitate fusion.[150,172]

Halifax Clamps. Halifax clamps are applied in a fashion similar to that of wires or cables in the Brooks procedure (Fig. 3-99). The clamps are placed over the C-1 arch and under the C-2 lamina and tightened with a posterior screw.[144,162,168] Several years ago, MRI-compatible clamps were introduced.[143]

Screw and Plate-Screw Fixation Techniques. The C-1 to C-2 fusion can be accomplished using transarticular screws (Fig. 3-100). Anterior lag screws can be used for displaced odontoid fractures. The Knorenger screw is designed for this purpose. It is similar in design to the Herbert screw used for scaphoid fractures in the wrist. The threaded ends of the screw cause compression of the fracture fragments. This technique may be useful for type II odontoid fractures.[172]

Grob[162] modified the transarticular technique by using a Y plate (Fig. 3-101), transarticular screws, bone grafting, and occipital fusion. This technique avoids the problems of sublaminar wire passage.[162,172]

Lower Cervical Spine Injuries

The mechanisms of injury are similar for the upper and lower cervical spine. In adults, nearly 80% of cervical spine injuries occur from C-3 to C-7; most are at the C-5 to C-7 levels.[150,154,161] Routine radiographs (AP, lateral, and both oblique views) allow most injuries to be identified.[150] However, in some cases, CT or conventional tomography are required to determine the full extent of injury to the bony structures (Figs. 3-102 and 3-103). Also, MRI is useful for evaluating the spinal cord and canal (Fig. 3-104). In addition, radiographs of the thoracic and lumbar spine should also be obtained to exclude combination injuries. Cervical fractures are associated with fractures in the thoracic and lumbar spine in 15% of patients.[148–150]

Management of Lower Cervical Injuries

Treatment options for lower cervical spine injuries depend on the integrity of neurologic structures and a radiographic assessment of stability. The goals are to decompress neural structures and stabilize the spine. Decompression may be achieved by realignment, but in some cases, removal of bone fragments (most common anteriorly) from the canal may be necessary. Most often, stable lesions with no neurologic deficit require only external support for management. Unstable or potentially unstable lesions require more aggressive therapy. Instrumentation for traumatic cervical spine injuries is most often a posterior device. However, anterior or combined approaches may be necessary.[150,162,168,173]

The indications for posterior procedures are mainly related to ligament instability.

Posterior Instrumentation

Wire-cable instrumentation. Posterior tension-band wiring or cables can be used in conjunction with bone grafting to achieve arthrodesis for unstable posterior soft tissue (ligament sprains) or osseous injuries (Fig. 3-105). Fracture-dislocations may require traction tongs for realignment prior to wire or cable fixation. Spinous process wiring is most commonly used to avoid dural injury associated with sublaminar wires.[162] Halo fixators or collars are used to support the operative site until healing has occurred. The type of device used depends on the injury, type of fixation, and reliability of the patient. This device is usually required for 3 or more months.[150]

Plate-screw systems. There are multiple plate and screw systems. Plates are contoured to fit the cervical lordosis. Screws are introduced into the articular masses (Figs. 3-106 and 3-107). Following the plane of the facets and using lateral deviation helps avoid inadvertent entry into the spinal canal or injury to the vertebral arteries, nerve roots, or facet joints. Both stainless steel and titanium implants are available. Titanium instrumentation causes less artifact on MRI scans but is more expensive and may fail because of notch sensitivity.[150] A key difference between implants is the ability to place the screw in the proper position to avoid injury to the vertebral artery, nerve root, cord, or facet, without being constrained by the location of the holes in the plate. Newer rod-screw systems are currently being evaluated to overcome this problem.

Hook plates have also been used for discoligamentous instability from C-2 to C-7. The plates are hooked under the lamina of the lower vertebra and attached to the lateral masses of the upper vertebra with screws (Figs. 3-108 and 3-109). Interspinous bone grafting is used.[166]

Clamp Instrumentation. Posterior laminar clamps (Halifax) are designed with two J-shaped ends to attach to adjacent lamina and a draw screw that tightens the clamps in a manner similar to compression rod-hook instruments (Fig. 3-99). These clamps are relatively simple to use and theoretically result in less chance of neurologic injury compared with passing sublaminar wires or cables.[144,162,172]

Anterior Instrumentation. Anterior instrumentation of the cervical spine can be used for arthrodesis following hyperextension injuries with disruption of the anterior column structures (anterior longitudinal ligament or anterior vertebra and disc).[154] Also, anterior instrumen-

(text continues on page 185)

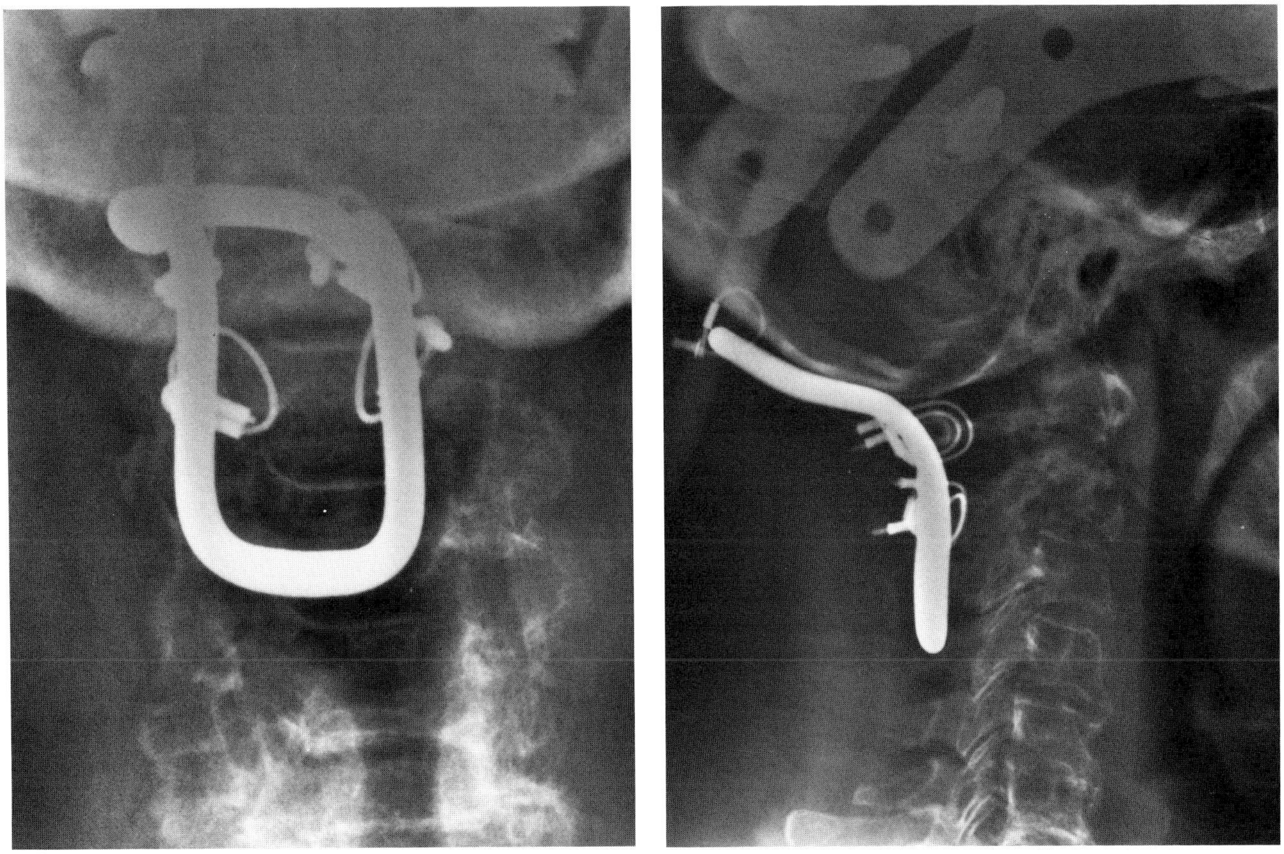

A B

FIG. 3-98. The AP **(A)** and lateral **(B)** radiographs demonstrate a contoured Luque rectangle and cables for occipital to C-2 fusion. Immediate postoperative support added using a halo vest.

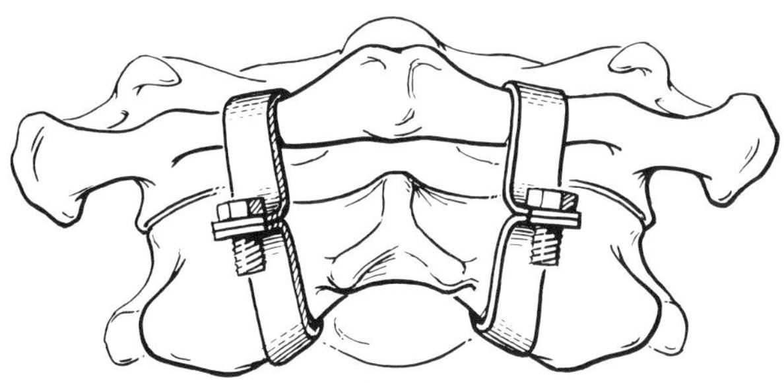

FIG. 3-99. Paired Halifax clamps for C-1 to C-2 fusion.

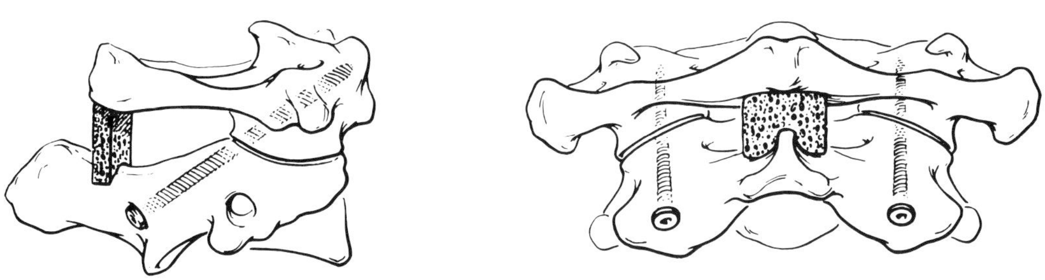

FIG. 3-100. Transarticular screw fixation.[162] The Magerl technique with two transarticular screws and a central graft between the arch of C-1 and C-2 spinous process.

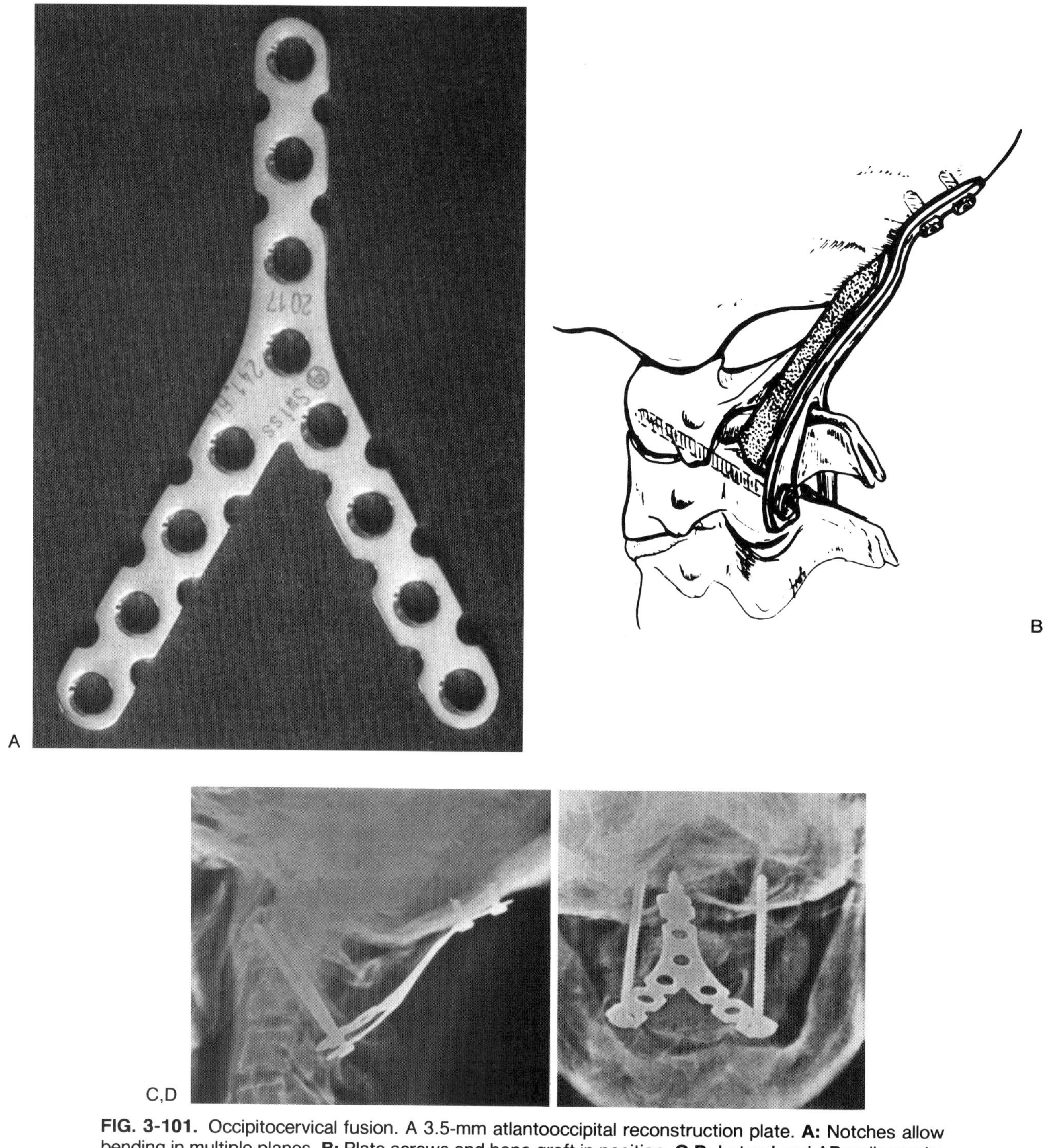

FIG. 3-101. Occipitocervical fusion. A 3.5-mm atlantooccipital reconstruction plate. **A:** Notches allow bending in multiple planes. **B:** Plate screws and bone graft in position. **C,D:** Lateral and AP radiographs demonstrating the transarticular screws, plate, bone graft, and two short occipital bone screws. (From Grob D, Dvorak J, Gschwend N, Froehlich M. Posterior occipitocervical fusion in rheumatoid arthritis. *Arch Orthop Trauma Surg* 1990;110:38–44.)

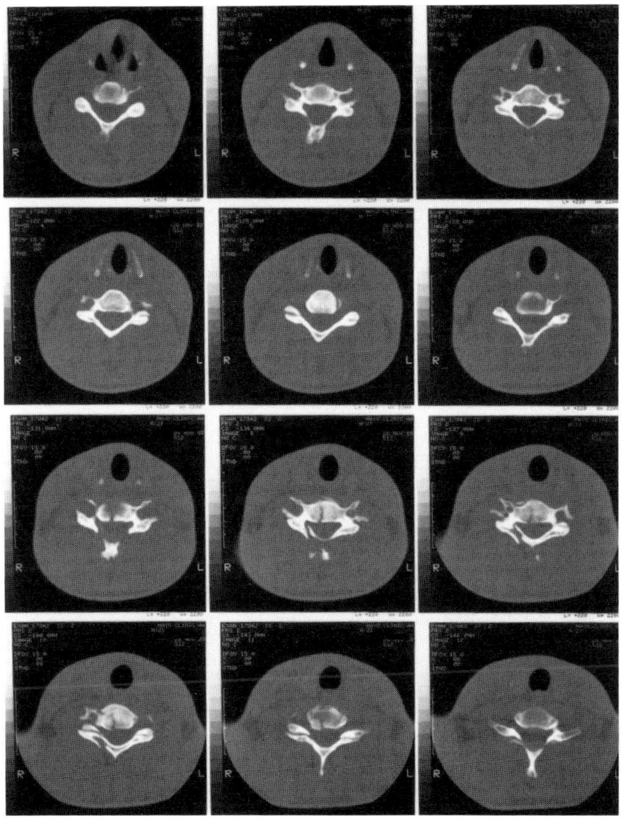

FIG. 3-102. Axial CT images demonstrating a complex lower cervical spine fracture with a sagittal body fracture and slight posterior displacement into the spinal canal (*lower left*). There are also multiple neural arch fractures.

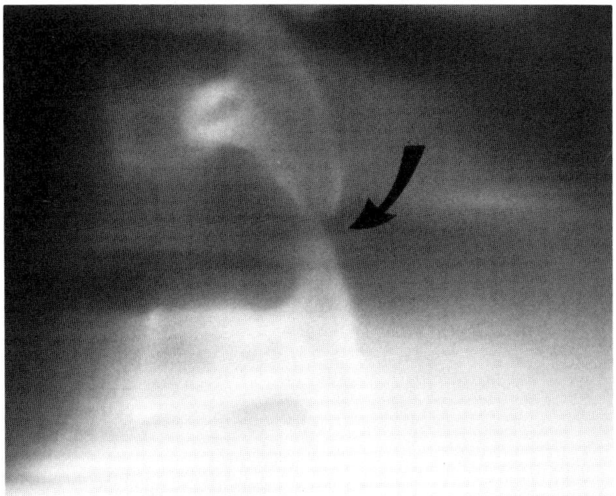

FIG. 3-103. Lateral tomogram demonstrating a perched facet (*arrow*).

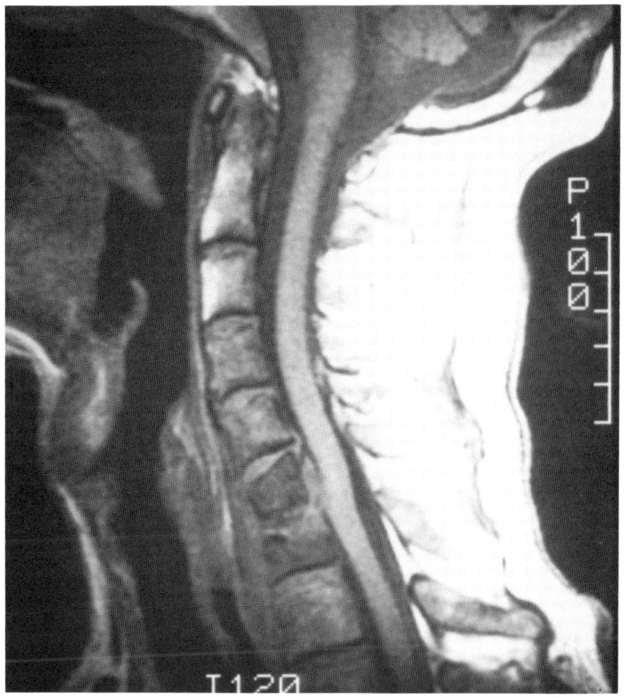

FIG. 3-104. Sagittal spin-echo (SE) 500/20 MRI scan demonstrating a C-6 to C-7 compression injury with slight cord deviation caused by the posterior hematoma.

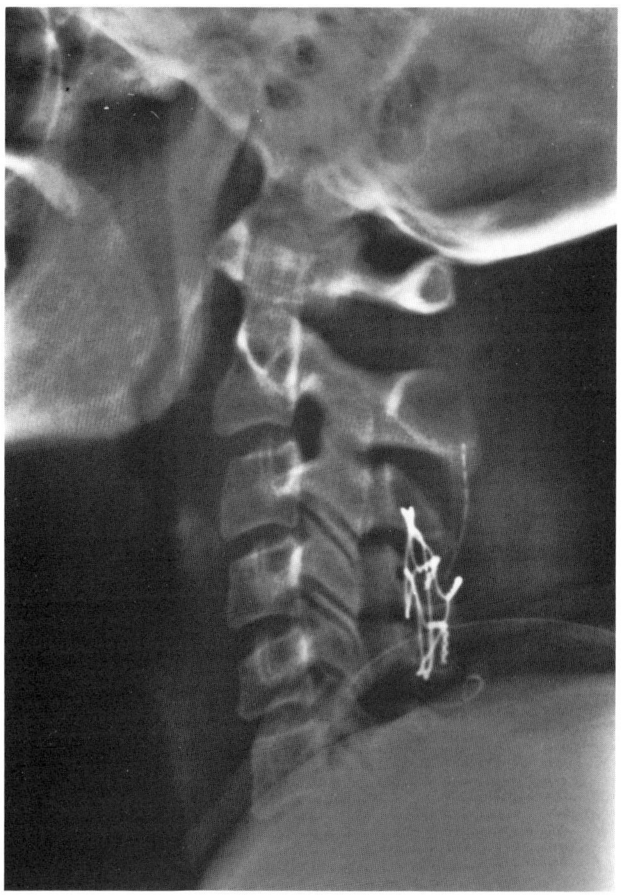

FIG. 3-105. Flexion-distraction injury with posterior ligament instability. Lateral radiograph shows normal alignment with spinous process wire and long graft from C-3 to C-5.

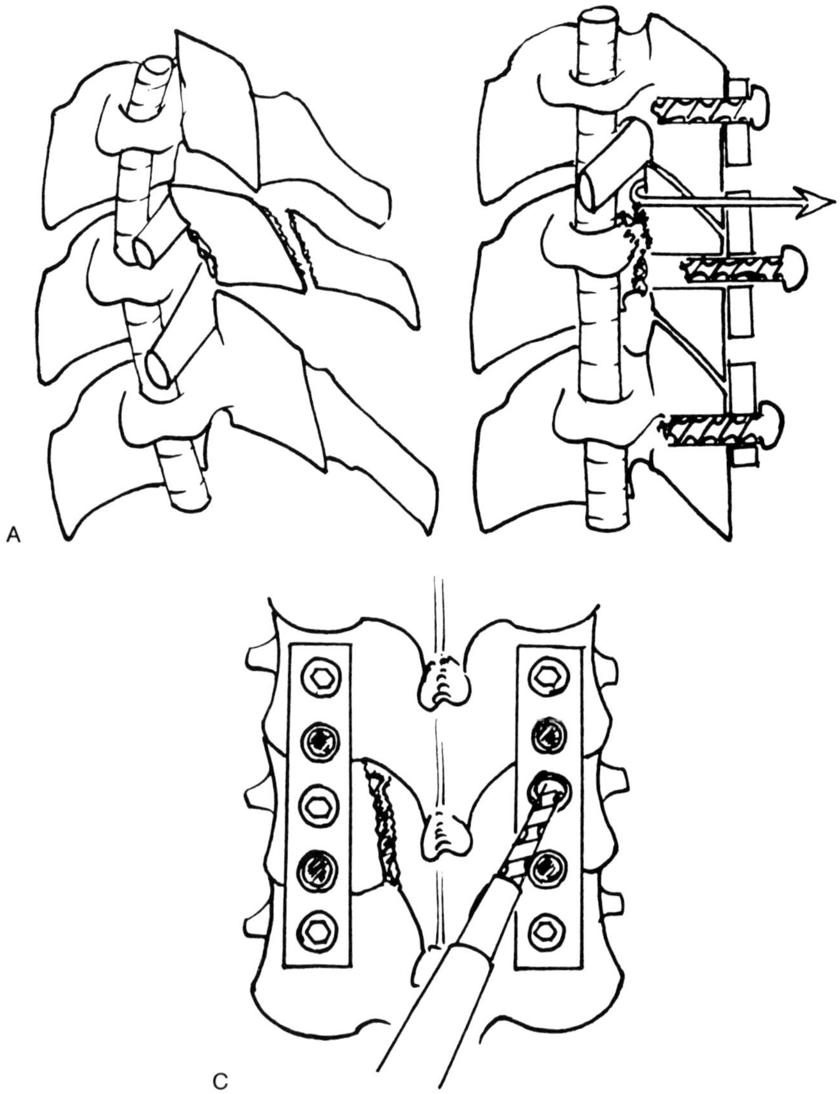

FIG. 3-106. Reduction of articular mass fracture **(A)** using plate and screw technique **(B,C)**. (From Nazarian SM, Louis RP. Posterior internal fixation with screw plates in traumatic lesions of the cervical spine. *Spine* 1991;16:564–571.)

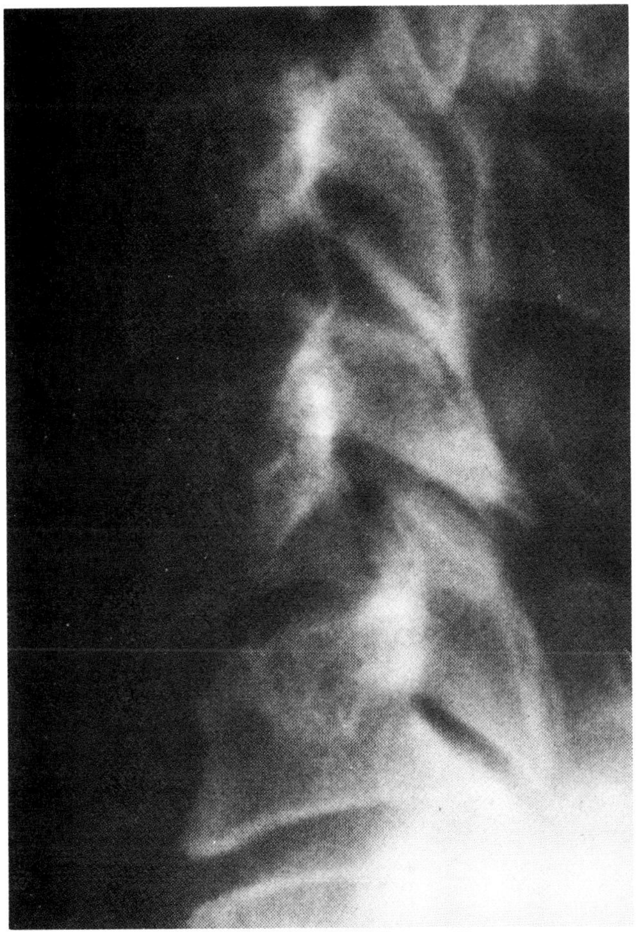

A

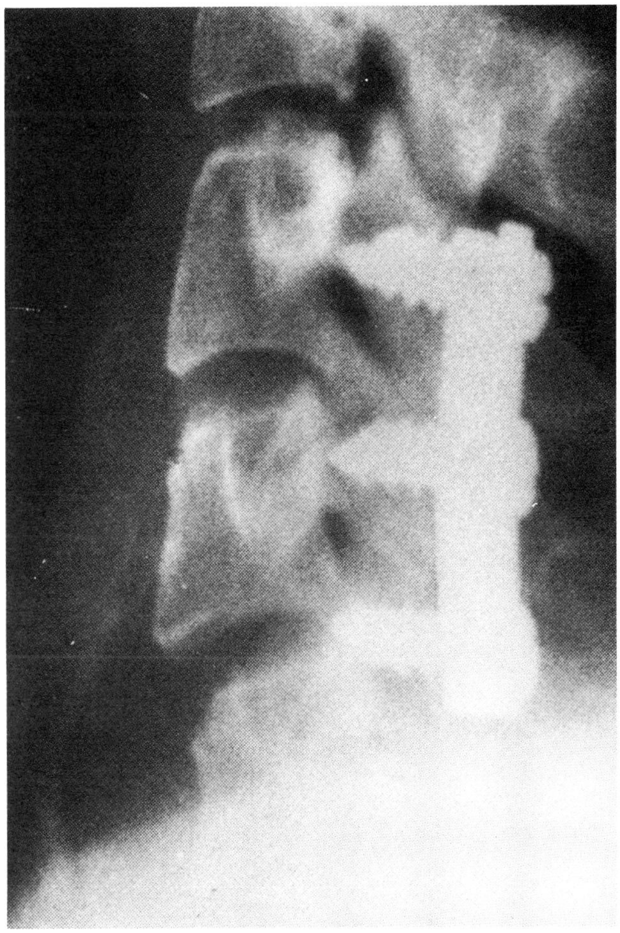

B

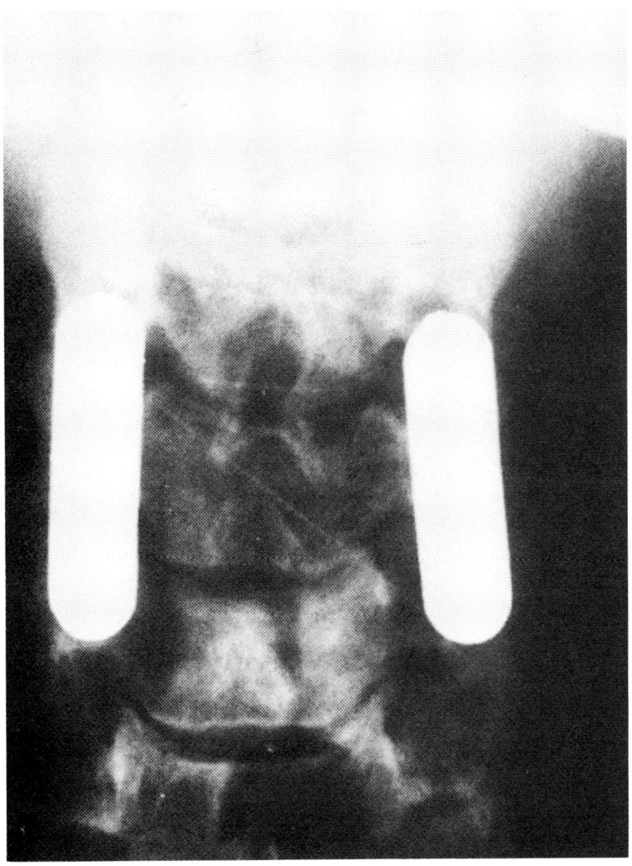

C

FIG. 3-107. A: Lateral radiograph of fractured articular mass. Lateral **(B)** and AP **(C)** radiographs after plate and screw instrumentation. (From Nazarian SM, Louis RP. Posterior internal fixation with screw plates in traumatic lesions of the cervical spine. *Spine* 1991;16:564–571.)

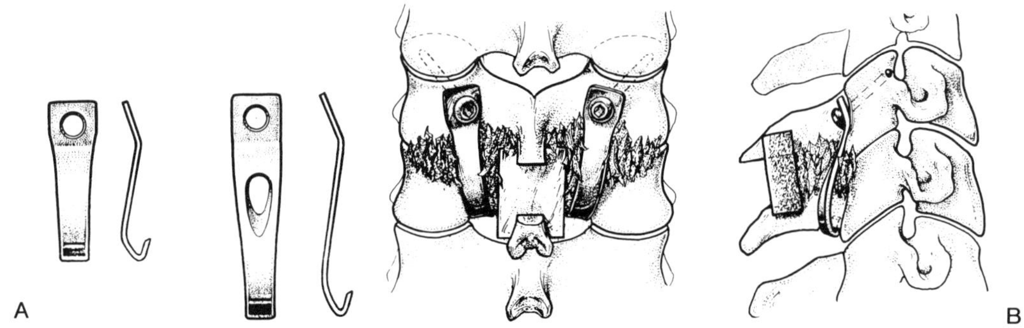

FIG. 3-108. **A:** Hook plate. **B:** Posterior and lateral views with hook plate and bone graft in position. (From Jeanneret B, Magerl F, Ward EH, Ward JCL. Posterior stabilization of the cervical spine with hook plates. *Spine* 1991;16:556–563.)

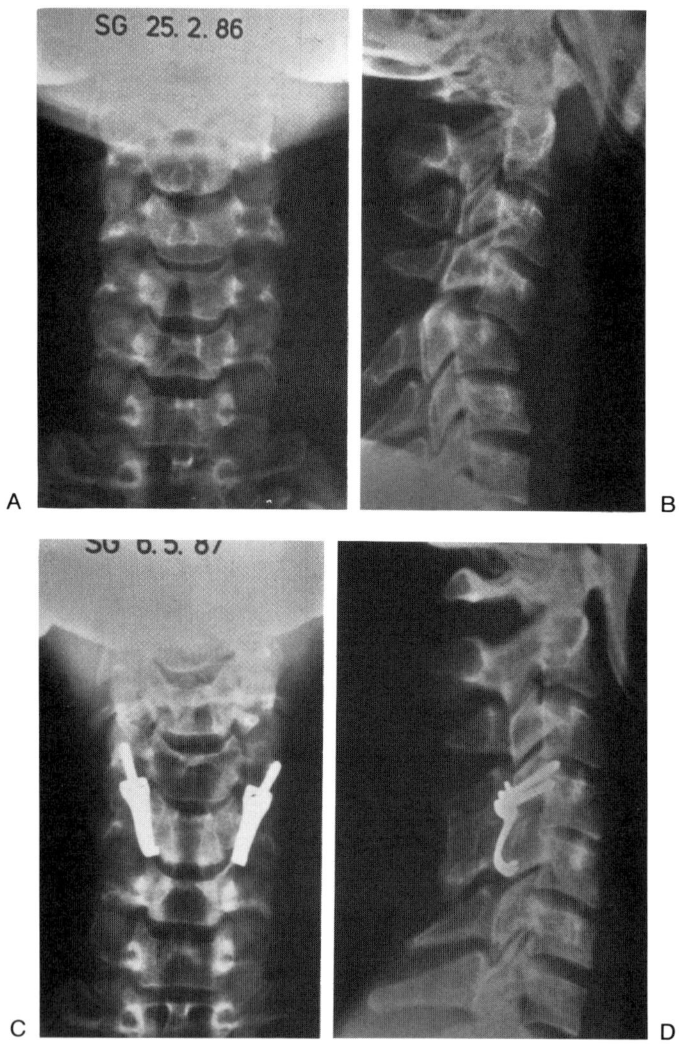

FIG. 3-109. The AP **(A)** and lateral (**B**) radiographs of flexion rotation injury at C-4 to C-5 with locking of one facet. **C,D:** Solid fusion is demonstrated at 14 months using hook plates and bone graft. (From Jeanneret B, Magerl F, Ward EH, Ward JCL. Posterior stabilization of the cervical spine with hook plates. *Spine* 1991;16:556–563.)

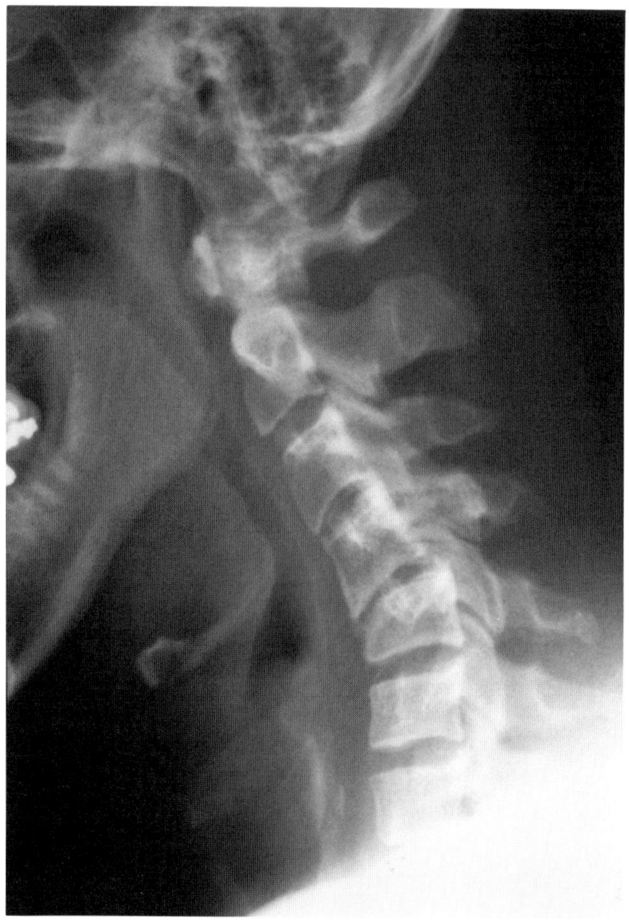

FIG. 3-110. C-4 to C-5 fracture subluxation. The posterior ligaments were disrupted leading to kyphosis with healing.

tation may be used after anterior decompression of flexion-compression injuries. Preoperatively, the surgeon must be certain to evaluate the posterior structures completely because anterior repairs may be less effective with posterior ligament disruption (Fig. 3-110).[150,173] Instrumentation is usually combined with one of several bone graft options.[169,173]

Anterior bone grafting can be accomplished with iliac, fibular, or rib grafts. Longer segments often require midfibular grafts. Iliac bone grafts are an excellent source of cortical and cancellous bone and are frequently used for interbody fusion plugs or with partial corpectomy (Fig. 3-111).[163,172]

Plate-screw instrumentation. Anterior fusion with plate, screw, and when necessary, bone grafts can be accomplished with several types of plate and screw systems.[160,167,172,173] Single-segment fusion with an interbody bone graft or plug is performed for degenerative disease or trauma (Smith-Robinson fusion, Fig. 3-111). Multiple levels can also be approached. Cloward described a technique that involves grafting with partial corpectomy (Fig. 3-111).[162,172]

Anterior fusion plates are thin to reduce prevertebral soft tissue irritation. Casper plates (Fig. 3-112) are configured with two rows of screw holes and wider at the bottom. H plates are stainless steel and expanded at screw hole sites. Cortical screws are used that are designed to pass through both the anterior and posterior cortex. The Morscher plate (Fig. 3-113) is a modification of the H plate.[172] The screw has an expanded head that locks it to the plate by virtue of a small set screw. The added stability allows the use of shorter screws that only engage the anterior cortex and, therefore, avoid the risks associated with penetrating the posterior vertebral cortex. Ingrowth screws, such as those seen in Figure 3-106, have been removed from the market.[172]

Combined Anterior and Posterior Instrumentation. Techniques described earlier can be used in combination for complex injuries or when bone loss and posterior support structures occur together. A second posterior procedure is required in some patients if instability occurs or posterior injuries are initially overlooked (Fig. 3-114).[150]

Thoracolumbar Spine Trauma

Anatomic differences have an impact on the diagnosis, classification, and management of thoracic and lumbar spine injuries.[178,183] There is normally a slight kyphotic curve in the thoracic spine. This is in contrast to the lordotic curves in the cervical and lumbar regions. Also, the spinal canal is smaller and more circular in the thoracic spine compared with the larger, more triangular configuration in the lumbar segments. As one progresses inferiorly, the vertebral bodies increase in size, and the discs increase in height, resulting in an increasing resistance to vertical compression forces.[178]

Because of differences in the range of motion, transition in the facet joints, and other anatomic factors, the thoracolumbar junction is the area that is most susceptible to injury. Nicoll[206] reported that 66% of thoracolumbar injuries occurred between T-12 and L-2.

Mechanism of Injury

The mechanisms of thoracolumbar injury are similar in some respects to those of cervical spine injury. A thorough understanding of the mechanism of injury, specifically which columns are involved, and the degree of stability is essential in selecting the appropriate treatment.[183]

The Denis[183] three-column approach is commonly used in classifying and evaluating the stability of thoracolumbar injuries (Fig. 3-115). The involvement of one column, even the posterior column, may not be sufficient to cause instability. However, posterior and middle column involvement is unstable, at least in flexion.[183]

Ferguson and Allen[189] classified thoracolumbar injuries into eight categories based on the mechanism of injury (Table 3-11). Most injuries involve flexion forces, with either rotational or compression forces in combination (76%, Table 3-11).[180,189] The rate of neurologic complications approaches 71% with torsion flexion injuries.[180] A similar incidence of neurologic injury occurs with flexion-distraction injuries at the thoracolumbar junction.[178]

The Frankel scale is commonly used to assess neurologic injury pre- and postoperatively.[180,190] This system is based on motor and sensory deficits below the level of thoracolumbar injury.[185]

A: no motor or sensory activity below the level of injury
B: sensory intact but no motor function below the level of injury
C: ineffective motor function
D: motor function effective but weak
E: sensory and motor function normal

TABLE 3-11. *Thoracolumbar fractures: the Ferguson-Allen classification*[180,189]

Type of injury	Incidence rates (%)
Compression-flexion	49
Torsion-flexion	16
Lateral-flexion	11
Translation	9
Vertical compression	7
Distraction-flexion	5
Distraction-extension	3
Minor injuries[a]	

[a] Not included in incidence; isolated transverse process fractures, etc.

(text continues on page 189)

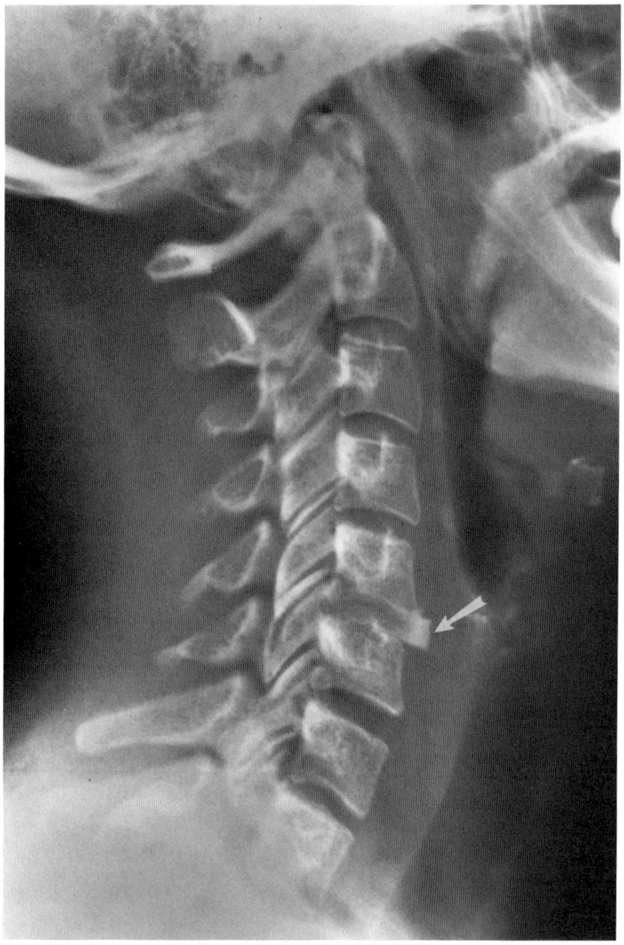

FIG. 3-111. Lateral view of the cervical spine following anterior discectomy and insertion of an iliac bone plug at C-5 to C-6 (*arrow*). The graft is partially extruded.

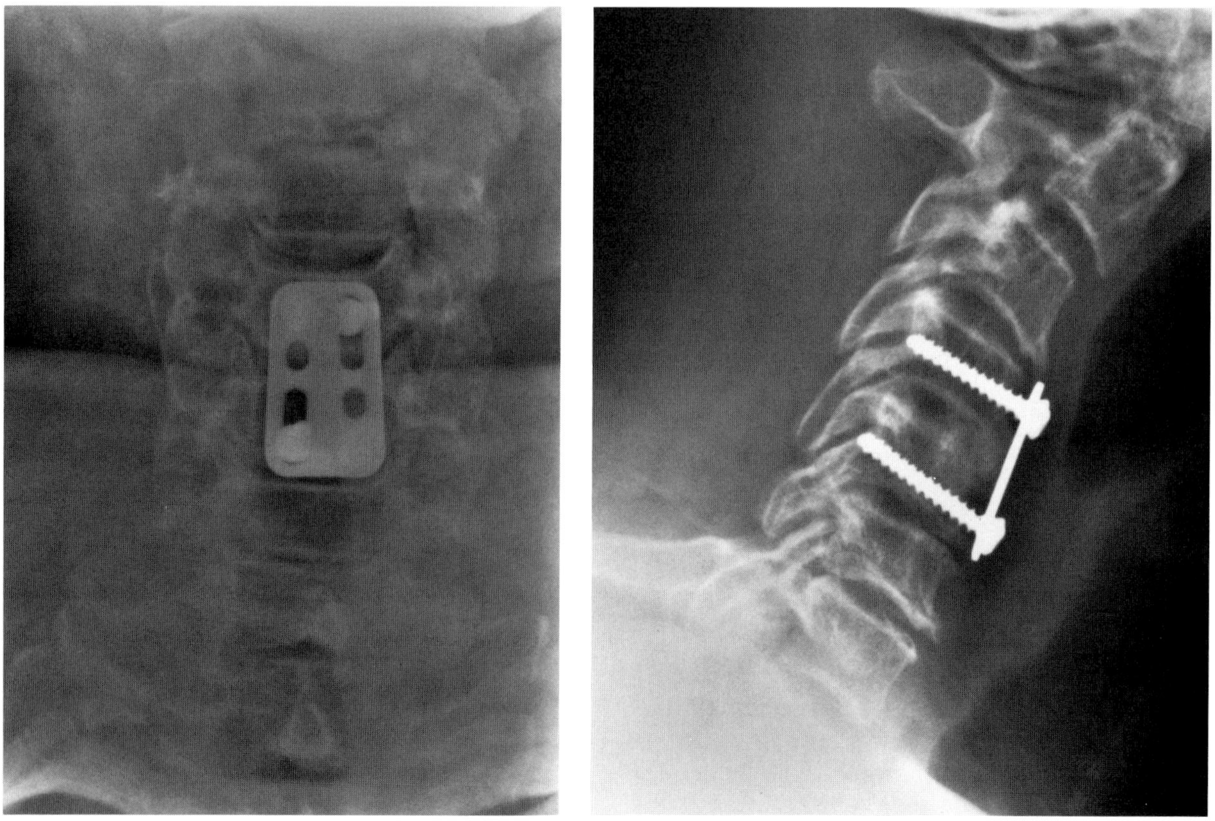

A B

FIG. 3-112. The AP **(A)** and lateral **(B)** radiographs demonstrating anterior fusion using a Casper plate, four bone screws, and iliac graft for C-4 to C-5 anterior fusion. The tips of the screws penetrate to at least the level of the posterior cortex. C-3 to C-6 posterior decompression.

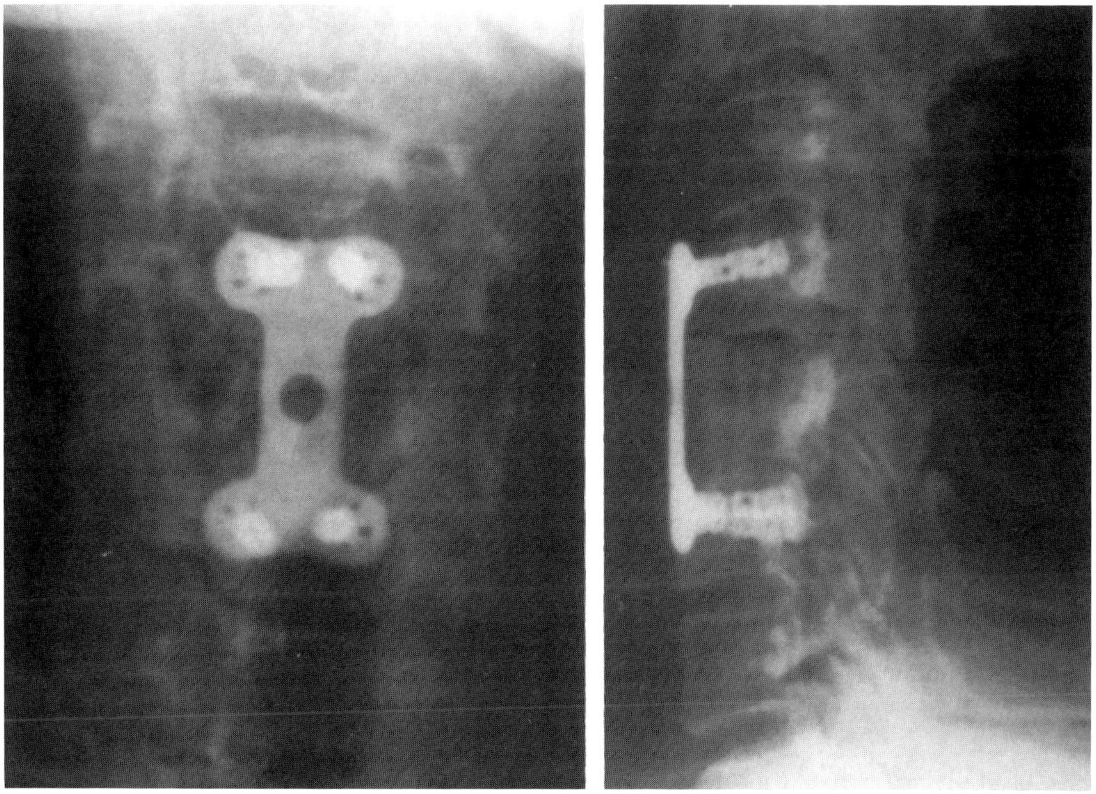

A B

FIG. 3-113. The AP **(A)** and lateral **(B)** radiographs of the cervical spine with a Morscher cervical spine plate and four ingrowth screws for anterior fusion at C-4 to C-5. (From Slone RM, MacMillan M, Montgomery WJ. Principles, basic hardware and fixation techniques for the cervical spine. *Radiographics* 1993; 13:341–356.)

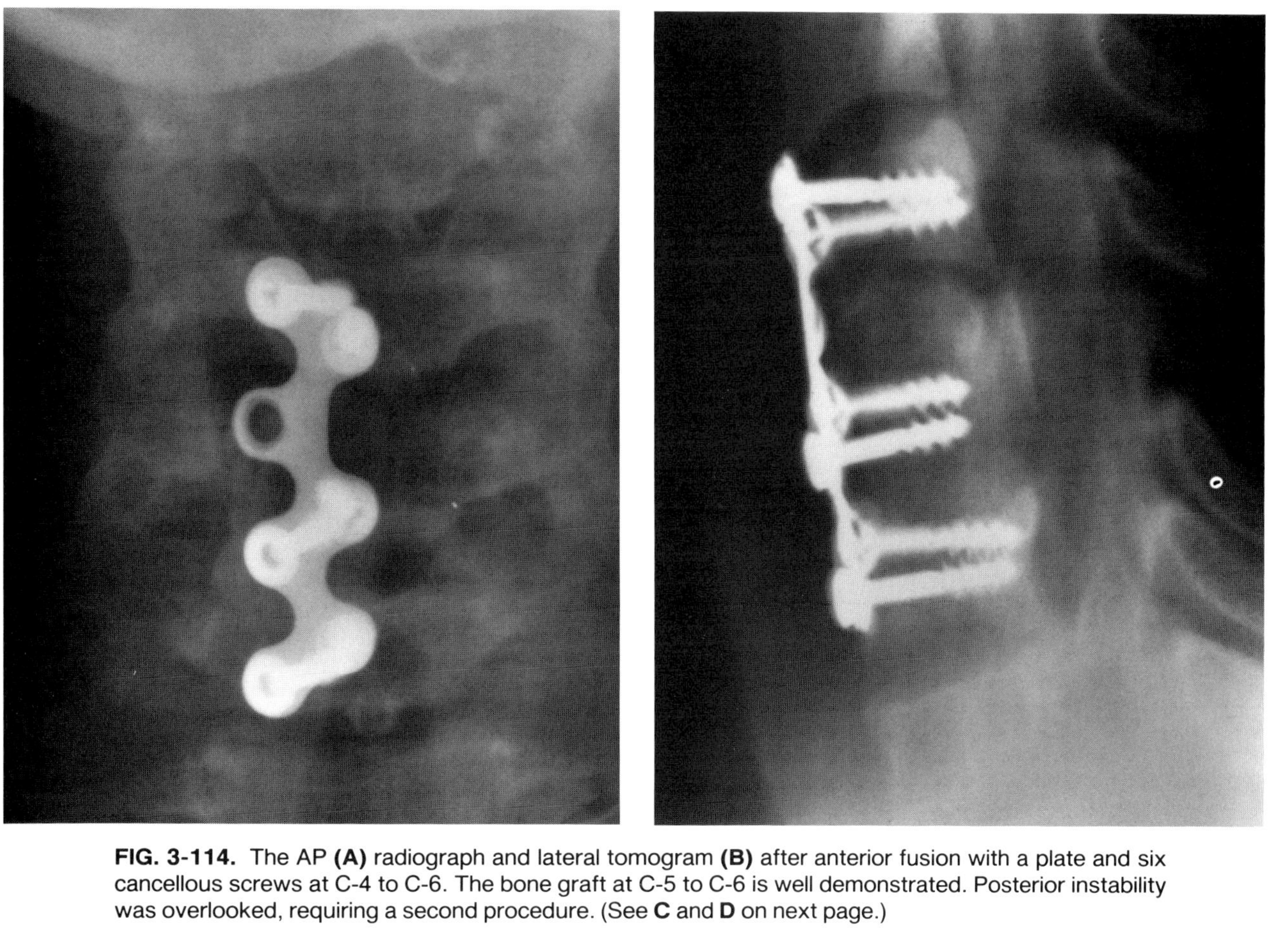

A B

FIG. 3-114. The AP **(A)** radiograph and lateral tomogram **(B)** after anterior fusion with a plate and six cancellous screws at C-4 to C-6. The bone graft at C-5 to C-6 is well demonstrated. Posterior instability was overlooked, requiring a second procedure. (See **C** and **D** on next page.)

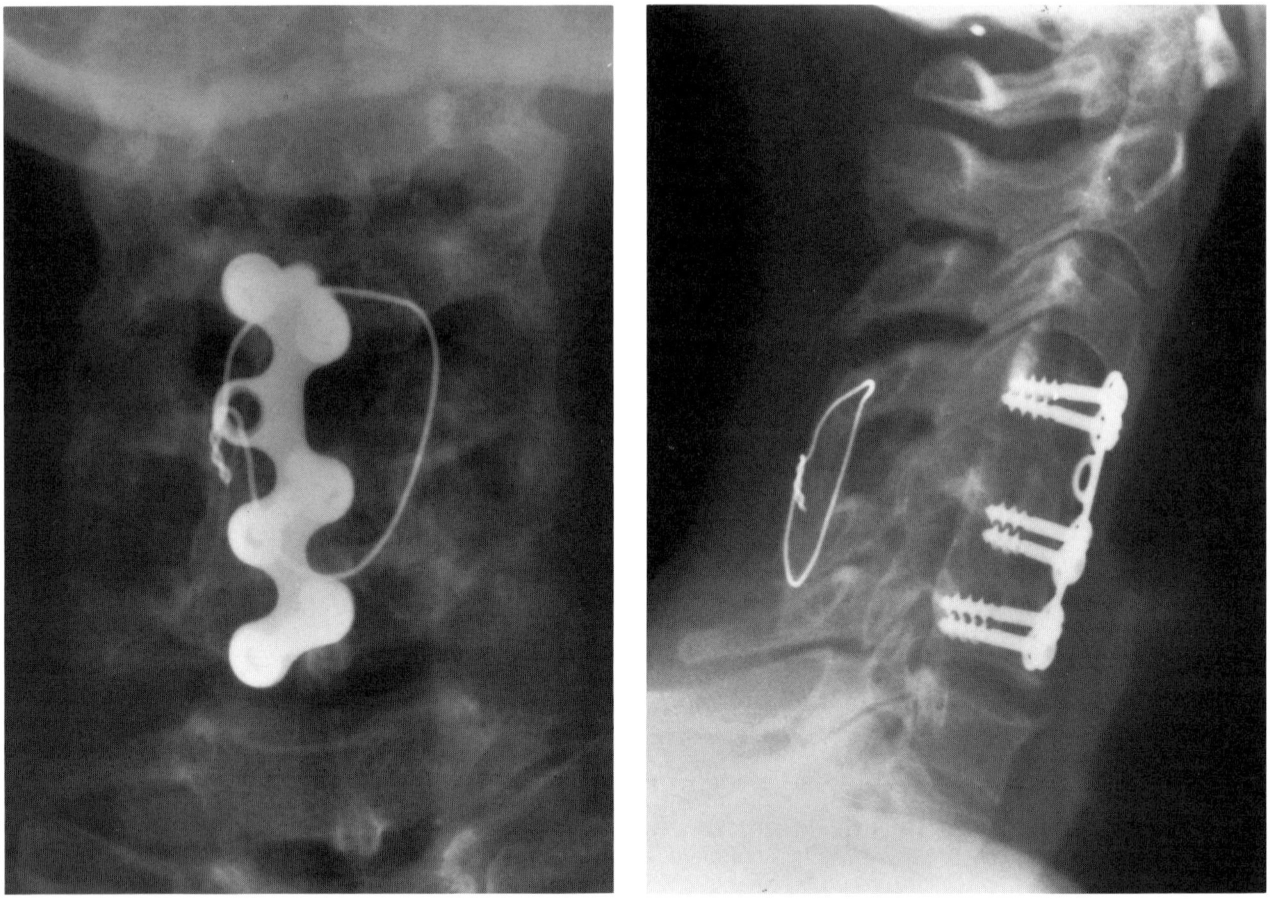

C D

FIG. 3-114. *Continued.* The AP **(C)** and lateral **(D)** radiographs demonstrate bone graft and wire fusion at C-4 to C-6. The C-5 spinous process was partially removed.

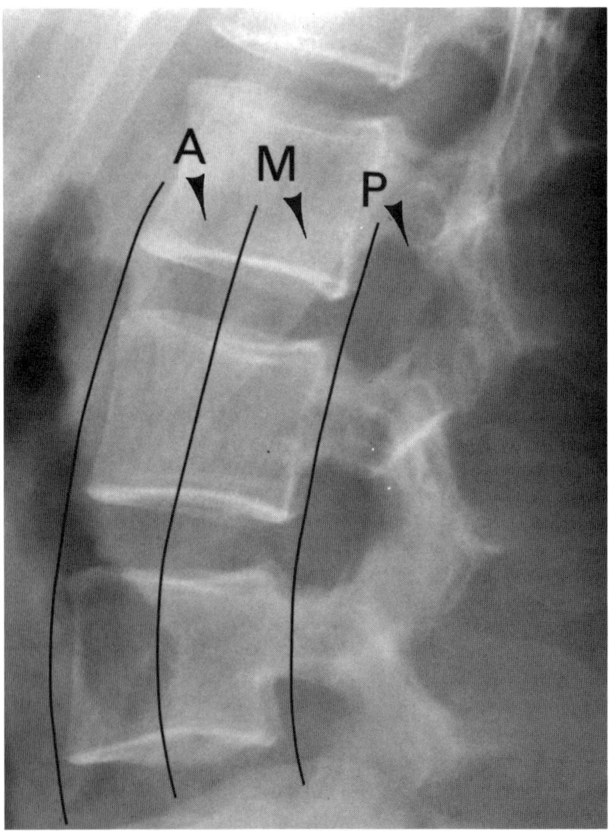

FIG. 3-115. Lateral view of the lumbar spine demonstrating the three columns used for the evaluation of thoracolumbar injury. *A,* anterior column: anterior vertebral one-half of the body anterior longitudinal ligament and anterior disc; *M,* middle column: posterior one-half of the vertebral body and disc and the posterior longitudinal ligament; *P,* posterior column: posterior bony arch ligamentum favium, capsule, anterospinous ligament, and supraspinous ligament.

Preoperative Imaging

Routine AP (Fig. 3-116) and lateral (Fig. 3-117) radiographs fulfill the minimal requirement for the detection and classification of spinal injuries. Much valuable information can and should be obtained on AP and lateral radiographs. The transverse processes, paraspinal soft tissues, posterior arch, and configuration of the vertebral body should be carefully assessed.[178] The three-column approach must be considered in determining the stability and mechanism of injury.[178,183] Measuring the change in lordosis or kyphotic deformity is important in completely assessing the injury and providing a baseline for operative correction (Fig. 3-117C).

For the evaluation of subtle injuries and bony involvement of the spinal canal, CT is especially useful.[134,184] Compromise of the spinal canal commonly occurs with flexion-compression and vertical-compression forces. Denis[183] and Denis et al.[184] classified burst fractures based on the radiographic appearance (Fig. 3-118). The CT features are most useful in this regard.[178] Type A burst fractures (Fig. 3-118B) account for approximately 23% of fractures. These fractures have posterior fragments at the superior and inferior vertebral margins with multiple small fragments.[177] Axial loading is the mechanism of injury. Type B fractures (Fig. 3-118B) are the most common (55% of burst fractures). This injury involves the superior end plate. There is often a single fracture line extending to the inferior end plate. Axial loading with compression is the likely mechanism of injury.[177,183] Type C burst fractures (Fig. 3-118B) are rare. Injuries associated with translation, type D, are divided according to the direction of translation. Lateral translation (type D1) is the most common. Anterior translation or subluxation (type D2) is less common. Axial loading with lateral compression can result in unilateral burst injuries (type E). These injuries are also uncommon.

The extent of spinal canal involvement in the lumbar spine is important in management planning. Here, CT images can be used to grade the degree of spinal canal compromise. Ferguson and Allen[189] categorized the involvement as follows:

A: 0% to 25% reduction in spinal canal by bone fragments
B: 25% to 50% canal compromise (Fig. 3-119A)
C: 50% to 75% canal compromise (Fig. 3-119B)
D: 75% to 100% canal compromise

Takata et al.[212] described an uncommon posterior rim fracture, which is also important to define with CT preoperatively. Three categories of fracture have been described (Fig. 3-120). Type I fractures (33%) are posterior rim fractures. Type II (29%) are larger rim fractures, and Type III (38%) are small localized fractures.

Thoracolumbar Instrumentation

The incidence of neurologic injury is significant with incomplete injuries, which have increased as a result of improved emergency systems.[178] Initially, the critical questions involve the extent of neurologic deficit and spinal stability. Complete injury at the T-10 level or above usually indicates irreversible cord injury.[178,183] Lesions below T-10 may involve the cauda equina or nerve roots and have a better prognosis for recovery.[178]

A careful evaluation of radiographic and CT features is useful in determining the extent of injury and columns involved. These factors, along with the level of injury, are important in selecting the appropriate instrumentation. The goals of therapy should be spinal canal decompression, improving the deformity with the relief of pain and maintenance of motion, and early mobilization.[134,175]

Basic concepts for treatment are used, depending on the site and type of injury. Anterior compression fractures with no middle or posterior column involvement may not require surgery, although stabilization is more likely to be required in fractures of the upper thoracic region.[178,203] Either Harrington rods, Cotrel-Dubousset, ISOLA, or TSRH systems can be used to reduce or prevent kyphotic deformity. Harrington-rod systems depend on an intact posterior ligament complex; therefore, they are not appropriate for flexion-distraction injuries.[203] Harrington rods are simple to use, have a low risk, and are satisfactory for most T-2 to T-11 fractures. Luque rods with sublaminar wires are useful for rotational stability but do not assist in distraction or axial loading.[202]

Instrumentation techniques should preserve lumbar lordosis and reduce kyphotic deformity. In the lumbar spine, attempts should be made to fuse as few segments as possible to retain flexibility and prevent long-term low-back pain.[203]

Posterior Instrumentation

Rod-Hook Systems. The rod-hook systems described earlier can be used, depending on the location and extent of injury.[176,205] Harrington rods are particularly well suited for thoracic injuries from T-2 to T-12.[201,203] There are several disadvantages to the use of conventional Harrington distraction rods. Generally, rods are extended three levels above and two to three vertebral segments below the level of the injury (Figs. 3-121 and 3-122). This includes numerous uninvolved segments and can reduce function. System failure due to hook loosening is also a problem.[175,182,191]

Several additional procedures can be performed to improve the fixation. These include additional sublaminar wires (Fig. 3-123), rod sleeves, and locking hooks.[175,182,188,195,196]

(text continues on page 195)

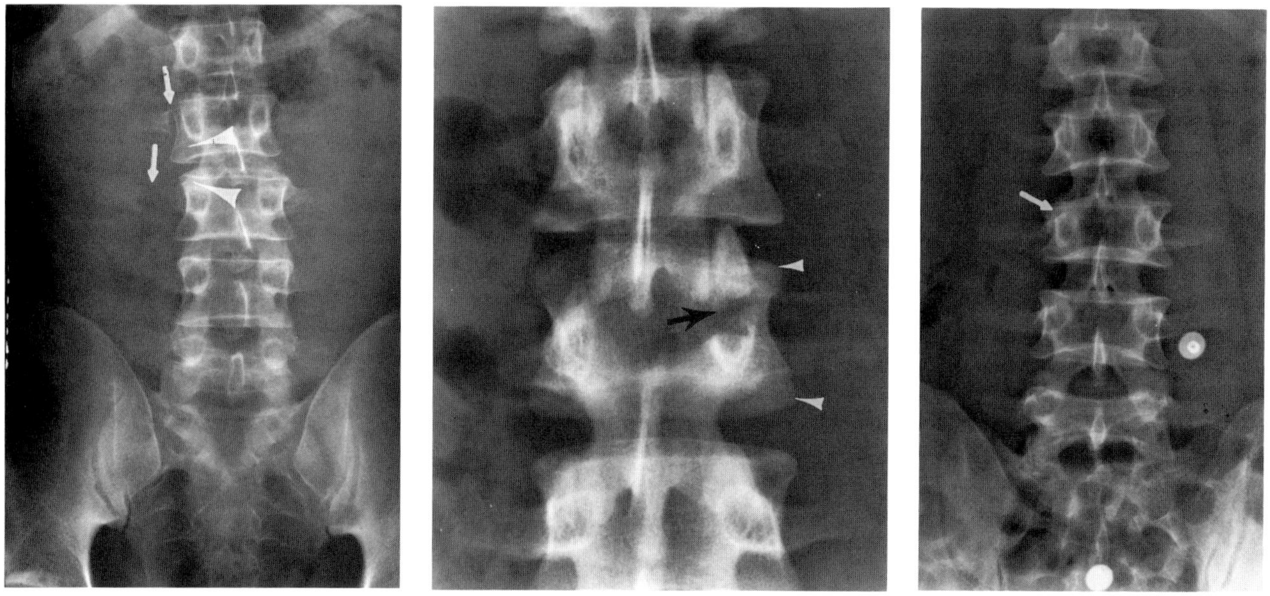

A B,C

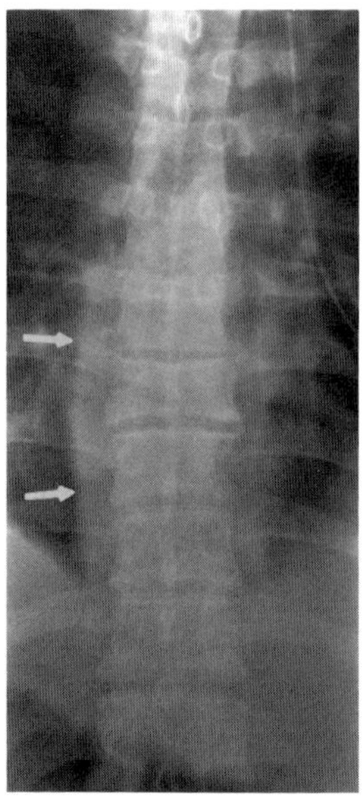

D

FIG. 3-116. The AP radiographs demonstrating features of spinal injury. **A:** Minor fracture: multiple transverse process fractures (*arrows*). Major injury: subtle translation (*arrowheads*) of L-2 on L-3. **B:** Pedicle and laminar fracture (*arrow*) with lateral compression (*arrow*) of L-3. **C:** Lateral compression (*arrow*) of L-3. **D:** Lower thoracic compression fractures with paraspinal swelling (*arrows*).

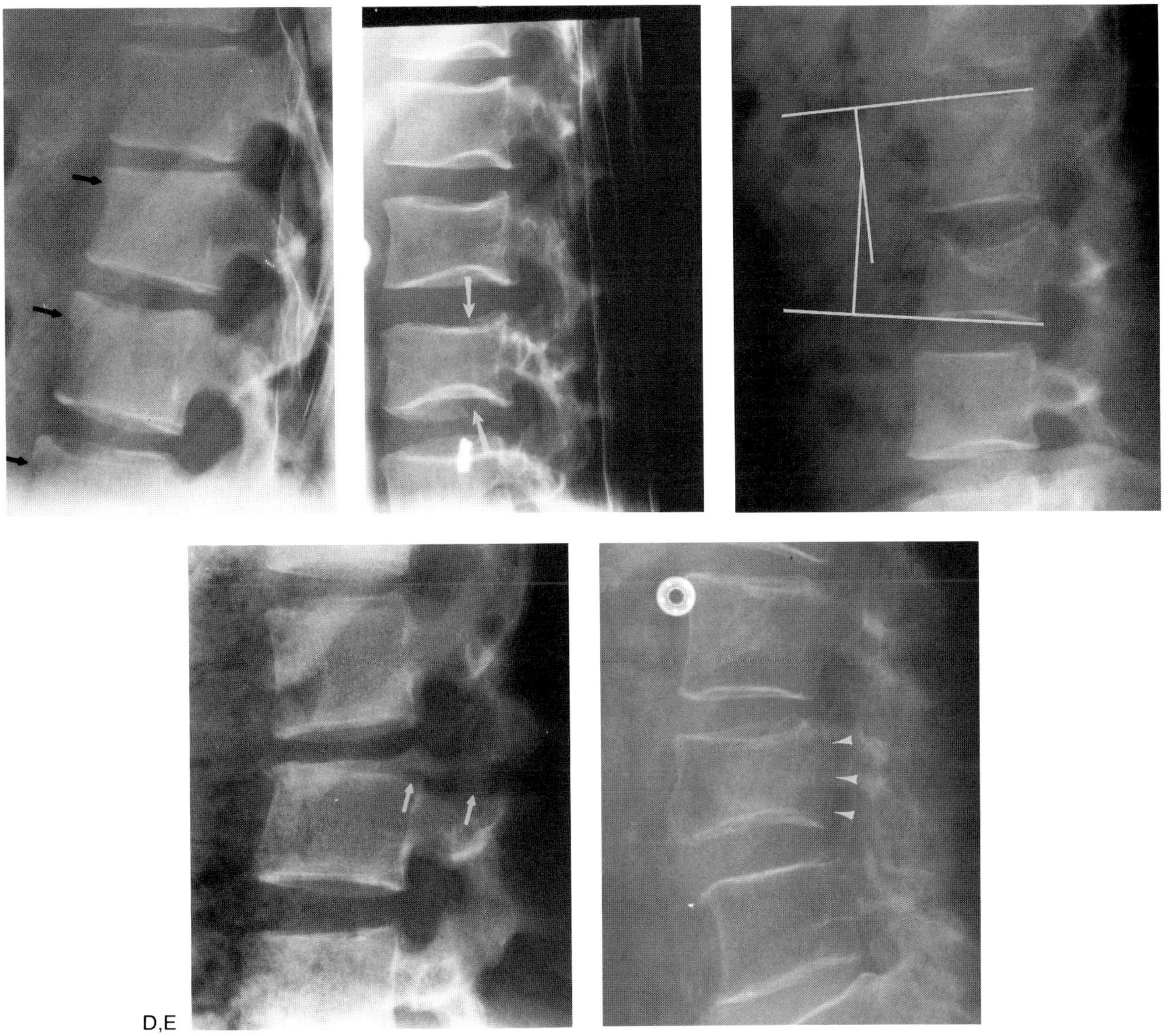

A B,C D,E

FIG. 3-117. Lateral views of the lumbar spine. **A:** Subtle anterior cortical compression fracture at T-12 to L-2 (*arrows*). **B:** Vertical compression injury with end-plate fractures (*arrows*) at L-4. **C:** L-3 compression fracture with kyphotic deformity. **D:** L-1 Chance fracture with extension into the pedicle and lamina (*arrows*). **E:** Burst fracture of L-3 with posterior bulging of the cortex (*arrowheads*).

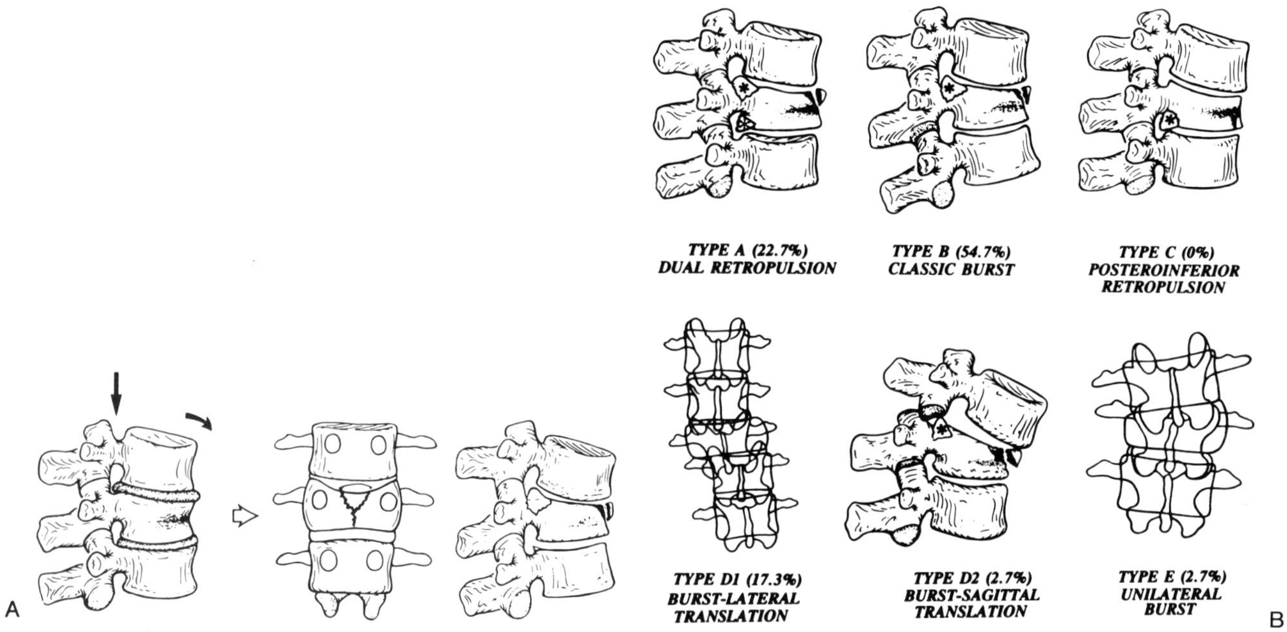

FIG. 3-118. Mechanism of injury **(A)** and classification **(B)** of burst fractures. (From Atlas SW, Regenbogen V, Rogers PF, Kina KS. The radiographic characterization of the burst fractures of the spine. *AJR* 1986;147:575–582.)

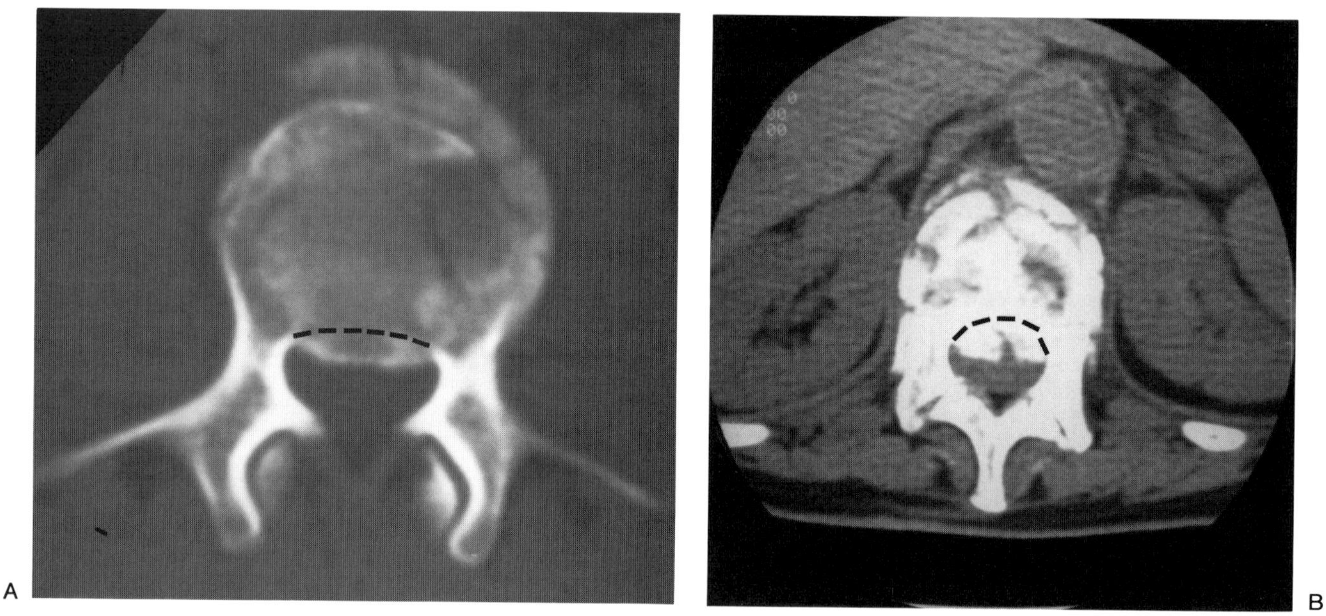

FIG. 3-119. The CT images of the lumbar spine demonstrating 25% canal compromise **(A)** and 50% canal compromise **(B)**.

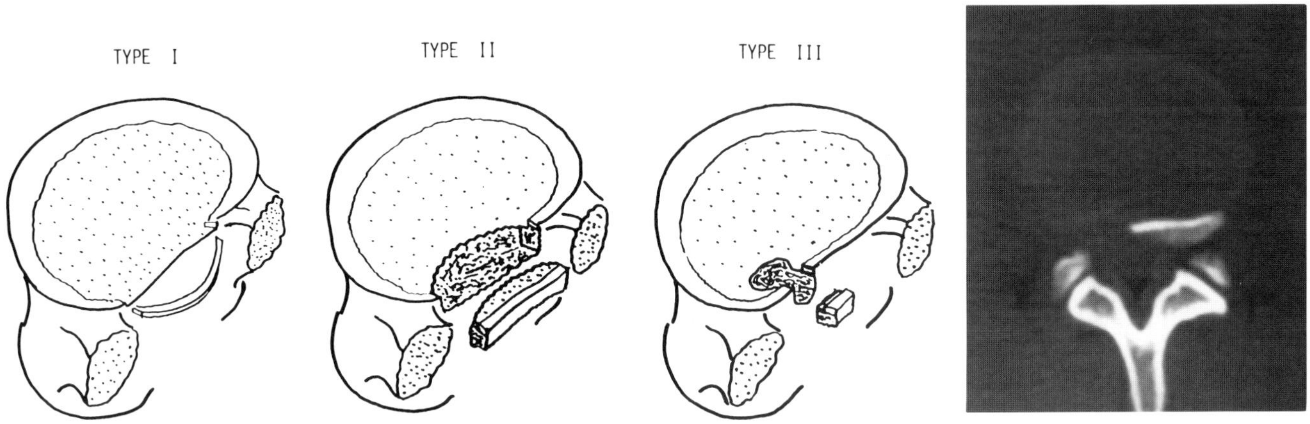

A B

FIG. 3-120. A: Posterior rim fractures. (From Takata K, Insue S, Takalioski K, Ohtsuka Y. Fracture of the posterior margin of the lumbar vertebra. *J Bone Joint Surg* [*Am*] 1988;70A:589–594.) **B:** Posterior lumbar margin fractures with fragment inversion.

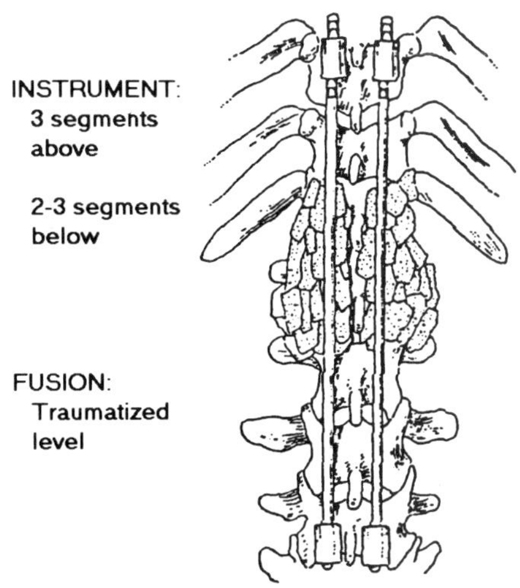

FIG. 3-121. Harrington rod fusion for limited arthrodesis in thoracolumbar trauma. Instrumentation at three segments above and two to three segments below the fracture. (From Dekutoski MB, Conlan ES, Salciccioli GG. Spinal mobility and deformity after Harrington rod stabilization and limited arthrodesis of thoracolumbar fractures. *J Bone Joint Surg* [*Am*] 1993;75A:168–176.)

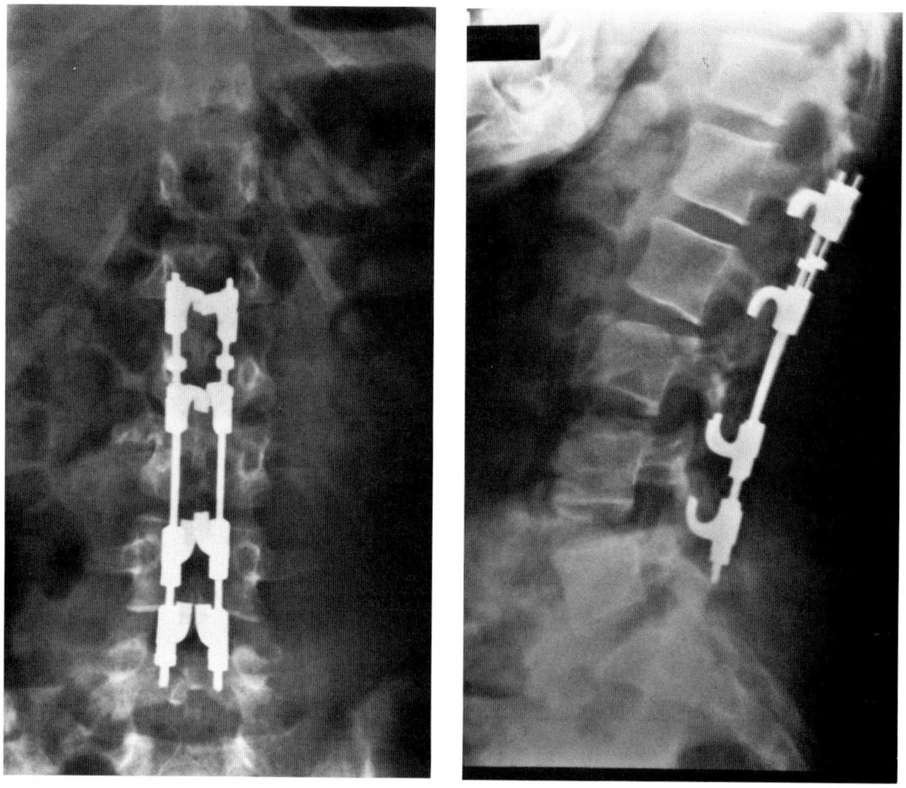

FIG. 3-122. The AP **(A)** and lateral **(B)** radiographs of a L-3 compression-distraction injury with separation of the posterior column. Threaded Harrington compression rods with laminar hooks.

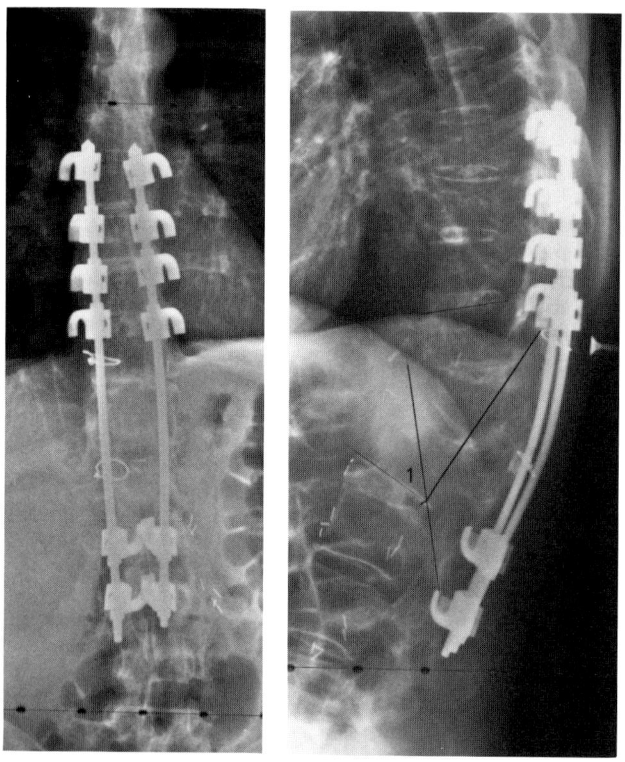

FIG. 3-123. The AP **(A)** and lateral **(B)** radiographs of a T-12 compression fracture-dislocation with kyphotic deformity. Harrington compression rods, hooks, and two sublaminar wires used with bone grafting.

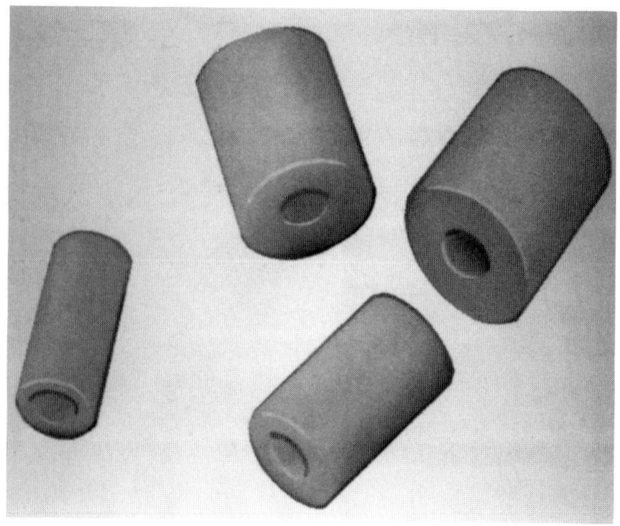

FIG. 3-124. Edwards™ rod sleeves, which are used with rod systems to facilitate reduction while reducing anterior impingement. (Courtesy of Zimmer, Warsaw, IN.)

Rod sleeves (Fig. 3-124) come in various sizes and are positioned to fill the void between the rod and posterior elements (Fig. 3-125). The sleeves are made of high-density polyethylene and impregnated with barium to make them radiopaque. The sleeves provide improved medial, lateral, and anterior stability in addition to pushing the vertebral body anteriorly and improving alignment (reduced kyphotic deformity).[188] Anatomic hooks (Fig. 3-126) are used for broad laminar contact.

Locking hooks reduce the incidence of hook pullout (Fig. 3-127) and improve rotational stability.[192,196]

Luque rods are also designed to include multiple segments above and below the level of injury.[202] Rods with sublaminar wire systems are not optimal for distraction and increasing vertebral height.[175,200,201]

Cotrel-Dubousset instrumentation is also more useful over longer segments.[200,203] When rod-hook systems are extended to the sacrum, screws may be selected for sacral attachment (Fig. 3-128). Fusion of too many segments can increase the incidence of iatrogenic flat back syndrome.[200,205]

Pedicle Screw Systems. Multiple pedicle screw systems (discussed previously) are available. Rigid short-segment fixation can be achieved. Pedicle screws can be used with rods (e.g., AO fixator, VSF, Wiltse system, Rogozinski rods, ISOLA, and TSRH; Fig. 3-129) or plates (e.g., AO plates or Steffee plates; Fig. 3-130).[175,181,195,199,200,211]

The Dick spinal internal fixator instrumentation was modified after the Magerl system and consists of 7-mm diameter threaded rods with square ends for clamp and serrated washer attachments (Fig. 3-131).[185] Schanz screws (Figs. 3-132 and 3-133) with a 5-mm diameter are used for transpedicular attachment.[175,185] This system controls lordosis and kyphosis and provides rotational stability. The system is designed to fix fewer segments, typically only the vertebra above and below the injury.[185,198]

The system is effective from T-8 to S-1 and is most commonly used for burst fractures. The Ölerud system[198,207] is similar in appearance and function.

Anterior Instrumentation

Anterior instrumentation can be used for hyperextension injuries or load sharing or when there are significant anterior bone voids.[187,201,203] There are several devices more commonly used in trauma. These include the Kaneda, Rezaian, and anterior plate-screw systems.

Kaneda Device. The Kaneda device was introduced in 1984. This system consists of two curved plates with staples (similar to Dwyer instrumentation) attached to the vertebral bodies with screws. The plates are connected by threaded rods that attach to screw heads with nuts (Fig. 3-134).[200,210]

Anterior Plate-Screw Instrumentation. The major indication for this technique is narrowing of the spinal canal that cannot be approached posteriorly.[195,210] Plates are available in several configurations (Fig. 3-135). A portion of the vertebra is removed, and the bone graft is positioned prior to plate and screw placement (Figs. 3-136 and 3-137).[195]

The ZPlate-ATL™ system (Fig. 3-138) was developed for thoracolumbar burst fractures and neoplasms. This system designed by Dr. T.A. Zdeblick has improved CT and MRI compatibility.

Some authors believe burst fractures and kyphotic deformities are better approached anteriorly. More complete decompression is possible.[195]

Anterior Rod-Screw Systems. Anterior rod-screw systems using Harrington rods and screws may be used to correct kyphotic deformities (Fig. 3-139).[197,203] Bi- or tricortical iliac grafts are used, which are similar to plate-screw techniques (Figs. 3-140 and 3-141).[197]

Rezaian System. This system is unique in that there are no screws or plates and only the involved segment is bridged by the device.[186,208] The system is designed to replace the compressed vertebra, achieve anterior decompression of the neural tissues, restore vertebral height, and correct kyphosis.[208] The turn-buckle device is currently available in four sizes, from 25 to 60 mm (Figs. 3-142 and 143). Rib grafts are used to connect the vertebra above and below the fixator (Fig. 3-142B).

Complications

The complications of spinal injury are usually considered to be related to the degree of injury or treatment. However, problems can occur during the evaluation period (leading to incorrect selection of treatment), during reduction (open or closed), and during the postoperative period.[201]

During the pretreatment phase, it is important for the radiologist and orthopedic surgeon to communicate so that the extent of injury, stability, and associated injuries are identified prior to selecting treatment options.[178] Failure to identify subtle unstable injuries (Fig. 3-144) or combination injuries must be avoided. For example, up to 20% of upper cervical spine injuries have associated lower cervical injuries (Fig. 3-145), and distant multilevel injuries occur in up to 15% of patients.[178,179]

Complications may also occur as a result of improper implant selection. For example, Luque rods do not counteract axial load, which can result in failure to correct vertebral height. Harrington rods alone may not correct thoracolumbar kyphosis.[201,202]

Also, when laminectomies are performed to decompress the spinal canal, proper fixation must be provided to prevent increasing neurologic deficits and deformity.[201]

(text continues on page 211)

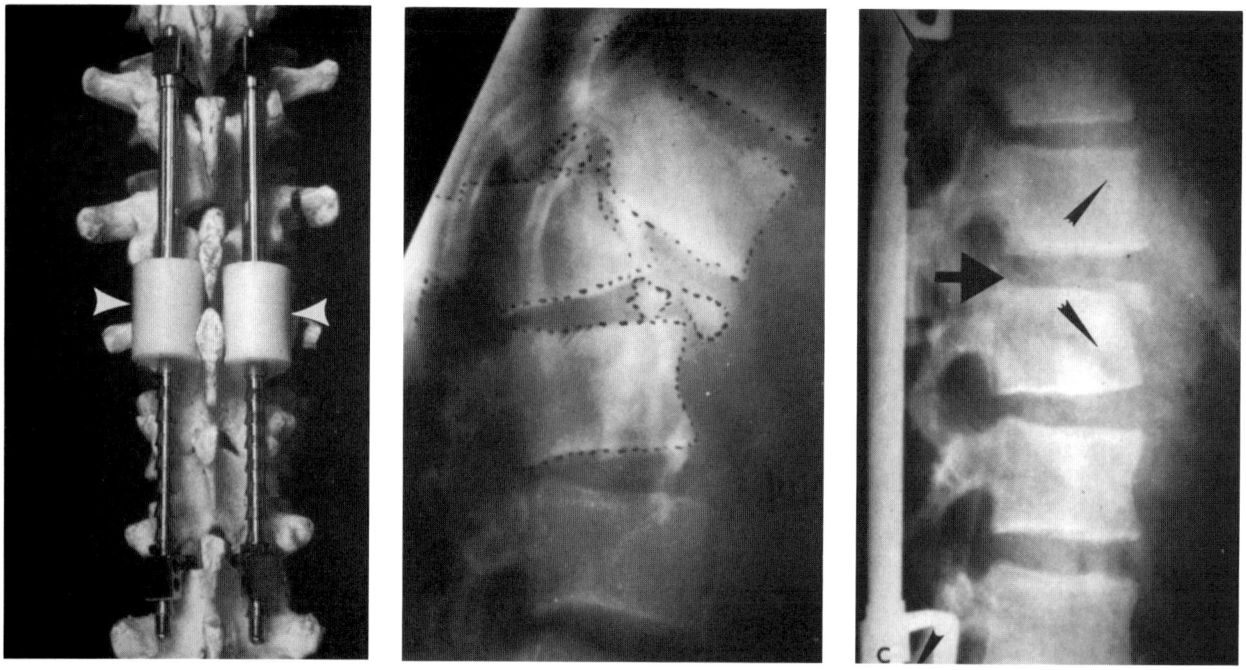

A B,C

FIG. 3-125. Flexion-compression injury with severe displacement and kyphotic deformity. **A:** Harrington distraction rods and rod sleeves (*arrows*). Pre- and postoperative radiographs demonstrating fracture-dislocation **(B)** and reduction **(C)**. The rod sleeves (*arrow*) cause a posterior-anterior force moment, with anterior distraction (*arrows*) working in concert with the distraction hooks. (From Edwards CC, Levine AM. Early rod-sleeve stabilization of the injured thoracic and lumbar spine. *Orthop Clin North Am* 1986;17:121–145.)

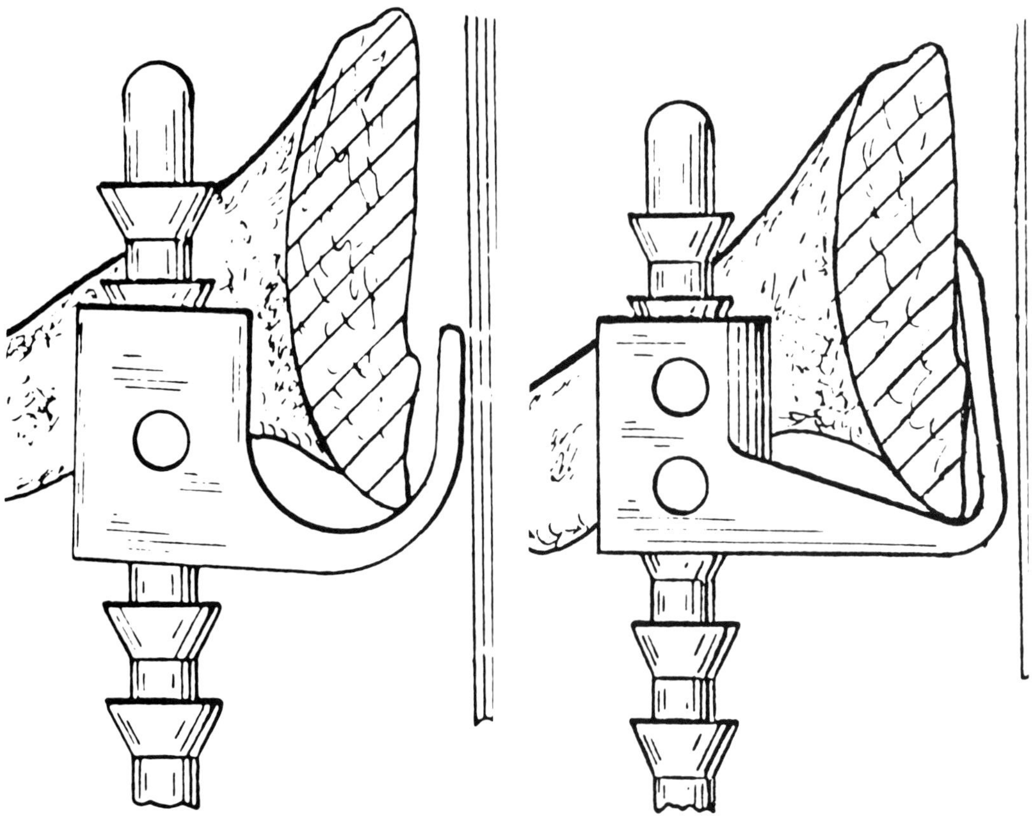

A B

FIG. 3-126. Conventional C hook **(A)** and anatomic hook **(B)** to improve lamina contact. (From Edwards CC, Levine AM. Early rod-sleeve stabilization of the injured thoracic and lumbar spine. *Orthop Clin North Am* 1986;17:121–145.)

A

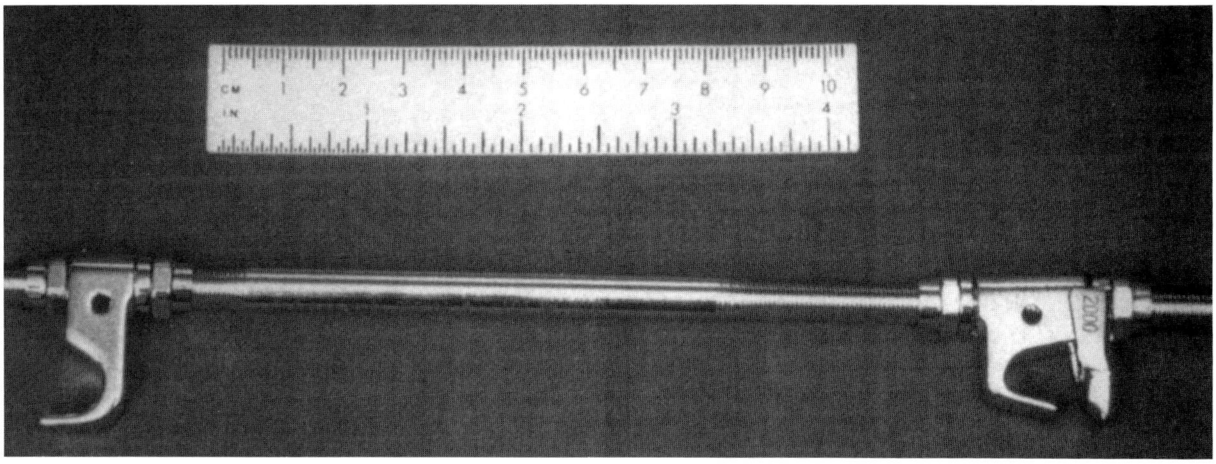

B

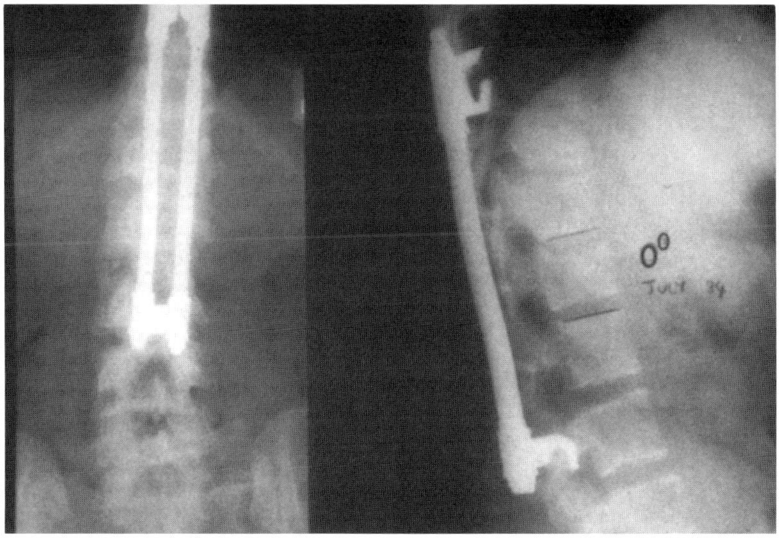

FIG. 3-127. **A:** Locking 7-mm spinal rod. The lower hook (*left*) is fixed by nuts in any position of rotation. The upper hook (*right*) has an upper cap to encircle the lamina and reduce pull out. **B:** Reduction of a marked compression fracture with locking hooks and rods. (From Gertzbein SD, Jacobs RR, Stoll J, et al. Results of a locking-hook spinal rod for fractures of the thoracic and lumbar spine. *Spine* 1990;15:275–280.)

A

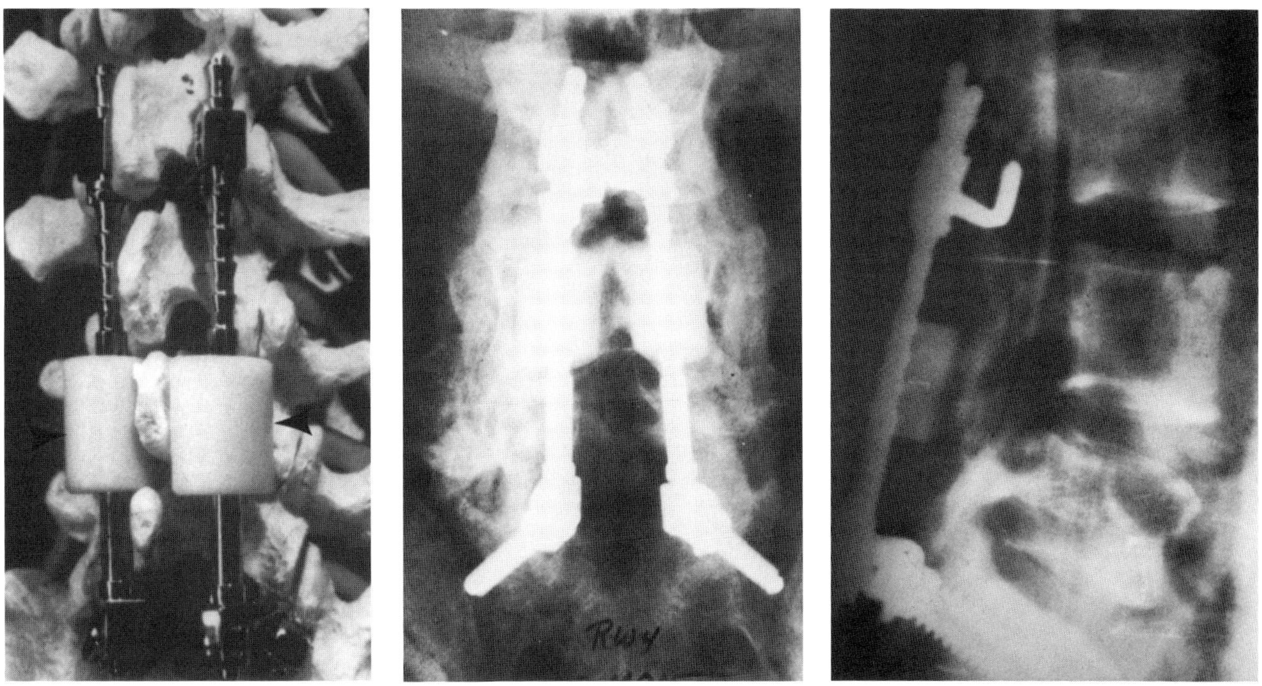

B,C

FIG. 3-128. A: Harrington distraction rods, rod sleeves (*arrows*), and sacral screws. The AP **(B)** and lateral **(C)** radiographs of short-segment Harrington rod, rod sleeve, and sacral alar screws for fixation. (From Edwards CC, Levine AM. Early rod-sleeve stabilization of the injured thoracic and lumbar spine. *Orthop Clin North Am* 1986;17:121–145.)

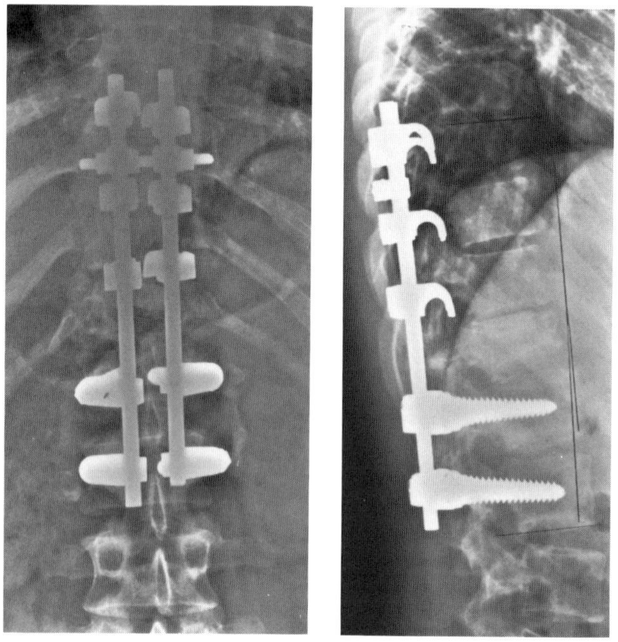

A B

FIG. 3-129. The AP **(A)** and lateral **(B)** radiographs of a T-12 burst fracture with ISOLA rods, six hooks, four pedicle screws with straight rod connectors, and one transverse stabilizer at the upper end of the system. There is minimal residual kyphosis.

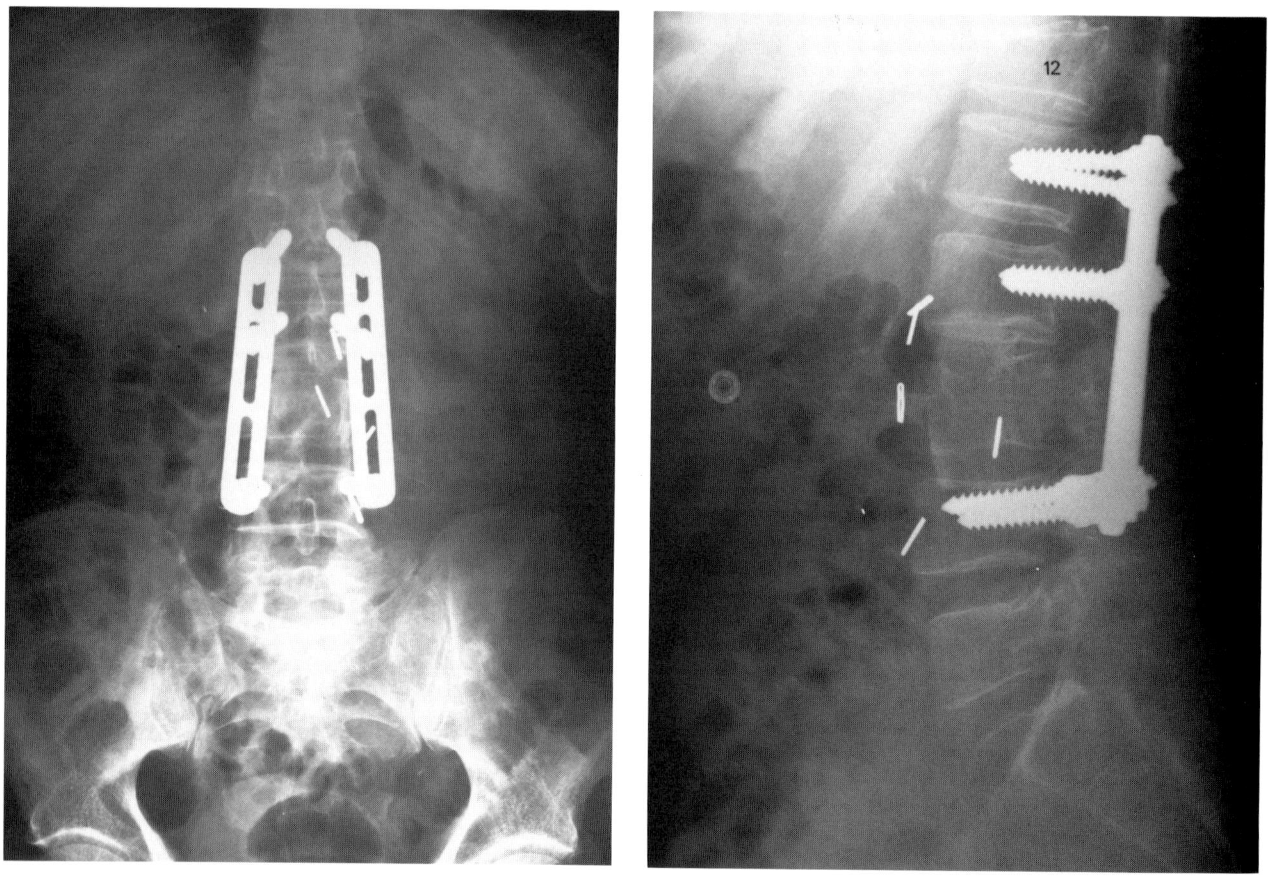

A B

FIG. 3-130. The AP **(A)** and lateral **(B)** radiographs of a L-3 fracture with anterior iliac bone graft and Steffee-type plates with six pedicle screws for fixation.

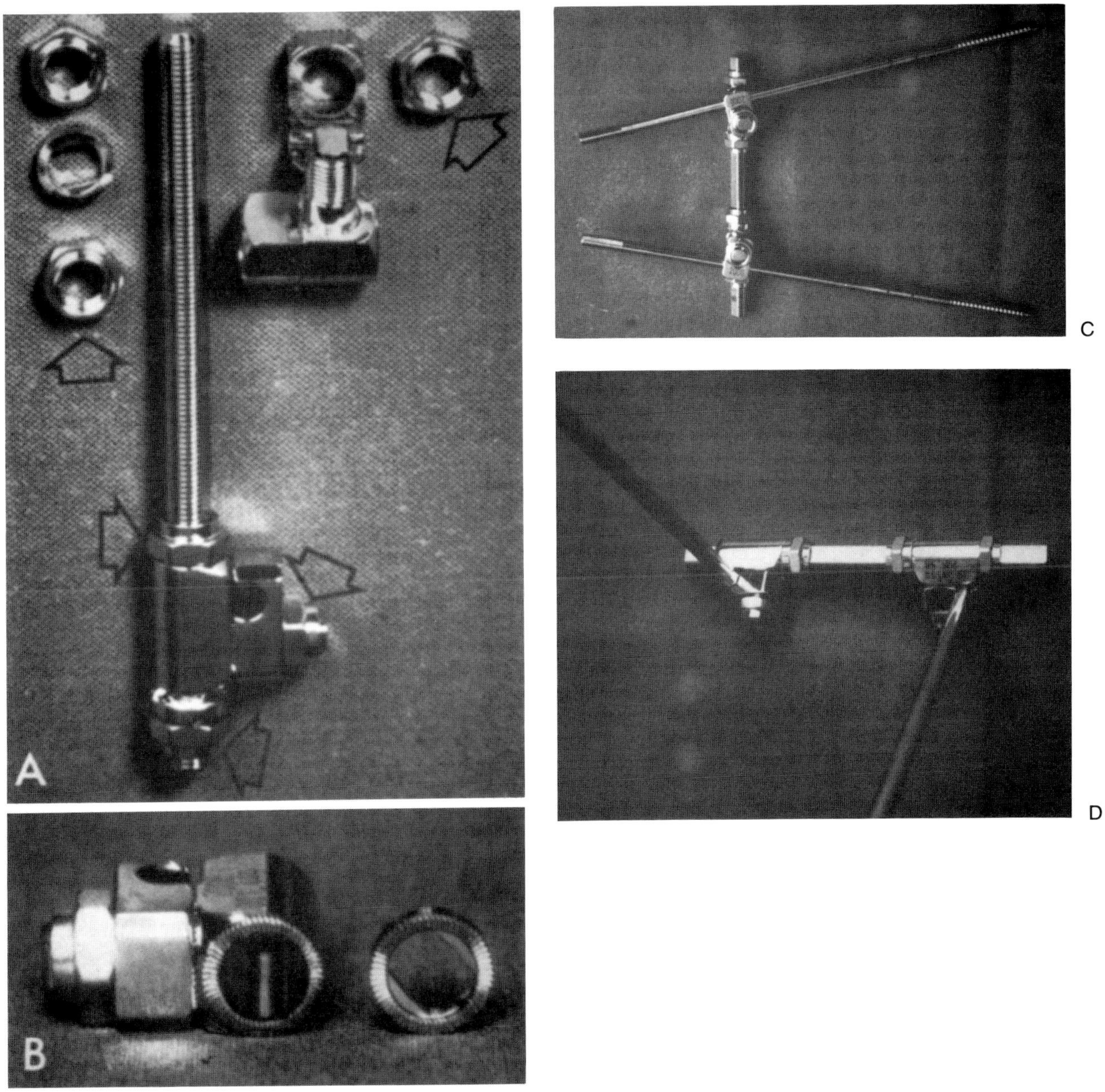

FIG. 3-131. Internal skeletal fixation system (Dick).[174] **A:** Threaded rod with mounted hinge clamp at the lower end. **B:** Serrated end of the hinge clamp and serrated washer. **C:** System assembled in lordotic position. **D:** Clamps rotated around the rod. (From Aebi M, Etter C, Kehl T, Thagott J. The internal skeletal fixation system: a new treatment of thoracolumbar fractures and other spinal disorders. *Clin Orthop* 1988;227:30–43.)

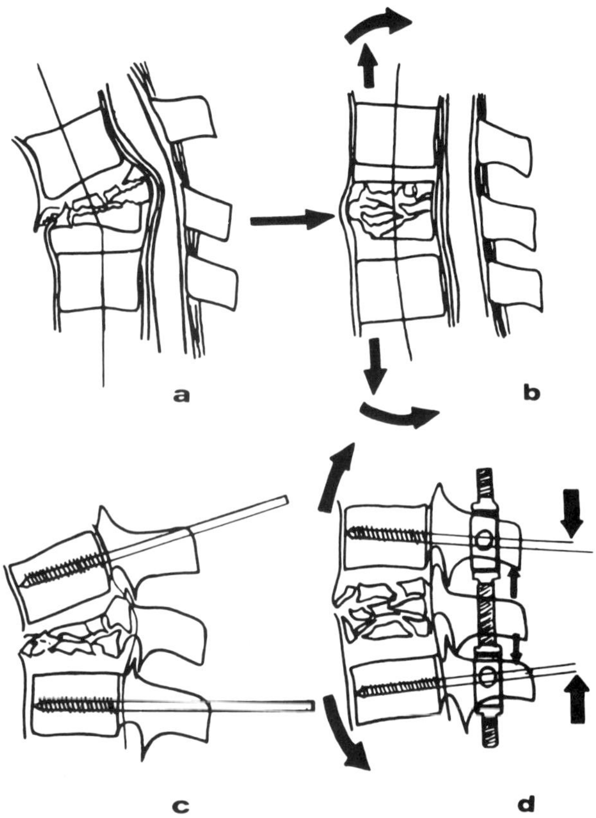

FIG. 3-132. Reduction of a burst fracture using the Dick internal fixator. **A,B:** Lordosis and distraction open anteriorly and reduce the posterior vertebral body. **C,D:** Schanz screws used to apply principles in A and B. (From Aebi M, Etter C, Kehl T, Thaggot J. The internal skeletal fixation system: a new treatment of thoracolumbar fractures and other spinal disorders. *Clin Orthop* 1988;227:30–43.)

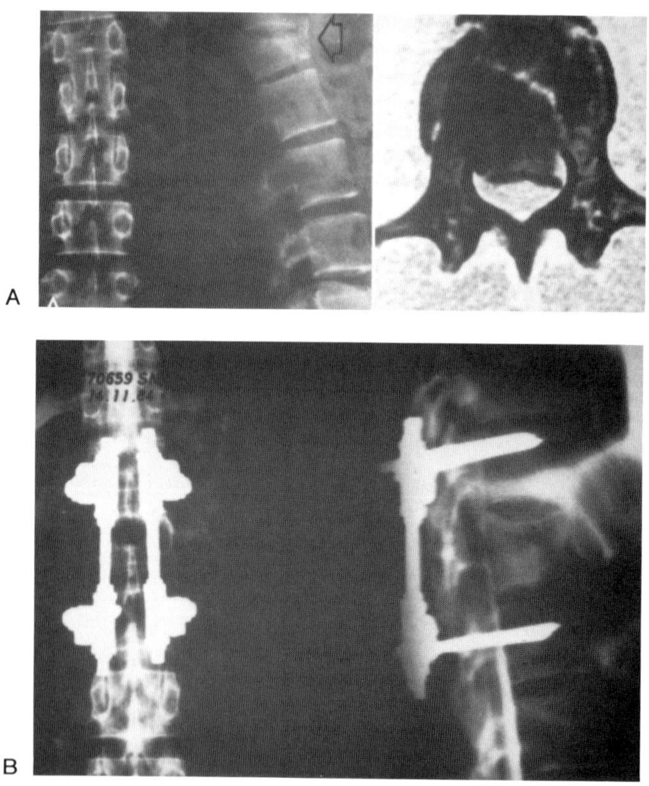

FIG. 3-133. A: The AP and lateral radiograph and CT image of a L-1 burst fracture. **B:** Postoperative AP and lateral radiographs after reduction. (From Aebi M, Etter C, Kehl T, Thaggot J. The internal skeletal fixation system: a new treatment of thoracolumbar fractures and other spinal disorders. *Clin Orthop* 1988;227:30–43.)

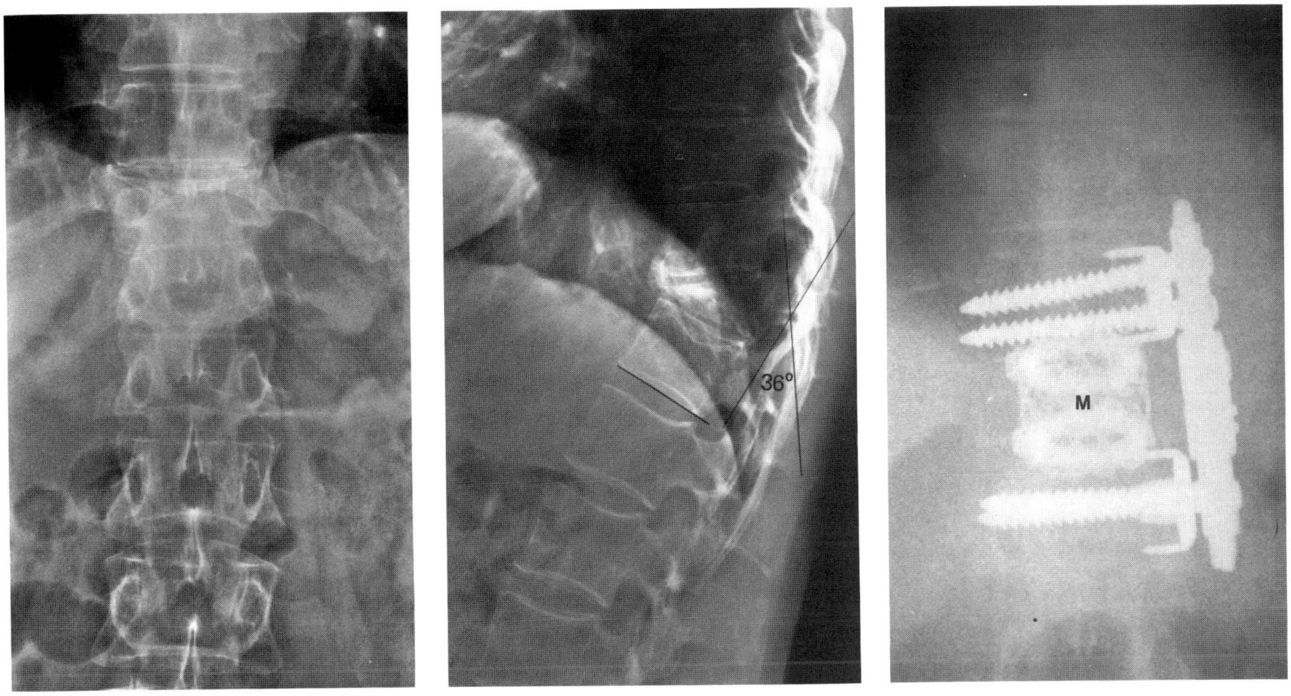

A B,C

FIG. 3-134. The AP **(A)** and lateral **(B)** radiographs of a T-11 burst fracture with 36° kyphosis. **C:** Corpectomy of T-11 with bone grafts, Moss titanium cage (*M*), and a Kaneda device with two paraspinal bars, rod couplers, two staples, and four vertebral screws.

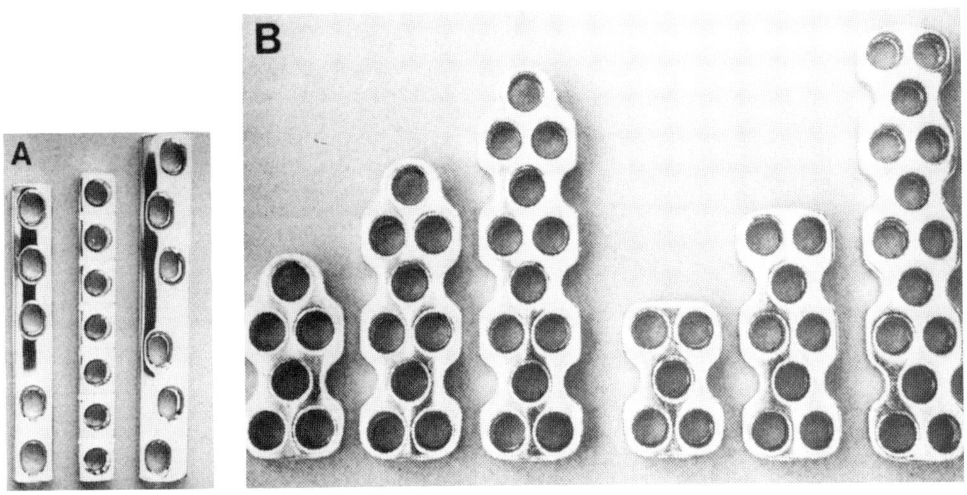

FIG. 3-135. Plates used for anterior instrumentation. **A:** Narrow DC plate (*left*), notch plate (*center*), and broad dynamic compression (DC) plate (*right*). **B:** Specially contoured spinal plates (Synthes, Paoli, PA). (From Haas N, Blauth M, Tscherne H. Anterior plating in thoracolumbar spine injuries. Indications, technique, and results. *Spine* 1991;16:S100–111.)

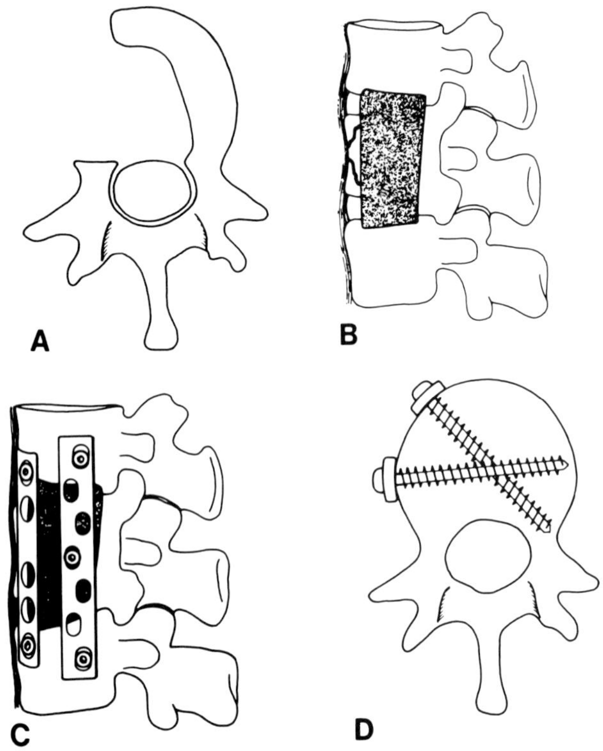

FIG. 3-136. Anterior plate-screw fixation. **A:** A portion of the vertebra is resected, and the dural sac is decompressed. **B:** Cortical bone graft in position. Lateral **(C)** and axial **(D)** dynamic compression (DC) plate and screw in position. (From Haas N, Blauth M, Tscherne H. Anterior plating in thoracolumbar spine injuries. Indications, technique, and results. *Spine* 1991;16: S100–111.)

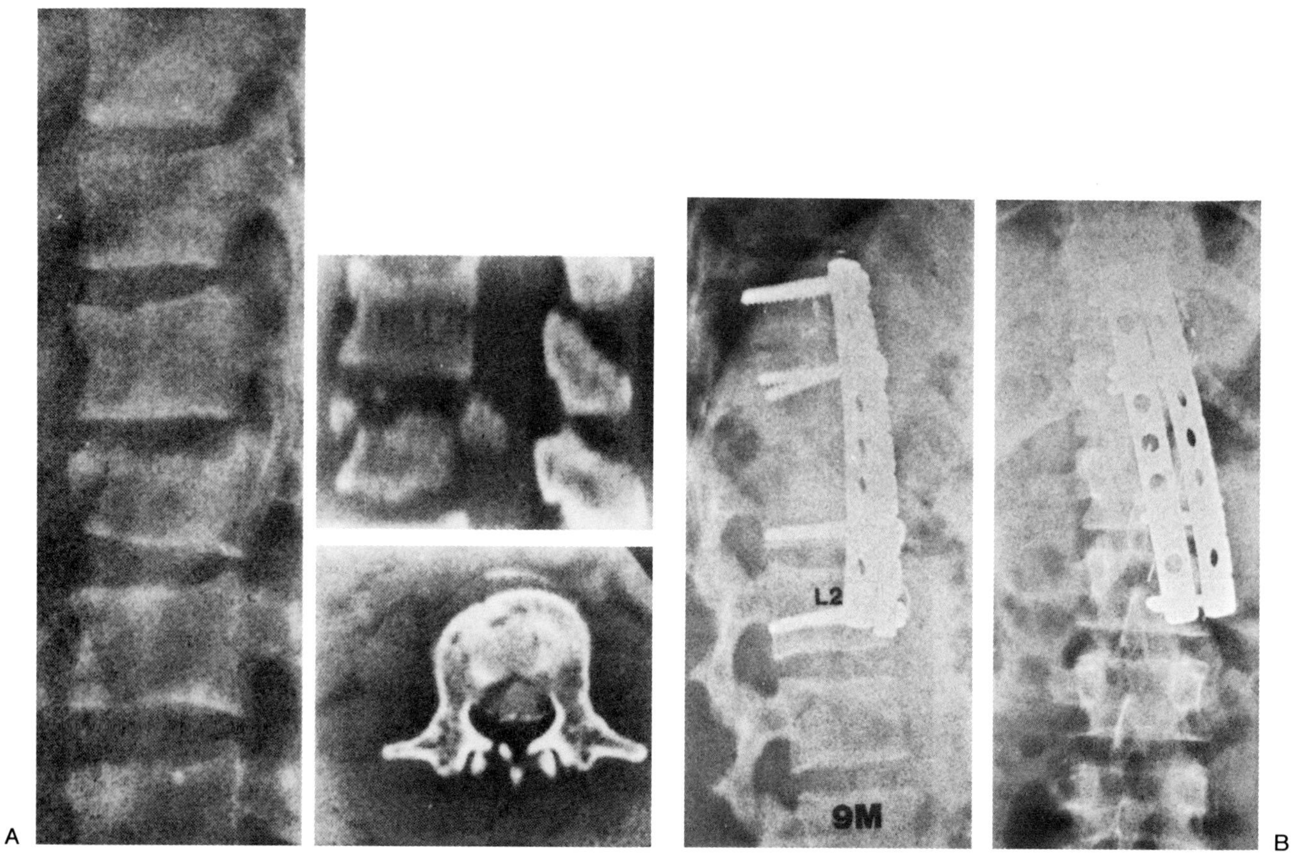

FIG. 3-137. A: Flexion-compression injury in an 18-year-old man demonstrated with lateral radiograph and CT images. **B:** Lateral and AP views 9 months after plates and screw fixation with notched plates. (From Haas N, Blauth M, Tscherne H. Anterior plating in thoracolumbar spine injuries. Indications, technique, and results. *Spine* 1991;16:S100–111.)

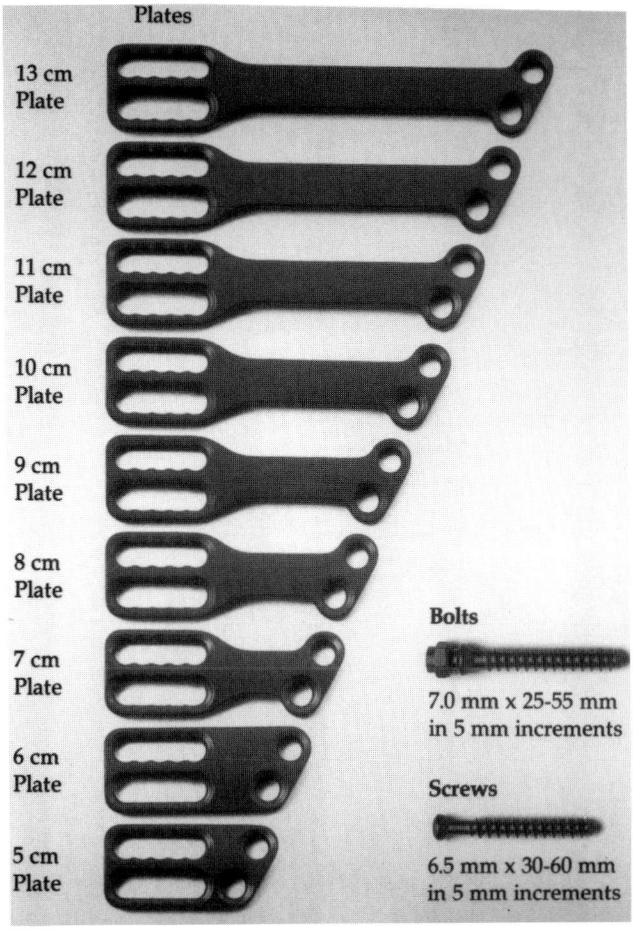

A

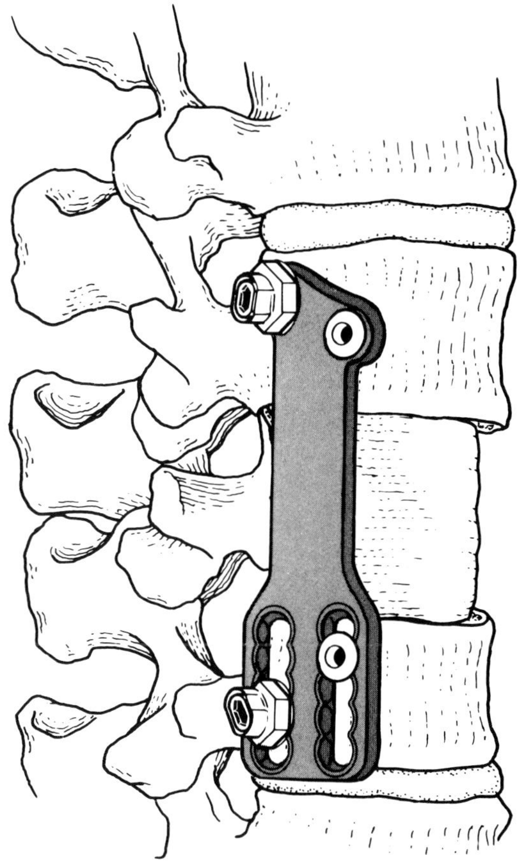

B

FIG. 3-138. **A:** Z plate-ATL™ plate, bolts, and screws. **B:** Corpectomy with bone graft and Z plate-ATL™ in place (Courtesy of Danek Medical, Memphis, TN.)

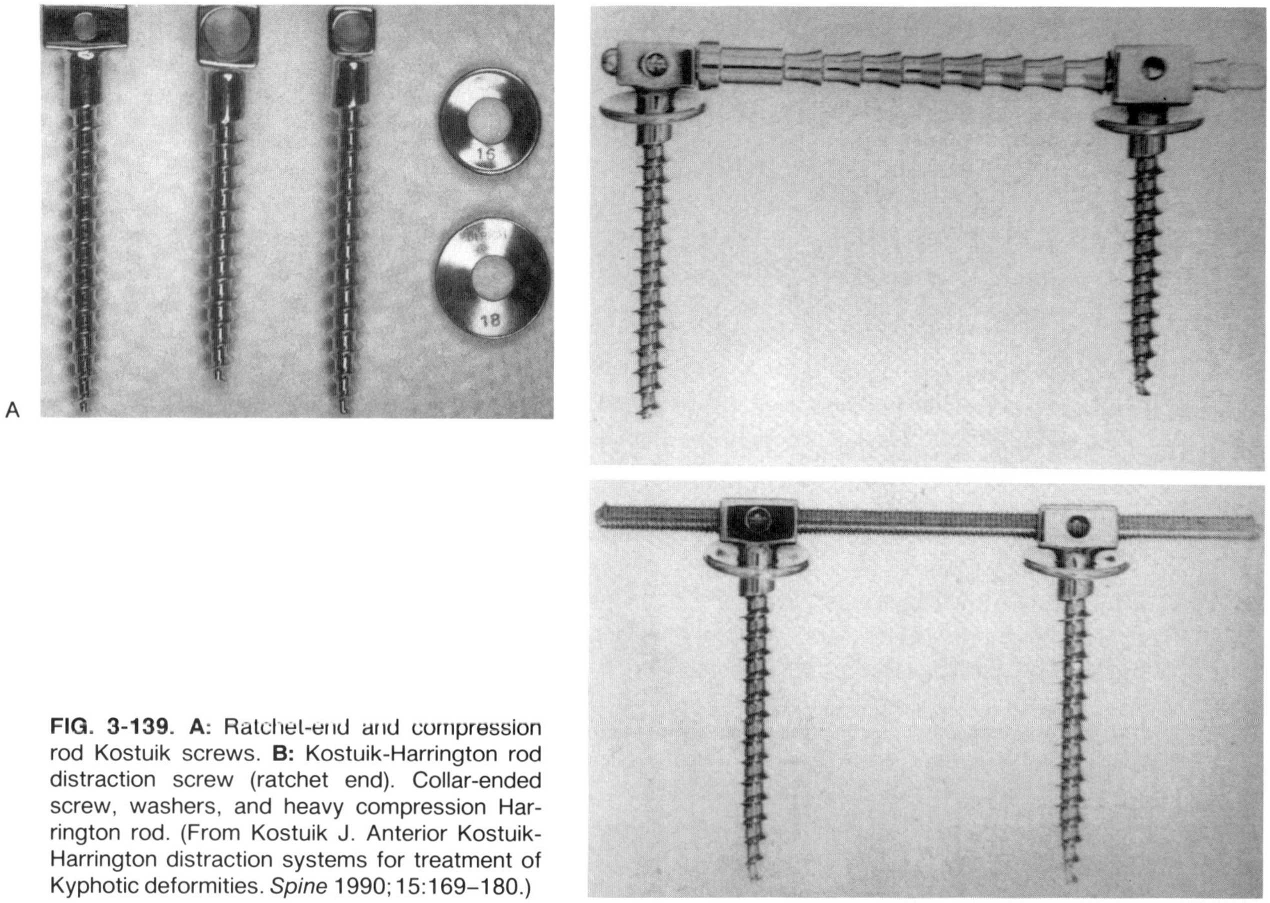

FIG. 3-139. **A:** Ratchet-end and compression rod Kostuik screws. **B:** Kostuik-Harrington rod distraction screw (ratchet end). Collar-ended screw, washers, and heavy compression Harrington rod. (From Kostuik J. Anterior Kostuik-Harrington distraction systems for treatment of Kyphotic deformities. *Spine* 1990;15:169–180.)

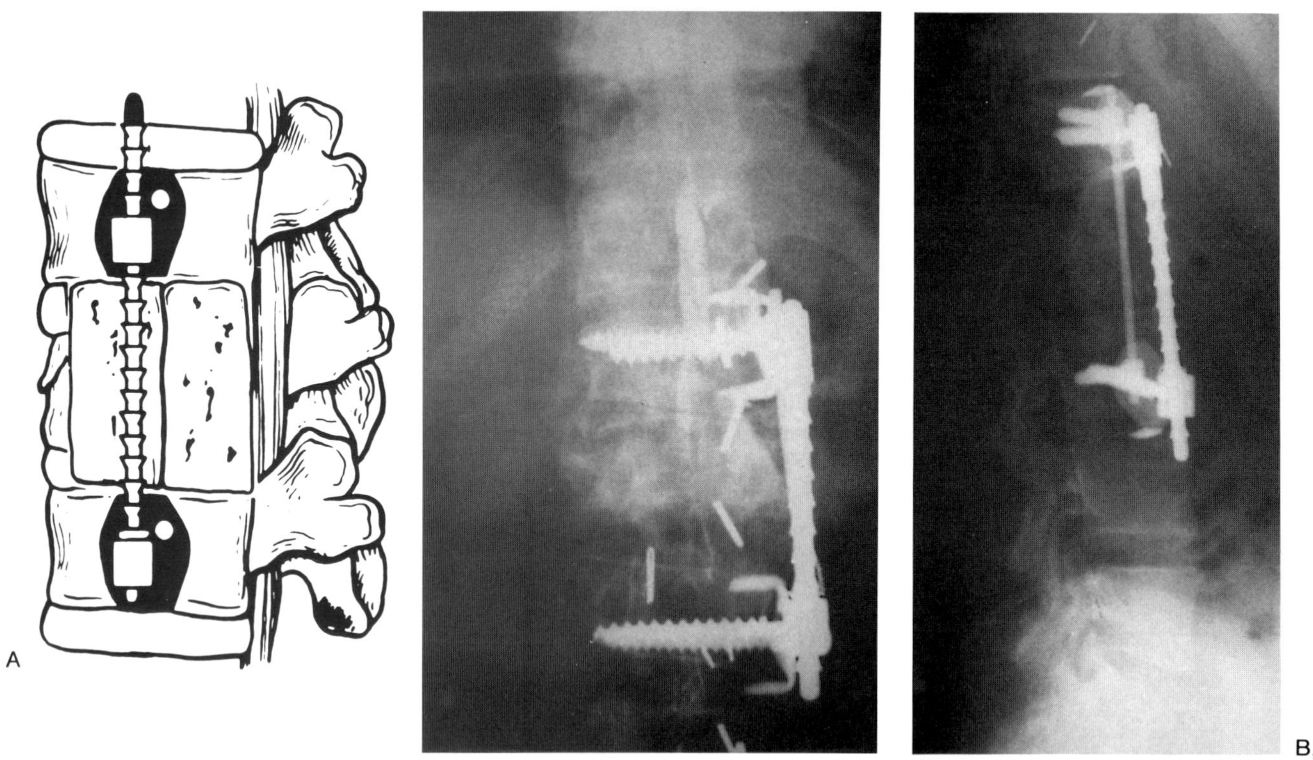

FIG. 3-140. A: Anterior lateral distraction rod with iliac bone graft. Harrington distraction and compression rods with bone graft seen on AP **(B)** and lateral **(C)** radiographs. (From Kostuik J. Anterior Kostuik-Harrington distraction systems for treatment of Kyphotic deformities. *Spine* 1990;15:169–180.)

A 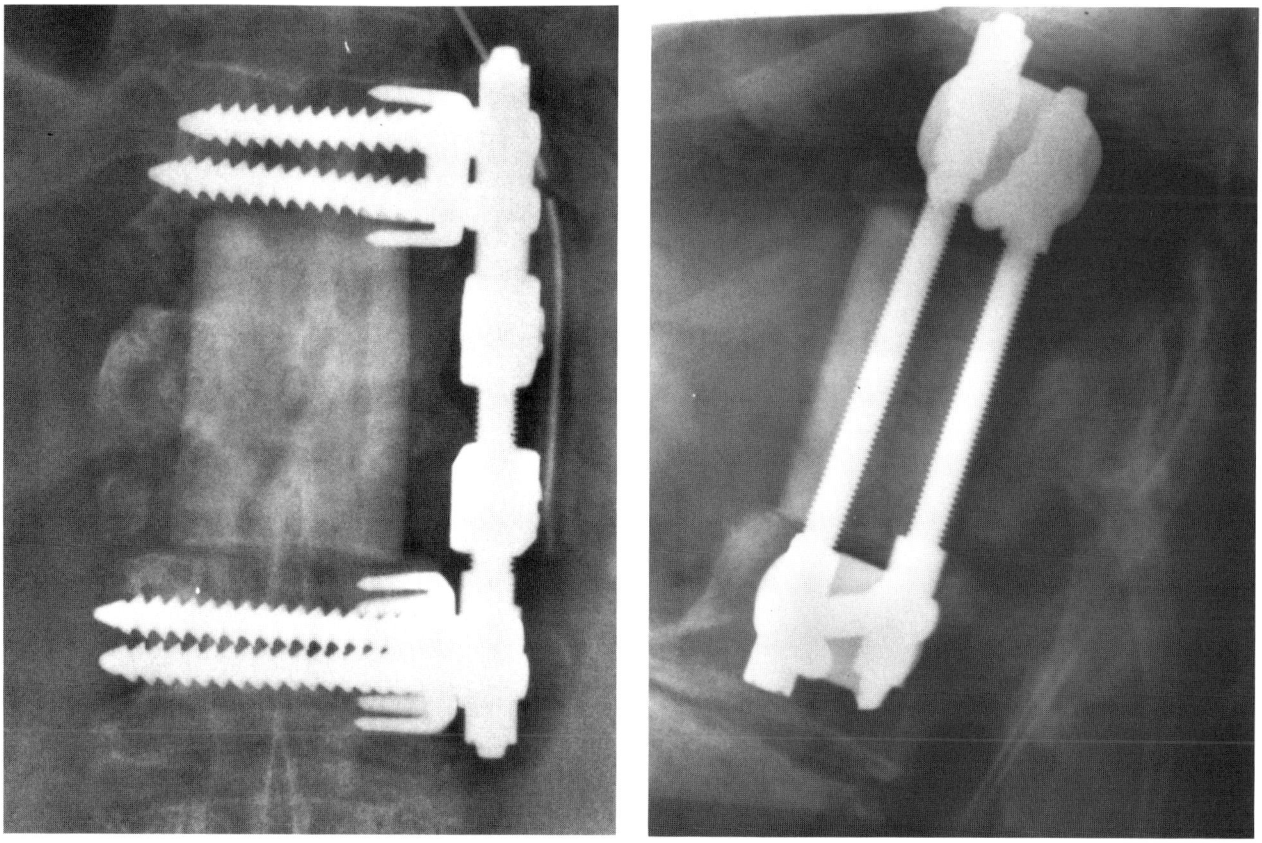 B

FIG. 3-141. The AP **(A)** and lateral **(B)** radiographs of anterior Kaneda rod and screw fixation with vertebral screws and staples and bone graft in place.

A 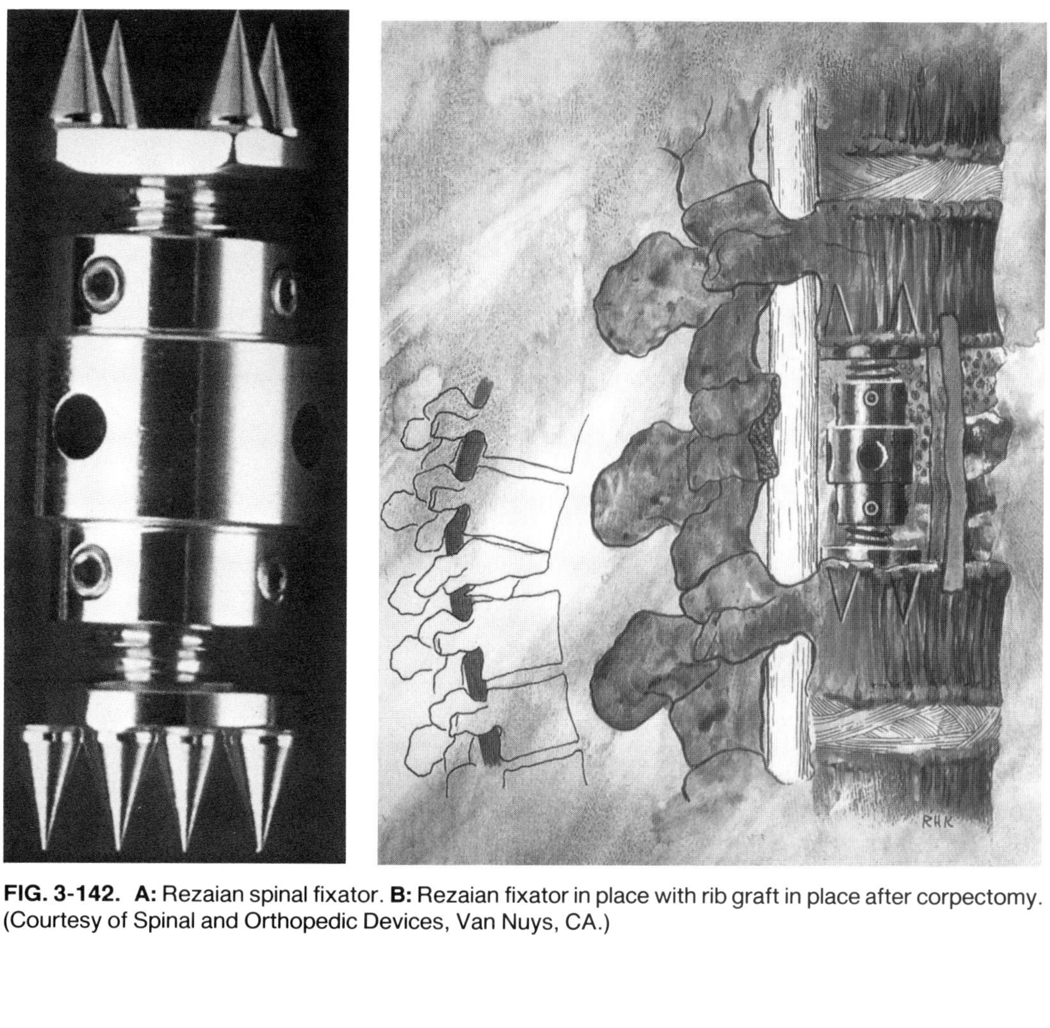 B

FIG. 3-142. A: Rezaian spinal fixator. **B:** Rezaian fixator in place with rib graft in place after corpectomy. (Courtesy of Spinal and Orthopedic Devices, Van Nuys, CA.)

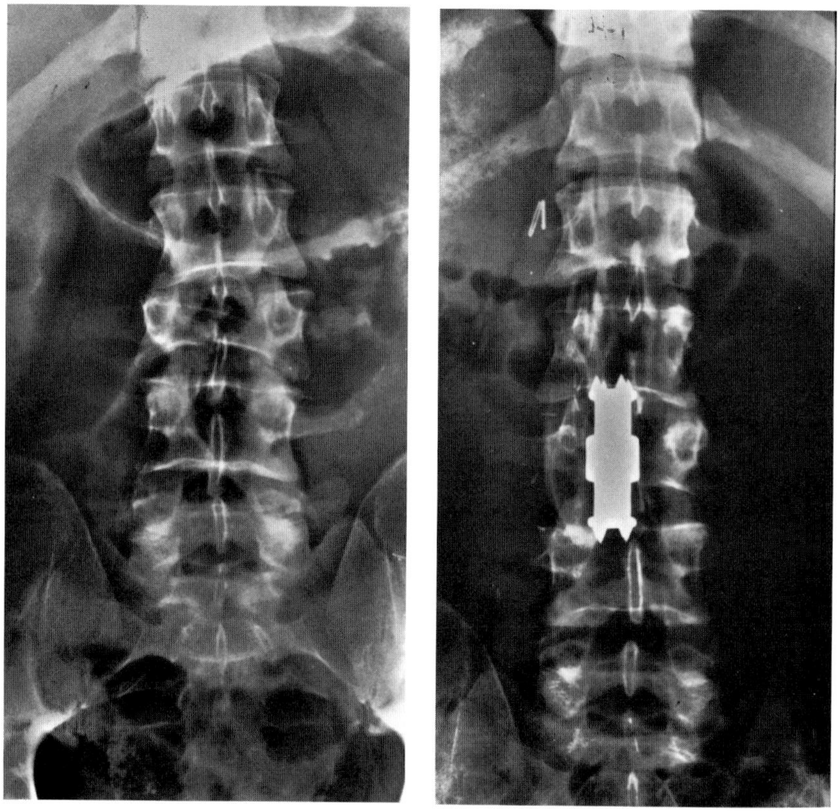

A B

FIG. 3-143. **A:** An AP radiograph of a L-3 burst fracture. **B:** An AP radiograph of Rezaian fixator after partial corpectomy. There is a bone graft on the right. (Courtesy of Spinal and Orthopedic Devices, Van Nuys, CA.)

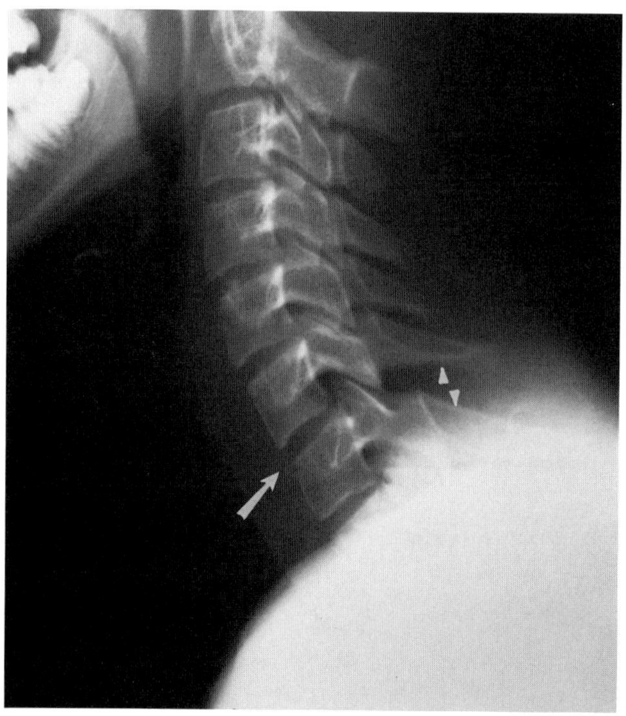

FIG. 3-144. Lateral view of the cervical spine demonstrating a mild anterosuperior fracture of the C-7 vertebral body (*arrow*). There is also widening of the interspinous distance (*arrowheads*) because of a posterior ligament injury (unstable).

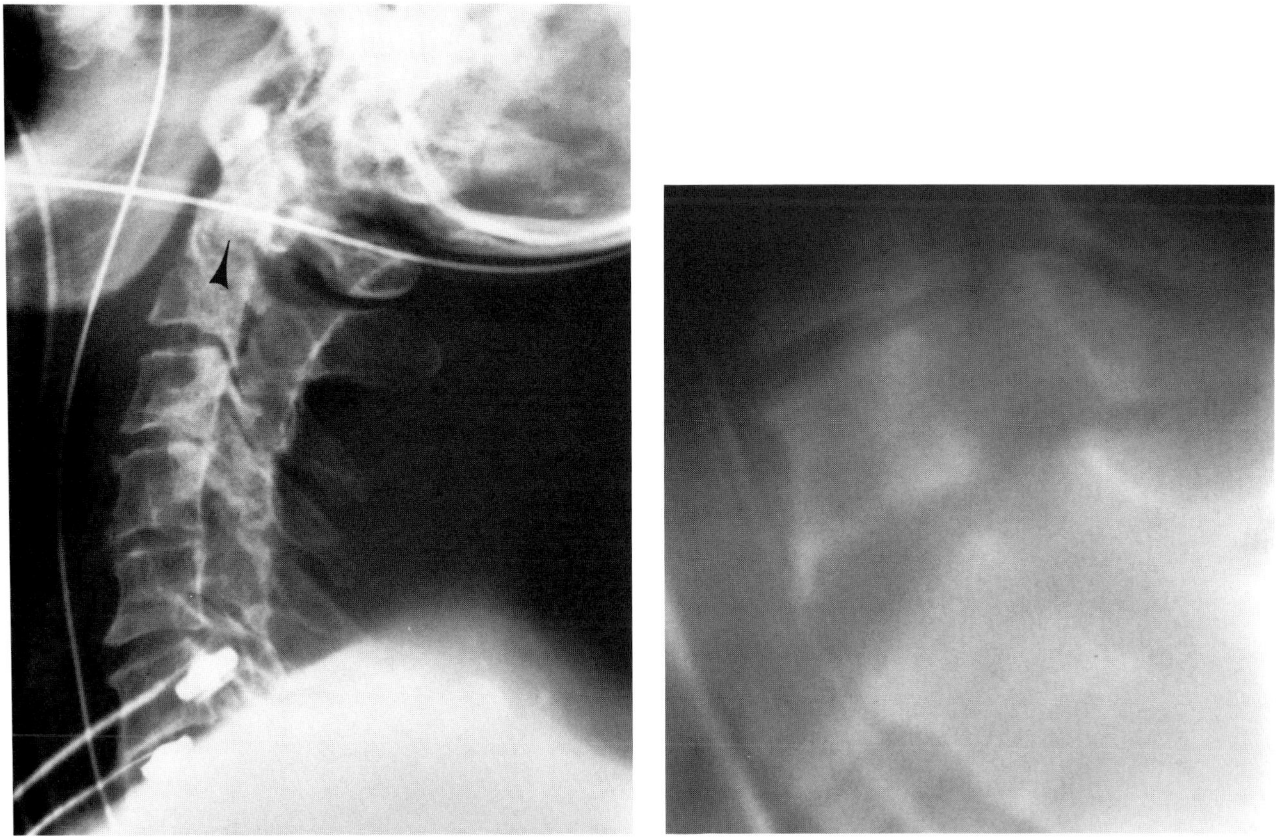

A B

FIG. 3-145. A: Lateral view of the cervical spine with a subtle odontoid fracture (*arrow*). C-7 was not seen, requiring further imaging studies. **B:** A lateral tomogram demonstrates a C-6 to C-7 hyperextension injury involving all three columns.

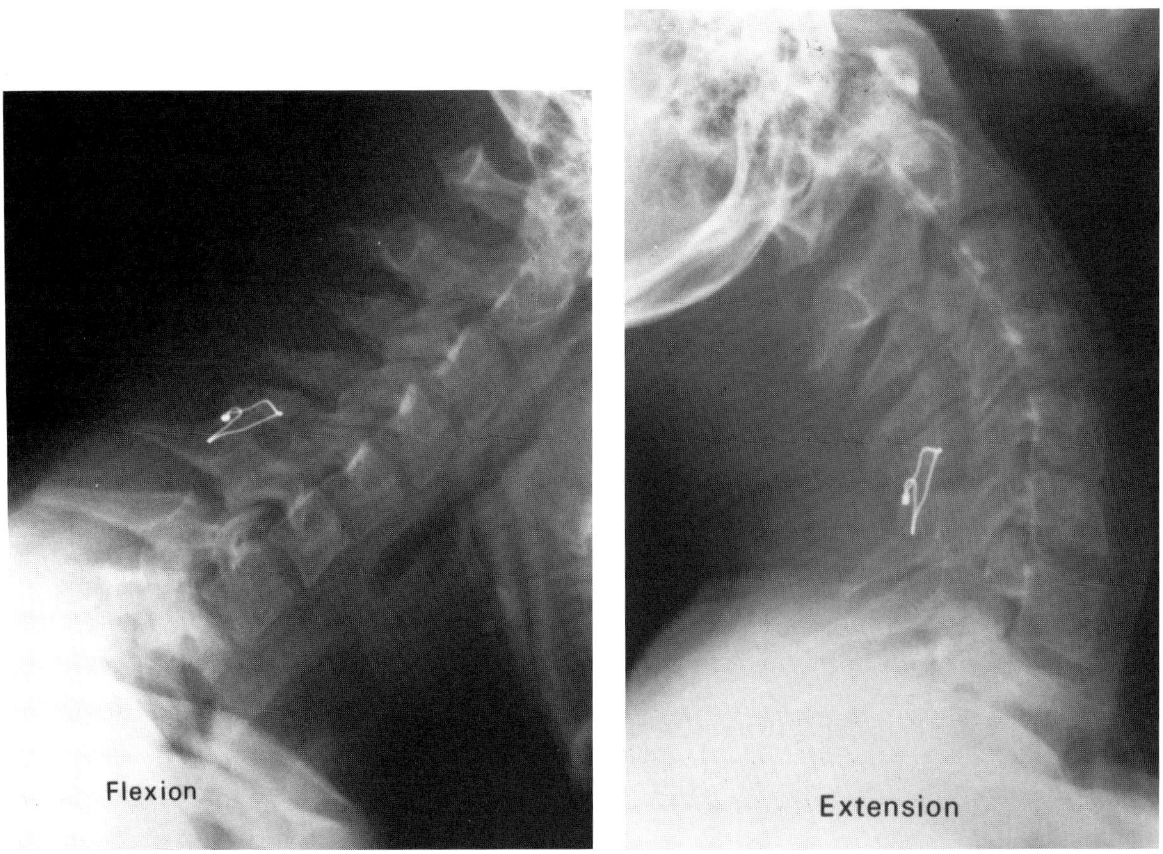

A B

FIG. 3-146. Distractive hyperflexion injury with posterior ligament disruption and instability at C-5 to C-6. Postoperative radiographs in flexion **(A)** and extension **(B)** show a solid posterior fusion with bone graft and spinous process curving. No motion at the fusion site. No lucent areas around the bone graft to suggest pseudarthrosis or fibrous union.

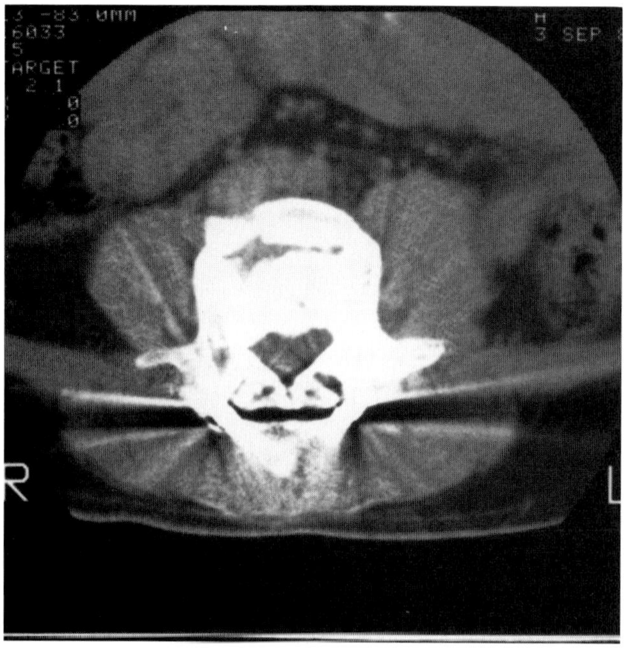

FIG. 3-147. Axial CT following Harrington compression rod fixation. The artifact degrades the image quality so that the spinal canal and bone graft are difficult to evaluate.

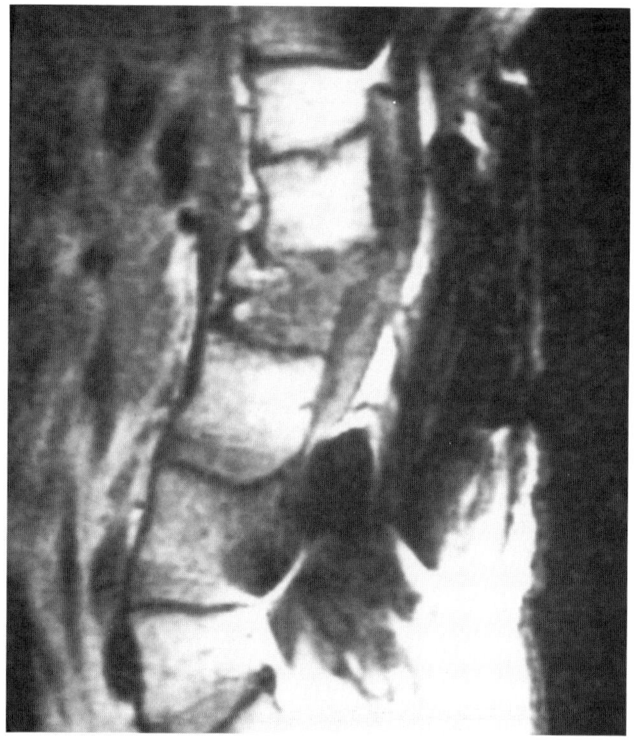

FIG. 3-148. Sagittal SE 500/20 MRI scans show a L-2 compression fracture. The Harrington rods make it difficult to evaluate the neural arch and spinal canal.

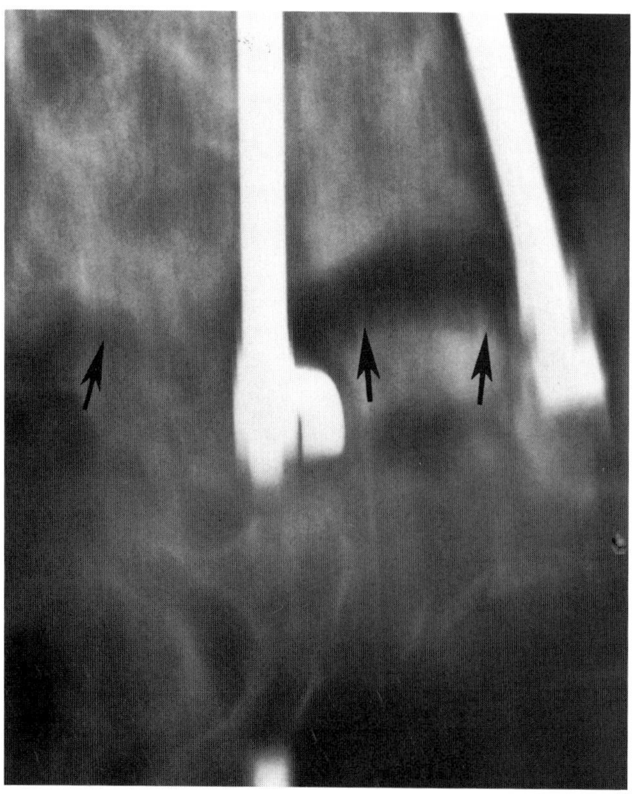

FIG. 3-149. An AP tomogram demonstrating a pseudarthrosis or fibrous union (*arrows*) after rod-hook instrumentation. Motion should be demonstrated with motion studies or flexion-extension tomography to confirm pseudarthrosis.[177]

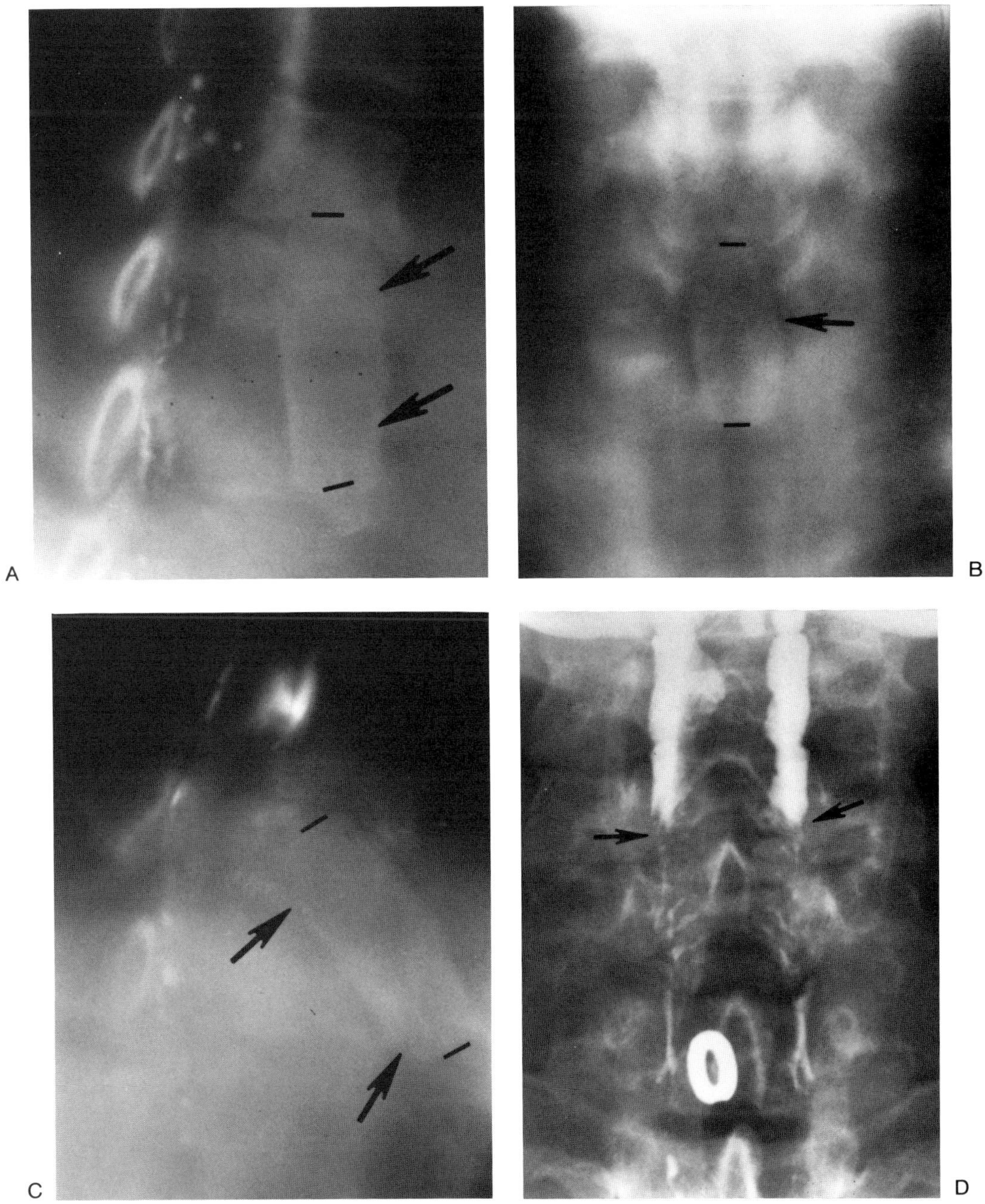

FIG. 3-150. **A:** Lateral tomogram after anterior bone block fusion without instrumentation. The AP **(B)** and lateral **(C)** tomograms 2 weeks later demonstrate displacement of the bone graft (*arrows*) and obstruction of the spinal canal on this view and the PA myelogram (*arrows*) **(D)**.

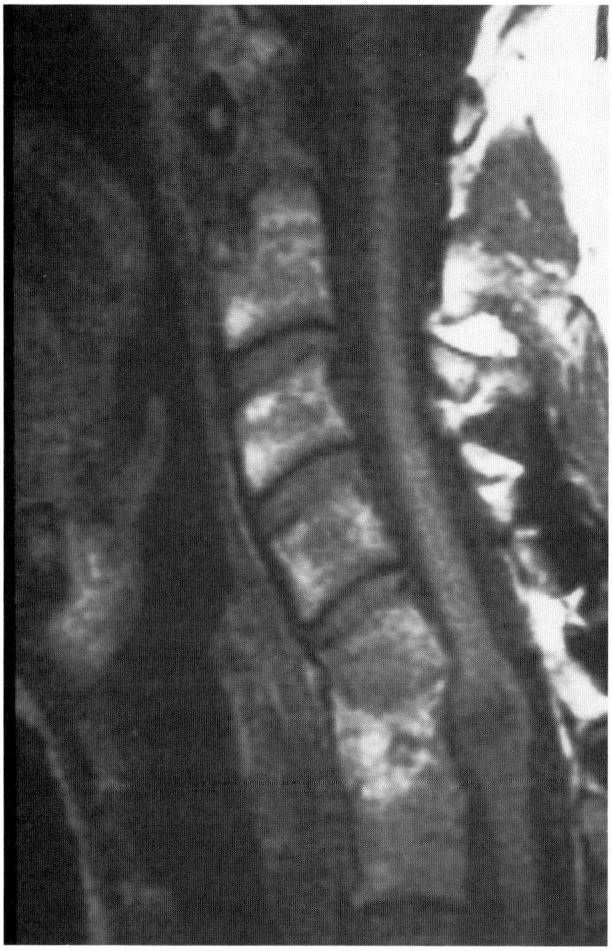

FIG. 3-151. Sagittal MRI scan after C-5 to C-6 flexion compression injury. There is a posttraumatic syrinx at this level.

A,B

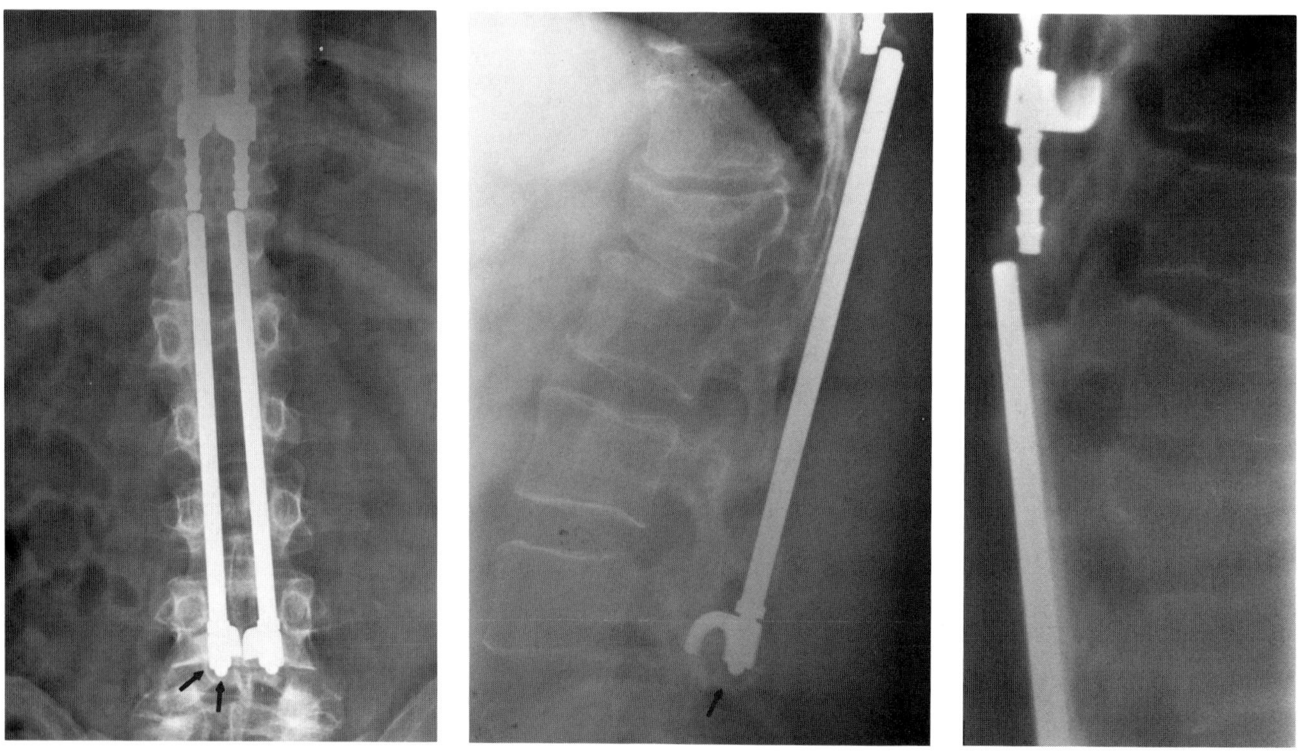

C

FIG. 3-152. The AP **(A)** and lateral **(B)** radiographs of a patient with T-12 to L-1 compression fractures treated with Harrington distraction rods and local bone graft. There are fractures of both rods at the ratchet-rod junction. No bone graft is visible. There is lucency at the tip of the lower end of the rods (*arrows*) caused by motion. **C:** Lateral tomogram shows widened facet joints at this level.

Postoperative complications may be related to the initial injury or surgical reduction or be extraspinal in nature. The complications are similar (Table 3-7) to those seen with spinal instrumentation for other abnormalities.[193,201]

Baseline radiographs in the AP and lateral projections are required postoperatively to assess the position of the instrumentation and to measure the correction in deformity compared with that in the preoperative studies.[178,209] Factors to consider include the change in height, translation or subluxation, kyphosis, and lumbar lordosis. Standing films should be used when possible because they are more physiologic and provide more functional information. When indicated, flexion-extension (Fig. 3-146) and lateral bending views may be added. More sophisticated imaging techniques may be difficult to use (MRI and CT) because of the artifact created by metal components (Figs. 3-147 and 3-148).[178,204] Therefore, conventional tomography may be used to evaluate bone graft healing (Fig. 3-149).

Complications related to the spine vary with the location, instrumentation, and surgical approach. Anterior procedures in the cervical spine are associated with the following problems:[193]

Transient recurrent nerve paresis caused by retraction during surgery
Vertebral and carotid artery tears
Airway obstruction (postoperative edema)
Esophageal tears
Bone graft extrusion (Fig. 3-150)

Posterior cervical fusions are more often associated with pseudarthrosis and infection.[197]

Anterior procedures in the thoracolumbar spine have a higher incidence of complications locally and at the bone graft donor site. More grafting is used to replace partial corpectomy sites. Also, vascular injuries occur more frequently.[195]

Neural injury is also more common with posterior procedures (cord), and nerve root injury is more common with anterior procedures. Implant migration hypertrophy of the bone graft or implant failure can also lead to changes in the neurologic deficit.[193,195,209] Pedicle screws may cause neural injury or anterior vascular injury if not properly positioned.[213,214]

Imaging of neural structures can be difficult in the presence of metal implants. Although MRI is safe, the artifact is often too great to obtain sufficient information. Titanium implants cause less artifact (Fig. 3-151).[178]

Instrument failure may be related to pseudarthrosis. The latter is more common with longer segment fusion and in older patients (Fig. 3-152).[211] Implant failures include hook pull out; plate, screw, wire, and rod fractures (Fig. 3-152); and implant loosening.[193,209,211]

Nonspinal or medial complications are also common. Genitourinary tract infections occur in up to 20% of patients and deep venous thrombosis, in up to 25%. These problems are most often seen in patients with posttraumatic paralysis or those who require prolonged hospitalization.[178,200] Ultrasonography is the most effective screening method for venoocclusive disease in the thigh and knee region.

Decubitus ulcers and local pin tract infections in patients with halo devices are also common. The incidence of gastrointestinal hemorrhage may reach 40% in patients receiving steroid therapy.[193]

REFERENCES

Scoliosis

1. Akbornia BA. Selection of methodology in surgical treatment of adolescent idiopathic scoliosis. *Orthop Clin North Am* 1988;19:313–329.
2. Allen BL, Ferguson RL. The Galveston experience with L-rod instrumentation for adolescent idiopathic scoliosis. *Clin Orthop* 1988;229:59–69.
3. Applegren G, Willner S. End vertebral angle—a roentgenographic method to describe scoliosis. *Spine* 1990;15:71–74.
4. Asher M, Carson W, Heinig C, Strippgen W, Arendt M, Lark R, Hartley M. A modular spinal rod linkage system to provide rotational stability. *Spine* 1988;13:272–277.
5. Asher M, DeSmet A, Cook L, Orrick J. Classification of adolescent idiopathic scoliosis curve patterns. A 3-dimensional analysis. *Orthop Trans* 1988;12:260.
6. Ashman RB, Herring JA, Johnston CE II, Lowery GL, Sutherlin CE III. *TSRH universal spinal instrumentation.* Dallas: Hudley & Assoc.; 1993.
7. Bauer R, Mostegl A, Eichenauer M. An analysis of the results of Dwyer and Zielke instrumentations in the treatment of scoliosis. *Arch Orthop Trauma Surg* 1986;105:302–309.
8. Birch JG, Herring JA, Roach JW, Johnston CE. Cotrel-Dubousset instrumentation in idiopathic scoliosis. A preliminary report. *Clin Orthop* 1988;227:24–29.
9. Bradford DS. Instrumentation of the lumbar spine. An overview. *Clin Orthop* 1986;203:209–218.
10. Bradford DS. Adult scoliosis. Current concepts of treatment. *Clin Orthop* 1988;229:70–87.
11. Cobb JR. Outline for the study of scoliosis. In: *Instructional course lecturers. The American Academy of Orthopaedic Surgeons.* Vol. 5. Ann Arbor: JW Edwards; 1948:261–275.
12. Cotrel Y, Dubousset J, Guillaumet M. New universal instrumentation in spinal surgery. *Clin Orthop* 1988;227:10–23.
13. Cundy PJ, Paterson DC, Hillier TM, Sutherland AD, Stephen JP, Foster BK. Cotrel-Dubousset instrumentation and vertebral rotation in adolescent idiopathic scoliosis. *J Bone Joint Surg [Br]* 1990;72B:670–674, 1990.
14. Dawson EG, Clader TJ, Bassett LW. A comparison of different methods used to diagnose pseudarthrosis. *J Bone Joint Surg [Am]* 1985;67A:1153–1159.
15. Dickson JH, Erwin WD, Rossi D. Harrington instrumentation and arthrodesis for idiopathic scoliosis. *J Bone Joint Surg [Am]* 1990;72A:678–683.
16. Drummond DS, Keene JS. Spinous process segmental spinal instrumentation. *Orthopedics* 1989;11:1403–1410.
17. Ferguson AB. *Roentgen diagnosis of the extremities and spine.* New York: Paul B. Hoeber; 1945.
18. Fitch RD, Turi M, Bowman BE, Hardaker WT. Comparison of Cotrel-Dubousset and Harrington rod instrumentation in idiopathic scoliosis. *J Pediatr Orthop* 1990;10:44–47.
19. Foley MJ, Calenoff L, Hendryx RW, Schafer MF. Thoracic and lumbar spine fusion: post-operative radiographic evaluation. *AJR Am J Roentgenol* 1983;141:373–380.
20. Goldstein LA, Waugh TR. Classification and terminology of scoliosis. *Clin Orthop* 1973;93:131–157.

21. Gray JE, Hoffman AD, Peterson HA. Reduction of radiation exposure during radiography for scoliosis. *J Bone Joint Surg [Am]* 1983;65A:5–12.
22. Hall JD. Dwyer instrumentation in anterior fusion of the spine. *J Bone Joint Surg [Am]* 1981;63A:1188.
23. Harrington PR. Technical details in relation to the successful use of instrumentation in scoliosis. *Orthop Clin North Am* 1972;3: 49–67.
24. Hayes MA, Tompkins SF, Herndon WA, Gruel CR, Kopta JA, Howard TC. Clinical and radiological evaluation of lumbosacral motion below fusion levels in idiopathic scoliosis. *Spine* 1988;13: 1161–1167.
25. Horton WC, Holt RT, Johnson JR, Leatherman KD. Zielke instrumentation in idiopathic scoliosis: late effects and minimizing complications. *Spine* 1988;13:1145–1149.
26. Kaneda K, Fujiya N, Satoh S. Results with Zielke instrumentation for idiopathic thoracolumbar and lumbar scoliosis. *Clin Orthop* 1986;205:195–203.
27. Keene JS, Drummond DS. The Wisconsin system. *Spine* 1982;7: 83.
28. King HA. Selection of fusion levels for posterior instrumentation and fusion in idiopathic scoliosis. *Orthop Clin North Am* 1988;19: 247–255.
29. King HA, Moe JH, Bradford DS, Winter RB. Selection of fusion levels in thoracic idiopathic scoliosis. *J Bone Joint Surg [Am]* 1983;65A:1302–1313.
30. Kohler R, Galland O, Mechin H, Michel CR, Onimus M. The Dwyer procedure in the treatment of idiopathic scoliosis. *Spine* 1990;15:75–80.
31. Korovessis P. Combined VDS and Harrington instrumentation for treatment of idiopathic double major curves. *Spine* 1987;12: 244–250.
32. Kostuik JP. Anterior Kostuik-Harrington distraction systems. *Orthopedics* 1988;11:1379–1391.
33. Kostuik JP. Adult scoliosis. In: Rothman RH, Simeone FA, eds. *The spine.* 3rd ed. Philadelphia: WB Saunders; 1992:879–911.
34. Lenke LG, Bridwell KH, Baldus C, Blanke K, Schoenecker PL. Cotrel-Dubousset instrumentation for adolescent idiopathic scoliosis. *J Bone Joint Surg [Am]* 1992;74A:1056–1066.
35. Matsuzaki H, Tokuhashi Y, Matsumoto F, Hoshino M, Kiuchi T, Toriyama S. Problems and solutions of pedicle screw plate fixation of lumbar spine. *Spine* 1990;15:1159–1165.
36. McAlister WH, Shackelford GD. Classification of spinal curvatures. *Radiol Clin North Am* 1975;13:93–121.
37. McAlister WH, Shackelford GD. Measurement of spinal curvatures. *Radiol Clin North Am* 1975;13:113–121.
38. McCarthy RE, McCullough FL, Peek RD, Harrison BH. A locking collar for Luque rods. *Orthopedics* 1988;11:921–926.
39. Mehdian H, Eisenstein S. Segmental spinal instrumentation using short closed wire loops. *Clin Orthop* 1989;247:90–96.
40. Moe JH. A critical analysis of methods of fusion for scoliosis. An evaluation of two hundred and sixty-six patients. *J Bone Joint Surg [Am]* 1958;40A:529–554.
41. Moe JH, Purcell GA, Bradford DS. Zielke instrumentation (VDS) for correction of spinal curvature: analysis of results in 66 patients. *Clin Orthop* 1983;180:133–153.
42. Nash CL, Moe JH. A study of vertebral rotation. *J Bone Joint Surg [Am]* 1969;51A:223–229.
43. Panjabi MM, Abumi K, Duranceau J, Crisco JJ. Biomechanical evaluation of spinal fixation devices. II. Stability provided by eight fixation devices. *Spine* 1988;13:1135–1140.
44. Phillips WA, Hensinger RN. Wisconsin instrumentation for posterior spinal fusion. *Clin Orthop* 1988;229:44–51.
45. Ponseti IV, Friedman B. Prognosis of idiopathic scoliosis. *J Bone Joint Surg [Am]* 1950;32A:381–395.
46. Puno RM, Johnson JR, Ostermann PAW, Holt RT. Analysis of the primary and compensatory curvatures following Zielke instrumentation for idiopathic scoliosis. *Spine* 1989;14:738–743.
47. Resina J, Ferreira-Aloes A. A technique of correction and internal fixation for scoliosis. *J Bone Joint Surg [Am]* 1977;59A:159–165.
48. Richards BS, Johnston CE II. Cotrel-Dubousset instrumentation for adolescent idiopathic scoliosis. *Orthopedics* 1987;10:649–654.
49. Shufflebarger HL, Clark CE. Cotrel-Dubousset instrumentation. *Orthopedics* 1988;11:1435–1440.
50. Shufflebarger HL, Clark CE. Fusion levels and hook patterns in thoracic scoliosis with Cotrel-Dubousset instrumentation. *Spine* 1990;15:916–920.
51. Slone RM, MacMillan M, Montgomery WJ, Heare M. Spinal fixation. Part 2: Fixation techniques and hardware for the thoracic and lumbosacral spine. *Radiographics* 1993;13:521–543.
52. Slone RM, MacMillan M, Montgomery WJ. Spinal fixation. Part 3: complications of spinal instrumentations. *Radiographics* 1993;13:797–816.
53. Thometz JG, Emans JB. A comparison between spinous process and sublaminar wiring combined with Harrington distraction instrumentation in the management of adolescent idiopathic scoliosis. *J Pediatr Orthop* 1988;8:129–132.
54. Weatherley CR, Draycott V, O'Brien JF, et al. The rib deformity of adolescent idiopathic scoliosis: a prospective study to evaluate changes after Harrington distraction and posterior fusion. *J Bone Joint Surg [Br]* 1987;69B:179–182.
55. Whitecloud TS, Skalley T. Roentgenographic measurement of pedicle screw penetration. *Clin Orthop* 1989;245:57–68.
56. Winter RB, Lonstein JE. Juvenile and adolescent scoliosis. In: Rothman RH, Simeone FA, eds. *The spine.* 3rd ed. Philadelphia: WB Saunders; 1992:373–430.
57. Wojcik AS, Webb JK, Burwell RG. Harrington-Luque and Cotrel-Dubousset instrumentation for idiopathic thoracic scoliosis. A postoperative comparison using segmental radiologic analysis. *Spine* 1990;15:424–431.
58. Wu K. Posterior vertebral instrumentation for correction of scoliosis. *Clin Orthop* 1987;215:40–46.

Lumbar Fusion

59. Allen BL, Ferguson RL. The Galveston experience with L-rod instrumentation for adolescent idiopathic scoliosis. *Clin Orthop* 1988;229:59–69.
60. Amato M, Totty WG, Gilula LA. Spondylolysis of the lumbar spine: demonstration of defects and laminar fragmentation. *Radiology* 1984;153:627–629.
61. Amundson G, Edwards CC, Garfin SR. Spondylolisthesis. In: Rothman RH, Simeone FA, eds. *The spine.* 3rd ed. Philadelphia: WB Saunders; 1992:913–969.
62. Beattie FC. Distraction rod fusion. *Clin Orthop* 1969;62:218–222.
63. Berquist TH. *Imaging of orthopedic trauma.* New York: Raven Press; 1992.
64. Gillespie HW. Vertebral retroposition (reversed spondylolisthesis). *Br J Radiol* 1951;24:193–197.
65. Bradford DS. Instrumentation of the lumbar spine. *Clin Orthop* 1986;203:209–218.
66. Burkus K, Loustein JE, Winter RB, Denis F. Long term follow-up of adolescents treated operatively for spondylolisthesis. *J Bone Joint Surg [Am]* 1992;74A:693–704.
67. Cabot JR, Fairen M, Roca J, Tur J, Blaimont P, VanElegein P, Libotte M. La pan orthrodese lumbosacrei avec la plaque crabe. *Acta Orthop Belg* 1981;47:657–666.
68. Dove J. Internal fixation of the lumbar spine. The Hartshill rectangle. *Clin Orthop* 1986;203:135–140.
69. Dubuc F. Knodt rod grafting. *Orthop Clin North Am* 1975;6:283–287.
70. Esses SI. The AO spinal internal fixator. *Spine* 1989;14:373–378.
71. Esses SI, Bednar DA. The spinal pedicle screw: techniques and systems. *Orthop Rev* 1989;18:676–682.
72. Farcy JP, Roye DP, Weidenbaum M. Cotrel-Dubousset instrumentation technique for revision of failed lumbosacral fusion. *Bull Hosp Jt Dis Orthop Inst* 1987;47:1–12.
73. Guyer DW, Wiltse LL, Peek RD. The Wiltse pedicle screw fixation system. *Orthopedics* 1988;11:1455–1460.
74. Harrington PR, Tullos RS. Reduction of severe spondylolisthesis in children. *South Med J* 1969;62:1–7.
75. Horowitch A, Peek RD, Thomas JC, Widell EH, DiMartino PP, Spencer CW, Weinstein J, Wiltse LL. The Wiltse pedicle screw fixation system. *Spine* 1989;14:461–467.
76. Kälebo P, Kadziolka R, Swärd L, Zaibresson BE. Stress views

in the comparative assessment of spondylotic spondylolisthesis. *Skeletal Radiol* 1989;17:570–575.
77. Kamioka Y, Yamamoto H. Lumbar trapezoid plate for lumbar spondylolisthesis. *Spine* 1990;15:1198–1203.
78. Kaneda K, Kazama H, Satoh S, Fujya M. Follow-up study of medial facetectomies and posterolateral fusion with instrumentation in unstable degenerative spondylolisthesis. *Clin Orthop* 1986;203:159–167.
79. Kinnard P, Ghibely A, Gordon D, Trias A, Basora J. Roy-Camille plates in unstable spinal conditions. A preliminary report. *Spine* 1986;11:131–135.
80. Kostuik JP, Errico TJ, Gleason TF. Luque instrumentation in degenerative conditions of the spine. *Spine* 1990;15:318–321.
81. Kostuik JP, Errico TJ, Gleason TF. Techniques of internal fixation for degenerative conditions of the lumbar spine. *Clin Orthop* 1986;203:219–231.
82. Krag MH. Spinal fusion: overviews of options for posterior internal fixation. In: Frymoyer JW, ed. *The adult spine: principles and practice.* New York: Raven Press; 1991:1919–1945.
83. Krag MH. Vermont spinal fixator. *Spine* 1992;6:121–145.
84. Krag MH, Beynnon BD, Pope MH, DeCoster TA. Depth of insertion of transpedicular vertebral screws into human vertebrae: effect upon screw-vertebra interface strength. *J Spine Disord* 1989;1:287–294.
85. Krag MH, Beynnon BD, Pope MH, Frymoyer JW, Haurgh LD, Weaver DL. An internal fixator for posterior application to short segments of the thoracic, lumbar and lumbosacral spine. *Clin Orthop* 1986;203:75–98.
86. Lee CK, deBare A. Lumbosacral fusion with Knodt distraction rods. *Spine* 1986;11:373–375.
87. Luque ER. Segmental spinal instrumentation of the lumbar spine. *Clin Orthop* 1986;203:126–134.
88. MacNab E. Spondylolisthesis with an intact neural arch—so called pseudospondylolisthesis. *J Bone Joint Surg [Br]* 1950;32B: 325–333.
89. Maldaque BE, Malghem JJ. Unilateral arch hypertrophy with spinous process tilt: a sign of arch deficiency. *Radiology* 1976;121: 574–576.
90. Mandell GA, Harke HT. Scintigraphy of spinal disorders in adolescents. *Skeletal Radiol* 1993;22:393–401.
91. Matsuzaki H, Tokuhashi Y, Matsumoto F, Hoshino M, Kiuchi T, Toriyama S. Problems and solutions of pedicle screw plate fixation of lumbar spine. *Spine* 1990;15:1159–1165.
92. Mehdian H, Jaffray D, Eisenstein SM. Dwyer-Hartshill transpedicular fixation for spinal fusion. *J Bone Joint Surg [Br]* 1989;71B:689–691.
93. Meyerding HW. Spondylolisthesis as an etiologic factor in backache. *JAMA* 1938;111:1972–1976.
94. Nathan H. Spondylolysis: its anatomy and mechanism of development. *J Bone Joint Surg [Am]* 1959;41A:303–320.
95. Neugebauer FL. A new contribution to the history and etiology of spondylolisthesis. *New Syndeham Soc Selected Monogr* 1988;121B:1–64.
96. Newman PH. The etiology of spondylolisthesis. *J Bone Joint Surg [Br]* 1963;45B:39–59.
97. Newman PH, Stone KH. The etiology of spondylolisthesis. *J Bone Joint Surg [Br]* 1963;45B:39–59.
98. Ogilvie JW, Schendel M. Comparison of lumbosacral fixation devices. *Clin Orthop* 1986;203:120–125.
99. Phillips WA, Hensinger RN. Wisconsin and other instrumentation for posterior spinal fusion. *Clin Orthop* 1988;229:44–51.
100. Pietruazka I. Early rehabilitation after fracture fixation with Daab's serrate plate and cancellous autotransplants. *Chir Nazzadow Ruchu Ortop Pol* 1980;45:507–510.
101. Rogozinski C, Rogozinski A. The Rogozinski spinal rod system: a new internal fixation of the spine. *Spine* 1992;6:107–120.
102. Rosenberg NJ. Degenerative spondylolisthesis. *J Bone Joint Surg [Am]* 1975;57A:467–474.
103. Roy-Camille R, Saillant G, Mazel C. Internal fixation of the lumbar spine with pedicle screw plating. *Clin Orthop* 1986;203:7–17.
104. Selby D. Internal fixation with Knodt's rods. *Clin Orthop* 1986;203:179–184.
105. Simmons EH, Capicotto WN. Posterior transpedicular Zielke instrumentation of the lumbar spine. *Clin Orthop* 1988;236:180–191.
106. Slone RM, MacMillan M, Montgomery WJ, Heare M. Spinal fixation. Part 2: fixation technique and hardware for the thoracic and lumbosacral spine. *Radiographics* 1993;13:521–543.
107. Slone RM, MacMillan M, Montgomery WJ. Spinal fixation. Part 3: complications of spinal instrumentation. *Radiographics* 1993;13:797–816.
108. Steffee AD, Biscup RS, Sitkowski DJ. Segmental spine plates with pedicle screw fixation: a new internal fixation device for disorders of lumbar and thoracolumbar spine. *Clin Orthop* 1986;203:45–53.
109. Steffee AD, Sitkowski DJ. Reduction and stabilization of grade IV spondylolisthesis. *Clin Orthop* 1988;227:82–89.
110. Steffee AD, Sitkowski DJ. Posterior lumbar interbody fusion and plates. *Clin Orthop* 1988;227:99–102.
111. Tillard WF. Etiology of spondylolisthesis. *Clin Orthop* 1976;117: 30.
112. West JL, Ogilivie JW, Bradford DS. Complications of the variable screw plate pedicle screw fixation. *Spine* 1991;16:576–579.
113. White AH, Zucherman JF, Hsu K. Lumbosacral fusions with Harrington rods and intersegmental wire. *Clin Orthop* 1986;203: 185–190.
114. Whitecloud TS, Skalley T. Roentgen measurement of pedicle screw penetration. *Clin Orthop* 1989;245:57–68.
115. Wilson PD, Straub LR. Lumbosacral fusion with metallic fixation. *Instr Course Lect* 1952;9:53–57.
116. Wiltse LL. The etiology of spondylolisthesis. *J Bone Joint Surg [Am]* 1962;44A:539–560.
117. Wiltse LL, Newman DH, MacNab I. Classification of spondylolysis and spondylolisthesis. *Clin Orthop* 1976;117:23–29.
118. Wiltse LL, Winter RB. Terminology and measurement of spondylolisthesis. *J Bone Joint Surg* 1983;65A:768–772.
119. Zdeblick TA. A prospective, randomized study of lumbar fusion. *Spine* 1993;18:983–991.

Introduction to Trauma

120. Acheson MB, Livingston RR, Richardson ML, Stunach GK. High resolution CT scanning in the evaluation of cervical spine fractures: comparison with plain film examinations. *AJR Am J Roentgenol* 1987;140:1179–1185.
121. Angtieaco EJC, Binet EF. Radiology of thoracic and lumbar fractures. *Clin Orthop* 1984;189:43–57.
122. Atlas RW, Regenbogen V, Rogers LF, Kim KS. The radiologic characterization of burst fractures of the spine. *AJR Am J Roentgenol* 1986;147:575–582.
123. Berquist TH. Imaging of adult cervical spine trauma. *Radiographics* 1988;8:667–694.
124. Berquist TH. *Imaging of orthopedic trauma.* New York: Raven Press; 1992.
125. Brand-Zawadzki M, Miller EM, Federle MP. CT in evaluation of spine trauma. *AJR Am J Roentgenol* 1981;136:369–375.
126. Calenoff L, Chessare RW, Rogers LF, et al. Multiple level spinal injuries. Importance of early recognition. *AJR Am J Roentgenol* 1978;130:665–669.
127. Denis F, Armstrong GW, Searls, BA, Motta L. Acute thoracolumbar burst fracture in the absence of neurological deficit. *Clin Orthop* 1984;189:142–149.
128. Daffner RH. *Imaging of vertebral trauma.* Rockville,MD: Aspen Press; 1988.
129. Daffner RH, Deeb ZL, Goldberg AK, Kordabarow A, Rothfus WE. The radiologic assessment of post-traumatic vertebral stability. *Skeletal Radiol* 1990;14:103–108.
130. Foley WF, Calenoff L, Hendrix RW, Schafer MF. Thoracic and lumbar spine fusion: postoperative radiographic evaluation. *AJR Am J Roentgenol* 1983;141:373–380.
131. Freedy MR, Midler KD, Erck JJ, Granke DS. Traumatic lumbosacral nerve root avulsion: evaluation with MR imaging. *J Comput Assist Tomogr* 1989;13:1052–1057.
132. Gehweiler JA, Osborne RL, Becker RE. *The radiology of vertebral trauma.* Philadelphia: WB Saunders; 1980.
133. Golimbu C, Firooznia H, Raffia M, et al. Computed tomography of thoracic and lumbar spine fractures that have been treated with Harrington instrumentation. *Radiology* 1984;151:731.

134. Guerra J, Gorfen SR, Resnick D. Vertebral burst fractures: CT analysis of the retropulsed fragment. *Radiology* 1984;153:769–772.
135. Harris JH. Radiographic evaluation of spine trauma. *Orthop Clin North Am* 1986;17:75–86.
136. Keene JS, Goletz TH, Lilleas F, et al. Diagnosis of vertebral fractures: a comparison of conventional and computed tomography. *J Bone Joint Surg [Am]* 1982;64A:586–594.
137. Levine AM. Surgical techniques for thoracic and lumbar trauma. In: Rothman RH, Simeone FA, eds. *The spine.* 3rd ed. Philadelphia: WB Saunders; 1992:1104–1133.
138. McAfee PC, Bohlman HH. Complications following Harrington instrumentation for fractures of the thoracolumbar spine. *J Bone Joint Surg [Am]* 1986;67A:672–686.
139. Nicoll EA. Fractures of the dorsolumbar spine. *J Bone Joint Surg [Br]* 1949;31B:376–394.
140. Steffee AD, Biscup RS, Sitkowski DJ. Segmental spinal plates with pedicle screw fixation. A new device for disorders of the lumbar and thoracolumbar spine. *Clin Orthop* 1986;203:45–53.
141. Villen J, Lindahl S, Irstain L, Nordwall A. Unstable conventional roentgenography of the reduction effect of Harrington instrumentation. *Spine* 1984;9:214–219.
142. White RR, Newberg A, Seligson D. Computerized tomographic assessment of the traumatized dorsolumbar spine before and after Harrington instrumentation. *Clin Orthop* 1980;146:150–156.
143. Wojcik WG, Edeiken-Monroe BS, Harris JH. Three dimensional computed tomography in acute cervical spine trauma. Preliminary report. *Skeletal Radiol* 1987;16:261–269.

Cervical Spine Trauma

144. Aldrich EF, Crow WN, Weber PB, Spagnolice TN. Use of MR imaging-compatible Halifax interlaminar clamps for posterior cervical fusion. *J Neurosurg* 1991;74:185–189.
145. Anderson LD, D'Alonzo RT. Fractures of the odontoid process of the axis. *J Bone Joint Surg [Am]* 1978;56A:1663–1674.
146. Atlas SW, Regenbogen V, Rogers LF, Kim KS. Radiographic characterization of burst fractures of the spine. *AJR Am J Roentgenol* 1986;147:575–582.
147. Babcock JL. Cervical spine injuries: diagnosis and classification. *Arch Surg* 1976;116:646–651.
148. Bedbrook GM. Spinal injuries with tetraplegia and paraplegia. *J Bone Joint Surg [Br]* 1979;61B:267–284.
149. Bedbrook GM. Stability of spinal fractures and fracture dislocations. *Paraplegia* 1971;9:23–32.
150. Berquist TH. *Imaging of orthopedic trauma.* New York: Raven Press; 1992.
151. Brooks AL, Jenkins EB. Atlanto-axial arthrodesis by wedge compression method. *J Bone Joint Surg [Am]* 1978;60A:279–284.
152. Burke JH, Harris JH. Acute injuries of the axis vertebra. *Skeletal Radiol* 1989;18:335–446.
153. Clintron E, Gilula LA, Murphy WA, Gehweiler JA. The widened disk space. A sign of cervical hyperextension injury. *Radiology* 1981;141:639–644.
154. Daffner RH. *Imaging of vertebral trauma.* Rockville,MD: Aspen Press; 1988.
155. Denis F. Spinal stability as defined by the three column spine concept in acute spinal trauma. *Clin Orthop* 1984;189:65–76.
156. Effendi B, Roy D, Cornish B, Dussault RG, Lauren CA. Fractures of the ring of the axis. *J Bone Joint Surg [Br]* 1988;63B:319–327.
157. Fielding JW. The status of arthrodesis of the cervical spine. *J Bone Joint Surg [Am]* 1988;70A:1571–1574.
158. Fielding JW, Hawkins RJ. Atlantoaxial rotary fixation. *J Bone Joint Surg [Br]* 1977;59B:37–44.
159. Gallie WE. Fractures and dislocations of the cervical spine. *Am J Surg* 1939;46:495–499.
160. Gassman J, Selingson D. The anterior cervical plate. *Spine* 1983;8:700–707.
161. Gehweiler JA, Osborne RL, Becker RF. *The radiology of vertebral trauma.* Philadelphia: WB Saunders; 1980.
162. Grob D. Internal fixation of the cervical spine. *Spine* 1991;16:281–301.
163. Grob D, Dvorak J, Gschwend N, Froehlich M. Posterior occipitocervical fusion in rheumatoid arthritis. *Arch Orthop Trauma Surg* 1990;110:38–44.
164. Grob D, Dvorak J, Panjabi M, Froehlich M, Hayek J. Posterior occipitocervical fusion: a preliminary report of a new technique. *Spine* 1991;16:517–523.
165. Holdsworth F. Fractures, dislocations and fracture/dislocations of the spine. *J Bone Joint Surg [Am]* 1970;52A:1534–1551.
166. Jeanneret B, Magerl F, Ward EH, Ward JCL. Posterior stabilization of the cervical spine with hook plates. *Spine* 1991;16:556–563.
167. Jonsson H, Cesarini K, Petren-Mallmin M, Rauschning W. Locking screw-plate fixation of cervical spine fractures with and without ancillary posterior plating. *Arch Orthop Trauma Surg* 1991;111:1–12.
168. Karasick D. Anterior cervical spine fusion: struts, plugs and plates. *Skeletal Radiol* 1993;22:85–94.
169. Krag MH, Beynnon BD. A new halo vest: rationale, design and biomechanical comparisons to standard halo vest designs. *Spine* 1988;13:228–235.
170. Levine AM, Edwards CC. The management of traumatic spondylolisthesis of the axis. *J Bone Joint Surg [Am]* 1985;67A:217–226.
171. Rabassa AE, Guinto FC, Crow WN, Chaljub G, Wright GD, Storey GS. CT of the spine: value of reformatted images. *AJR Am J Roentgenol* 1993;161:1223–1227.
172. Slone RM, MacMillan M, Montgomery WJ. Principles, basic hardware and fixation techniques for the cervical spine. *Radiographics* 1993;13:341–356.
173. Ulrich C, Wördsdörfer O, Claes L, Mugerl F. Comparative study of the stability of anterior and posterior cervical spine fixation procedures. *Arch Orthop Trauma Surg* 1987;106:226–231.
174. White AA. Biomechanical analysis of clinical stabilization of the cervical spine. *Clin Orthop* 1975;109:85–96.

Thoracolumbar Spine Trauma

175. Aebi M, Etter C, Kehl T, Thagott J. The internal skeletal fixation system: a new treatment of thoracolumbar fractures and other spinal disorders. *Clin Orthop* 1988;227:30–43.
176. Asher M, Carson W, Heinig C, Strippgen W, Arendt M, Lark R, Hartley M. A modular spinal rod linkage system to provide rotational stability. *Spine* 1988;13:272–277.
177. Atlas SW, Regenbogen V, Rogers PF, Kina KS. The radiographic characterization of the burst fractures of the spine. *AJR Am J Roentgenol* 1986;147:575–582.
178. Berquist TH. *Imaging of orthopedic trauma.* 2nd ed. New York: Raven Press; 1992.
179. Calenoff L, Chessare RW, Rogers LF, et al. Multiple level spinal injuries. Importance of early recognition. *AJR Am J Roentgenol* 1978;130:665–669.
180. Colter JM, Vernace JV, Michalski JA. The use of Harrington rods for thoracolumbar fractures. *Orthop Clin North Am* 1986;17:87–103.
181. Daniaux H, Seykora P, Genelin A, Lang T, Kathrein A. Application of posterior plating and modifications in thoracolumbar spine injuries: indications, techniques, and results. *Spine* 1991;16:1255–1335.
182. Dekutoski MB, Conlan ES, Salciccioli GG. Spinal mobility and deformity after Harrington rod stabilization and limited arthrodesis of thoracolumbar fractures. *J Bone Joint Surg [Am]* 1993;75A:168–176.
183. Denis F. The three-column spine and its significance in the classification of acute thoracolumbar spinal injuries. *Spine* 1983;8:817–831.
184. Denis F, Ruiz H, Searls K. Comparison between square-ended distraction rods and standard round-ended rods in the treatment of thoracolumbar injuries. A statistical analysis. *Clin Orthop* 1984;189:162–167.
185. Dick W, Kluger P, Margerl F, Wörsdorfer O, Zach G. A new device for internal fixation of thoracolumbar and lumbar spine fractures, the "fixateur interne." *Paraplegia* 1985;23:225–232.

186. Dombrowski ET. Rezaian fixator in the anterior stabilization of the unstable spine. *Orthop Rev* 1986;15:65–69.
187. Dunn HK. Anterior stabilization of thoracolumbar injuries. *Clin Orthop* 1984;189:116.
188. Edwards CC, Levine AM. Early rod-sleeve stabilization of the injured thoracic and lumbar spine. *Orthop Clin North Am* 1986;17:121–145.
189. Ferguson RL, Allen BL. A mechanistic classification of thoracolumbar spine fractures. *Clin Orthop* 1984;189:77.
190. Frankel HL, Hancock DO, Hyslop G, et al. The value of postural reduction in the initial management of closed injuries of the spine with paraplegia and tetraplegia. *Paraplegia* 1969;7:179–192.
191. Gardner VO, Armstrong GWD. Long-term lumbar facet joint changes in spinal fracture patients treated with Harrington rods. *Spine* 1990;15:479–484.
192. Gertzbein SD, Jacobs RR, Stoll J, Martin C, Marks P, Zazl M, Rowed D, Schwartz M. Results of a locking-hook spinal rod for fractures of the thoracic and lumbar spine. *Spine* 1990;15:275–280.
193. Grob D. Internal fixation of the cervical spine. *Spine* 1991;16:281–301.
194. Guyer DW, Wiltse LL, Peek RD. The Wiltse pedicle screw fixation system. *Orthopedics* 1988;11:1455–1460.
195. Haas N, Blauth M, Tscherne H. Anterior plating in thoracolumbar spine injuries. Indications, technique, and results. *Spine* 1991;16:S100–111.
196. Jacobs RR, Montesano PX. Development of the locking hook spinal rod system. *Orthopedics* 1988;11:1415–1421.
197. Kostuik JP. Anterior Kostuik-Harrington distraction systems for treatment of kyphotic deformities. *Spine* 1990;15:169–180.
198. Krag MH. Spine fusion: overview of options and posterior fixation devices. In: Frymoyer JW, ed. *The adult spine: principles and practice.* New York: Raven Press; 1991:1919–1945.
199. Krag MH, Weaver DL, Beynnon BD, Harigh LD. Morphometry of the thoracic and lumbar spine related to transpedicular screw placement for surgical spinal fixation. *Spine* 1988;13:27–32.
200. Levine AM. Surgical techniques for thoracic and lumbar trauma. In: Rothman RH, Simeone FA, eds. *The spine.* 3rd ed. Philadelphia: WB Saunders; 1992:1104–1133.
201. Levine AM, Edwards CC. Complications of treatment of acute spinal injury. *Orthop Clin North Am* 1986;17:183–203.
202. Luque ER, Cassis N, Romirez-Wiella G. Segmental spinal instrumentation in the treatment of fractures of the thoracolumbar spine. *Spine* 1982;7:312–317.
203. McAfee PC. Spinal instrumentation for thoracolumbar fractures. In: Rothman RH, Simeone FA, eds. *The spine.* 3rd ed. Philadelphia: WB Saunders; 1992:1135–1165.
204. McAfee PC, Yuon HA, Freedrubson BE, Lubecky JP. The value of computed tomography in thoracolumbar fractures: an analysis of 100 consecutive cases. *J Bone Joint Surg* [*Am*] 1983;65A:461–473.
205. McLain RF, Sparling E, Benson DR. Early failure of short-segment pedicle instrumentation for thoracolumbar fractures. *J Bone Joint Surg* [*Am*] 1993;75A:162–167.
206. Nicoll EA. Fractures of the dorsolumbar spine. *J Bone Joint Surg* [*Br*] 1949;31B:376–394.
207. Olerud S, Karlstrom G, Sjostrom L. Transpedicular fixation of thoracolumbar vertebral fractures. *Clin Orthop* 1988;227:44–51.
208. Rezaian SM. Rezaian spinal fixator for management of fractures of the thoracolumbar spine. *J Neurol Orthop Med Surg* 1991;12:307–314.
209. Slone RM, MacMillan M, Montgomery WJ. Spinal fixation. Part 3: complications of spinal instrumentation. *Radiographics* 1993;13:797–816.
210. Slone RM, MacMillan M, Montgomery WJ, Heare M. Spinal fixation. Part 2: fixation techniques and hardware for the thoracic and lumbosacral spine. *Radiographics* 1993;13:521–543.
211. Steffee AD, Biscup RS, Sitkowski DJ. Segmental spinal plates with pedicle screw fixation. A new device for disorders of the lumbar and thoracolumbar spine. *Clin Orthop* 1986;203:45–53.
212. Takata K, Insue S, Takalioski K, Ohtsuka Y. Fracture of the posterior margin of the lumbar vertebra. *J Bone Joint Surg* [*Am*] 1988;70A:589–594.
213. West JL, Bradford DS, Ogilvie JW. Result of spinal arthrodesis with pedicle screw-plate fixation. *J Bone Joint Surg* [*Am*] 1991;73A:1179–1184.
214. West JL, Ogilvie JW, Bradford DS. Complications of the variable screw plate pedicle screw fixation. *Spine* 1991;16:576–579.

Imaging Atlas of Orthopedic Appliances and Prostheses,
edited by T.H. Berquist.
Mayo Clinic Foundation © 1995.
Published by Raven Press, Ltd., New York.

CHAPTER 4

The Pelvis and Hips

Thomas H. Berquist, David G. Lewallen, and Barbara L. McComb

There are numerous orthopedic implants and protheses used for repair or joint replacement in the pelvis and hips. This chapter reviews basic clinical and imaging concepts as they apply to orthopedic problems in the pelvis and hips. Trauma, arthroplasty, and other common orthopedic procedures are stressed. Emphasis is placed on adult disorders.

IMAGING TECHNIQUES

New imaging techniques have dramatically changed approaches to evaluating disorders of the pelvis and hips.[4,7,11] Despite these advances, routine radiography remains the primary screening technique for evaluating pathologic conditions and obtaining measurements or templates for hip arthroplasty procedures.[1,7]

Radiographs, fluoroscopically positioned spot views, stress views, and occasionally, conventional tomography play valuable roles for evaluating disorders of the pelvis and hips. A minimum of two views are required to provide adequate information for diagnoses and classification.[2,7]

Pelvis

The anteroposterior (AP) view of the pelvis should include the lower lumbar spine, iliac crests, and upper femurs. This view demonstrates significant soft tissue and osseous anatomy. Most fractures can be identified on this view, and as is demonstrated later in the Arthroplasty section, measurements for reconstructive or joint-replacement procedures can be obtained.[7,19,24,36,38,39] The feet should be rotated internally 15° to ensure proper positioning of the greater and lesser trochanter.[2,5] Figure 4-1 demonstrates some of the important features to be evaluated carefully on the AP view of the pelvis.

In addition, AP angled views (inlet and tangential) are useful in traumatized patients to identify fractures and the degree of displacement more clearly (Fig. 4-2). The inlet view is obtained by angling the tube 40° to the feet. The tangential view is angled in the opposite direction (toward the head), using 25° of angulation for males and 40° for females.[2,5,7,37] These views are obtained without moving the patient.

Hips

The AP, oblique, lateral, and Judet views of the hips may be required in a given clinical situation to evaluate proximal femoral and acetabular anatomy completely.[5,7,22]

The AP view of the hip normally includes most of the innominate bone and proximal femur (Fig. 4-3). Centering improves the measurement's accuracy and assessment of the joint compared with the AP views of the pelvis.[1,2,3] More of the femur can be included with magnification markers prior to prosthetic joint replacements.[7]

Judet views are useful for evaluating the acetabular margins, anterior and posterior columns, iliac wing, and obturator foramen (Fig. 4-4).[7,23,28] These views are taken with the involved side rotated anteriorly 45° (Fig. 4-4B) and posteriorly 45° (Fig. 4-4C). The iliac and obturator oblique views are the equivalent of extremity AP and lateral views obtained at 90° with respect to the structure of interest. These obliquely oriented views of the acetabulum and iliac wing are helpful in revealing acetabular

(*text continues on page 220*)

T. H. Berquist: Mayo Medical School and Department of Diagnostic Radiology, Mayo Clinic Jacksonville, Jacksonville, Florida 32224.

D. G. Lewallen: Mayo Medical School and Department of Orthopedic Surgery, Mayo Clinic, Rochester, Minnesota 55903.

B. L. McComb: Department of Diagnostic Radiology, Mayo Clinic Jacksonville, Jacksonville, Florida 32224.

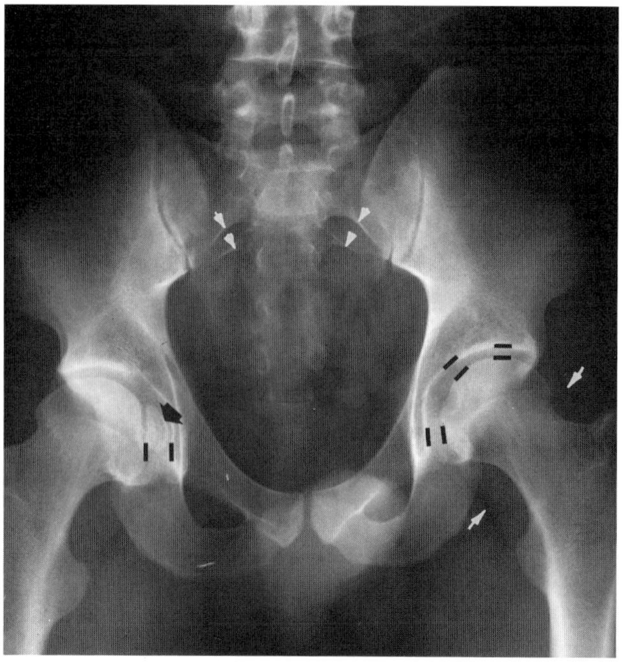

FIG. 4-1. An AP view of the pelvis. The normal joint space is marked on the left (*lines*), and the fat stripes are identified in the normal position (*white arrows*). The joint space on the right is widened (*lines*) medially because of the large osteochondral fragment (*arrow*) in the joint space. The arcuate lines (*arrowheads*) should be carefully evaluated to avoid overlooking subtle fractures. Both sacroiliac joints are normal and symmetric.

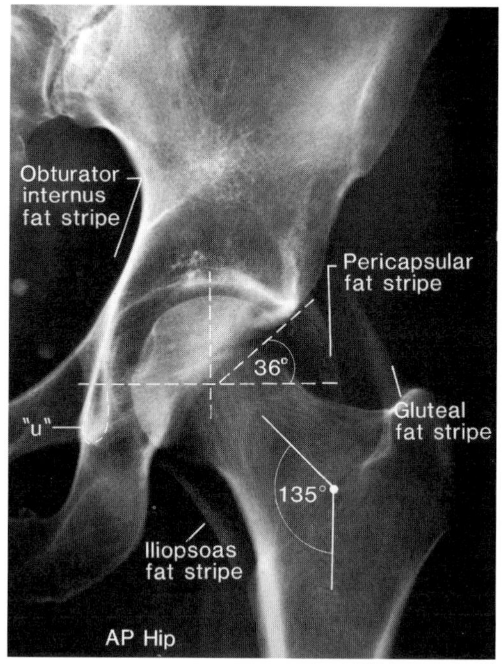

FIG. 4-3. An AP view of the hip demonstrating the pericapsular fat stripes, acetabular angle (36°), femoral neck angle, and teardrop line ("u") of the medial acetabulum. (From Berquist TH. Imaging atlas of orthopedic trauma, 2nd ed. New York: Raven Press, 1992.)

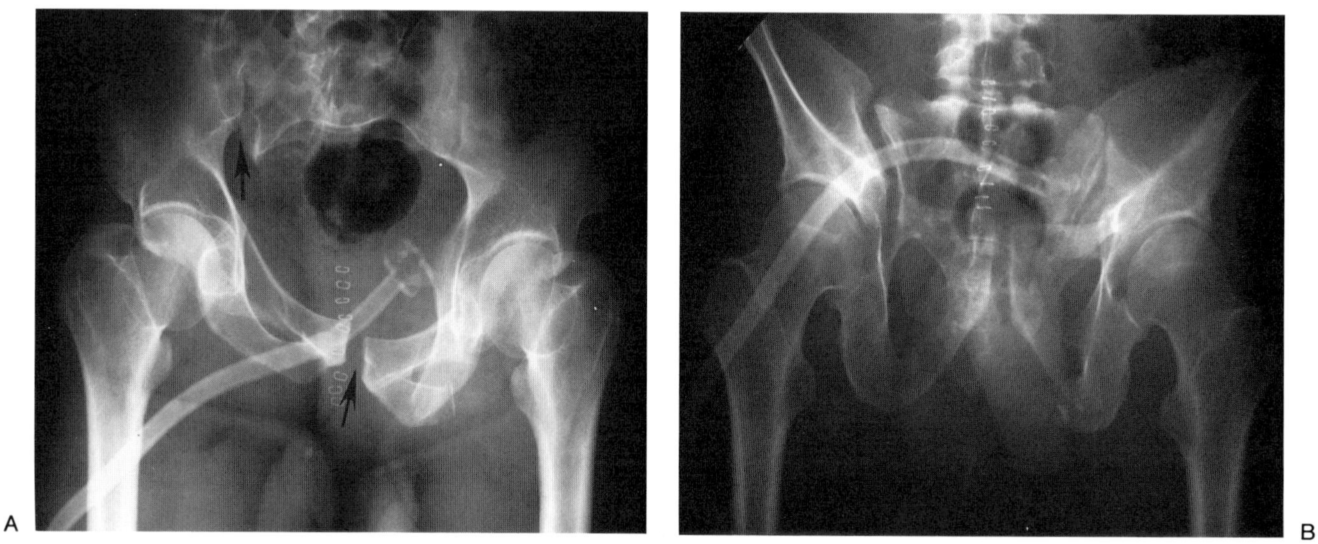

FIG. 4-2. Class III pelvic fracture with diastasis of the pubic symphysis and right sacroiliac joint (*arrows*). **A:** The degree of step off at the joint is most easily appreciated on the inlet view. **B:** The sacroiliac joint widening is more easily evaluated on the tangential view. Suprapubic cystostomy tube in place as a result of bladder and urethral injury. There are also pubic rami fractures on the left.

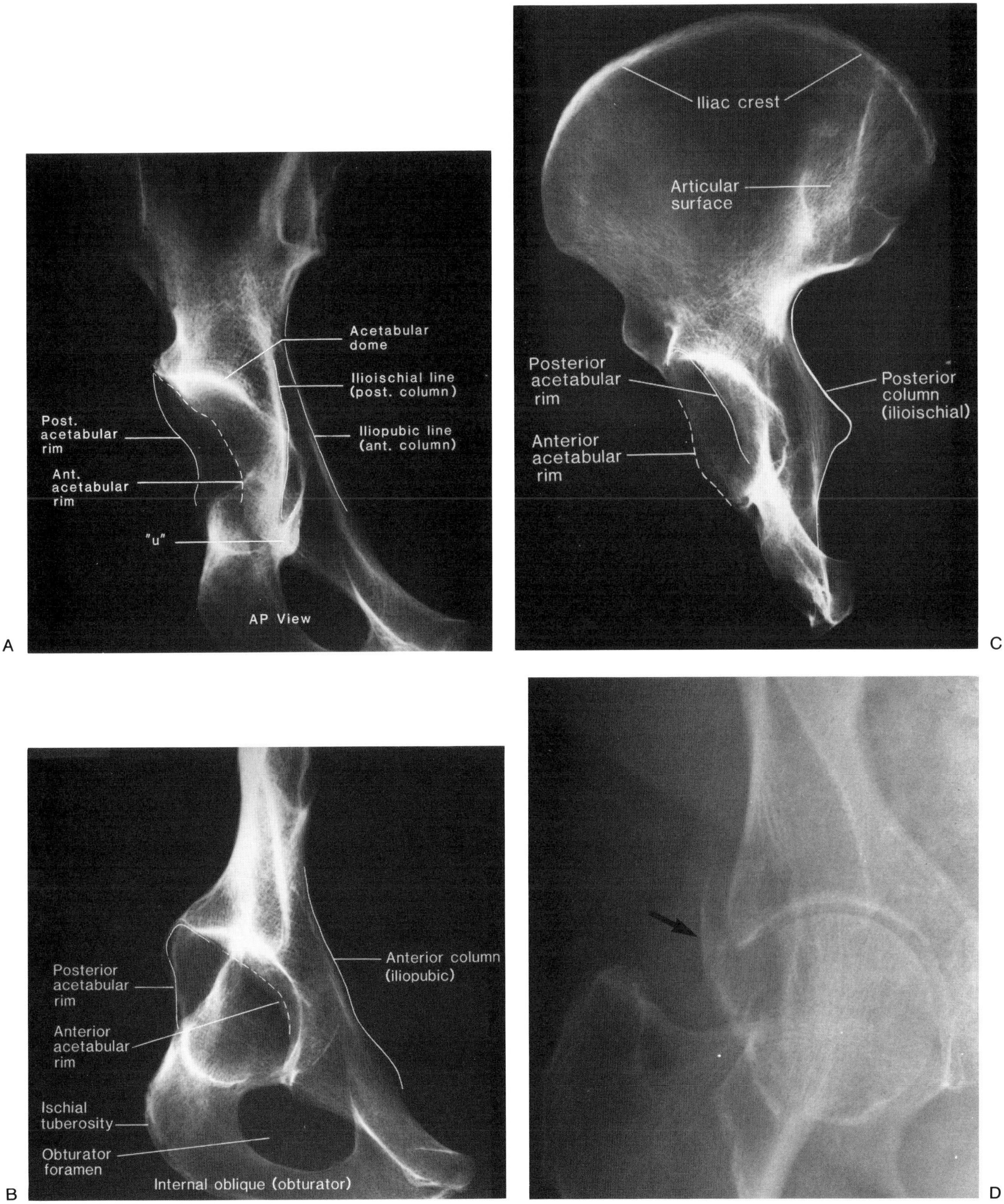

FIG. 4-4. Judet views: Bone with anatomy labeled in the AP projection **(A)**, 45° anterior oblique (obturator) projection **(B)**, and 45° posterior iliac oblique projection **(C)**. **D:** Posterior acetabular rim fracture demonstrated on the anterior (obturator) oblique.

fracture anatomy and subtle pubic rami fractures, which are otherwise easily misunderstood or overlooked if these views are not obtained. The patient should be rotated 45° rather than angling the x-ray tube to prevent distortion of anatomy; careful log-rolling maneuvers are used for patients with gross pelvic instability or polytrauma.[7,23,28]

The routine lateral view of the hip is useful for evaluating the femoral head and neck and acetabulum.[3,20,21,22] However, in injured patients, a modified technique is often required because of the inability to position the patient properly (Fig. 4-5A). The Johnson[22] technique can be used in this setting. The patient does not have to be moved. The cassette (10 × 12 inches) is placed next to the hip to be examined and angled 65° with the table. The tube is angled 25° (Fig. 4-5B) to be perpendicular to the cassette. Both hips are actually seen clearly with this technique (Fig. 4-5C).[7,22]

Oblique views provide an additional view of the femoral neck, the trochanter, and the femoral head. This view is particularly useful for an evaluation of articular changes in avascular necrosis (AVN, Fig. 4-6).[7,29]

Computed Tomography (CT)

In the evaluation of a number of disorders in the pelvis and hips, CT plays a major role.[9–11,13,16,30,32] Some authors proceed directly to CT after an AP view of the pelvis in trauma patients. In addition, CT is useful to assess subtle trauma (Fig. 4-7) and complex bone and soft tissue injury (Fig. 4-8).[9,10,13,16] Conventional reconstructed images (coronal and sagittal) and three-dimensional images are useful for surgical planning and evaluating bone stock prior to reconstructive procedures.[7,9,10]

Radionuclide Scintigraphy

Radionuclide scans are used for the detection of subtle fractures (Fig. 4-9), especially in the femoral neck.[7,15] Combined technetium-99m–gallium-67 or technetium-99m–indium-111-labeled white blood cell scans are commonly used in patients with suspected infection after total hip replacement.[7] This is discussed more completely under Arthroplasty.

Although radionuclide imaging can also be used to detect AVN, magnetic resonance imaging (MRI) is more often used in this setting today.[12,14,17]

Both MRI and ultrasonography are more commonly used for complications and are discussed in the appropriate sections later.[6,18,31,33,40] Angiography (diagnostic and therapeutic), arthrography, and diagnostic and therapeutic injections also play important roles in the imaging of trauma and orthopedic complications following surgery and hip arthroplasty.[8,25,26,27,34,35]

TRAUMA

Imaging plays an important role in the detection, classification, and evaluation of complications of injuries to the pelvis and hips. This section reviews common orthopedic classifications used to assist typical treatment planning and the appearance of the image and the potential complications of implants used for treatment.

Pelvic Fractures

Pelvic fractures represent only 2% to 3% of all skeletal fractures. Minor pelvic fractures (undisplaced ring fracture or fractures not involving the ring) are fairly common in elderly patients. Severe pelvic fractures with instability usually result from high-velocity motor vehicle accidents or industrial injuries. Complex pelvic fractures tend to occur in younger individuals (50%, < 50 years of age). Morbidity and mortality rates can be significant with severe injuries.[41,45,71,85–88]

Proper management requires thorough radiographic evaluation, which may be compromised by hemodynamic instability.[78,85,86,108,117] Proper classification of the injury is essential for planning the treatment of the pelvic and associated injuries.[41,50,63,89,111,112,119] In addition to standard x-ray views, a push-pull test under fluoroscopic control or using AP radiographs while applying first axial traction and then proximal (upward) pressure on the injured leg and hemipelvis has been shown to be both safe and effective in diagnosing occult vertical instability following pelvic injury.[45]

Classification

Numerous classification systems have been proposed for pelvic fractures.[50,64,67,89,90,110–113] These systems are usually based on the stability, location, and mechanism of injury of the fracture and whether the injury is open or closed.[60] Three commonly used systems are reviewed here.

Tile[111,112] modified the Pennal et al.[90] system, which was based on mechanism of injury (Table 4-1).[59] As in our experience, fractures displaced greater than 1 cm are potentially unstable, and when they involve the ring, they nearly always have associated second fractures or diastases of the symphysis or sacroiliac joint.[41,96,97] Young et al.[118–120] described radiographic patterns that are useful for therapeutic planning based on lateral compression, anteroposterior compressions, and vertical shearing injuries. Most injuries occur with lateral compression (41% to 72%, Fig. 4-10). The AP compression injuries account for 15% to 25% of pelvic fractures (Fig. 4-11); vertical shearing, for 6% (Fig. 4-12); and combination injuries, for 14% of pelvic fractures.[60,64,118,119,120] The

(*text continues on page 227*)

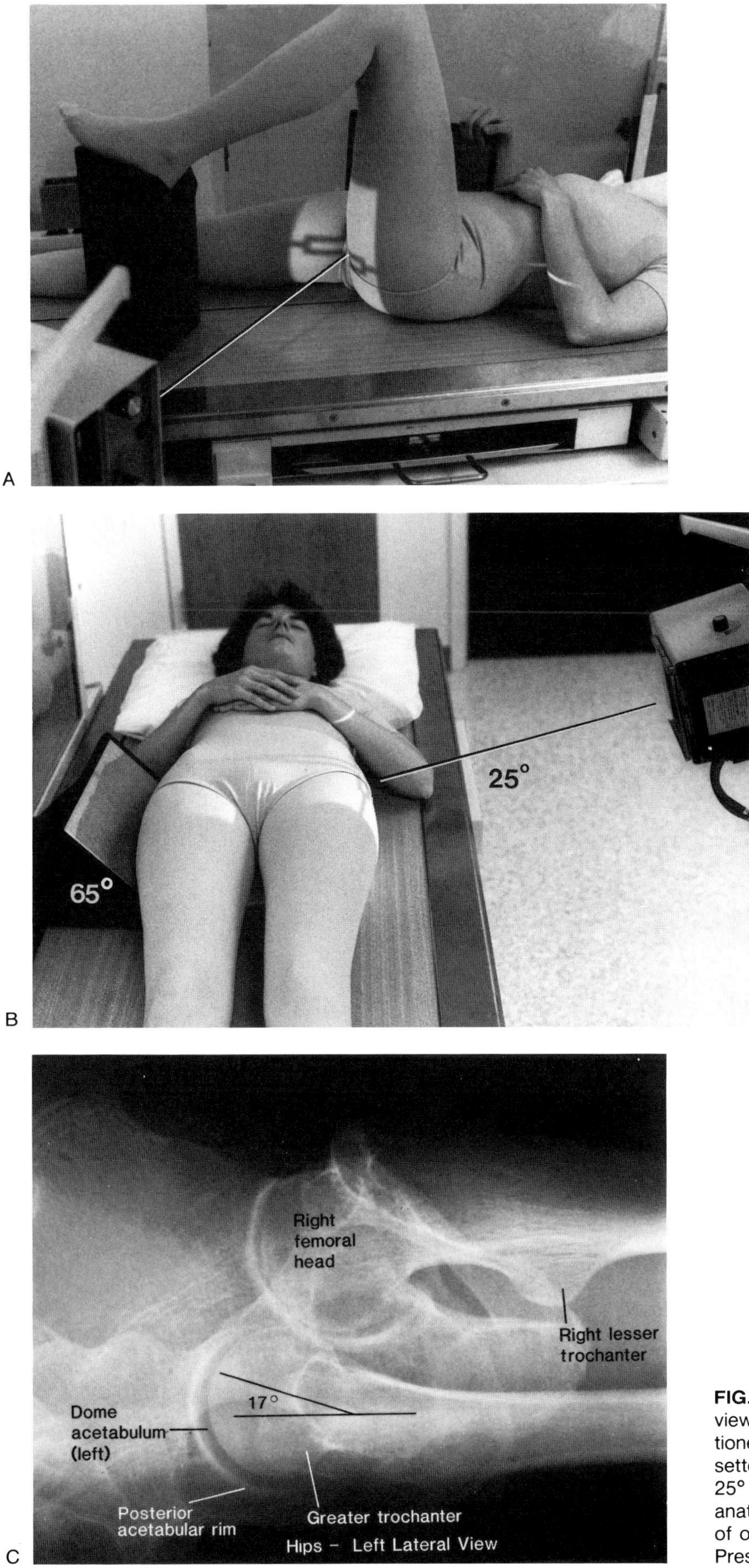

FIG. 4-5. A: Patient positioned for routine lateral view of the hip (*line, central beam*) **B:** Patient positioned for angled cross-table technique. The cassette is 65° to the table and the central beam (*line*), 25° off the horizontal. **C:** Lateral radiograph with anatomy labeled (From Berquist TH. Imaging atlas of orthopedic trauma. 2nd ed. New York: Raven Press, 1992.)

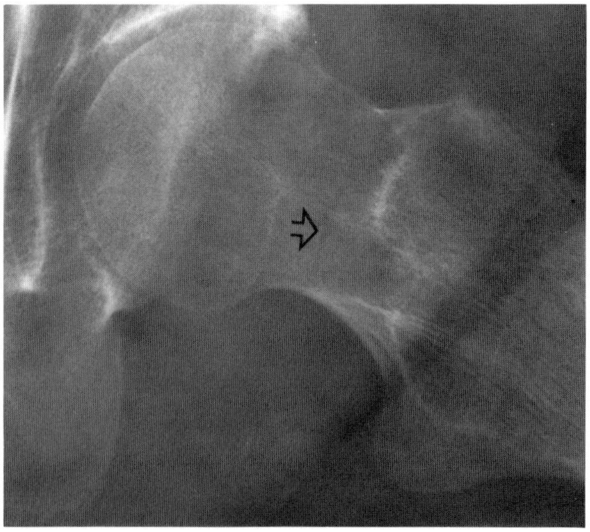

A

FIG. 4-6. Oblique views of the hip. **A:** Oblique radiograph demonstrating an undisplaced femoral neck fracture (*arrow*). The AP **(B)** and oblique **(C)** views of the hip in a patient with AVN and articular collapse (*arrow*, C).

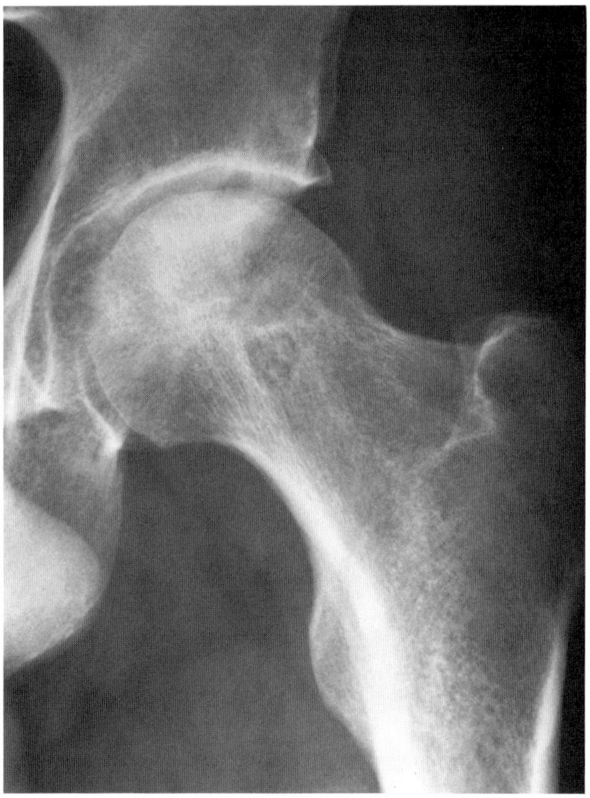

B

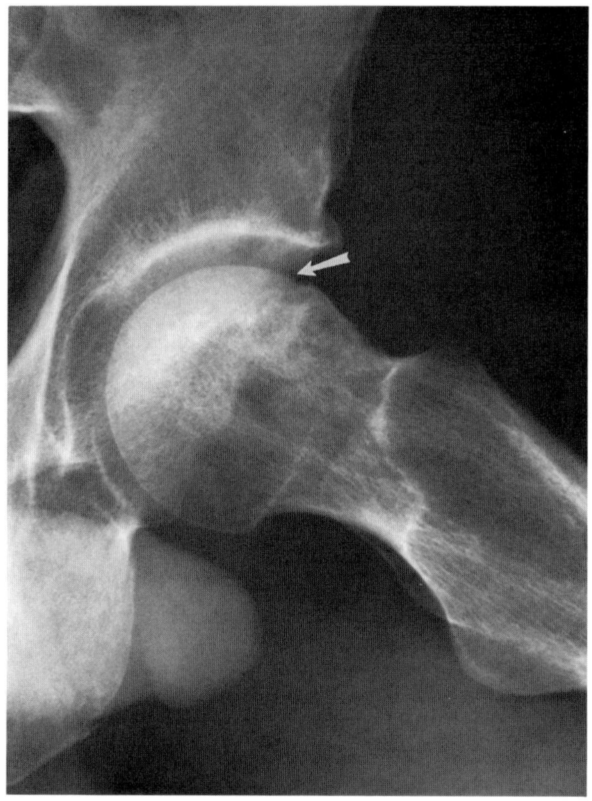

C

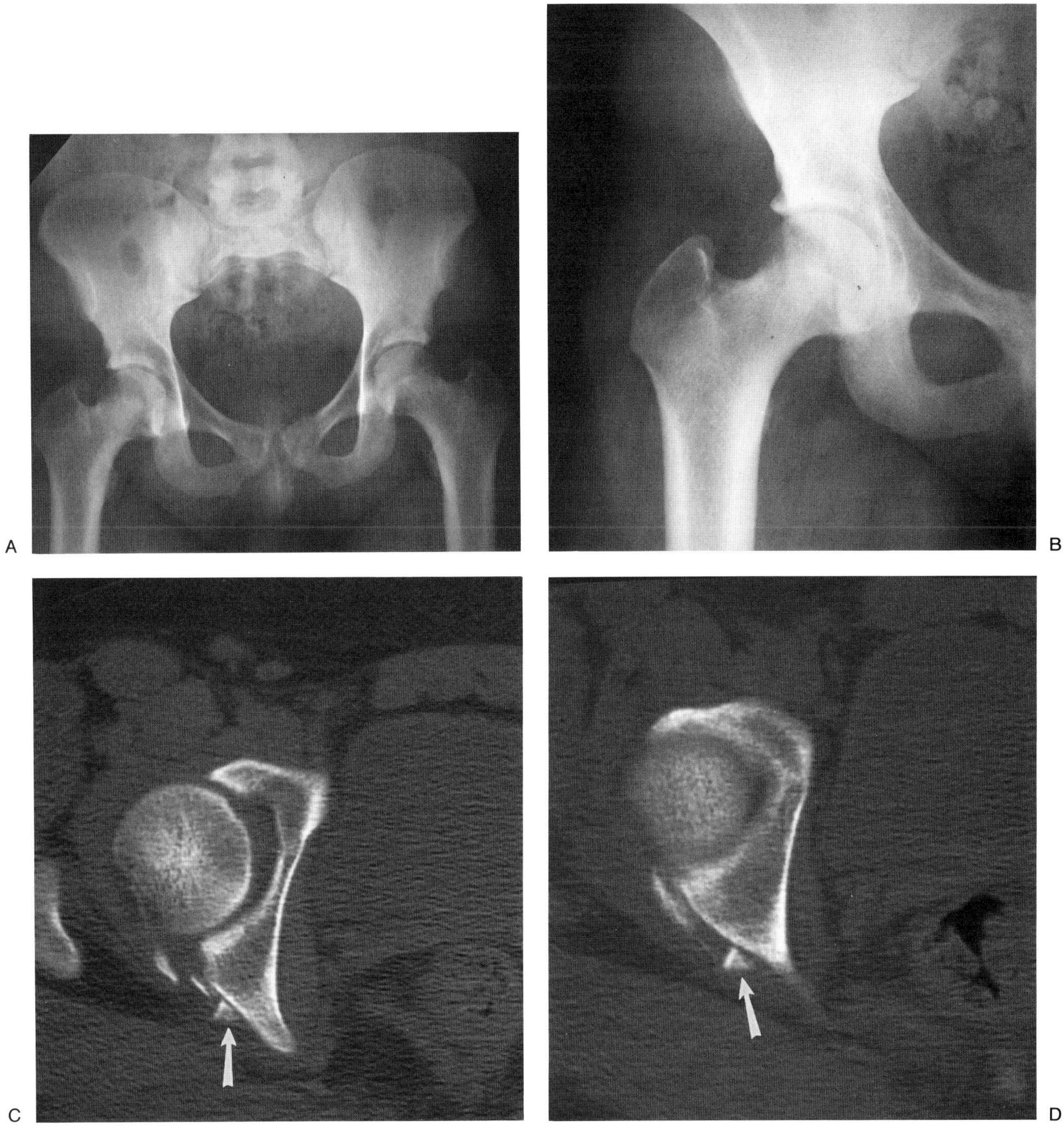

FIG. 4-7. The AP views of the pelvis **(A)** and right hip **(B)** are unremarkable. There is a questionable bony density behind the femoral head on the AP view of the hip (B). **C,D:** The CT images clearly demonstrate a posterior wall fracture with a displaced articular fragment (*arrow*) caused by a posterior dislocation, which has been reduced.

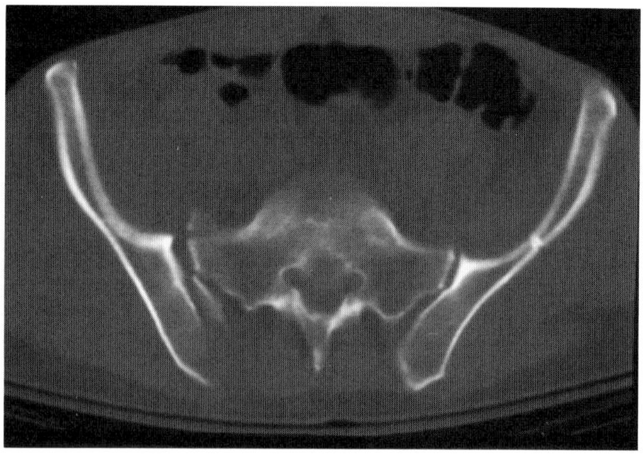

A

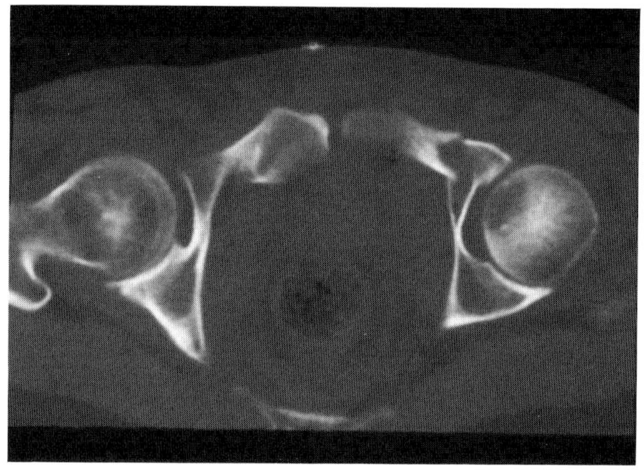

B

FIG. 4-8. Class III pelvic fracture: CT images of the sacral region **(A)** and pubic bone **(B)** with bone settings clearly demonstrate the fractures.

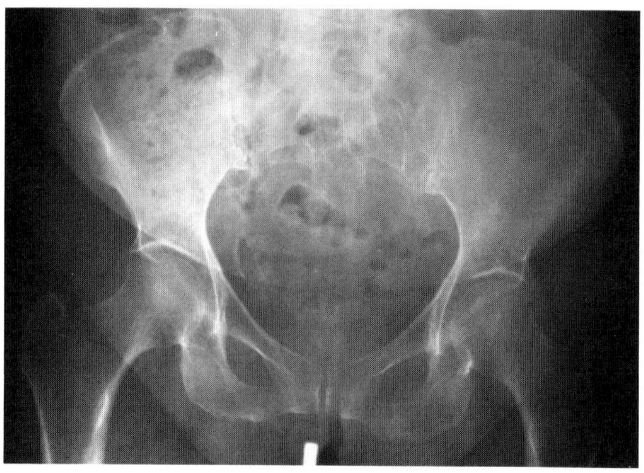

A

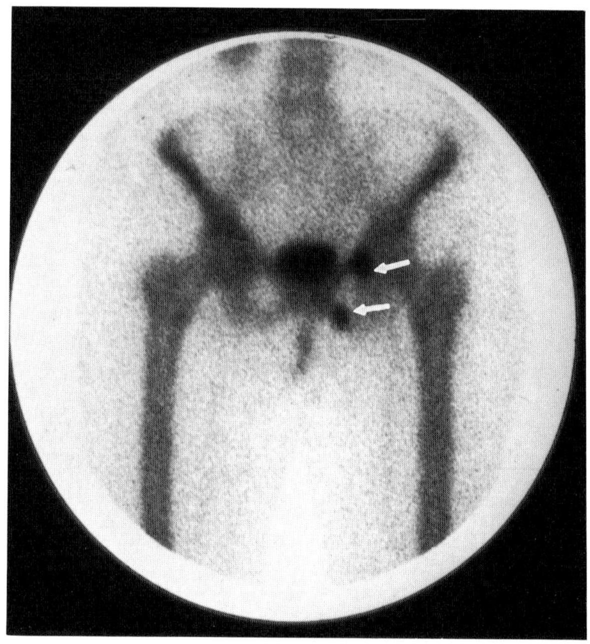

B

FIG. 4-9. An AP view of the pelvis (**A**) and technetium-99m scintigram (**B**) of the pelvis in a patient with left hip pain. The undisplaced pubic rami fractures are easily identified on the bone scan (*arrows*).

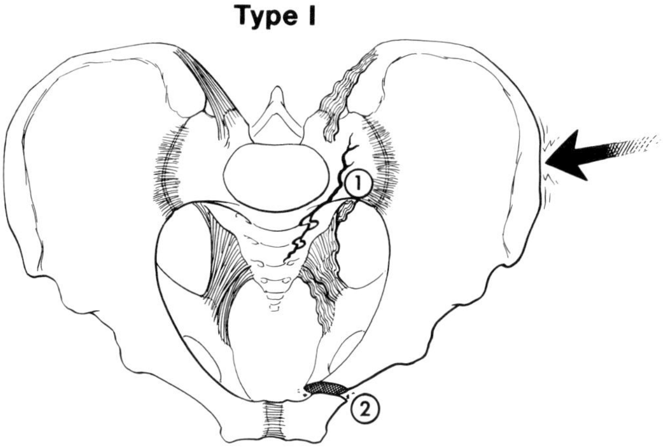

A

FIG. 4-10. Lateral compression injuries (41% to 72%) of pelvic fractures.[118–120] **A:** Type I: oblique or horizontal pubic rami fractures (*2*) with a crush injury (*1*) of the sacrum, ilium, or sacroiliac joint caused by lateral compression force. The force is directed toward the posterior pelvis, and the ligaments are intact; therefore, this is usually stable. **B:** Type II: force is directed anterolaterally, leading to oblique or horizontal rami fractures with either diastasis of the sacroiliac joints (IIA) or an iliac wing fracture (IIB). **C:** Type III: anterolateral force with pubic rami fractures and diastasis of sacroiliac ligaments bilaterally (IIIA) or sacroiliac ligaments and ipsilateral iliac wing (IIIB).

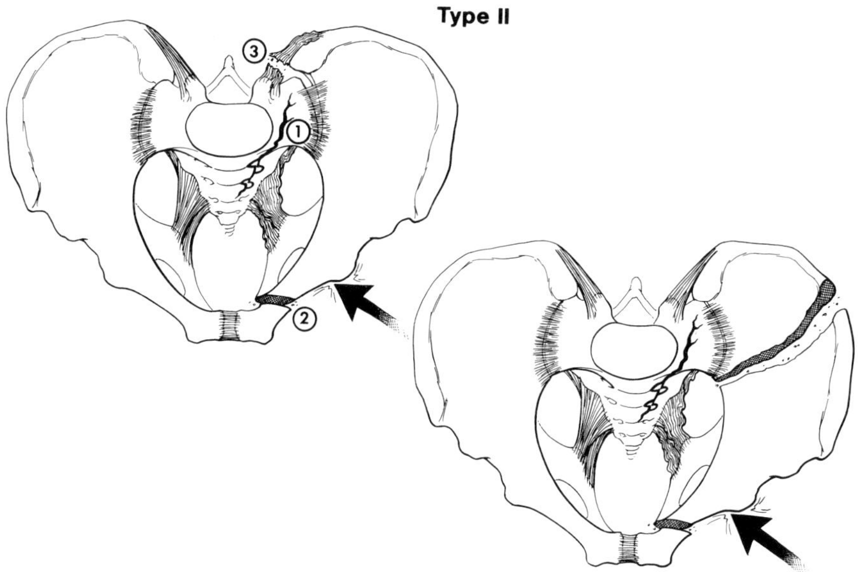

B

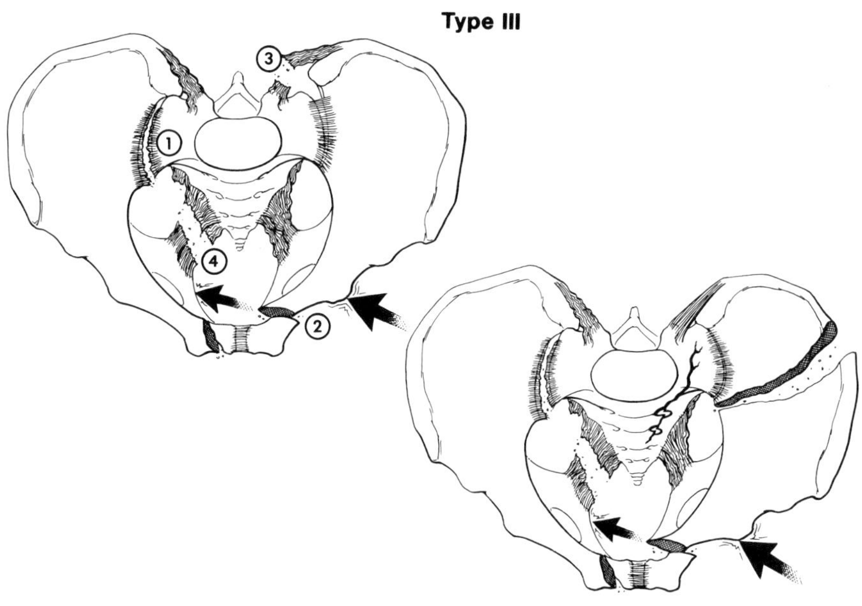

C

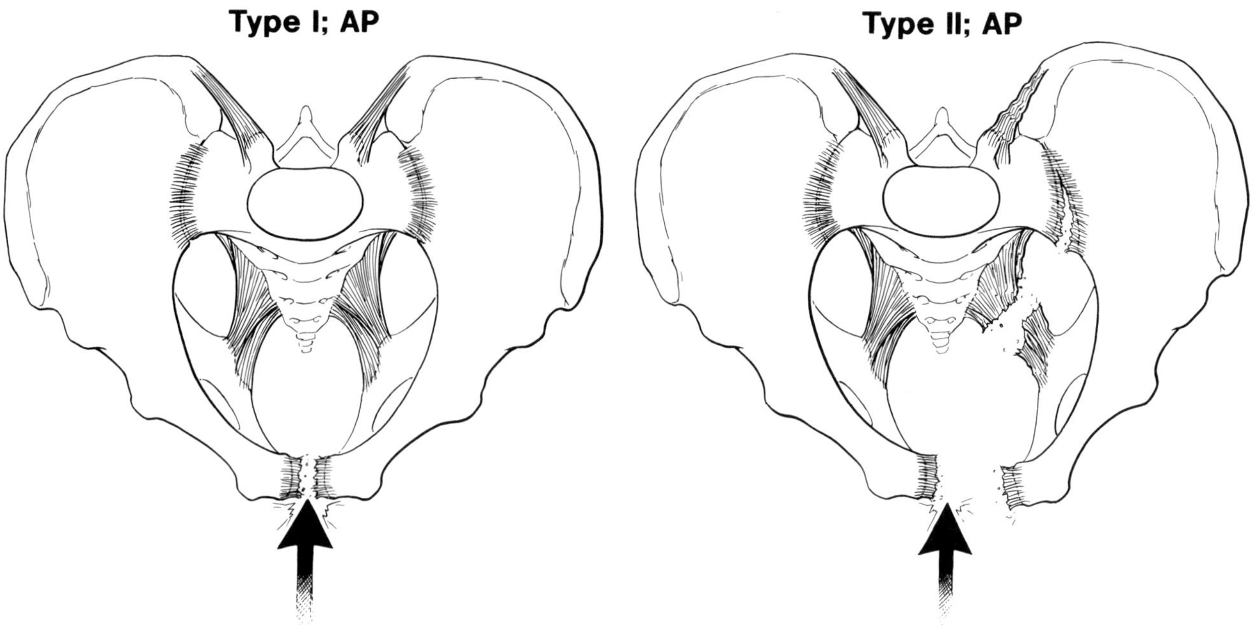

A

B

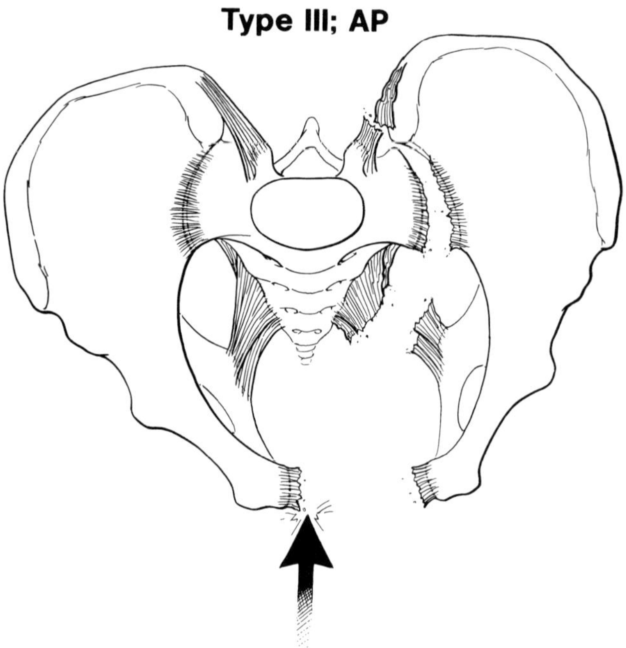

C

FIG. 4-11. Examples of AP compression injuries (15% to 25% of pelvic fractures).[118–120] **A:** Type I: vertical pubic rami fractures or diastasis of the pubic symphysis. **B:** Type II: pubic rami fractures or wider diastasis of the symphysis. **C:** Type III: wide symphysis diastasis with disruption of anterior and posterior sacroiliac ligaments, which corresponds to Tile B1.

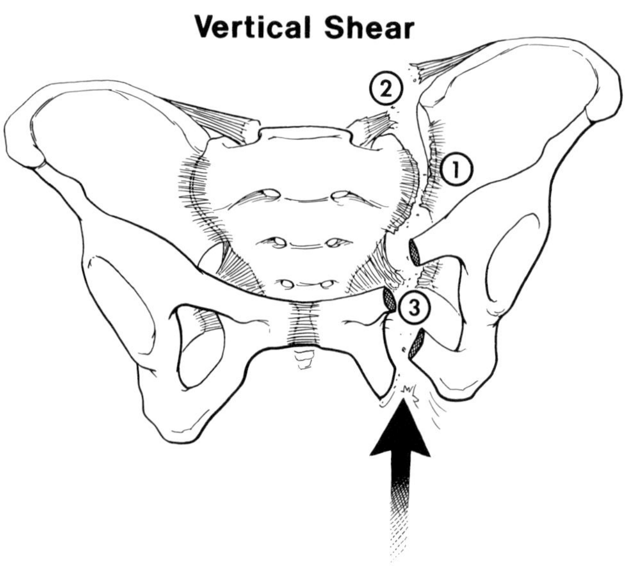

FIG. 4-12. Vertical shear injuries (6% of pelvic fractures).[118–120] Forces are transmitted vertically through the femur or laterally to the midline. A vertical step off is often apparent radiographically.

TABLE 4-1. *Tile classification*[60,95,111,112]

Category		Fractures (example)
A		Stable injuries
	A1	Fracture does not involve the ring (avulsion, transverse sacral fractures)
	A2	Stable, minimally displaced fractures of the ring (isolated pubic ramus fracture)
B		Rotationally unstable, vertically stable
	B1	Open book (diastasis of pubic symphysis ± sacroiliac diastasis)
	B2	Lateral compression: ipsilateral (pubic ramus fracture with ilium or sacroiliac involvement)
	B3	Lateral compression: contralateral (bucket-handle fracture)
C		Unstable rotationally and vertically
	C1	Unilateral
	C2	Bilateral
	C3	Associated acetabular fracture

Key and Conwell[69] classification modified by Kane[68] is a simple system that lends itself to a discussion of imaging and complications (Table 4-2).[41] Class I fractures (28% of injuries) are breaks that do not involve the pelvic ring, which are similar to Tile A1 injuries. These include avulsion fractures, transverse sacral fractures, and Duverney fractures (Fig. 4-13).[41,58] Class II fractures are single breaks in the pelvic ring (pubic ramus fractures, usually near the symphysis), and they accounted for 36% of injuries in our series. If undisplaced, a second fracture in the pelvis is not likely.[41] Insufficiency fractures could be included in this group.[52,53,104] Class III fractures are double breaks in the pelvic ring, which are unstable and associated with significant complications (Fig. 4-14).[41,66,85,86,103,107] Hemorrhage is the most frequent problem. Orthopedic fixation and stabilization is required. Class IV fractures are acetabular fractures, which if displaced, have complications similar to those of class III fractures.[41,46,57,68–70,72,102,103,106] The complications and imaging techniques are discussed following the treatment options.

Treatment

The treatment of pelvic fractures may be simple and conservative for undisplaced pubic rami fractures or Class I and II (Key and Conwell) and type A (Tile) fractures.[68,69,110,114,115,121] Associated complications are usually minimal with these injuries.[41,79] Unstable fractures are a different matter. Hemodynamic instability and associated injuries can create an emergency situation with high morbidity and significant mortality rates.[41,59,85,86,94,97] For the purposes of this atlas, we concentrate on the orthopedic aspects of treatment of pelvic fractures.

External Fixation

External fixation is a common method of the treatment for hemodynamically unstable patients. Generally, these patients have shear (Fig. 4-14) or anterior compression injuries (Fig. 4-11).[97] In general, some type of posterior fixation is often required after the patient has been stabilized because anterior fixators do not effectively stabilize the sacroiliac complex.[79,83,84,95,105] External fixators have the ability to maintain reduction during healing in rotationally unstable injuries (Tile type B) but not in vertically unstable injuries (Tile type C).[60,81,112] Figure 4-14 demonstrates a vertically unstable injury with an external fixator and posterior internal fixation.

In summary, the indications for external fixation include decreasing pelvic volume for hemorrhage control, temporary stabilization, and definitive treatment of rotationally unstable open book injuries, which are nonetheless vertically stable because of the preservation of the posterior sacroiliac ligament complex.[60,112] Most authors prefer large (5-mm) external fixation pins to add stability. The effectiveness of the fixator and the forces applied depends on its ability to reverse the forces of the mechanism of injury (Figs. 4-15 through 4-18).[60,65,81,84,112] Radiographically, it may be difficult to evaluate pin position on the single AP view. Angled views, especially the

TABLE 4-2. *Key and Conwell classification with Kane modification, 750 patients, Mayo Clinic*[41,58,68,97]

Class	% Patients	Description
I	25	Fractures of individual bones without interruption of the pelvic ring
		Single pubic ramus fracture
		Avulsion fracture
		Duverney fracture
		Transverse sacral fracture
		Coccyx fracture
II	36	Single break in the pelvic ring
		Fracture of two ipsilateral rami
		Fracture near or subluxation of pubic symphysis or sacroiliac joint
III	16	Double breaks in the pelvic ring
		Straddle fracture
		Sprung pelvis
		Malgaigne fracture
		Bucket-handle fracture
		Complex fracture
IV	24	Acetabular fractures
		Undisplaced
		Displaced

From Berquist,[7] with permission.

(*text continues on page 231*)

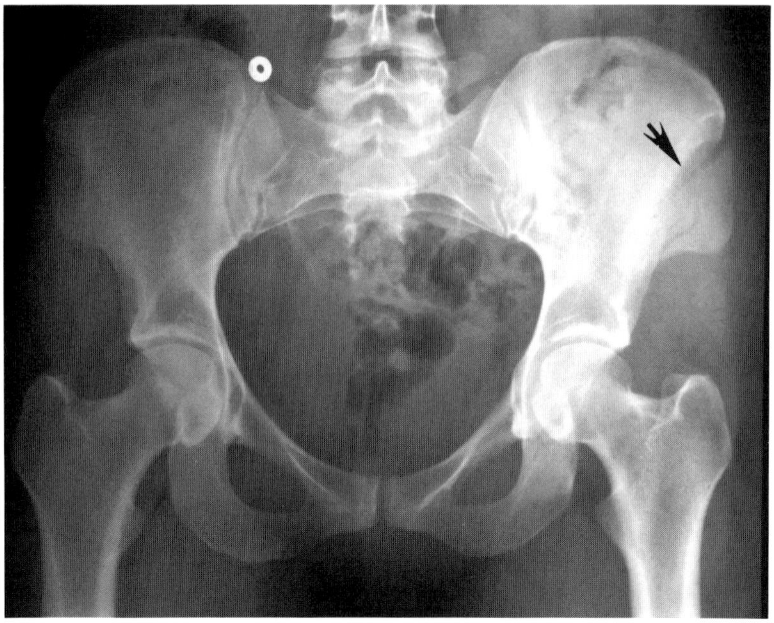

FIG. 4-13. An AP view of the pelvis demonstrating a fracture of the left ilium (Duverney fracture) (*arrow*).

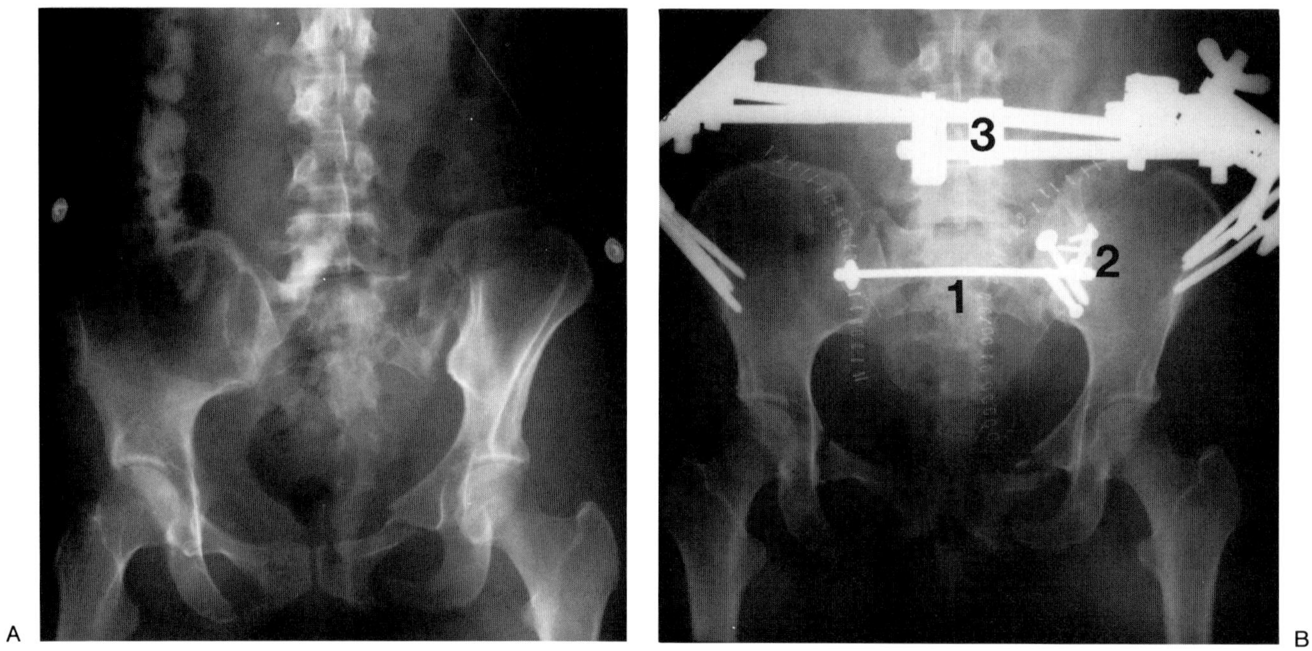

FIG. 4-14. A: An AP view of the pelvis demonstrating a vertical shear injury (Class III injury) with pubic rami fractures and disruption of the left sacroiliac joint. The fracture was reduced using a transiliac threaded rod and nuts (*1*), posterior interfragmentary screws (*2*), and a miniplate. There is an Ace-Fischer (*3*) external fixator for anterior stability (**B**).

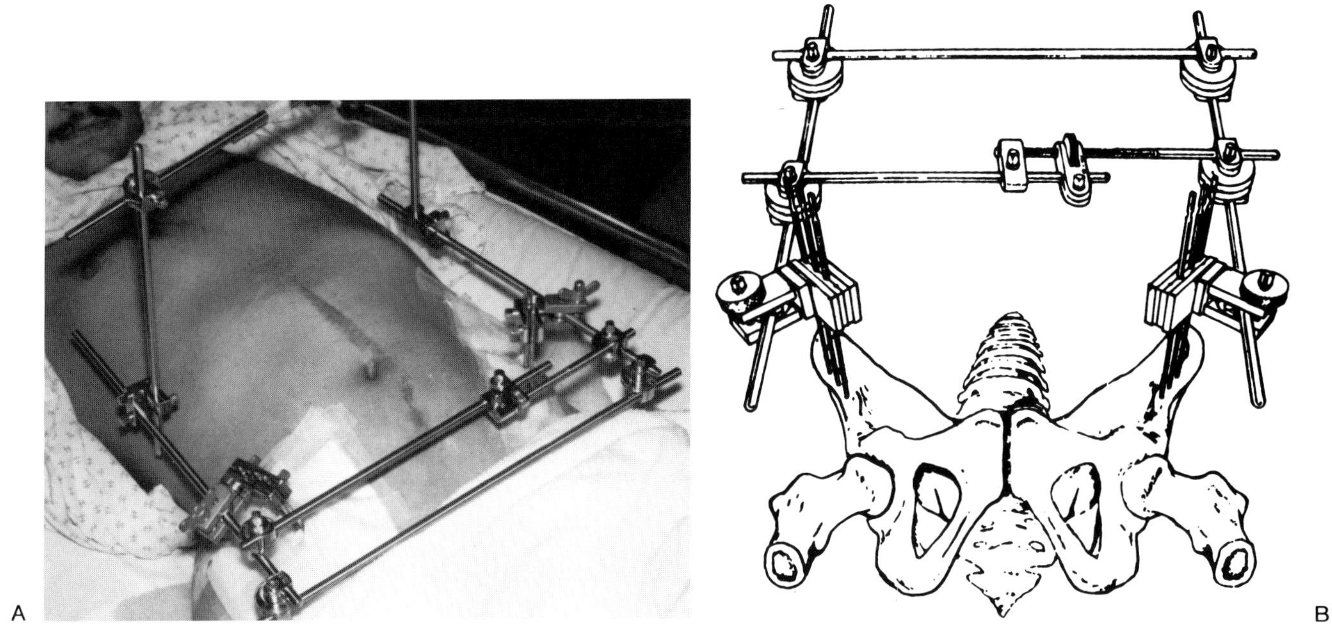

FIG. 4-15. A: Patient with Hoffman-Vidal external fixation in position. **B:** Hoffman fixation for bipolar fixation assembly. (B, Courtesy of Zimmer, Warsaw, IN.)

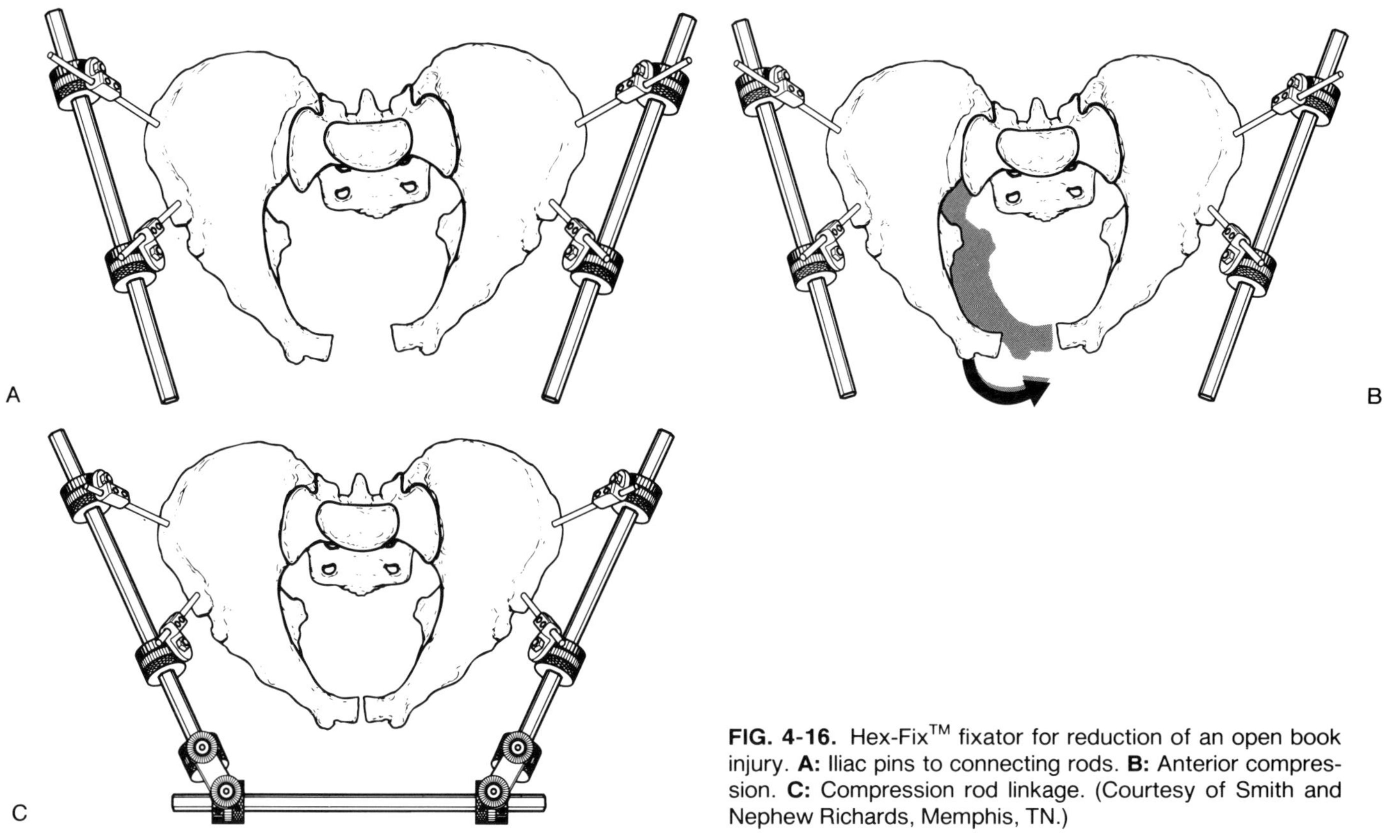

FIG. 4-16. Hex-Fix™ fixator for reduction of an open book injury. **A:** Iliac pins to connecting rods. **B:** Anterior compression. **C:** Compression rod linkage. (Courtesy of Smith and Nephew Richards, Memphis, TN.)

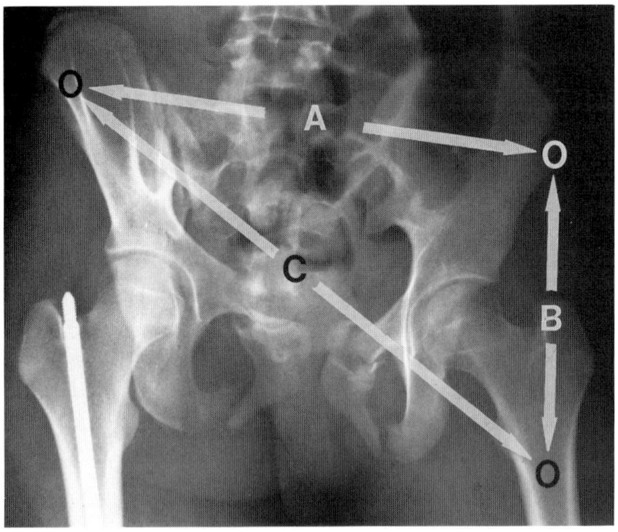

FIG. 4-17. Some potential assemblies for reduction of pelvic fractures.[65,84,105,116] (0 = pin placement, → = forces). **A:** Transverse bipolar assembly: forces can be used for compression or distraction. **B:** Vertical bipolar assembly using iliac wing and the ipsilateral femur. This can increase or decrease the distance. Care must be taken not to distract the hip joint excessively. **C:** Oblique bipolar assembly using the iliac wing and contralateral femur. A–C: Tripolar using three connecting rods with two iliac and one femoral pin site.

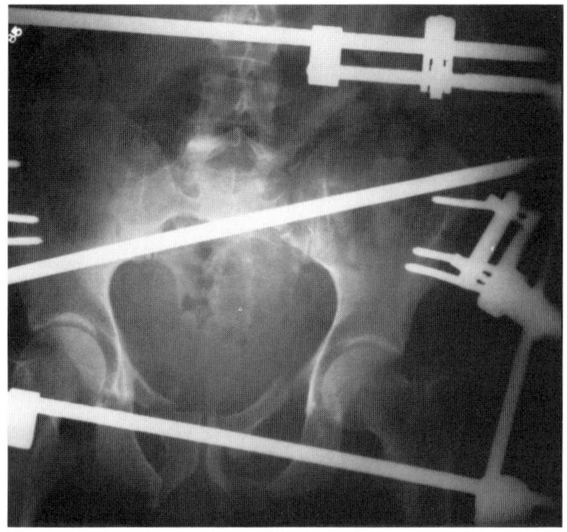

FIG. 4-18. An AP view of the pelvis with an anterior straddle fracture (pubic rami bilaterally) and left sacroiliac injury reduced using transverse and oblique assembly configuration with a Hoffman-Vidal fixator.

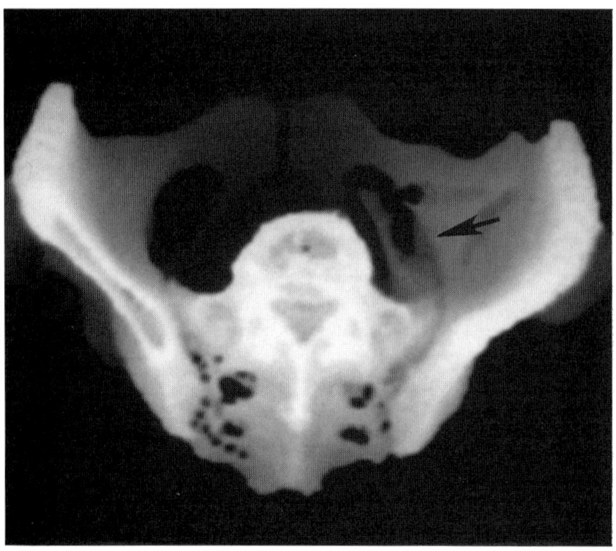

A

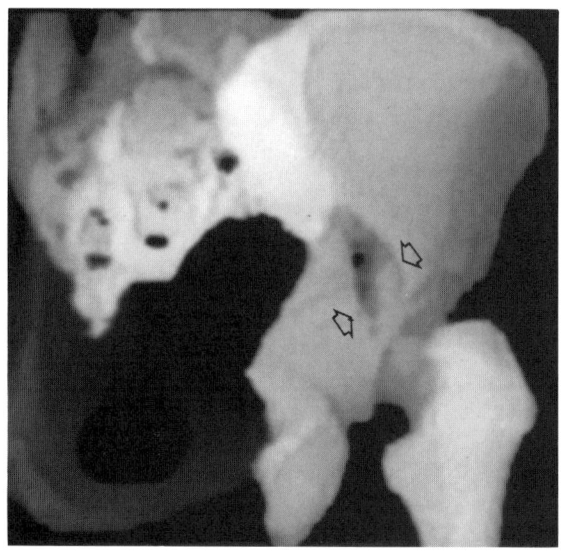

C

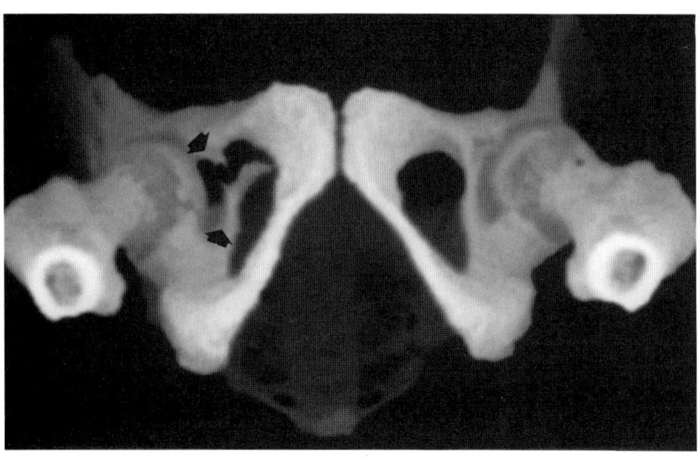

B

FIG. 4-19. A–C: Three-dimensional reconstruction in three different views of an acetabular fracture. The positions of the central and posterior column fragments are clearly defined (*arrows*).

obturator oblique (which shows the wing of the ilium in profile), can be obtained without moving the patient in this instance. When pins are positioned in the iliac wing, they should lie between the cortices of the ilium, with the pin tips between or just through the inner cortex.[195]

Internal Fixation

Conservative treatment with traction, pelvic slings, or external fixation devices may be suitable for the acute treatment phase while patients are being evaluated and stabilized. However, these methods are not sufficient for unstable injuries and must not delay treatment in patients with polytrauma. When used as definitive treatment of isolated injuries, nonoperative treatment may lead to an increased risk of complications. Matta and Saucedo[81] reported malunion or nonunion in more than 50% of patients treated with pelvic slings or traction. External fixation alone was initially satisfactory, but fractures healed in only one of nine patients with unstable injuries. Twenty-five of 29 patient treated with internal fixation healed, despite unstable fractures.

Indications for Internal Fixation[60,81,112]

- Posterior sacroiliac ligament disruptions
- Failed closed reduction
- Residual deformity after external fixation
- Multiple injuries (to allow rapid mobilization)
- Acetabular fractures
- Certain open wounds
- Vertically unstable injuries

Operative intervention may be performed electively up to 2 to 3 days after the injury in medically stable patients with isolated pelvic injuries, but many, alternatively, may need to be done urgently within 24 hours of admission in certain unstable patients, expecially in polytrauma to allow rapid mobilization and reduced mortality rates.[41,79] Because most unstable pelvic injuries involve anterior and posterior structures, stabilization likewise must be performed in general both anteriorly and posteriorly.[54,59,79] Conventional or three-dimensional CT images are useful in planning the operative approach, especially when complex acetabular fractures are to be included in the operative procedure (Fig. 4-19).[41,91]

Posterior stabilization can be achieved using cancellous screws and washers or threaded $^{3}/_{16}$-inch compression rods with washers and bolts (Figs. 4-20 and 4-21).[54,60,95] Double cobra-head plates and anterior sacroiliac plates and screws can also be used for posterior pelvic fixation.[95]

Anterior stabilization can be achieved with either an anterior external fixation frame or with interal fixation devices. Symphysis separation of > 2 cm can be reduced using a single plate and screws or a simple two-hole plate with vertical screws (Fig. 4-22).[54] Vertical shear injuries are difficult to stabilize anteriorly with one plate (Fig. 4-23). Therefore most authors prefer two plates at a 90° angle (superior and anterior).[60,95,112] Fractures of the acetabulum are reviewed separately, but they are usually reduced using reconstruction plates and screws (Fig. 4-24).[67,73,74]

Complications and Postoperative Imaging

Table 4-3 summarizes the complications associated with pelvic fracture and the potential sequelae of orthopedic treatment. In the acute setting, hemorrhage is the most significant and potentially life-threatening problem. In our patients with class III pelvic fractures, the mortality rate was 22%, due to hemorrhage.[41,76,97] Secondary problems, such as renal failure, which is caused by shock and volume loss, compound this problem. Hematomas can become infected in open fractures (3% of our cases). The mortality rate from infected hematomas is reported to reach as high as 50%.[44,85–87,91,93]

Angiography may be required to diagnose and control hemorrhage. Various embolic materials can be used to stabilize the patient and control bleeding.[80,82,86,88,101,103] Today, most pelvic bleeding can be controlled with external fixators or antishock garments.[41,85,86] Angiography is only required in 3% to 5% of cases.[85,86,92,109]

Neurologic complications, predominantly in the sacral plexus, occur in up to 21% of complex pelvic fractures.[41,62] Leg weakness, incontinence, and impotence may result. Sciatic nerve injury was noted in only 4% of

TABLE 4-3. *Complex pelvic fracture complications*[41,55,68,95,97,112]

Complication	Incidence rates (%)
Primary trauma	
Significant hemorrhage (required transfusion)	71 (required transfusion)
Associated fractures	65 (average, 2.2/patient)
Neurologic	21
Genitourinary	19
Head injury	11
Abdominal injury	11
Chest injury	11
Orthopedic complications	
Nonunion	
Malunion	
Leg-length discrepancy	
Instability (symphysis and sacroiliac)	
AVN (femoral head)	
Myositis ossificans	
Implant failure	
Infection	
Deep: internal fixation	
Superficial: pin tracts (external fixators)	

(*text continues on page 235*)

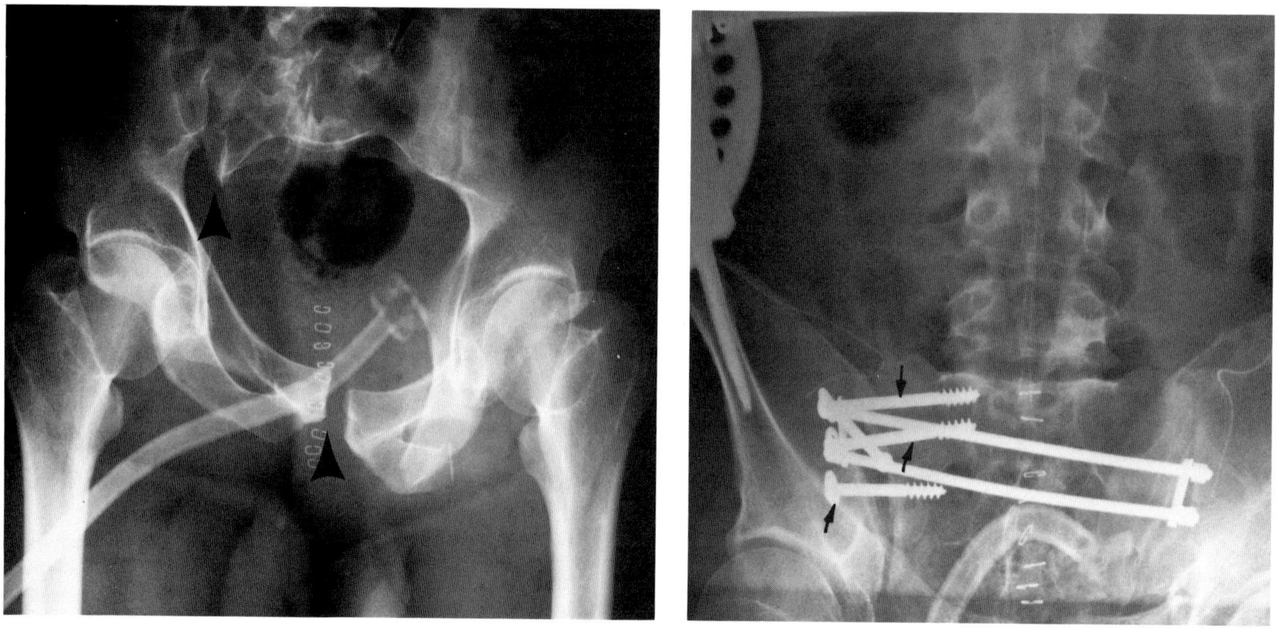

A B

FIG. 4-20. A: Vertical shearing injury seen on the AP view of the pelvis with a step off of the pubic symphysis and right sacroiliac joint (*arrowheads*). Suprapubic tube in place because of bladder and urethral injury. **B:** Anterior stabilization with a transverse bipolar assembly fixator. The sacroiliac joint was repaired using three cancellous screws with washers (*small arrows*), a lag screw, and two transverse iliac compression rods and nuts.

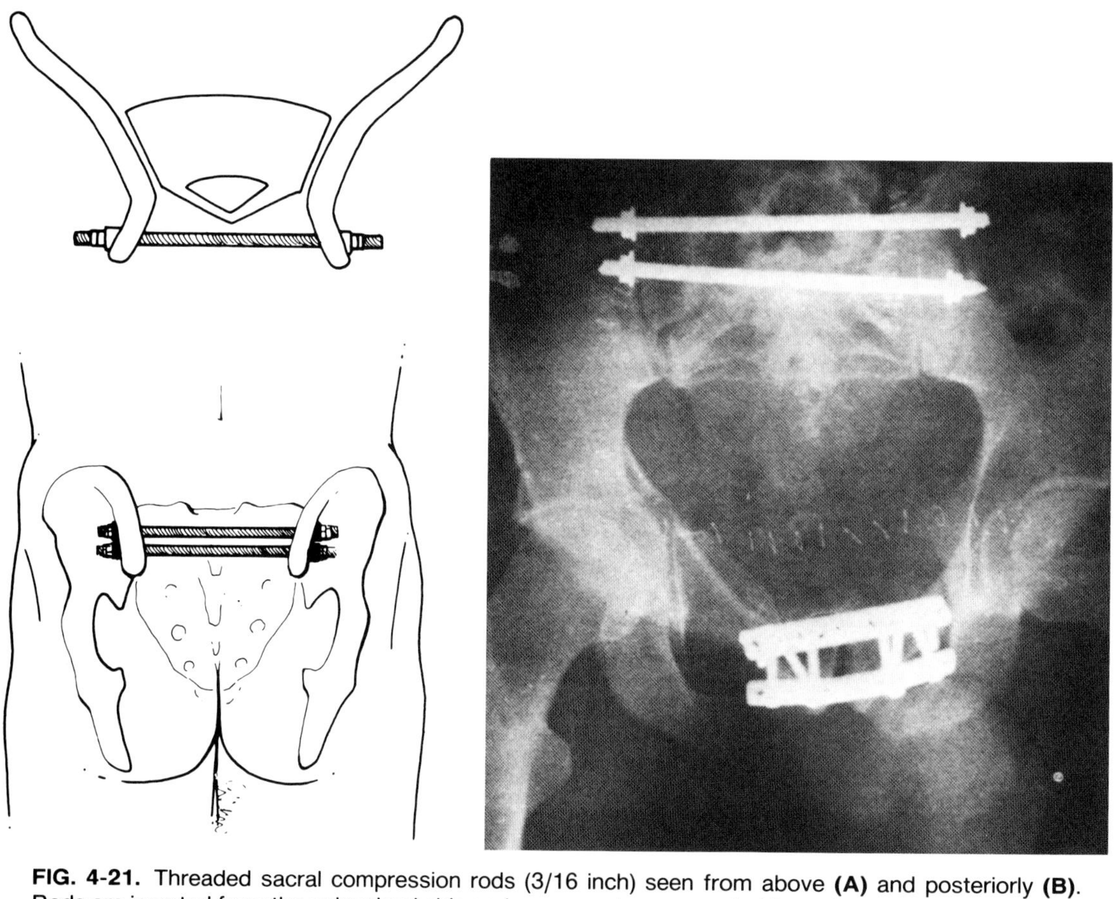

A B C

FIG. 4-21. Threaded sacral compression rods (3/16 inch) seen from above **(A)** and posteriorly **(B)**. Rods are inserted from the uninvolved side and compression secured with washers and nuts. **C:** An AP radiograph after posterior transsacral rod placement with dual anterior plates to reduce a vertical shear injury. (From Dabezies E, Millet CUJ, Murphy CP, Acker JH, Robicheaux RE, d'Ambrosia RD. Stabilization of sacroiliac joint disruption with threaded compression rods. *Clin Orthop* 1989;246:165–171.)

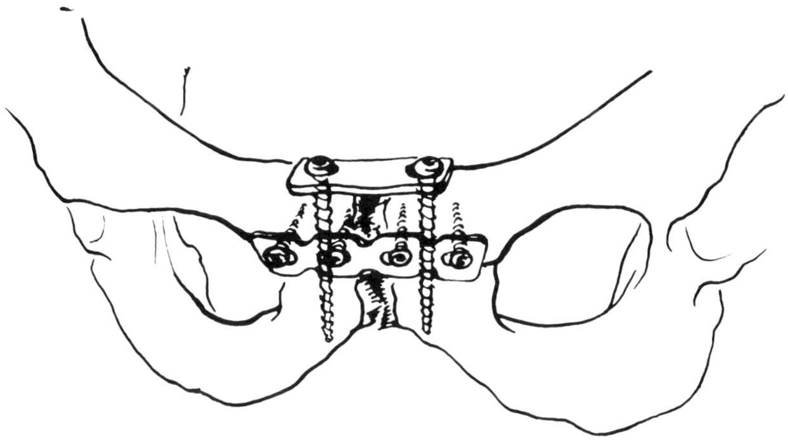

FIG. 4-22. Two-hole plate with screws to fix the pubic symphysis internally. (From Tile M. Pelvic ring fractures. *J Bone Joint Surg [Br]* 1988;70B:1–12.)

A
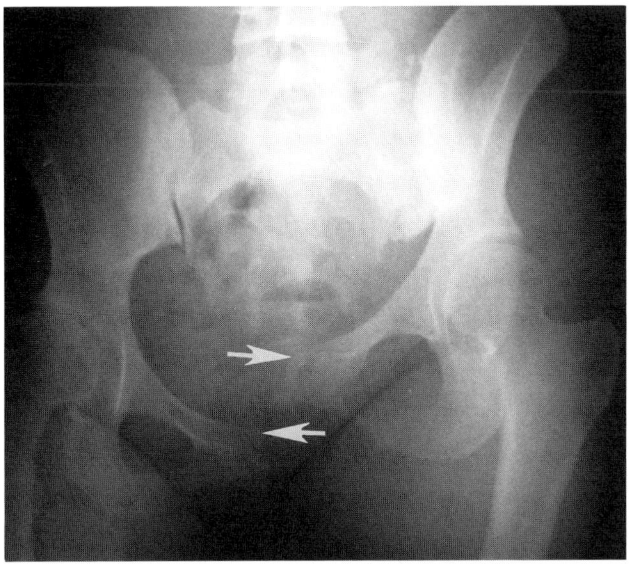

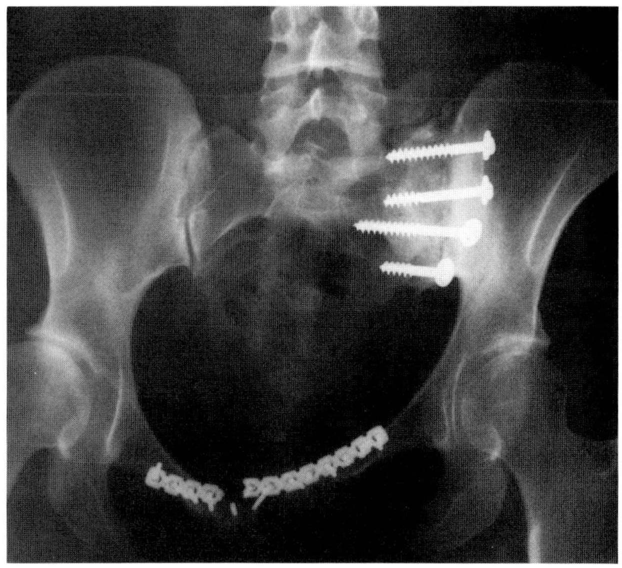
B

C
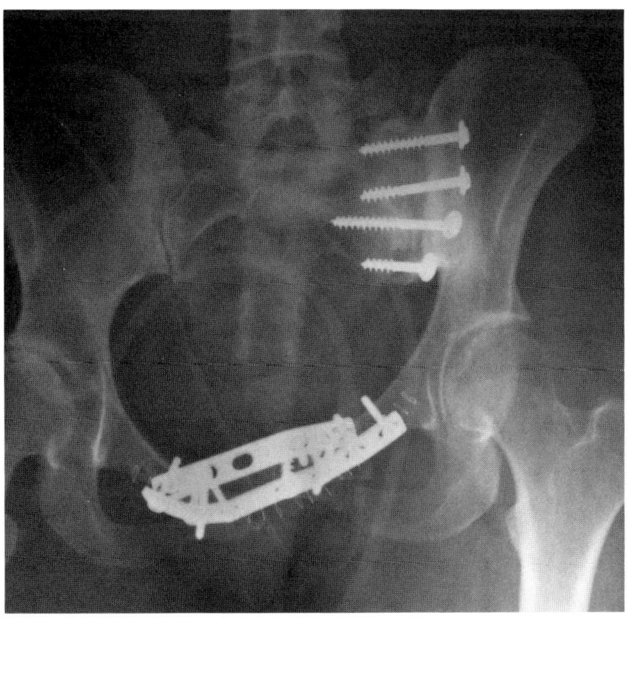

FIG. 4-23. A: The AP view of the pelvis demonstrating a vertical shear injury with marked displacement of the pubic symphysis (*arrows*). **B:** Initial reduction of the sacroiliac joint was achieved with four cancellous screws and washers. A single reconstruction plate and screws were used anteriorly. The plate fractured, and reduction was lost. **C:** The symphysis was reduced and internally fixed using two plates and cortical screws.

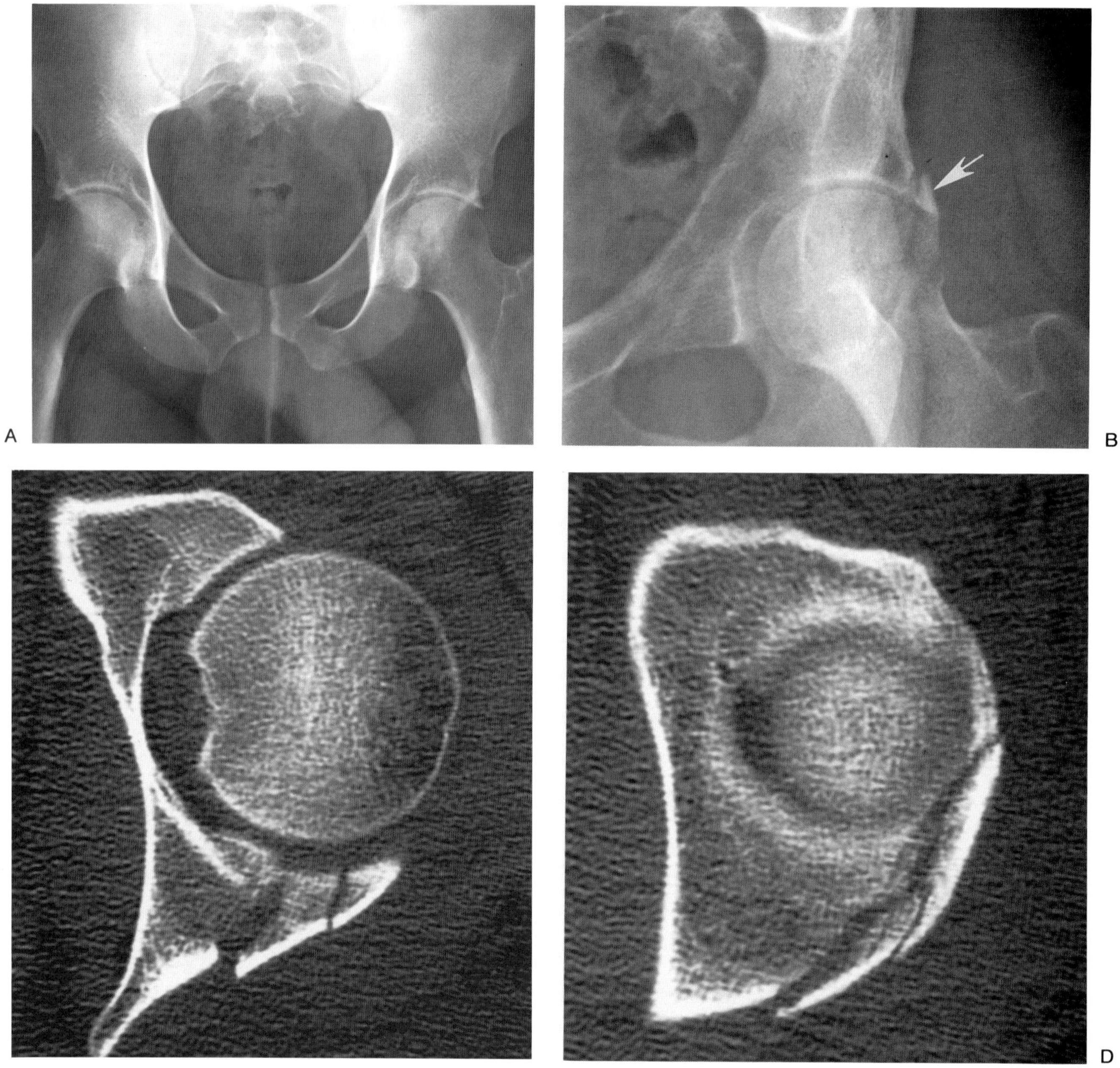

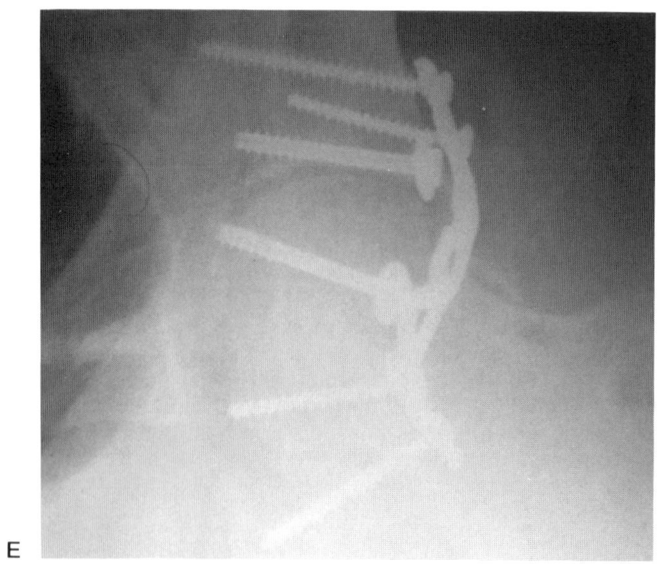

FIG. 4-24. A: The AP view of the pelvis is normal. **B:** Judet view demonstrates a posterior acetabular rim fracture (*arrow*). **C,D:** The CT images demonstrate the posterior of the fragments. **E:** The fracture was reduced using a reconstruction plate and screws with washers.

our patients.[41,42,97] These injuries are more common with acetabular fractures or posterior dislocations (10% to 13%).[61]

Genitourinary injuries are most often associated with straddle fractures or unstable injuries about the symphysis.[41,43,47,51,56,60,98–100] Of the 19% incidence of genitourinary complications in our series, most involved the posterior urethra (50%), followed by the bladder (25%), kidney (15%), and vagina.[41,97] The evaluation of the urethra and bladder should be accomplished with care, and only after hemodynamic stability has been achieved or the need for angiography has been excluded. In the presence of a ruptured urethra or bladder, contrast extravasation can interfere with the interpretation of angiograms until the contrast has been reabsorbed. We prefer to perform a gentle retrograde urethrogram using a Foley catheter and fluoroscopic guidance. The catheter can be slowly advanced; if no defects are identified, it can be safely positioned in the bladder for cystography and fluid monitoring.[41,48,49]

Eleven percent of patients experienced head, chest, or abdominal injuries. In some cases, these injuries required attention before the pelvic injuries.[41,75,92,97]

Complications related to orthopedic management and the devices used may require a radiographic assessment for delineation. Certain complications (Table 4-3) require an evaluation in the acute setting, such as appropriate imaging to confirm proper pin positioning following external fixator application. This may be made difficult by an inability to position the patient properly. In some cases, C-arm fluoroscopy is used to define the problem better; using nonstandard projections may help.[60,95]

Some orthopedic complications occur following the initial treatment. Sitting, weight bearing, and a return to increasing levels of function may make certain problems, such as instability or recurrent deformity, occur or become more obvious (Fig. 4-23). Pain is often associated with these problems. Confirming the site of pain (i.e., sacroiliac or symphysis instability) may require several imaging techniques and diagnostic injection to confirm the problem prior to instituting further therapy.[41]

Late instability can be evaluated with standing alternate weight-bearing spot views. Fluoroscopic imaging is also useful for evaluating motion in suspected nonunions. Even in the presence of metal implants, CT is useful to evaluate bone and soft tissue pathologic conditions (Fig. 4-25). With MRI, AVN is most effectively studied when there is no metal in the femoral head.

Acetabular Fractures

Fractures of the acetabulum have been previously briefly discussed (class IV, Key and Conwell). However, because of the complexity of these injuries further discussion is necessary.

Acetabular fractures comprise 24% of pelvic injuries.[122] Anatomically, the acetabulum is similar to an inverted "Y" with anterior and posterior columns (Fig. 4-26). Fracture patterns may be simple or complex and are generally related to the degree and direction of force produced against the femur or femoral head. The position of the femur at the time of injury dictates the size of the fragments and columns affected (Fig. 4-27).[122,127,133,134]

Classifications

There are numerous acetabular fracture classifications, all of which describe simple (undisplaced, Fig. 4-28) and complex (T type, transverse, and anterior and posterior column combinations) patterns. Complex fractures (Fig. 4-29) may involve both columns and the femoral head or neck. Three commonly used classification schemes are reviewed. The classification of Tile et al.[133,134] is a modification of the AO and other classifications.[130] This classification is based on the direction of force that created the injury, which is useful for surgical planning. This system is summarized in Table 4-4. The AO classification system is based on single column, both columns, or variations of transverse fracture patterns (Table 4-5, Fig. 4-30).[130] Table 4-6 presents the third and

TABLE 4-4. *Acetabular fractures: Tile classification*[110,112]

Undisplaced		
Displaced		
Type I		Posterior fractures with or without associated posterior dislocation
	A	Posterior column
	B	Posterior acetabular rim 1. Associated posterior column 2. Associated transverse fracture
Type II		Anterior column fracture with or without associated anterior dislocation
	A	Anterior column
	B	Anterior acetabular rim
	C	Associated anterior or transverse fracture
Type III		Anterior fracture with or without central dislocation
	A	Transverse fracture
	B	T-type fractures
	C	Associated transverse and acetabular rim fractures
	D	Both columns fractured

(*text continues on page 238*)

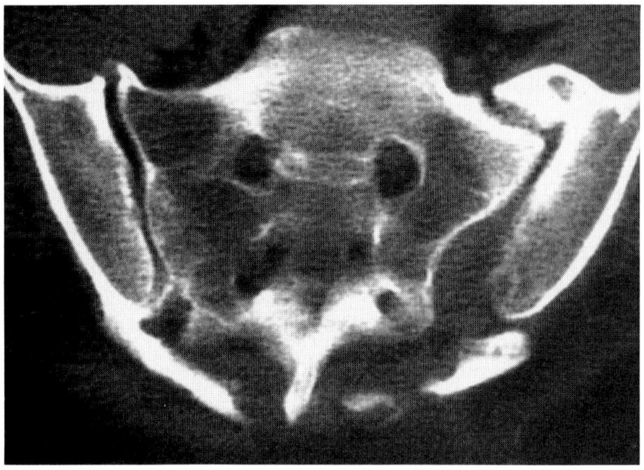

FIG. 4-25. The CT image of the sacrum and sacroiliac joints demonstrating soft tissue ossification after pelvic fracture with posterior ligament disruption.

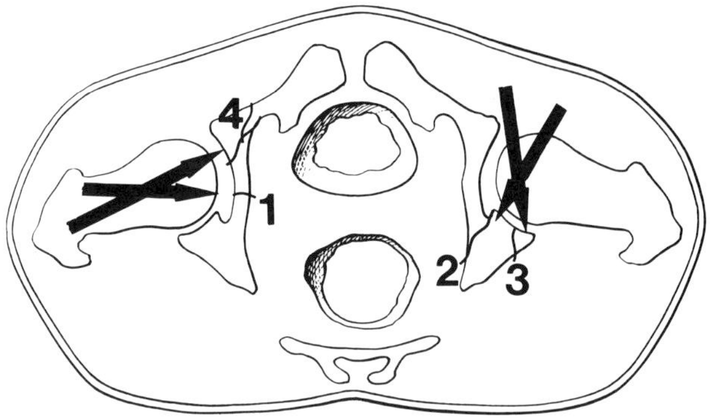

FIG. 4-27. The pelvis and hips demonstrating force direction (→) and fractures (~) of the acetabulum. *1,* Central fracture; *2,* posterior wall and column; *3,* posterior rim; *4,* anterior wall fracture.

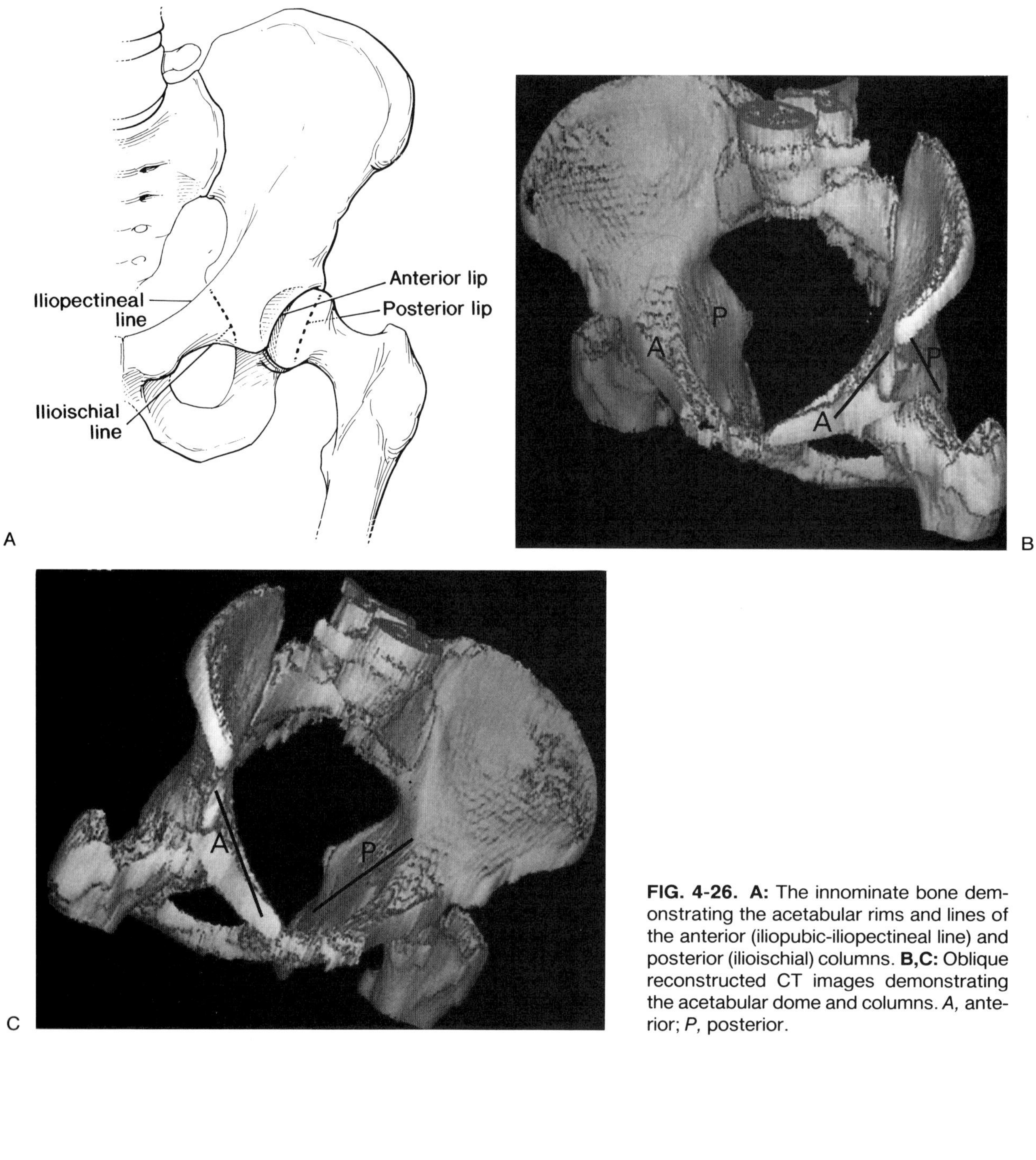

FIG. 4-26. A: The innominate bone demonstrating the acetabular rims and lines of the anterior (iliopubic-iliopectineal line) and posterior (ilioischial) columns. **B,C:** Oblique reconstructed CT images demonstrating the acetabular dome and columns. *A,* anterior; *P,* posterior.

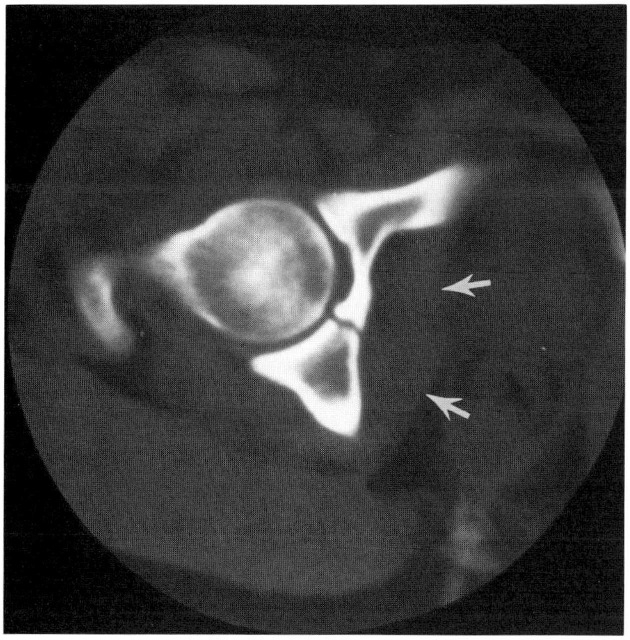

FIG. 4-28. Axial CT image of an undisplaced central acetabular fracture. There is marked swelling of the obstructor internus (*arrows*).

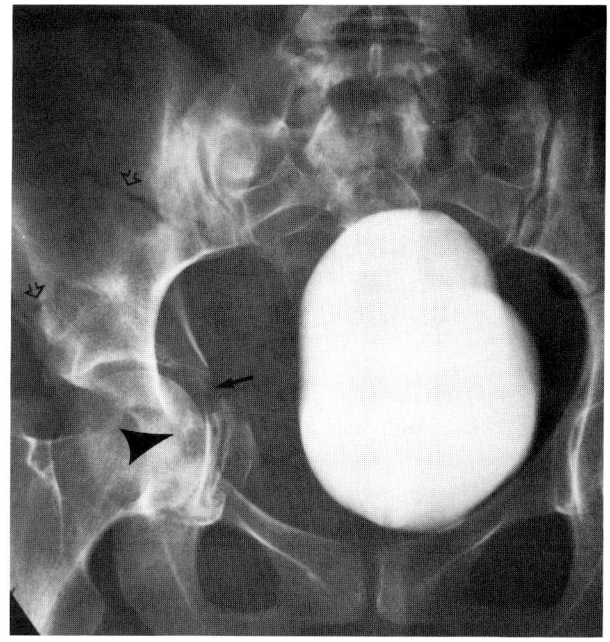

FIG. 4-29. An AP view of the pelvis demonstrating a central dislocation (*small black arrow*) with fractures of the posterior ilium (*open arrows*) and anterior column (*back arrowhead*). The bladder is displaced by hematoma.

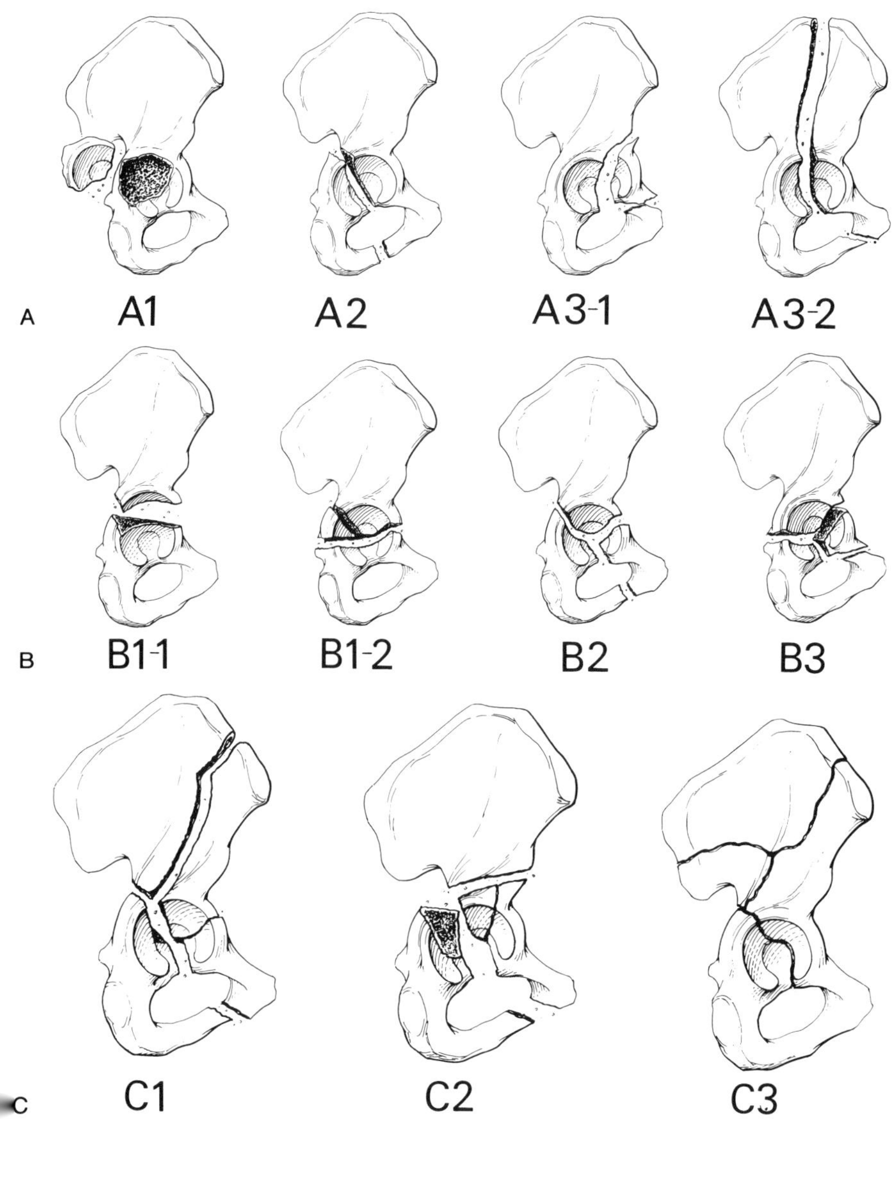

FIG. 4-30. AO fracture patterns. **A:** Type A: A1, posterior wall fracture; A2, posterior column; A3.1, anterior wall; A3-2, anterior column. **B:** Type B: B1-1, transverse; B1-2, transverse with posterior wall fragment; B2, T fracture; B3, anterior column with posterior transverse fracture. **C:** Type C: C1, both columns with fracture extending to iliac crest; C2, anterior column extending to inferior iliac spine; C3, both columns with fracture extending to the sacroiliac joint.

TABLE 4-5. *AO classification of acetabular fractures*[130]

Type A		One column involved
	A1	Posterior wall
	A2	Posterior column
	A3	Anterior wall and/or column
Type B		Transverse
	B1	Transverse with posterior acetabular involvement
	B2	T-type fracture
	B3	Anterior column with posterior involvement (Y-type fracture)
Type C		Both columns fractured and articular segments, including the dome, separated from ilium
	C1	Both columns with the anterior column extending to iliac crest
	C2	Both columns with anterior fracture involving anterior ilium
	C3	Both columns fractured with posterior fracture extending to the sacroiliac joint

most widely used classification scheme for acetabular fractures, as described by Judet et al.[126] in 1964. This system, although detailed and allowing subcategorization of the various complex fracture patterns seen, is rooted in the concept that the acetabulum rests between an anterior column and a posterior column, both of which have walls of the acetabulum associated with them. The naming procedure then is related to how the procedure patterns involve either the AP wall and anterior or posterior columns. It has gained wide acceptance in the orthopedic community because it assists in planning the surgical approach and operative treatment of these challenging problems.[126,127]

Treatment

The goal for treating acetabular fractures is to reestablish the articular anatomy.[124,126,127] Treatment selection is based on the fracture pattern and obviously patient status.[130] Patient weight, age, and activity must be considered. Minimally displaced fractures, even when the roof or dome of the acetabulum is involved, may be treated conservatively if the displacement is not greater than 2 to 5 mm. Anterior-column and transverse fractures may also be treated with closed techniques.[123–135]

Indication for Open Reduction and Internal Fixation
- Unstable posterior fragment (Figs. 4-19 and 4-24)
- Displaced acetabular dome fractures (Fig. 4-31)
- High T fractures
- Displaced two-column fractures
- Retained joint fragments causing joint incongruence
- Femoral head or Garden III or IV neck fractures

Although these are controversial, at least in the past, most authors report good results with open reduction and internal fixation for these indications. Judet et al.[126] reported good results in 90% of their patients treated with internal fixation. Matta[128] and Matta and Merritt[129] also stress the need for open reduction for displaced acetabular fractures.

If we assume there is no femoral neck or femoral shaft fracture, traction may be used initially in patients with an isolated injury, with the definitive procedure done several days later. Interfragmentary screws alone or with washers or cortical screws with 3.5-mm reconstruction plates are often used to reconstruct the fracture fragments (Fig. 4-24).[127,128,133]

Complications associated with displaced acetabular fractures are similar to those described with class III or complex pelvic fractures. There are several complications that are more frequent, including sciatic nerve injury (16% to 33%), superior gluteal nerve injury, and heterotopic ossification (3% to 69%); AVN of the femoral head is reported in 6% of acetabular fractures. Posttraumatic chondrolysis may also occur following acetabular fractures.[121,133]

Routine radiographs and CT are sufficient for revealing most complications[77,78]; MRI is useful for the detection of early AVN or neural injury, depending on the position of metallic implants.[121]

Dislocations and Fracture Dislocations of the Hip

Dislocations of the hip account for only about 5% of articular dislocations.[136,157] Significant and, generally, high-velocity trauma (motor vehicle accidents, motor cycle accidents, and falls from significant heights) is responsible for most dislocations.[139] Because of the severity of trauma, multiple injuries occur in 75% of patients.[153]

Dislocations may be central, anterior, or posterior. "Central dislocations" were discussed previously (class IV pelvic fractures) because they are always associated with displaced acetabular fractures and are better de-

TABLE 4-6. *Classification of acetabular fractures*

Elementary fractures	Associated fractures
Posterior wall	Posterior column + posterior wall
Posterior column	Transverse + posterior wall
Anterior wall	Anterior column + posterior hemitransverse
Anterior column	T-shaped
Transverse	Both column

Classification of acetabular fractures was originally described by Judet et al.[126] in their review of a clinical series of acetabular fractures treated with open reduction and internal fixation. This method of classification has recently been validated by Letournel and Judet's[27] review of 960 fractures, 90% of which were treated surgically, as a useful means of not only understanding fracture anatomy, but also guiding the surgical approach and operative treatment.

scribed as such. Therefore, this section concentrates on anterior and posterior dislocations.

Posterior Dislocations

Posterior dislocations occur seven- to tenfold more frequently than do anterior dislocations.[139,157] The injury occurs with trauma to the knee or foot with the hip in the flexed position.[139] Associated posterior acetabular wall or column fractures are common. The size and location of the fracture fragments depend on the position of the femur at the time of injury. The more the femur is abducted, the larger is the fragment (Figs. 4-32 and 4-33).

Posterior dislocations have been classified by Stewart and Milford,[155] Epstein,[145] and Thompson and Epstein.[158] These systems are based on associated acetabular and femoral fractures and correlate the injuries with the prognosis.[145,154,157] The Thompson-Epstein classification is most often used (Table 4-7).[145,158] Pipkin[150] further classified type V fractures into four subtypes (Table 4-7, Fig. 4-34).[150,152] Femoral head fractures occur with up to 63% of posterior dislocations, usually when the hip is flexed less than 90°.[152,156]

Anterior Dislocations

Anterior dislocations account for 13% to 18% of hip dislocations (Fig. 4-35).[139,140,146,157] The injury occurs with forced abduction and external rotation of the hip.

TABLE 4-7. *Posterior dislocations of the hip: Thompson-Epstein with Pipkin subclassification (V)*[145,146,150,152,157]

Type	Description
I	Posterior dislocation with no or only minor acetabular fracture (Fig. 4-32)
II	Posterior dislocation with a single large acetabular fragment
III	Posterior dislocation with comminution of the acetabular rim
IV	Posterior dislocation with fracture of the acetabular floor
V	Posterior dislocation with fracture of the femoral head (Fig. 4-33)
Pipkin (type V) subclassification	
I	Posterior dislocation with femoral head fracture inferior to fovea (Fig. 4-34A)
II	Posterior dislocation with femoral head fracture cephalad to fovea (Fig. 4-34B)
III	Type I or II with femoral neck fracture (Fig. 4-34C)
IV	Type I, II, or III with acetabular fracture (Fig. 4-34D)

TABLE 4-8. *Anterior hip dislocations: Epstein classification*[146]

Type	Description
I	Superior dislocation with femoral head in pubic or supraspinous position
A	Simple dislocation with no associated fracture
B	Associated fracture of the femoral head and neck
C	Associated acetabular fracture
II	Inferior dislocation with femoral head over the obturator foramen (Fig. 4-35) or perineum
A	No associated fracture
B	Associated fracture of the femoral head or neck
C	Associated acetabular fracture

The Epstein[146] classification is commonly used for anterior dislocations (Table 4-8). Associated fractures of the femoral head occur in 70% to 75% of cases.[140,142] Both shearing osteochondral and impacted fractures of the superior lateral femoral head are common.

Imaging of Hip Dislocations

Routine radiographs (AP and lateral) and Judet views are essential for the evaluation of the acetabulum and femoral head and neck. In most cases, CT is required to evaluate the dislocation completely, but it is usually done following reduction to avoid delay. When there is no obvious fracture on routine prereduction views, CT after reduction may reveal unrecognized subtle injuries, which were initially overlooked.[147–149,151] This is especially important in patients with joint incongruency after reduction (Figs. 4-36 and 4-37).

Treatment

As soon as possible, dislocations with no associated fracture should be reduced using closed techniques. The incidence of AVN is high if reduction is not obtained within 12 hours. Crutches can be used until the pain subsides and soft tissue healing has occurred.[139,144]

When there are associated fractures, the treatment varies with the type (femur, femoral head, femoral neck, or acetabulum) and degree of injury. Open reduction and internal fixation is indicated if more than one third of the femoral head is fractured, or if there are any significantly displaced fragments involving the weight-bearing surface or preventing joint congruence. Large fragments can be repositioned and held with one or more screws.[139,144,152]

Small posterior acetabular fragments may, at times, be ignored. Larger posterior wall fragments must be reduced to prevent joint subluxation. Internal fixation with screws or reconstruction plate-screw techniques are generally used.[139,148,149] Displaced acetabular fractures

(*text continues on page 242*)

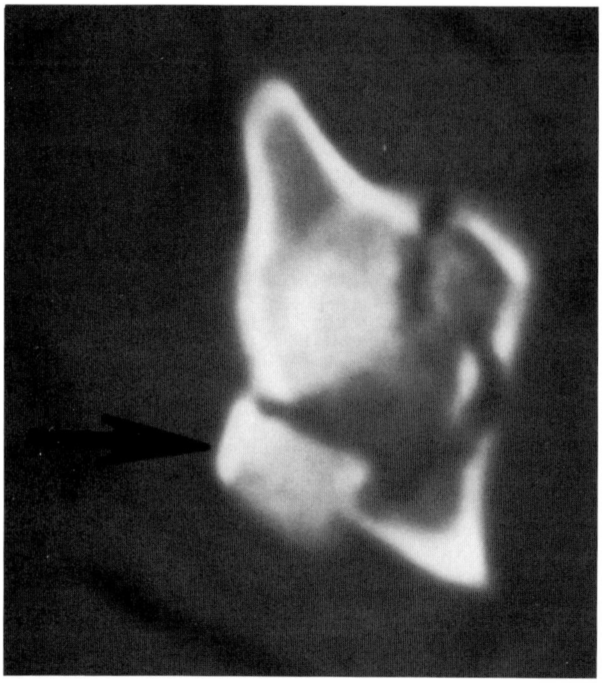

FIG. 4-31. Axial CT image demonstrating fragmentation of the acetabular dome with displaced rotated lateral fragment (*arrow*).

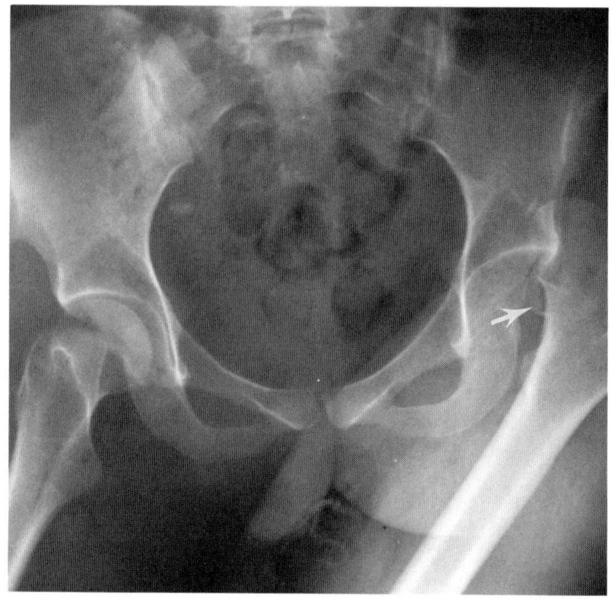

FIG. 4-32. The AP views of the pelvis demonstrating a Thompson-Epstein type I posterior dislocation with a small rim fragment (*arrow*).

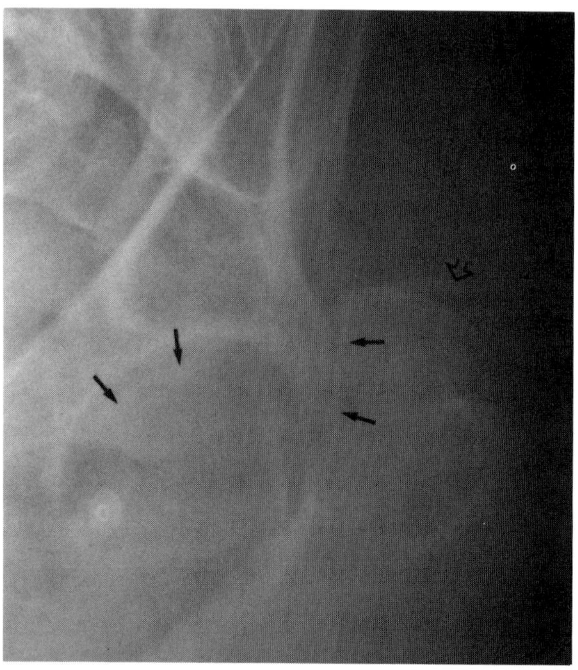

FIG. 4-33. Anterior Judet view demonstrating a posterior dislocation with a large femoral head fragment (*black arrows*) remaining in the joint. There is also a small osteochondral fracture (*open arrow*).

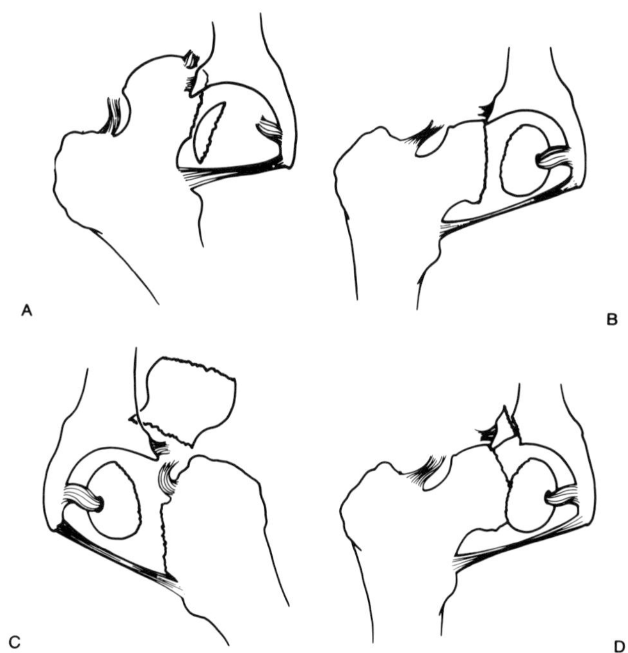

FIG. 4-34. Pipkin classification of posterior dislocation with femoral head fractures.[150,152] **A:** Type I: fracture caudad to fovea. **B:** Type II: fracture cephalad to fovea. **C:** Type III: type I or II with femoral neck fracture. **D:** Type IV: type I, II, or III with associated acetabular fracture. (From Roeder LF, DeLee JC. Femoral head fractures associated with posterior hip dislocation. *Clin Orthop* 1980;147:121–130.)

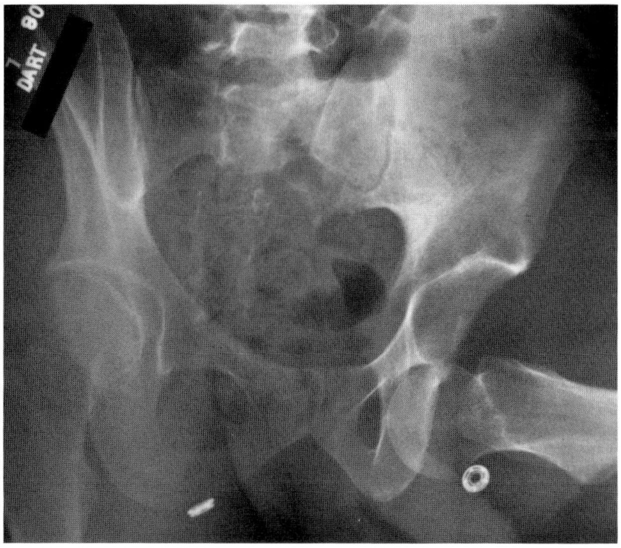

FIG. 4-35. Oblique view of the pelvis demonstrating an anterior dislocation on the left.

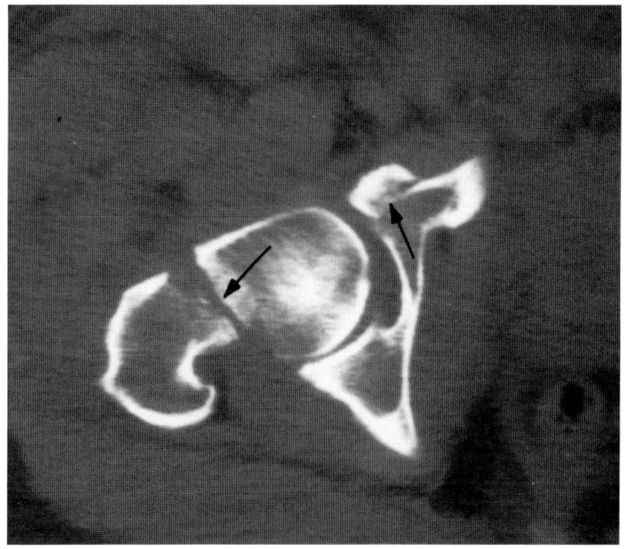

FIG. 4-37. The CT image after reduction of an anterior dislocation showing associated acetabular and femoral neck fractures (*arrows*).

A 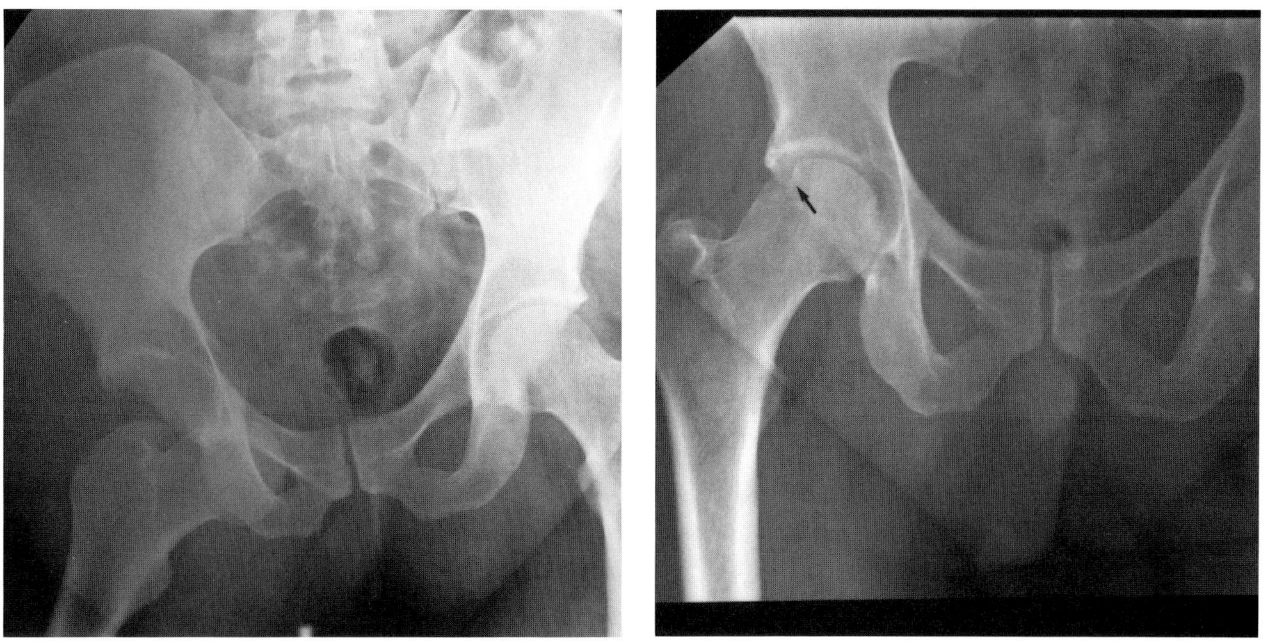 B

FIG. 4-36. **A:** An AP view of the pelvis demonstrating an anterior dislocation. **B:** Postreduction AP radiograph shows an impacted osteochondral fracture (*arrow*), the superolateral femoral head.

involving the posterior column also need to be reduced as anatomically as possible.[139]

Treatment of associated femoral neck fractures is a more complicated problem. Any acetabular fragments should be reduced with internal fixation. The femoral neck fracture can be pinned, depending on the clinical situation (e.g., the patient's age and joint status preinjury) and whether the fracture's configuration does not present an unduly increased risk for AVN (see Femoral Neck Fractures). In some cases of older patients and/or marked displacement, an endoprothesis should be used for the initial treatment to restore function and avoid AVN and/or nonunion.[139,147]

Complications

The complications associated with fracture-dislocation of the hip are summarized in Table 4-9. Regardless of the type of dislocation, early reduction is important. The incidence of AVN of the femoral head is 5% to 26%, but if the dislocation is not reduced within 48 hours, the results are uniformly poor. The incidence of AVN is slightly lower (8%) with anterior dislocation;[137,138,139,152] MRI is the most sensitive and specific technique for the detection of femoral head necrosis. Image degradation can be significant when there are metal implants in or adjacent to the femoral head. In this setting, radionuclide scans or even conventional tomography could be considered.

Sciatic nerve injury occurs in 10% to 17% of posterior dislocations.[139,140] Prompt reduction is indicated when sciatic nerve injury is suspected.[144,146]

Associated fractures are usually easily identified on routine radiographs. Associated femoral shaft fractures present a unique problem because they may mask the dislocation. Rosenthal and Coker[153] reported ipsilateral femoral and patellar fractures in 4% of their patients.

Osteoarthritis is a common complication, which may not be manifested for years after the injury.[146,152] Epstein[146] reported posttraumatic arthritis in 23% of patients. The incidence is even higher (35%) in patients treated with closed reduction. This complication is more common with associated acetabular fractures and in heavy active patients.[152,159]

Less common complications (Table 4-9) include myositis ossificans and redislocation.[149,152,153] Thrombophlebitis and pulmonary embolus may occur during the initial hospitalization phase of treatment.[141,153]

TABLE 4-9. *Fracture-dislocation of the hip complications*[139,140,143,152]

Common complications
Osteoarthritis
Associated fractures
AVN of the femoral head
Sciatic nerve injury
Uncommon complications
Infection
Myositis ossificans
Redislocation
Thrombophlebitis
Pulmonary embolus

Femoral Neck Fractures

Femoral neck fractures occur most commonly in elderly patients. They are more common in women than in men.[169,171] The bone mineral content is frequently diminished so that spontaneous fatigue fractures and low-energy trauma, such as falls from a standing height, are responsible for most injuries.[169,180] Hypotheses to explain femoral neck fractures include (1) direct trauma; (2) microfractures, which become complete with minor trauma; and (3) fractures resulting from rotational forces during a fall.[176]

Classification

Femoral neck fractures may be subcapital (most common), transcervical, or basicervical (Fig. 4-38). The fractures may be complete or incomplete. Stress fractures and insufficiency fractures are common in young athletes and elderly patients, respectively (Fig. 4-39).[169,176,180]

There are several orthopedic classification systems for femoral neck fractures. The Pauwel[186] classification is based on the angle of the fracture. This measurement is most easily assessed on the AP radiograph by using the distal fracture fragment because the femoral head may shift after the fracture.[169] Using this classification, type I fractures form an angle of 30° or less (Fig. 4-40A) with the horizontal. Type II fractures (Fig. 4-40B) have an angle of 30° to 70°, and type III fractures have a more vertical plane, with angles greater than 70° (Fig. 4-40C).[186] The more vertical the fracture is, the more likely it is to be unstable. More horizontal fractures tend to undergo impaction, which improves stability and facilitates healing.

The Garden[174,175] classification is based on the degree of displacement on prereduction radiographs (Table 4-10).[172] Stage I fractures are incomplete, involving the lateral cortex (abduction-impaction) with intact medial trabeculae (Fig. 4-41A). Stage II fractures are complete (both cortices involved), but there is no displacement (Fig. 4-41B). Stage III fractures are partially displaced (Fig. 4-41C), and stage IV fractures are completely displaced (Table 4-9).[172,174,175]

Because of observer error in properly classifying these injuries, some authors would prefer to group stages I and II (undisplaced) and stages III and IV (displaced)

(text continues on page 245)

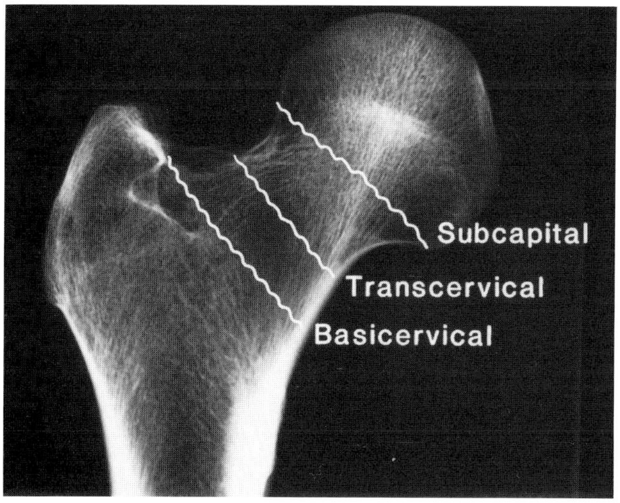

FIG. 4-38. Skeletal specimen demonstrating the levels of femoral neck fractures. (From Berquist TH. Imaging of orthopedic trauma. 2nd ed. New York: Raven Press, 1992.)

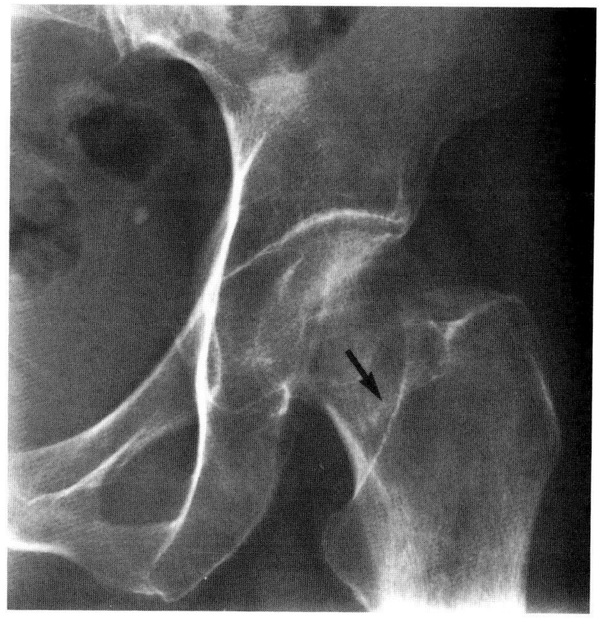

FIG. 4-39. An AP view of the hip in an elderly patient with bony condensation (*arrow*) caused by an insufficiency fracture.

A

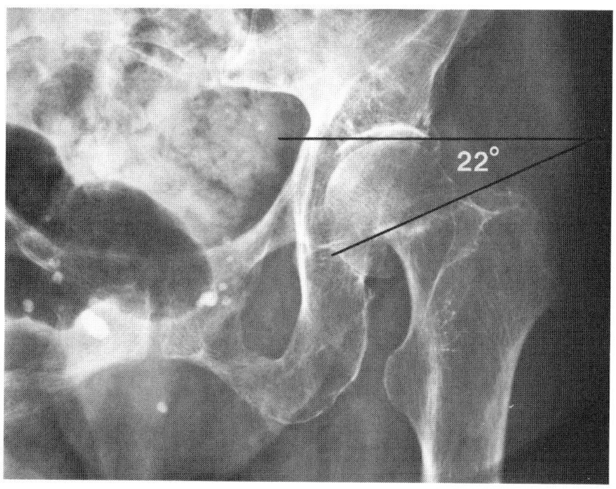

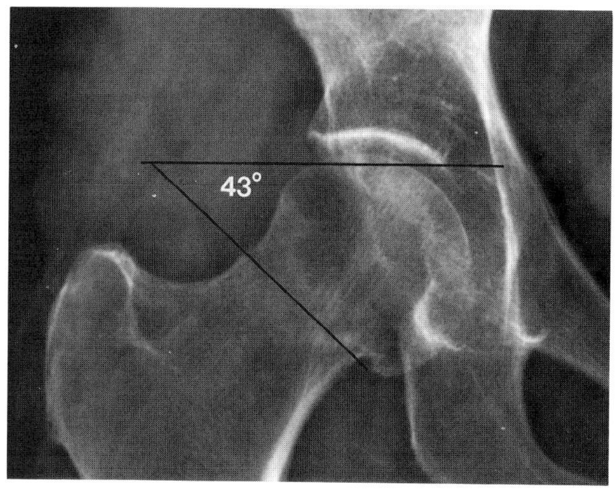

B

C

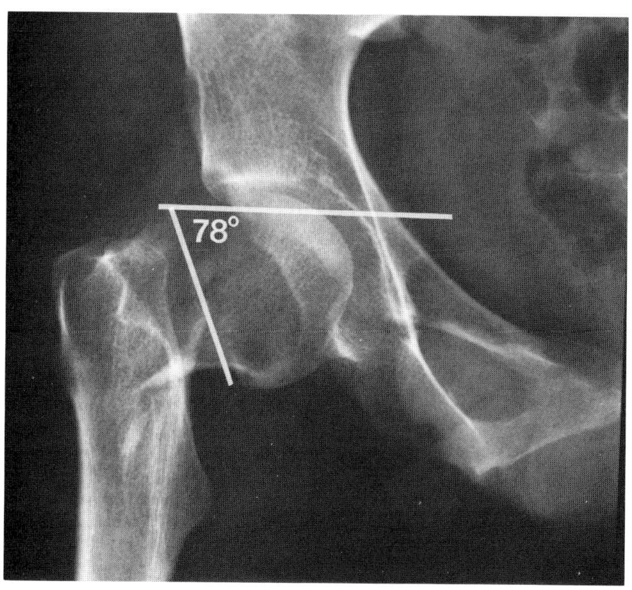

FIG. 4-40. Femoral neck fractures. Pauwel classification. **A:** The AP radiograph of the left hip demonstrating a Pauwel type I fracture (< 30°), which measures 22°. **B:** The AP radiograph of the right hip demonstrating a Pauwel type II fracture (30° to 70°) measuring 43° with the horizontal. **C:** The AP radiograph of the right hip demonstrating a Pauwel type III fracture (measuring 78°).

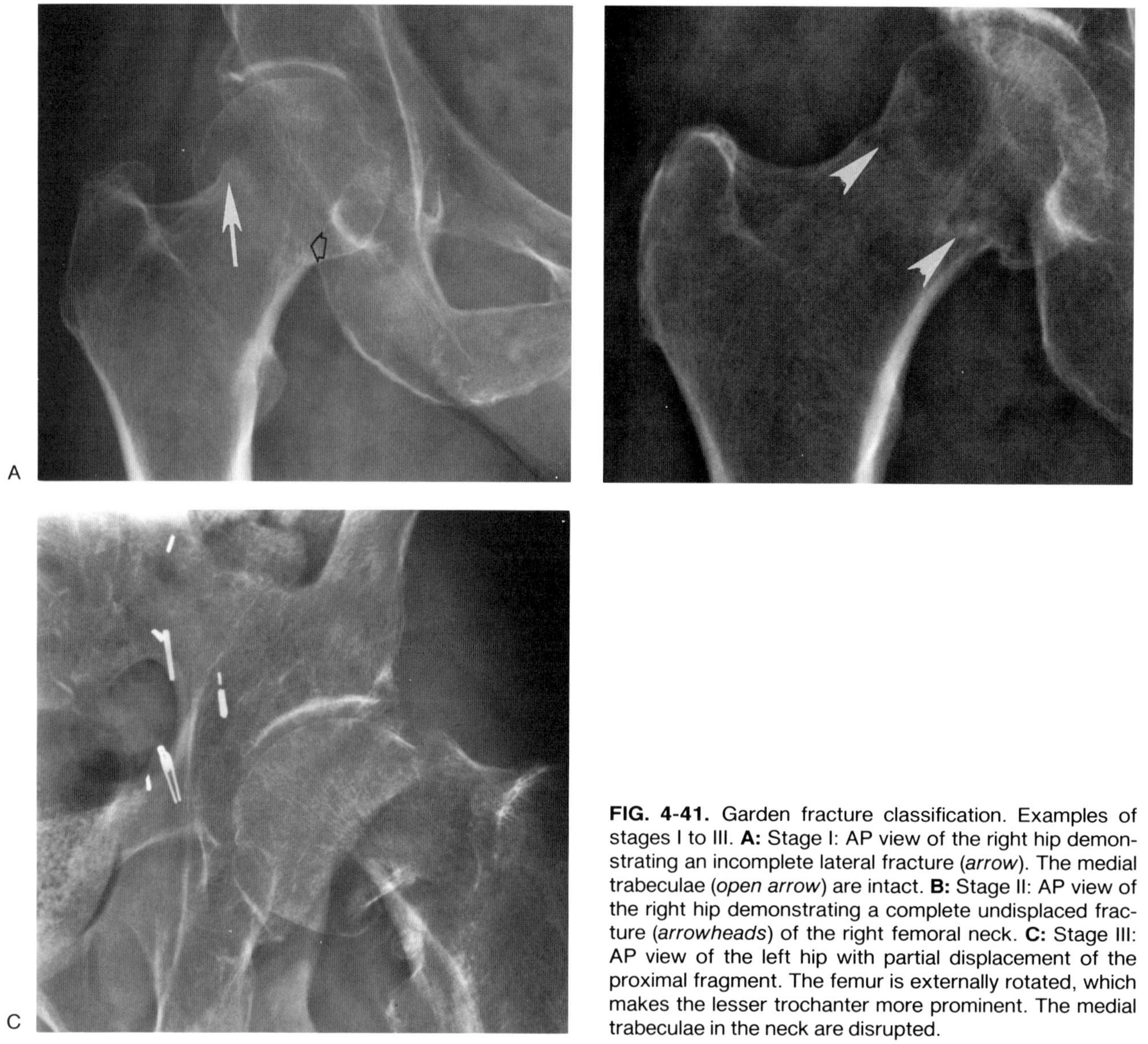

FIG. 4-41. Garden fracture classification. Examples of stages I to III. **A:** Stage I: AP view of the right hip demonstrating an incomplete lateral fracture (*arrow*). The medial trabeculae (*open arrow*) are intact. **B:** Stage II: AP view of the right hip demonstrating a complete undisplaced fracture (*arrowheads*) of the right femoral neck. **C:** Stage III: AP view of the left hip with partial displacement of the proximal fragment. The femur is externally rotated, which makes the lesser trochanter more prominent. The medial trabeculae in the neck are disrupted.

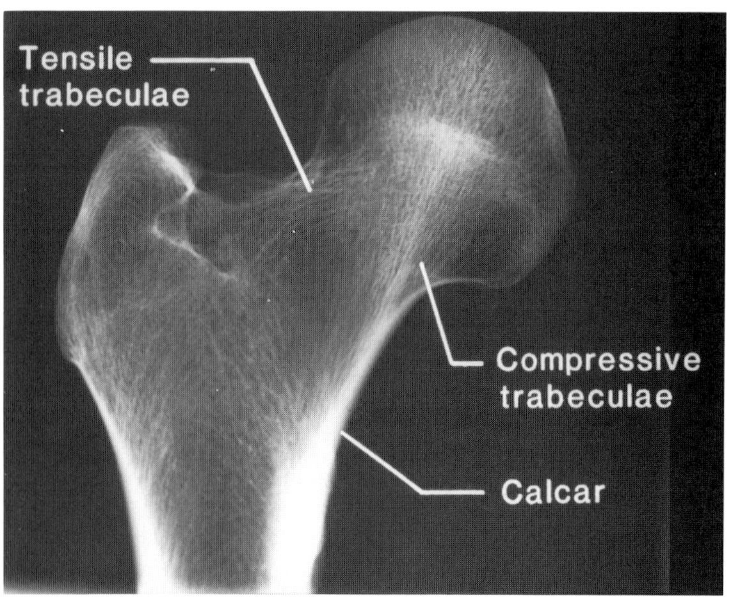

FIG. 4-42. Specimen radiograph of the upper femur demonstrating the trabeculae pattern of the femoral neck (From Berquist TH. Imaging of orthopedic trauma. 2nd ed. New York: Raven Press, 1992.)

TABLE 4-10. *Femoral neck fractures: Garden classification*[169,172,174,175]

Stage	Description
I	Incomplete or impacted fracture with no displacement of the medial trabeculae (Fig. 4-41A).
II	Complete fracture without displacement (Fig. 4-41B).
III	Complete fracture with partial displacement and varus angulation of the femoral head, shortening, and external rotation of the femur (Fig. 4-41C).
IV	Complete fracture with total displacement. The femoral head trabeculae align with the acetabulum.

together because the treatment options are similar for stages I and II and for stages III and IV injuries.[169,172,185,192]

Imaging

Preoperative imaging with AP and lateral radiographs is sufficient to make the diagnosis in most patients. Careful attention to the trabecular pattern on the AP view (Fig. 4-42) and cortical contact on the lateral view (Fig. 4-43) is important for classification and treatment planning.[169,191] Subtle stress fractures or insufficiency fractures may require radionuclide imaging for early detection. Equally effective, MRI is, however, more costly.[169,188]

Treatment

The treatment of femoral neck fractures depends on the stability of the injury, the patient's status (i.e., age, activity, weight, and general health factors), and the patient's compliance.[163,165,166,169,172,185,197] Stable fractures include incomplete stress fractures, fatigue fractures, and Garden stage I (abduction with impaction) injuries.[172] Garden stage II fractures are undisplaced but not impacted; therefore, they tend to become unstable.[172,181] Garden stage III and IV fractures are unstable and have a higher incidence of AVN. Comminution of the posterior femoral neck is even more difficult to manage.[172,187]

Stages I and II

The treatment of impacted (Garden stage I) or stress fractures is controversial. If the patient can walk without pain or raise the involved leg without assistance in the supine position, especially within 2 days of the injury, up to 80% of patients may heal without intervention.[169,177] Patient compliance is important. Therefore, some authors prefer to pin stage I and, certainly, stage II fractures. The latter is less controversial because displacement is more likely.[162,169,172,177,182]

Fixation can be accomplished using Hagie, Knowles, or Moore pins or cannulated hip screws (Figs. 4-44 to 4-46).[182,189,194,195]

Dynamic hip screws (Fig. 4-47) or sliding nails can also be used. However, when fractures are impacted or stable, they may disimpact with placement of this device.[172,178] Some prefer a dynamic hip screw with a Knowles pin for stage II fractures to reduce the chances of fragment rotation.[172]

Stages III and IV

Treatment options for stages III and IV unstable injuries include reduction and internal fixation, hemiarthroplasty, and total hip replacement.[169,172,181,197] Simple pin fixation techniques are generally inadequate, with nonunion reported in up to 14% of cases.[192] The incidence of AVN is also higher with stages III and IV fractures (34.5%) compared with that in undisplaced fractures (5.9%). This leads to a consideration of hemiarthroplasty as initial treatment by some authors.[172,181,192,197] However, all agree that a well-reduced united femoral head is preferable to a prosthesis. This is not easily achieved in stage IV or comminuted osteopenic femurs.[169] Lu-Yao et al.,[181] reported nonunion in 33% and AVN in 16% of patients treated with internal fixation followed for ≤ 2 years. Therefore, in older patients (> 70 years old), debilitated patients, and those with fracture dislocation (Fig. 4-48), hemiarthroplasty is preferred.[172,190,193,196,197] The indications for endoprothesis summarized by DeLee[172] are listed in Table 4-11. Figures 4-49 through 4-51 demonstrate examples of unipolar and bipolar prostheses.

Complications

The complications of femoral neck fractures depend on whether they are intra- or extracapsular, whether they are comminuted, their stability, and whether the circulation to the femoral head is impaired. Mortality rates in elderly patients may exceed 20% during the first year after fracture.[196] The most significant and common complications are AVN of the femoral head

TABLE 4-11. *Femoral neck fractures: indications for hemiarthroplasty*[172]

Displaced fracture in patients > 75 years
Debilitated patients
Pathologic fractures
Fractures with dislocation of the femoral head (Fig. 4-48)
Failed internal fixation
Poor patient compliance

(*text continues on page 250*)

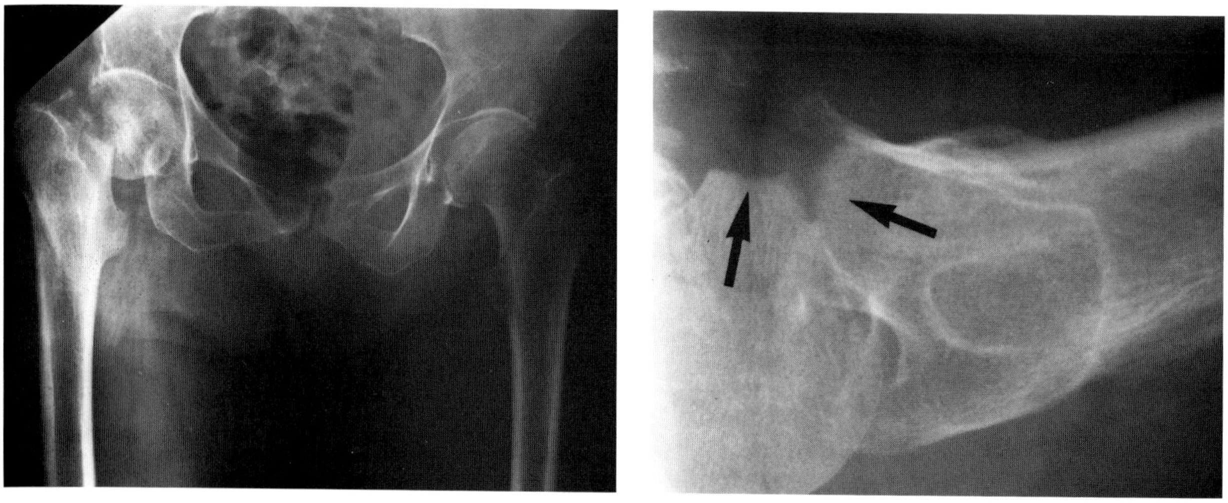

A B

FIG. 4-43. The AP **(A)** and lateral **(B)** radiographs of a Garden stage III fracture. There is no anterior cortical contact. *Arrows* define the degree of rotation of the femoral head on the lateral view (B).

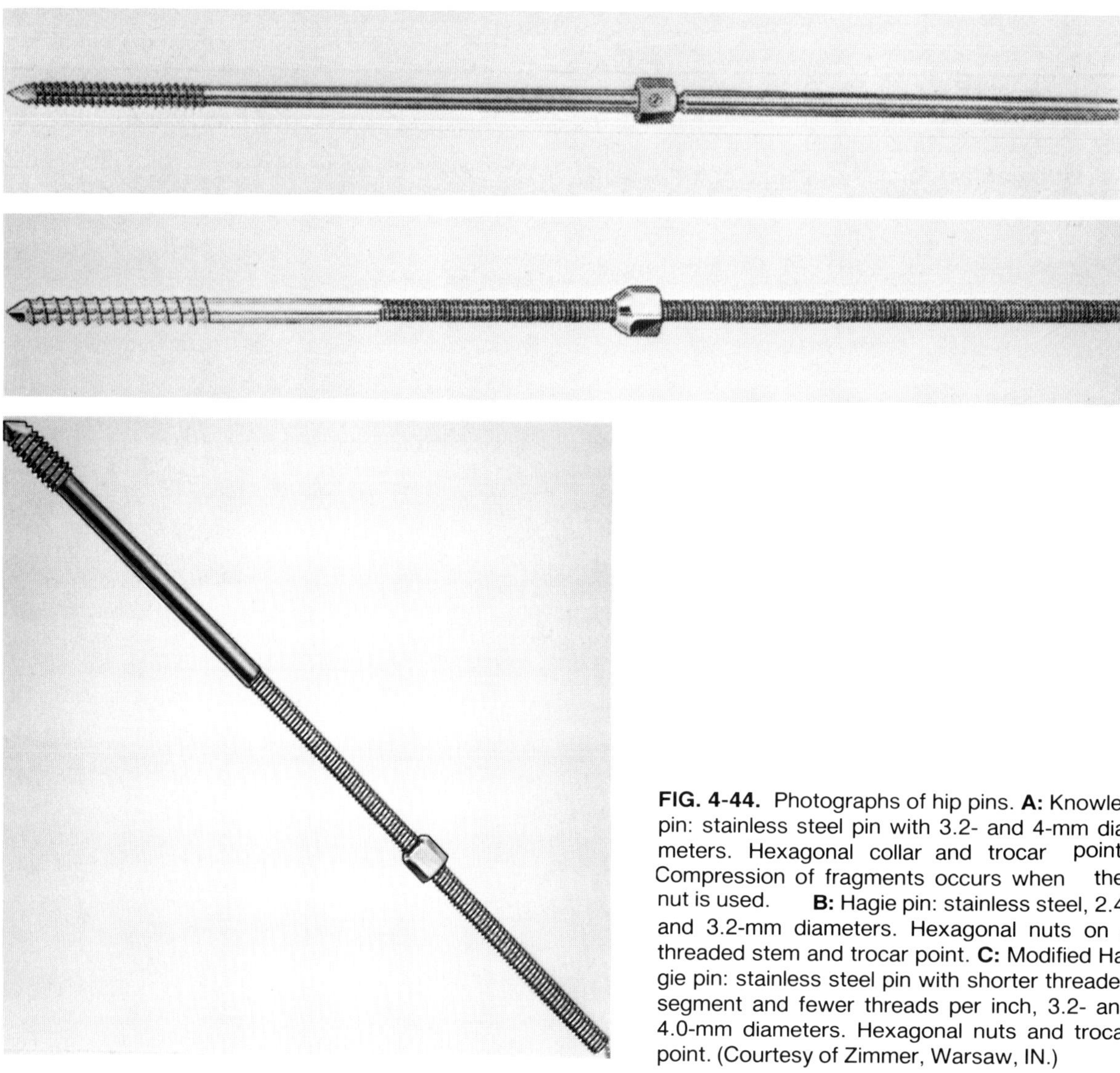

A B C

FIG. 4-44. Photographs of hip pins. **A:** Knowles pin: stainless steel pin with 3.2- and 4-mm diameters. Hexagonal collar and trocar point. Compression of fragments occurs when the nut is used. **B:** Hagie pin: stainless steel, 2.4- and 3.2-mm diameters. Hexagonal nuts on a threaded stem and trocar point. **C:** Modified Hagie pin: stainless steel pin with shorter threaded segment and fewer threads per inch, 3.2- and 4.0-mm diameters. Hexagonal nuts and trocar point. (Courtesy of Zimmer, Warsaw, IN.)

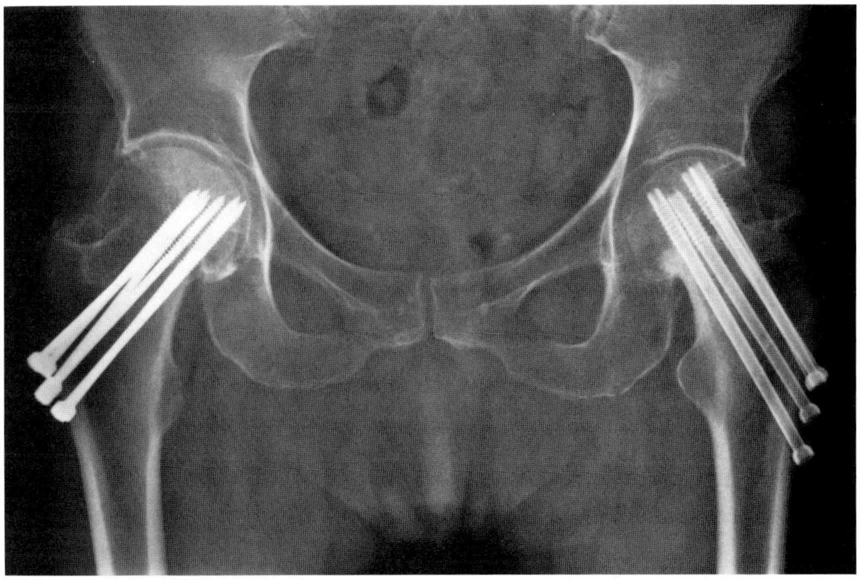

FIG. 4-45. The AP views of the pelvis with bilateral Garden stage II fractures. The fracture on the right is internally fixed with five Knowles pins and the fracture on the left, with four cannulated Ace screws.

A 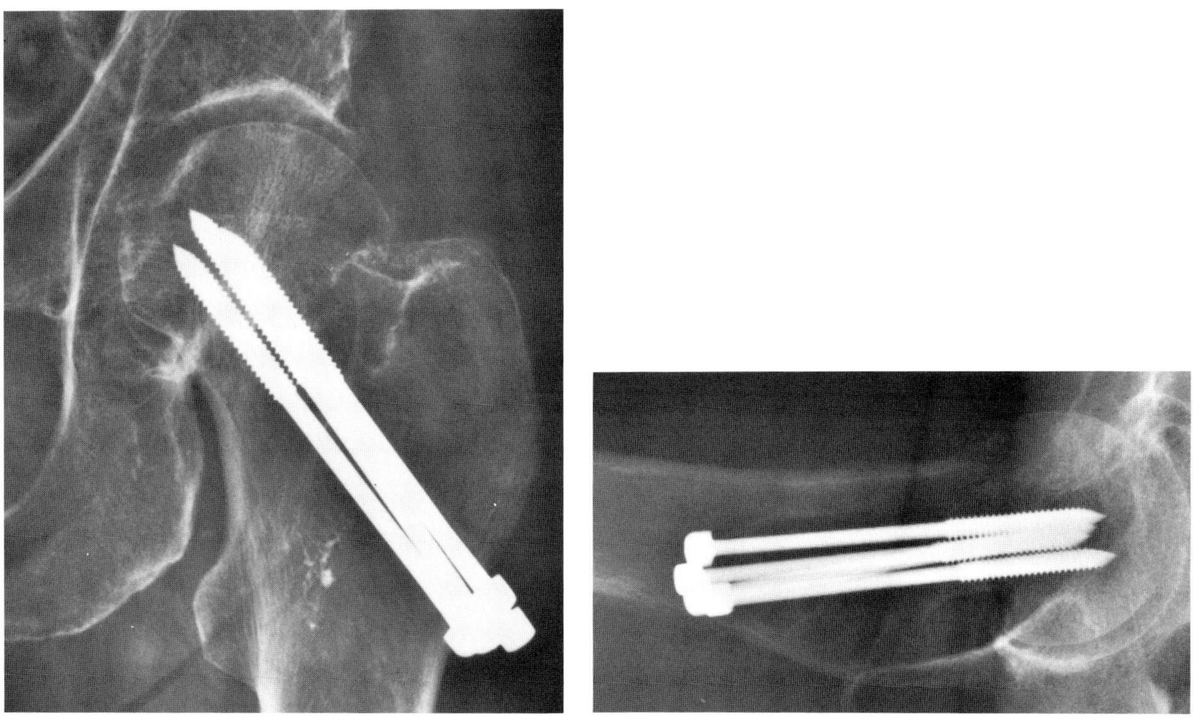 B

FIG. 4-46. The AP **(A)** and lateral **(B)** radiographs demonstrating an impacted femoral neck fracture internally fixed with four Knowles pins.

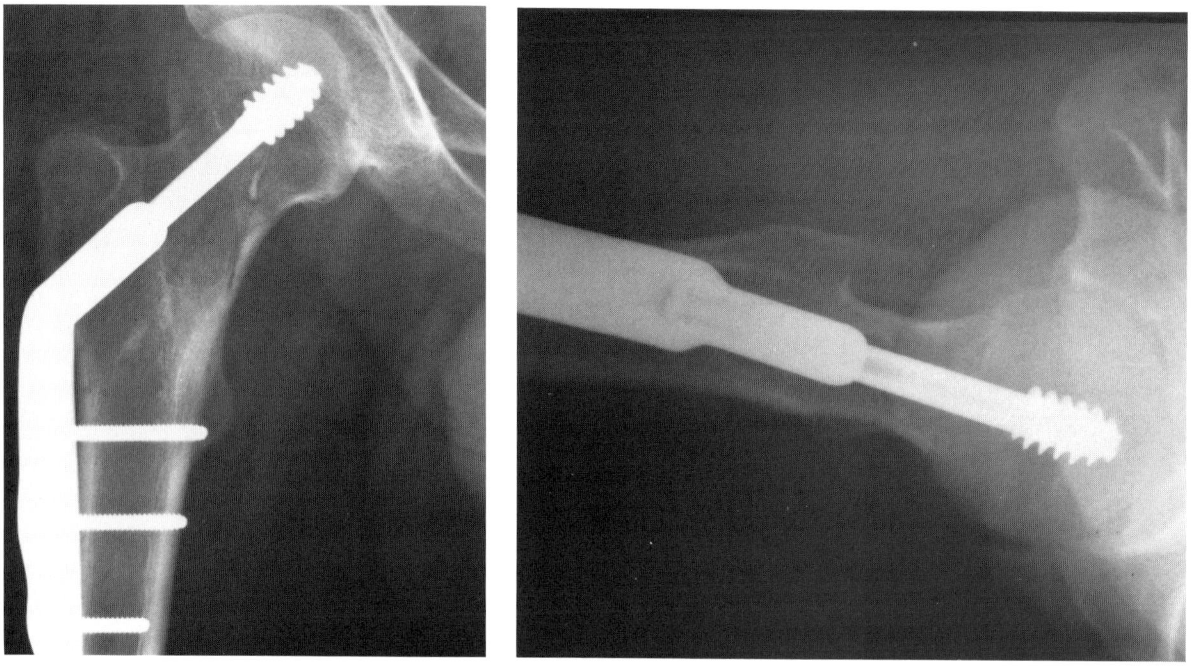

A B

FIG. 4-47. The AP **(A)** and lateral **(B)** radiographs of a comminuted right femoral neck fracture internally fixed with a cannulated dynamic hip screw and four-hole side plate (see Chapter 2).

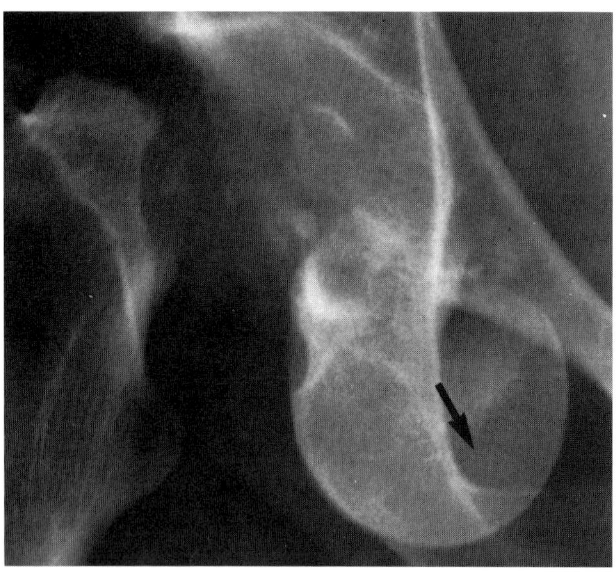

FIG. 4-48. The AP radiograph of the hip with femoral neck fracture and anterior dislocation of the femoral head (*arrow*).

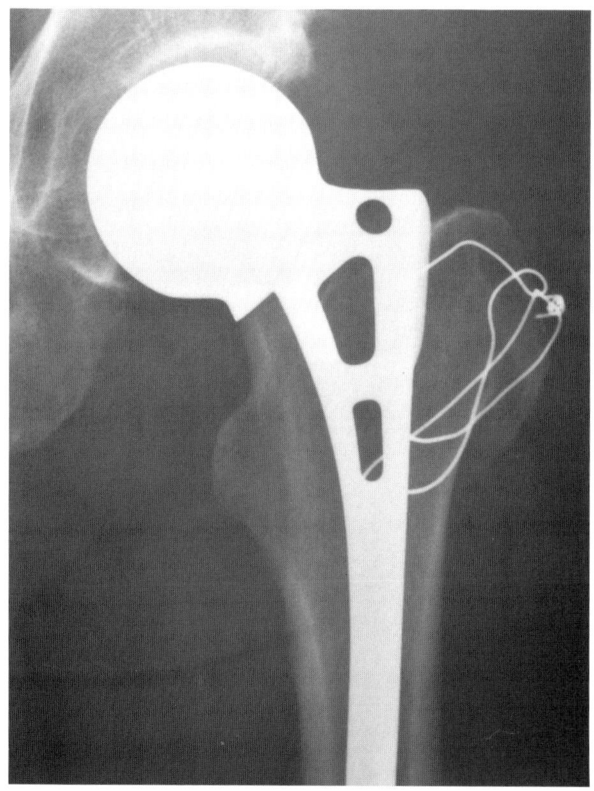

FIG. 4-49. An AP radiograph of the left hip with an Austin-Moore endoprostheses and wiring of the greater tuberosity for treatment of a Garden III femoral neck fracture.

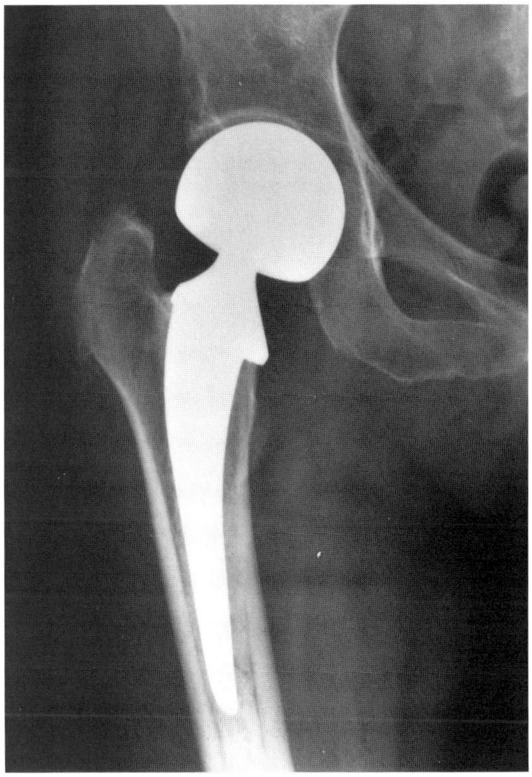

FIG. 4-50. Bateman bipolar endoprosthesis with cemented femoral component for treatment of a Garden IV femoral neck fracture.

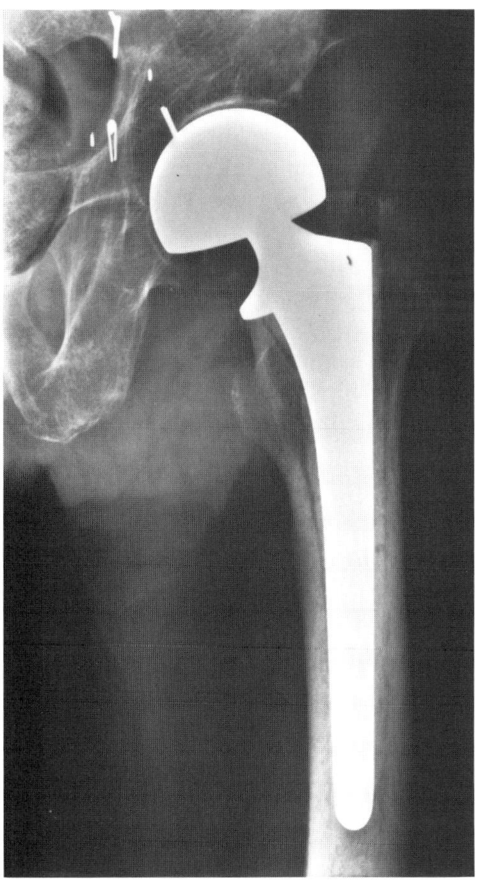

A

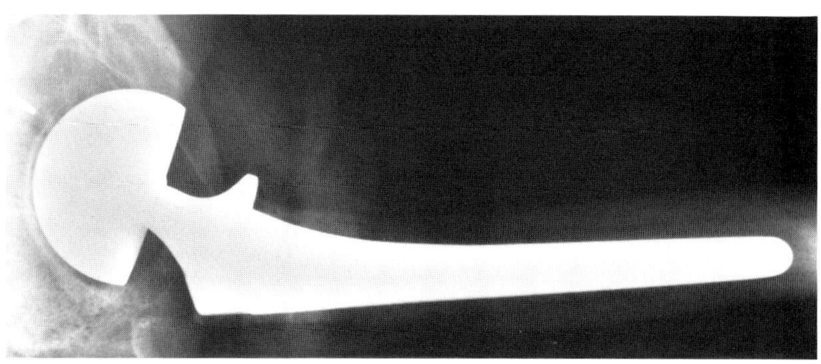

B

FIG. 4-51. The AP **(A)** and lateral **(B)** radiographs of an Osteonics OCD bipolar component system for a stage III femoral neck fracture (Osteonics, Allendale, NJ.)

and nonunion.[160,168,170,179] Other complications include malunion, infection, deep venous thrombosis, and pulmonary emboli.[169,172]

With Garden stages III and IV fractures, AVN is the most common. The incidence is slightly higher in female than in male patients.[160] The blood supply to the femoral head can be significantly diminished, especially with displaced and rotated fractures. The foveal artery only provides sufficient vascular supply in about 4% of patients (Fig. 4-52).[163] After fracture, AVN may become clinically apparent as early as 3 to 5 months or as late as 17 years.[172]

Radiographic evaluation is useful, especially in the presence of metal fixation devices. Although MRI is usually preferred, a metal artifact can degrade the image quality, making the diagnosis difficult.[167,169,183] Ficat and Arlet[173] defined the radiographic stages of AVN. Initially, the radiographs are normal (stage I). Over 3 to 36 months (average, 10 months), areas of increased density develop (stage II). Structural collapse or the crescent sign can be identified in stage III, which can be seen between 5 and 24 months. Stage IV is more easily detected because of articular collapse and joint space narrowing or secondary osteoarthritis (Fig. 4-53).[169,173,184] Radionuclide scintigraphy is still a useful technique. Metal implants cause photopenic areas, which must be taken into consideration when interpreting images.[164,169]

Nonunion is the second most common complication after femoral neck fracture. Nonunion is rare when fractures are undisplaced, but it occurs in 20% to 30% of displaced fractures (Fig. 4-54).[161,172] Treatment of nonunions can be accomplished using bone grafts or endoprostheses.[169]

Radiographs or fluoroscopically positioned spot views should also be obtained to be certain the pins have not penetrated the femoral head. Figure 4-55 demonstrates a healed femoral neck fracture with three modified Hagie pins (Fig. 4-44C). The threaded stems project laterally into the soft tissues. Soft tissue irritation may require implant removal.

Trochanteric Fractures

There are basically three categories of trochanteric fractures. Intertrochanteric fractures follow the intertrochanteric line. Subtrochanteric fractures and avulsion fractures of the greater or lesser trochanter complete the three categories.[198]

Intertrochanteric Fractures

Intertrochanteric fractures are extracapsular, and thus, there is less problem with nonunion and AVN than with femoral neck fractures.[198,200,206,219] The fractures follow the intertrochanteric line (Fig. 4-56) and may be displaced, undisplaced, or comminuted with lesser and greater trochanteric fragments (Figs. 4-57 and 4-58). They occur most commonly in elderly patients as a result of falls or other minor trauma.[206]

Multiple classification systems have been used for trochanteric fractures. The Jensen[215] modification of the Evans[210] system is commonly used (Fig. 4-59).[206] This system is based on the prognosis for anatomic reduction and the likelihood of postreduction instability. The degree of calcar comminution and greater trochanteric involvement are the primary considerations. Stable fractures follow the intertrochanteric line. Type 1 and 2 fractures are stable and can be reduced in 94% of cases. The remaining types are unstable. Table 4-12 summarizes the Jensen[215] modification of the Evans[210] system.[198,206]

Subtrochanteric Fractures

Subtrochanteric fractures involve the cortical bone below the lesser trochanter. The femoral shaft and intertrochanteric region are frequently involved. These fractures tend to occur in a younger population and are usually related to high-velocity trauma, such as motor vehicle accidents.[200]

Fielding[211] classified subtrochanteric fractures according to the zones involved (Fig. 4-60). The Boyd and Griffin[200] classification was based on the prognosis and the ease of obtaining and maintaining reduction (Fig. 4-60). Type I fractures are simple intertrochanteric fractures. Types III and IV fractures (Fig. 4-61) were unstable and prone to loss of reduction.[200]

The Seinsheimer[230] classification (Fig. 4-62, Table 4-13) is more complex. Implant failure and nonunion problems are more likely with type IIIA and type V fractures.[206,230] For treatment purposes, stable subtrochanteric fractures are those in which the posterior and medial cortex can be brought back into contact.

TABLE 4-12. *Intertrochanteric fractures: Jensen modification of Evans classification*[206,215]

Type	Description
1	Undisplaced two-part fracture, stable (Fig. 4-56)
2	Displaced two-part fracture (Fig. 4-57)
3	Three-part fracture with greater trochanter displaced
4	Three-part fracture with displaced calcar and lesser trochanter
5	Four-part fracture with medial and posterior cortex fractures (Fig. 4-58)

(text continues on page 257)

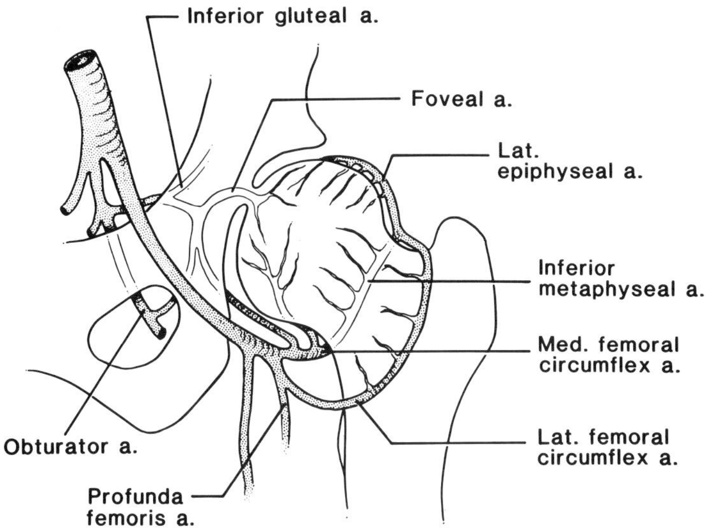

FIG. 4-52. The vascular supply of the femoral head. (From Berquist TH. Imaging atlas of orthopedic trauma. 2nd ed. New York: Raven Press, 1992.)

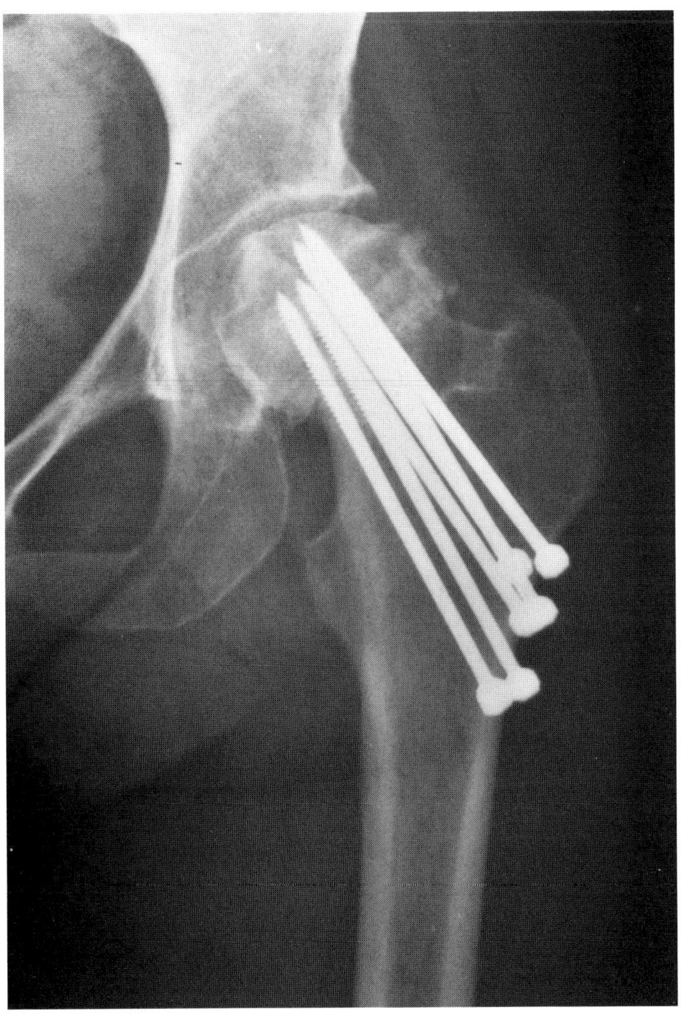

FIG. 4-53. An AP radiograph of the hip after pinning with six Knowles pins. There is stage IV AVN with associated degenerative changes.

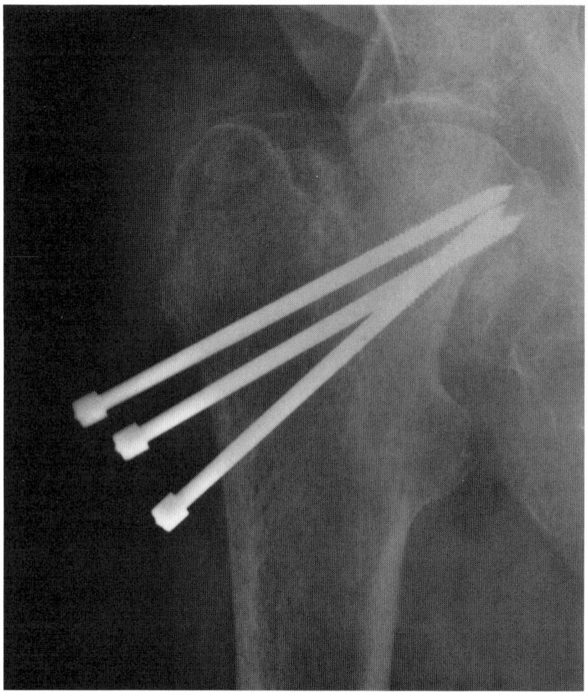

A

FIG. 4-54. **A:** An AP radiograph of the right hip with an old femoral neck fracture with subsidence of the Knowles pins and collapse of the fracture. **B,C:** The AP tomographs clearly demonstrate the nonunion.

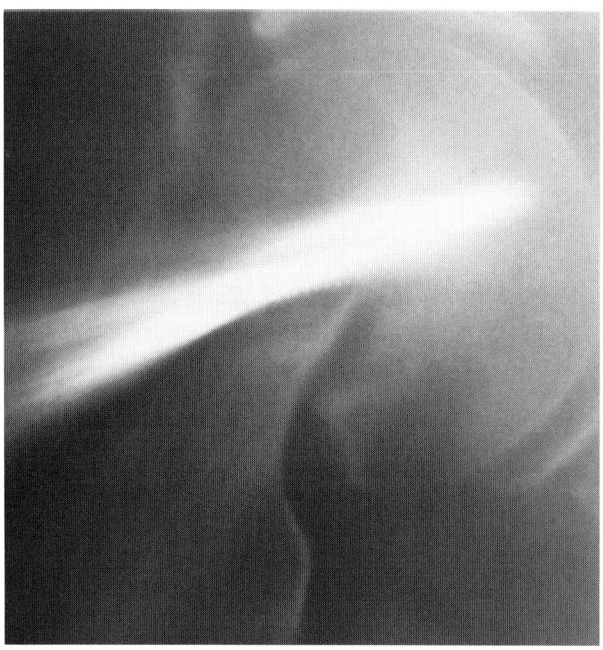

B

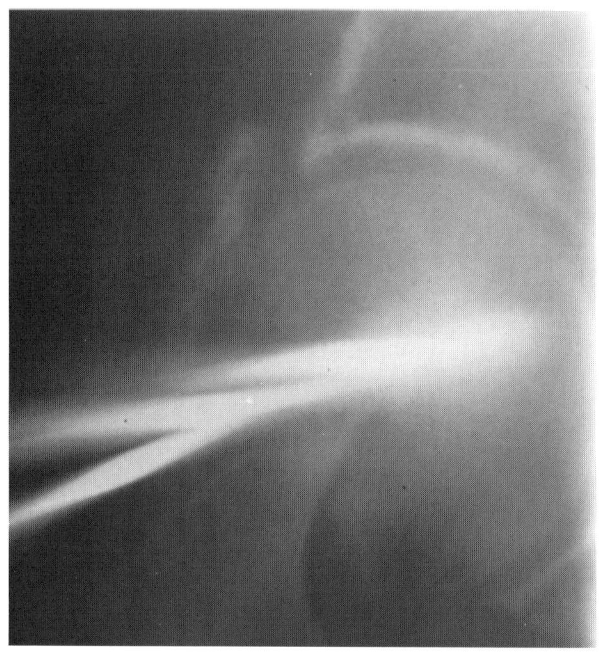

C

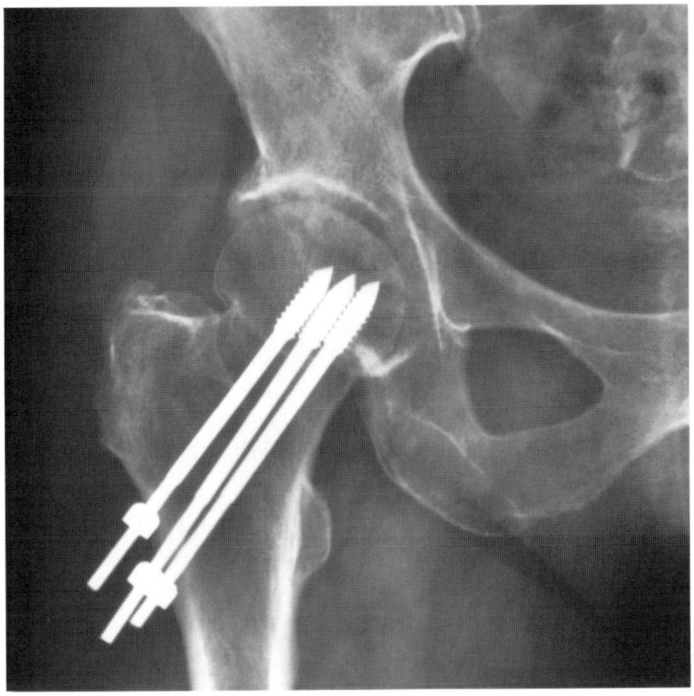

FIG. 4-55. An AP view of the right hip demonstrating a healed femoral neck fracture with three modified Hagie pins. The threaded stems project laterally, which led to soft tissue irritation in this patient.

A

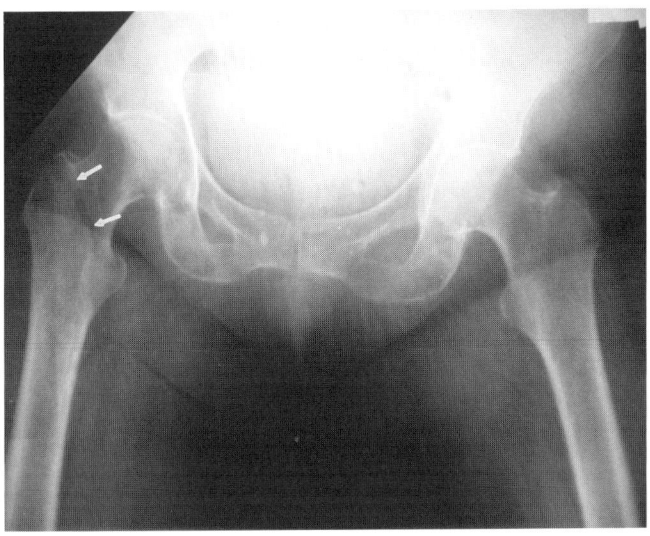

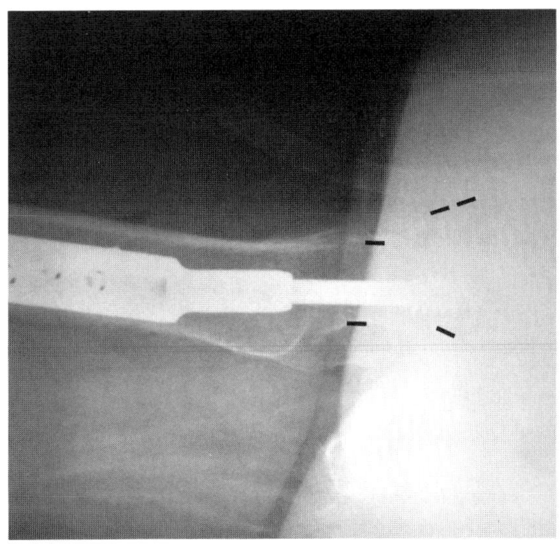

C

B

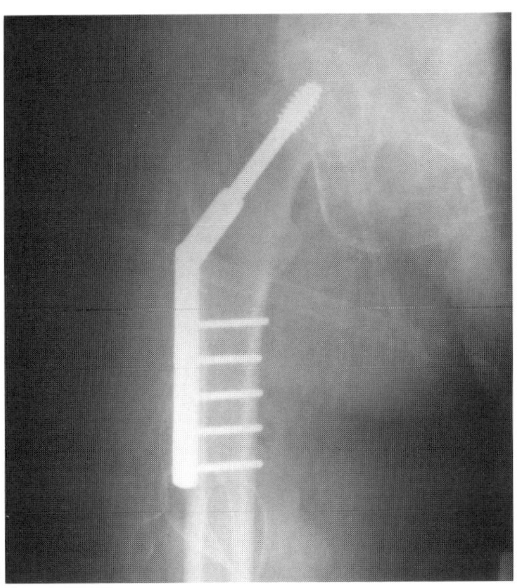

FIG. 4-56. **A:** Stable type 1 intertrochanteric fracture. The fracture is undisplaced and follows the intertrochanteric line (*arrows*). **B:** Postoperative AP radiograph after internal fixation with a dynamic hip screw with 150° five-hole side plate and cortical screws. The screw is slightly superior in the femoral head on the AP view. **C:** Lateral view shows slight posterior positioning of the screw head. Lines mark the outline of the femoral head and neck.

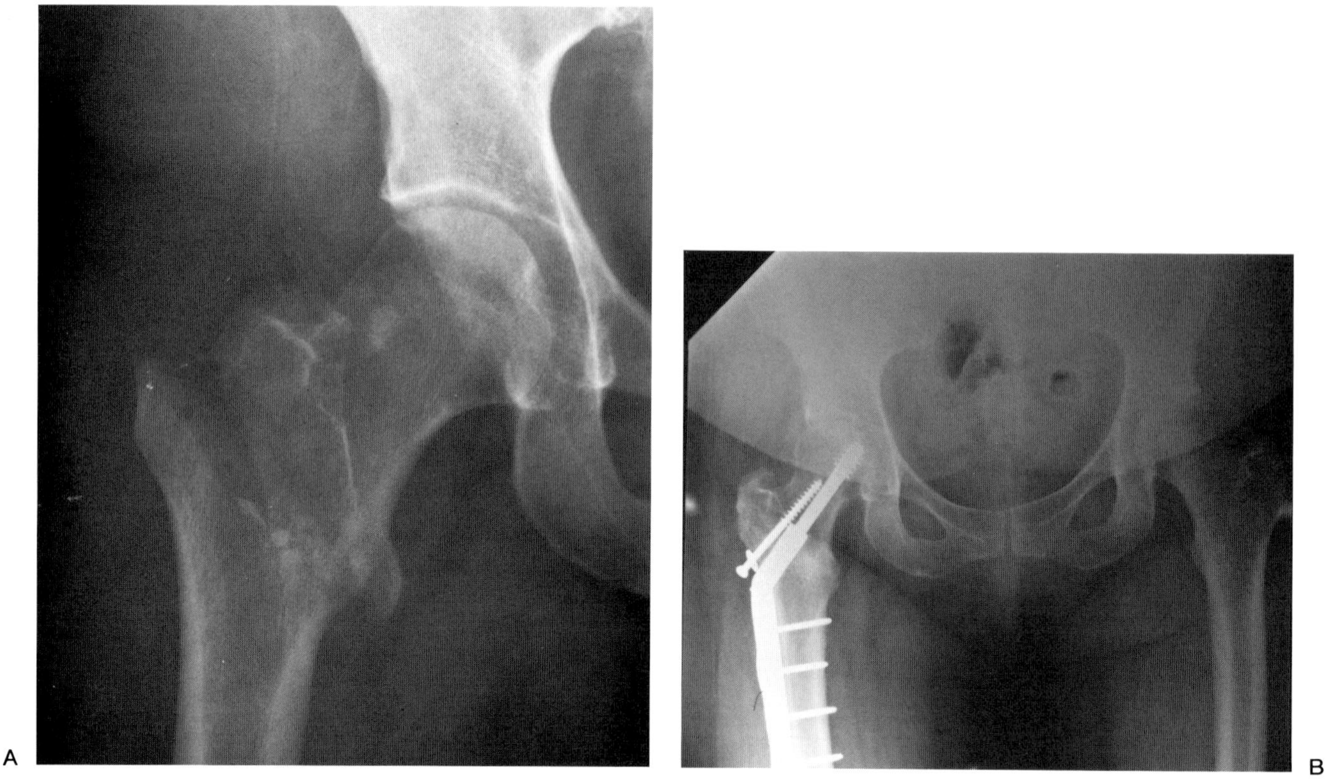

FIG. 4-57. **A:** An AP view of a displaced two-part intertrochanteric fracture (type 2). **B:** Internal fixation with a dynamic hip screw. A second cancellous screw and washer were used to reduce the likelihood of rotation.

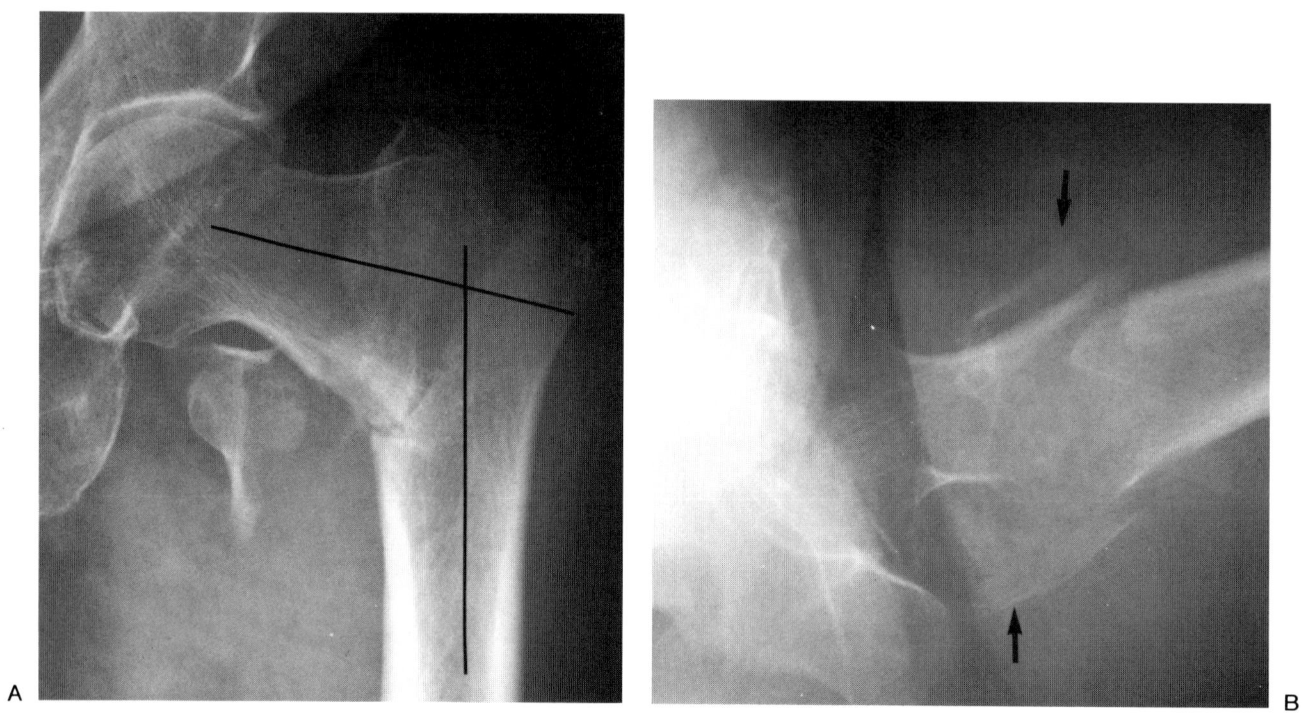

FIG. 4-58. The AP **(A)** and lateral **(B)** radiographs of a displaced four-part intertrochanteric fracture (type 5). Note the varus deformity of the femoral neck.

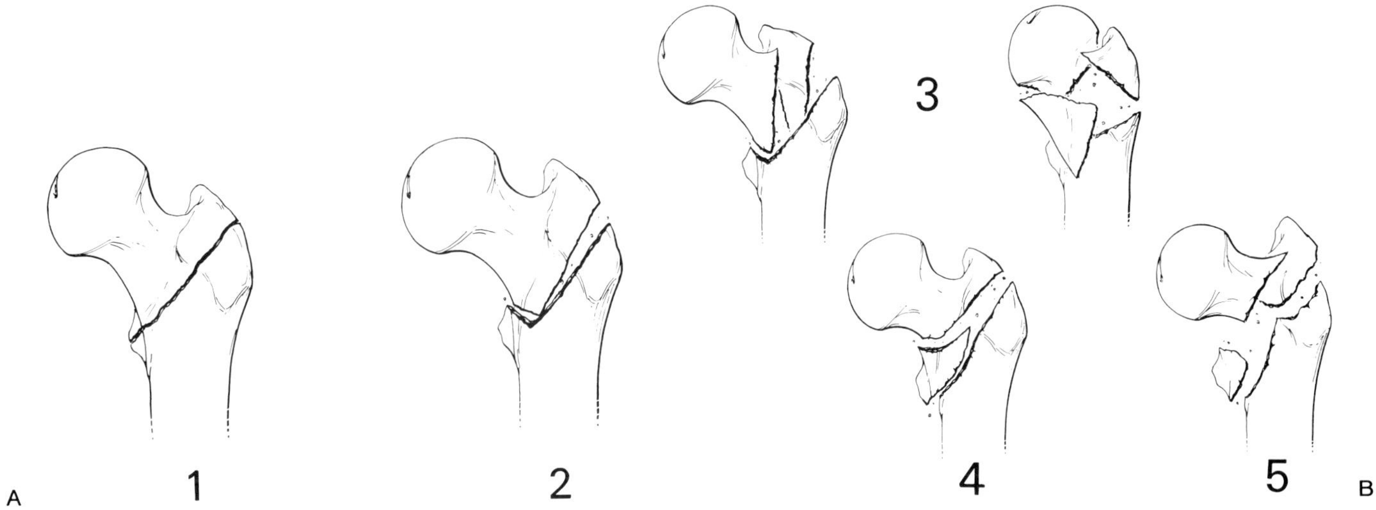

FIG. 4-59. The Jensen modification of the Evans system for intertrochanteric fractures. **A:** Type 1: undisplaced two-part fracture, type 2: displaced two-part fracture. **B:** Type 3: three fragments without posterolateral support, type 4: three fragments without medial support, type 5: four-fragment fractures.

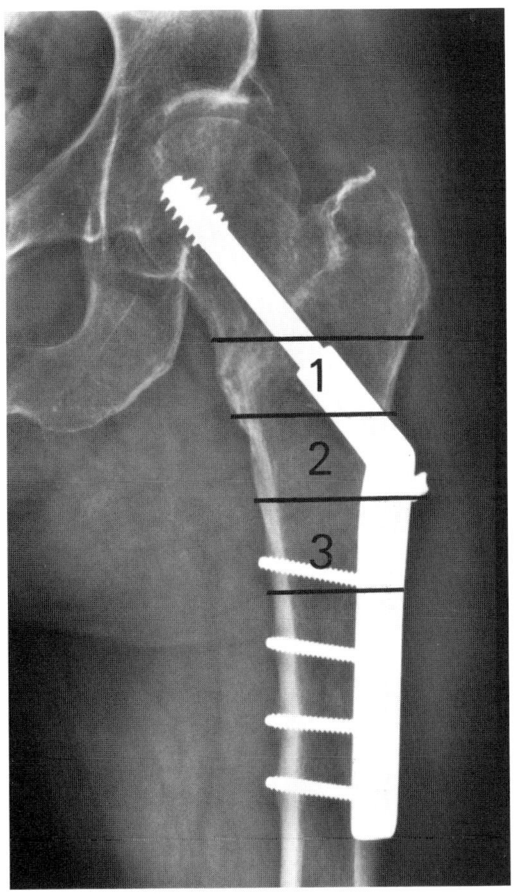

FIG. 4-60. An AP view of the hip with dynamic hip screw for fracture fixation demonstrating the Fielding zones of subtrochanteric fractures. Zone 1: lesser trochanteric region. Zone 2: 1 to 2 inches distal to the lesser trochanter. Zone 3: 2 to 3 inches below the lesser trochanter.

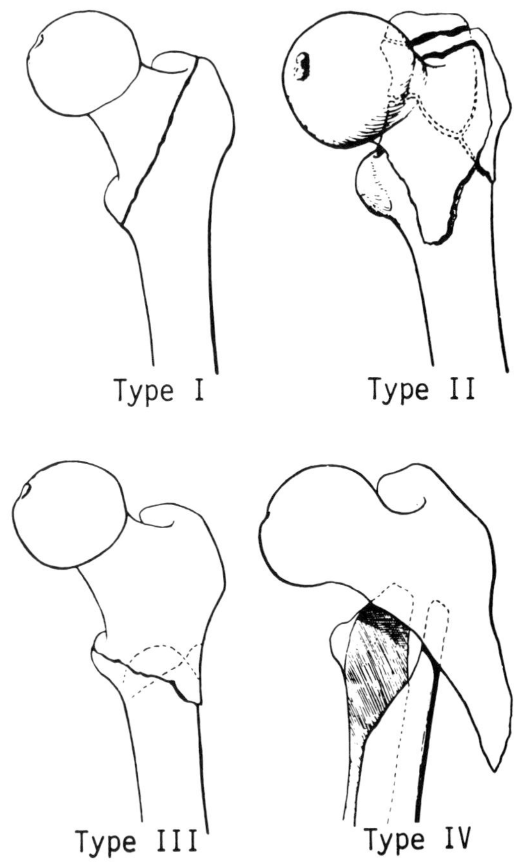

FIG. 4-61. The Boyd and Griffin classification. Type I: stable undisplaced trochanteric fracture. Type II: stable, minimally displaced comminuted fractures. Type III: posteromedial comminution, unstable. Type IV: intertrochanteric with subtrochanteric extension, unstable (From Boyd HB, Griffin LL. Classification and treatment of trochanteric fractures. *Arch Surg* 1949;58:853–866.)

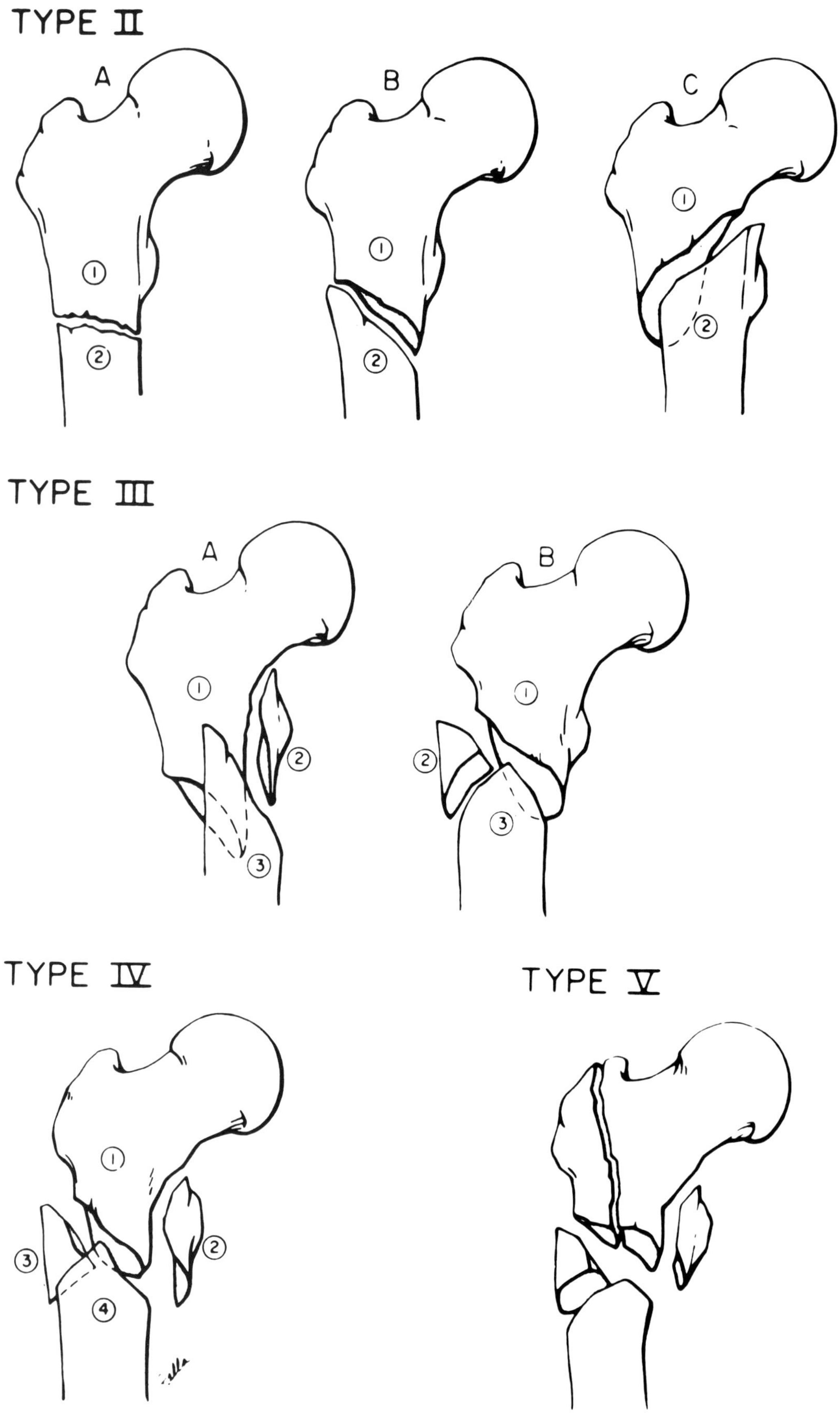

FIG. 4-62. The Seinsheimer classification (see Table 4-13). (From Seinsheimer F. Subtrochanteric fractures of the femur. *J Bone Joint Surg [Am]* 1978;60A:300–306.)

TABLE 4-13. *Subtrochanteric fractures: Seinsheimer classification*[206,230]

Type	Description
I	Undisplaced, any fracture with <2 mm displacement
II	Two-part fractures
A	Transverse subtrochanteric fracture
B	Spiral subtrochanteric fracture
C	Spiral fracture with lesser trochanteric involvement
III	Three-part fractures
A[a]	Spiral three-part fractures with lesser trochanter displaced
B	Spiral three-part fractures with lateral butterfly fragment
IV	Four or more fragments
V[a]	Subtrochanteric fracture that extends into the greater trochanter

[a] All implant failures and nonunions are in groups IIIA and V.[230]

Avulsion Fractures

Isolated avulsion fractures of the greater or lesser trochanter are uncommon. Greater trochanteric avulsion fractures occur with abrupt gluteal muscle contractions and are more common in elderly patients. However, this injury without an associated intertrochanteric fracture is unusual.[198,206] Lesser trochanteric fractures occur with abrupt iliopsoas contraction. This injury more commonly occurs in young athletes.[198]

Imaging

In most cases, intertrochanteric, subtrochanteric, and avulsion injuries can be detected and properly classified on AP and lateral radiographs. Careful attention must be paid to the medial cortex (lesser trochanter and calcar) and posterior cortex, both on initial and reduction views, to determine stability and treatment planning (Fig. 4-58).[200,206,214,230] Complex injuries may require further evaluation with conventional tomography, CT, or three-dimensional reconstruction techniques (Fig. 4-63).[198]

Treatment

The treatment of avulsion fractures is usually conservative. Surgical reduction is usually not indicated for isolated avulsion injuries unless the fragment is displaced ≥ 2 cm.[198,199,206]

Intertrochanteric fractures occur most commonly in elderly patients. Therefore, early treatment and mobilization is important.[208,212,213,217,223] Anatomic reduction of the fractures, in which the posterior and medial corteices are is brought back into contact, is ideal to achieve stability and reduce the chances of varus and posterior deformities.[206,219,227,231]

Stable nonanatomic reductions may also be acceptable. Generally, radiographs are reviewed after closed manipulation to determine the treatment best suited for a given injury.[206,217,223,232] When necessary, medial bone grafts or methyl methacrylate can be used to reinforce the cortex and fill in bone defects.[229]

There are four basic internal fixation options for intertrochanteric fractures.[203,206,207,220,224] These are summarized as follows:

1. Fixed nail plate or blade plate.[201,206,214,233] Pugh, Holt, or Jewett nails are mainly of historical interest. They do not allow controlled impaction of fragments; therefore, penetration of the femoral head or neck can occur (Figs. 4-64 to 4-66). These devices are adequate for undisplaced fractures, but they are not commonly used today.[206,221]
2. Sliding nail or screw-plate systems.[201,206,214,221,224] There are many sliding hip nail or screw-plate devices (Figs. 4-67 to 4-69). Most authors prefer this technique today. The nail or screw can be positioned deeper in the head, and controlled impaction of the fragments occurs. Newer screws (Fig. 4-69) are cannulated so they can be inserted over a guide.
3. Intramedullary systems.[204,209,216,225] Intramedullary nails and interlocking systems were discussed in Chapter 2. Ender, Küntscher, and short interlocking intramedullary nails can be used (Figs. 4-70 to 4-74). Ender nailing (Fig. 4-70) has been suggested for very elderly patients who may require early mobilization and minimal surgical trauma.[206,208,216,225] New modular systems are commonly used with subtrochanteric fractures (discussed subsequently).
4. Hemiarthroplasty.[203,206,218] Bipolar or unipolar hemiarthroplasty can be selected, but these devices are not well suited to these lower fractures because they depend on bone in the trochanteric area for support and stability is often impaired by the fracture that is present.

The approaches used for the treatment of subtrochanteric fracture are similar in many respects. In fact, discussions of these two categories of injury often overlap, as do the classification systems.[198] Earlier more aggressive treatment is indicated for young active individuals injured in high-velocity motor vehicle accidents than for elderly individuals who sustain injuries caused by minor trauma.

The same categories described with intertrochanteric fractures can be applied to the treatment of subtrochanteric fractures.[224–236] However, interlocking full-length or short intramedullary devices are gaining popularity. Stress on the implants is reduced compared

(*text continues on page 266*)

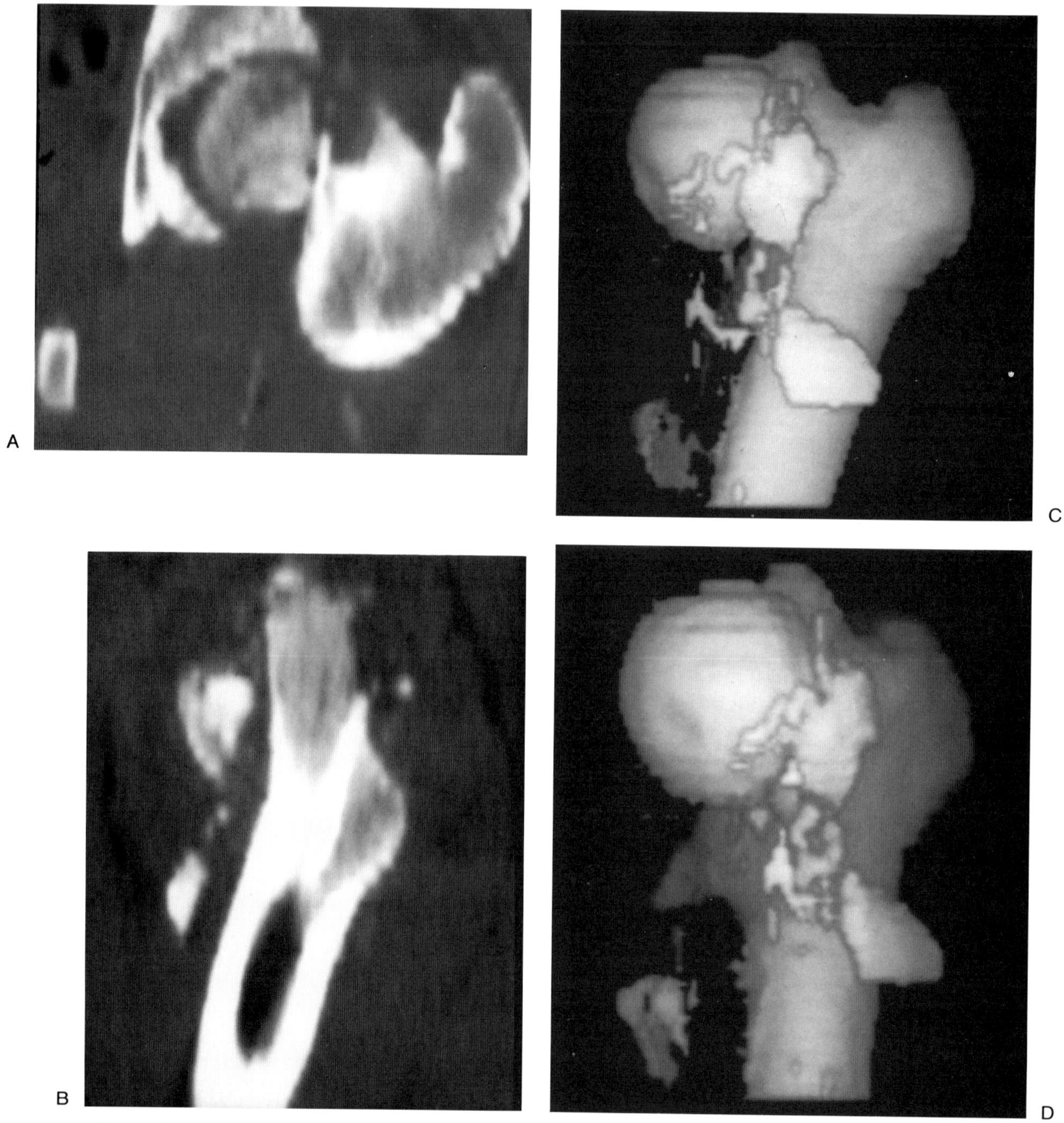

FIG. 4-63. Complex fracture of the left femoral neck and trochanteric region. Reformatted coronal images **(A,B)** and three-dimensional images in two different degrees of obliquity **(C,D)** improve the assessment of fracture fragments.

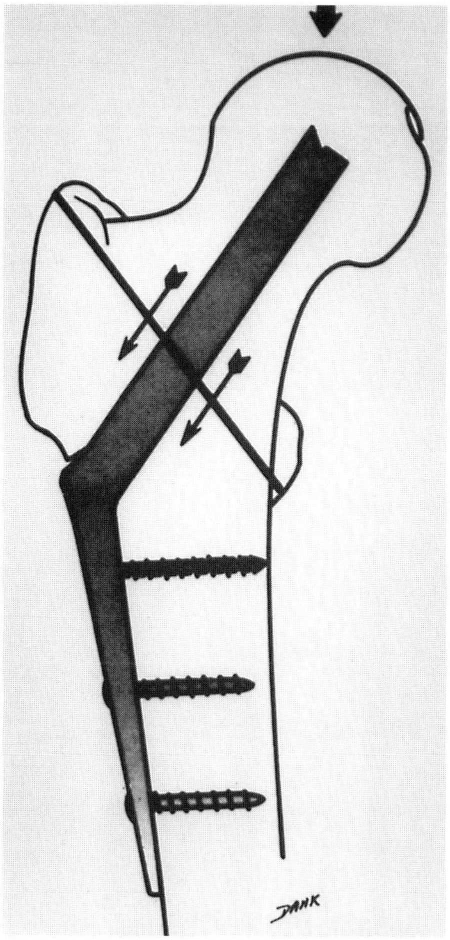

FIG. 4-64. A nonsliding nail-plate fixation of an undisplaced intertrochanteric fracture. *Arrows* in the fracture region demonstrate forces with weight-bearing forces transmitted from above (*upper arrow*). (From Zickel RE. Fractures of the adult femur excluding the femoral head and neck. A review and evaluation of current therapy. *Clin Orthop* 1980;147:93–106.)

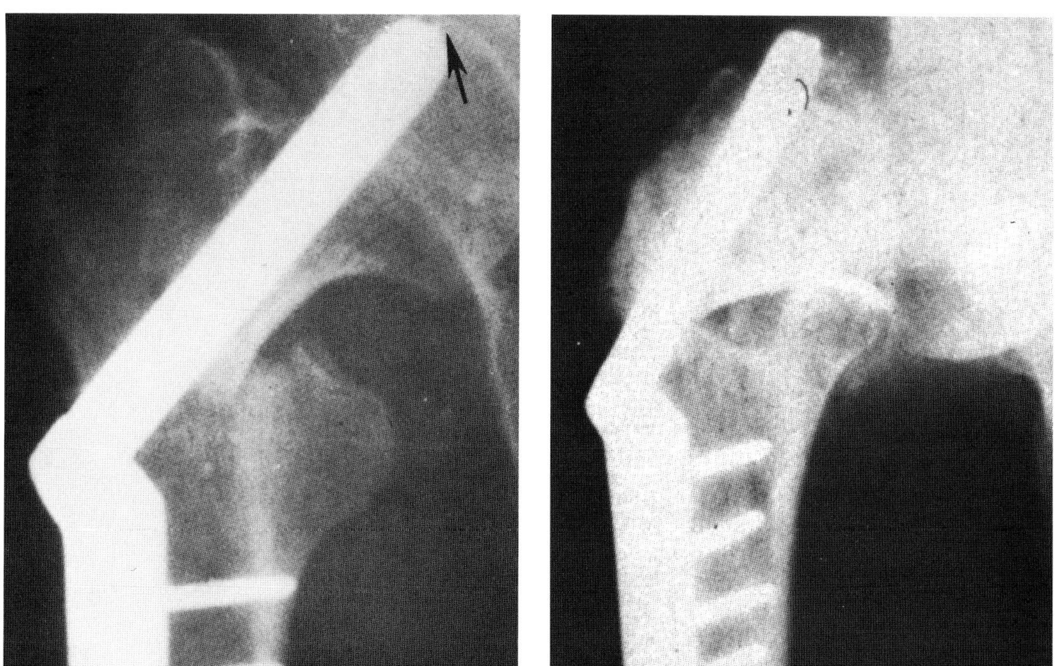

A B

FIG. 4-65. A: Varus reduction and a poorly positioned Jewett nail. Note the superior position with nail tip near the articular surface (*arrow*). **B:** Later, the nail cut through the femoral head and neck. (From Zickel RE. Fractures of the adult femur excluding the femoral head and neck. A review and evaluation of current therapy. *Clin Orthop* 1980;147:93–106.)

A 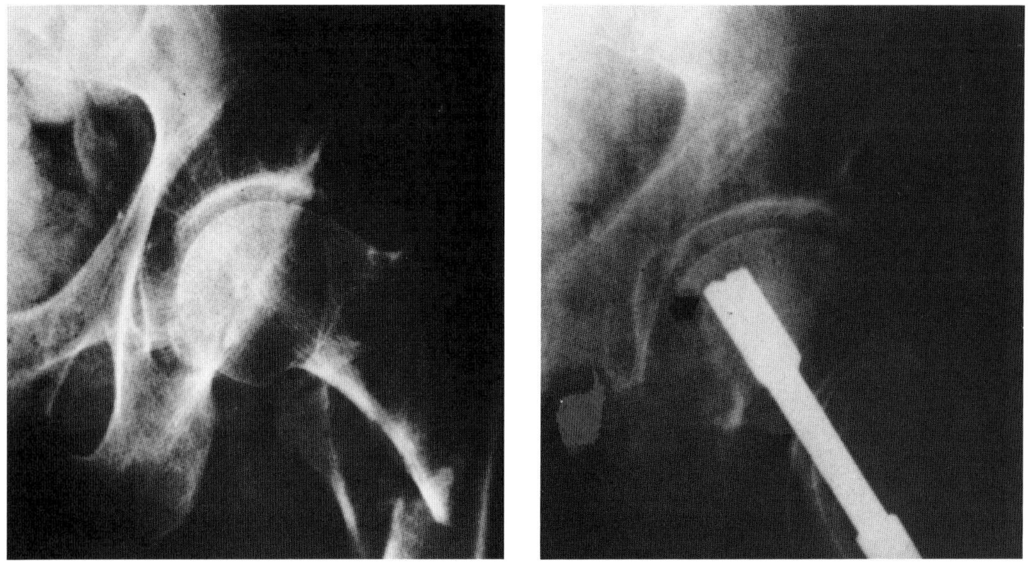 B

FIG. 4-66. **A:** Comminuted four-part intertrochanteric fracture in varus position. **B:** Internal fixation with a sliding Massie nail with 150° angled side plate. (From Zickel RE. Fractures of the adult femur excluding the femoral head and neck. A review and evaluation of current therapy. *Clin Orthop* 1980;147:93–106.)

A 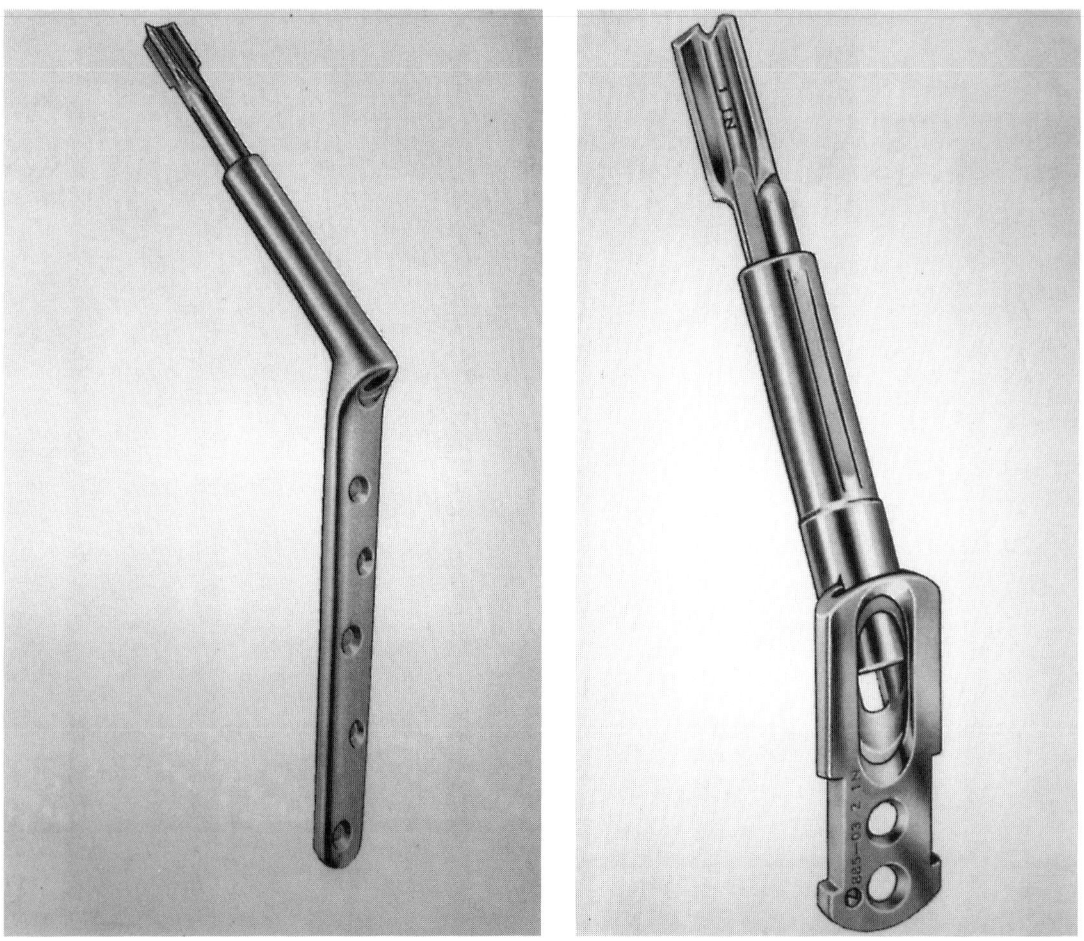 B

FIG. 4-67. Sliding nail-screw plate systems. (Courtesy of Zimmer, Warsaw, IN.) **A:** Massie sliding triflanged nail with five-hole side plate with 150° angle. **B:** Hagie sliding triflanged nail and side plate.

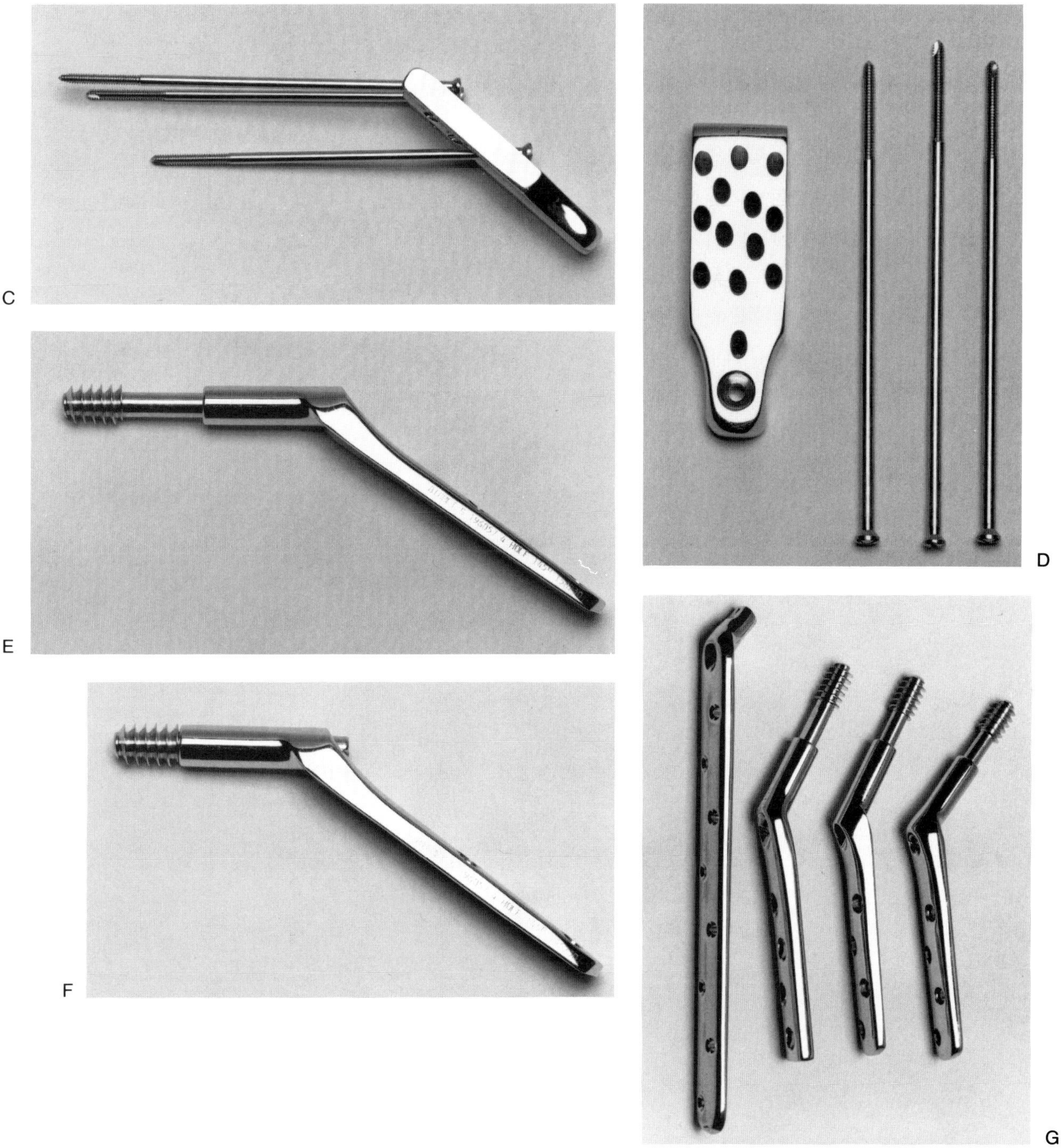

FIG. 4-67. (*Continued.*) Deyerle side plate and screws seen from the side **(C)** and separated **(D)**. Dynamic hip screw seen from the side **(E)** and with screw impacted in the side plate, variable-angled four-hole side plates **(F)**, and a long eight-hole side plate on the left **(G)**.

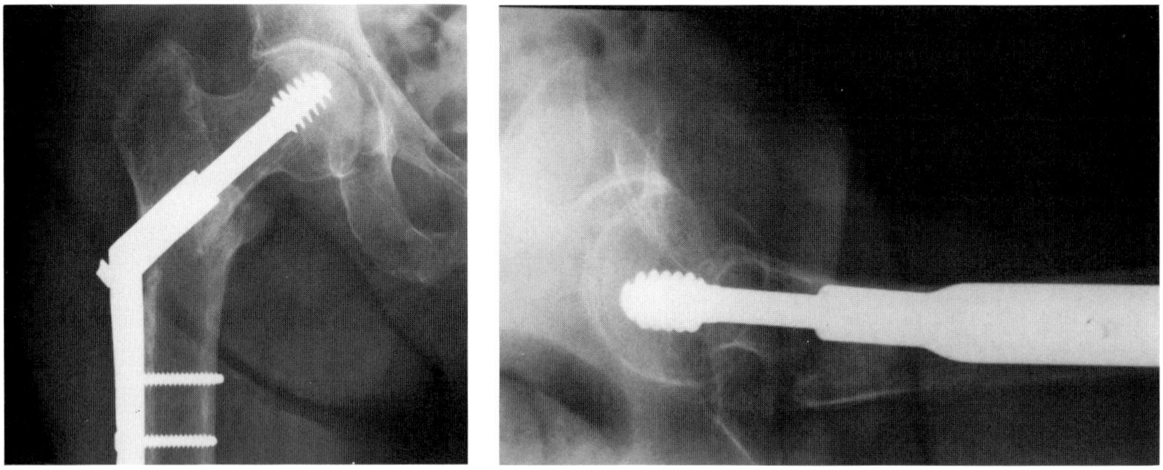

A B

FIG. 4-68. The AP **(A)** and lateral **(B)** radiographs of an intertrochanteric fracture internally fixed with a dynamic hip screw and five-hole 135° side plate. The screw is properly positioned in the subchondral central portion of the head. The cortical screws have proper purchase in the opposite cortex.

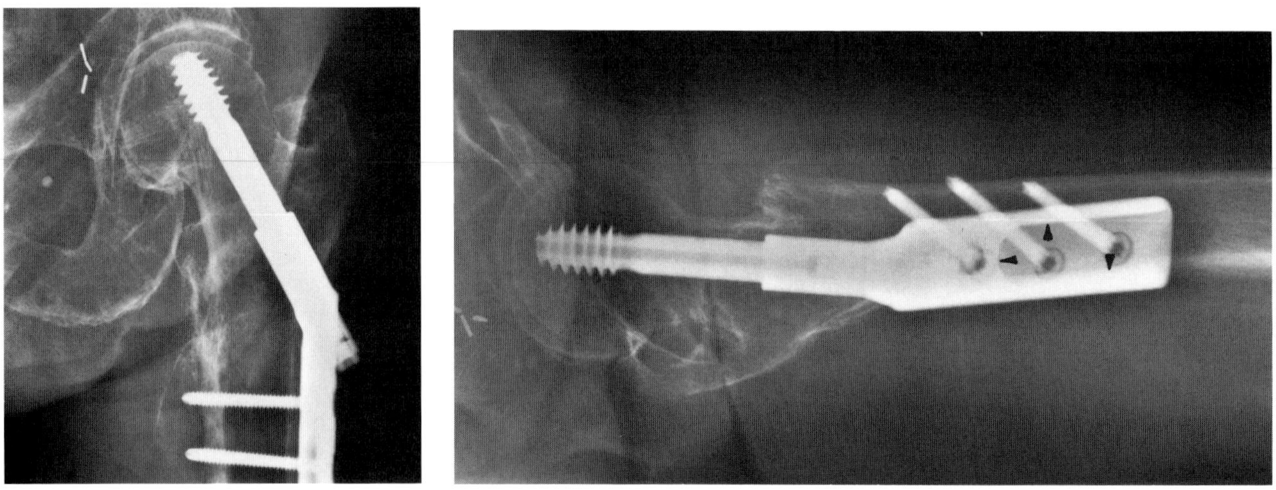

A B

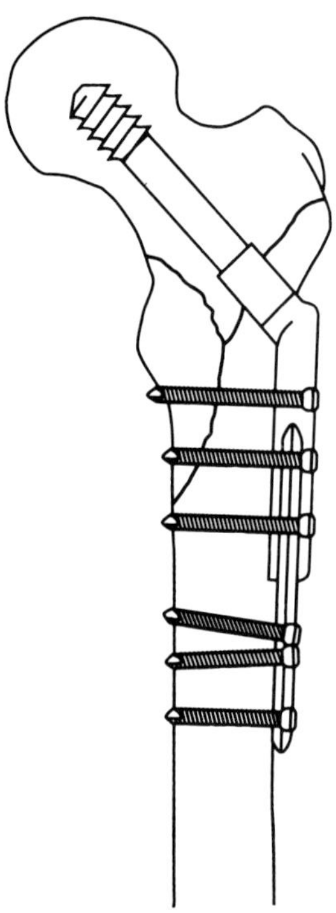

C

FIG. 4-69. The AP **(A)** and lateral **(B)** radiographs of an internally fixed intertrochanteric fracture using a cannulated sliding screw with a three-hole modular side plate. The slot (*arrows*) allows the addition of extra length. **C:** Alta^{TM} modular trauma system with additional side plate. (Courtesy of Howmedica, Rutherford, NJ.)

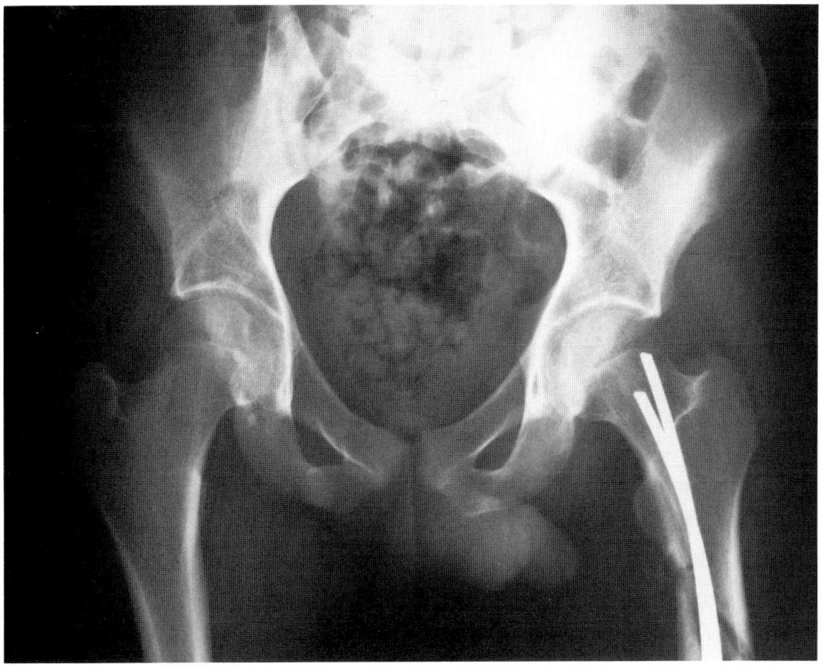

FIG. 4-70. Elderly patient with a proximal femoral fracture treated with two Ender nails.

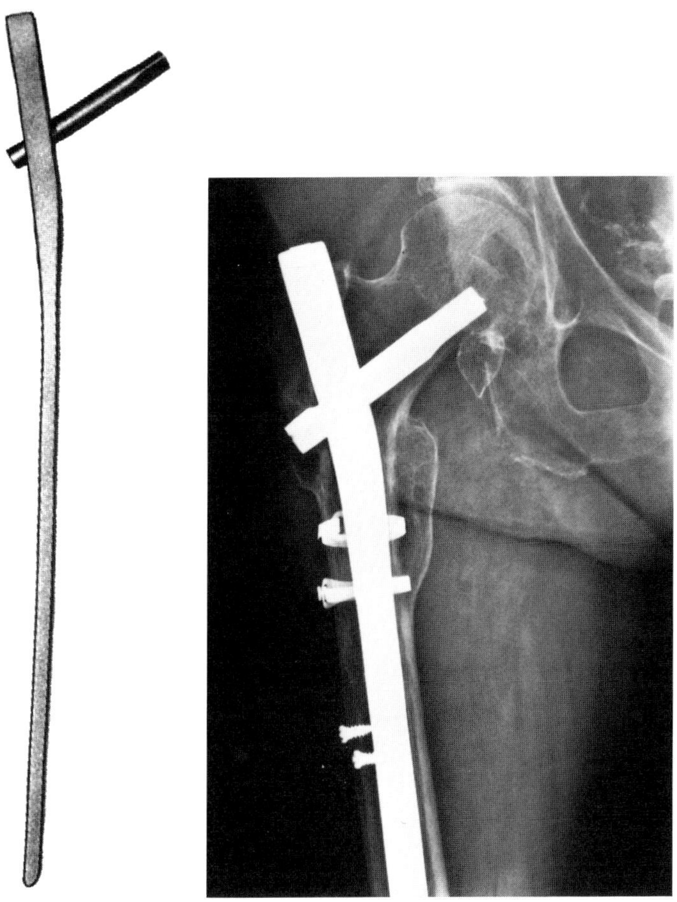

A,B

FIG. 4-71. A: Zickel intramedullary nail. (Courtesy of Howmedica, Rutherford, NJ.) The AP views of the upper femur **(B)**, lower femur **(C)**, and lateral femur **(D)**, demonstrating a healed subtrochanteric fracture treated by Zickel intramedullary nail. (See **C** and **D** on next page.)

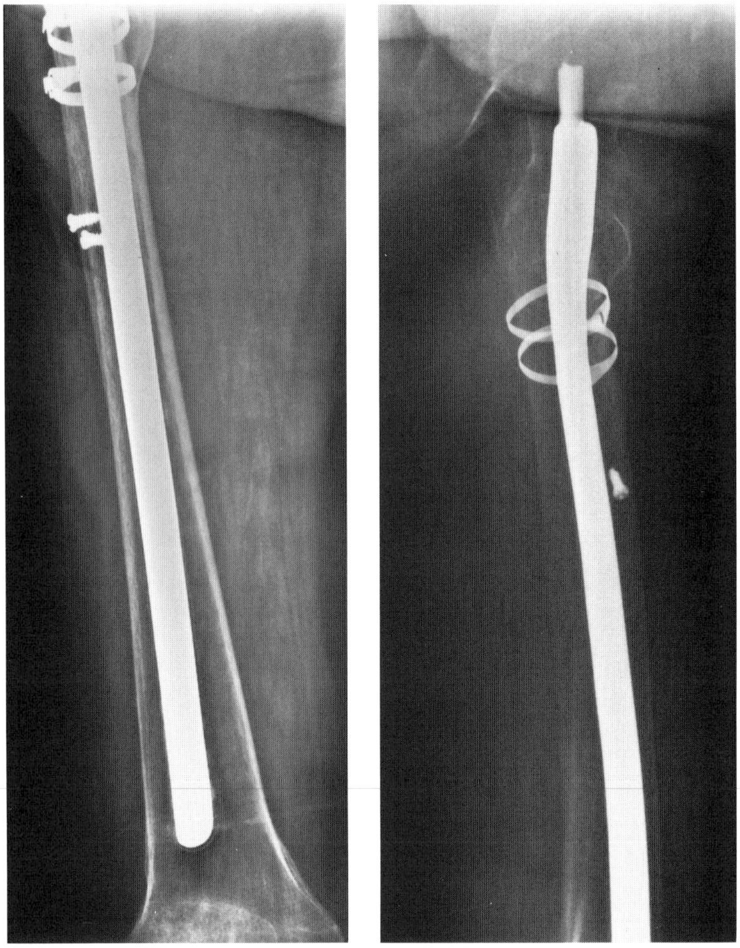

C,D

FIG. 4-71. *Continued.*

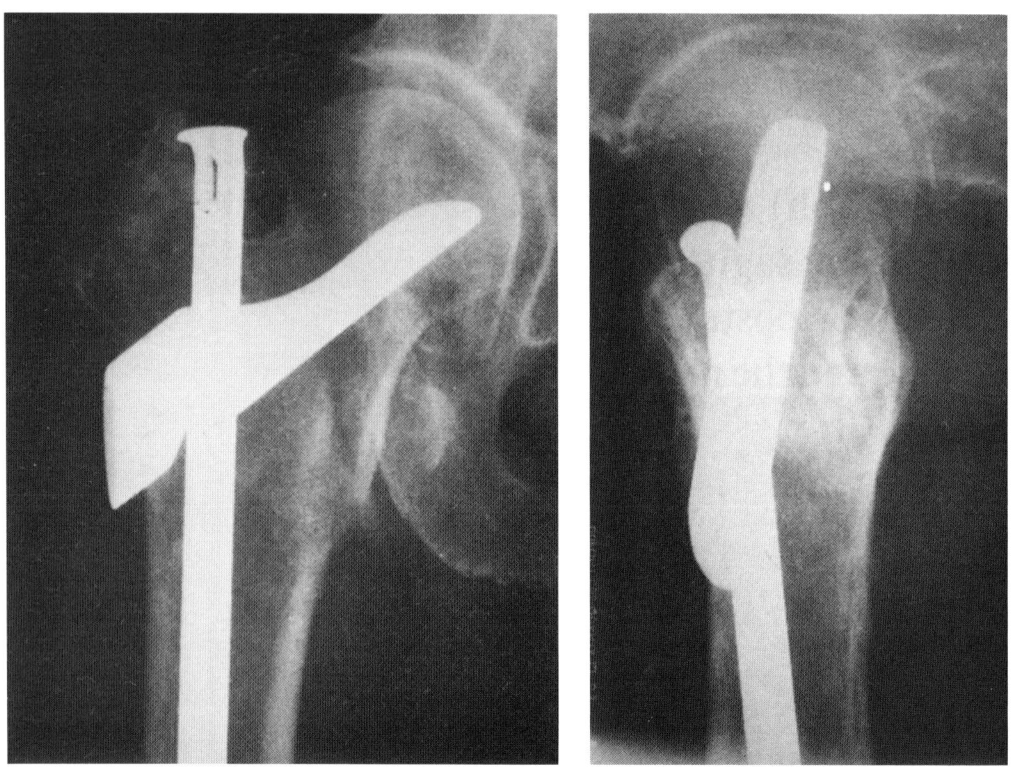

A B

FIG. 4-72. The AP **(A)** and lateral **(B)** radiographs of a Küntscher Y-nail for fixation of an intertrochanteric fracture. (From Davis TRC, Sher JL, Horsmon A, et al. Intertrochanteric fractures: mechanical failure after internal fixation. *J Bone Joint Surg [Br]* 1990;72B:26–31.)

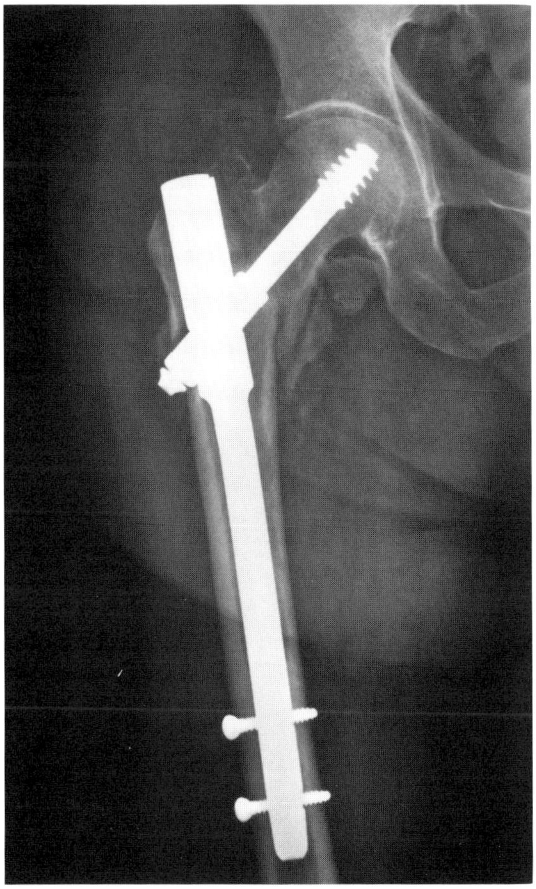

FIG. 4-73. Comminuted intertrochanteric fracture with subtrochanteric involvement treated with an interlocking Russell-Taylor™ nail and dynamic hip screw. (Courtesy of Smith and Nephew Richards, Memphis, TN.)

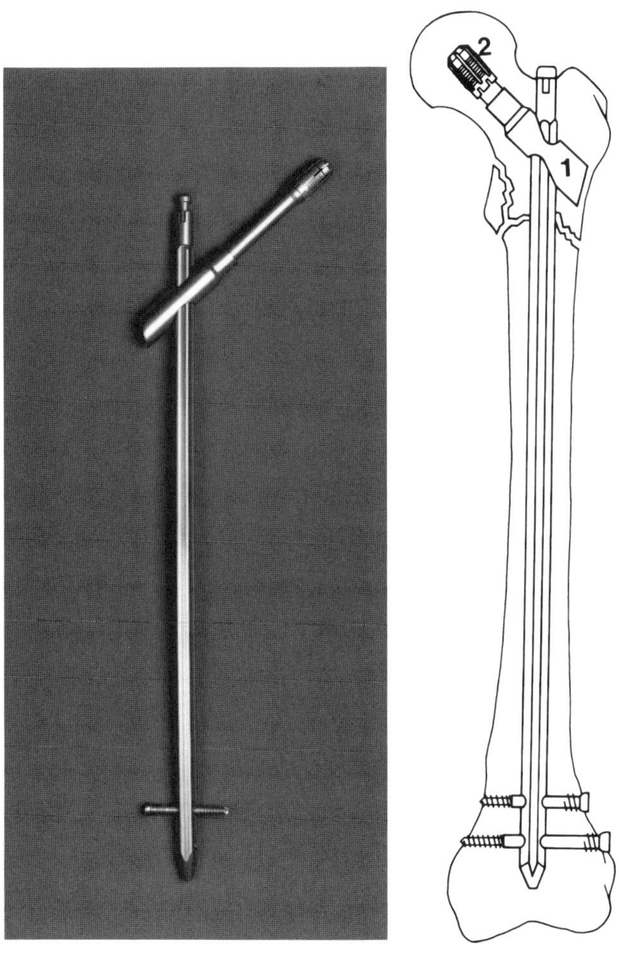

A,B

FIG. 4-74. Photograph **(A)** and illustration **(B)** of the femoral Alta™ modular intramedullary locking rod with rod connector (*1*) and hip blot with the Alta™ dome (*2*) instead of a screw.

with that of the more common sliding hip screw or fixed nail plate devices.[206] Figures 4-71 through 4-75 demonstrate examples of subtrochanteric fracture treatment options.[198,206,233–236]

Postoperative Imaging and Complications

The complications of trochanteric fractures, specifically intertrochanteric and subtrochanteric, are similar to those of other fractures. Nonunion, malunion, and infection occur to varying degrees, depending on the injury and fixation required. Major differences compared with other fractures are the higher incidence of implant failure, loss of reduction, and significant mortality rate. Kyle et al.[217] reported 10% to 30% mortality rates in the first year after fracture.

Implant failure or a loss of reduction is greater with unstable fractures and those treated with rigid or nonsliding fixation devices.[198,202] Brien et al.[201] compared subtrochanteric fractures treated with Zickel nails (Fig. 4-76), 95° blade plates, and interlocking medullary nails (Figs. 4-73 and 4-74). The former two devices require an open reduction. Ninety-four percent of intramedullary nails were inserted using closed techniques and were believed to reduce blood loss potentially, minimize soft tissue stripping, and shorten operating time. The incidence of malunion was 48% with the Zickel nail, 24% with the blade-plate technique but only 3% with intramedullary nailing. There were no infections with intramedullary nails. Deep infection occurred in 4% to 5% of patients treated with blade-plate and Zickel nail techniques.

The incidence of implant cut out from the femoral head or neck is also higher with fixed or nondynamic systems (16.5%).[205] Although this technique is controversial, 75% of implant cut outs (Fig. 4-76) occurred when the nail or screw was not positioned in the central portion of the femoral head and neck.

A loss of reduction or varus displacement may be accepted if union occurs.[206] In some cases (Fig. 4-77), traction can be used to prevent increasing displacement, or reoperation may be necessary.[205,206,223,226]

Because of the extracapsular location of these fractures, AVN is an uncommon (0.08%) complication.[217]

Imaging for the detection of most complications can be accomplished with AP and lateral radiographs. The position of the fragments, especially the posterior and medial cortex, should be followed and the location of the implants noted.[228] As discussed previously, it would be ideal for the implant in the femoral head and neck to be centrally located (Fig. 4-78). Most problems occur with eccentric positioning, especially when the nails are too superior in the femoral head (Fig. 4-76).[198,206]

Metal implants can cause significant image degradation with CT or MRI. Conventional tomography is still useful to evaluate healing or suspected nonunion (Fig. 4-79). Radionuclide studies or joint aspiration can be used when infection is suspected.[198]

HIP ARTHROPLASTY

Hip arthroplasty techniques have progressed dramatically over the past 20 years, providing valuable stimulation and background data for the development of joint replacements in other areas.[324]

The first documented attempts to improve hip function were early osteotomies described by Barton in 1826 and, later, by Ollier in 1885 and Murphy in 1915. Arthroplasties were originally performed with soft tissue interpositions, using fascia and other soft tissues. Cup arthroplasties were performed as early as 1923 by Smith-Peterson.[364] Various materials were used, progressing to metal alloys, which were used into the 1970s (Fig. 4-80).[259,364]

In the 1930s and 1940s, metal balls were attached to triflanged nails for femoral head replacement, leading the way for the development of intramedullary femoral stems. An evaluation of the unipolar endoprosthesis resulted in the development of the Moore prosthesis constructed of vitallium, being developed in 1950 (Fig. 4-81).[259,331]

The bipolar endoprosthesis, which combined a femoral stem with a free-riding acetabular cup, was developed by Bateman in 1974.[241,259,318] The femoral component could be either press fitted or cemented (Fig. 4-82).[241,260,331] Bipolar prostheses have evolved and continue to be used today.[248,331]

Total hip arthroplasty has evolved through many stages over the last 30 to 40 years.[242,259,285,367] Table 4-14 summarizes some of the early metal-to-metal, metal-to-polyethylene, and multiple part or modular de-

TABLE 4-14. *Early total hip arthroplasties*[285]

Metal-to-metal components
McKee-Farrar (Fig. 4-83)
Ring (Fig. 4-84)
Brist-Moore
McBride-Moore
Sbarbaro
Metal femoral-polyethylene acetabular
Charnley
Charnly-Müller
Bucholz-St. George
Stanmore
Aufranc-Turner
Trapezoidal-28
Multipart or modular
Frost
Harris
Tronzo
Deyerle

signs.[242,285,339,341] Early metal-to-metal components, such as the McKee and Watson-Farrar, were cemented (Fig. 4-83). The Ring metal-to-metal prosthesis (Fig. 4-84) was not cemented.[242] Significant progress occurred with development of the Charnley prosthesis (Fig. 4-85). The polyethylene acetabular component had wire incorporated to provide radiographic visibility. This system was modified by Müller. The Aufranc-Turner prosthesis (Fig. 4-86) had an expanded collar on the femoral component and an eccentric acetabular wall, which may create the appearance of an asymmetric femoral head position radiographically.[242]

Cemented components helped reduce loosening. Originally, the methyl methacrylate was not visible radiographically (Fig. 4-87). However, the cement was impregnated with barium, which makes it radiopaque and assists in the radiographic evaluation.[242,323,363,376–378]

Early techniques for the preparation of the acetabulum for cementation of the acetabular component frequently led to methyl methacrylate penetration into the pelvis. Although such complications were rare, wire mesh was often used to assist in the prevention of extension of cement into the pelvis (Fig. 4-88).[242,259]

The popularity of hip arthroplasty continues to evolve, with continued efforts to improve component design and longevity.[237,259,291] Thousands of these procedures are performed annually. The number of procedures performed in Olmsted County between 1987 and 1990 was approximately 60 per 100,000 population. Projected to the national population, this would be around 150,000 procedures in the United States per year.[237,329]

Patient Selection

Hip replacement arthroplasty is an elective procedure that is most often performed in patients older than 60 years of age. The patient selection is based on clinical features, radiographic features, and careful evaluation of the risks versus the benefits in each patient.[263]

The patient should not have other medical problems that increase the risk of surgery or contraindicate the procedure itself. Active infection, paralysis, and significant neuromuscular dysfunction are contraindications to total hip arthroplasty.[333]

Assuming no systemic contraindication, the clinical factors determining the feasibility for joint-replacement procedures are based on the clinical setting, pain pattern, patient's age, and radiographic features.[263,287,331]

The most common indications for joint-replacement arthroplasty are osteoarthritis, rheumatoid arthritis and other erosive arthropathies, traumatic arthritis, AVN, and congenital hip disorders.[279,290,291] Certain neoplasms may also be treated in this manner (see Chapter 14). If radiographs indicate a process correctable by hip replacement arthroplasty, the approach to the timing of the procedure varies with the patient's age and pain symptoms.[263,331]

DeOrio and Blasser[263] described indications by age category. Patients older than age 65 years are considered for joint replacement when pain interferes with activity or sleep and it is not improved with 3 to 6 months of conservative therapy. This might include antiinflammatory medication or hip injection with anesthetic and steroid.[239,244] Patients 55 to 65 years of age are usually given a longer trial of conservative therapy. For those younger than 55 years of age, their activity must be much more limited and their pain severe to consider arthroplasty. Also, osteotomy or arthrodesis may be reasonable alternatives to arthroplasty in younger patients.[263]

As with other joint-replacement procedures, there are scoring systems that can be used to evaluate improvement. The scores are usually calculated pre- and postoperatively. The Harris[297] hip score system[262] has four categories: (1) pain (0 to 44 points), (2) function (0 to 47 points), (3) deformity (0 to 4 points), and (4) range of motion (0 to 5 points).[331] Patients with severe pain are given 10 points (0, if totally disabled), and moderate pain is scored at 20 points. The functional categories include stair climbing, daily activities, walking ability, and the need for support (cane or crutches).[293,297]

Preoperative imaging plays a significant role in determining the site and cause of the symptoms and evaluating the bone and soft tissue anatomy. Imaging requires routine radiography and, in some cases, additional techniques to assist further in operative planning.[279,288,323,378]

Routine Radiographs

Standard radiographs include an AP view of the pelvis and AP and lateral views of the hip and upper femur, with magnification markers on each film. The patella should be anterior, with the leg internally rotated 15° (great toes usually touch), to ensure consistency and proper position of the femoral head and neck on the AP view. An oblique view is also included with the preoperative hip series. Certain features and measurements are made on the AP and lateral views that assist in operative planning. The features to be evaluated on the AP view are summarized in Fig. 4-89 and listed as follows:[263,284,378]

1. Ischial tuberosity line used to evaluate leg-length discrepancy (Fig. 4-89B) roughly
2. Ilioischial line (Kohler's line, Fig. 4-89A)
3. Acetabular angle and superior coverage (Fig. 4-89A)
4. Femoral canal (calcar-to-canal-isthmus ratio) (Fig. 89D)

(text continues on page 274)

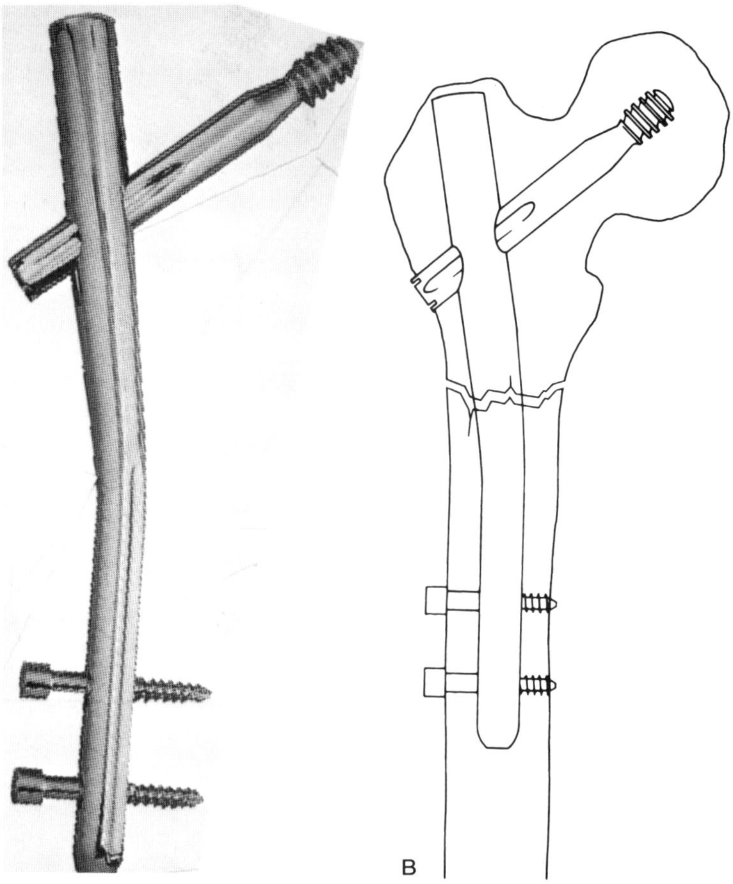

A B

FIG. 4-75. Photograph **(A)** and illustration **(B)** of the Gamma™ locking nail system for subtrochanteric fixation in this illustration. (Courtesy of Howmedica, Rutherford, NJ.)

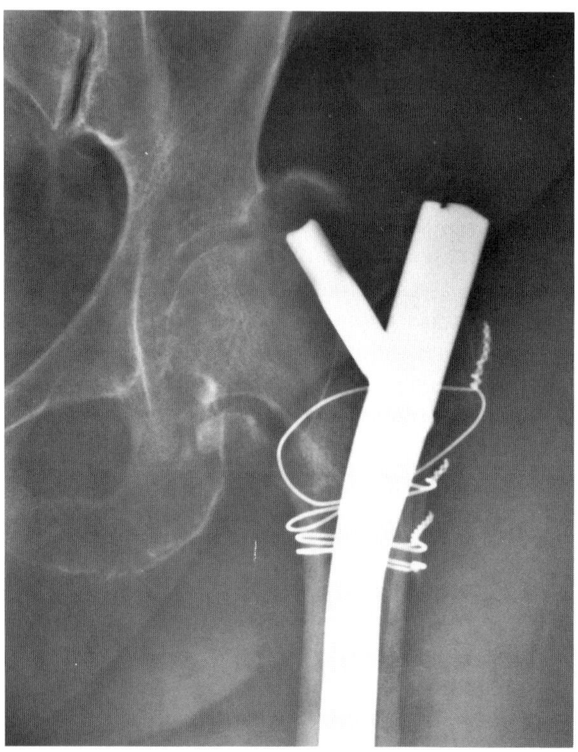

FIG. 4-76. An AP radiograph of the left hip after fixation of a comminuted trochanteric fracture with a Zickel nail. The nail has cut out of the femoral head and neck, and the fracture is in a varus position.

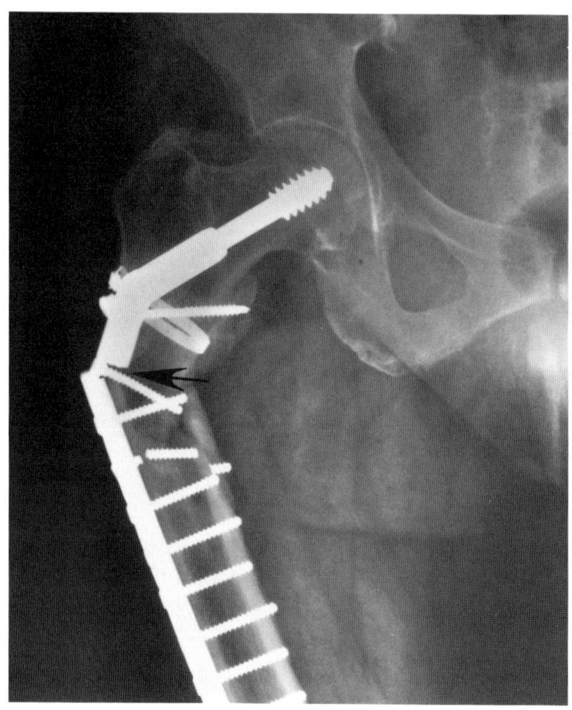

FIG. 4-77. Subtrochanteric fracture treated with a dynamic hip screw and long side plate. The plate has fractured through the second screw hole (*arrow*), resulting in marked deformity requiring revision.

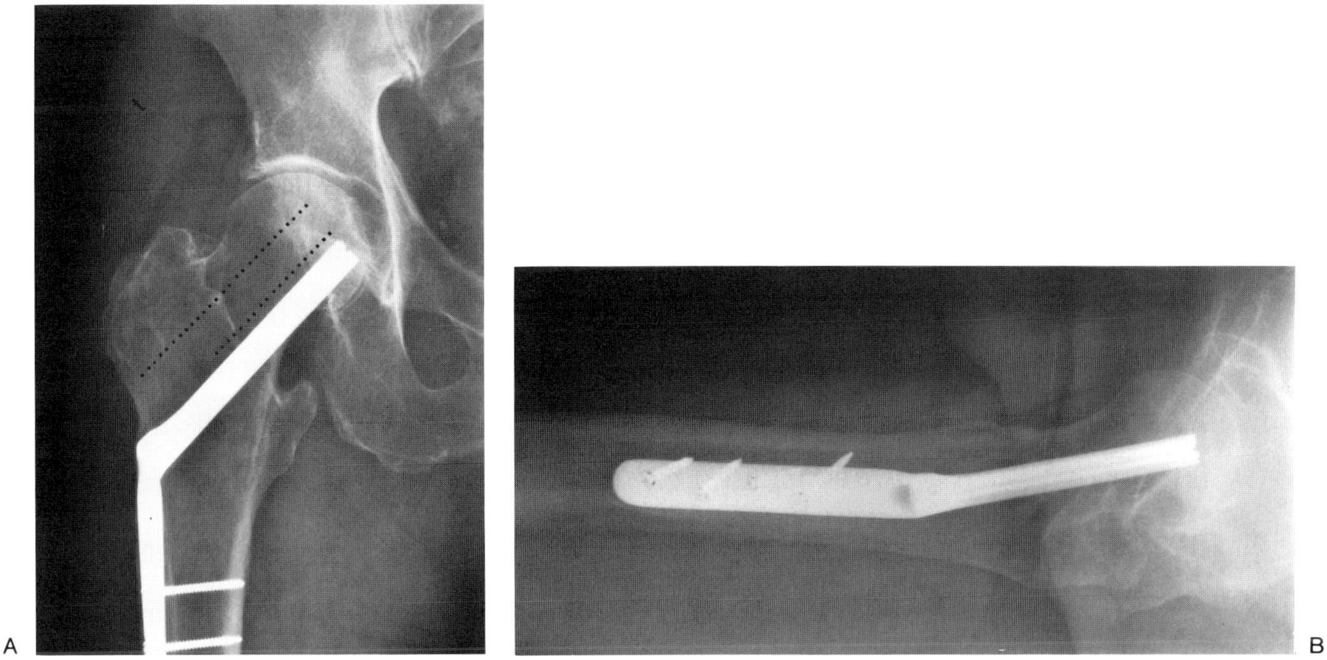

FIG. 4-78. Nail-plate fixation of the right femur with a healed fracture. The nail is placed through the inferior cortex of the femoral neck into the femoral head on the AP radiograph. **A:** The ideal position is marked (*dotted lines*). **B:** On the lateral view, the position appears satisfactory.

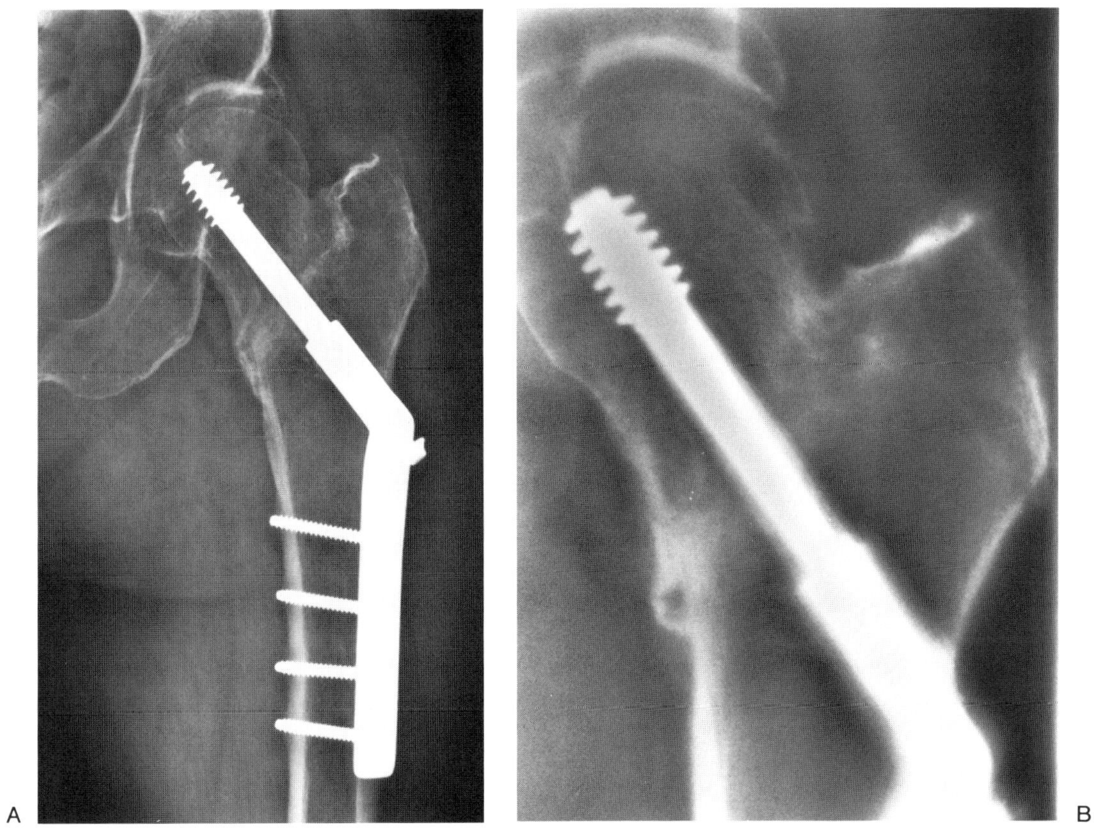

FIG. 4-79. Hip pain after internal fixation of a displaced two-part intertrochanteric fracture. **A:** An AP radiograph shows sclerosis along the fracture line. No loss of reduction and fixation with a dynamic hip screw. The AP tomograms **(B,C)** demonstrate a healed impacted fracture. (See **C** on next page.)

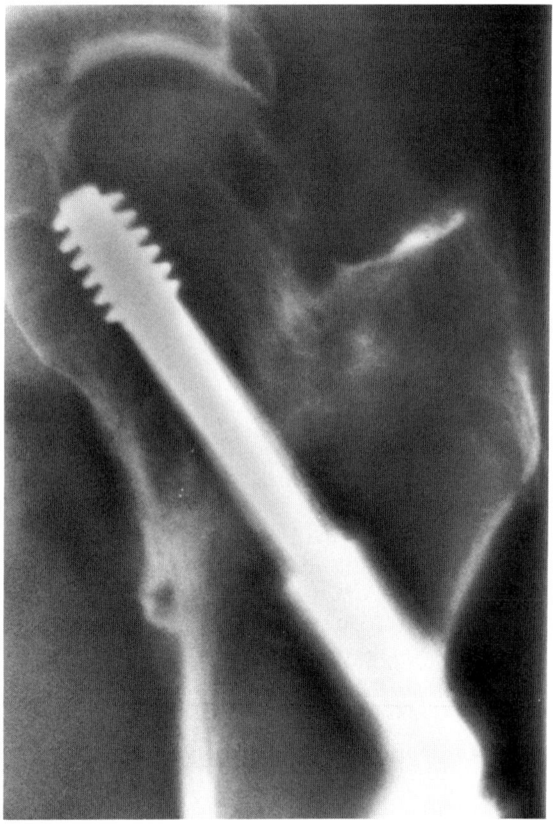

C

FIG. 4-79. *Continued.*

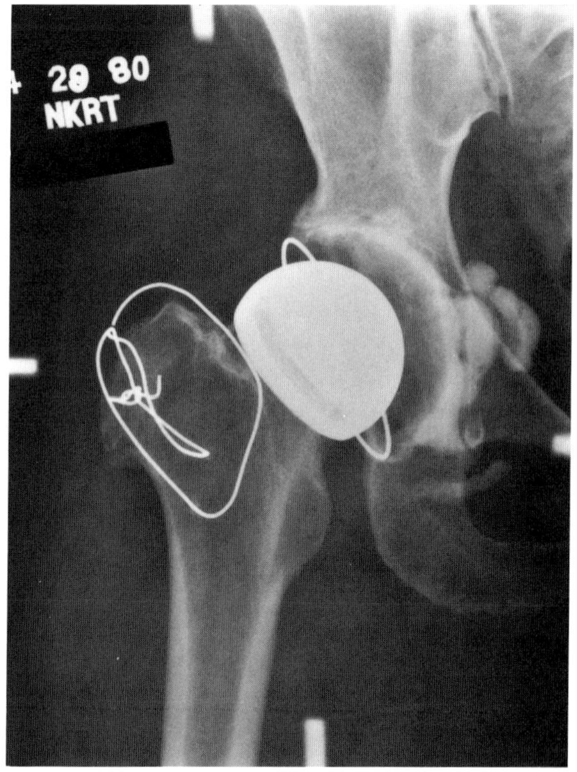

FIG. 4-80. An AP radiograph of the right hip with a resurfacing THARIES arthroplasty with cemented polyethylene acetabular component.

A,B

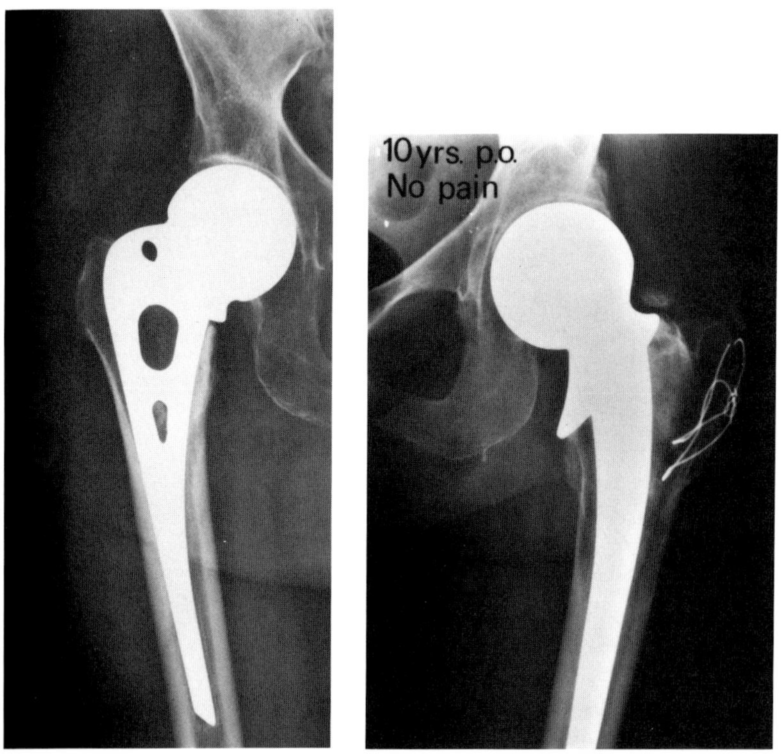

FIG. 4-81. A: An AP radiograph of a Moore prosthesis. **B:** An AP radiograph of a cemented Thompson prosthesis with no pain 10 years after implantation. (Courtesy of Mark B. Coventry, Mayo Clinic, Rochester, MN.)

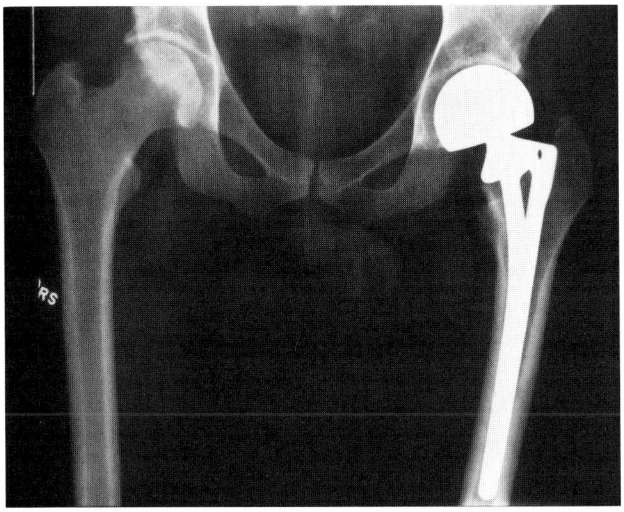

FIG. 4-82. An AP radiograph of the hip with a bipolar prostheses on the left.

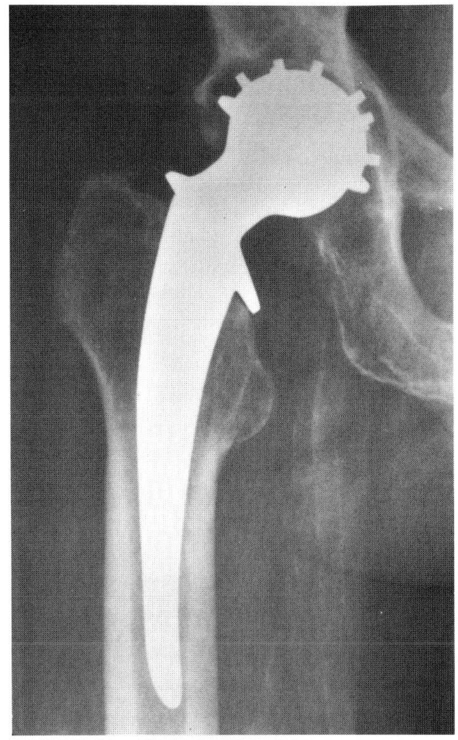

FIG. 4-83. An AP radiograph of a metal-to-metal McKee-Farrar prosthesis. Note the osteolysis around the superolateral aspect of the acetabular component likely due to metal particulate debris. (Courtesy of Dr. Jack Beabout, Rochester, MN.)

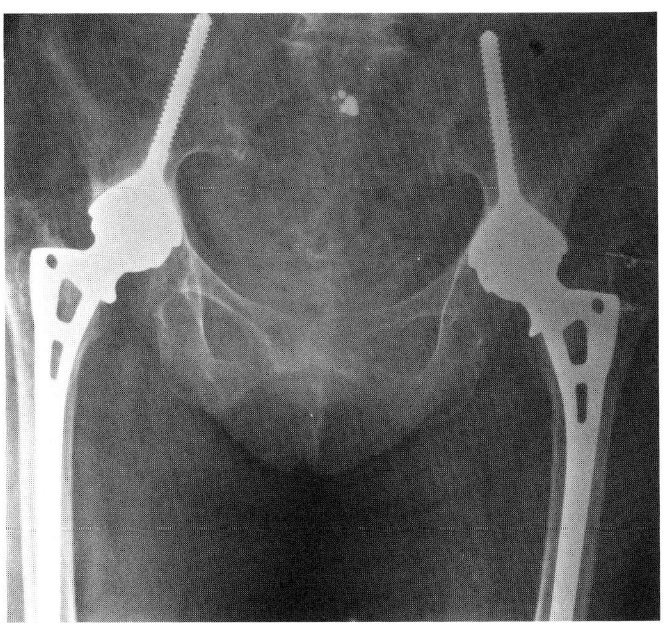

FIG. 4-84. An AP radiograph of the pelvis demonstrating bilateral metal-to-metal Ring hip prostheses. There are long fixation screws on the acetabular components. The femoral component is essentially a Moore endoprosthesis. (Courtesy of Dr. Jack Beabout, Rochester, MN.)

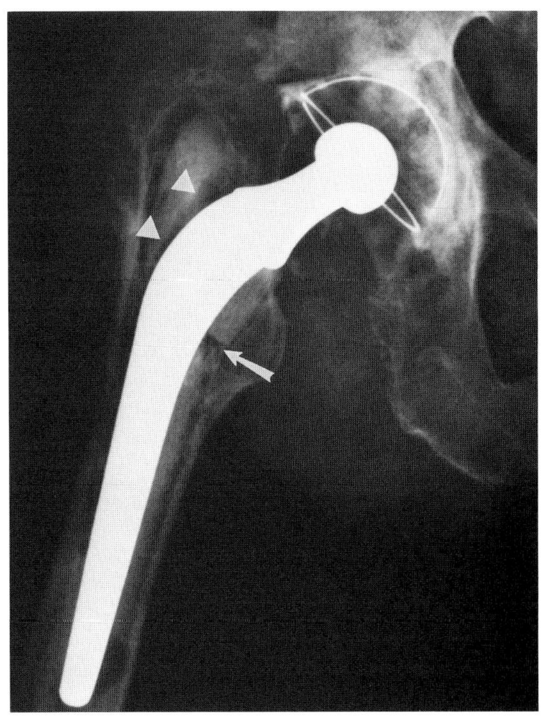

FIG. 4-85. Cemented Charnley hip prosthesis with loosening of the femoral component. Note the cement fracture medially (*arrow*) and metal cement gap laterally (*arrowheads*). The wire in the polyethylene acetabular component is clearly seen.

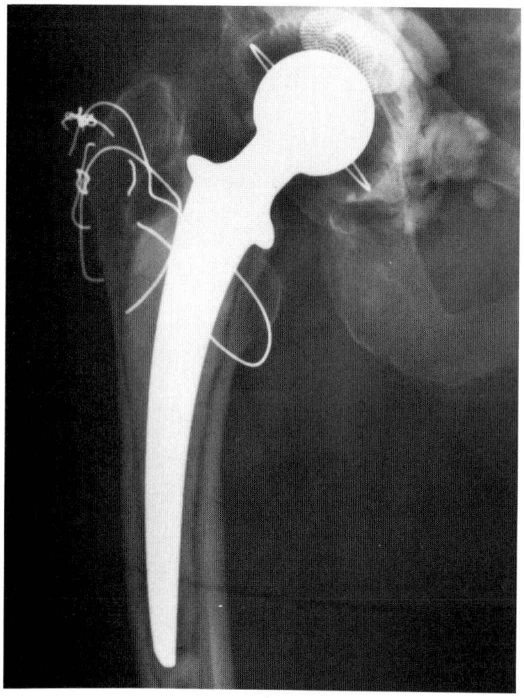

FIG. 4-86. Aufranc-Turner hip prosthesis with varus migration and distal cement fracture caused by femoral component loosening. There is a wire cement restrictor in the acetabulum, but cement still entered the pelvis.

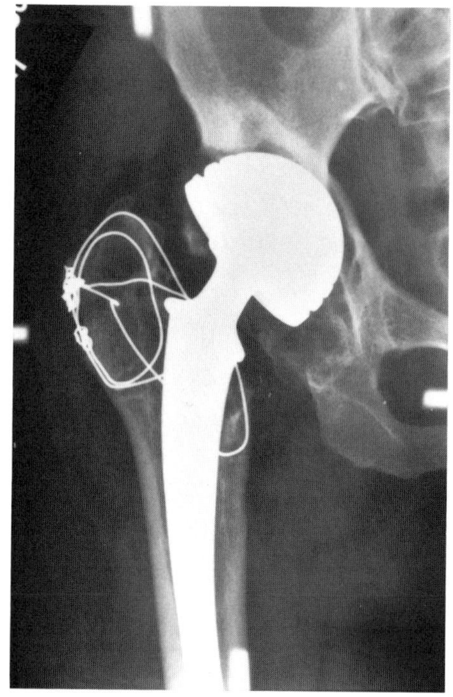

FIG. 4-87. Harris prosthesis with cemented components but no barium in the methyl methacrylate. This makes it more difficult to evaluate loosening.

A

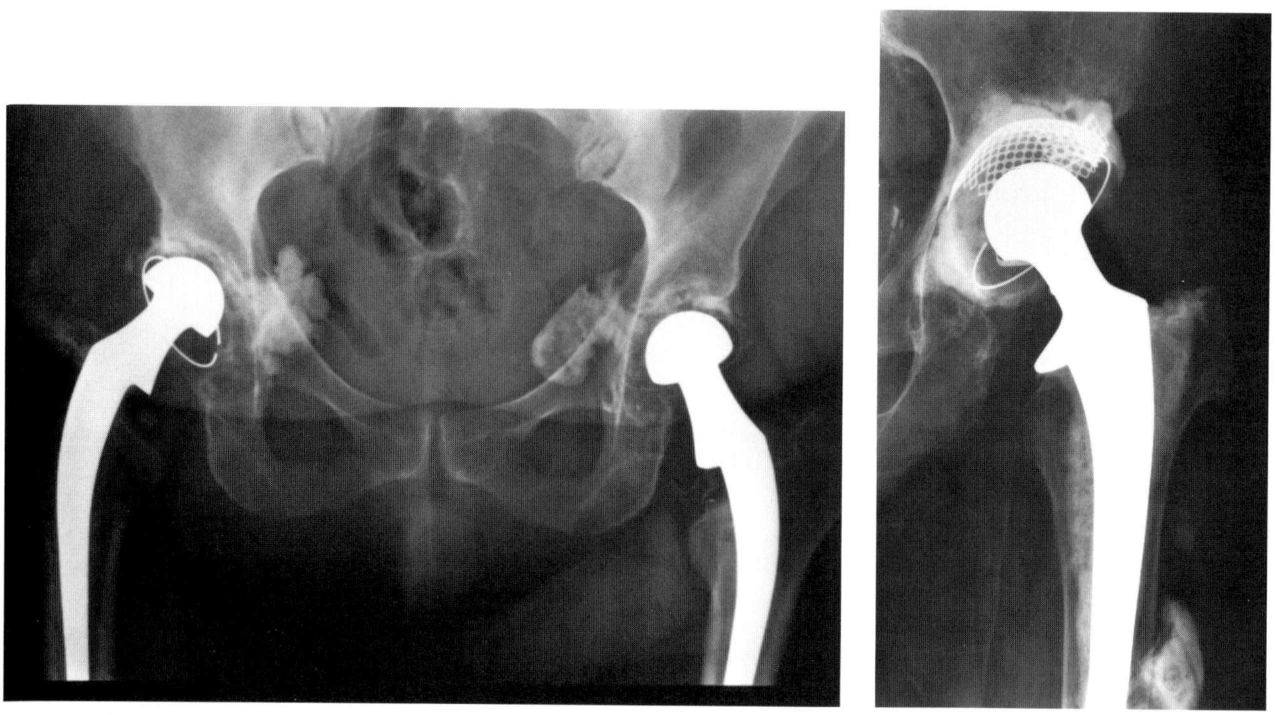

B

FIG. 4-88. A: An AP radiograph of the pelvis with bilateral arthroplasties. The methyl methacrylate protrudes into the pelvis bilaterally. **B:** Left hip arthroplasty with a large wire mesh in the upper acetabular region.

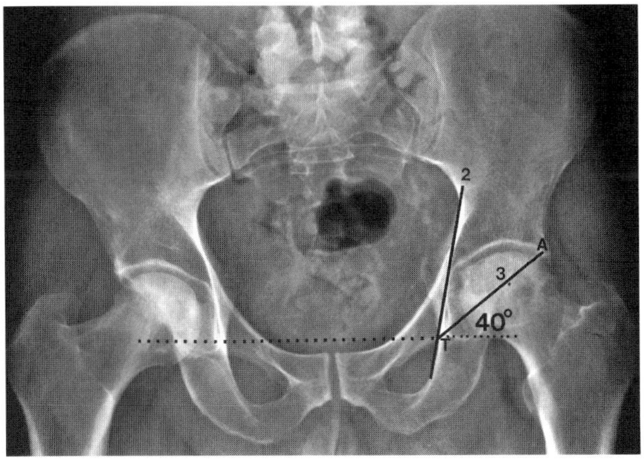

A

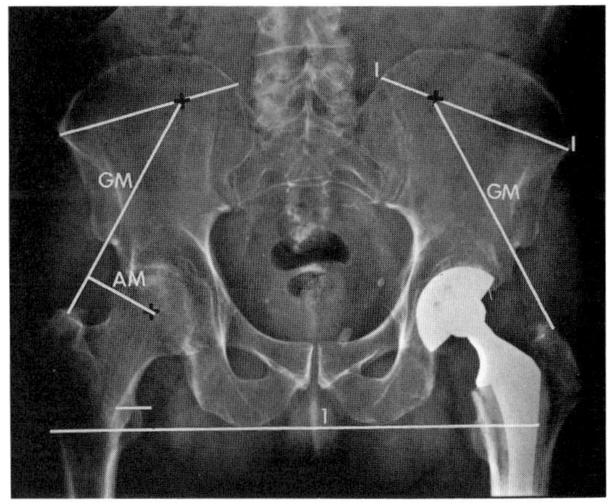

B

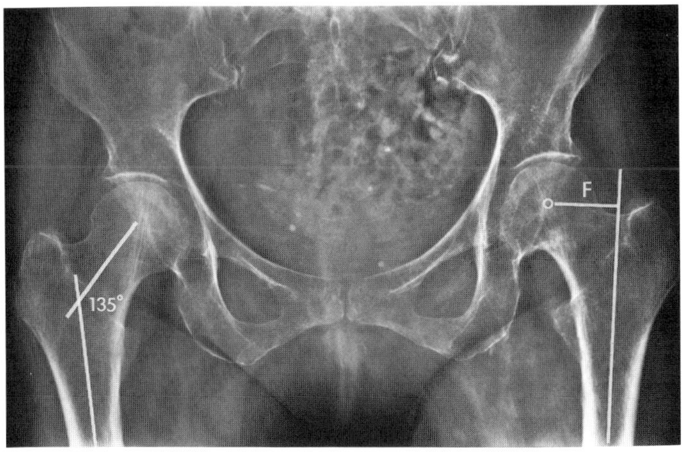

C

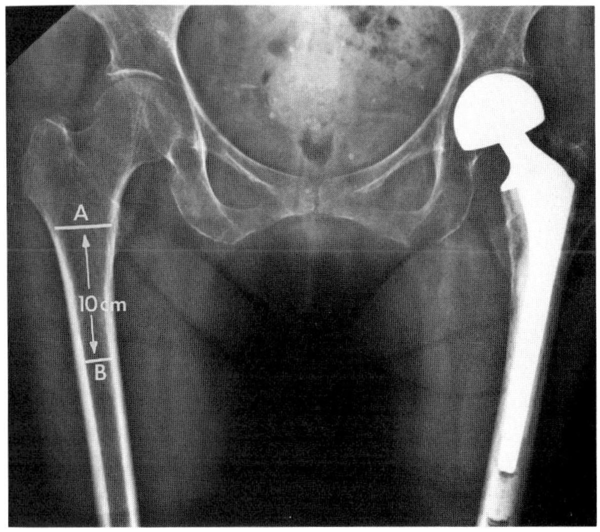

D

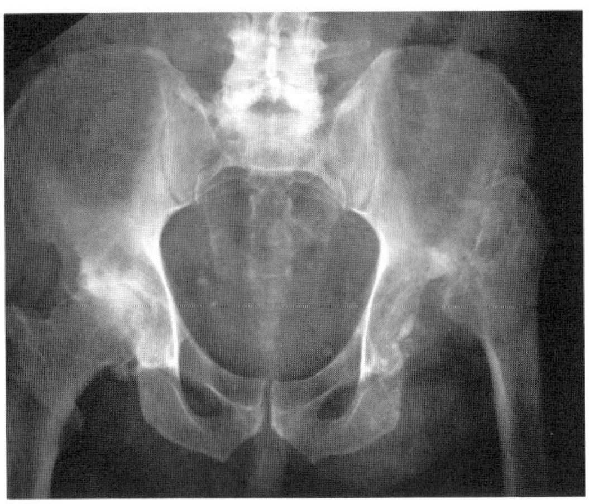

E

FIG. 4-89. Radiographic features and measurements on the AP view. **A:** An AP radiograph of the pelvis demonstrating stage III (articular collapse) AVN of the left femoral head. The right femur is not properly positioned (lesser trochanter not visible). The film does not include enough of the femoral shaft to evaluate the calcar-to-canal-isthmus ratio (CC ratio). At least 10 cm of the femur below the lesser trochanter must be included on the radiograph. Certain data can be obtained. *2,* Ilioischial line (Kohler's line). A line from the pelvic border of the sciatic notch to the lateral inferior edge of the obturator foramen. This is used to evaluate acetabular protrusion. *3,* Superior acetabular margin (*A*) to the inferior tear drop (*T*). This line is used to evaluate superior coverage. Angle formed with the horizontal teardrop line (*dotted line*) ≤ 45°. The teardrop line is drawn along the inferior margin of the acetabular "teardrop." This line can also be used to measure leg-length discrepancy by comparing distances to the lesser trochanter. **B:** An AP view of the pelvis with left hip replacement. *1,* Ischial tuberosity line. Note the superior position of the right lesser trochanter (*white line*) compared with the left. Gluteal muscle tract: this is determined by drawing one line connecting the anterior and posterior superior iliac spines (*I*). A second line is drawn from the greater tuberosity to the junction of the posterior and middle thirds (+) of the iliac (*I*) line. The second line (*GM*) defines the gluteal muscle plane. The abductor moment arm (*AM*) measured on the right is a perpendicular from the center of the femoral head (+) to the gluteal muscle tract (*GM*). **C:** An AP radiograph of the pelvis demonstrating the femoral offset. Coxa valga and vara are judged by the distance from the center of the femoral head *via* a perpendicular line (*F*) to a line through the center of the femoral shaft. The actual angle can also be measured as shown on the right hip (normal, 135°). **D:** An AP radiograph of the pelvis and upper femur to include sufficient femoral shaft to measure the femoral canal (CC ratio) and include the entire stem and cement for the left long-stem bipolar endoprosthesis. The CC ratio is obtained by measuring the marrow canal at the midlesser trochanter (*A*) and a second measurement 10 cm below (*B*) B/A × 100% = 50%. If the ratio is greater than 75%, a porous-coated femoral component may not be usable.[263,291] The normal ratio in young patients is 50%. This increases with age and bone loss.[264,291] **E:** An AP radiograph of the pelvis with destruction of the left femoral head and superior subluxation of the left femur. There is advanced osteoarthritis on the right with osteophytes and superior acetabular subchondral bone loss.

5. Gluteal muscle tract (Fig. 4-89A)
6. Abductor moment (Fig. 4-89A)
7. Coxa vara and valga (Fig. 4-89C)
8. Osteophytes, diffuse idiopathic skeletal hyperostosis (DISH), bone loss (Fig. 4-89E)

To evaluate all these features, it is often necessary to center the x-ray cassette for a pelvic radiograph, which includes the iliac crests (Fig. 4-89B) and a second AP view centered lower (Fig. 4-89C,D) to evaluate more of the femur.

Additional imaging studies may be required in some cases. Bone loss or deformity is often optimally evaluated with CT. Isotopic studies and MRI are useful in certain patients.[244,292] We find diagnostic injections with aspiration to be a useful preoperative technique in selected patients. This is useful for joint aspiration to exclude infection in some, but more importantly, it allows injection of the hip or, in some cases, the lumbar facet joint(s) or knee to confirm that the hip is the source of pain.[238,244]

Orthopedic vendors provide femoral and acetabular templates (Fig. 4-90). These provide valuable preoperative information for component selection and sizing. Adequate space for cement must be kept in mind when the femoral component will be cemented with methyl methacrylate.[242,263,285]

Component Selection and Design

Prostheses have evolved significantly over the years, with numerous femoral and acetabular component designs, new alloys, and surface coatings in use and under evaluation.[242,243,285,331,350,359,366]

Biomaterials for Implants

Orthopedic prostheses are configured using various metal alloys, high-density or ultrahigh molecular weight polyethylene (UHMWPE), and ceramic components.[256,283,284,320] Components are designed in an attempt to provide low friction, strength, and minimal local and systemic effects.[280,281,320]

Metal Alloys

Today, most metal components are composed of cobalt-chromium-molybdenum or titanium. Alloys are designed for strength, wear resistance, and inert properties. An oxidized state is used to provide resistance to corrosion. Alloys of iron or cobalt have a chromium oxidized surface.[320] Surface hardness of the metal is important and assists in maintaining a smooth surface and reducing wear. Hardness can be enhanced by placing a nitrogen surface on the metal or by ion implantation of the surface.[266,280,291,331]

Cobalt-chromium alloys are usually preferred over titanium for bearing surfaces because the latter is associated with more significant particulate metal debris. This problem is reduced by using a nitride coating on the titanium.[280,291]

A porous coating is used with many types of femoral components to facilitate bone ingrowth. The coating techniques include sintering, diffusion-bonding, and plasma-spray techniques.[249]

Sintering

This is a high-temperature process that allows particle-to-particle and particle-to-substrate bonding at contact points. This technique reduces fatigue strength by 20% to 40%. The strength of the noncoated portion of the stem is also reduced (Fig. 4-91).[249,291]

Diffusion Bonding

Relatively low temperatures are used in diffusion bonding compared with the sintering process. Pressure is used with titanium fiber metal, which also causes some weakening (Fig. 4-91).[249]

Plasma Spray

Metal powder is partially melted in a plasma flame and placed on the implant through a carrier gas with an applied electrical field in the plasma-spray technique. There is less surface porosity than with sintered beads or fiber mesh coating.[249,291,320]

Bone ingrowth on porous surfaces is dependent on the surface area of the porous coating, pore size, and implant stability (motion at bone-component interface).[249,273,291] Small pore size (< 100 μm) is suboptimal. Most agree that a pore size of 100 to 400 μm is optimal. Larger pore sizes and/or motion frequently lead to fibrous ingrowth.[248,320] Bone ingrowth can also be enhanced by calcium phosphate or hydroxyapatite coating.[249,262,370]

The different metal alloys have varying wear resistance. Titanium is less wear resistant than are cobalt alloys, especially if it is not treated with surface coating.[320,362]

Wear debris can result in local and potentially systemic changes. Although such changes have not yet been clearly identified as a clinical problem at this time, systemic reactions, such as hypersensitivity and carcinogenic effects, have been sought.[320]

It is known that a small percentage of the population may react to cobalt or nickel alloys, especially after cutaneous exposure, because these metals serve as haptens, leading to a type IV delayed hypersensitivity reaction.[280] Implant loosening or an increased porous surface area

(*text continues on page 277*)

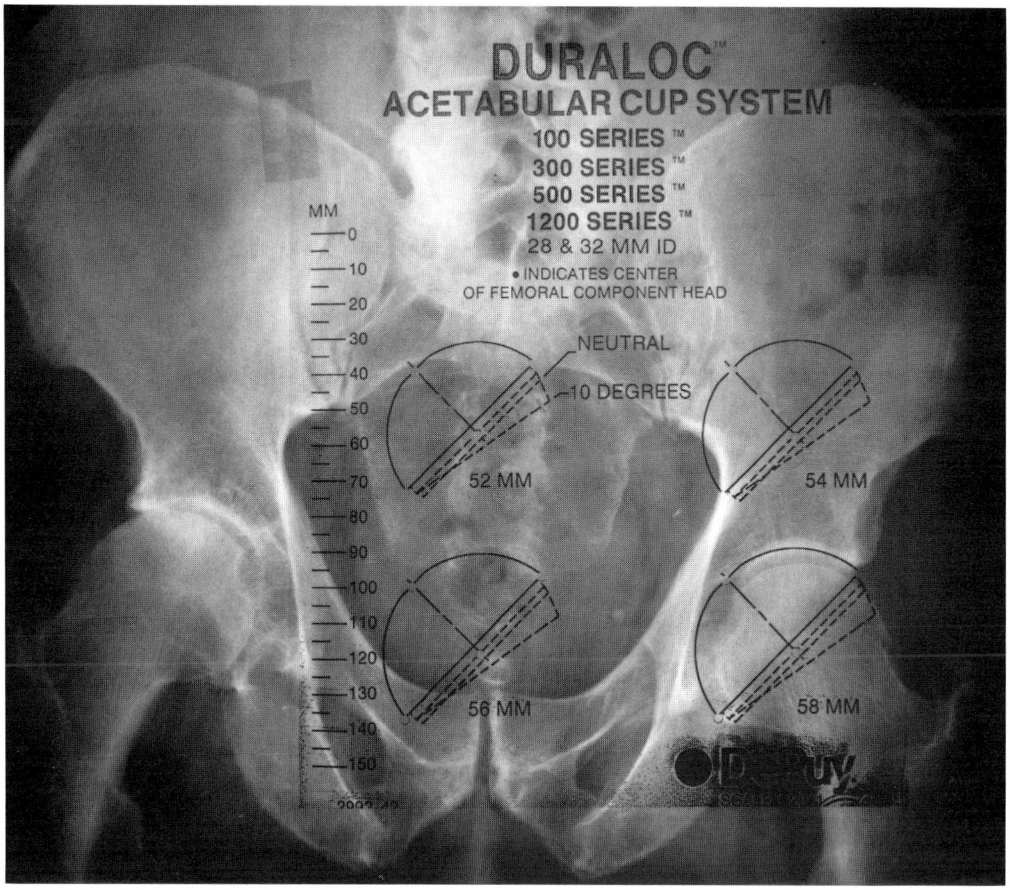

FIG. 4-90. An AP radiograph of the pelvis with an acetabular template in position on the left.

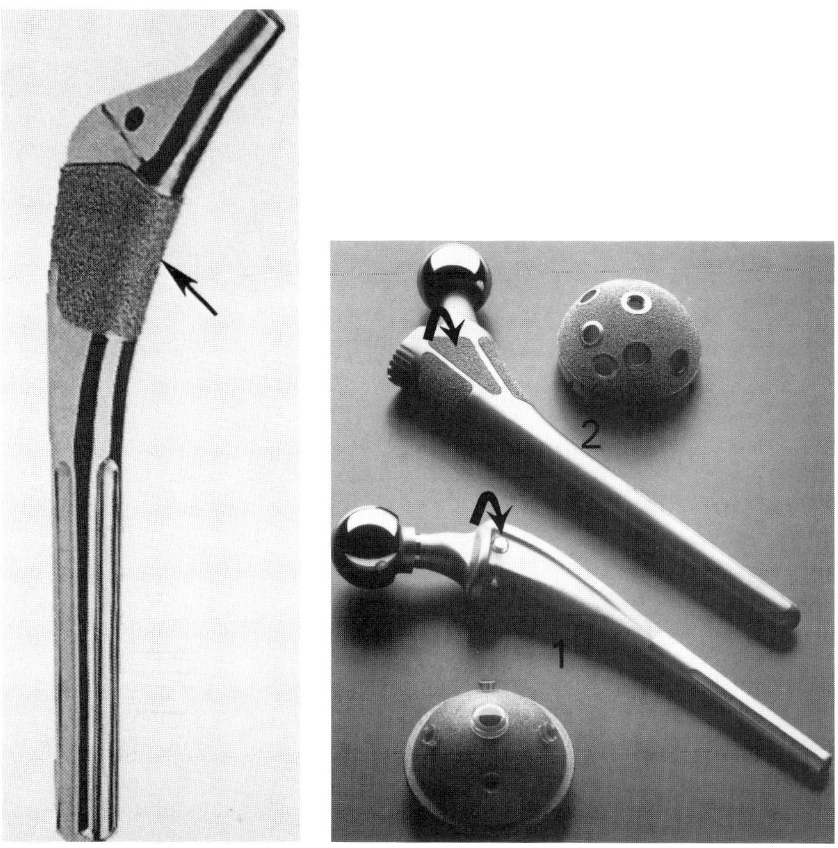

FIG. 4-91. Femoral components with different alloys and surfaces. **A:** Zimmer anatomic femoral component. Titanium Ti-6Al-4V alloy with Ti-nidium surface. Titanium fiber mesh pads on the neck (*arrow*). (Courtesy of Zimmer, Warsaw, IN.) **B:** P.F.C.™ arthroplasty components. The cemented stem (*1*) with proximal spacers (*arrow*) to optimize cement mantle thickness. The porous-coated stem (*2*) with 290-μm pore size (*arrow*). (See **C** on next page.) (Courtesy of Johnson and Johnson Orthopedics, Raynham, MA.)

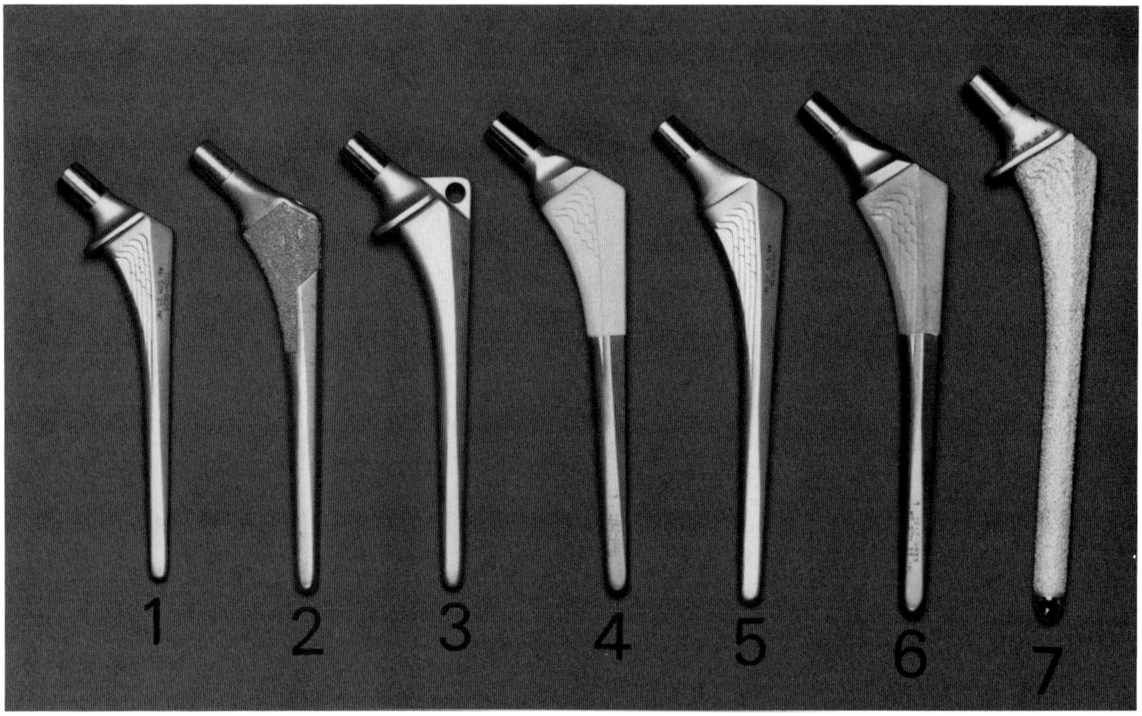

C

FIG. 4-91. (*Continued.*) **C:** Osteonics femoral component stems. (Courtesy of Osteonics, Allendale, NJ.) The Omnifit™ specialty stem (*7*) has a roughed surface over its entire length, except for the distal bullet tip. The Omnifit-HA™ (*6*) has a proximal hydroxyapatite surface.

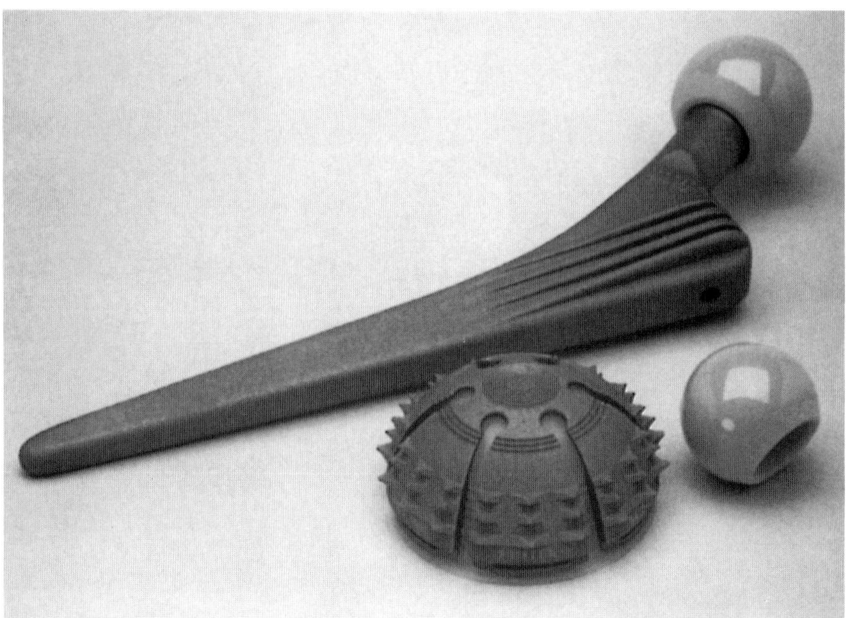

FIG. 4-92. CLS uncemented total hip replacement system. (Courtesy of Protek AG, Berne, Switzerland.) Three-dimensional TiGAl7N6 alloy femoral stem with a ceramic (BIOLOX™-Al_2O_3) modular head and titanium threaded acetabular component.

may increase the metal ion release rates.[280,320] Haynes et al.[300] demonstrated that cobalt-chromium particles cause a more local toxic response; titanium-aluminum-vanadium particles are more likely to stimulate systemic mediators, such as prostaglandin E_2.[280]

Ceramic Implants

Ceramic surfaces are hard, smooth, and wet under the physiologic conditions within the joint.[285] These features facilitate smooth articulation with UHMWPE acetabular components. Ceramic implants are used selectively in our practice in younger active patients in whom long-term wear is the greatest concern (Fig. 4-92).[272,285,336]

Polyethylene Components

The normal articular surface provides a smooth low-friction joint. To reproduce this with prosthetic components has been a challenge. Several combinations (metal to metal, ceramic, and metal to polyethylene) have been researched over the past few decades. Today, the most widely used articulation is polished metal on UHMWPE.[256,280,320,351]

Component Selection

There are numerous designs (unipolar, bipolar, total joint replacement, and modular) for hip arthroplasty components. The choice depends on the indications; anatomy; patient's age, weight, and activity; and of course, the surgeon's preference.[263,331]

Femoral Components

The femoral component may be unipolar or bipolar, a primary or standard total joint replacement component, or a special customized or revision design.

Unipolar Implants

Unipolar implants are used primarily for the treatment of fractures or femoral head abnormalities, such as AVN in the elderly population (Fig. 4-93).[318,321,354,382] Figures 4-94 to 4-96 illustrate examples of other types of endoprostheses. Newer modular designs with a wider selection of stem and head sizes may improve the survival of unipolar components.[318,382]

Bipolar Implants

Bipolar implants were designed to improve function and decrease acetabular wear, which were problems with unipolar endoprosthesis. Bipolar components have either a press fit or cemented femoral component. Femoral components may either be monolithic (with a single solid implant stem, head, or neck) or modular (with separate head and neck assemblies placed on the stem for flexibility in head size selection and neck length). The free-riding acetabular cup has a central polyethylene bearing with an outer metal shell cup. The original design was developed by Bateman (Fig. 4-82) in 1974.[241,318,321,352,375] Numerous series indicate success in pain relief and implant survival using bipolar prostheses.[284,318] A reduction in acetabular wear with bipolar implants compared with that in fixed-head unipolar devices has been documented.

Bipolar implants are most often used for femoral neck fractures or, occasionally, for patients with AVN, fractures, or other femoral head and neck pathologic findings. Implants have been reported to survive up to 15 years.[241,318] Figures 4-97 to 4-99 demonstrate examples of several types of bipolar prostheses.

Femoral Components for Total Hip Replacement

Modular systems today are frequently designed so that femoral stems can be more precisely sized to the patient's dimensions, e.g., femoral head, neck offset, and even the deformity caused by the underlying hip pathologic condition. Adjustment in leg length and soft tissue tension across the hip can be accomplished by designing the length of the modular head used with a bipolar configuration or for total joint replacement. This section further defines the variations of femoral components and their design.

Femoral component considerations and variations include the following:

1. Head size (modular or fixed to stem)
2. Neck geometry, angle, offset
3. Collar versus noncollar design
4. Stem configuration and length
5. Stem sleeves
6. Medullary canal plugs
7. Cemented versus uncemented (porous and press fit)

Femoral Head

The femoral head should provide a hard smooth articulating surface. Many sizes are available, but four standard dimensions are used widely: 22-, 26-, 28-, and 32-mm diameters. The original Charnley prosthesis (Fig. 4-100) had a 22-mm head. Larger head sizes theoretically increase hip stability and the range of motion, but acetabular wear is also increased. Larger head sizes require thinner polyethylene (Fig. 4-101) acetabular surfaces within a given cup size. Today, most prefer 22- to 28-mm head diameters.[330,366]

(*text continues on page 283*)

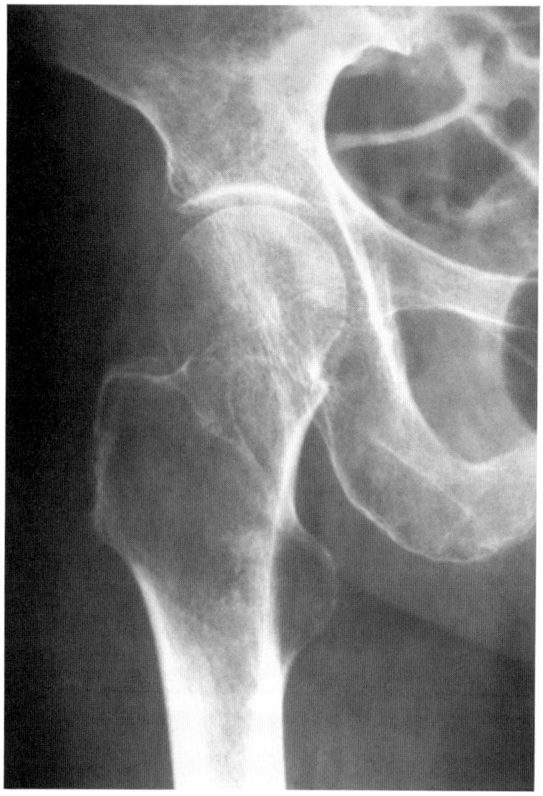

A

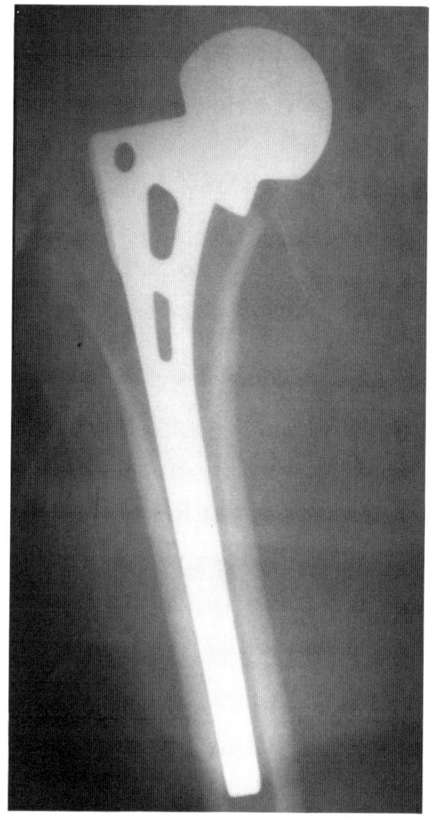

B

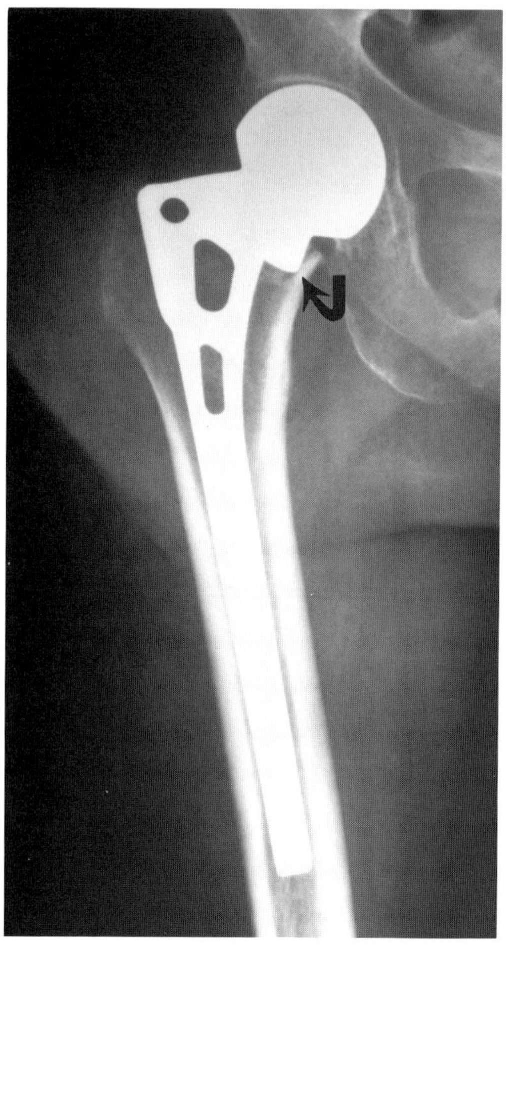

C

FIG. 4-93. A: Right femoral neck fracture demonstrated on AP radiograph. **B:** Postoperative radiograph demonstrating a straight fenestrated narrow-stem Moore endoprosthesis. **C:** Five days later, the component has subsided so the collar (*arrow*) is below the calcar.

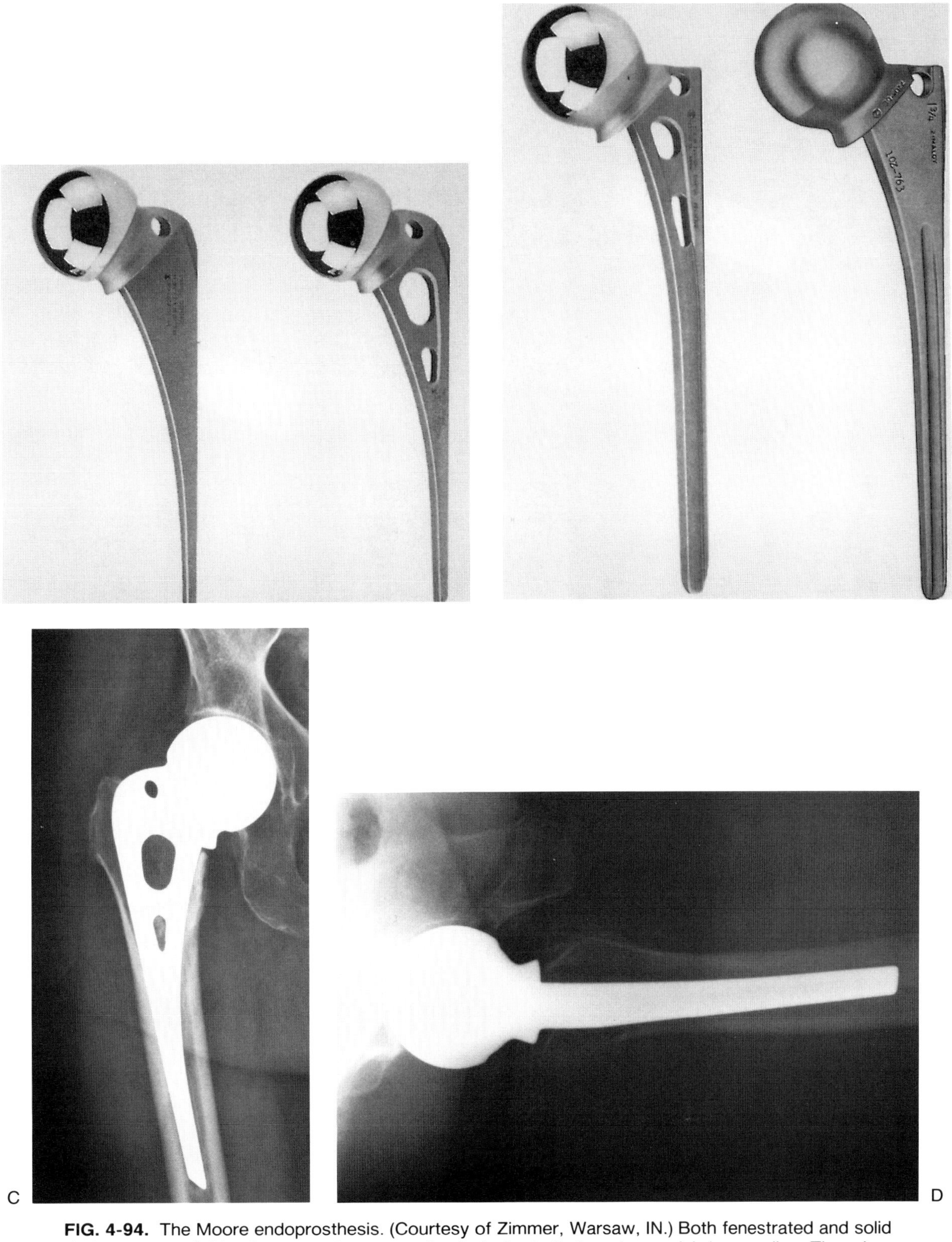

FIG. 4-94. The Moore endoprosthesis. (Courtesy of Zimmer, Warsaw, IN.) Both fenestrated and solid designs are available. Components are constructed of cobalt-chromium-molybdenum alloy. There is a hole in the lateral neck to facilitate impaction and removal. **A:** Solid left and fenestrated right standard design: head sizes, 38 to 63 mm; stem lengths, 127 to 152 mm. **B:** Straight solid right and fenestrated left design: head sizes, 38 to 63 mm; stem length, 165 to 191 mm. The AP **(C)** and lateral **(D)** radiographs of a standard Moore prosthesis.

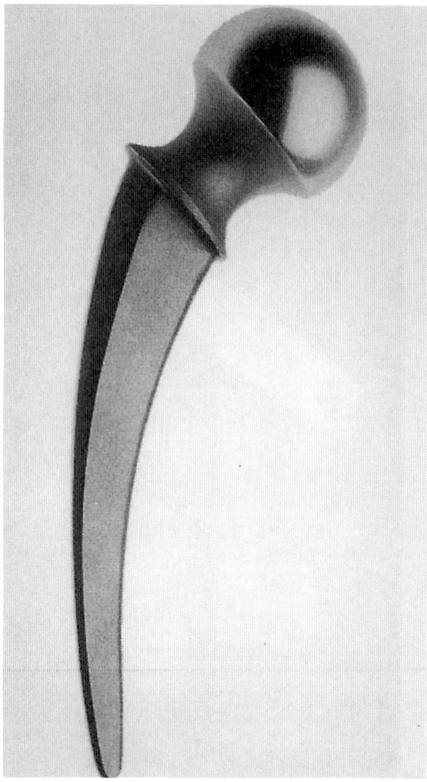

FIG. 4-95. Müller endoprosthesis. (Courtesy of Zimmer, Warsaw, IN.) Designed for cement use. Head size, 41 to 54 mm; cobalt-chromium-molybdenum alloy.

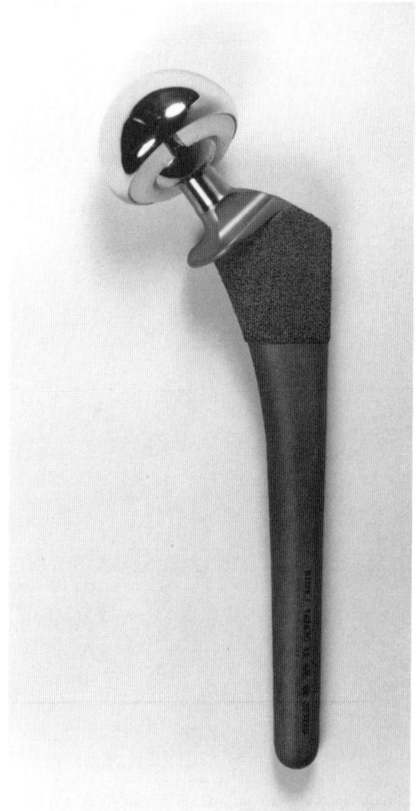

FIG. 4-97. A Biomet porous-coated femoral prosthesis with modular head and bipolar cup attached. (Courtesy of Biomet, Warsaw, IN.)

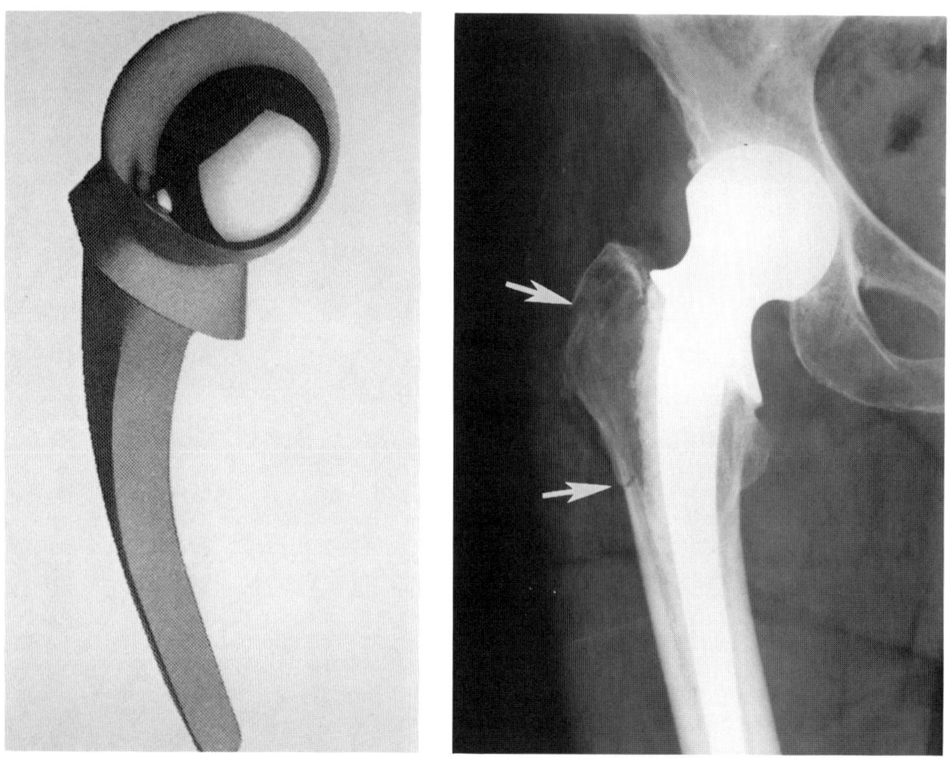

A B

FIG. 4-96. A: Thompson endoprosthesis. (Courtesy of Zimmer, Warsaw, IN.) Cobalt-chromium-molybdenum alloy. Head sizes, 38 to 63 mm; stem length, 105 mm. **B:** An AP radiograph of a cemented Thompson endoprosthesis. There are fractures of the greater trochanter and shaft (*arrows*).

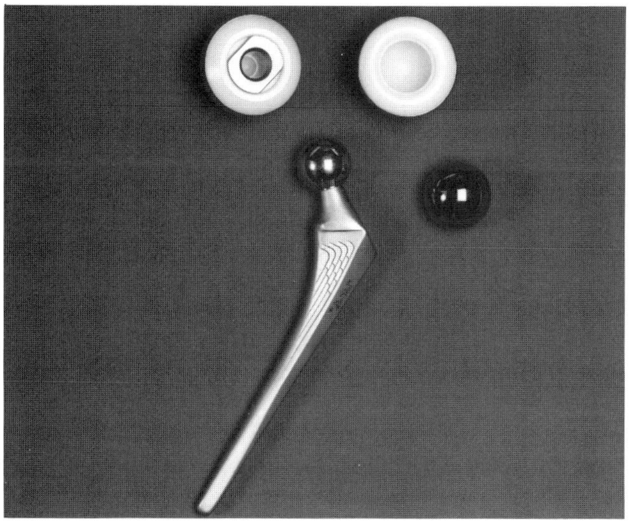

FIG. 4-98. Osteonics Omnifit^{TM} modular bipolar component. (Courtesy of Osteonics, Allendale, NJ.)

A

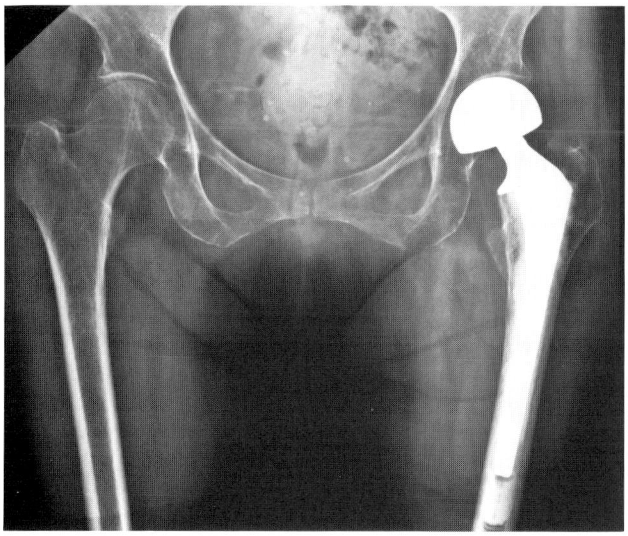

B,C

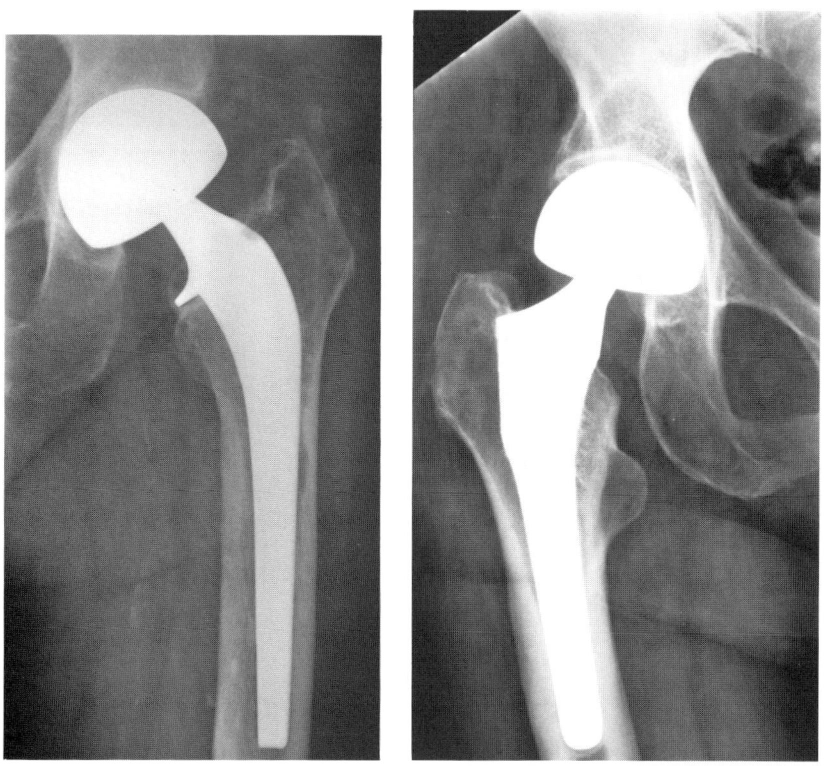

FIG. 4-99. The AP radiographs of cemented **(A)**, press fit **(B)**, and porous-coated **(C)** bipolar components, all inserted in patient younger than 65 years of age for femoral neck fractures or AVN of the femoral head.

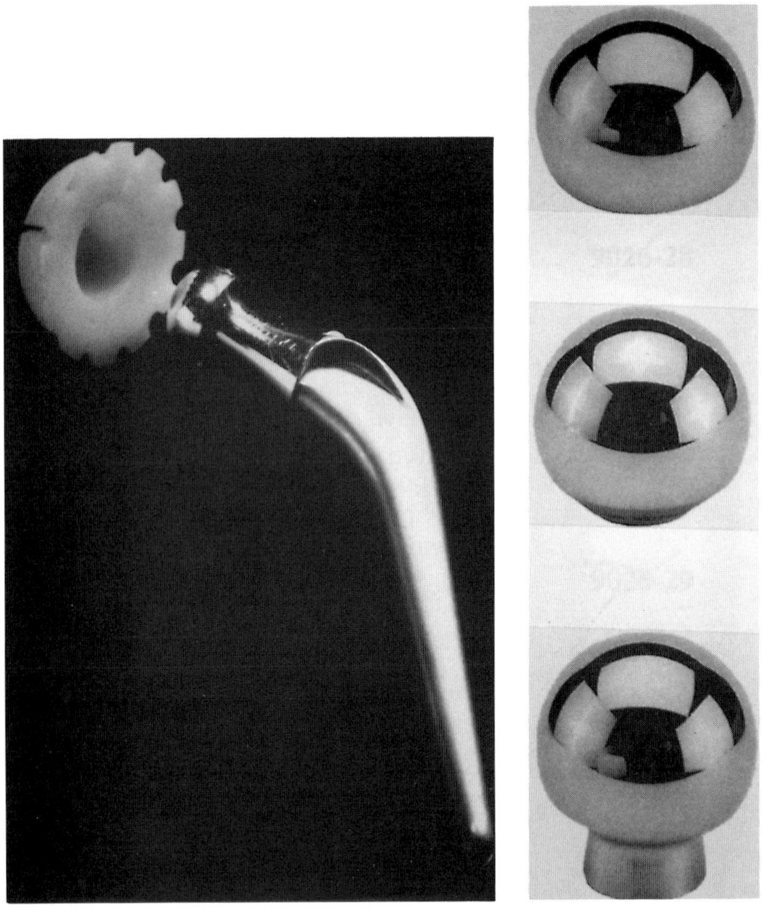

A,B

FIG. 4-100. A: The Charnley total hip with a 22-mm head and polyethylene acetabular component. (From Bentley E, Dowd G. Surgical treatment of arthritis in the elderly. *Rheum Dis Clin North Am* 1986;12:290–313.) **B:** Modular femoral head components with different neck lengths. These modular heads are available in 22-, 26-, 28-, and 32-mm diameters. (Courtesy of Zimmer, Warsaw, IN.)

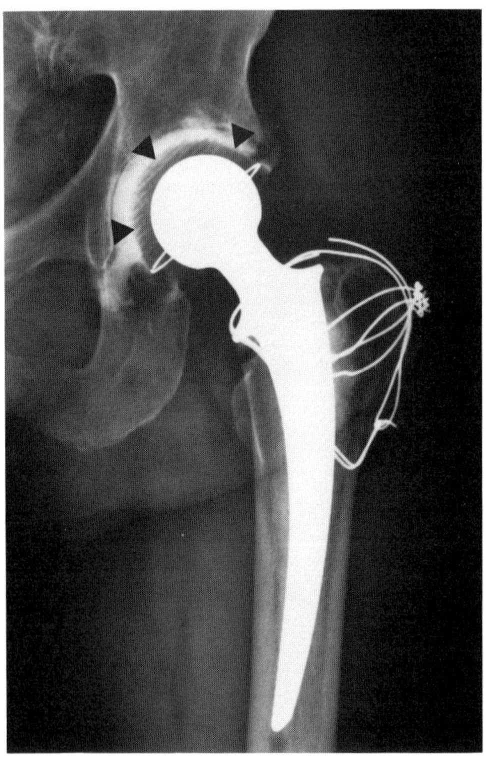

FIG. 4-101. An AP view of the left hip with a cemented Charnley-Müller total hip. Note the thinner acetabular polyethylene (*arrowheads*) and larger head size (32 mm) compared with the Charnley prosthesis with a 22-mm head in Figs. 4-85 and 4-100. Note, coincidentally, that there is x-ray evidence of superolateral polyethylene wear (narrowing) and acetabular loosening at the cement bone interface.

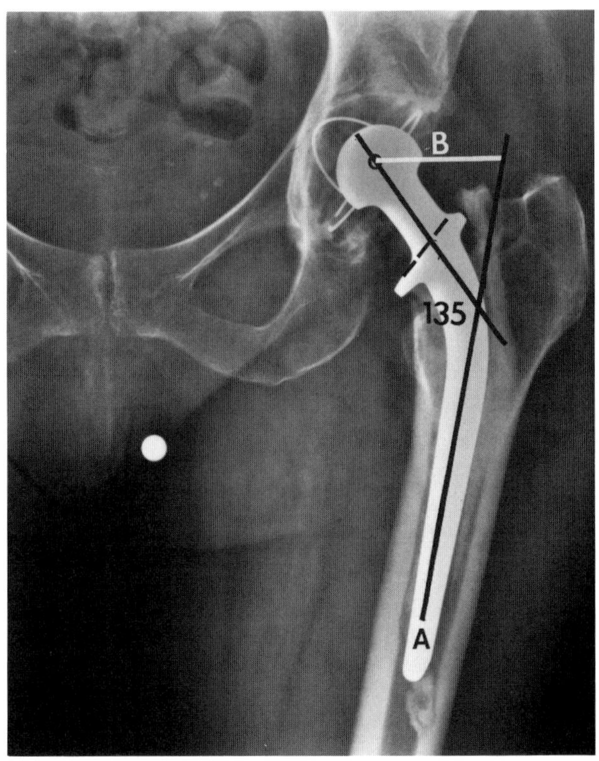

FIG. 4-102. An AP view of the pelvis demonstrating a trapezoidal-28 (T-28) left hip arthroplasty. The neck angle is 135°. The neck offset is measured from the line longitudinal to the stem (*A*) to the center of the femoral head (*line B*). The neck length is measured from the center of the femoral head (*O*) to the base of the neck (*dotted line*).

Femoral Neck

There is significant load distributed through the neck region. Although numerous variations of the geometry, stem angle length, and offset (Fig. 4-102) have been attempted, certain aspects of the neck of the femoral component are fairly standard. The angle is fairly well established (Fig. 4-102) at 135°, which is similar to the normal femur.[280,366] Most prosthetic femoral necks are 30- to 40-mm wide, with an average diameter of 35 mm. The necks of some modular components are thinner (Fig. 4-99). Device breakage caused by fatique failure at head-neck modular connections has occurred with several different designs.

Collars

The use of collars on the femoral component has been debated. Most collars extend medially to contact the calcar (Figs. 4-103 and 4-104). Some collars also extend anteriorly and posteriorly. When used with cement, the collar limits distal subsidence on the cement mantle. However, the cement mantle often fragments, and calcar resorption (Fig. 4-105) is common. Decreased loosening problems have been reported with cement and collared components in some series. The utility of collars without cement is not as well documented. Collars theoretically reduce subsidence, which decreases motion and enhances bone ingrowth. On the other hand, if no collar is present, slight subsidence may improve the fit.[331,366] Figure 4-106 demonstrates one system with a modular collar, which may be used or not used, as desired by the operating surgeon.

Femoral Stems

Femoral components continue to evolve as engineers strive to improve the survival of hip implants and prevent loosening. Variations in the head, neck, and collar have been noted previously. However, there are multiple other variations in the femoral component. These differences include shape, length, alloy, and coatings. Most femoral components are constructed of titanium or cobalt-chromium-molybdenum alloys. Titanium is more often used uncemented and cobalt-chromium-molybdenum, with cement.[249,306]

Curved stems with sharp edges, such as the Müller implant (Fig.4-101), are rarely used today because the cement mantle is subjected to excessive stress and can be too difficult to maintain uniformly around the implant.[379] Today, straight tapered stems, such as the Harris-Galante (Fig. 4-107), or anatomic femoral components (Fig. 4-108) and curved press-fit components are most commonly used for primary implants.[250] Straight-stem components may require more bone modification proximally to accept the component because curved anatomic stems more closely fit the anatomy of the normal upper femur.[250,331,366]

The length of the stem is variable (120 to 160 mm for primary and longer, > 200 mm, for revision stems), and length has implications with regard to survival and stress patterns. Shorter stems create higher stress proximally. Longer stems increase stem stress and transfer stress distally while shielding the bone proximally.

Femoral components may be coated with various substances and porous materials. Titanium stems are often coated with titanium nitride (Fig. 4-108) to increase surface hardness and reduce metal debris.[280] Porous coating, precoating with methyl methacrylate, hydroxyapatite, and other surface-roughing techniques are used to enhance cement technique or bone ingrowth.[249,261,269,370,371] These designs are basically developed for components to be cemented and press fitted. Press-fit components are often used in younger patients to reduce cement failures, with the hope that they may be more durable. Either smooth or porous stems can be used.

Cement techniques have improved significantly since the original work by Charnley in 1962.[252,254,261,351] Cement is effective but may be one of the weak links in hip arthroplasty.[269,311] Modifications in methyl methacrylate have occurred over the years. Low-viscosity methyl methacrylate more easily extrudes into bone, but its fatigue strength is reduced. The addition of carbon fibers increases the strength of the cement but decreases its protrusion into bone.[261,269,311] Cement spacers (Fig. 4-109) and distal plugs (Fig. 4-110) are used to improve and control the distribution of cement.[249,269,311] The distribution and thickness are important to prevent implant loosening. The femoral stem should be central and neutral, specifically not in > 5° varus position, with cement distributed without voids around the component. Ebramzadeh et al.[269] evaluated cement thickness and component-canal ratios in 836 cemented femoral components. When the medial cement mantle measured at the upper medial margin (Fig. 4-111) was 2 to 5 mm, the outcomes were superior to those with a thinner or thicker mantle. Less than 2 mm of residual cancellous bone medially was also superior for survival. Stems that filled greater than 50% of the canal (Fig. 4-111) also had superior results.

Stem Sleeves

Stem sleeves are also available for the proximal and distal stem. Distal sleeves are available in several sizes and lengths (Fig. 4-112) to improve fit and reduce the transfer to bullet tips or centralizers (Fig. 4-106).

Proximal sleeves and stem modifications are also

(*text continues on page 289*)

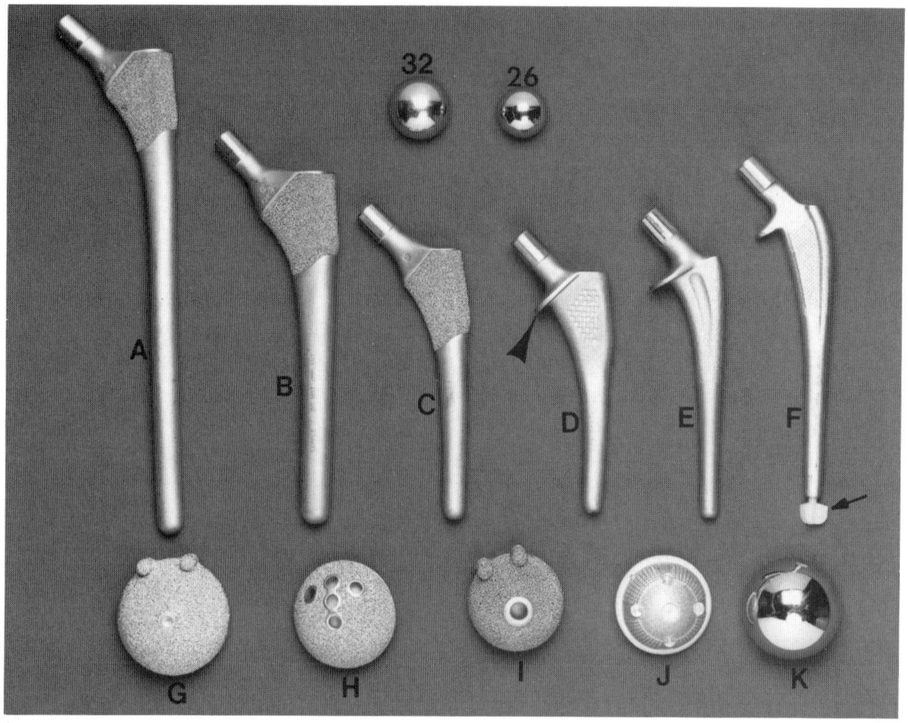

FIG. 4-103. Hip systems with and without collars. (Courtesy of Howmedica, Rutherford, NJ.) Stem is Vitallium alloy. **A:** Porous-coated anatomic (PCA) device with long stem. **B:** PCA with medium stem. **C:** PCA with short stem. **D:** Precision series E with textured stem and medial collar (*arrow*). **E,F:** Precision stems with distal centralizer on F (*arrow*). *Top:* The 32- and 26-mm modular heads. *Bottom:* Acetabular components seen from attachment side **(G–J)** and bipolar component **(K)**.

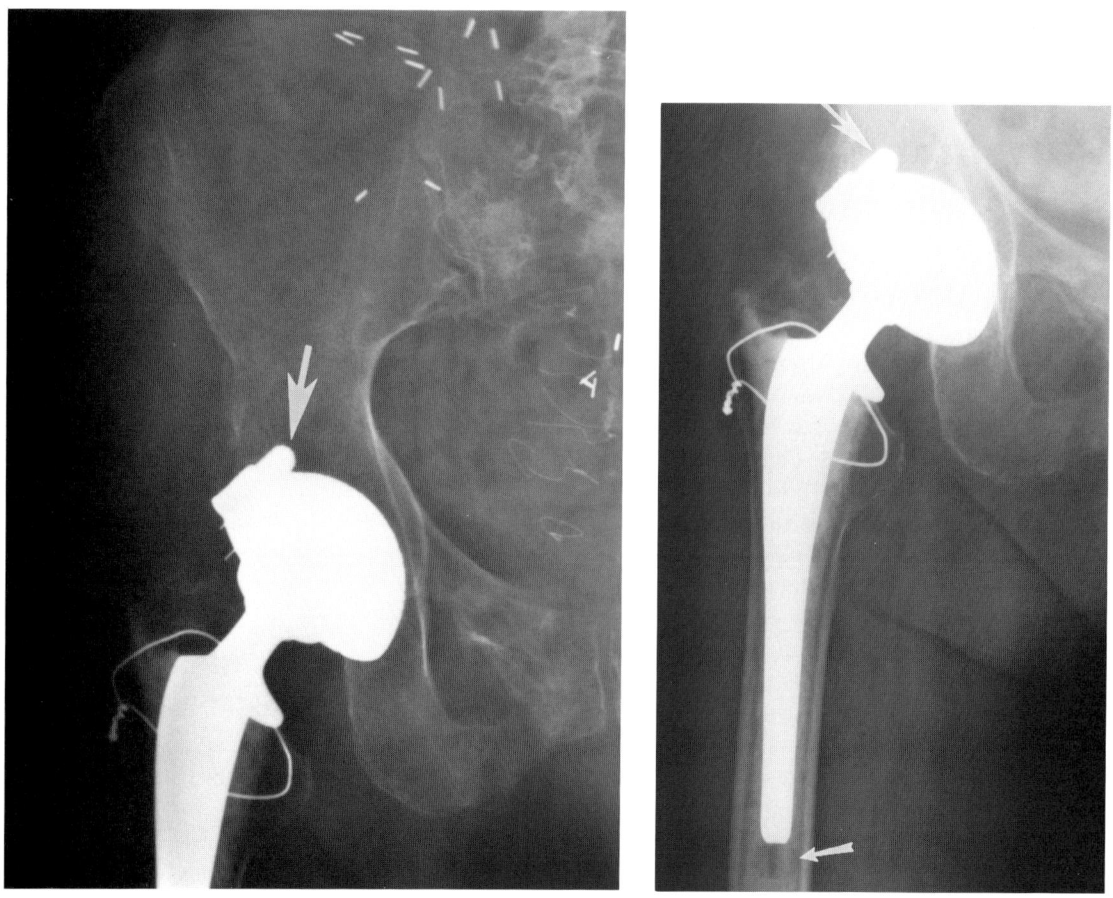

A B

FIG. 4-104. Howmedica hip arthroplasty on the right. The AP views of the pelvis **(A)**, upper femur **(B)**, and lateral view **(C)** demonstrate a PCA acetabular component. (Note the lateral porous-coated peg, *arrow*). The femoral component is a cemented Precision^{TM} stem (collar) with a distal centralizer (*lower arrow* in B).

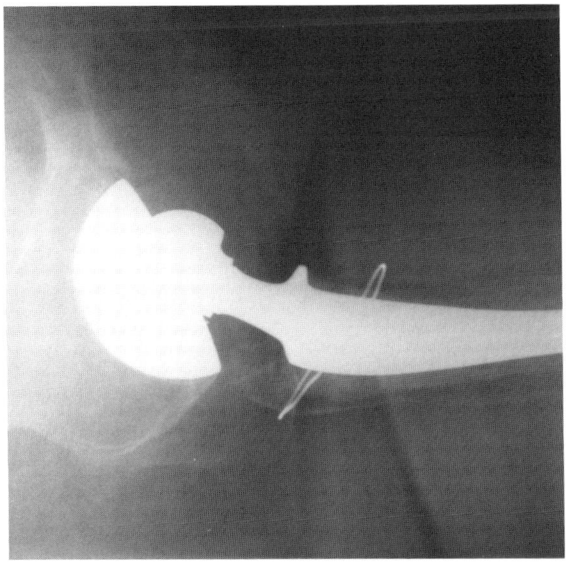

C

FIG. 4-104. *Continued.*

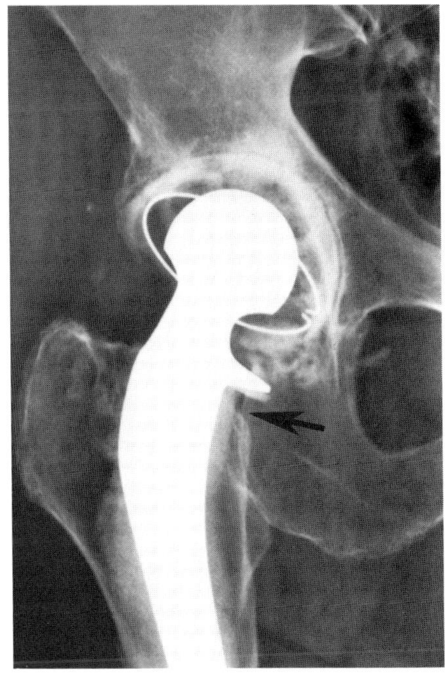

FIG. 4-105. Cemented total hip arthroplasty. The cement mantle under the medial collar is fragmented and the calcar resorbed (*arrow*).

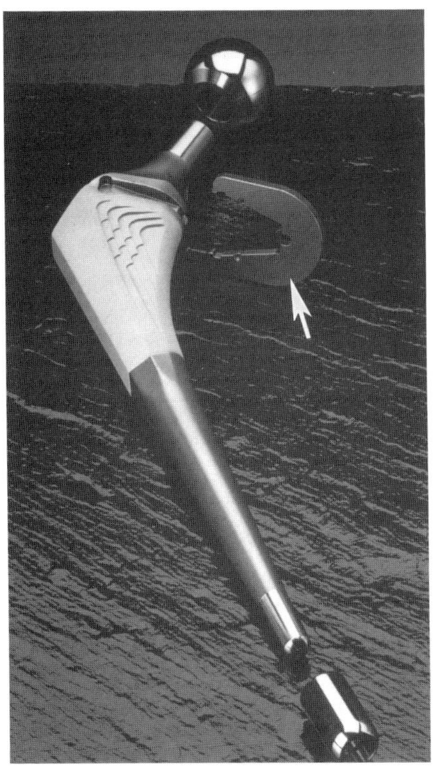

A

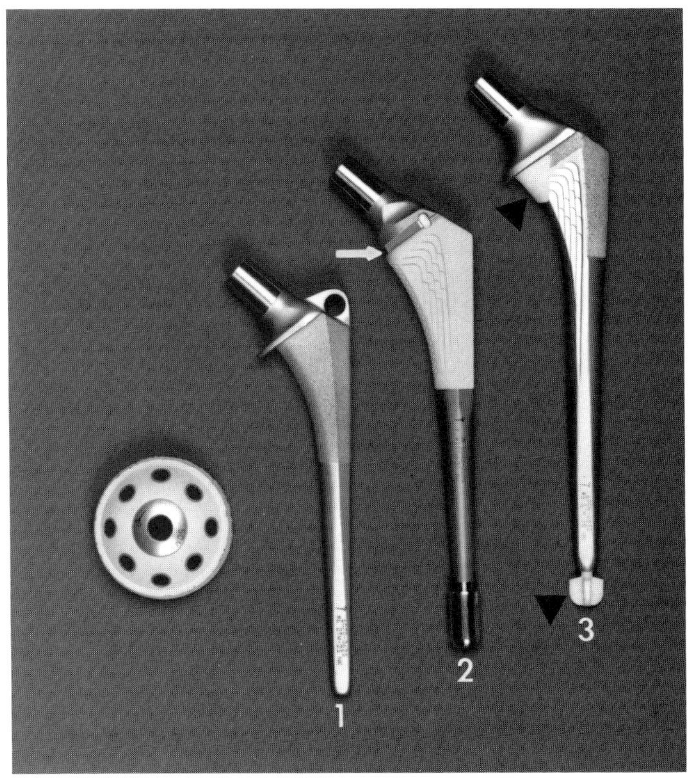

B

FIG. 4-106. Osteonics hip systems. (Courtesy of Osteonics, Allendale, NJ.) **A:** The Omniflex-HA™ system with modular collar (*arrow*) and distal tip (sizes, 8 to 25 mm). **B:** Osteonics femoral stems (*1–3*) and DUAL geometry hydroxyapatite acetabular component. *1,* Osteonics Hemihip; *2,* Omniflex-HA™ without collar (*arrow*), but with modular tip; *3,* Omnifit "C" stem with modular upper spacer and lower centralizer (*arrowheads*). The AP **(C)** and lateral **(D)** radiographs of an Osteonics Omniflex-HA™ femoral component without the collar (*arrow*). The modular tip is in place. This system has a fairly characteristic radiographic appearance. There is no cement used with this component. (See **C** and **D** on next page.)

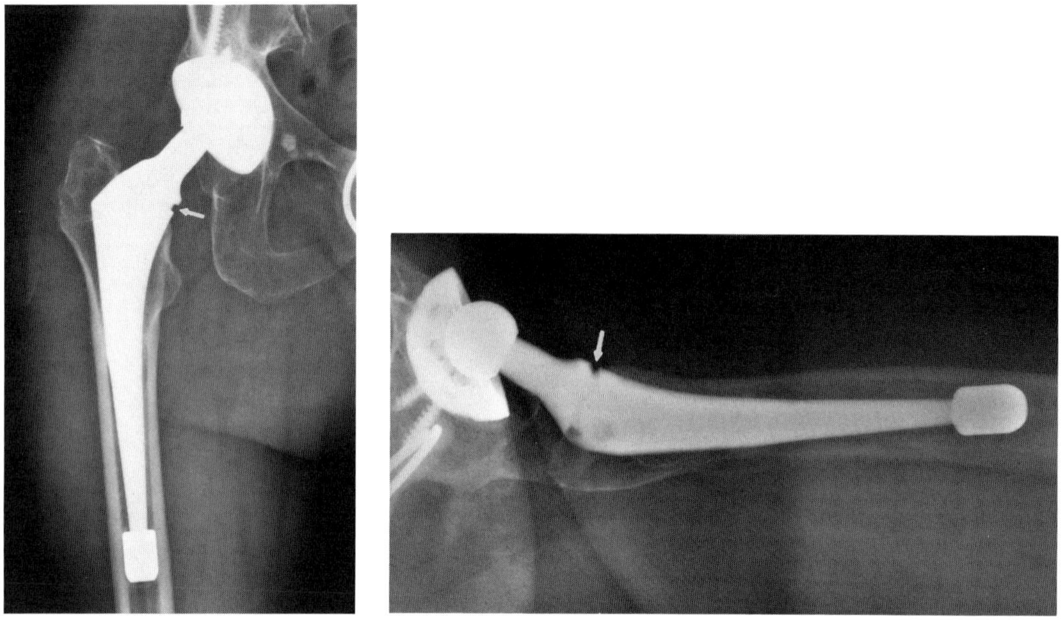

C

D

FIG. 4-106. *Continued.*

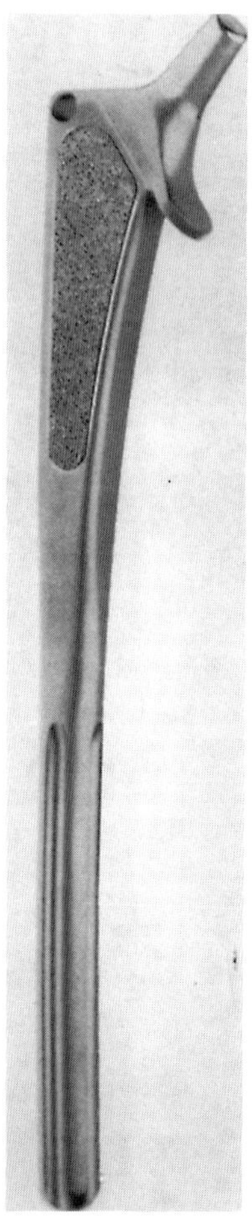

FIG. 4-107. BIAS total hip femoral component configured with a straight stem and upper taper plus a medial collar. The prosthesis is titanium (Ti-6Al-4V) with titanium fiber metal pads proximally. The Morse taper neck allows four different head sizes to be used. (Courtesy of Zimmer, Warsaw, IN.)

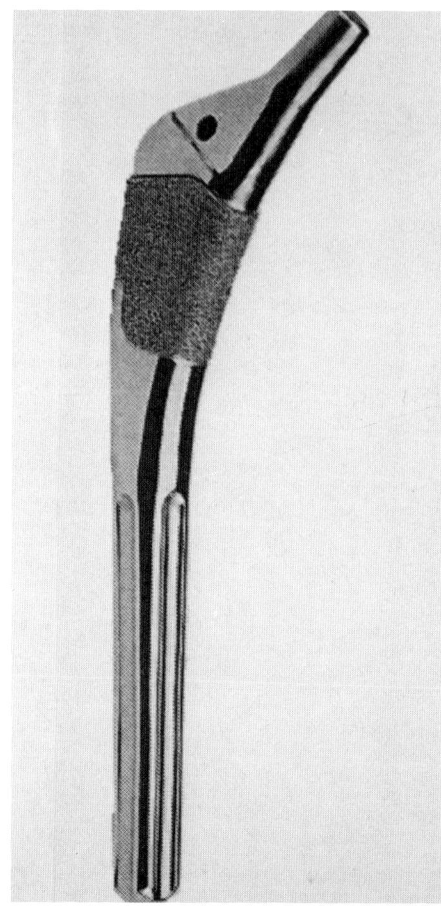

FIG. 4-108. Anatomic curved stem prosthesis of titanium Ti-6Al-4V alloy with curves to match femoral anatomy. The neck is antiverted 12°, and there is a proximal titanium fiber mesh surface. (Courtesy of Zimmer, Warsaw, IN.)

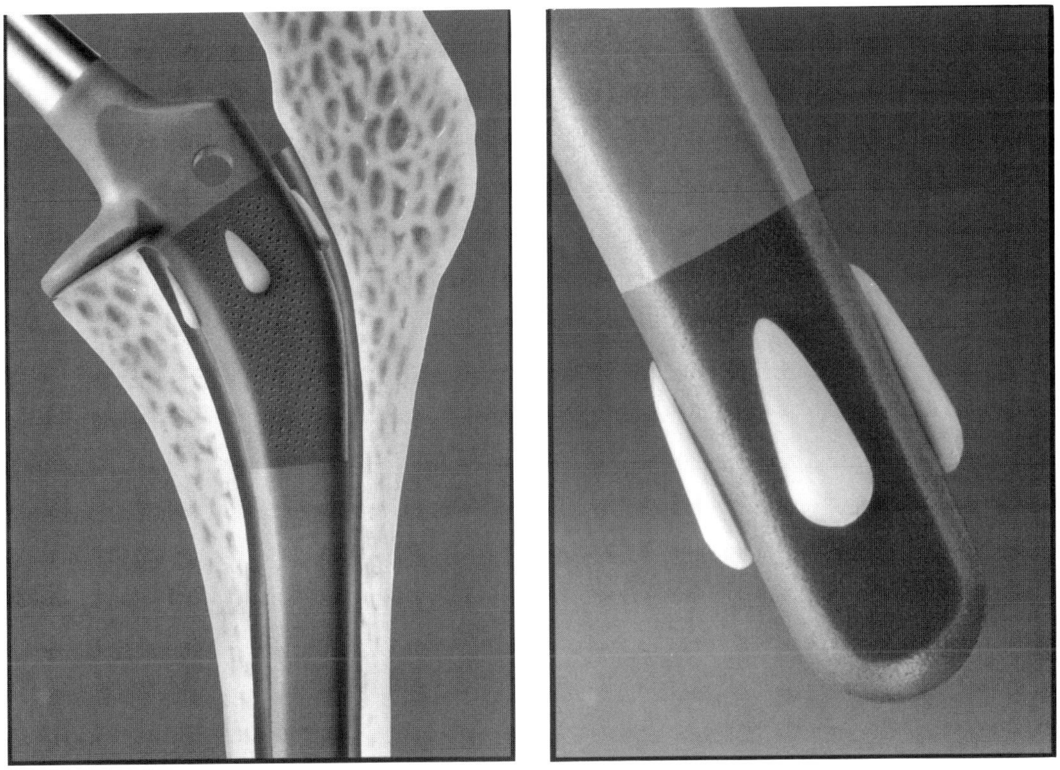

A B

FIG. 4-109. Centralign^{TM} precoat prosthesis. (Courtesy of Zimmer, Warsaw, IN.) The component is precoated with polymethyl methacrylate proximally and distally. There are polymethyl methacrylate centralizers proximally **(A)** and distally **(B)** to assist in positioning and cement mantle formation.

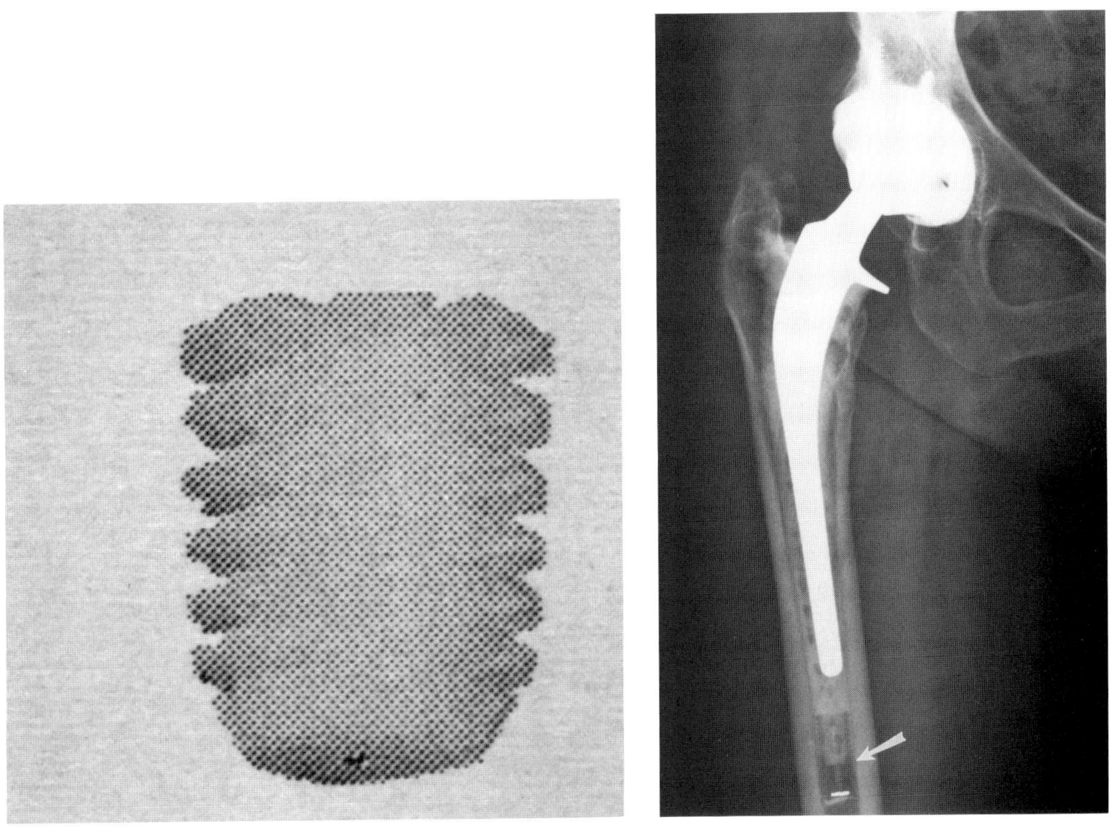

A B

FIG. 4-110. A: Cement restrictor, which is positioned in the canal below the femoral component tip to restrict cement flow. (Courtesy of DePuy, Warsaw, IN.) **B:** An AP radiograph of the femur with cemented femoral component and distal nonopaque cement restrictor (*arrow*) with opaque marker.

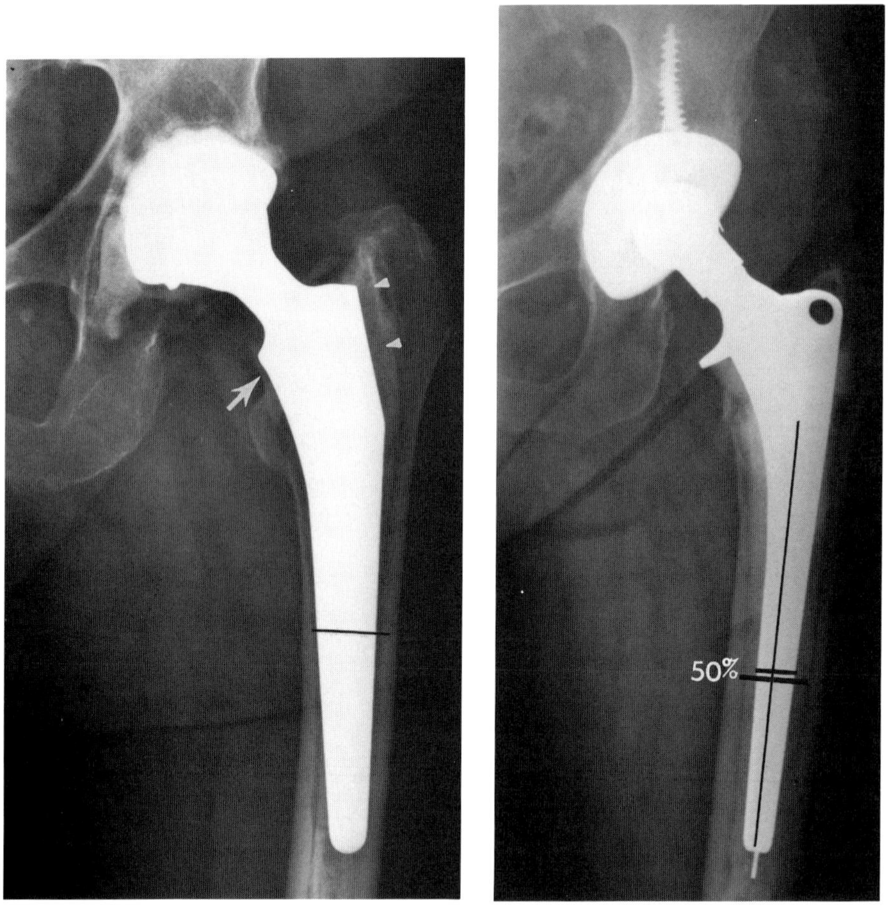

A,B

FIG. 4-111. A: Cemented femoral component with little if any cement medially (*arrow*). The femoral component measured at the junction of the mid and distal thirds (*line*) fills >50% of the narrow space. The component has shifted into varus position (note metal cement gap (*arrowheads*) superiorly. **B:** Osteonics cemented femoral component in neutral position (*line*) with good cement mantle The component fills 50% of the canal.

FIG. 4-112. A: Stem sleeves with 2- (*left*) and 4-mm thicknesses (*right*). (Courtesy of Intermedics Orthopedics, Austin, TX.) The AP **(B)** and lateral **(C)** radiographs of an Intermedics APR II^{TM} hip system with full-length sleeve (*1*, *arrow*), a modular head (*2*), and a fully coated titanium acetabular component with two 6.5-mm cancellous screws for fixation.

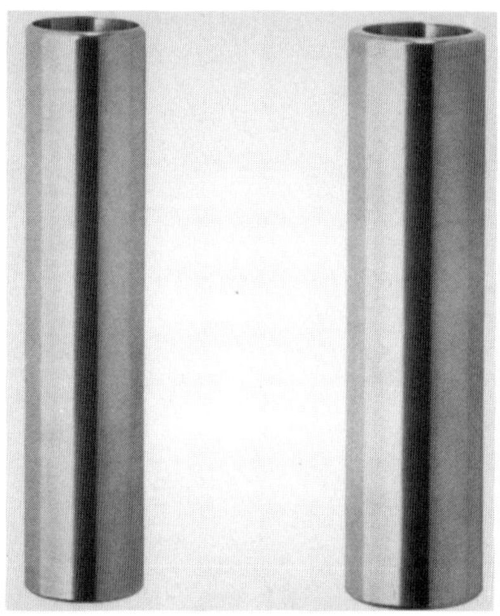

A

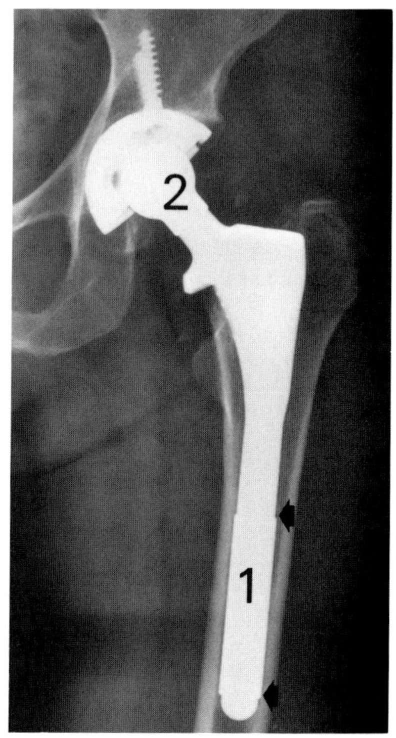

B

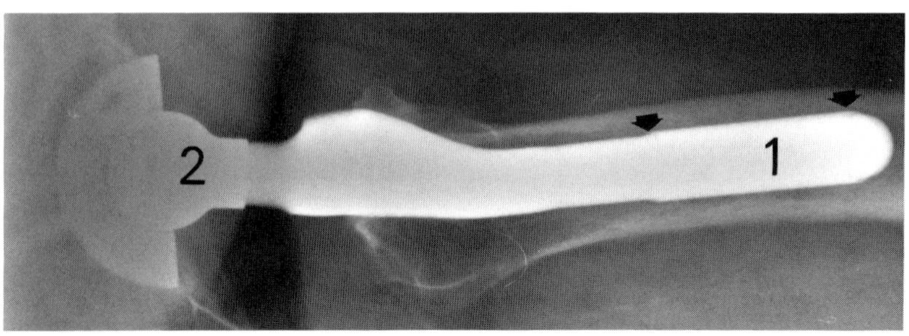

C

available in several configurations. Those that are easily identified radiographically give a significantly different appearance to the femoral component (Fig. 4-113).

Figures 4-114 to 4-122 demonstrate features of other hip systems and femoral components.

Acetabular Components

The initial hip arthroplasty components were metal on metal (Figs. 4-83 and 4-84).[242] The Charnley prosthesis and its later Müller modification (Figs. 4-85, 4-91, and 4-101) converted to cemented high-density polyethylene acetabular components.[242,277,319,333,348,369] In 1971, Harris[296] introduced the metal-backed acetabular component. This was originally considered to allow the replacement of the inner polyethylene liner.[348] Since that time, the metal backing has also been demonstrated to decrease and improve the distribution of stress to the acetabular bone.[331,349] There is some controversy concerning the failure rates of all polyethylene and metal-backed components.[331,349,383] Many still prefer metal-backed components, but there has been a dramatic resurgence in the use of polyethylene cups when cementing total hip arthroplasties in elderly low-demand patients.[331,383]

With the addition of porous-coated metal backing, additional questions arose in regard to the need for cement with metal-backed acetabular components. Uncemented designs may be a simple shell, may be threaded, have pegs or projections, or use cancellous screws to improve fixation. Some authors prefer porous implants without cement. Decreased bone lysis and heterotopic bone formation have been reported with uncemented systems.[249] Most acetabular components currently inserted in the United States are uncemented designs.[326,342,343,365] Figures 4-123 to 4-125 demonstrate common variations in acetabular components. Other systems were demonstrated in Figs. 4-114 to 4-122.

Special Primary Designs

There have been several special primary hip arthroplasty designs developed in recent years. Morrey,[332] at the Mayo Clinic, developed a short-stem femoral component (60 mm) with 150° valgus neck. The femoral component design (Fig. 4-126) requires less bone removal and, therefore, should be better suited to later revision if necessary. This technique may be particularly useful in young patients with small bones or congenital disorders.

Huo et al.[307] reported on a cemented low-offset femoral stem (Fig. 4-127) and conventional acetabular components for dysplastic hips. The diagnoses included coxa vara, congenital dislocation, achondrodysplasia, and spondyloephiphyseal dysplasia (Fig. 4-127).

Postoperative Imaging and Complications

The evaluation of cemented and uncemented hip components can usually be accomplished with serial radiographs and clinical evaluation. Pre- and postoperative hip scores can be used for comparison. When implant failure is suspected, imaging techniques and diagnostic injections with or without associated arthrography play a valuable role in defining the nature of the patients symptoms (i.e., intraarticular or implant related versus periarticular or unrelated to the arthroplasty components). This section outlines the normal radiographic features and the evaluation of specific complications using imaging techniques.

Normal Postoperative Radiographs

Radiologists should be familiar with normal measurements, zones for the evaluation of femoral and acetabular components, and the radiographic features that are significant (i.e., indicate loosening or infection) and insignificant.[240,251,267,292,308,310,323] Cemented and uncemented components may be used. An awareness of normal and abnormal radiographic features in either setting is important. Today, it is not unusual to have cemented femoral and uncemented acetabular components.

Certain measurements are used to evaluate the femoral and acetabular components and provide baseline information for follow-up (Fig. 4-128). The position of both components should be carefully assessed on AP and lateral radiographs. It is essential to exclude the entire femoral component on both the AP and lateral view. The femur should be included to several centimeters below the cement plug or 4 to 5 cm distal to the tip of an uncemented femoral component (Fig. 4-129).

An evaluation of the cement technique or fit with uncemented femoral components should also be considered on postoperative baseline studies.[269,292,382] For uncemented components, the stem below the lesser trochanter on the AP view is considered an optimal fit if it is within 1 mm of the cortex (Fig. 4-130). When less than 10% of the stem is within 1 mm of the cortex (calculated against the stem length), the fit is considered poor; when 10% to 40%, fair; and when greater than 40%, good.[292,302] On the lateral radiograph, the stem should be within 2 mm of the cortex at two of three possible contact points [(1) proximal anterior, (2) distal anterior, or (3) posterior; Fig. 4-131)].[302]

Current techniques have improved both because of new component designs (Fig. 4-132; see also Figs. 4-109, 4-110, and 4-120B,C) and better cement placement procedures (cement guns, cement restrictions, and centralizers and spacers on components).[269,270,336,340] Early studies demonstrated increased failure rates when there was

(text continues on page 313)

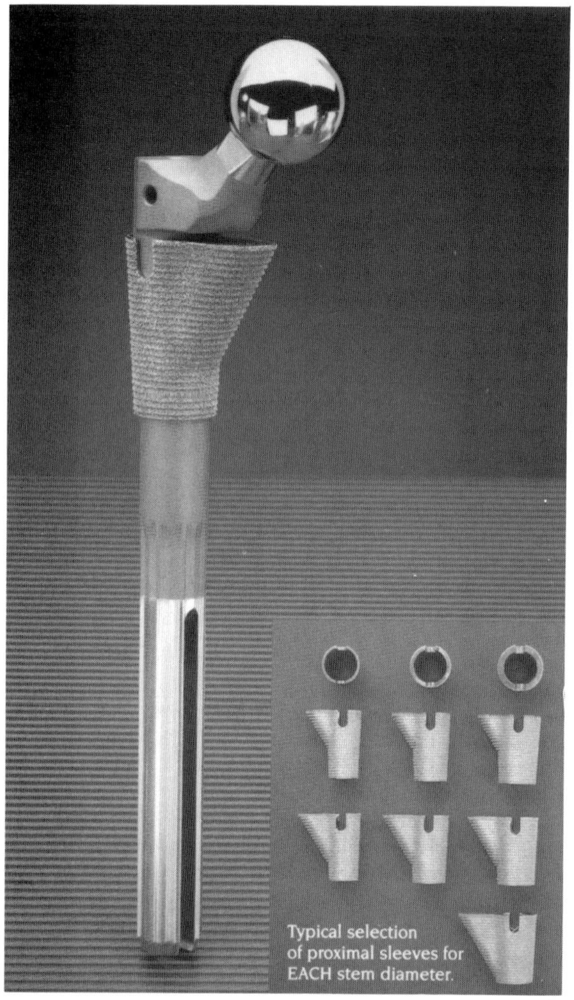

A

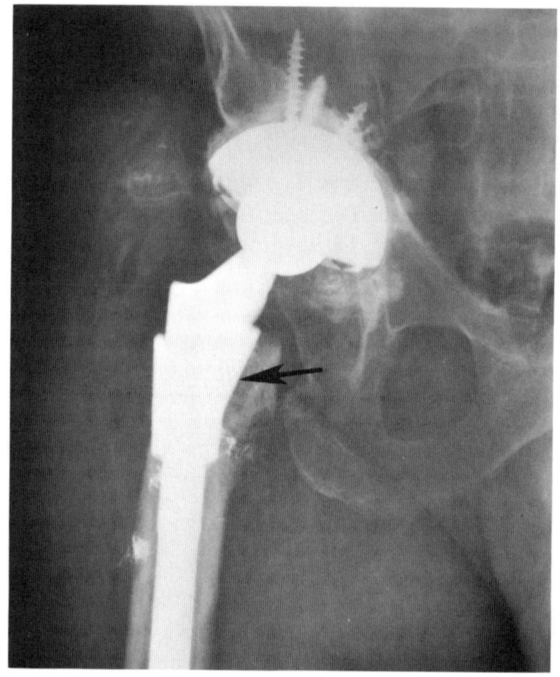

C

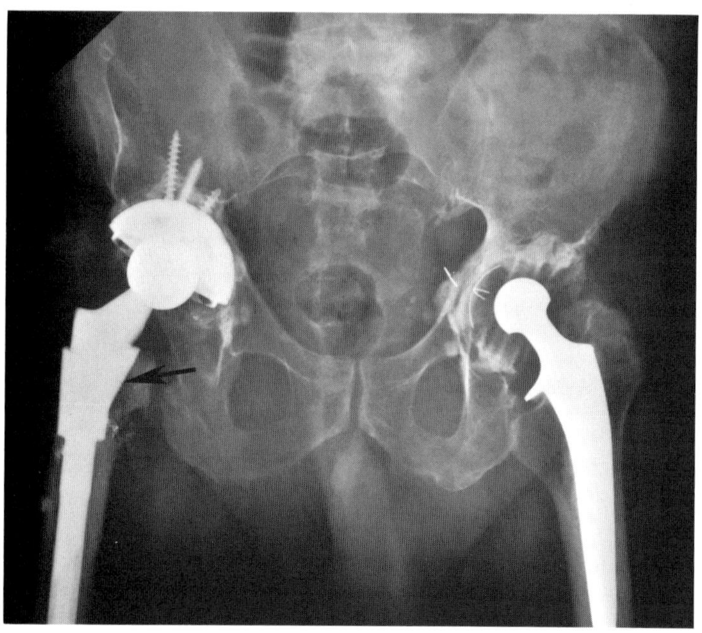

B

FIG. 4-113. A: The S-ROM™ system with proximal femoral stem modular sleeves, which allows flexibility at time of surgery (specifically, revision surgery) to deal with proximal femoral deficiency. (Courtesy of Joint Medical Products, Stamford, CT.) The AP radiographs of the pelvis **(B)** and femur **(C)** after revision of the right hip with the S-ROM™ modular system. Note the characteristic appearance of the proximal ZT™ sleeve (*arrow*).

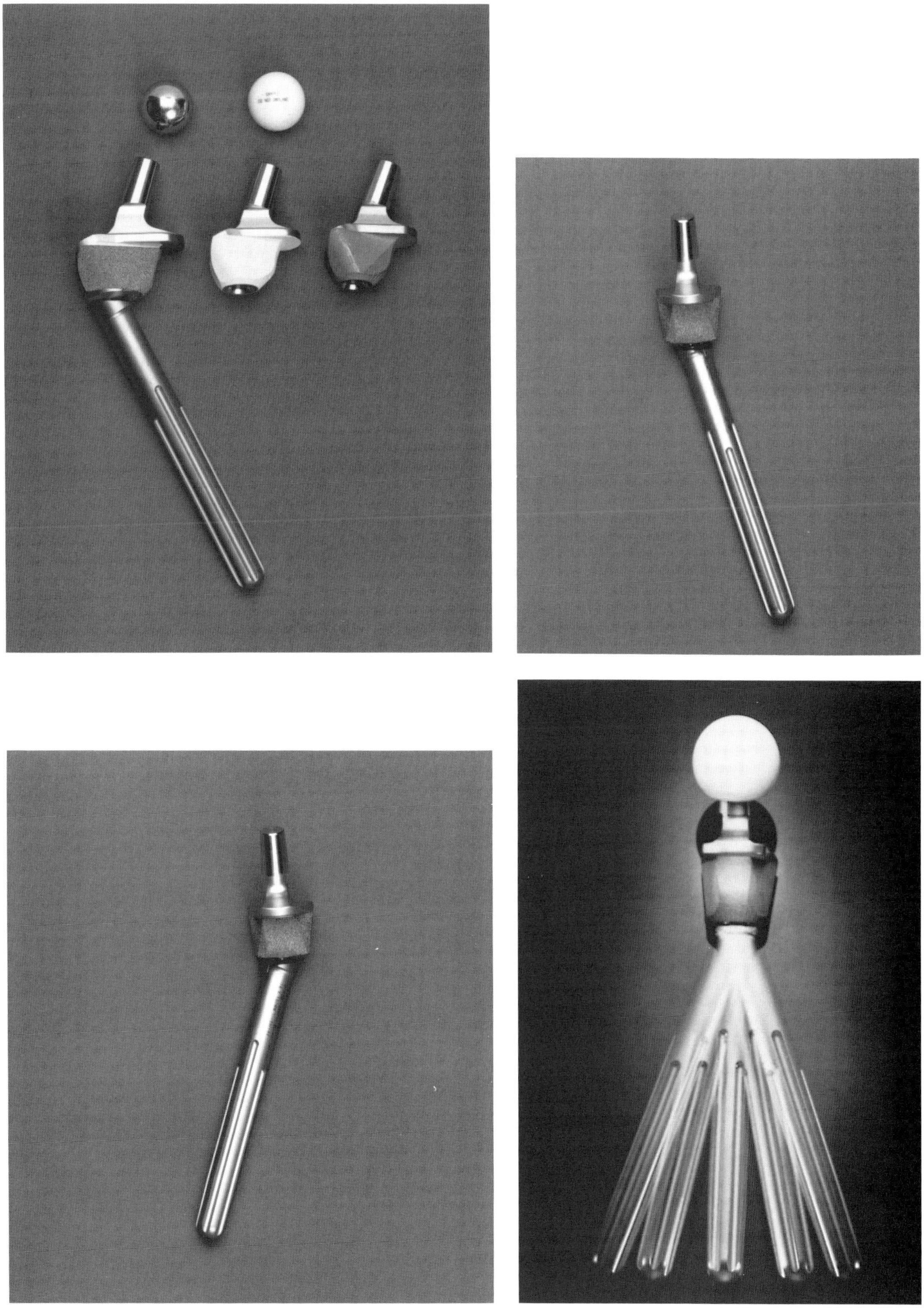

A B C D

FIG. 4-114. Infinity™ modular hip system. (Courtesy of Wright Medical Technology, Arlington, TN.) Femoral head: cobalt-chromium or ceramic in 28- and 32-mm sizes. **A–D:** Modular femoral component allows different coronal and sagittal plane positions to improve proximal contact. Titanium alloy.

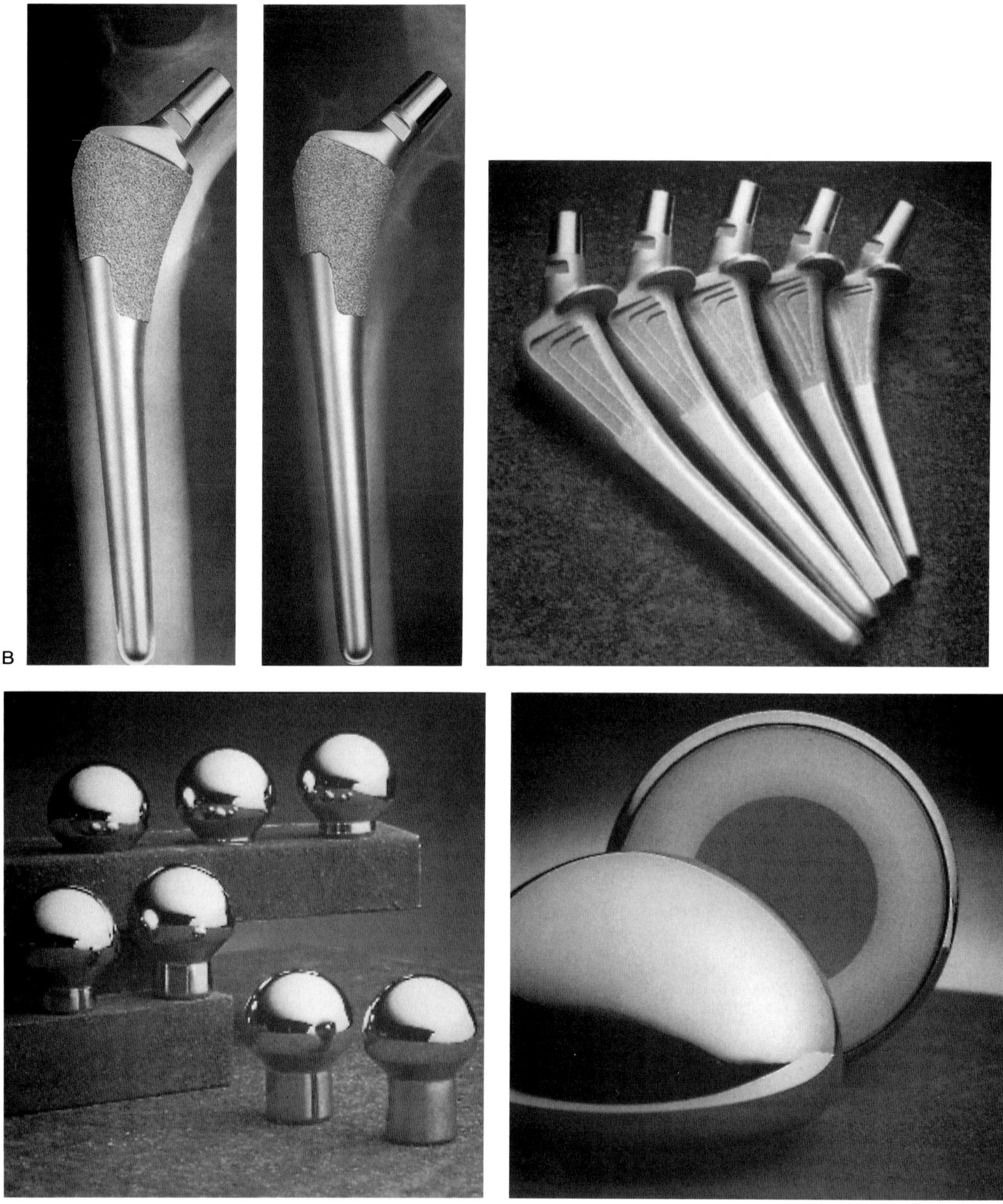

A,B C D E

FIG. 4-115. Perfecta™ total hip system. (Courtesy of Orthomet, Minneapolis, MN.) Porous-coated (plasma-spray) titanium standard-flare **(A)** and reduced-flare **(B)** femoral components. **C:** Nonporous-coated cobalt-chromium Perfecta™ femoral components with collars. **D:** Femoral head components with neck lengths of 0 to 15 mm. Head diameters: 28 to 32 mm. Bipolar **(E)** mantle acetabular component with polymethyl methacrylate spaces (*arrow*, **F**), porous-coated domed acetabular component with cancellous screws **(G)**.

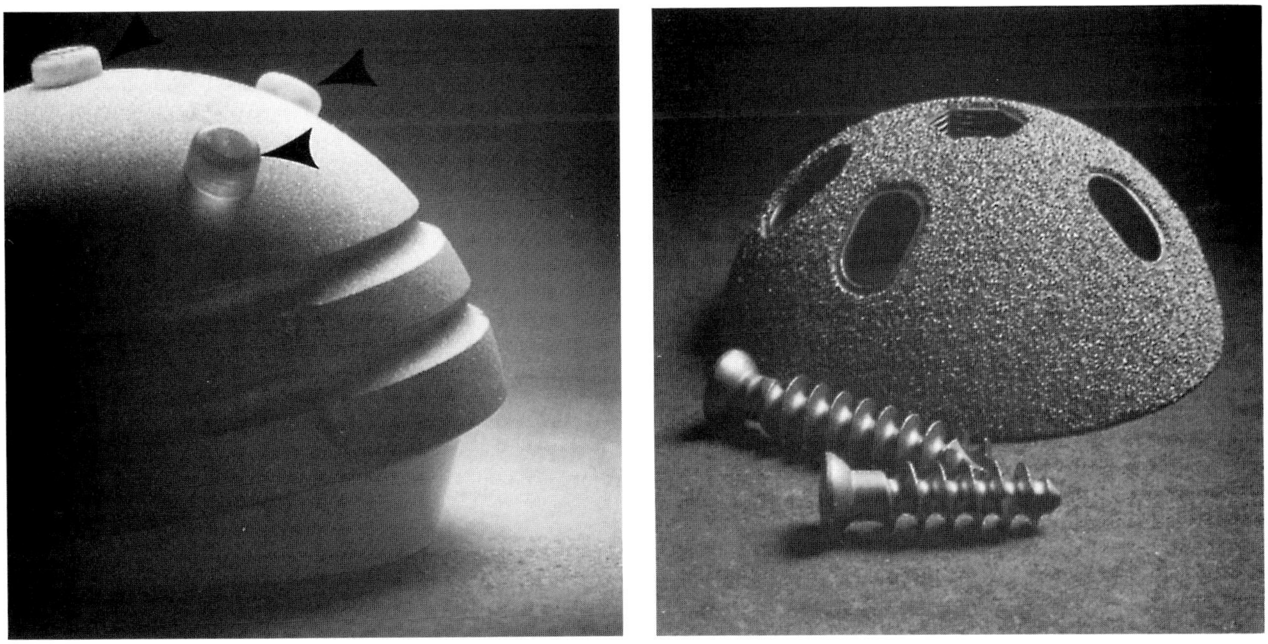

F G

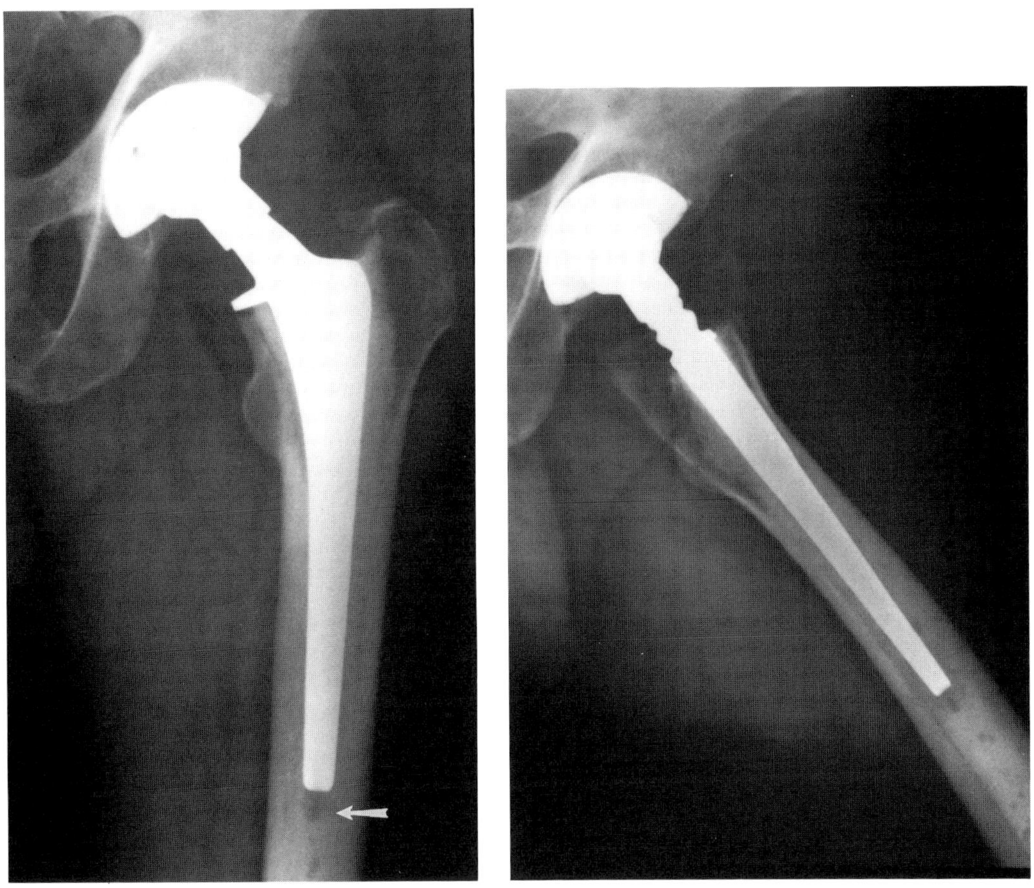

H I

FIG. 4-115. (*Continued.*) The AP **(H)** and oblique **(I)** radiographs of a Perfecta^{TM} hip system on the left. The system is modular; a domed acetabulum component and cemented nonporous stem with distal centralizer (*arrow*) were used. (Courtesy of Dr. William L. Overdylee, Minneapolis, MN.)

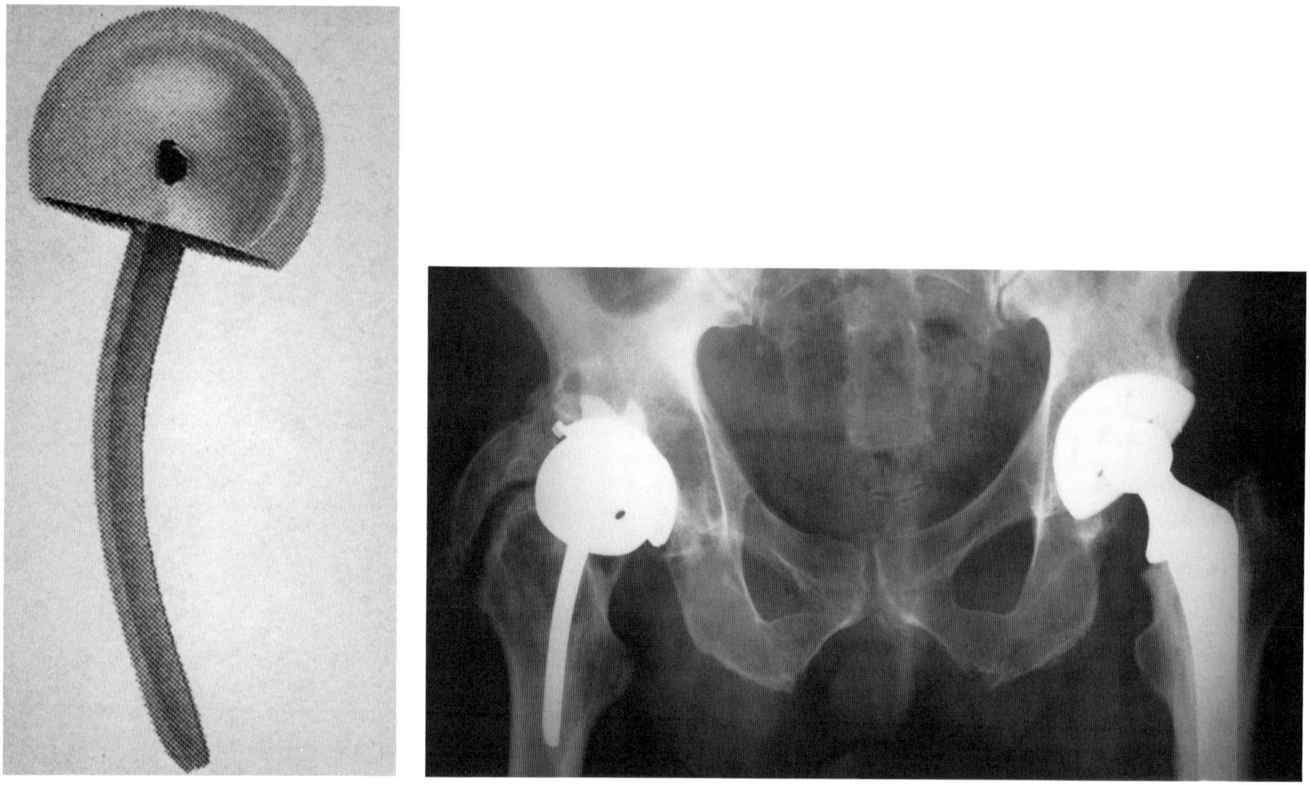

FIG. 4-116. A: The T.A.R.A. hip with a porous-coated femoral stem. (Courtesy of DePuy, Warsaw, IN.) **B:** The AP radiographs of the pelvis with a T.A.R.A. prosthesis on the right. There is extensive heterotopic bone laterally.

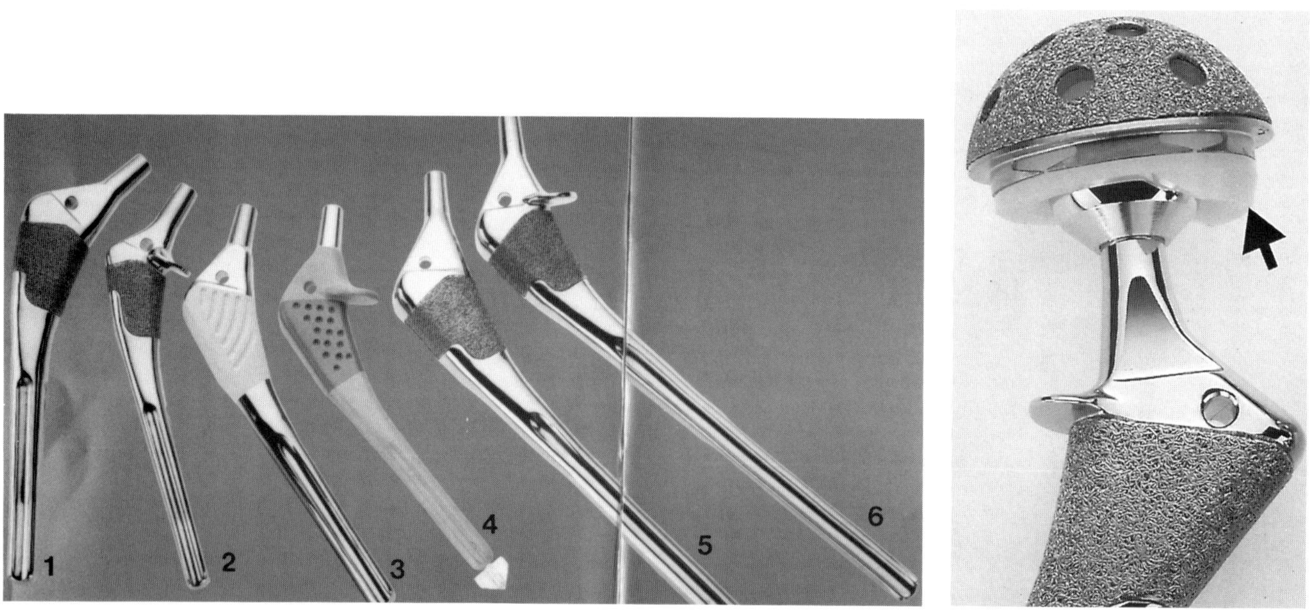

FIG. 4-117. Zimmer total hip systems (Courtesy of Zimmer, Warsaw, IN.) **A:** Anatomic™ femoral stems: titanium hardened with Ti-nidium™, except Anatomic CC™ (cobalt-chromium-molybdenum alloy). *1,* Anatomic™: proximal porous coat, no collar; *2,* Anatomic CP™: similar to Anatomic but with collar; *3,* Anatomic HA™: no collar, hydroxyapatite proximal surface; *4,* Anatomic CC™: collar, polymethyl methacrylate proximal surface with distal centralizer; *5,* Anatomic LS™: Anatomic™ with a long stem; *6,* Anatomic BR™: long stem with a collar. **B:** HG multilock stem and HGP II acetabular component with augmented lateral (*arrow*) polyethylene liner.

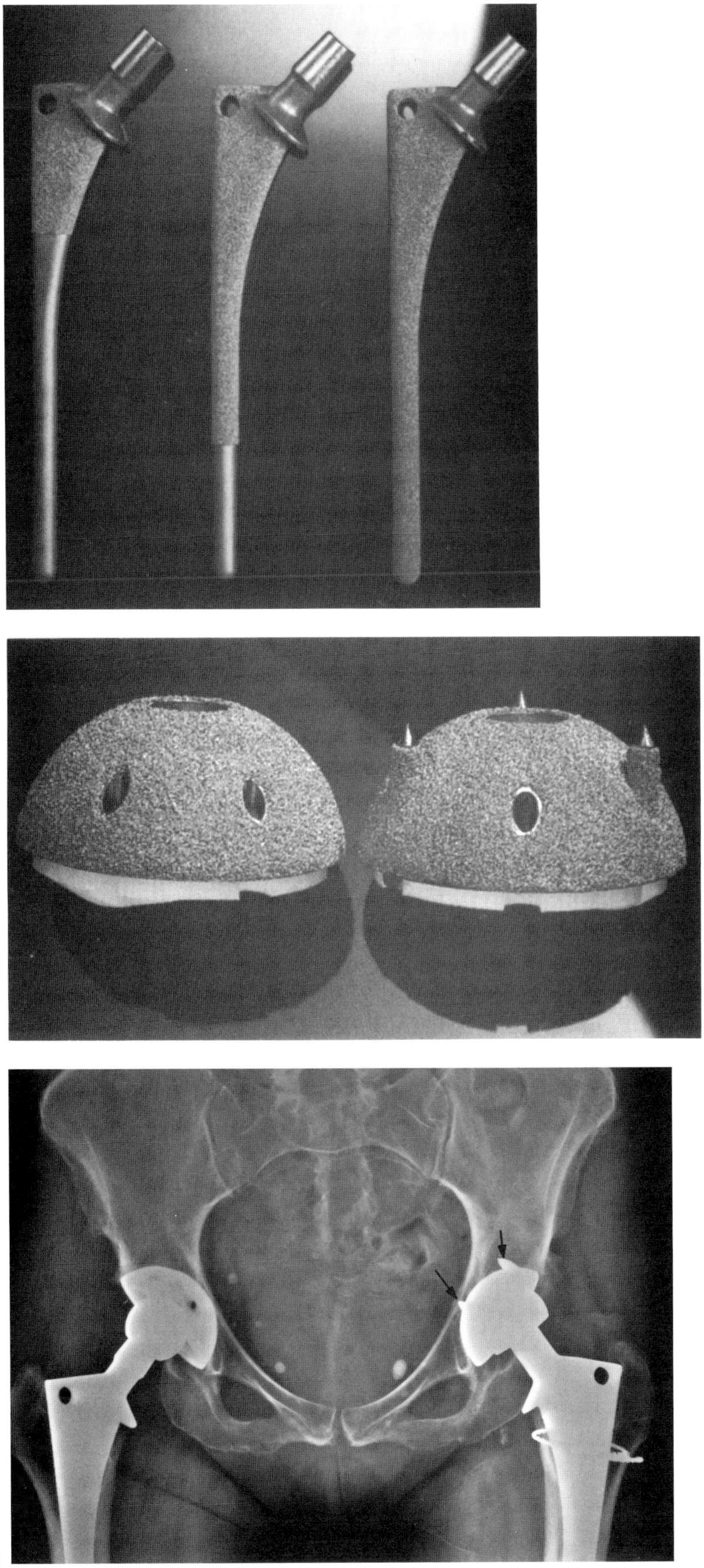

A

B

C

FIG. 4-118. DePuy hip systems. Anatomic medullary locking (AML) systems. (Courtesy of DePuy, Warsaw, IN.) **A:** AML femoral stems with porous coating over the proximal stem (*left*), proximal three fourths of the stem (*middle*), and fully coated (*right*). **B:** Coated acetabular components. Standard left, three pegs right. **C:** An AP radiograph of the pelvis with bilateral DePuy AML prostheses. The acetabular component on the right is press fitted. The left acetabular component is spiked (*arrows*). (See **D–F** on next page.)

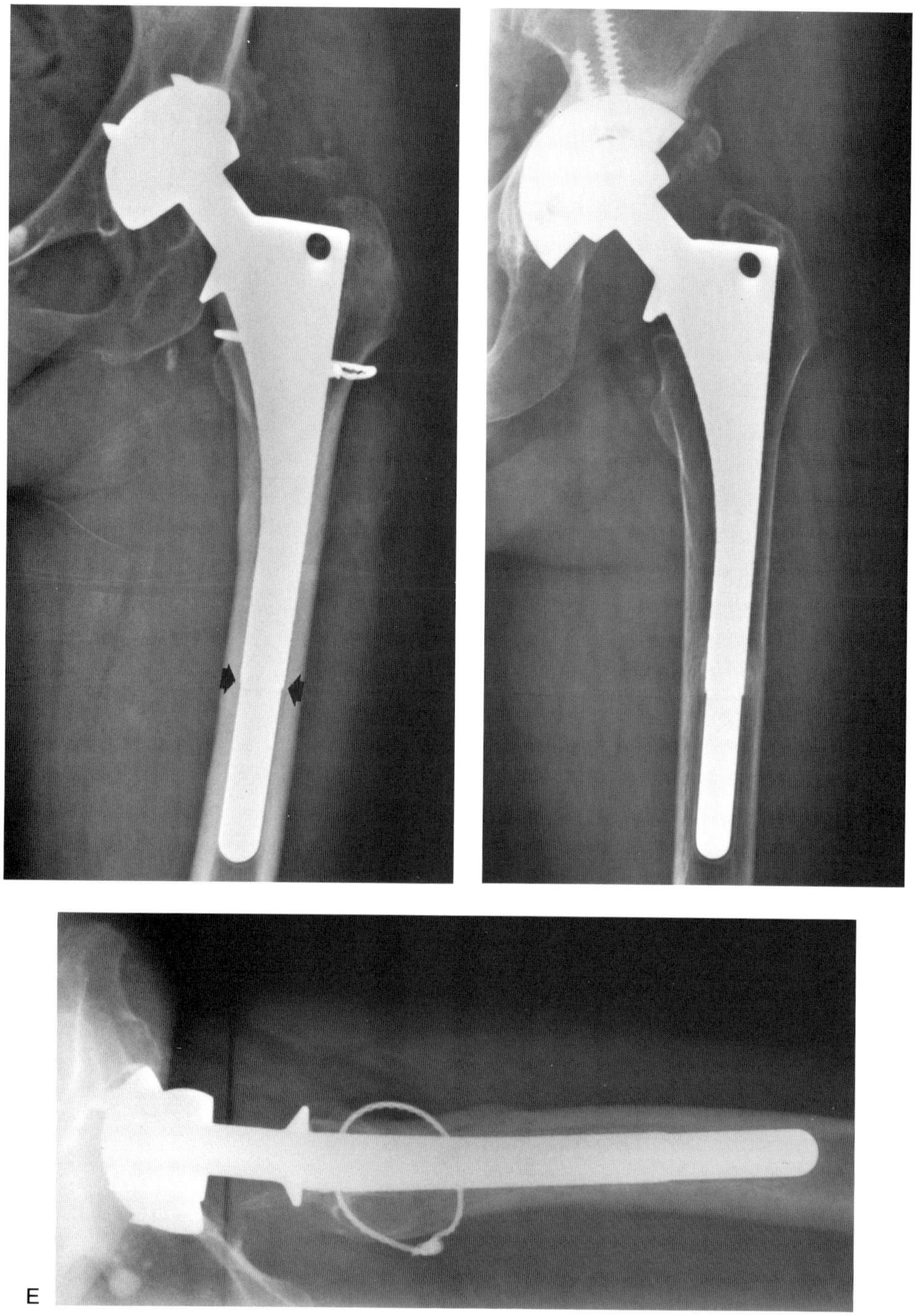

D

F

E

FIG. 4-118. (*Continued.*) The AP **(D)** and lateral **(E)** radiographs of the femur show the entire component with the porous coating extending three fourths of the length of the stem (*arrows*). **F:** An AP view of the left upper femur with an AML system with a standard porous-coated acetabular component with two screws for fixation.

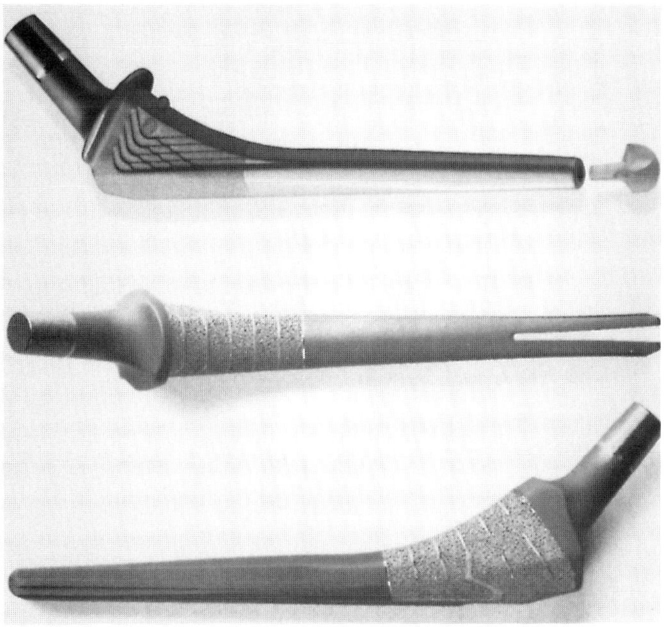

A

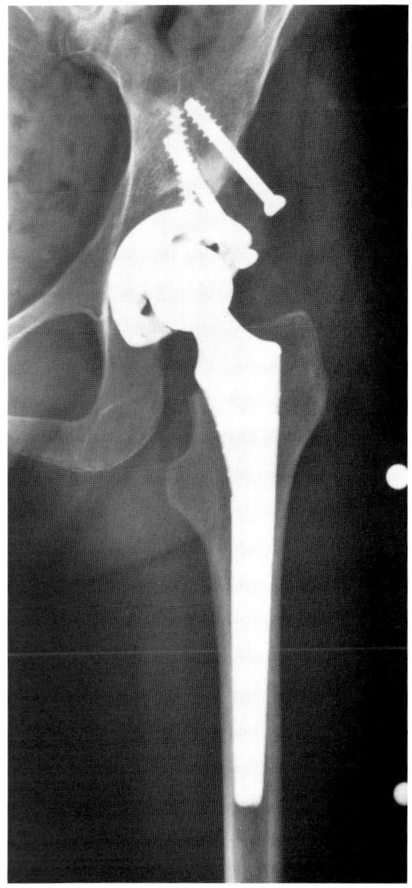

C

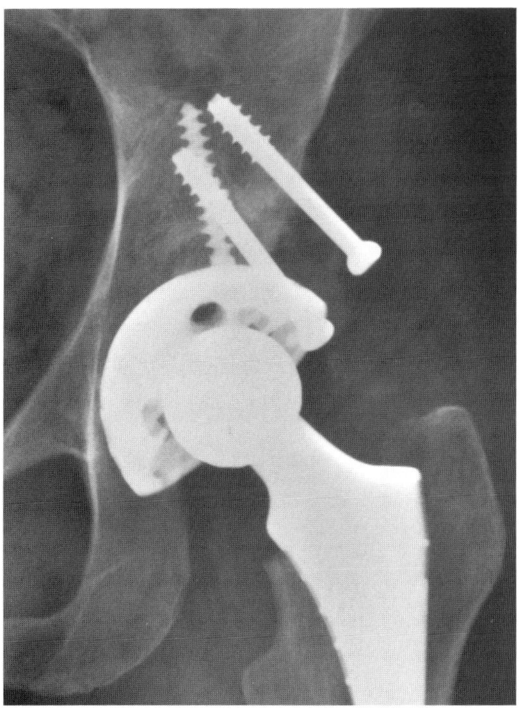

B

FIG. 4-119. Intermedics Natural hip system. (Courtesy of Intermedics Orthopedics, Austin, TX.) **A:** Intermedics femoral stems with centralizer (*top*), flared self-adjusting slot (*middle*), and fluted stem (*below*). The upper component is cobalt-chromium with a collar, and the lower two stems are titanium with proximal porous coating. The AP views of the pelvis **(B)** and femur **(C)** demonstrating an Intermedics Natural hip with a distal slot in the femoral component. (See **D–G** on next page.)

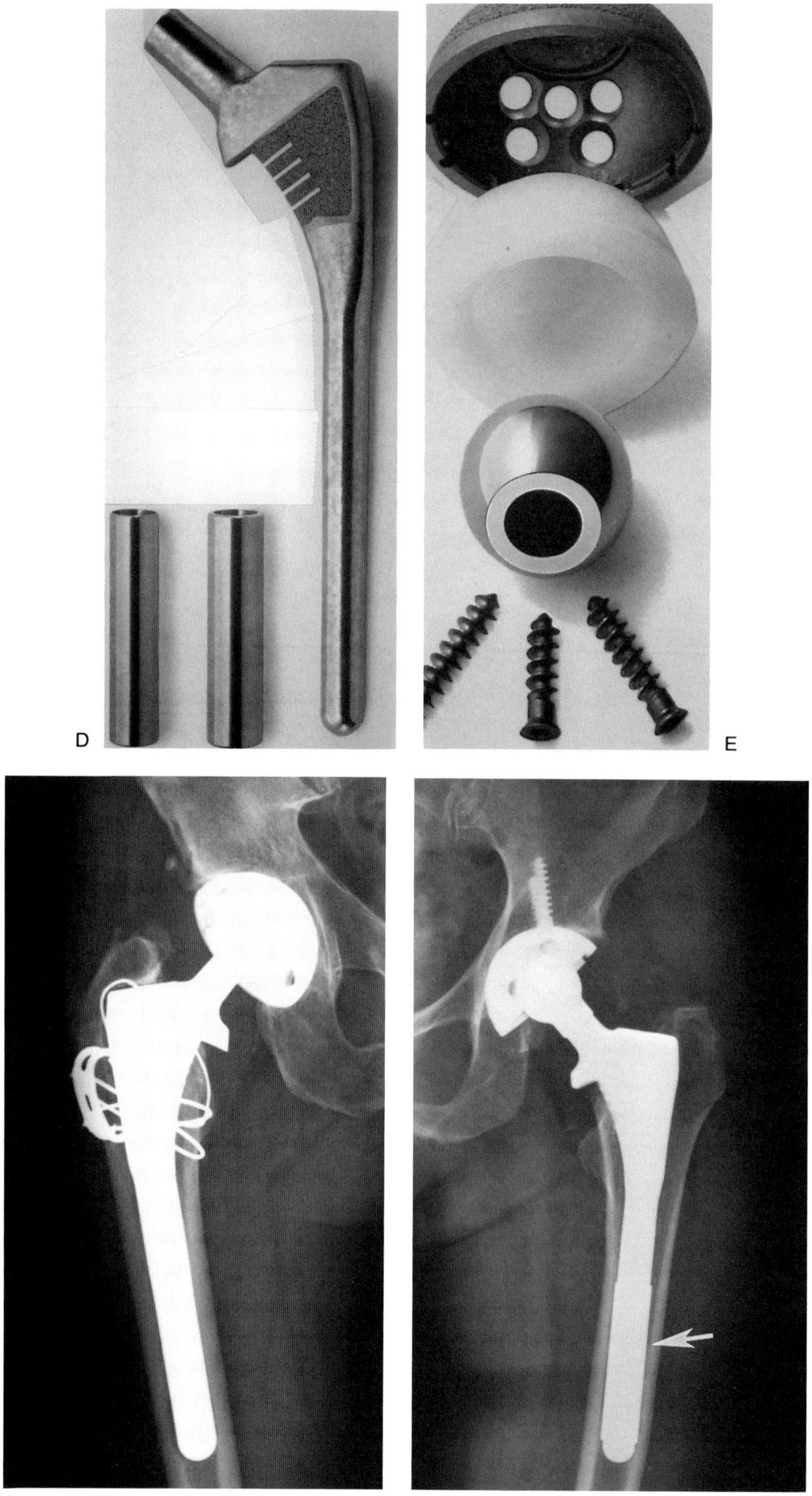

FIG. 4-119. (*Continued.*) **D:** APR II femoral stem with two sleeve sizes (2 and 4 mm). **E:** Titanium hemispheric acetabular component with liner, modular head, and screws. **F,G:** An AP radiograph of an Intermedics APR II without the sleeve (F) and with the sleeve (*arrow,* G). There is a Dall-Miles cable-claw system around the upper femur in F. The collar and proximal femoral component have a fairly unique radiographic appearance.

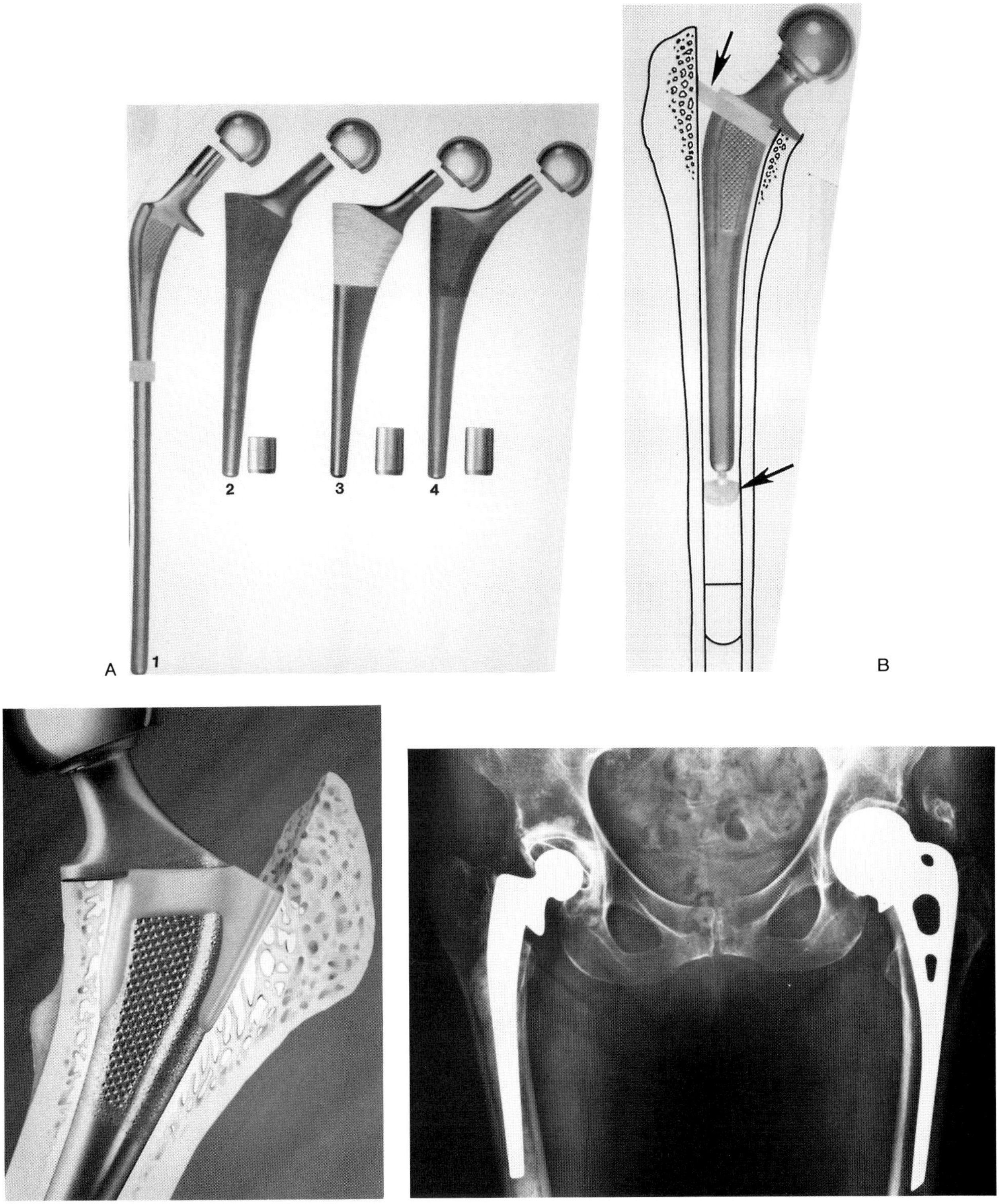

FIG. 4-120. Howmedica hip systems. (Courtesy of Howmedica, Rutherford, NJ.) **A:** Femoral stems: *1,* long stem; *2,* Precision™; *3,* Osteolock™; *4,* primary femoral. Modular heads above and sleeves below. **B:** Distal centralizer and upper spacer (*arrow*) to assist with positioning during cementation. **C:** Precision STRATA™ system with upper spacer for cemented hip systems. **D:** An AP radiograph of the pelvis with cemented hip arthroplasty on the right and a Moore endoprosthesis on the left. (See **E–H** on next page.)

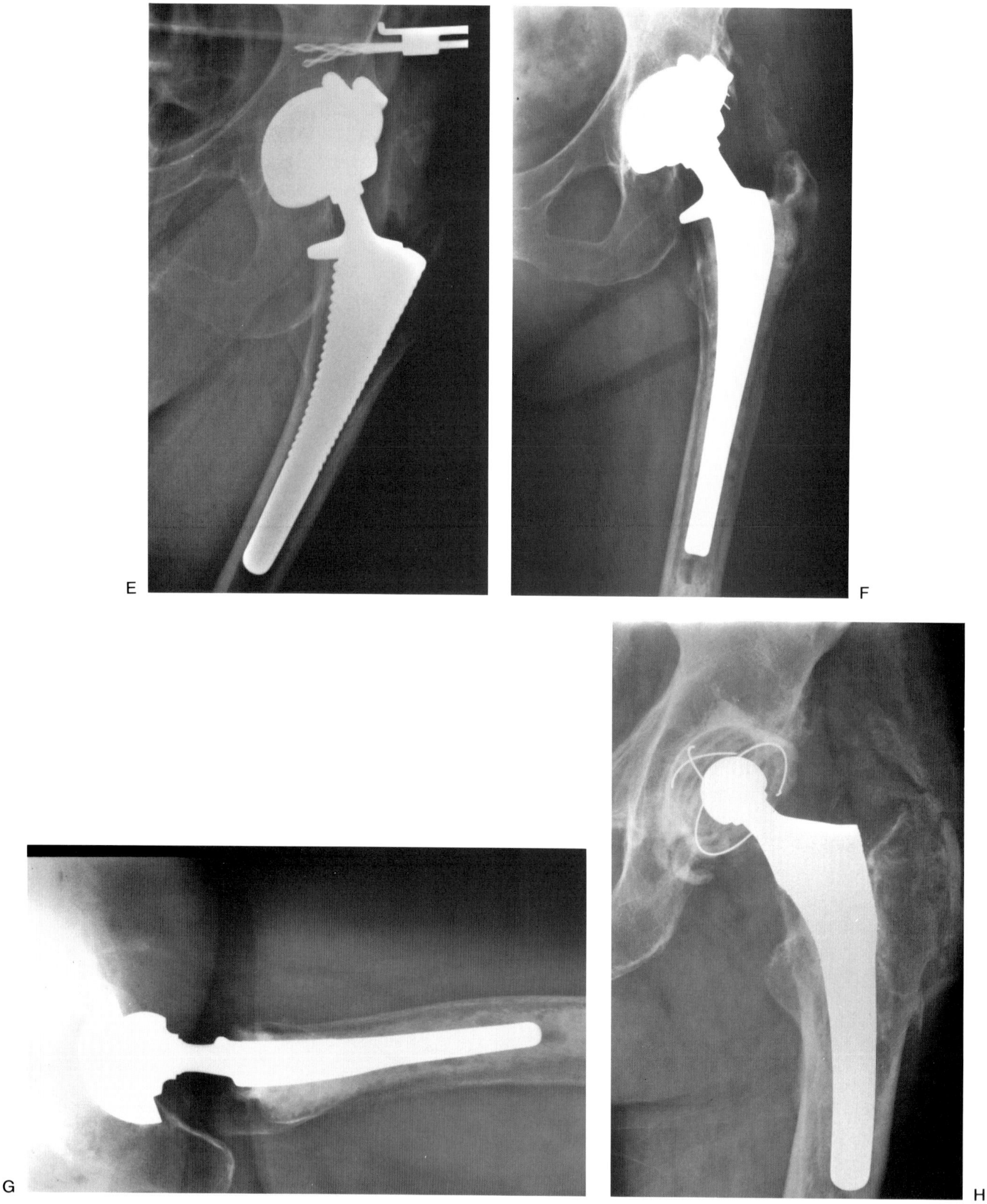

FIG. 4-120. (*Continued.*) **E:** PCA acetabular component with femoral broach in place. The AP **(F)** and lateral **(G)** radiographs after placement of a number 3 Precision^{TM} stem. **H:** Howmedica PCA femoral component and cemented acetabular component without metal backing. The femoral component is undersized for the large proximal femur and is in the varus position.

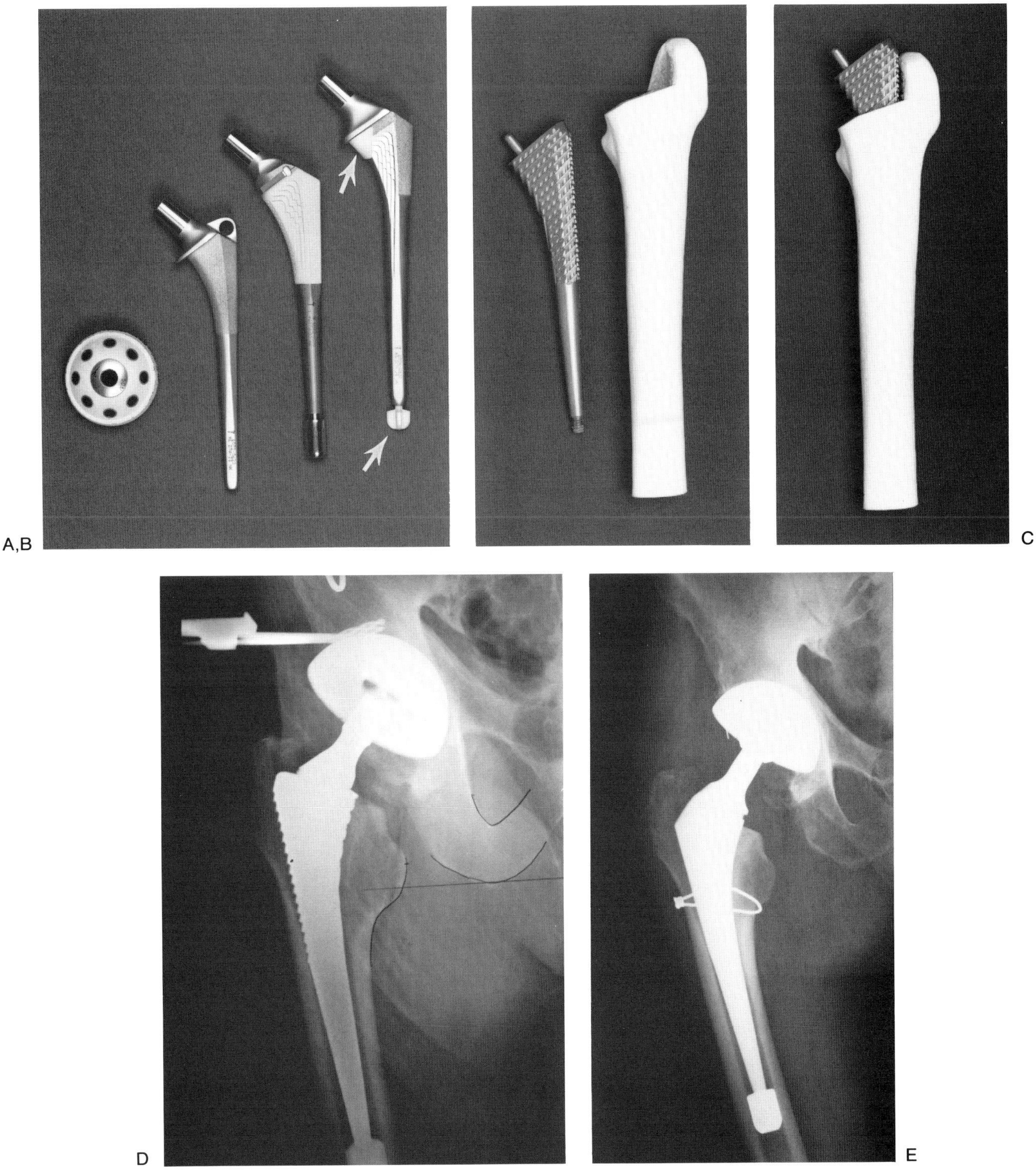

FIG. 4-121. Osteonics hip systems. (Courtesy of Osteonics, Allendale, NJ.) **A:** DUAL geometry hydroxyapatite-coated acetabular component with Hemi™ stem (*left*), Omniflex-HA™ without collar but with distal centralizer (*middle*), and Omnifit "C" stem with proximal and distal spacers (*arrows, right*). Broach adjacent to bone model **(B)**, in bone **(C)**, and during preparation of the femur with broach and distal bullet in place **(D)**. **E:** An AP radiograph of an Omniflex-HA™ stem with modular head and uncemented femoral component. Single Dall-Miles cable around the upper femur.

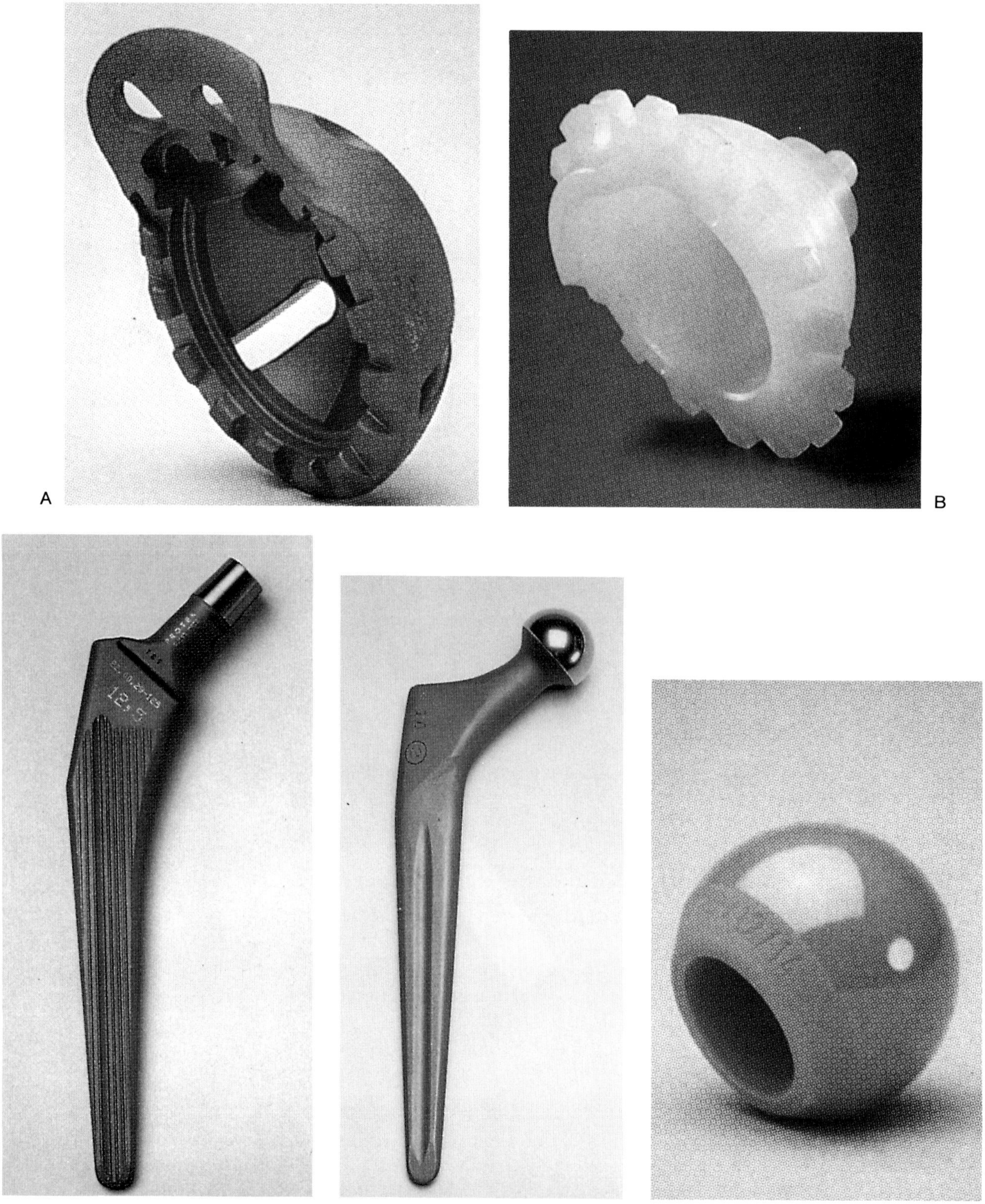

A B C,D E

FIG. 4-122. PROTEK™ hip system. (PROTEK AG, Berne, Switzerland. Courtesy of Techmedica, A. Sulzermedica, Camarillo, CA.) Acetabular components. Titanium shell **(A)** and SL polyethylene insert **(B)**. Note upper acetabular screw holes. Femoral components **(C)**, cemented straight SL stem **(D)**, cemented SL CDH stem, and ceramic modular BIOLOX™ head **(E)**.

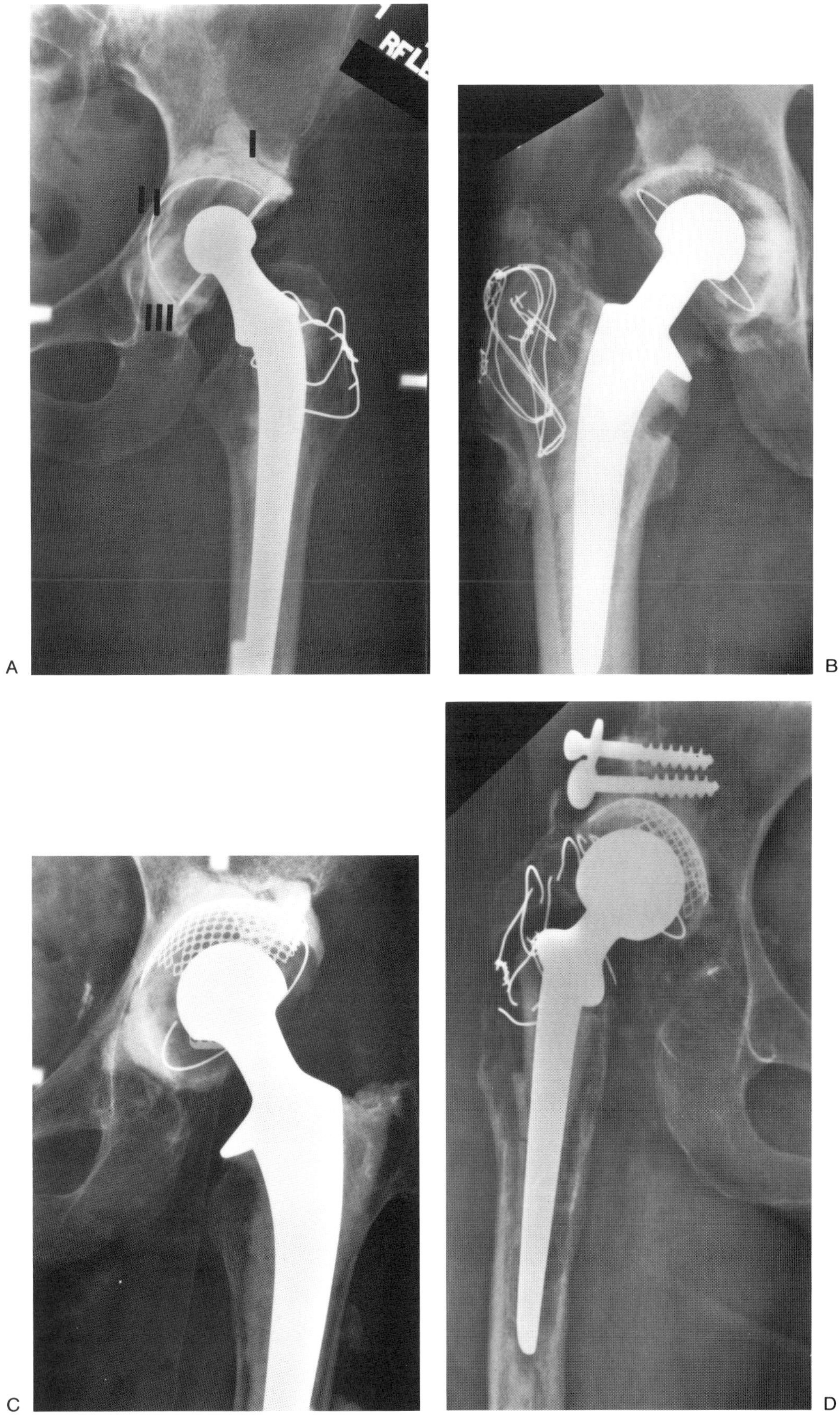

FIG. 4-123. Radiographs of all polyethylene acetabular components with opaque wire markers. **A:** Cemented left hip arthroplasty with polyethylene acetabular component. The cement mantle is thick in zones I and III and thin in zone II. **B:** Cemented polyethylene acetabular component with less cement superiorly than medially. **C:** Cemented polyethylene component with acetabular mesh and reconstruction of a new acetabular roof. **D:** There is a cement fracture and poor cement technique around the femoral component with femoral component loosening. (See **E–G** on next page.)

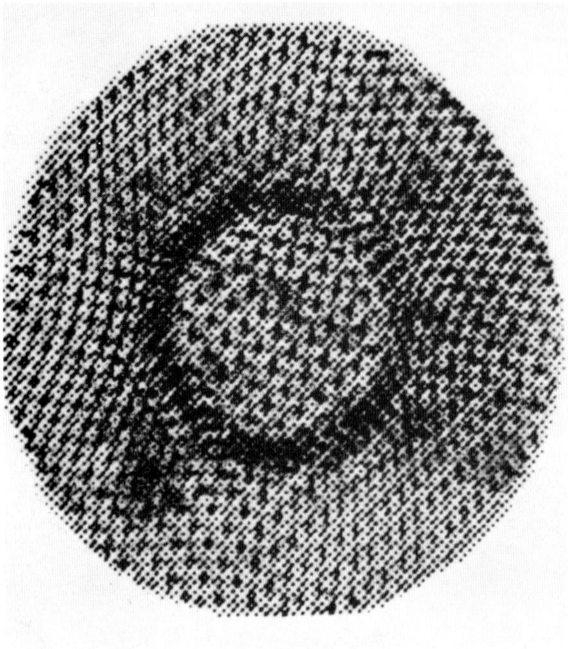

E

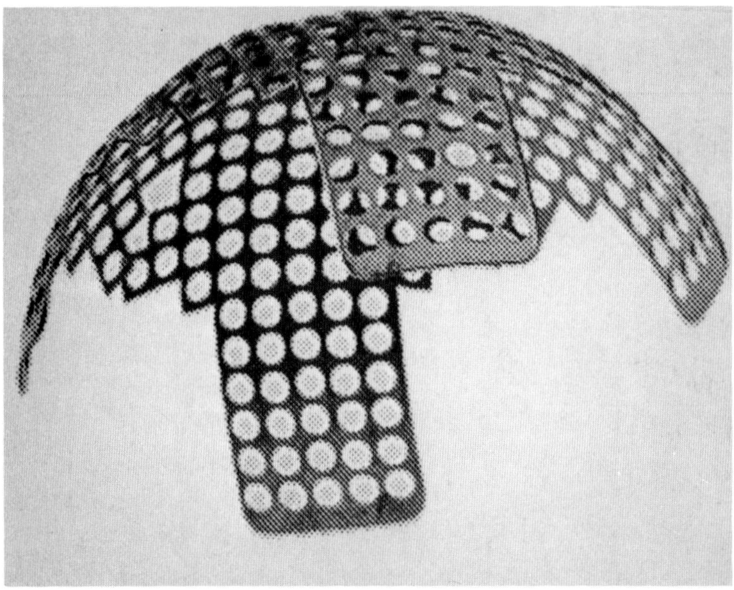

F

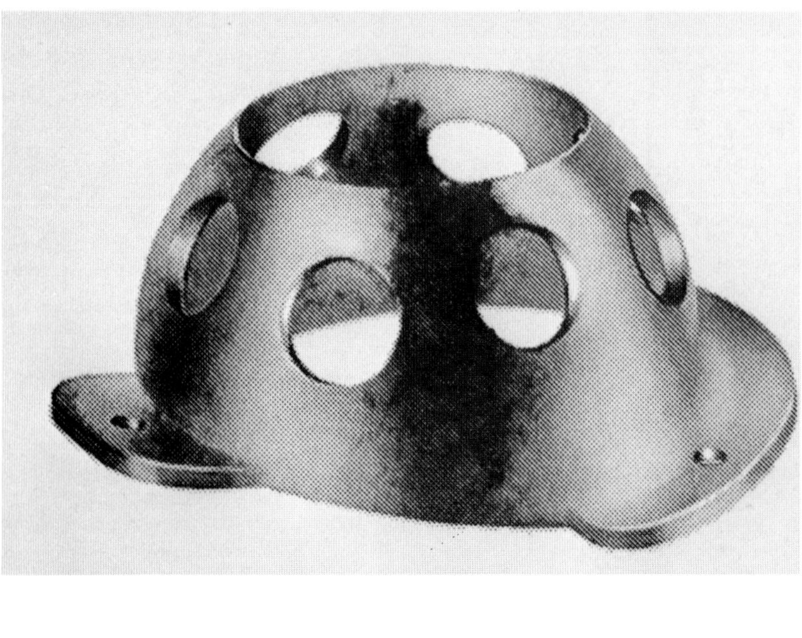

G

FIG. 4-123. (*Continued.*) **E–G:** Charnley cement restrictor (E), acetabular mesh (F), and Oh-Harris protrusio shell. (Courtesy of Howmedica, Rutherford, NJ.)

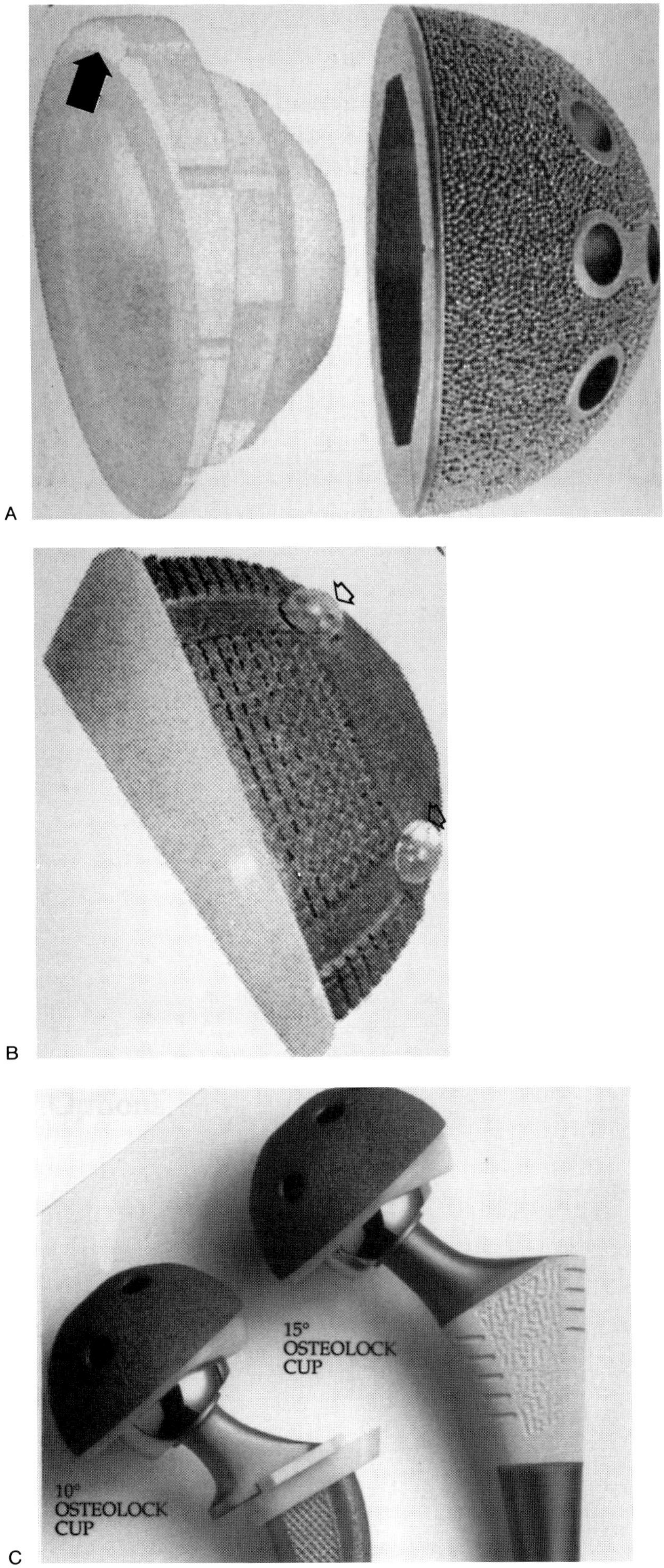

FIG. 4-124. Acetabular shells and polyethylene inserts. (Courtesy of Howmedica, Rutherford, NJ.) **A:** P.C.A.™ acetabular component with exaggerated or augmented upper lip on the polyethylene liner (*arrow*). **B:** Ridged Precision™ acetabular shell with cement spacers (*arrows*). **C:** Steolock™ cups with 10° and 15° lines for augmentation.

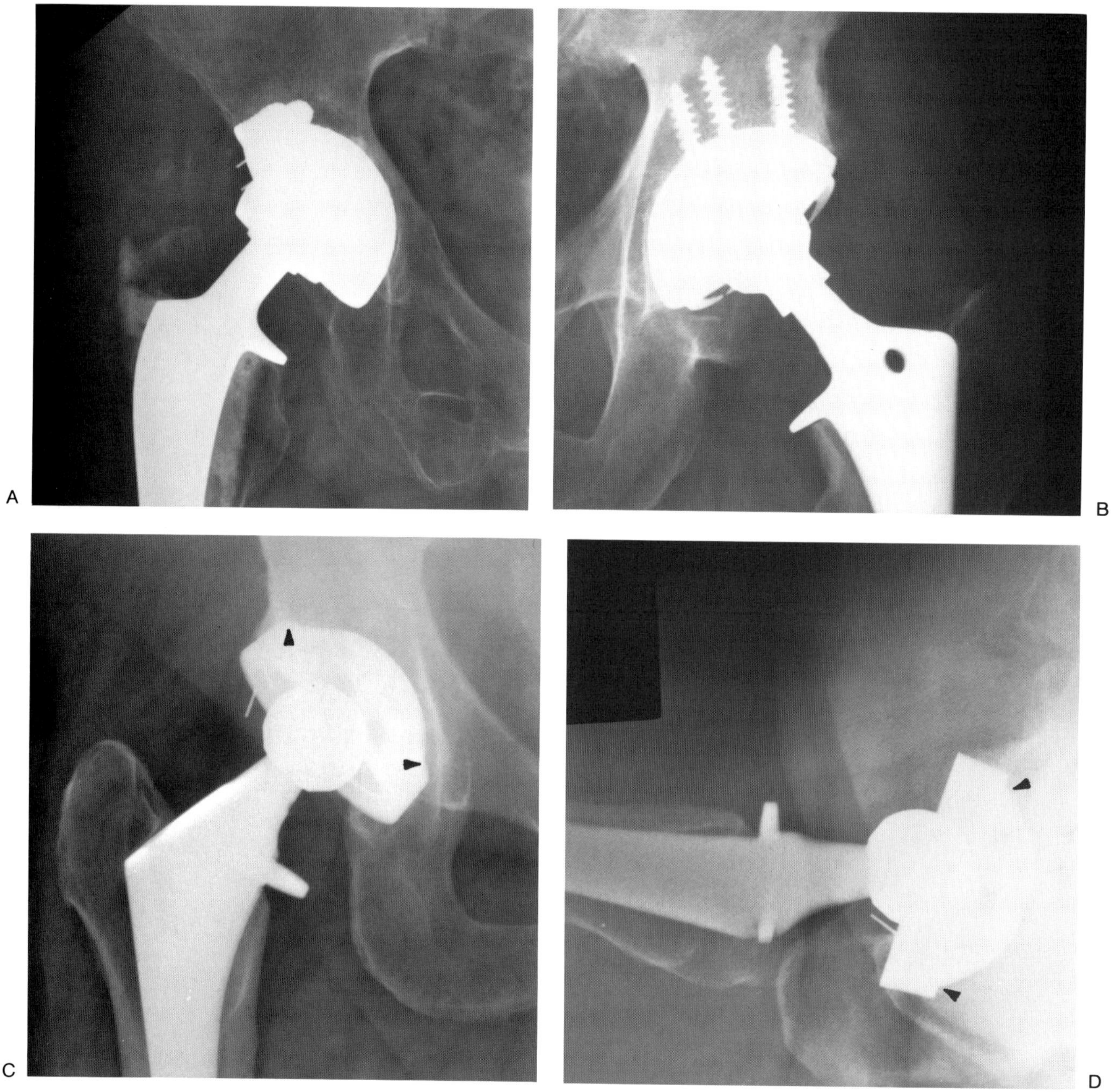

FIG. 4-125. Radiographs of uncemented acetabular components. **A:** P.C.A.™ acetabular component with two lateral porous-coated pegs. (Courtesy of Howmedica, Rutherford, NJ.) **B:** Harris-Galante uncemented acetabular component with three cancellous screws. (Courtesy of Zimmer, Warsaw, IN.) The AP **(C)** and lateral **(D)** DUAL geometry acetabular component. Note the peripheral lip (*small arrows*). (Osteonics, Allendale, NJ.)

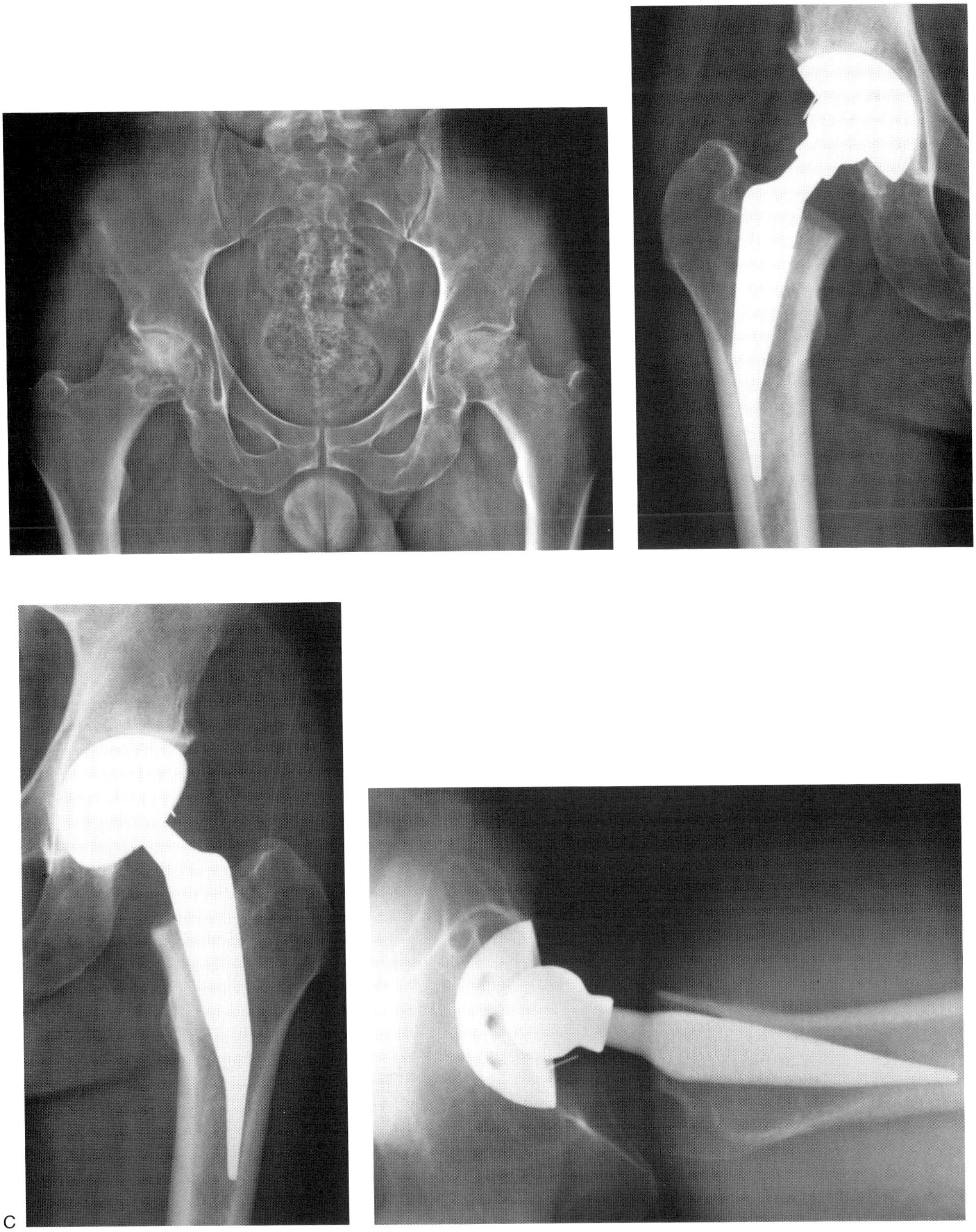

FIG. 4-126. A: An AP radiograph of the pelvis in a 28-year-old man with bilateral stage IV AVN (articular deformity and joint space narrowing). The AP views of both upper femurs demonstrating the unique short-stem design of the Morrey femoral component. **D:** Lateral view of the right hip demonstrating the tapered tip in a second projection. Uncemented acetabular components with screw holes and modular heads bilaterally.

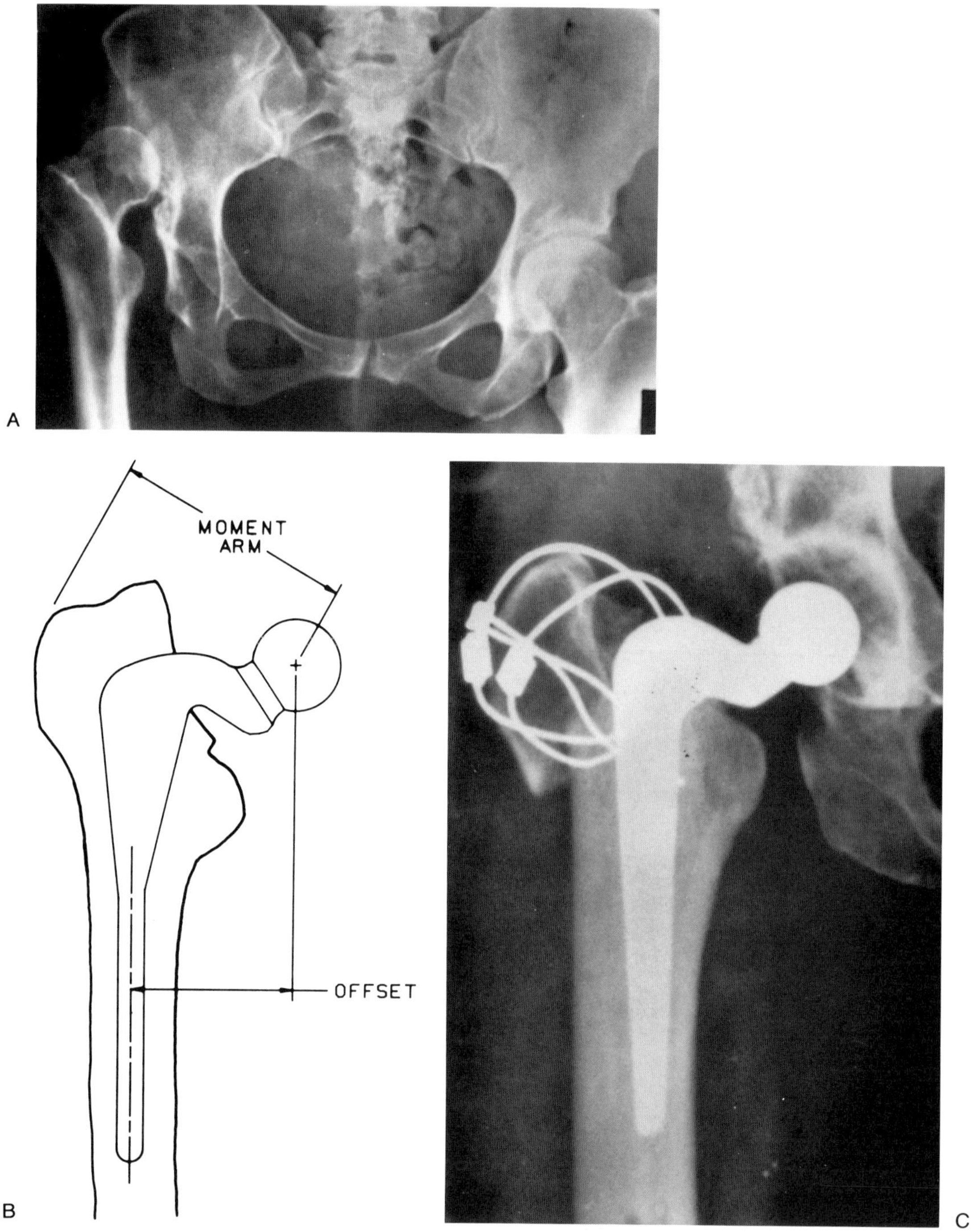

FIG. 4-127. Custom-designed femoral prosthesis to match femoral head offset length in patients with congenital hip or other dysplasias. **A:** An AP view of the pelvis and hips showing dislocation and acetabular dysplasia on the right. **B:** Femoral offset measurement and component configuration. **C:** An AP radiograph of the hip demonstrating the custom-designed femoral component and standard cemented polyethylene acetabular component. (From Huo MH, Salvati EA, Lieberman JR, Burstein AH, Wilson PD. Custom-designed femoral prostheses in total hip arthroplasty done with cement for severe dysplasia of the hip. *J Bone Joint Surg [Am]* 1993;75A:1497–1504.)

A

B

C

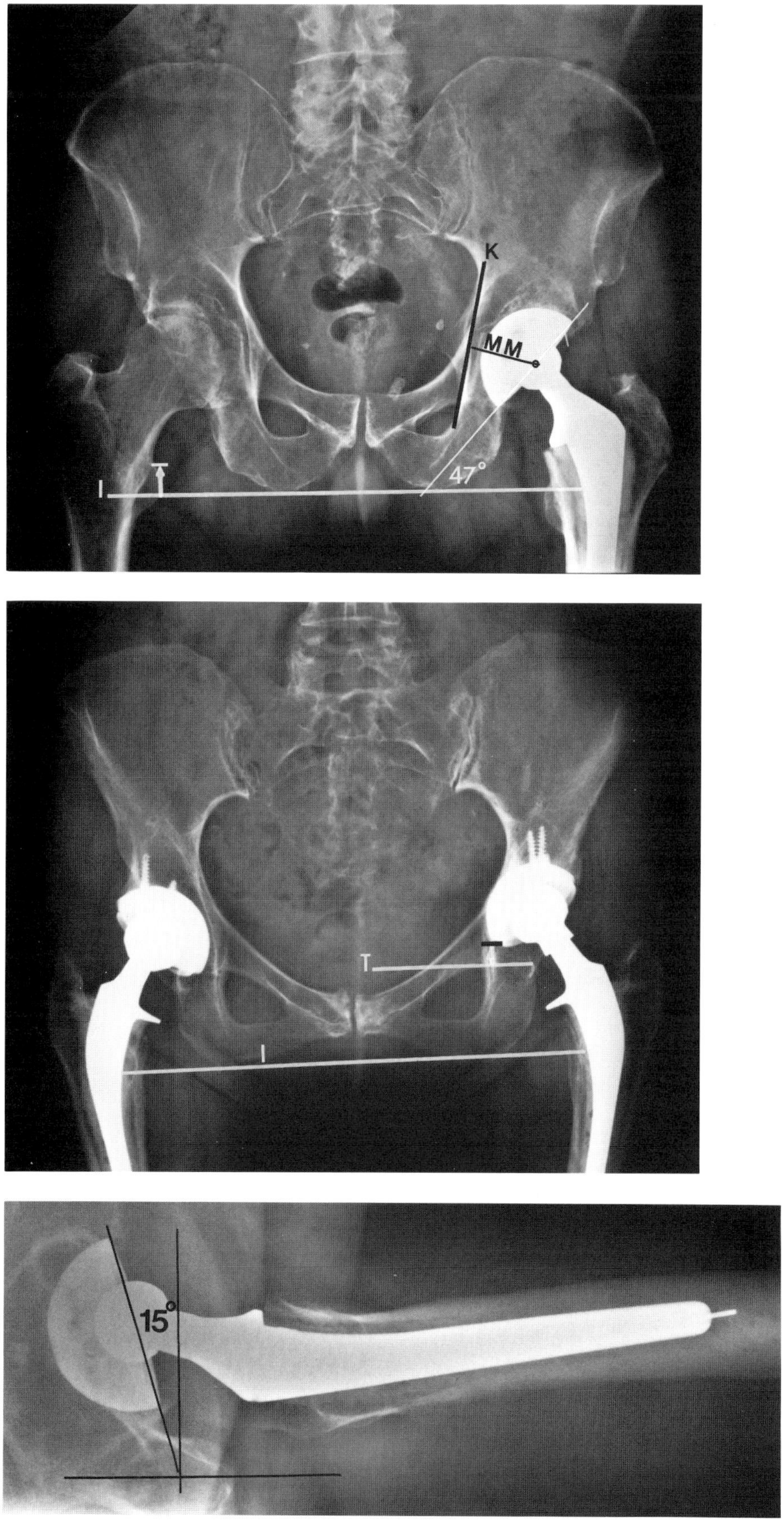

FIG. 4-128. Measurements after hip arthroplasty. **A:** An AP radiograph after insertion of a cemented femoral and uncemented 56-mm acetabular component. The biischial line is drawn across the ischial tuberosities (*I*). This line is used to evaluate the acetabular angle and leg-length differences.[279,376–378] The acetabular angle is formed by a line along the metal margin of a metal shell component or the marker ring in a polyethylene component.[279,377] The angle is generally around 45°, but the optimal angle can vary, depending on component design. Greater than 55° or less than 35° is considered poor technique.[293] Leg length can be compared using the upper margin of the lesser trochanter and the biischial line. A true AP position of the femurs (patella anterior and legs internally rotated 15°) is important for consistency. In this example, there is slight shortening of the operated side (*line,* lesser trochanter on right). Kohler's line (Fig. 4-89) (*K*) is used to evaluate protrusion or medial migration. The line extends from the margin of the sciatic notch to the lower lateral margin of the obturator foramen. Medial migration is assessed by measuring variations in distance from Kohler's line (K) to the center of the femoral head (*line* mm).[278,282] **B:** Additional measurements on the AP view of the pelvis may also be useful. A baseline comparison for superior acetabular migration can be made using the distance from the teardrop (*T*) line or biischial line (*I*) to the base of the acetabular component (*dark line*).[279] The acetabular angle can also be measured from the teardrop line,[325] but the ischial line is easier to constrict if the teardrop is not clearly seen. **C:** Lateral radiograph demonstrating measurements of acetabular anteversion. This angle is measured from a line perpendicular to horizontal because the femoral position is inconsistent. This angle is typically neutral to 15°.[323] The femoral stem should be neutrally positioned in the femoral canal.

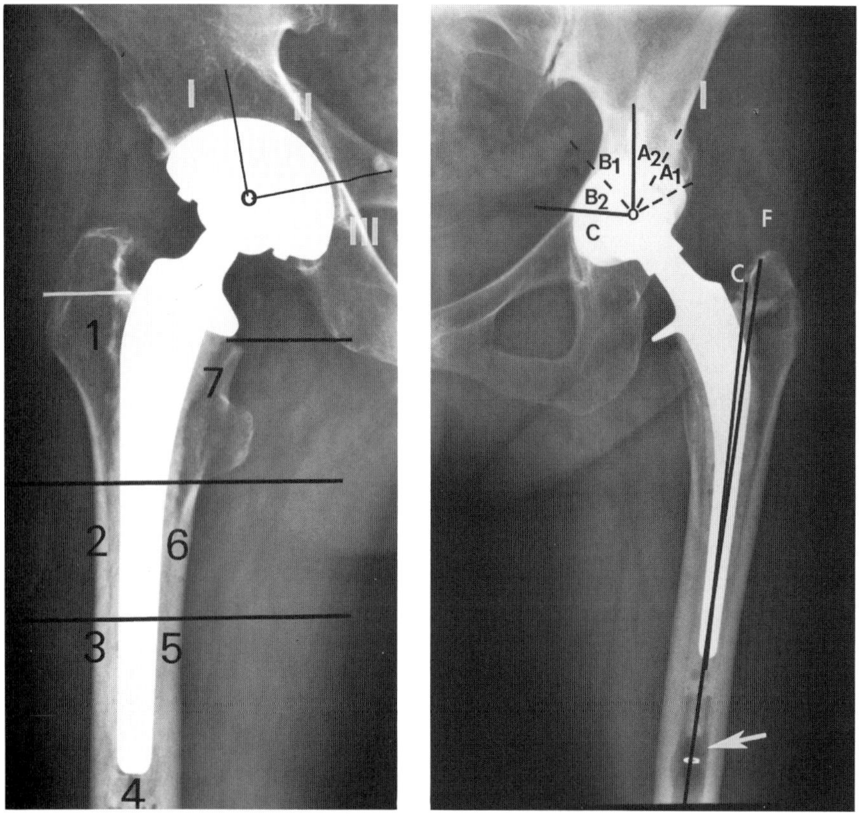

A,B

FIG. 4-129. A: An AP radiograph of the right hip with cemented femoral and uncemented acetabular components. The zone for acetabular component evaluation is demonstrated. Dividing the acetabular component into three zones is simple to work with. A five-zone technique is demonstrated here. The femoral component is evaluated using seven zones, as described by Gruen et al.[290,382] The zones are numbered *1* to *7*, extending from proximal lateral to the proximal medial around the entire component. Zone *4* is the tip. Note that the radiograph does not include enough of the femur distal to the tip of the femoral component. **B:** The appropriate length of femur is included on the film. The femur is visible below the cement restrictor (*arrow*). An alternative acetabular zone method, described by Martell et al.,[325] is demonstrated. Zone I and II were divided into two zones (A1 and A2 for zone I and B1 and B2 for zone II). The axis of the femoral component (*C*) should be neutral or in slight valgus compared with the femoral shaft (*F, lines*).[376–378,382]

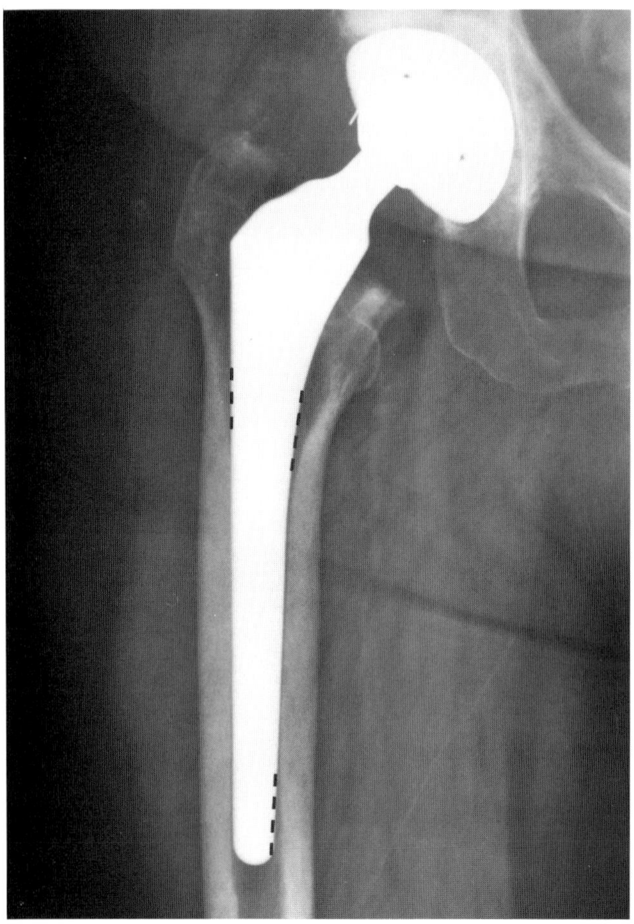

FIG. 4-130. An AP radiograph of the right femur with uncemented components. The stem of the femoral component is within 1 mm of the cortex for more than 50% of its length below the lesser trochanter, indicating a good fit.[298] Exceptions are marked with *broken lines*.

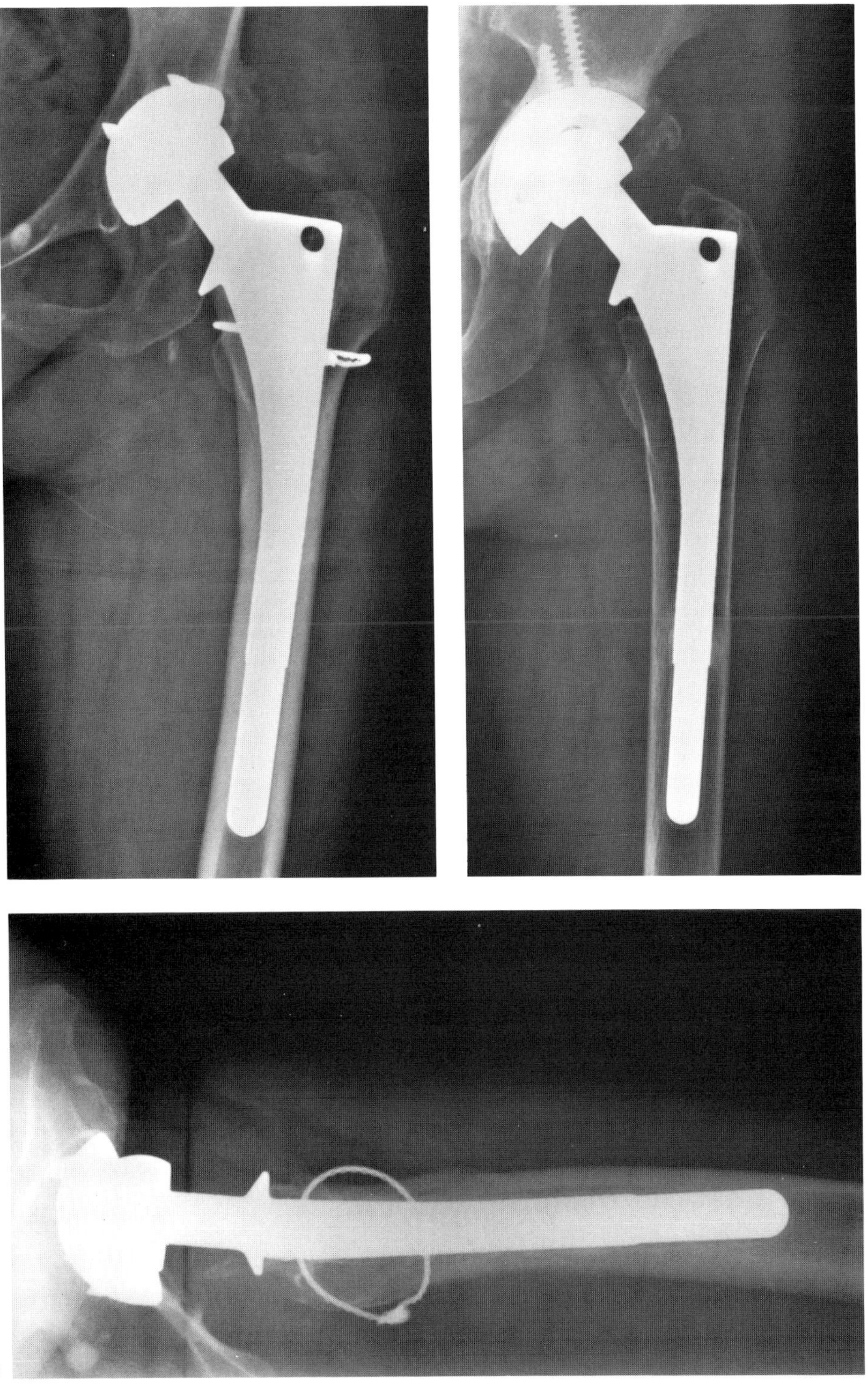

A C

B

FIG. 4-131. The AP **(A)** and lateral **(B)** radiographs of a DePuy AML prosthesis with porous coating, except for the distal fourth of the stem. The fit is excellent on the AP radiograph, and on the lateral view, there is good contact proximally and distally anteriorly and posteriorly. **C:** The same femoral implant in an osteoporotic femur with > 3 mm between the stem and cortex. However, with this extent of cortical thinning, a larger component might cause intraoperative fracture as a result of three-point bending during insertion. There is a lucent halo with a sclerotic margin around the tip, which is of no clinical significance in most cases.

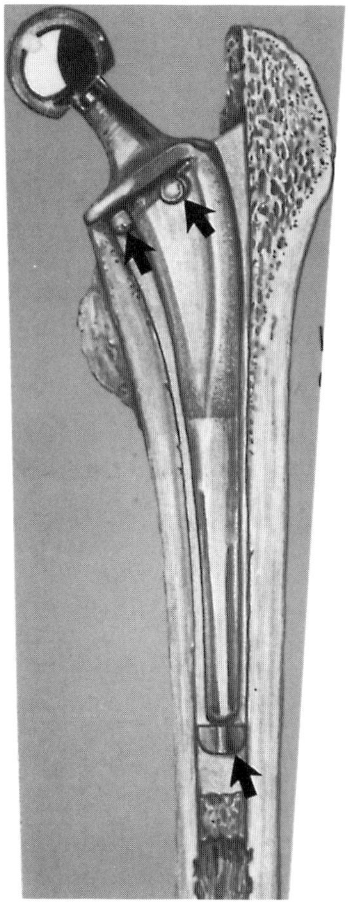

A

FIG. 4-132. A: A P.F.C.™ femoral component with collar, proximal spacers (*arrows*), and a distal centralizer (*arrows*) to improve cement distribution and the formation of optimal mantle thickness. (Courtesy of Johnson and Johnson Orthopedics, Raynham, MA.) **B:** Radiograph of a cemented femoral component with an excellent cement mantle proximally along the stem and distal to the component. **C:** Radiograph of a cemented femoral component with uneven distribution, little cement medially (*arrow*), and voids around the component type (*arrows*).

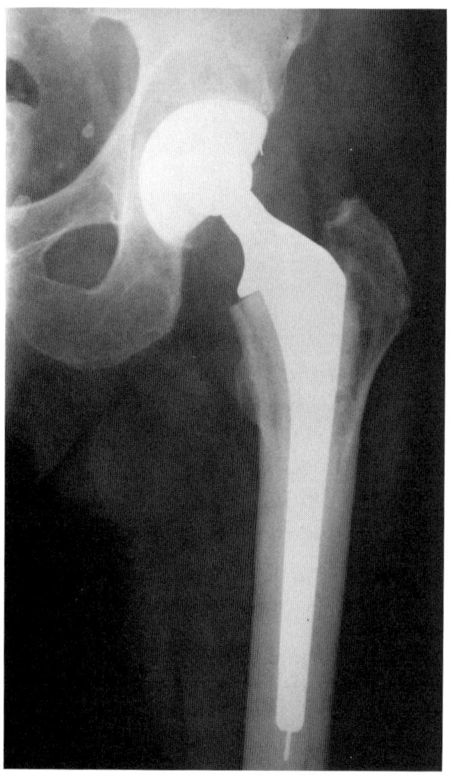

B

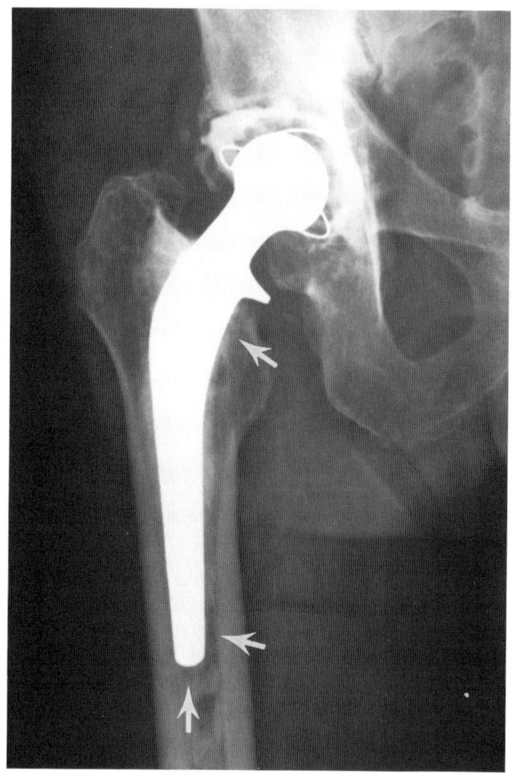

C

insufficient cement medially or around the femoral component tip (Fig. 4-132).[243,270] The cement mantle in zone 7 (Fig. 4-129) should be 2 to 5 mm.[269]

Radiographic changes occur over time in asymptomatic patients, which should not be overinterpreted or considered precursors to component loosening. Kaplan et al.[309] and others have emphasized the findings that are especially useful when evaluating uncemented components.[292,302,334,335] These radiographic features and their incidence in 85 patients with ingrowth components are as follows:[309]

1. Proximal stress shielding (bone loss caused by the loss of normal stress), 98% (Fig. 4-133)
2. Lucent lines with sclerotic margins, especially in zones 1 and 7, 79% (Fig. 4-133)
3. Endosteal sclerosis at the tip and laterally, 36%
4. Heterotopic bone lateral to the neck, 24%
5. Cortical thickening at the femoral tip, 12%
6. Benign periosteal reaction, 4%

Complications

The number of variations in hip components continues to expand; therefore, radiologists must keep pace with the evaluation of all types, either cemented or uncemented. Positive clinical results have been achieved with both.[250,271,311,314,325] Charnley's original or slightly modified designs with cement technique have demonstrated survival rates of near 90% at 20 years.[254,311,351,360]

Uncemented components have also developed an impressive track record, especially in younger more active patients. Hip scores postoperatively are typically well above 95 (Harris).[262] Although follow-up data are still evolving, 95% survival rates have been demonstrated at 5 years.[325]

Patients with symptoms after surgery may have any number of etiologic explanations. The symptoms are not always related to the hip. This must be kept in mind when imaging patients and selecting the most appropriate techniques. Pain is probably the most common symptom, but decreased function, limp, and other signs may also be present. The imaging of patients with hip symptoms postoperatively is most easily discussed by categories of complications.[244,245]

Loosening

Component loosening is one of the most common complications following total hip replacement.[243–245,282] Early results suggested failure might be related to cement or cement techniques.[311,312,377,378] Improved cement techniques have dramatically reduced loosening from rates as high as 57% to 15% to 18% with new metal-backed components.[376–378] However, other factors have also been implicated in loosening in both cemented and uncemented components. Biologic reactions in periprosthetic tissues have been demonstrated with both techniques; polyethylene wear and the release of micron to submicron particles are now a major concern with all hip systems. Macrophages in the membrane around components have been studied and found to contain polyethylene cement and metal debris, resulting in the release of bone resorption products.[301,302,304,305,308] Tumor necrosis factor, interleukin-1β, platelet-derived growth factor, and prostaglandin E_2 have all been implicated in bone resorption and fibrous proliferation, which are implicated in component loosening.[301,317,319,340,346] Uncemented titanium implants have been associated with more wear debris than have cobalt-chromium-molybdenum alloys (especially when beads of titanium were used). However, the release of bioactive products seems to be similar with both alloys.[317,356–359]

Imaging of patients with suspected component loosening has been primarily performed using routine radiographs, subtraction arthrography, and radionuclide scintigraphy.[238,242,244,276,287,313,323,326,338]

Routine Radiograph. Routine radiographs in the AP and lateral projections are useful.[272,274] Serial examinations to evaluate changes in a component's position or periprosthetic changes are accurate. Most data in the current literature describe the radiographic evaluation of cemented components because confidence levels are highest in this setting. Lyons et al.[323] reported that loosening of acetabular components and femoral components could be accurately predicted on routine radiographs in 69% and 84% of patients, respectively. Table 4-15 summarizes the routine radiographic features of cemented component loosening.

TABLE 4-15. *Total hip arthroplasty: cemented component loosening on routine radiographs*[254,300,323,376,378,379]

Acetabular component
Lucent zone at bone cement interface > 2 mm, especially in zone II
Progressive widening or irregularity of lucent zone (Fig. 4-136)
Migration (Fig. 4-134)
Cement fracture (Fig. 4-135)
Acetabular fracture or protrusion
Femoral component
Varus migration
Femoral-stem fracture
Cement fracture
Endoseal resorption
Lucent zones at bone cement interface > 2 mm or progressing
Cement voids > 50% around stem
Subsidence

In our experience, acetabular component loosening can be diagnosed with confidence (100%) on routine radiographs if, on serial radiographs (Fig. 4-134), cement fracture or protrusion (Fig. 4-135) or progressive widening of the lucent zone to > 2 mm can be demonstrated (Fig. 4-136). Thin (< 2 mm) lucent lines at the bone-cement interface in zones I and III are common and can be seen as early as 6 months after surgery.[299,323,376–378]

The evaluation of cemented femoral components is somewhat easier. Progression of lucent lines (Fig. 4-136), cement fracture (Fig. 4-135), and endosteal scalloping are reliable signs of loosening. Infection should also be considered with endosteal scalloping. Varus migration (Fig. 4-137) indicated loosening of the femoral component in all our cases.[323] Fracture of the femoral component is easily detected (Fig. 4-138) on routine radiographs.

Uncemented components are more difficult to evaluate with routine radiographs.[309] Lucent lines are fairly common, and even with some progression, the components may not be clinically loose (Fig. 4-139).[298,302,309] Sight subsidence, indicated by sclerosis at the femoral tip or a radiographic measurement, does not necessarily indicate loosening of uncemented femoral components. Acetabular migration on serial radiographs is a useful sign of acetabular loosening.[282,298,309,323] We could make the argument for fluoroscopically positioning uncemented components for follow-up studies to be certain that the positioning is consistent and the components are aligned to optimal advantage for detecting periprosthetic bone changes.

Arthrography. Arthrography has many uses following hip arthroplasty.[238,303,323,347] Contrast injection is useful for the identification of loosening and other causes of pain, such as pseudobursae, infection, nonunion of the greater trochanter, and adhesive capsulitis.[244,245,323,326,337,345] Fluid can be aspirated for culture and anesthetic injected to assist in confirming that the pain is intraarticular. The latter is especially useful in difficult cases.[244,245]

Some patients have obvious signs of loosening on routine radiographs (Figs. 4-135 and 4-136). In this setting, aspiration to exclude infection, which is commonly seen with loosening, is the more important portion of the study. The technique was discribed briefly in Chapter 1. However, further discussion is warranted in this section. We prefer the subtraction technique in patients with cemented (barium in methyl methacrylate) and uncemented components.[245,323,326] This technique can be performed using conventional film techniques or digital subtraction equipment.[337,345]

Patients are supine on the arthrographic table with the leg supported by bolsters or sandbags to reduce motion. The groin is prepared using sterile technique, and the entry site is anesthetized using a local anesthetic. We typically enter the joint anteriorly or anterolaterally, being careful to avoid the femoral vessels and nerve (Fig. 4-140). Other approaches, such as lateral, may be necessary in patients with extensive heterotopic bone formation.[316]

After the 22- or 18-gauge spinal needle is in place (metal neck felt at the needle tip), fluid is aspirated, or the joint is flushed with nonbacteriostatic sterile saline to send for culture. At this point, a mask film is taken to use for subtraction after the injection of contrast agent. We mix 5 ml of Marcaine™ (Sanofi Winthrop, New York, NY) with 20 ml of Hypaque M-60™ (Squibb Diagnostics, New Brunswick, NJ) for injection. The injections are monitored fluorscopically, and the contrast agent is injected until lymphatic feeling is detected or pressure makes the injection difficult. We also question the patient regarding discomfort, which can also be used as an end point for the injection. When the injection is completed, the second film is taken for subtraction prior to removing the needle. Moving the needle may lead to patient motion. After the needle is removed, we take AP, internal, external, and oblique radiographs. Stress, traction, and lateral views should also be obtained. Postambulation views are useful in subtle or difficult cases to improve the chances that the contrast agent will extend around the component when loosening is present.[240,295,376–378]

The accuracy of this technique is better with cemented femoral components than with acetabular components. We noted a sensitivity of 96% and a specificity of 92% for the femoral component (Fig. 4-141). Large pseudocapsules (>20 ml) decompress the joint, making extravasation around the acetabulum more difficult (Fig. 4-142). Small capsules (≤10 ml), on the other hand, allow the clinician to force small amounts of contrast agent into zones I and III.[326] The two most reliable indications of loosening are contrast detection at the bone-cement interface in zone II or a thick irregular area of the contrast agent (>2 mm) in any zone. These factors were 95% accurate in diagnosis. Thin contrast lines (<2 mm) in zones I and III are only 50% accurate (Fig. 4-141).[142,326]

Data on subtraction arthrography are still being generated for noncemented components. Early experience has been disappointing compared with the positive results with cemented components (Figs. 4-143 and 4-144). Frequently, markedly loose implants (as in revisions) did not show residence or dye dissection at the implant bone interface on arthrography. However, combining routine radiographic features with an x-ray-guided response to the intraarticular anesthetic injection still is a useful tool. In addition, other pathologic findings, such as adhesive capsulitis or large pseudobursae or fistulae, can be identified. Obviously, joint fluid can be studied to assist in patients with suspected infections.

Radionuclide Scans. Bone scanning with technetium-

(text continues on page 323)

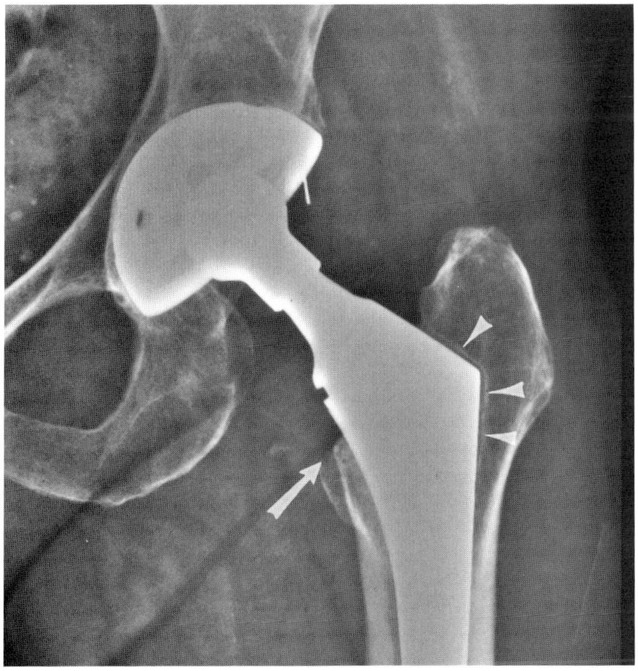

FIG. 4-133. An AP radiograph demonstrating a well-defined 1- to 2-mm lucent area in zone I (*arrowheads*) and rounding of the medial cortex as a result of stress shielding (*arrow*). These findings are of no clinical significance.

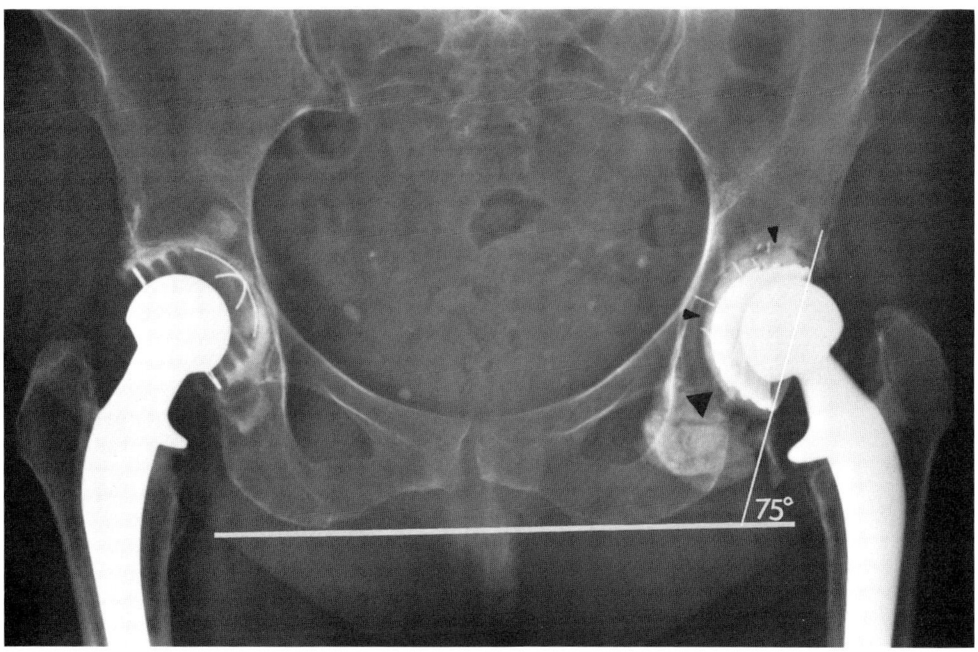

FIG. 4-134. An AP radiograph of the pelvis demonstrating bilateral hip arthroplasties with cemented components. There is a thin lucent zone around the left acetabular component. Zone III is wider (*larger arrow*), and the component has shifted, indicating loosening. The acetabular angle measures 75°.

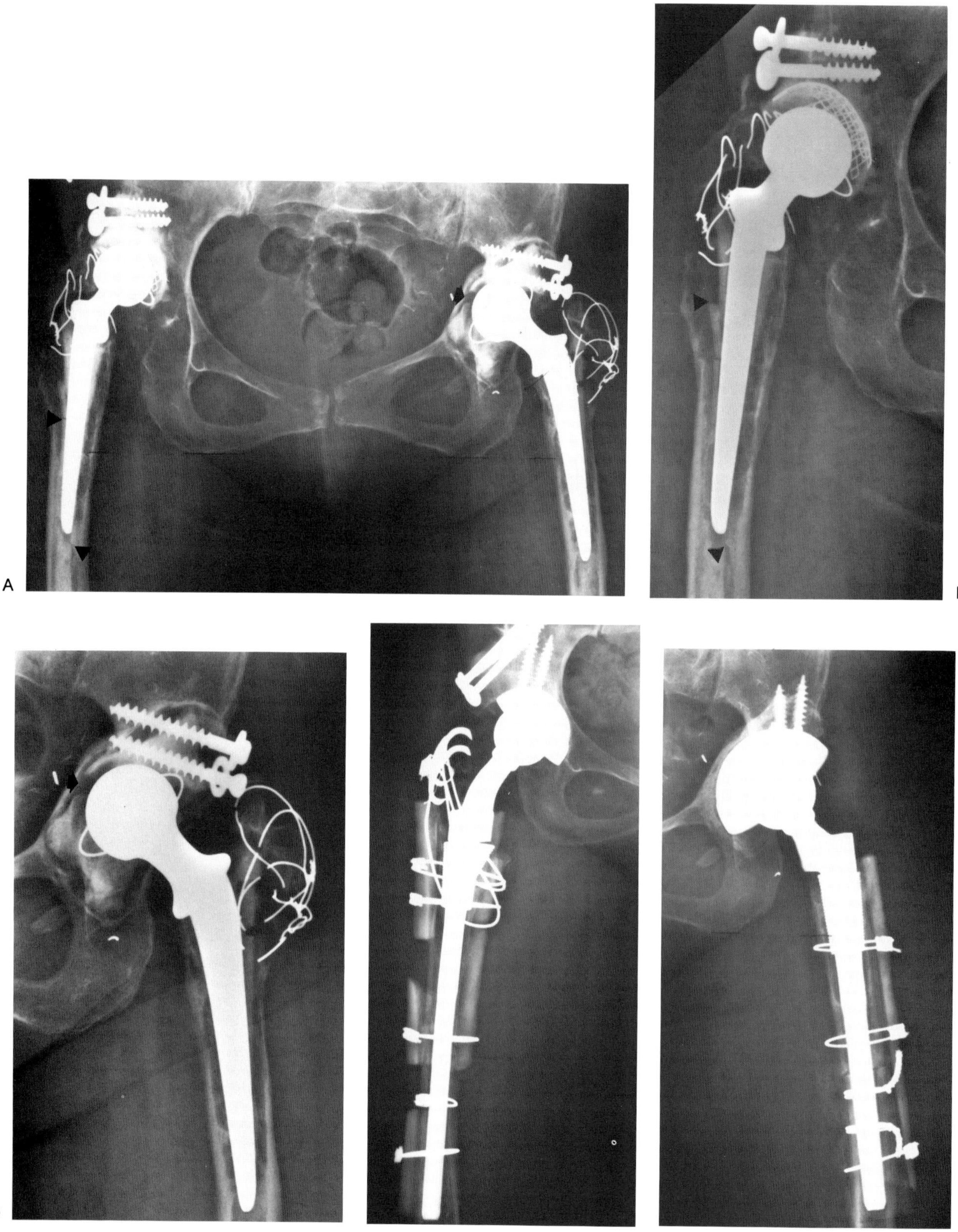

FIG. 4-135. An AP radiograph of the pelvis **(A)** and AP views of the right hip **(B)** and left hip **(C)**. There are bilateral cemented components with acetabular augmentation and bilateral cancellous screws and washers. The acetabular cement on the left is fractured (*arrow*), and there is also a wide lucent zone. There is also endosteal scalloping around the femoral component, which was also loose. The cement around the femoral component on the right is fractured as a result of loosening (*arrows*). **D,E:** Both components were revised using S-ROM™ femoral components. (Note the typical upper sleeve, Fig. 4-113). The femurs were reinforced with cortical bone graft and Dall-Miles cables. There is a Dall-Miles trochanteric claw-cable system on the right.

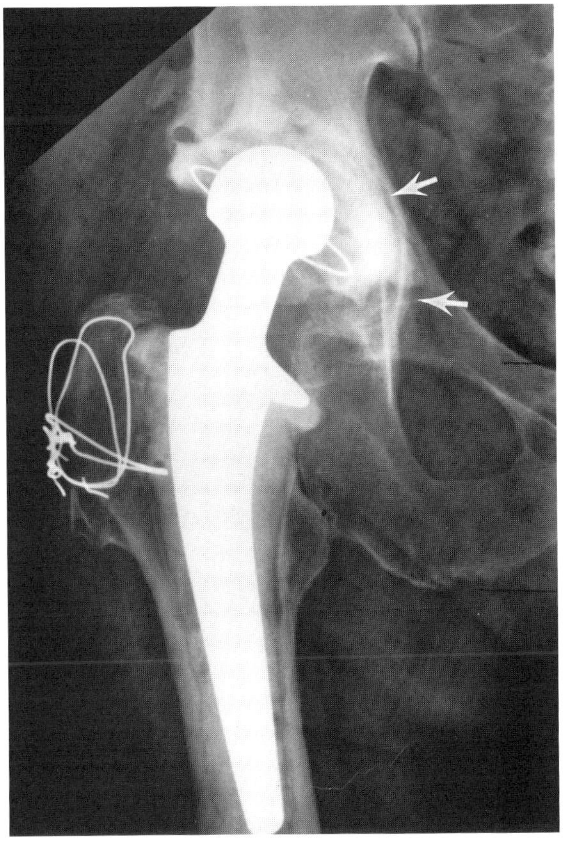
A

FIG. 4-136. **A:** Radiograph of the right hip demonstrates a cemented arthroplasty with a slight lucent zone at the bone-cement interface of the acetabular component in zones II and III (*arrows*). There are also thin lucent areas around the femoral component. **B:** Two years later, a lucent area with osteolysis has developed in zone I (*arrow*) of the acetabular component. There has been marked progression of the lucent area around the femoral component (*arrows*). **C:** Right hip revised using a S-ROM™ femoral component (Fig. 4-113) and uncemented acetabular component.

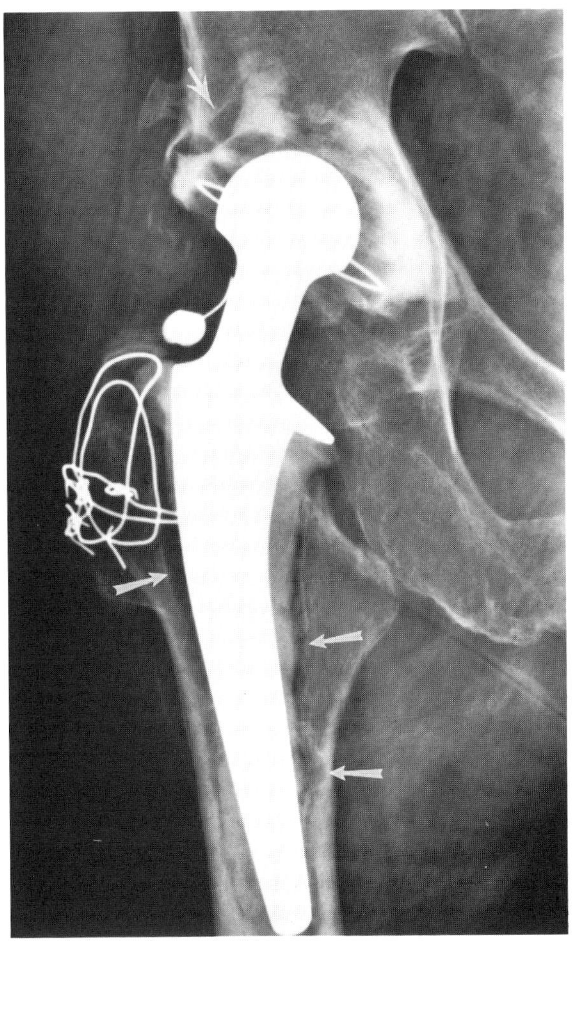
B

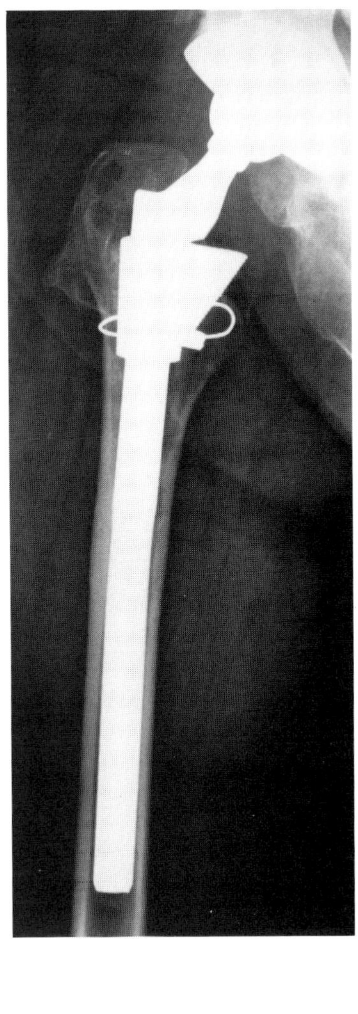
C

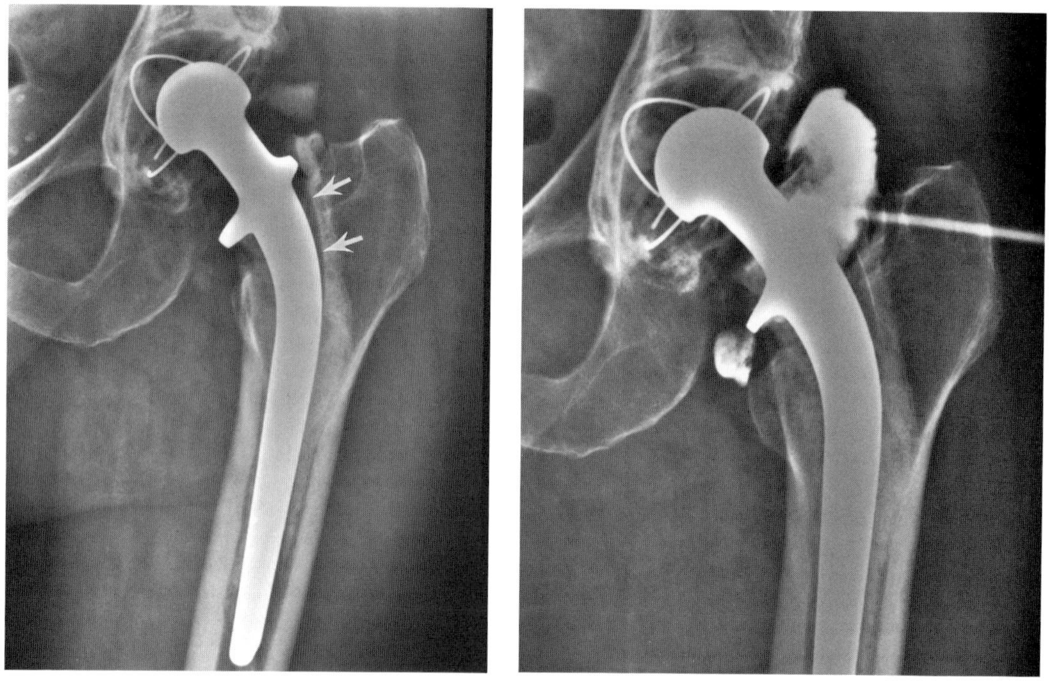

A

B

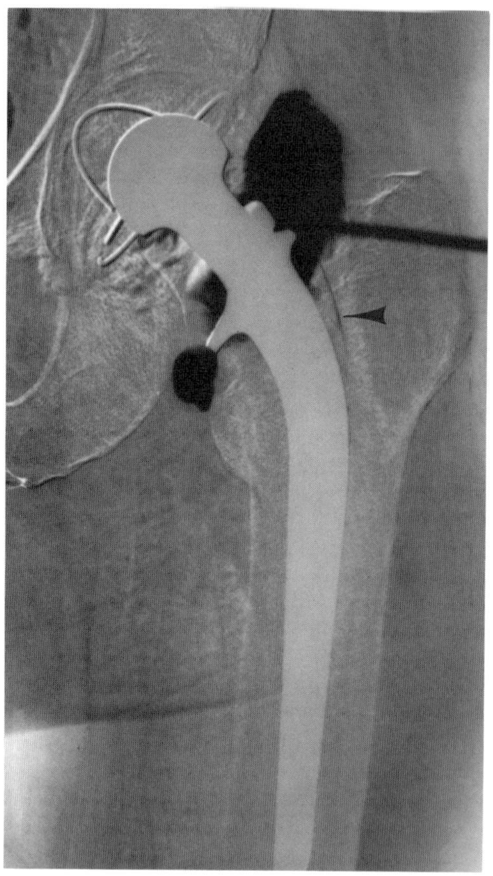

C

FIG. 4-137. A: An AP radiograph of the left hip and femur demonstrating gross migration with a wide lucent area at the metal-cement interface along the upper lateral T-28 component (*arrows*). The cement is fractured at the tip. Subtraction arthrogram (**B**, pre-; **C,** postsubtraction) shows contrast agent along the upper interface with no evidence of acetabular loosening.

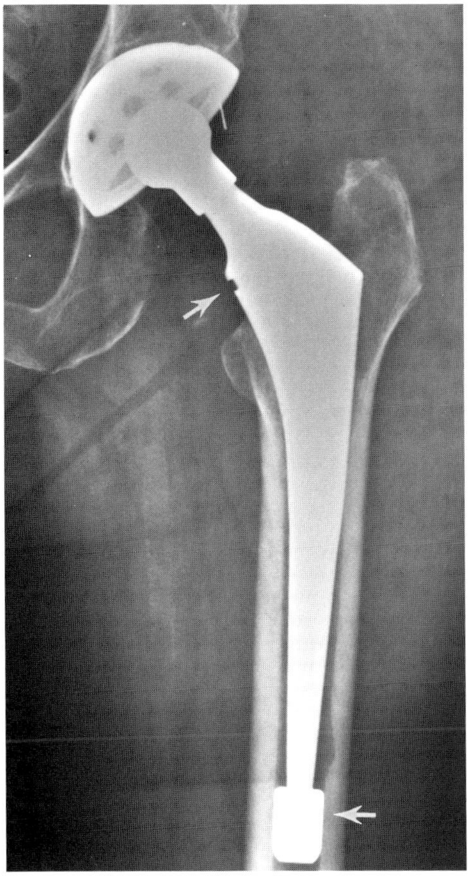

D

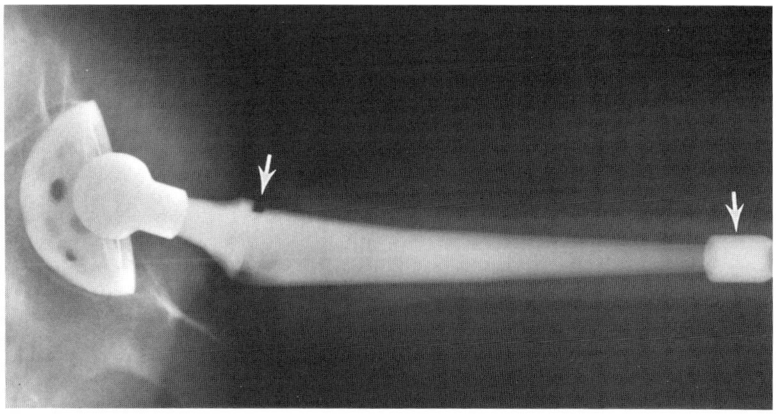

E

FIG. 4-137. (*Continued.*) **D,E:** Both components were revised using an Osteonics Omniflex^{TM} component without the modular collar (*upper arrow*) and a 14-mm bullet tip (*lower arrow*). See also Figs. 4-106 and 4-121.

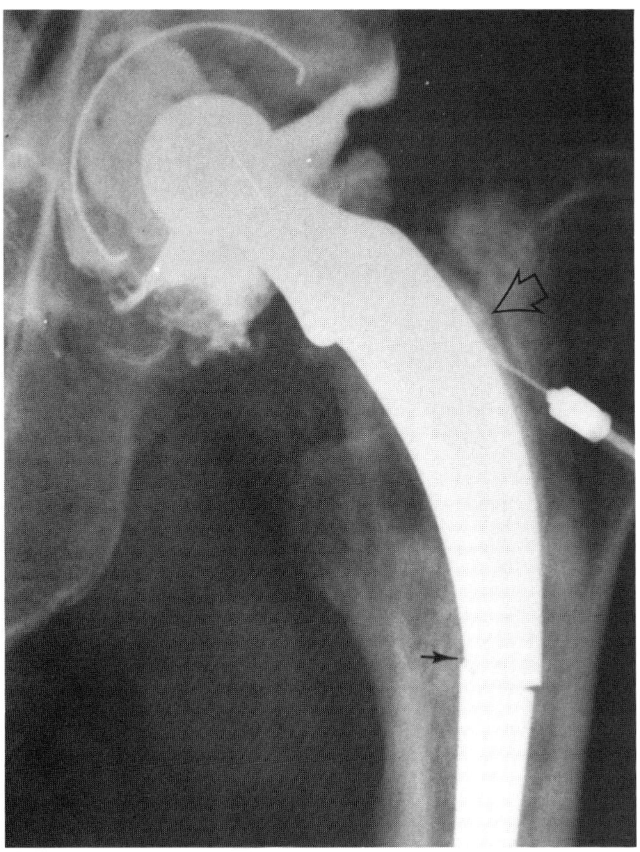

FIG. 4-138. An AP radiograph taken during arthrography. The femoral stem is fractured (*lower black arrow*). There is migration of the upper fragment (*open arrow*).

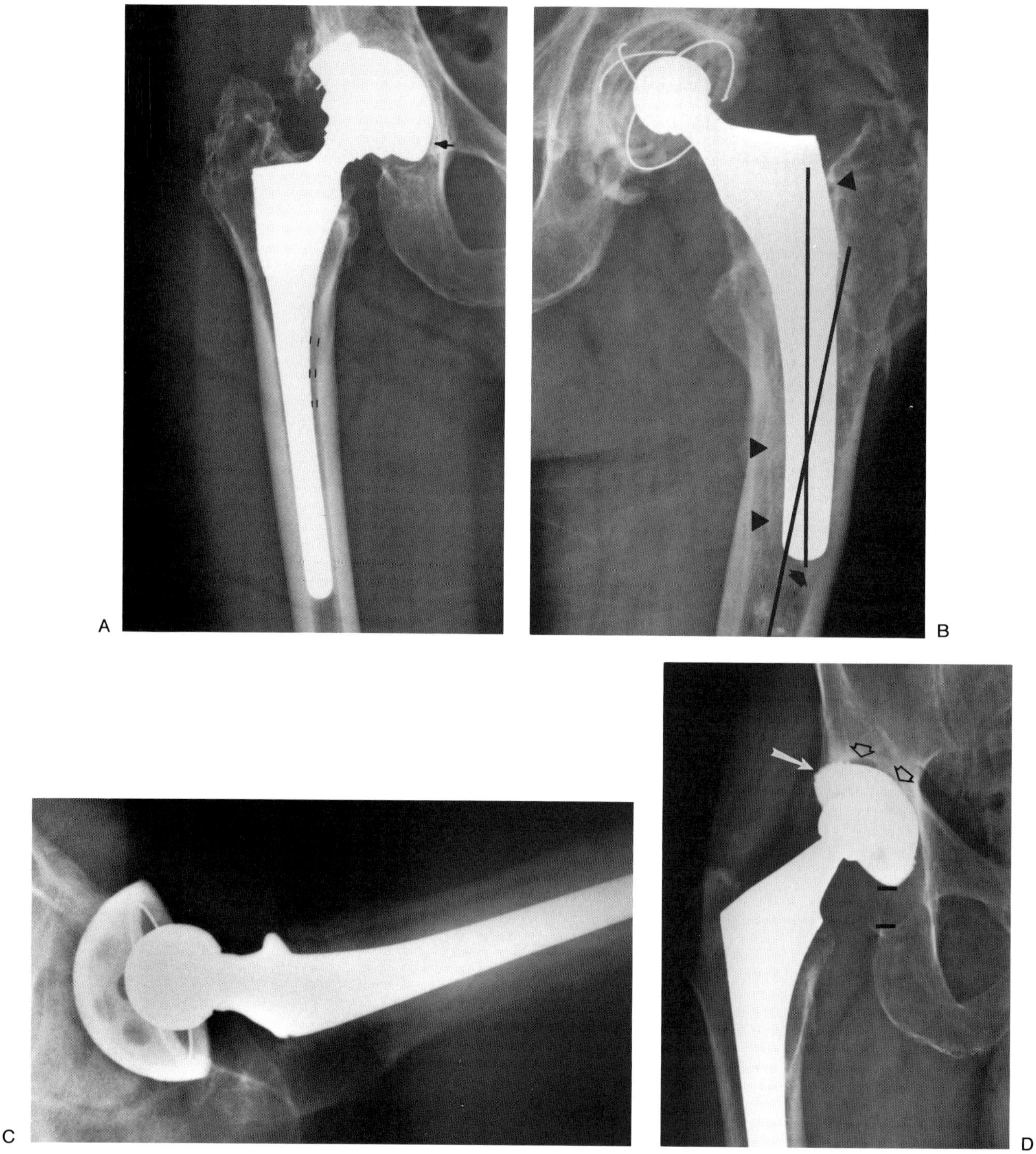

FIG. 4-139. Routine radiographs of uncemented components. **A:** P.C.A.™ hip arthroplasty on the right (Howmedica, Rutherford, NJ.) There is a thin lucent line in zone III of the acetabular component (*arrow*), which is of no significance. No lucent lines are noted around the femoral component. Note the stem fit in the femur. There is greater than 2 mm of marrow along the upper medial stem (*lines*). The fit is still good overall. **B:** Cemented acetabular component with porous-coated femoral component. The component is in varus position, with a wide lucent zone along the lower component medially (*arrows*). There is sclerosis at the tip, indicating subsidence (*arrow*), and a lucent zone superolaterally. This component was loose. **C:** Lateral view of an uncemented acetabular component with a poorly defined lucent zone around the component. No clinical evidence of loosening. **D:** Uncemented right total hip arthroplasty with a loose threaded acetabular component. There is irregular lucency in zones I and II (*open arrows*), and the component has shifted so the upper threads are incompletely covered by bone (*white arrow*). Lower lines show the degree of superior migration.

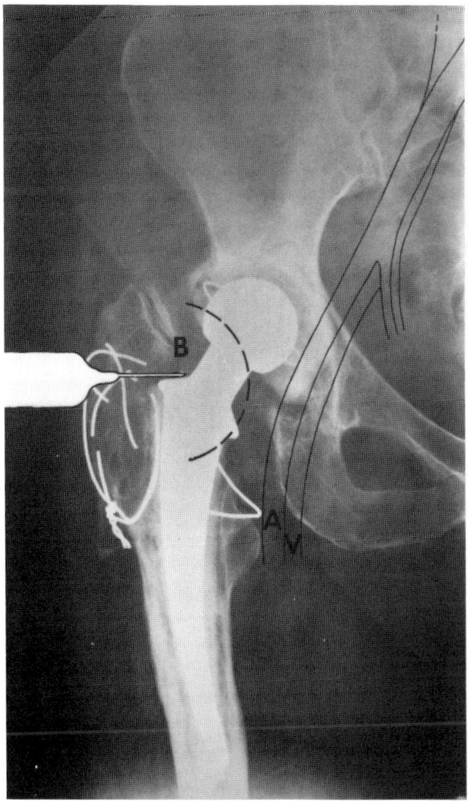

FIG. 4-140. Radiograph with vessels (artery, *A*; vein, *V*) and entry zone (*B*) marked. We prefer to place the needle along the lateral component neck so we can move up and down slightly in the pseudocapsule. (From Lyons CW, Berquist TH, et al. Evaluation of radiographic findings in painful hip arthroplasties. *Clin Orthop* 1985;195:239–251.)

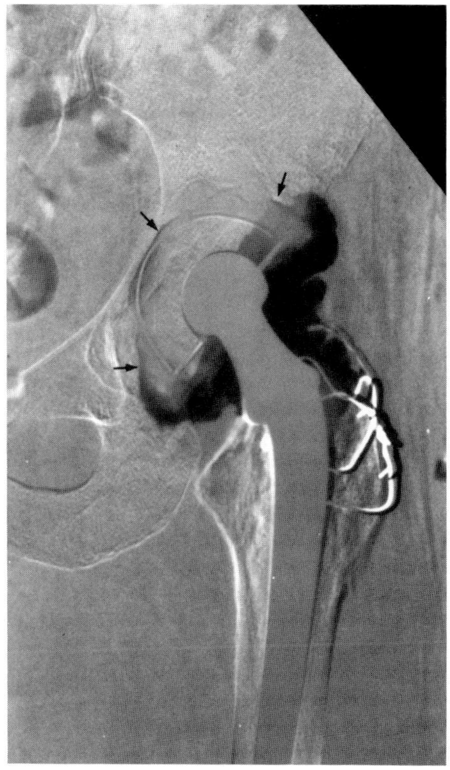

FIG. 4-142. An AP subtraction arthrogram with a large (20 ml) pseudocapsule and contrast agent around the bone cement interface (*arrows*) in all three zones caused by loosening.

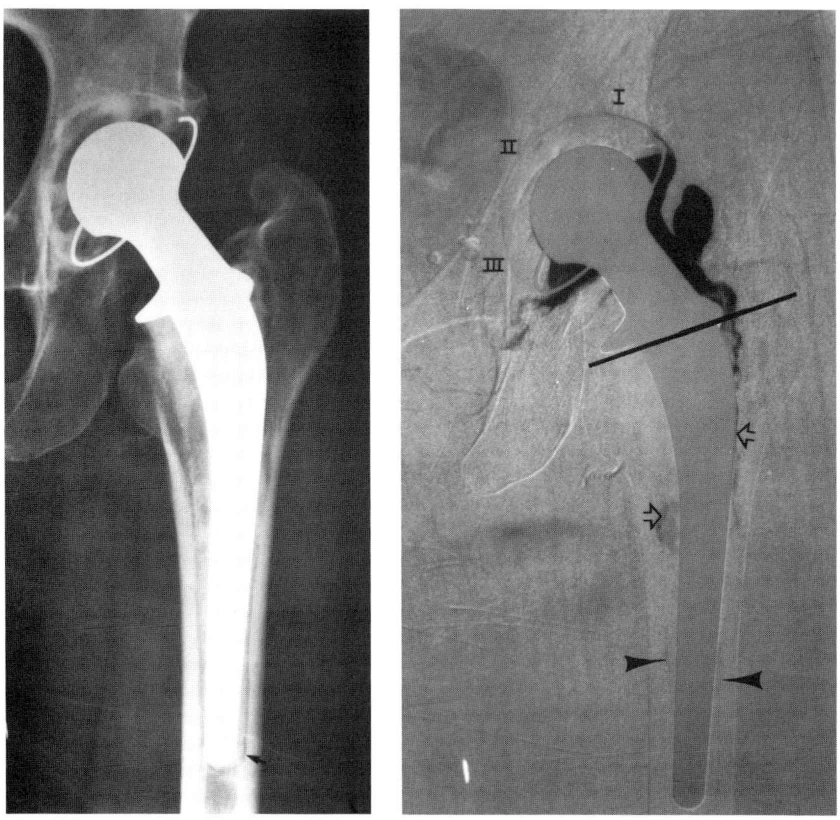

,B

FIG. 4-141. A: Prearthrogram AP radiograph demonstrates a thin lucent zone at the tip of the femoral component (*arrow*). Proximally, there is lucency along the lateral aspect of the cement. Is this marrow or loosening? **B:** Subtraction arthrogram demonstrates irregular contrast agent along the upper stem (*open arrows*) and distally (*black arrows*) caused by loosening. There is also a thin irregular line of contrast agent around the acetabular component in all three zones. Both components were loose. Contrast agent along the upper femoral component greater than 1 cm below the neck (*line*) indicates loosening of conventional length components. Long-stem or revision components are more difficult. We prefer to note contrast agent along the upper 50% before considering the component loose radiographically.

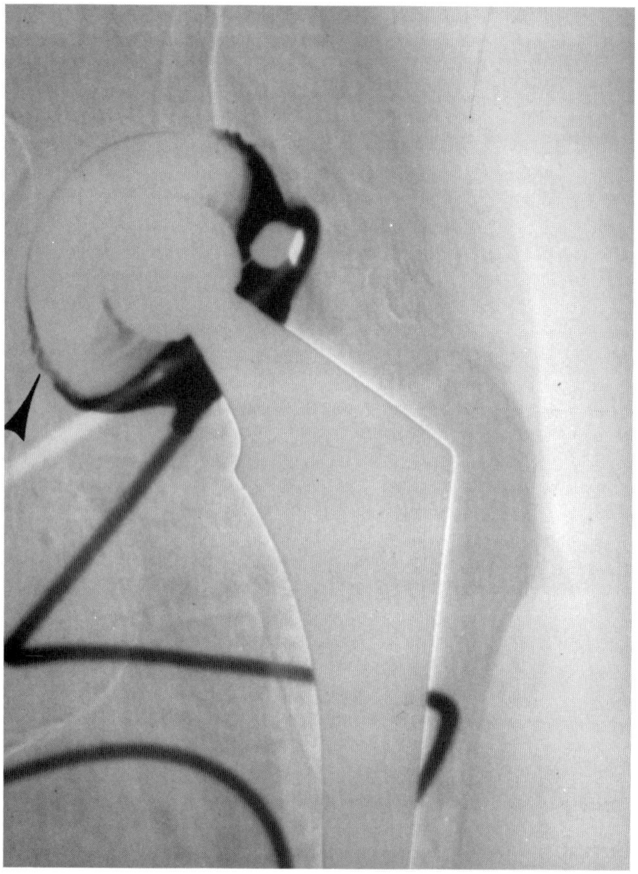

FIG. 4-143. Uncemented left hip arthroplasty. Subtraction arthrogram with anesthetic shows contrast agent in all three zones of the acetabular component with irregularity in zone III (*arrow*). No femoral component loosening. The acetabular component was loose and revised.

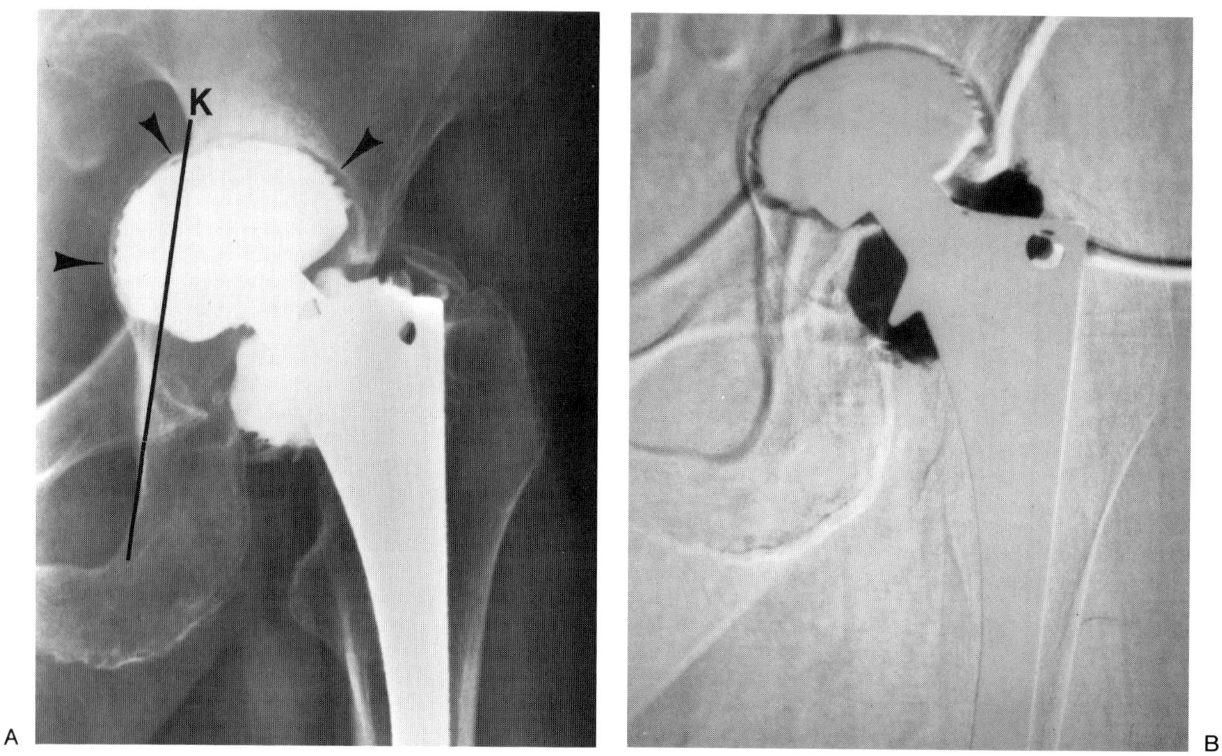

FIG. 4-144. Pre- **(A)** and postsubtraction **(B)** radiographs with a threaded acetabular component with protrusion (Kohler's line) and a wide lucent zone (*arrows*) on the presubtraction image (A). The subtraction view is misregistered; therefore, it is difficult to be sure the dark line around the acetabular is contrast agent. Anesthetic injection completely relieved the symptoms, and based on routine film findings, the component was revised.

99m methylene diphosphonate (MDP) has been used to evaluate lossening and infection.[288,323,338,355] Utz et al.[374] demonstrated increased activity with regions of the lesser trochanter and shaft for up to 6 months following surgery. Increased tracer activity is typically not seen after 1 year. However, in some asymptomatic patients, the activity remains increased in the acetabular region, greater trochanter, and at the tip of the femoral component for up to 2 years (Figs. 4-145 and 4-146).

Radionuclide arthrography has also been used to improve the specificity of detecting component loosening A dose of 1 mCi of technetium-99m sulfur colloid is injected intraarticularly during arthrography. Imaging is performed 1.5 hours later. Increased tracer along the component indicates loosening. Experience with this technique is limited to date. However, its utility may be particularly suited to porous-coated or uncemented components.[349,373]

Infection

The rate of infection with total hip replacement has decreased significantly with improved techniques and the use of prophylactic antibiotics.[368] Early results reported infections in 8% to 11% of patients. However, deep infection is currently reported in the 1% to 2% range for revisions and less than 0.5% for primary hip arthroplasties.[315,312,331]

The radiographic diagnosis of infection is somewhat imprecise. Two findings on routine radiographs are associated with infection in more than 80% of patients. The most useful is endosteal scalloping (Fig. 4-147). A laminated periosteal reaction is also seen with infection. The sensitivity of endosteal scalloping is only 47%, but the specificity is 96%. Periosteal new bone formation is only 25% sensitive but 92% specific.[323]

Arthrography adds certain imaging criteria, but more importantly, it allows needle access for fluid aspiration for culture. Although the technique is controversial, with false-negative and false-positive results, we found that fluid aspiration correctly identified the organism in 71% of patients.[326] An irregular pseudocapsule or sinus tracts with or without cavities also indicate infection (Figs. 4-148 and 4-149).[244,323,368] Lymphatic filling is nonspecific and not a useful finding (Fig. 4-149).[323]

Conventional technetium scans alone are not as effective as combined studies. However, a negative technetium-99m MDP study result does effectively exclude loosening, infection, or other osseous pathologic findings.[323,374] Focal uptake is also unusual in an infected hip arthroplasty. The changes are more frequently diffuse (Fig. 4-150).[374]

Gallium-67 and indium-111-labeled white blood cell studies are also used in patients with suspected infections. Gallium accumulates in tumors, abscesses, normal marrow, and areas of bone remodeling. Therefore, it must be used in conjunction with technetium-99m MDP to exclude uptake caused by simple bone turnover.[323,338,374] We prefer indium-111-labeled white blood cells because the results indicate that this technique is more specific and sensitive, especially when combined with bone scan results.[323,338]

Dislocations

Dislocation of hip components is uncommon (3%) but usually occurs during the early postoperative period or with the initiation of weight bearing.[242,247,260,331,381] There are numerous factors that increase the risk of dislocation, including smaller head size (a 22-mm head is more likely to dislocate than a larger one), previous surgery, surgical approach (posterior more likely than arterolateral), component malposition, avulsion of the greater trochanter, and the patient's age and preoperative diagnosis.[260,331]

Imaging of dislocations is easily accomplished on AP and lateral radiographs (Fig. 4-151). In the early postoperative period, other views, such as the frog-leg oblique view, should be avoided, or a dislocation can be created. Dislocation of the acetabular liner has also been reported.[381]

Pseudobursae

Pseudobursae are identified in up to 43% of patients after hip arthroplasty. These most commonly occur in the greater trochanteric, supraacetabular, and iliopsoas regions. Up to one third of patients have had previous dislocations. Pain can occur with these bursae, without loosening or other complications. Unlike infected cavities, these bursae are smooth walled and frequently large (Fig. 4-152). Anesthetic injection with aspiration should be considered in this situation.[245]

Greater Trochanteric Avulsion or Nonunion

When an osteotomy of the greater trochanter is performed, it is generally reattached with wire or, more recently, a Dall-Miles cable-claw system. Union occurs in 6 to 12 weeks in 95% of cases.[240,349] Routine radiographs are usually adequate for diagnosis. When union cannot be judged, subtraction arthrograms (Fig. 4-153) may be indicated. Wire fracture is common and does not indicate a bad result.[240,378] Wire fracture may occur years after the osteotomy has healed. Wire fragments can cause bursitis.[378] Concerns about cable breakage have emerged, but the frequency of this problem is still not clear.

An uncemented or avulsed greater trochanter does not always need repair. If displaced less than 2 cm, function can remain acceptable. When there is significant displacement and pain or a limp, reoperation may be necessary.[378]

(*text continues on page 330*)

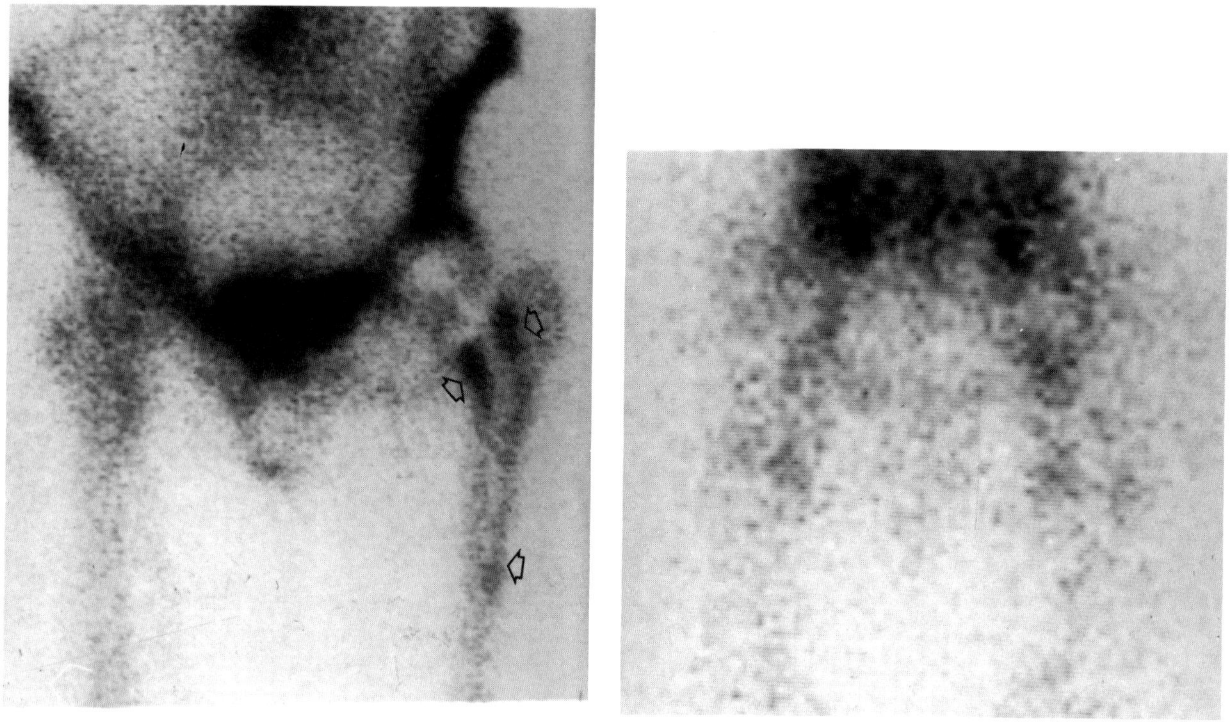

A B

FIG. 4-145. Combined technetium-99m MDP image **(A)** and indium-111-labeled white blood cell study **(B)** in a patient 2 years after surgery with suspected loosening and possible infection. There is increased tracer at the upper and lower aspect of the stem (*arrows*) on the technetium scan because of loosening. The indium scan is normal. No infection at time of revision.

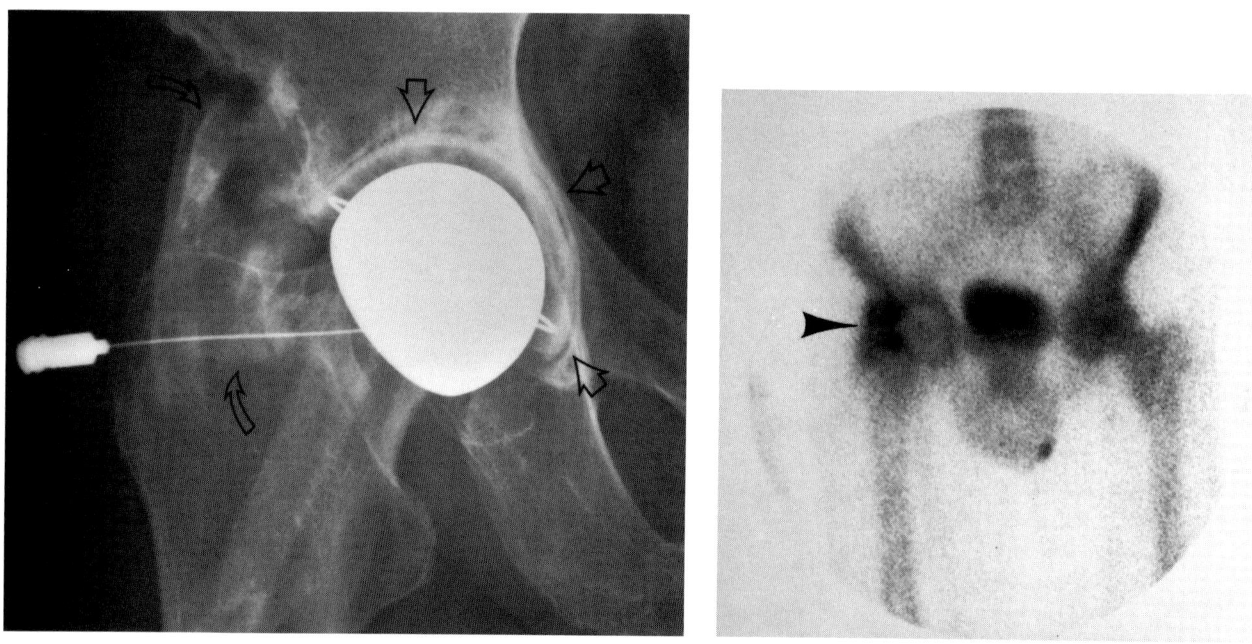

A B

FIG. 4-146. A: Preinjection arthrogram radiograph demonstrating lucency around the acetabular component (*open arrows*) and heterotopic bone (*curved arrows*). **B:** Technetium-99m MDP scan shows increased uptake within the region of the heterotopic bone (*arrow*). The acetabular component is not clearly loose.

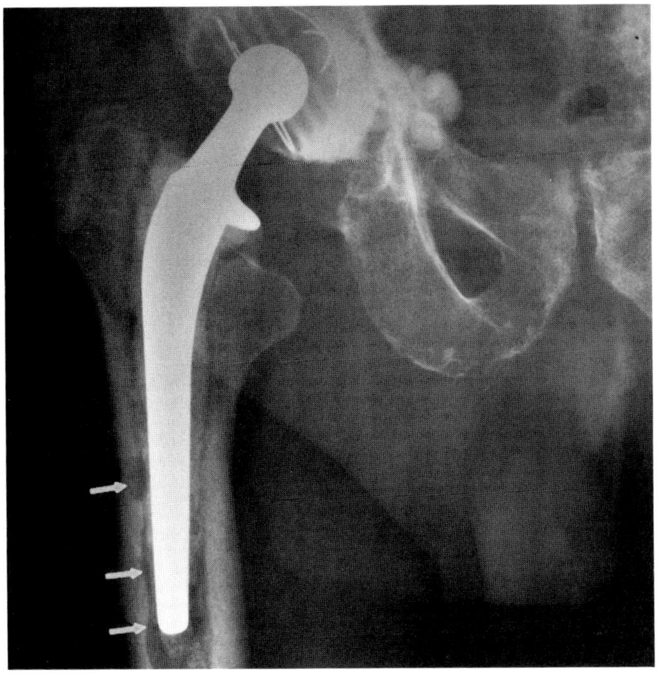

FIG. 4-147. An AP radiograph of the right femur demonstrating endosteal scalloping (*arrows*) caused by loosening and infection.

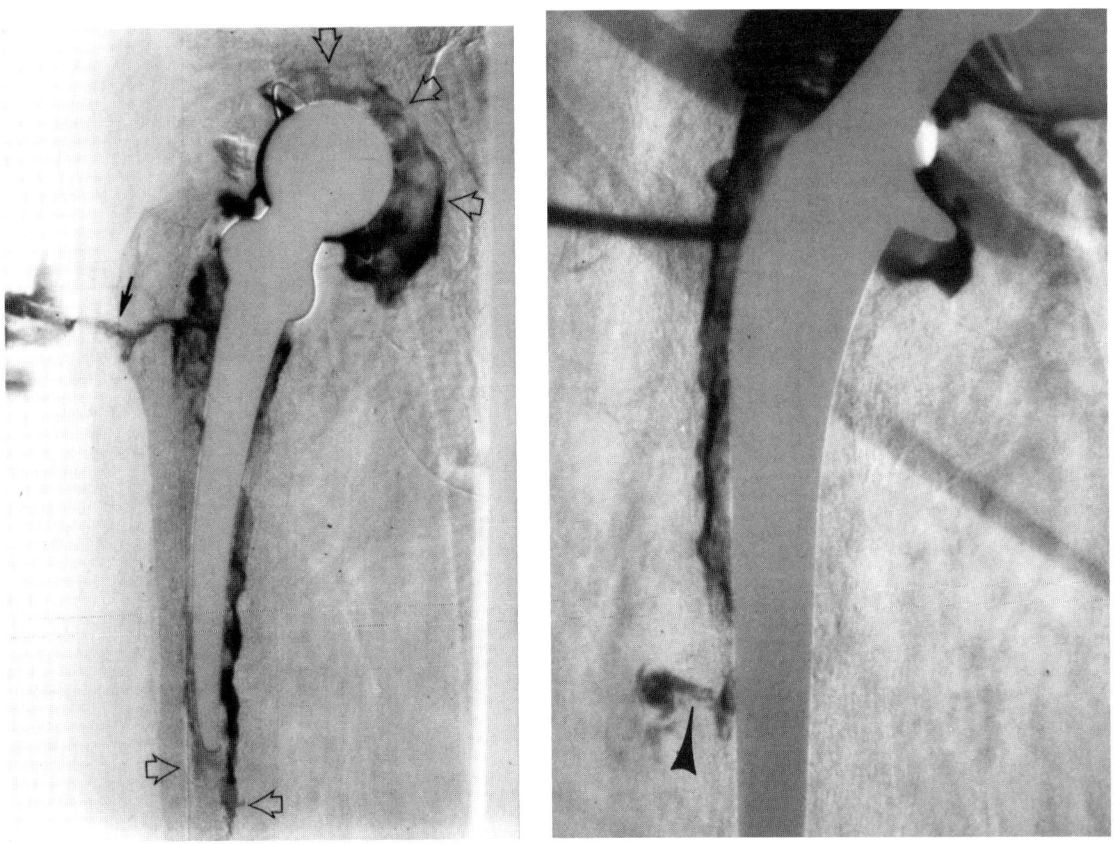

A B

FIG. 4-148. Arthrograms demonstrating features seen with infection. **A:** Subtraction arthrogram of the right hip demonstrated thick irregular contrast agent collections along the femoral and acetabular components, indicating obvious loosening (*open arrows*). There is a fistula and abscess laterally (*black arrow*). **B:** Subtraction arthrogram demonstrating loosening of the femoral component with a distal fistula (*arrow*) caused by infection. (See **C** and **D** on next page.)

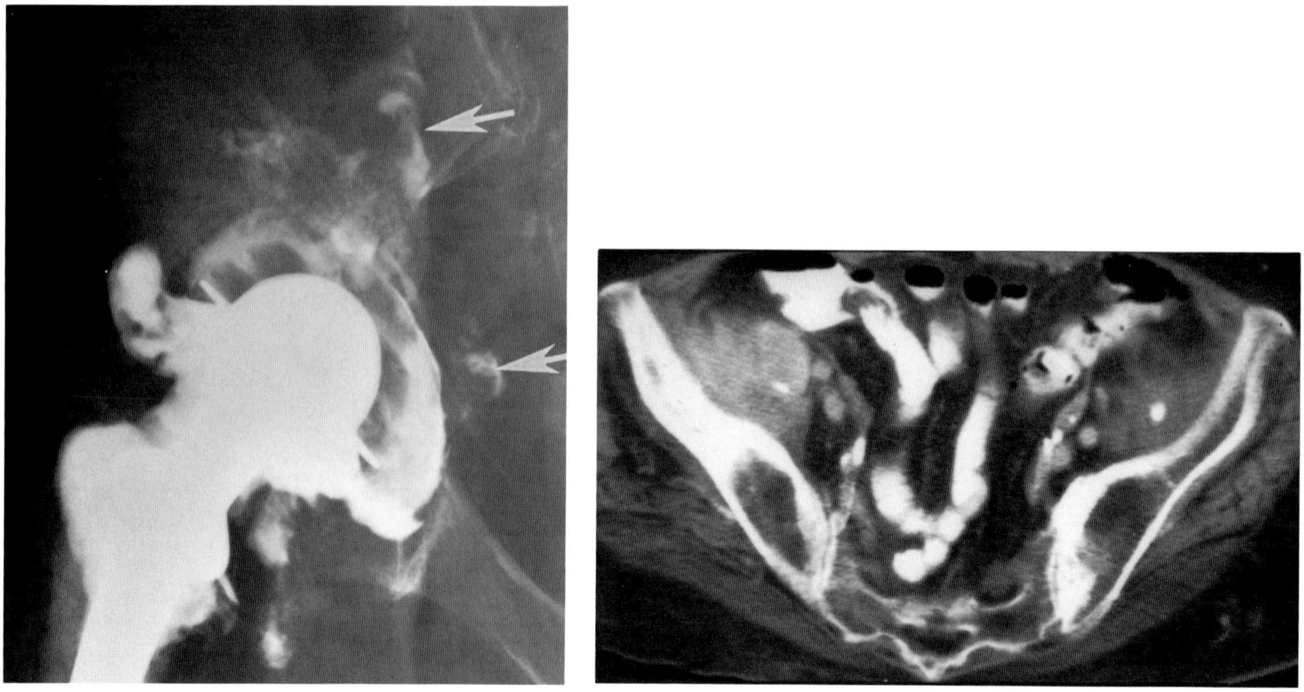

C D

FIG. 4-148. (*Continued.*) Arthrogram **(C)** and CT scan **(D)** demonstrate irregular contrast agent extending into the pelvis (*arrows,* C) with a psoas abscess.

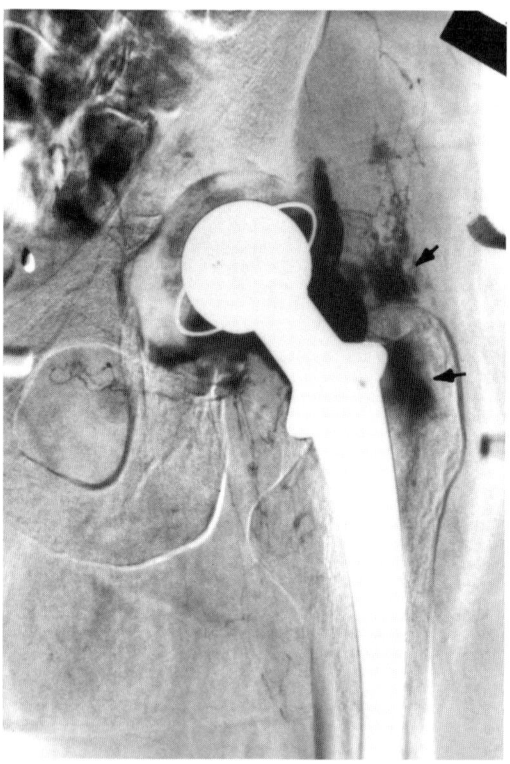

FIG. 4-149. Subtraction arthrogram of the left hip demonstrating capsular irregularities (*arrows*), which is consistent with infection. The lymphatic filling can be seen with many conditions, including capsular distention.

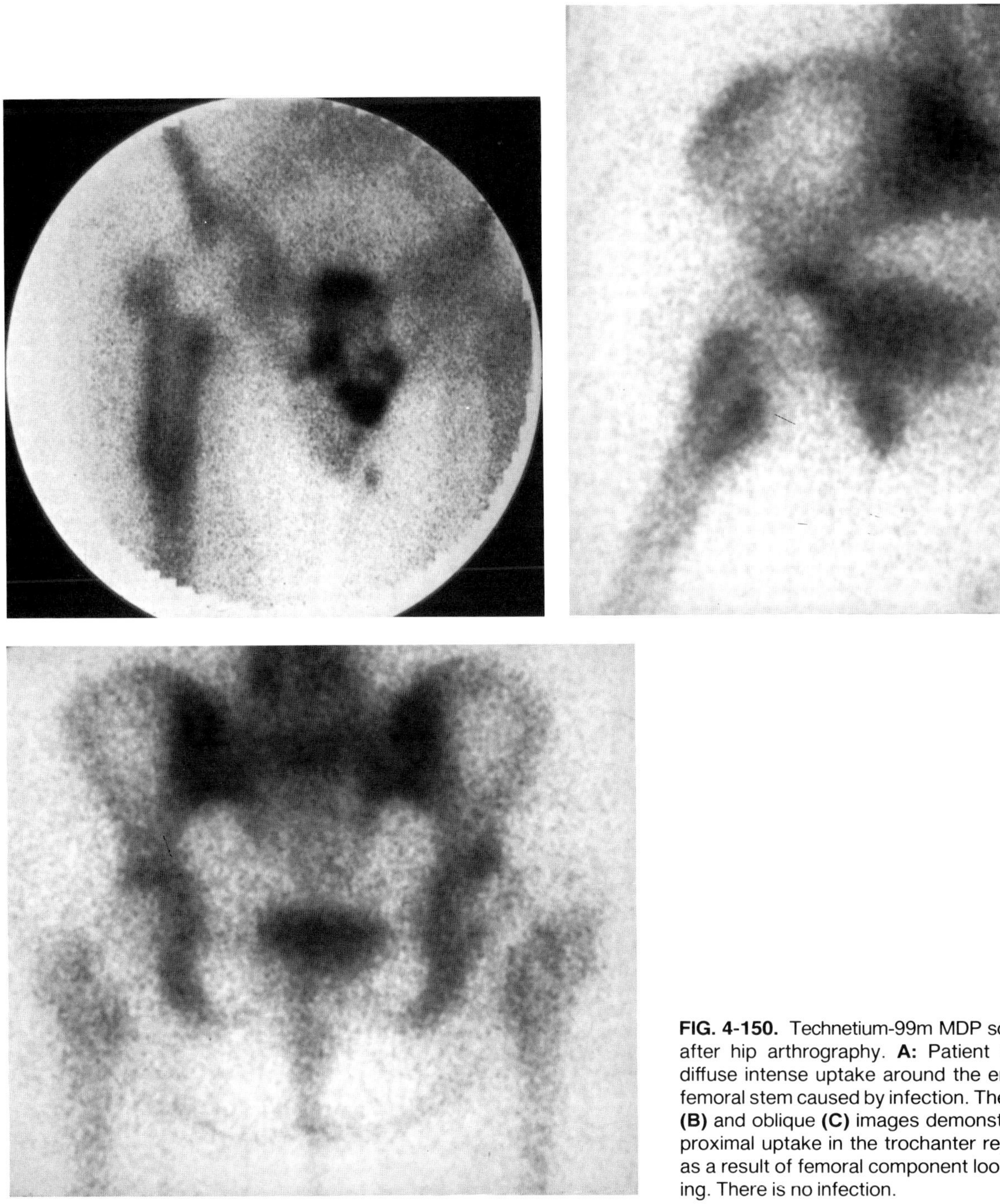

FIG. 4-150. Technetium-99m MDP scans after hip arthrography. **A:** Patient with diffuse intense uptake around the entire femoral stem caused by infection. The AP **(B)** and oblique **(C)** images demonstrate proximal uptake in the trochanter region as a result of femoral component loosening. There is no infection.

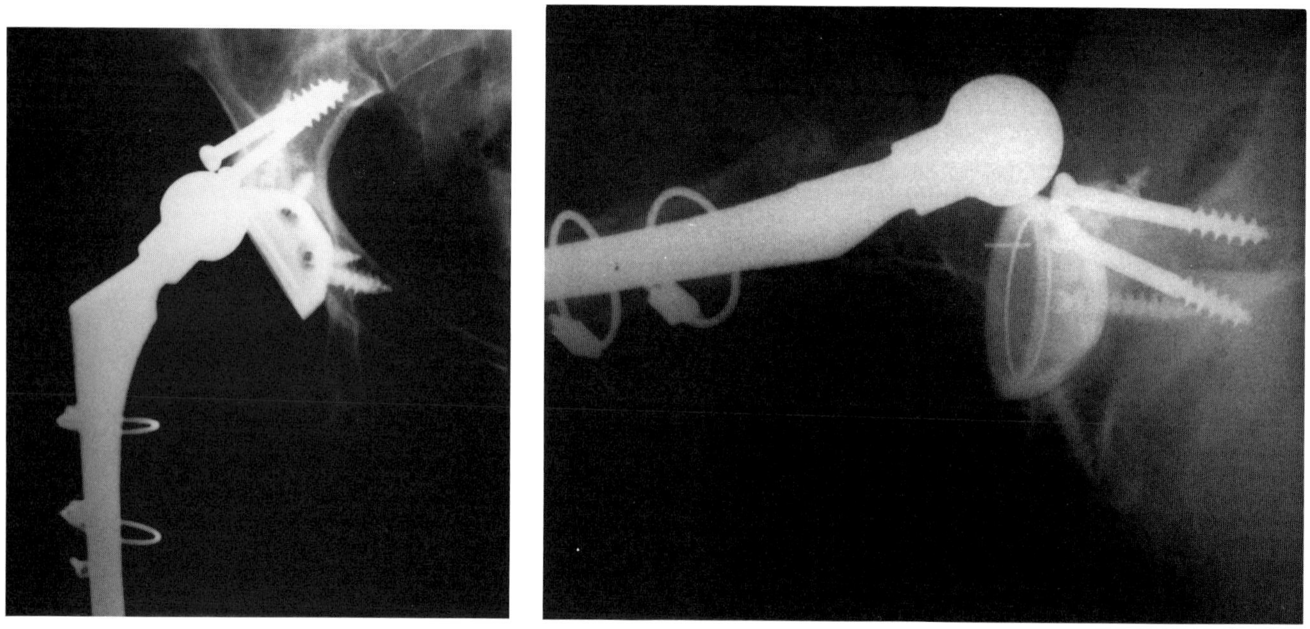

A B

FIG. 4-151. The AP **(A)** and lateral **(B)** radiographs of a revision modular system on the right. The femur dislocated anterosuperiorly several days after surgery.

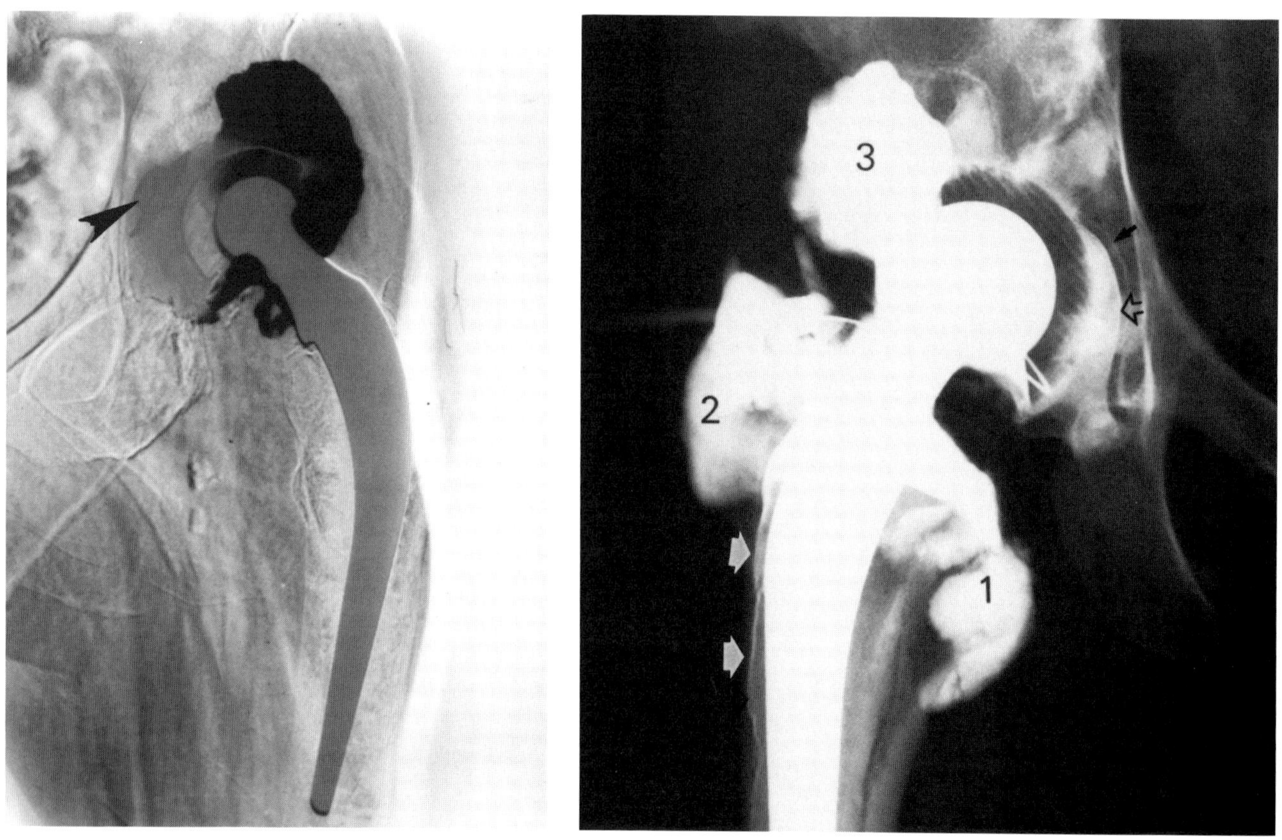

A B

FIG. 4-152. Pseudobursae. **A:** Subtraction arthrogram in a patient with previous dislocations and a large supraacetabular pseudobursa. Charnley prosthesis with cement restrictor in the acetabulum (*arrow*). **B:** Patient with loosening (*arrows*) and three pseudobursae. *1,* lesser trochanteric; *2,* greater trochanteric; *3,* supraacetabular.

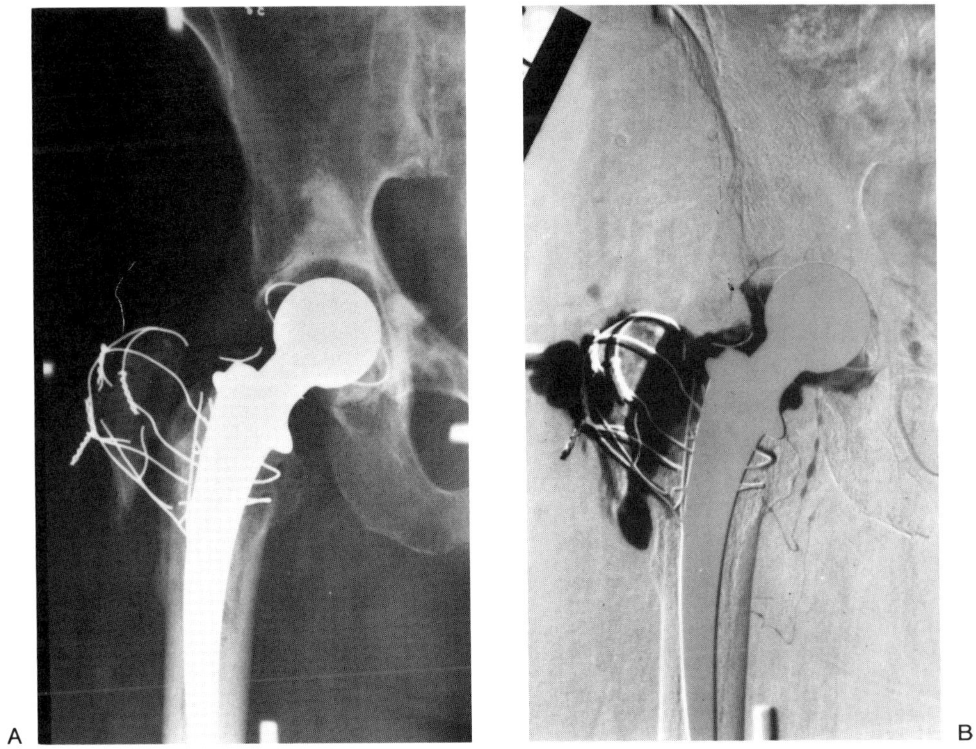

FIG. 4-153. **A:** An AP radiograph of the right hip demonstrating wire fragmentation and a displaced greater trochanter. The patient had pain with a limp. **B:** Subtraction arthrogram demonstrates contrast agent extending between the femur and greater trochanter as a result of nonunion. There is also a trochanteric bursa laterally.

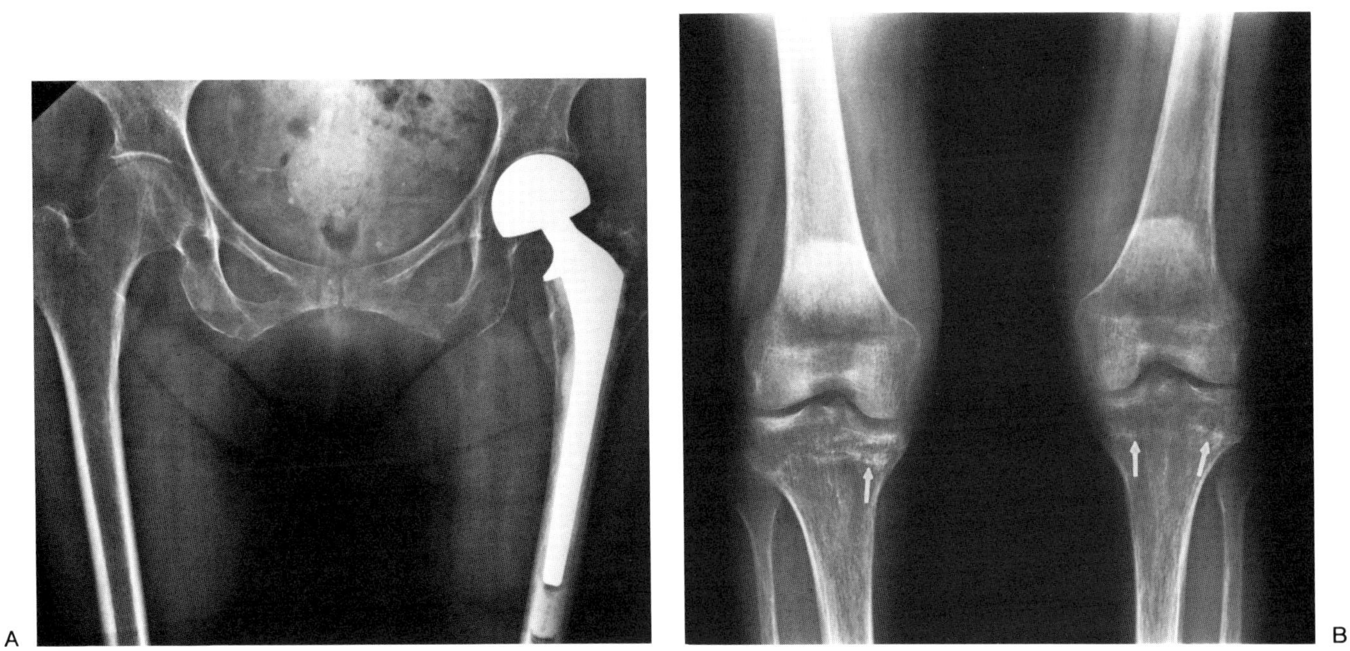

FIG. 4-154. A 70-year-old inactive woman with a recently implanted left bipolar arthroplasty for a femoral neck fracture (**A**). Knee pain developed with activity, and a standing radiograph of the knees (**B**) demonstrated bilateral tibial insufficiency fractures (*arrows*).

Heterotopic Bone Formation

Heterotopic ossification occurs to some degree after hip arthroplasty on most patients. This is usually of little consequence clinically.[242] Heterotopic bone is more likely to develop in patients with DISH, male patients with osteoarthritis, ankylosing spondylitis, previous surgery, or extensive surgical trauma.[331,361]

Morrey[331] classified heterotopic bone on the AP radiograph. Grade I is less than 5 mm of bone between the greater trochanter and acetabulum. Grade II bone formation is < 50% of the distance; grade II, > 50%; and Grade IV, ankylosis. Extensive ectopic bone formation can restrict motion and reduce function. In high-risk patients, there are three basic techniques to reduce the bone formation. These include antiinflammatory medication, diphosphonates, and low-dose radiation several days after surgery. Most prefer low-dose radiation.[361]

Fractures

Fractures may occur intraoperatively, postoperatively, or at a distant site (lower extremity, pubic rami, or sacrum) as a result of stress in a previously inactive patient (Fig. 4-154).[242,344] Intraoperative fractures can occur during cement removal, during dislocation of the femoral head from the acetabular component, or during reaming.[331,344] Fractures that are identified during surgery can be managed using a longer stem or with cerclage wire or cable. Some intraoperative fractures are overlooked until postoperative radiographs are obtained. Postoperative fractures may occur after minimal trauma (cement windows or screw tracts) or with motor vehicle accidents.[331]

Osteolysis and Arthropathy

The local tissue response to cement, metal, and especially, polyethylene debris can lead to aggressive synovitis and arthropathy (Fig. 4-155) or osteolysis.[356–359,379] Bone resorption may occur as a small focal area of endosteal scalloping, a longer linear area of resorption, or a large local area resembling a tumor (Fig. 4-156). This has been referred to as a granulomatous pseudotumor.[253,289] Histologic evaluations of periprosthetic tissues have demonstrated macrophages containing polyethylene, metal, or methyl methacrylate debris.[255,356–359,379,380]

Radiographic features may be subtle or aggressive (Figs. 4-155 and 4-156). Loosening and component failure or polyethylene wear should be searched for carefully on radiographs. Early detection will assist in revision before extensive bone loss and further component deterioration occurs.[289,353]

Revision Arthroplasty

Revision arthroplasty is most frequently performed for aseptic loosening, infection, and instability.[246,258,327,372,384] Problems with cement removal (when the components were cemented) and inadequate bone stock can lead to recurrent loosening. This was a particular problem with cemented revision components in which loosening is reported in 50% of patients at 5 years.[372,376]

For the purposes of this atlas, we discuss acetabular and femoral problems separately, followed by treatment options for infection.

Acetabular Components

The high loosening rates with cemented revision components have resulted in a shift toward uncemented acetabular revisions with bone grafting and cancellous screw augmentation, as necessary.[258,326,372] Diminished bone stock and protrusion are a particular problem in the acetabulum (Figs. 4-157 and 4-158).[258,326] The acetabulum can be reinforced with autogenous bone grafts or allografts. Protrusion shells have also been used in this setting (Fig. 4-157).[258,326,372]

Either autogenous grafts or allografts can be used to fill bone defects after thorough preparation of the acetabulum. All cement and membranous material should be removed. Smaller defects can be filled with autogenous bone or allografts. Cortical grafts may be required for larger defects. Some authors advocate a two-stage procedure when there is significant bone loss. This allows the bone graft to heal; therefore, in theory, it is better prepared to facilitate ingrowth in uncemented porous components when the revision is performed. Up to 12 months is allowed for healing with two-stage procedures.[327,372]

When significant bone loss is suspected, it may be useful to obtain CT images prior to revision. Although the metal artifact causes image degradation, sufficient information is usually obtained to plan the procedure (Fig. 4-159). Reformatting CT images in the coronal or sagittal planes may actually reduce the artifact and provide additional information.[275] Titanium implants also tend to cause less artifact than do stainless steel.[268] Early results with uncemented revision components and bone grafting show failure rates as low as 1%.[372]

Femoral Component

Revision of the femoral component can be equally difficult, especially if the original component was cemented. The revision technique depends on what is being revised, i.e., endoprosthesis fracture fixation devices (Fig. 4-160), cemented component, conventional or

(*text continues on page 335*)

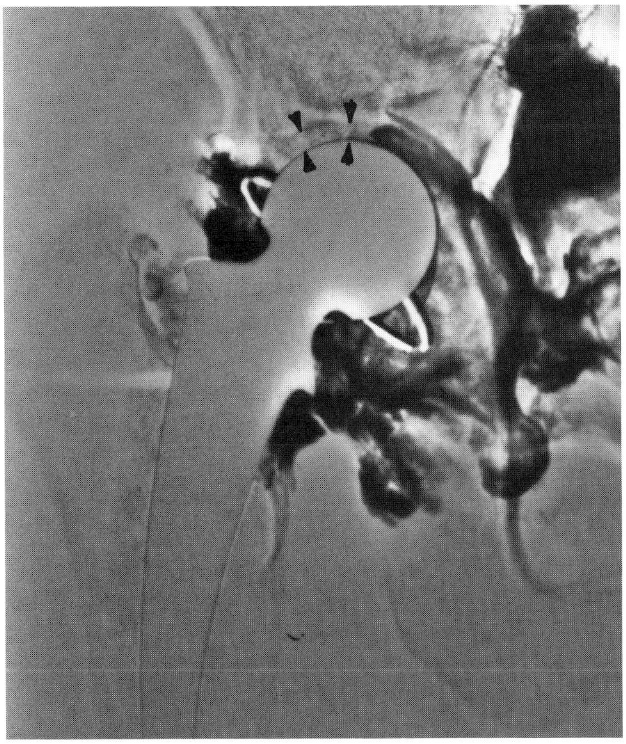

FIG. 4-155. Subtraction arthrogram in a patient with advanced synovitis with irregularity of the pseudocapsule. The osteolysis has disrupted the acetabulum. Contrast agent enters the pelvis and pelvic nodes. Note the thin rim of polyethylene in the upper acetabulum (*arrows*) caused by polyethylene wear.

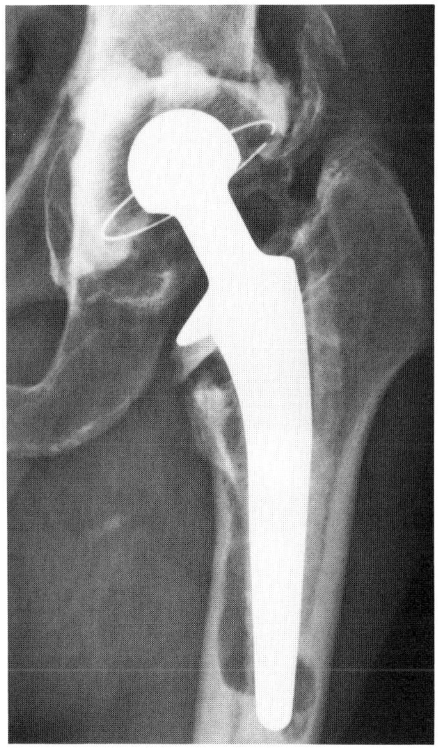

FIG. 4-156. An AP radiograph of the left hip with osteolysis at the femoral tip and along the medial component. The component has loosened and migrated into varus position. There is grade III (> 50%) heterotopic bone laterally.

A

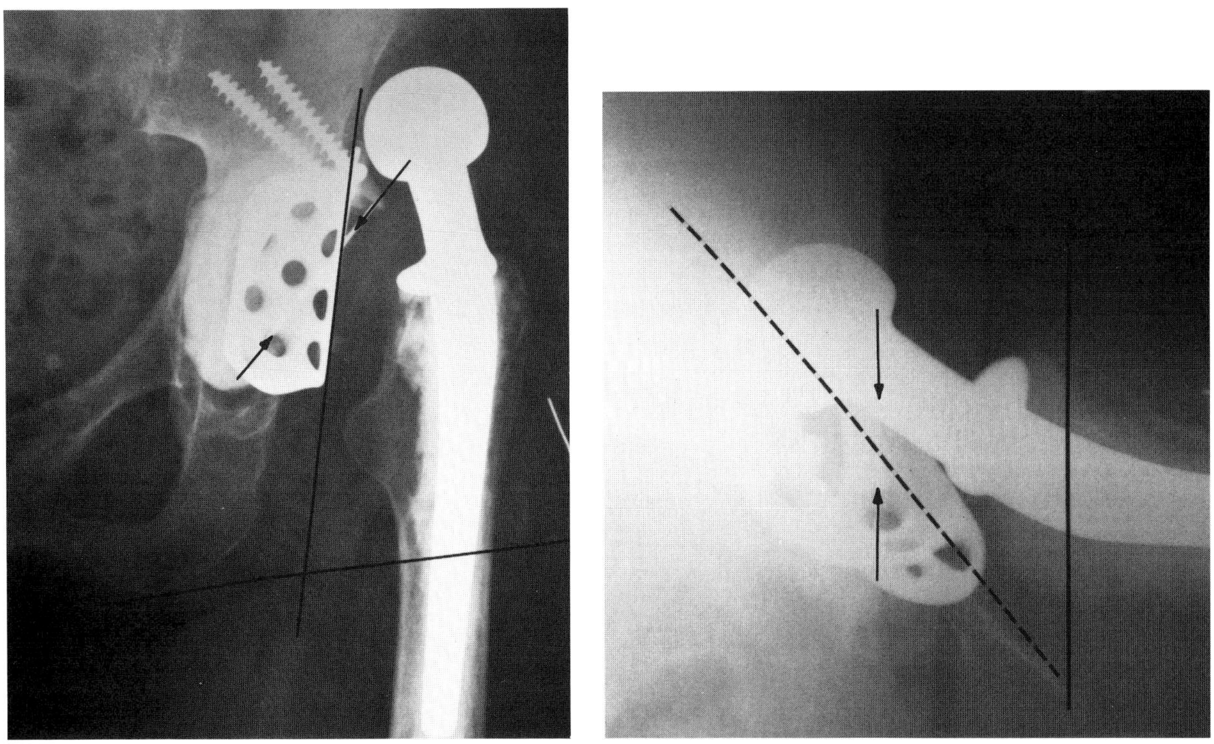

B

FIG. 4-157. Revision of a left hip arthroplasty using cement and a protrusio shell with cancellous screws. The protrusio shell is vertically oriented. The marker (*arrows*) of the acetabular component is oriented 45° on the AP radiograph **(A)**, and the protrusio shell is anteverted 43° on the lateral view **(B)** with the marker ring (*arrows*) in neutral position. The femoral component has dislocated superiorly.

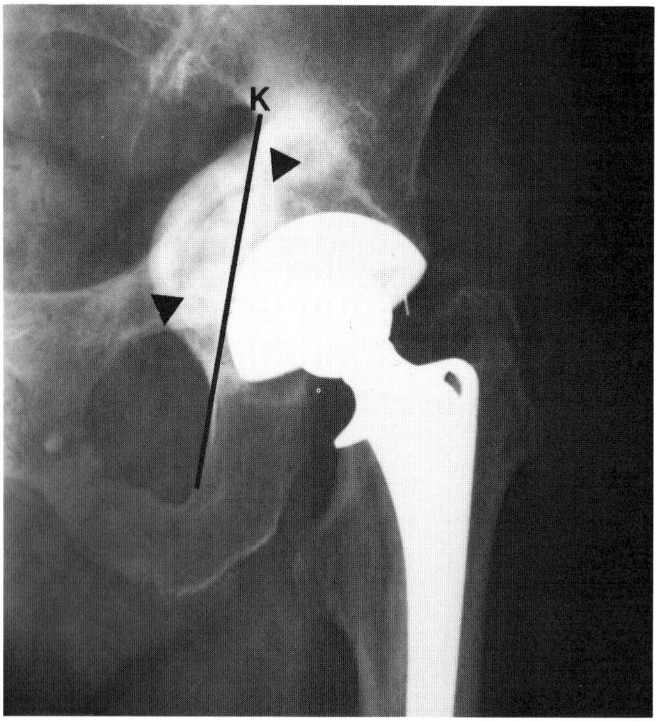

FIG. 4-158. Marked acetabular protrusion (note Kohler's line, *K*) with bone grafting with morselized graft and femoral head segment (*arrows*). An uncemented hemispheric acetabular component without screws was used for revision.

A
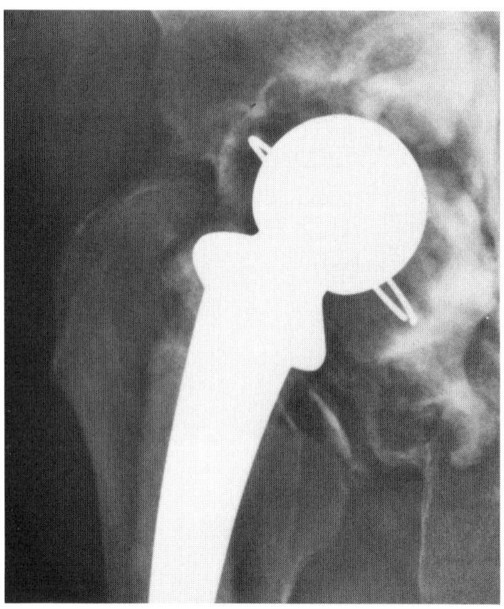

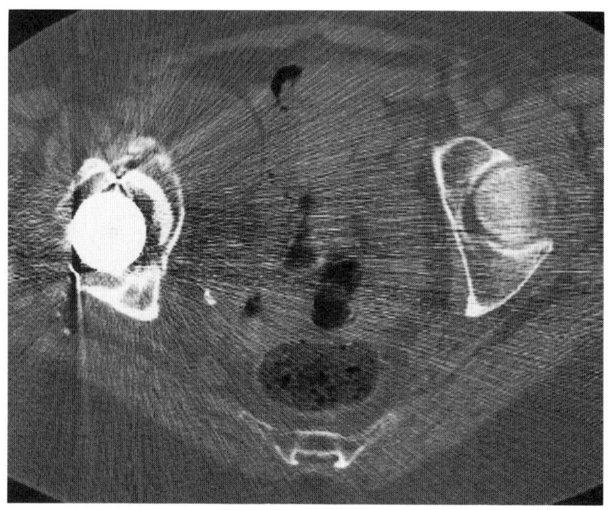
B

C
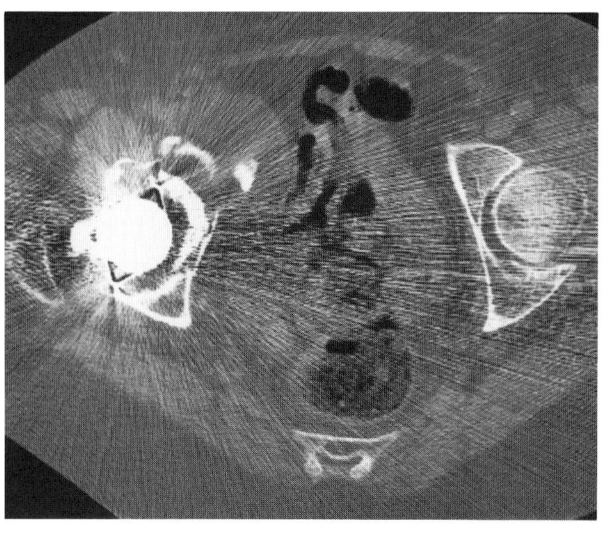

FIG. 4-159. A: Cemented hip arthroplasty with gross loosening cement fracture and acetabular bone loss. **B,C:** Preoperative CT images are degraded by metal artifact, but the bone around the component can be easily evaluated. There is significant bone loss medially and anteriorly.

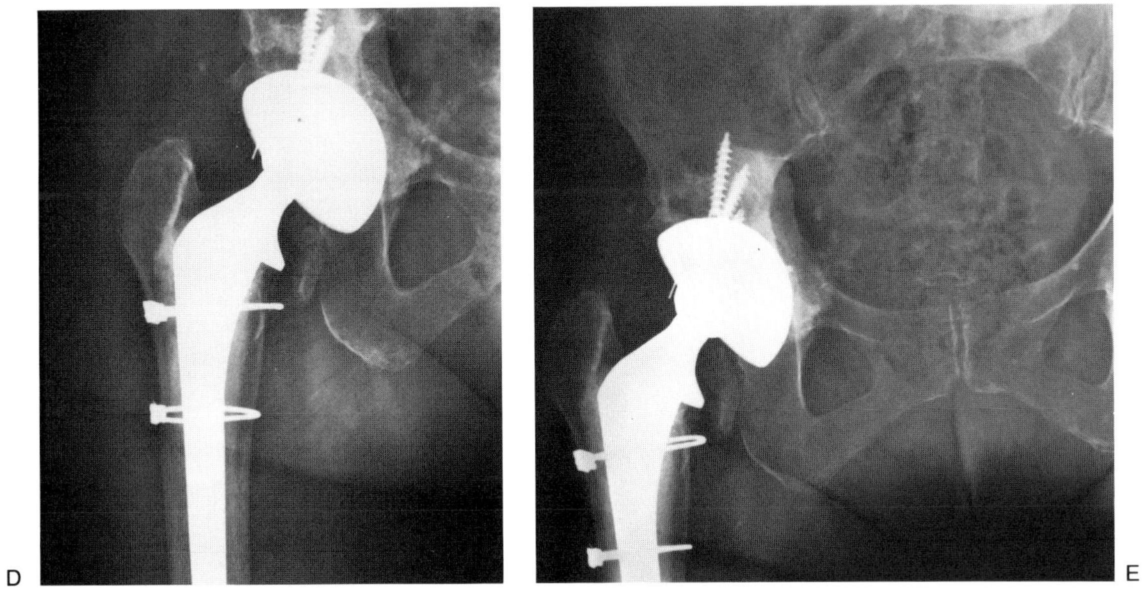

FIG. 4-159. (*Continued.*) The AP radiographs of the upper femur **(D)** and pelvis **(E)** after revision with morselized graft medially and superiorly and cortical graft anteriorly. Cancellous screws were used in the acetabular component. The femoral revision component was cemented and the upper femur prophylactically supported with two Dall-Miles cables.

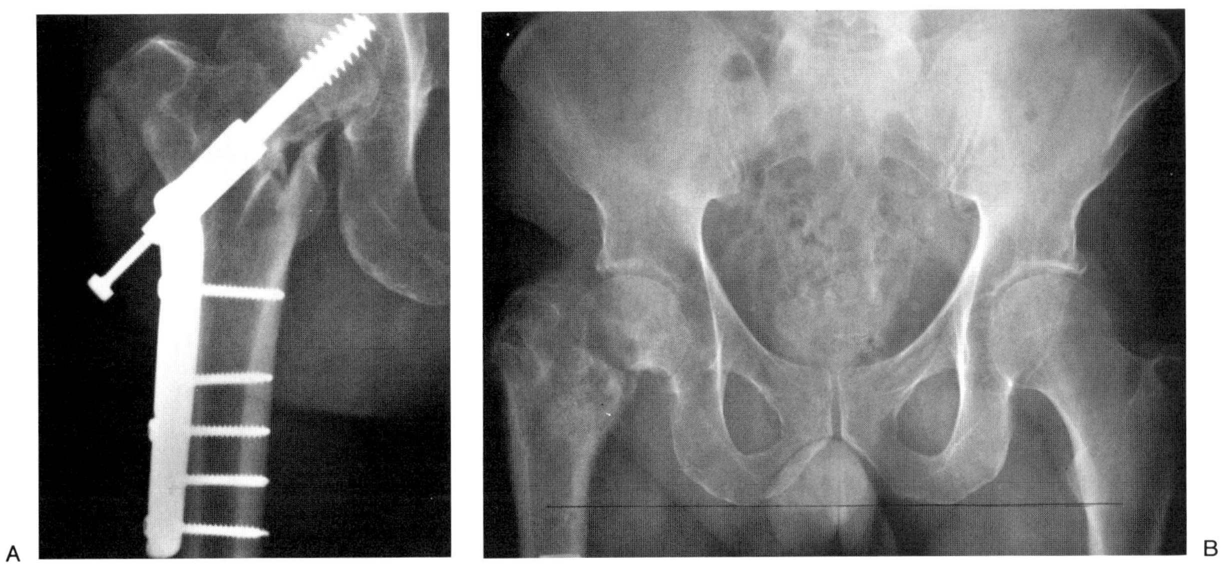

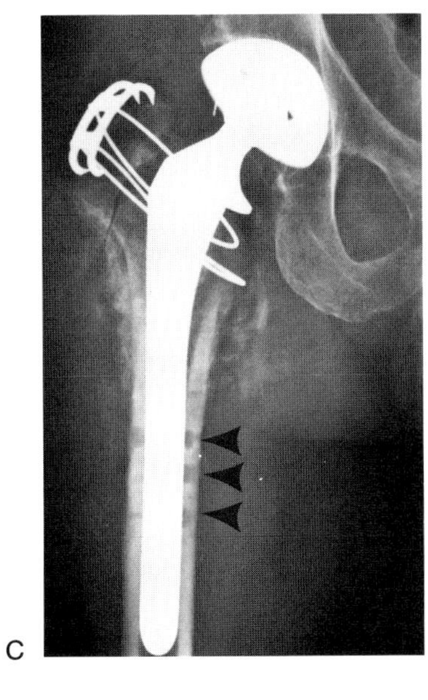

FIG. 4-160. **A:** An AP radiograph of the right hip with a comminuted intertrochanteric fracture treated with a dynamic hip screw and five-hole (135° angle side plate). **B:** The fracture went on to nonunion. A hip prosthesis was positioned using a long coated Osteonics specialty femoral component (Osteonics, Allendale, NJ) and a Dall-Miles cable system. **C:** Note the stem extends well below the screw tracts (*arrows*). (See **D** and **E** on next page.)

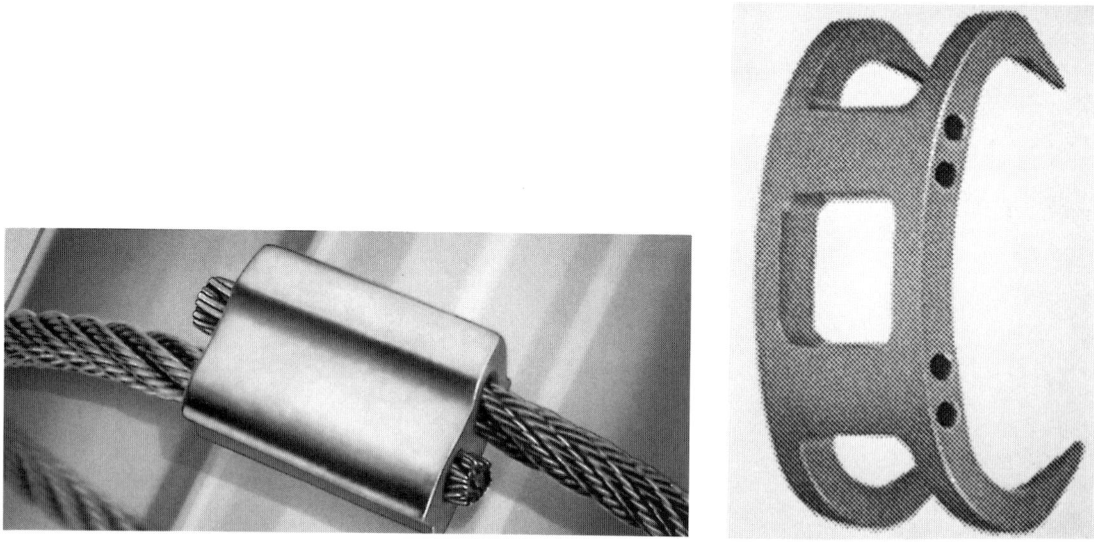

D E

FIG. 4-160. (*Continued.*) Dall-Miles cable and clamp **(D)** and claw **(E)** with holes for cable. (Courtesy of Howmedica, Rutherford, NJ.)

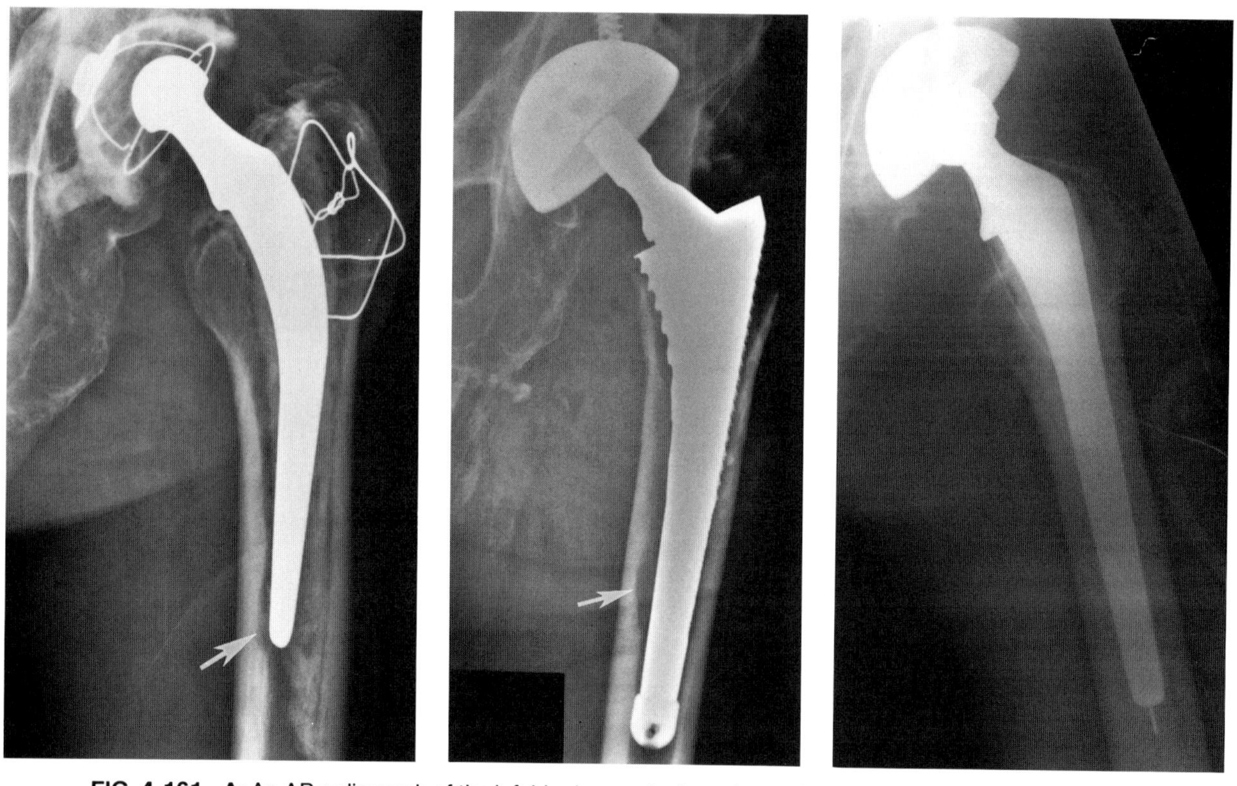

A,B C

FIG. 4-161. A: An AP radiograph of the left hip demonstrating a loose Charnley femoral component with slight endosteal scalloping at the femoral component tip (*arrow*). **B:** Operative radiograph with a broach in the femoral canal extending beyond the cortical defect (*arrow*). A 15-mm distal bullet on the broach, which was sized to a 12 press-fit component. **C:** Revision was accomplished with an Omnifit™ component.

long-stem component, and femoral bone stock. Proximal fit is important for immediate stability, but the length of the stem need not be longer, depending on the bone stock and presence of cortical thinning or defects (Figs. 4-161 and 4-162). When cortical defects are present from the previous surgery or created during cement removal or reaming, a longer stem should be used to extend 2 to 2.5 diameters below the defect.[312,315]

Bone grafts may also be required with femoral revisions (Figs. 4-163 and 4-164). Autografts are preferred to allografts, but when large areas require grafting, the latter is more commonly used. Long-segment femoral-section allografts (see Chapter 14) can be used with customized femoral components when long segments of upper femur need to be replaced.

Special components, including modular calcar replacement stems (Figs. 4-164 to 4-167) or proximal sleeves (Fig. 4-164), can also be used to improve proximal fit and stability.[312,315]

Infection

The treatment and revision of patients with infected hip arthroplasties vary with the patient's age, activity, and general health; the virulence of the organism; and the extent of the infection.[312,327] These decisions are generally made with the culture of preoperative aspirates or tissue culture during the component is removed. The revision may be performed as a one-, two-, or three-stage procedure.[312,327,384] One-stage revisions may be performed with organisms of low virulence, using antibiotic-impregnated cement. More virulent organisms or purulent low-grade infections are usually treated in two stages (Fig. 4-167). Patients are treated with parenteral antibiotics for 6 weeks or longer, and the revision is generally performed in 12 months.[312,327] We frequently reaspirate the unoccupied joint prior to the revision to increase our confidence level that the infection has cleared. Some authors advocate the use of a femoral antibiotic spacer during this time interval.[384]

Three-stage procedures are usually reserved for aggressive infections with bone loss or for younger patients.[327] This method involves resection arthroplasty with the identification and treatment of the organism (stage 1); bone grafting of the acetabulum and femur, as indicated, 3 to 6 months later (stage 2); and revision with uncemented components in another 9 to 12 months (stage 3).[312,327,384]

ARTHRODESIS AND OSTEOTOMIES OF THE HIP

Arthrodesis and several types of osteotomy are performed about the hip in adults and children.[385–392] Imaging plays a significant role in operative treatment planning and follow-up of these procedures.

Arthrodesis

Hip arthrodesis was initially performed in the late 1800s. In the early 1900s, the procedure was commonly used to treat tuberculosis of the hip. Early problems with pseudarthrosis (15% to 30%) have been improved with new fixation techniques so that pseudarthrosis rates are now 10% or less.[386,388,394]

Arthrodesis is best suited for the young active patient with monarticular hip disease, usually infectious or posttraumatic.[386,387,395] This procedure remains an alternative to arthroplasty because of the high failure rates of total hip or cup arthroplasty in younger patients. Even in patients younger than 60 years of age, revision rates for hip arthroplasty reach 9%.[394]

Hips are usually fused in 30° of flexion, 0° to 5° of adduction, and 10° to 15° of external rotation. This may be more easily assessed clinically than radiographically. In children, the angles of flexion and adduction increase with age which may require a second procedure.[386,387,395]

There are numerous surgical approaches to hip arthrodesis. Intraarticular, extraarticular, and combined approaches may be selected, depending on the cause. Patients with tuberculosis were treated with intraarticular removal of cartilage and synovium with fusion using plate and screw or threaded Steinmann pin techniques (Fig. 4-168).[168,386,387,395] More extensive techniques may require bone grafting with fixation using cobra-head plates, threaded rods, and nuts or compression screws (Fig. 4-169).[388]

Postoperative complications include pseudarthrosis, deep infection, and pain in the ipsilateral knee, spine, and contralateral hip.[386,387] Pseudarthrosis (Fig. 4-170) is less common with new fixation techniques but still occurs in up to 10% of patients.[386,388,395] Routine radiography with fluoroscopic stress views (abduction and adduction), conventional tomography, or reformatted CT may be required for diagnosis.

Pain in the ipsilateral knee occurs in 60% of patients, low-back pain in 60%, and contralateral hip pain in 25% of patients.[386] This occurs as a result of stress shifting with a solid hip fusion. Hip and knee pain are more likely in patients with the hip fused in slight abduction instead of the recommended neutral to 5° of adduction. Callaghan et al.[386] reported excellent function (70% of patients could walk 1 mile, and all but 1 of 28 were able to work) in most of the 28 patients followed an average of 35 years. Conversion to arthroplasty can be accomplished in the fused hip and knee if necessary.[386,394]

The hip, knee, and spine can usually be evaluated with routine radiographs, including flexion and extension

(*text continues on page 344*)

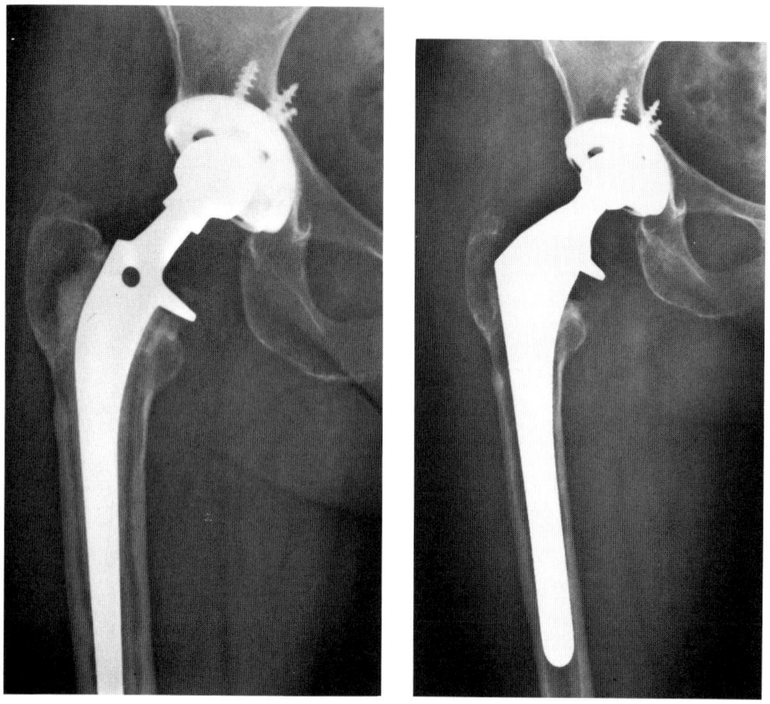

A,B

FIG. 4-162. A: An AP radiograph of a Zimmer Harris Precoat Plus cemented component, which has loosened. **B:** The metal acetabular cup was in a good position with only slight polyethylene wear. The polyethylene liner was replaced with a 10° build-up liner to accommodate the specialty femoral component. Note the fit of the component proximally and distally.

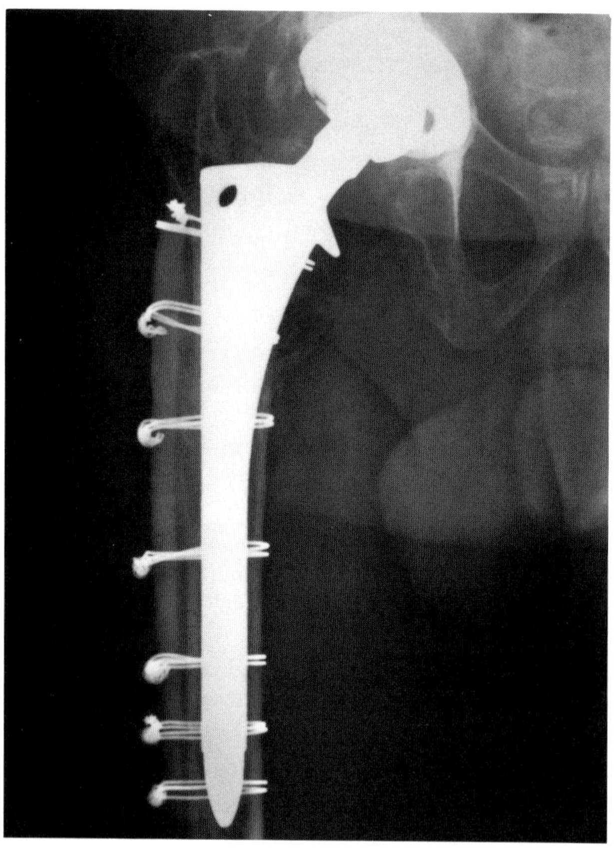

FIG. 4-163. An AP radiograph of the right upper femur after revision with a long cortical graft and cerclage wire. Note the extensive upper medial bone loss.

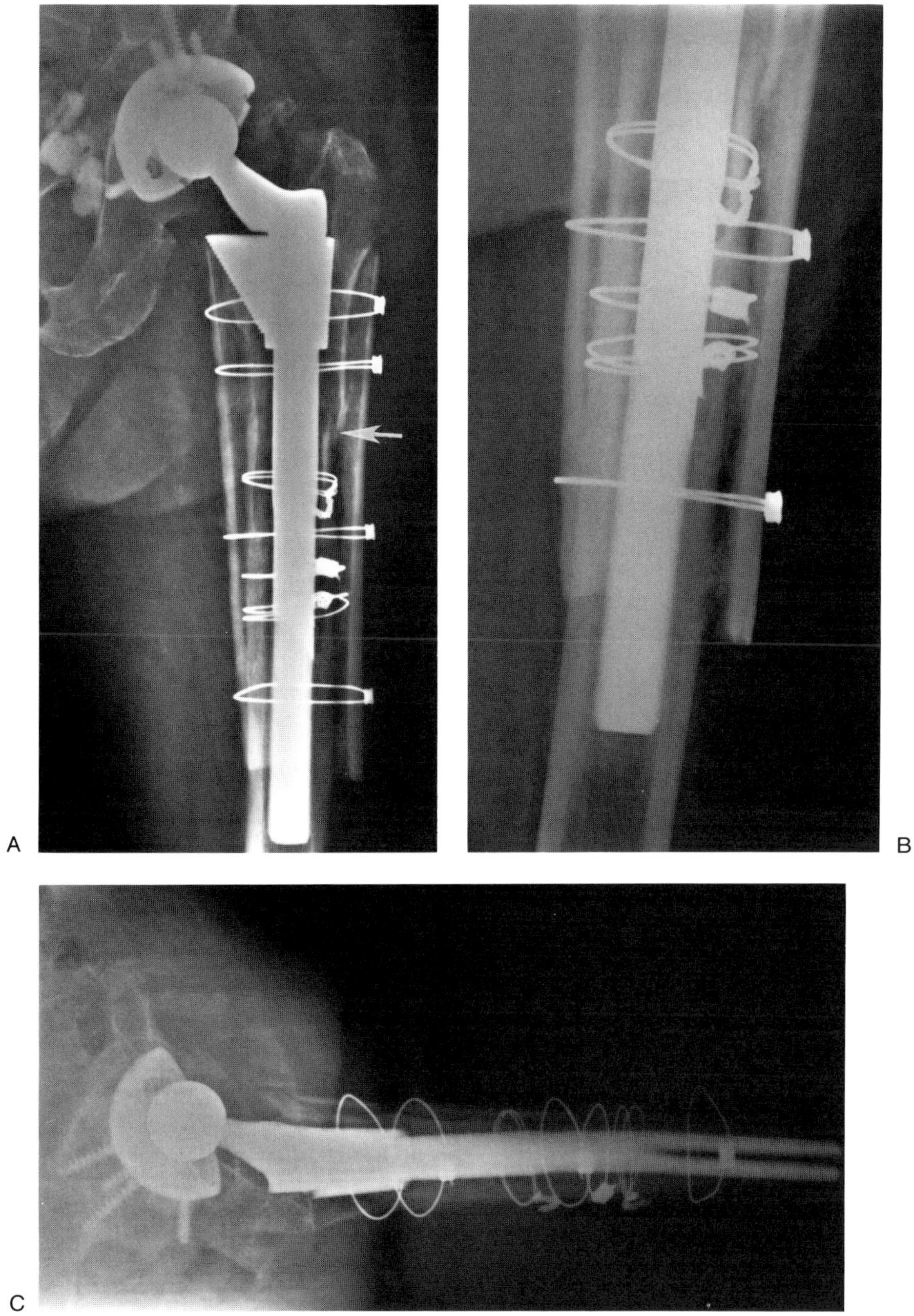

FIG. 4-164. The AP radiographs of the upper **(A)**, lower femur **(B)**, and lateral view (**C**) of a left hip revision using a S-ROM™ system with cortical allograft onlay struts and multiple Dall-Miles cables. Note the femoral osteolysis and fracture (*arrow*). The acetabulum also required considerable morselized grafting.

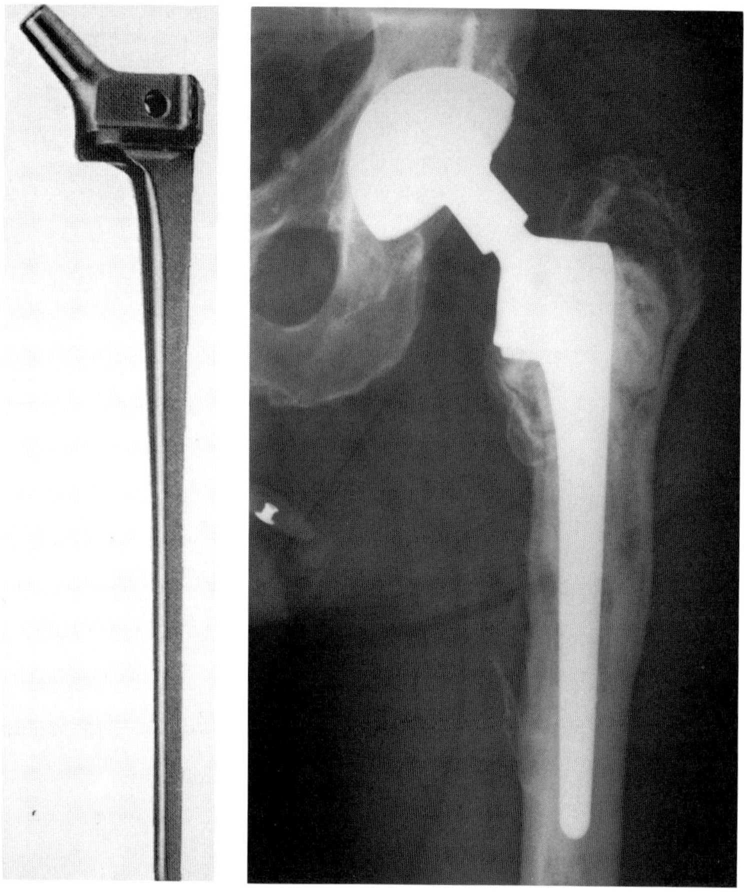

A,B

FIG. 4-165. **A:** Modular calcar femoral component. (Courtesy of Zimmer, Warsaw, IN.) **B:** An AP radiograph demonstrating a modular calcar revision component.

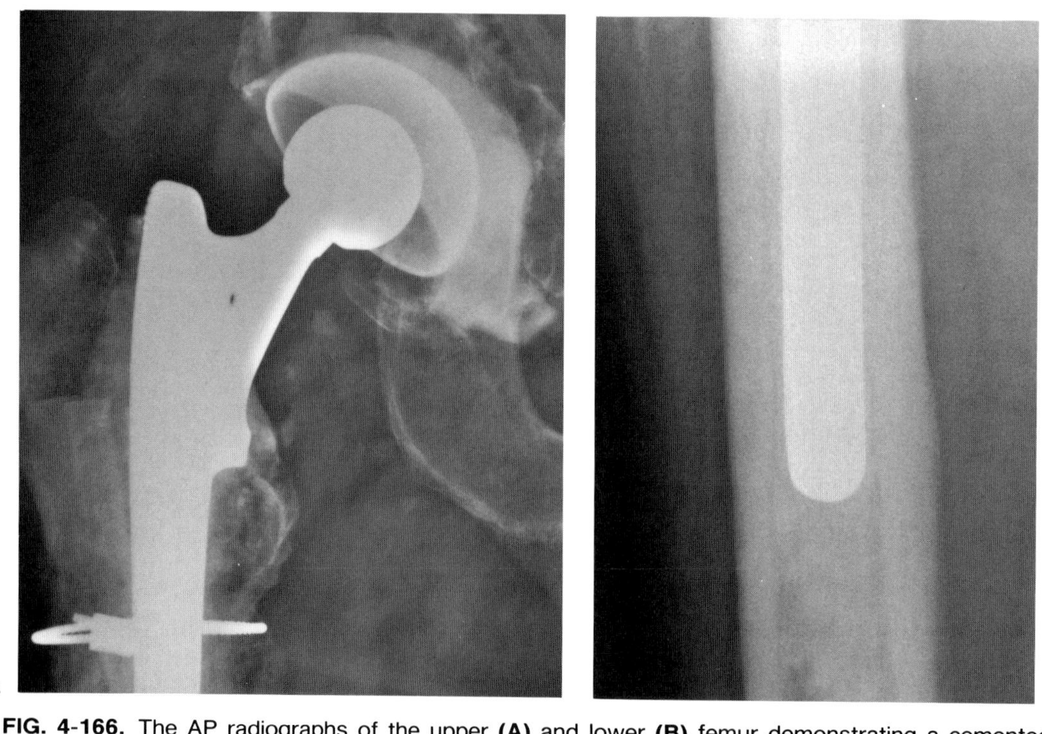

A B

FIG. 4-166. The AP radiographs of the upper **(A)** and lower **(B)** femur demonstrating a cemented custom-designed head and neck component with proximal bone graft and Dall-Miles cable.

A

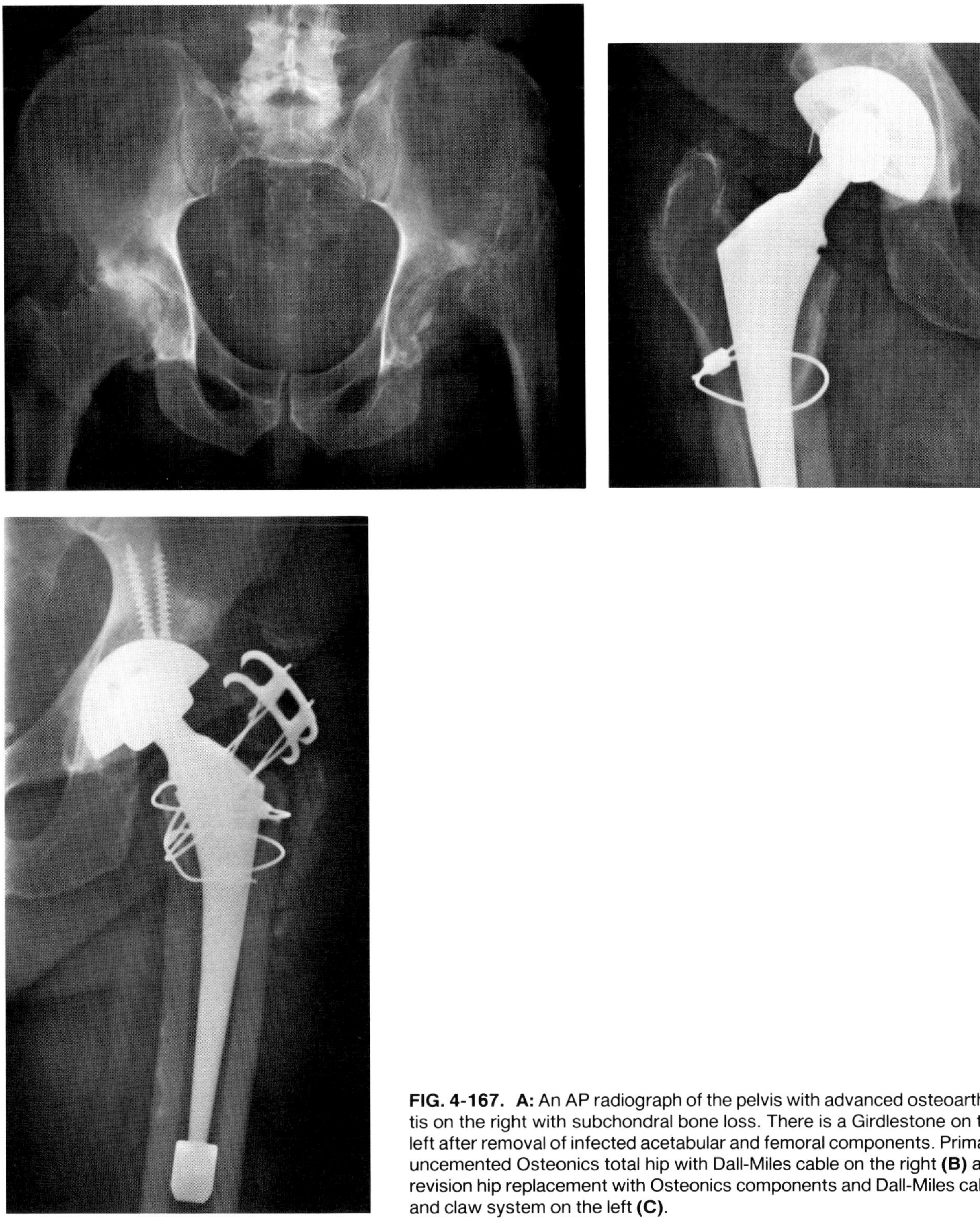

B

C

FIG. 4-167. A: An AP radiograph of the pelvis with advanced osteoarthritis on the right with subchondral bone loss. There is a Girdlestone on the left after removal of infected acetabular and femoral components. Primary uncemented Osteonics total hip with Dall-Miles cable on the right **(B)** and revision hip replacement with Osteonics components and Dall-Miles cable and claw system on the left **(C)**.

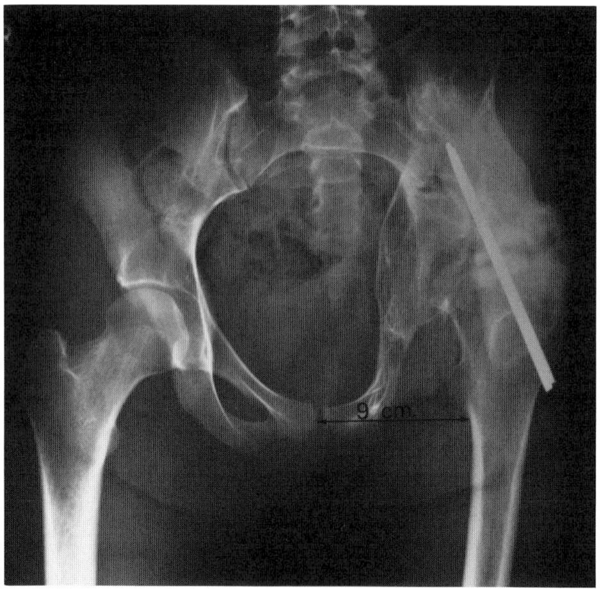

FIG. 4-168. The AP radiographs of the pelvis and hips demonstrating an arthrodesis on the left with bone graft and Steinmann pin fixation. Note the adducted position of the femur compared with the right hip. (Courtesy of Mark B. Coventry, Mayo Clinic, Rochester, MN.)

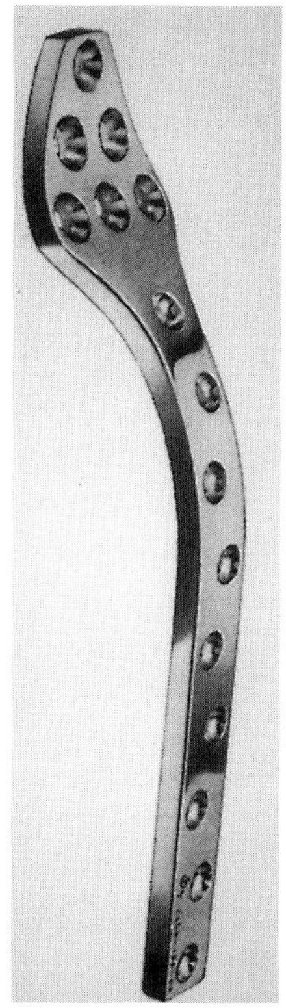

FIG. 4-169. A cobra-head plate. (Courtesy of Zimmer, Warsaw, IN.)

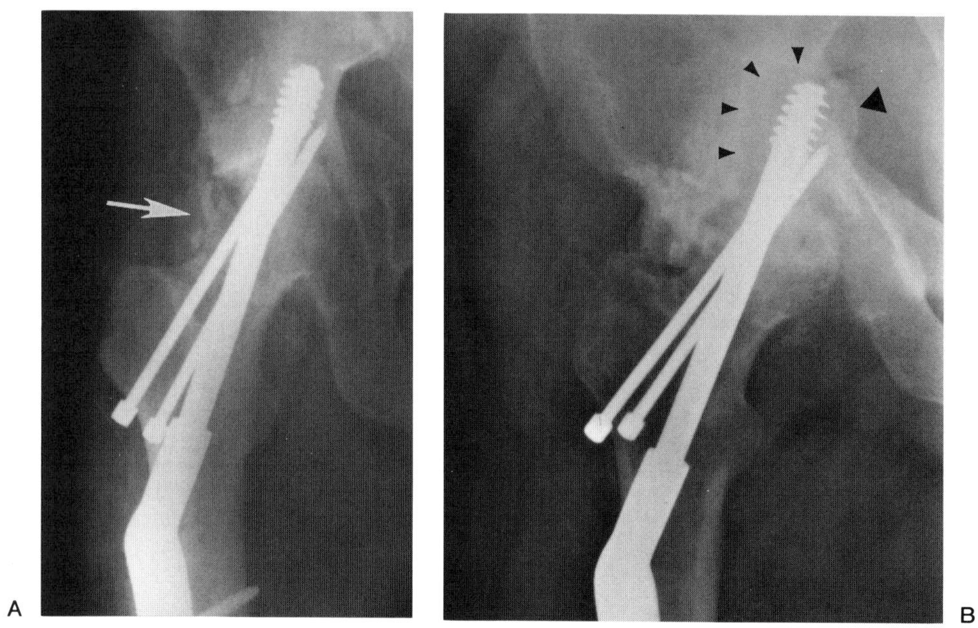

FIG. 4-170. A: An AP radiograph of the right hip after arthrodesis with a dynamic hip screw with 150° angled side plate and two Knowles pins. There is a cancellous bone graft along the lateral joint space (*arrow*). **B:** Six months later, the bone graft is incorporated superiorly but not inferiorly. The screw is toggling (*small arrows*) and has fractured through the acetabulum (*large arrow*).

A

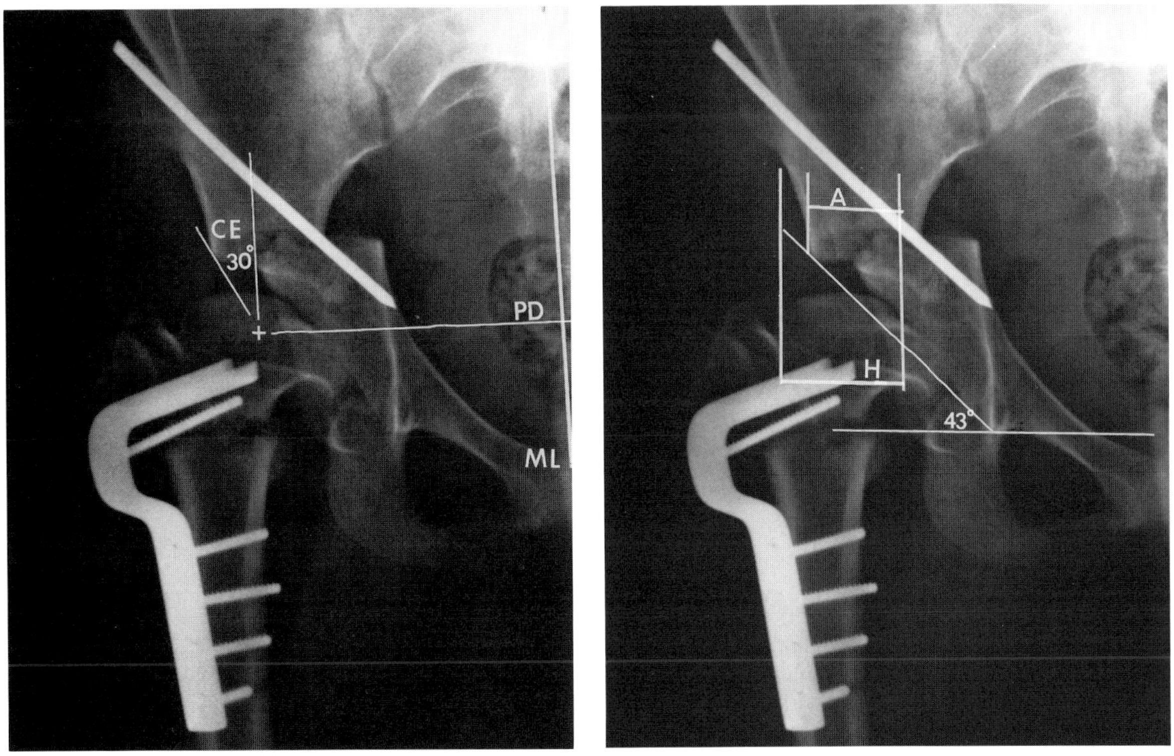

B

FIG. 4-171. A: An AP radiograph of the right hemipelvis demonstrating a Salter osteotomy with pin fixation and a varus femoral osteotomy with a 90° blade plate and screws for fixation. Midline (S-1 to pubic symphysis): white vertical line (*ML*). Perpendicular distance from midline to center of femoral head (*PD*). Wiberg center-edge (CE) angle = 30°. **B:** Same patient with additional measurements used to evaluate osteotomies. Acetabular angle (Sharp). Teardrop line (line along the inferior teardrop bilaterally) to the acetabular margin. In this case, the angle measures 43°. Acetabular head index: width of head covered (*A*) divided by width of head (*H*) × 100%. In this case, the index is 70%.

A

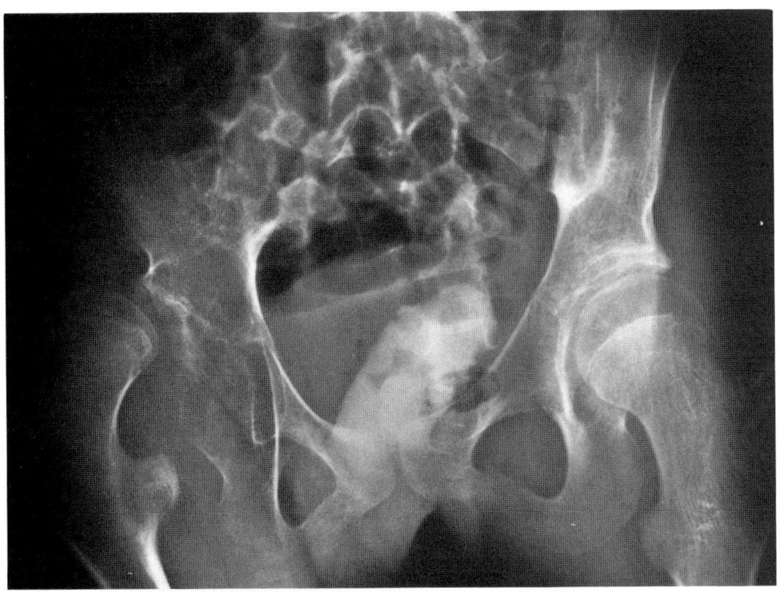

FIG. 4-172. A: An AP radiograph of the pelvis with congenital hip dislocation on the right. (See **B** and **C** on next page.)

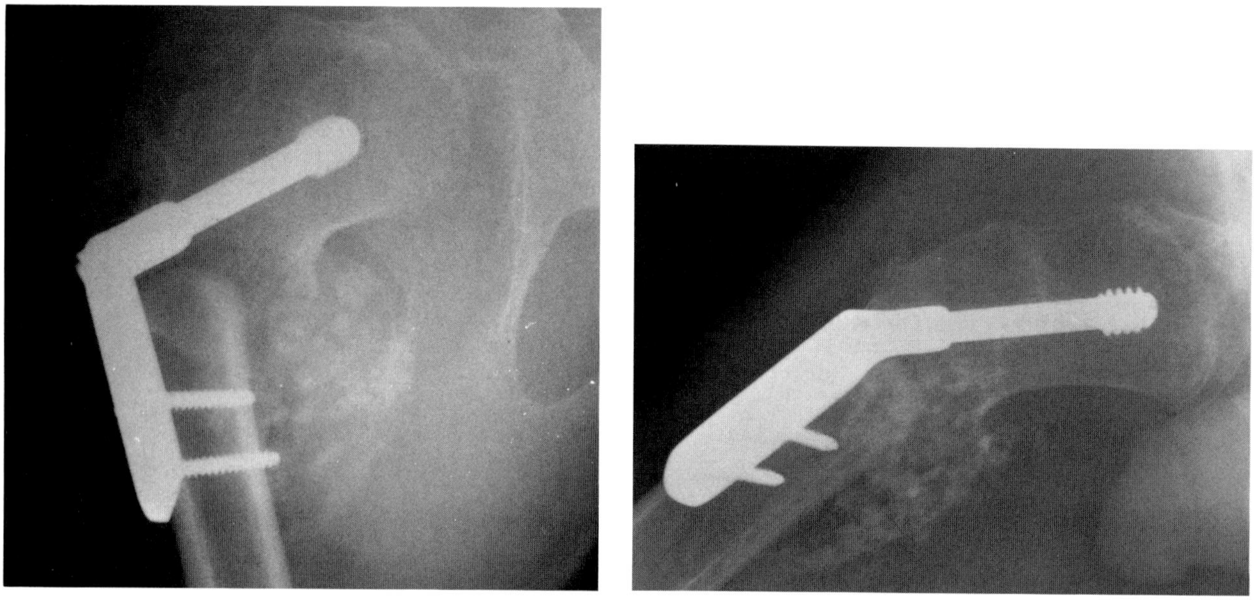

B C

FIG. 4-172. (*Continued.*) Postoperative AP **(B)** and oblique **(C)** radiographs demonstrating a proximal femoral osteotomy with pediatric dynamic hip screw and medial bone graft.

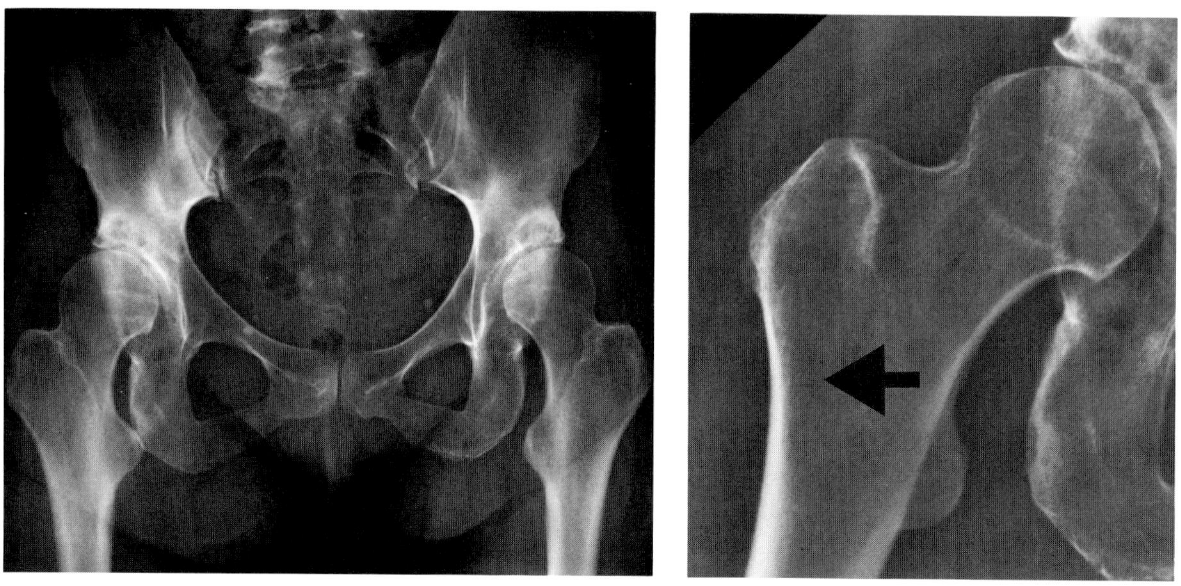

A B

FIG. 4-173. **A:** An AP radiograph of the pelvis demonstrating osteoarthritis with coxa valga deformities in both femoral necks. Abduction **(B)** and adduction **(C)** views show limited motion.

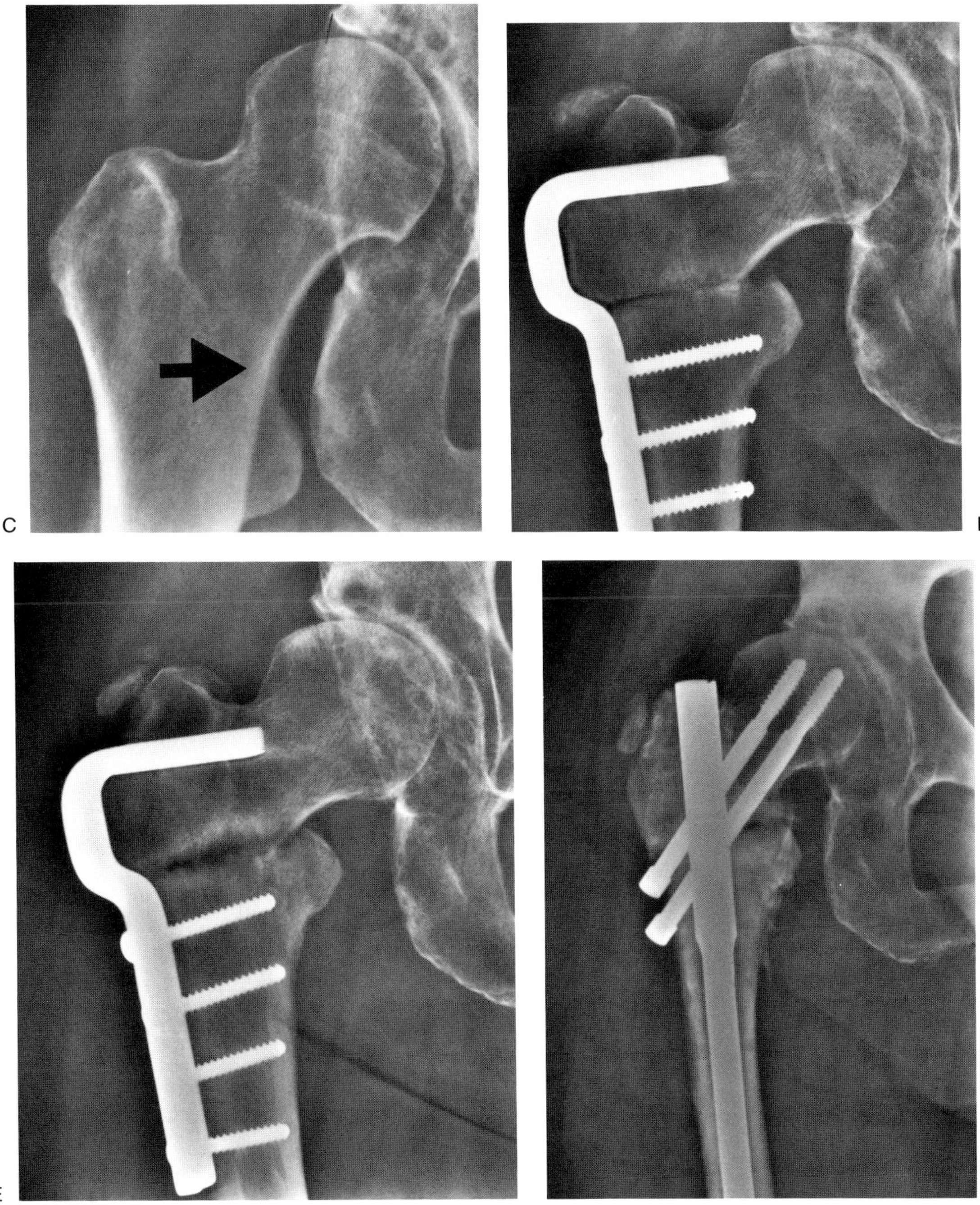

C D

E F

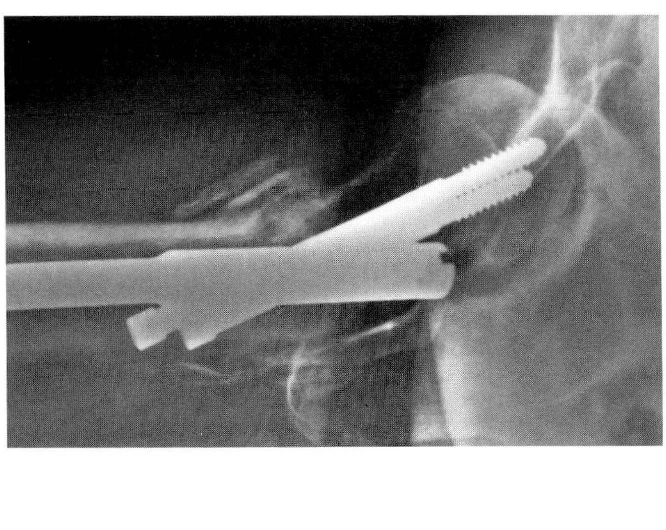

G

FIG. 4-173. (*Continued.*) **D:** A varus osteotomy was performed using a 90° blade plate for fixation (see Chapter 2 for photographs of blade plates). **E:** Three months later, the fracture line is widening and irregular, indicating nonunion. **F,G:** The osteotomy was revised using a Russell-Taylor™ nail and femoral two neck screws. The bone graft is better demonstrated on the lateral view (G).

views of the spine. Diagnostic anesthetic or therapeutic (anesthetic and corticosteroid) injections can be helpful in localizing symptoms in difficult cases.

Osteotomies

Osteotomies about the hip are most often performed to improve femoral head coverage and correct rotational or anteversion deformities with femur.[385,388,391,393,396]

Pelvic osteotomies are most commonly performed for congenital hip dysplasia or Perthes disease.[385,388,390] Several techniques have been commonly used, depending on the age and extent of correction required.[385,388] The Salter and Pemberton osteotomies are designed to treat children in the 18-months- to 6-years-old and 18-months- to 10-years-old age ranges, respectively.[385,388,390] The Pemberton technique redirects the acetabular roof by placing the osteotomy in the cove above the acetabulum and uses the triradiate cartilage to rotate the acetabular roof anteriorly and laterally. Using the Salter technique, the cut is directed from the sciatic notch to the anterior inferior iliac spine (Fig. 4-171). The fragments and a triangular bone graft arc hcld in place by a Kirschner wire (K wire) or Steinmann pin.[388,390,396]

The Chiari osteotomy is used more often in children older than 6 years of age.[385,390] A transverse iliac osteotomy is performed, shifting the inferior innominate bone medially to improve coverage of the femoral head.

Pre- and postoperative evaluations are most often measured on standard AP radiographs. The measurements and angles are summarized as follows:[385,388,390]

Midline: vertical line from the spinous process of S-1 to the pubic symphysis (Fig. 4-171)
Perpendicular distance: distance from the midline to the center of the femoral head (PD in Fig. 4-171)
Wiberg angle: angle formed by vertical line to the center of the femoral head and acetabular margin (CE, center-edge angle); the greater the coverage, the larger the angle (Fig. 4-171)
Acetabular angle (Sharp): teardrop line to acetabular margin (Fig. 4-171B)
Acetabular-head index: distance from the medial margin of the femoral head to the acetabulum divided by the transverse width of the femoral head

Radiologists should be familiar with these measurements in the pre- and postoperative setting.

Femoral osteotomies are performed for pain relief and to improve the stability of a number of congenital and acquired disorders.[385,388] Preoperative AP and lateral radiographs and abduction-adduction AP views are used to determine the type of procedure and the extent of correction required. For rotational osteotomies or more accurate calculations, femoral neck anteversion CT may be required.

The indications include congenital hip dysplasia (Fig. 4-172), slipped capital femoral epiphysis, coxa vara or valga deformities, degenerative arthritis, and AVN (Fig. 4-173).[385,388,390] In adults, hip replacement procedures are usually performed when possible.

The complications include pseudarthrosis or nonunion (Fig. 4-173), deep infection, AVN, and implant failure. Routine radiography may be adquate for detecting most early problems with union or instrument failure. Metal generally degrades MRI scans, which makes detection of AVN more difficult. Reformatted CT images, conventional tomography, or radionuclide scans may be helpful in this setting.[385,388,390,396]

REFERENCES

Imaging Techniques

1. Armbuster TG, Guerra J, Resnick D, Goergen TG, Feingold ML, Niwayama G, Danzig LA. The adult hip: an anatomic study. *Radiology* 1978;128:1–10.
2. Ballinger PW. *Merrill's atlas of radiographic positions and radiologic procedures.* 5th ed. St. Louis: CV Mosby Co; 1982.
3. Berkebile RD, Fisher DL, Albrecht LF. The gull-wing sign: valuc of the lateral view of the pelvis in fracture-dislocations of the acetabular rim and posterior dislocation of the femoral head. *Radiology* 1965;84:937–939.
4. Berman L, Catterall A, Meiere HB. Ultrasound of the hip: a review of the applications of a new technique. *Br J Radiol* 1986;59: 13–17.
5. Bernau A, Berquist TH. *Orthopaedic positioning in diagnostic radiology.* Baltimore: Urban and Schwarzenberg; 1983.
6. Berquist TH. *Magnetic resonance of the musculoskeletal system.* 2nd ed. New York: Raven Press; 1990.
7. Berquist TH. *Imaging of orthopedic trauma.* 2nd ed. New York: Raven Press; 1992.
8. Berquist TH. Diagnostic and therapeutic injections as an aid to musculoskeletal diagnosis. *Semin Intervent Radiol* 1993;4:326–343.
9. Burk DL, Mears DC, Herbert DL, Straub WH, Cooperstein LA, Beck EA. Pelvic and acetabular fractures: examined by angled CT scanning. *Radiology* 1984;153:548.
10. Burk DL, Mears DC, Kennedy WH, Cooperstein LA, Herbert DL. Three dimensional computed tomography of acetabular fractures. *Radiology* 1985;155:183–186.
11. Dihlmann W, Nebel G. Computed tomography of the hip joint capsule. *J Comptut Assist Tomogr* 1983;7:278–285.
12. Dodig D, Ugarkovic B, Orlic D. Bone scintigraphy in idiopathic aseptic femoral head necrosis. *Eur J Nucl Med* 1983;8:23–25.
13. Drebin RA, Magid D, Robertson DD, Fishman EK. Fidelity of three dimensional CT for imaging of fracture gaps. *J Comput Assist Tomogr* 1989;13:487–489.
14. Gelman MI, Coleman RE, Stevens PM, Davey BW. Radiography, radionuclide imaging, and arthrography in evaluation of total hip and knee replacement. *Radiology* 1978;128:677–682.
15. Geslin JE, Thrall JH, Espinosa JL, Older RA. Early detection of stress fractures using Tc-99m polyphosphate. *Radiology* 1976; 121:683–687.
16. Glynn TP, Kreipke DL, DeRosa GP. Computed tomography arthrography in traumatic hip dislocation. *Skeletal Radiol* 1989;18:29–31.
17. Greiff JE, Laung S, Hoilurd-Carlsen PF. Early detection by Tc-99m-Sm-pyrophosphate of femoral head necroses following medial femoral neck fractures. *Acta Orthop Scand* 1980;51:119.
18. Harcke HT, Grissom LF, Furkelstein MS. Evaluation of the musculoskeletal system with sonography. *AJR Am J Roentgenol* 1988;150:1253–1261.

19. Harris JH, Loh CK, Perlman HC, Rotz CT Jr. The Roentgen diagnosis of pelvic extraperitoneal effusion. *Radiology* 1977;125: 343–350.
20. Hickey PM. Value of the lateral view of the hip. *AJR Am J Roentgenol* 1916;3:308–309.
21. Janes L. Lateral roentgenography of the neck of the femur. *AJR Am J Roentgenol* 1935;33:504.
22. Johnson CR. A new method for Roentgen examination of the upper femur. *J Bone Joint Surg* 1932;30:859–866.
23. Judet R, Judet J, Letournel E. Fractures of the acetabulum: classification and surgical approaches to open reduction. *J Bone Joint Surg [Am]* 1964;46A:1615–1646.
24. Kalman MA. Radiology of soft tissue shadows in the pelvis: another look. *AJR Am J Roentgenol* 1978;130:493–498.
25. Kam J, Jackson H, Ben-Menachem Y. Vascular injuries in blunt pelvic trauma. *Radiol Clin North Am* 1981;19:171–186.
26. Lancaster SJ, Cummings RJ. Hip aspiration: verification of needle position by air arthrography. *J Pediatr Orthop* 1987;7:91–92.
27. Lang EK. The role of angiography in trauma. *Radiol Clin North Am* 1976;14:353–370.
28. Letournel E. Acetabular fractures: classification and management. *Clin Orthop* 1980;151:81–106.
29. Phillips HB. New Roentgen demonstration of the neck of the femur. *Am J Surg* 1928;5:392–393.
30. Pritchard RS, Shah HR, Nelson CL, Fitzrandolph RL. MR and CT appearance of iliopsoas bursal distension secondary to diseased hips. *J Comput Assist Tomogr* 1990;14:797–800.
31. Robinson HJ, Hartleben DD, Lund G, Schreman J. Evaluation of magnetic resonance imaging in the diagnosis of osteonecrosis of the femoral head. *J Bone Joint Surg [Am]* 1989;71A:650–663.
32. Saks BJ. Normal acetabular anatomy for acetabular fracture assessment: CT and plain film correlation. *Radiology* 1986;159: 139–145.
33. Speer KP, Spritzer CE, Harrelson JM, Nunley JA. Magnetic resonance imaging of the femoral head after acute intracapsular fracture of the femoral neck. *J Bone Joint Surg [Am]* 1990;72A:98–103.
34. Staple TW. Arthrographic demonstration of iliopsoas bursa extension of the hip joint. *Radiology* 1972;102:515–516.
35. Staple TW, Jung D, Mork A. Snapping tendon syndrome: hip tenography with fluoroscopic monitoring. *Radiology* 1988;166: 873–874.
36. Sweeney JP, Helms CA, Minagi H, Louie KW. The widened teardrop distance: a plain film indicator of hip joint effusion in adults. *AJR Am J Roentgenol* 1987;149:117–119.
37. Taylor R. Modified AP projection of the anterior bones of the pelvis. *Radiogr Clin Photo* 1941;17:67.
38. Young JWR, Burgess AR, Brumback RJ, Poke A. Pelvic fractures: value of plain radiography for early assessment and management. *Radiology* 1986;160:445–451.
39. Young JWR, Burgess AR, Brumback RJ, Poke A. Lateral compression fractures of the pelvis: the importance of plain radiographs in the diagnosis and surgical management. *Skeletal Radiol* 1986;15:103–109.
40. Zieger MM, Dorr U, Schulz RD. Ultrasonography of hip joint effusions. *Skeletal Radiol* 1987;16:607–611.

Pelvic Fractures

41. Berquist TH. *Imaging of orthopedic trauma.* 2nd ed. New York: Raven Press; 1992.
42. Bonnin JG. Sacral fractures and injury to the cauda equina. *J Bone Joint Surg* 1945;27:113–127.
43. Brosman SA, Paul JG. Trauma of the bladder. *Surg Gynecol Obstet* 1976;143:605–608.
44. Buchanan TI. Bowel entrapment by pelvic fracture fragments: a case report and review of the literature. *Clin Orthop* 1980;147: 164–166.
45. Bucholz RW. The pathologic anatomy of Malgaigne fracture dislocations of the pelvis. *J Bone Joint Surg [Am]* 1981;63A:400–404.
46. Caudel RJ, Crawford AH. Avulsion fracture of the acetabular margin. *J Bone Joint Surg [Am]* 1988;78A:1568–1570.
47. Clark SS, Prudencio RF. Lower urinary tract injury associated with pelvic fractures. *Surg Clin North Am* 1972;52:183–201.
48. Colapinto V. Trauma of the pelvis: urethral injury. *Clin Orthop* 1980;151:46–55.
49. Colapinto V, McCallum RW. Injury to the male posterior urethra in fractures of the pelvis: a new classification. *J Urol* 1977;118: 575–580.
50. Connally WB, Hedberg EA. Fractures and dislocations of the pelvis. *J Trauma* 1969;9:104–111.
51. Cooke CP, Levinsohn EM, Baker BE. Septic hip in pelvic fracture with urologic injury. *Clin Orthop* 1980;147:253–257.
52. Cooper KL, Beabout JW, McLeod RA. Supra-acetabular insufficiency fracture. *Radiology* 1985;157:15–17.
53. Cooper KL, Beabout JW, Swee RG. Insufficiency fractures of the sacrum. *Radiology* 1985;156:15–20.
54. Dabezies E, Millet CUJ, Murphy CP, Acker JH, Robicheaux RE, d'Ambrosia RD. Stabilization of sacroiliac joint disruption with threaded compression rods. *Clin Orthop* 1989;246:165–171.
55. Daffner RH. Pelvic trauma. In: McCort JJ, ed. *Trauma radiology.* New York: Churchill Livingstone; 1990.
56. Dunn W, Morris HD. Fractures and dislocation of the pelvis. *J Bone Joint Surg [Am]* 1968;50A:1634–1648.
57. Dunn WA, Russo CL. Central acetabular fractures. *J Trauma* 1973;13:695–705.
58. Duverney JG. *Traite des maladies des os.* Vol. 1. Paris: De Bure l'Aine; 1751.
59. Eichenholtz SN, Stark RM. Central acetabular fractures: a review of 35 cases. *J Bone Joint Surg [Am]* 1964;46A:695–714.
60. Failinger S, McGanity PL. Unstable fractures of the pelvic ring. *J Bone Joint Surg [Am]* 1992;74A:781–791.
61. Fassler PR, Siviontkowski MF, Kilroy AW, Routt ML. Injury of the sciatic nerve associated with acetabular fractures. *J Bone Joint Surg* 1993;75A:1157–1166.
62. Goodell CL. Neurologic deficits associated with pelvic fractures. *J Neurosurg* 1966;24:837–842.
63. Harley JD, Mack LA, Winquist RA. CT of acetabular fractures: comparison with conventional radiography. *AJR Am J Roentgenol* 1982;138:413–417.
64. Holdsworth EW. Dislocations and fracture-dislocations of the pelvis. *J Bone Joint Surg [Br]* 1948;30B:461–466.
65. Holm CL. Treatment of pelvic fractures and dislocations. Skeletal traction and dual pelvic traction sling. *Clin Orthop* 1973;97:97–107.
66. Jackson H, Kam J, Harris JH, Harle TS. The sacral arcuate lines in upper sacral fractures. *Radiology* 1982;145:35–39.
67. Judet R, Judet J, Letournel E. Fractures of the acetabulum: classification and surgical approaches to reduction. *J Bone Joint Surg [Am]* 1964;46A:1615–1646.
68. Kane WJ. Fractures of the pelvis. In: Rockwood CA, Green DP, eds. *Fractures in adults.* 2nd ed. Vol. 2. Philadelphia: JB Lippincott; 1984:1093–1209.
69. Key JA, Conwell HE. *Management of fractures, dislocations, and sprains.* St. Louis: CV Mosby; 1951.
70. Knight RA, Smith H. Central acetabular fractures. *J Bone Joint Surg [Am]* 1958;49A:1–16.
71. Kvarstein B, Riska EB, Slatis P. Pelvic fractures. *Ann Chir Gynaecol* 1981;70:256–263.
72. Lansinger O. Fractures of the acetabulum: a clinical, radiological, and experimental study. *Acta Orthop Scand* 1977;165:1–94.
73. Letournel E. Surgical repair of acetabular fractures more than three weeks after injury, apart from total hip arthroplasty. *Int Orthop* 1979;2:305–313.
74. Letournel E. Acetabular fractures. Classification and management. *Clin Orthop* 1980;151:81–106.
75. Levine JI, Crampton RS. Major abdominal injury associated with pelvic fractures. *Surg Gynecol Obstet* 1963;116:223.
76. Looser KJ, Crombie HD. Pelvic fracture: an anatomic guide to the severity of injury. A review of 100 cases. *Am J Surg* 1976;132: 638–641.
77. Mack LA, Duesdieker GA, Harley JD, Bach AW, Winquist RA. CT of acetabular fractures: postoperative appearances. *AJR Am J Roentgenol* 1983;141:891–894.

78. Mack LA, Harley D, Winquist RA. CT of acetabular fractures. Analysis of fracture patterns. *AJR Am J Roentgenol* 1982;138:407–412.
79. Majeed SA. External fixation of the injured pelvis. Functional outcome. *J Bone Joint Surg [Br]* 1990;72B:612–614.
80. Margolies MN, Ring EJ, Waltman AC, Kerr WS Jr, Baum S. Arteriography in the management of hemorrhage from pelvic fractures. *N Engl J Med* 1972;287:317–321.
81. Matta JM, Saucedo T. Internal fixation of pelvic ring fractures. *Clin Orthop* 1989;242:83–97.
82. McAvoy JM, Cook JH. A treatment plan for rapid assessment of the patient with massive blood loss and pelvic fractures. *Arch Surg* 1978;113:986–990.
83. McMurtry R, Walton D, Dickinson D, Kellam J, Tile M. Pelvic disruption in the polytraumatized patient. A management protocol. *Clin Orthop* 1980;151:22–30.
84. Mears DC, Fu F. External fixation of pelvic fractures. *Orthop Clin North Am* 1980;11:465–479.
85. Mucha P, McGanity PLJ. Recognizing and avoiding complications with pelvic fractures. *Inf in Surg Jan* 1985;:53–62.
86. Mucha P, Welch TJ. Hemorrhage in major pelvic fractures. *Surg Clin North Am* 1988;68:757–773.
87. O'Keefe TJ. Retroperitoneal abscess: a potentially fatal complication of closed fracture of the pelvis. *J Bone Joint Surg [Am]* 1978;60A:1117–1121.
88. Paster SB, Van Houten FX, Adams DF. Percutaneous balloon catheter. A technique for control of arterial hemorrhage caused by pelvic fractures. *JAMA* 1974;230:573–575.
89. Peltier LF. Complications associated with fractures of the pelvis. *J Bone Joint Surg [Am]* 1965;47A:1060–1064.
90. Pennal GF, Tile M, Waddell JP, Garside H. Pelvic disruption: assessment and classification. *Clin Orthop* 1980;151:12–21.
91. Perry JF. Pelvic open fractures. *Clin Orthop* 1980;151:41–45.
92. Roberts JL, Dalen K, Bosanko CM, Jafir SZH. CT in abdominal and pelvic trauma. *Radiographics* 1993;13:735–752.
93. Rothenberger DA, Kellam J, McGonigal D. Open pelvic fractures: a lethal injury. *J Trauma* 1978;18:184–187.
94. Rowe CR, Lowell JD. Prognosis of fractures of the acetabulum. *J Bone Joint Surg [Am]* 1961;43A:30–59.
95. Russell TA. Fractures of the pelvis and hips. In: Crenshaw AH, ed. *Campbell's operative orthopedics.* 8th ed. Vol. 2. St. Louis: Mosby Year Book; 1992:895–987.
96. Saks BJ. Normal acetabular anatomy for acetabular fracture assessment: CT and plain film correlation. *Radiology* 1986;159:139–145.
97. Sampson J, Berquist TH. Pelvic fractures: a review of 750 cases. Presented at the American Roentgen Ray Society, Las Vegas, NV, 1981.
98. Sandler CM, Hall JT, Rodriquez MB, Corsure JN. Bladder injury in blunt pelvic trauma. *Radiology* 1986;156:633–638.
99. Sandler CM, Harris JH, Corriere JN, Toombs BD. Posterior urethral injury after pelvic fracture. *AJR Am J Roentgenol* 1981;137:1233–1237.
100. Sandler CM, Phillips JM, Harris JD, Toombs BD. Radiology of the bladder and urethra in blunt pelvic trauma. *Radiol Clin North Am* 1981;19:195–211.
101. Sclafani SJA, Becker JA, Traumatic presacral hemorrhage: angiographic diagnosis and therapy. *AJR Am J Roentgenol* 1982;138:123–126.
102. Scott WW, Fishman EK, Magid D. Acetabular fractures: optimal imaging. *Radiology* 1987;165:537–539.
103. Sheldon GF, Winestock DP. Hemorrhage from open pelvic fracture controlled intraoperatively with balloon catheter. *J Trauma* 1978;18:68–70.
104. Silakŏvich W, Love L. Stress fracture of the pubic ramus. *J Bone Joint Surg [Am]* 1954;36A:573–576.
105. Slatis P, Karaharju E. External fixation of unstable pelvic fractures. *Clin Orthop* 1980;171:75–80.
106. Stewart MJ, Milford LW. Fracture-dislocation of the hip. An end result study. *J Bone Joint Surg [Am]* 1954;36A:315–341.
107. Taylor RG. Pelvic dislocation. *Br J Surg* 1942;39:126–132.
108. Thaggard A III, Harle TS, Carlson V. Fractures and dislocations of the bony pelvis and hip. *Semin Roentgenol* 1978;13:117–134.
109. Thompson KR, Goldin AR. Angiographic technique in interventional radiology. *Radiol Clin North Am* 1980;17:375–391.
110. Tile M. Fractures of the acetabulum. *Orthop Clin North Am* 1980;11:481–506.
111. Tile M. Pelvic fractures: operative vs. non-operative treatment. *Orthop Clin North Am* 1980;11:423–464.
112. Tile M. Pelvic ring fractures. *J Bone Joint Surg [Br]* 1988;70B;1–12.
113. Watson-Jones R. Dislocations and fracture-dislocations of the pelvis. *Br J Surg* 1938;25:773–781.
114. Webb LX, Gristina AG, Wilson JR, Rhyne AL, Meredith JH, Hansen ST Jr. Two hole plate fixation. *J Trauma* 1988;28:813–817.
115. Weil GC, Price EM, Rusbridge HW. The diagnosis and treatment of fractures of the pelvis and their complications. *Am J Surg* 1939;44:108–116.
116. Wild JJ, Hanson GJ Jr, Tullos HL. Unstable fractures of the pelvis treated by external fixation. *J Bone Joint Surg [Am]* 1982;64A:1010–1019.
117. Young JWR, Burgess AR, Brumback RJ, Poka A. Pelvic fractures: value of plain radiography in early assessment and management. *Radiology* 1986;160:445–451.
118. Young JWR, Burgess AR. *Radiologic management of pelvic ring fractures.* Baltimore: Urban and Schwarzenberg; 1987.
119. Young JWR, Burgess AR, Brumback RJ, Poka A. lateral compression fractures of the pelvis: importance of plain radiographs in diagnosis and surgical management. *Skeletal Radiol* 1986;15:103–109.
120. Young JWR, Resnick CS. Fractures of the pelvis: current concepts of classification. *AJR Am J Roentgenol* 1990;155:1169–1175.
121. Zorn G. Beckenbrüche mit Harnröhrenverletzungen ihre Behanalung und Ergebnisse. *Beitr Klin Chir* 1960;201:147.

Acetabular Fractures

122. Berquist TH. *Imaging of orthopedic trauma.* 2nd ed. New York: Raven Press; 1992.
123. Bosse, MJ, Poka A, Reinert CM, Brumback RJ, Bathon H, Burgess AR. Preoperative angiographic assessment of the superior gluteal artery in acetabular fractures requiring extensile exposure. The American Academy of Orthopaedic Surgeons Annual Meeting, Atlanta, Feb. 4–9. *J Orthop Trauma* 1988;2:303–307.
124. Carnesale PG, Stewart MJ, Barnes SN. Acetabular disruption and central fracture-dislocation of the hip. *J Bone Joint Surg [Am]* 1975;57A:1054–1059.
125. Henderson MR, Apyan PM. Both-column acetabular fracture in a multiple trauma patient. *J Tenn Med Assoc* 1988;81:516–518.
126. Judet R, Judet J, Letournel RE. Fractures of the acetabulum: classification and surgical approaches for open reduction. *J Bone Joint Surg [Am]* 1964;46A;1615–1647.
127. Letournel E, Judet R. *Fractures of the acetabulum.* 2nd ed. New York: Springer-Verlag, 1994.
128. Matta J. Operative indications and choice of surgical approach for fractures of the acetabulum. *Tech Orthop* 1986;1:13–22.
129. Matta J, Merritt PO. Displaced acetabular fractures. *Clin Orthop* 1988;230:83–97.
130. Müller ME. *Manual of internal fixation.* 3rd ed. Heidelberg: Springer-Verlag; 1990.
131. Pennal GF, Davidson J, Garside H, Plewes J. Results of treatment of acetabular fractures. *Clin Orthop* 1980;151:115–123.
132. Rowe CR, Lowell JD. Prognosis of fractures of the acetabulum. *J Bone Joint Surg [Am]* 1961;43A:30–59.
133. Tile M. Fractures of the acetabulum. In: Rockwood CA, Green DP, Bucholz RW, eds. *Rockwood and Green's fractures in adults.* 3rd ed. Philadelphia: JB Lippincott; 1991:1442–1479.
134. Tile M, Kellam J, Joyce M. Fractures of the acetabulum: classification, management protocol and results of treatment. *J Bone Joint Surg [Br]* 1985;67B:324–325.
135. Ylinen P, Santavirta S, Slatis P. Outcome of acetabular fractures: a 7-year follow-up. *J Trauma* 1989;29:19–24.

Dislocations and Fracture: Dislocations of the Hip

136. Armstrong JR. Traumatic dislocation of the hip joint. *J Bone Joint Surg [Br]* 1948;30B:430–445.
137. Charkraborti S, Miller IM. Dislocation of the hip associated with fracture of the femoral head. *Injury* 1975;7:134–142.
138. Dehne E, Immerman EW. Dislocation of the hip combined with fracture of the shaft of the femur on the same side. *J Bone Joint Surg [Am]* 1951;33A:731–745.
139. DeLee JC. Fractures and dislocations of the hip. In: Rockwood CA, Green DP, Bucholz RW. *Fractures in adults*. Vol. 2. Philadelphia: JB Lippincott; 1991:1481–1652.
140. DeLee JC, Evans JA, Thomas J. Anterior dislocation of the hip associated with femoral head fractures. *J Bone Joint Surg [Am]* 1980;62A:960–964.
141. Dorfman GS, Froelich HA, Groman JJ, Urbanek PJ. Herndon JH. Lower extremity venous thrombosis in patients with acute hip fractures. *AJR Am J Roentgenol* 1990;154:851–855.
142. Dussault RG, Beauregard G, Fauteaux P, Lauren C, Boisjoly A. Femoral head fracture following anterior hip dislocation. *Radiology* 1980;135:627–629.
143. Ehtisham SMA. Traumatic dislocation of the hip joint with fracture of the femoral shaft on the same side. *J Trauma* 1976;16: 196–205.
144. Epstein HC. Posterior fracture-dislocation of the hip—comparison of open and closed methods of treatment in certain types. *J Bone Joint Surg [Am]* 1961;43A:1079–1098.
145. Epstein HC. Posterior fracture-dislocation of the hip. *J Bone Joint Surg [Am]* 1974;56A:1103–1127.
146. Epstein HC. Traumatic dislocation of the hip. *Clin Orthop* 1973;92:116–142.
147. Ghormley RK, Sullivan R. Traumatic dislocation of the hip. *Am J Surg* 1953;85:298–301.
148. Hougaard K, Thomsen PB. Traumatic posterior fracture dislocation of the hip with fracture of the femoral head, neck or both. *J Bone Joint Surg [Am]* 1988;70A:233–238.
149. Keigh JE, Brashear HR, Guilford WB. Stability of posterior fracture-dislocations of the hip. *J Bone Joint Surg [Am]* 1988;70A: 711–714.
150. Pipkin G. Treatment of grade IV fracture-dislocations of the hip. *J Bone Joint Surg [Am]* 1957;39A:1027–1042.
151. Richardson P, Young JWR, Porter D. CT detection of cortical fracture of the femoral head associated with posterior hip dislocation. *AJR Am J Roentgenol* 1990;155:93–94.
152. Roeder LF, DeLee JC. Femoral head fractures associated with posterior hip dislocation. *Clin Orthop* 1980;147:121–130.
153. Rosenthal RE, Coker WL. Fracture-dislocations of the hip: an epidemiological review. *J Trauma* 1979;19:572–581.
154. Smith GR, Loop JW. Radiological classification of posterior hip dislocation. *Radiology* 1976;119:569–574.
155. Stewart MJ, Milford LW. Fracture-dislocations of the hip. *J Bone Joint Surg [Am]* 1954;36A:315–342.
156. Tehranzadeh J, Vanarthos W, Pais MJ. Osteochondral impaction of the femoral head with associated hip dislocation: CT study in 35 patients. *AJR Am J Roentgenol* 1990;155:1049–1052.
157. Thaggard A III, Harle TS, Carlson V. Fractures and dislocations of the bony pelvis and hips. *Semin Roentgenol* 1978;13:117–134.
158. Thompson VP, Epstein HC. Traumatic dislocation of the hip. *J Bone Joint Surg [Am]* 1951;33A:747–778.
159. Urist MR. Fracture-dislocation of the hip joint. *J Bone Joint Surg [Am]* 1948;30A:699–727.

Femoral Neck Fractures

160. Ambrose GB, Garcia A, Neer CS. Displaced intracapsular fractures of the neck of the femur. *J Trauma* 1963;3:361–369.
161. Anonymous. Femoral neck fractures (adult). *AAOS Bull* 1989; : 11–12.
162. Arnold WD. The effect of early weight bearing on the stability of femoral neck fractures treated with Knowles pins. *J Bone Joint Surg [Am]* 1984;66A:847–852.
163. Arnoldi CC, Lemperg RK. Fractures of the femoral neck. *Clin Orthop* 1977;129:217–222.
164. Asnis SE, Shoji H, Bohne WHO. Scintimetric evaluation of complications of femoral neck fractures. *Clin Orthop* 1976;121:149–156.
165. Banks HH. Factors influencing the results in fractures of the femoral neck. *J Bone Joint Surg [Am]* 1962;44A:931–946.
166. Barnes R, Brown J, Garden RS, Nicoll EA. Subcapital fractures of the femur. A prospective review. *J Bone Joint Surg [Br]* 1976;58B:2–24.
167. Bassett LW, Mirra JM, Craccholo A, Gold RH. Ischemic necrosis of the femoral head. Correlation of magnetic resonance imaging and histologic sections. *Clin Orthop* 1987;233:181–187.
168. Berquist TH. *Magnetic resonance of the musculoskeletal system*. 2nd ed. New York: Raven Press; 1990.
169. Berquist TH. *Imaging of orthopedic trauma*. 2nd ed. New York: Raven Press; 1992.
170. Bobechko WP, Harris WR. The radiographic density of avascular bone. *J Bone Joint Surg [Br]* 1960;42B:626–632.
171. De Haas W, Macnab I. Fractures of the neck of the femur. *S Afr Med J* 1956;30:1005–1010.
172. DeLee JC. Fractures and dislocations of the hip. In: Rockwood CA, Green DP, Bucholz RW, eds. *Rockwood and Green's fractures in adults*. 3rd. ed. Vol. 2. Philadelphia: JB Lippincott; 1991: 1481–1651.
173. Ficat P, Arlet J. Diagnostic de l'ostéo-necrose fémorocapitale primitive au stade I (stade pré-radiologique). *Rev Chir Orthop* 1968;54:637.
174. Garden RS. Stability and union of subcapital fractures of the femur. *J Bone Joint Surg [Br]* 1964;46B:630–712.
175. Garden RS. Reduction and fixation of subcapital fractures of the femur. *Orthop Clin North Am* 1974;5:683–712.
176. Griffiths WEG, Swanson SA, Freeman MAR. Experimental fatigue fractures of the femoral neck. *J Bone Joint Surg [Br]* 1971;54B:136–143.
177. Hanson BA, Solgaard S. Impacted fractures of the femoral neck treated by early mobilization and weight-bearing. *Acta Orthop Scand* 1978;49:180–185.
178. Harper M, Neustorf J. Fractures of the femoral neck associated with technical errors in closed medullary nailing of the femur. *J Bone Joint Surg [Am]* 1986;68A:624–626.
179. Hungerford DS. Pathogenic consideration in ischemic necrosis of bone. *Can J Surg* 1981;24:583–586.
180. Jeffrey CC. Spontaneous fracture of the femoral neck. *Orthop Clin North Am* 1974;5:713–727.
181. Lu-Yao GL, Keller RB, Littenberg B, Wennberg JE. Outcomes of displaced fractures of the femoral neck. *J Bone Joint Surg [Am]* 1994;76A:15–25.
182. Meyers MH. Impacted and undisplaced femoral neck fractures. In: *The hip. Proceedings of the Tenth Open Scientific Meeting of the Hip Society*. St. Louis: CV Mosby Co; 1982.
183. Mitchell DG, Kressel HY, Arger PH, Dalinka M, Spritzer CE, Steinberg ME. Avascular necrosis of the femoral head: morphologic assessment by MR imaging with CT correlation. *Radiology* 1986;161:739–742.
184. Norman A, Bullough P. The radiolucent crescent sign. An early diagnositc sign of necrosis of the femoral head. *Bull Hosp Jt Dis Orthop Inst* 1963;24:99–104.
185. Olerud C, Hellquist E. Internal fixation of femoral neck fractures. *J Bone Joint Surg [Br]* 1991;73B:16–19.
186. Pauwel F. *Der Schenkelausbruch: ein mechanishes Problem. Grundlagen des heilungsvorganges Prognose und kausale Therapie*. Stuttgart: Ferdinande Enke; 1935.
187. Phemister DB. Bone growth and repair. *Ann Surg* 1935;102:261.
188. Rizzo PF, Gould ES, Lyden JP, Asnis SE. Diagnosis of occult fractures about the hip. *J Bone Joint Surg [Am]* 1993;75A:395–402.
189. Rubin R, Trent P, Arnold W, Burstein A. Knowles pinning of experimental femoral neck fractures: Biomechanical study. *J Trauma* 1981;21:1036–1039.
190. Salvati EA, Wilson PD. Long-term results of the femoral-head replacement. *J Bone Joint Surg [Am]* 1972;55A:1355–1356.
191. Scheck M. Intracapsular fractures of the femoral neck. Commi-

nution of the posterior cortex as a cause of unstable fracture. *J Bone Joint Surg [Am]* 1959;41A:1187–1200.
192. Shih C, Wang K. Femoral neck fractures: 121 cases treated by Knowles pinning. *Clin Orthop* 1991;271:195–200.
193. Sikorski JM, Barrington R. Internal fixation versus hemiarthroplasty for the displaced subcapital fracture of the femur: a prospective, randomized study. *J Bone Joint Surg [Br]* 1981;63B: 356–361.
194. Springer ER, Lachiewicz PF, Gilbert JA. Internal fixation of femoral neck fractures. A comparative study of Knowles pins and 6.5 mm cancellous screws. *Clin Orthop* 1991;267:85–92.
195. Turner A, Taylor JF, Casty H, Owen R. The radiographic evaluation of multiple pin fixation of the femoral head. *Br J Radiol* 1984;57:887–890.
196. White BL, Fisher WD, Laurin CA. Rate of mortality for elderly patients after fracture of the hip in the 1980's. *J Bone Joint Surg [Am]* 1987;69A:1335–1340.
197. Yamagata M, Chao EY, Ilstrup DM, Melton LJ III, Coventry MB, Stauffer RN. Fixed-head and bipolar hip endoprostheses. A retrospective clinical and roentgenographic study. *J Arthroplasty* 1987;2:327–341.

Trochanteric Fractures

198. Berquist TH. *Imaging of orthopedic trauma.* 2nd ed. New York: Raven Press; 1992.
199. Bertin KC, Horstman J, Coleman SS. Isolated fracture of the lesser trochanter in adults: an initial manifestation of metastatic disease. *J Bone Joint Surg [Am]* 1984;66A:770–773.
200. Boyd HB, Griffin LL. Classification and treatment of trochanteric fractures. *Arch Surg* 1949;58:853–866.
201. Brien WW, Wiss DA, Becker V Jr, Lehman T. Subtrochanteric fractures: a comparison of the Zickel nail, 95° blade plate, and interlocking nail. *J Orthop Trauma* 1991;5:458–464.
202. Brodell JD, Leve AR. Disengagement and intrapelvic protrusion of the screw from a sliding screw-plate device. *J Bone Joint Surg [Am]* 1983;65A:697–700.
203. Broos PL, Rommeus PM, Delgyn PRJ, Greens VR, Stappaerts KH. Pertrochanteric fractures in the elderly: are these indications for primary prosthetic replacement? *J Orthop Trauma* 1991;5: 446–451.
204. Chapman MW, Bowman WE, Csongradi JJ, Day LJ, Trafton PG, Bovidl EG. The use of Ender's pins in extracapsular fractures of the hip. *J Bone Joint Surg [Am]* 1981;63A:14–28.
205. Davis TRC, Sher JL, Horsmon A, Simpson M, Porter BB, Checketts RG. Intertrochanteric fractures: mechanical failure after internal fixation. *J Bone Joint Surg [Br]* 1990;72B:26–31.
206. DeLee JC. Fractures and dislocations of the hip. In: Rockwood CA, Green DP, Bucholz RW, eds. *Fractures in adults.* Vol. 2. Philadelphia: JB Lippincott; 1991:1481–1651.
207. DenHartog BD, Bartal E, Cooke F. Treatment of unstable intertrochanteric fracture. *J Bone Joint Surg [Am]* 1991;73A:726–733.
208. Dimon JH, Hughston JC. Unstable intertrochanteric fractures of the hip. *J Bone Joint Surg [Am]* 1967;49A:440–450.
209. Ender HG. Treatment of trochanteric and subtrochanteric fractures of the femur with Ender pins. In: *The hip. Proceedings of the Sixth Open Scientific Meeting of the Hip Society.* St. Louis: CV Mosby; 1978.
210. Evans EM. The treatment of trochanteric fractures of the femur. *J Bone Joint Surg [Br]* 1949;31B:190–203.
211. Fielding JW. Subtrochanteric fractures. *Clin Orthop* 1973;92: 86–99.
212. Haentjens P, Castileyn PP, DeBoeck H, Handelberg F, Opdecain P. Treatment of unstable intertrochanteric and subtrochanteric fractures in elderly patients. *J Bone Joint Surg [Am]* 1989;71A: 1214–1224.
213. Hafner RHV. Trochanteric fractures of the femur. *J Bone Joint Surg [Br]* 1951;33B:513–516.
214. Heyse-Moore GH, MacEachern AG, Evans DC. Treatment of intertrochanteric fractures of the femur. A comparison of the Richards screw-plate with the Jewett nail-plate. *J Bone Joint Surg [Br]* 1983;65B:262–267.
215. Jensen JS. Classification of trochanteric fractures. *Acta Orthop Scand* 1980;51:803–810.
216. Kuderna H, Böhler N, Collon DJ. Treatment of intertrochanteric and subtrochanteric fractures of the femur by the Ender method. *J Bone Joint Surg [Am]* 1976;58A:604–611.
217. Kyle RF, Gustilo RB, Premer RF. Analysis of 622 intertrochanteric hip fractures. *J Bone Joint Surg [Am]* 1979;61A:216–221.
218. Lord G, Marotte JH, Blantard JP, Guillamon JL, Hannoun L. Head and neck arthroplasty in treatment of intertrochanteric fractures after age 70. *Rev Chir Orthop* 1977;63:135–148.
219. May JMB, Chacha PB. Displacement of trochanteric fractures and their influence on reduction. *J Bone Joint Surg [Br]* 1968;50B:318–323.
220. McLaren CAN, Buckely JR, Rowley DI. Intertrochanteric fractures of the femur: a randomized prospective trial comparing the Pugh nail with the dynamic hip screw. *Injury* 1991;22:193–196.
221. Mulholland RC, Gunn DR. Sliding screw-plate fixation of intertrochanteric femoral fractures. *J Trauma* 1975;12:581–591.
222. Müller ME, Nazarian S, Koch P. *Classification AO des fractures I.* Berlin: Springer-Verlag; 1987:120–121.
223. Naimark A, Kossoff J, Schepsis A. Intertrochanteric fractures: current concepts on an old subject. *AJR Am J Roentgenol* 1979;133:889–894.
224. Nangu S, Olerud C, Rehnberg L. Treatment of intertrochanteric fractures: comparison of Ender nails and sliding screw plates. *J Orthop Trauma* 1991;5:452–457.
225. Pankovich AM, Tarabishy I. Ender nailing of intertrochanteric and subtrochanteric femoral fractures. *J Bone Joint Surg [Am]* 1980;62A:635–645.
226. Rasmussen K. McLaughlin osteosynthesis in trochanteric fractures. *Acta Chir Scand* 1953;108:246.
227. Sarmiento A, Williams EM. Unstable trochanteric fracture: treatment with valgus osteotomy and I-beam nail-plate: Preliminary report of 100 cases. *J Bone Joint Surg [Am]* 1970;52A:1309–1318.
228. Sartoris DJ, Kerr R, Goergen T, Resnick D. Sliding-screw plate fixation of proximal femoral fractures. *Skeletal Radiol* 1985;14: 104–110.
229. Schatzker J. Methyl methacrylate as adjunct in internal fixation of intertrochanteric fractures of the femur. *Can J Surg* 1979;22: 179–182.
230. Seinsheimer F. Subtrochanteric fractures of the femur. *J Bone Joint Surg [Am]* 1978;60A:300–306.
231. Sernbo I, Johnell O, Gentz C, Nelsson J. Unstable intertrochanteric fractures of the hip. *J Bone Joint Surg [Am]* 1988;70A:1297–1303.
232. Wade PA, Campbell RD, Kerin RJ. Management of intertrochanteric fractures of the femur. *Am J Surg* 1959;97:634–643.
233. Whatley JR, Garland DE, Whitecloud T III, et al. Subtrochanteric fracture of the femur: treatment with ASIF blade-plate fixation. *South Med J* 1978;71:1372–1375.
234. Yelton C, Low W. Iatrogenic subtrochanteric fracture: a complication of Zickel nails. *J Bone Joint Surg [Am]* 1986;68A:1237–1240.
235. Zickel RE. Fractures of the adult femur excluding the femoral head and neck. A review and evaluation of current therapy. *Clin Orthop* 1980;147:93–106.
236. Zickel RE, Bercik MJ, Licciardi LM. A continuing study on the use of the Zickel intramedullary appliances in fractures and lesions of the proximal femur. In: *The hip. Proceedings of the Sixth Open Scientific Meeting of the Hip Society.* St. Louis: CV Mosby; 1978.

Hip Arthroplasty

237. Barber TC, Healy WH. The hospital cost of total hip arthroplasty. A comparison between 1981 and 1990. *J Bone Joint Surg [Am]* 1993;75A:321–330.
238. Barentsz, JO, Lemmens JM, Slooff TJJH. The use of subtraction

arthrography in total hip arthroplasties. *Fortschr Röntgenstr* 1986;144:440–446.

239. Barrack RL, Harris WH. The value of aspiration of the hip joint before revision total hip arthroplasty. *J Bone Joint Surg [Am]* 1993;75A:66–76.
240. Barrack RL, Tanzer R, Kattaparam SV, Harris WH. The value of contrast arthrography in assessing loosening of symptomatic uncemented total hip components. *Skeletal Radiol* 1994;23:37–41.
241. Bateman JE, Berenji AR, Bayne O, Greyson ND. Long-term results of bipolar arthroplasty in osteoarthritis of the hip. *Clin Orthop* 1990;251:54–66.
242. Beabout JW. Radiology of total hip arthroplasty. *Radiol Clin North Am* 1975;13:3–19.
243. Beckenbaugh RD, Ilstrup DM. Total hip arthroplasty: a review of three hundred and thirty-three cases with long follow-up. *J Bone Joint Surg [Am]* 1978;60A:306–313.
244. Berquist TH. Diagnostic and therapeutic injections as an aid to musculoskeletal diagnosis. *Semin Intervent Radiol* 1993;10:326–343.
245. Berquist TH, Bender CE, Maus TP, Ward EM, Rand JA. Pseudobursae: a useful finding in patients with painful hip arthroplasty. *AJR Am J Roentgenol* 1987;148:103–106.
246. Brentlinger A, Hunter JR. Perforation of the external iliac artery and ureter presenting as acute hemorrhagic cystitis after total hip replacement: report of a case. *J Bone Joint Surg [Am]* 1987;69A:620–622.
247. Brien WW, Salvati EA, Wright TM, Nelson CL, Hungerford DS, Gilliam DL. Dissociation of acetabular components after hip arthroplasty: report of four cases. *J Bone Joint Surg [Am]* 1990;72A:1548–1550.
248. Butler JC, Skalley TC, Cook SD, Brinker MR, Haddad RJ, Sackett JR, Cheramie JB. Clinical and roentgenographic evaluation of bipolar prostheses with noncemented anatomic medullary locking femoral stems. *Clin Orthop* 1990;254:180–188.
249. Callaghan JJ. The clinical results and basic science of total hip arthroplasty with porous-coated prostheses. *J Bone Joint Surg [Am]* 1993;75A:299–310.
250. Callaghan JJ, Fulghum CS, Glisson RR, Stranne SK. The effect of femoral stem geometry on interface motion in uncemented porous-coated total hip prostheses. *J Bone Joint Surg [Am]* 1992;74A:839–848.
251. Chafetz N, Baumrind S, Murray WR, Genant HR. Femoral prosthesis subsidence in asymptomatic patients: a stereophotogrammetric assessment. *Invest Radiol* 1984;19:235–241.
252. Chan KH, Ahined AM. Polymethylmethracrylate. In: Morrey BF, ed. *Joint replacement arthroplasty.* New York: Churchill Livingstone; 1991:23–36.
253. Chandler HP, Reineck FT, Wixson RL, McCarthy JC. Total hip replacement in patients younger than thirty years old. *J Bone Joint Surg [Am]* 1981;63A:1426–1434.
254. Charnley J. Total hip replacement. *JAMA* 1974;230:1025.
255. Chew FS, Lev MH. Polyethylene osteolysis. *AJR Am J Roentgenol* 1992;159:1254.
256. Collier JP, Mayor MB, Surprenant VA, Surprenant HP, Dauphinais LA, Jensen BA. The biomechanical problems of polyethylene as a bearing surface. *Clin Orthop* 1990;261:107–113.
257. Cone RO, Yaru N, Resnick D, Gershuni D, Guerra J Jr. Intracapsular pressure monitoring during arthrographic evaluation of painful hip prostheses. *AJR Am J Roentgenol* 1983;141:885–889.
258. Convery FR, Minteer-Convery M, Devine SD, Meyers MH. Acetabular augmentation in primary and revision total hip arthroplasty with cementless prostheses. *Clin Orthop* 1990;252:167–175.
259. Coventry MB. Historical perspective of hip arthroplasty. In: Morrey BF, ed. *Joint replacement arthroplasty.* New York: Churchill Livingstone; 1996:491–499.
260. Coventry MB. Late dislocations in patients with Charnley total hip arthroplasty. *J Bone Joint Surg [Am]* 1985;67A:832–841.
261. Daly PJ, Morrey BF. Operative correction of an unstable total hip arthroplasty. *J Bone Joint Surg [Am]* 1992;74A:1334–1343.
262. D'Antonio JA, Capello WM, Crothers OD, Jaffe WL, Manley MT. Early clinical experience with hydroxyapatite-coated femoral implants. *J Bone Joint Surg [Am]* 1992;74A:995–1008.
263. DeOrio JK, Blasser KE. Indications and patient selection. In: Morrey BE, ed. *Joint replacement arthroplasty.* New York: Churchill Livingstone; 1991:547–559.
264. Dorr LD. Total hip replacement using the APR system. Bone ingrowth hip arthroplasty. *Tech Orthop* 1986;1:22–34.
265. Dorr LD, Sakimura I, Mohler JG. Pulmonary emboli following total hip arthroplasty: incidence study. *J Bone Joint Surg [Am]* 1979;61A:1083–1086.
266. Draenert K, Draenert Y. Possibilities and limitations of the cementless fixation of endoprosthetic components. In: Morscher E, ed. *The cementless fixation of hip endoprostheses.* New York: Springer-Verlag; 1984.
267. Dumbleton JH. Wear and prosthetic joints. In: Morrey BF, ed. *Joint replacement arthroplasty.* New York: Churchill Livingstone; 1991:47–59.
268. Ebraheim NA, Coombs R, Rusin JJ, Jackson WT. Reduction of postoperative CT artifacts of pelvic fractures by use of titanium implants. *Orthopedics* 1990;13:1357–1358.
269. Ebramzadeh E, Sarmient OA, McKelloys HA, Llinas A, Gogan W. The cement mantle in total hip arthroplasty. *J Bone Joint Surg [Am]* 1994;76A:77–86.
270. Egund N, Lidgren L, Önnerfält R. Improved positioning of the femoral stem with a centralizing device. *Acta Orthop Scand* 1990;61:236–239.
271. Engh CA, Griffin WL, Marx CL. Cementless acetabular components. *J Bone Joint Surg [Br]* 1990;72B:53–59.
272. Engh CA, Massin P, Suthers KE. Roentgenographic assessment of the biologic fixation of porous-surfaced femoral components. *Clin Orthop* 1990;257:107–128.
273. Engh CA, McGovern TF, Bobyn JD, Harriw WH. A quantitative evaluation of periprosthetic bone-remodeling after cementless total hip arthroplasty. *J Bone Joint Surg [Am]* 1992;74A:1009–1020.
274. Engh CA, Zettl-Schaffer KF, Kukita Y, Sweet D, Jasty M, Bragdon C. Historical and radiographic assessment of well functiong porous-coated acetabular components. *J Bone Joint Surg [Am]* 1993;75A:814–824.
275. Fishman E, Magid D, Robertson DD, Brooker AF, Weiss P, Sieglman SS. Metallic hip implants: CT with multi reconstruction. *Radiology* 1986;160:675–681.
276. Földes K, Gaal M, Balint P, Nemenyi K, Kiss C, Balint GP, Buchanan WW. Ultrasonography after hip arthroplasty. *Skeletal Radiol* 1992;21:297–299.
277. Fox GM, McBeath AA, Heiner JP. Hip replacement with a threaded acetabular cup. A follow-up study. *J Bone Joint Surg [Am]* 1994;76A:195–201.
278. Freedman MT. Radiologic aspects of femoral head replacements and cup mold arthroplasties. *Radiol Clin North Am* 1975;13:45–56.
279. Freiberger RH. Evaluation of hip prostheses by imaging methods. *Semin Roentgenol* 1986;21:20–28.
280. Friedman RJ, Black J, Galante JO, Jacobs JJ, Skinner HB. Orthopedic biomaterials and implant fixation. *J Bone Joint Surg [Am]* 1993;75A:1086–1109.
281. Galante JO. Overview of current attempts to eliminate methyl methacrylate. In: *The hip. Proceedings of the Eleventh International Open Scientific Meeting of the Hip Society.*; 1983.
282. García-Cimbrelo E, Munuera L. Early and late loosening of the acetabular cup after low-friction arthroplasty. *J Bone Joint Surg [Am]* 1992;74A:1119–1128.
283. Gilbert JH, Buckley CA, Jacobs JJ, Bertan KC, Zernick MR. Intergranular corrosion-fatigue failure of cobalt-alloy femoral stems. *J Bone Joint Surg [Am]* 1994;76A:110–115.
284. Gilberty R. Hemiarthroplasty of the hip using a low-friction bipolar endoprostheses. *Clin Orthop* 1983;175:86–92.
285. Gilula LA, Staple TW. Miniature atlas of total hip prostheses. *Radiol Clin North Am* 1975;13:21–44.
286. Goldring SR, Jasty M, Roelke MS Rourke CM, Bringhurst FR, Harrisu A. Formation of a synovial-like membrane at the bone-cement interface. *Arthritis Rheum* 1986;29:836–842.
287. Goldring SR, Schiller AL, Roelke M, Rourke CM, O'Neil DA, Harris WH. The synovial-like membrane at the bone-cement interface in loose total hip replacements and its proposed role in bone lysis. *J Bone Joint Surg [Am]* 1983;65A:575–584.

288. Goldstein HA. Bone scintigraphy. *Orthop Clin North Am* 1983;14:243–256.
289. Griffiths HJ, Burke J, Bonfiglio TA. Granulomatous pseudotumors in total joint replacement. *Skeletal Radiol* 1987;16:146–152.
290. Gruen TA, McNiece GM, Amstutz HC. Modes of failure of cemented stem-type femoral components. A radiographic analysis of loosening. *Clin Orthop* 1979;141:17–27.
291. Habermann ET. Total joint replacement: an overview. *Semin Roentgenol* 1986;21:7–19.
292. Haddad RJ Jr, Skalley TC, Cook SD, Brinker MR, Cheramil J, Meyer R, Missry J. Clinical and roentgenographic evaluation of noncemented porous-coated anatomic medullary locking (AML) and porous-coated anatomic (PCA) total hip arthroplasties. *Clin Orthop* 1990;258:176–182.
293. Haddad RJ, Cook SD, Brinker MR. A comparison of three varieties of noncemented porous-coated hip replacement. *J Bone Joint Surg* [*Br*] 1990;72B:2–8.
294. Hansen AD, Lewallen DG. Cemented hip replacement: techniques. In: Morrey BF, ed. *Joint replacement arthroplasty.* New York: Churchill Livingstone; 1991:601–618.
295. Hardy DC, Reinus WR, Totty WG, Keyser CK. Arthrography after total hip arthroplasty: utility of postambulation radiographs. *Skeletal Radiol* 1988;17:20–23.
296. Harris WH. A new total hip implant. *Clin Orthop* 1971;81:105–113.
297. Harris WH. Traumatic arthritis of the hip after dislocation and acetabular fractures: treatment by mold arthroplasty: an end result study using a new method of result evaluation. *J Bone Joint Surg* [*Am*] 1969;51A:737–755.
298. Harris WH, McCarthy JC Jr, O'Neill DA. Femoral component loosening using contemporary techniques of femoral cement fixation. *J Bone Joint Surg* [*Am*] 1982;64A:1063–1067.
299. Harris WH, Schiller AL, Scholler JM, Freiberg RA, Scott R. Extensive localized bone resorption in the femur following total hip replacement. *J Bone Joint Surg* [*Am*] 1976;58A:612–618.
300. Haynes DR, Rogers SD, Hay S, Pearcy MJ, Howie DW. The differences in toxicity and release of bone-resorbing mediators induced by titanium and cobalt-chromium-alloy wear particles. *J Bone Joint Surg* [*Am*] 1993;75A:825–834.
301. Hedley AK. Present state, problems, and future implications of porous-coated implants. In: Reiley LH Jr, ed. *Proceedings of the Eighth Open Scientific Meeting of the Hip Society.* St. Louis: CV Mosby; 1980.
302. Heekin RD, Callaghan JJ, Hopkinson WJ, Savory CG, Xenos JS. The porous-coated anatomic total hip prosthesis, inserted without cement: results after five to seven years in a prospective study. *J Bone Joint Surg* [*Am*] 1993;75A:77–91.
303. Hendrix RW, Wixson RL, Rana NA, Rogers LF. Arthrography after total hip arthroplasty: a modified technique used in the diagnosis of pain. *Radiology* 1983;148:647–652.
304. Horowitz SM, Doty SB, Lane JM, Burstein AH. Studies of the mechanism by which mechanical failure of polyethylene leads to bone resorption. *J Bone Joint Surg* [*Am*] 1993;75A:802–813.
305. Huddleston HD. Femoral lysis after cemented hip arthroplasty. *J Arthroplasty* 1988;3:285–297.
306. Huiskes R. The various stress patterns of press-fit, ingrown, and cemented femoral stems. *Clin Orthop* 1990;261:27–38.
307. Huo MH, Salvati EA, Lieberman JR, Burstein AH, Wilson PD. Custom-designed femoral prostheses in total hip arthroplasty done with cement for severe dysplasia of the hip. *J Bone Joint Surg* [*Am*] 1993;75A:1497–1504.
308. Jiranek WA, Machadom, Jasty M, Jevsevar D, Wolfe HJ, Goldring SR, Goldberg MJ, Harris WH. Production of cytokines around loosened cemented acetabular components. *J Bone Joint Surg* [*Am*] 1993;75A:863–878.
309. Kaplan PA, Montesi SA, Jardon OM, Gregory PR. Bone-ingrowth hip prostheses in asymptomatic patients: radiographic fractures. *Radiology* 1988;169:221–227.
310. Kavanagh BF. Evaluation of the painful total hip arthroplasty. In: Morrey BF, ed. *Joint replacement arthroplasty.* New York: Churchill Livingstone; 1991:779–788.
311. Kavanagh BF, Hassen AD, Coventry MB. Cemented hip replacement. Results. In: Morrey BF, ed. *Joint replacement arthroplasty.* New York: Churchill Livingstone; 1991:639–646.
312. Kavanagh BF, Ilstrip DM, Fitzgerald RH Jr. Revision total hip arthroplasty. *J Bone Joint Surg* [*Am*] 1985;67A:517–526.
313. Kavanagh BF, Mariani EM, Cabanela ME Ilstrup DM, Morrey DB. Uncemented hip replacement. Results. In: Morrey BF, ed. *Joint replacement arthroplasty.* New York: Churchill Livingstone; 1991:647–662.
314. Kavanagh BF, Morrey BF, Mariani EM, Cabanela ME. Uncemented hip replacement: technique. In: Morrey BF, ed. *Joint replacement arthroplasty.* New York: Churchill Livingstone; 1991:619–638.
315. Kavanagh BF. Revision hip arthroplasty: techniques. In: Morrey BF, ed. *Joint replacement arthroplasty.* New York: Churchill Livingstone; 1991:789–795.
316. Kilcoyne RF, Kaplan P. The lateral approach for hip arthrography. *Skeletal Radiol* 1992;21:239–240.
317. Kim KJ, Rubash HE. In vivo and in vitro analysis of membranes from hip prosthesis inserted without cement. *J Bone Joint Surg* [*Am*] 1994;76A:172–180.
318. Kummer FJ. Bipolar prostheses: a critical review. *Bull Hosp Jt Dis Orthop Inst* 1990;50:70–76.
319. Kummer FJ, Jaffe WL, Steiner GC. Wear-caused failure of a polyethylene acetabular cup with associated granuloma: a case report. *Bull Hosp Jt Dis Orthop Inst* 1990;50:196–199.
320. Lemons JE. Metallic alloys. In: Morrey BF, ed. *Joint replacement arthroplasty.* New York: Churchill Livingstone; 1991:13–21.
321. Lestrange NR. Bipolar arthroplasty for 496 hip fractures. *Clin Orthop* 1990;251:7 19.
322. Lewellan DG, Cabanela ME. Inadequate acetabular bone: techniques. In: Morrey BF, ed. *Joint replacement arthroplasty.* New York: Churchill Livingstone; 1991:797–808.
323. Lyons CW, Berquist TH, Lyons JC, Rand JA, Brown ML. Evaluation of radiographic findings in painful hip arthroplasties. *Clin Orthop* 1985;195:239–251.
324. Madhok R, Lewallen DG, Wallrichs SL, Ilstrup DM, Kurland RL, Melton JL. Trends in the utilization of primary total hip arthroplasty, 1969 through 1990: a population-based study in Olmsted County, Minnesota. *Mayo Clin Proc* 1993;68:11–18.
325. Martell JM, Pierson RH, Jacobs JJ, Rosenberg AG, Maley M, Galente JO. Primary total hip reconstruction with a titanium fiber-coated prostheses inserted without cement. *J Bone Joint Surg* [*Am*] 1993;75A:554–571.
326. Maus TP, Berquist TH, Bender CE, Rand JA. Arthrographic study of painful total hip arthroplasty: refined criteria. *Radiology* 1987;162:721–727.
327. Mayer G, Harseil K. Acetabular reinforcement of total hip replacement. *Arch Orthop Trauma Surg* 1986;105:227–231.
328. McDonald DJ, Fitzgerald RH Jr, Ilstrup DM. Two-stage reconstruction of a total hip arthroplasty because of infection. *J Bone Joint Surg* [*Am*] 1989;71A:828–834.
329. Mjöberg F, Franzén H, Selvik G. Early detection of prosthetic-hip loosening: comparison of low- and high-viscosity bone cement. *Acta Orthop Scand* 1990;61:273–274.
330. Morrey BF. Femoral head size. In: Morrey BF, ed. *Joint replacement arthroplasty.* New York: Churchill Livingstone; 1991:587–599.
331. Morrey BF. *Joint replacement arthroplasty.* New York: Churchill Livingstone; 1991.
332. Morrey BF. Short-stemmed uncemented femoral replacement component. In: Morrey BF, ed. *Joint replacement arthroplasty.* New York: Churchill Livingstone; 1991:663–672.
333. Morrey BF. Acetabulum. In: Morrey BF, ed. *Joint replacement arthroplasty.* New York: Churchill Livingstone; 1991:561–572.
334. Morscher EW. Cementless total hip arthroplasty. *Clin Orthop* 1983;181:76.
335. Morscher EW. *The cementless fixation of hip endoprostheses.* New York: Springer-Verlag; 1984.
336. Mulroy RD Jr, Harris WH. The effect of improved cementing techniques on component loosening in total hip replacement: an 11-year radiographic review. *J Bone Joint Surg* [*Br*] 1990;72B:757–760.

337. Newberg AH, Wetzner SM. Digital subtraction arthrography. *Radiology* 1985;154:238–239.
338. Oates E. Scintigraphic diagnoses of infection and inflammation. *Appl Radiol* 1992;21:48–53.
339. Ohlin A. Failure of the Christiansen hip: survival analysis of 265 cases. *Acta Orthop Scand* 1990;61:7–11.
340. Ohlin A, Johnell O, Lerner UH. The pathogenesis of loosening of total hip arthroplasties: the production of factors by periprosthetic tissues that stimulate in vitro bone resorption. *Clin Orthop* 1990;253:287–296.
341. Ohlin A, Önsten I. Loosening of the Lubinus hip: 202 cases followed for 3–6 years. *Acta Orthop Scand* 1990;61:244–247.
342. Önsten I, Carlsson AS, Ohlun A, Nilsson JA. Migration of acetabular components inserted with and without cement, in one-stage bilateral hip arthroplasty. *J Bone Joint Surg [Am]* 1994;76A:185–194.
343. Padgett DE, Kull L, Rosenberg A, Sumner DR, Galante JO. Revision of the acetabular component without cement after total hip arthroplasty. *J Bone Joint Surg [Am]* 1993;75A:663–672.
344. Pellicci PM, Inglis AE, Salvati EA. Perforation of the femoral shaft during total hip replacement: report of twelve cases. *J Bone Joint Surg [Am]* 1980;62A:234–240.
345. Phillips WC, Kattapuram SV. Prosthetic hip replacements: plain films and arthrography for component loosening. *AJR Am J Roentgenol* 1982;138:677–682.
346. Quale JL, Murphey MD, Huntrakoon M, Reckling FW, Neff JR. Titanium-induced arthropathy associated with polyethylene-metal separation after total joint replacement. *Radiology* 1992;182:855–858.
347. Resnick D, Kerr R, Andrè M, Guerra J, Cone RO, Atkinson D, Pineda C. Digital arthrography in the evaluation of painful joint prostheses. *Invest Radiol* 1984;19:432–437.
348. Ritter MA, Keating EM, Faris PM, Brago G. Metal-backed acetabular cups in total hip arthroplasty. *J Bone Joint Surg [Am]* 1990;72A:672–677.
349. Rosenthall L, Addis AE, Hill RO. Combined radionuclide and radiocontrast arthrography for evaluating hip arthroplasty. *Nucl Med* 1985;10:531–534.
350. Rothman RH, Cohn JC. Cemented versus cementless total hip arthoplasty: a critical review. *Clin Orthop* 1990;254:153–169.
351. Salvati EA, Wilson PD Jr, Jolley MN, Vakili F, Aglietti P, Brown GC. A ten-year follow-up study of our first one hundred consecutive Charnley total hip replacements. *J Bone Joint Surg [Am]* 1981;63A:753–767.
352. Salzer M, Knahr K, Frank P. Radiologic and clinical follow-ups of uncemented femoral endoprostheses with and without collars. In: Morscher E, ed. *The cementless fixation of hip endoprostheses.* New York: Springer-Verlag; 1984.
353. Santavirta S, Hoikka V, Eskola A, Konttinen YT, Paavilainen T, Tallroth K. Aggressive granulomatous lesions in cementless total hip arthroplasty. *J Bone Joint Surg [Br]* 1990;72B:980–984.
354. Sarmiento A. Austin Moore prosthesis in the arthritic hip. *Clin Orthop* 1972;82:14.
355. Schauwecker DS. The scintigraphic diagnoses of osteomyelitis. *AJR Am J Roentgenol* 1992;158:9–18.
356. Schenk RK, Herrmann W. Histologic studies on the incorporation of uncemented implants. In: Morscher E, ed. *The cementless fixation of hip endoprostheses.* New York: Springer-Verlag; 1984.
357. Schmalzried TP, Harris WH. The Harris-Galante porous-coated acetabular component with screw fixation. *J Bone Joint Surg [Am]* 1992;74A:1130–1139.
358. Schmalzried TP, Jasty M, Harris WH. Periprosthetic bone loss in total hip arthroplasty. *J Bone Joint Surg [Am]* 1992;74A:849–867.
359. Schulte KR, Callaghan JJ, Kelley SS, Johnston RC. The outcome of Charnley total hip arthroplasty with cement after a minimum twenty year follow-up. *J Bone Joint Surg [Am]* 1993;75A:961–975.
360. Scott WW, Riley LH, Dorfman HD. Focal lytic lesions associated with femoral stem loosening in total hip prosthesis. *AJR Am J Roentgenol* 1985;144:977–982.
361. Seegenschmiedt MH, Goldman AR, Martus P, Wolfel R, Hohmann D, Sauer R. Prophylactic radiation therapy for prevention of heterotopic ossification after hip arthroplasty. Results in 141 high-risk hips. *Radiology* 1993;188:257–264.
362. Skinner HB. Porous coatings in total joint arthroplasty: the wave of the future? *Am Coll Surg Bull* 1985;70:14–15.
363. Sledge CB. Total hip replacement: current concepts of fixation and prosthetic design. In: *Harvard Medical School Orthopedic Radiology Course Syllabus.* Boston: Brigham and Women's Hospital Department of Continuing Education; 1986.
364. Smith-Peterson MN. Arthroplasty of the hip. A new method. *J Bone Joint Surg [Am]* 1939;21A:269–288.
365. Snorrason F, Kärrholm J. Primary migration of fully-threaded acetabular prostheses: a Roentgen stereophotogrammetric analysis. *J Bone Joint Surg [Br]* 1990;72B:647–652.
366. Stauffer RN, Chao EYS. The femur. In: Morrey BF, ed. *Joint replacement arthroplasty.* New York: Churchill Livingstone; 1991:573–586.
367. Stauffer RM. Ten-year follow-up study of total hip replacement. With particular reference to roentgenographic loosening of the components. *J Bone Joint Surg [Am]* 1982;64A:983.
368. Steinbach LS, Schneider R, Goldman AB, Ranawat CS, Ghelman BJ. Bursae and abscess cavities communicating with the hip. *Radiology* 1985;156:303–307.
369. Tanzer M, Drucker D, Jasty M, McDonald M, Harris WH. Revision of the acetabular component with an uncemented Harris-Galante porous-coated prosthesis. *J Bone Joint Surg [Am]* 1992;74A:987–994.
370. Tisdel CL, Goldberg VM, Parr JA, Bensusan JS, Starkoff LS, Stevenson S. The influence of hydroxyapatite and tricalcium-phospate coating in bone growth into titanium fiber-metal implants. *J Bone Joint Surg [Am]* 1994;76A:159–171.
371. Turner TM, Sumner DR, Urban RM, Rivéro DP, Galante JO. A comparative study of porous coatings in a weight-bearing total hip-arthroplasty model. *J Bone Joint Surg [Am]* 1986;68A:1396–1408.
372. Turner TM, Urban RM, Summer DR, Galante JO. Revision without cement of aseptically loose, cemented hip arthroplasty. *J Bone Joint Surg [Am]* 1993;75A:845–862.
373. Uri G, Wellman H, Capello W, Robb I, Greenman G. Scintigraphic and x-ray arthrographic diagnosis of femoral prosthesis loosening: concise communication. *J Nucl Med* 1984;25:661–663.
374. Utz JA, Lull RJ, Galvin EG. Asymptomatic total hip prosthesis: natural history determined using Tc-99m MDP bone scans. *Radiology* 1986;161:509–512.
375. Vázquez-Vela E, Váquez-Vela G. Acetabular reaction to the Bateman bipolar prosthesis. *Clin Orthop* 1990;251:87–91.
376. Weissman BN. The radiology of total joint replacement. *Orthop Clin North Am* 1983;14:171–191.
377. Weissman BN. Current topics in the radiology of joint replacement surgery. *Radiol Clin North Am* 1990;28:1111–1134.
378. Weissman BN, Sledge CG. *Orthopedic radiology.* Philadelphia: WB Saunders; 1986.
379. Willert H-G, Buchhorn GH. Biocompatability of endoprosthetic materials. In: Morscher E, ed. *The cementless fixation of hip endoprostheses.* New York: Springer-Verlag; 1984.
380. Willert H-G, Ludwig J, Semlitsch M. Reaction of bone to methacrylate after hip arthroplasty. A long-term gross, light-microscopic, and scanning-electron microscopic study. *J Bone Joint Surg* 1974;56A:1368–1382.
381. Wilson AJ, Monsees B, Blair V III. Acetabular cup dislocation: a new complication of total joint arthroplasty. *AJR Am J Roentgenol* 1988;151:133–134.
382. Wilson-McDonald J, Morscher E. Comparison between straight- and curved-stem Müller femoral prostheses: 5- to 10-year results of 545 total hip replacements. *Arch Orthop Trauma Surg* 1989;109:14–20.
383. Wilson-McDonald J, Morscher E, Masar Z. Cementless uncoated polyethylene acetabular components in total hip replacement: review of five- to 10-year results. *J Bone Joint Surg [Br]* 1990;72B:423–430.
384. Zilbens KW, Casser HR, Ohnsorge J. Treatment of an old infection in a total hip replacement with an interim spacer prostheses. *Acta Orthop Trauma Surg* 1990;109:94–96.

Arthrodesis and Osteotomies of the Hip

385. Cahuzac JPN, Nimus M, Trottman F, Clement JL, Laurain JM, Lebarbcer P. Chiari pelvic osteotomy in Perthes disease. *J Pediatr Orthop* 1990;10:163–166.

386. Callaghan JJ, Brand RA, Pedersen DR. Hip arthrodesis: a long term follow-up. *J Bone Joint Surg* [*Am*] 1985;67A:1328–1335.

387. Canesale PG. Arthrodeses of the ankle, knee and hip. In: Crenshaw AH, ed. *Campbell's operative orthopedics*. 8th ed. St. Louis: Mosby-Year Book; 1992:317–370.

388. Dutkowsky JP. Miscellaneous non-traumatic disorders. In: Crenshaw AH, ed. *Campbell's operative orthopedics*. 8th ed. St. Louis: Mosby-Year Book; 1992:2005–2057.

389. Fish JB. Cuniform osteotomy of the femoral neck in treatment of slipped crystal femoral epiphysis. *J Bone Joint Surg* [*Am*] 1994;76A:46–58.

390. Ford LT. Osteotomies: nomenclature and uses. *Radiol Clin North Am* 1973;13:79–92.

391. Grant AD, Lehman WB, Strongwater AM, Atar D. Cannulated blade plate for proximal femoral varus osteotomy. *Clin Orthop* 1990;259:111–113.

392. Matsuno T, Ichioka Y, Kaneda K. Modified Chiari pelvic osteotomy: a long term follow-up study. *J Bone Joint Surg* [*Am*] 1992;74A:470–478.

393. Price CT, Lovell WW. Thompson arthrodeses of the hip in children. *J Bone Joint Surg* [*Am*] 1980;62A:1118–1123.

394. Ranawat CS, Atkinson RE, Salvati EA, Wilson PD Jr. Conventional hip arthroplasty for degenerative joint disease in patients of 45 to 60 years. *J Bone Joint Surg* [*Am*] 1984;66A:745–751.

395. Watson-Jones R, Robinson WC. Arthrodeses of the osteoarthritic hip joint. *J Bone Joint Surg* [*Br*] 1956;38B:353–377.

396. Wong-Chung J, Ryan M, O'Brien TM. Movement of the femoral head after Salter osteotomy for acetabular dysplasia. *J Bone Joint Surg* [*Br*] 1990;72B:563–567.

Imaging Atlas of Orthopedic Appliances and Prostheses,
edited by T.H. Berquist.
Mayo Clinic Foundation © 1995.
Published by Raven Press, Ltd., New York.

CHAPTER 5

The Femoral Shaft

Thomas H. Berquist and Mark P. Brodersen

The femur is the longest, largest, and strongest bone in the body. Because of its length, width, and weight-bearing role, it must tolerate extremes of axial loading and angular and rotational stresses. The femur is surrounded by large muscle groups, and a large blood supply is provided for fracture healing. Therefore, the main problem with the treatment of femoral fractures is not healing, as much as maintaining length and alignment.[3,11,55]

Fractures and fixation techniques for the upper femur (femoral head-subtrochanteric region) were discussed in Chapter 4. This section concentrates on fixation devices for the femoral shaft. Intercondylar fractures are discussed in Chapter 6. Limb salvage procedures for neoplasms are included in Chapter 14.

TRAUMA

Femoral shaft fractures are usually associated with high-velocity injuries, such as automobile accidents, and they are frequently associated with significant soft tissue injury.[4,11,15,19,36,37] Most fractures occur in children and young adults. In patients with hip or knee arthroplasties, fractures tend to occur at the end of the component.[4,21,44,46]

Classifications of Femoral Shaft Injuries

Femoral shaft fractures may be open or closed. Open injuries may result from external trauma or internal extrusion of fracture fragments.[4,15,65]

T. H. Berquist: Mayo Medical School and Department of Diagnostic Radiology, Mayo Clinic Jacksonville, Jacksonville, Florida 32224.

M. P. Brodersen: Mayo Medical School and Department of Orthopedic Surgery, Mayo Clinic Jacksonville, Jacksonville, Florida 32224.

Soft tissue injuries are difficult to classify radiographically.[5] However, understanding the soft tissue injury classification is useful as it applies to the selection of fixation devices for management.[4,37,38]

Gustilo and Anderson[37] and Gustilo et al.[38] classified open fractures.[12] Grade I and II open fractures have less tissue destruction and wound contamination; therefore, internal nailing can still be accomplished without a risk of postoperative infection as long as the wounds are properly débrided. Grade IIIA and B open fractures have extensive soft tissue injury with periosteal and bone exposure. This results in a higher incidence of infection, regardless of the type of fixation selected.[4,12,37,38,65]

Several fracture classifications have also been defined, which aid in the selection of appropriate management. Winquist and Hansen[79] and Winquist et al.[80] devised a commonly used femoral shaft fracture classification. Their classification is based on circumferential cortical contact. Type I (Fig. 5-1) fractures have a small comminuted fragment with greater than 50% cortical contact of the main fragments. Type II (Fig. 5-2) fractures have a larger fragment but maintain 50% cortical contact. With Type III fractures (Fig. 5-3), there is less than 50% cortical contact. Type IV fractures (Fig. 5-4) are severely comminuted with no cortical contact.

Fractures may also be characterized by their location and segment involvement (Figs. 5-5 through 5-13).[72,73] Most fractures occur in the middle third of the shaft. Shortening and overriding of fragments commonly occurs. The proximal fragment may be rotated outward as a result of the force exerted by the external rotators. In fractures of the upper third of the femur, the proximal fragment may be flexed by the iliopsoas, abducted by the gluteal muscles, and rotated by the external rotators (Fig. 5-14). Distal fragments may angulate posteriorly because of forces exerted by the gastrocnemius, popliteus, and plantaris, with fractures of the distal femoral shaft.[4,15,79,80]

(*text continues on page 357*)

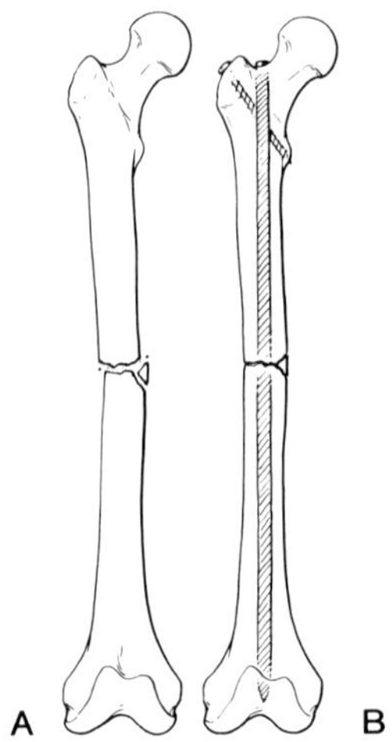

FIG. 5-1. Type I fracture (small comminuted fragment with greater than 50% cortical contact of main fragments) preoperatively **(A)** and after intramedullary nail fixation **(B)**. (From Winquist RA, Hansen ST. Closed medullary nailing of femoral fractures. *J Bone Joint Surg [Am]* 1984; 66A:529–539.)

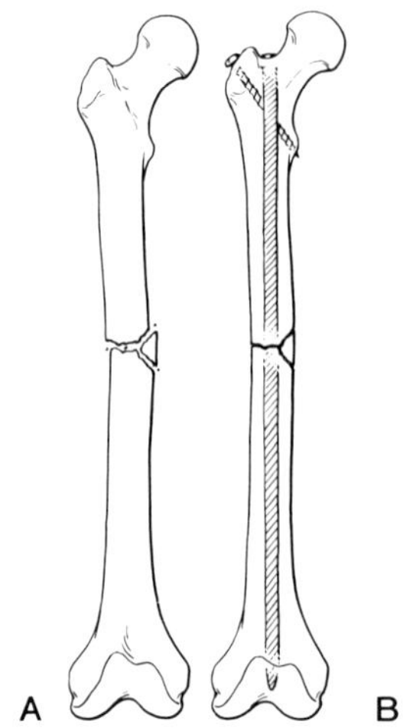

FIG. 5-2. Type II fracture (larger comminuted fragment with greater than 50% cortical contact of main fragments) preoperatively **(A)** and after intramedullary nailing **(B)**. (From Winquist RA, Hansen ST. Closed medullary nailing of femoral fractures. *J Bone Joint Surg [Am]* 1984;66A:529–539.)

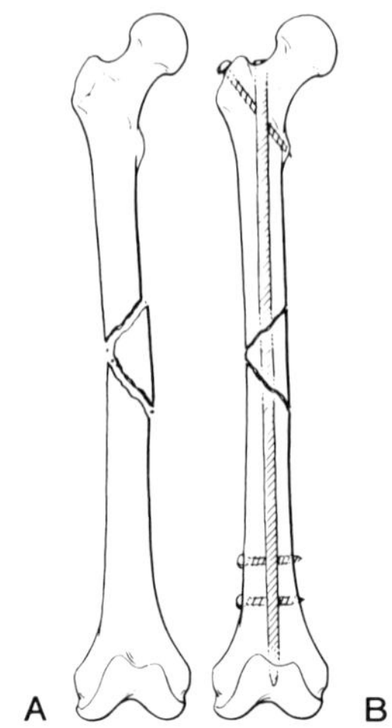

FIG. 5-3. Type III fracture (less than 50% cortical contact) preoperatively **(A)** and after intramedullary nailing **(B)**. (From Winquist RA, Hansen ST. Closed medullary nailing of femoral fractures. *J Bone Joint Surg [Am]* 1984;66A:529–539.)

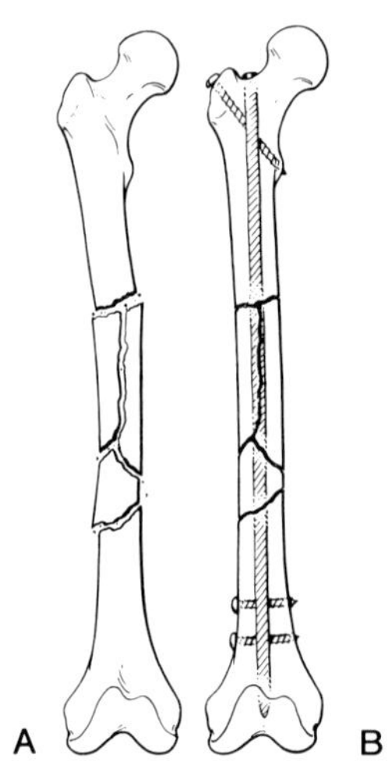

FIG. 5-4. Type IV fracture (severely comminuted with no cortical contact) preoperatively **(A)** and after intramedullary nailing **(B)**. (From Winquist RA, Hansen ST. Closed medullary nailing of femoral fractures. *J Bone Joint Surg [Am]* 1984;66A:529–539.)

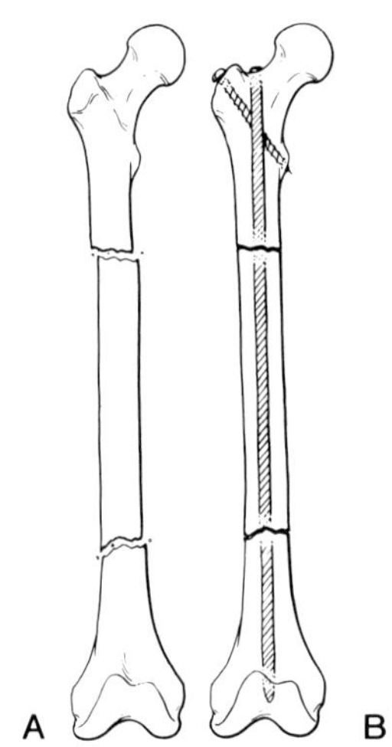

FIG. 5-5. Comminuted segmental transverse fractures preoperatively **(A)** and postoperatively **(B)**. (From Winquist RA, Hansen ST. Closed medullary nailing of femoral fractures. *J Bone Joint Surg [Am]* 1984;66A:529–539.)

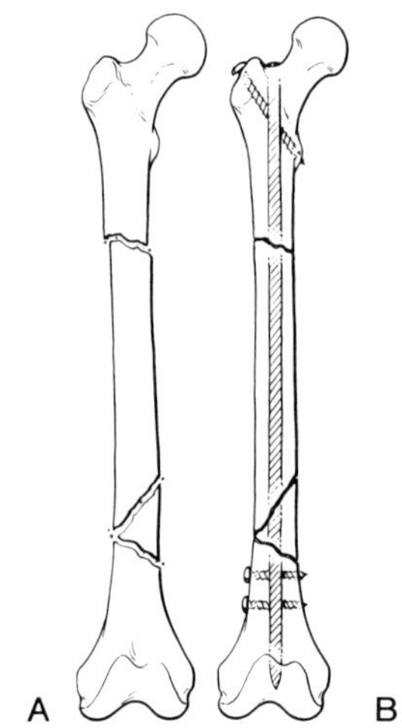

FIG. 5-6. Segmental oblique and comminuted fractures preoperatively **(A)** and after intramedullary nailing **(B)**. (From Winquist RA, Hansen ST. Closed medullary nailing of femoral fractures. *J Bone Joint Surg [Am]* 1984;66A:529–539.)

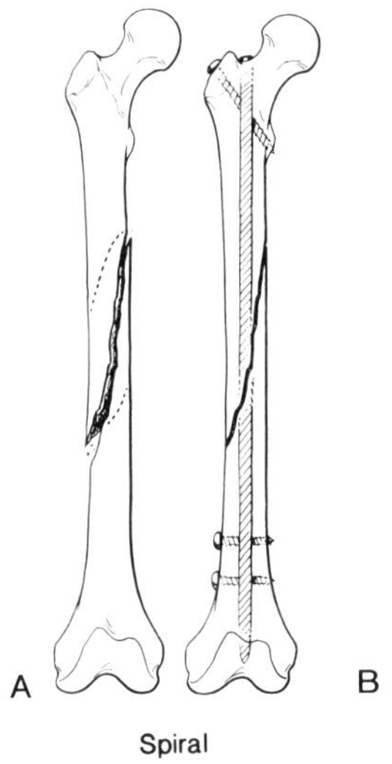

FIG. 5-7. Midshaft spiral fracture preoperatively **(A)** and after intramedullary nailing **(B)**. (From Winquist RA, Hansen ST. Closed medullary nailing of femoral fractures. *J Bone Joint Surg [Am]* 1984; 66A:529–539.)

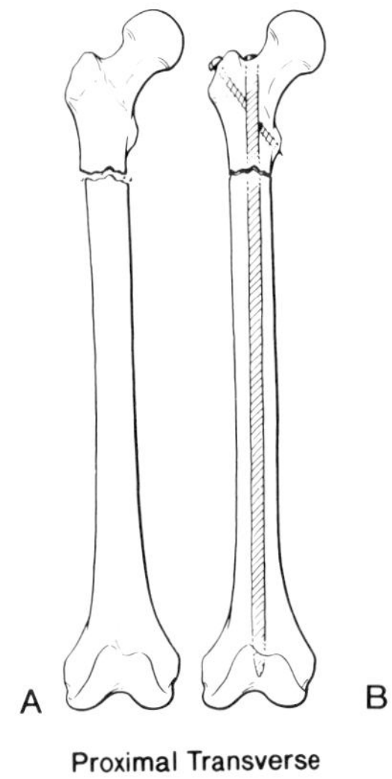

FIG. 5-8. Proximal transverse fracture preoperatively **(A)** and postoperatively **(B)**. (From Winquist RA, Hansen ST. Closed medullary nailing of femoral fractures. *J Bone Joint Surg [Am]* 1984; 66A:529–539.)

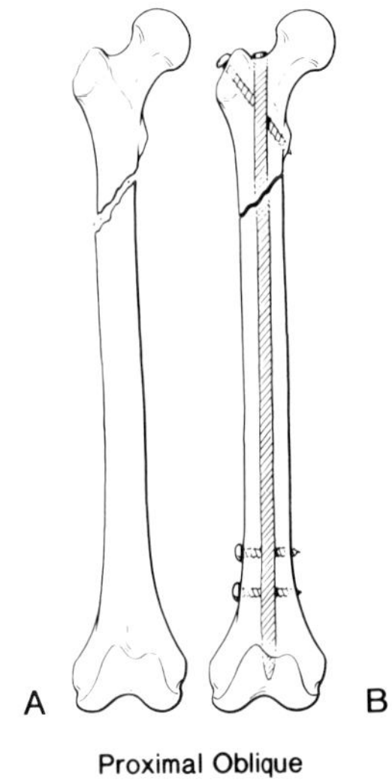

FIG. 5-9. Proximal oblique fracture preoperatively **(A)** and after intramedullary nailing **(B)**. (From Winquist RA, Hansen ST. Closed medullary nailing of femoral fractures. *J Bone Joint Surg [Am]* 1984;66A:529–539.)

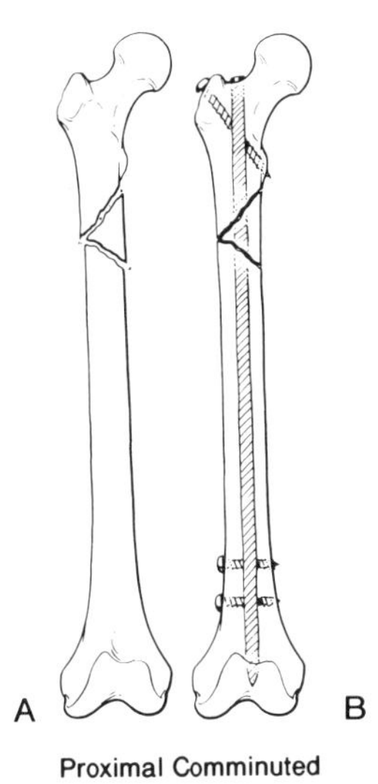

FIG. 5-10. Proximal comminuted fracture preoperatively **(A)** and postoperatively **(B)**. (From Winquist RA, Hansen ST. Closed medullary nailing of femoral fractures. *J Bone Joint Surg [Am]* 1984; 66A:529–539.)

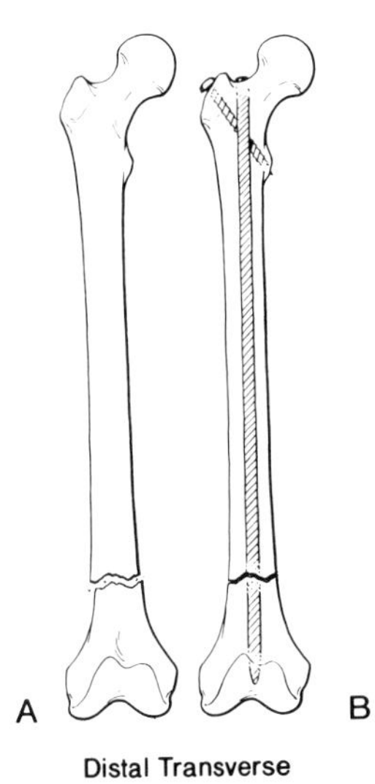

FIG. 5-11. Distal transverse fracture preoperatively **(A)** and postoperatively **(B)**. (From Winquist RA, Hansen ST. Closed medullary nailing of femoral fractures. *J Bone Joint Surg [Am]* 1984; 66A:529–539.)

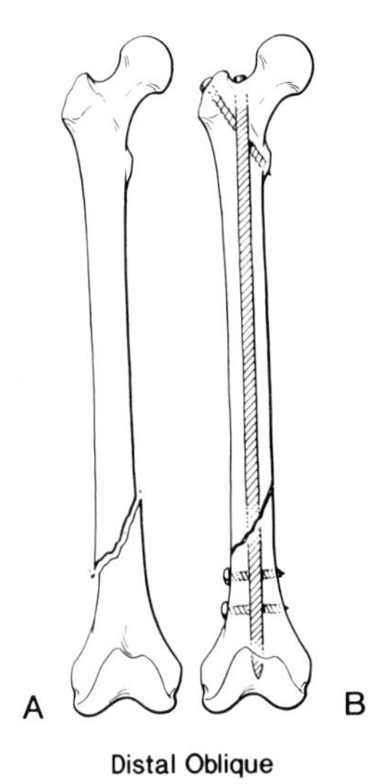

FIG. 5-12. Oblique distal fracture preoperatively **(A)** and postoperatively **(B)**. (From Winquist RA, Hansen ST. Closed medullary nailing of femoral fractures. *J Bone Joint Surg [Am]* 1984;66A:529–539.)

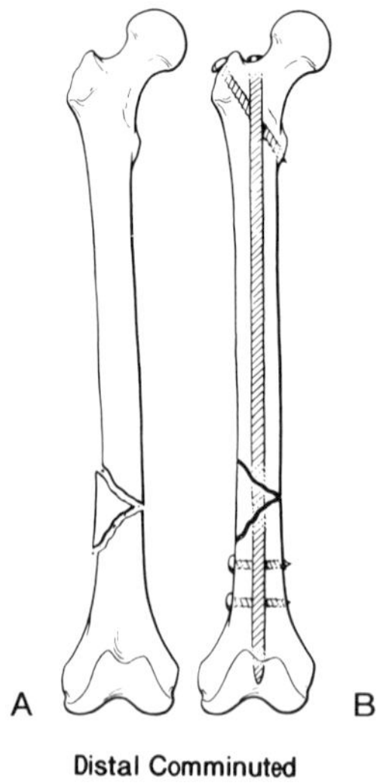

FIG. 5-13. Distal comminuted fracture preoperatively **(A)** and after interlocking medullary nail fixation **(B)**. (From Winquist RA, Hansen ST. Closed medullary nailing of femoral fractures. *J Bone Joint Surg [Am]* 1984;66A:529–539.)

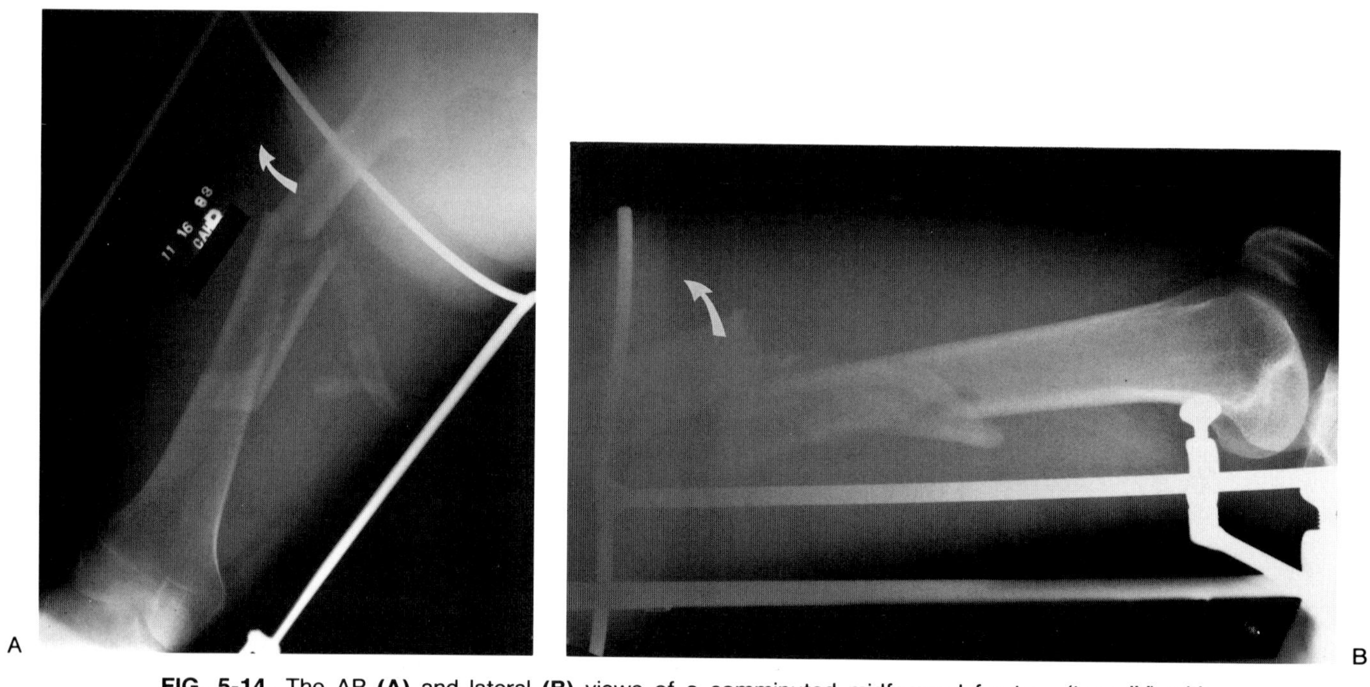

FIG. 5-14. The AP **(A)** and lateral **(B)** views of a comminuted midfemoral fracture (type IV) with the proximal fragment flexed (*arrow,* B) and abducted (*arrow,* A) by the glutei, external rotators, and iliopsoas.

Preoperative Imaging

Standard routine views of the femur include anteroposterior (AP) and lateral projections. The hip and knee should be included on these views or with additional films if necessary. This is required to determine the type of fixation necessary, to evaluate optimal traction pin placement, and most importantly, to exclude ipsilateral femoral neck and knee injuries.[4,15,24,65] The tibia, fibula, foot, and ankle should be carefully examined to exclude multiple injuries. When indicated, AP and lateral views of these structures should also be obtained.[4,5]

Additional techniques, such as computed tomography (CT), conventional tomography, or magnetic resonance imaging (MRI) are usually not required. These techniques are reserved for subtle injuries or the evaluation of complex fractures or the extent of soft tissue injury.[5,6] Angiography may be required in cases in which vascular injury is suspected.[4,5,15,64]

Treatment Options

The basic principles in the treatment of femoral shaft fractures are the restoration of position and alignment, maintenance of length, immobilization until union occurs, and restoration of normal function. Apposition of bone fragments is required for union, and acceptable alignment is necessary to minimize deformity. Shortening of 1 to 1.5 cm is acceptable without hip or knee disability.[4,8–18]

Definitive treatment should begin as soon as possible to optimize the chances for union. Fracture management has evolved from traction, hip spica body casts, and bracing to the widespread use of internal fixation devices.[11,15,65,66] Important considerations before instituting therapy include the severity or comminution of the fracture, soft tissue damage (vascular and nerve included), the patient's age and medical and physical condition, and associated injuries (femoral neck and tibial fracture).[6,15,40,48,73] Various treatment methods, specifically involving hardware or fixation devices, are reviewed.

Traction

Skeletal traction is useful for the early treatment of a fracture of the femoral shaft when an operation must be delayed by the severity of the injury and/or additional injuries preclude early management by other methods.[15–18,38] Traction is the treatment of choice for highly comminuted fractures in which fixation or immobilization cannot be achieved.[5] The goal of early traction is to restore length in the first 24 hours. After this period, a hematoma around the fracture begins to organize, which may require more traction to maintain femoral length.[15,18,55]

Both skin and skeletal traction techniques can be used. The former is mainly used for acute emergencies. Skeletal traction is usually achieved by placing a Steinmann pin (threaded or smooth) or Kirschner wire (K wire; Fig. 5-15A,B) through the upper tibia (Fig. 5-16C,D) or distal femur (Fig. 5-16). Steinmann pins are larger, especially if threaded, and cause more soft tissue injury than do the smaller K wires. The threaded Steinmann pins reduce the motion of the pin in bone.[15] The K wires tend to cut through bone and loosen with time.[42]

Traction through the tibia is contraindicated with associated ligament injuries of the knee. Distal femoral pins (Fig. 5-16) allow more direct force to be applied. However, soft tissue scarring may cause stiffness in the vastus medialis and lateralis.[15,42] In addition, a femoral pin is usually not used if internal fixation of the femur is planned in the near future because of the chance of infection.

There are several types of traction used (Fig. 5-17).

Böhler-Braun frame: combined femoral and calcaneal pins.[42]

Thomas splint: half ring for traction pin with thigh sling to prevent soft tissue sag and leg support with Pearson attachment (Fig. 5-15A,B and 5-17C–E). This is one of the most common devices.[42]

Newfeld roller traction: Steinmann pin in plaster to permit early knee motion with traction applied to plaster.[15,42,48,74]

90-90 traction: both hip and knee flexed 90° with vertical traction on femur. Used for subtrochanteric or proximal femoral fractures to reduce flexion of proximal fragment.[15]

Perkin's traction:[18] a traction pin is placed in the upper tibia with traction applied by two pulleys at the end of the bed (~approximately 20 pounds for an adult). The bed is "split" to allow knee flexion. This reduces the knee stiffness often associated with other traction techniques. Length and weight adjustments are made using a measure so that radiographs are not taken as frequently.

Advantages[15,17,42,74]
- Early treatment of complex injuries
- Alternative when surgery not possible

Disadvantages[15,17,38]
- Requires frequent radiographs in the first 24 hours to check position
- Increased incidence of nonunion, delayed union (~approximately 30%), shortening, and malunion
- Loss of knee motion
- Pin tract infections
- Prolonged immobilization and bed rest (cost and medical complications)

(text continues on page 360)

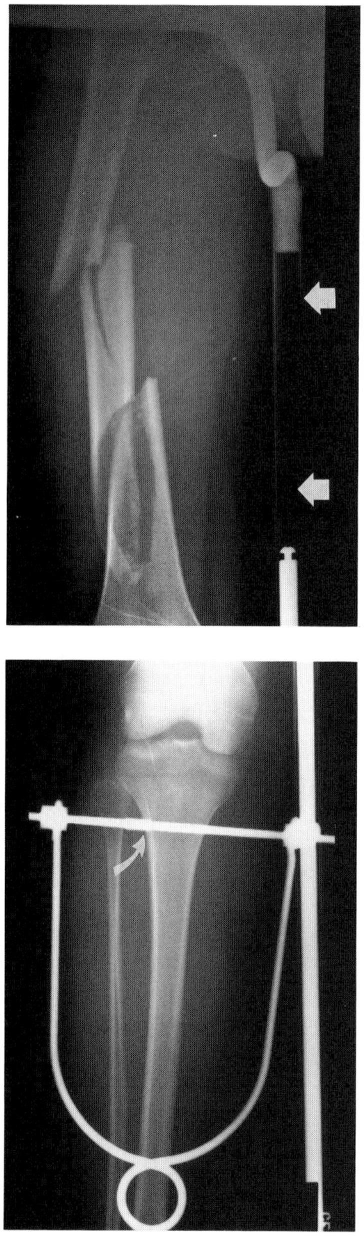

A

C

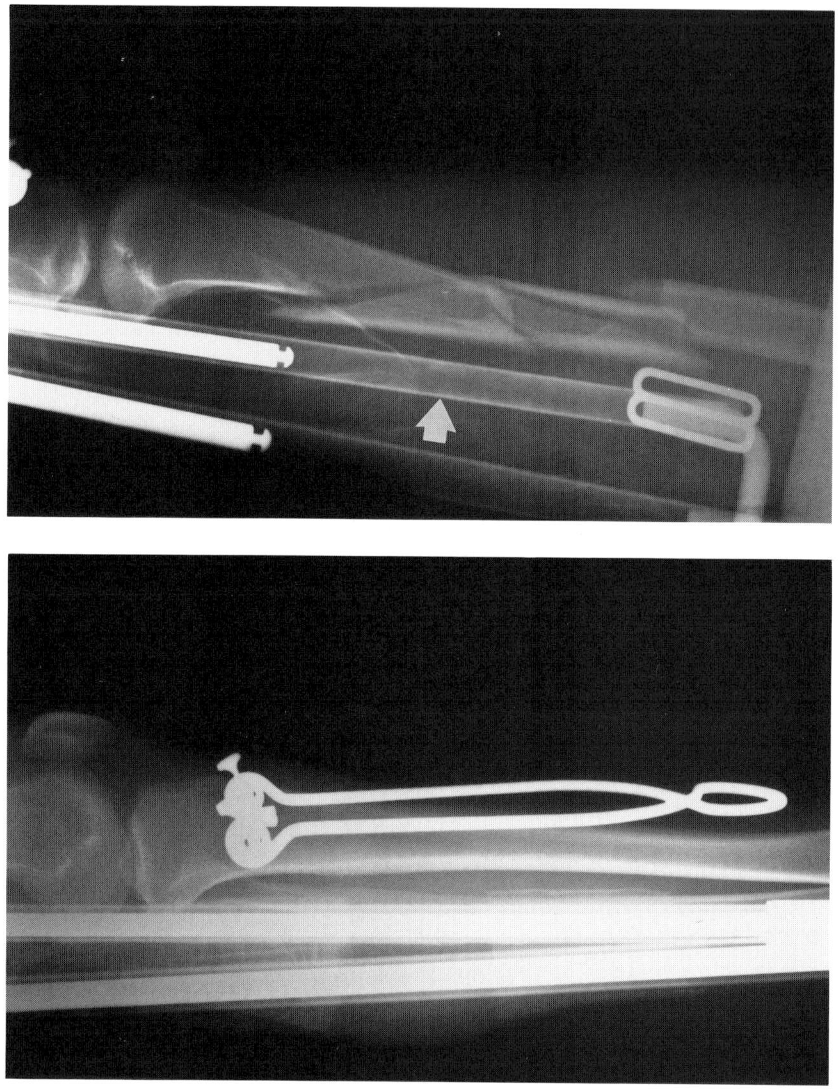

B

D

FIG. 5-15. Comminuted fracture of the left midfemur (Winquist-Hansen type IV) seen on AP **(A)** and lateral **(B)** views. Note the thigh-support portion of the traction device (*arrows*) is radiolucent through most of its length. The AP **(C)** and lateral **(D)** views of the tibia and knee showing the position of the Steinmann pin in the tibia. Note the threads just enter the lateral tibial cortex (*arrow*). The pin is parallel to the articular surface to allow balanced traction. The Steinmann pin is held in a Böhler holder.

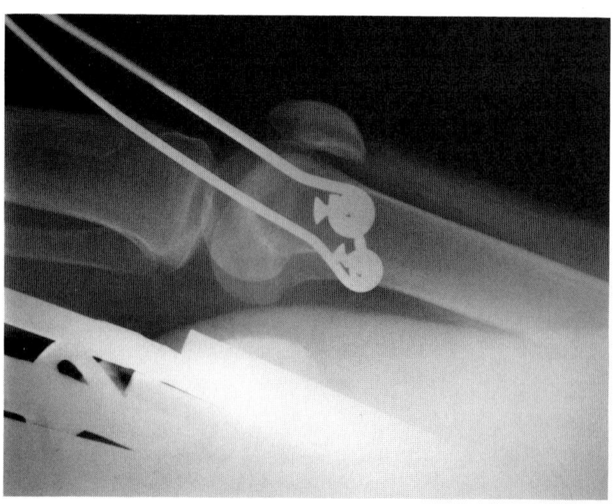

FIG. 5-16. Lateral view of the knee demonstrating traction pin the distal femur.

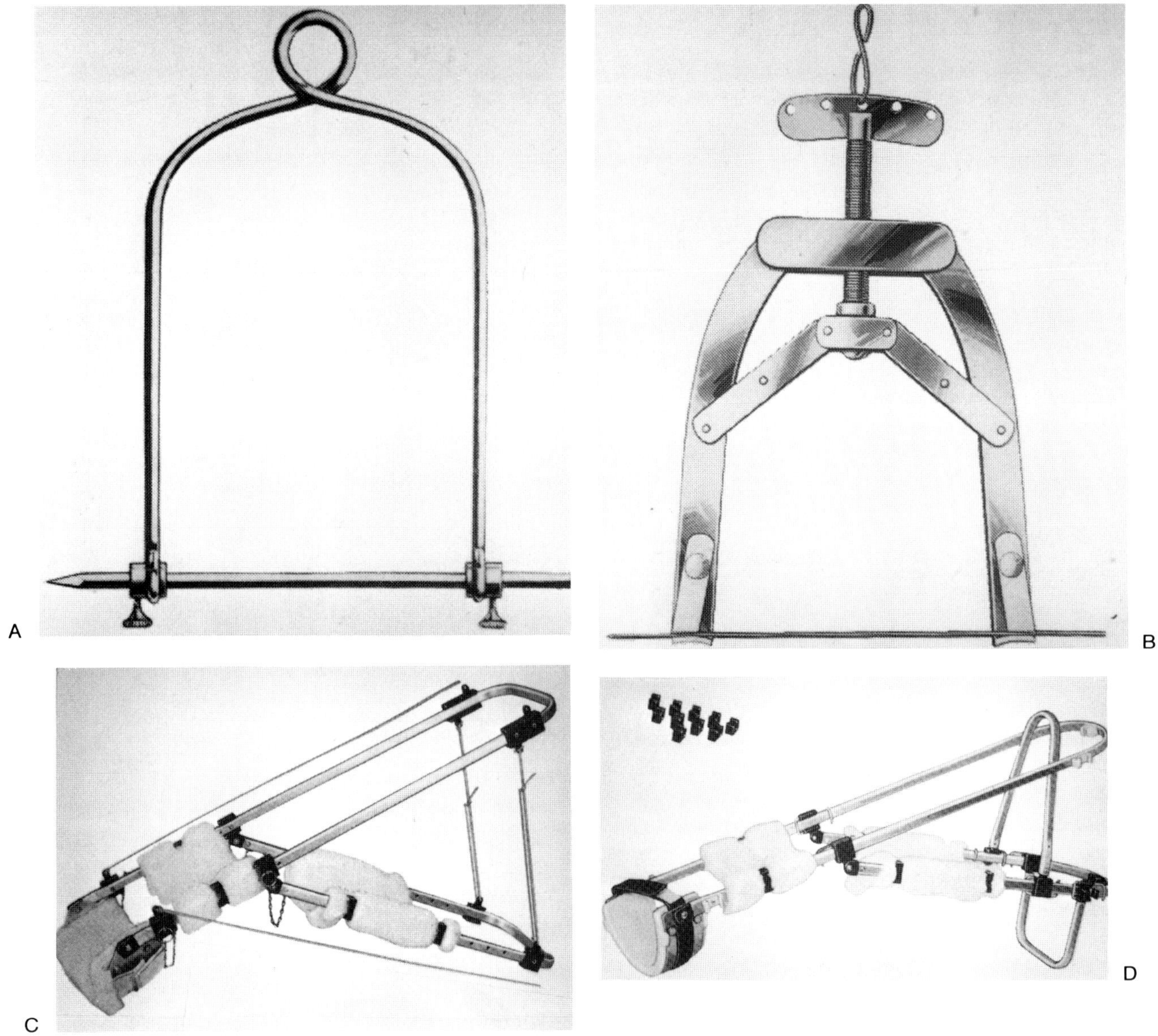

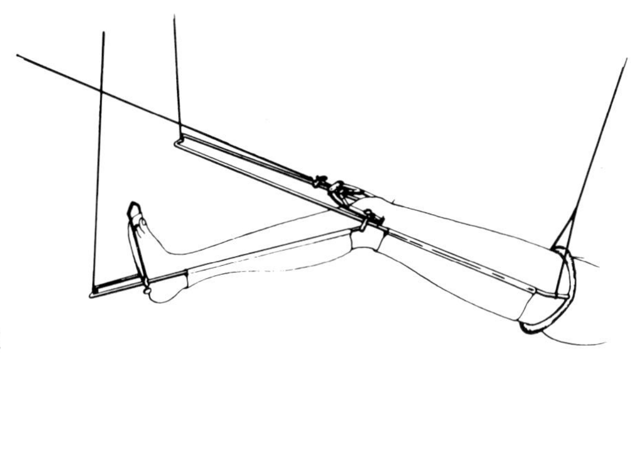

FIG. 5-17. Traction devices. **A:** Böhler-Steinmann pin holder with an unthreaded Steinmann pin (see Fig. 5-15). **B:** K-wire tractor. **C:** Brady suspension system for femoral-shaft and lower-extremity fractures. This radiolucent system is the same as the Thomas system. **D:** Radiolucent Thomas splint. **E:** Illustration of Thomas splint with Pearson attachment. Converts Thomas splint to balanced suspension and allows passive knee motion.

Cast-Brace Fixation

Preliminary skeletal traction is often used prior to cast-brace treatment.[5,15,16] The indications for cast-brace treatment include open fractures, distal third fractures, and comminuted fractures. This technique is not appropriate for simple transverse oblique fractures or proximal third fractures (Fig. 5-18). The cast-brace technique provides a contact capsule about the thigh, allowing muscles to provide a dynamic stabilizing effect on the fracture.[15,31,41]

Advantages[4,5,15,41]
- Allows early ambulation
- Improved muscle function
- Avoid surgical complications
- Reduced knee stiffness compared with that in internal fixation

Disadvantage
- Shortening more common than that with internal fixation

External Fixation

External fixation is not commonly used today. However, frame fixators (Fig. 5-19) do allow fracture fixation and wound access.[4,15,34,63] Steinmann pins and plaster (Fig. 5-20) can be used in a similar fashion.[31] The indications for external fixation include open fractures, highly comminuted fractures, bone lengthening, and treatment of nonunion.[10,15,42] External fixators (see Chapter 2) are categorized by their design as simple, clamp, and ring fixators.[5,42,74]

Simple Fixators

Simple fixators provide more latitude for pin placement but allow little adjustment after application,[42] for example, the Roger-Anderson apparatus (Fig. 5-21A).

Clamp Fixators

Clamp fixators allow further or final reduction after application. Pin spread and angle are directed by the clamp,[42] for example, the Hoffmann fixator (Fig. 5-21B).

Ring Fixators

These devices allow a more precise correction of angulation and rotation but limit wound access,[42] for example, the Ace-Fischer and Ilizarov systems (Fig. 5-21C–F).

Multiple variations of external fixation devices are available (Figs. 5-22 to 5-26), which are suited to specific injuries and clinical settings. Radiographically, AP and lateral views are important to ensure the proper position. Repeat studies should be obtained following frame adjustments and during the healing process (Figs. 5-25 to 5-27).

The disadvantages of external fixation include pin tract infections (at a rate up to 50%) and quadriceps tethering, and scarring by pins can lead to decreased knee motion.[11,55]

Internal Fixation

Internal fixation is a common means of treating femoral shaft fractures. The techniques include intramedullary nailing, double-plate fixation, and occasionally, supplementation with wires, cables, or bone grafting.[5,15,26,42,74] The geometry of the fracture is important in selecting the optimal fixation technique.

Plate Fixation

Plate fixation is useful in certain situations but has largely been replaced by medullary nail fixation.[15,65,66] Advocates include the location and unusual comminution as indications.[15,65] Generally, two plates at 90° angles are used.[66] This provides additional rigid fixation, especially for rotational stability. Plating permits anatomic reduction (Figs. 5-28 and 5-29). However, a large operative site is required, and bone exposure reduces the vascular supply. Bone fragments may become devitalized, increasing the incidence of infection and delaying healing. The plate also functions as a load-bearing device and is thus susceptible to fatigue fracture (Fig. 5-30).[15,42]

Advantages[15,65]
- Early ambulation
- Improved anatomic reduction compared with closed techniques
- Applicable to certain proximal and distal fractures

Disadvantages[11,47]
- Lost fixation secondary to nonunion ~(9%)
- Infections more common (up to 6%)
- Instrument failure

Intramedullary Fixation

Intramedullary nailing was introduced by Küntscher in 1940 but did not gain popularity in North America until the 1970s. Intramedullary nails may be introduced using closed or open techniques. Standard, flexible, and interlocking rods are available.[43,60,61,74] Intramedullary nails are not used in young children because of possible growth plate injury.[15,74]

Closed intramedullary nailing can be performed without operative exposure of the fracture site. This reduces

(text continues on page 369)

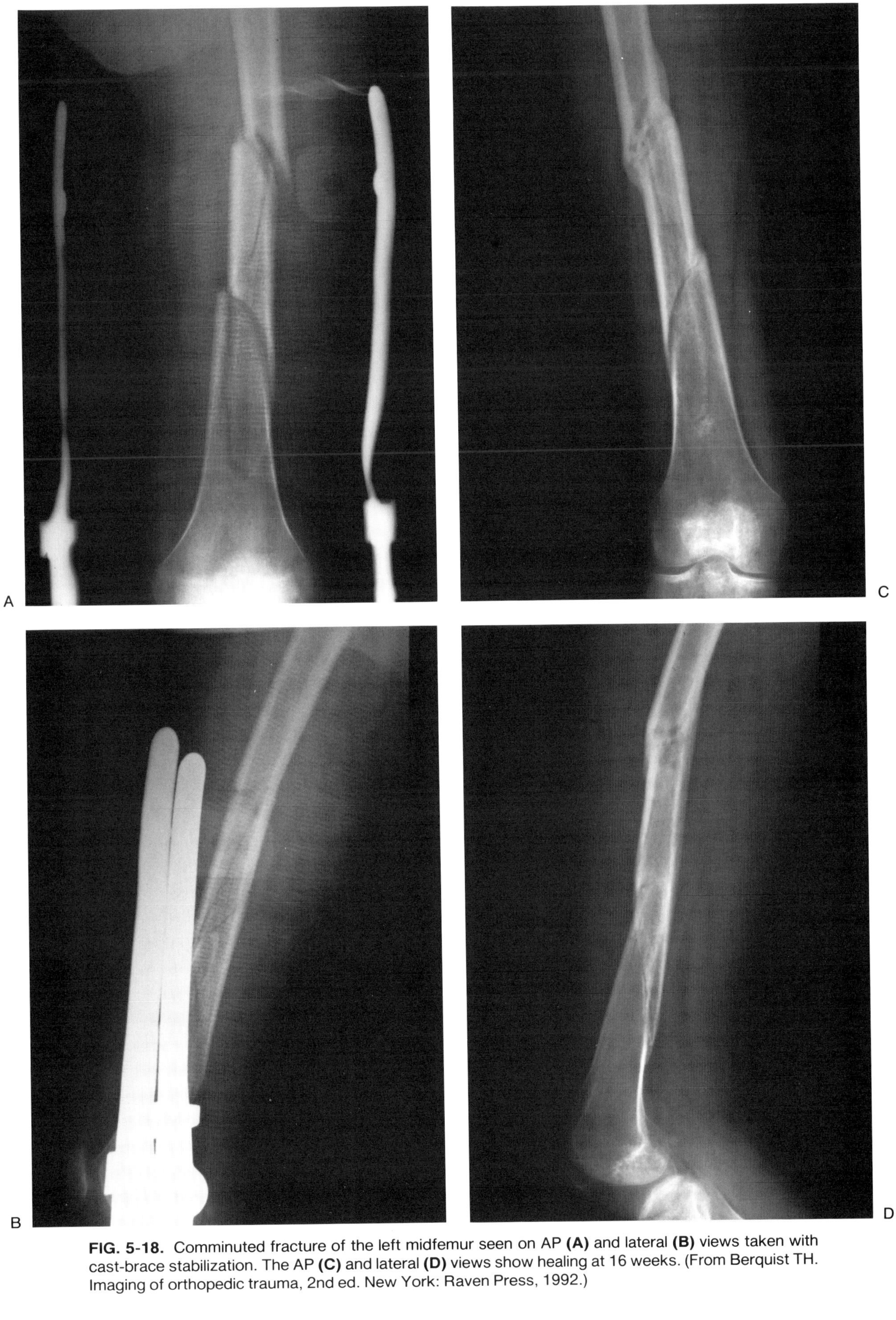

FIG. 5-18. Comminuted fracture of the left midfemur seen on AP **(A)** and lateral **(B)** views taken with cast-brace stabilization. The AP **(C)** and lateral **(D)** views show healing at 16 weeks. (From Berquist TH. Imaging of orthopedic trauma, 2nd ed. New York: Raven Press, 1992.)

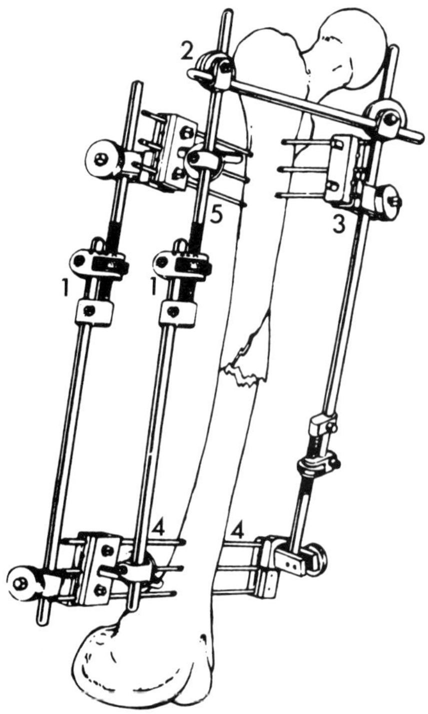

FIG. 5-19. External fixation of a midfemoral fracture (Winquist-Hansen type II). There are adjustable rods (*1*), couplings (*2*), pin clamps (*3*), transfixation pins (*4*), and half pins (*5*). (Courtesy of Zimmer, Warsaw, IN.)

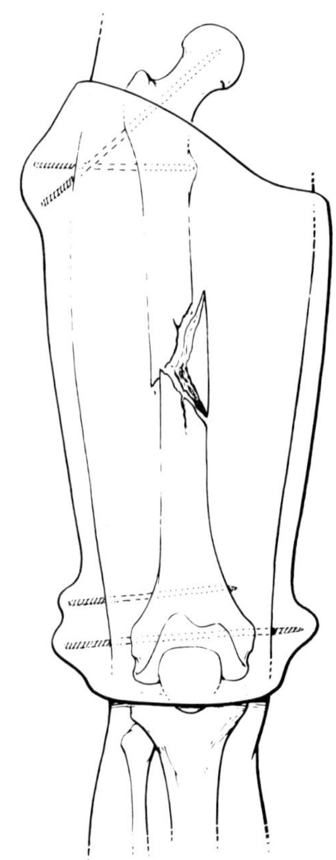

FIG. 5-20. Pin-plaster fixation of a comminuted midfemoral fracture.

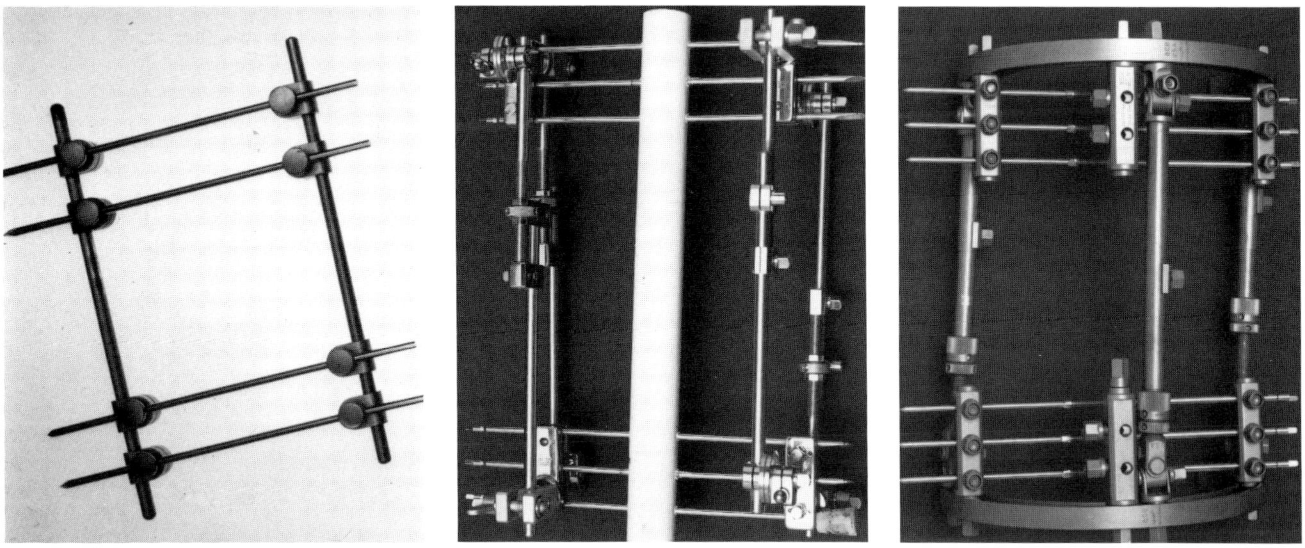

A,B C

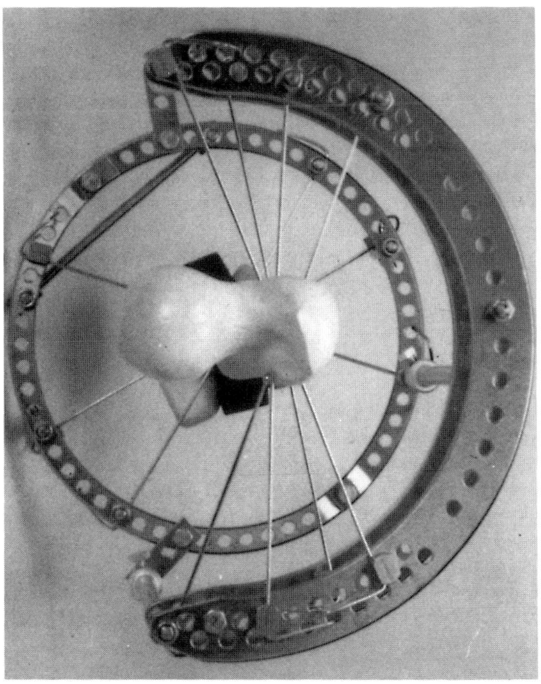

D

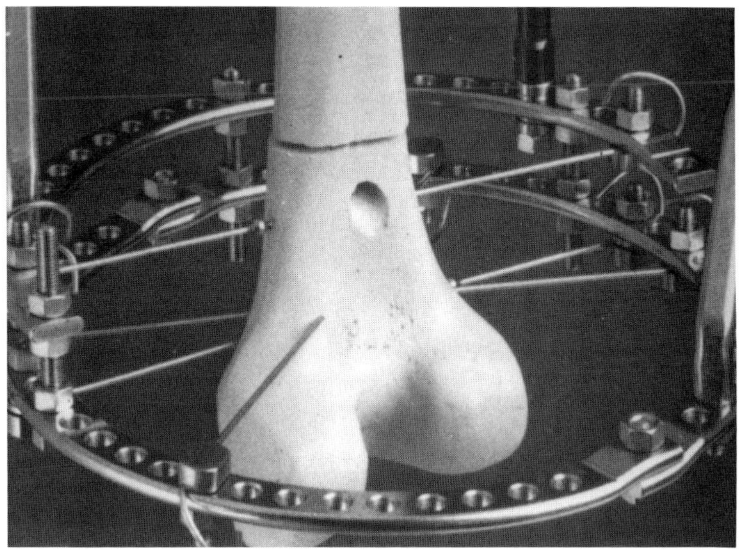

E

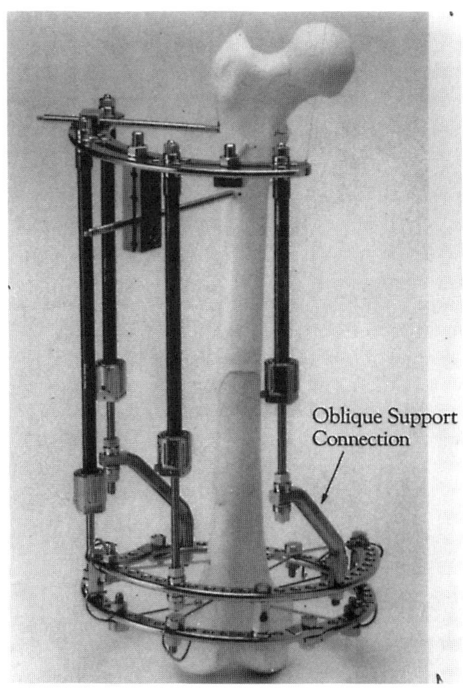

F

FIG. 5-21. External fixators used for femoral fractures. **A:** Roger-Anderson apparatus. **B:** Hoffmann fixator with bilateral adjustable rods and transfixation pins. **C:** Ace-Fischer apparatus rings connected by rods with universal joints. Ilizarov apparatus seen from above **(D)**, distally **(E)**, and with the entire femur **(F)** demonstrating the telescopic rods and oblique support connection. (D–F: Courtesy of Smith and Nephew Richards, Memphis, TN.)

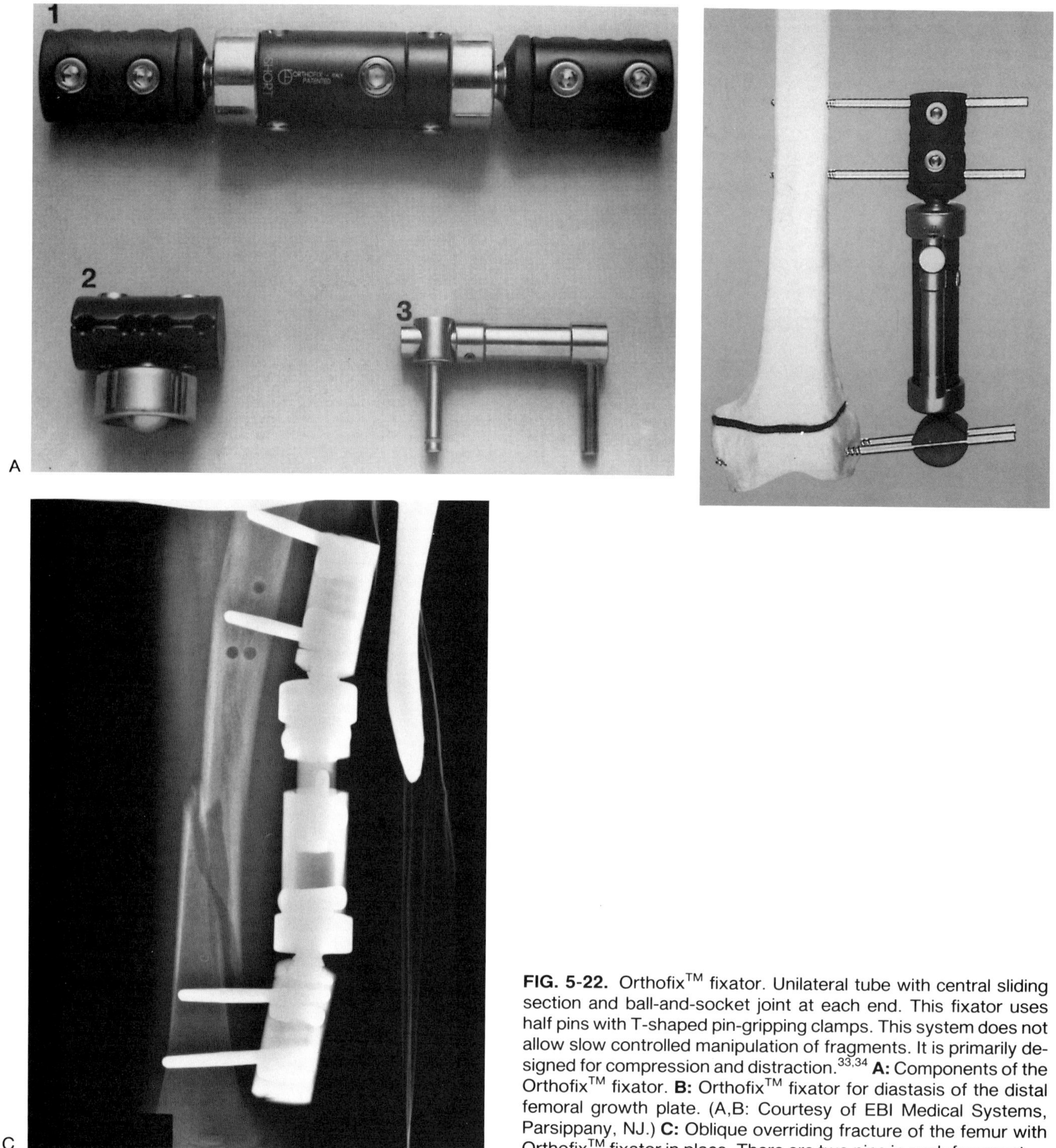

FIG. 5-22. Orthofix™ fixator. Unilateral tube with central sliding section and ball-and-socket joint at each end. This fixator uses half pins with T-shaped pin-gripping clamps. This system does not allow slow controlled manipulation of fragments. It is primarily designed for compression and distraction.[33,34] **A:** Components of the Orthofix™ fixator. **B:** Orthofix™ fixator for diastasis of the distal femoral growth plate. (A,B: Courtesy of EBI Medical Systems, Parsippany, NJ.) **C:** Oblique overriding fracture of the femur with Orthofix™ fixator in place. There are two pins in each fragment.

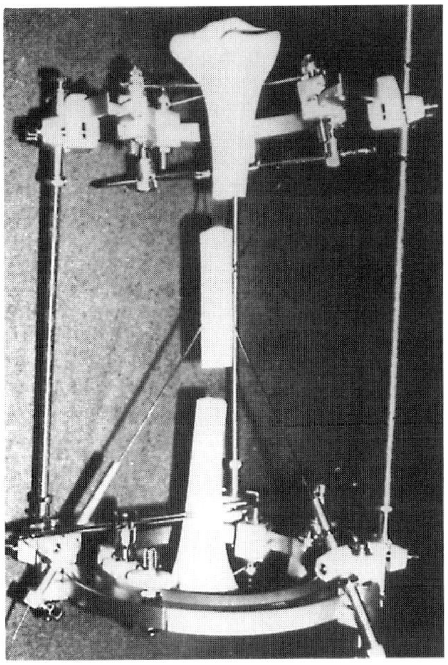

FIG. 5-23. Spinelli-Monticelli fixator set up for bone transport with oblique directional wires. This system is a modification of the Ilizarov and primarily used for leg lengthening. (From Green SA. The Ilizarov method: Raudio technique. *Orthop Clin North Am* 1991;22:677–688.)

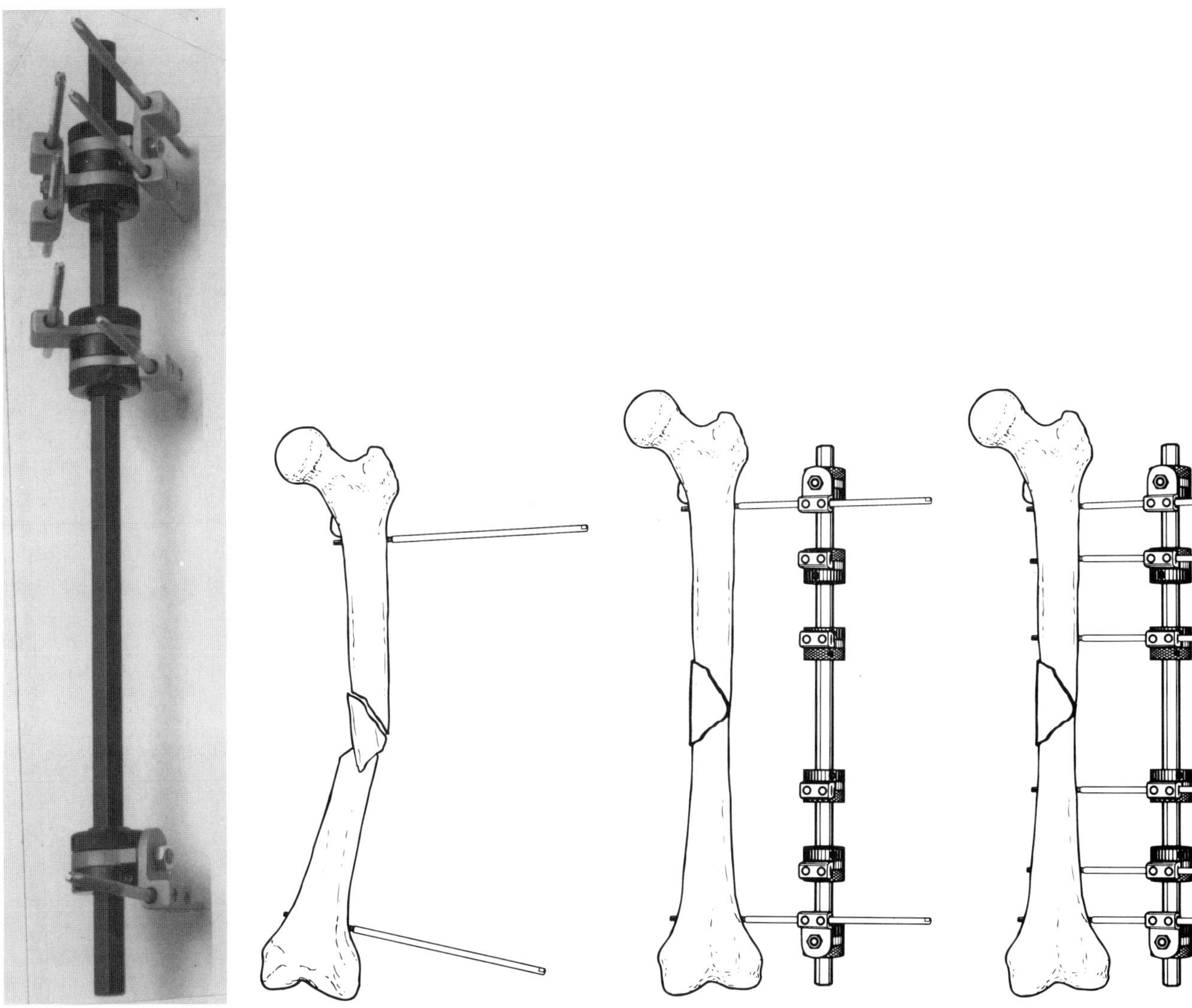

A,B C,D

FIG. 5-24. Hex-Fix™ fixator. Single hexagonal bar designed to stabilize segmentally comminuted fractures with half pins from multiple angles. Spools are used to secure the pin clamps in the proper plain. **A:** Hex-Fix™ fixator. **B:** Midshaft femoral fracture with two half pins in place. **C:** Manipulation of spools and pin clamp allows alignment of the fragments. **D:** Additional pins added so that three half pins are in position in both fragments. (Courtesy of Smith and Nephew Richards, Memphis, TN.)

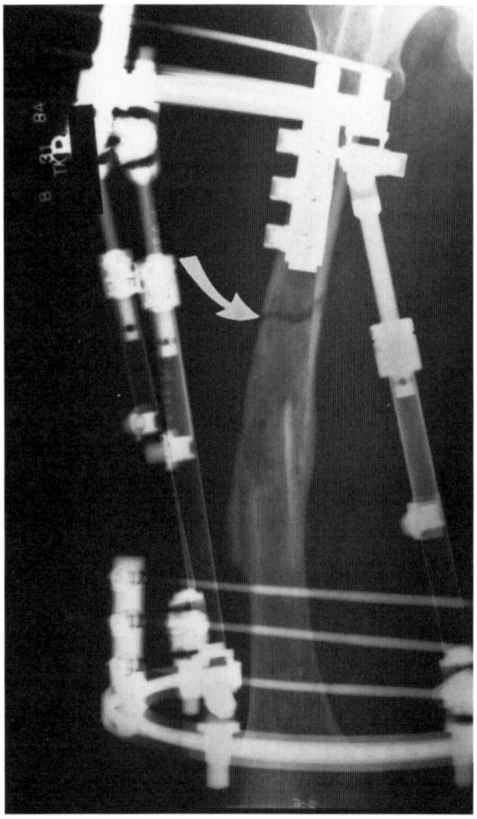

FIG. 5-25. An AP view of the femur with an old fracture deformity and refracture (*arrow*) treated with an Ace-Fischer external fixator.

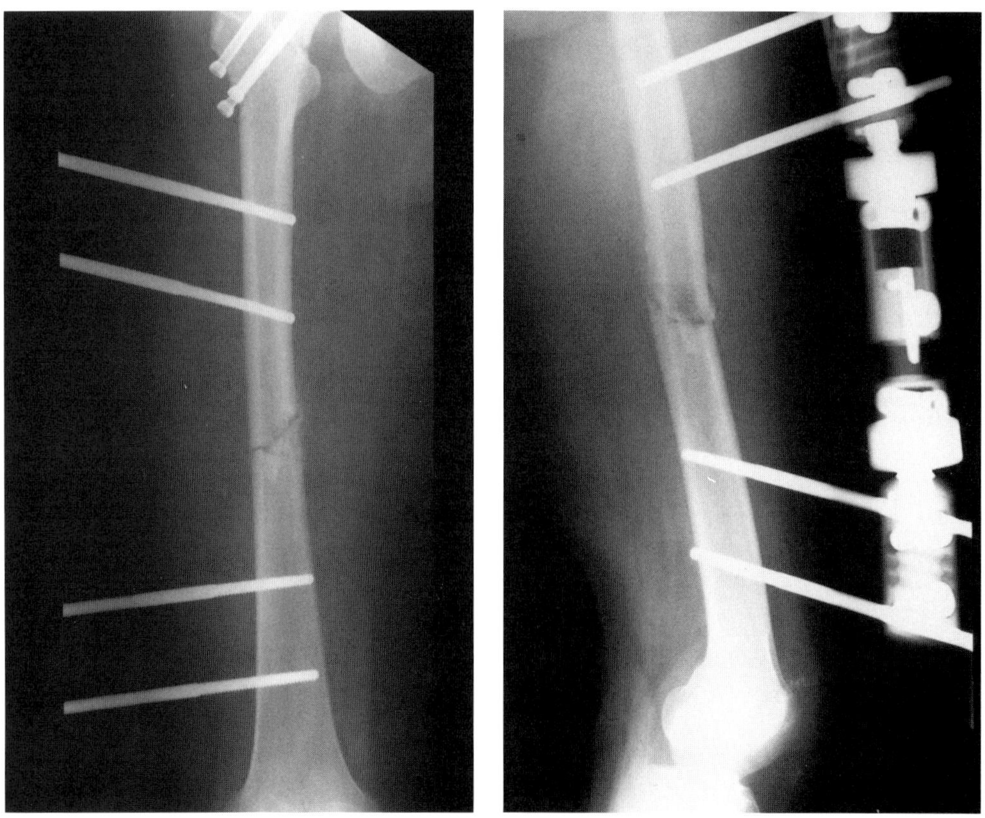

A B

FIG. 5-26. Femoral neck fracture and Winquist-Hansen type I midfemoral fracture. **A:** The AP radiograph shows cannulated Ace pins for fixation of the femoral neck and two threaded half pins above and below the fracture. **B:** Lateral view shows good alignment with a unilateral Orthofix™ fixator.

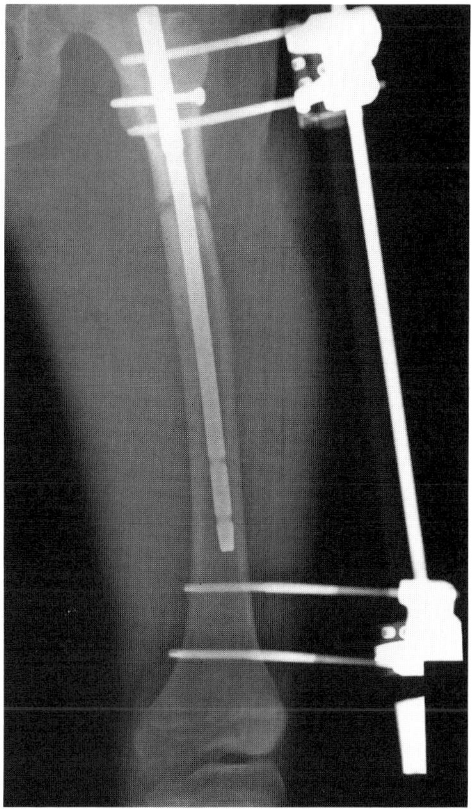

FIG. 5-27. Transverse fracture of the upper femur. The AP view of the femur demonstrating a Russell-Taylor™ nail and upper locking screw. There is also external fixation with a Hex-Fix™ fixator using two pins in each fragment.

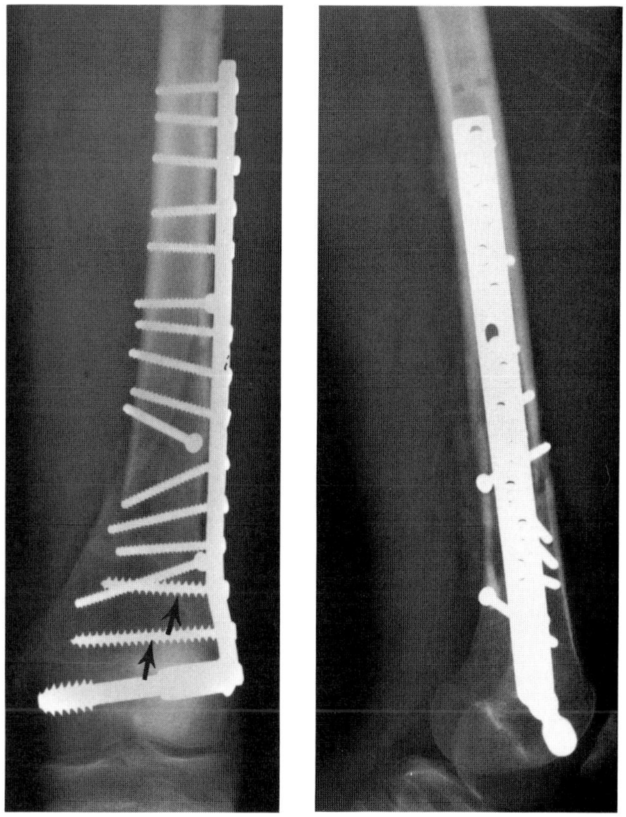

A,B

FIG. 5-29. The AP **(A)** and lateral **(B)** views of a distal femoral fracture internally fixed with a dynamic condylar screw and a long 15-hole side plate. There are fully threaded cancellous screws distally (*arrows*) and several lag screws.

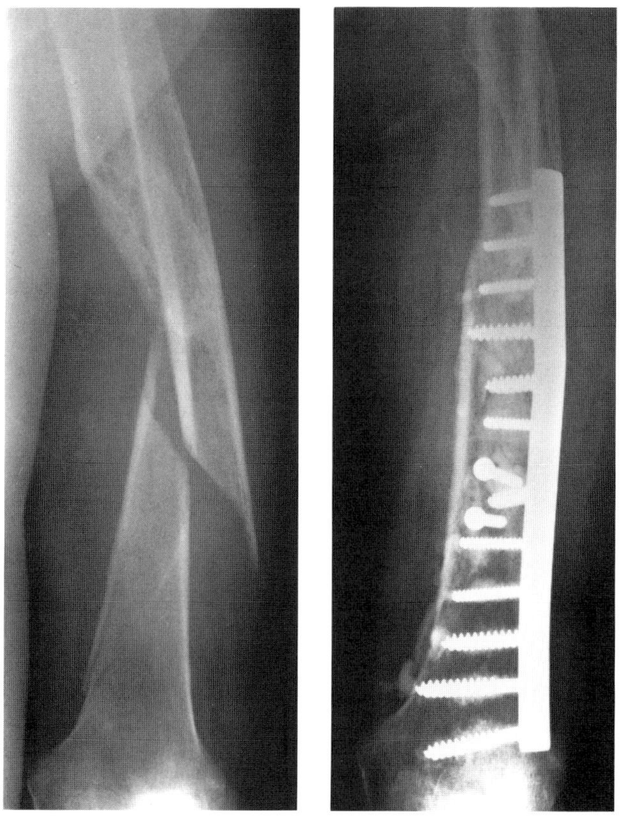

A,B

FIG. 5-28. A: The AP view of a comminuted fracture of the midfemur. **B:** Reduction was achieved with a 12-hole dynamic compression (DC) plate and several additional lag screws. Methyl methacrylate was used to assist holding the screws.

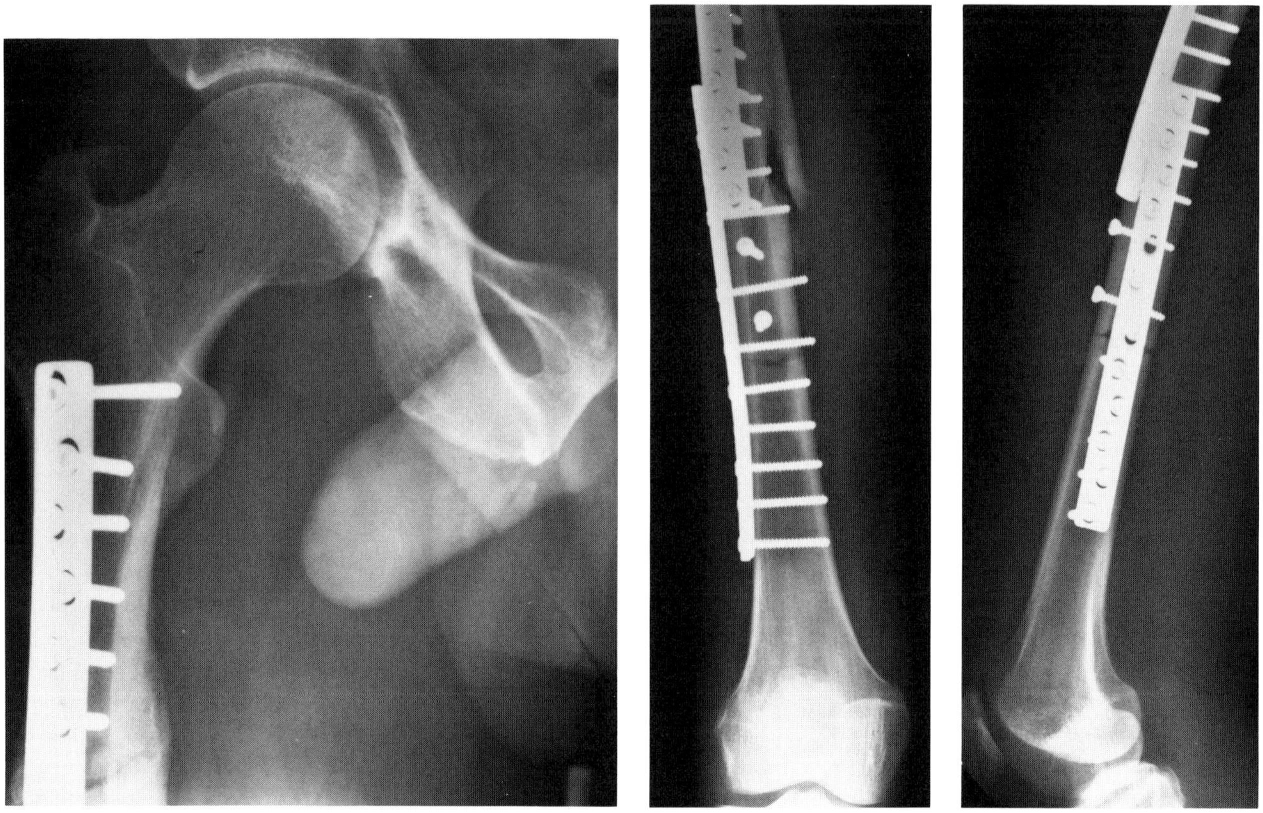

A B,C

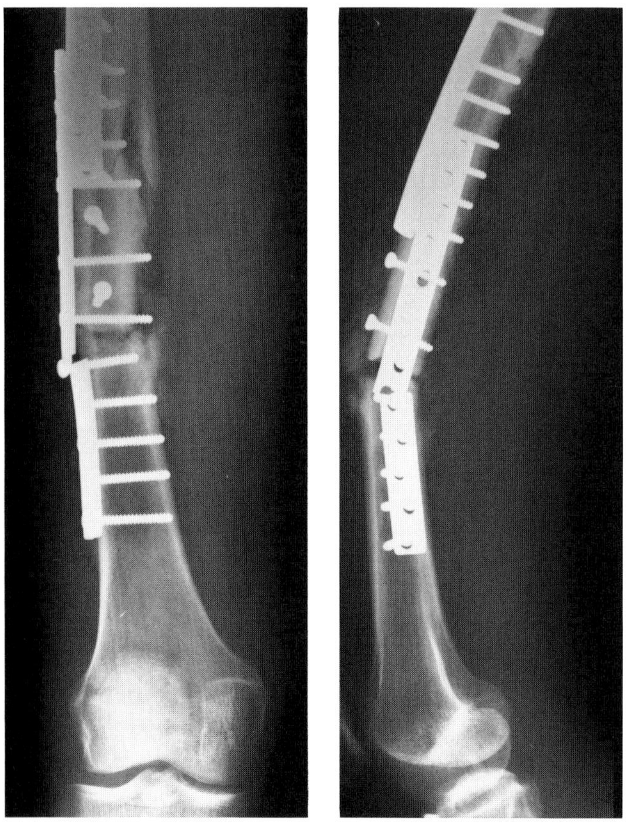

D,E

FIG. 5-30. Fracture of the femur fixed with two DC plates and screws. The AP **(A,B)** and lateral views **(C)**. A plate fracture occurred at the lower transverse fracture **(D,E)** 12 weeks later.

soft tissue damage and decreases the incidence of infection.[2,11,71] The technique provides the early use of the affected limb and reliable union and alignment.[5,71] Reaming of the canal is necessary to permit the insertion of a nail 13 mm in diameter. The nails have different cross-sectional configurations (discussed later), including diamond, fluted, open cloverleaf, and square (Fig. 5-31).[11,15,74] Today, most prefer to use nails with an open-section cloverleaf cross-sectional appearance. This design permits insertion over a guide, and when inserted unreamed, the configuration may preserve endosteal vascularity.[11,71] The rod length is selected by measuring the rod radiographically adjacent to the uninvolved femur (Fig. 5-32) or by an intramedullary guide wire. The nail should be long enough to extend from the upper edge of the patella to 1.3 to 1.9 cm above the lateral margin of the femoral neck. The diameter is most accurately selected at the time of surgery.[15,71,74]

Closed reduction requires a special table and fluoroscopic guidance. It is more difficult to perform in the presence of significant comminution.[11,70,79,80]

Open medullary nailing is accomplished by exposing the fracture site. The advantages include (1) less expensive equipment and no special table, (2) no preliminary traction required, (3) anatomic reduction easier to accomplish, (4) large middle fragments can be stabilized, (5) better for nonunions, and (6) rotational malalignment rare. The disadvantages include disruption of the hematoma around the fracture and an increased incidence of infection.[11,74]

The specific hardware is demonstrated in the next few sections.

Flexible Nails

Ender Rod. Flexible Ender rods (Fig. 5-33) can be used with a closed technique to fix femoral shaft fractures internally. The rods can be prebent to fit the canal (Fig. 5-34). Typically, the rods are inserted either posteromedially or posterolaterally 2 to 3 cm above the superior pole of the patella. They are directed cephalad through the fracture.[11,60,74,78] The rods can also be inserted through the greater trochanter, which reduces problems with knee function (Fig. 5-34). The number of rods used is determined by measuring the medullary canal at its narrowest diameter on AP and lateral radiographs. One rod is inserted for each 5 mm of diameter.[78] Ender rods are best suited to fractures with good cortical contact and minimal comminution (Winquist-Hansen types I and II, Fig. 5-35). Long oblique or bicortical comminuted fractures are difficult to treat with Ender rods.[60,74,78]

Hospital stays with Ender rod treatment average 27 days. When used with appropriate fractures, the results are excellent.[11,74,78]

Rush Rod. Rush rods are flexible and can be prebent similar to Ender rods (Fig. 5-36). These devices do not prevent rotation. Shortening is also a significant problem with oblique or comminuted fractures.[5,11]

Standard Intramedullary Nails

Standard intramedullary nails may require reaming of the medullary canal prior to insertion. The largest diameter nail is used to reduce rotational deformity.[3,15,43,46]

Hansen-Street Nail. The Hansen-Street nail is a noncannulated solid nail with a diamond-shaped cross-sectional configuration (Fig. 5-37). This device was introduced in 1947.[42] The nail is used for midfemoral fractures and does not require reaming. A closed technique is typically used. The mean hospital stay with Hansen-Street nailing is 32 days. Crutches are required with initial weight bearing.[46]

Radiographically, this nail can be identified by its solid diamond configuration and threaded upper end (Fig. 5-38).

Schneider Nail. The Schneider nail (Fig. 5-39) is a flanged, double I-beam nail with graduated saw-toothed ends, which allow the nail to be inserted without reaming. The ends of this nail allow it to be easily identified on radiographs (Fig. 5-39). This nail is infrequently used since the introduction of hollow interlocking nails.

Sampson Fluted Rod. The Sampson fluted rod is not frequently used today (Fig. 5-40).[3,5,15] This rod was designed to correct certain problems experienced with other early intramedullary devices. The fluted intramedullary rod has a circular cross-section for maximal bending strength and external fluting to increase coupling with the bone above and below the fracture site to prevent rotation (Fig. 5-40). The system includes extenders, which allows flexibility in length during insertion.[3,15] These features improve bending strength rigidity and rotational control.[3] The rods are available in straight and curved configurations (Fig. 5-40). This device is primarily used for comminuted midshaft fractures and nonunions.

Zickel Nail. The Zickel nail is used primarily for subtrochanteric fractures and pathologic fractures of the upper femur (see Chapter 4). This solid nail is combined with a Smith-Peterson nail for the femoral neck (Fig. 5-41).[82]

Zickel Supracondylar Device. This intramedullary fixation device is designed for distal femoral fractures. It consists of two rods that are rigid distally and flexible proximally (Fig. 5-42A). Two cancellous screws are used for distal fixation (Fig. 5-42B). The device is inserted distally with a percutaneous technique.[83]

Küntscher Nail. This nail is commonly used for the general treatment of femoral fractures. The open cloverleaf cross-sectional design permits insertion over a guide (Fig. 5-43). The cloverleaf configuration permits endosteal revascularization. The risk of bone damage is sig-

(*text continues on page 377*)

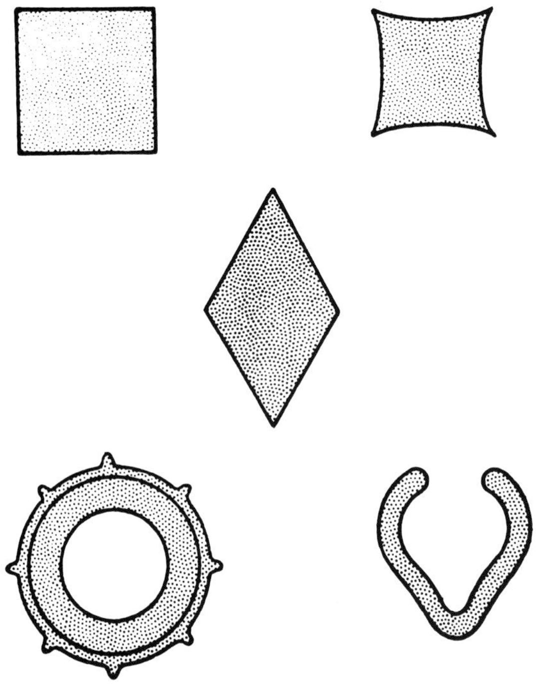

FIG. 5-31. Cross-sectional appearances of standard early femoral nails. (From Zickel RE. Fractures of the adult femur excluding femoral head and neck. *Clin Orthop* 1980;147:93–114.)

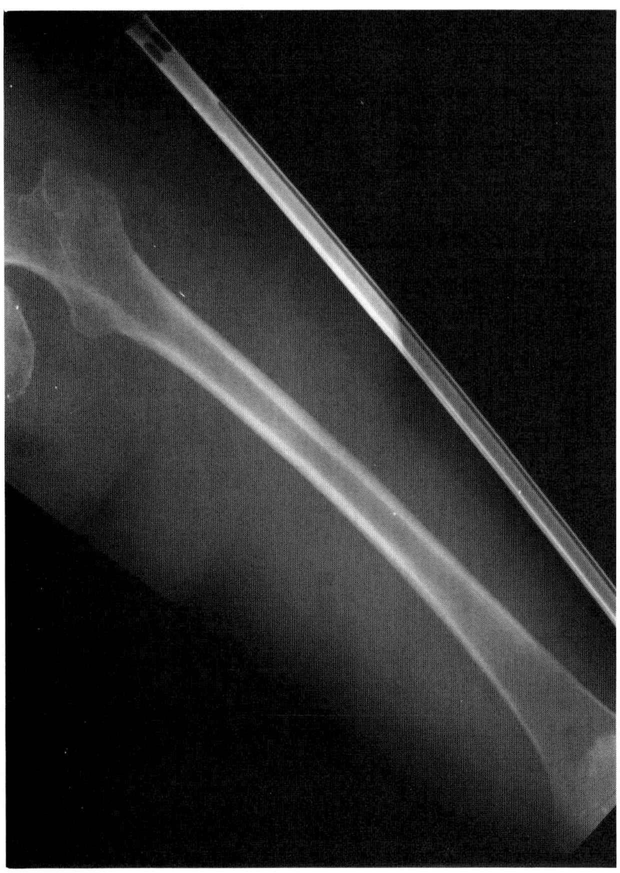

FIG. 5-32. Operative AP radiograph with femoral nail aligned along the normal femur.

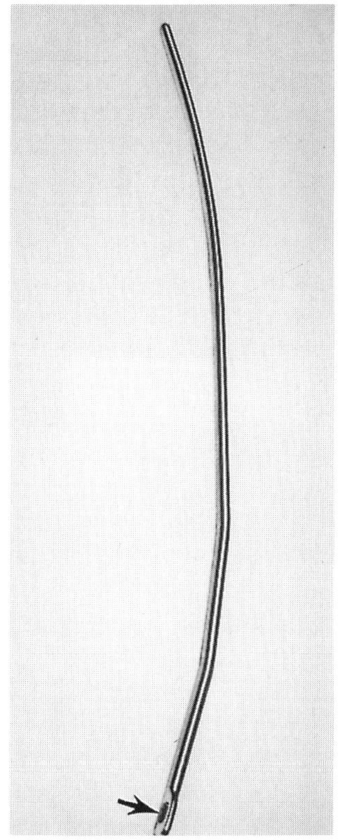

FIG. 5-33. Ender rod with hold at the distal end (*arrow*), which can be used for sutures.

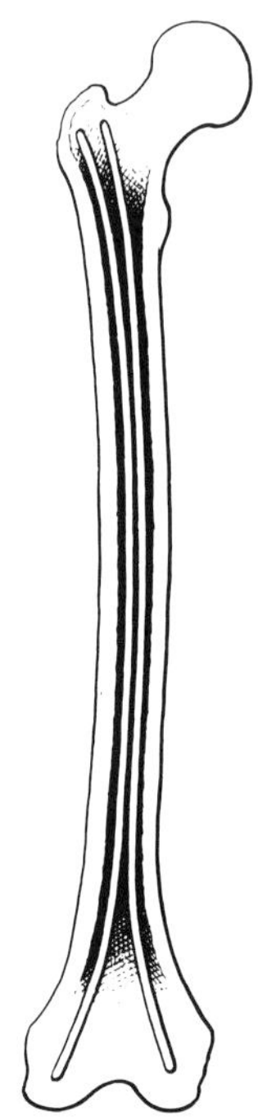

FIG. 5-34. Prebent Ender rods inserted from the greater trochanter. The medullary canal is measured in the narrowest portion on AP and lateral radiographs. Generally, one rod is inserted for each 5 mm of distance.

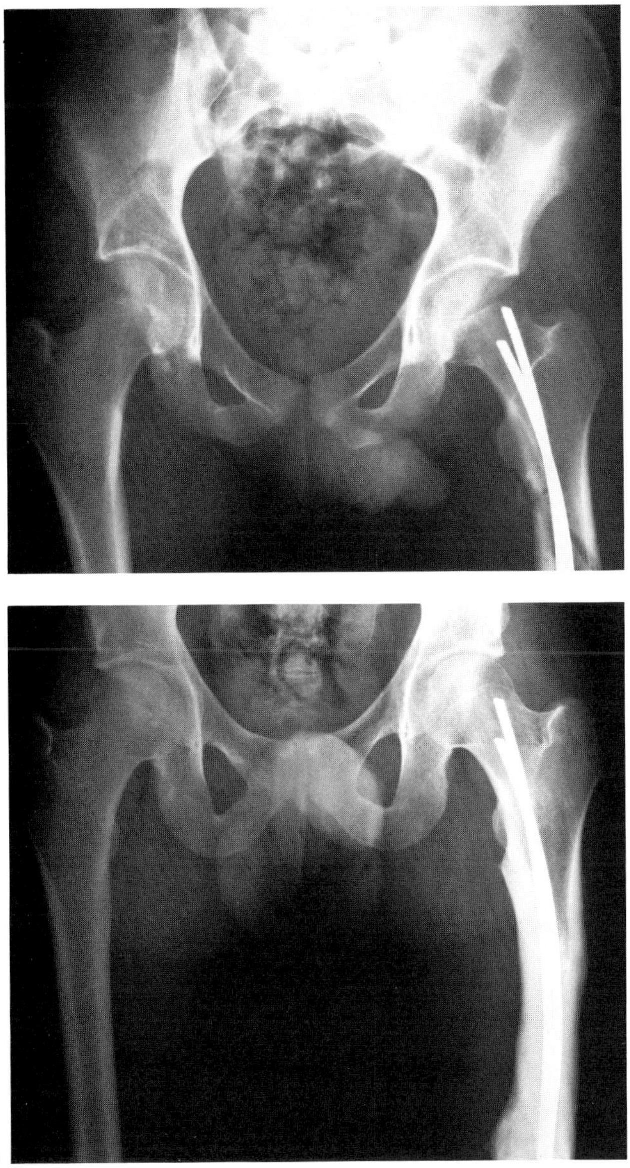

A

D

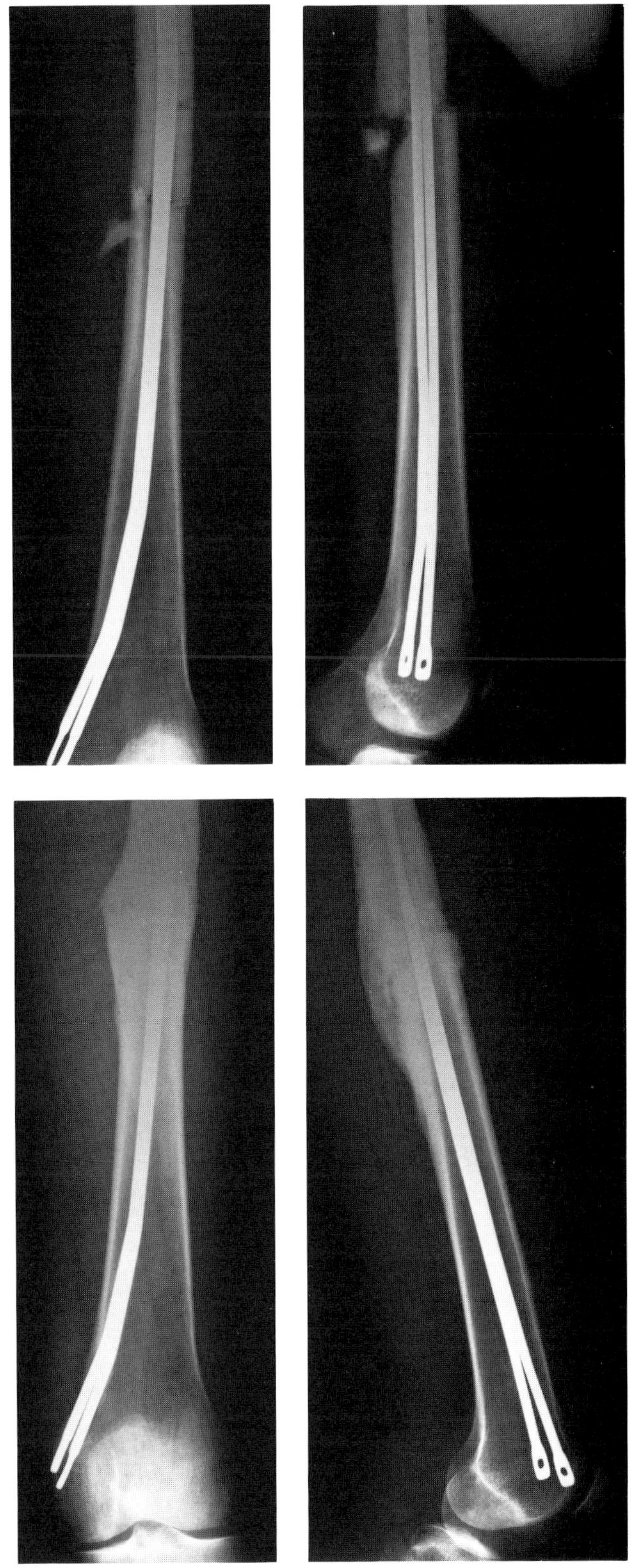

B,C

E,F

FIG. 5-35. The AP view of the pelvis **(A)** and left femur **(B)** and lateral view of the femur **(C)** in a patient with a comminuted femoral fracture treated with two Ender rods. **D–F:** One year, follow-up shows the fractures are healed.

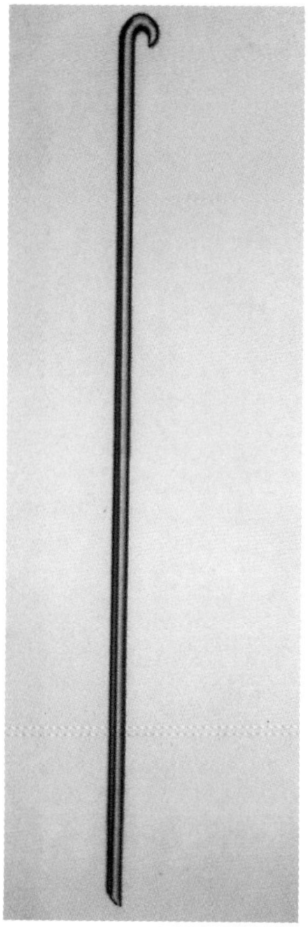

FIG. 5-36. A Rush rod.

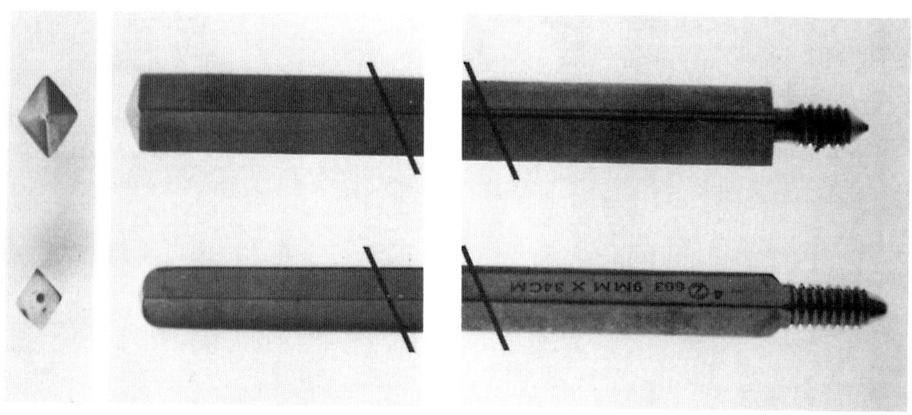

A B

FIG. 5-37. Nine- and 11-mm diameter Hansen-Street nails **(A)** on end and **(B)** shown longitudinally with threaded end. (From Hogh J, Mikkelson P. Hansen-Street nailing of fractures of the femoral shaft. A study of 70 cases. *Injury* 1983;4:440–446.)

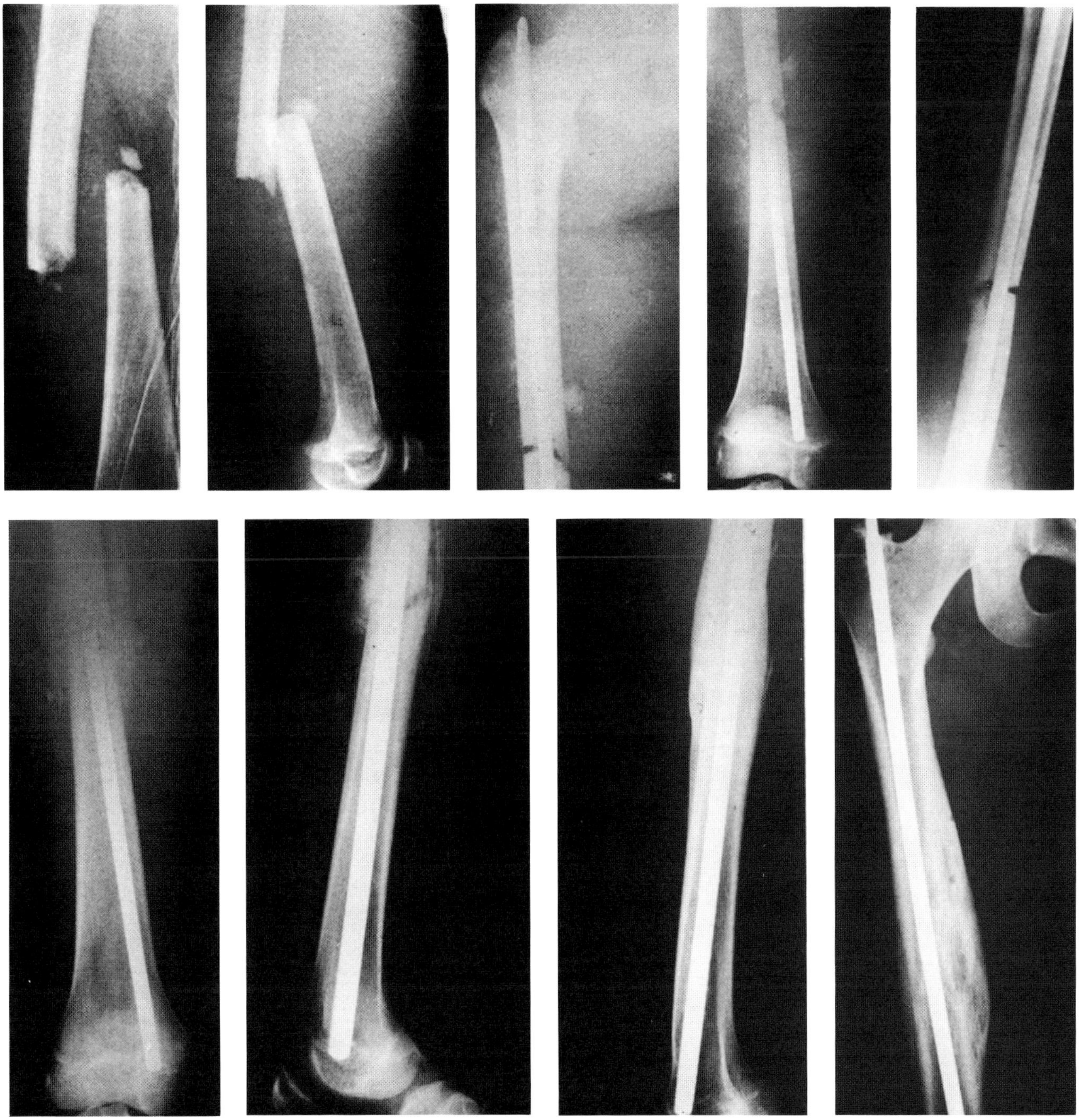

A,B C

D E

FIG. 5-38. The AP **(A)** and lateral **(B)** radiographs of a comminuted right midfemur fracture. Radiographs taken after surgery **(C)** and at 12 weeks **(D)** and 18 months **(E)** with the fracture healed. (From Hogh J, Mikkelson P. Hansen-Street nailing of fractures of the femoral shaft. A study of 70 cases. *Injury* 1983;4:440–446.)

A,B

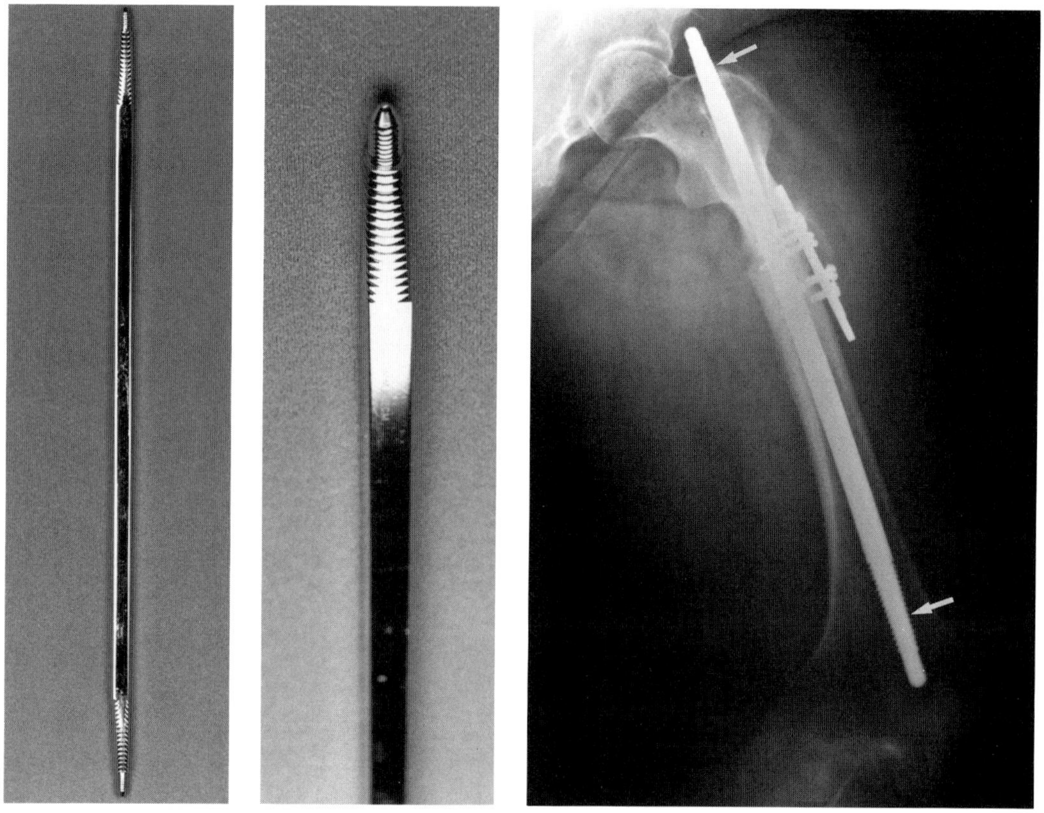

C

FIG. 5-39. A Schneider nail **(A)** and a close-up of the end **(B)**. **C:** The AP radiograph of the femur with a nonunited upper shaft fracture and Schneider nail in place. Note the tapered threaded ends (*arrows*).

A

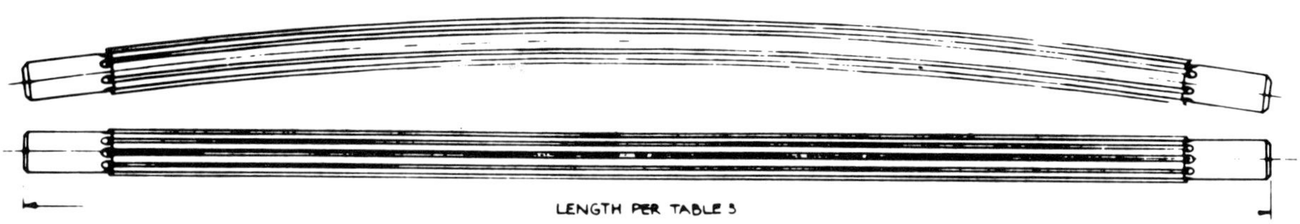

B

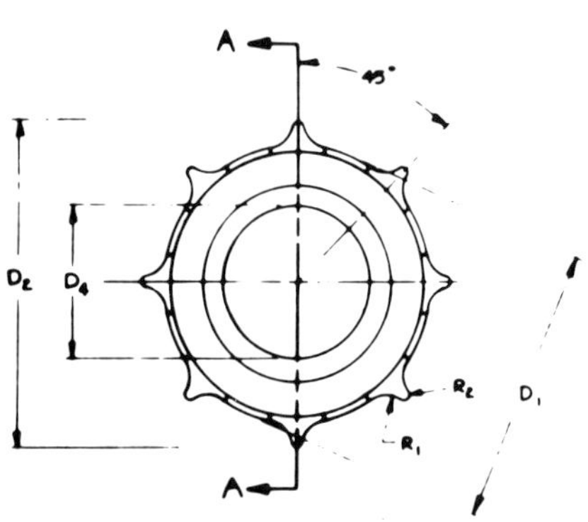

FIG. 5-40. Fluted medullary rod. **A:** Shown from the side. **B:** Cross-sectional configuration. (From Allen WC, Piotruwski G, Burstein A. A fluted femoral intramedullary rod: biomechanical analysis and preliminary clinical results. *J Bone Joint Surg [Am]* 1978;60A:500–515.)

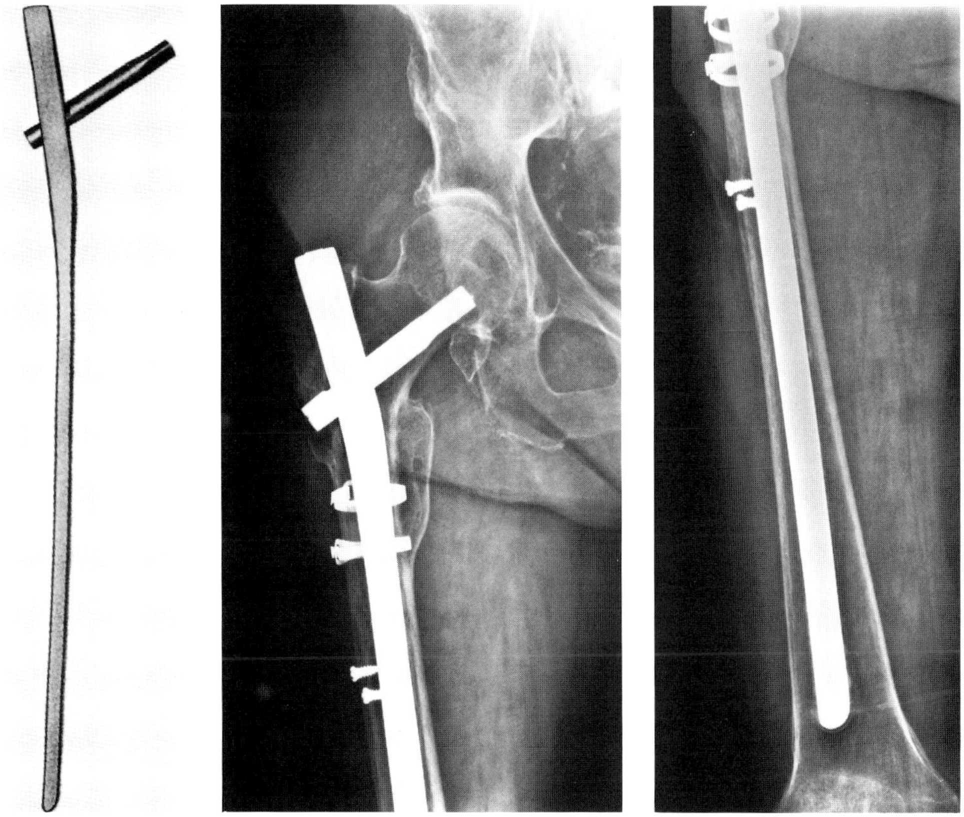

A B,C

FIG. 5-41. **A:** Zickel nail. (Courtesy of Howmedica, Rutherford, NJ.) The AP radiograph of the hip **(B)** and femur **(C)** showing a healed upper femoral fracture with Zickel nail fixation.

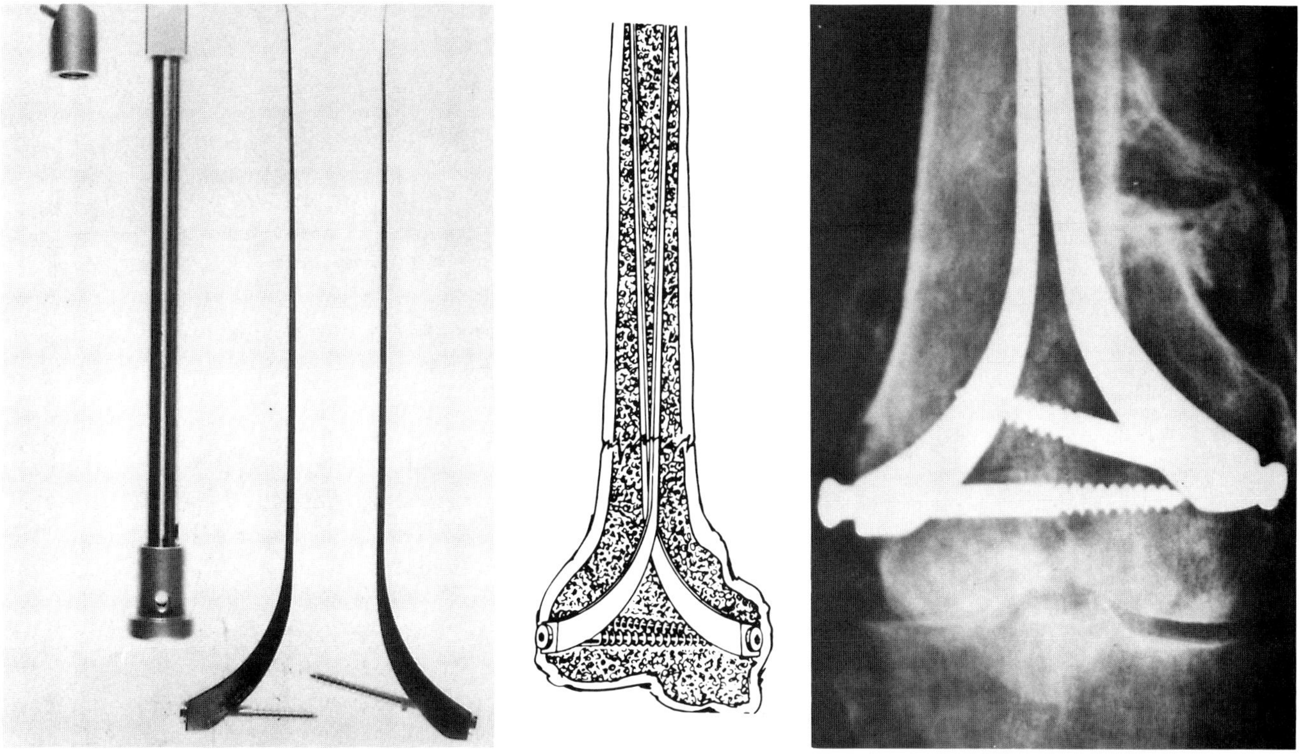

A,B C

FIG. 5-42. Zickel supracondylar fixator. **A:** The two rods and impactor on the left. **B:** Appliance in place with cancellous cross-screws. **C:** The AP radiograph with Zickel fixation and healed fracture at 13 weeks. (From Zickel RE, Fietti VG, Lawsing JF III, Cochran GVB. A new intramedullary fixation device for distal third of the femur. *Clin Orthop* 1977;125:185–191.)

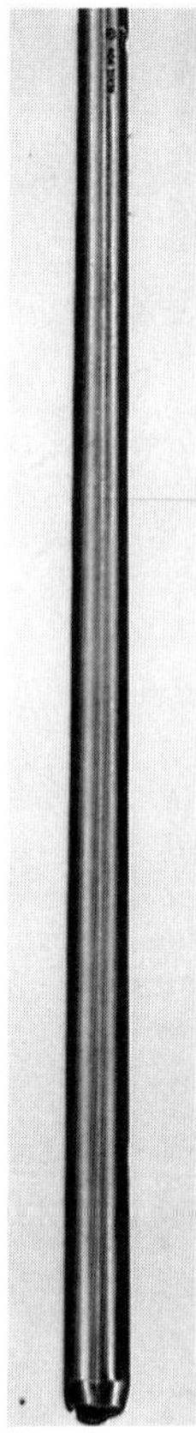

FIG. 5-43. Küntscher rod. Note the open cloverleaf tip. This straight rod is available in variable lengths and 8- to 17-mm diameters. (Courtesy of Zimmer, Warsaw, IN.)

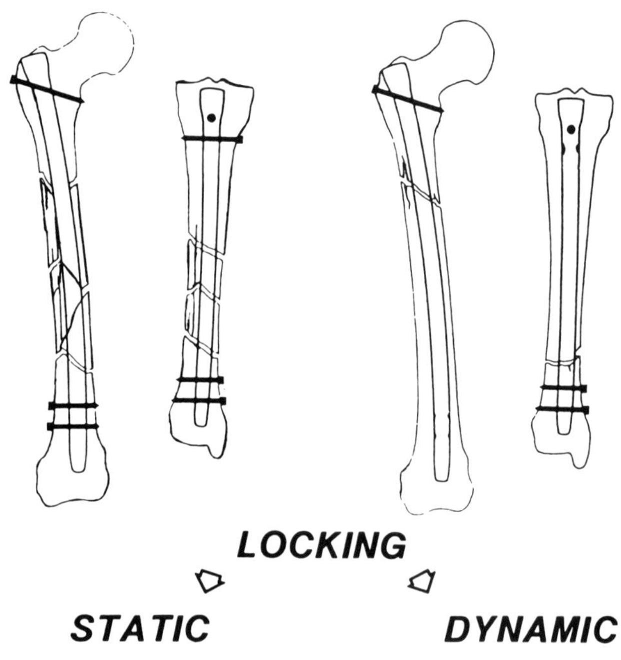

FIG. 5-44. Static and dynamic intramedullary nailing. (From Kempf I, Grosse A, Beck G. Closed locked intramedullary nailing: its application to comminuted fractures of the femur. *J Bone Joint Surg [Am]* 1985;67A:709–720.)

nificantly reduced compared with that of the fluted nail. Shortening and rotation can occur using the standard nonlocking nail.[15]

Locking Intramedullary Nails. Interlocking medullary nails are basically modifications of the original Küntscher nail or other open-nail variations.[23,71,74,75] Although most nails are open, a solid nail that does not require reaming is available.[64,74]

Although the basic concept is similar, several types of interlocking medullary nails are available.[2,5,11–13,29,49,50,52,53,64,68,81] Both static (Figs. 5-44 to 5-46) dynamic configurations are possible using the interlocking systems. Placing screws in only the proximal or distal rod holes results in a dynamic configuration because the fragments can compress with weight bearing. In the static configuration, screws are placed at both ends of the nail (Fig. 5-47).

AO-ASIF Nail. This nail is a thin-walled open nail with a cloverleaf cross-section similar to the Küntscher nail. The upper end has a conical threaded inner surface (Figs. 5-46 and 5-48) for use with threaded bolts for insertion and removal. There are two proximal holes (one oval) and two holes distally (Fig. 5-48). The nail is tapered distally, and the open portion and conical proximal end are easily identified radiographically.[68,74]

Grosse-Kempf Nail. This nail was designed after the Küntscher nail and is slotted in a manner similar to the AO-ASIF nail. The hole system is similar to that of the other nails.[27,61,71] The upper end differs from the AO-ASIF nail in that it is less conical and the slot is less apparent (Fig. 5-49).

Uniflex™ System. The Uniflex femoral nail is a hollow slotted nail configured of titanium alloy. This interlocking nail (Fig. 5-50) may be identified radiographically by its longitudinal slot and straight upper end (compare with Figs. 5-48 and 5-49).

Russell-Taylor™ Nail. The Russell-Taylor™ (stainless steel) nail differs from the AO-ASIF, Grosse-Kempf, and Uniflex™ nails in that it is not slotted (Fig. 5-51).[23] There are three configurations: standard, delta, and reconstruction nails. The standard nail is expanded in the proximal 15 cm to provide additional strength for proximal screw fixation. The delta nail is expanded in its upper 7 cm. There are two oblique proximal holes and two distal holes (Fig. 5-51B,C). Fully threaded self-tapping screws are used for locking. The reconstruction nail has a longer (8 cm) expanded upper portion.

Brooker-Wills Nail. The Brooker-Wills nail differs from the previous systems primarily in that blades are used distally for stability (Fig. 5-52). There are screw holes proximally, which is similar to the other systems.[7,77]

ZMS™ Nail. This nail has a conical tip and straight upper end with threads for use with the targeting instrument (Fig. 5-53). The nail has a more unique cross-sectional configuration (Fig. 5-53A) than do other hollow or slotted hollow nails.

Alta™ Modular Femoral Nail. This interlocking femoral nail also has a unique appearance (Fig. 5-54). It has a rigid appearance with a tapered tip and proximal and distal screw holes. The proximal rod connector can be used with a lag screw (Figs. 5-54B and 5-55) or plunger with an Alta™ dome. This system has a unique radiographic appearance compared with that of other interlocking nails (Figs. 5-54 and 5-55).

Combination Techniques

In certain cases, multiple internal or external fixation systems are used simultaneously. The selection of systems varies with the extent of soft tissue injury and fracture pattern and whether multisystem injury is present (Figs. 5-56 and 5-57).[28,39,56,69]

LENGTH DISCREPANCY

Discrepancy in lower extremity length is a common problem with numerous causes (Table 5-1).[21,25–27,55,59] The tibia and femur have primary diaphyseal and secondary epiphyseal ossification centers. The physeal regions contribute most significantly to extremity growth and overall length. The femur contributes 54% and the tibia, 46% of the overall lower extremity growth. The distal femoral and upper tibial growth plates are most important in this regard.[21,59]

A determination of whether intervention is necessary is based on multiple factors (Table 5-2). Minimal differences in extremity length are not unusual. Differences of up to 2 cm can be managed conservatively (shoe lift).[21,25,55,59] Length discrepancy of ≤5 cm can be approached with epiphysodesis of the uninvolved extremity. Other factors and more significant deformity may require extremity lengthening procedures.[25,27]

TABLE 5-1. *Lower extremity length discrepancy: cause*[21,25–27,55,59]

Congenital
Focal femoral deficiency
Congenitally short femur
Congenital hip dislocation
Paralysis
Infection
Trauma
Shortening
Physeal injury
Malunion, overriding
Lengthening
Diaphyseal: growth acceleration
Neoplasms
Bone disease
Osteogenesis imperfecta
Fibrous dysplasia (shepherd's crook deformity)

(*text continues on page 387*)

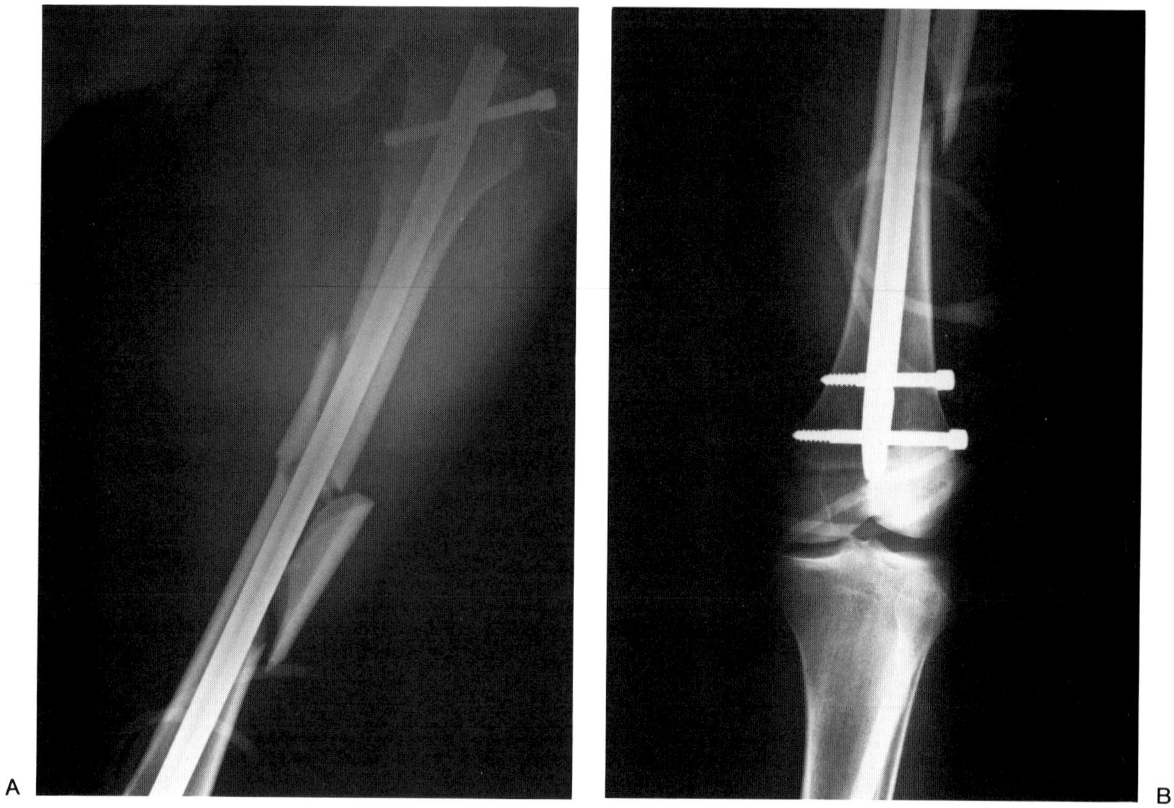

FIG. 5-45. The AP views of the upper (A) and distal (B) left femur demonstrating a comminuted midshaft fracture with proximal and distal screws (static interlocking).

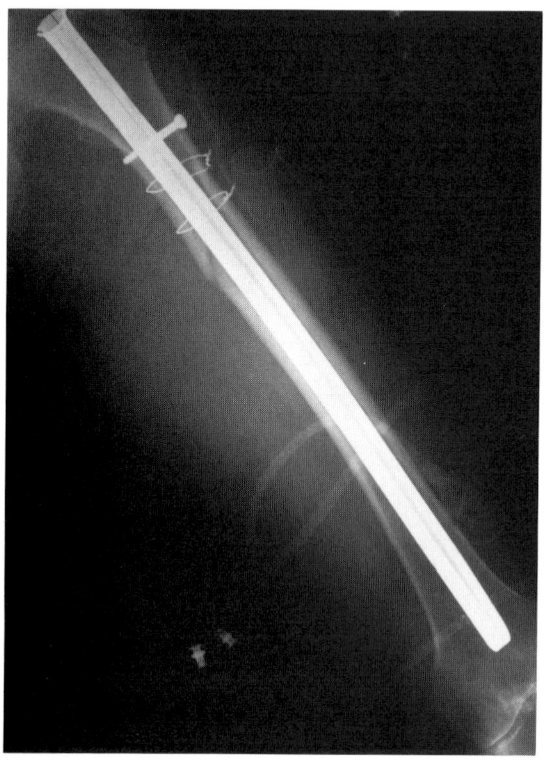

FIG. 5-46. The AP view of the femur with a fracture of the upper femur. AO-ASIF nail with a single screw in the upper fragment and two cerclage wires for dynamic interlocking.

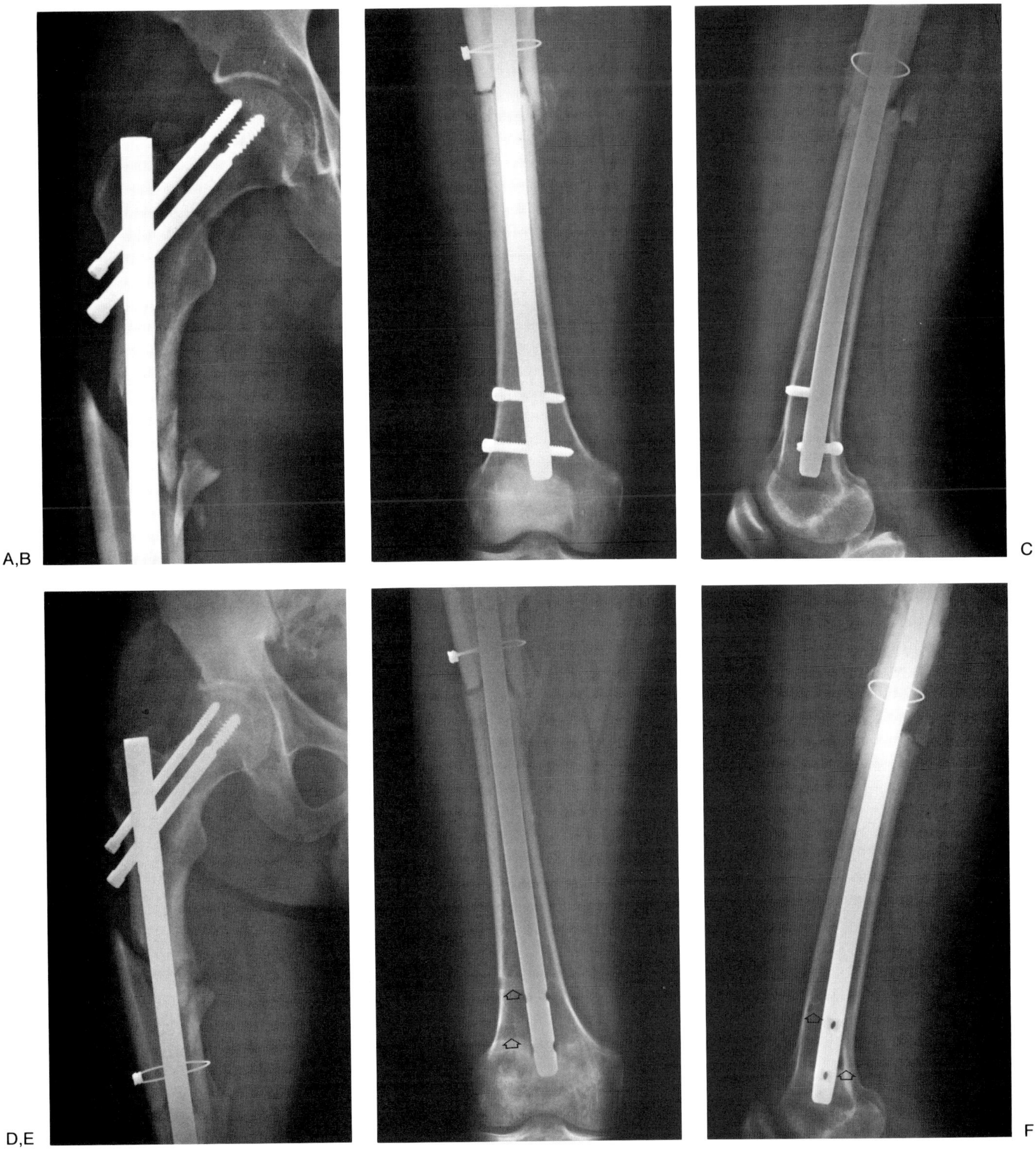

FIG. 5-47. The AP **(A,B)** and lateral **(C)** views of the femur with a comminuted upper femoral shaft and femoral neck fracture. A Russell-Taylor™ nail with upper lag screws and distal screws was used for static fixation. There is a Dall-Miles cable around the comminuted fragment. Three months later, the distal screws were removed, creating a dynamic system. The AP **(D,E)** and lateral **(F)** radiographs show the fracture has impacted. Note the change in position (*arrows*) of the screw tracts compared with the holes.

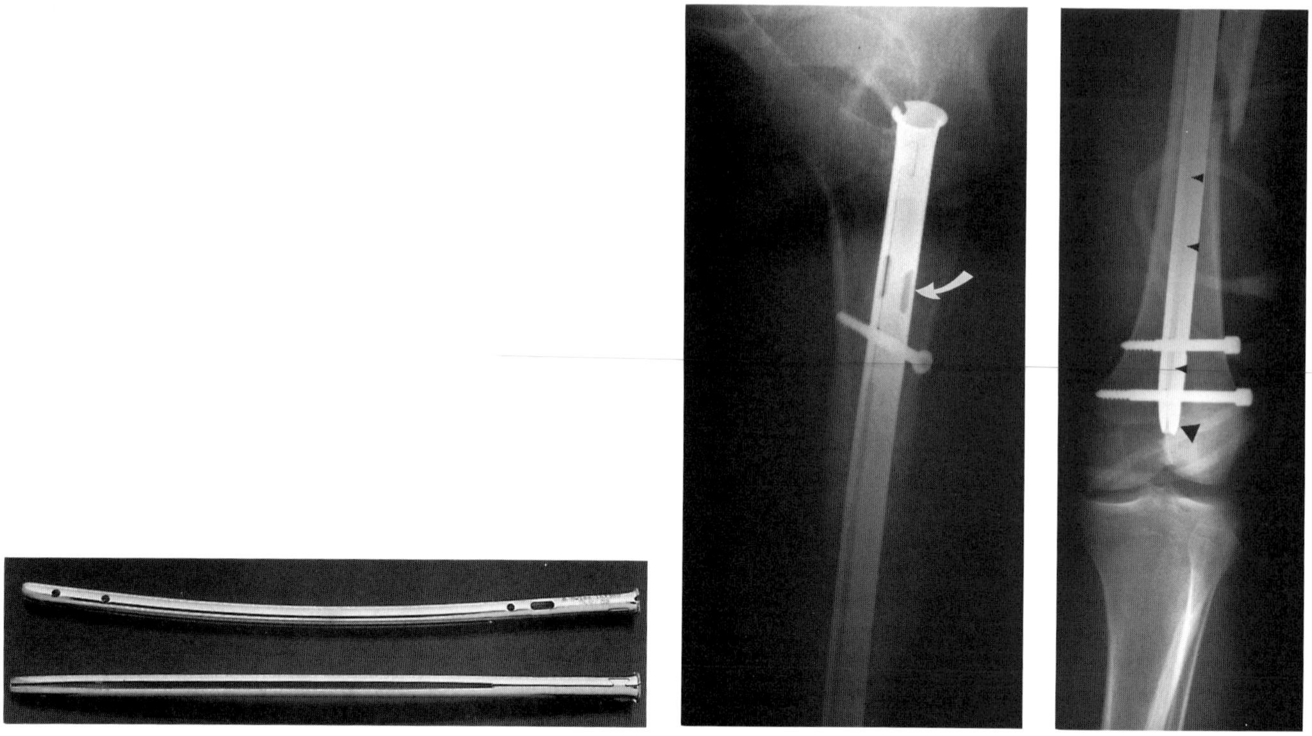

A B,C

FIG. 5-48. **A:** AO femoral nail with femoral curve (*top*). (From Rüedi,[64] with permission.) **B:** Lateral view of the upper femur with the AO nail demonstrating the conical upper end, long oval hole (*arrow*), and a screw in the round hole. **C:** The AP view of the distal femur demonstrating the slot (*small arrows*) and tip (*large arrow*). Two distal screws.

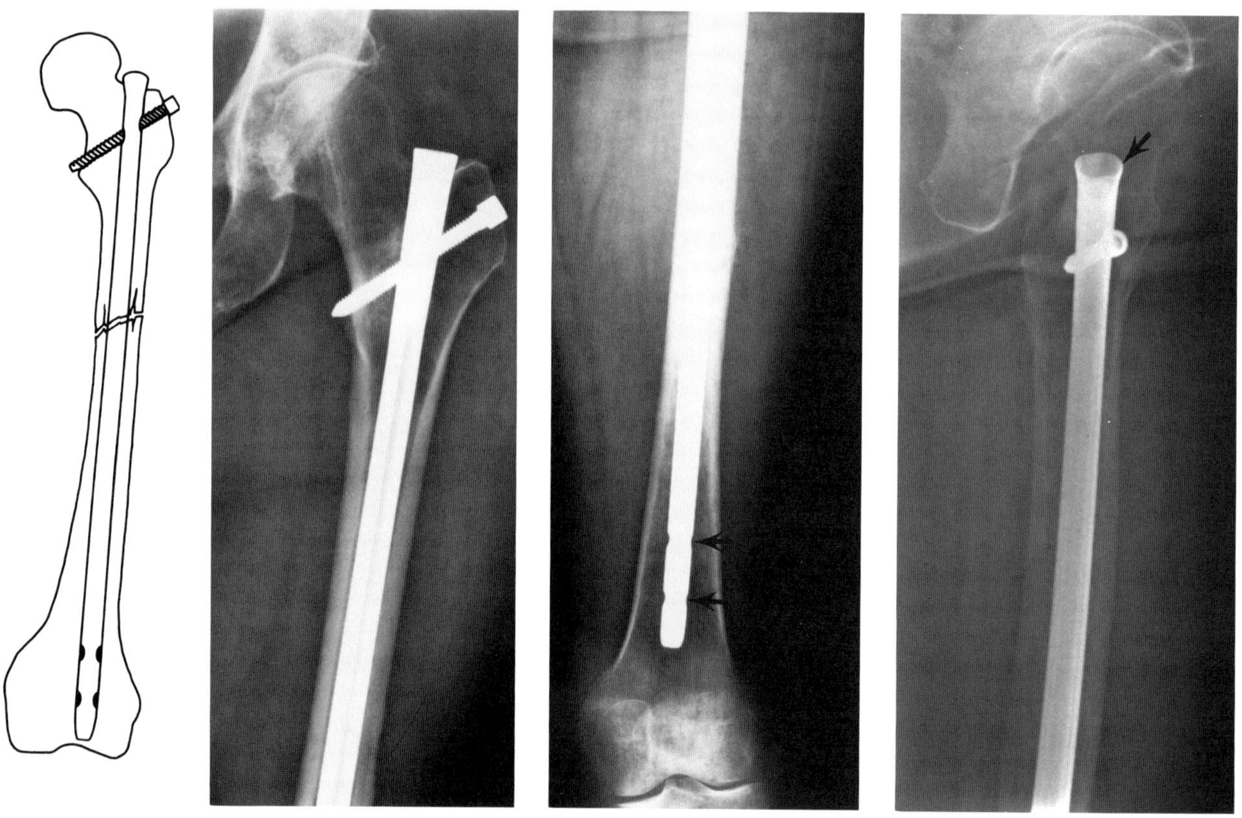

A,B C,D

FIG. 5-49. Grosse-Kempf nail. **A:** A Grosse-Kempf nail with upper screw for midfemoral fracture fixation. (Courtesy of Howmedica, Rutherford, NJ.) **B,C:** The AP views of the femur with a dynamic Grosse-Kempf nail and a single proximal screw. There are two distal holes (*arrows*). The upper end and tip differ significantly from those of the AO-ASIF nail (Fig. 5-47) radiographically. **D:** Lateral view of the upper femur demonstrating the slight upper tapering (*arrow*).

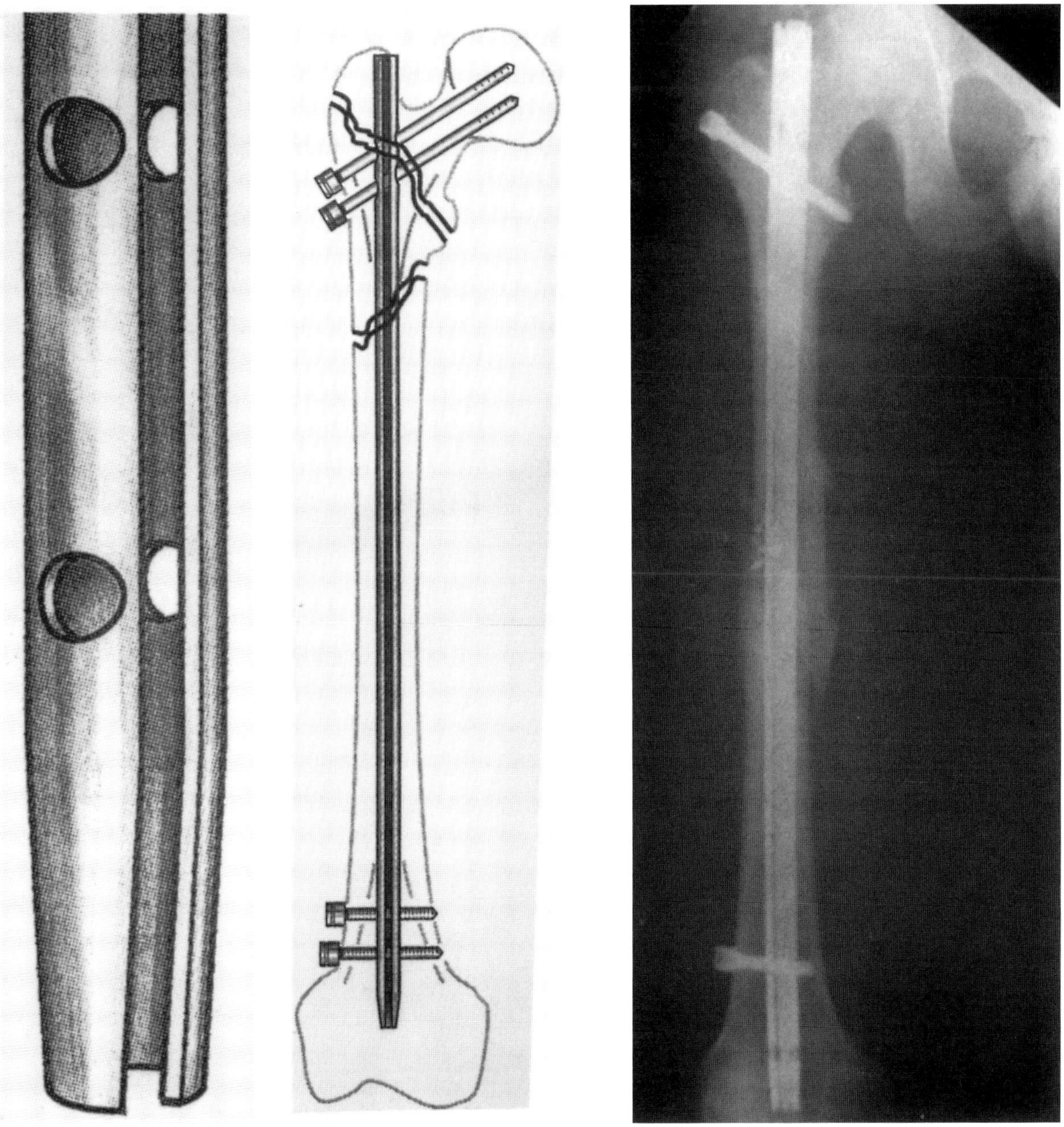

A,B C

FIG. 5-50. Uniflex™ femoral system. **A:** The slotted tip of the Uniflex™ nail with two screw holes. **B:** Uniflex™ nail with upper lag screws and two distal locking screws for fixation of a comminuted femoral fracture. **C:** An AP radiograph of a Uniflex™ nail with proximal and distal screws for fixation of a comminuted femoral fracture. (Courtesy of Biomet, Warsaw, IN.)

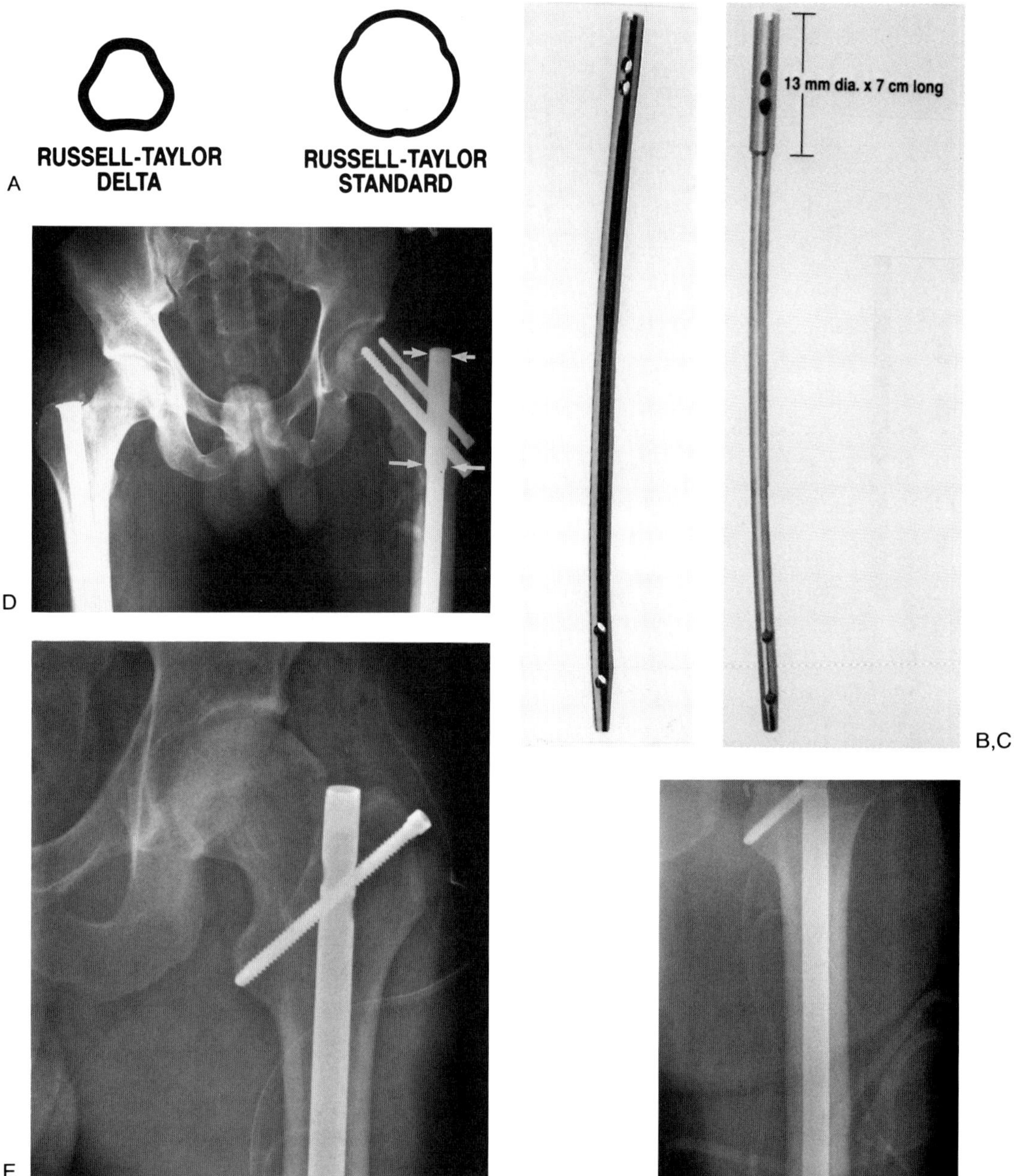

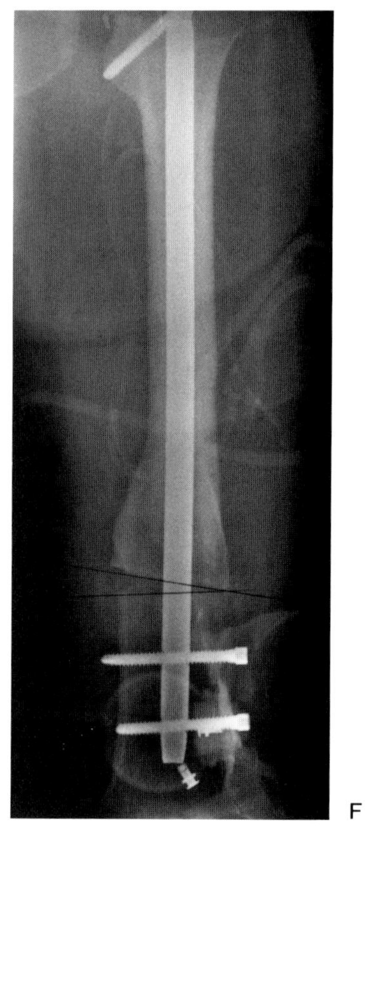

FIG. 5-51. Russell-Taylor™ nail. **A:** Cross-sectional configuration of the nonslotted standard and delta configurations of the Russell-Taylor™ nail. **B,C:** Russell-Taylor™ delta femoral nail and delta nail. **D:** An AP view of the pelvis with bilateral femoral fractures. There is an AO nail on the right and a Russell-Taylor™ reconstruction nail with two femoral neck lag screws on the left. Note the expanded upper portion (*arrows*). The AP views of the upper femur **(E)** and lower femur **(F)** with a standard Russell-Taylor™ nail for fixation after a distal femoral osteotomy. (A–C: Courtesy of Smith and Nephew Richards, Memphis, TN.)

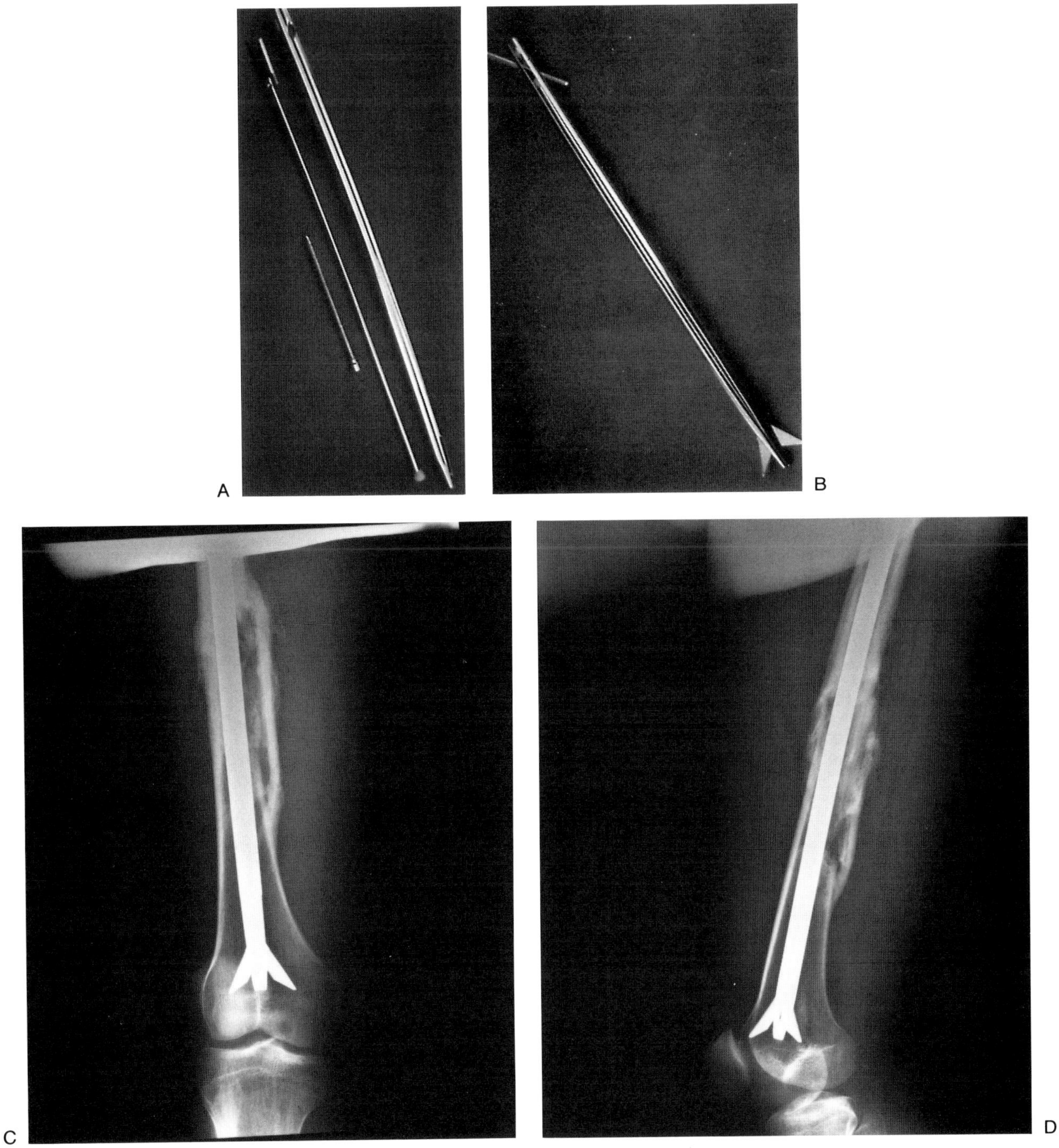

FIG. 5-52. Brooker-Wills nail. **A:** Unassembled components of Brooker-Wills system. **B:** Assembled components with distal fixator displayed and a proximal screw in place. (From White EM, Healy WL, Brumback RJ, Burgess AR, Brooker AF. The treatment of fractures of the femoral shaft with the Brooker-Wills distal locking intramedullary nail. *J Bone Joint Surg [Am]* 1986;68A:865–876.) The AP **(C)** and lateral **(D)** radiographs of the distal femur with a healed midshaft fracture, which was internally fixed with a Brooker-Wills nail.

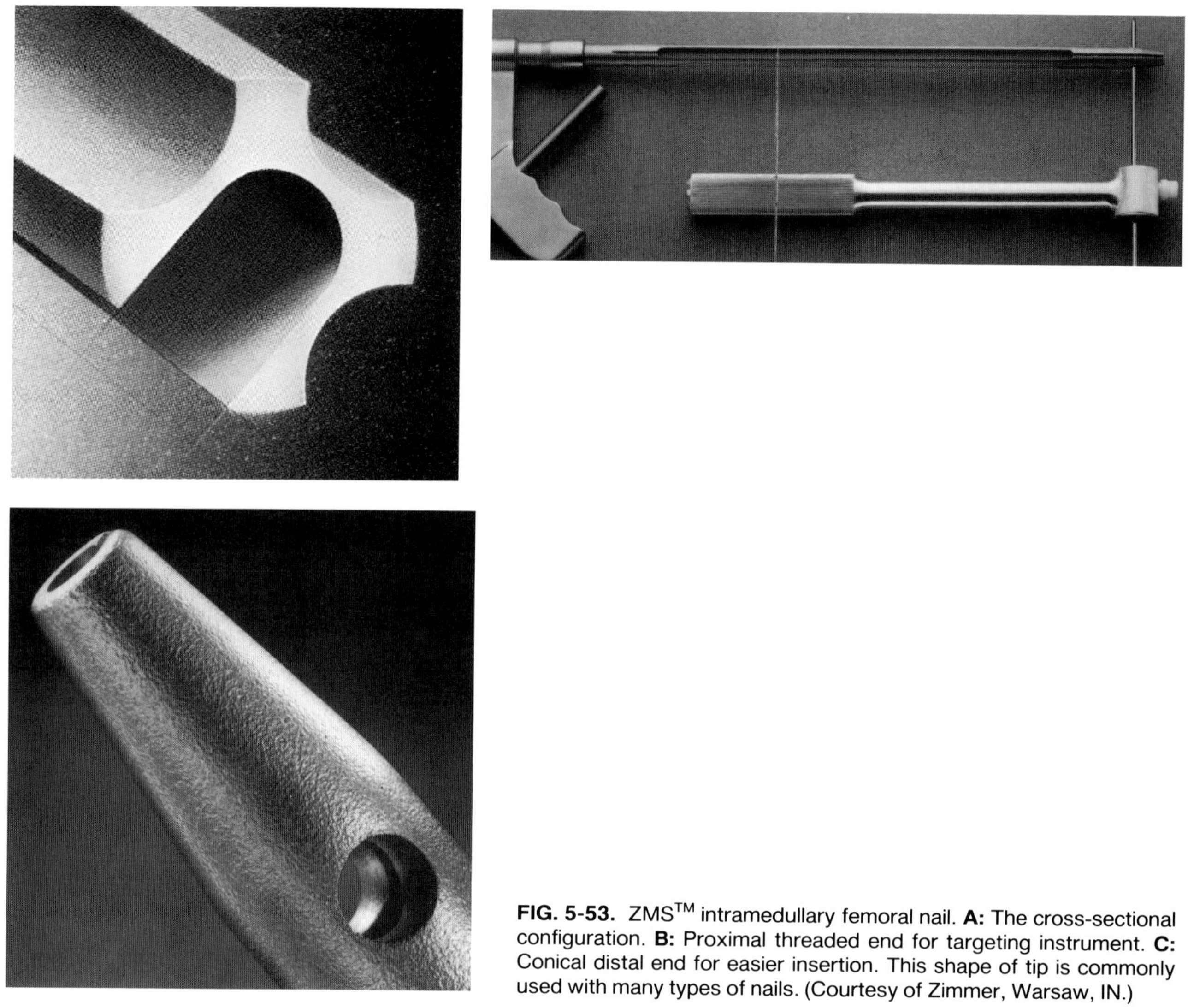

A B C

FIG. 5-53. ZMS^{TM} intramedullary femoral nail. **A:** The cross-sectional configuration. **B:** Proximal threaded end for targeting instrument. **C:** Conical distal end for easier insertion. This shape of tip is commonly used with many types of nails. (Courtesy of Zimmer, Warsaw, IN.)

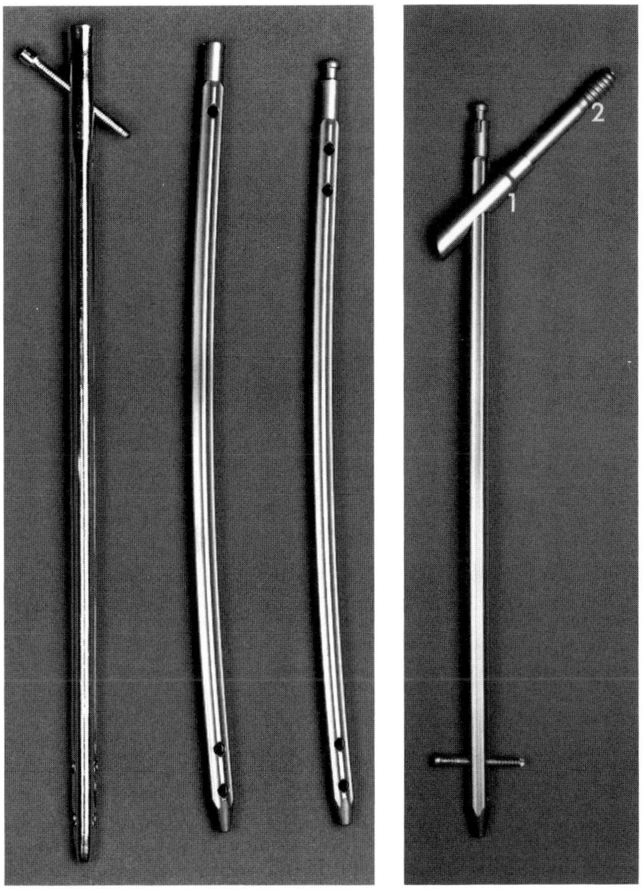

A B

FIG. 5-54. Alta™ modular interlocking femoral nail. **A:** A hollow Grosse-Kempf nail with proximal screw (*left*) and the Alta™ intramedullary nails (*middle* and *right*). **B:** Alta™ interlocking nail with a single distal screw and a proximal rod connector (*1*) and lag screw (*2*). (Courtesy of Howmedica, Rutherford, NJ.)

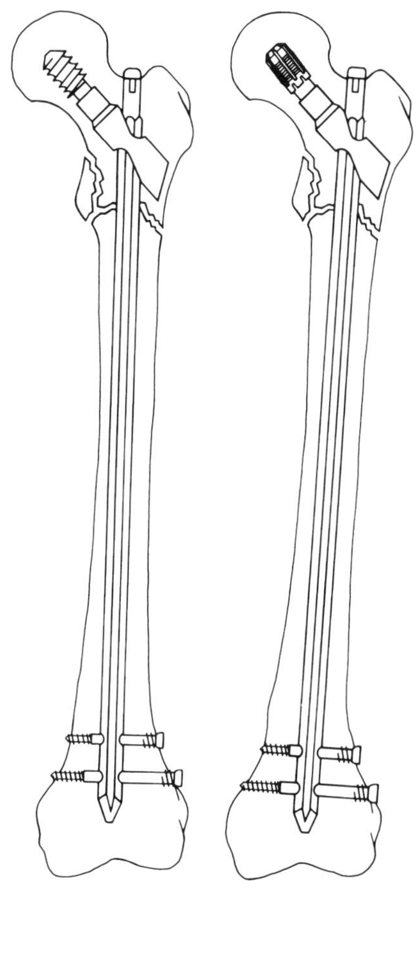

A B

FIG. 5-55. Alta™ modular interlocking femoral nail for fixation of a subtrochanteric fracture using a lag screw **(A)** and dome **(B)**.

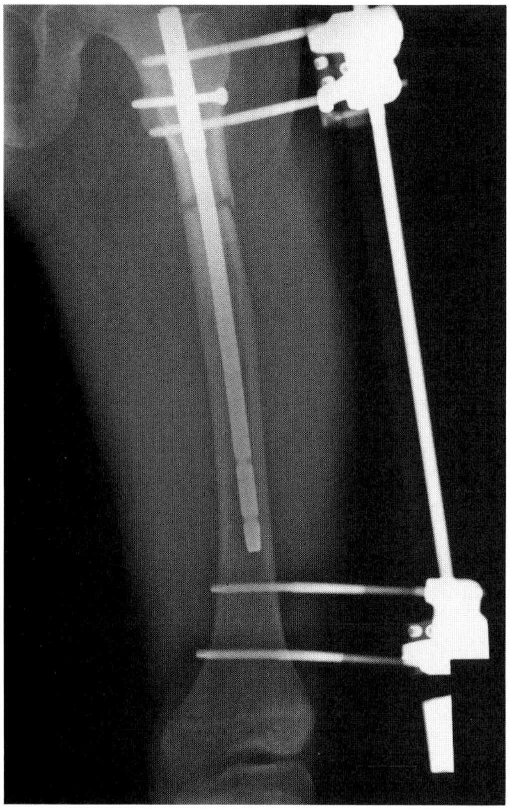

FIG. 5-56. The AP view of the left femur with a transverse proximal femoral fracture. Fixation was accomplished using a Hex-Fix™ external fixator and a short Russell-Taylor™ intramedullary reconstruction nail.

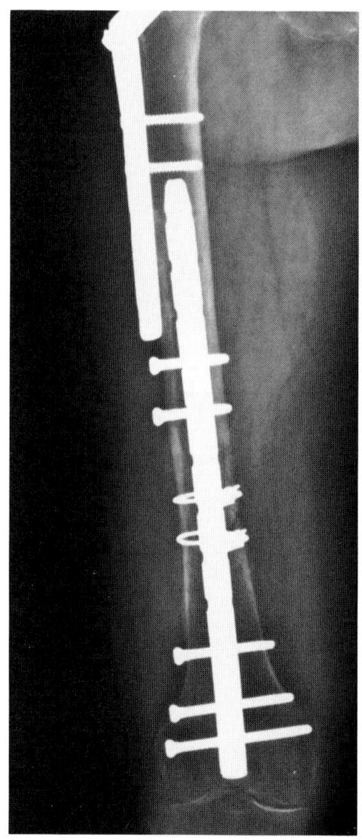

FIG. 5-57. Distal and proximal femoral fractures with a dynamic hip screw for fixation of the neck fracture and a reconstruction nail with screws and two Dall-Miles cables distally.

TABLE 5-2. *Extremity length discrepancy: considerations for operative intervention*[21,59]

Cause
Length discrepancy
Age
Anticipated height or growth potential
Sex
Patient requirements

Preoperative Imaging

Preoperative imaging can usually be accomplished with routine radiographs of the lower extremities, including the foot and ankle, scanograms (Fig. 5-58A) and CT.[1,22,32,35,45,54,62] The latter is particularly useful for length and rotational deformities.[32,45]

Length discrepancies > 2 cm and < 18 cm can be considered for reconstructive procedures.[26,27] An absolute discrepancy is measured between the iliac crest and tibiotalar joint. An apparent discrepancy can occur with contractures or neurologic disorders. From a radiographic standpoint, length measurements can be obtained using conventional scanograms or CT.[32,45,62]

Orthoroentgenography is a commonly used technique that uses three separate exposures centered over the hips, knees, and ankles with a metal rule placed along the extremity.[22,35,54] Variations in technique include a moving radiographic tube with collimated beam and long exposure times (Fig. 5-58A).[64] More recently, biplanar lateral and frontal CT have been used.[1,32,45] The measurements are accurate, the patient does not have to remain motionless as long as with conventional techniques, and the radiation exposure is actually less with CT.[32] Lateral CT images are preferred in patients with knee flexion deformities.

A demonstration of a serial measurement change on scanograms or no change is also important in determining whether the discrepancy can be corrected.[21] Whichever technique is selected should be performed consistently on the same patient.

Preoperative skeletal age determinations using a routine posteroanterior view of the left hand and wrist are essential to correlate the chronologic age with the skeletal age. Foot and ankle abnormalities must also be evaluated prior to a consideration of surgical management. Generally, AP, lateral, oblique, and standing views are adequate for this purpose.[5,21,25] After the extent and location of the discrepancy are determined, the appropriate therapy can be considered.

Surgical Options

Epiphysodesis-Ephiphyseal Plate Stapling

This technique is designed to cause physeal growth arrest. The distal femur or proximal tibia and fibular epiphyses are most often used. If successful, the opposite extremity will continue to grow, reducing the length discrepancy in the extremities. This procedure is usually reserved for discrepancies of 5 cm or less. Bone blocks can also be placed across the physis.

Epiphyseal stapling can also be used to fuse the growth plate symmetrically or asymmetrically.

Femoral Shaft Shortening or Lengthening

Femoral shortening or lengthening can be used to reduce the discrepancy. In the former, a segment of bone is resected and internally fixed with a plate and screw technique.

There are several lengthening techniques (Figs. 5-58B and 5-59).[25,26] Using the Wägner technique, an osteotomy is performed, and initial lengthening of 1.5 cm is generally obtained initially.[21,26,27] Radiographs are used to follow the position of the fragments and the degree of separation. Each day, the fragments are separated an additional 1.5 mm by using an external fixator, such as a Wägner, Orthofix™, or Ilizarov external fixator (Fig. 5-58C).[26] When the desired length is obtained, the bone gap is grafted, and lengthening plates are used for fixation (Figs. 5-58D and 5-59).[21,26,27] The third or final stage is plate removal.

The other technique that can be used is callotasis (Fig. 5-58E). Either a uniplanar (Fig. 5-60) or circular external fixator is used. A percutaneous osteotomy is performed after applying the fixator. The osteotomy is distracted 1 mm per day using four 0.25-mm distractions per day. The callus that forms is distracted in this manner until the desired length is attained. The frame is left in place until solid union is achieved.[25,26]

Complications and Postoperative Imaging

The procedures described here have similar complications in some respects. However, slight differences make it simpler to discuss the complications and imaging based on the cause and type of fixation used.

Trauma

Complications can be related to the extent of bone and soft tissue injury and the type of procedure.[37,38,40,58] Local and systemic complications are not uncommon (Table 5-3).[5]

Fractures may not unite as a result of inadequate fixation, insufficient immobilization, excessive traction with distraction of the fracture fragments, and soft tissue interposition and infection. Delayed union is usually defined as nonhealing by 6 months.[15] Malunion or angulation deformities are more likely to occur with traction or less rigid forms of fixation. Nonunion may require reoperation.[15]

(text continues on page 390)

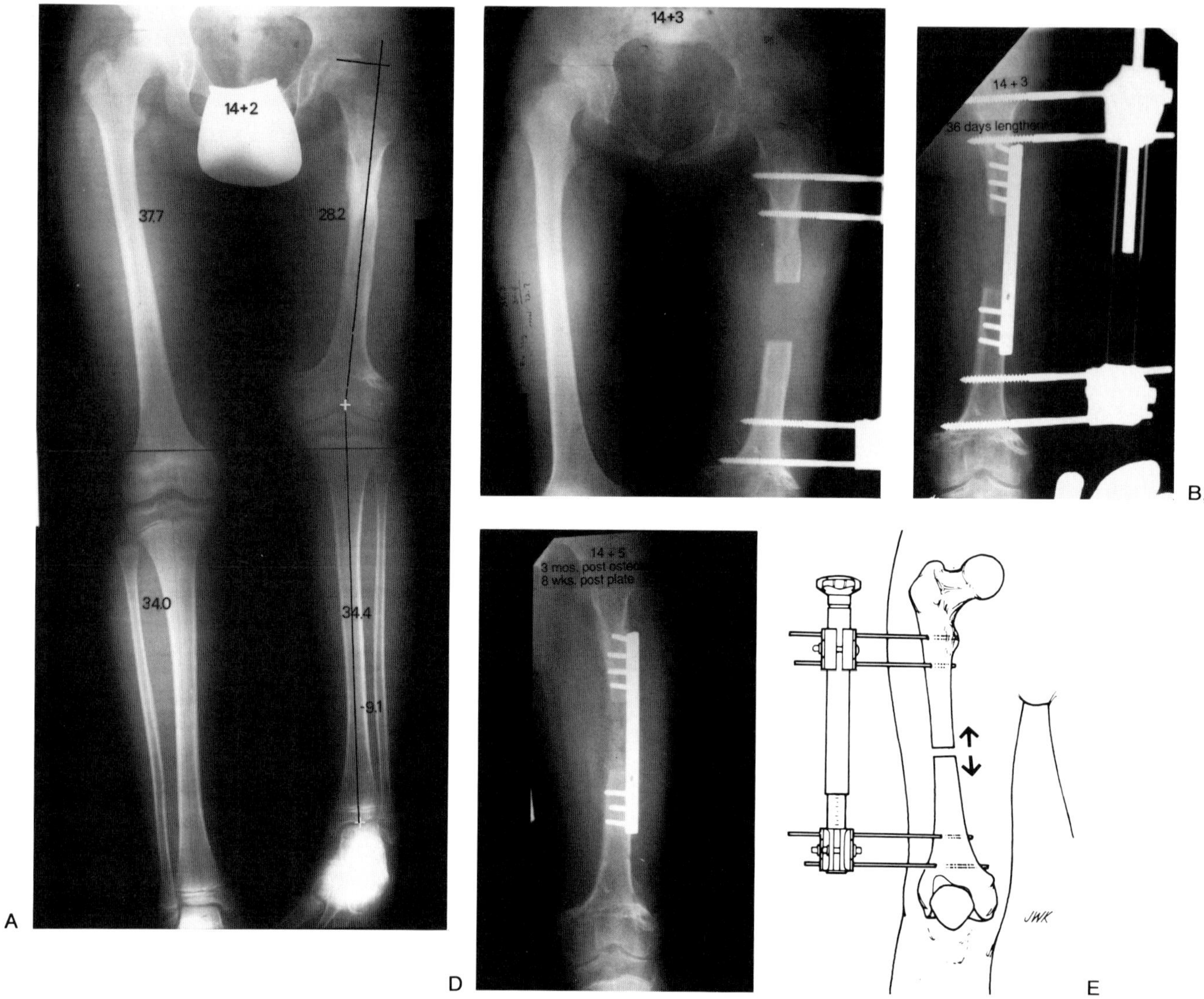

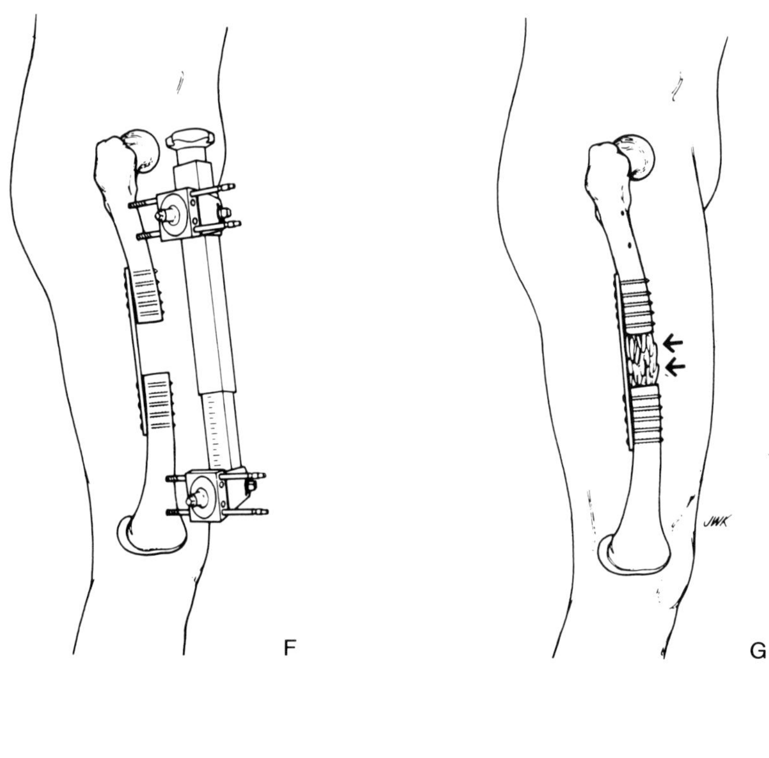

FIG. 5-58. Leg lengthening in a child with congenital shortening of the left femur. (Courtesy of HA Peterson, Mayo Clinic, Rochester, MN.) **A:** AP scanogram demonstrating shortening of the left femur. Lines are drawn along the shaft and a perpendicular connector from the top of the femoral head. The femoral notch and tibial articular surface at the ankle are used for end points.[62] **B:** The AP view following osteotomy and separation of the fragments with a Wägner apparatus. **C:** The AP view following bone grafting of the gap and lengthening plate fixation (36 days). **D:** Three months postosteotomy and 8 weeks after plating with Wägner apparatus removal. Wägner apparatus for leg lengthening **(E)** and technique with plating **(F)** and insertion of bone graft in the bone gap **(G)**.

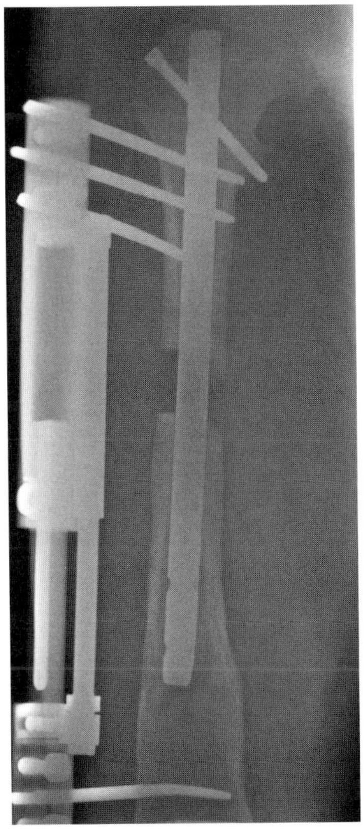

FIG. 5-59. Old fracture deformity of the right femur with femoral shortening. Lengthening was accomplished using a midfemoral osteotomy with intramedullary reconstruction nail and Orthofix™ external fixator.

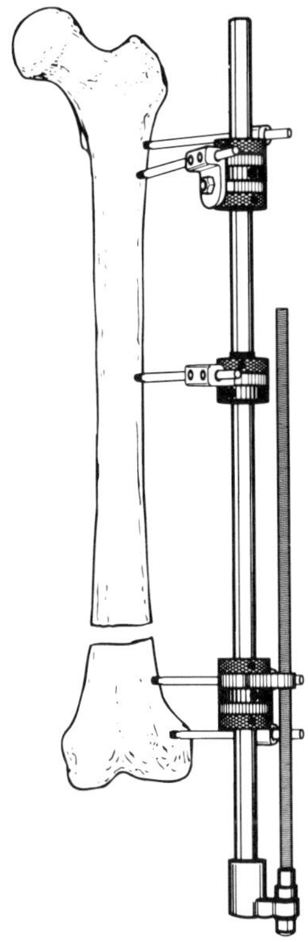

FIG. 5-60. Illustration of distal femoral osteotomy for lengthening using a Hex-Fix™ external fixator. (Courtesy of Smith and Nephew Richards, Memphis, TN.)

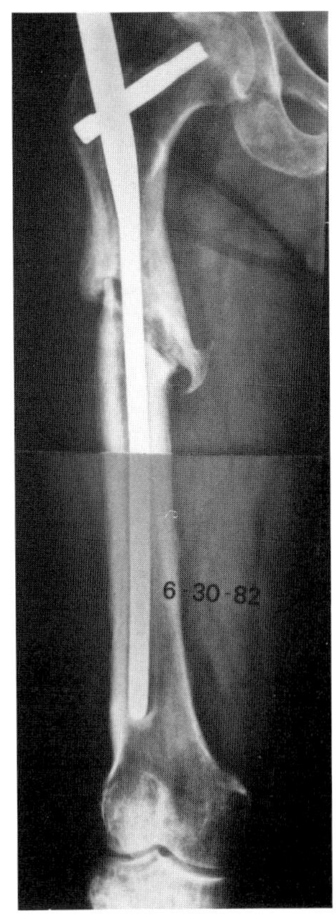

FIG. 5-61. The AP view of the femur with a Zickel nail for fixation. There is hypertrophic nonunion of the upper femoral fracture.

TABLE 5-3. *Femoral shaft fractures: complications*[7,11,15,20,30,44,53,60,76]

Local
Osseous
Refracture
Nonunion
Malunion
Delayed union
Associated fractures
Infection
Avascular necrosis of femoral head
Length discrepancy
Instrument failure
Soft tissue
Compartment syndrome
Venous thrombosis
Arterial injury
Neural injury
Knee stiffness (reduced range of motion)
Systemic
Distance fractures
Fat emboli
Pulmonary emboli
Adult respiratory distress syndrome
Pneumonia
Head injury
Abdominal Injury

From Berquist,[5] with permission.

Malunion is more common than nonunion. This is partially caused by muscle forces, which tend to angulate fragments. Malunion is more frequently associated with skeletal traction and closed cast treatment techniques.[5,15,33,51] However, shortening and rotation also occur with nonlocking intramedullary nails in up to 8% of cases.[15,42,74,75]

Delayed union, malunion, and nonunion can generally be evaluated with clinical findings and routine serial radiographs taken in at least two projections, typically AP and lateral views (Fig. 5-61).[5] Metallic implants may cause too much artifact for MRI or CT.[6] However, conventional tomography can still be useful, even in the presence of significant metal (Fig. 5-62).

A serious complication of femoral shaft fracture is unrecognized fracture of the ipsilateral hip, knee, tibia, and fibula. Ligament injuries of the knee must also be excluded if traction is considered for initial therapy.[5,15,57] Routine radiographs are usually adequate for an evaluation of ipsilateral combined injuries (Fig. 5-26).[5,24]

Refracture occurs infrequently with internal fixation (Fig. 5-63). It occurs most commonly in the initial 3 to 4 weeks during quadriceps exercises. Stress-induced remodeling reduces the risk of refracture after 8 to 12 weeks.[15]

Infection is a significant problem, which is and related to the extent of injury and treatment technique.[5,15,37,38] Infection occurs in ≥24% of Gustilo type III fractures. Further categorization of type III injuries (A, B, and C) was established to grade the degree of soft tissue injury. Type IIIA injuries demonstrate significant soft tissue injury, but the bone is still adequately covered. There is exposure of bone and periosteal stripping with type IIIB injuries. Type IIIC injuries have exposed bone and vascular injury.[38] Traction or external fixation may be best initially with these complex open wounds because wound access is enhanced.[15,33,37,38]

Infection can also be related to open surgical techniques.[5,15] Pin tract infections, which may involve the bone or soft tissues, occur with traction pins and external fixators.[4,5] Routine radiographs may not be effective for the early detection of infection, but MRI is sensitive and, in this setting, specific. However, significant metal artifact, especially from screws, reduces its usefulness.[6] Radionuclide studies are useful in subtle cases.[5] Combined technetium-99m methylene diphosphonate and gallium-67 or indium-111-labeled leukocytes are most useful.[5]

Instrument failure can occur with any fixation device (Figs. 5-62 and 5-64). Broken intramedullary nails occur more commonly with comminuted fractures and when the nail is too small for the femoral canal.[15,30] Nail fracture also occurs more commonly when distal femoral fractures are within 5 cm of the more proximal of the lower two holes (Fig. 5-65).[17] The fixation device may remain intact but fracture through the bone (Fig. 5-66).

Soft tissue complications (Table 5-3) include compartment syndrome, deep venous thrombosis, arterial, neural injury, and infection.[7,11,19,31,53,67] Reduced knee function may occur with femoral traction as a result of quadriceps scarring. External fixation pins can cause similar problems. This complication is less likely to occur with medullary nailing, especially using the closed technique.[5,11,15]

Soft tissue symptoms may be related to hardware positioning, such as screws that project too far into the soft tissues (Fig. 5-67). The proximal end of an intramedullary nail should protrude 1.3 to 1.9 cm above the femoral neck. It is not unusual to detect heterotopic ossification in this region (Fig. 5-68).[15]

Venous abnormalities in the thigh are generally easily evaluated with ultrasonography. Arterial injury requires angiography (Fig. 5-69). Subtle soft tissue or neural injury is most effectively evaluated with MRI if there is not too much metal in the region of interest (Fig. 5-70).6

Systemic complications (Table 5-3) occur more commonly with multisystem trauma or when treatment delays and prolonged hospitalization are required. The use of interlocking intramedullary nailing permits early exercise and mobilization, reducing the likelihood of these complications.[5,15]

Complications of Leg Lengthening

Many of the previously mentioned complications can also occur with leg-lengthening procedures. However,

(*text continues on page 396*)

A

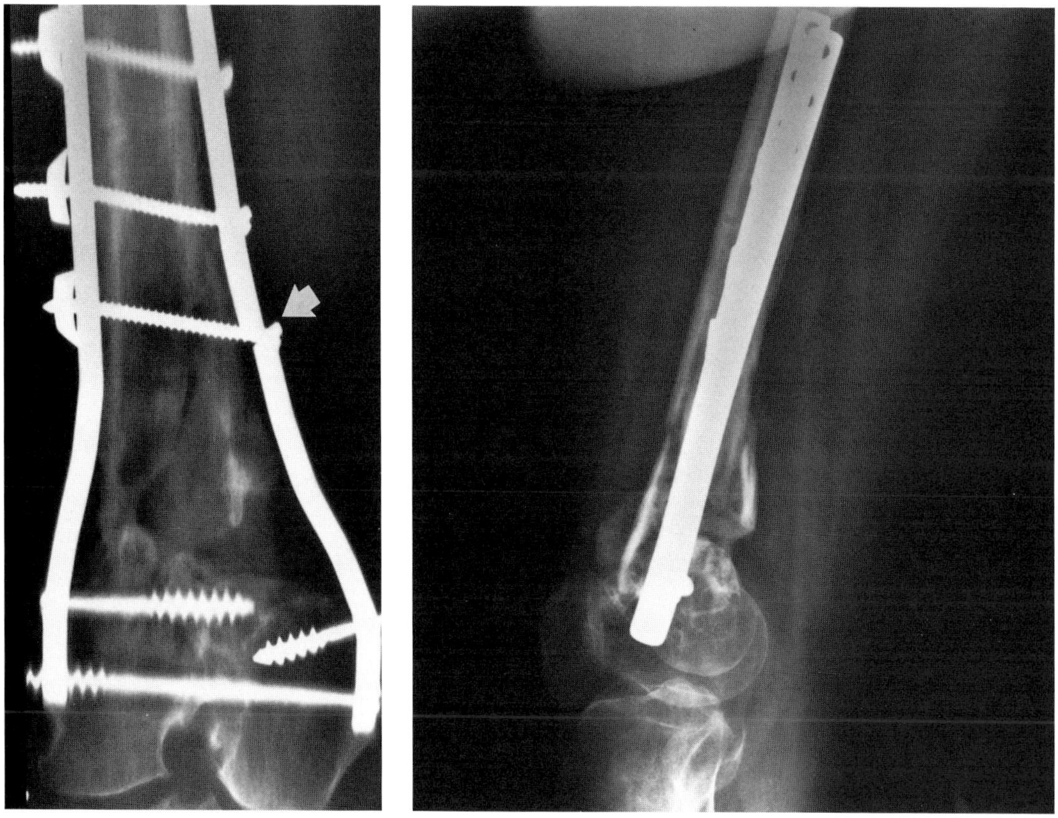

B

FIG. 5-62. The AP **(A)** and lateral **(B)** tomograms of a partially united distal femoral fracture with double-plate and screw fixation. There is a fracture (*arrow*) in the medial plate.

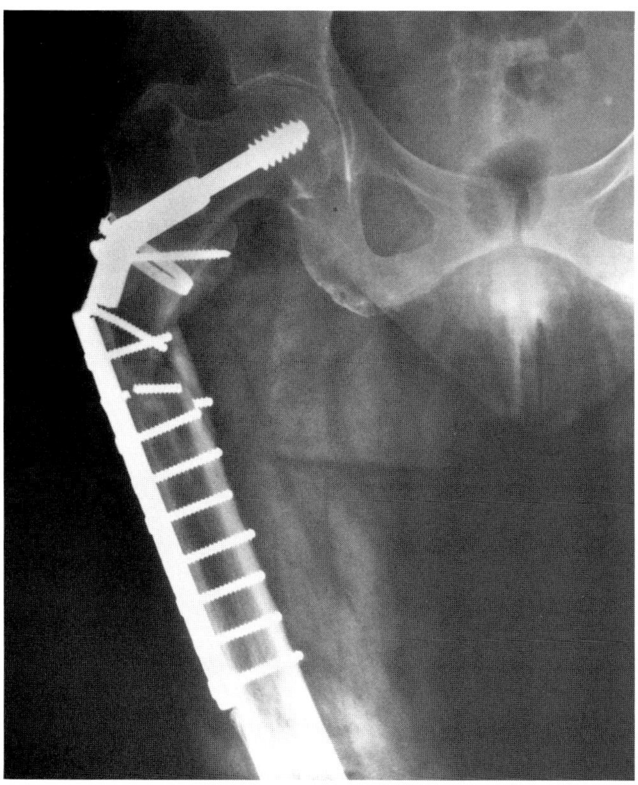

FIG. 5-63. An AP view of the femur demonstrating fracture of the side plate in an upper femoral fracture.

A

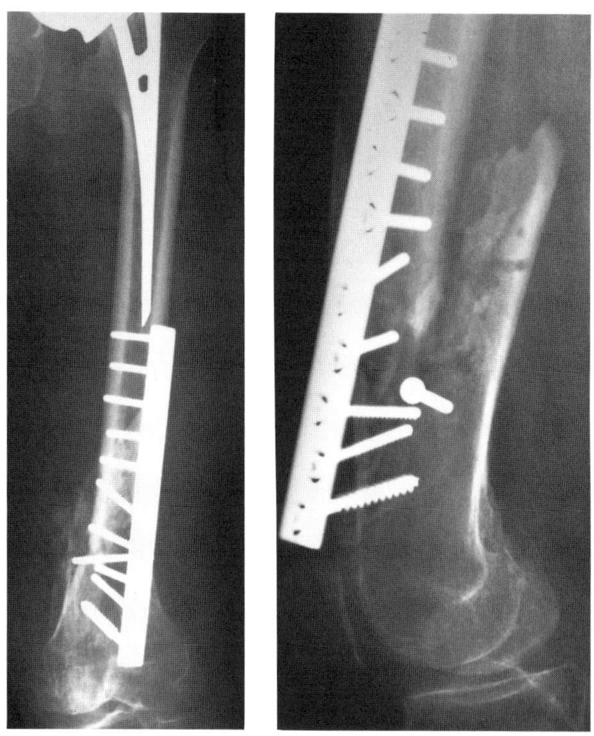

B

FIG. 5-64. A: An AP view of the femur demonstrating a proximal endoprosthesis with DC plate fixation of the comminuted distal femoral fracture. **B:** The lateral view shows pulling free of the distal fragment from the plate and screws.

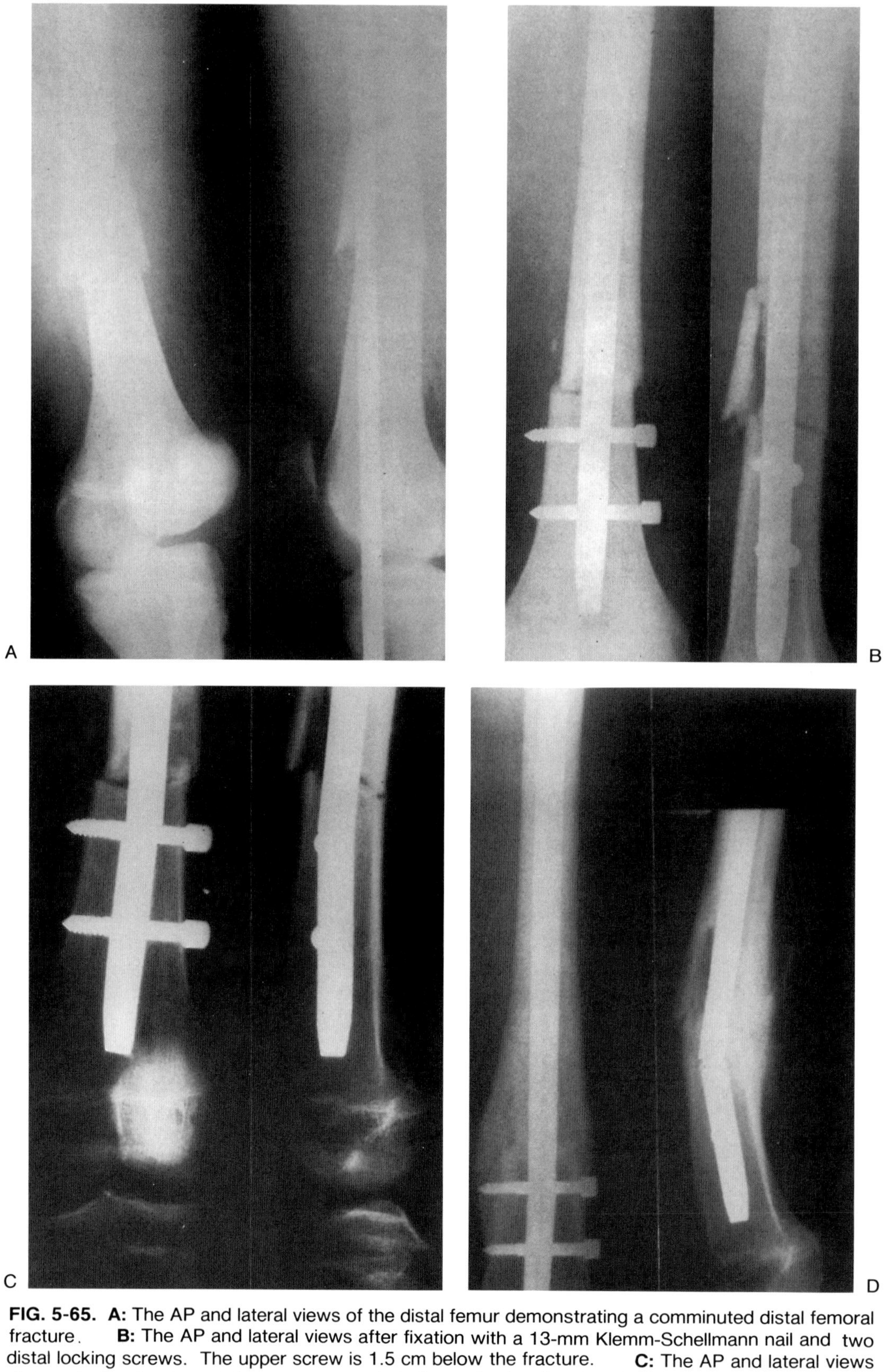

FIG. 5-65. **A:** The AP and lateral views of the distal femur demonstrating a comminuted distal femoral fracture. **B:** The AP and lateral views after fixation with a 13-mm Klemm-Schellmann nail and two distal locking screws. The upper screw is 1.5 cm below the fracture. **C:** The AP and lateral views demonstrating fracture at the upper screw hole 1 month after fixation. **D:** The AP and lateral views 6 months after fixation show healing with 15° of angulation. (From Bucholz RW, Ross SE, Lawrence KL. Fatigue fracture of the interlocking nail in the treatment of fractures of the distal part of the femoral shaft. *J Bone Joint Surg [Am]* 1987;69A:1391–1399.)

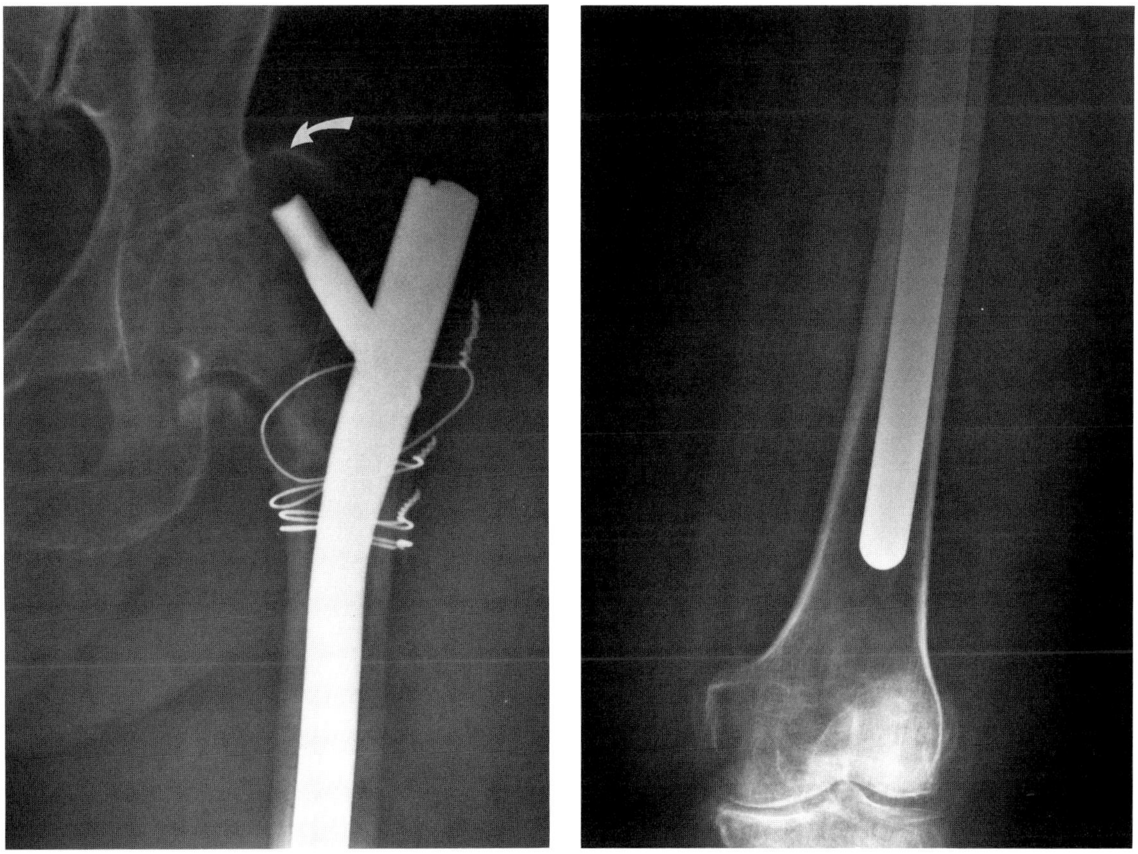

A B

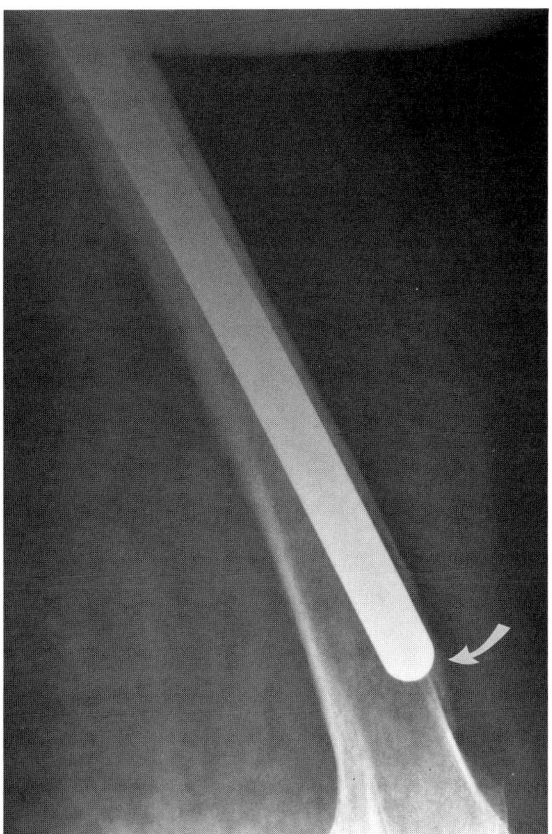

C

FIG. 5-66. Subtrochanteric fracture of the left femur with Zickel nail and cerclage wires proximally. **A:** The triphalangeal neck nail has fractured through and eroded the acetabular margin (*arrow*). The AP **(B)** and lateral **(C)** views show that the distal portion of the nail has broken through the anterior cortex (*arrow*).

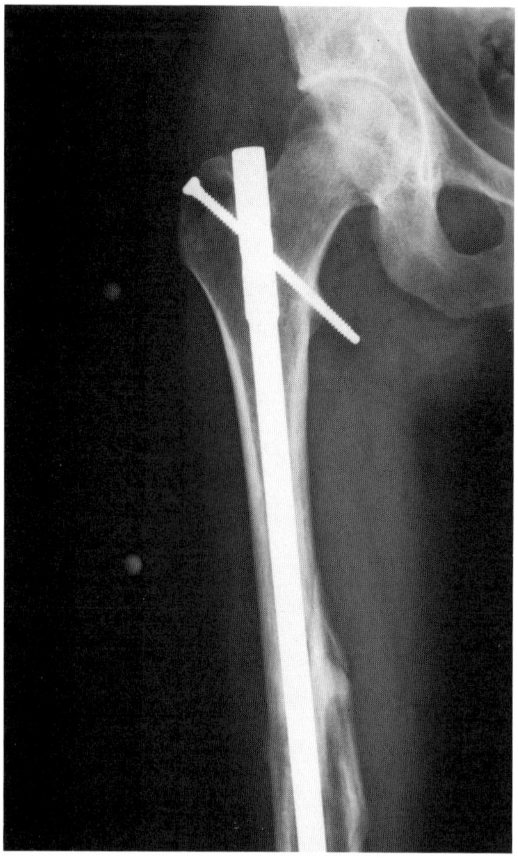

FIG. 5-67. An AP view of the right hip with a Russell-Taylor™ nail and proximal locking screw. The screw protrudes medially into the soft tissues. This may be of no consequence. If symptoms occur, fluoroscopic positioning should be used to detect the exact location of the screw tip. Either CT or ultrasonography can be used to evaluate adjacent soft tissues and vasculature.

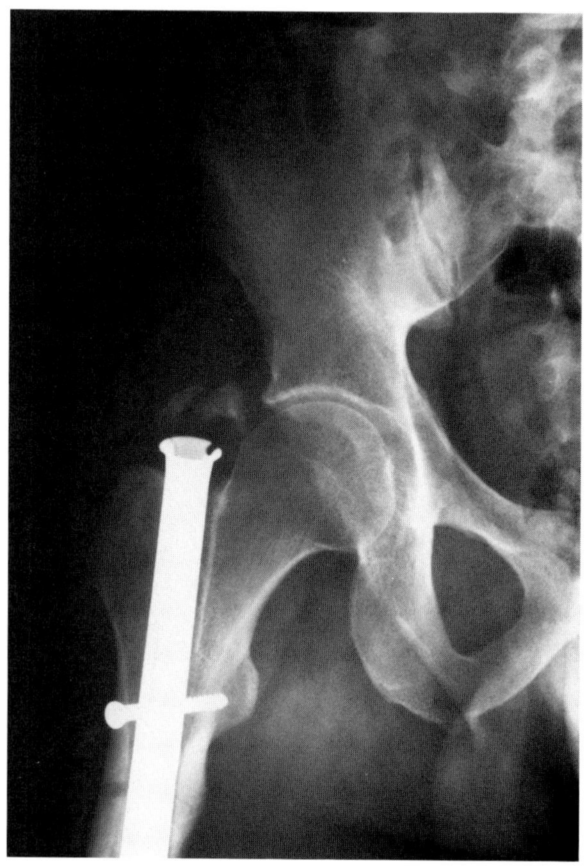

FIG. 5-68. The AP view of the hip demonstrating heterotopic bone over the upper end of the nail.

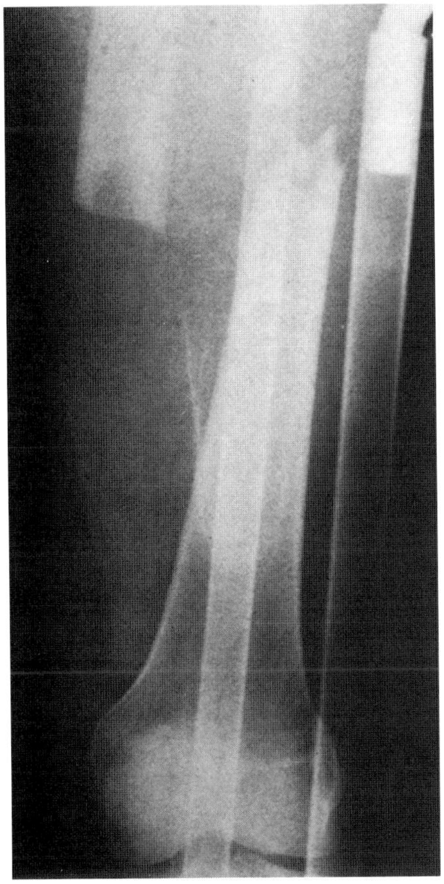

A

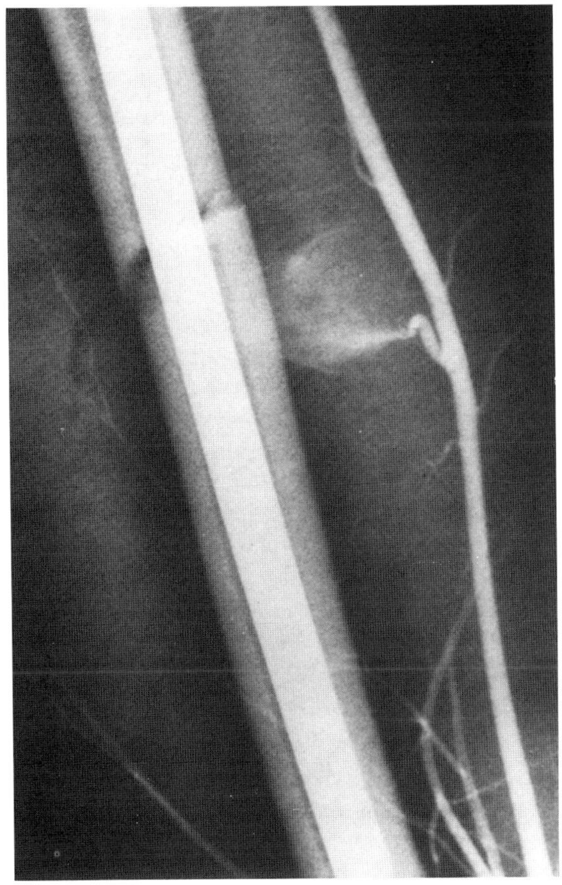

B

FIG. 5-69. Arterial injury with compartment syndrome. **A:** An AP view demonstrating a displaced femoral fracture. **B:** Arteriogram demonstrating bleeding from a branch of the superficial femoral artery. (From Tarlow SD, Achterman CA, Hayburst J, Ovida DN. Acute compartment syndrome in the thigh complicating fracture of the femur. *J Bone Joint Surg [Am]* 1986;68A:1439–1443.)

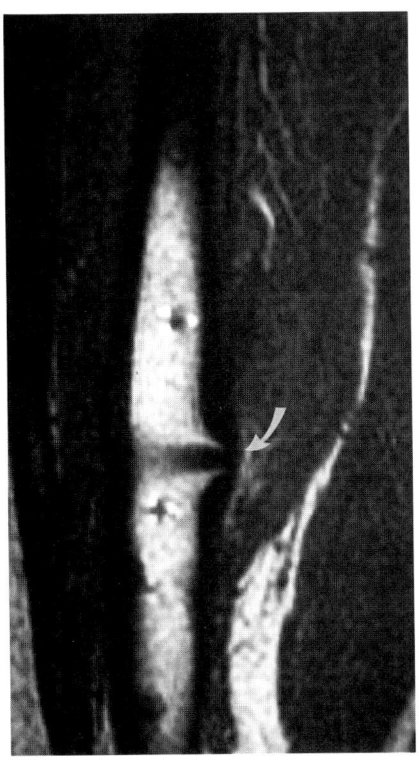

A

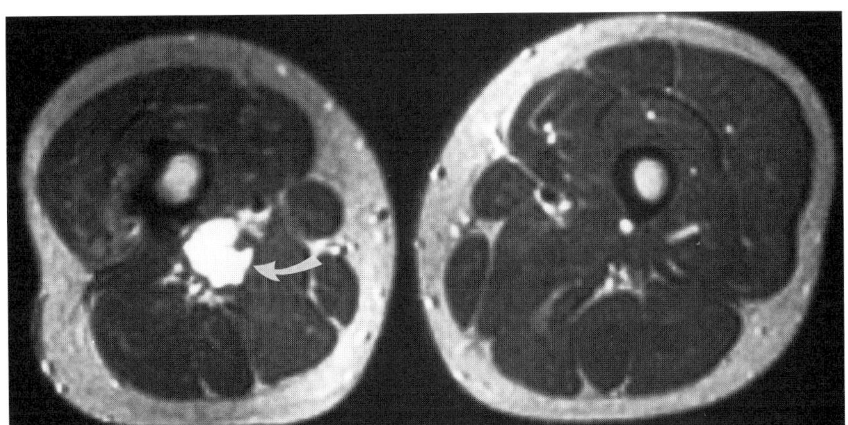

B

FIG. 5-70. Previous right femur fracture. The plate and screws were removed because of persistent pain. **A:** Sagittal spin-echo (SE) 500/20 image shows the pin tracts with cortical deformity (*arrow*). **B:** Axial SE 2,000/60 image shows a well-defined high-intensity lesion (*arrow*) caused by a posttraumatic neuroma.

TABLE 5-4. *Complications of leg lengthening*[25,26]

Complication	Techniques	
	Wägner (%)	Callotasis[a] (%)
Pin tract infection	22	2–10
Deep infection	7	2
Nonunion	10	1
Malunion	22	1–3
Premature consolidation	—	1–7
Compartment syndrome	3	0
Implant failure	2	0
Late fracture	11	3

[a] Includes both circular and uniplanar frame techniques. Premature healing only occurs with callotasis technique.

there are some variations, and the incidence of complications is much higher with lengthening procedures. Complications have been reported in 29% to 81% of cases.[25]

Minor sepsis around the pin tracts and pin tract loosening are the most common. Skin slough at the osteotomy site, fracture, premature consolidation, and angular deformities also occur.[25] Table 5-4 summarizes complications using Wägner and callotasis techniques.[26]

REFERENCES

1. Aaron A, Weinstein D, Thickman D, Elbert R. Comparison of orthoroentgenography and computed tomography in measurement of limb-length discrepancy. *J Bone Joint Surg* [*Am*] 1992;74A: 897–902.
2. Alho A, Stromsoe K, Ekeland A. Locked intramedullary nailing of femoral shaft fractures. *J Trauma* 1991;31:49–59.
3. Allen WC, Piotruwski G, Burstein A. A fluted femoral intramedullary rod: biomechanical analysis and preliminary clinical results. *J Bone Joint Surg* [*Am*] 1978;60A:500–515.
4. Barquet A, Manaferro J, Dubra A, Nin F. Ipsilateral open fracture of the femur and tibia treated by using the dynamic ASIF-BM tubular external fixator. *J Trauma* 1991;31:1312–1315.
5. Berquist TH. *Imaging of orthopedic trauma.* 2nd ed. New York: Raven Press; 1992.
6. Berquist TH. *MRI of the musculoskeletal system.* 2nd ed. New York: Raven Press; 1990.
7. Blumberg KD, Foster WC, Blumberg JF, Adelaar RS, Deblois ME, Hussey RW, Loughran TP, Cardea JA. A comparison of the Brooker-Wills and Russell-Taylor nails for treatment of patients who have fractures of the femoral shaft. *J Bone Joint Surg* [*Am*] 1990;72A:1019–1024.
8. Bone LB, Johnson KD, Weigelt J, Scheinberg R. Early versus delayed stabilization of femoral fractures. *J Bone Joint Surg* [*Am*] 1989;71A:336–340.
9. Brien WW, Wiss DA, Becker V, Lehman T. Subtrochanteric femur fractures: a comparison of Zickel nail, 95° blade plate and interlocking nail. *J Orthop Trauma* 1991;5:458–464.
10. Broekhuizen AH, Boxma H, van der Meulen PA, Snijders CJ. Performance of external fixation devices in femoral fractures; the ultimate challenge? A laboratory study with plastic rods. *Injury* 1990;21:145–151.
11. Brumback RJ, Ellison PS, Poka A, Lakatos R, Bathon GH, Burgess AR. Intramedullary nailing of open fractures of the femoral shaft. *J Bone Joint Surg* [*Am*] 1989;71A:1324–1330.
12. Brumback RJ, Reilly JP, Poka A, Lakatos RP, Bathon GH, Burgess AR. Intramedullary nailing of femoral shaft fractures. Part I: decision-making errors with interlocking fixation. *J Bone Joint Surg* [*Am*] 1988;70A:1441–1452.
13. Brumback RJ, Uwagie-Ero S, Lakatos RP, Poka A, Bathon GH, Burgess AR. Intramedullary nailing of femoral shaft fractures. Part II: fracture-healing with static interlocking fixation. *J Bone Joint Surg* [*Am*] 1988;70A:1453–1462.
14. Brumback RJ, Wells JD, Lakatos R, Poka A, Bathon GH, Burgess AR. Heterotopic ossification about the hip after intramedullary nailing for fractures of the femur. *J Bone Joint Surg* [*Am*] 1990;72A:1067–1073.
15. Bucholz RW, Brumback RJ. Fractures of the shaft of the femur. In: Rockwood CA, Green DD, Bucholz RW, eds. *Fractures in adults.* 3rd ed. Vol. 2. New York: JB Lippincott; 1991:1653–1724.
16. Bucholz RW, Jones A. Current concepts review. Fractures of the shaft of the femur. *J Bone Joint Surg* [*Am*] 1991;73A:1561–1566.
17. Bucholz RW, Ross SE, Lawrence KL. Fatigue cture of the interlocking nail in the treatment of fractures of tne distal part of the femoral shaft. *J Bone Joint Surg* [*Am*] 1987;69A:1391–1399.
18. Buxton RA. The use of Perkins traction in treatment of femoral shaft fractures. *J Bone Joint Surg* [*Br*] 1981;63B:362–366.
19. Clancey GJ. Acute posterior compartment syndrome in the thigh. *J Bone Joint Surg* [*Am*] 1985;67A:1278–1280.
20. Clancey GJ, Smith RF, Madenwald MB. Fractures of the distal end of the femur below hip implants in elderly patients. *J Bone Joint Surg* [*Am*] 1983;65A:491–494.
21. Coleman SS. Lower limb length discrepancy. In: Lovell WW, Winter RB, eds. *Pediatric orthopedics.* Vol. 2. Philadelphia: JB Lippincott; 1986:281–864.
22. Cooke TDV, Scudamore RA, Bryant JT, Sorbie C, Siu D, Fisher D. A quantitative approach to radiography of the lower limb. *J Bone Joint Surg* [*Br*] 1991;73B:715–720.
23. Covey DC, Saha S, Lipka JM, Albright JA. Biomechanical comparison of slotted and nonslotted interlocking nails in distal femoral shaft fractures. *Clin Orthop* 1990;252:246–251.
24. Daffner RH, Reuner BL, Butterfield SL. Ipsilateral femoral neck and shaft fractures: an overlooked associated. *Skeletal Radiol* 1991;20:251–254.
25. Dahl MT, Fischer DA. Lower extremity lengthening by Wagner's method and by callus distraction. *Orthop Clin North Am* 1991;22: 643–649.
26. Elridge JC, Bell DF. Problems with substantial limb-lengthening. *Orthop Clin North Am* 1991;22:625–631.
27. Faber FWM, Keescen W, Van Roermund PM. Complications of leg lengthening. *Acta Orthop Scand* 1991;62:327–332.
28. Fitzgerald JAW, Southgate GW. Cerclage wiring in the management of comminuted fractures of the femoral shaft. *Injury* 1987;18:111–116.
29. Folleràs G, Ahlo A, Strømsøe K, Ekeland E, Thoresen BO. Locked intramedullary nailing of fractures of femur and tibia. *Injury* 1990;21:385–388.
30. Franklin JL, Winquist RA, Benirschke SK, Hansen ST Jr. Broken intramedullary nails. *J Bone Joint Surg* [*Am*] 1988;70A:1463–1471.
31. Garland DE, Chick R, Taylor J, Salisbury RB. Treatment of proximal third femoral fractures with pins and thigh plaster. *Clin Orthop* 1981;160:86–93.
32. Glass RBJ, Poznauski AK. Leg-length determination with biplanar CT scanograms. *Radiology* 1985;156:833–834.
33. Green SA. Complications of external skeletal fixation. *Clin Orthop* 1983;180:109–115.
34. Green SA. The Ilizarov method: Raudio technique. *Orthop Clin North Am* 1991;22:677–688.
35. Green WT, Wyatt GM, Anderson M. Orthoroentgenography as a method of measuring the bones of the lower extremities. *J Bone Joint Surg* 1946;28:60–65.
36. Guichet JM, Spivak JM, Trouilloud P, Grammont PM. Lower limb-length discrepancy. An epidemiologic study. *Clin Orthop* 1991;272:235–241.
37. Gustilo RB, Anderson JT. Prevention of infection in treatment of 1025 open fractures of long bones. Retrospective and prospective analysis. *J Bone Joint Surg* [*Am*] 1976;58A:453–458.
38. Gustilo RB, Mendoza RM, Williams DN. Problems in management of type III (severe) open fractures. A new classification of type III open fractures. *J Trauma* 1984;24:742–746.
39. Hajek PD, Bidnell HR, Brouson WE, Albright JA, Saha S. The use of one compared to two distal screws in the treatment of femoral

shaft fractures with interlocking intramedullary nailing. *J Bone Joint Surg [Am]* 1993;75A:519–525.

40. Hanks GA, Handal JA, Evarts CM. Deep venous thrombosis after trauma to the lower extremity in patients who had a previous arthrodesis of the hip. A report of three cases. *J Bone Joint Surg [Am]* 1989;71A:1414–1417.
41. Hardy AE. The treatment of femoral fractures by cast-brace application and early ambulation. *J Bone Joint Surg [Am]* 1983;65A: 56–64.
42. Harkness JW, Ramsey WC, Harkness JW. Principles of fractures and dislocations. In: Rockwood CA, Green DP, Bucholz RW, eds. *Rockwood and Green's fractures in adults.* 3rd ed. Vol. 1. Philadelphia: JB Lippincott;1991:1–180.
43. Harper MC. Fractures of the femur treated by open and closed intramedullary nailing using fluted rod. *J Bone Joint Surg [Am]* 1985;67A:699–708.
44. Hely WL, Siliski JM, Incavo SJ. Operative treatment of distal femoral fractures proximal to total knee replacements. *J Bone Joint Surg [Am]* 1983;75A:27–34.
45. Helms CA, McCarthy S. CT scanograms for measuring leg length discrepancy. *Radiology* 1984;151:802.
46. Hogh J, Mikkelson P. Hansen-Street nailing of fractures of the femoral shaft. A study of 70 cases. *Injury* 1983;4:440–446.
47. Johansson JE, McBroom R, Barrington TW, Hunter GA. Fracture of the ipsilateral femur in patients with total hip replacement. *J Bone Joint Surg [Am]* 1981;63A:1435–1442.
48. Johnson KD, Johnston DWC, Parker B. Comminuted femoral shaft fractures: treatment by roller traction, cerclage wire and intramedullary nail or interlocking medullary nail. *J Bone Joint Surg* [Am] 1984;66A:1222–1235.
49. Kempf I, Grosse A, Beck G. Closed locked intramedullary nailing: its application to comminuted fractures of the femur. *J Bone Joint Surg [Am]* 1985;67A:709–720.
50. Knudsen CJM, Grobler GP, Close REW. Inserting distal screws in a locked femoral nail. *J Bone Joint Surg [Br]* 1991;73B:660–661.
51. Kretfek C, Haas N, Walker J, Tscherne H. Treatment of femoral shaft fractures in children by external fixation. *Injury* 1991;4:263–266.
52. Leung KS, Shen WY, So WS, Mui LT, Grosse A. Interlocking intramedullary nailing for supracondylar fractures of the distal part of the femur. *J Bone Joint Surg [Am]* 1991;73A:332–340.
53. Majkowski RS, Baker AS. Interlocking nails for femoral fractures: 28 patients followed for 1–2 years. *Acta Orthop Scand* 1991;62: 342–345.
54. Merrill OE. A method for the roentgen measurement of long bones. *AJR Am J Roentgenol* 1942;48:405–406.
55. Moseley CF. Leg lengthening: the historical perspective. *Orthop Clin North Am* 1991;22:555–561.
56. Murphy CP, D'Ambrosia RD, Dabezies EJ, Acker JH, Shoji H, Chuinard RG. Complex femur fractures: treatment with the Wagner external fixation device or the Grosse-Kempf interlocking nail. *J Trauma* 1988;28:1553–1561.
57. Neumann L. Subtrochanteric fractures following Gouffon pinning of subcapital femoral fractures. *Injury* 1990;21:366–368.
58. Nichols PJR. Rehabilitation after fracture of the shaft of the femur. *J Bone Joint Surg [Br]* 1965;45B:96–102.
59. Österman K, Merikanto J. Diaphyseal bone lengthening in children using Wagner device: long-term results. *J Pediatr Orthop* 1991;1:449–451.
60. Pankovich AM, Goldflies ML, Pearson RL. Closed Ender nailing of femoral-shaft fractures. *J Bone Joint Surg [Am]* 1979;61A:222–232.
61. Pasqualini M, Murena PF. The Grosse-Kempf nail in femoral and tibial shaft fractures. *Int Orthop Traumatol* 1991;17:321–336.
62. Pugh DG, Winkler NT. Scanography for leg length measurement: an easy satisfactory method. *Radiology* 1966;87:130–133.
63. Rööser B, Bengtson S, Herrlin K, Önnerfält R. External fixation of femoral fractures: experience with 15 cases. *J Orthop Trauma* 1990;4:70–74.
64. Rüedi T. Intramedullary nailing with interlocking. *Arch Orthop Trauma Surg* 1990;109:317–320.
65. Rüedi TP, Lüscher JN. Results after internal fixation of comminuted fractures of the femoral shaft with DC plates. *Clin Orthop* 1979;138:74–76.
66. Sanders R, Swiontkowski M, Rosen H, Helfet D. Double-plating of comminuted, unstable fractures of the distal part of the femur. *J Bone Joint Surg [Am]* 1991;73A:341–346.
67. Schwartz JT, Brumback RJ, Lakatos R, Poka A, Gathon H, Burgess AR. Acute compartment syndrome of the thigh. *J Bone Joint Surg [Am]* 1989;71A:392–400.
68. Seiler JG III, Swiontkowski MF. A prospective evaluation of the AO/ASIF universal femoral nail in the treatment of traumatic and reconstructive problems of the femur. *J Trauma* 1991;131:121–126.
69. Seligson D, Kristiansen TK. Use of the Wagner apparatus in complicated fractures of the distal femur. *J Trauma* 1978;18:795–799.
70. Star AM, Whittaker RP, Shuster HM, Duda J, Menkowitz E. Difficulties during removal of fluted femoral intramedullary rods. *J Bone Joint Surg [Am]* 1989;71A:343–344.
71. Strømsøe K, Alho A, Ekeland A. The Grosse-Kempf nail for distal femoral fractures. 2-year follow-up of 25 cases. *Acta Orthop Scand* 1990;61:512–516.
72. Styf JR, Körner LM. Chronic anterior compartment syndrome of the leg. *J Bone Joint Surg [Am]* 1986;68A:1338–1352.
73. Tarlow SD, Achterman CA, Hayburst J, Ovida DN. Acute compartment syndrome in the thigh complicating fracture of the femur. *J Bone Joint Surg [Am]* 1986;68A:1439–1443.
74. Taylor JC. Fractures of the lower extremity. In: Crenshaw AH, ed. *Campbell's operative orthopedics.* 8th ed. St. Louis: CV Mosby; 1992:785–893.
75. Thoresen BO, Alho A, Ekeland A, Strømsøe K, Follerås G, Haukebø A. Interlocking intramedullary nailing in femoral shaft fractures. A report of 48 cases. *J Bone Joint Surg [Am]* 1985;67A: 1313–1320.
76. Velazquez RJ, Bell DF, Armstrong PF, Babyn P, Tibshirani R. Complications of the use of the Ilizarov technique in correction of limb deformities in children. *J Bone Joint Surg [Am]* 1993;75A: 1148–1156.
77. White EM, Healy WL, Brumback RJ, Burgess AR, Brooker AF. The treatment of fractures of the femoral shaft with the Brooker-Wills distal locking intramedullary nail. *J Bone Joint Surg [Am]* 1986;68A:865–876.
78. Walters J, Shepherd-Wilson W, Lyons T, Close R. Femoral shaft fractures treated by Ender nails using a trochanteric approach. *J Bone Joint Surg [Br]* 1990;72B:14–18.
79. Winquist RA, Hansen ST Jr. Comminuted fractures of the femoral shaft treated by intramedullary nailing. *Orthop Clin North Am* 1980;11:633–648.
80. Winquist RA, Hansen ST Jr, Clawson DK. Closed intramedullary nailing of femoral fractures. A report of 520 cases. *J Bone Joint Surg [Am]* 1988;66A:529–539.
81. Wu CC, Shih CH, Lee ZL. Subtrochanteric fractures treated with interlocking nailing. *J Trauma* 1991;31:326–333.
82. Zickel RE. Fractures of the adult femur excluding femoral head and neck. *Clin Orthop* 1980;147:93–114.
83. Zickel RE, Fietti VG, Lawsing JF III, Cochran GVB. A new intramedullary fixation device for distal third of the femur. *Clin Orthop* 1977;125:185–191.

Imaging Atlas of Orthopedic Appliances and Prostheses,
edited by T.H. Berquist.
Mayo Clinic Foundation © 1995.
Published by Raven Press, Ltd., New York.

CHAPTER 6

The Knee

Thomas H. Berquist and Kurt E. Blasser

The knee is a complex anatomic structure. Osseous, cartilaginous, and passive and dynamic restraints must be preserved to ensure optimal function. To this end, numerous orthopedic procedures and devices have been designed to maintain a knee that is functional and pain free. This chapter demonstrates orthopedic devices and imaging techniques used for trauma, arthroplasty, and other common surgical procedures used in the knee.

TRAUMA

Preoperative Imaging

Routine radiographic techniques remain the most useful screening technique for skeletal injuries about the knee. Soft tissue changes on routine films are also useful in suggesting associated ligament injuries.[4,6,16,46] We routinely obtain anteroposterior (AP), lateral, and oblique views of the knee in the acute setting (Fig. 6-1). Standing views are not normally required to evaluate trauma.[46] However, ideally, the lateral view should be obtained using cross-table technique. A lipohemarthrosis may be the only clue to a subtle intraarticular fracture (Fig. 6-2).[23] The presence of an effusion or hemarthrosis may indicate anterior cruciate ligament (ACL) injury (Fig. 6-3).6,46 Additional views, such as the notch view (Fig. 6-4) and patellar views (Fig. 6-5), may be useful for the detection of subluxation, dislocation, osteochondral fractures, and patellar fractures.[19,28,31,33,35,38,40]

Stress views are useful for soft tissue evaluation (Fig. 6-6). However, they can be difficult to perform, inaccurate, and harmful when done by inexperienced persons.[6,33] Magnetic resonance imaging (MRI) is more frequently used to evaluate soft tissue and articular injuries if the patient's status will allow the procedure to be performed (Fig. 6-7).[5]

Subtle or complex injuries may require conventional or computed tomography (CT) for complete evaluation.[1,6,46] These techniques are discussed more fully later as they apply to specific injuries.

Supracondylar Fractures of the Femur

Supracondylar fractures of the femur are those fractures involving the distal 9 to 15 cm, as measured from the articular surface of the femoral condyles.[6,22,54] These fractures may be impacted, undisplaced, displaced, or comminuted (Fig. 6-8).[26] When such fractures are intraarticular (Fig. 6-9), they present an even more difficult treatment challenge than do the supracondylar fractures that do not involve the articular surface. When comminution is severe, preoperative CT or conventional tomography may be useful to assist in treatment planning.[46] Associated injuries of the tibial plateau, knee, and hip are frequent.[50] Therefore, the entire femur, hip, and knee should be evaluated to exclude associated injuries.[46]

The mechanism of injury is usually varus or valgus stress, with associated axial or rotary forces. The injuries are usually related to high-velocity trauma, such as occurs in motor vehicle accidents.[26,46,50]

Classification

The general configuration of supracondylar fractures was noted earlier (Fig. 6-8). Several classification

(*text continues on page 405*)

T. H. Berquist: Mayo Medical School and Department of Diagnostic Radiology, Mayo Clinic Jacksonville, Jacksonville, Florida 32224.

K. E. Blasser: Department of Orthopedics, Mayo Clinic Jacksonville, Jacksonville, Florida 32224.

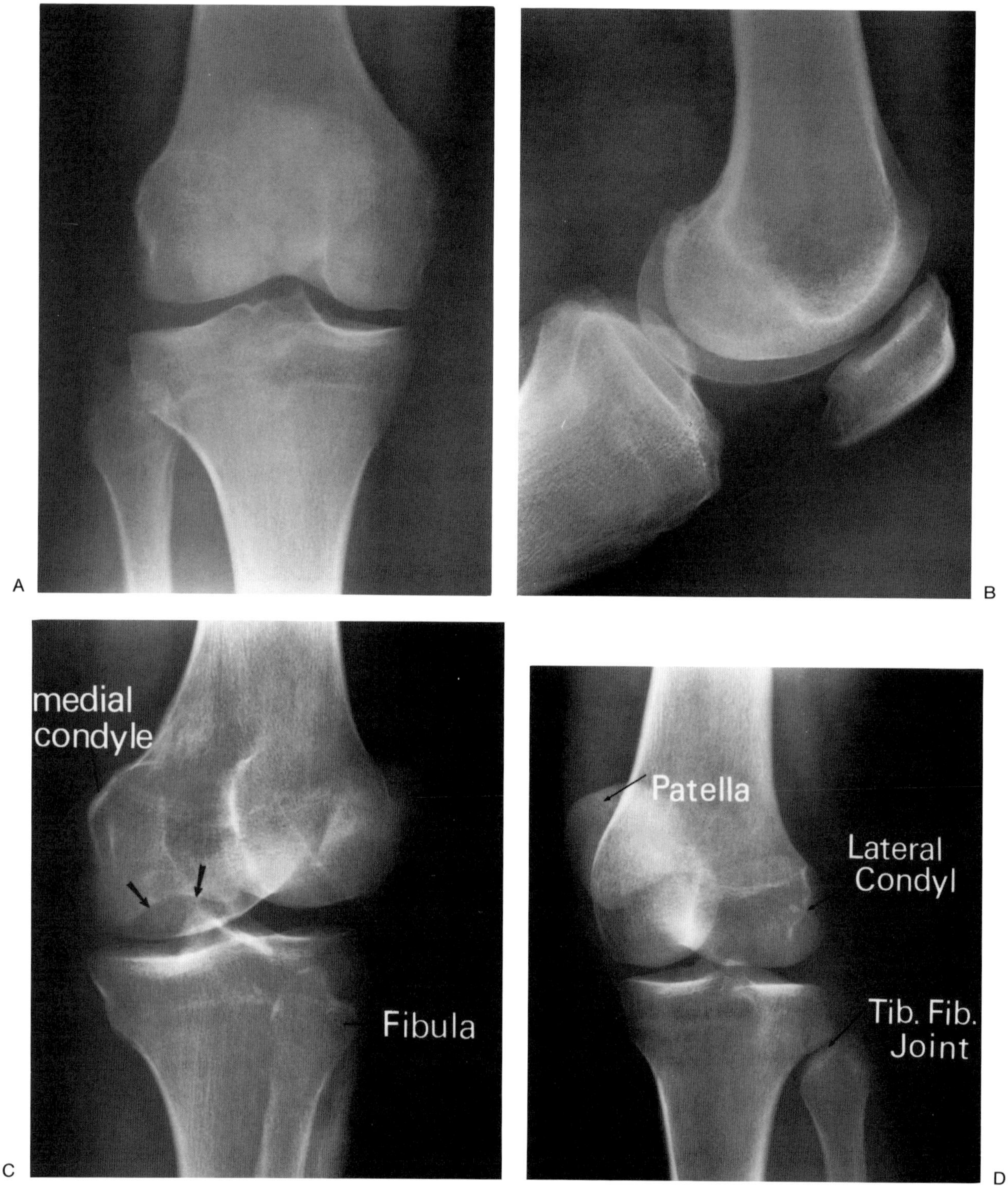

FIG. 6-1. Normal AP **(A)** and lateral **(B)** views of the knee. External **(C)** and internal **(D)** oblique views. The external oblique (C) demonstrates the medial joint and osseous structures to better advantage. Note the femoral condyle fracture (*arrows*). The internal oblique view (D) demonstrates the lateral compartment and tibiofibular articulation.

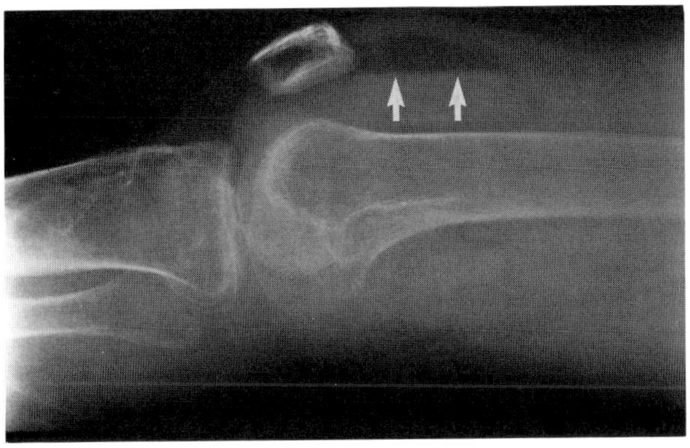

FIG 6-2. Cross-table lateral view of the knee demonstrating a lipohemarthrosis (*arrows*).

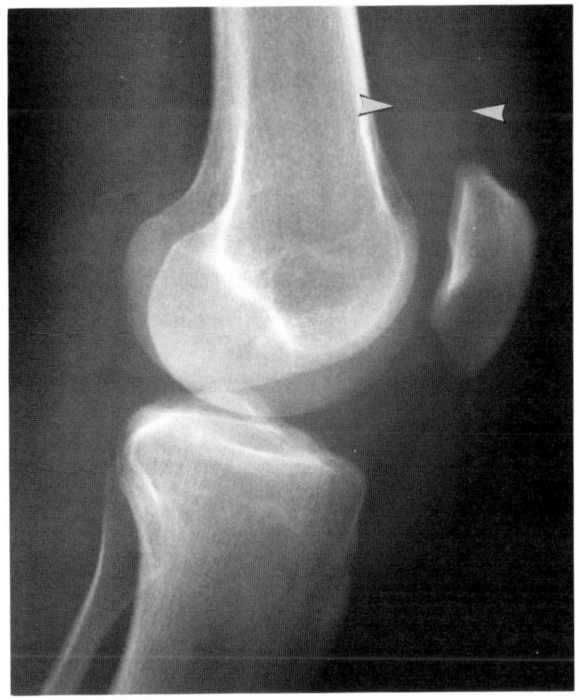

FIG. 6-3. Lateral view of the knee demonstrating a large effusion (*arrows*) in a patient with an acute ACL tear.

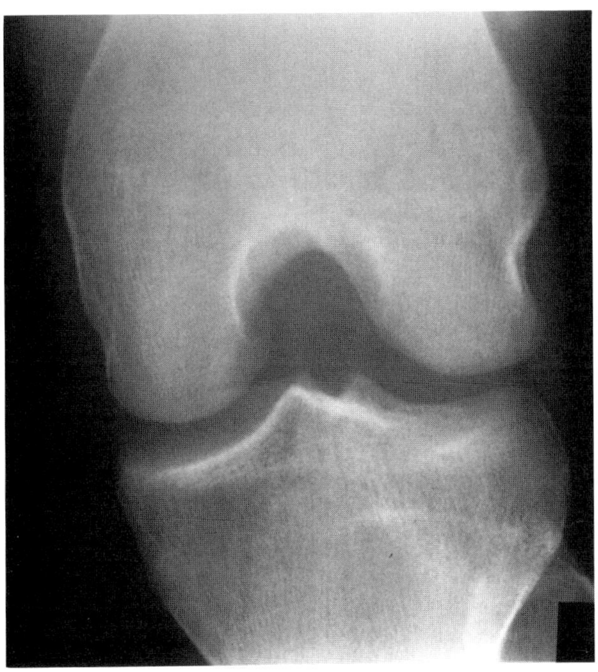

A

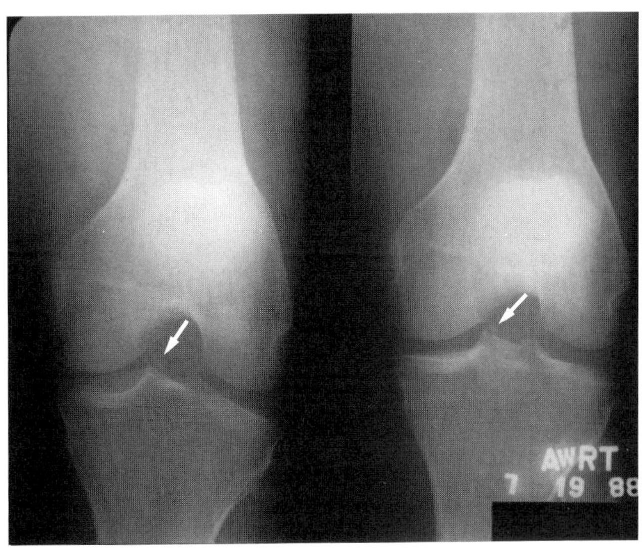

B

FIG. 6-4. Notch views. Normal notch view **(A)** and notch view **(B)** demonstrating a tibial spine fracture (*arrow*).

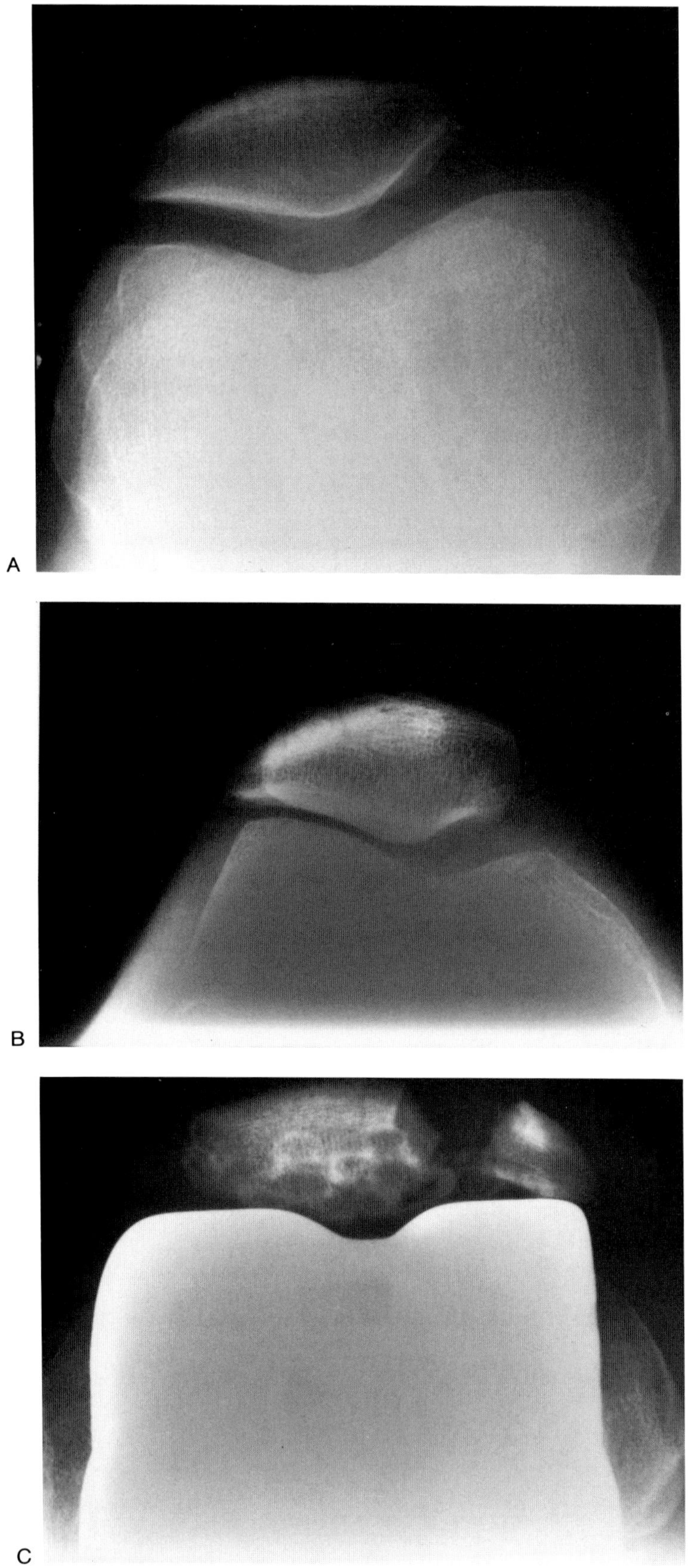

FIG. 6-5. Patellar views. **A:** Normal view. **B:** Lateral subluxation with joint space narrowing. **C:** Knee arthroplasty with all-polyethylene patellar component complicated by a lateral fracture.

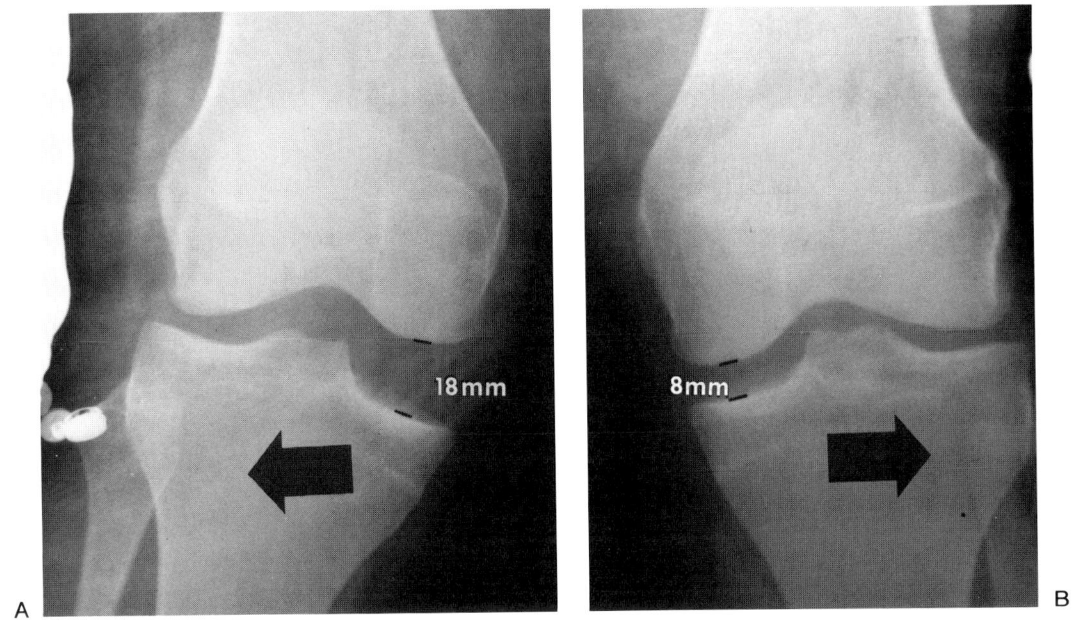

FIG. 6-6. Stress views include AP, varus, and valgus. Stress is applied to both knees for comparison. The examination should be performed with fluoroscopic guidance. Valgus stress views of the right **(A)** and normal left knee **(B)** demonstrate a 10-mm difference on the right in a patient with MCL and ACL disruptions.

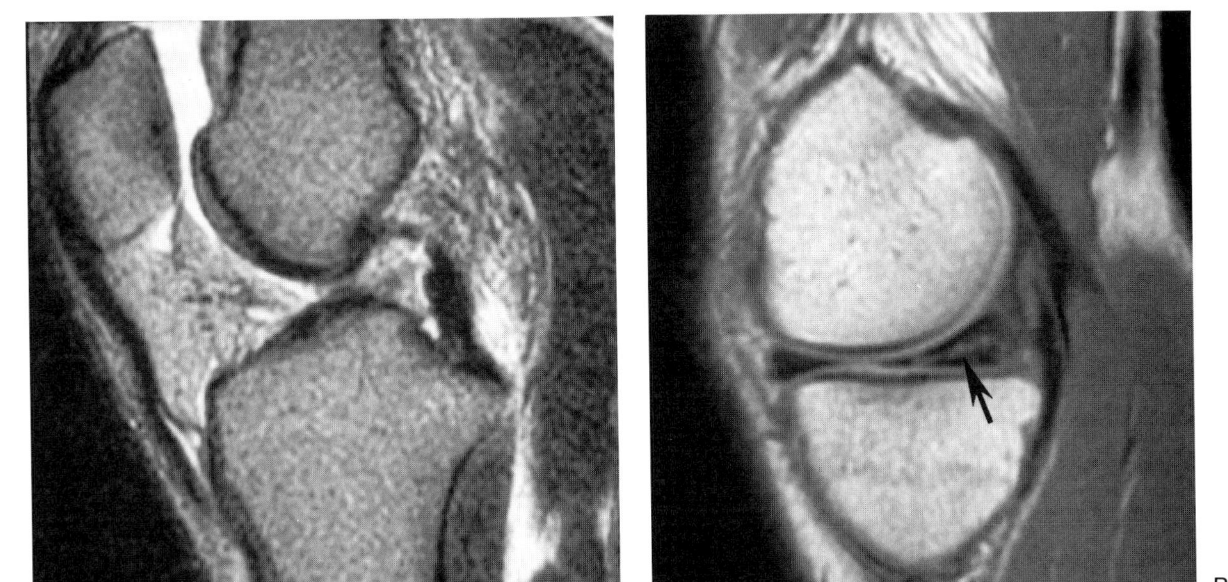

FIG. 6-7. The MRI scans of soft tissue injuries of the knee. **A:** Sagittal SE 2,000/60 image demonstrating an effusion and complete tear of the ACL. **B:** Sagittal SE 2,000/30 image demonstrating an oblique tear (*arrow*) of the posterior horn of the medial meniscus.

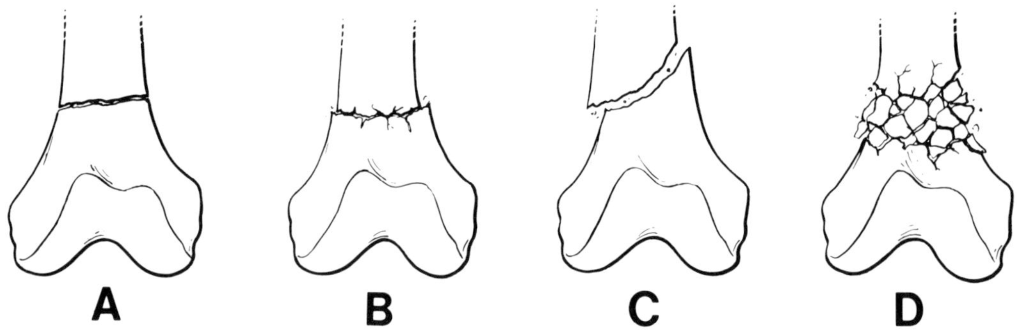

FIG. 6-8. General categories of nonintraarticular supracondylar fractures. **A:** Undisplaced. **B:** Impacted. **C:** Displaced. **D:** Comminuted.

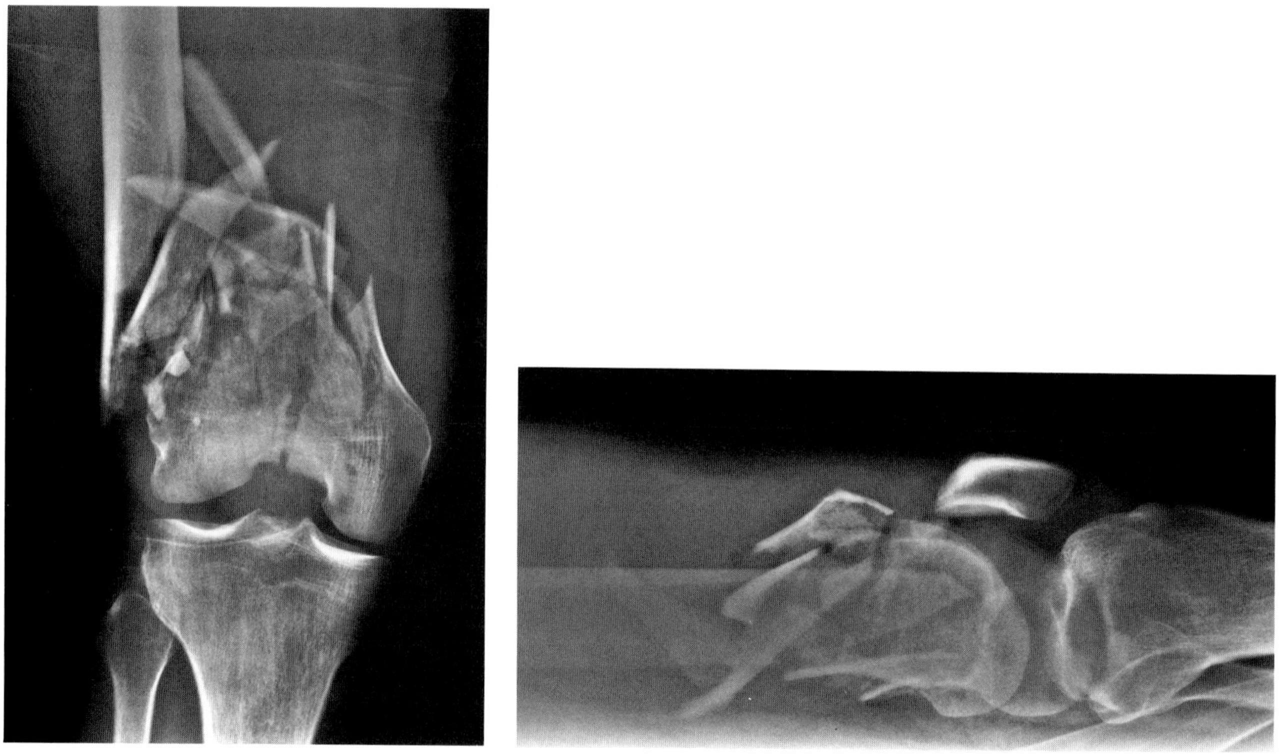

FIG. 6-9. The AP **(A)** and lateral **(B)** radiographs of a severely comminuted intraarticular supracondylar fracture.

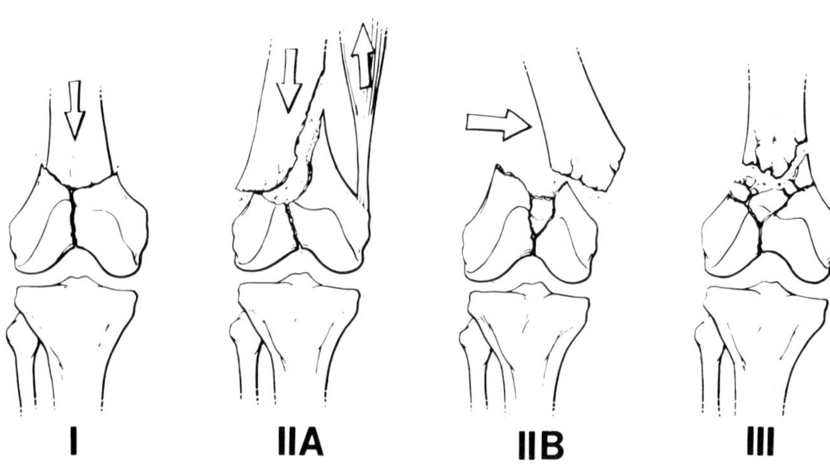

FIG. 6-10. The Neer[43] classification for supracondylar fractures of the femur. A type I fracture is Y- or T-shaped intraarticular fracture with minimal displacement. Type IIA has condylar segments that are displaced medially. Type IIB has condylar segments that are displaced laterally. Type III has comminution of the distal shaft with intraarticular involvement.

schemes have been suggested for supracondylar fractures. The two most frequently used were described by Neer et al.[43] (Fig. 6-10) and Seinsheimer[52] (Fig. 6-11). Using the Neer system, type I fractures are minimally displaced (Fig. 6-10). These fractures comprised 31% of cases in their series.[43] Type II fractures were divided into two subgroups. The condyles are medially displaced in type IIA (29%) and laterally displaced in type IIB (21%). The distal shaft is comminuted in type III fractures (Fig. 6-10).

Four categories are recognized using the Seinsheimer classification.[52] A type 1 fracture (Fig. 6-11) is nondisplaced. Type 2 fractures have two subgroups (A, two part; B, comminuted), and the fracture does not extend into the intraarticular region. Type 3 fractures are divided into three subgroups, depending on whether the medial (A), lateral (B), or both condyles (C) are separated (Fig. 6-11). Type 4 fractures involve the articular surface of the condyles (Fig. 6-11) and, like type 3 fractures, are subdivided, depending on whether medial (A), lateral (B), or more complex articular surface involvement (C and D) is present.

Treatment

The treatment options are similar for intraarticular and nonarticular supracondylar fractures. The treatment goal for nonintraarticular fractures is to restore axial alignment. The goal for treating intraarticular fractures is to restore the anatomy of the articular surface. The treatment options include closed and open techniques.[24,41] Reduction can be difficult to obtain or maintain because of the muscle forces acting on the fragments. Impacted fractures may be treated with long leg casting.[46] Traction is commonly used for comminuted fractures, at least during the initial stages of treatment.[26,43,46,52] Although single- or double-pin traction is commonly used (Figs. 6-12 and 6-13), a single traction pin can be placed in the upper tibia. A second pin in the distal fragment adds to fragment stability, but additional complications must be considered (see Chapter 2).

Open treatment can be accomplished using Ender nails, Rush rods, interlocking medullary nails, or the Zickel intramedullary appliances (Fig. 6-14).[26,58] More commonly, blade plates (Fig. 6-15) (Elliot, Jewett, or AO) or dynamic condylar screws (Fig. 6-16) are used. These have largely replaced plate and screw techniques. Ipsilateral shaft and distal fractures can be treated with interlocking medullary nails in some cases (Fig. 6-17).[13] The thin cortex in the condylar and metaphyseal region makes it difficult to obtain optimal screw purchase.[58] Most supracondylar fractures heal in 3 to 4 months, but delayed union (Fig. 6-18) is fairly common.[26]

Relative contraindications to internal fixation include severe comminution and osteoporotic bone in elderly patients.[46]

Patellar Fractures

Patellar fractures comprise about 1% of skeletal injuries.[10] Its superficial anterior position over the knee places the patella at risk for direct trauma. Indirect trauma frequently results in a greater degree of separation (Fig. 6-19).[10,46]

Classification

Patellar fractures are classified according to the location and plane of the fractures.[32,46] In 34% to 80% of cases, the fractures are transverse or oblique. Stellate or comminuted fractures make up 16% to 30% and vertical fractures, 12% to 28% of patellar fractures.[10,26,46]

Radiographs

The AP, lateral, and axial or Merchant views (Fig. 6-20) are required to identify patellar fractures and evaluate the articular surfaces. The lateral view is most useful for evaluating separation (Fig. 6-19), and both the axial and lateral views are useful for evaluating the articular surface.[4,6,46] Bipartite patella should not be confused with a fracture. A bipartite patella is frequently bilateral, and the ossicle is located in the upper outer quadrant of the patella (Fig. 6-21).[6,7]

Treatment

The treatment goals include anatomic reduction, restoration of soft tissues (specifically the retinacula and anterior extensor mechanism), and accurate articular restoration.[46]

Simple fractures with minimal (2 to 4 mm) displacement and articular irregularity may be treated with a cylinder cast for 3 to 6 weeks.[8,10,26] Open or percutaneous pin reduction is recommended for fractures (transverse or oblique) with > 4 mm of separation (Fig. 6-22).[8,10,26,45,46] Simple tension-band wiring (see Chapter 2) is usually modified by the addition of two vertical Kirschner wires (K wires, Figs. 6-19 and 6-22). The compression forces of the quadriceps assist in reducing the articular separation postoperatively.[8,46] Cerclage wiring may also be used (Fig. 6-23). This technique provides stronger support than do tension-band or modified tension-band techniques. Cerclage wiring is especially useful for comminuted fractures.[15]

Percutaneous pins with external clamps (Fig. 6-24) can also be used, but this technique is not common in North America.[45]

Vertical fractures or severely comminuted fractures or small inferior pole fractures may require partial or complete patellectomy.[10]

(*text continues on page 418*)

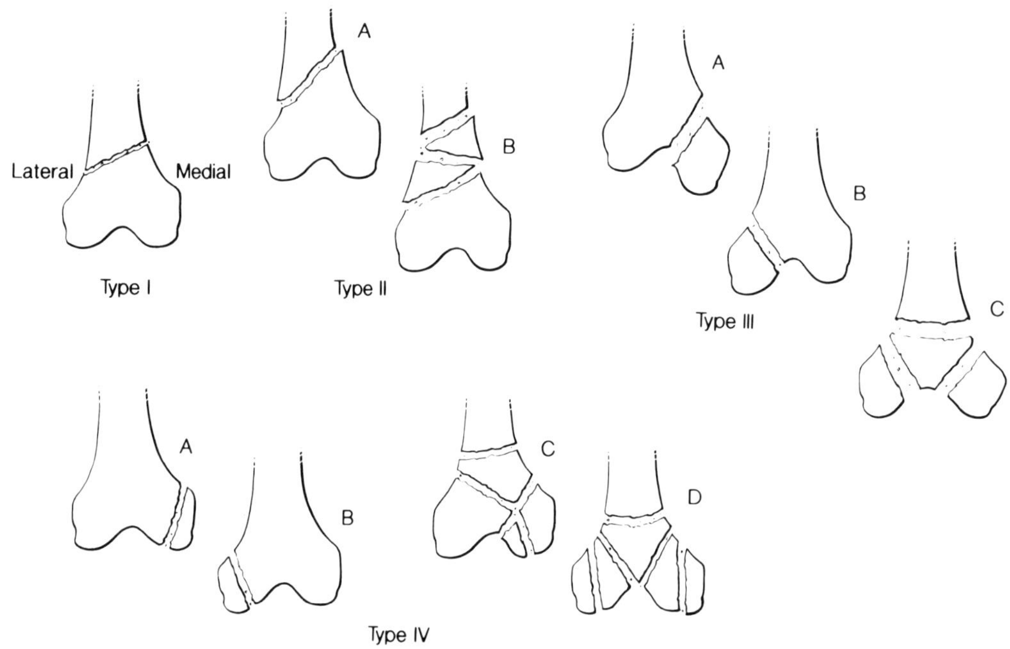

FIG. 6-11. Seinsheimer[52] classification. Type 1 is an undisplaced supracondylar fracture. Type 2A is a displaced two-part fracture with no intraarticular component. Type 2B is a displaced comminuted fracture with no intraarticular involvement. Type 3A is an isolated medial condylar fracture. Type 3B is an isolated lateral condylar fracture. In type 3C, both condyles are fractured with a supracondylar fracture. Type 4A is a fracture of the articular surface of the medial condyle. Type 4B is a fracture of the lateral condylar articular surface. In a type 4C, there is comminution of one or, in type 4D, both condylar articular surfaces.

A

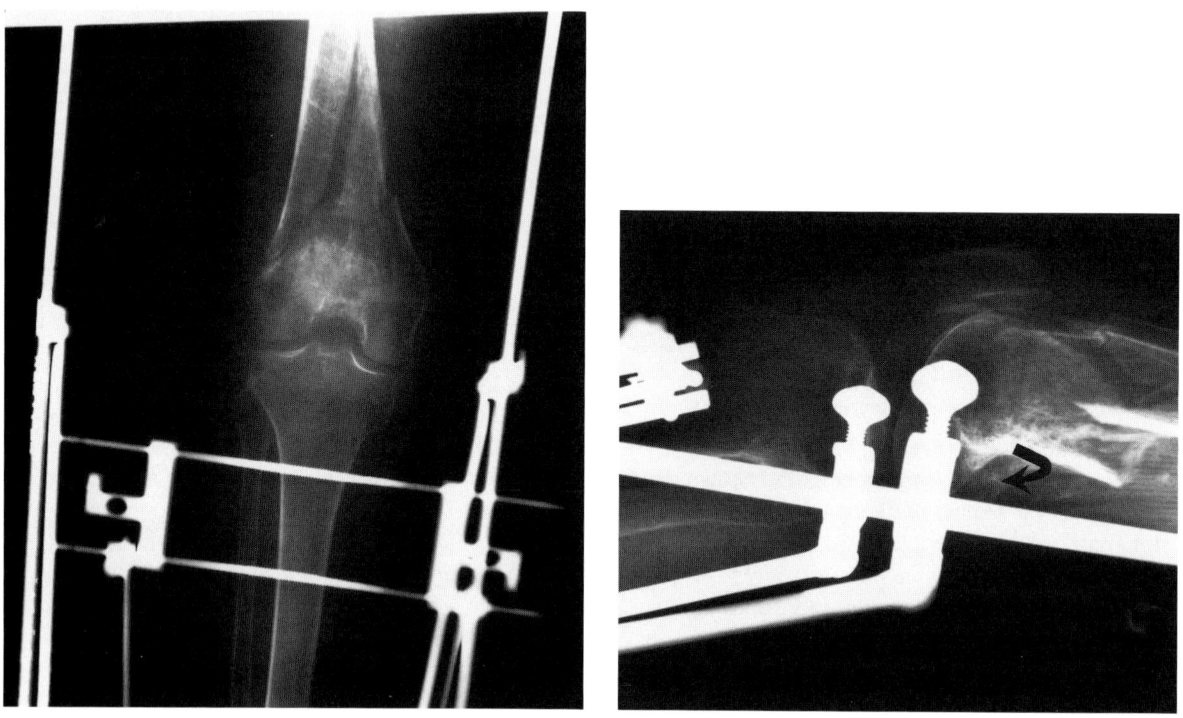

B

FIG. 6-12. Supracondylar fracture in traction with double tibial pins. **A:** The AP view of the comminuted supracondylar fracture of the right femur. Two threaded Steinmann pins are in the upper tibia. **B:** Lateral view demonstrates posterior rotation of the distal fragment as a result of gastrocnemius muscle forces (*arrow*).

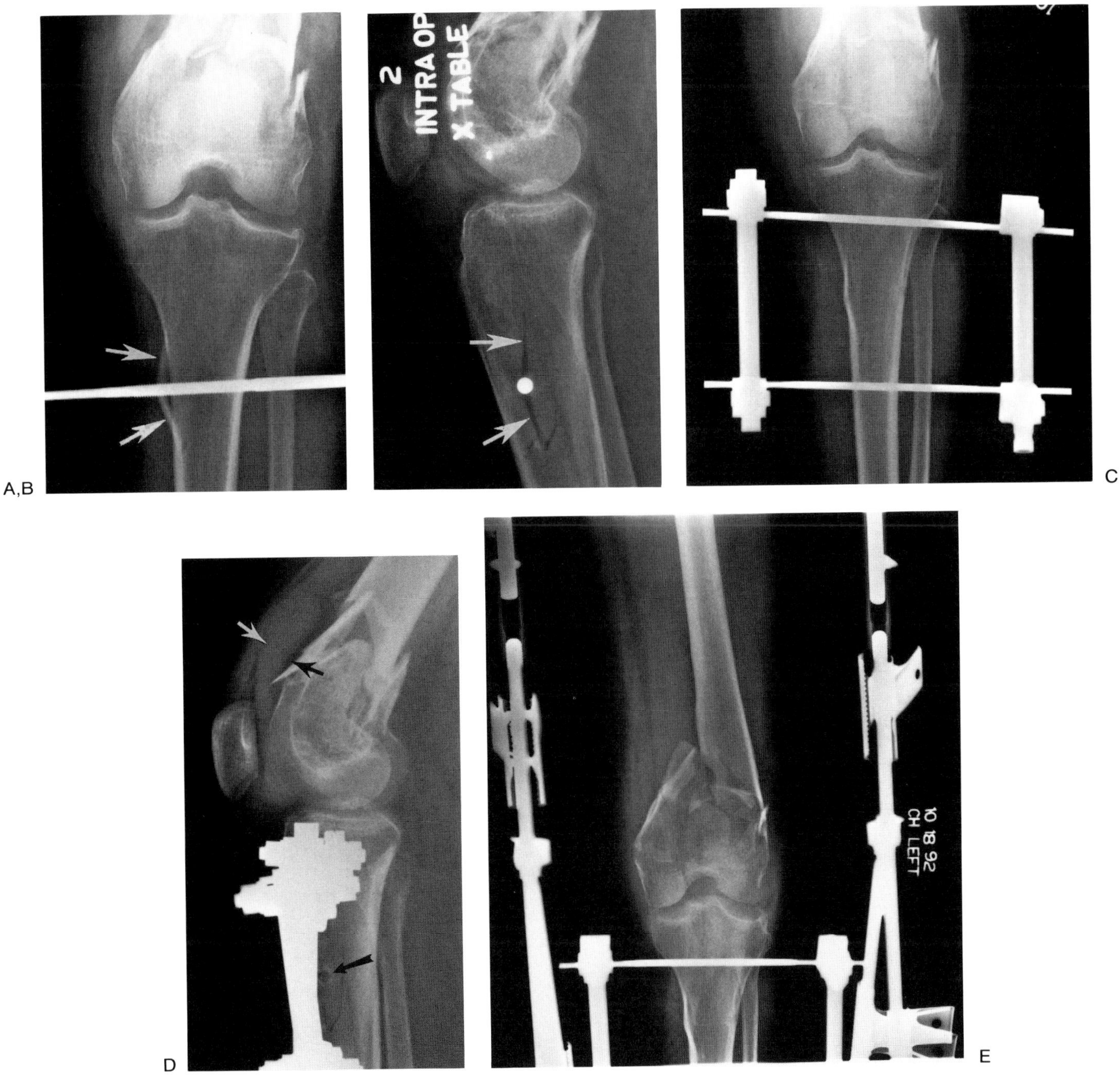

FIG. 6-13. Badly comminuted supracondylar fracture. The AP **(A)** and lateral **(B)** radiographs taken after insertion of a threaded tibial traction pin. The pin fractured the medial cortex (*arrows*). The pin tract was bypassed with a pin proximally and distally with an AO frame attached as shown on AP **(C)** and lateral **(D)** radiographs. Note the old pin tract (*lower arrow*) and the large knee effusion (*upper arrows*). AP **(E)** and lateral **(F)** radiographs after traction was applied. Traction was converted to a cast brace **(G** and **H)** 4 weeks later. The brace obscures the fracture on the lateral view **(H)**. AP radiograph at 6 months **(I)** shows the fracture has healed. (See **F–I** on next page.)

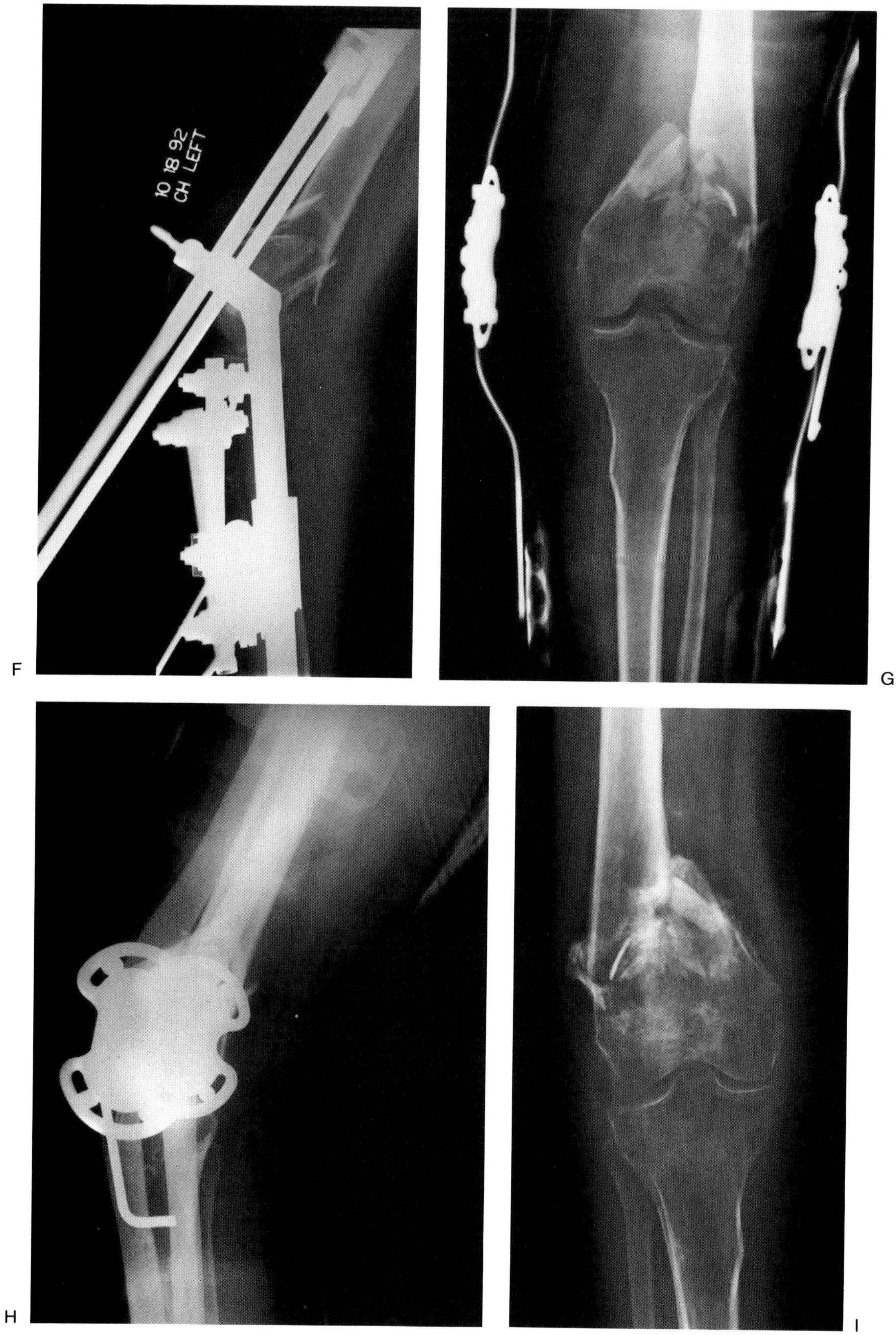

FIG. 6-13. *Continued.*

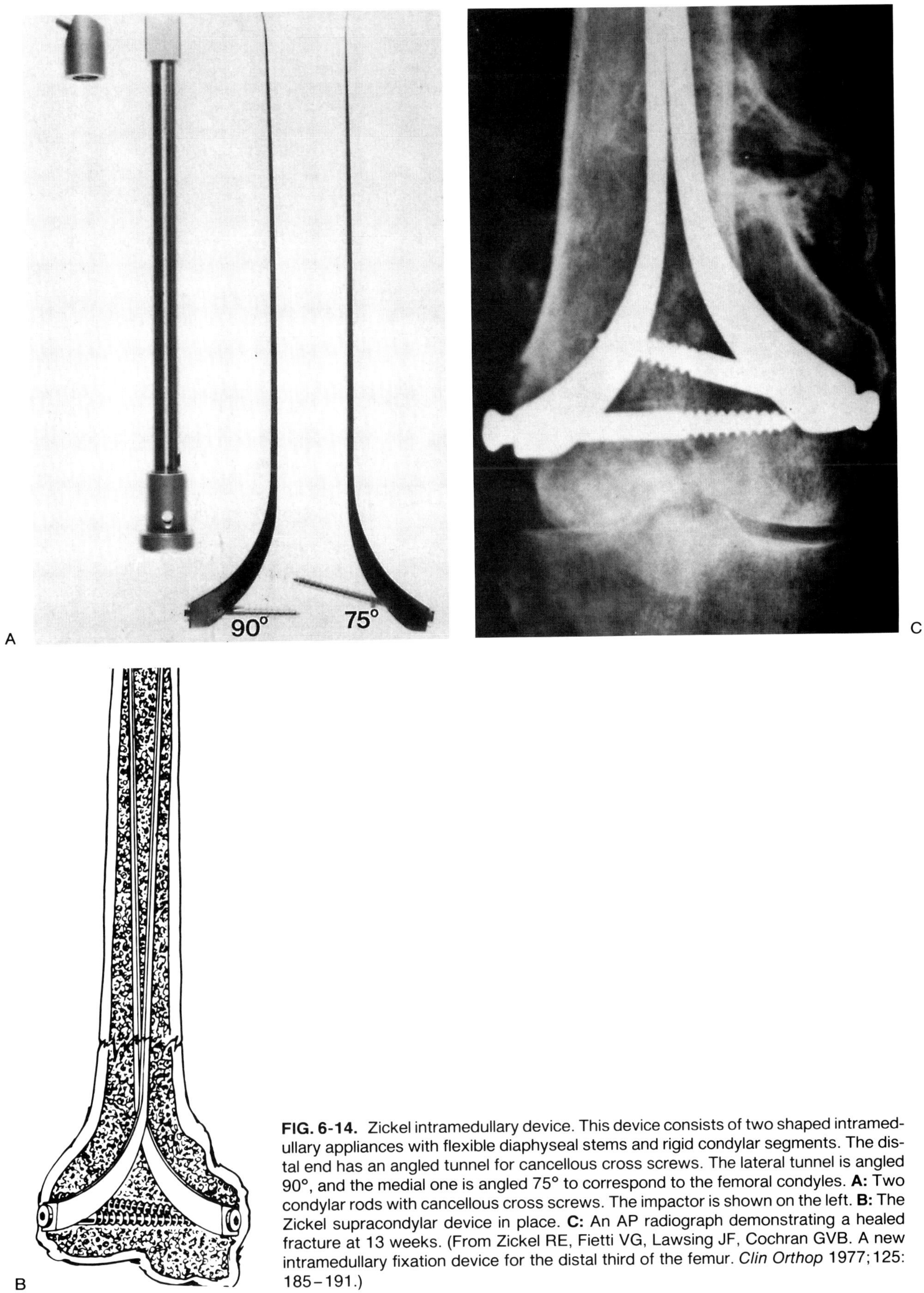

FIG. 6-14. Zickel intramedullary device. This device consists of two shaped intramedullary appliances with flexible diaphyseal stems and rigid condylar segments. The distal end has an angled tunnel for cancellous cross screws. The lateral tunnel is angled 90°, and the medial one is angled 75° to correspond to the femoral condyles. **A:** Two condylar rods with cancellous cross screws. The impactor is shown on the left. **B:** The Zickel supracondylar device in place. **C:** An AP radiograph demonstrating a healed fracture at 13 weeks. (From Zickel RE, Fietti VG, Lawsing JF, Cochran GVB. A new intramedullary fixation device for the distal third of the femur. *Clin Orthop* 1977;125: 185–191.)

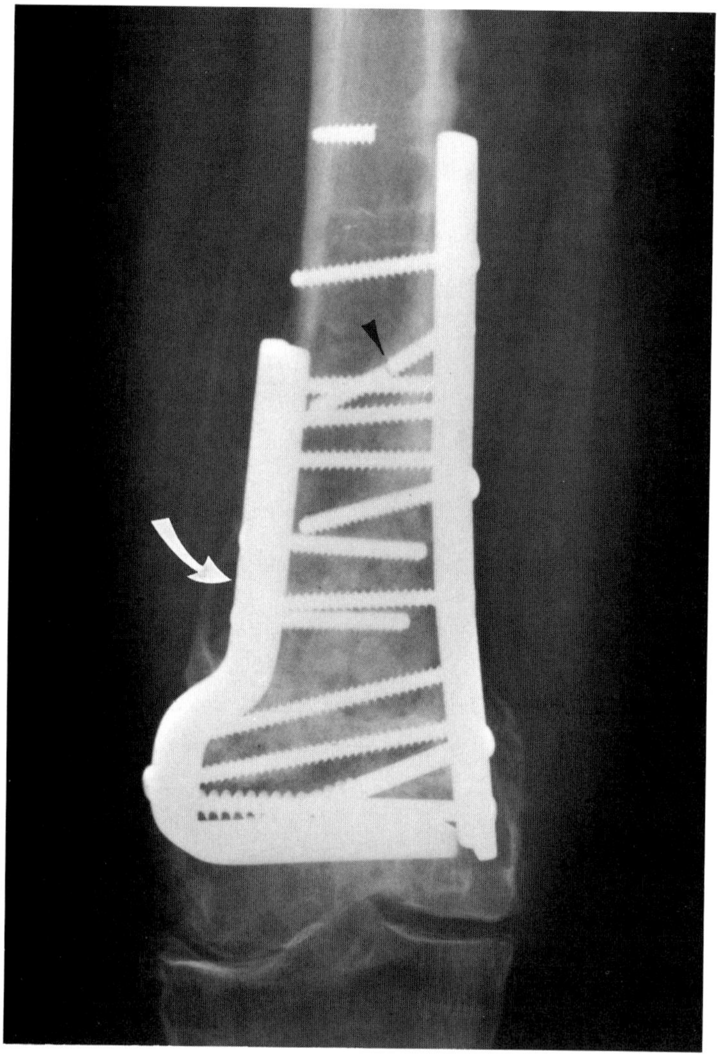

FIG. 6-15. The AP view of the distal femur demonstrating a healed supracondylar fracture with a dynamic compression plate (DCP) and condylar blade plate (*curved arrow*) for fixation. Both cortical and cancellous screws were used distally. There is a fracture of one of the upper cortical screws (*arrowhead*) and a screw remnant superiorly from an initial fixation plate that failed.

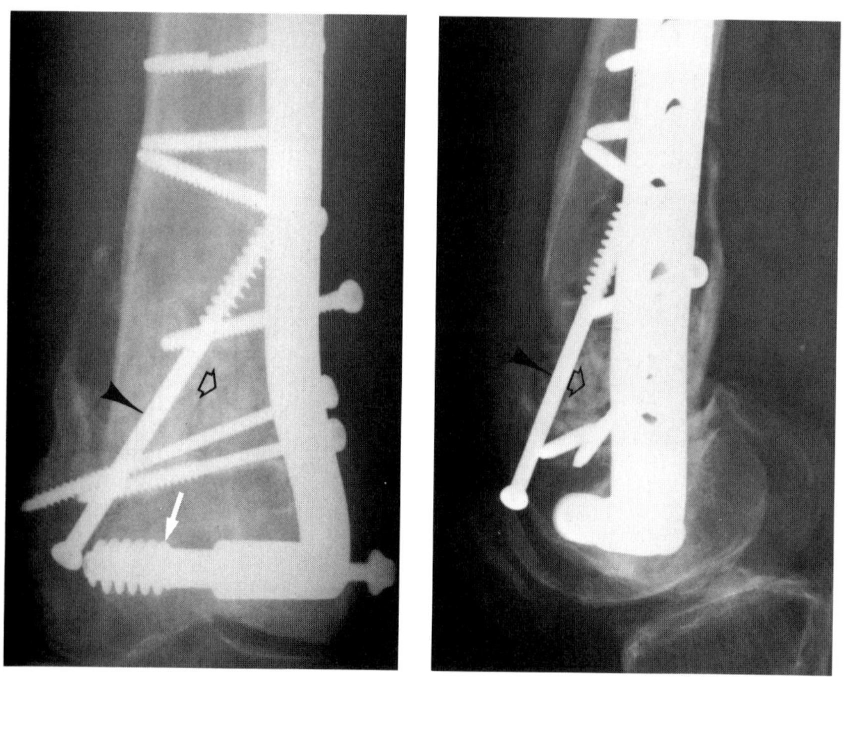

A,B

FIG. 6-16. The AP **(A)** and lateral **(B)** radiographs of the distal femur in a patient with delayed union. Internal fixation was achieved with a dynamic condylar screw and side plate with proximal cortical screws and two cancellous screws above the dynamic compression screw (*white arrow*). There is also a cancellous lag screw (*black arrowhead*) and bone graft (*open black arrow*) to fill in a region of bone loss.

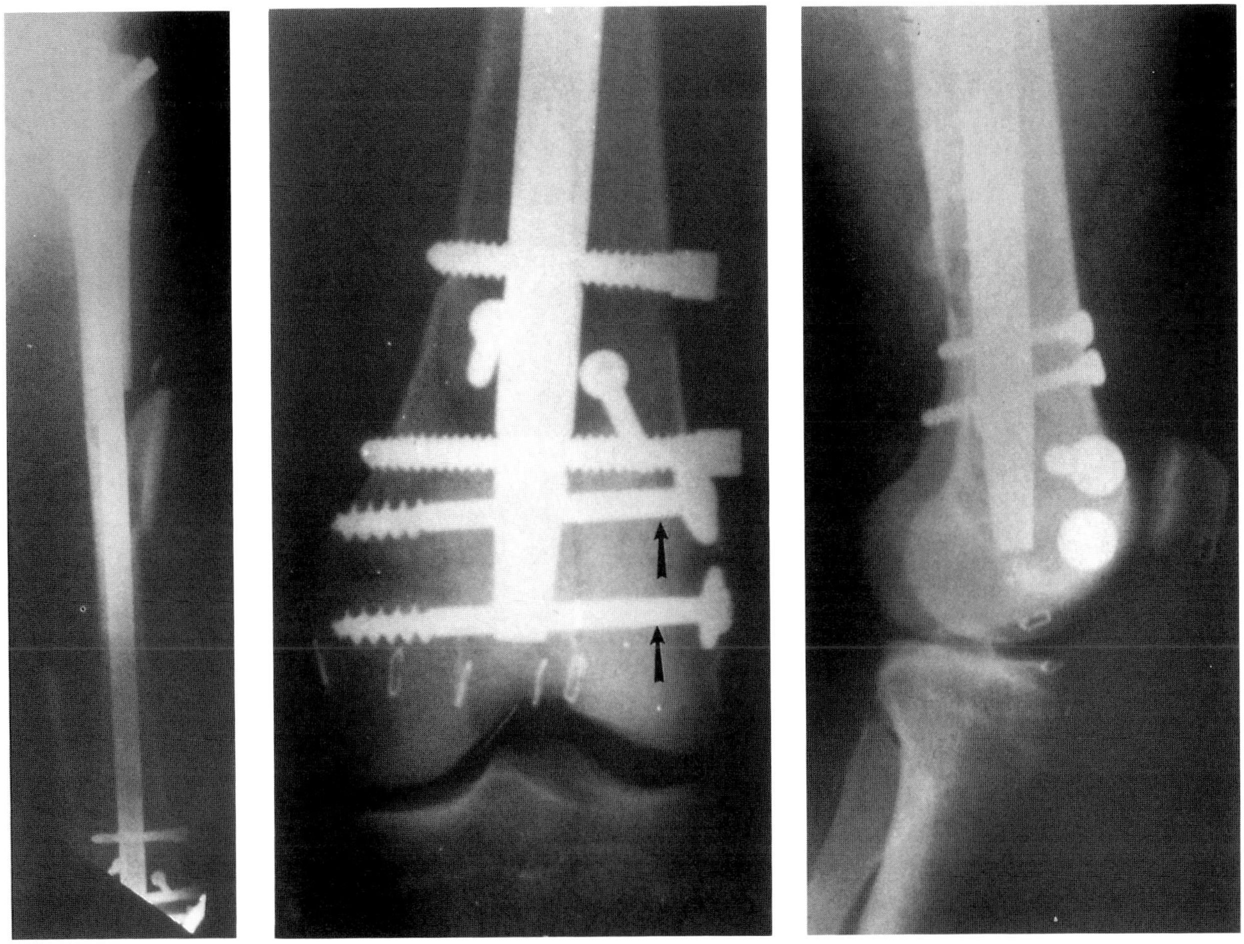

A,B C

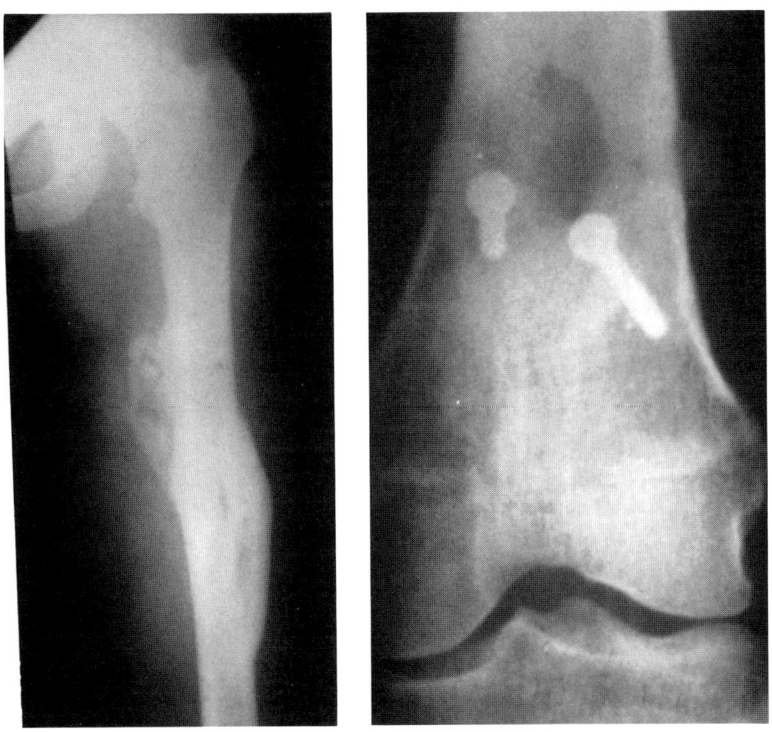

D,E

FIG. 6-17. Ipsilateral fractures of the shaft and supracondylar regions. The AP views of the shaft **(A)** and distal femur **(B)** with intramedullary nail and distal lag screws and locking screws. There are also two cancellous screws with washers (*arrows*). **C:** Lateral view of the knee. **D,E:** The AP views after healing and intramedullary nail removed. Only two lag screws remain. (From Butler MS, Brumback RJ, Ellison T, Poka A, Bathon GH, Burgess AR. Interlocking nailing for ipsilateral fractures of the femoral shaft and distal part of the femur. *J Bone Joint Surg* [*Am*] 1991;73A:1492–1502.)

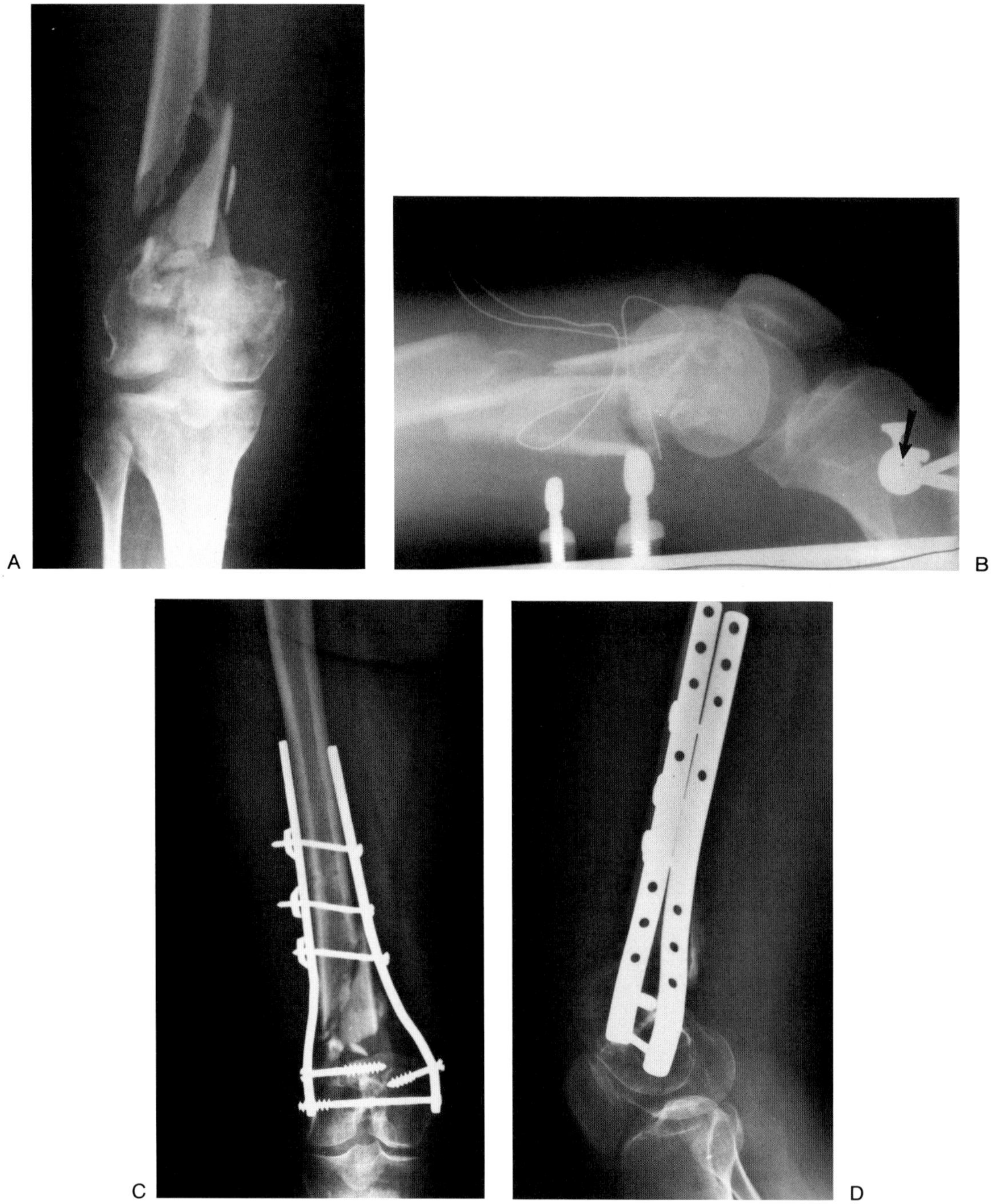

FIG. 6-18. Comminuted supracondylar intraarticular fracture (Neer type III or Seinsheimer type 3C) of the right femur. The AP **(A)** and lateral **(B)** views taken in traction using a single tibial pin (*arrow*). The AP **(C)** and lateral **(D)** views at 1 year and the AP tomograms.

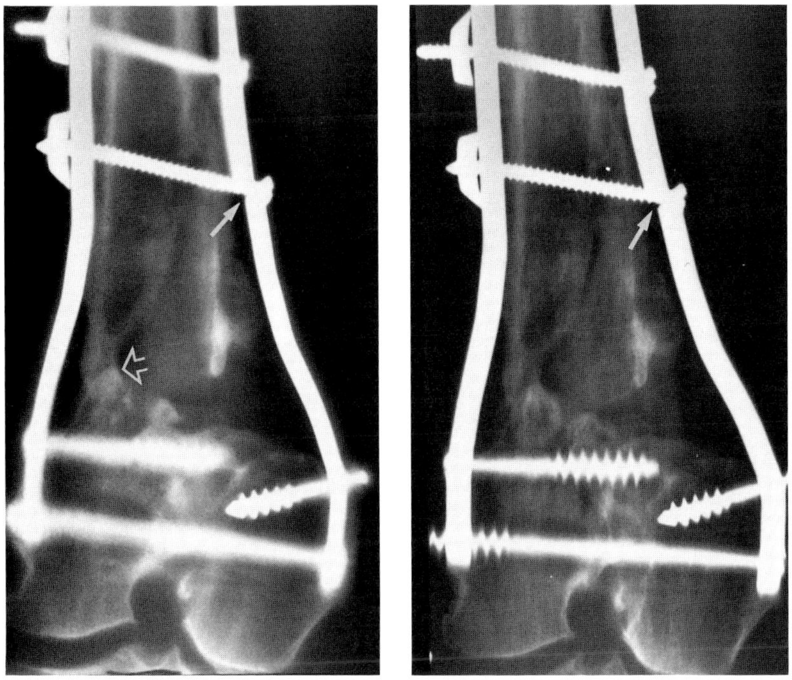
E,F

FIG. 6-18. (*Continued.*) **(E,F)** obtained 1 year later show a large area of central bone void. The fracture was internally fixed with double DCPs and distal cancellous screws with three upper bolts. The tomograms (E,F) demonstrate a plate fracture through the screw hole (*arrow*) with bone union at the lateral margin (*open arrow*) and a large gap medially.

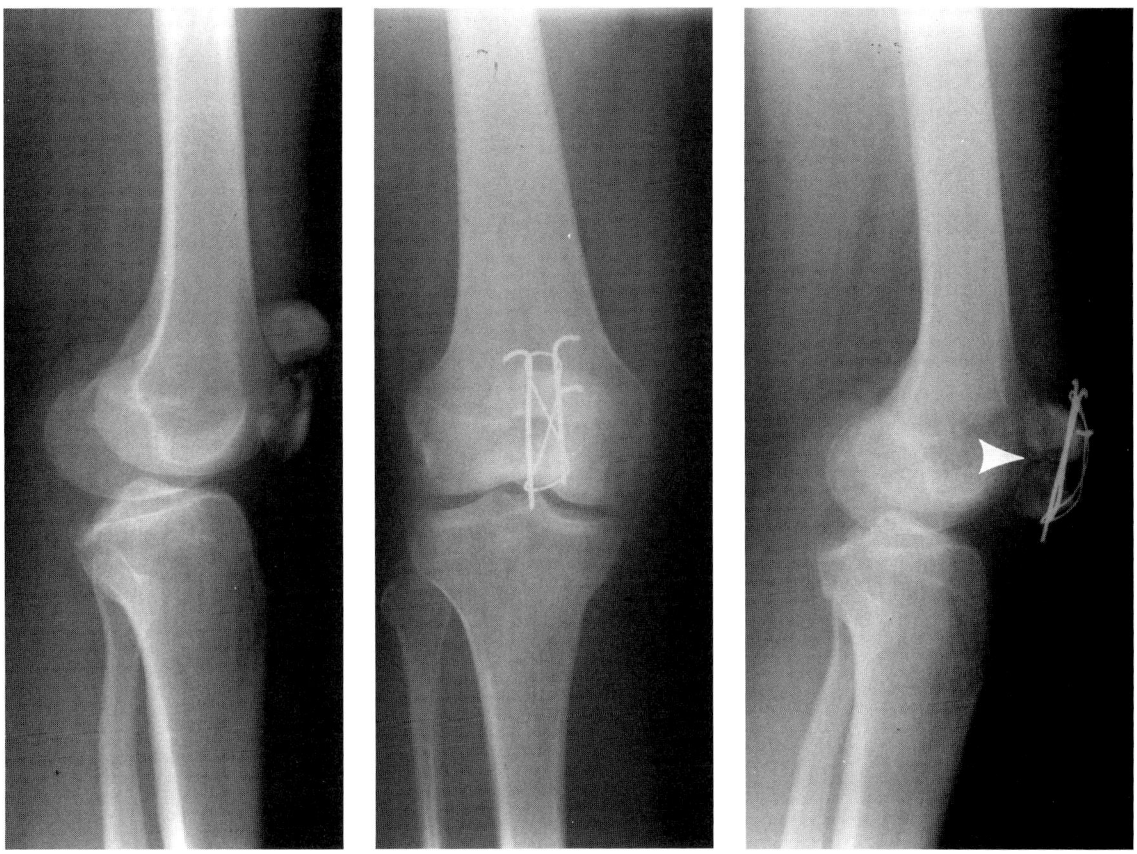
A,B C

FIG. 6-19. A: Lateral view of the knee demonstrating a comminuted transverse fracture of the patella. The AP **(B)** and lateral **(C)** views following modified tension-band fixation with two vertical K wires. There is still 3 to 4 mm of separation of the articular surface (*arrowhead*).

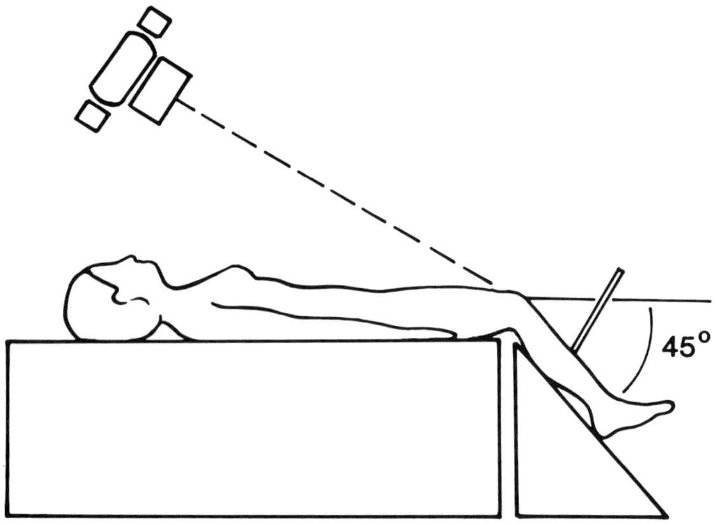

FIG. 6-20. Positioning and tube angle for the Merchant view.

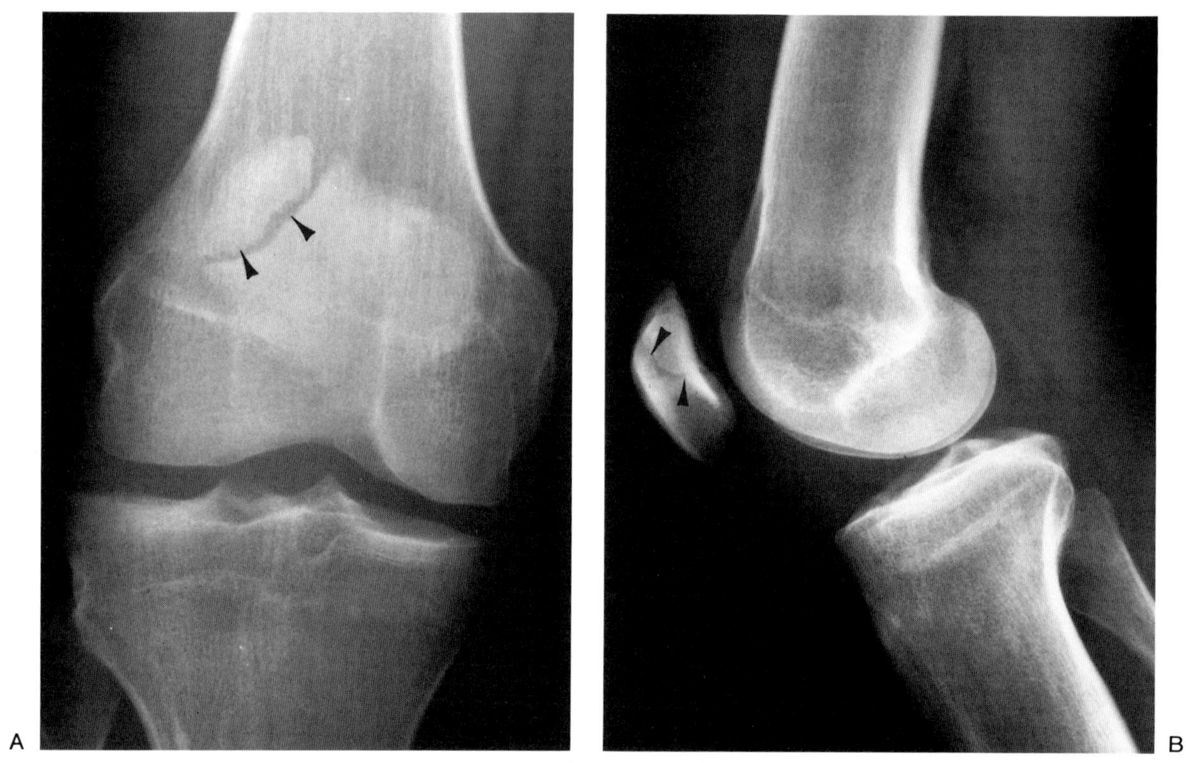

FIG. 6-21. Bipartite patella. The AP **(A)** and lateral **(B)** views of a bipartite patella. The defect is in the upper outer quadrant (*arrows*).

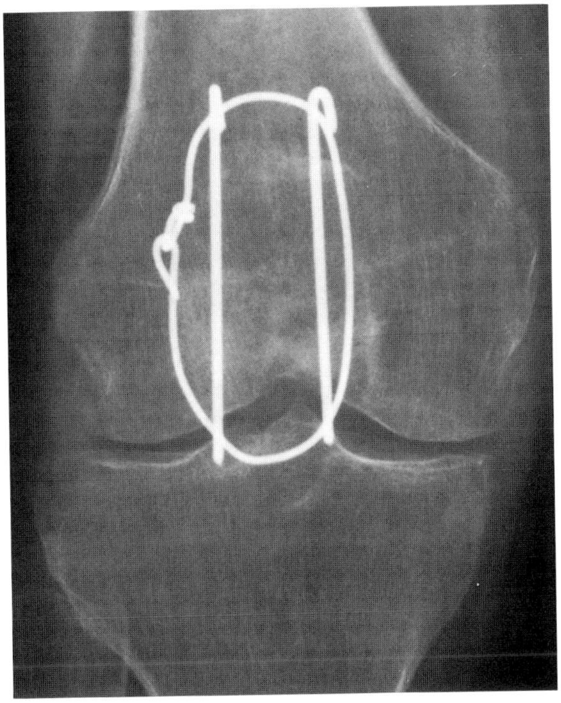

A

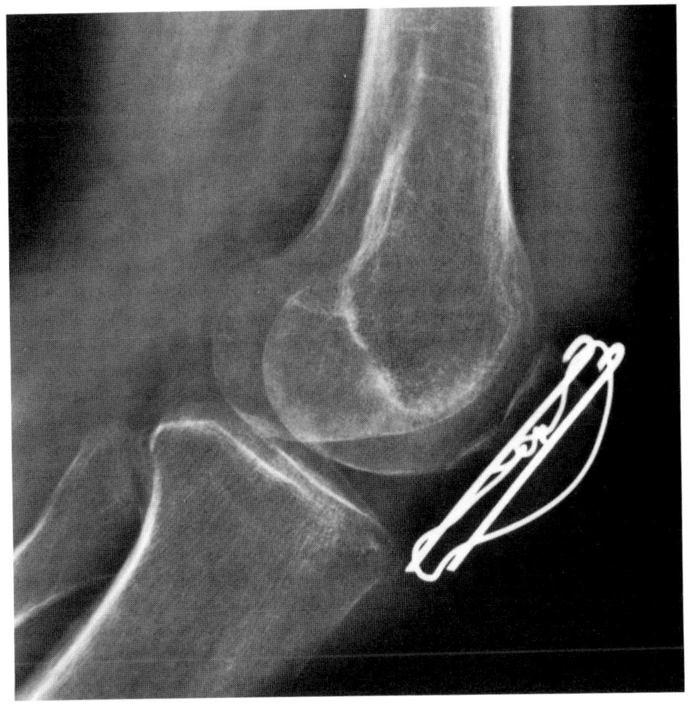

B

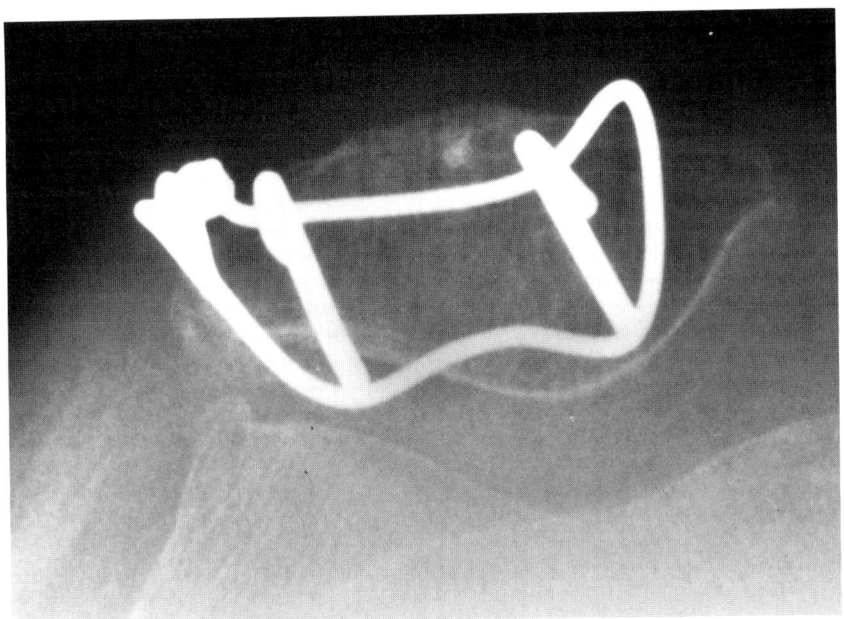

C

FIG. 6-22. The AP **(A)**, lateral **(B)**, and Merchant views **(C)** of patellar fixation with tension-band wiring and two vertical K wires.

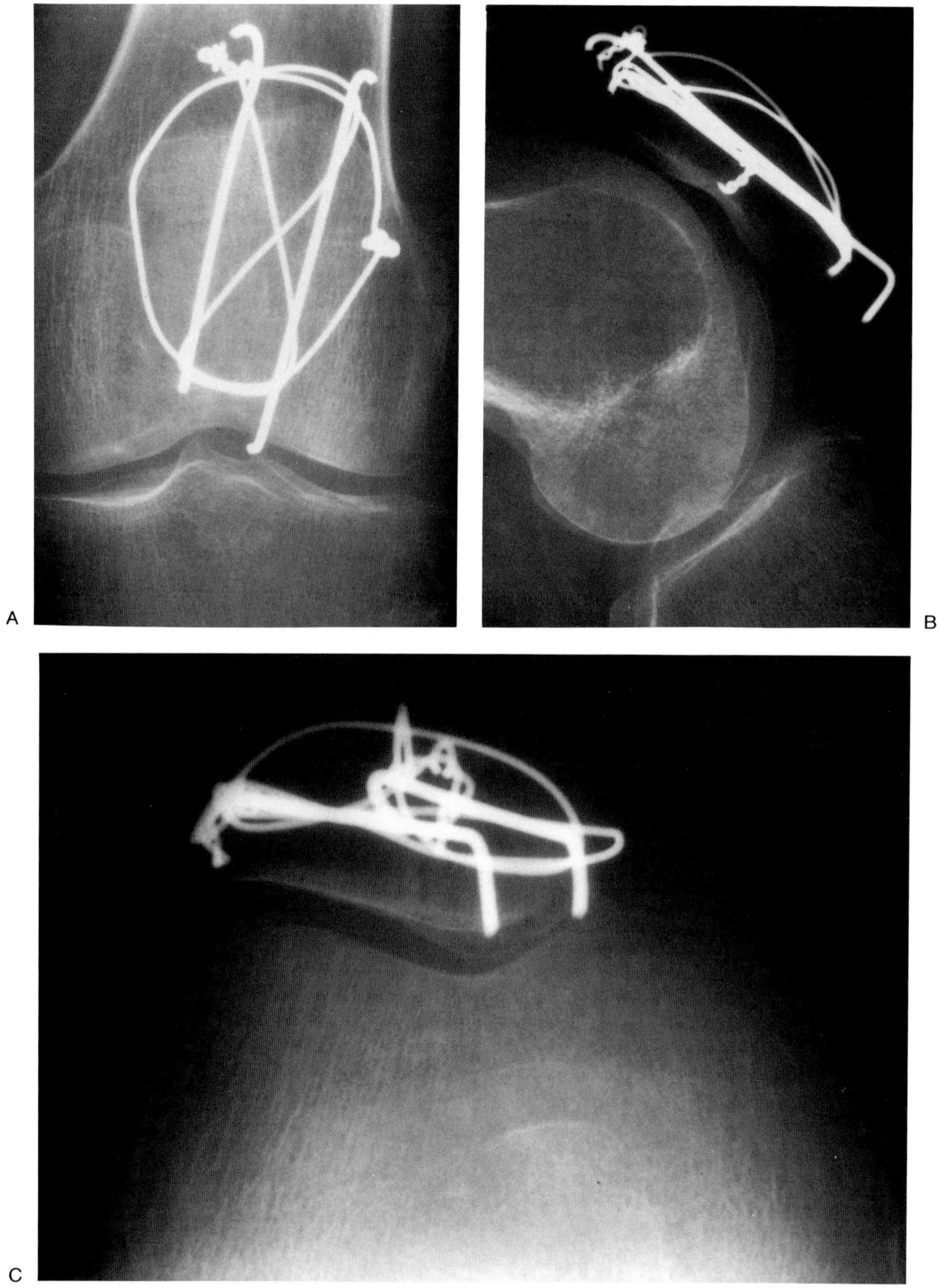

FIG. 6-23. Wire and K wire with cerclage. The AP **(A)**, lateral **(B)**, and Merchant views **(C)**.

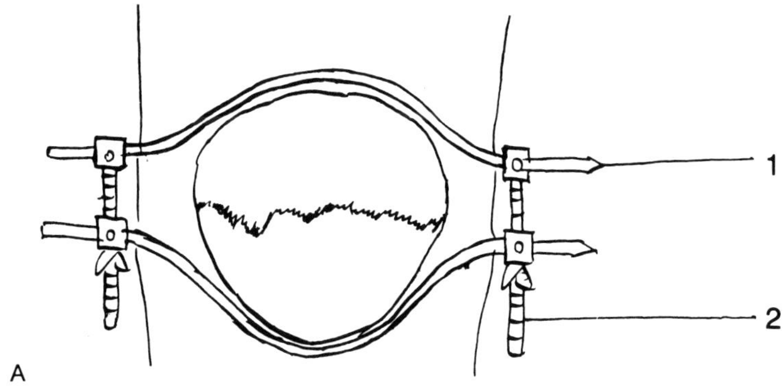

FIG. 6-24. External fixation of patellar fractures. **A:** The entry points and exits of percutaneous pins. The pins are compressed with external fixation clamps. Lateral **(B)** and AP **(C)** views of percutaneous pin and external clamp fixation of a transverse patellar fracture. (From Quan-Yi L, Jia-Wen W. Fracture of the patella treated by open reduction and external compressive skeletal fixation. *J Bone Joint Surg* [*Am*] 1987;69A:83–89.)

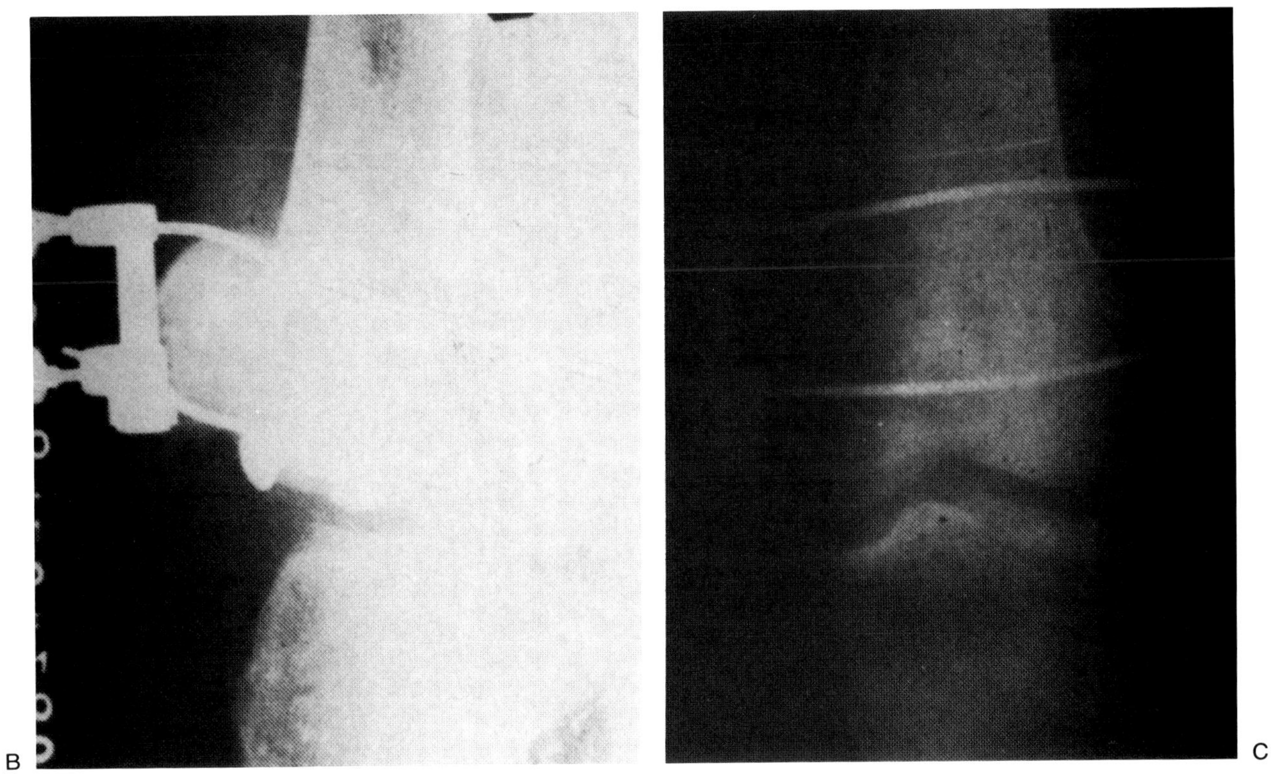

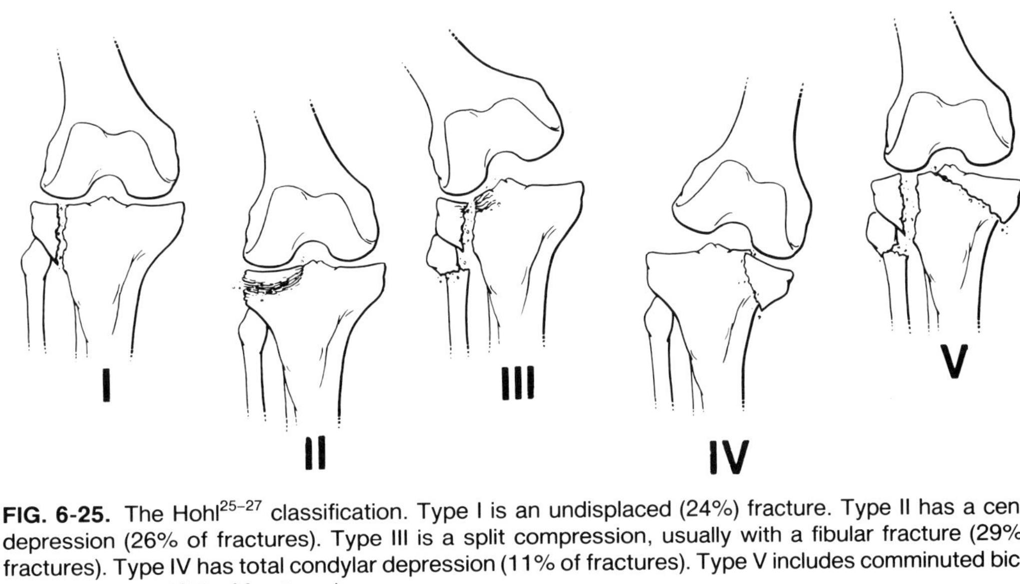

FIG. 6-25. The Hohl[25–27] classification. Type I is an undisplaced (24%) fracture. Type II has a central depression (26% of fractures). Type III is a split compression, usually with a fibular fracture (29% of fractures). Type IV has total condylar depression (11% of fractures). Type V includes comminuted bicondylar fractures (10% of fractures).

Proximal Tibial Fractures

Fractures of the proximal tibia in adults may involve the articular surface (osteochondral fractures, condyle, and plateau fractures), metaphysis, or tuberosity without articular involvement.[26,46] In children and adolescents, the fractures involve the tibial spine, tibial tuberosity, or physis.[11,44] The latter are rare and account for <5% of physeal fractures.[44] We will discuss the fractures treated with internal fixation devices.

Tibial Condyle Fractures

Tibial condyle fractures result from significant falls or motor vehicle accidents. Vertical compression forces may lead to T or Y fractures. Varus and valgus forces involve the medial and lateral tibial plateaus, respectively. Injuries of the ligament also commonly occur with varus and valgus forces. Rotational or twisting forces can produce a variety of fracture patterns.[26,36,46]

Classification

Numerous classification schemes have been devised for tibial condyle fractures.[12,18,25–27,36,46] The Hohl[25–27] classification is commonly used (Fig. 6-25). Type I fractures are undisplaced; type II fractures have a central depression of the lateral plateau. Type III fractures are split with a fibular neck fracture, type IV fractures demonstrate total condylar depression, and type V fractures involve both condyles (Fig. 6-25)[25,27]

Moore[42] developed a modified classification (Fig. 6-26), dividing such injuries into fractures and fracture-dislocations. Fracture-dislocations are unstable and require open reduction.[26,42]

Soft tissue injuries commonly accompany tibial condyle fractures. Injury to the ligaments and menisci occur most frequently. These injuries, specifically ligamentous, can result in an unsatisfactory response to therapy if not recognized preoperatively.[46] Neurovascular injury, especially to the peroneal nerve, is also fairly common.[12]

Preoperative Imaging

Most fractures are easily detected on AP and lateral views of the knee (Figs. 6-27 and 6-28). Subtle undisplaced fractures may be overlooked if oblique or cross-table lateral (lipohemarthrosis) views are not obtained.[46] Also, angling the tube 10° caudad on the AP view parallels the joint surface, making it easier to identify subtle fractures.

Conventional tomography (Fig. 6-29) or CT with reconstruction is frequently required to evaluate fracture configuration and the degree of separation or depression of the fragments.[1,18,36,46] Depression of 5 to 8 mm and separation of the fragments by ≥4 mm generally indicate the need for internal fixation.[26,46] Subtle marginal avulsions (Fig. 6-30) of the tibia or fibula may be the only clues to an injury to the ligament in a painful swollen knee.[26,46] Certain fracture patterns (i.e., split or depressed fractures) are more likely to have associated ligament injuries.[5,46] The most useful imaging technique to confirm suspected soft tissue injuries is MRI.[5]

Stress testing can be useful. This is particularly important with the knee in extension. Demonstration of > 5° of lateral instability in extension is an indicator for operative fixation.[26] Rasmussen[47] demonstrated that 70% of split fractures, 52% of bicondylar fractures, 45% of medial condylar fractures, and 24% of fractures with local compression were unstable in extension.

Treatment

The type of treatment selected depends on the extent of bone and soft tissue injury, the patient's age, the knee function required for the patient's activity or profession, and whether there are associated injuries.[26,46]

Minimally displaced fractures can be treated conservatively with cast immobilization, cast bracing, or traction and early mobilization.[18,26,46] Generally, no weight bearing is permitted for 12 to 16 weeks (Fig. 6-30).[18]

Unstable fractures with depression of 5 to 8 mm or separation of fragments usually require open reduction. Elevation of fragments can be accomplished, but their position is difficult to maintain.[26] Bone grafting is often necessary to fill the defects prior to instrumentation. The type of fixation depends on the degree of injury. K wires, cancellous screws, tibial bolts, and buttress plates may be used alone or in combination (Figs. 6-31 to 6-35). Bicondylar fractures may require double plates or combined internal and external fixation (Fig. 6-35).[25,26,37,48]

Miscellaneous Proximal Tibial Fractures

Other isolated fractures and fractures with soft tissue injury also occur. These include avulsion fractures, tibial spine fractures, stress fractures, and tuberosity and physeal fractures. Fractures of the proximal tibial physis are rare, accounting for 0.5% to 3% of physeal injuries.[11] Femoral physeal injuries occur more frequently because of the ligamentous supporting structures. The ligaments extend below the tibial physis but attach below the femoral physis (Fig. 6-36). Most physeal injuries are Salter-Harris type I (32%) and type IV (29%). Detection of these injuries may be difficult with routine radiographs. Gentle fluoroscopically controlled stress views are useful in patients with instability to differentiate a physeal injury

(*text continues on page 424*)

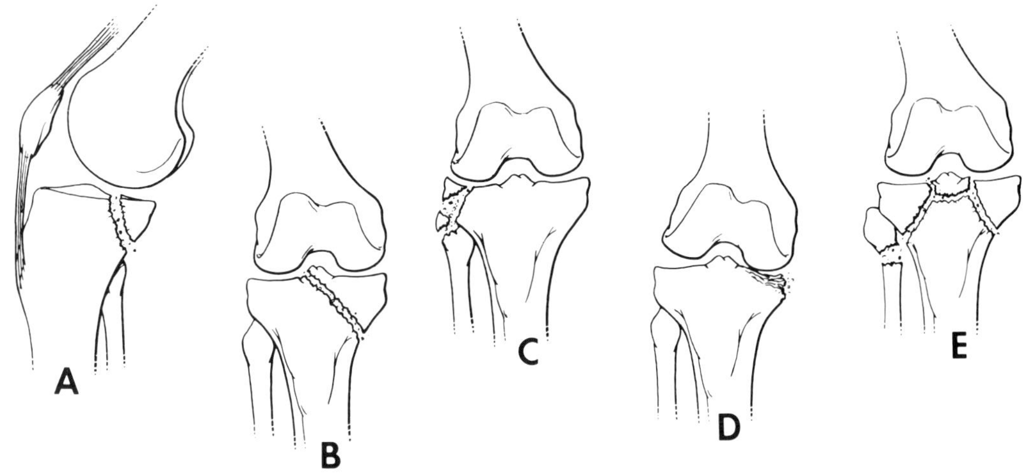

FIG. 6-26. The Moore classification. **A:** Split fracture. **B:** Total plateau fracture. **C:** Marginal avulsion. **D:** Marginal depression. **E:** Bicondylar four-part fracture.

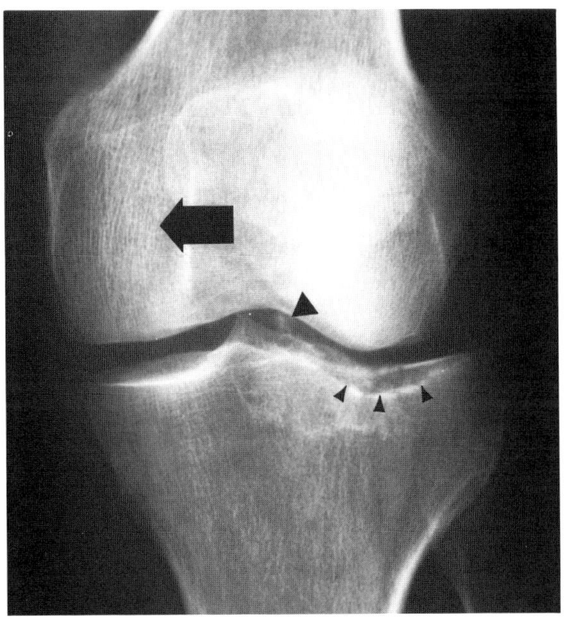

FIG. 6-27. An AP view of the knee demonstrating a type II (Hohl) fracture of the lateral tibial plateau (*small arrowheads*). There is also a tibial spine fracture (*arrowhead*) and medial shift (*large arrow*) caused by a medial ligament injury.

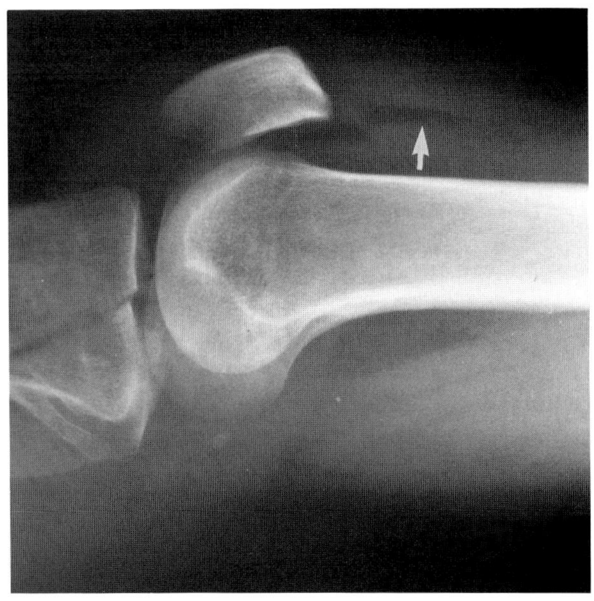

FIG. 6-28. Cross-table lateral view of the knee demonstrating a split fracture. There is a lipohemarthrosis (*arrow*).

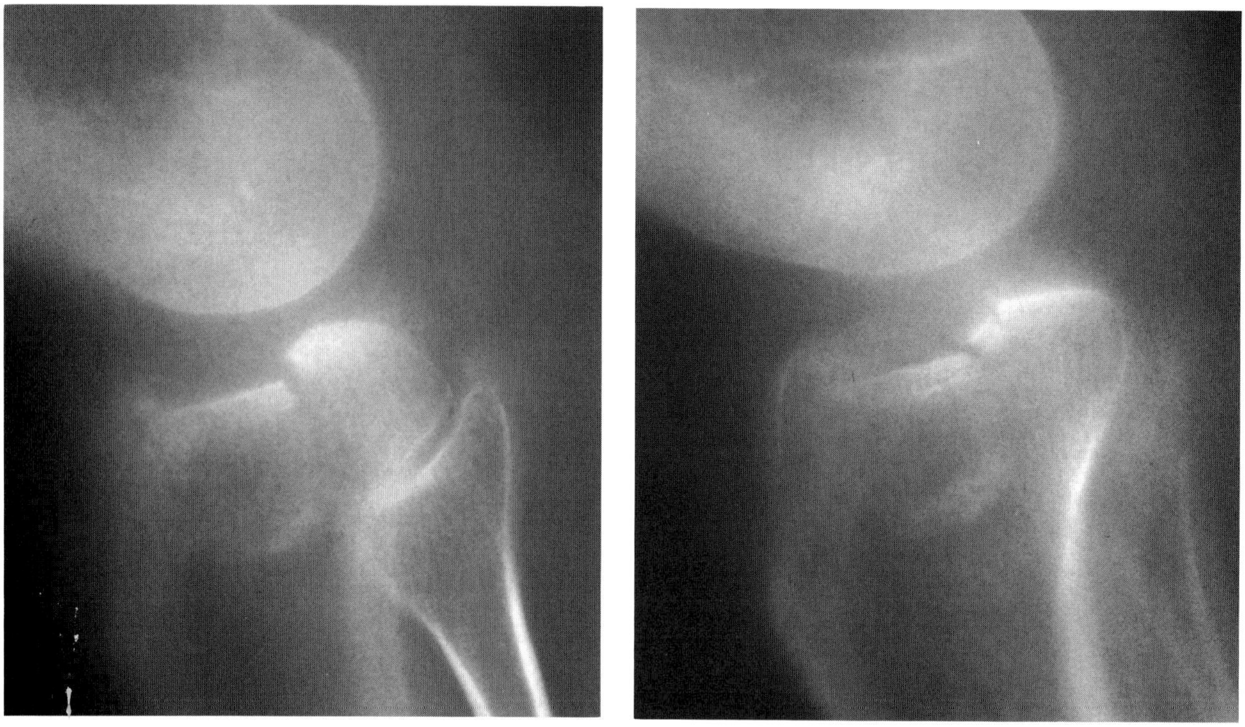

A B

FIG. 6-29. A,B: Lateral tomograms demonstrating the fragments and degree of depression in the lateral tibial plateau.

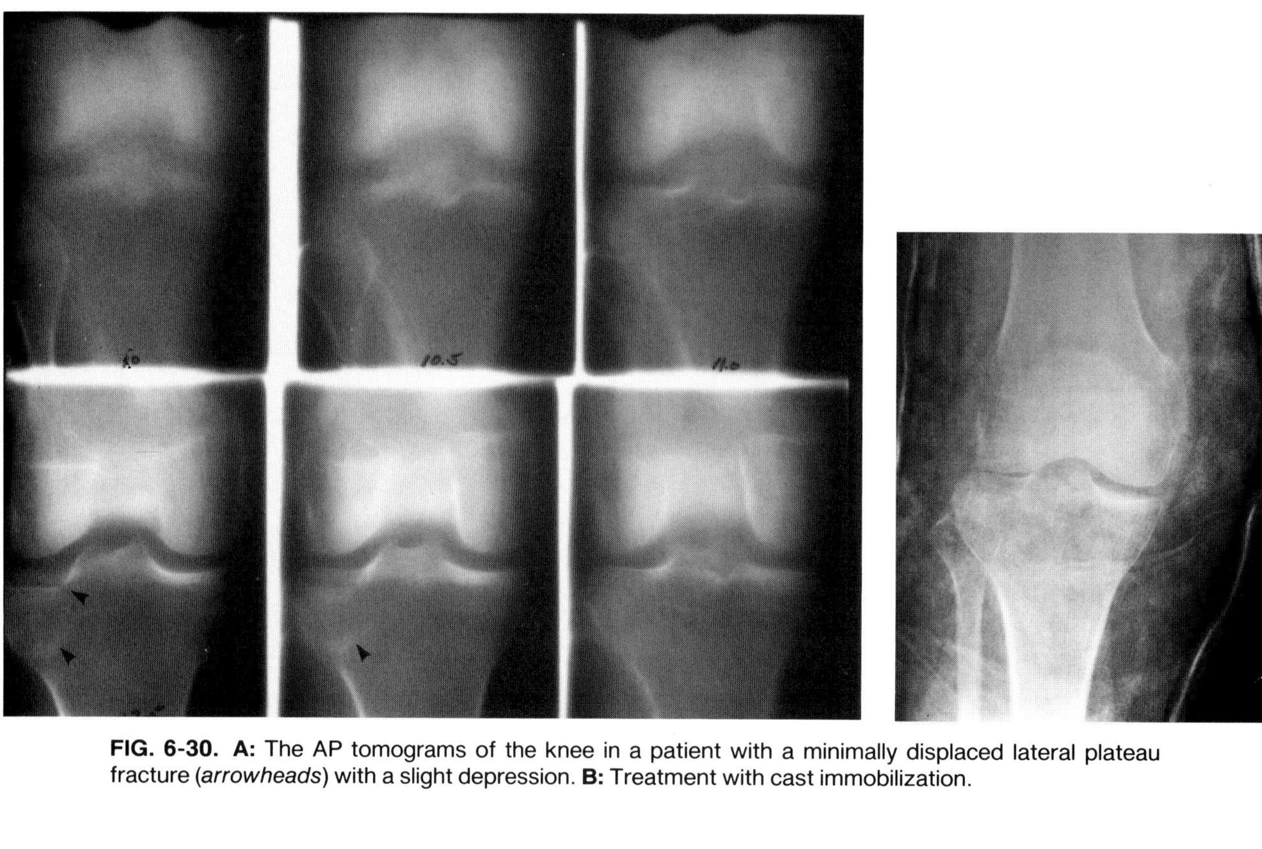

A B

FIG. 6-30. A: The AP tomograms of the knee in a patient with a minimally displaced lateral plateau fracture (*arrowheads*) with a slight depression. **B:** Treatment with cast immobilization.

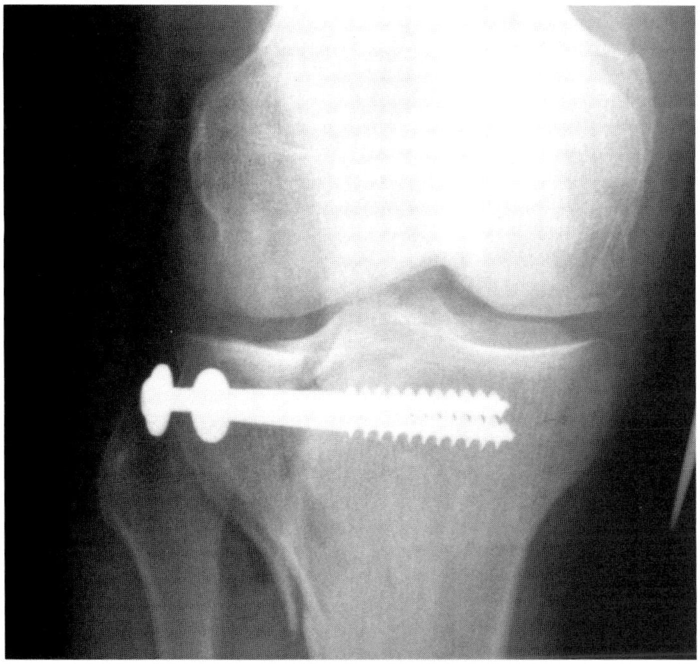

FIG. 6-31. Lateral tibial plateau fracture fixed with two cancellous screws and washers to protect the thin bone under the screw heads.

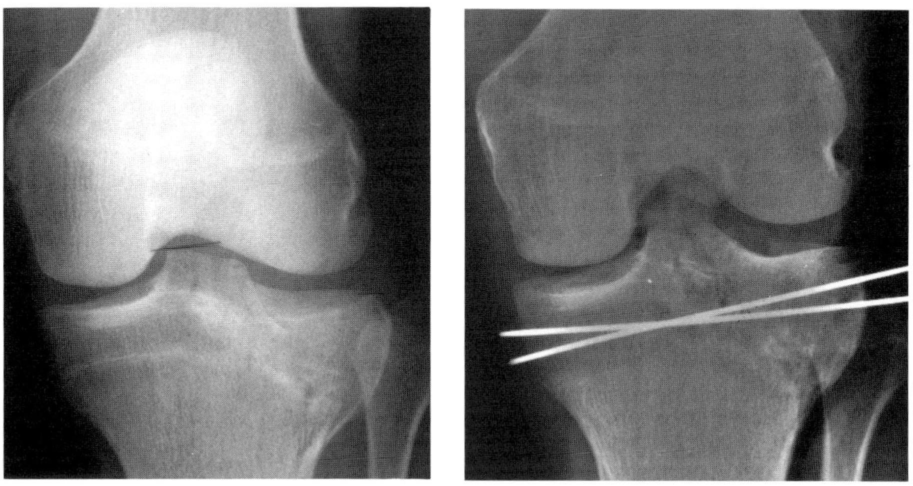

A B

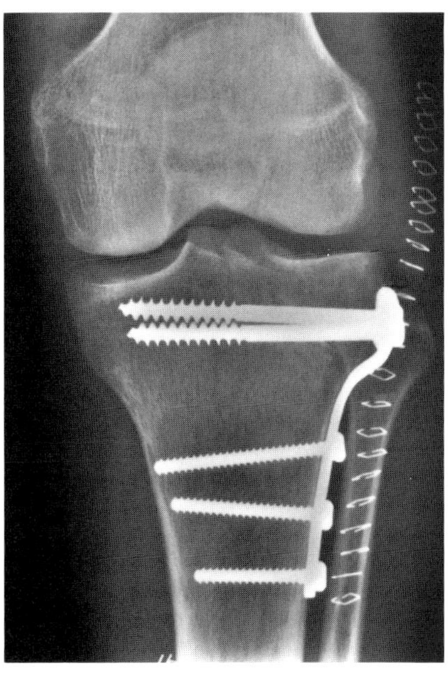

C

FIG. 6-32. Lateral plateau fracture. **A:** The AP radiograph demonstrating a Hohl type IV lateral plateau fracture. **B:** Fragments were reduced with bone graft to reconstitute the height and then stabilized with two K wires. **C–E:** A "T" buttress plate (C) was contoured to the metaphysis and fixed with two 6.5-mm cancellous screws and three 4.5-mm cortical screws. Note the oblong hole in the plate (D,E) to allow adjustment after this screw is placed (*arrow*, D). (See **D** and **E** on next page.)

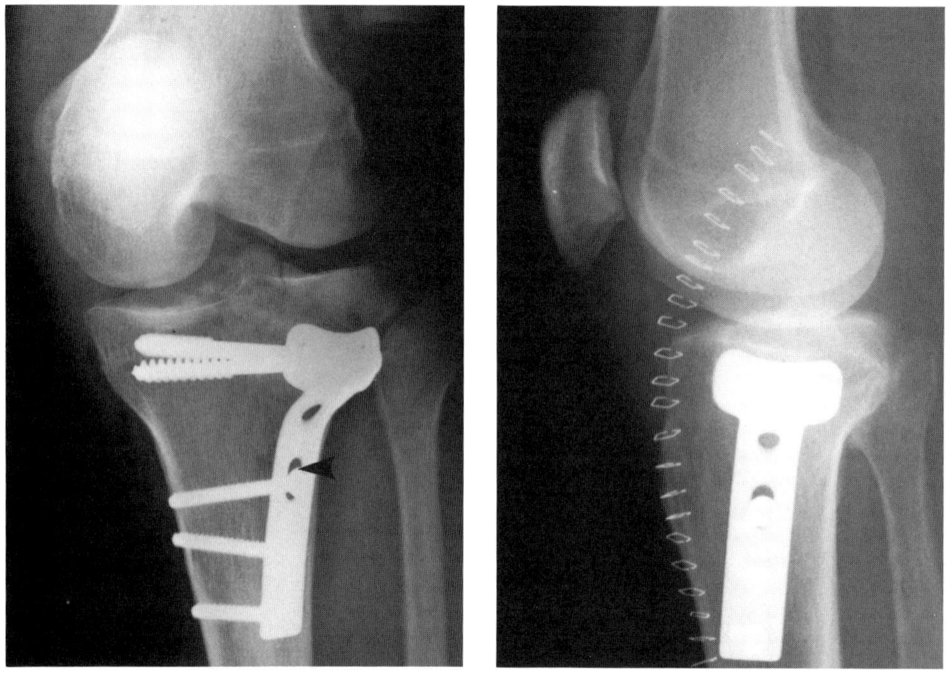

D E

FIG. 6-32. *Continued.*

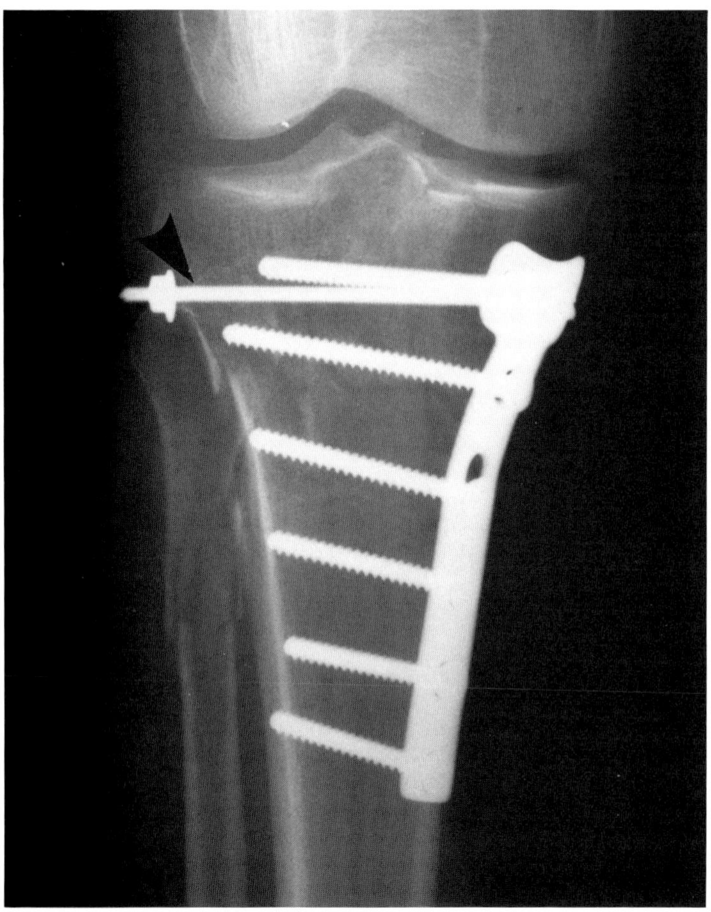

FIG. 6-33. An AP view of the knee demonstrating an upper tibial fracture involving the medial plateau. Internal fixation with a T buttress plate and tibial bolt (*arrow*). There is also a minimally displaced fibular fracture.

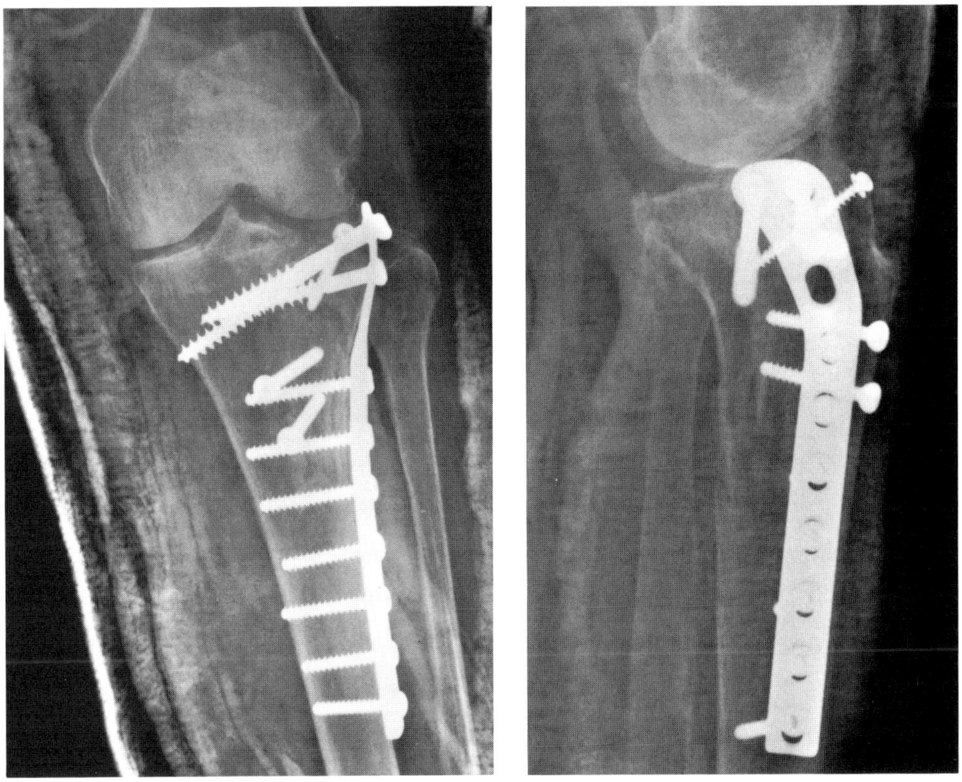

A B

FIG. 6-34. Lateral tibial plateau fracture with upper tibial involvement. The AP **(A)** and lateral **(B)** radiographs demonstrate internal fixation with a ten-hole lateral buttress plate. There are seven cortical screws distally, and two cancellous screws in the proximal plate. Four interfragmentary screws were also used.

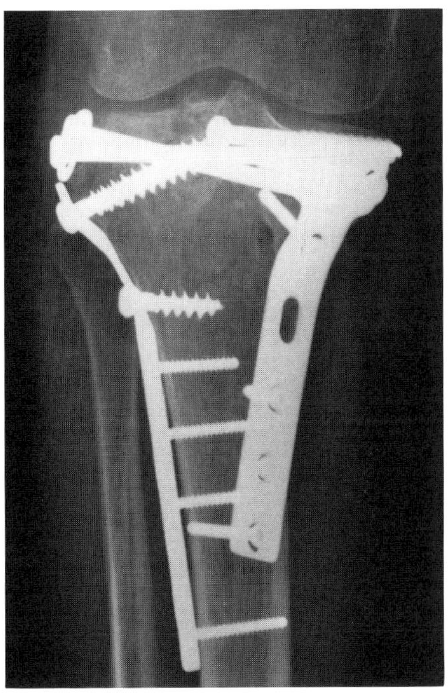

FIG. 6-35. Bicondylar fracture (Hohl type V) internally fixed with bilateral buttress plates. There are two cancellous screws with washers in the lateral condyle.

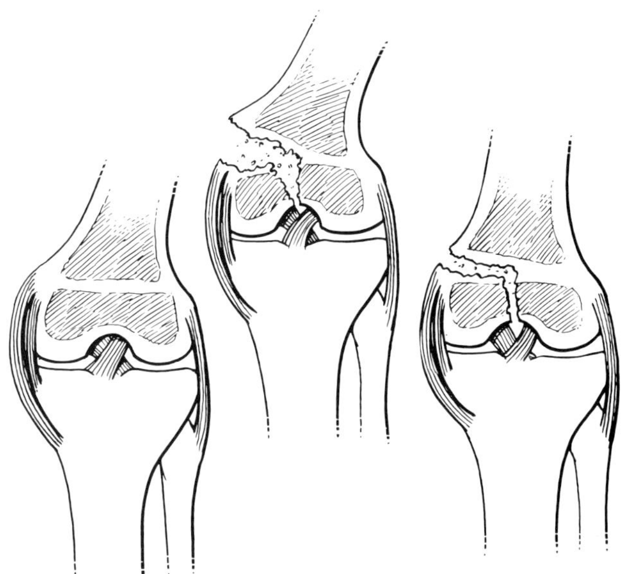

FIG. 6-36. Ligaments and growth plates of the knee. The femoral physis is more susceptible to injury. (From Berquist TH. *Imaging in sports injuries.* Rockville, MD: Aspen Press, 1992.)

from an injury to the ligament (Fig. 6-37). However, MRI is an easier and safer method for evaluating both physeal and ligament injuries (Fig. 6-38).[7,15]

The Segond fracture (small vertical fracture of the lateral aspect of the tibia just distal to the plateau) is associated with ACL and medial meniscal injury.[15] Most of the miscellaneous injuries previously mentioned are not treated with fixation devices. However, Polakoff et al.[44] described the use of tension-band wiring for tibial tuberosity fractures in adolescents.

Ipsilateral Fractures of the Tibia and Femur

Ipsilateral fractures of the tibia and femur present significant problems in management. This injury has been called "floating knee."[9] The injuries occur most frequently with high-velocity trauma, such as motor vehicle accidents.[9,26,46] Local and distant associated injuries are common. Neurovascular and knee ligament injuries are reported in 7% and 8% of patients, respectively. Nearly 60% of fractures are open, causing further problems with management.[21]

Two classification schemes are commonly used for these combination injuries. Blake and McBryde[9] classified type 1 injuries as fractures of the tibia and femur that isolated the knee. A type 2A injury involves the knee joint, and type 2B injuries involve the hip or ankle. Fraser et al.[21] classified type I fractures (71% of cases) as shaft fractures of the tibia and femur without knee involvement. Type IIA fractures extend into the tibial plateau (16.5%), and type IIB fractures involve the femoral articular surface. Type IIC fractures (8%) involve both articular surfaces (Fig. 6-39).

Treatment of these injuries can be accomplished with nonoperative treatment of both or surgical fixation of one or both injuries, using the techniques described previously and in Chapter 5 (Fig. 6-40).[46]

Soft Tissue Injuries

Injuries to the ligaments and supporting structures of the knee are common clinical problems.[46] The ACL is the most frequently injured soft tissue (39%). This injury is present in 70% of patients with acute hemarthrosis.[2,46] Combined injuries of the ACL and medial collateral ligament (MCL) occur in 30% of injuries with medial capsular injuries in 12%.[2] The remaining 19% of injuries involve the lateral collateral ligament (LCL), posterior cruciate ligament (PCL, 5%), or other combination injuries.[2,46]

Imaging of soft tissue injuries has been greatly enhanced with MRI. However, routine radiography should still be the initial screening technique to evaluate osseous injury. In addition, valuable clues to associated injuries can be detected. The presence of an effusion (Fig. 6-41) on the lateral radiograph following acute injury may suggest an ACL disruption.[46] Small osteophytes on the inner aspect of the medial femoral condyle near the medial tibial spine have also been described with ACL insufficiency. This finding is most easily identified on a notch view with the knee flexed 30° (Fig. 6-42).[20] The AP and varus-valgus stress views are also useful when done by experienced persons. Local anesthesia is often required.[29,46]

Arthrography is rarely indicated today, except for joint aspiration; MRI is an excellent technique for the identification of meniscal, ligament, and tendon injuries about the knee. Osseous injuries are also easily identified. Even subtle bone bruises or stress fractures are easily detected (Fig. 6-43). Double-echo MPGR or T2-weighted spin-echo (SE) sequences are the most useful because the abnormality or tear has a high signal intensity compared with the normal low signal intensity of menisci, ligaments, and tendons (Fig. 6-44). The MRI definition of ligament or meniscal injury and the extent of injury is useful in therapeutic planning.[46]

Treatment

The treatment options include nonoperative treatment, early repair, or a rehabilitation program with delayed repair.[3,46,53,57] For the purposes of this atlas, we emphasize the techniques that can be evaluated radiographically.

Repairs of the ACL, PCL, MCL, and LCL are performed alone or in combination.[3,6] Until recently, soft tissue repairs required long periods of rehabilitation, and imaging was of little value for evaluating results. Newer techniques for ACL and PCL repair use iliotibial band, patellar tendon with bone attachments, allografts (Fig. 6-45), and Goretex (polytetraflouroethylene) or polypropylene braid augmentation with interference screws or staples.[3,17,39,53,57] Isometric positioning of these grafts is important and can be evaluated with routine radiography.[39] Figure 6-46 demonstrates the isometric tunnel sites for the ACL, PCL, MCL, and LCL attachments. Isometric points allow the ligaments to maintain consistent length with flexion and extension.[39,46] The screw (Fig. 6-47) and/or staple positions do not necessarily indicate the position of the ligament. Screws compress the bone plug at the tendon ends in the tunnel (Figs. 6-47 and 6-48) and staples (Fig. 6-48) are more peripheral at the edge of the tunnel. The course of the bony tunnel is, therefore, more easily followed when an interference screw is used. The artifact caused by screws decreases the ability to evaluate tunnels using MRI. The tendon or graft between the screws is more easily assessed.[46]

(*text continues on page 434*)

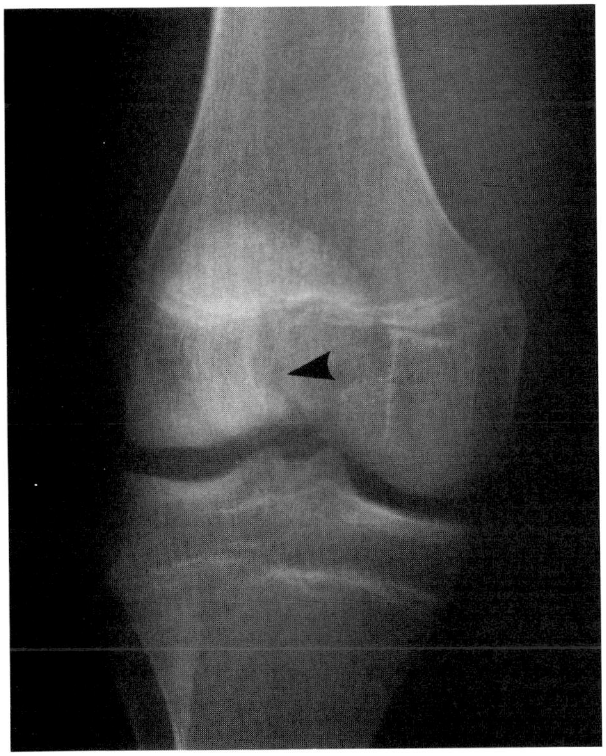

A

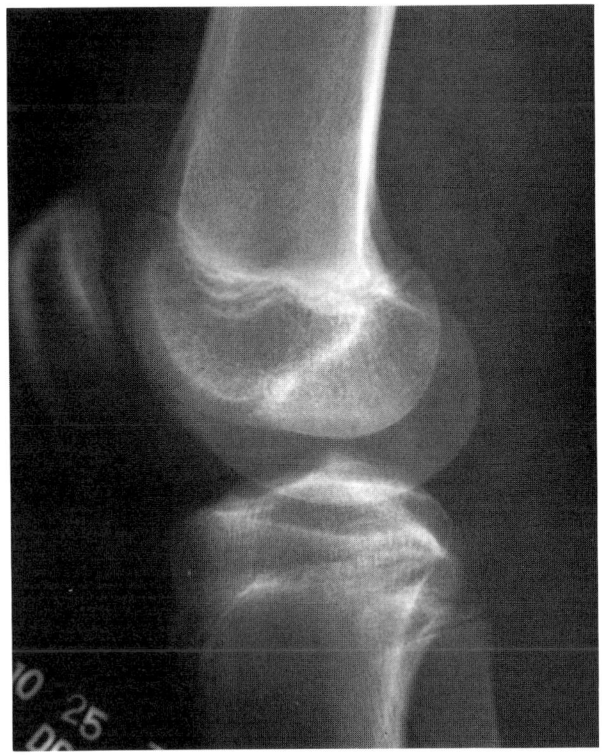

B

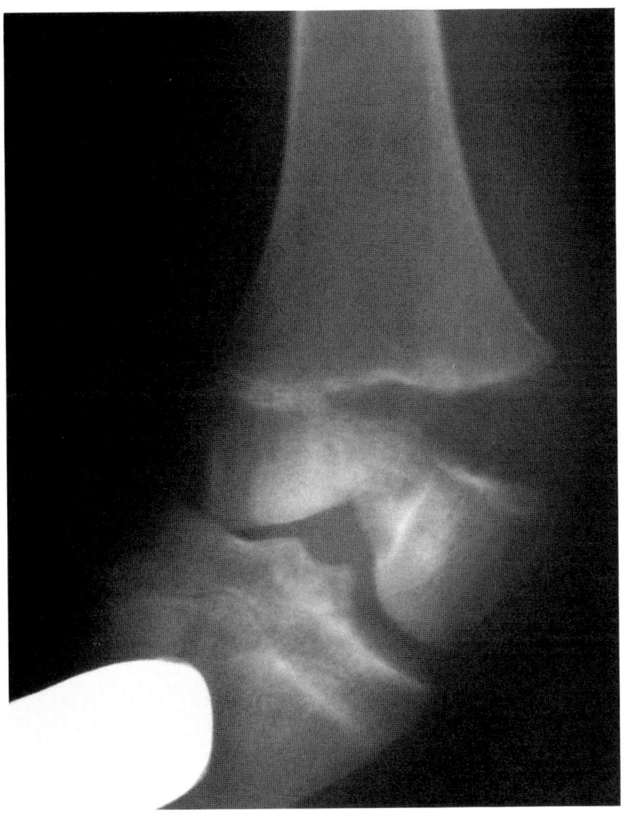

C

FIG. 6-37. The AP **(A)** and lateral **(B)** views of the knee. There is a subtle (*arrow*) Salter-Harris type III fracture, which was overlooked. **C:** Stress view widely separated the physis. Gentle fluoroscopic stress should have been performed. (From Berquist TH. *Imaging in sports injuries*. Rockville, MD: Aspen Press, 1992.)

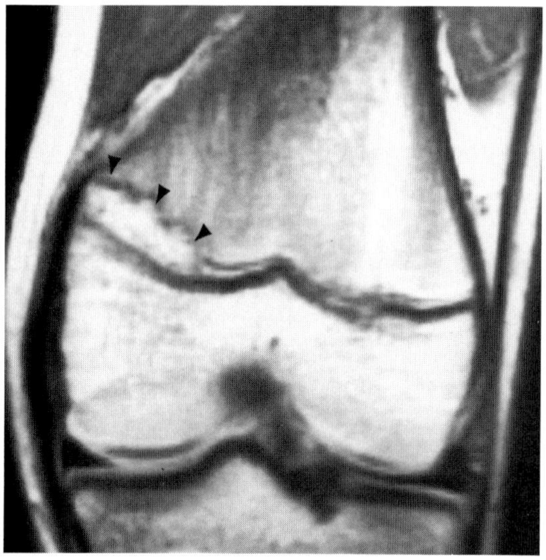

FIG. 6-38. The SE 2,000/30 coronal image of the knee in a baseball player with medial joint line pain. There is a partial physeal fracture (*arrows*) medially. The meniscus and medial collateral ligament are normal.

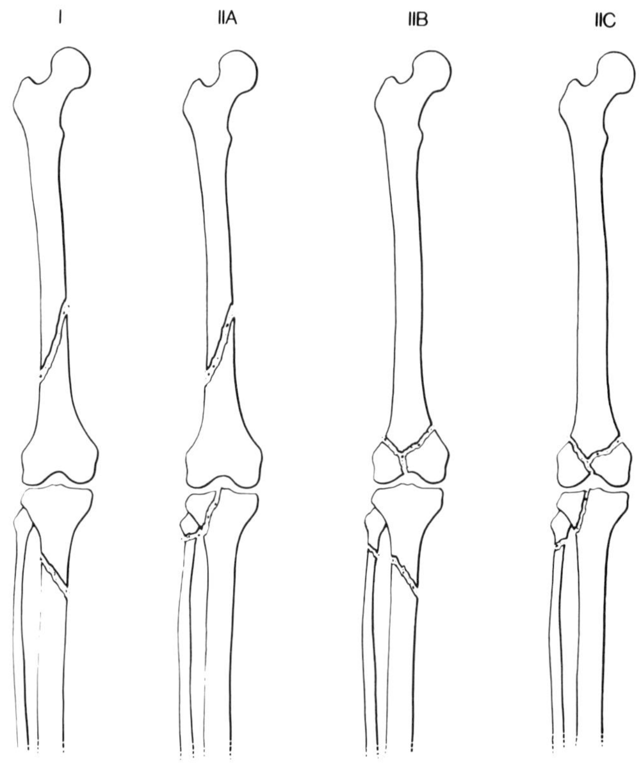

FIG. 6-39. The Fraser et al.[21] classification of ipsilateral femur and tibial fractures. Type I are fractures of the tibia and femur without knee involvement. Type IIA is a fracture of the tibial plateau with a femoral shaft fracture. Type IIB is a fracture of the tibial shaft and an intraarticular fracture of the femur. Type IIC are intraarticular fractures of the tibia and femur.

A,B

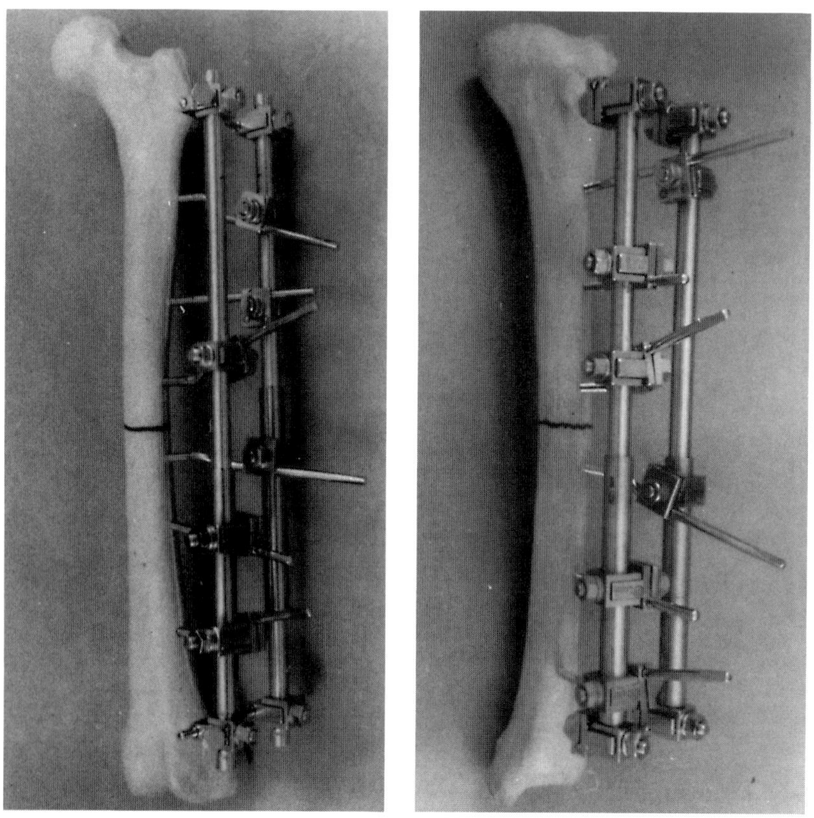

FIG. 6-40. Unilateral ASIF-BM frame on the femur **(A)** and tibia **(B)**.

C,D

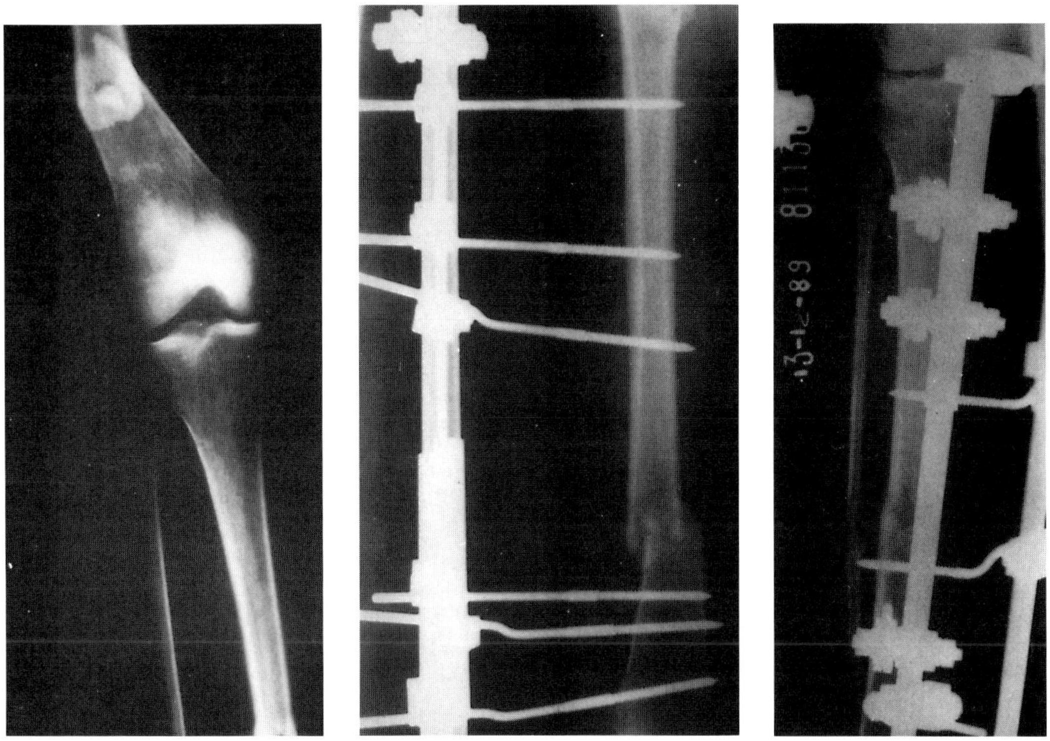

E

FIG. 6-40. (*Continued.*) **C:** The AP view of the leg demonstrating distal femoral and tibia-fibular fractures. Radiographs of the femur **(D)** and tibia **(E)** after ASIF-BM external fixation. (From Barquet A, Massaferro J, Dubra A, Nun F. Ipsilateral open fracture of the femur and tibia treated using dynamic ASIF-BM tubular external fixation: case reports. *J Trauma* 1991;31:1312–1315.)

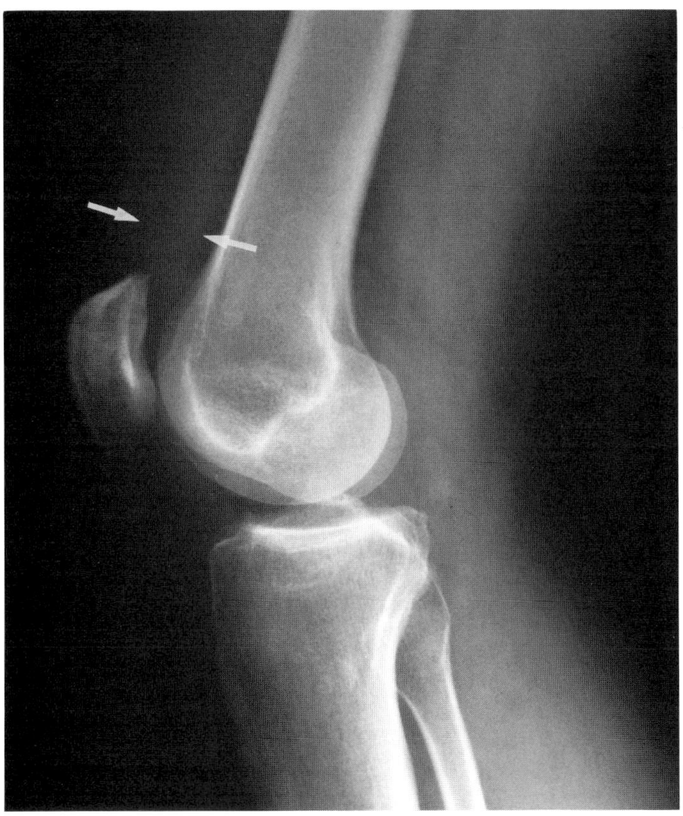

FIG. 6-41. Lateral radiograph of the knee after acute injury demonstrating an effusion (*arrows*). An ACL tear was also present.

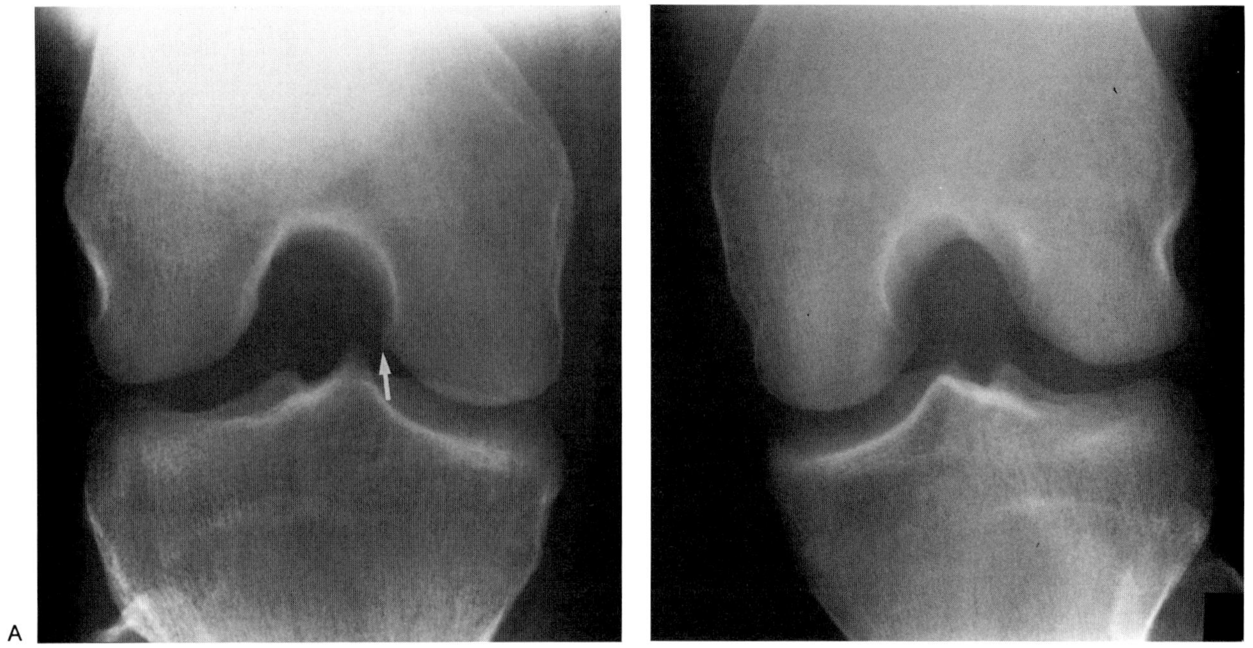

FIG. 6-42. A: Notch view of the knee in a patient with ACL deficiency. Note the medial osteophyte (*arrow*) on the femoral condyle. B: Normal notch view.

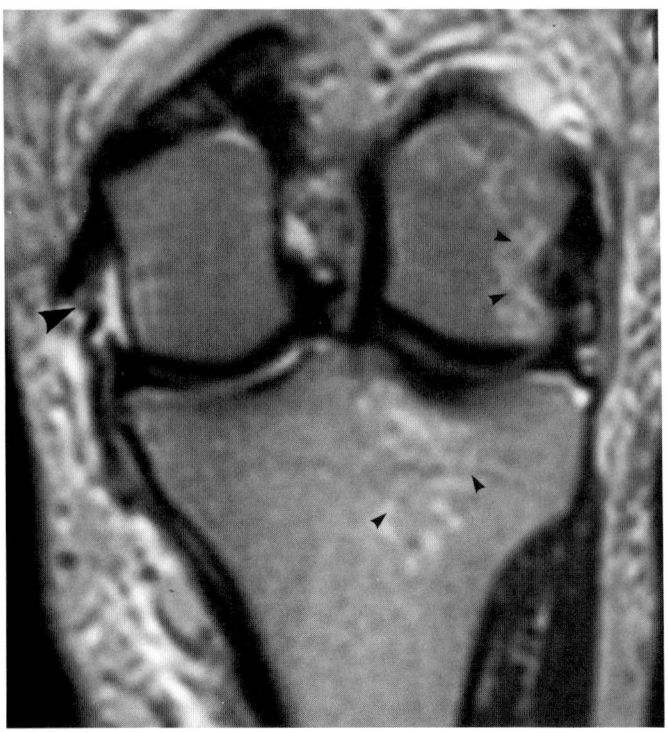

FIG. 6-43. Coronal SE 2,000/60 image of the knee following a valgus injury in football. There is a tear of the medial collateral ligament (*large arrowhead*) and condylar bone bruises in the femur and tibia (*small arrowheads*) laterally.

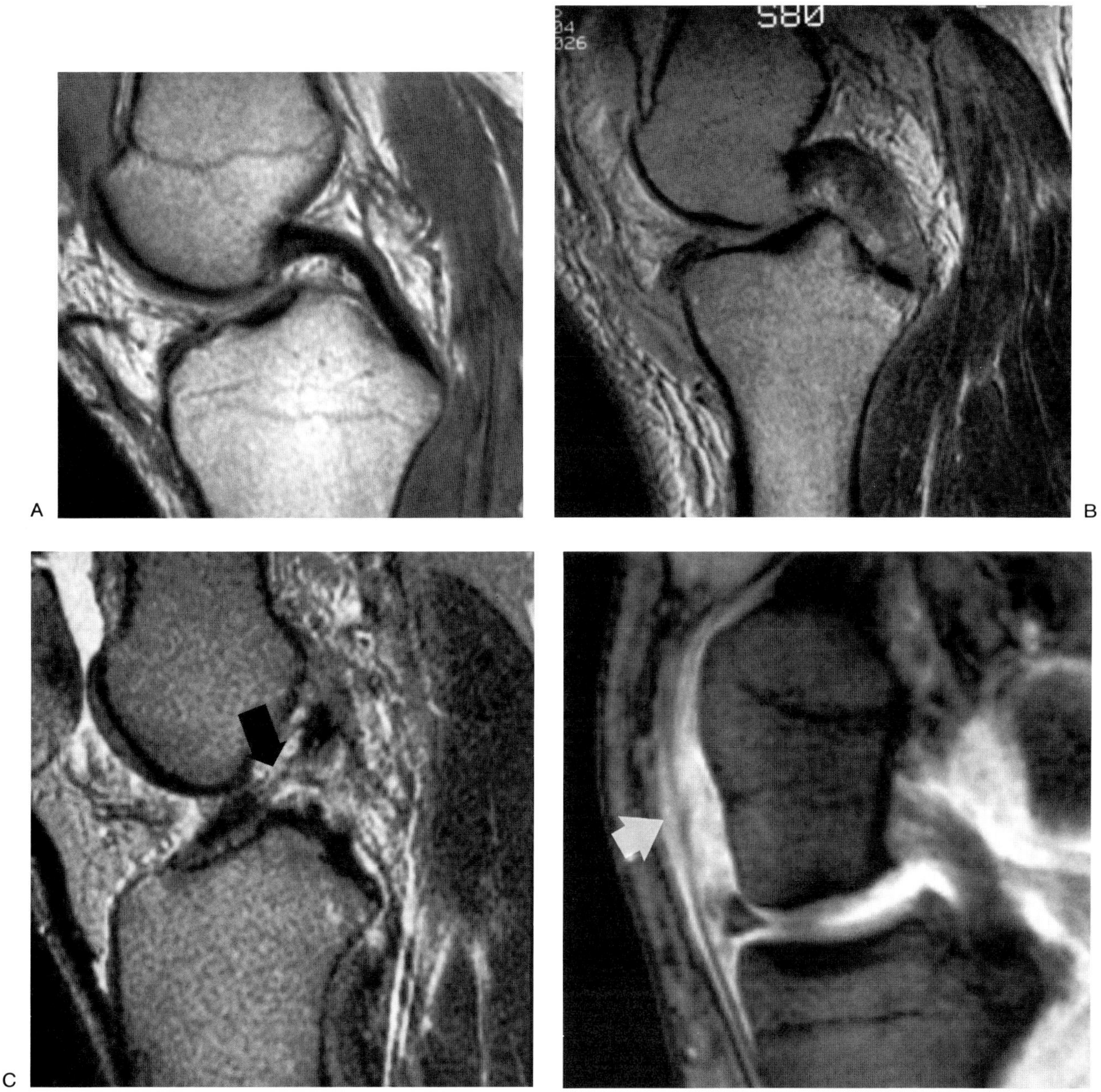

FIG. 6-44. Soft tissue injuries of the knee. Normal **(A)** and partially torn **(B)** thickened PCL. **C:** Effusion and mid-ACL tear (*arrow*). **D:** Partially torn MCL (MPGR sequence).

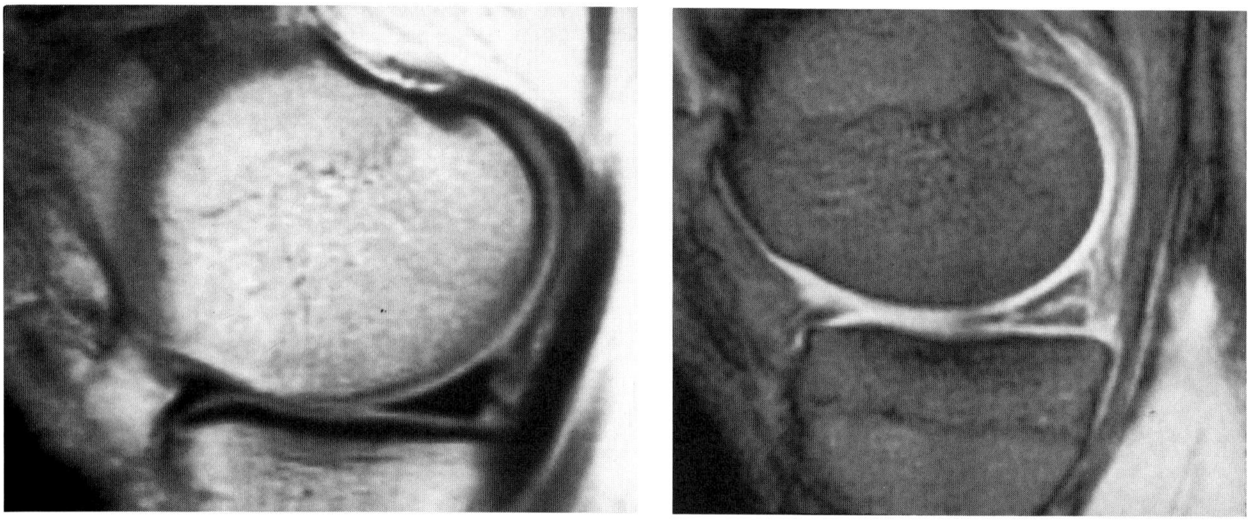

E F

FIG. 6-44. (*Continued.*) Normal **(E)** and torn **(F)** posterior horn of the medial meniscus.

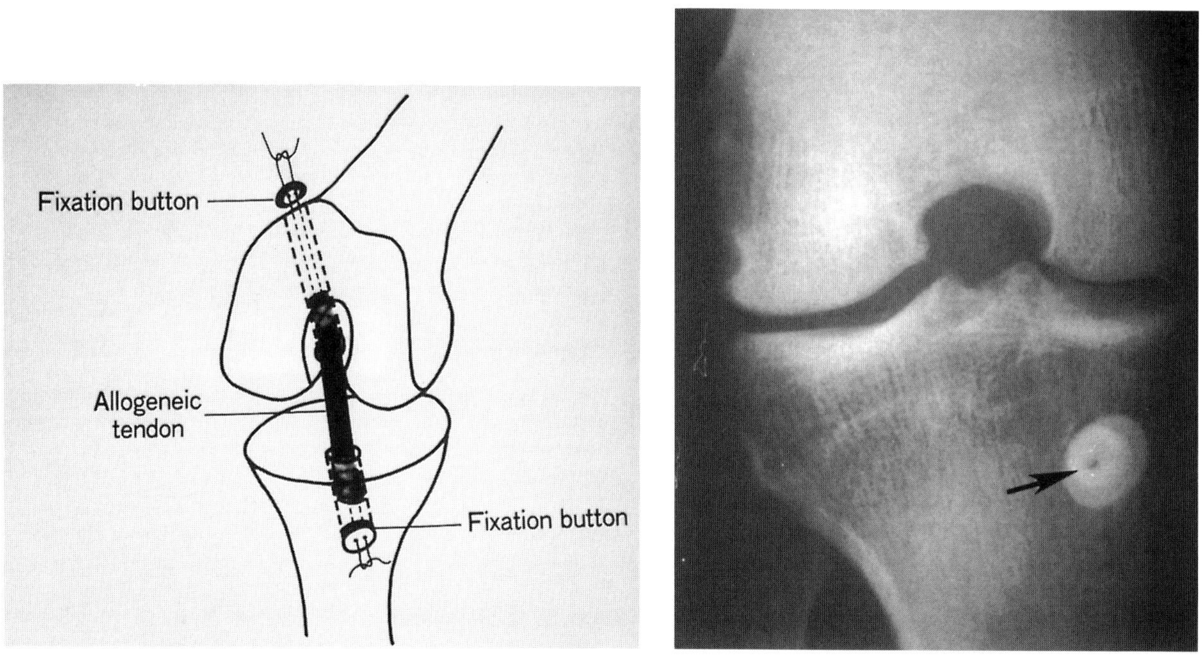

A B

FIG. 6-45. A: Operative technique for fresh-frozen tendon allograft reconstruction of the ACL. **B:** The AP radiograph with lateral compartment arthrosis. The tibial button (*arrow*) is visible. (From Shino K, Inoue M, Horibe S, Hamada M, Ono K. Reconstruction of the anterior cruciate ligament using allogenic tendon: long term followup. *Am J Sports Med* 1990;18:457–465.)

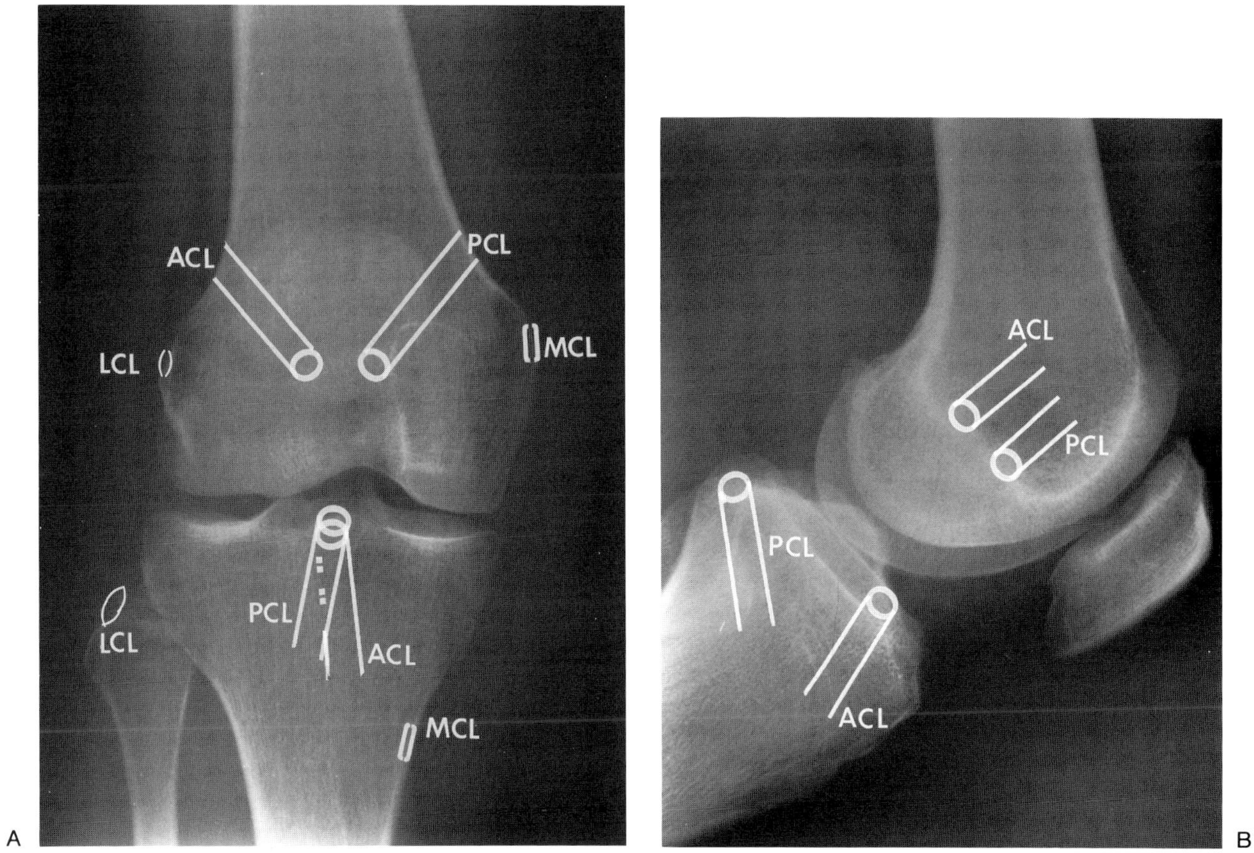

FIG. 6-46. Isometric points for knee reconstruction. **A:** An AP radiograph demonstrating femoral and osseous drilled tunnels for ACL and PCL grafts. Isometric points for MCL and LCL are also demonstrated. **B:** Lateral radiograph demonstrates ACL and PCL tunnel. (From Manaster BJ, Remley K, Newman AP, Mann FA. Knee ligament reconstruction: plain film analysis. *AJR* 1988;150:337–342.)

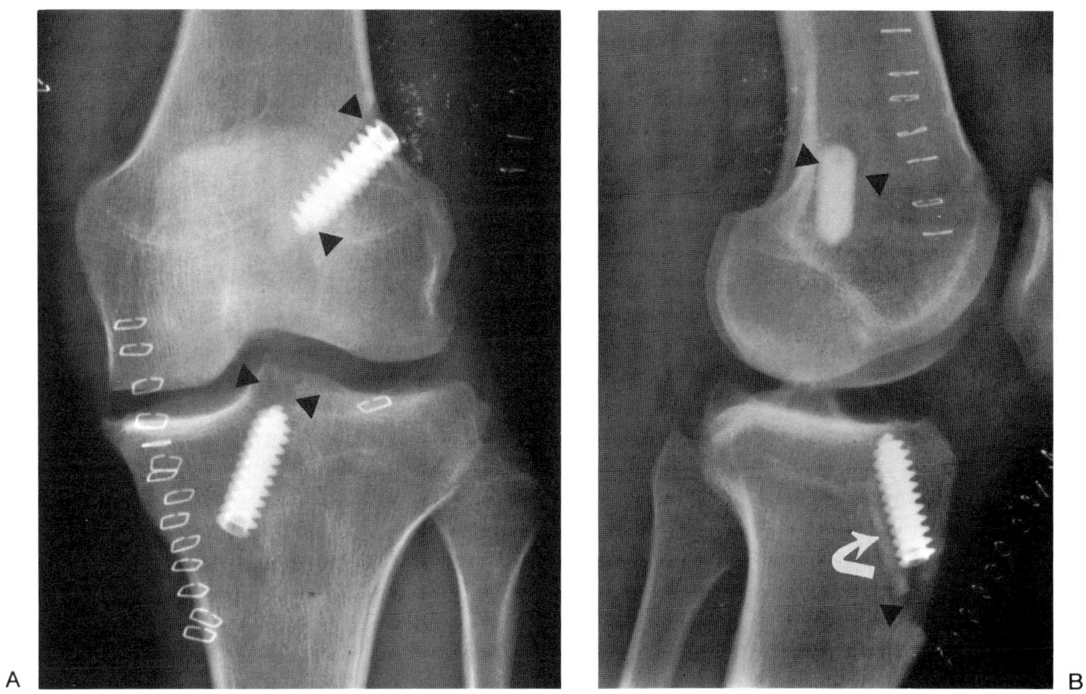

FIG. 6-47. The ACL repair. **A:** An AP view of the knee demonstrates the tunnels (*small arrows*), which are more easily appreciated with interference screw fixation. **B:** Lateral radiograph demonstrates the tunnels (*small arrows*) and the screw compressing the bone at the lower end of the patellar graft (*curved arrow*).

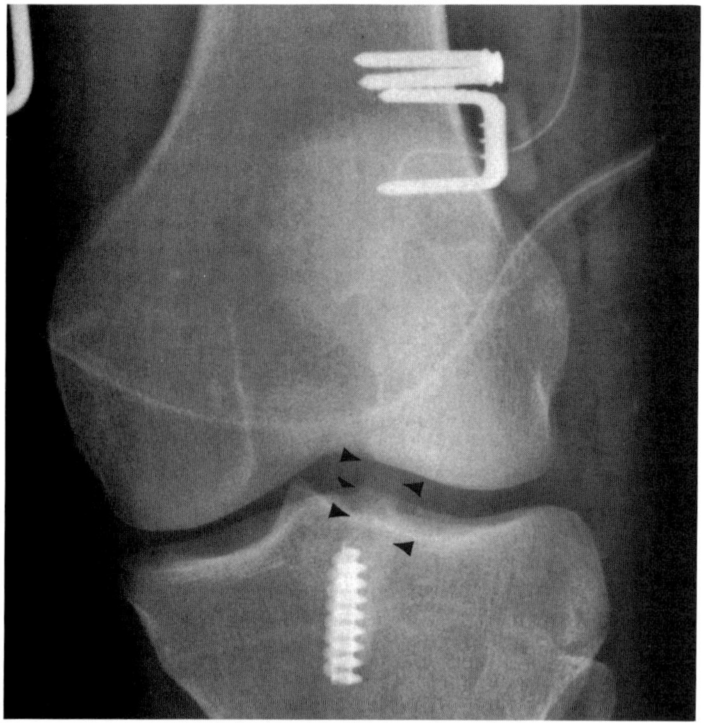

FIG. 6-48. An ACL repair with interference screw distally and staple fixation proximally. The graft can be seen passing through the joint (*arrows*), but the femoral tunnel is not easily detected on the AP view.

A

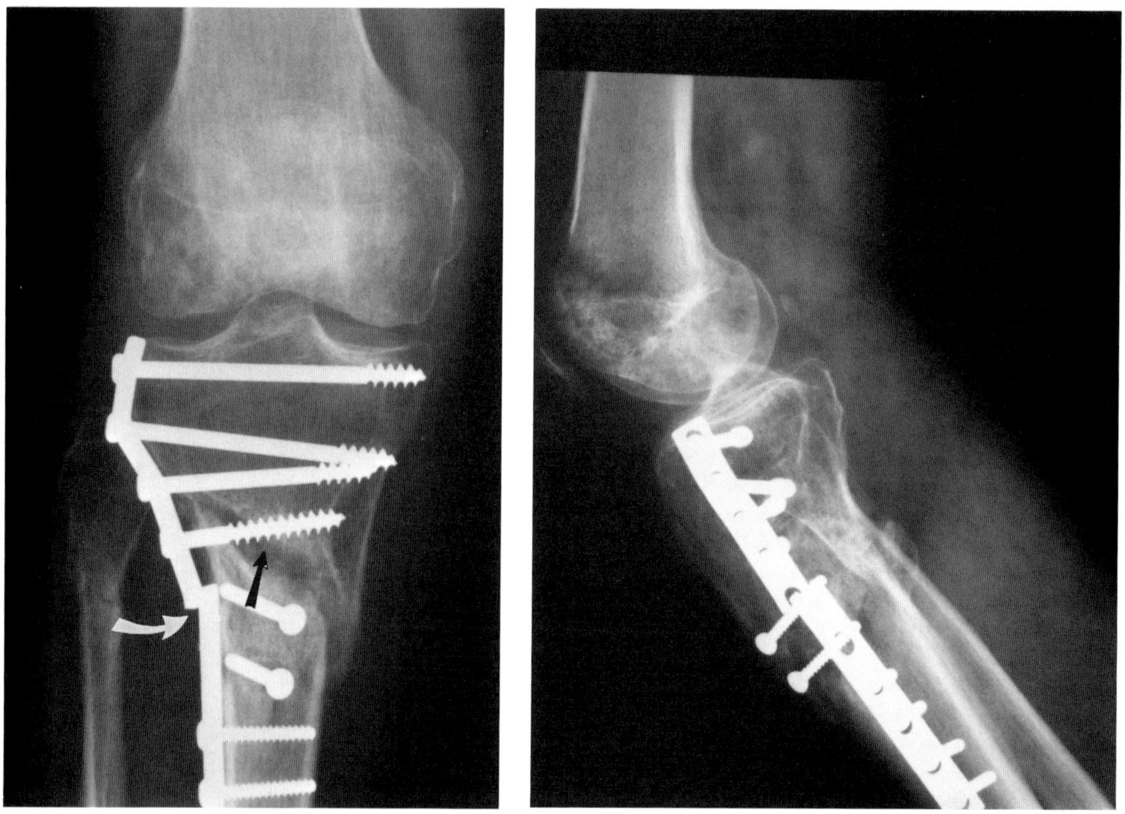

B

FIG. 6-49. The AP **(A)** and lateral **(B)** views several months after DCP fixation of a comminuted upper tibial fracture with bone loss (*black arrow*). The plate fractured (*white arrow*) just distal to the fracture line and through a screw hole. The fracture was reoperated, and bone graft was used to fill in gaps in the bone.

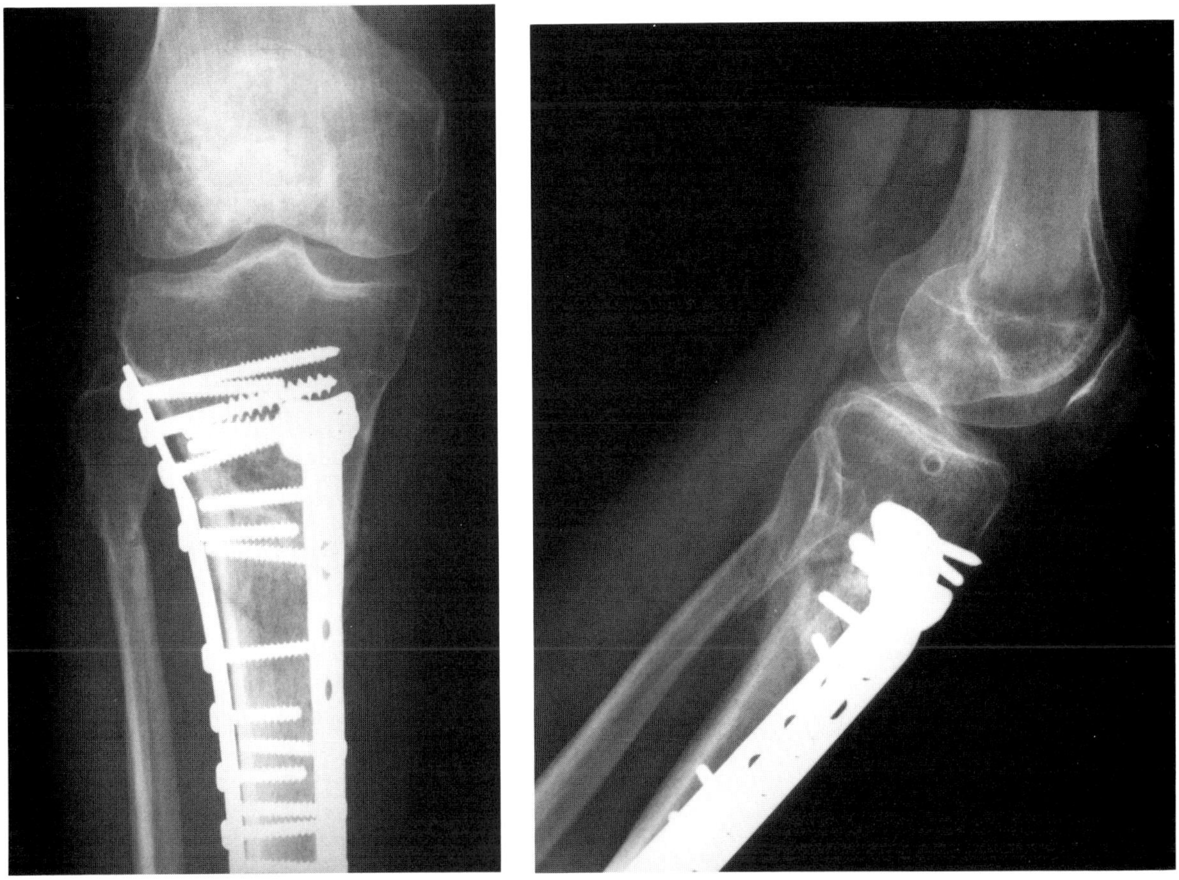

C D

FIG. 6-49. (*Continued.*) **C,D:** A long T buttress and lateral condylar buttress plate with cortical and cancellous screws were used for fixation.

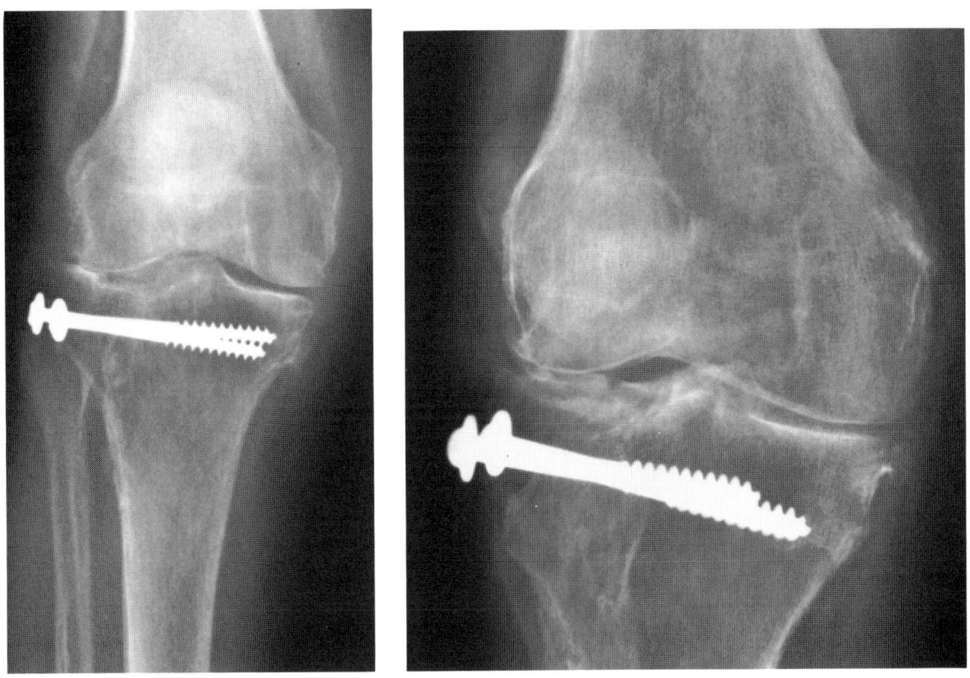

A B

FIG. 6-50. The AP **(A)** and oblique **(B)** radiographs of the knee after internal fixation of lateral tibial plateau with two cancellous screws and washers. There is residual joint deformity and bicompartmental arthritis with cartilage loss.

Postoperative Imaging and Complications

The complications related to osseous injury may be related to the mechanism of injury and associated trauma or treatment. The more significant the trauma (comminuted fractures, fracture-dislocation, or ipsilateral femoral and tibial fractures), the more likely there are to be local or systemic complications.[14,18,26,46,56]

During the acute phases of injury and treatment, the significant distant complications include associated chest and abdominal trauma, fat emboli, and pulmonary emboli.[14,26,46] For purposes of this atlas, we concentrate on the imaging of local problems directly related to the knee injury or treatment instituted.

Local osseous changes, such as a loss of reduction, delayed union, nonunion, and instrument failure, can be evaluated with routine radiography or, in some cases, tomography. Supracondylar fractures generally heal in 3 to 4 months.[26] Other fractures about the knee typically heal within this time, depending on the severity of injury.

Internal fixation results in success in more than 75% of patients.[26,46,51] Failures, when they occur, are commonly related to incomplete reduction, failure to achieve interfragment compression, failure to use bone grafts to fill gaps and incorrect type or length of implants, and patient noncompliance (Fig. 6-49).[51]

Articular deformity is a significant problem, resulting in a chronic painful joint, laxity, and arthrosis. Tibial plateau fractures are particularly likely to result in articular deformity if articular alignment and height are not restored. Varus (71%) and valgus (31%) alignment problems occur most frequently (Fig. 6-50).55 Similar alignment problems occur with physeal injuries and partial growth plate closure (Fig. 6-51).[11]

Avascular necrosis is unusual, although this can occur with patellar fractures. This complication most often affects the proximal pole. Generally, healing occurs with time.[46,49] Tension-band and K-wire fixation interfere with MRI images to some degree. However, depending on the type of fixation, MRI is best suited to identify this problem.

Soft tissue injuries may complicate the initial injury or occur during the repair or the posttreatment period. Vascular injury must be diagnosed prior to therapy and monitored properly in the postoperative period. Arterial injury can occur with proximal tibial physeal injury (Fig. 6-52) and with other fracture dislocations of the knee.[34,46] Arteriography is the most accurate technique used to determine the extent of injury (e.g., intimal tear, occlusion, or disruption). Significant bleeding may lead to compartment syndrome.[34] Venous thrombosis is fairly common in the postoperative period. Cohen et al.[14] reported thrombophlebitis in 20 of 35 patients following knee surgery. Ultrasonography is useful in the thigh and popliteal region and should be the first technique in patients with suspected deep vein thrombosis. The calf is more difficult to evaluate. Venography may be required in questionable or difficult cases.[46]

Neural injuries about the knee are particularly common to the peroneal nerve. The sartorial and infrapatellar branches of the saphenous nerve may also be injured. The injuries may occur from the initial trauma or during surgical intervention. More severe injuries may require months to resolve. Most neural injuries are stretch related and heal with time (3 to 4 weeks). Posttraumatic neuromas also occur. In this setting, MRI is the most useful to identify and characterize the type of injury. Minor stretch injuries may show normal neural structure with little adjacent or internal signal intensity. Significant injury may reveal enlargement and increased signal intensity in the nerve. Neuromas are also well-defined high-signal-intensity masses. These injuries are most easily identified with T2-weighted sequences.[5]

An injury to the supporting structures may result in instability. Routine stress views, if properly performed, are useful to evaluate new or overlooked ligament injuries. Varus, valgus, and AP stress views should be obtained; MRI is also useful if there is no excessive hardware in place. Screws create significant local artifacts, which may interfere with ligament assessment. Routine films should be reviewed to determine if the metal is too close to the region of interest before considering MRI.[5] In the case of surgical reconstruction, the appearance of the tunnel and interference screws and staples can be evaluated on routine views.

Figure 6-46 demonstrates the normal position of the tunnels for ACL and PCL repair. Isometric positions for MCL and LCL are also demonstrated. The ACL takes an oblique course from the lateral femoral condyle to the tibial eminence (Fig. 6-53).[5,39,46] Manaster et al.[39] reported that, for purposes of isometric positions, the femoral tunnel is more important than the tibial tunnel. On the lateral radiograph (Fig. 6-54B), the ACL tunnel is posterior near the cortex and enters at the intercondylar shelf. On the AP view (notch), the tunnel begins just superior to the femoral condyle and enters the joint at the superolateral aspect of the notch. The tibial tunnel for the ACL enters below the tubercle and extends into the joint anterior to the tibial spine (Fig. 6-46).[39] The PCL originates below the tibial joint line and extends in a near-sagittal plane to the lateral side of the medial femoral condyle (Fig. 6-53).[39,46] On the lateral view, the femoral PCL tunnel is anterior to the ACL tunnel, with the tibial tunnel found posteriorly. On the AP notch view, the femoral tunnel begins above the medial femoral condyle, entering the superomedial aspect of the notch. The collateral ligaments (Fig. 6-46) can be evaluated by staple placement at the isometric points.[39]

(*text continues on page 437*)

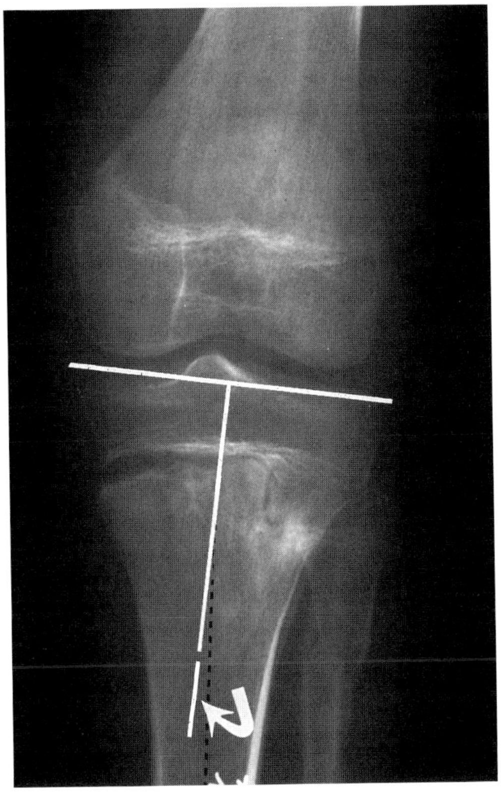

FIG. 6-51. An AP view of the knee demonstrating a physeal fracture with partial closure laterally and asymmetry medially. This results in a tilt (*white lines*) off the tibial axis.

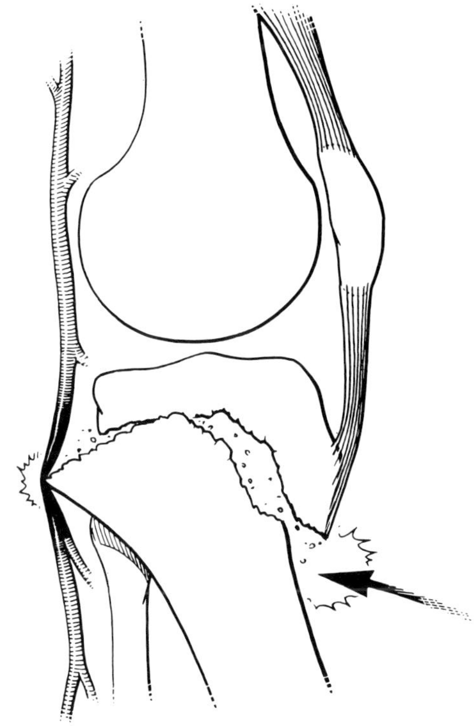

FIG. 6-52. Popliteal artery injury associated with displaced fracture of the proximal tibial physis. (From Berquist TH. *Imaging in sports injuries.* Rockville, MD: Aspen Press, 1992.)

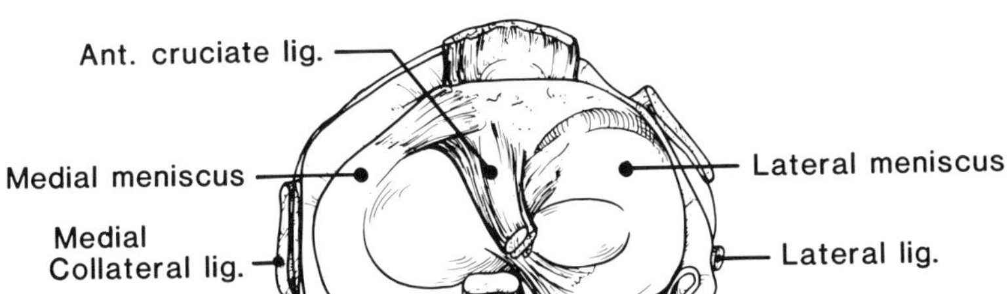

A

FIG. 6-53. The ligament anatomy of the knee. **A:** Axial. (See **B** on next page.)

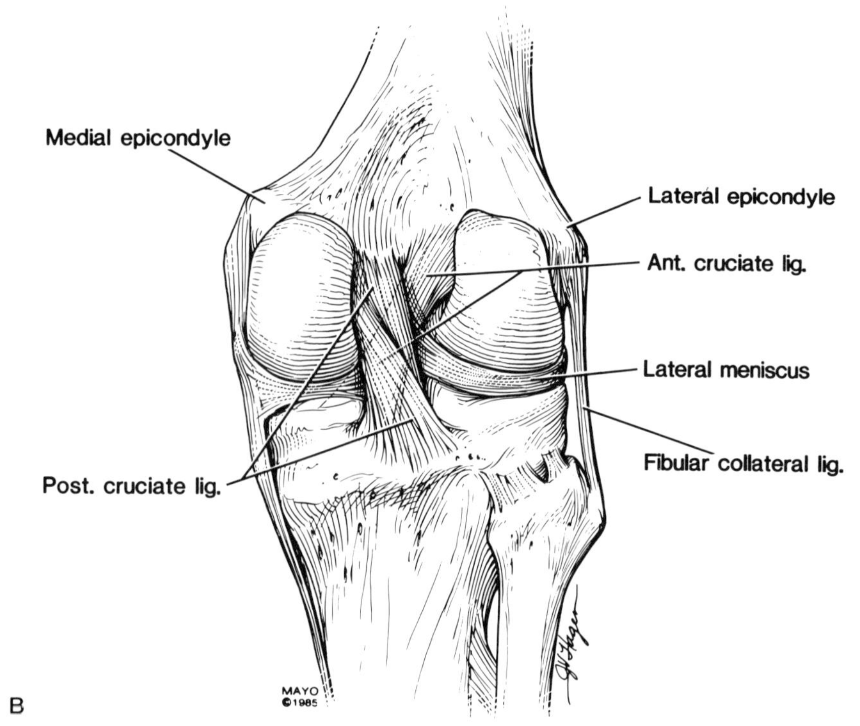

FIG. 6-53. (*Continued.*) **B:** Coronal. (From Berquist TH. *MRI of the musculoskeletal system*, 2nd ed. New York: Raven Press, 1990.)

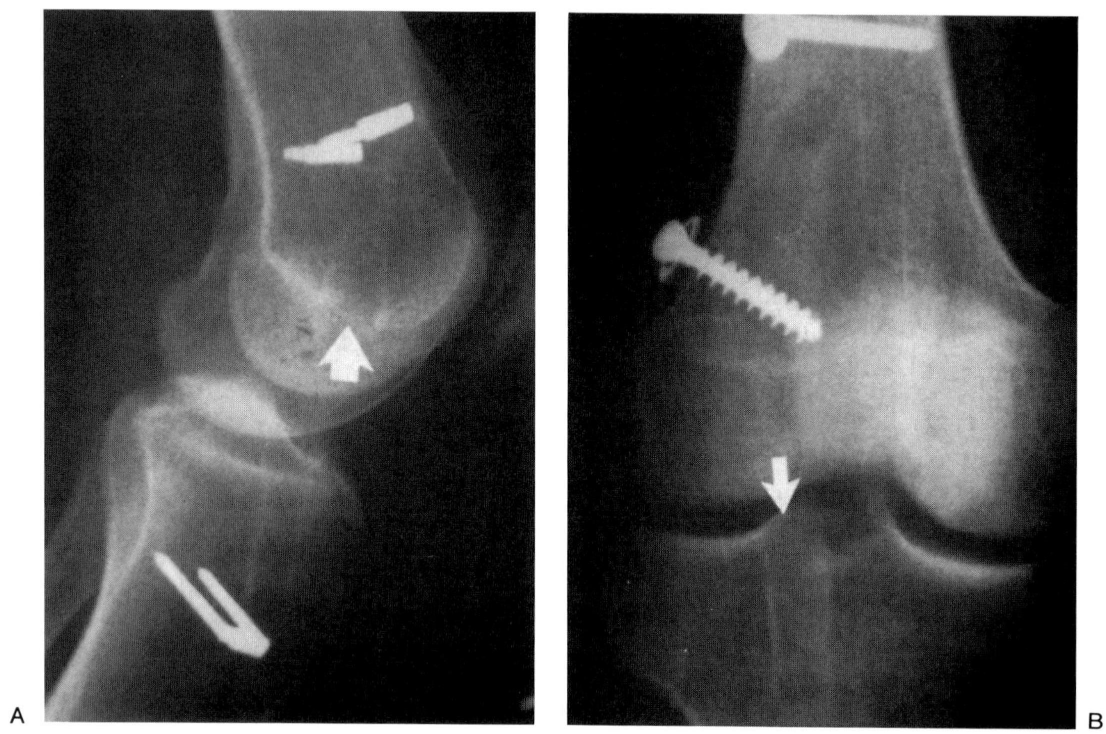

FIG. 6-54. Nonisometric reconstruction. **A:** The femoral tunnel (*arrow*) is anterior to its isometric position on the lateral view (compare with Fig. 6-46). **B:** An AP view of the knee demonstrating failed ACL repair caused by the incorrect (too lateral) positioning of the tibial tunnel (*arrow*). Failure repair was attempted with a prosthetic ligament (screws). (From Manaster BJ, Remley K, Newman AP, Mann FA. Knee ligament reconstruction: plain film analysis. *AJR* 1988;150:337–342.)

The lack of isometric placement can be evaluated on routine radiographs (Figs. 6-54 and 6-55). Other complications reported by Manaster et al.[39] include fractures of the patella, bone plug fracture, and graft fracture. Impingement of the intercondylar roof on the ACL may also create failure after reconstruction.[30] Effusions are not unusual and generally clear spontaneously. In addition, MRI can be used to evaluate the tunnel and graft. However, artifacts along the staple or screw may decrease its ability to evaluate the bone plugs (Fig. 6-56).

Infection can occur with open fractures or following internal fixation. Metal implants may interfere with CT and MRI results. Routine radiographic changes occur late. However, sequestra and other findings may be defined by tomography or fluoroscopically positioned spot views of pin tracts. When there is no open wound or sinus tract for culture, radionuclide studies with technetium-99m and gallium-67 or indium-111-labeled leukocytes may be the best technique for the early detection of osteomyelitis. Joint space aspiration and culture of synovial fluid is useful for suspected joint space infections.[46]

KNEE ARTHROPLASTY

Knee arthroplasty arose as an alternative to arthrodesis.[81,126,149] Hemiarthroplasty with femoral resurfacing began in the 1930s, followed by the use of metal components to reconstruct the knee in the 1940s.[100,114,169] Hinged prosthesis followed, but because of the high failure rates, numerous modifications have been made and continue to be made to improve the results of knee arthroplasty procedures.[113,159] Continued refinements now provide good to excellent results in up to 90% of patients.[113,169]

The total condylar designs were developed in the 1970s and remain the "gold standard" to which modifications and component variations are compared.[137,150] This section presents examples of knee arthroplasty components and their radiographic appearance. Preoperative evaluation and decision making are stressed, along with the techniques for postoperative evaluation. General concepts are stressed (e.g., cemented versus cementless and basic design concepts) because it is beyond the scope of this text to discuss every possible system or system combination that could be used.

Indications and Contraindications

The goals of knee arthroplasty include pain relief and improved range of motion, function, and stability.[169]

Knee arthroplasty is contraindicated in patients with active infections or arthrodeses. Reduced strength in the extension mechanism, neurotrophic arthropathy, prior osteomyelitis, and vascular insufficiency are relative contraindications. However, neurotrophic arthropathies and even previous arthrodeses are repaired by some authors. Patients with excessive occupational or physical demands and markedly obese patients are also not good candidates for knee replacement.[65,90,91,139]

Basic Biomechanics and Component Design

Normal knee motion includes flexion-extension (hinge) along with sliding, rolling, and spinning motions. Sliding motion results in high friction and wear. Spinning motion has no change in the position of the contact point. Moderate friction and wear occur. With rolling motion, the areas of contact for the two surfaces are similar, and the degree of wear and friction is the least.[144,145]

Prostheses are designed to mimic certain knee motions, depending on the extent of the constraint of the prosthesis. Constraint refers to the stability afforded to the knee by the contour of the components.[159] An unconstrained prosthesis (nonconstrained or minimally constrained) is a resurfacing prosthesis (i.e., polycentric prosthesis) that relies on intact collateral and cruciate ligaments (Fig. 6-57). The tibial components are relatively flat.[106,118] Relatively normal knee motion is maintained.[68,145,159]

Semiconstrained prostheses add some stability by using concave surfaced tibial components (Figs. 6-58 and 6-59). Instability is reduced by selecting a tibial component that is thick enough to keep the collateral ligaments at proper tension. The ACL is sacrificed in most cases (total condylar prosthesis). The PCL may be preserved, in which case, the tibial component has a notch posteriorly (Fig. 6-59). The posterior-stabilized condylar prosthesis is a semiconstrained prosthesis used with absent or resected PCLs (Fig. 6-60B). A central post is placed between the tibial and femoral components, which adds a degree of constraint over the nonposteriorly constrained knee.[145,159]

Constrained prostheses are used in patients with inadequate soft tissue support or bone loss or for revision arthroplasty. Metal-on-metal hinged prostheses had disadvantages, including metal wear with release of metal particles, more bone resection required, and failure to permit rotation, which increased the incidence of loosening.[159,175] Both linked and nonlinked designs are available (Fig. 6-61).[99,121] The initial hinged designs (Guepar and Walldius) frequently failed, and a more recent constrained prosthesis allows rotation and distraction (Kinematic™ rotating hinge, Howmedica, Rutherford, NJ; Fig. 6-60A).[145,159,175]

Component Structure

Considerable effort and research has gone into developing the most suitable alloys and plastic for joint components. Stainless steel components are adequate for el-

(*text continues on page 442*)

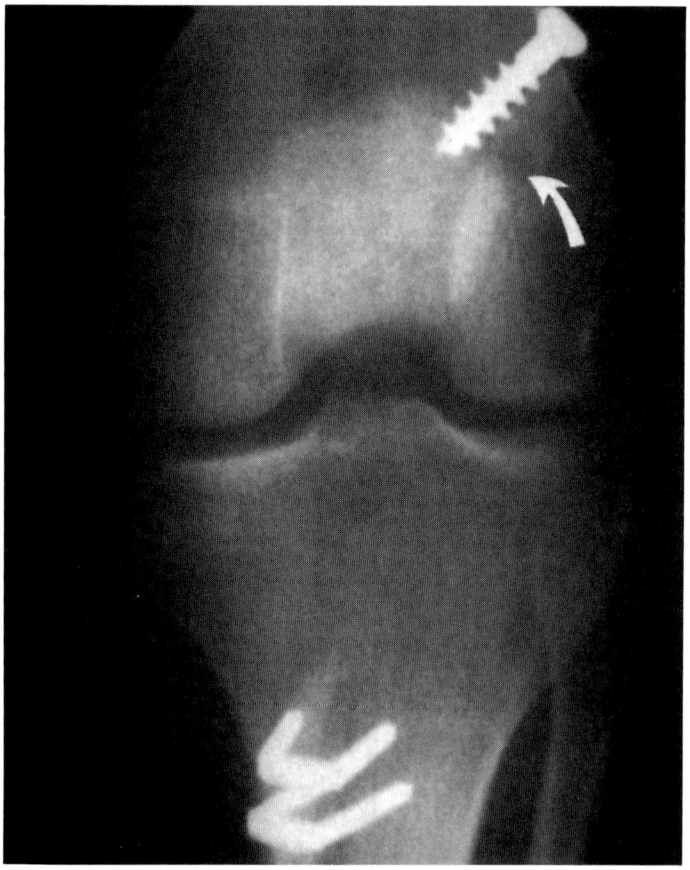

FIG. 6-55. An AP view of the knee after ACL repair. The femoral bone plug is fractured (*arrow*) and displaced slightly distally. (From Manaster BJ, Remley K, Newman AP, Mann FA. Knee ligament reconstruction: plain film analysis. *AJR* 1988;150:337–342.)

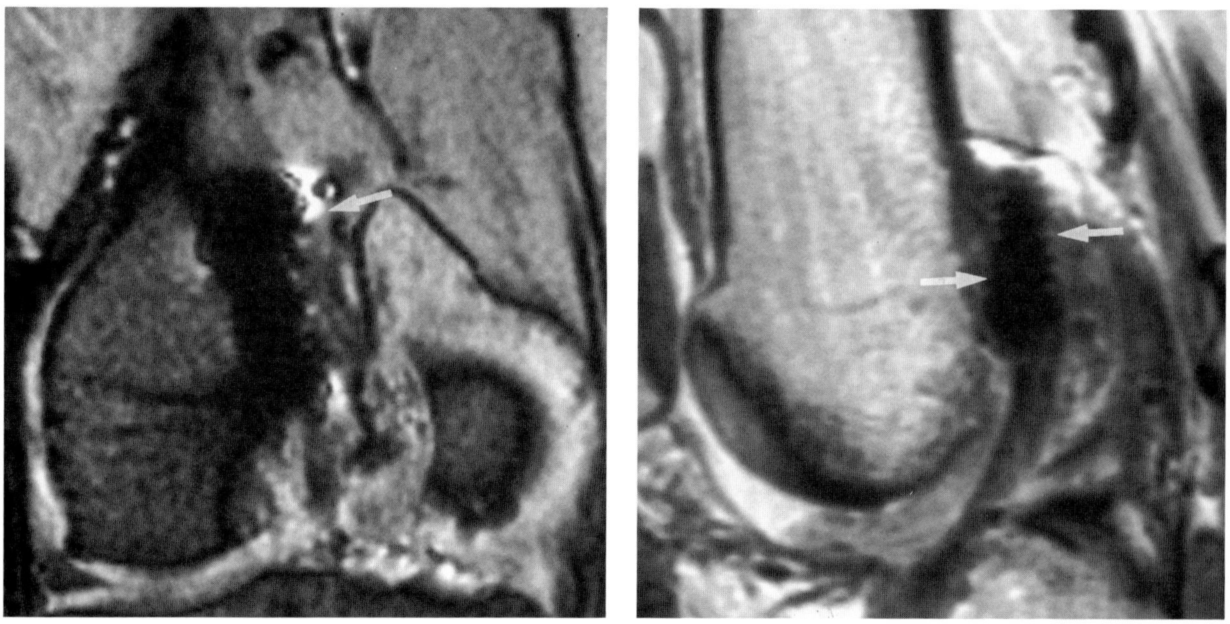

A B

FIG. 6-56. The MRI scan of the knee following ACL repair with a tendon graft and interference screws. **A:** Coronal gradient-echo image (400/31, FA 30°) demonstrating artifact from the screw in the femoral tunnel (*arrow*). **B:** Sagittal SE 2,000/30 image demonstrates the graft in good position. There is less artifact from the femoral screw (*arrows*). Note the effusion, which is not unusual after cruciate repairs.

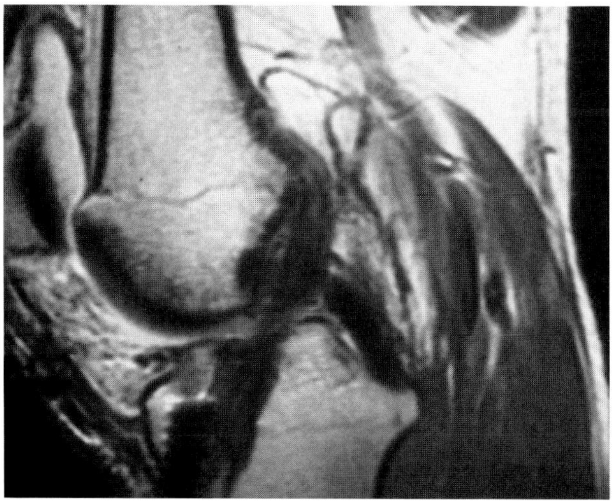

C

FIG. 6-56. (*Continued.*) **C:** Sagittal SE 2,000/30 image demonstrating the tibial tunnel and screw with slight artifact.

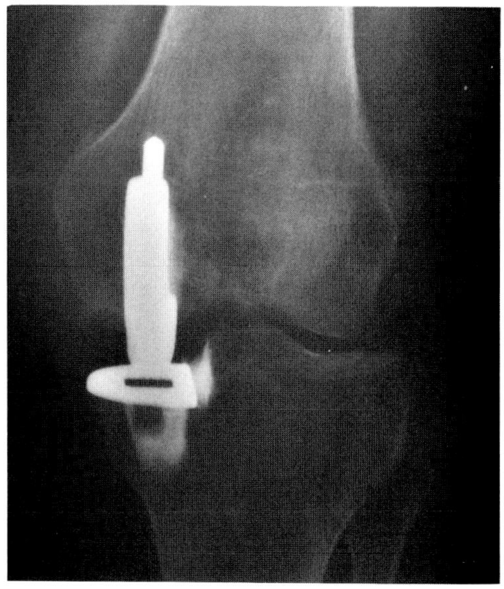

FIG. 6-57. Nonconstrained prosthesis. An AP view of the knee following unicompartmental arthroplasty with polycentric components.

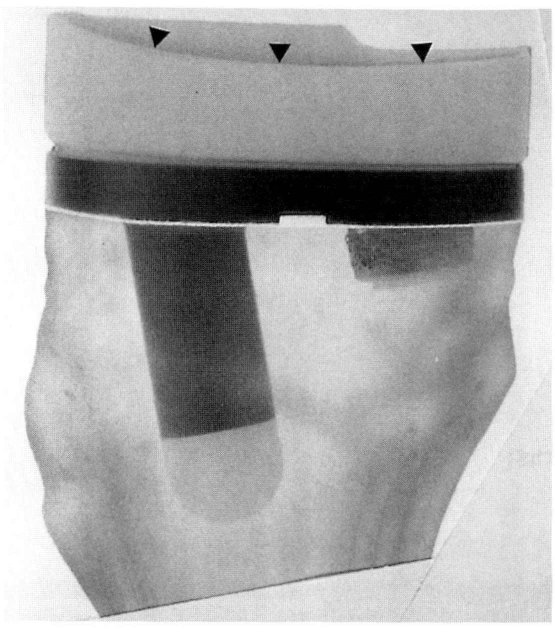

A

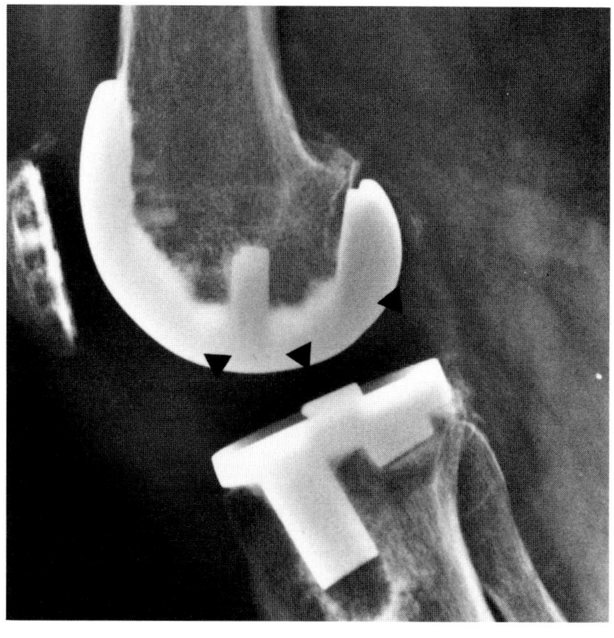

C

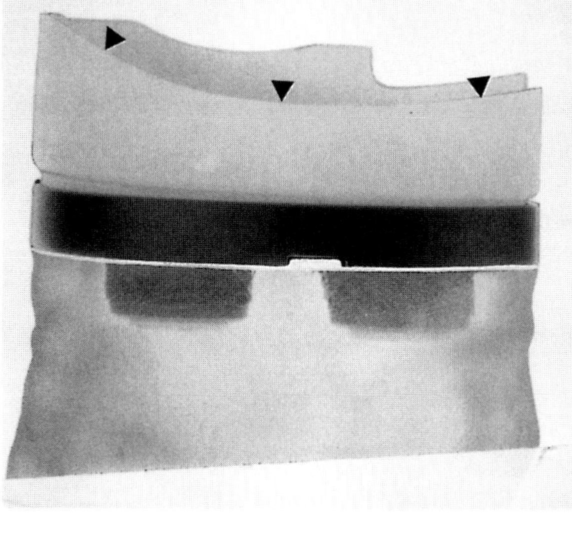

B

FIG. 6-58. Lateral illustrations of ultrahigh molecular weight polyethylene tibial components (*arrows*) with a relatively flat surface **(A)** for minimal constraint and a more concave option **(B)** providing more constraint in patients with less soft tissue support. (Courtesy of Zimmer, Warsaw, IN.) **C:** Lateral radiograph demonstrating a concave polyethylene tibial component (*arrowheads*) with metal tray. Miller-Galante II with all-polyethylene patellar component. Cemented tibial and femoral components.

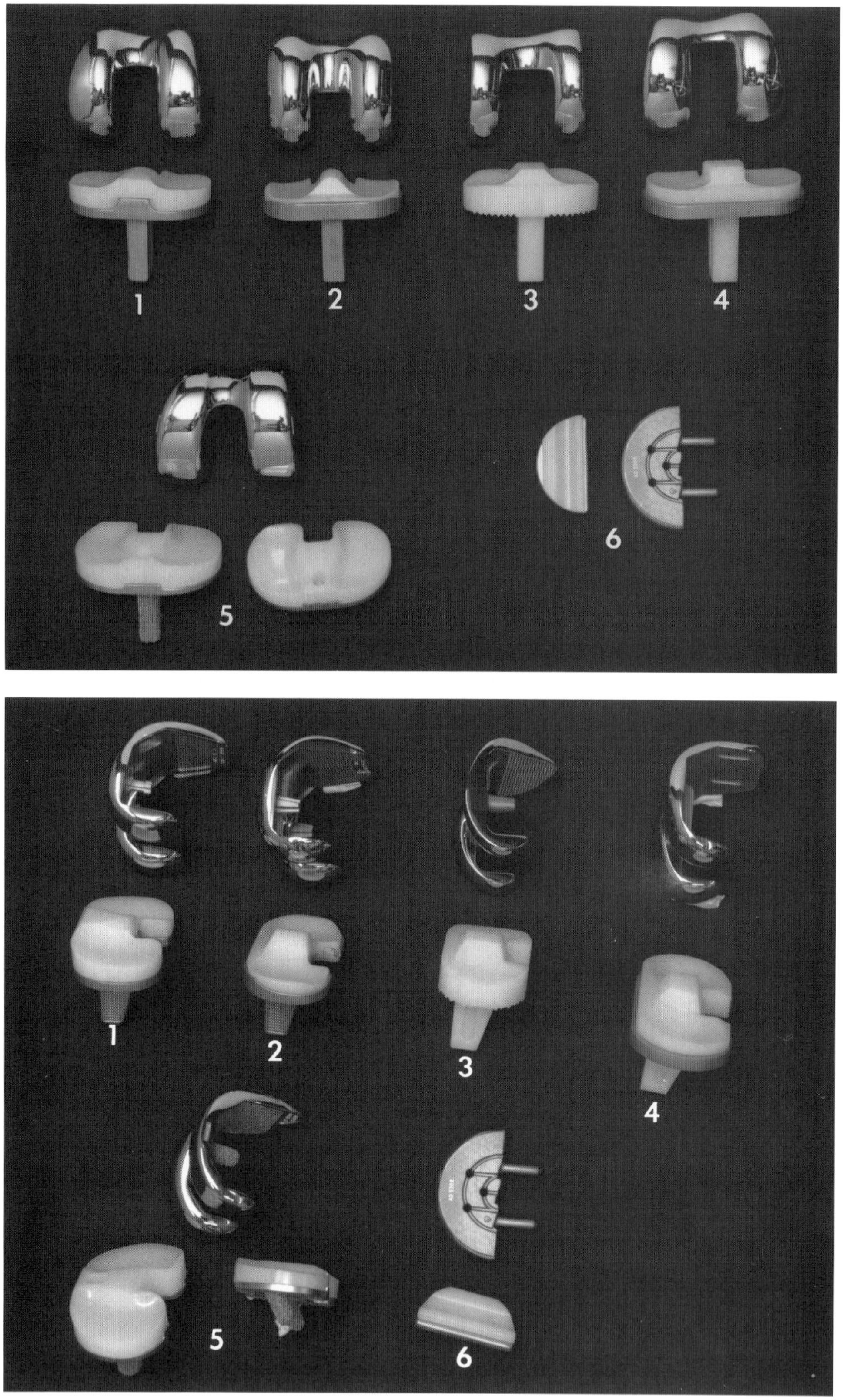

A

B

FIG. 6-59. The AP **(A)** and lateral **(B)** views of semi- and unconstrained prostheses. *1,* Kinematic condylar; *2,* cruciate condylar; *3,* anatomic; *4,* Townley-Botham; *5,* PCA; 6, polycentric. (From Rand JA, Berquist TH. The knee. In: Berquist TH, ed. *Imaging of orthopedic trauma and surgery.* Philadelphia: WB Saunders, 1986;293–391.)

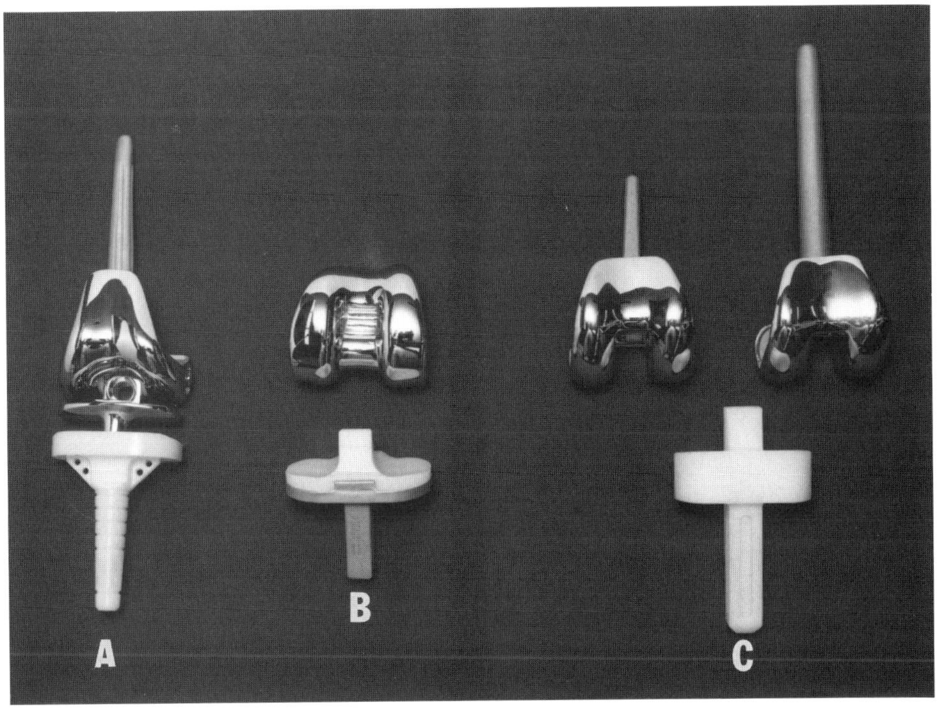

FIG. 6-60. The AP views of constrained and moderately constrained prostheses. **A:** Kinematic rotating hinge (constrained, used for knee revisions). **B:** Kinematic stabilizer (moderately constrained). **C:** Total condylar III with augmented stem (moderately constrained).

A,B

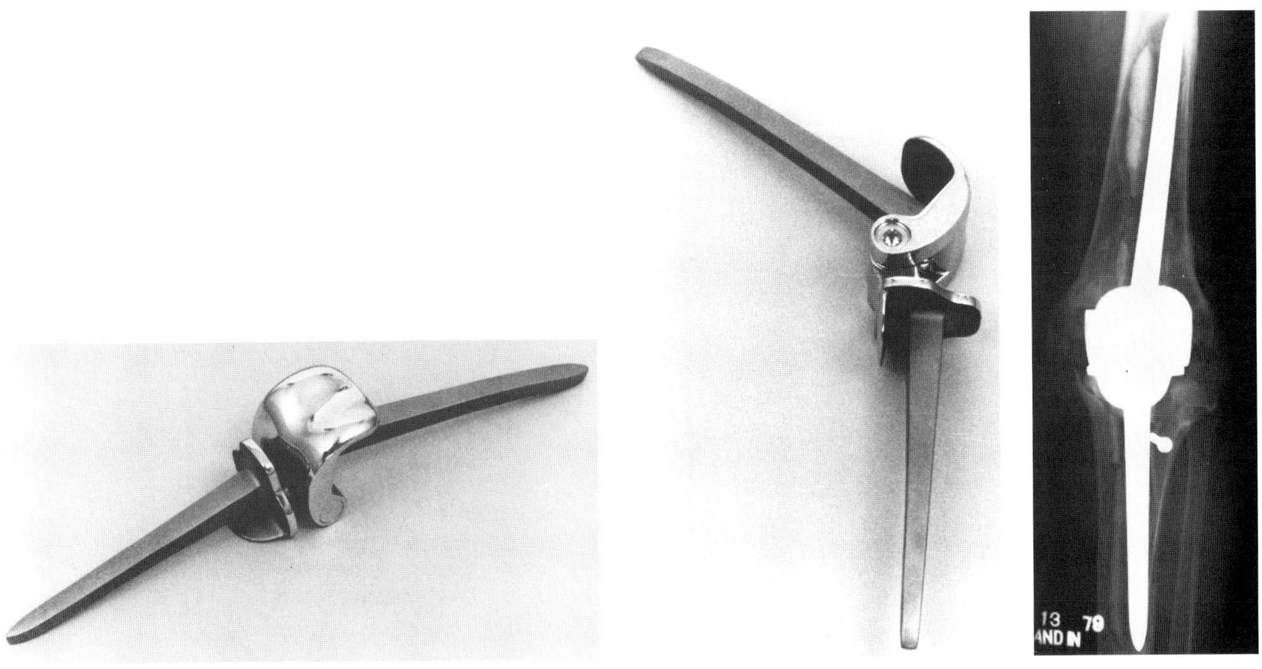

C

FIG. 6-61. Guepar prosthesis. The AP **(A)** and lateral **(B)** views. **C:** An AP view of the knee in a patient with a loose Guepar prosthesis. Note the obvious cement fractures and advanced lucency around both femoral and tibial stems. (From Rand JA, Berquist TH. The knee. In: Berquist TH, ed. *Imaging of orthopedic trauma and surgery*. Philadelphia: WB Saunders, 1986;293–391.)

derly patients or those with a low activity level. However, stainless steel has largely been abandoned because of problems with corrosion, bioincompatibility, fatigue fractures, and difficulty with creating porous surfaces.[87,175]

Metal alloys are more commonly used with ultrahigh molecular weight polyethylene or, in some cases, ceramic articular surfaces. The two most common metal alloys are titanium and cobalt based.[87] Cobalt-chromium or cobalt-chromium-molybdenum alloys and titanium-aluminum-vanadium alloys are commonly used. The addition of nitrogen ions improves the hardness and surface wear of the metals.[79,84,87,144] Cobalt-chromium alloys resist fatigue and corrosion but are theoretically more toxic to the surrounding tissues. Titanium-based alloys are less toxic but create increased release of inflammatory mediators, e.g., prostaglandin E_2, interleukin-6 and -1, and tumor necrosis factor.[94] Whatever the drawbacks of these alloys may be, they tend to have increased survival when used with polyethylene surfaces compared with metal-on-metal prostheses.[175]

Preoperative Clinical Evaluation

As noted earlier, the patient's condition, weight, age, activity level, and occupation and the cause of the knee symptoms (i.e., osteoarthritis versus erosive arthritis) are major considerations. A more definitive scoring system has been used for years. This system was developed by the Hospital for Special Surgery during the early years of knee replacement surgery. Their system incorporates a functional component; therefore, the scores naturally tend to deteriorate with age.[102] The Knee Society has developed a new system that separates the knee rating and functional assessment. The knee assessment portion contains three essential parameters: pain, stability, and range of motion. A well-aligned knee with 125° of motion, no pain, and negligible instability is awarded 100 points.[102,169] The maximal score for walking or stair climbing is also 100 points for patients whose walking distance is unlimited and stair climbing is normal or accomplished without railing support.[102]

The following point system is a summary of the table provided by Insall et al.[102] (Table 6-1).

There are point deductions for contractures, extensor function loss, and poor alignment in the knee category and for cane or crutch support requirements in the functional group.[102] These scores are used pre- and postoperatively to assess the results of arthroplasty. They appear frequently in the orthopedic literature; therefore, radiologists should be familiar with these scoring methods.[113,116,150,160,181]

Preoperative Imaging

Preoperative radiographic evaluation is important to assess the local bone and soft tissue anatomy and the entire lower extremity.[159,169] Routine preoperative radiographs include full-length standing AP, lateral, and Merchant views of the patella. The accuracy of the joint space evaluation may be increased by using the PA 45° flexed-knee technique described by Rosenberg et al.[153] However, in most cases, the full-length standing AP is adequate for the joint space evaluation and allows the necessary measurements to be calculated.[144,169]

The standing full-length radiograph should be reviewed to detect any fracture, malunion, bowing of the long bones, length discrepancy, or incongruence of the hip and ankle joints that may have an impact on knee replacement (Fig. 6-62). Measurements are important. The mechanical axis is determined by drawing a line from the center of the femoral head (Fig. 6-62) to the

(text continues on page 444)

TABLE 6-1. *Point system for knee rating*

Knee rating (maximum, 100 points[a])		Functional[a]	
Parameter	Points	Task	Points
Pain		Walking	
None	50	Unlimited	50
Moderate	25	>10 blocks	40
Severe	0	5–10 blocks	20
		Housebound	0
Range of motion [maximum, 25 points (125°)]			
5° = 1 point		Stairs	
Stability		Normal	50
AP <5 mm	10	Descending with railing	40–15
>10 mm	0	Unable to climb stairs	0
Medial-lateral <5°	15		
6–9°	10		
10–14°	5		
15°	0		

[a] More categories in each section.

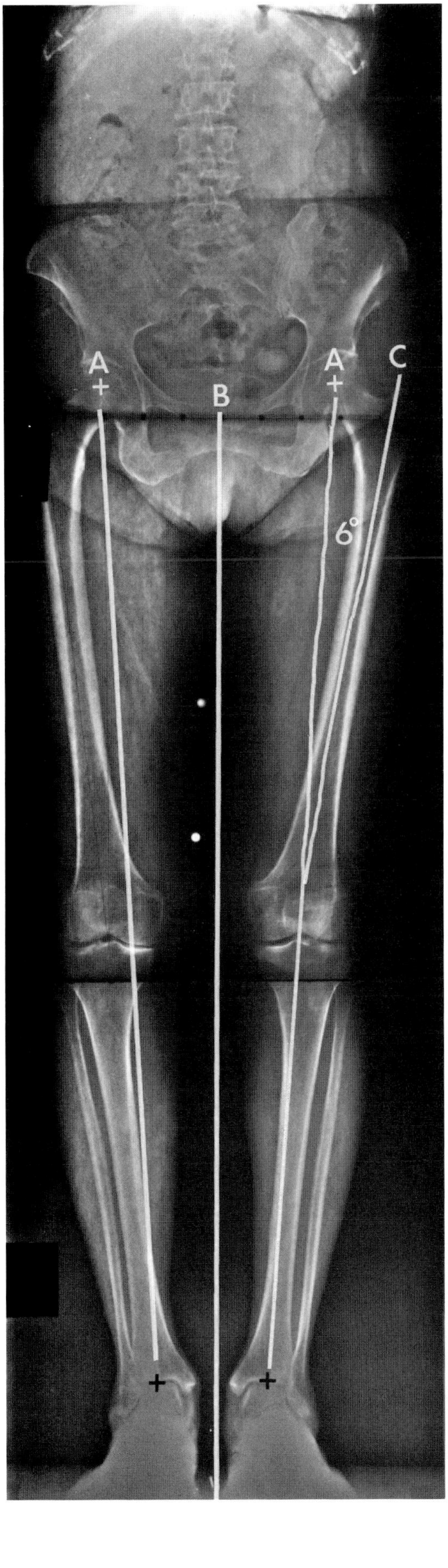

FIG. 6-62. Preoperative full-length radiographs demonstrating the mechanical axis **(A)** (*white line* from the center of the femoral head (+) to the center of the knee and ankle [+]) and vertical axis **(B)**. Note that the mechanical axis on the right passes slightly medially to the midknee because of osteoarthritis with medial compartment narrowing and slight varus deformity. The mechanical axis is through the center of the normal left knee. The mechanical axis of the femur **(C)** is about 6° valgus from the mechanical axis (A). The normal femorotibial angle is 5° to 7° valgus.

center of the ankle. This line should pass through or near the center of the knee. The mechanical axis is generally 3° off the vertical axis (vertical line, Fig. 6-62). The anatomic axis is the angle formed by the lines drawn along the femur and tibia. The knee and ankle angles are also calculated as shown in Figure 6-62.[169]

The degree of osteoarthritis can also be graded on the standing AP view by using the Kellgren-Lawrence system (Fig. 6-63), which is based on osteophytes and secondary changes, or a system based on joint space narrowing that was devised by Brandt et al.[67] (Table 6-2).

The degree of involvement is especially important if unicompartmental procedures are being considered. Osteoarthritic change in both tibiofemoral compartments, subluxation, or chondrocalcinosis are contraindications for unicompartmental replacement.[68]

All three views should be assessed for the degree of arthritic involvement, bone loss, avascular necrosis, and other bone changes (Fig. 6-64).[129,159] Subtle changes may require additional studies, such as radionuclide imaging or MRI, to evaluate early avascular necrosis.[169] In addition, MRI is more sensitive than routine radiographs for the detection of early bone and cartilage abnormalities (Fig. 6-65),[64] and CT can also be used to evaluate the bone stock preoperatively.

Ligaments can be evaluated clinically in most cases. However, when the results are questionable, stress views or MRI (Fig. 6-66) may be required to define the ligamentous anatomy and instability more accurately.[64,72]

Joint aspiration may also be indicated in patients with effusions to exclude infections or define the nature of the arthropathy better.[159,169]

Component Selection

Clinical features (age, weight, symptoms, and activity level) and preoperative image studies are considered when selecting the type of prosthesis that will best suit the patient. In general, the least constrained prosthesis should be used for primary reconstruction.[129] There are numerous minor variations in current condylar designs. When cruciate ligaments are intact and retained, more anatomic designs are used. When the cruciate ligaments are sacrificed or more constrained components are considered, less anatomic components are required.[141] Some institutions use the posterior-stabilized designs for their primary knee replacements.

Deficiency of the collateral ligaments is usually not a significant problem with modern condylar designs.[141,159] Preserving the PCL has several advantages, including (1) improving lever-arm quadriceps function, (2) assisting in tibial-femoral load transfer, (3) preserving proprioceptive nerves, and (4) aiding in the normal tibial "roll back" mechanism of the knee. The PCL is preserved in patients with a weak extensor mechanism or patellectomy. Surgery is slightly more difficult when the PCL is preserved because the soft tissue balance must be more precise.[141]

Bone deficiency and angular deformities from old fractures must be considered and plans for their correction developed. These corrections may include tibial wedges, longer intramedullary component stems, custom components, bone grafting, or the use of methyl methacrylate with or without screws.[129,141]

Tibial Components

Loosening problems with the early designs, retention or sacrifice of the cruciate ligaments, stability problems requiring a more constrained design, and other factors have resulted in numerous variations to assist with postoperative function and increase the survival of tibial components. Tibial components may be symmetric (i.e, both medial and lateral surfaces have the same shape) or anatomic (i.e., medial and lateral surfaces are configured to the different shapes of the tibial condyles). The components may be all polyethylene, or metal backed with variable-height polyethylene spacers. The tibial compo-

(*text continues on page 448*)

TABLE 6-2. *Classification schemes for osteoarthritis*

Grade	Kellgren-Lawrence classification	Joint space narrowing system[67]
0	Normal	<25% narrowing without secondary changes (geodes, sclerosis, osteophytes, Fig. 6-63)
I	Doubtful narrowing with possible osteophytes	<25% narrowing with secondary features or moderate narrowing without secondary features
II	Definite osteophytes with possible joint space narrowing	25–50% joint space narrowing and secondary features or 50–75% narrowing without secondary features
III	Moderate multiple osteophytes, definite narrowing, some sclerosis, and possible bone contour abnormalities (Fig. 6-63C)	50–75% narrowing with secondary features or >75% narrowing with no secondary features (Fig. 6-63B)
IV	Large osteophytes, marked narrowing, sclerosis, and deformity (Fig. 6-63D)	>75% narrowing with secondary features

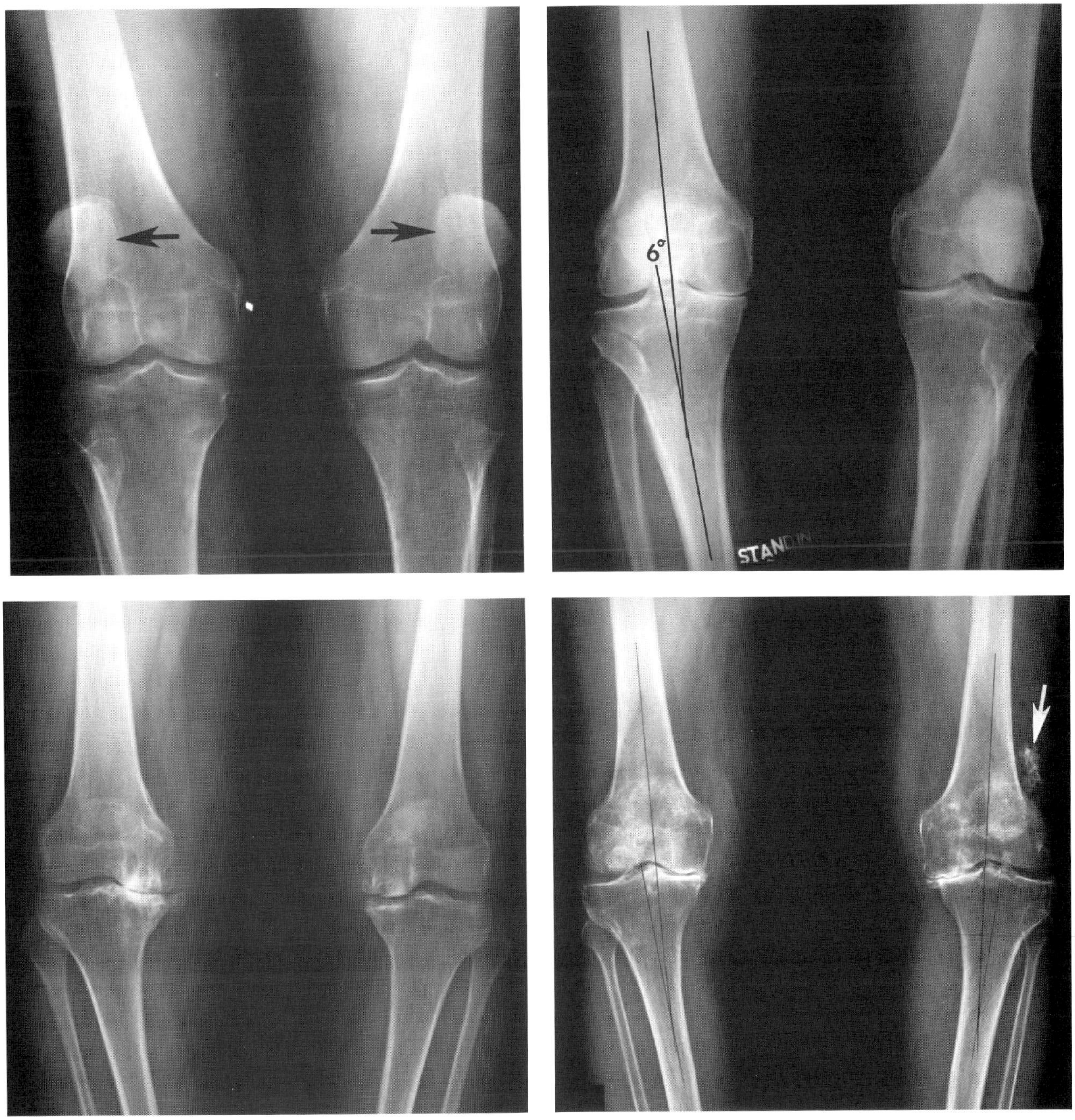

A B C D

FIG. 6-63. Osteoarthritis, standing AP views. **A:** The joint spaces are preserved in both knees. Note the lateral subluxation of both patellae (*arrows*). **B:** Medial joint space narrowing more marked on the right. Femorotibial angle on the right, 6° varus. **C:** Advanced osteoarthritis with secondary sclerosis and osteophyte formation (Kellgren-Lawrence grade III). **D:** Advanced osteoarthritis with more extensive deformity and medial subluxation on the left, 7° to 8° varus deformity bilaterally (*lines*). Note the osteocartilaginous loose body in the left suprapatellar bursa (*arrow*).

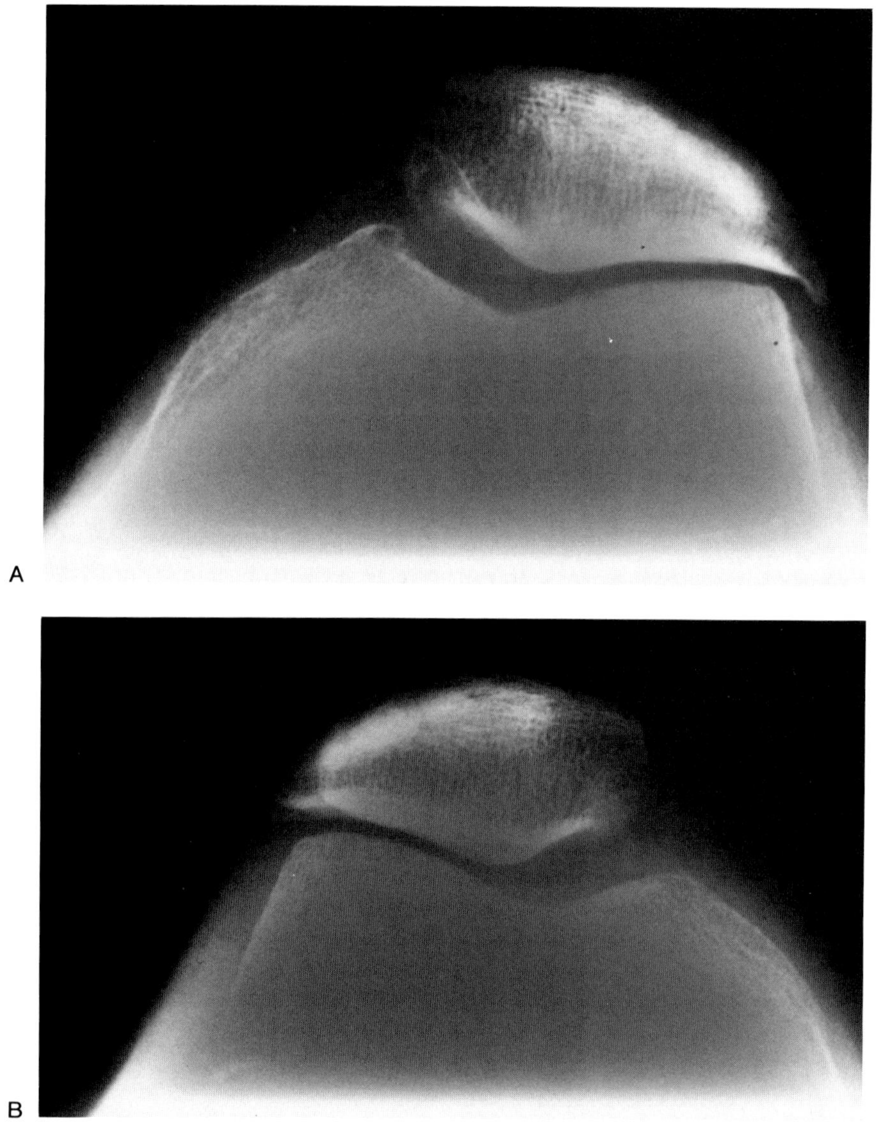

FIG. 6-64. A,B: Bilateral patellar views demonstrating patellofemoral arthrosis with lateral patellar subluxation.

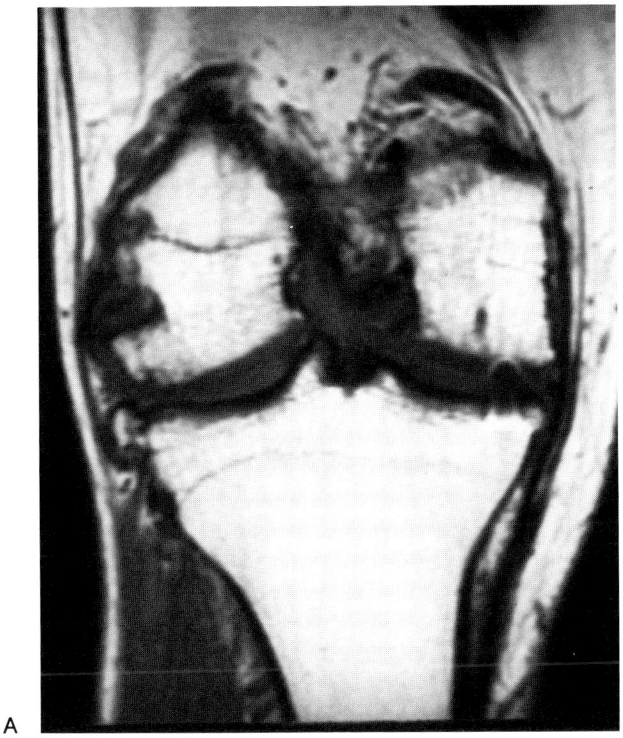
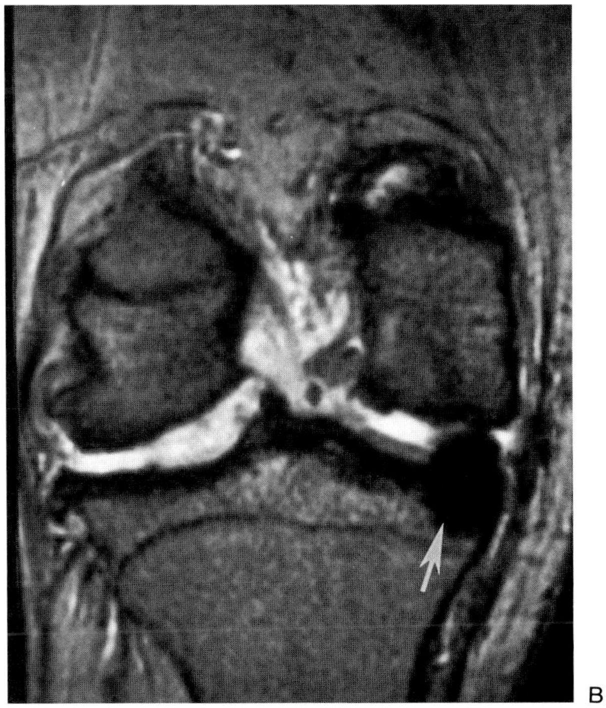

FIG. 6-65. Coronal T1 (SE 500/20, A) and T2 (SE 2,000/60; B) images of the knee demonstrating large osteophytes and marked cartilage loss. Note metal artifact (*arrow*) from previous arthroscopy.

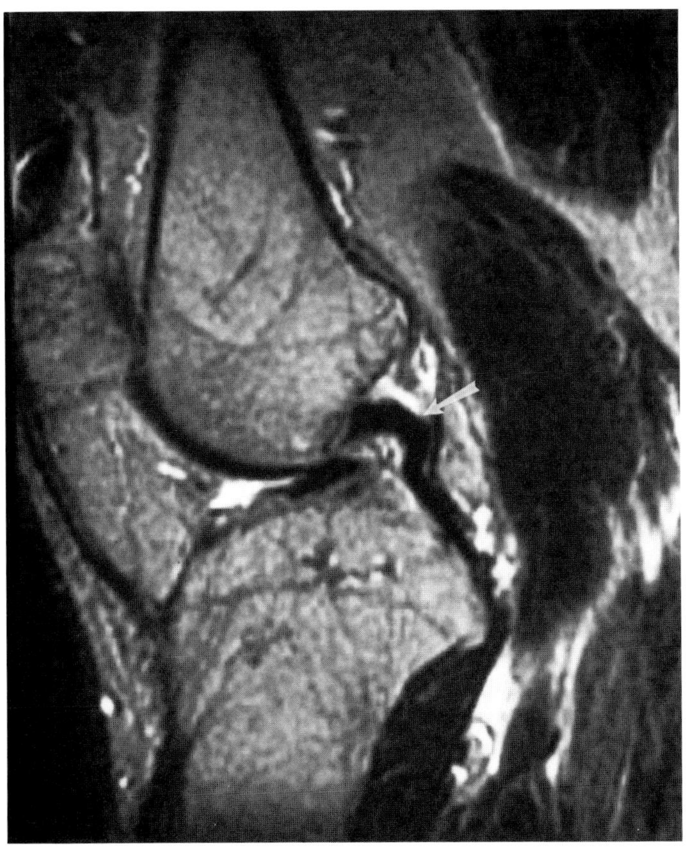

FIG. 6-66. Sagittal SE 2,000/60 image demonstrating a complete ACL tear with secondary hooking of the PCL (*arrow*).

nents may be designed for ingrowth, in which case screws may be used for additional fixation, or cement fixation. Additional considerations include augmented stems and wedges for bone loss. This section demonstrates common variations in tibial components. These changes are often subtle, and the differentiation of the types or specific manufacturer may not always be possible radiographically. However, when possible, the identification should be as specific as possible because the results and complications vary with some types of components, which is important in the postoperative evaluation.[63]

Unicompartmental

Early polycentric tibial components were all polyethylene and cemented into a trough created in the tibial condyle (Figs. 6-57, 6-59, and 6-67).[69,118] Newer designs (Figs. 6-68 and 6-69) have metal-backed tibial components, which can be cemented or screwed in place.[112,118]

Bicompartmental

Bicompartmental tibial components vary considerably. The initial designs used cemented polyethylene components. These included the polycentric (Fig. 6-59) and geometric systems (Fig. 6-70).[69,118] Sixty-six percent of polycentric replacements survived 10 years.[118] The total condylar knee design was initiated in 1974 and remains the "gold standard." Modifications of this system have evolved since that time.[150] The tibial component of the total condylar knee is cemented. The tibial component is nonopaque radiographically with a central stem (Fig. 6-71).[145] The total condylar III (Zimmer, Warsaw, IN) was designed in the 1970s (Fig. 6-60C). The tibial component has a tibial post that fits into the femoral component to provide posterior constraint and limit varus and valgus stress. This design provided stability without a hinge (see Guepar prosthesis, Fig. 6-61). The total condylar III system was designed for patients with instability or bone loss and was commonly used for revision surgery.[152] The tibial component is cemented but does not contain opaque metal (Fig. 6-72).

An all-polyethylene, cementless tibial component was designed in 1977 by the Imperial College, London Hospital (ICLH knee, Fig. 6-73). This component can be identified radiographically by its lack of metal and well-defined polyethylene pegs extending into the tibia.[159] There were problems with polyethylene wear and subsidence of the medial portion of the component. Despite such problems, 87% of these knee replacements survived 7 to 9 years.[157] Other polyethylene tibial components were also devised (Figs. 6-74 and 6-75).

Metal backing for the polyethylene tibial components (Fig. 6-76) improved the load distribution to bone and cold deformation of the polyethylene. These components are more commonly used today. The tibial trays come in a variety of configurations. The metal designs of other tibial components also allow a better radiographic identification and determination of the degree of constraint.[145,159] Metal hinged (constrained) knee replacements are obvious radiographically (Fig. 6-59).[99,109,117,121,165,176,182] The appearance of the Kinematic rotating hinge prosthesis is also characteristic (Fig. 6-60A and 6-77). The tibial component has a notched polyethylene outer core with a large central metal stem and a metal tray, which is elevated above the condyles. There is a posterior metal post with a central hole seen on the AP view (Fig. 6-77). This hinged cemented knee system is not commonly used, except in debilitated patients or for revision arthroplasty with the loss of soft tissue constraints.[144,165]

Today, most knee systems are variations of the condylar design, with cemented or uncemented tibial components using metal-backed polyethylene tibial resurfacing.[60,65,66,77,83,92,96,116,140,155,157,163,178] Thicker polyethylene spacers (≥6 mm) are preferred to reduce wear.[66]

The tibial tray may be smaller laterally than medially to improve the match with the tibial surface, provide maximum coverage, and reduce overhang problems (Fig. 6-78). Most symmetric components cover approximately 85% of the tibial surface. Except for the identification of prosthesis overhang (Fig. 6-79), the two variations may not be appreciated radiographically. Overhang of the component medially may lead to pes anserinus bursitis.[96] Lateral overhang of the tibial component is rarely a problem.

Variations that include cruciate retention, PCL retention (Fig. 6-59 and 6-60), or sacrifice of the cruciate ligaments are also designed (Fig. 6-80). These features may be difficult to identify; however, thickness and deformity (Fig. 6-81) can be evaluated and should be reviewed carefully to detect early polyethylene wear.

Therefore, there are several basic concepts with regard to the tibial systems and cruciate ligament retention. The total condylar design of the 1970s sacrificed the PCL and a tibial stem or post was used. The posterior-stabilized prosthesis was configured similarly (Fig. 6-80).[104] The Kinematic stabilized prosthesis was similar, except that the tibial post engages the femoral component in extension. The posterior cruciate condylar knee has a posterior tibial cutout to allow the PCL to be preserved.[144]

Additional metal differences include variations in the stem design and custom-designed components or tibial wedges to use in patients with bone loss (Figs. 6-74 to 6-85).[140,144]

Porous-coated components are designed for bone ingrowth and bone preservation. They were originally designed because of occasional devastating bone loss in cemented components, which was thought to be due to the cement. These components can also be used with cement.[107] Cementless components are often augmented

(*text continues on page 460*)

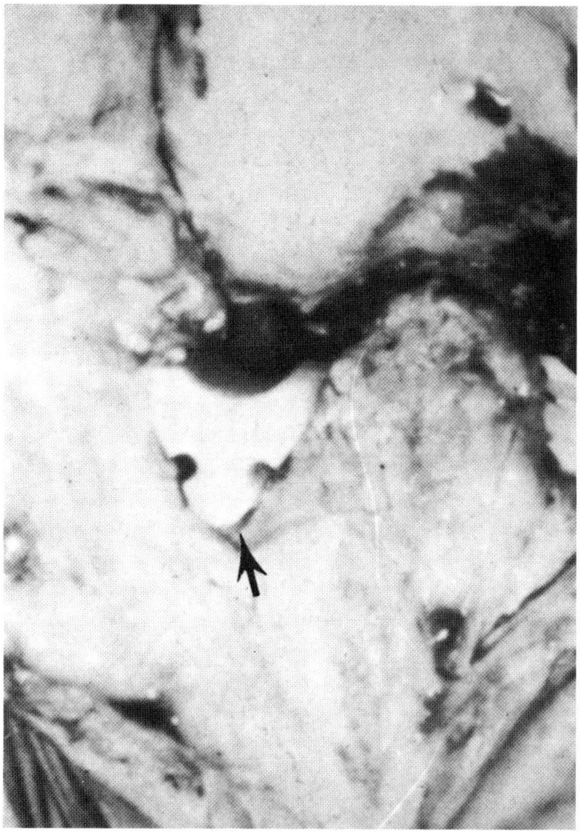

A

FIG. 6-67. Polycentric knee arthroplasty. **A:** An improperly seated medial track (*arrow*), which projects anteriorly. Lateral **(B)** and AP **(C)** views of bicompartmental polycentric reconstruction. There is a large cyst or area of osteolysis in the lateral femoral condyle. (From Bryan RS, Peterson LFA. Polycentric total knee arthroplasty. *Orthop Clin North Am* 1973;4:575–585.)

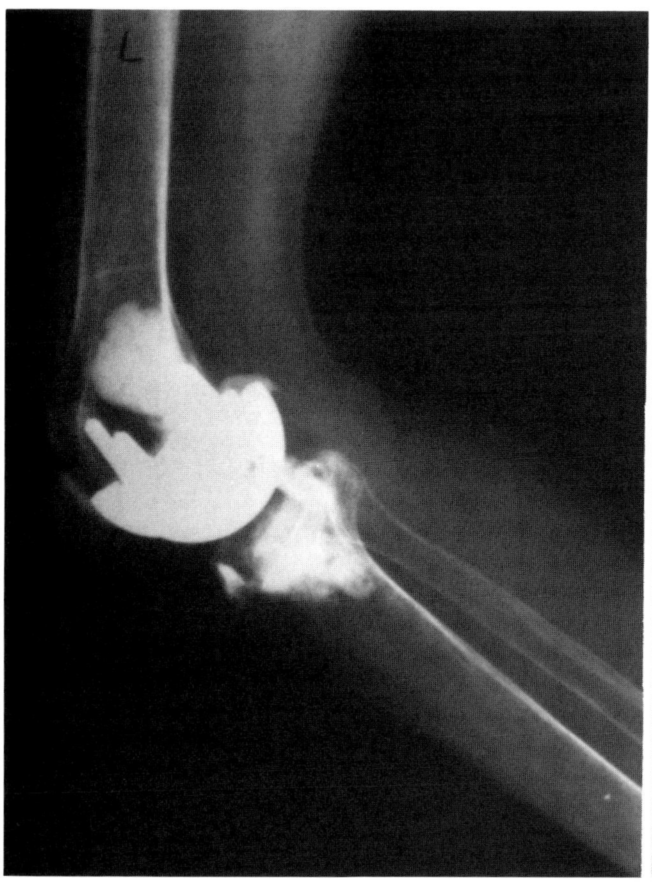

B

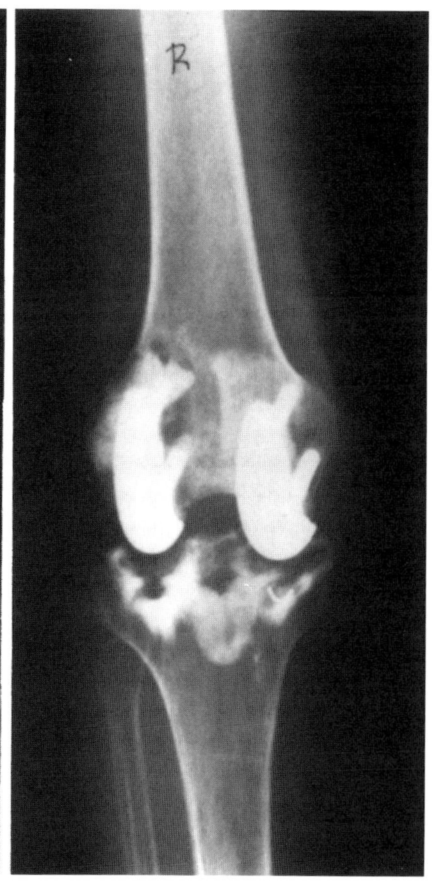

C

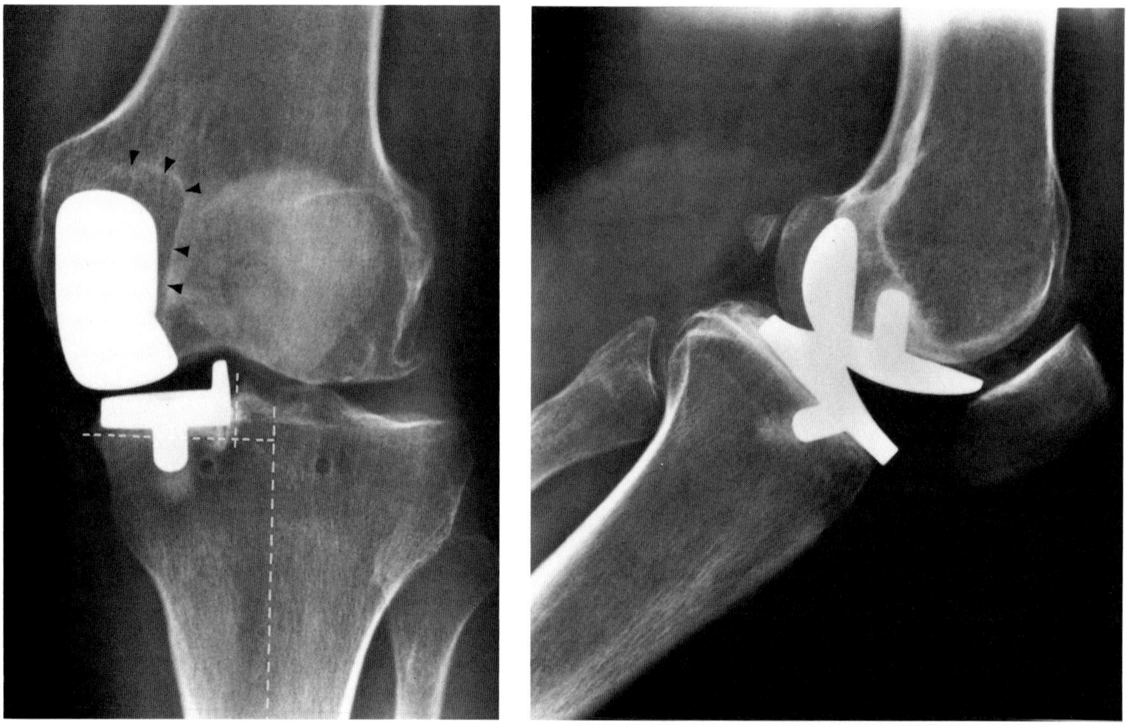

A B

FIG. 6-68. Unicompartmental arthroplasty. The AP **(A)** and lateral **(B)** views show a cemented metal-backed tibial component. The tibial cut should be perpendicular to the tibial axis (*dotted line*) and begin at the margin of the tibial spine.[161] Note the medial subluxation of the femur. The femoral component has migrated from its original position (*arrows*).

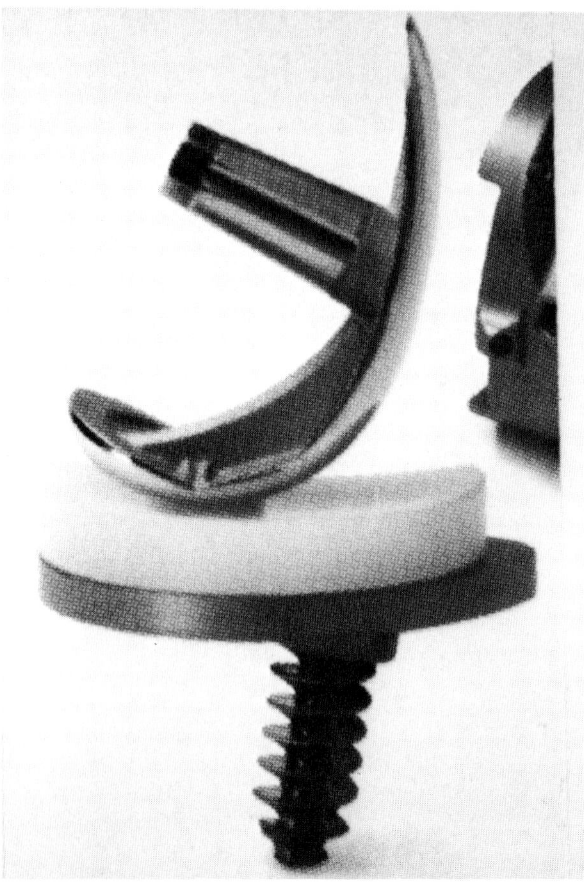

FIG. 6-69. The Genesis™ unicompartmental knee. The tibial component can be fixed with a cancellous screw. (Courtesy of Smith and Nephew Richards, Memphis, TN.)

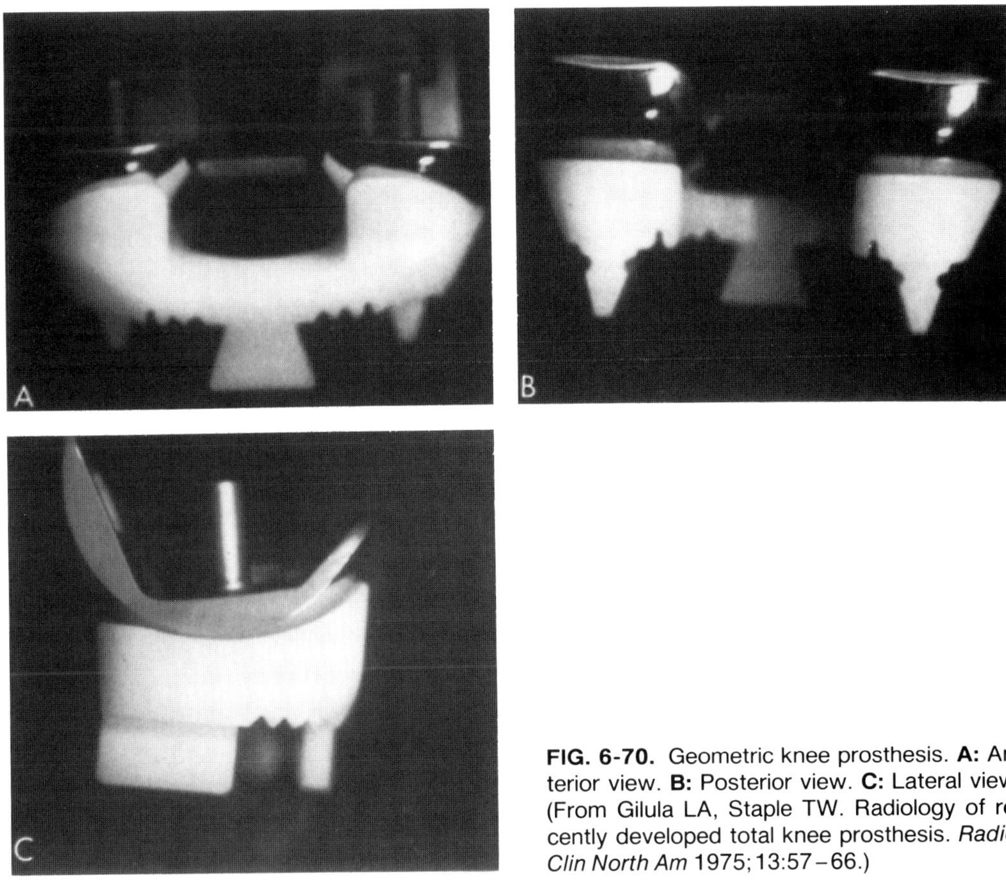

FIG. 6-70. Geometric knee prosthesis. **A:** Anterior view. **B:** Posterior view. **C:** Lateral view. (From Gilula LA, Staple TW. Radiology of recently developed total knee prosthesis. *Radiol Clin North Am* 1975;13:57–66.)

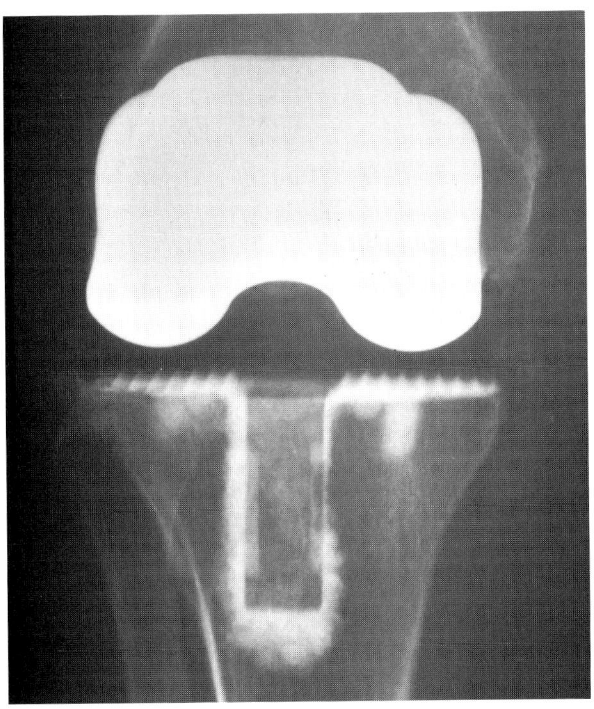

FIG. 6-71. An AP radiograph of a total condylar prosthesis with a cemented tibial component with a central stem.

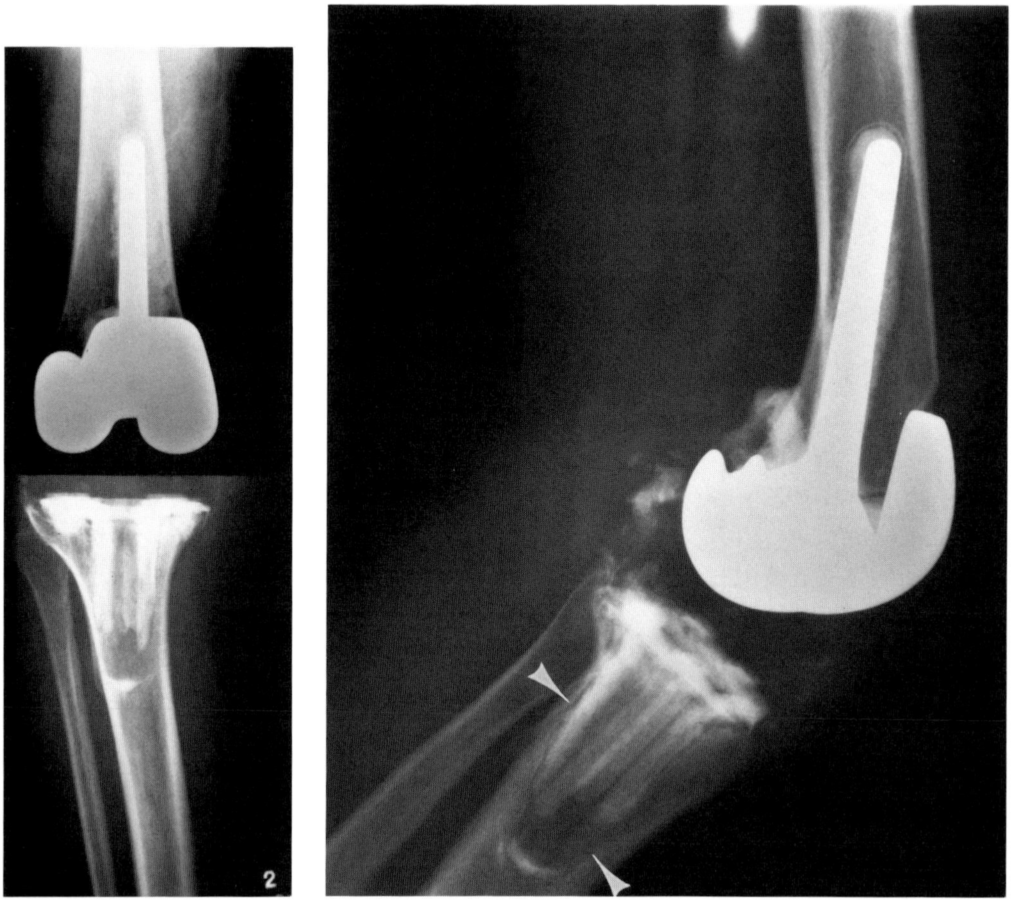

A B

FIG. 6-72. The AP **(A)** and lateral **(B)** views of a condylar III prosthesis. The femoral component has a long stem. Both components are cemented. The tibial component has no opaque metal parts. Note the lucency (*arrows*) at the bone cement interface caused by loosening. Also, note that the femoral component was not fluoroscopically positioned, making it difficult to evaluate the interfaces.

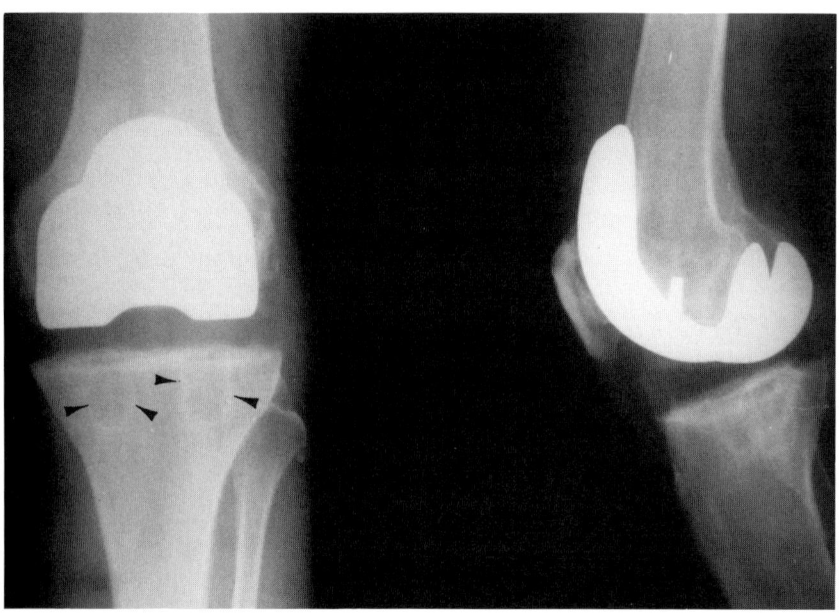

FIG. 6-73. The AP and lateral views of the knee with an ICLH knee. The tibial component is all polyethylene and has well-defined pegs (*arrows*).

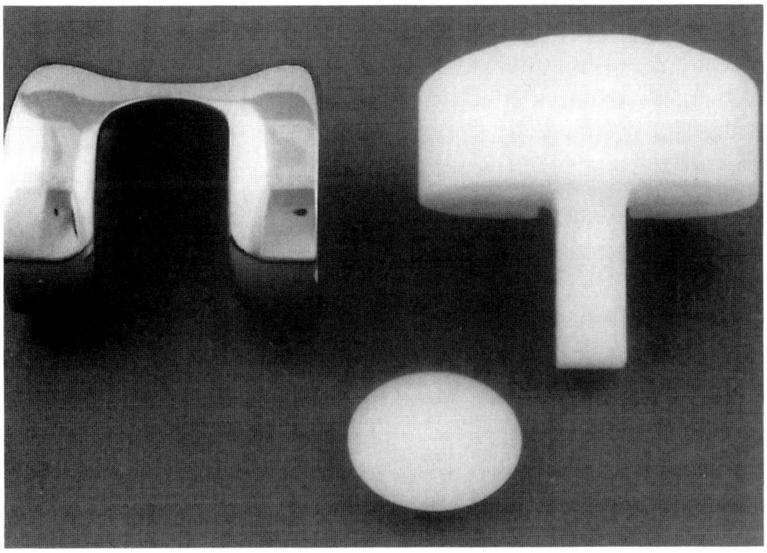

FIG. 6-74. The femoral, patellar, and all-polyethylene tibial components of a duopatellar knee system manufactured by Johnson and Johnson Orthopedics (Raynham, MA). (From Boyd AD, Ewald FC, Thomas WH, Poss R, Sledge CB. Long-term complications after total knee arthroplasty with or without patellar resurfacing. *J Bone Joint Surg* [*Am*]1993;75A:674–681.)

A 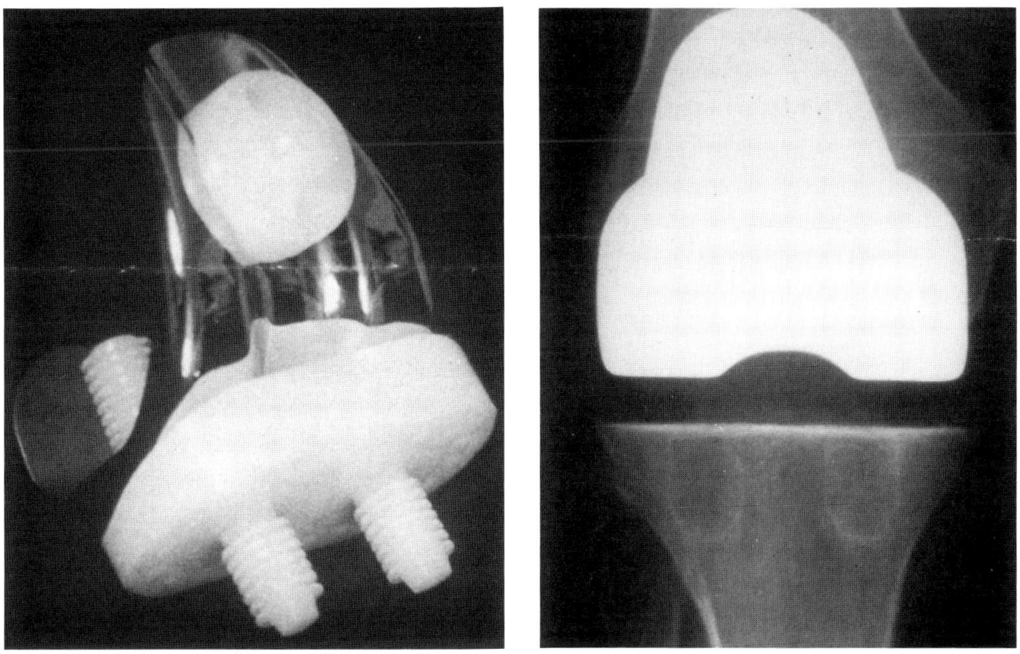 B

C 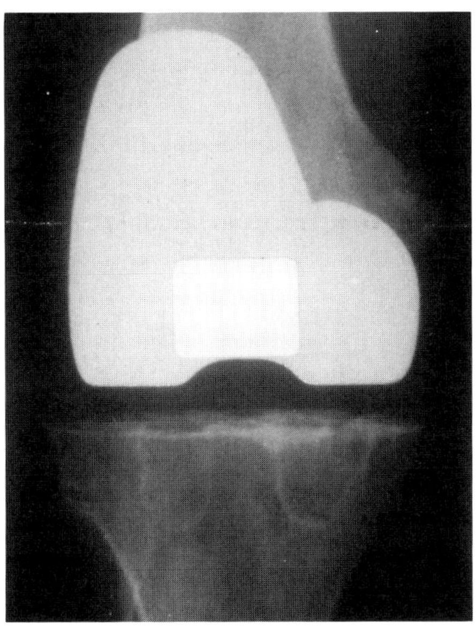

FIG. 6-75. A: The Freeman-Samuelson total knee system with a polyethylene tibial component and two finned polyethylene pegs. The AP radiographs postoperatively at 9 years **(B)** and 8 years **(C)** later show the component is well seated. The radiograph in C was not properly aligned. (From Samuelson K, Nelson L. An all-polyethylene cementless tibial component. A 5 to 9 year follow-up study. *Clin Orthop* 1990; 260:93–97.)

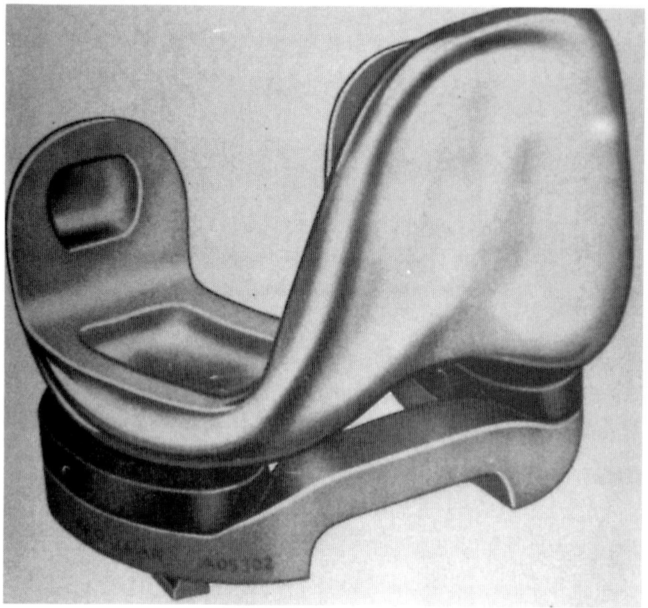

FIG. 6-76. The Cloutier knee. This is a total anatomic resurfacing prosthesis with asymmetric femoral components (different components required for right and left knee), a metal tibial retainer, and two polyethylene tibial articular components (*arrows*) that snap into the tibial retainer. (From Cloutier J. Long term results after non-constrained total knee arthroplasty. *Clin Orthop* 1991;273:63–65.)

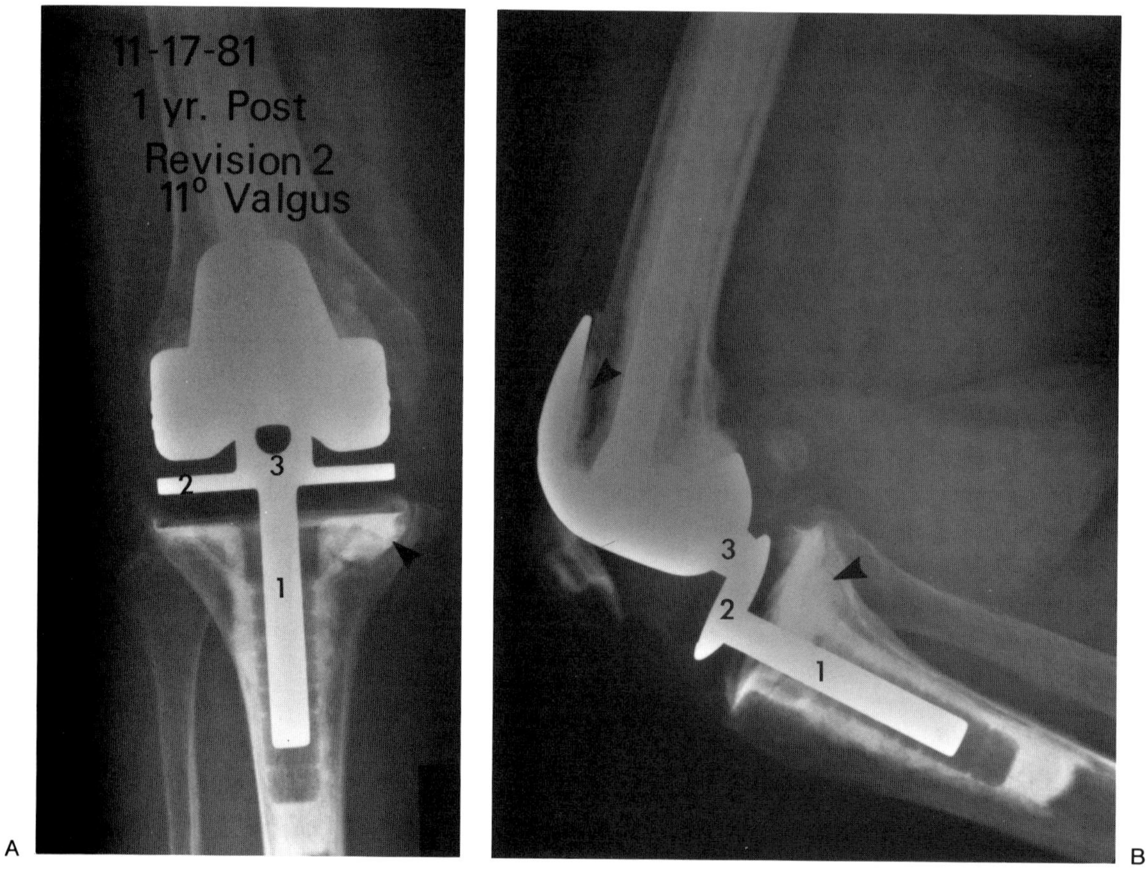

FIG. 6-77. The AP **(A)** and lateral **(B)** views of the Kinematic™ rotating hinge prosthesis. The tibial component has a distinct radiographic appearance with a large central stem (*1*), an elevated metal tray (*2*), and a posterior metal post with a central hole (*3*) on the AP view. There are several areas of lucency at the bone cement interface (*arrows*). (From Rand JA, Berquist TH. The knee. In: Berquist TH, ed. *Imaging of orthopedic trauma and surgery*. Philadelphia: WB Saunders, 1986;293–391.)

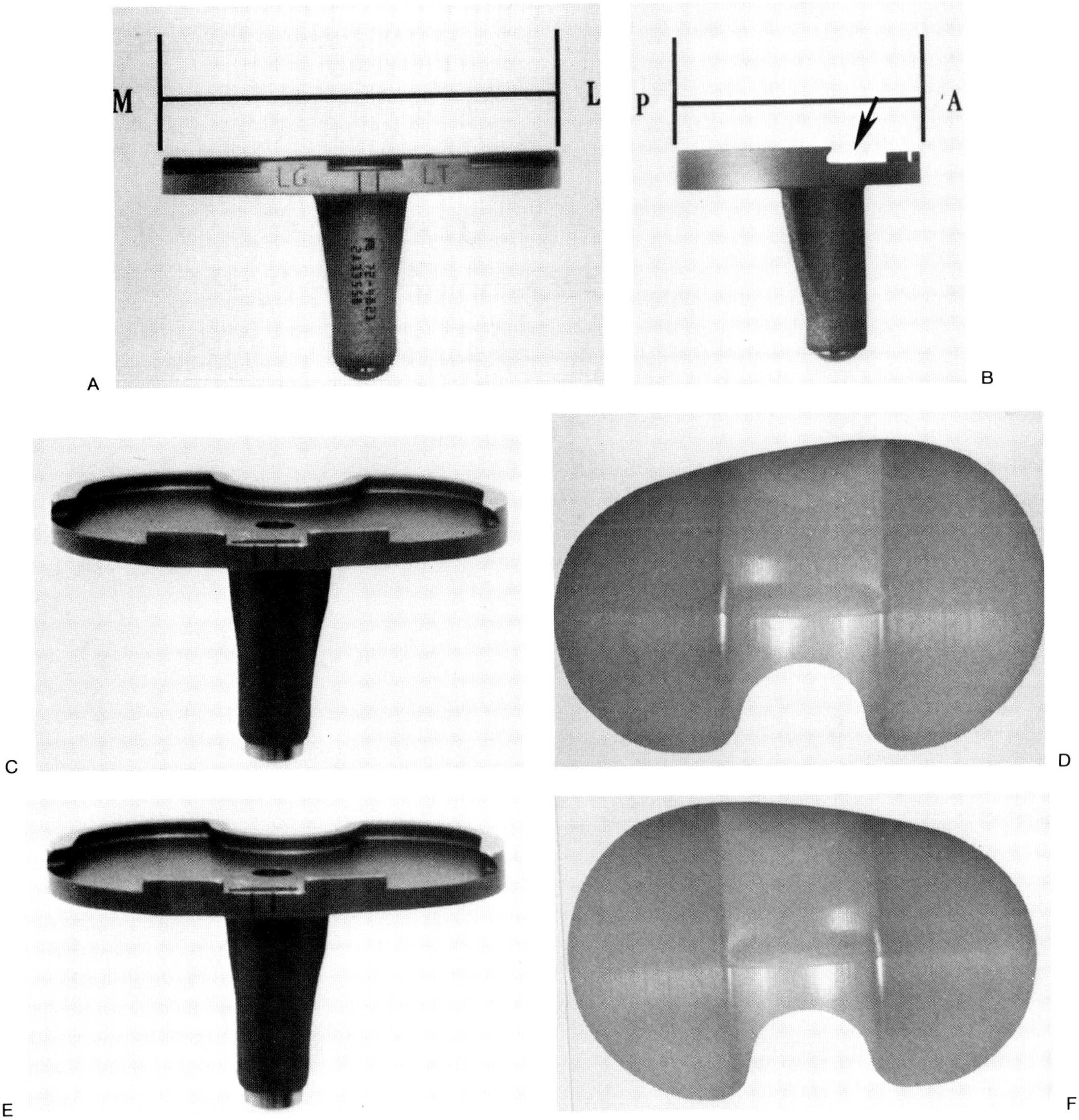

FIG. 6-78. The Genesis™ total knee system with tibial components designed to fit the tibial condyles more anatomically. Tibial tray shown from the front **(A)** and side **(B)**. *M*, medial; *L*, lateral; *A*, anterior; *P*, posterior. Note the configuration of the stem and anterior notch (*arrow*) of the tibial tray. Left tibial tray and polyethylene insert **(C,D)** and right tibial tray and polyethylene insert **(E,F)**. (See **G** and **H** on next page.)

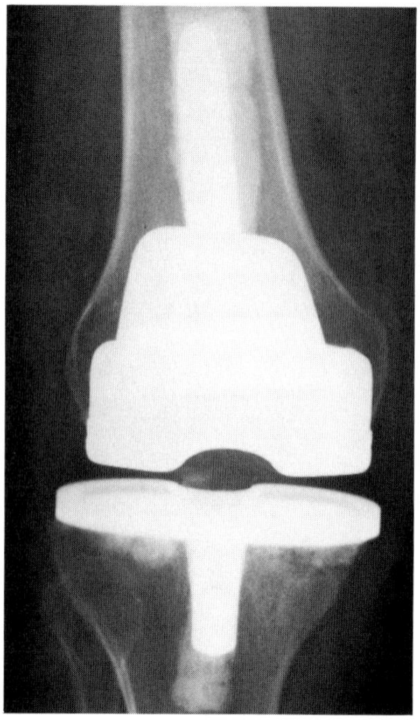

G

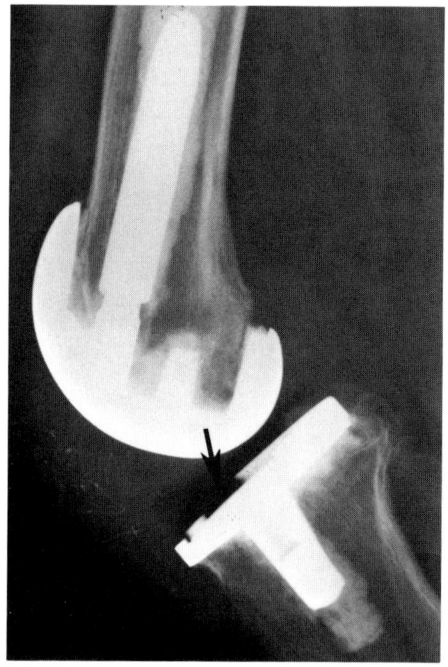

H

FIG. 6-78. (*Continued.*) The AP **(G)** and lateral **(H)** radiographs of a knee reconstruction with a patellectomy and Genesis™ tibial component. Note stem and anterior notch (*arrow*) and augmentation stem on the femoral component. Both components are cemented.

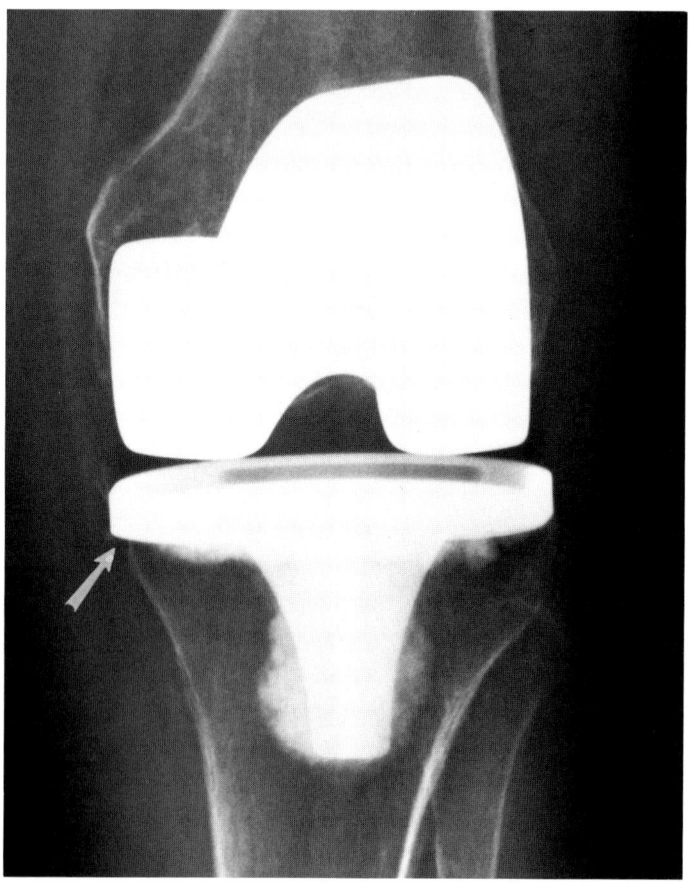

FIG. 6-79. Symmetric cemented tibial component with medial overriding of the component on the tibia (*arrow*).

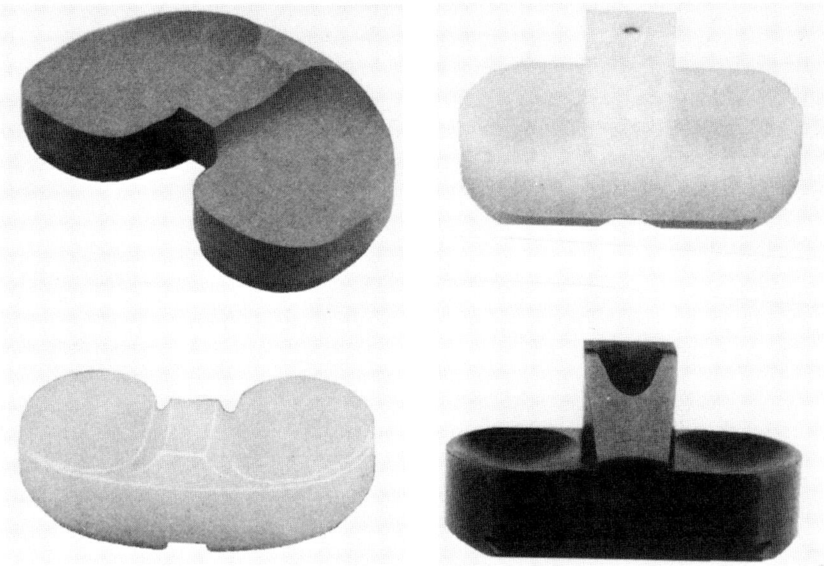

A,B

FIG. 6-80. Polyethylene spacers for metal tibial tray with PCL cutout **(A)** and large central post **(B)** for constrained tibial component of Insall-Burstein II modular knee system. (Courtesy of Zimmer, Warsaw, IN.)

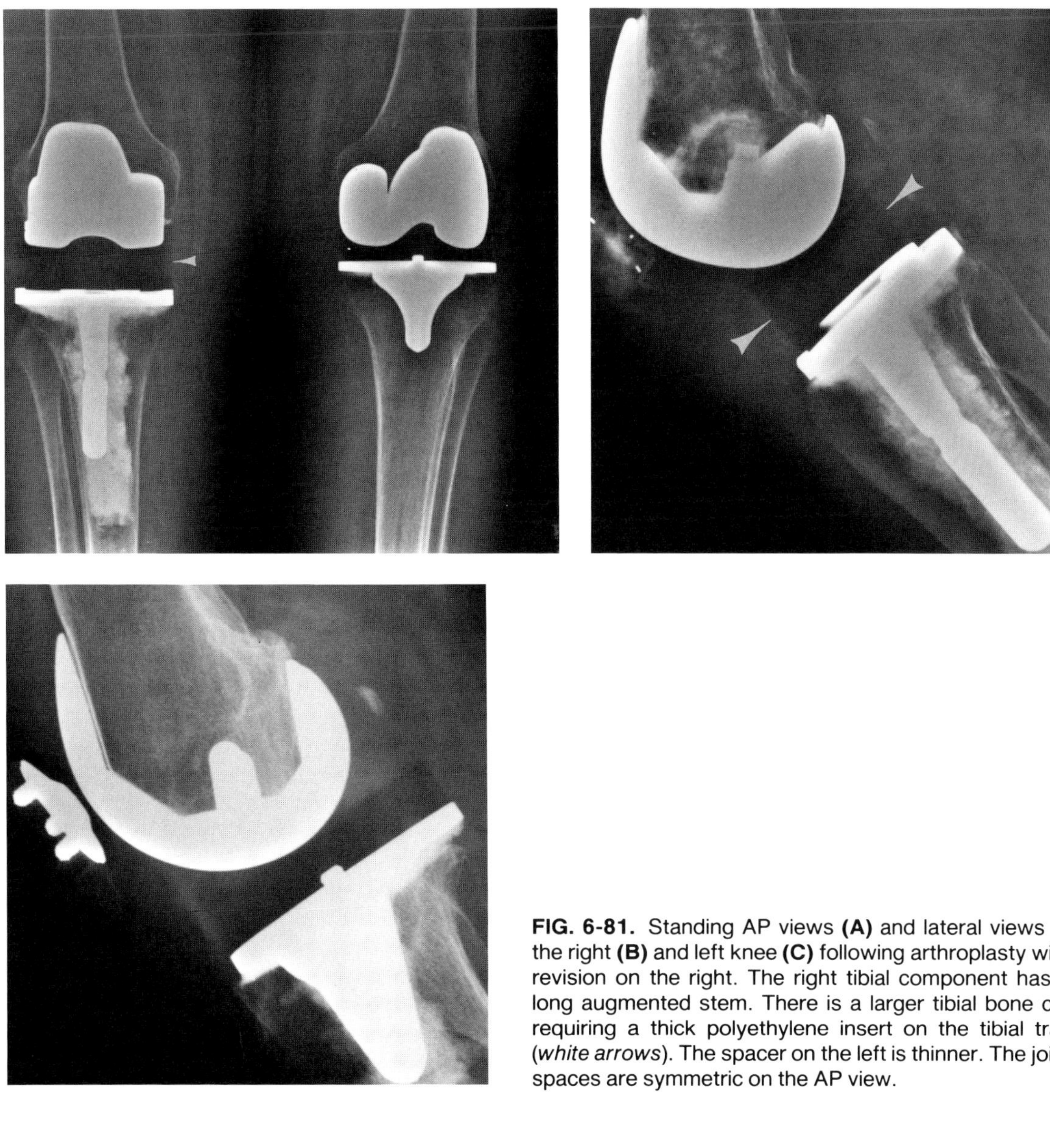

A B C

FIG. 6-81. Standing AP views **(A)** and lateral views of the right **(B)** and left knee **(C)** following arthroplasty with revision on the right. The right tibial component has a long augmented stem. There is a larger tibial bone cut requiring a thick polyethylene insert on the tibial tray (*white arrows*). The spacer on the left is thinner. The joint spaces are symmetric on the AP view.

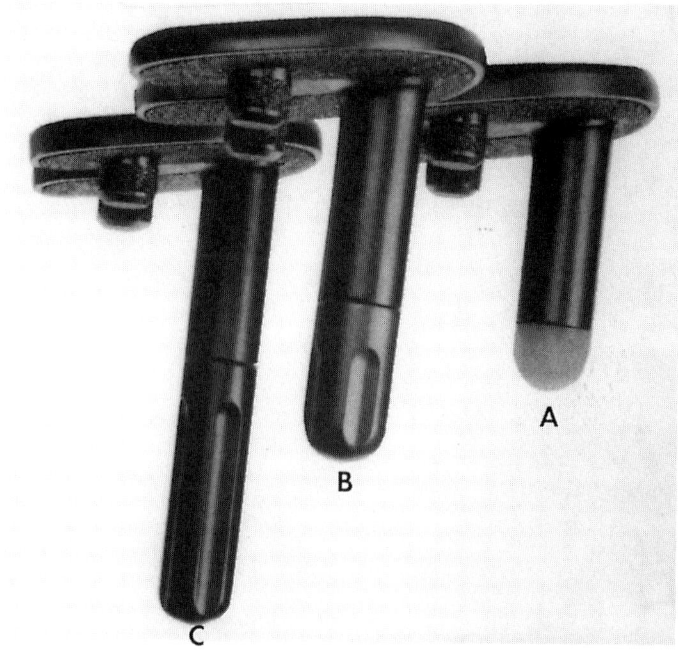

FIG. 6-82. Porous-coated Miller-Galante tibial trays with two porous-coated pegs and normal **(A)** and augmented **(B,C)** stems. (Courtesy of Zimmer, Warsaw, IN.)

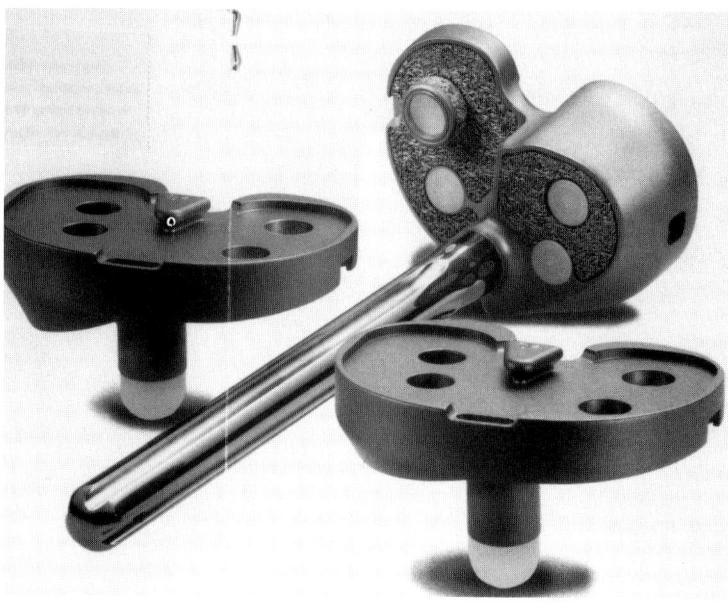

FIG. 6-83. Customized tibial components with built in tibial wedges and long revision stem. (Courtesy of Zimmer, Warsaw, IN.)

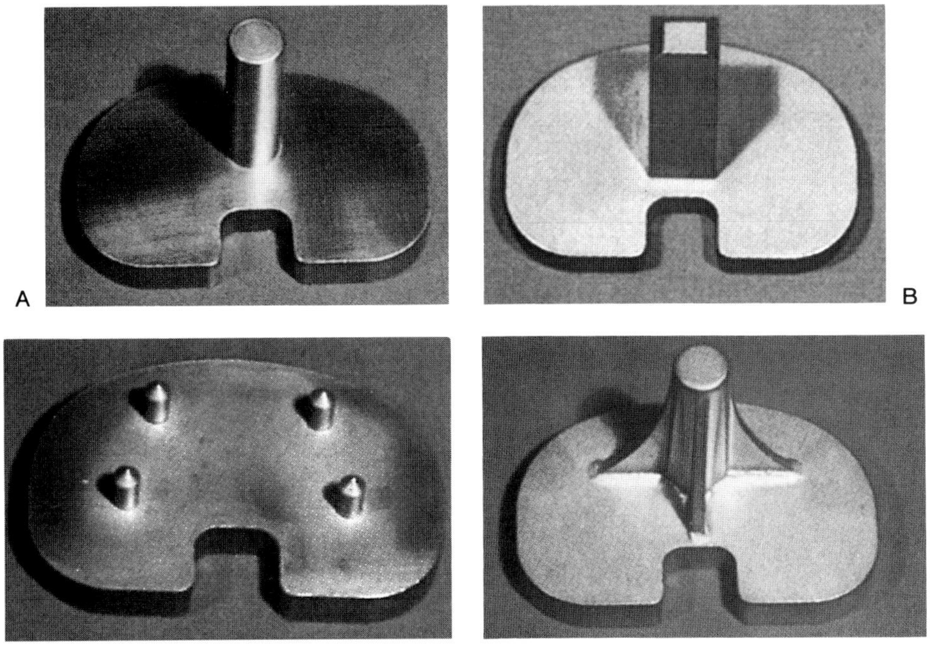

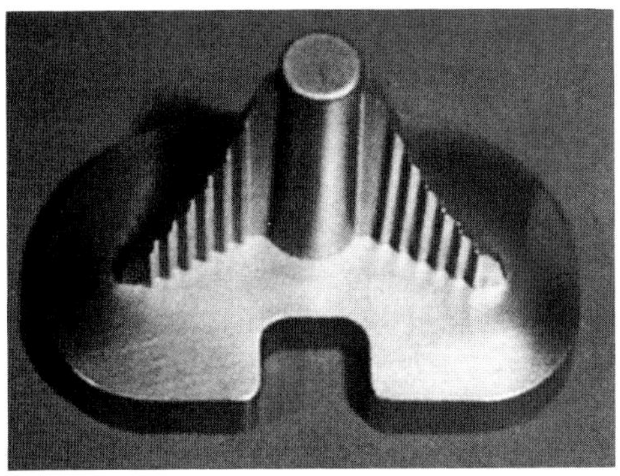

FIG. 6-84. Variations in metal tibial trays seen from below (tibial attachment). **A:** Single round post. **B:** Rectangular post. **C:** Four nonporous pegs. **D:** Cruciform heel. **E:** Deltafit heel. (Courtesy of Osteonics, Allendale, NJ.)

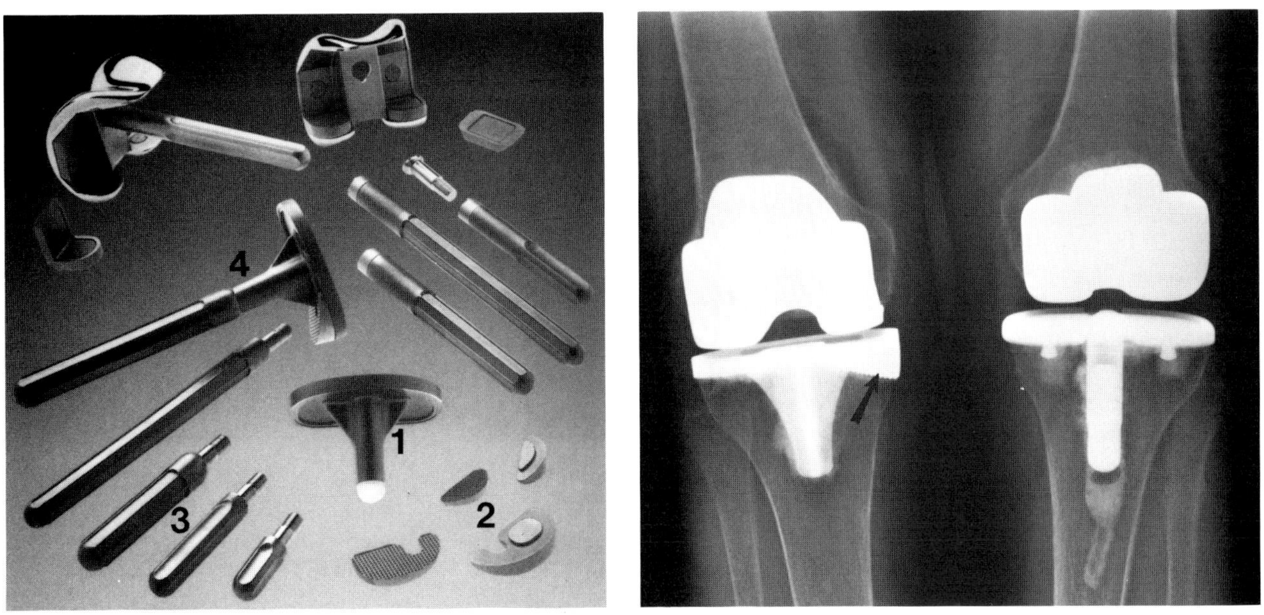

FIG. 6-85. **A:** The Johnson and Johnson P.F.C.™ modular knee with conventional tibial tray (*1*), augmentation wedges (*2*), stems (*3*), and components assembled (*4*). Femoral components and inserts are shown above. (Courtesy of Johnson and Johnson Orthopaedics, Raynham, MA.) **B:** Standing AP views of the knees with a Johnson and Johnson system with augmentation wedge (*arrow*) on the right and a Harris-Galante system with a long-stem tibial component on the left.

with cancellous screws (Fig. 6-86).[65,97,122,127,157,163,178] The type of porous coating varies. The porous-coated anatomic (PCA, Howmedica) prosthesis is coated with sintered cobalt-chromium beads (Fig. 6-87). The Natural Knee (NK, Intermedics Orthopedics, Austin, TX; Fig. 6-88) uses a network lattice of titanium.[65] Porous-coated components are used in young patients with tricompartment disease who have normal body weight and will cooperate in regard to activity postoperatively.[142,151,171] Figures 6-89 and 6-90 demonstrate examples of other porous-coated tibial components.[90]

Femoral Components

Femoral components are designed for ingrowth (porous coated) (Fig. 6-91) or cement fixation (Fig. 6-92). As in tibial components, cement can be used in either case. As little bone as possible is removed to fit the femoral component. The total condylar design with variations to adapt to a cruciate design (Figs. 6-84 and 6-93) is most often used. Symmetric and anatomic designs (i.e., fits the shape and size of the femoral condyle) are available. There are also variations in the configuration and length of the patellar articulating surface (Figs. 6-94 and 6-95). The type of stem (e.g., augmented porous-coated pegs or a single central post) also varies (Figs. 6-72A, 6-77, 6-93, and 6-96).[96,129,145] There are fewer problems with loosening with the femoral component compared with the tibial component.[96]

Patellar Components

Patellar surface replacement is nearly always performed today to decrease patellofemoral pain and reduce later complications.[75,125,131] Early patellar components were polyethylene (Fig. 6-97). Later, metal backing was added to provide more uniform load transfer (Fig. 6-98), to aid in the prevention of polyethylene deformity, and to provide a surface for porous coating.[129,138] Recent reports have indicated failure with metal-backed components caused by polyethylene wear. This may be related to the thinner polyethylene surface on metal-backed components. Wear varies with the type of alloy used. Cobalt-chromium backing is associated with the least wear compared with both titanium and nonimplanted titanium metal-backed components.[126] Most surgeons currently prefer cemented all-polyethylene patellar components.[70,126]

Radiographic analysis requires lateral and Merchant views.[109,118,132] Fluoroscopic positioning is recommended (Fig. 6-99).

Unicompartmental Joint Replacement

Reports of unicompartmental arthroplasty were disappointing initially (Fig. 6-100). However, this technique has regained popularity in recent years.[73,95,129,172] This technique is indicated as an alternative to tibial osteotomy or tricompartmental arthroplasty in patients with unicompartmental osteoarthritis.[73] Such patients should have unicompartmental pain, minimal patellar symptoms, normal cruciate and collateral ligaments, and normal hip motion.

The AP standing views, lateral views, and Merchant patellar views are required for the preoperative evaluation.[63] Some authors recommend the 45° flexion posteroanterior (PA) standing views to detect more subtle joint space narrowing.[73,153] The radiographic findings should be confined to one tibiofemoral compartment, with mild changes acceptable in the patellofemoral compartment. There should be no degenerative arthritis or chondrocalcinosis in the opposite tibiofemoral compartment.[73]

The advantages reported include reduced blood loss (no transfusions), preservation of the cruciate ligaments, greater flexion postoperatively, and reduced need for postoperative manipulation or physical therapy.[73] There is also less bone resection and soft tissue injury with this technique. The knee's kinematic characteristics remain closer to normal.[95] Although reduced bone loss was touted as a reason for unicompartmental replacement initially, there is often significant bone loss when these components are revised. In older patients, it may be better to proceed with a total knee replacement.

The revision of failed unicompartmental arthroplasty was originally thought to be simpler than tricompartmental arthroplasty. However, unicompartmental bone loss must still be corrected.[129]

Components

Today, better component design is available.[102,110,163,166,168] Both constrained and unconstrained designs are marketed (Fig. 6-101). The femoral components are broader, and the tibial components are more often metal backed currently. Precoating of the components provides a stronger bond with cement. Figures 6-102 to 6-104 demonstrate several component options (Figs. 6-67 to 6-69 also).

The results were good to excellent in 98% of unconstrained and 70% of constrained components, as reported by Hodge and Chandler.[95] Only 8% of unconstrained prostheses required revision to total knee arthroplasty compared with 27% for constrained components. The average follow-up was 53 months.

Scott et al.[160] reported on 130 knees followed for 8 to 12 years. Ninety percent survived 9 years; 85%, 10 years; and 82%, 11 years. Flexion of 115° was achieved, and 87% of patients had no pain. In their experience, there were fewer complications and a higher initial success rate compared with those in tibial osteotomy (Fig. 6-105).[160]

Patients of normal or lighter weight, lower activity levels, and older than 70 years of age are well suited for uni-

(*text continues on page 474*)

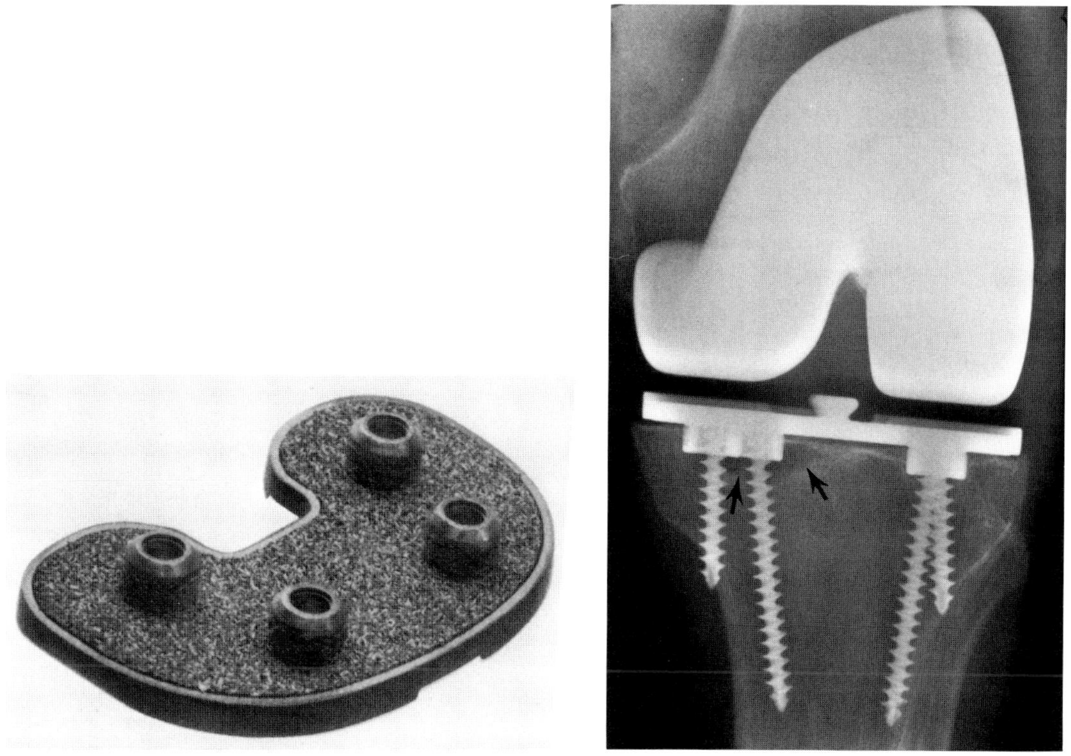

A B

FIG. 6-86. **A:** The porous surface of a Miller-Galante with four porous pegs (titanium fiber metal mesh). (Courtesy of Zimmer, Warsaw, IN.) **B:** An AP view of the knee with Miller-Galante porous tibial tray and four cancellous screws. There is poorly defined lucency medially (*arrows*) caused by infection.

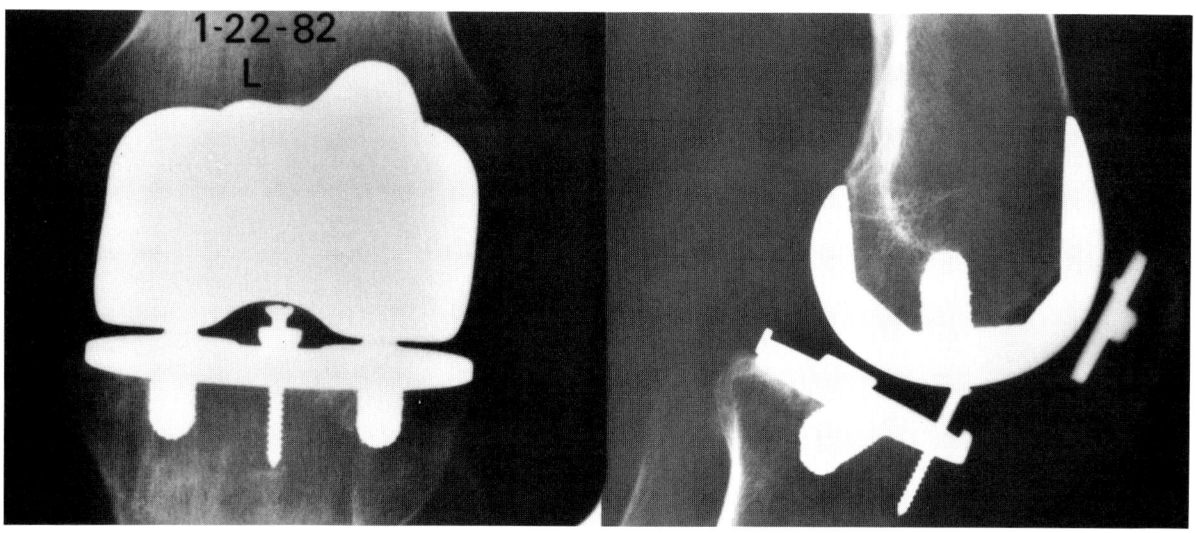

FIG. 6-87. The AP and lateral views of a PCA ingrowth knee arthroplasty. There is a single cancellous screw in the anterior tibial tray. The metal beads are obvious on the tibial and femoral pegs.

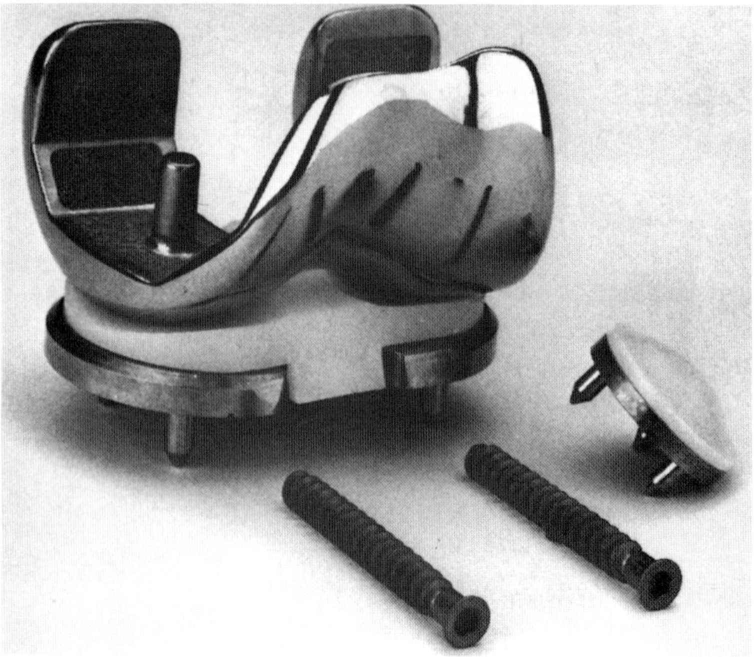

FIG. 6-88. Intermedics NK femoral, tibial, and patellar components. Two 6.5-mm cancellous screws are used for tibial tray fixation. (Courtesy of Intermedics Orthopedics, Austin, TX.) (From Hofmann AA, Murdock LE, Wyatt RWB, Alpert JP. Total knee arthroplasty: two-four year experience using an asymmetric tibial tray and a deep trochlear-grooved femoral component. *Clin Orthop* 1991;269:78–88.)

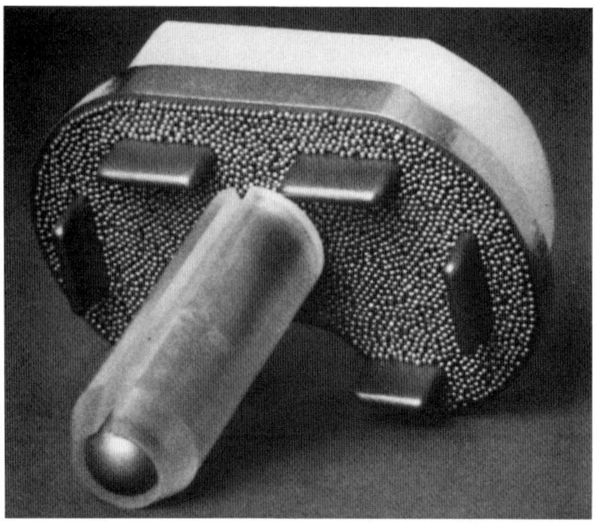

A

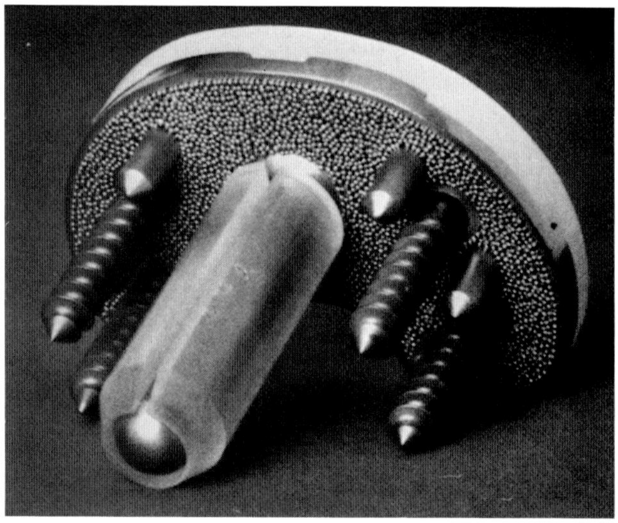

B

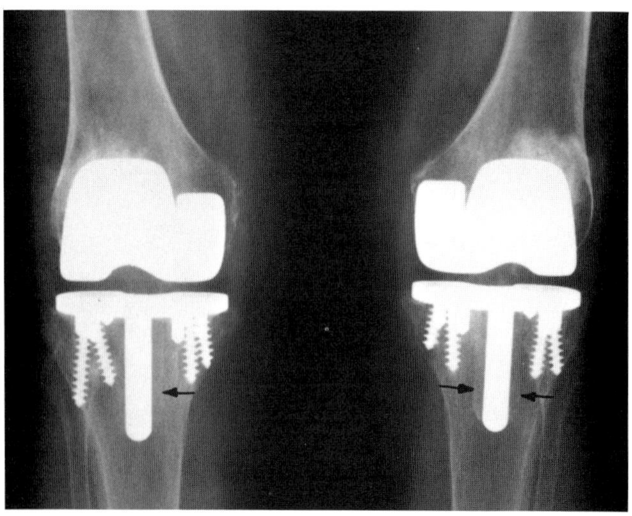

C

FIG. 6-89. A: The Ortholoc™ I tibial component with peripheral pegs or blades and a central stem. **B:** Screws and pegs were added to the Ortholoc™ II. Manufactured by Wright Medical Technology (Arlington, TN). (From Whiteside LA. The effect of patient age, gender, and tibial compoment fixation or pain relief after cementless total knee arthroplasty. *Clin Orthop* 1991;271:21–27.) The AP **(C)** and lateral **(D,E)** radiographs of an Ortholoc™ II knee. Note the lucent sleeve around the central stem.

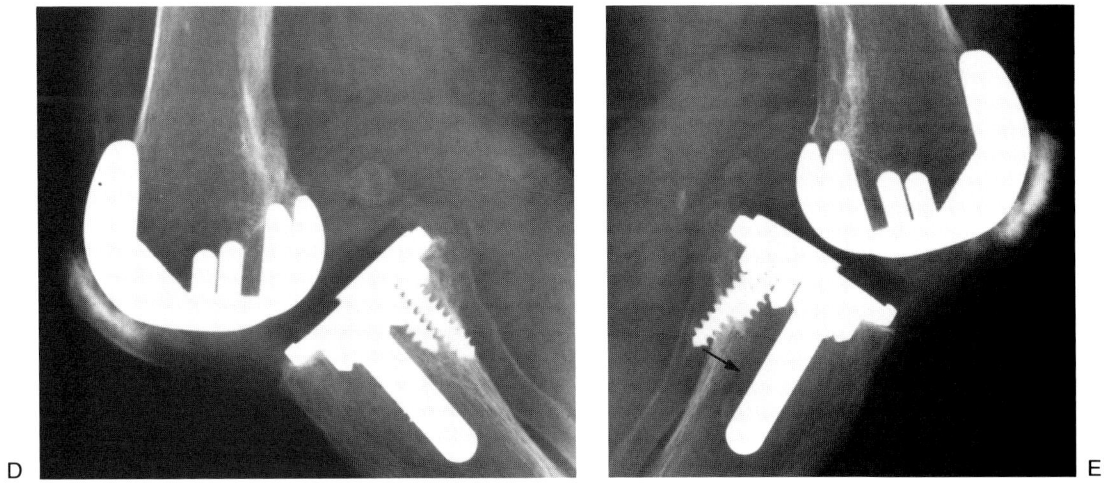

FIG. 6-89. *Continued.*

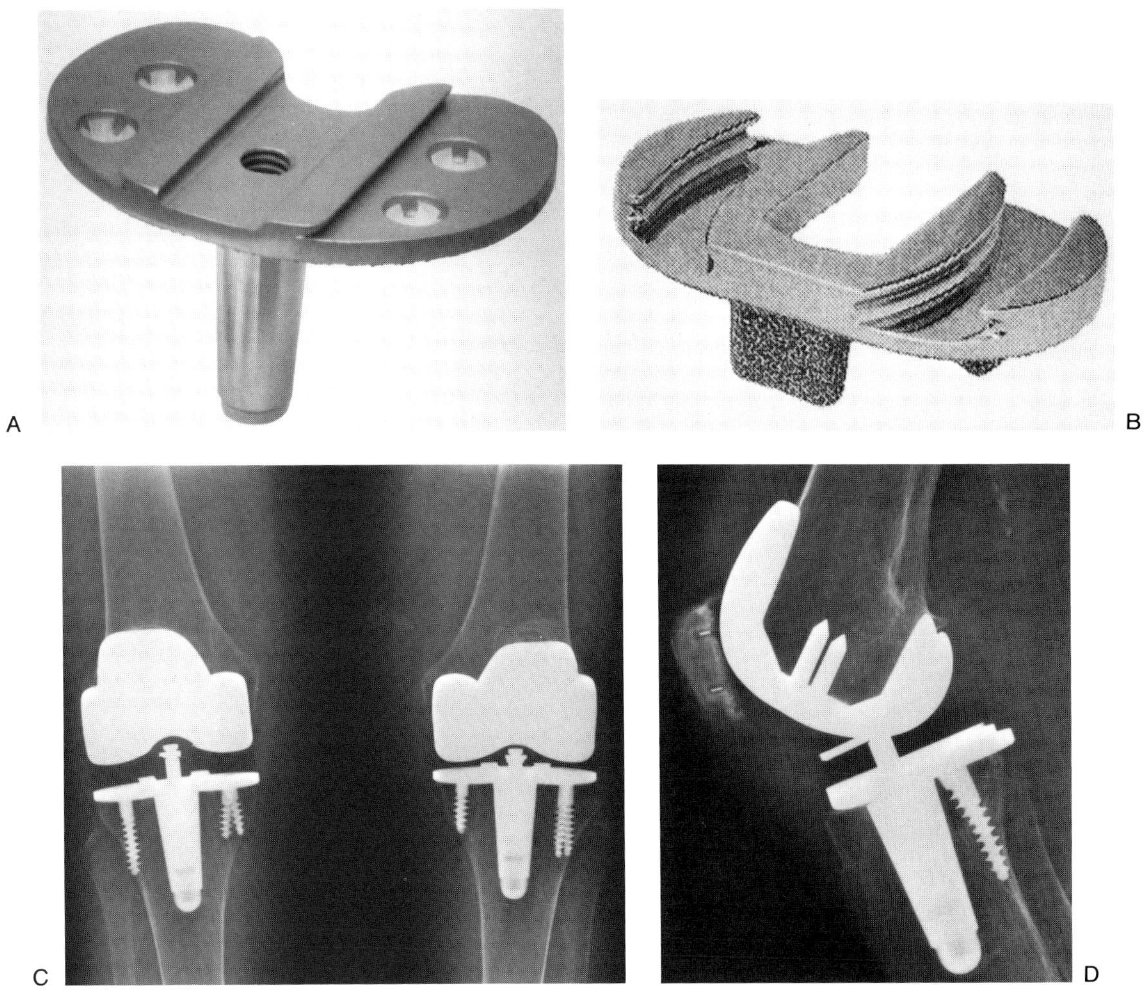

FIG. 6-90. DePuy knee components. **A:** Primary porous-coated tray. **B:** Bicruciate-retaining porous-coated tibial tray. Note the large central cruciate cutout. (A,B: Courtesy of DePuy, Warsaw, IN.) The AP standing **(C)** and lateral **(D)** radiographs of AMK™ knee system with a central stem and cancellous screws.

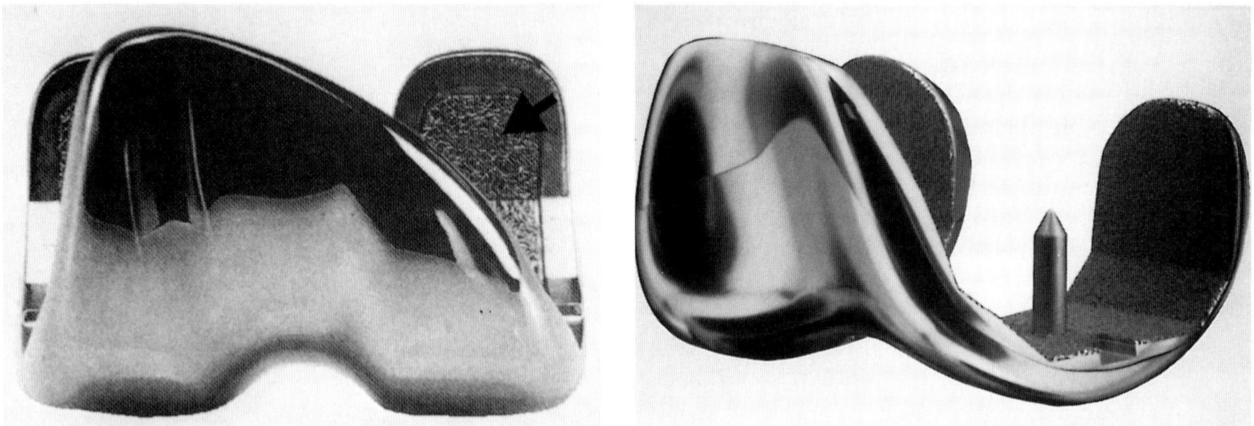

FIG. 6-91. Femoral components with porous coating. **A:** Miller-Galante II (right knee) femoral component with titanium fiber mesh (*arrow*) on the bone interface. (Courtesy of Zimmer, Warsaw, IN.) **B:** AMK™ porous-coated femoral component. (Courtesy of DePuy, Warsaw, IN.)

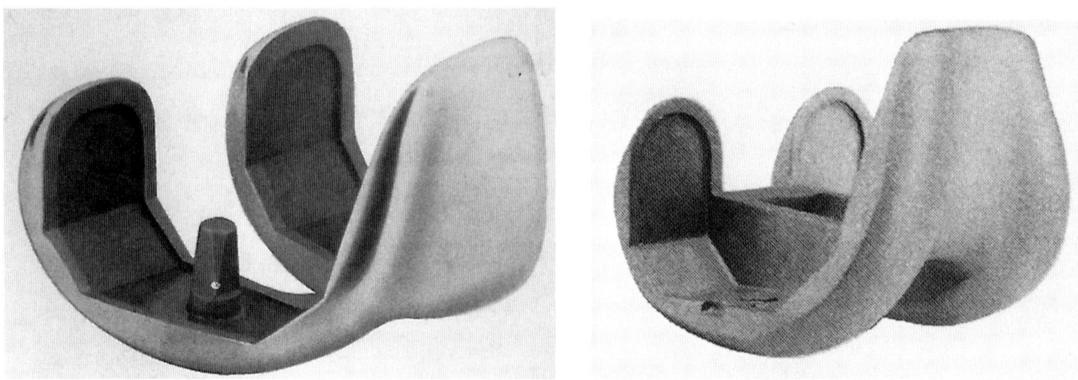

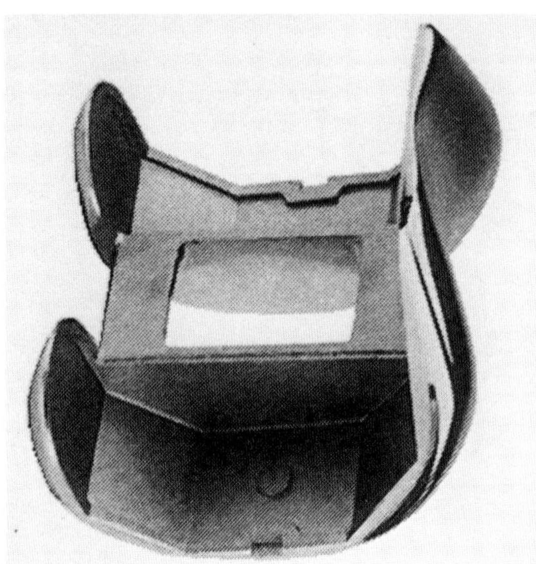

FIG. 6-92. Nonporous-coated femoral components. **A:** Standard Miller-Galante femoral component configured with cobalt-chromium-molybdenum alloy. Posterior-stabilized femoral component with a central rectangular cutout seen from the side **(B)** and above **(C)**. (Courtesy of Zimmer, Warsaw, IN.) Note there are no femoral pegs with the posterior-stabilized design.

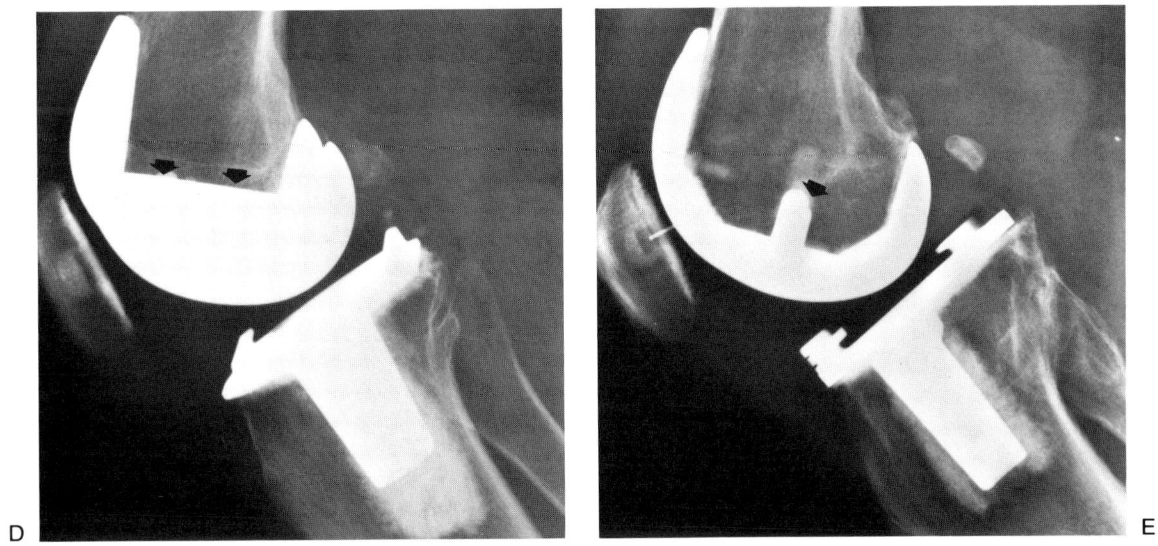

FIG. 6-92. (*Continued.*) **D:** Lateral radiographs of a posterior-stabilized femoral component with a flat surface (*arrows*) and no pegs. **E:** Lateral radiograph of a standard femoral component with pegs (*arrow*).

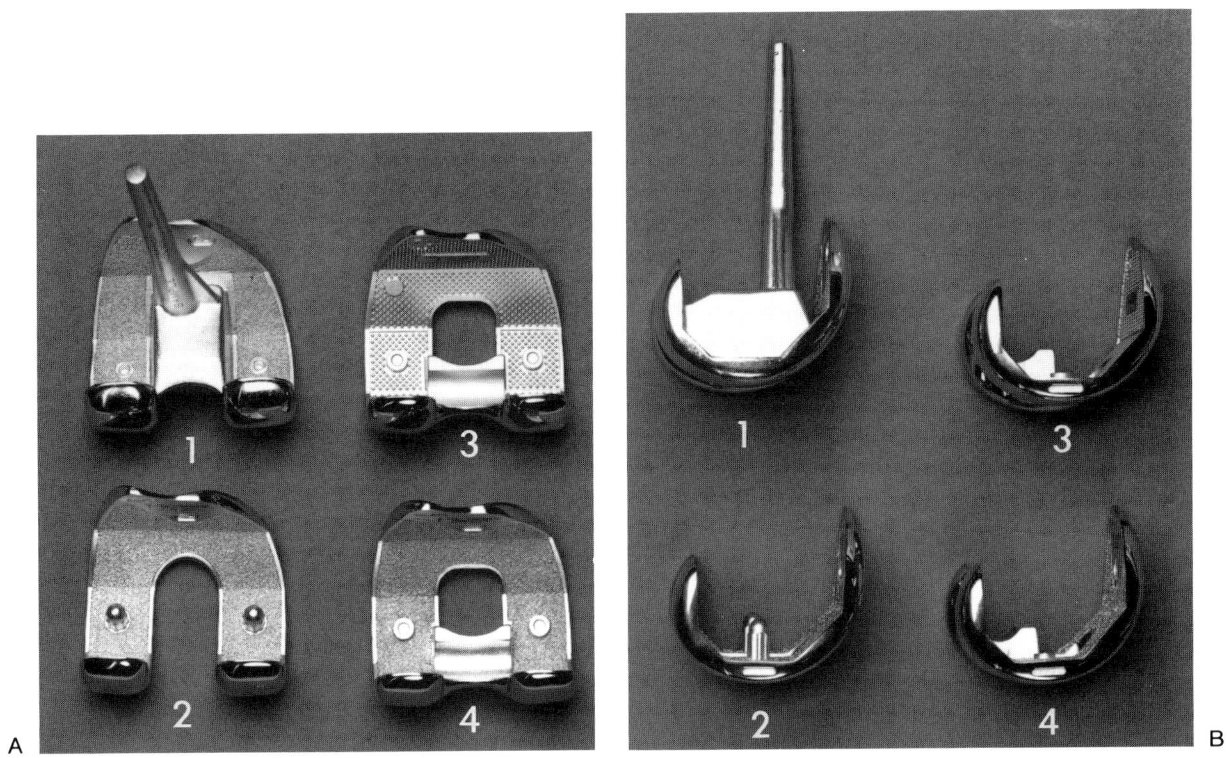

FIG. 6-93. Femoral components for revision (*1*), cruciate-sparing (*2*), and posterior-stabilized types with standard (*3*) and porous (*4*) coating shown from above **(A)**, the side **(B)**. and the front **(C)**. (See **C** on next page.) (Courtesy of Osteonics, Allendale, NJ.)

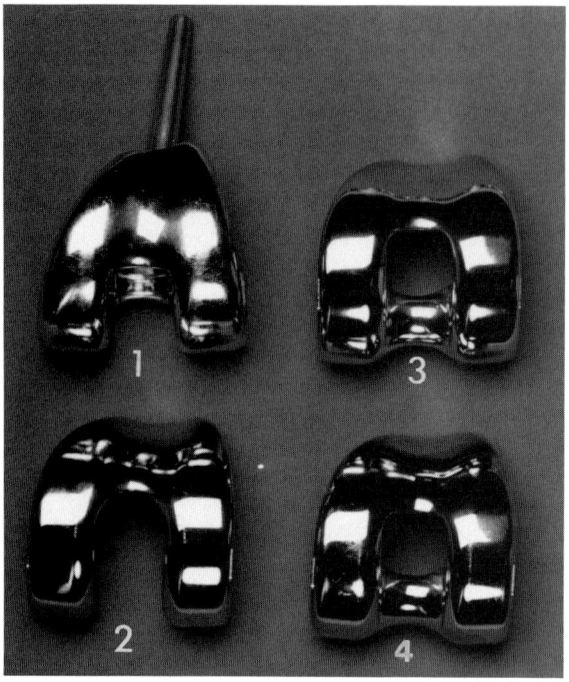

C

FIG. 6-93. *Continued.*

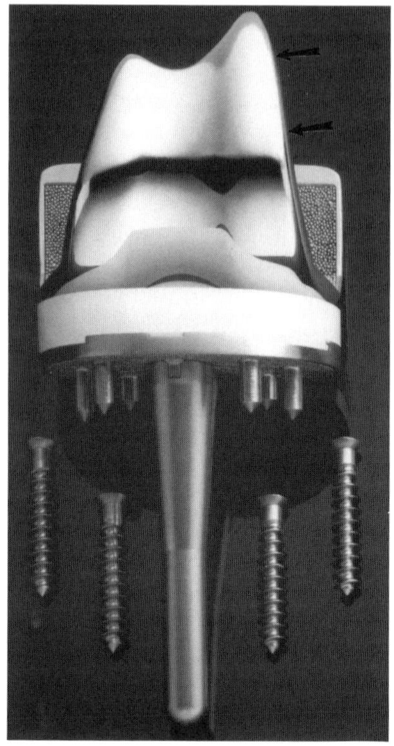

FIG. 6-95. The Whiteside Osteoloc™ modular knee system with a raised lateral condyle on the femoral component (*arrows*) for patellar tracking, (Courtesy of Wright Medical Technology, Arlington, TN.)

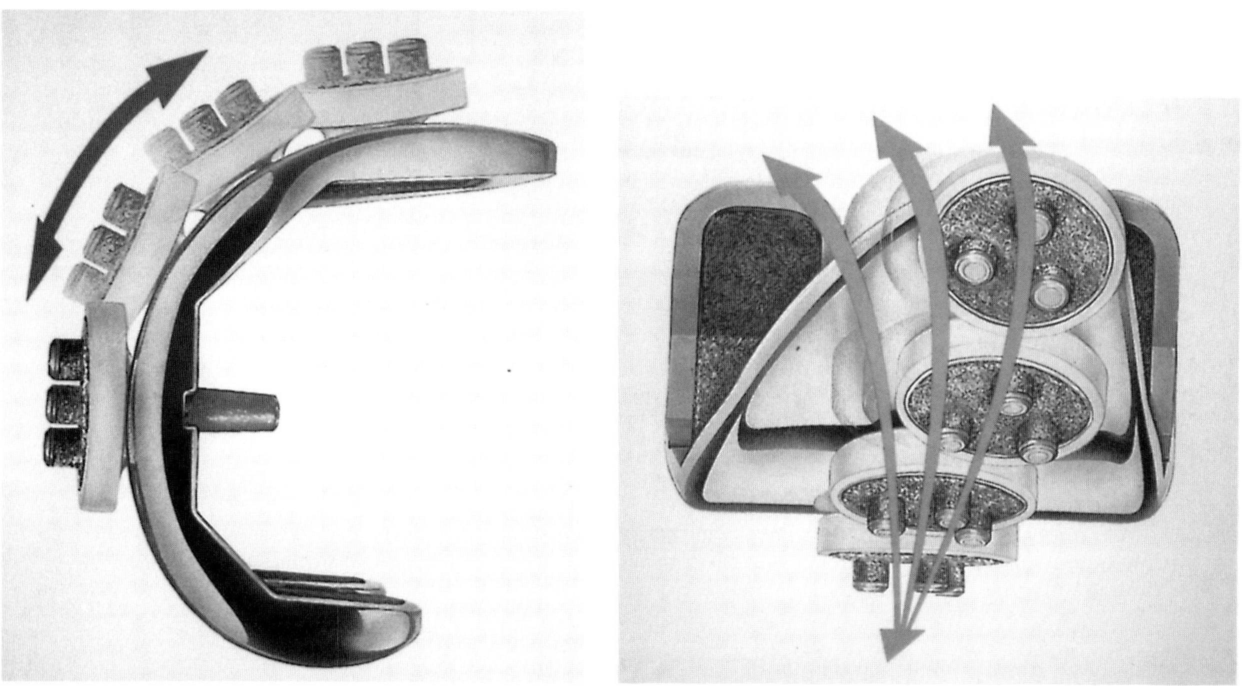

A B

FIG. 6-94. Patellar tracking. The lateral **(A)** and AP **(B)** view of patellar tracking on the femoral component of a Miller-Galante II knee system. (Courtesy of Zimmer, Warsaw, IN.)

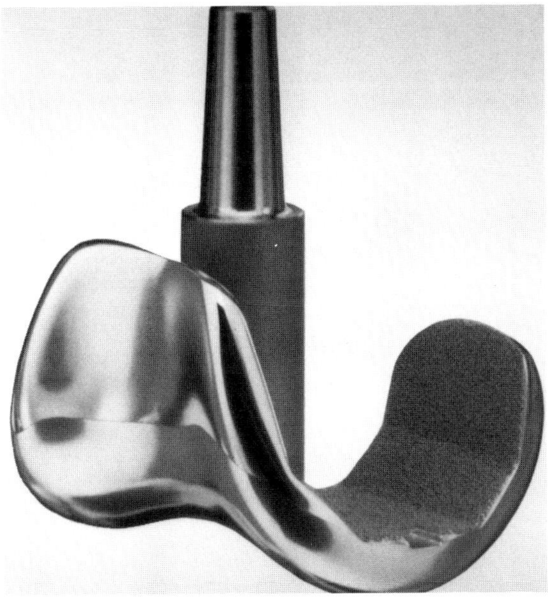

A

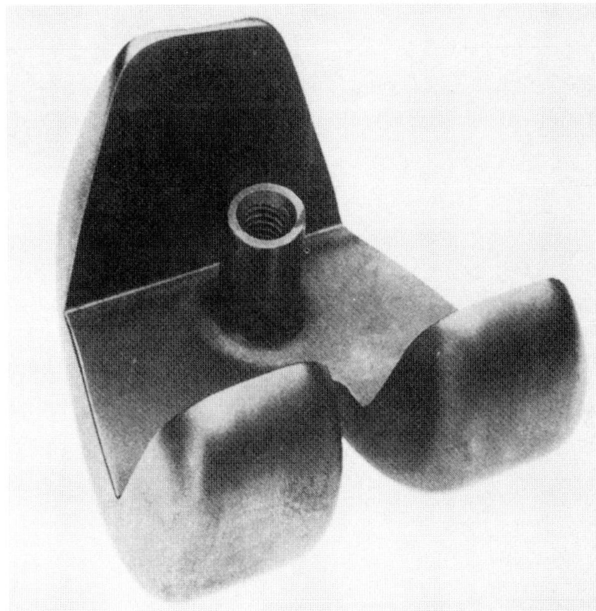

B

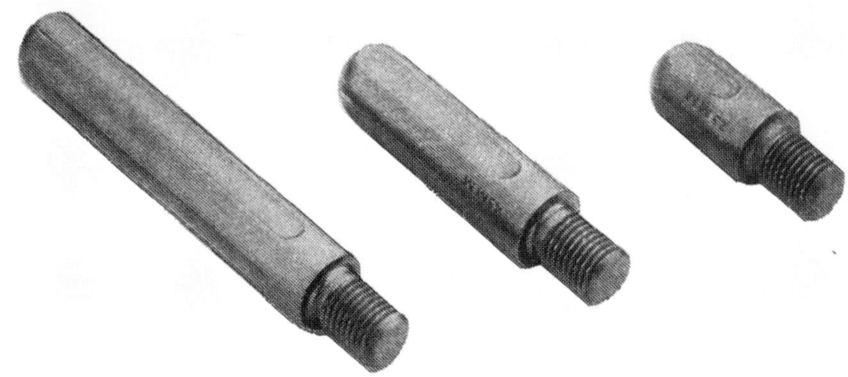

C

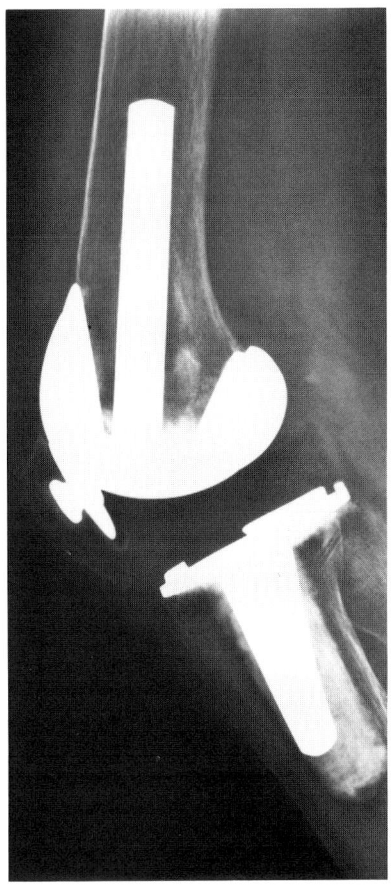

D

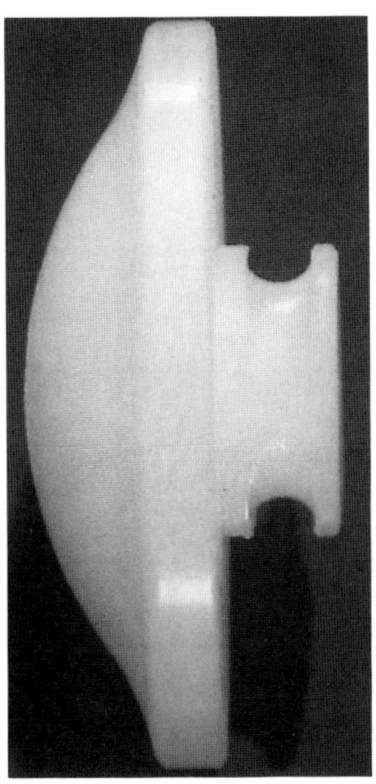

E

FIG. 6-96. Femoral stem variations. **A:** Revision porous femoral component (cobalt-chromium). (Courtesy of DePuy, Warsaw, IN.) Miller-Galante precoat revision femoral component (cobalt-chromium-molybdenum) **(B)** with stem adaptors **(C)**. (Courtesy of Zimmer, Warsaw, IN.) **D:** Lateral radiograph of the knee with a revision system. Compare this femoral component with Fig. 6-92D,E.

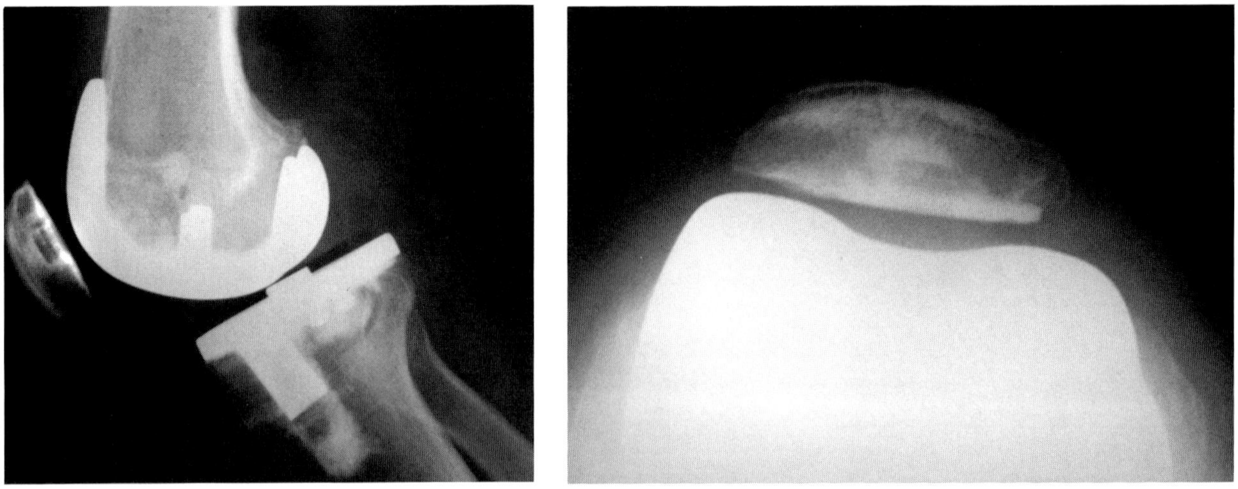

A B

FIG. 6-97. Lateral **(A)** and patellar **(B)** views of a cemented all-polyethylene patellar component in the Miller-Galante II knee system.

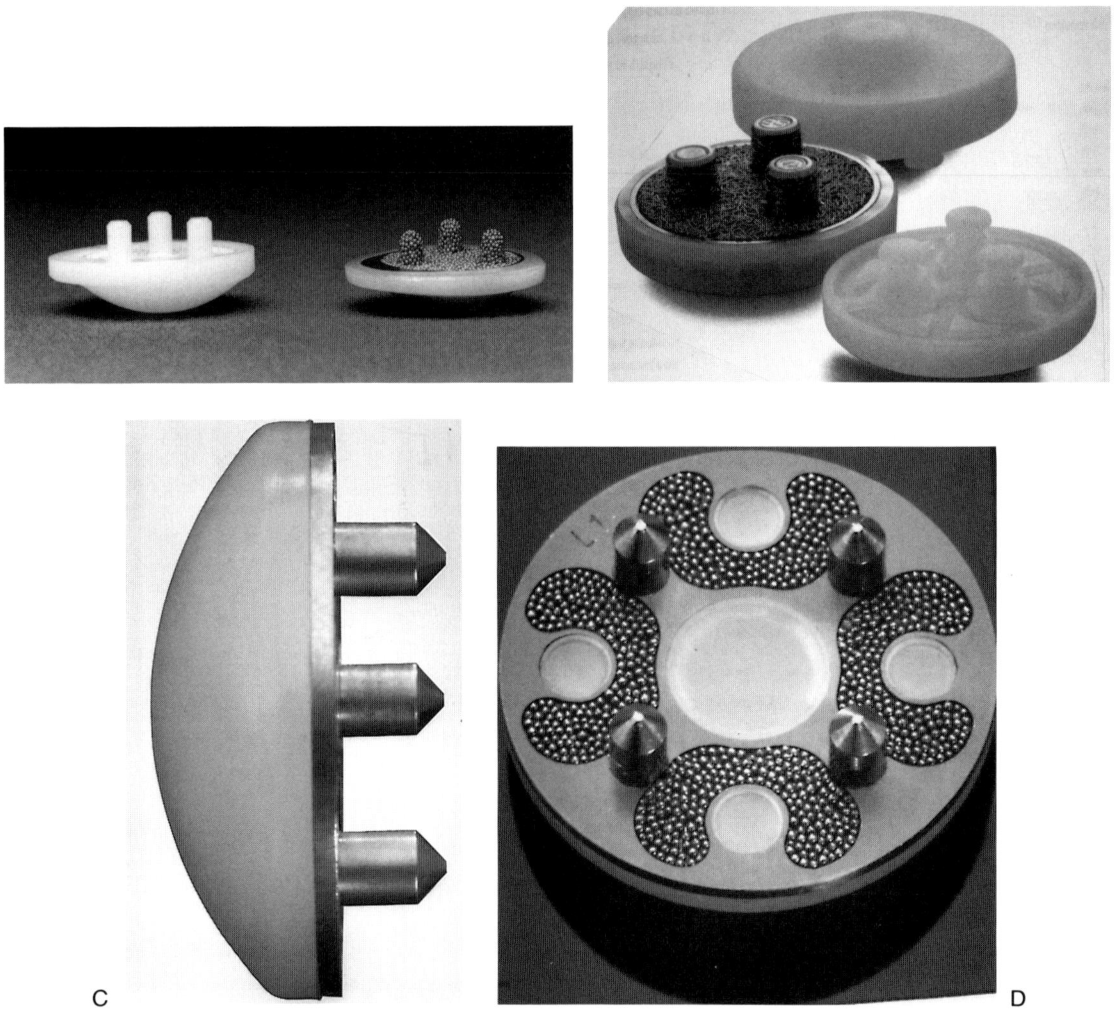

A B C D

FIG. 6-98. Patellar components. **A:** All-polyethylene (*left*) and porous-coated metal-backed patellar components. (Courtesy of Howmedica, Rutherford, NJ.) **B:** Fiber mesh metal-backed and anterior and posterior views of all-polyethylene patellar components. (Courtesy of Zimmer, Warsaw, IN.) Whiteside Ortholoc^{TM} patellar components with metal-backed components seen laterally **(C)** and from behind **(D)** and on an all-polyethylene component with a single central post **(E)**. (Courtesy of Wright Medical Technology, Arlington, TN.)

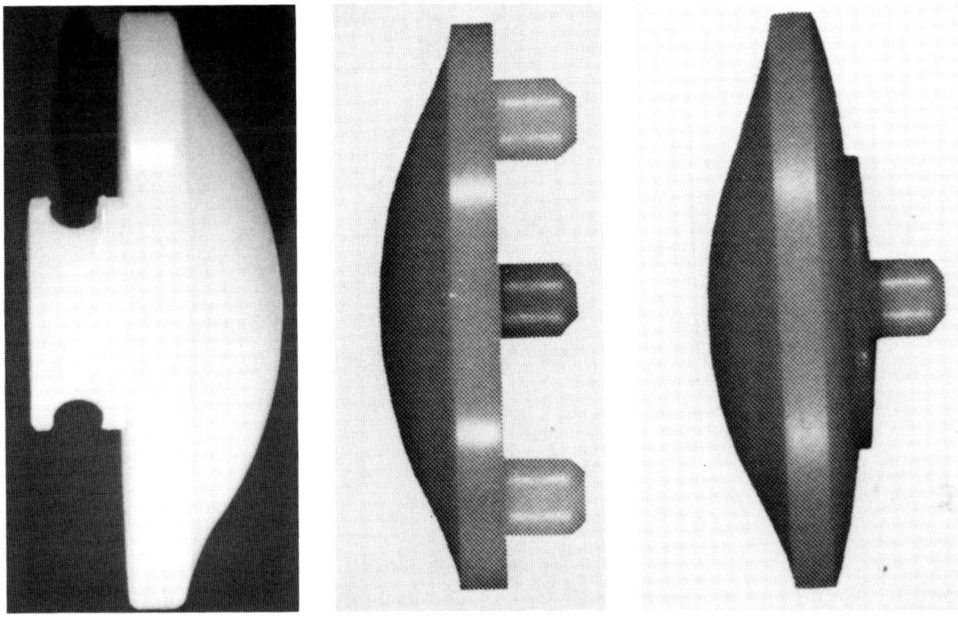

E,F G

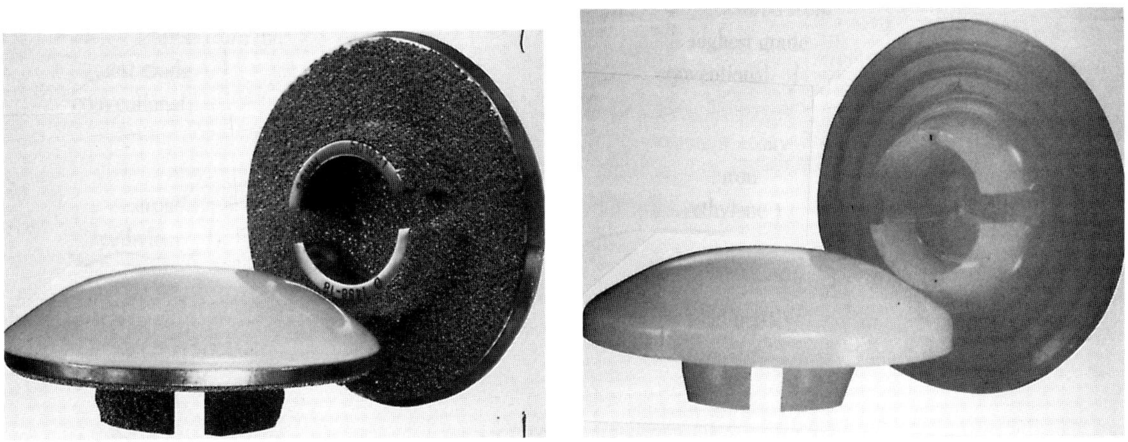

H I

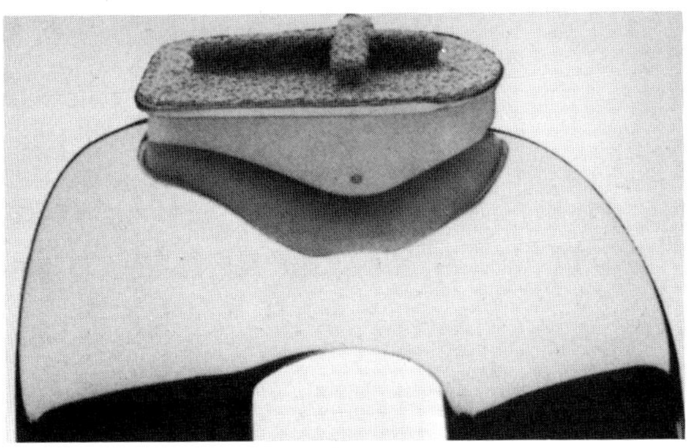

J

FIG. 6-98. (*Continued.*) Resurfacing **(F)** and biconvex **(G)** patellar components. (Courtesy of Smith and Nephew Richards, Memphis, TN.) Porous-coated metal-backed (AMK™) **(H)**, all-polyethylene (AMK™) **(I)**, and porous-coated metal backed (LCS™) **(J)** patellar components. (Courtesy of DePuy, Warsaw, IN.)

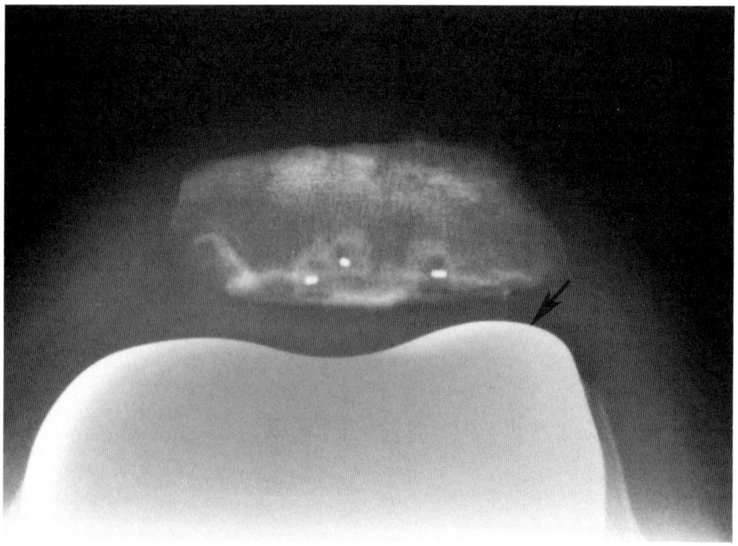

A

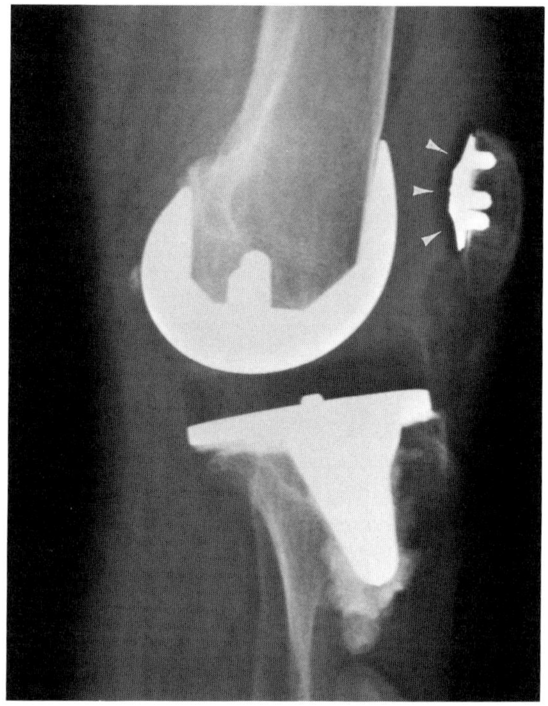

B

FIG. 6-99. **A:** Merchant view showing a cemented all-polyethylene patellar component. There is slight lateral tilt. Note the slightly more prominent lateral condylar portion (*arrow*) of the femoral component. **B:** Fluoroscopically positioned lateral in extension. The metal-backed patellar component is in profile, and the lucent polyethylene (*arrows*) is identified against the joint effusion.

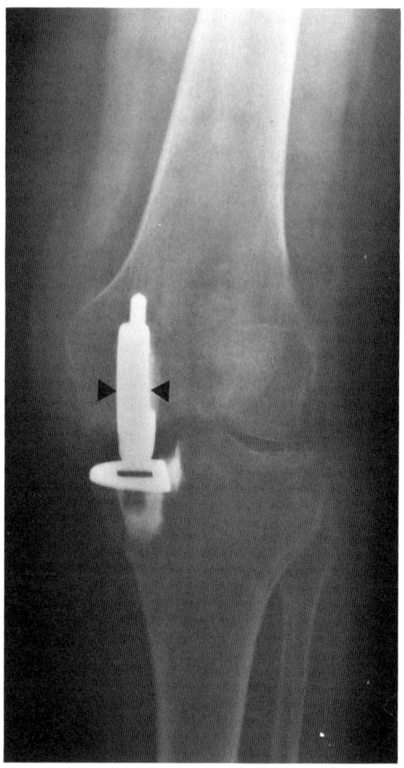

A

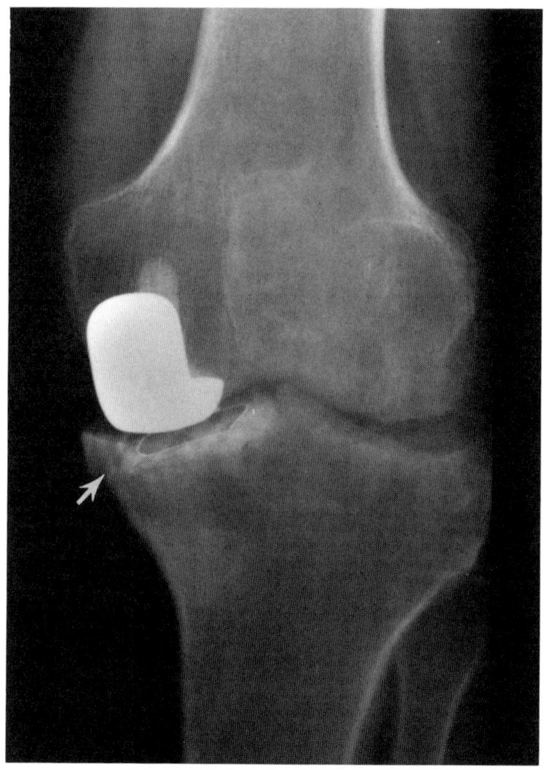

B

FIG. 6-100. Early unicompartmental arthroplasties. **A:** An AP view of the knee with medial compartment polycentric components. Note the narrow width (*arrows*) of the femoral component. The tibial component is metal backed. Both are cemented. **B:** An AP view of the knee with a medial compartment Marmor prosthesis. Note the subsidence of the tibial component with a tibial margin fracture (*arrow*). There is also obvious degenerative arthritis in the lateral compartment.

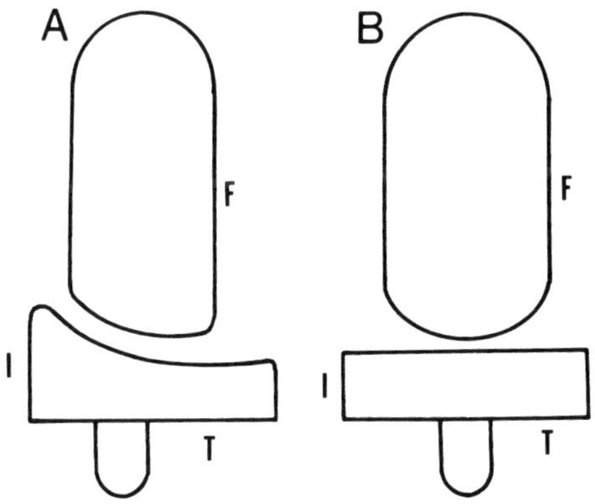

FIG. 6-101. The AP illustrations of constrained **(A)** and unconstrained **(B)** unicompartmental implants. *I,* side toward intercondylar spine; *F,* side opposite tibial spine; *T,* tibial surface. (From Hodge A, Chandler HP. Unicompartmental knee replacement: a comparison of constrained and unconstrained designs. *J Bone Joint Surg* [*Am*] 1992;74A:877–882.)

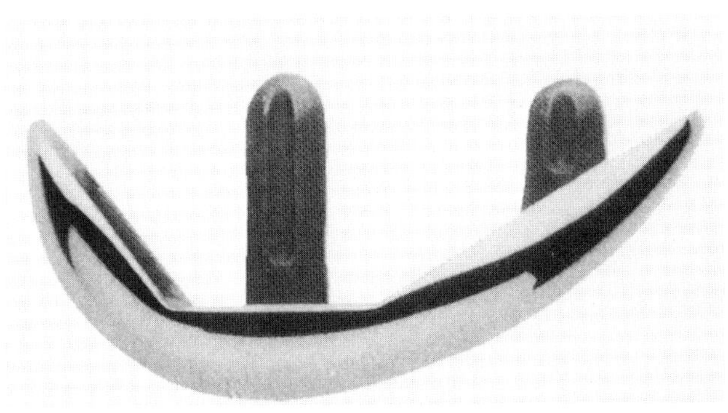

FIG. 6-102. Lateral view of the Zimmer unicompartmental Miller-Galante knee. There are two fluted posts (cobalt-chromium-molybdenum alloy). (Courtesy of Zimmer, Warsaw, IN.)

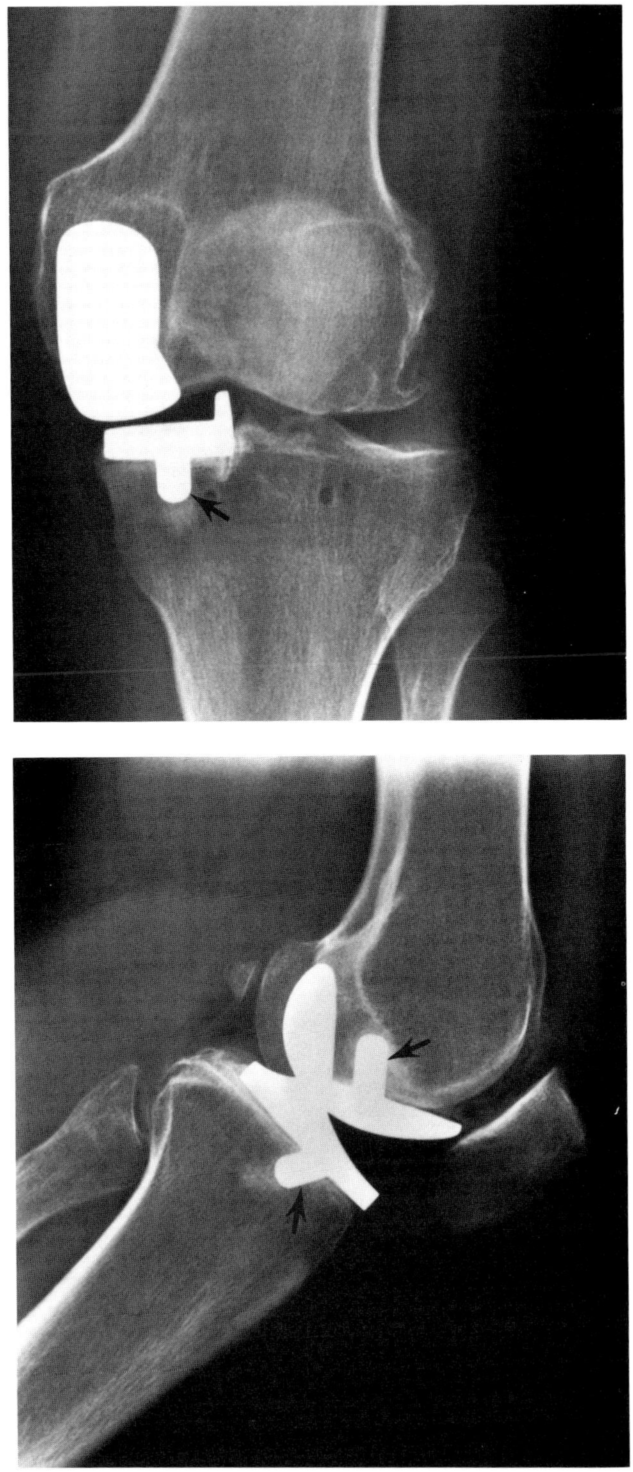

A

B

FIG. 6-103. The AP **(A)** and lateral **(B)** radiographs of a Howmedica P.C.A.™ unicompartmental arthroplasty. The components are Vitallium alloy with an ultrahigh molecular weight polyethylene tibial spacer. There is a single metal post in each component (*arrows*).

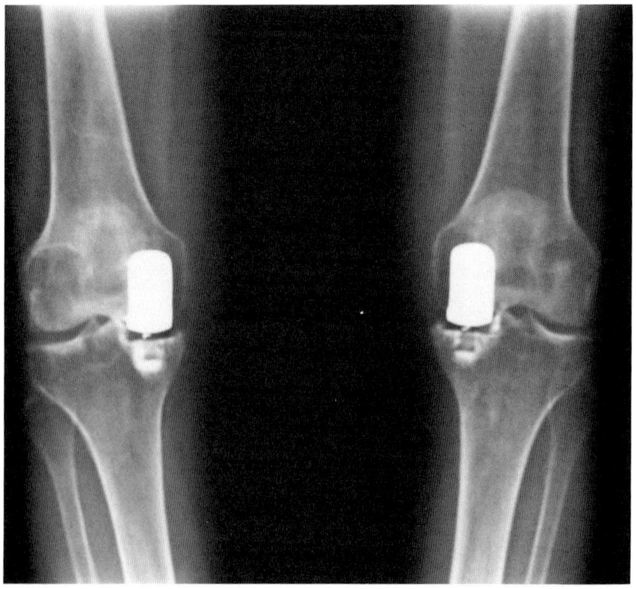
A

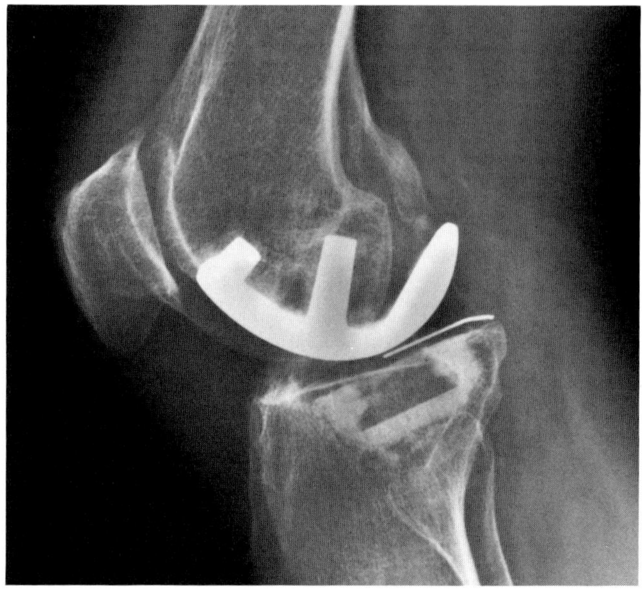
B

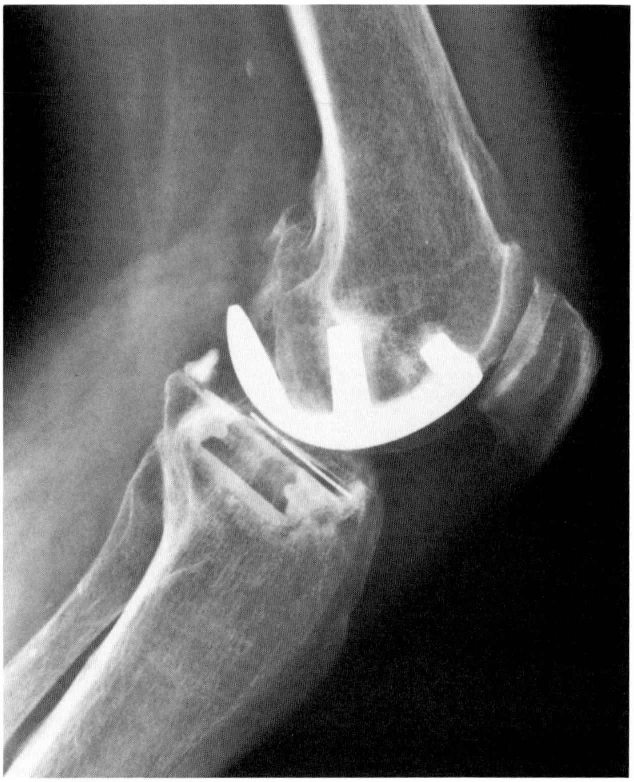
C

FIG. 6-104. The AP **(A)** standing and lateral **(B,C)** views of lateral medial compartmental arthroplasties with all-polyethylene tibial components, which contain a marker wire.

A
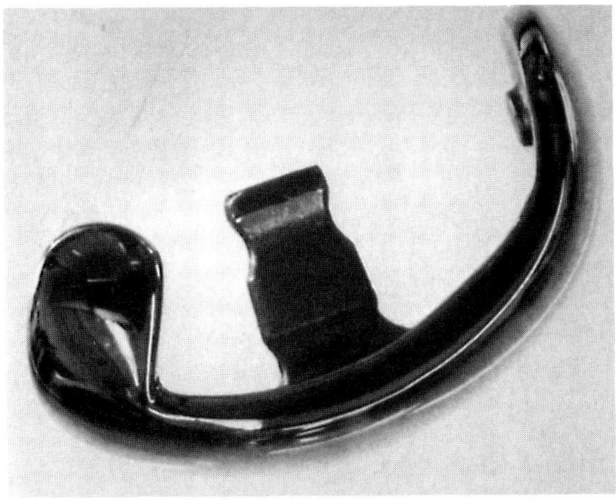

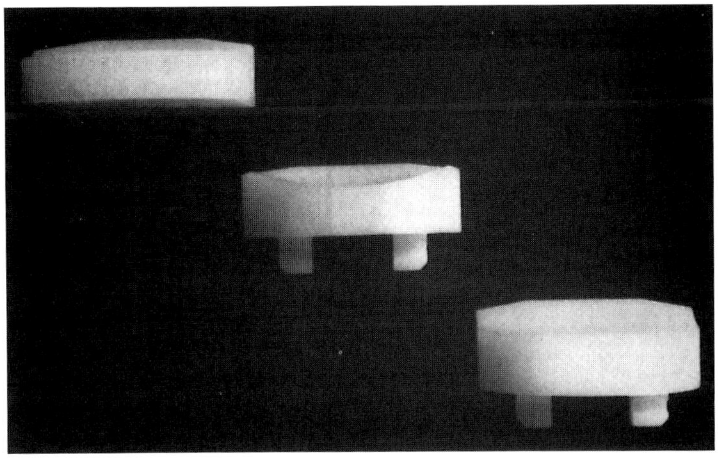
B

C,D
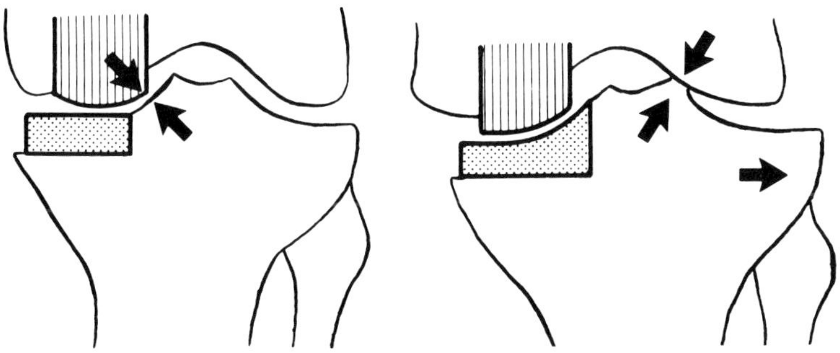

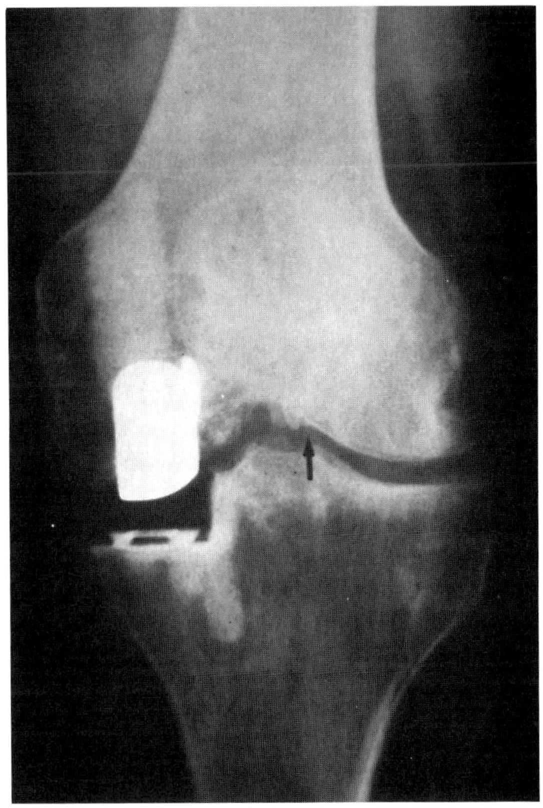
E

FIG. 6-105. Femoral **(A)** and tibial **(B)** components used in a series of 100 patients by Scott and Santore.[161] **C:** When the femoral component is placed too close to the intercondylar notch, it is mated with a flat tibial component that provides no constraint and impingement on the tibial spine (*arrows*) may occur. **D:** When the medial femoral component is placed too close to the intercondylar notch and is mated with a constrained tibial component, the lateral femoral condyle may impinge on the tibial spine (*arrows*). **E:** An AP radiograph with femoral impingement on the tibial spine (*arrow*). (From Scott RD, Santore RF. Unicondylar unicompartmental replacement for osteoarthritis of the knee. *J Bone Joint Surg* 1981;63:536–544.)

compartmental arthroplasty if the previously mentioned criteria are considered. Patients younger than 60 years of age with a higher activity demand and greater body weight may be better suited for osteotomy. Pain at rest is a contraindication to tibial osteotomy.[129,160]

Tricompartmental Arthroplasty

Attempts at knee arthroplasty really began in the 19th century, but it was not until the 1950s that workable prosthetic designs and consistent improvements with modifications in designs and component makeup (e.g., metal alloys and polyethylene) began.[159] The constrained designs, primarily hinged components, were developed from the 1950s through the 1970s by Walldius (Fig. 6-106)[176] in 1951, Shiers[164] in 1954, Young[182] in 1958 (Fig. 6-107), Stanmore (Fig. 6-108)[117] in 1969, and the Guepar group[98,121] in 1970 (Fig. 6-61). The original components were acrylic, and then designs using Vitallium were constructed.[98,121,182] The clinical follow-up of these designs over 1 to 9 years demonstrated satisfactory results in about 63% to 65% of patients. However, the incidence of loosening (16% to 30%) and deep infection (8% to 13%) were far too high.[86,100,103,106,134–136] Patellar complications, including instability, pain, and patellar tendon rupture, were also reported.[121] Today, hinged components are reserved for patients with significant bone loss, ligament instability, neurotrophic knees, or failed surface replacement arthroplasty. The incidence of complications is still higher than for more modern condylar designs or knee arthrodesis.[99]

The disappointing results with early hinged components were attributed to their size, metal-to-metal surfaces, and lack of rotational motion, which caused excessive torque to be transmitted to the bone-cement interface.[147] Modifications that allowed rotation were developed. The Kinematic rotating-hinge prosthesis (Fig. 6-60) allowed axial rotation and distraction between the inner tibial-bearing and outer sleeve. Seventy-two percent of the patients reported on by Rand et al.[147] had good or excellent results, based on their knee rating score. However, the rates of postoperative complications were still unacceptable. Infection occurred in 16%, patellar instability in 22%, and implant breakage in 6%.

The Attenborough knee was designed as a stabilized (constrained) gliding prosthesis with patellar resurfacing (Fig. 6-109).[109] The initial reports on this implant showed an 80% patient satisfaction rate. However, longer follow-up studies demonstrated wound healing problems in 20%, deep infections in 3% to 5%, and loosening requiring revision in 20% (Fig. 6-109).[109]

The Noiles prosthesis (Joint Medical Products, Stamford, CT) was introduced as a modified constrained hinge implant in the late 1970s.[165] The femoral component is cemented with methyl methacrylate. The tibial component inserts into a cemented polyethylene sleeve. The tibial and femoral components are hinged, but axial motion and 20° of medial and lateral rotation were allowed (Fig. 6-110). Satisfactory results were obtained in 44% of patients, and failure occurred in the remaining 56% of patients, as reported by Shindell et al.[165]

Resurfacing arthroplasties, which was more anatomic, preserved soft tissue support and required much less bone removal. In the early 1970s, the polycentric design (Figs. 6-59 and 6-111) was commonly used. This implant consisted of two separate Vitallium femoral components and two polyethylene tibial components. This prosthesis was technically difficult to position (Fig. 6-111).[69,129] Calculated success rates 10 years following surgery were only 66%.[118] Ligament instability (13%), loosening (7%), infection (3%), and patellofemoral syndromes in 4% were reported complications.

The geometric resurfacing prosthesis was designed in the early 1970s.[149] The femoral component was constructed of Vitallium with the condylar units joined by a crossbar (Figs. 6-70 and 6-112).[89] The tibial component consisted of one unit instead of the separate condylar trays used with the polycentric prosthesis. This single unit was high-density polyethylene with a crossbar uniting the weight-bearing portions (Fig. 6-112).[89,148] Wires were embedded in the polyethylene to allow better radiographic evaluation. Both components were cemented. The cruciate ligaments were retained. Rand and Coventry[148] reported on 102 knees followed for 11 years. The survival rates for the prosthesis were 78% at 10 years, with 83% of patients reporting no pain or only mild discomfort. Twenty percent of knees had to be revised in their series.

The concept of bicompartmental resurfacing is still used, although today most prefer uni- or tricompartmental reconstruction. Stockley et al.[168] reported on the St. Georg Sledge knee (Fig. 6-113) in 1990. The 5-year evaluation showed 92.3% survival of the components.

The condylar design was initiated at the Hospital for Special Surgery in 1973. All implants since that time are variations that differ in design (e.g., ligament retention or sacrifice, metal-backed versus all-polyethylene patellar and tibial components, stem variation for patients with bone loss, and cemented versus uncemented), depending on the problem with the implants that surgeons were trying to solved or the patient's needs in regard to reconstruction.

The total condylar design used metal femoral and polyethylene tibial components (Fig. 6-114), which could be used for most knee reconstructions.[105] The polyethylene tibial component was a one-piece device with cup-shaped articular zones and a central eminence to prevent translation of the femur on the tibia.[103,105] The patellar component was a dome-shaped polyethylene device with a single central lug for fixation.[103] Insall et al.[105] reported good to excellent results in 90% of 220 knees. The reoperation rate at 3 to 5 years was only 3.6%. Eighty-seven percent were satisfactory at 10 years.[103]

(text continues on page 480)

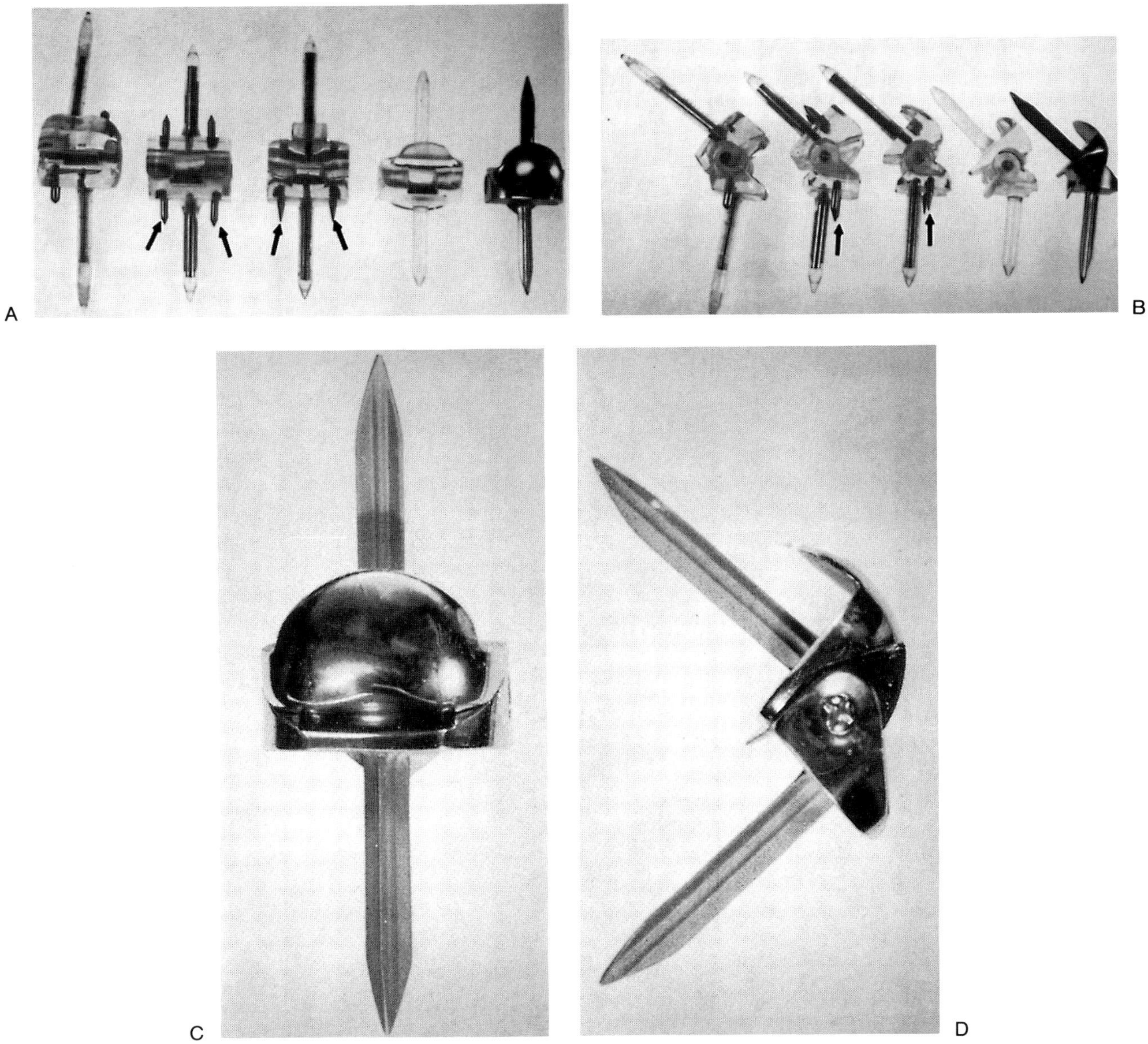

FIG. 6-106. The Walldius hinged prosthesis. The AP **(A)** and lateral **(B)** photographs of early designs with long medullary stems and constructed with acrylic resins. Stainless steel (*arrows*) pins were used to prevent rotation. The AP **(C)** and lateral **(D)** photographs of newer Vitallium designs modified with a Teflon^{TM} covering on the axis. (From Walldius B. Arthroplasty of the knee using endoprosthesis. *Acta Orthop Scand* 1960;30:137–148.)

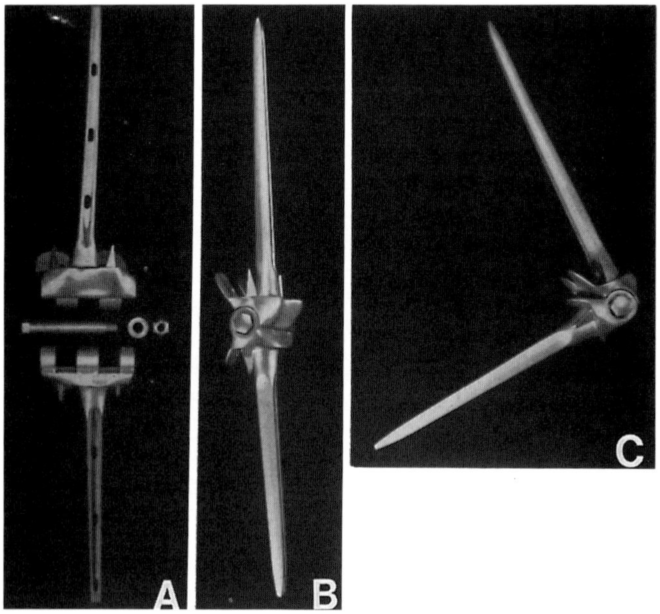

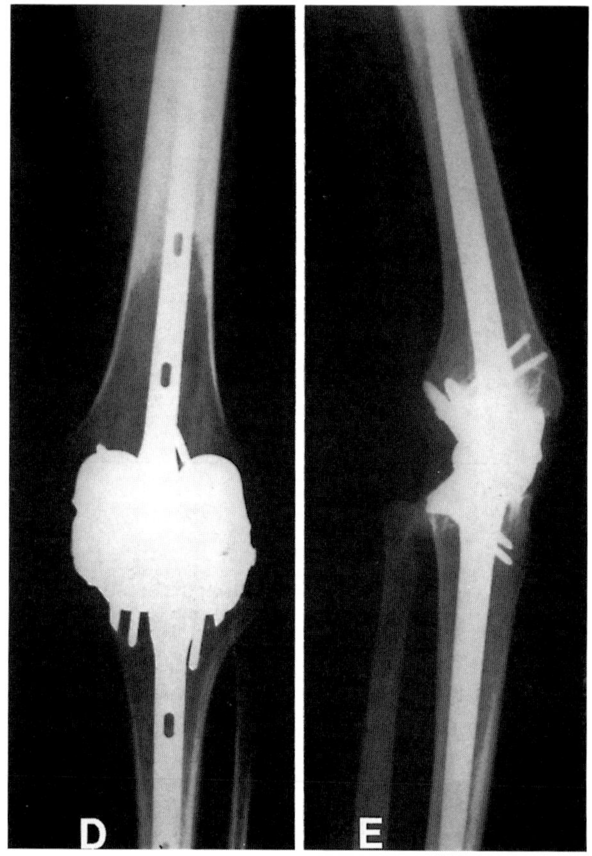

FIG. 6-107. The components **(A)** and appearance **(B,C)** of the Young prosthesis. The AP **(D)** and lateral **(E)** views of a Young prosthesis 5 years after implantation. (From Young HH. Use of a hinged Vitallium prosthesis for arthroplasty of the knee: a preliminary report. *J Bone Joint Surg* [*Am*]. 1963;45A:1627–1642.)

A

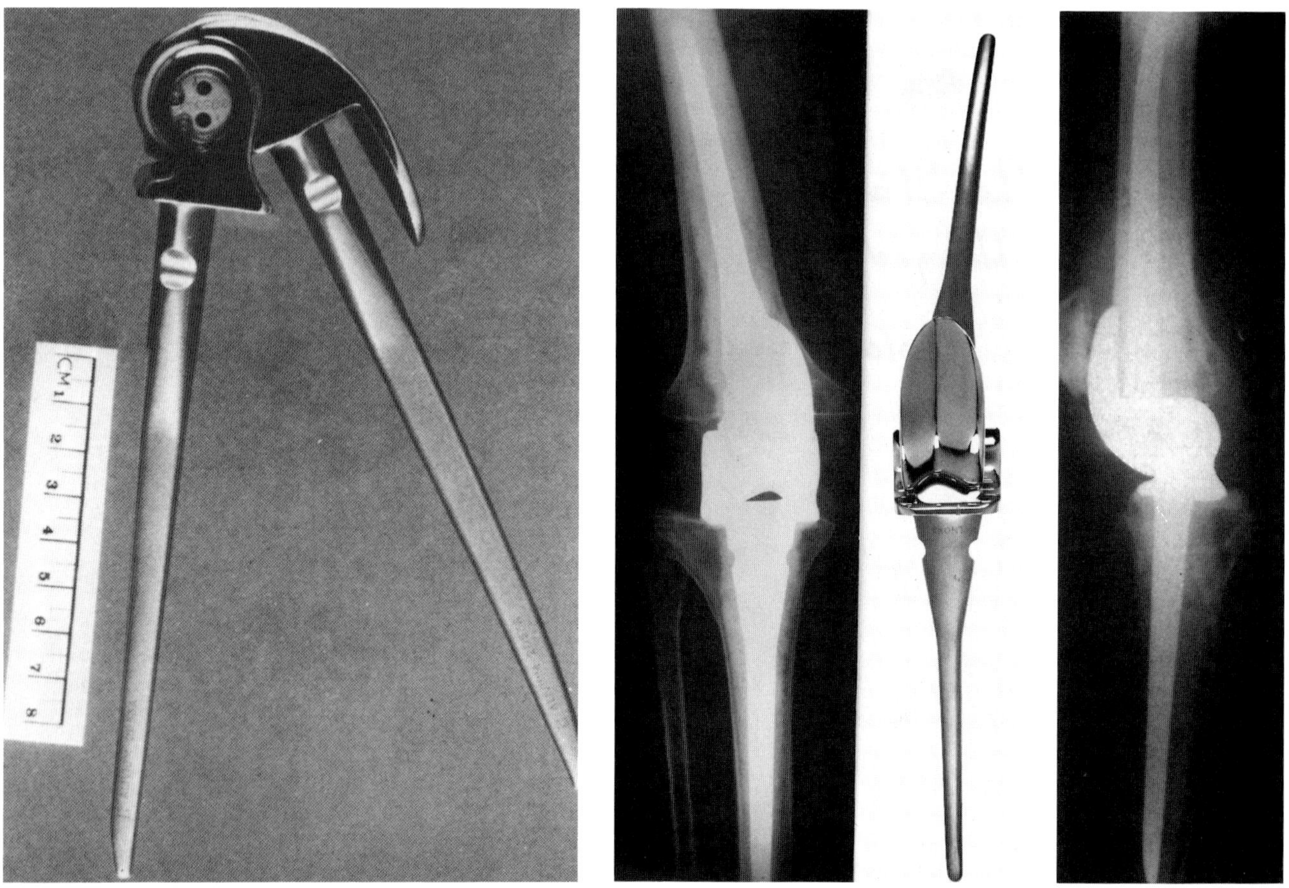

B,C

FIG. 6-108. A: A Mark 4 Stanmore prosthesis. Radiograph and prosthesis following surgery **(B)** and lateral view **(C)**. (From Lettin AWF et al. Assessment of survival and clinical results of Stanmore total knee replacement. *J Bone Joint Surg* [*Br*] 1984;66B:355–361.)

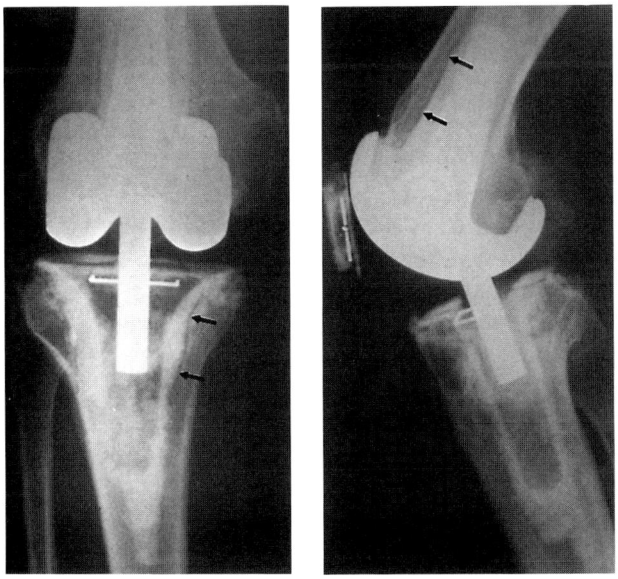

A,B

FIG. 6-109. The AP **(A)** and lateral **(B)** radiographs 2 years following surgery with an Attenborough implant. There is lucency at the bone cement interface (*arrows*) caused by infection and loosening. (From Kershaw CJ, Therman AEG. The Attenborough knee. A four to ten year review. *J Bone Joint Surg* [*Br*] 1988;70B:89–93.)

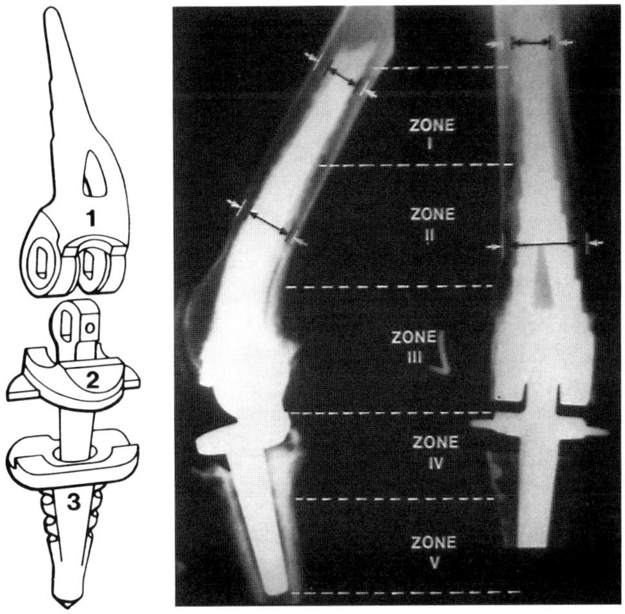

A B,C

FIG. 6-110. A: The components of the Noiles prosthesis. The femoral component (*1*) is hinged by a pin to the tibial component (*2*), which is positioned in a cemented polyethylene sleeve (*3*). Lateral **(B)** and AP **(C)** radiographs demonstrating the zones that were evaluated postoperatively. The medullary width (*white arrows*) and the cement mantle (*black arrows*) were measured where noted. (From Shindell R, Neumann R, Connolly JF, Jordon OM. Evaluation of the Noiles hinged knee prostheses. A 5 year study of 17 knees. *J Bone Joint Surg* [*Am*] 1986;68A:579–586.)

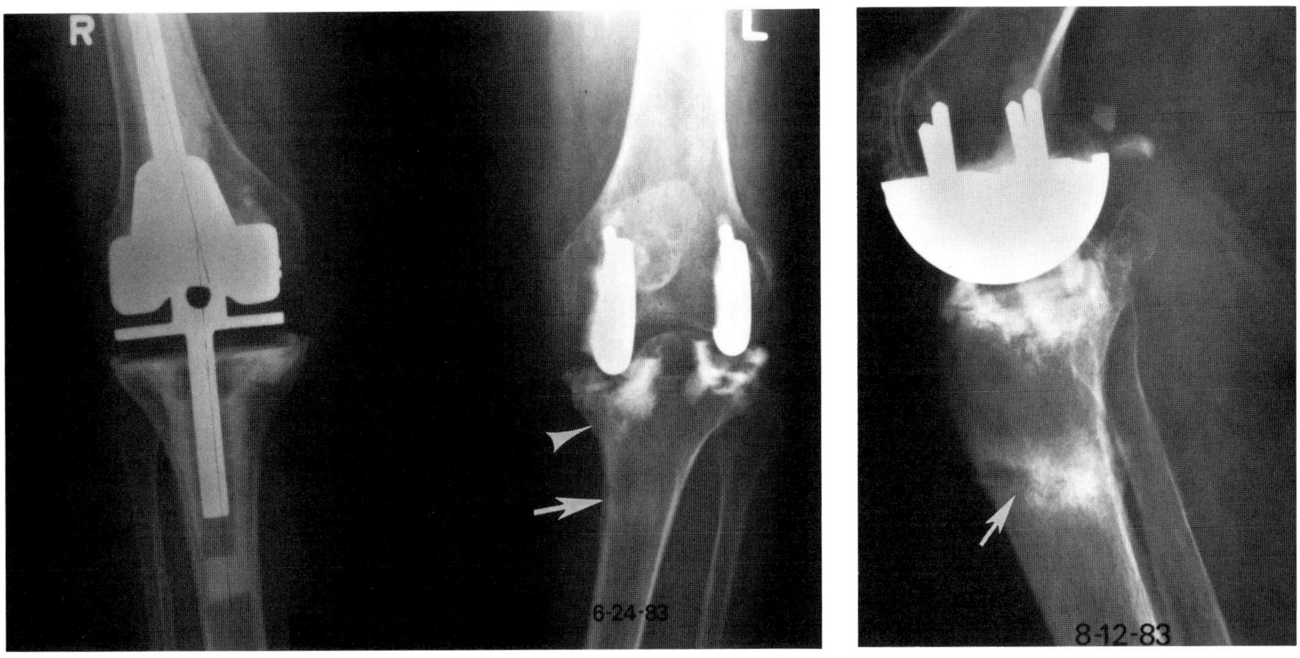

FIG. 6-111. Standing AP views of the knee with a Kinematic™ rotating hinge prosthesis on the *right* and polycentric arthroplasty on the *left*. There is collapse of the medial tibial plateau (*top arrowhead*) and a proximal shaft stress fracture (*arrows*) on the left.

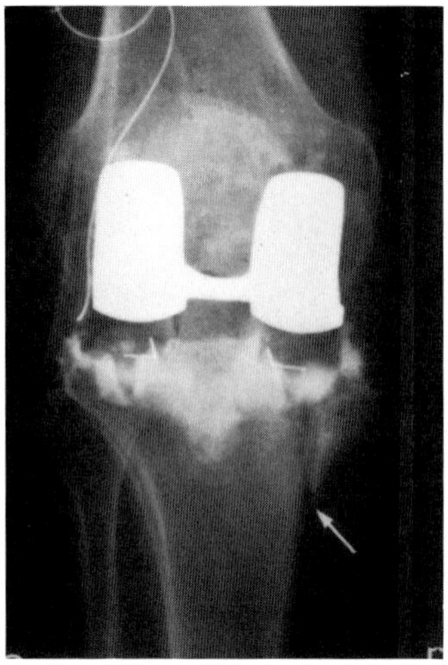

FIG. 6-112. An AP view of the knee demonstrating a geometric knee arthroplasty. Note the medial tibial fracture (*arrow*, Fig. 6-68).

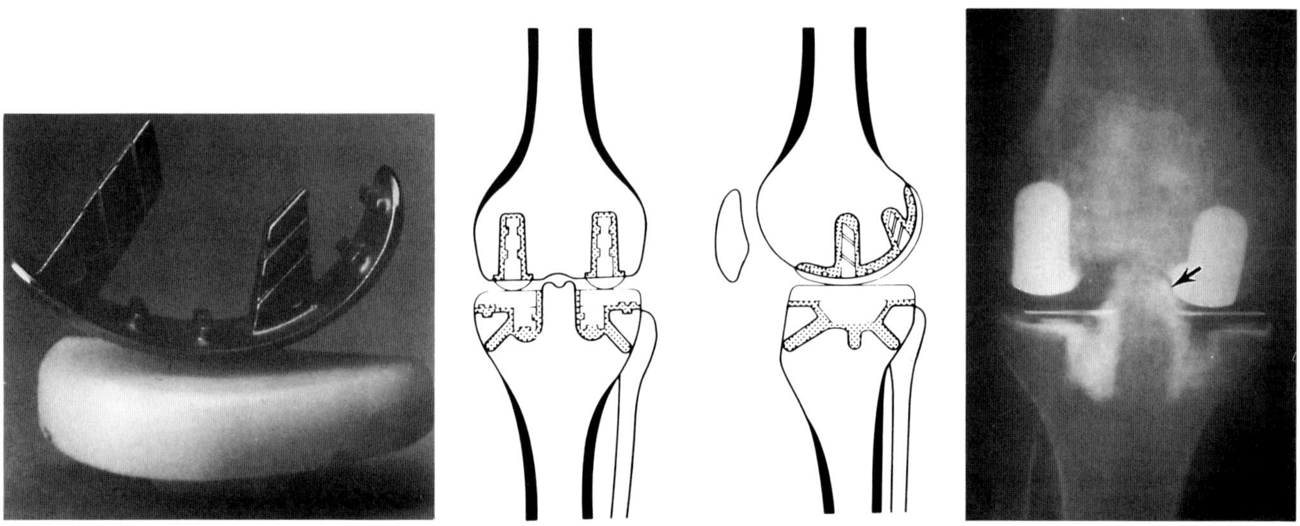

A B,C

FIG. 6-113. A: St. Georg Sledge knee prosthesis. **B:** Cemented tibial legs. **C:** An AP radiograph demonstrating impingement of the femoral component against the intercondylar imminence (*arrow*). (From Stockley L, Douglas DL, Elson RA. Bicondylar St. Georg Sledge knee arthroplasty. *Clin Orthop* 1990;225:228–234.)

A 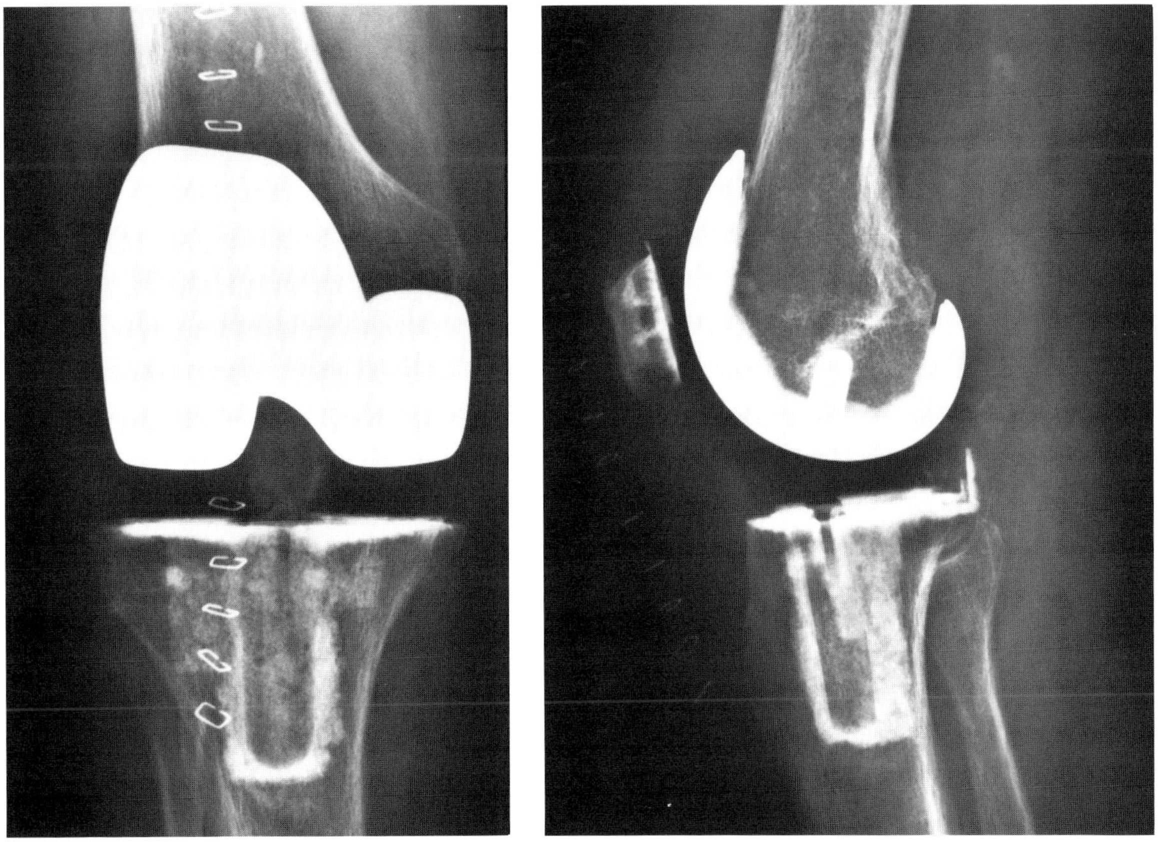 B

FIG. 6-114. The AP **(A)** and lateral **(B)** radiographs of a total condylar prosthesis with cemented polyethylene tibial component.

A 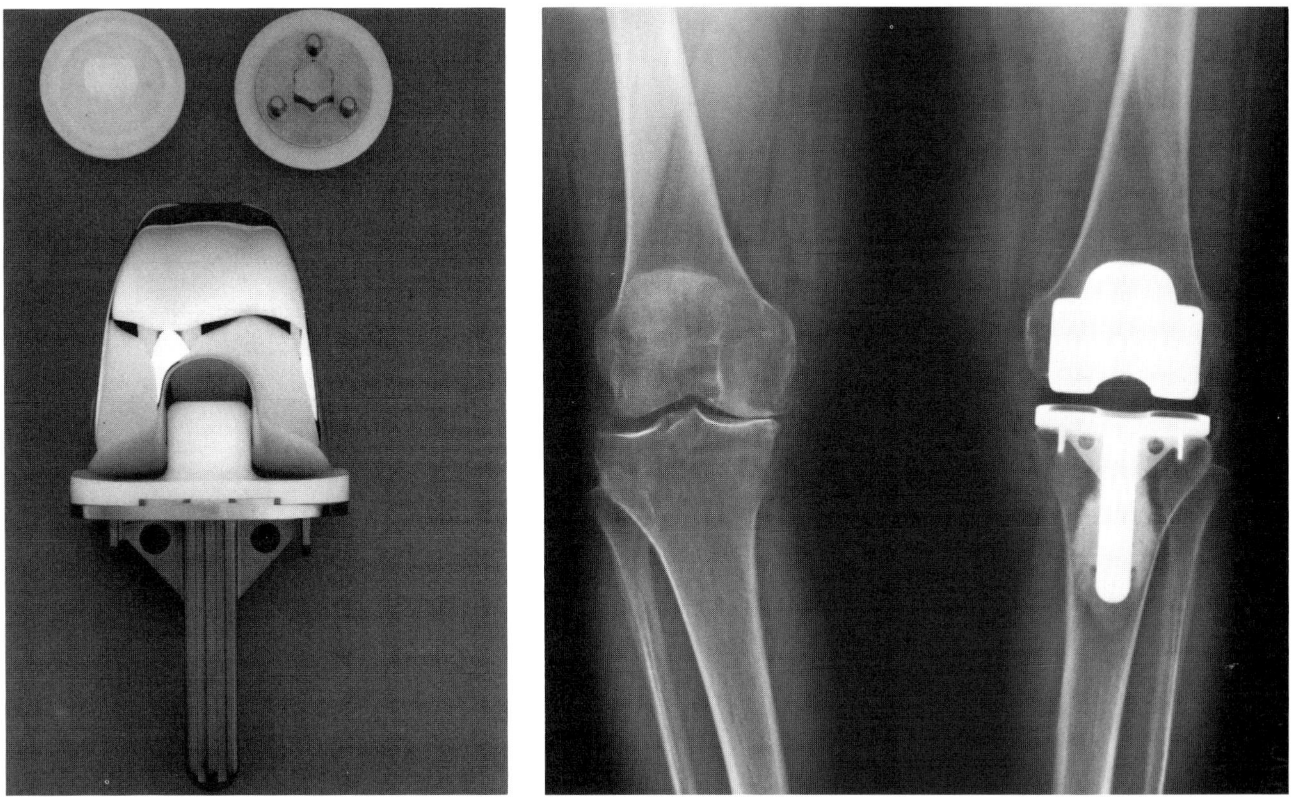 B

FIG. 6-115. A: Frontal illustration of the Lacey™ posterior-stabilized knee system. The articular (*left*) and metal-backed bone interface (*right*) of the patellar component are demonstrated. The long tibial stem and upper winged appearance makes this component easy to identify radiographically (*B*). (Courtesy of Wright Medical Technology, Arlington, TN.) **B:** Standing AP views of the knee with a Lacey™ knee replacement on the left.

The posterior cruciate condylar (Figs. 6-92 and 6-93) differs in that the tibial component is cut out posteriorly to allow retention of the PCL. Preserving the PCL was believed to improve the range of motion, stair climbing, tibial roll back, and posterior stability.[144] Most PCL-sparing condylar components have metal-backed tibial components. There is a deeper intercondylar cut in the femoral component posteriorly (Figs. 6-92A and 6-93A–C, number 1).

The Kinematic condylar knee was designed to resolve problems, which at least were perceived, with the PCL condylar design.[144] This system also spared the PCL.[86,181] The Kinematic-I uses cemented components. The tibial component is metal backed with a central fixation stem. The posterior tibial component is flatter to allow femoral roll back and more normal PCL function. The range of motion was improved by these changes.[144] The patellar component is all polyethylene and symmetric.[86,181] The results were good to excellent in 90% of cases, with 106° of flexion.

The posterior-stabilized condylar prosthesis (Fig. 6-115) is a cruciate-sacrificing system designed to increase posterior stability in flexion and improve stair climbing.[144,167] The tibial component has a central post (Fig. 6-115A), which fits into a rectangular cutout in the posteriorly closed femoral component. The posterior tibial articular surface is also more cupped than the cruciate-sparing components.[134,144] At our institution, we preserve the PCL whenever possible. When this cannot be accomplished, the posterior-stabilized prosthesis is usually selected.[129]

The Kinematic stabilized prosthesis differs from the posterior-stabilized design in that the central tibial post engages the femoral component in extension and provides medial-lateral stability.[144]

The PCA (Fig. 6-116) design became available in 1980.[78] This system was designed to reestablish kinematic knee function with minimal bone removal. The tibial component is metal backed with a posterior cutout for PCL preservation. The bone-metal interface is coated with chrom-cobalt beads. The patellar component was anatomically configured in a manner similar to the normal patellar articular surface. The NK (Intermedics Orthopedics, Austin, Texas) porous-coated system is coated with a cancellous structured titanium surface.[65] The Ortholoc™ design (Wright Medical Technology, Arlington, TN; Fig. 6-89) also used metal beads, but the tibial component has a central stem with lateral pegs and screws to ensure symmetric support and load bearing.[178] Porous-coated components can be used with and without cement.[144] Good (knee scores of 80 to 90) to excellent (knee score of 90 to 100) results were obtained in 78% to 100% of patients with average flexion of 103° to 106°.[78]

More recent advances include press-fit designs with removable polyethylene trays. Figures 6-117 to 6-128 demonstrate some of the other knee systems used currently.

Revision Arthroplasty

Revision arthroplasty is indicated for mechanical failure caused by loosening, instability, poor or reduced range of motion, and extensor dysfunction.[115,143] Revision surgery is more difficult because of the increased bone loss from the original procedure and other factors, such as infection and ligament instability.[85] Several stages may be required when infection is present. Contraindications for considering revision include soft tissue insufficiency, vascular disease, obesity, and uncorrectable bone loss.[143]

Revision surgery usually requires bone grafting and more customized components with longer stems, tibial wedges, or more constrained prostheses (Figs. 6-129 to 6-133). A hinged prosthesis may be indicated, especially when soft tissue support is inadequate (Fig. 6-134).[99,117,182] In some patients, arthrodesis may be the best solution (Fig. 6-135).[129] Fascial arthroplasty (components removed and cavity allowed to fill with scar tissue) is also a consideration today.

Postoperative Imaging and Complications

Routine radiographs should be taken immediately postoperatively. The AP and lateral views are obtained to check the alignment and component position and to exclude obvious problems, such as periprosthetic fracture.[129] When the patient can tolerate a complete knee series, this should be obtained. This should include standing AP (most surgeons prefer a full-length [hip to ankle] view), lateral, and Merchant or patellar views. The AP and lateral views should be optimally positioned with fluoroscopy to allow a more thorough evaluation of lucent lines and component position. Flexion and extension lateral views are also obtained in this manner (Fig. 6-136). After the initial studies, the patient is generally reevaluated radiographically at 6 months and 1 year. Yearly follow-up is adequate after this, unless otherwise indicated. Serial studies are the key to the detection of abnormal changes in lucent zones, subsidence, infection, polyethylene wear, and other complications. Serial examinations are especially useful with uncemented components.

For simplicity, it is best to describe the radiographic evaluation on each view.

Standing AP View

The mechanical axis, tibial and femoral component position, and area of tibia covered by the component should be evaluated. Figure 6-137 demonstrates the femoral (α) and tibial (β) angles. The ideal tibial angle is 90° (±5°). If the angle is greater than 90°, the component is in valgus position. If the angle is less than 90° (Figs. 6-137 and 6-138), the component is in varus position.[167]

(*text continues on page 505*)

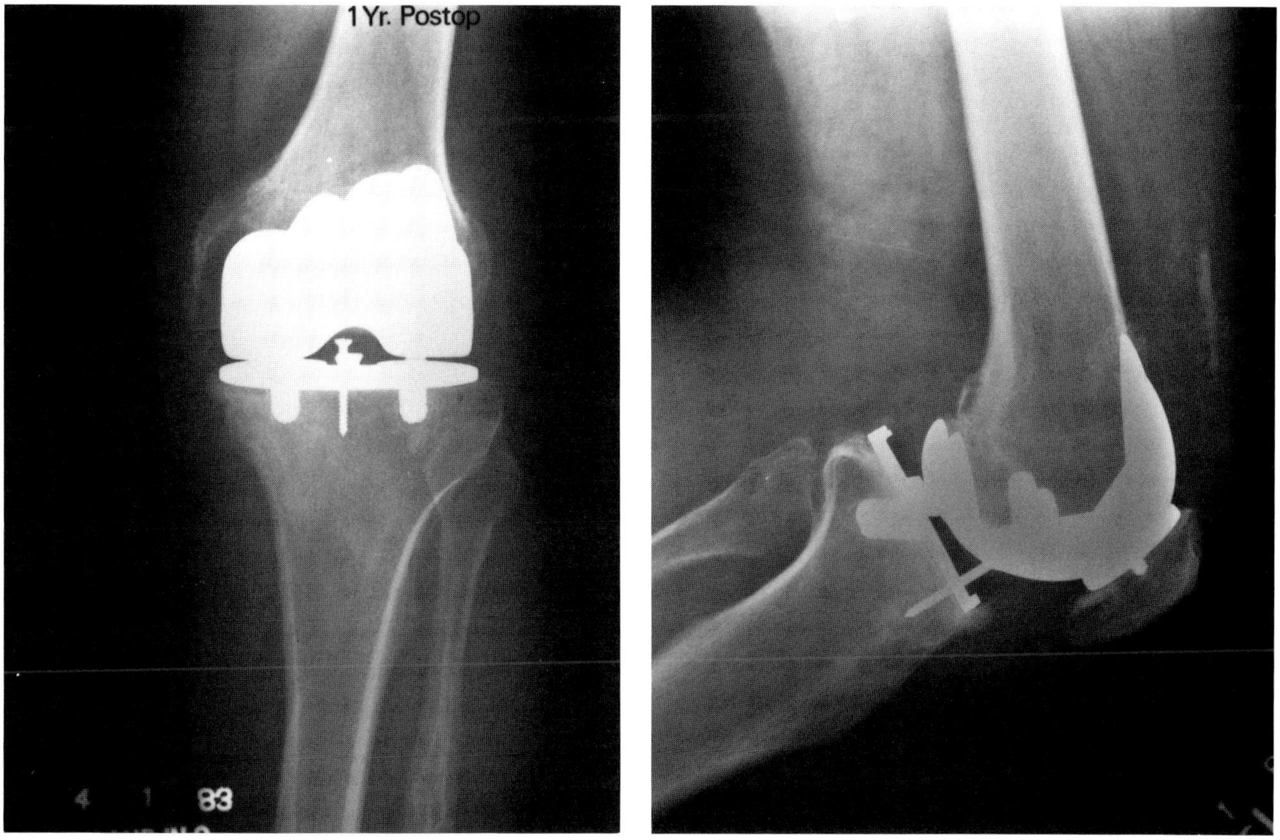

A B

FIG. 6-116. P.C.A.™ knee arthroplasty. The AP **(A)** and lateral **(B)** view of the knee with P.C.A.™ arthroplasty. There is a single anterior screw in the tibial component and a metal-backed patellar component. Note the old tibial and fibular fracture deformities.

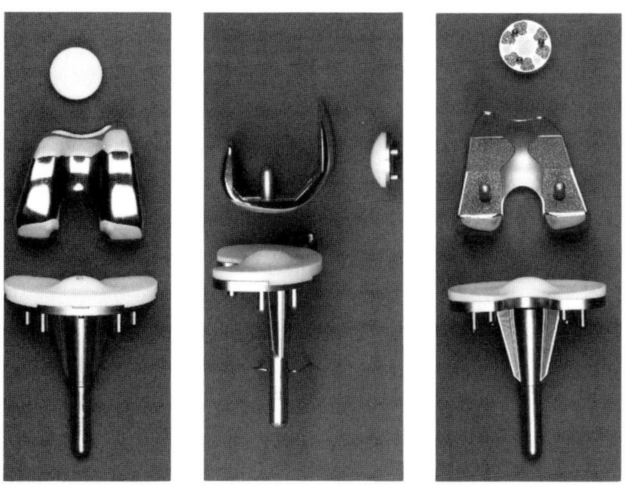

A,B C

FIG. 6-117. Ortholoc™ modular knee system with porous-coated tibial and femoral components. The metal-backed patellar component is configured with pegs and adjacent porous-coated segments. Components seen from the front **(A)**, side **(B)**, and back **(C)**. (Courtesy of Wright Medical Technology, Arlington, TN.)

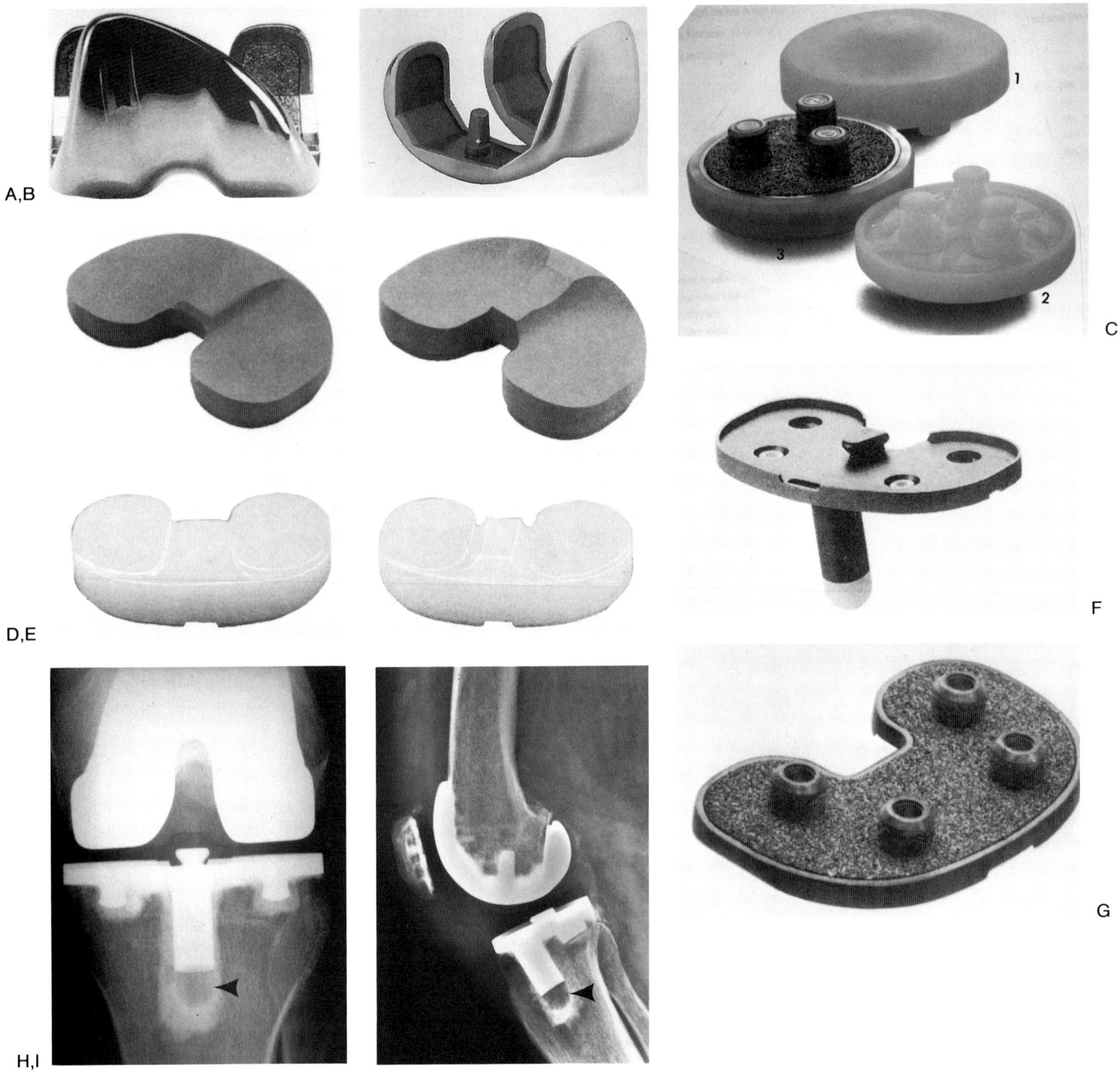

FIG. 6-118. Zimmer Miller-Galante knee systems. **A:** Femoral component (MGII) with porous-coated mesh. **B:** Kinematic™ condylar precoated femoral component. **C:** Patellar components with all-polyethylene (*1* and *2*) and titanium fiber mesh metal backing (*3*). Tibial components. **D:** Flat polyethylene tibial inserts. **E:** Lipped polyethylene tibial inserts. **F:** Porous stemmed tibial tray with two posterior pegs and two anterior holes for bone screws (MG-II). The tip of the stem is lucent radiographically (H,I). **G:** Titanium fiber mesh tibial tray with four bone screw holes seen from below. Notch view **(H)** and lateral view **(I)** of a Miller-Galante II with cemented components. All-polyethylene patellar component. Note the lucent bullet-shaped tip on the tibial stem (*arrow*). (A–G: Courtesy of Zimmer, Warsaw, IN.)

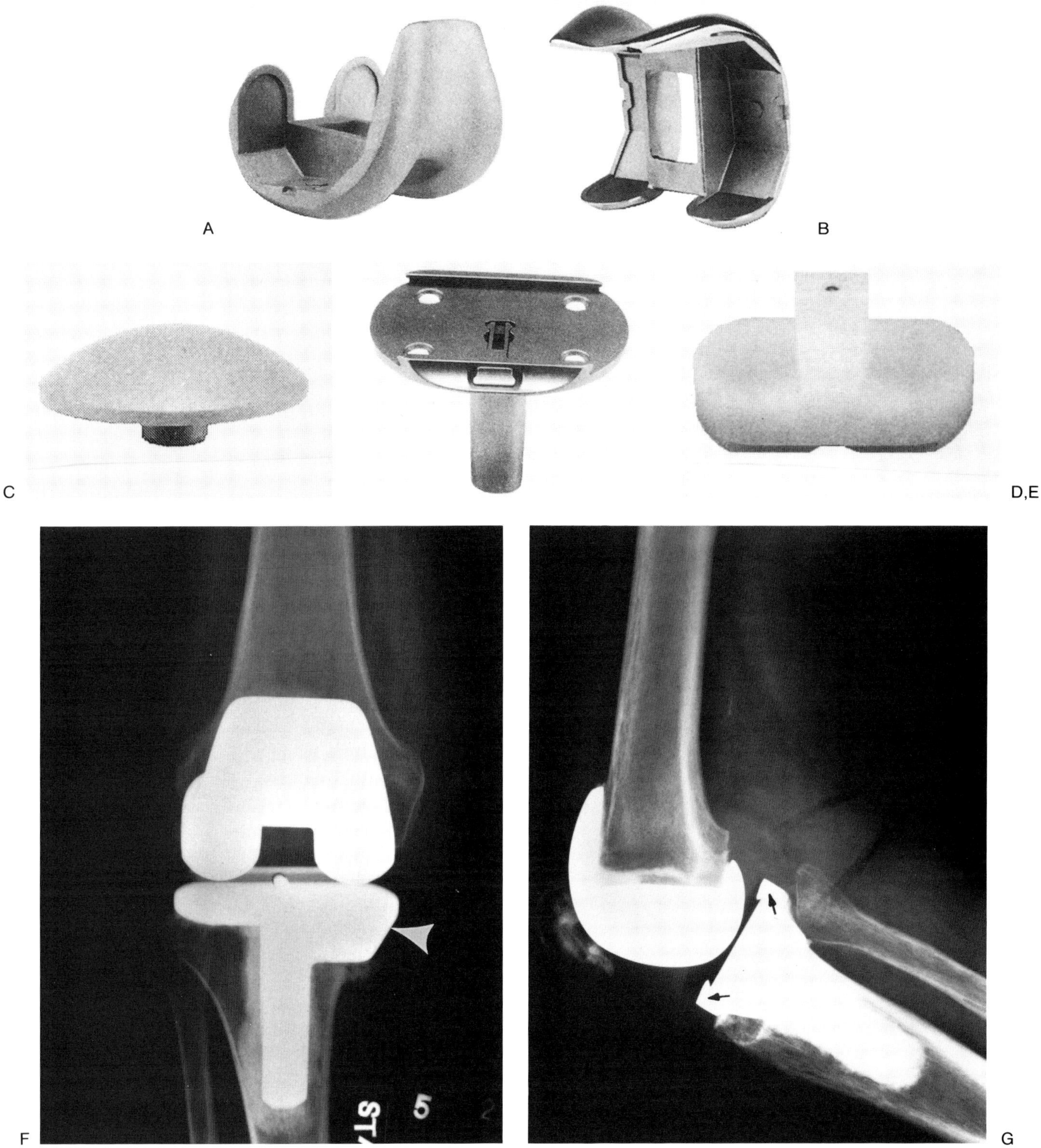

FIG. 6-119. Insall-Burstein II posterior-stabilized knee system. (A–E: Courtesy of Zimmer, Warsaw, IN.) Femoral components seen from the side **(A)** and top **(B)** with rectangular slot for the tibial post. The PCL is not retained. **C:** All-polyethylene patellar dome with a central peg. **D:** Tibial tray with anterior and posterior lips but no posterior notch (Fig. 6-118) and a central stem. **E:** Polyethylene tibial insert with a central post. Insall-Burstein modified with a medial tibial wedge (*arrow*) seen on AP **(F)** and lateral **(G)** radiographs. Note the lack of femoral posts (Fig. 6-118I) seen with most components. The tibial tray is best identified on the lateral view (*arrows* mark ridges). Compare D and F.

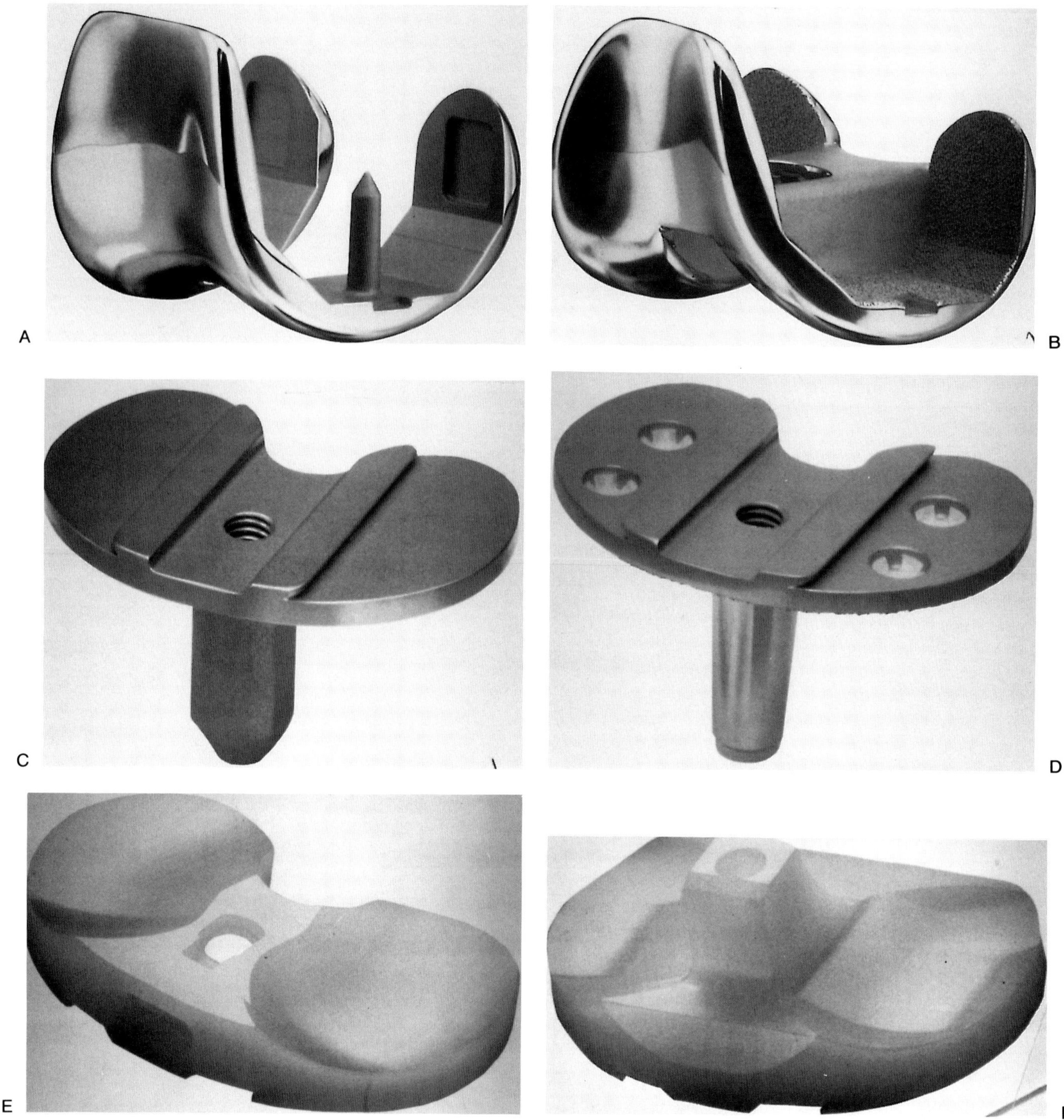

FIG. 6-120. AMK™ total knee system. The femoral components are cobalt-chromium alloy. **A:** Universal textured with single smooth pointed medial and lateral posts. **B:** Porous-coated posterior-stabilized femoral component with central cam and no medial or lateral posts. The tibial components are as follows. **C:** Tibial tray with single central 34-mm stem. **D:** Porous-coated tibial tray with holes for four cancellous screws plus a central stem. **E:** Standard polyethylene insert with condylar shape to match the femoral component. **F:** Posterior-stabilized tibial insert with prominent central post, which interacts with the femoral cam (Fig. 6-120B) to prevent subluxation. The patellar components are as follows.

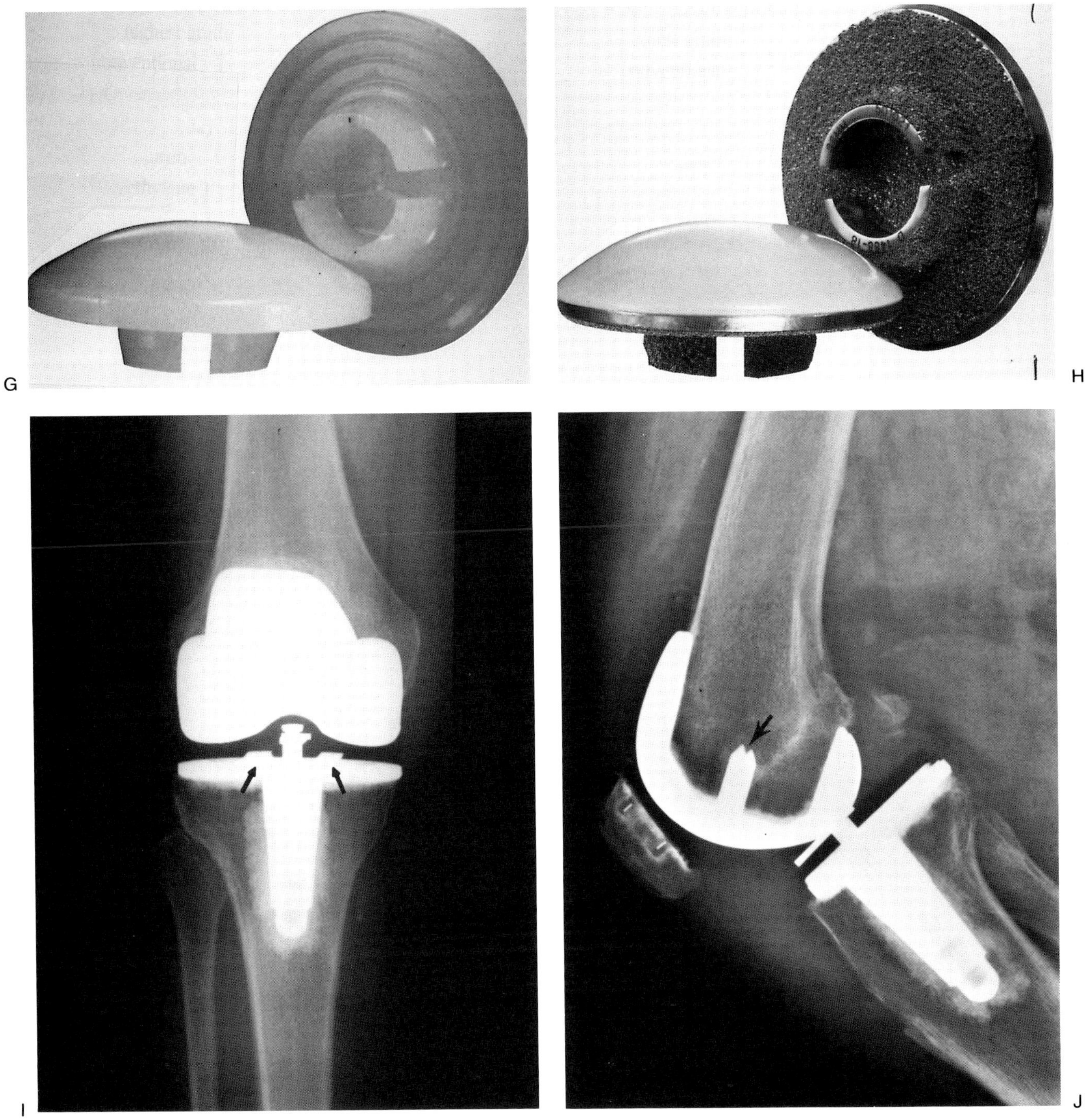

FIG. 6-120. (*Continued.*) **G:** All-polyethylene, note concentric grooves. **H:** Porous-coated metal-backed tibial components. The AP **(I)** and lateral **(J)** radiographs of a cemented AMK^{TM} total knee with an all-polyethylene tibial component. Note the smooth pointed posts of the femoral component (*arrow*, **J**) and the two metal tray ridges (*arrows*, **I**) and the metal insert holder anteriorly.(**A–H**: Courtesy of DePuy, Warsaw, IN.)

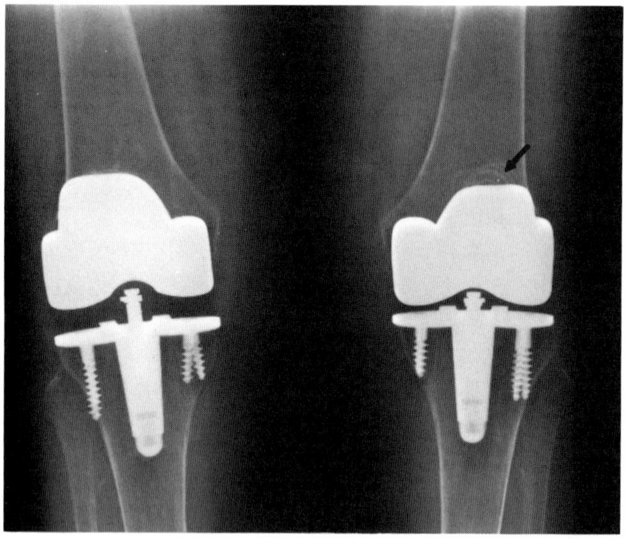

A

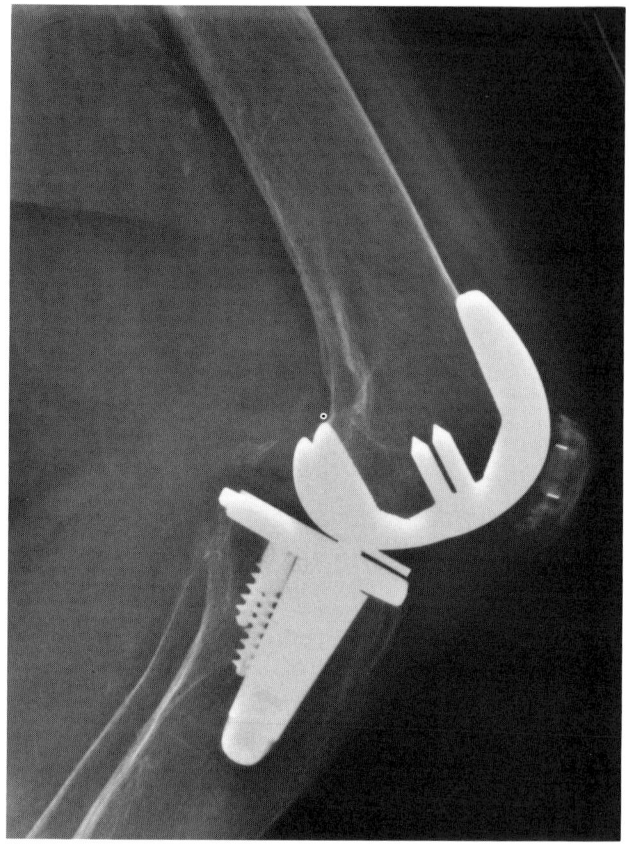

B

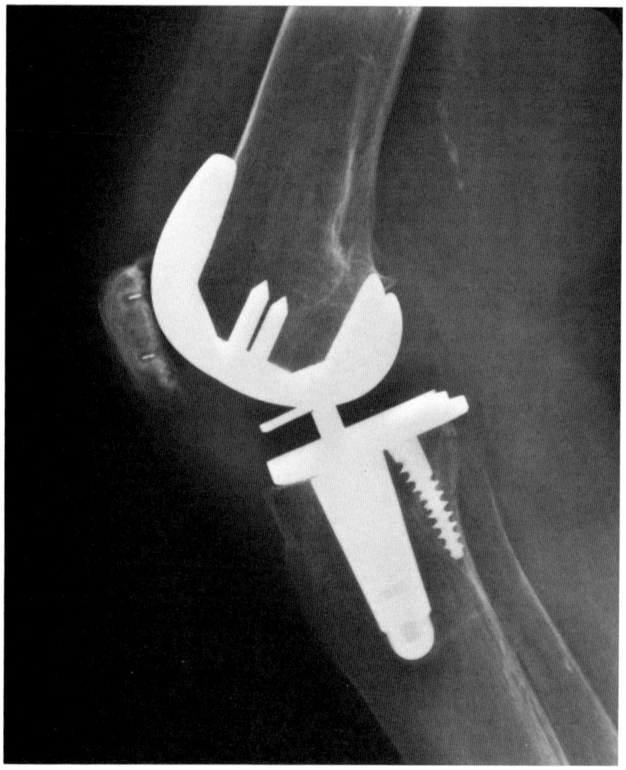

C

FIG. 6-121. The AP standing **(A)** and lateral **(B,C)** views of the knees after bilateral DePuy AMK™ arthroplasties with the addition of cancellous screws. The grooves (Fig. 6-120C) of the patellar component can be seen on the left (*arrow*).

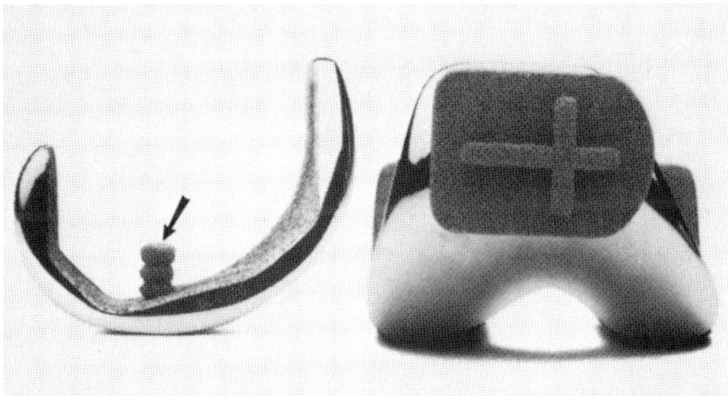

A

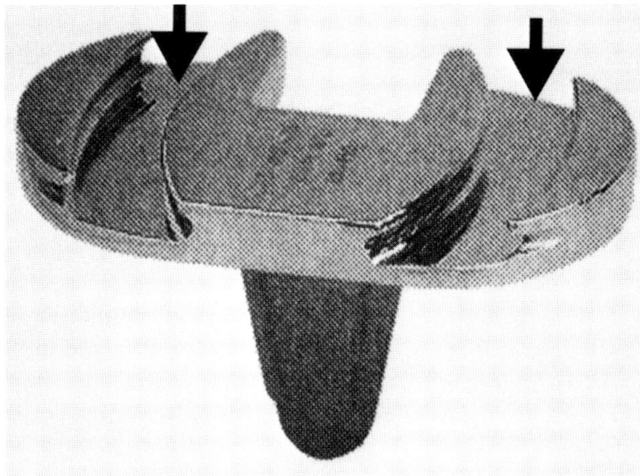

B

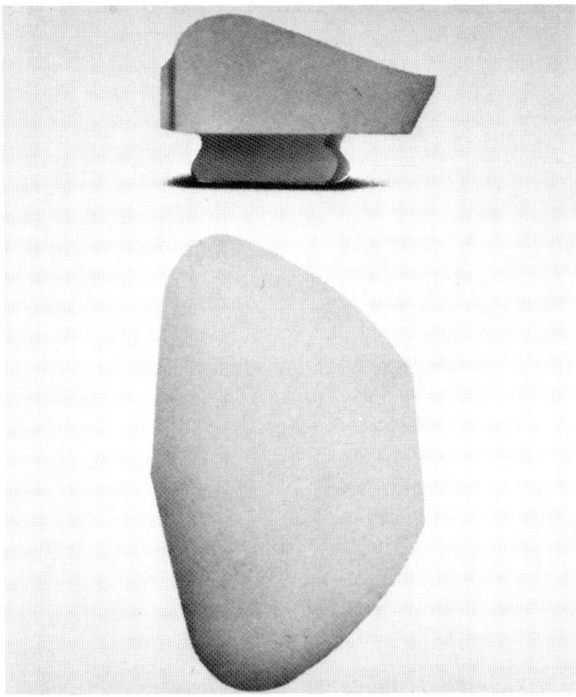

C

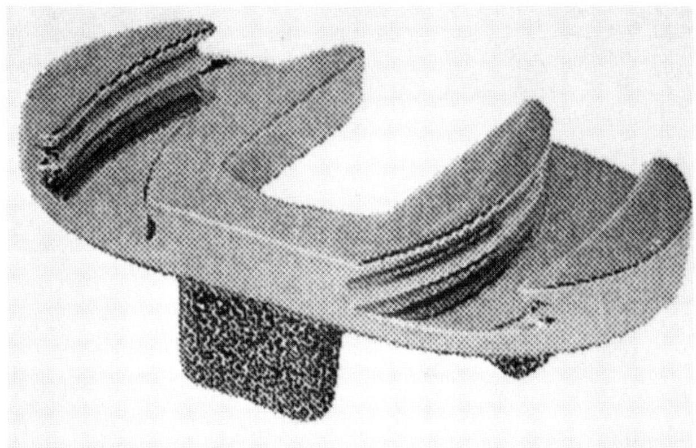

D

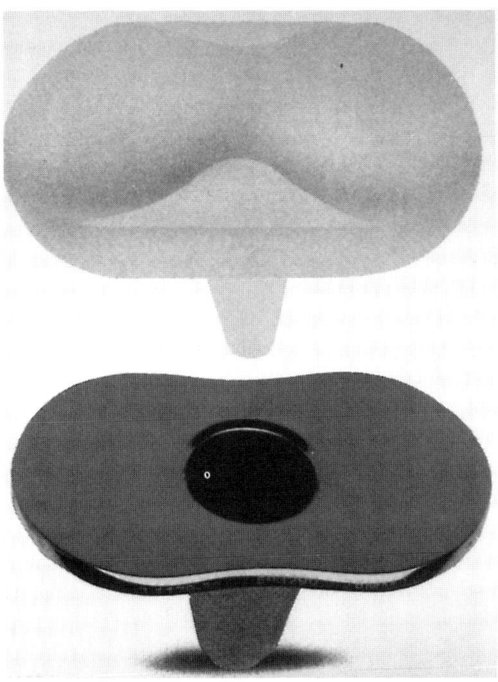

E

FIG. 6-122. New Jersey LCS™ DePuy (A–E: Courtesy of DePuy, Warsaw, IN.) The femoral components are as follows. **A:** Porous and nonporous surfaces with a single ridged femoral post (*arrow*) medially and laterally. Seen from the side and front with the patellar component in place. The tibial components include the following. **B:** A PCL-retaining component with insert tracks (*arrows*) for meniscal bearings (*c*). **C:** Tibial polyethylene meniscal bearing seen from the front and top. **D:** Tibial tray for preservation of both cruciates. **E:** Rotating tibial tray with polyethylene insert for noncruciate retention. This allows unrestricted axial motion and partial constraint against AP shearing forces. The patellar component is the following. (See **F–I** on next page.)

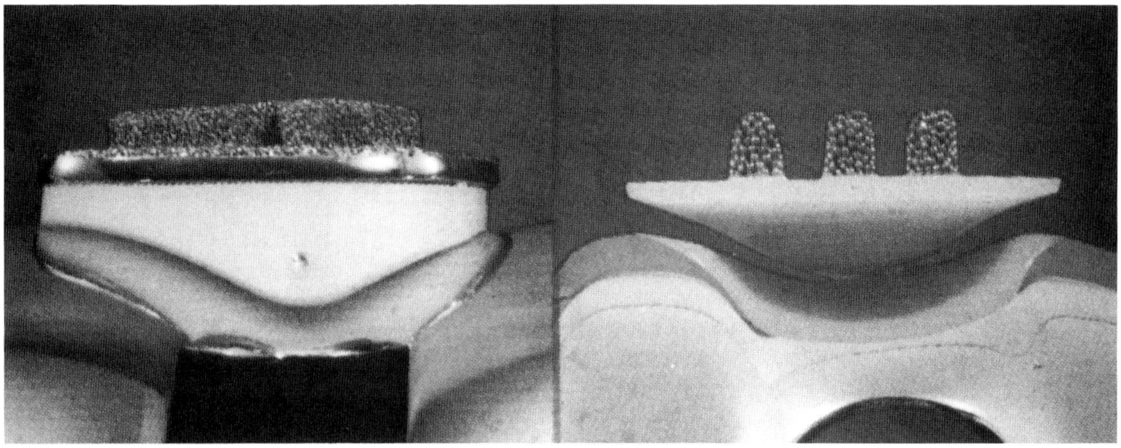

F

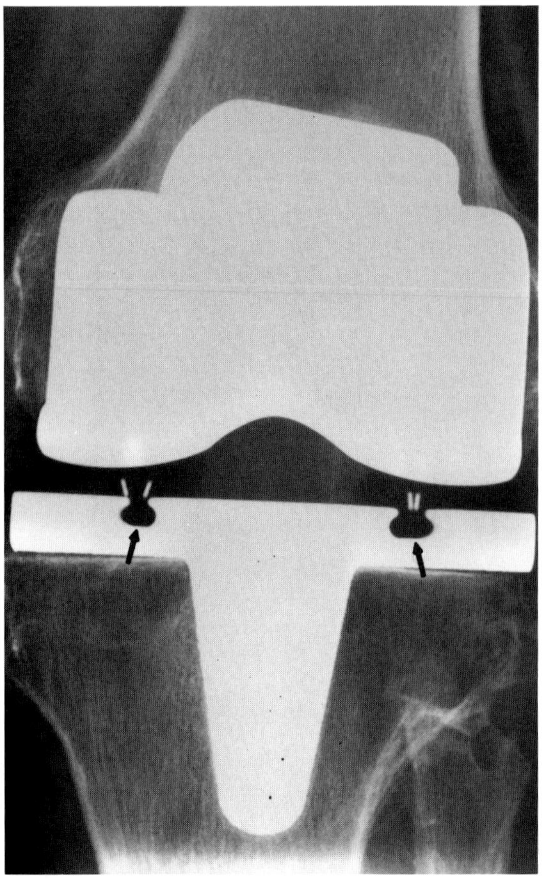

G

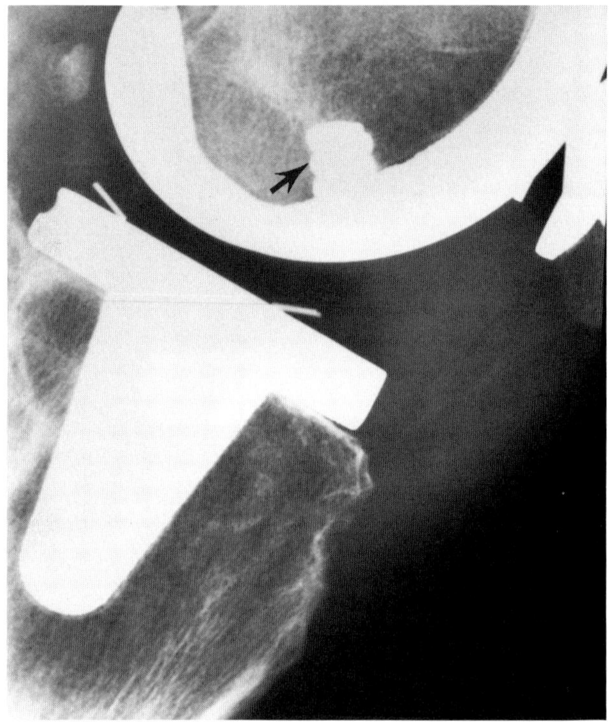

H

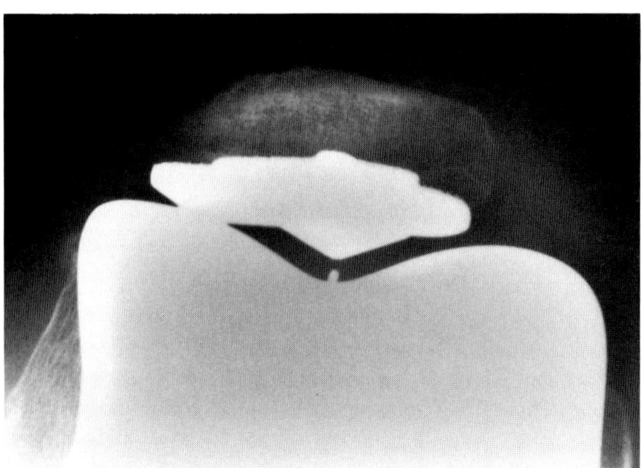

I

FIG. 6-122. (*Continued.*) **F:** LCS™, *left,* and conventional dome-shaped patellar component, *right.* **G–I:** Radiographs of the LCS™ total knee obtained with fluoroscopic positioning. G: The AP view shows the tracks for the polyethylene meniscal bearings (*arrows*). H: Lateral view showing the ridged femoral post (*arrow*). I: Merchant view of the patella with the asymmetric metal-backed patellar component.

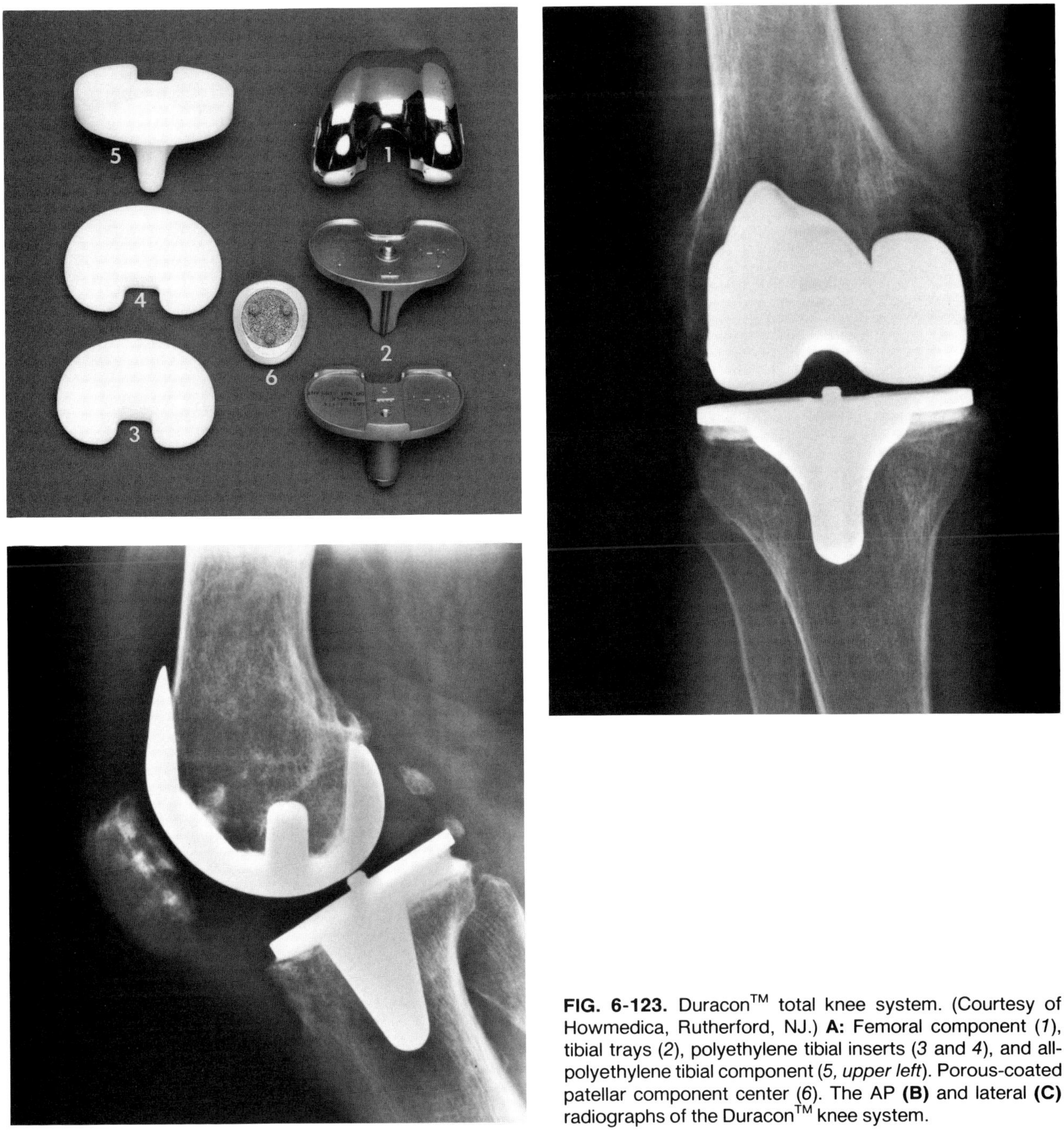

FIG. 6-123. Duracon^{TM} total knee system. (Courtesy of Howmedica, Rutherford, NJ.) **A:** Femoral component (*1*), tibial trays (*2*), polyethylene tibial inserts (*3* and *4*), and all-polyethylene tibial component (*5, upper left*). Porous-coated patellar component center (*6*). The AP **(B)** and lateral **(C)** radiographs of the Duracon^{TM} knee system.

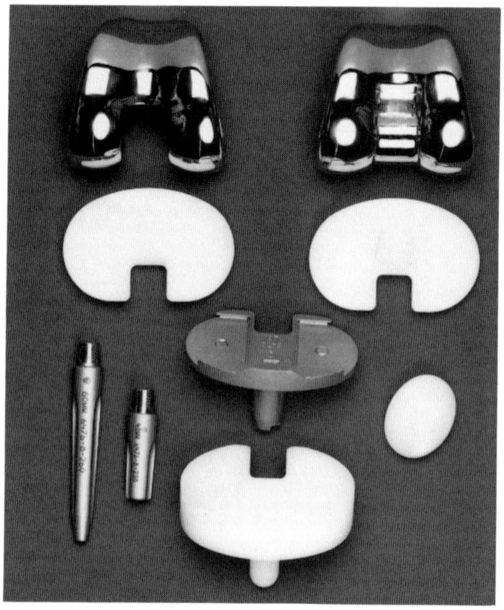

A

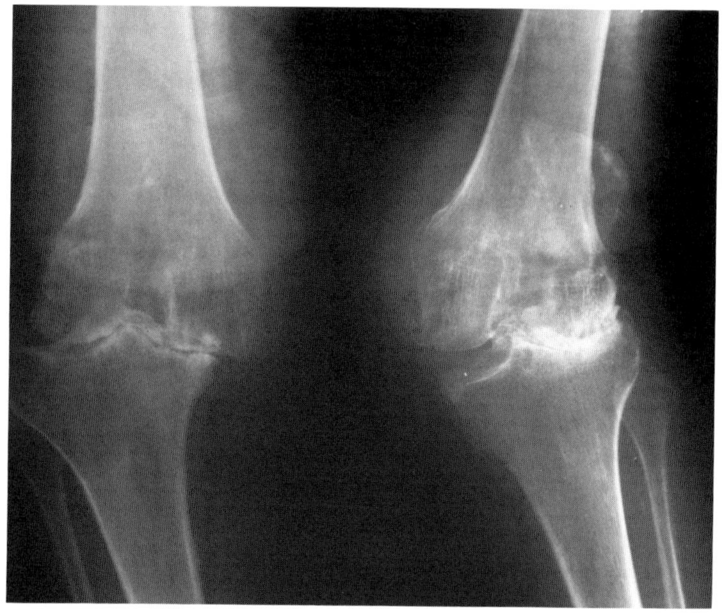

B

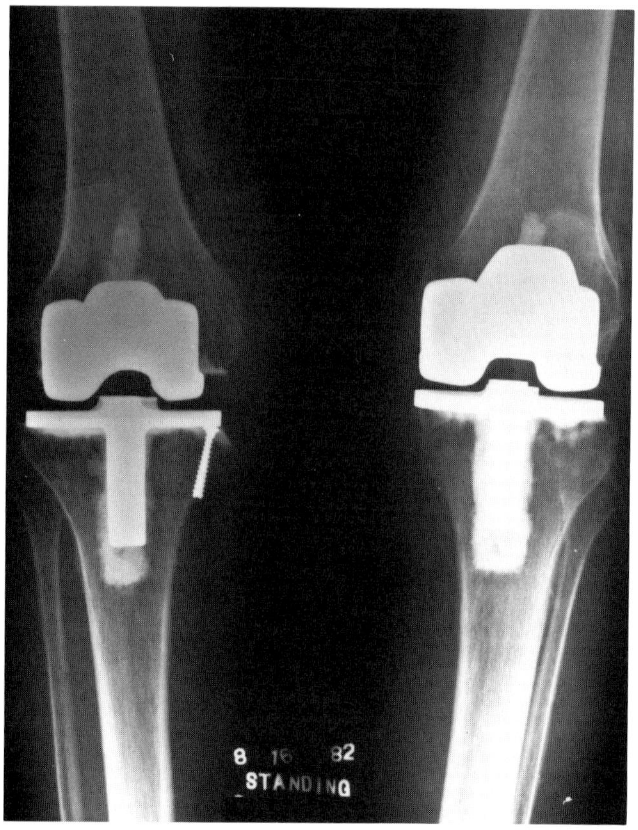

C

FIG. 6-124. Kinemax™ total knee system. (Courtesy of Howmedica, Rutherford, NJ.) **A:** Condylar (*left*) and stabilized femoral component (*right*), tibial inserts center with tibial tray, and all-polyethylene tibial component below. Augmentation stems, *left,* and polyethylene patellar component, *lower left.* **B:** Standing preoperative views of the knee demonstrating advanced arthrosis with medial instability on the left. **C:** Bilateral Kinematic™ implants. Note the cement and screws on the right to correct bone loss.

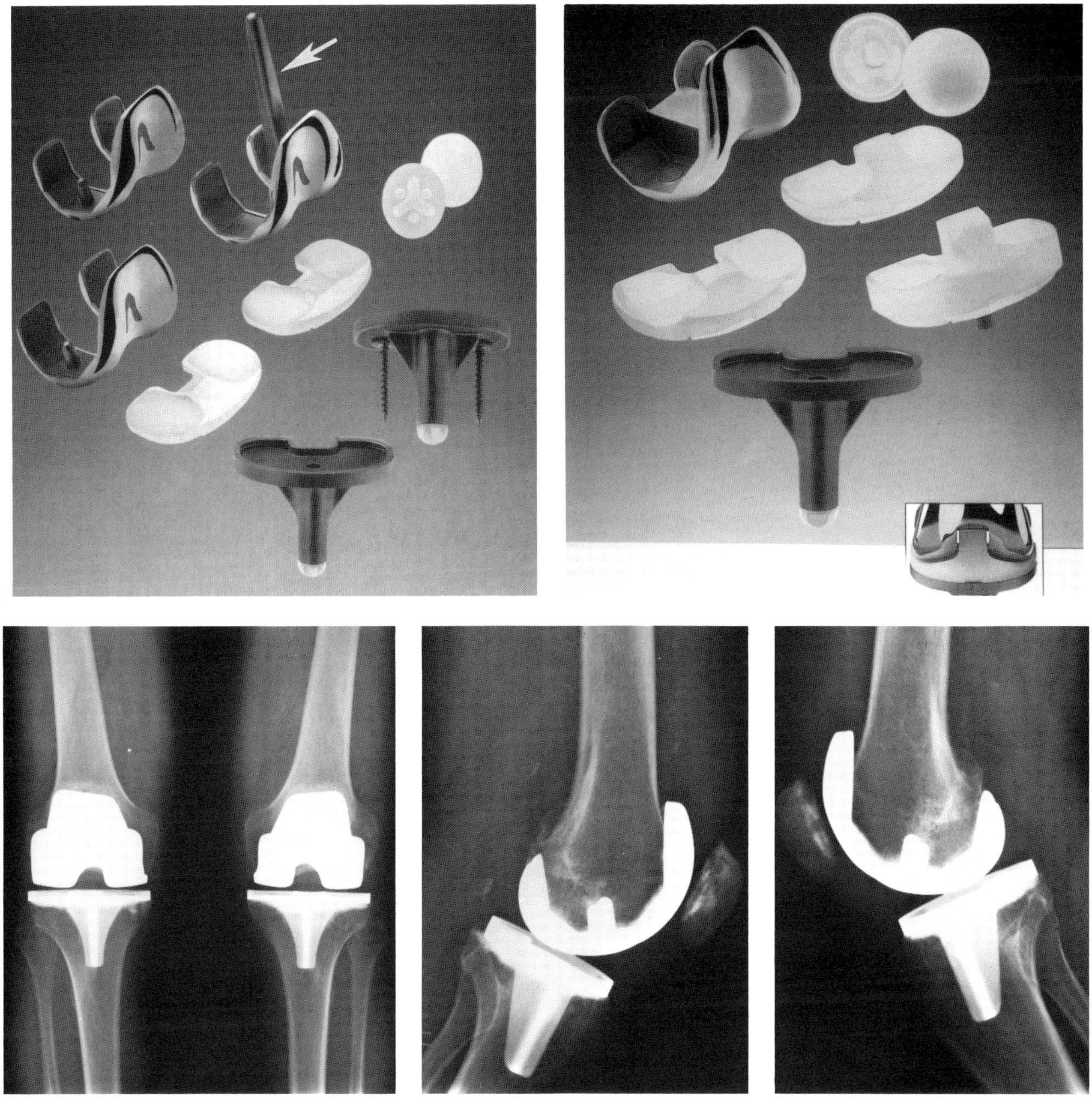

FIG. 6-125. P.F.C.™ modular knee system. (Courtesy of Johnson & Johnson Orthopedics, Raynham, MA.) **A:** Cruciate-retaining femoral and tibial components. Revision stem (*right, arrow*) and all-polyethylene patellar components. **B:** Posterior-stabilized femoral and tibial components. Standing AP **(C)** and lateral **(D,E)** radiographs of Johnson and Johnson total knee systems.

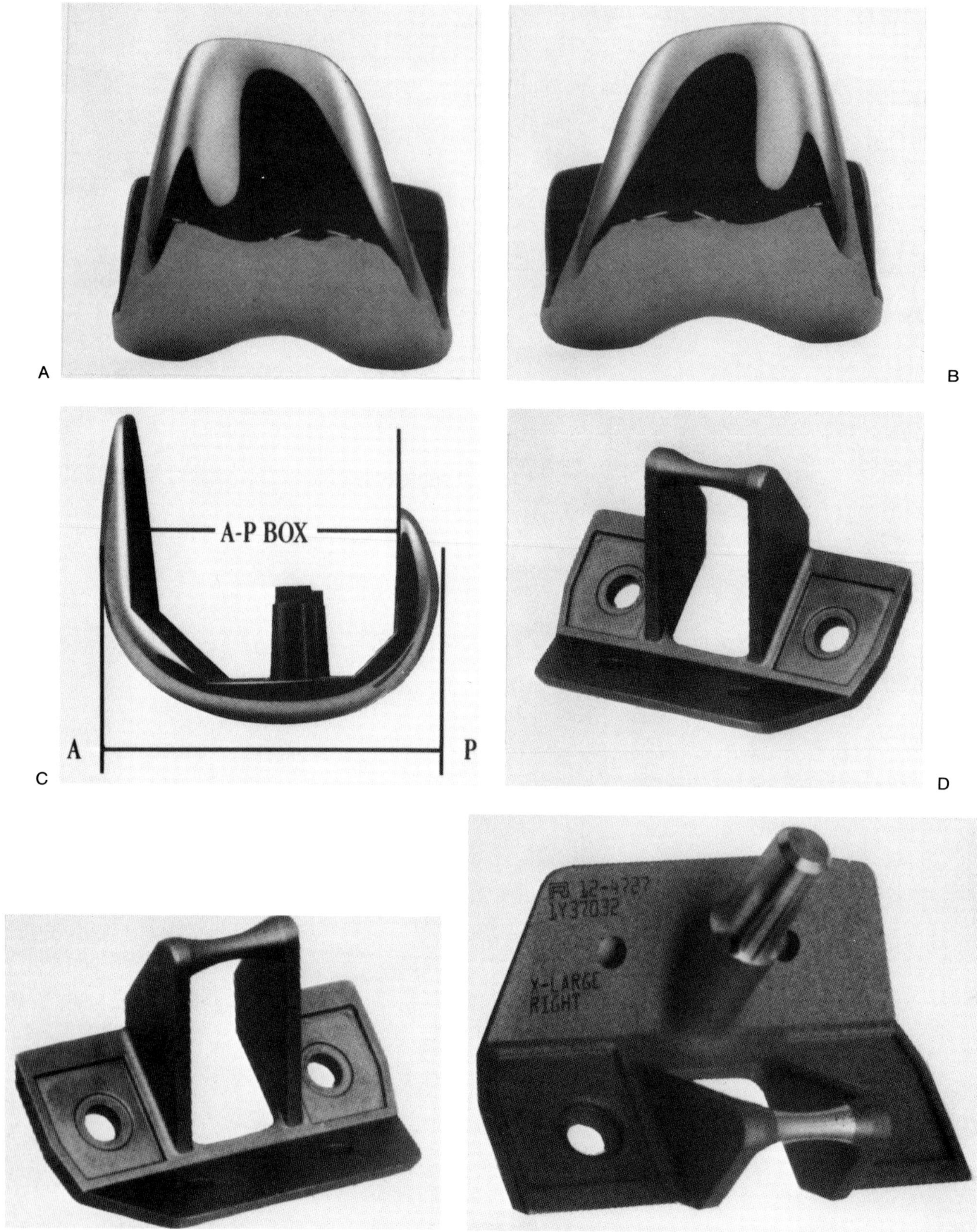

FIG. 6-126. Genesis™ knee system. (Courtesy of Smith and Nephew Richards, Memphis, TN.) **A:** Right femoral component seen from anteriorly. **B:** Left seen from anteriorly. **C:** Seen from the side with square-top femoral posts. Right **(D)** and left **(E)** femoral inserts for posterior-stabilized configuration. Revision nodule for posterior-stabilized **(F)** and cruciate-retaining.

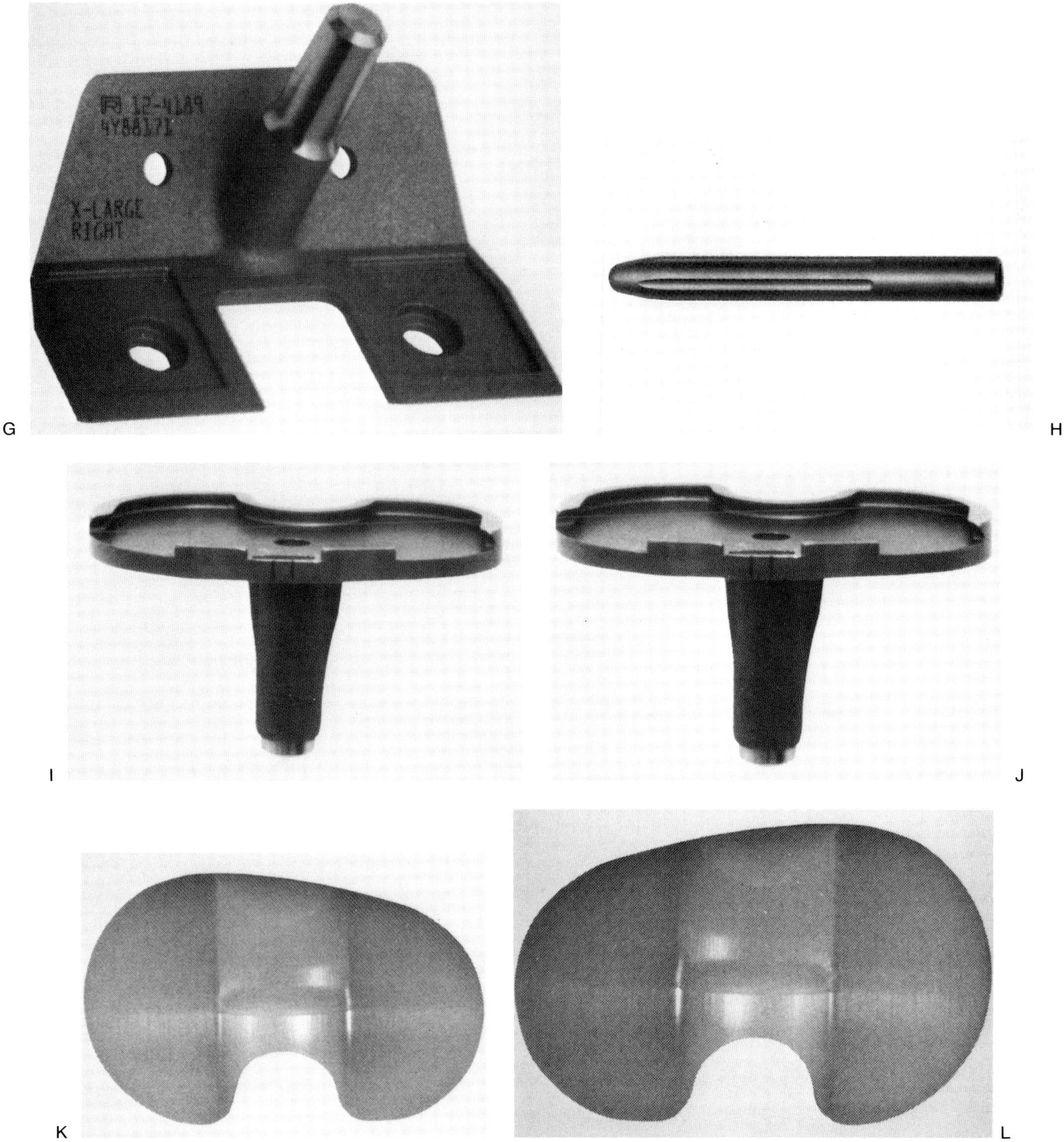

FIG. 6-126. (*Continued.*) **(G)** with augmentation stem **(H)**. Tibial components include right **(I)** and left **(J)** tibial trays with right **(K)** and left **(L)** polyethylene inserts. (See **M–R** on next page.)

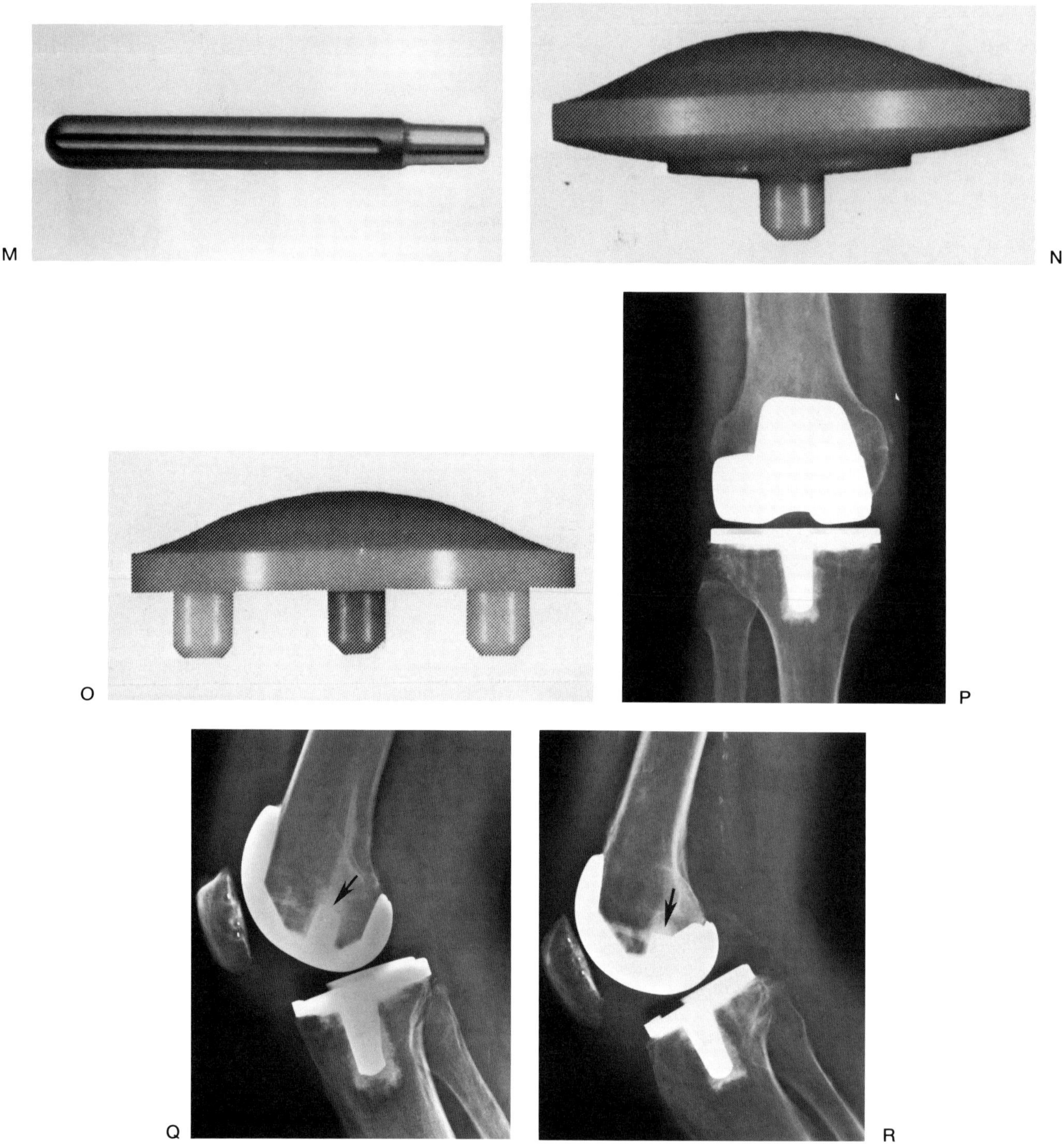

FIG. 6-126. (*Continued.*) **(M)** Augmentation tibial stem for revisions. Patellar components include biconvex with single peg **(N)** and conventional with three pegs **(O)**. Genesis™ cruciate-retaining **(Q)** and posterior-stabilized **(R)** components. The femoral pegs are just visible (*arrows*) on the posterior-stabilized systems.

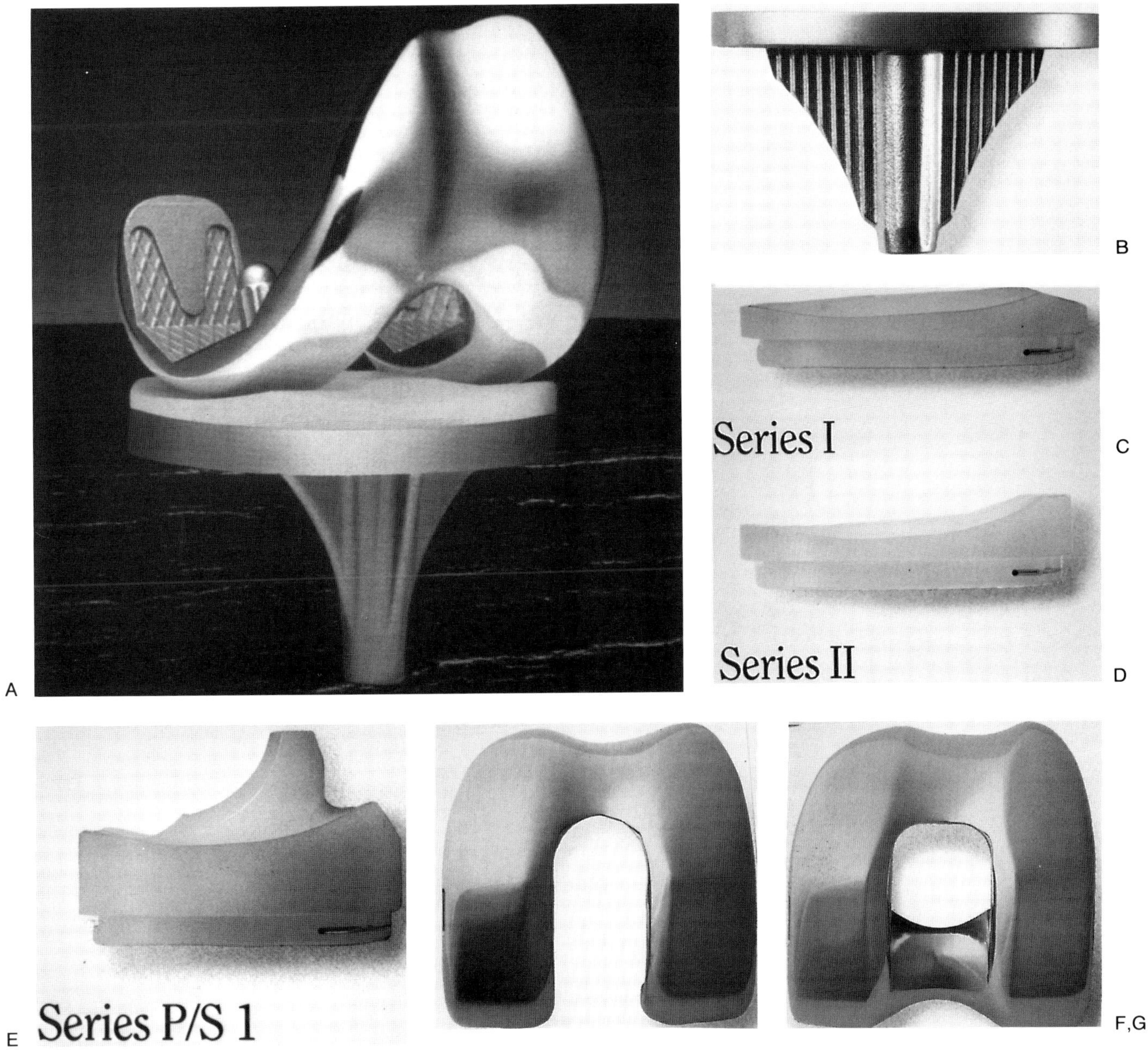

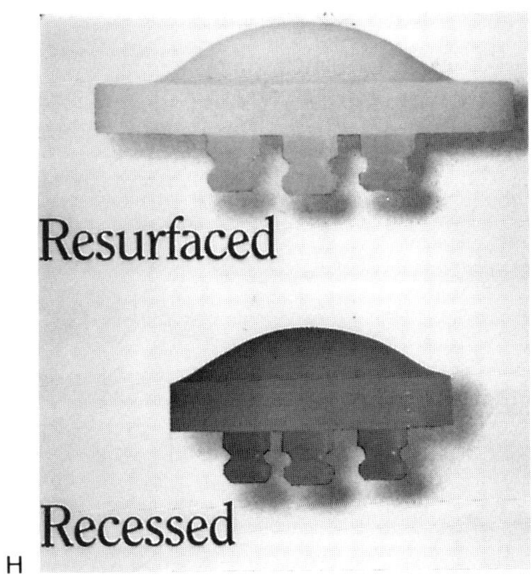

FIG. 6-127. Osteonics knee systems. (Courtesy of Osteonics, Allendale, NJ.) **A:** Omnifit^{TM} total knee system. **B:** Deltafit^{TM} tibial tray. Unconstrained **(C)**, constrained **(D)**, and posterior-stabilized **(E)** inserts. **F:** Cruciate-retaining femoral component. **G:** Posterior-stabilized femoral component. **H:** Resurfaced and recessed patellar components.

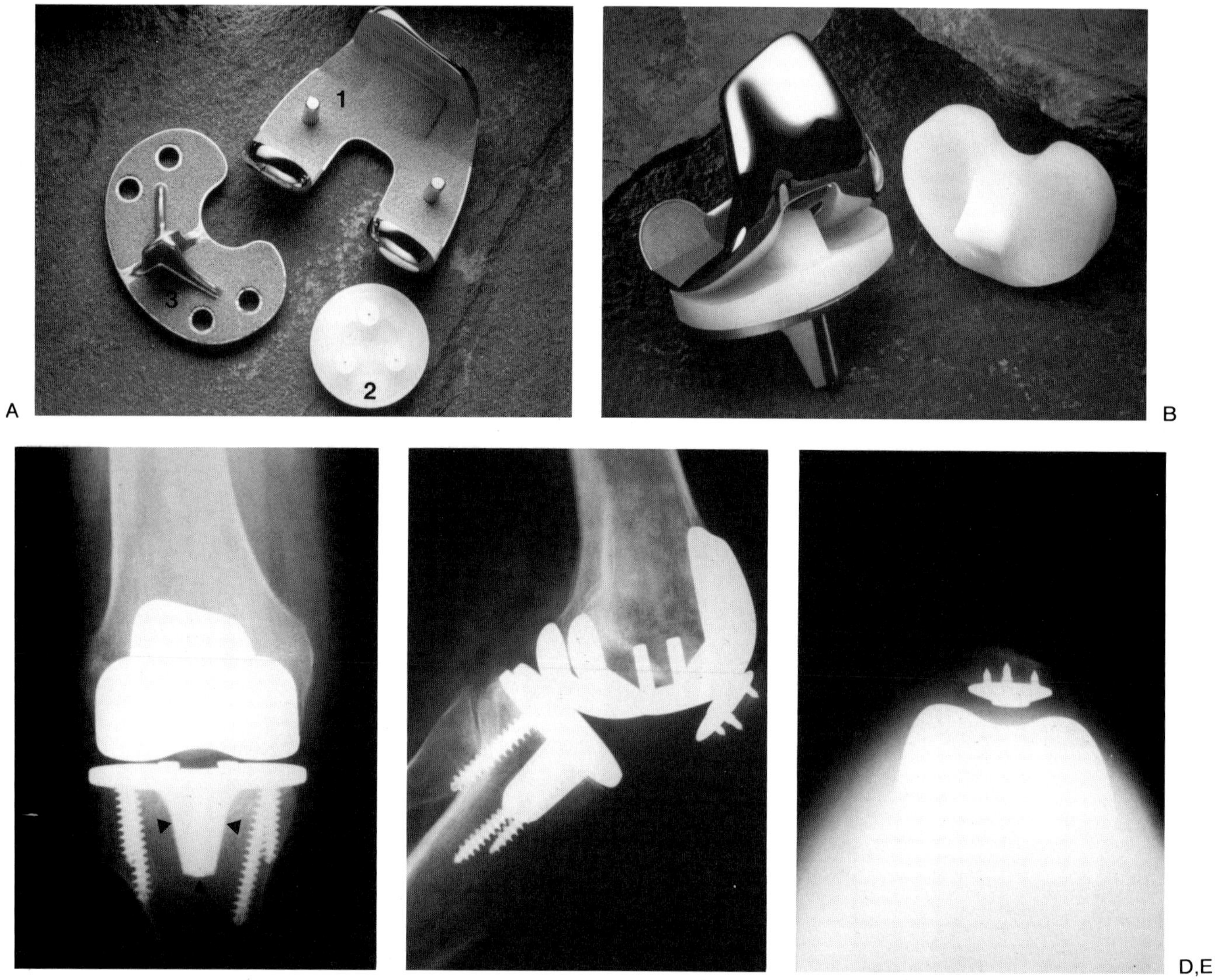

FIG. 6-128. Axiom™ total knee system. (Courtesy of Orthomet, Minneapolis, MN.) **A:** Proportionally designed porous-coated femoral (*1*), all-polyethylene patellar (*2*), and quadrafin keel tibial component with four screw holes (*3*) of the PCL-sparing system. **B:** Femoral and tibial components with tibial insert (*right*) for the posterior-stabilized system. The AP **(C)**, lateral **(D)**, and Merchant **(E)** views of an Axiom™ total knee with four cancellous screws in the tibial tray. Note keel configuration (*arrowheads,* **C**).

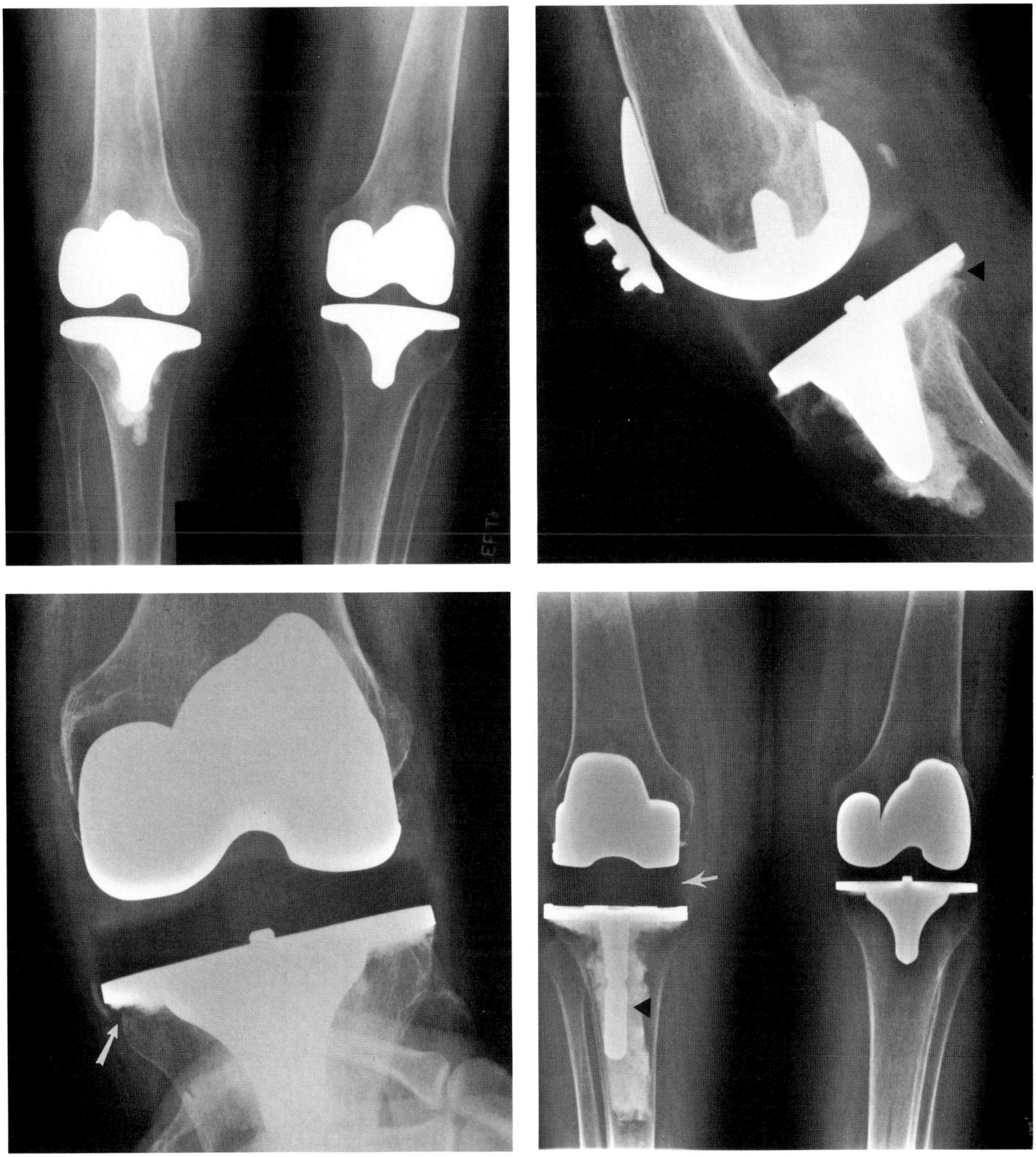

FIG. 6-129. Standing AP **(A)**, lateral **(B)**, and stress view **(C)** of a painful knee arthroplasty. The tibial component overhangs posteriorly (*black arrow,* B), and there is lucency medially (*white arrow,* C) and medial ligament laxity. On the standing view, the tibial component has subsided medially. The knee was revised using a Genesis™ knee system **(D)** (Smith and Nephew Richards, Memphis, TN) with an augmented tibial stem (*arrowhead*) and a thick polyethylene tibial insert (*arrow*).

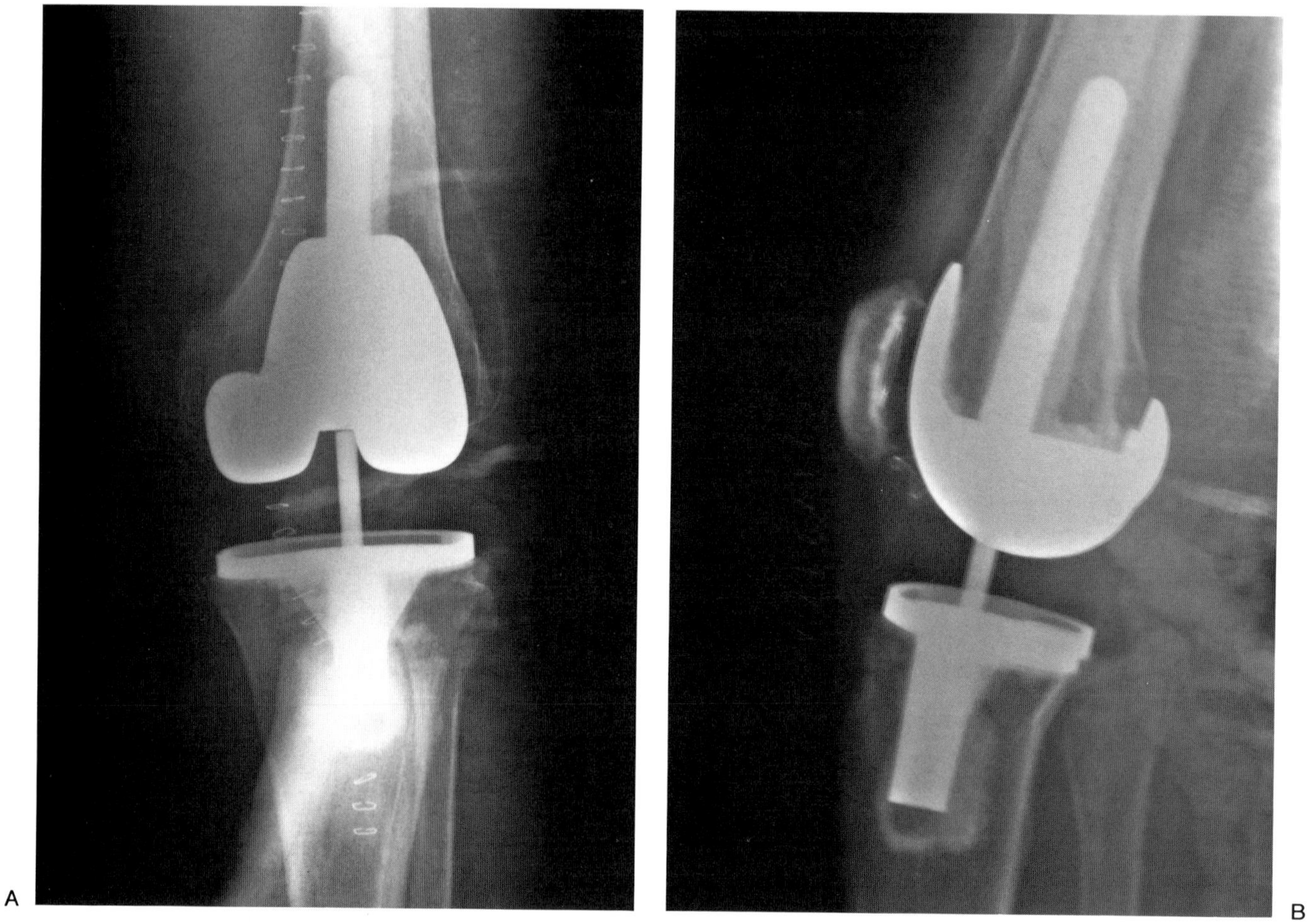

FIG. 6-130. Polyethylene failure. The knee was revised using a Johnson and Johnson augmented stem femoral component (posterior stabilized). A modular tibial tray with a constrained (generally thicker) tibial insert and a Genesis™ biconvex patellar component (Fig. 6-126). The AP **(A)** and lateral **(B)** radiographs.

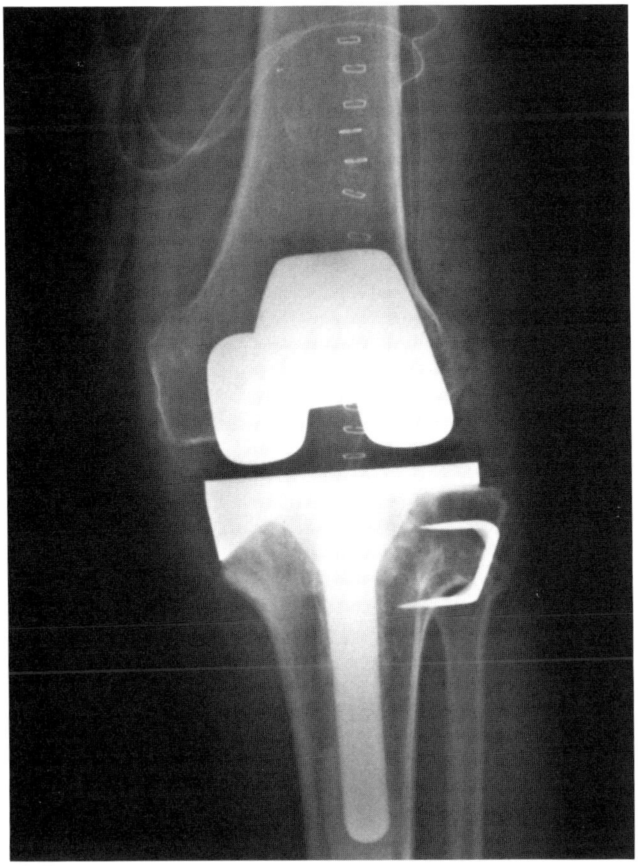

A

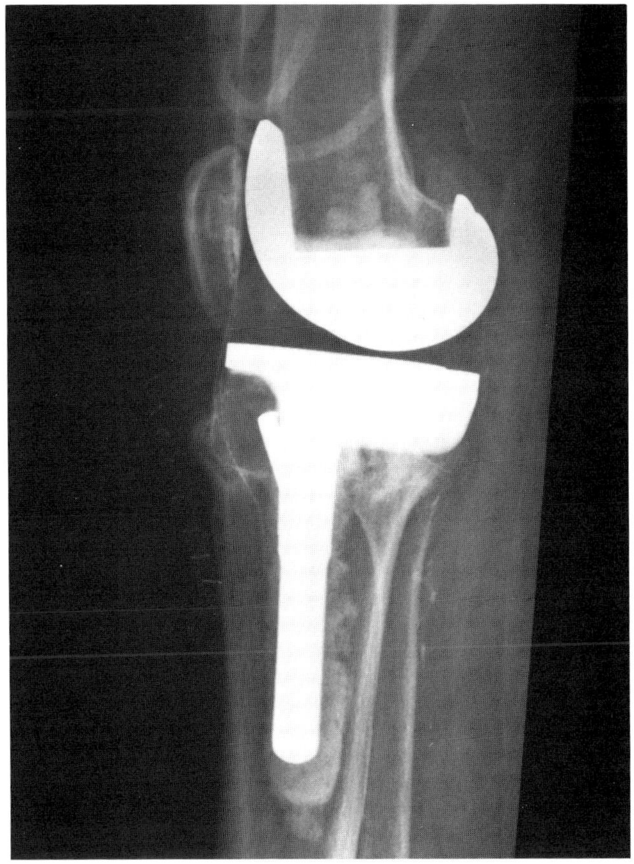

B

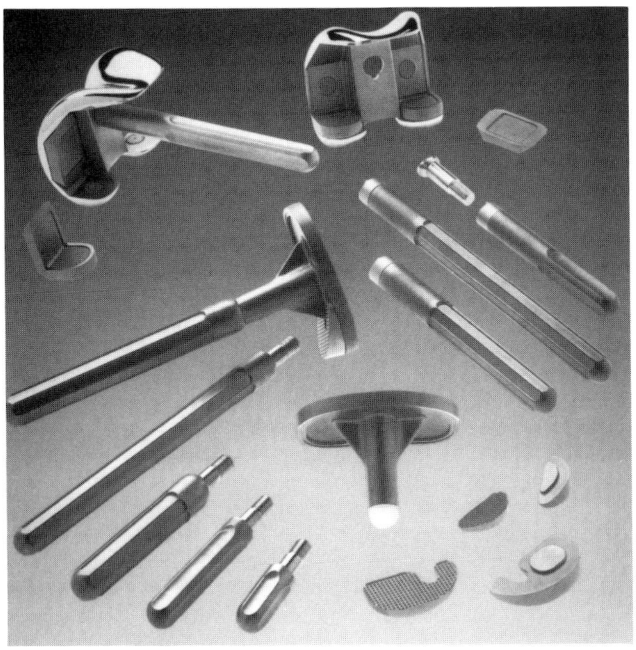

C

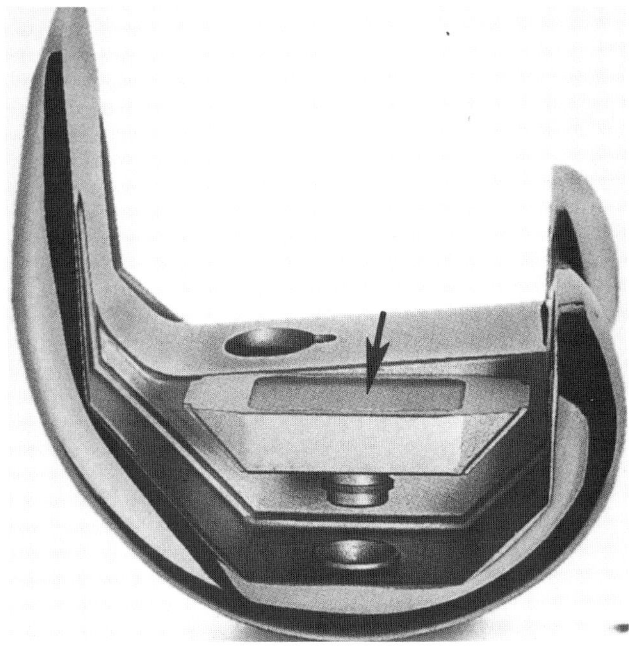

D

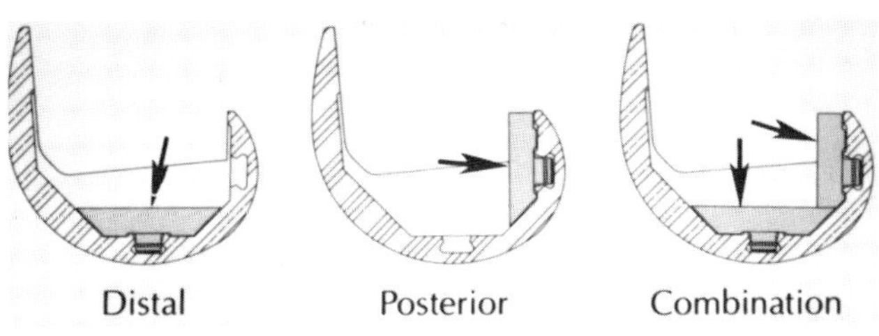

E

FIG. 6-131. The AP **(A)** and lateral **(B)** radiographs of a Johnson and Johnson P.F.C.™ modular knee with posterior-stabilized femoral component and a constrained tibial tray with medial wedge and augmented stem. The patellar component is all polyethylene with a central peg. **C:** Johnson and Johnson P.F.C.™ revision components. **D,E:** Side views of the posterior-stabilized femoral component (D) and variable positions for augmentation wedges (*arrows*). (Courtesy of Johnson and Johnson Orthopaedics, New Brunswick, NJ.)

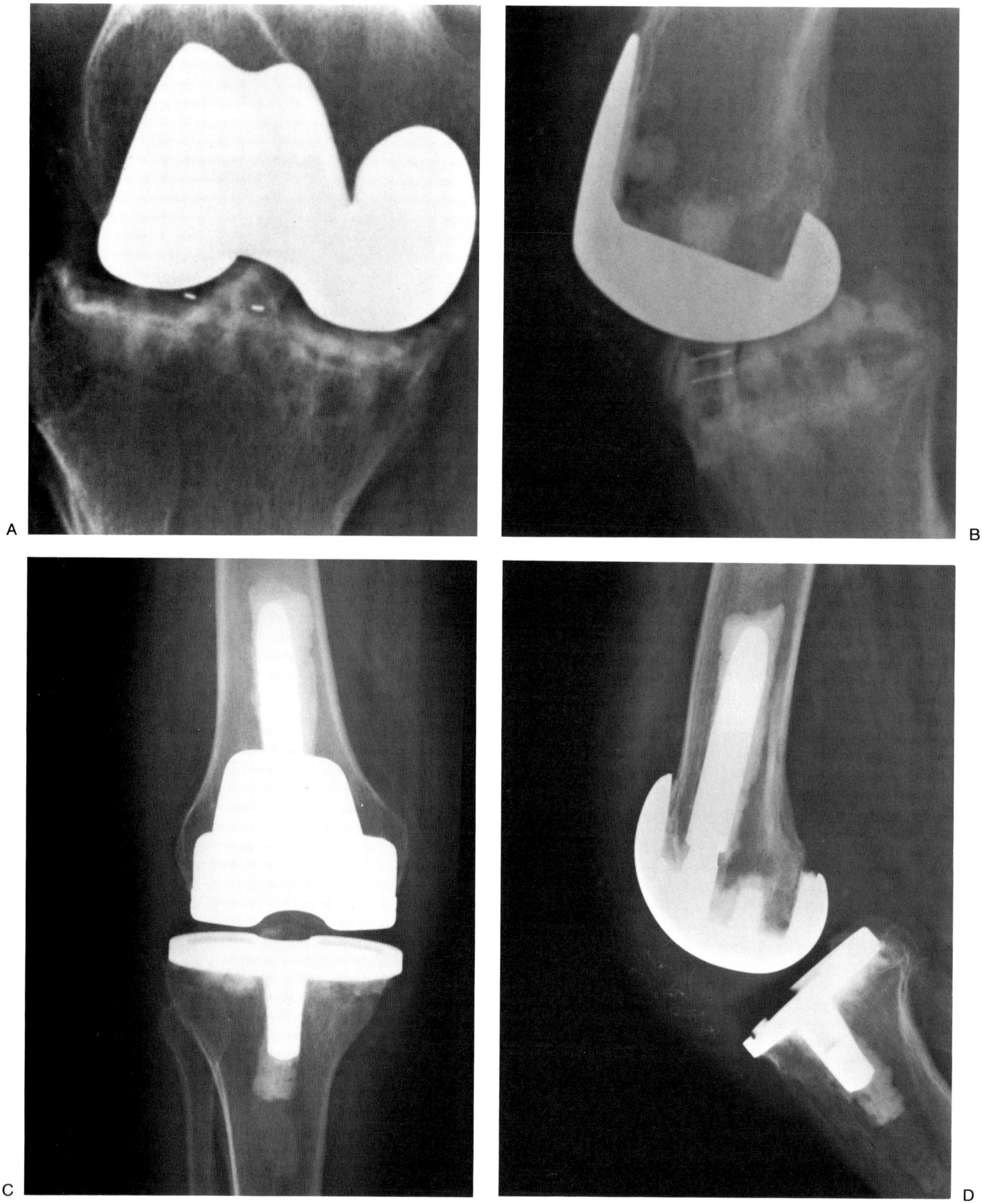

FIG. 6-132. The AP (A) and lateral (B) views of a failed knee arthroplasty with pain and instability. The knee was revised using a Genesis™ conventional tibial component and augmented stem on the femoral component demonstrated on AP (C) and lateral (D) radiographs.

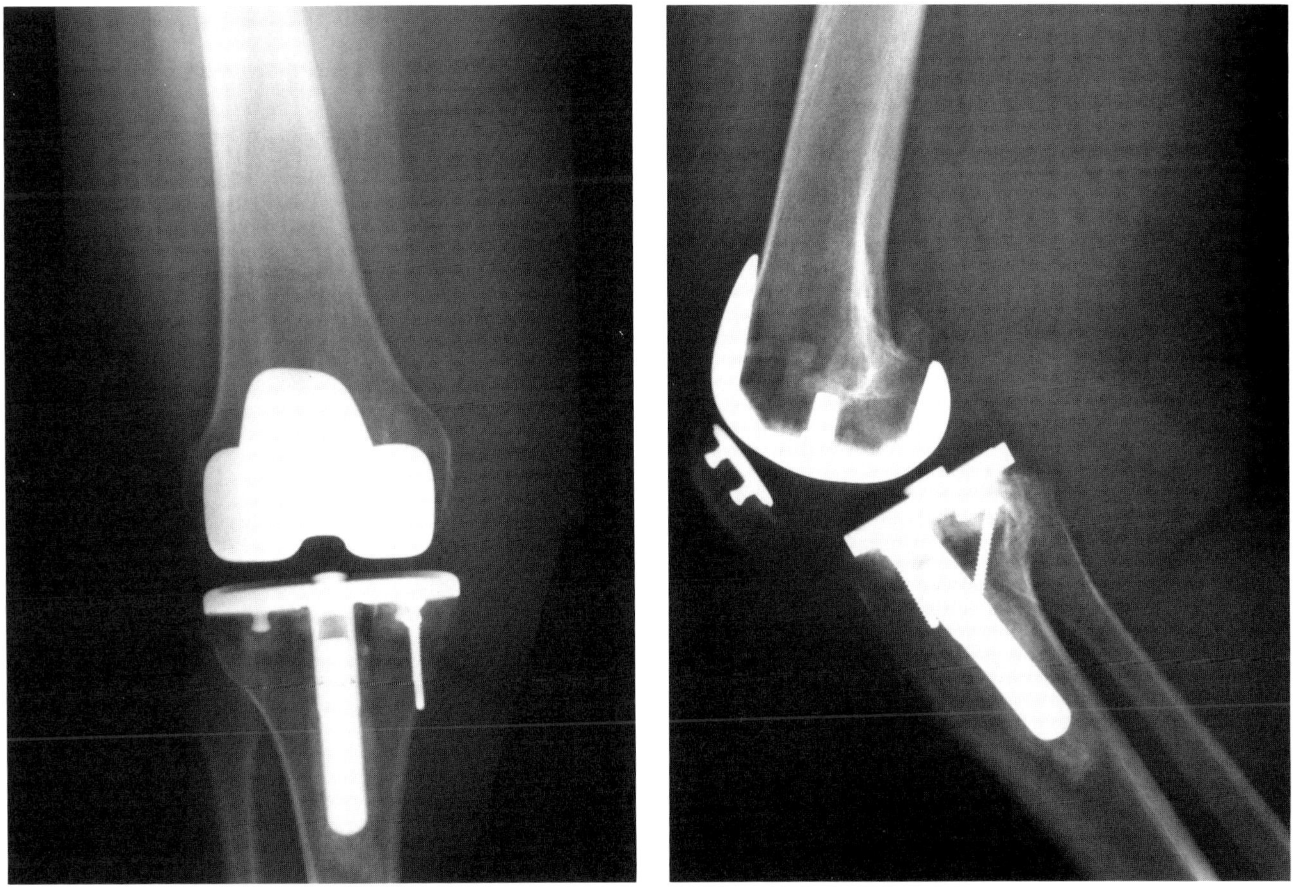

A B

FIG. 6-133. The AP **(A)** and lateral **(B)** radiographs of a revised knee using a Miller-Galante II tibial tray (Zimmer, Warsaw, IN) with augmented stem. Bone graft with screw fixation medially.

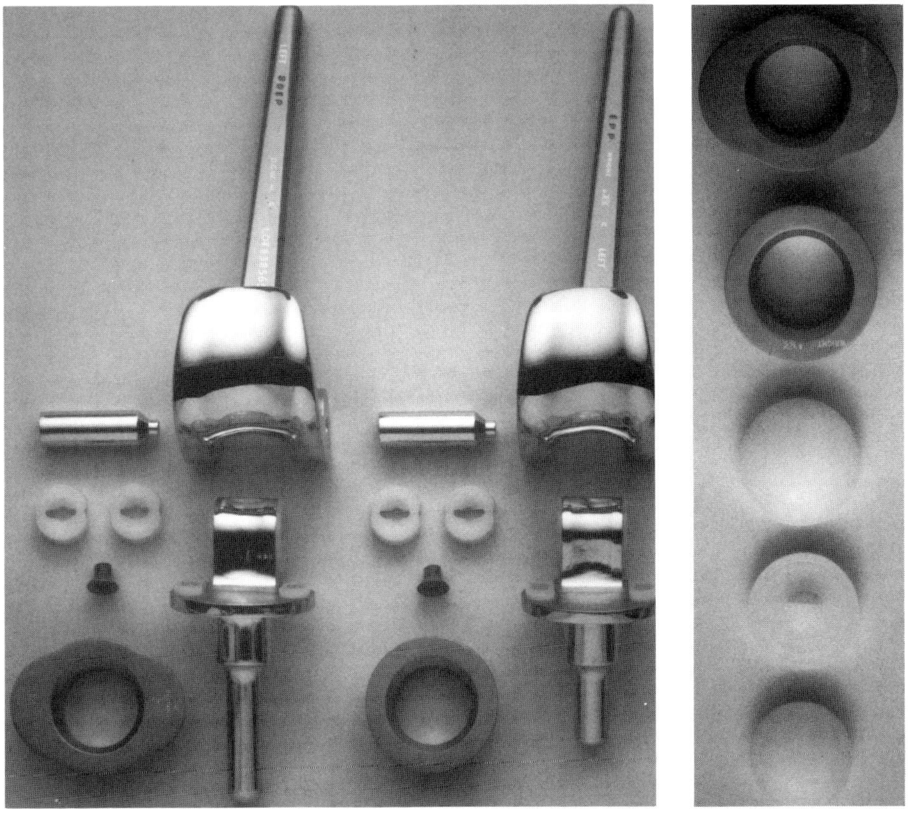

A B

FIG. 6-134. Lacey^{TM} rotating hinge knee system with femoral and tibial components **(A)** and patellar components **(B)**. (Courtesy of Wright Medical Technology, Arlington, TN.)

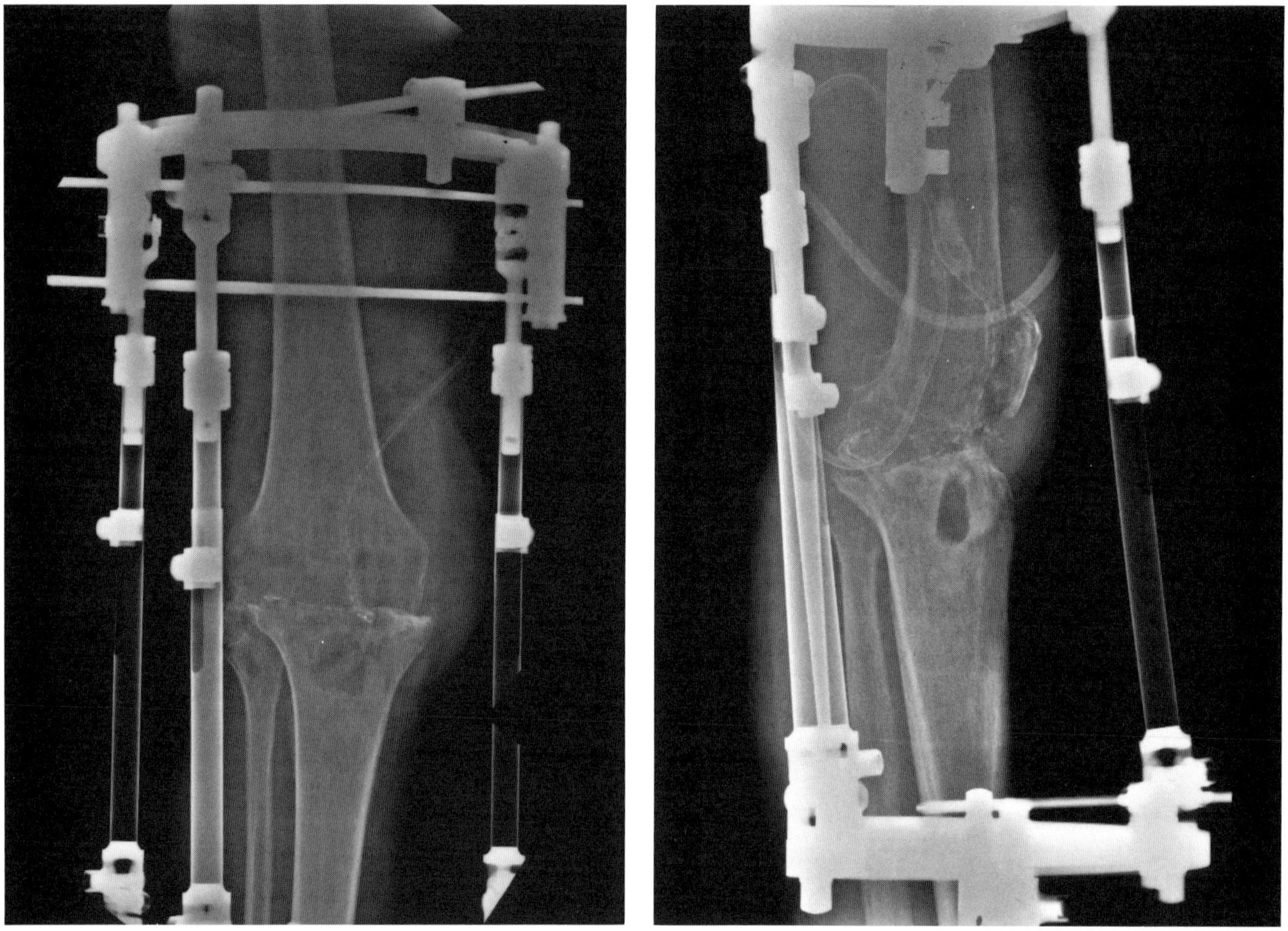

A B

FIG. 6-135. Failed right knee arthroplasty. The components have been removed. Arthrodesis with Fisher external fixation. The AP **(A)** and lateral **(B)** radiographs with drain in place.

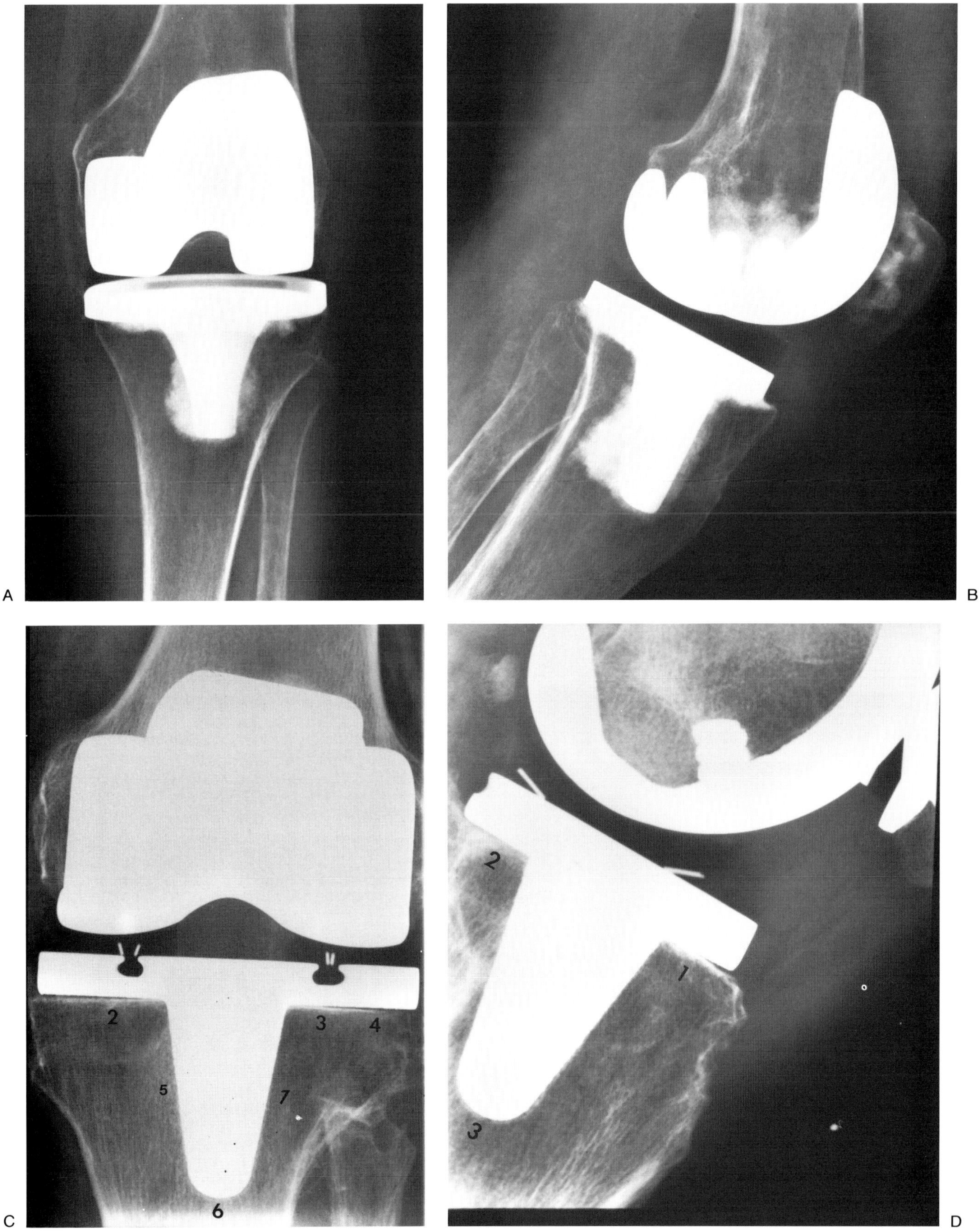

FIG. 6-136. Routine AP **(A)** and lateral **(B)** views of the knee obtained without fluoroscopic guidance. The components are not properly aligned; therefore, the normal measurements and interfaces cannot be adequately evaluated. Fluoroscopically positioned spot views of the tibial component (LCS™ knee system, DePuy, Warsaw, IN) in the AP **(C)** and lateral **(D)** views allow proper evaluation of the component interface zones. (Note numbers used to describe changes in different areas of the component interfaces.)

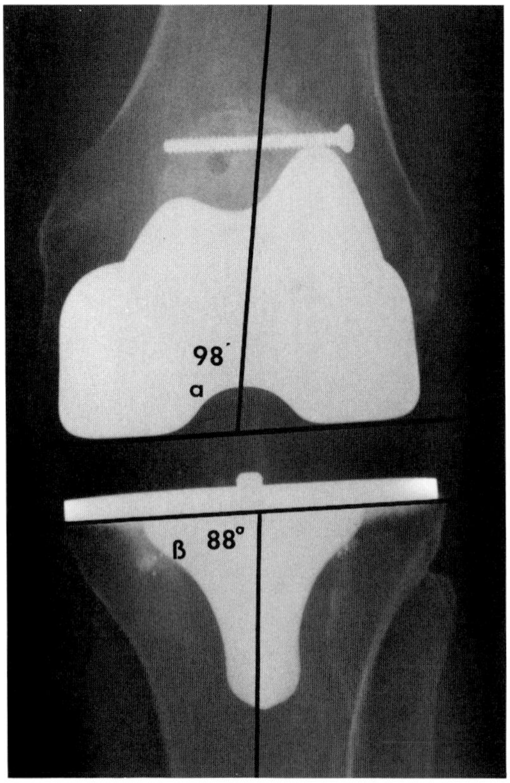

FIG. 6-137. An AP view of the knee (Howmedica Duracon™ knee system) demonstrating tibial (*a*) and femoral (*B*) angles. The tibial angle is measured by a component line along the tibial component and the tibial axis. The femoral angle is configured in a similar fashion. The tibial angle should be 90°. Angles less than 90° are varus and greater than 90°, valgus deflections. Both angles are measured on the medial side. In this case, the femoral component angle is 98°, which is optimal. The tibial component angle is 88°, which is in a slight varus position.

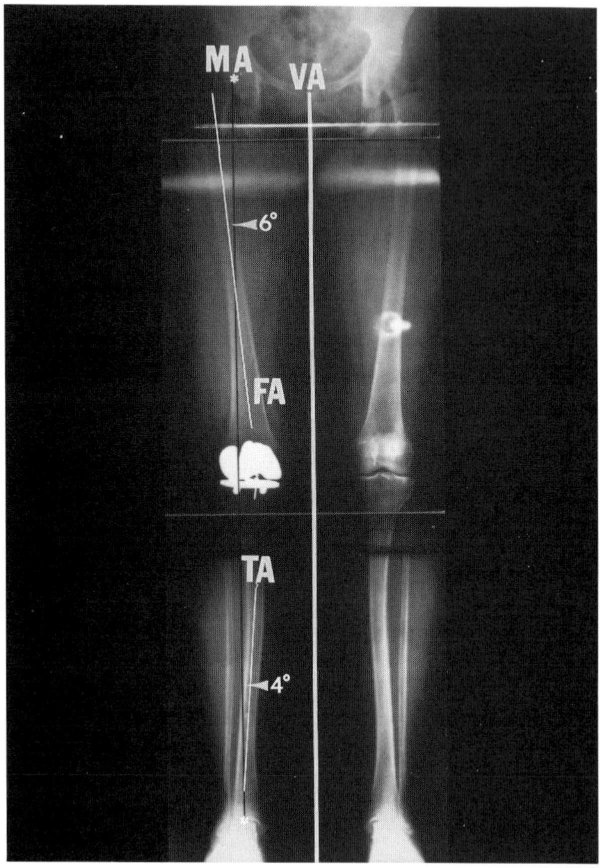

FIG. 6-138. Standing AP view of the lower extremities after right PCA knee replacement on the right. The mechanical axis (*MA, black vertical line*) is drawn from the midfemoral head to the midankle joint and should pass through or near the center of the knee.[125] The mechanical axis of the femur is normally about 6° valgus to the mechanical axis of the lower extremity. In this patient, the femoral axis is 6° valgus (*FA, white line*). The tibial axis (*TA, white line*) is normally along or slightly varus to the mechanical axis and 2° to 3° varus from the vertical axis (*VA*) of the body.[128]

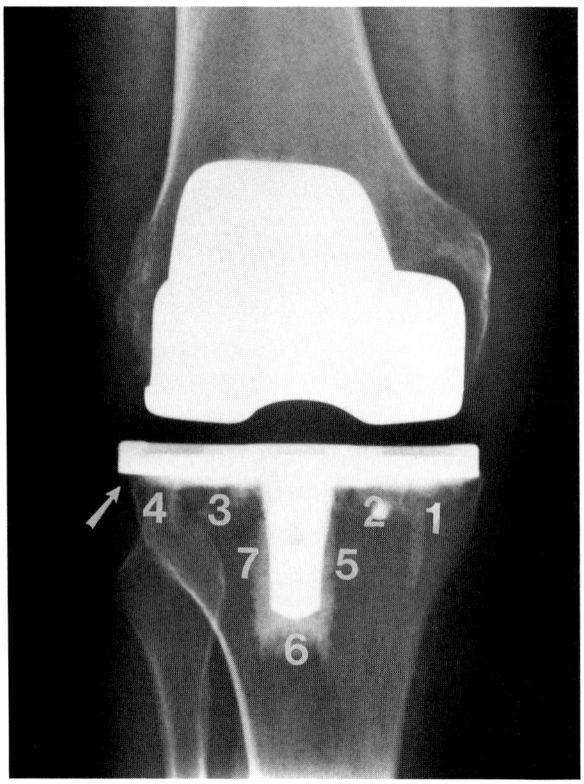

FIG. 6-139. Zones for evaluating lucency about the metal-bone (porous uncemented) or bone cement (cemented components) interface on the AP view (Genesis™ knee system). Fluoroscopically positioned AP for tibial component. Note the lateral overhang (*arrow*). The zones are numbered medially to laterally. Lucency is most commonly seen in the peripheral zones (1 and 4).[88,154,167] Lucency < 2 mm and incomplete or nonprogressive is usually of no significance.

The femoral angle should be 97° to 98° (Fig. 6-136). The femoral-tibial angle should be 5° to 7° (±5°) valgus, although 5° to 10° valgus angles have been used by some authors (Fig. 6-138).[78,86,134] Most use full-length (hip to ankle) views of this, but a variation of only 1.6° was demonstrated when comparing this technique with conventional standing knees on 18-inch film.[135] Figure 6-137 is a well-positioned AP view. On the standing full-length film (Fig. 6-138), the knee is rotated, which makes it difficult to measure these angles accurately.

The mechanical axis is a line drawn from the center of the femoral head to the center of the ankle joint (Fig. 6-138). In a normally aligned knee, this line should also pass through the knee joint near the center.[128] The anatomic axis of the femur (Fig. 6-138) is normally approximately 6° valgus to the mechanical axis. The tibial axis is generally about 2° to 3° varus to the central axis of the body and nearly in line with the mechanical axis (Fig. 6-138).

Standardized nomenclature lucent zones on the AP view are typically designed for components with a central stem; however, zones for more complex fixation systems have also been described (Fig. 6-139). When in doubt, label the radiograph with a wax pencil so the surgeon can relate what is seen on the patient to the zone described by the radiologist. The degree of tibial coverage and the medial-lateral position of the tibial component should also be assessed on the AP view (Fig. 6-139). Anatomic tibial trays (Fig. 6-126) that are designed to cover the plateau more uniformly are larger medially than laterally.[129]

Lateral View

Likewise, there are several compartment angles, positions of the components, and component interfaces that require evaluation on the lateral view (Fig. 6-140).

The tibial angle formed by the tibial axis and tibial component should be about 90°, but if the angle is slightly less than this, the results can be acceptable. If the angle is greater than 90°, the tibial component is considered hyperextended. If it is less than 90°, the tibial component is in flexion deformity. When the angle exceeds 90°, the tension on the PCL is reduced, and increased flexion is possible. The angle formed by the femoral component and femoral axis should be near zero (Fig. 6-140A).[86,169,170,173] The lower pole of the patella is normally about 9 to 10 mm superior to the anterior tibial component on the lateral view (Fig. 6-140C).

The lucent zones (Fig. 6-140B) should also be evaluated. Femoral lucent lines are most common in zones 1 and 4 and tibial, in zones 1 and 2. If these lucent lines are incomplete, < 2 mm, and not progressing, they are usually of no significance.[78,138] Lucent lines are reported in 15% to 20% of femoral compartments, and up to 65% of tibial components demonstrate incomplete lucent lines at the metal-bone or bone-cement interfaces.[71,88,101,154,167] With porous-coated components, progressive loss of beads or loosening of greater than 10 suggests loosening.[78,101]

The degree of motion can be assessed on the lateral view or clinically. The extent of flexion and extension is important and part of the knee scoring system described earlier. Approximately 65° of flexion is required to climb stairs and 70° of flexion for walking with a normal gait. Descending stairs (85° flexion) and rising from a setting position (105° flexion) requires a greater range of motion.[71,101]

Merchant View

The position, lucent zones, and femoropatellar relationship (subluxation or dislocation) are assessed on the Merchant or sunrise and lateral views (Fig. 6-141D). With metal-backed components, the polyethylene wear may be more easily assessed, and the area of the peg-metal interface should be assessed for fracture.[129,138]

Table 6-3 summarizes the features to assess on the radiographic views described. Additional techniques are often required to evaluate patients with suspected complications more fully.[63,108]

Complications

The follow-up evaluation of patients after knee arthroplasty incorporates clinical and imaging features. The knee score described earlier is used to evaluate the degree of improvement postoperatively.[102] The Knee So-

(*text continues on page 508*)

TABLE 6-3. *Postoperative radiographic assessment*[69,78,86,101,102,154,159,167,169,170]

Radiographic view	Features to study
AP standing (Figs. 6-137 and 6-138)	Mechanical axis Femoral axis Tibial axis Femorotibial angle (4–7° valgus) Tibial component angle (β) (90°, >90° = valgus, <90° = varus) Femoral angle (α) (97–98°) Lucent zones (Fig. 6-139) Polyethylene wear (Fig. 6-142)
Lateral view	Femoral component angle (δ) (0°) Tibial component angle (∞) (90°) Flexion-extension Lucent zones Patellar relationship Area of tibial coverage (AP and lateral combined, Fig. 6-136)
Merchant view (Fig. 6-141D)	Patella-prosthesis relationship Lucent zones Subluxation Dislocation

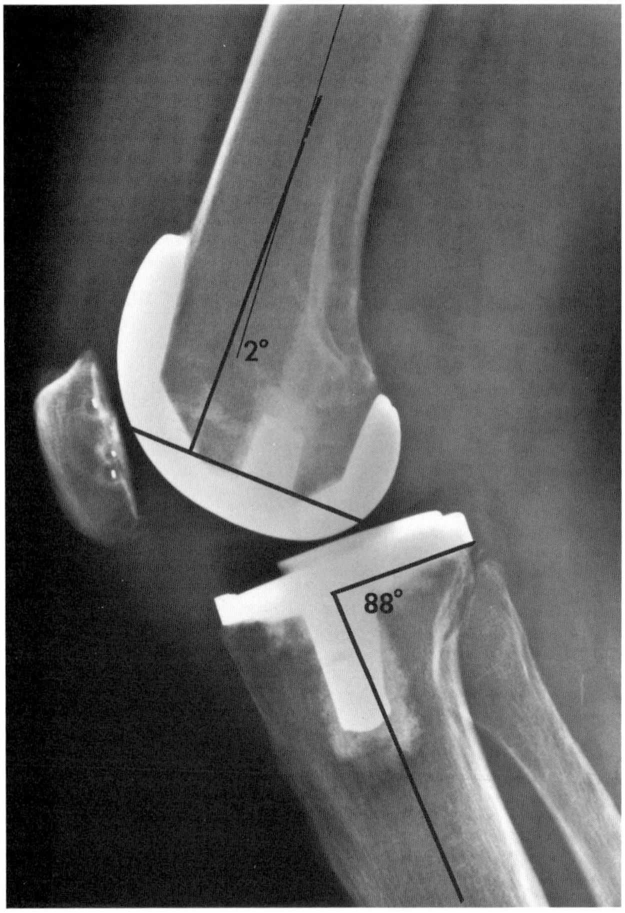

A

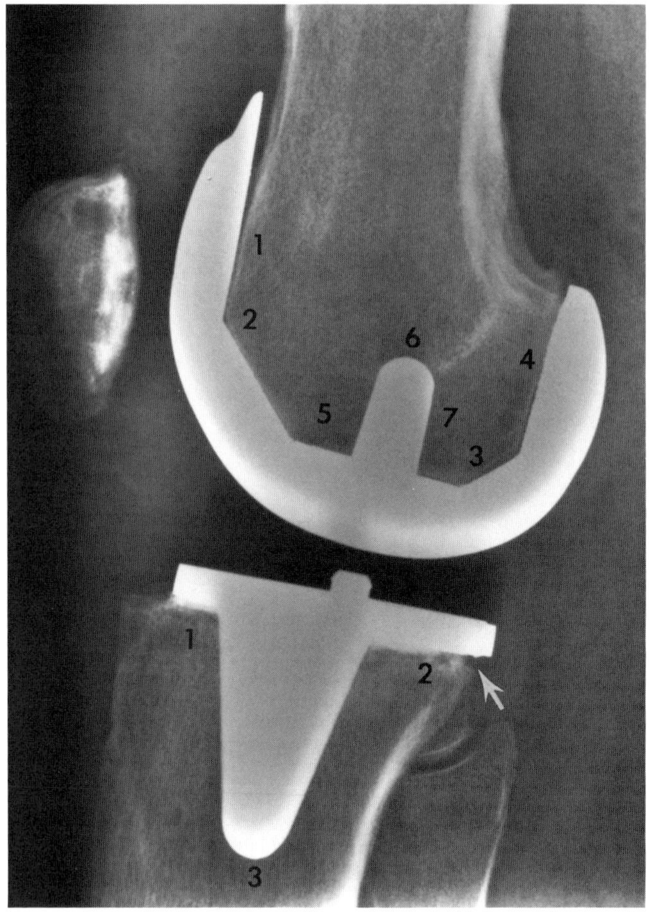

B

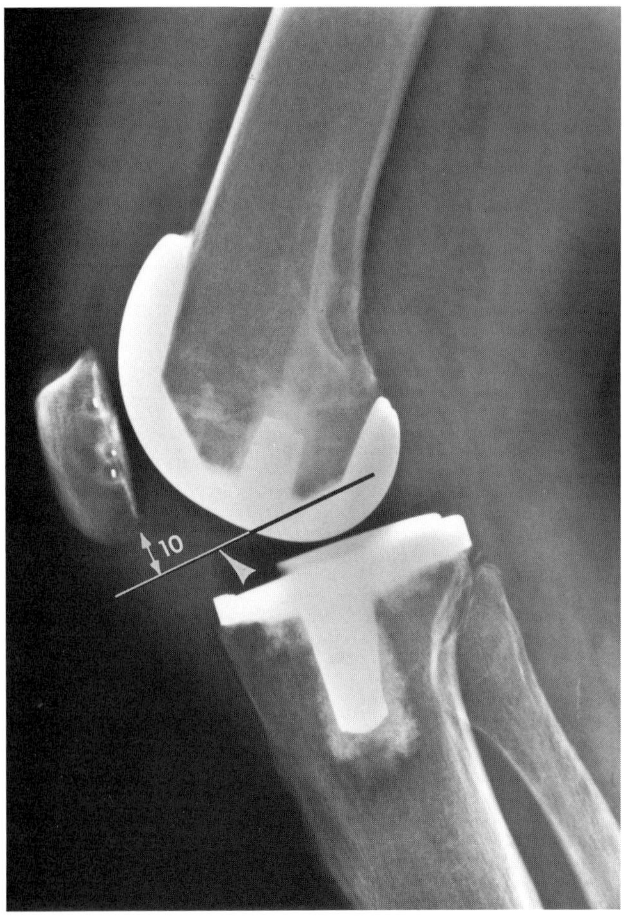

C

FIG. 6-140. A: Lateral view of the knee demonstrating the tibial angle (88°) and the femoral angle of the components. The tibial component should be at about 90° to the tibial axis and the femoral component, near 0°.[169,170] **B:** Lateral view following knee arthroplasty. There is posterior overhang of the tibial tray (*arrow*). There is incomplete lucency in zones 1 and 4 of the femoral component, which is commonly seen.[76,101] The irregular but incomplete lucency in zone 2 of the tibial component bears watching. **C:** The lower pole of the patella is normally about 9 to 10 mm above the anterior polyethylene lip (*arrow*) of the tibial component (*lines*) with the knee 20° to 30° flexed, as positioned for the normal lateral view.[134]

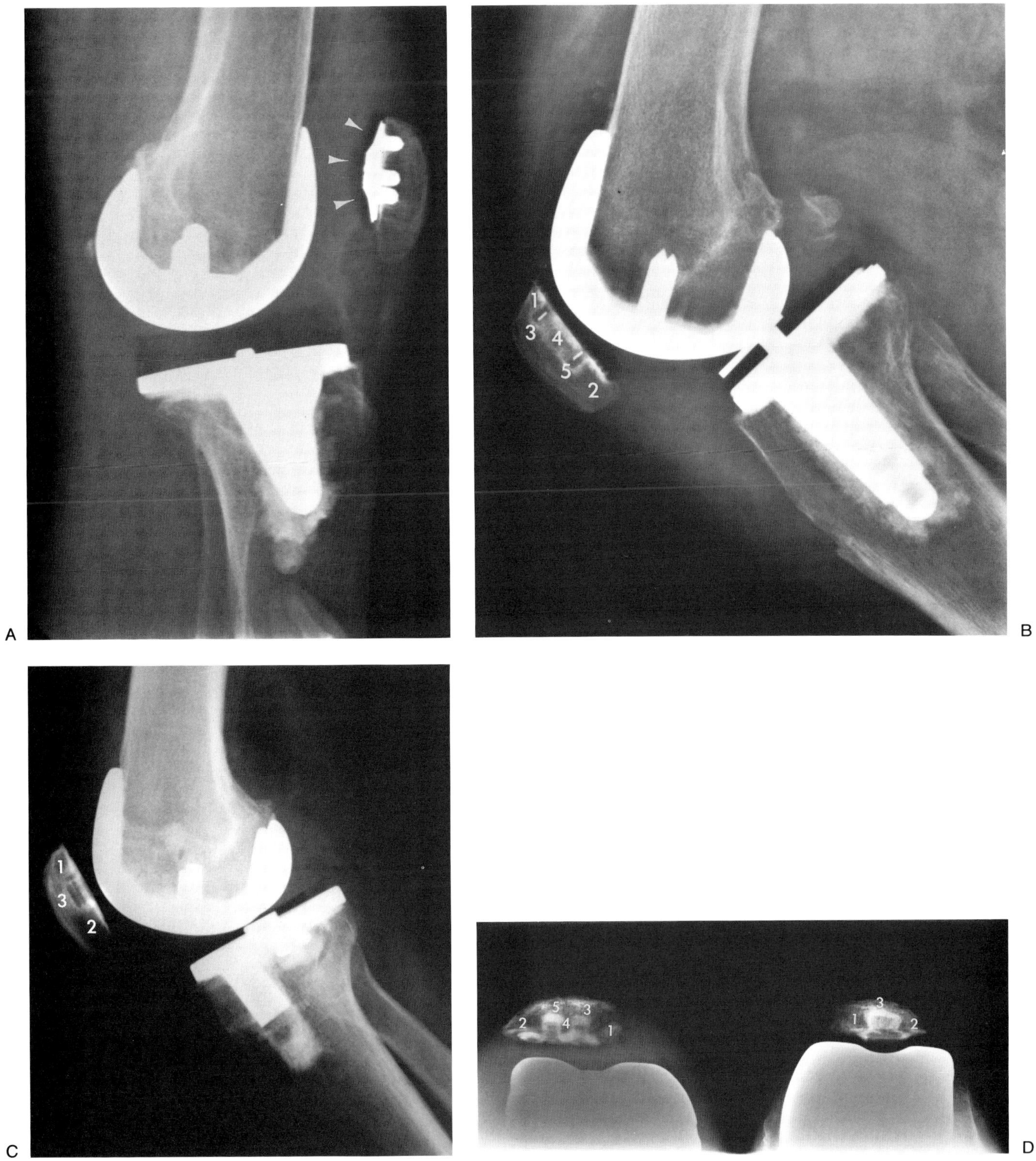

FIG. 6-141. Patellar assessment. **A:** Left lateral view taken in extension. There is slight posterior subluxation of the femur on the tibia. The patellar component is metal backed with three pegs. The polyethylene dome is clearly seen (*arrows*). **B,C:** Lateral views of all polyethylene patellar components with zones marked (B: DePuy, Warsaw, IN; C: Miller-Galante II, Zimmer, Warsaw, IN). **D:** Merchant views of bilateral polyethylene patellar components. There are multiple pegs on the left and a single peg on the right. Both are cemented. The left patella is subluxed laterally. There are no lucent zones at the component interfaces.

ciety system is based on pain (50 points for no pain), stability (25 points for no instability), and motion (maximum, 25 points; 1 point for each 5° of motion). An excellent result is 90 to 100 points; good, 80 to 90 points; fair, 70 to 80 points; and poor, less than 70 points.[78] Using today's condylar designs with patellar resurfacing, most authors report good to excellent results in more than 90% of patients.[88,102,129,130] The renewed interest sparked by unicompartmental components has led to comparable results in patients so treated.[95,161]

The complications of total knee arthroplasty are summarized in Table 6-4. Most patients with complications present with pain, swelling, and limited motion or instability.[159] Certain problems are minor and can be treated conservatively. Extensor mechanism dysfunction, infection, loosening, instability, and fracture require more aggressive therapy or revision (Fig. 6-142).[129,159]

Extension Mechanism Dysfunction

Problems with the extensor mechanism have replaced loosening as the number one problem following knee arthroplasty.[75,90] The incidence of this complication varies with the specific complication (< 5% to 30%) but accounts for up to 50% of revision procedures.[88,90,125,129] The onset of extensor mechanism complications varies, but most seem to occur 1 to 2 years after surgery.[75] The complications include patellar fracture (transverse or upper and lower pole), subluxation, dislocation, quadriceps tendon rupture, patellar ligament rupture, loosening, and component wear or failure.[66,75,91,125] The latter appears to be a more significant problem with metal-backed patellar components.[125,129] Many authors report switching to all-polyethylene components.[138,181]

Serial radiographs (AP, lateral, and Merchant views) are the best screening method for most extensor mechanism problems (Figs. 6-143 to 6-147). Flexion and extension lateral views and axial views in varying degrees of flexion may be useful in more subtle cases.

Loosening

Component loosening was far too common with the early hinged components (20% to 30%, Fig. 6-148).[99,109,182] The development of the condylar system and recent variations of this have reduced problems with loosening significantly. Today, the incidence of loosening is only a few percent.[129]

Patients with mechanical loosening usually present with pain. Preoperative factors, such as ligament instability, tibial bone loss, and obesity, can predispose the component to loosening if they are not corrected. Tibial component loosening occurs most frequently.[129,159]

Serial routine radiographs that are fluoroscopically positioned are most useful for evaluating the metal-bone (uncemented) or bone-cement interfaces (Fig. 6-149). Subtle changes in position are required to align each component properly. Flexion-extension lateral and fluoroscopically controlled stress views provide additional information regarding stability. Lucent lines are frequently seen in the peripheral zones of the tibial component (~ 65%) and the femoral component (15% to 20%).[71,154,159,167] Lucent lines less than 2 mm, which are incomplete, are usually not associated with loosening. The progression of lucent lines with widening and/or extension along the component (especially the stems or pegs) is more significant (Fig. 6-150).[71,88,154,167] Uncemented porous-coated components are more difficult to evaluate. Lucent lines, or progressive shedding of beads, indicate loosening.[78,101] Other factors that indicate tibial component loosening include subsidence (usually medially), collapse of the adjacent trabecular bone, and cement fragmentation (Fig. 6-151).[159]

Unless obvious (>2 mm and significant area involved), lucent lines and other routine radiographic features are often inconclusive. In the symptomatic patient, further imaging with radionuclide scans or subtraction arthrography may more clearly define the problem.[63] Technetium-99m bone scans are of little value for the first 8 to 10 months following surgery because uptake is normally present in the periprosthetic regions during this recovery period. Some activity may persist for more than 1 year. A positive scan finding after this time, coupled with normal or equivocal routine radiographs, is useful in confirming loosening.[63,145]

Subtraction arthrography is not as useful in the knee as it is in the hip. The joint space in the knee is large and decompresses the joint when it is distended with contrast medium (Fig. 6-152). Therefore, the filling of subtle areas between the bone-cement or metal-cement interface is more difficult. Also, two image planes would be ideal, but this is difficult to accomplish with the subtraction technique. Joint aspiration at the time of arthrography is useful when infection is suspected.[63]

TABLE 6-4. *Total knee arthroplasty: complications*[88,129,130,138,159,161,181]

Wound healing
Infection
Patellofemoral (extensor mechanism)
Loosening
Instability
Fracture-dislocation
Pain
Deep venous thrombosis
Pulmonary emboli
Pes anserinus bursitis
Synovitis

Infection

Superficial or wound infections and deep infection both occur. The former are usually seen in the immediate postoperative period, and they are less likely to require sacrifice of the components. Careful technique and

(text continues on page 516)

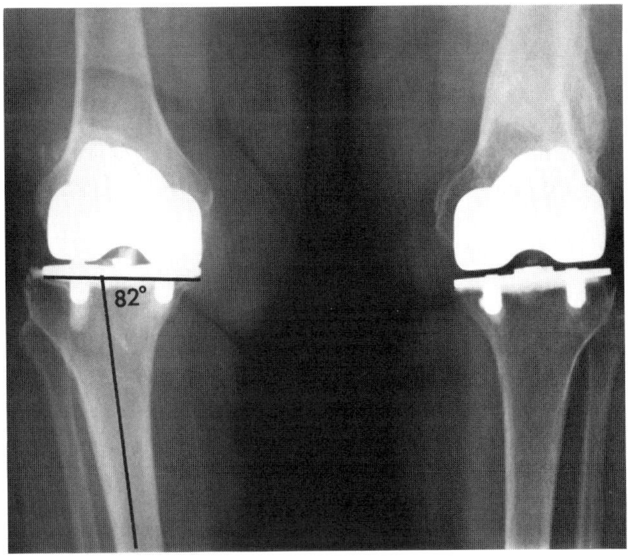

FIG. 6-142. Standing AP view of both knees following PCA cemented joint replacements. There is an old fracture of the left femur. Note the symmetric polyethylene space on the left and medial wear with joint space loss on the right medially. There is also medial overhang of the tibial component and subsidence with the component into varus position.

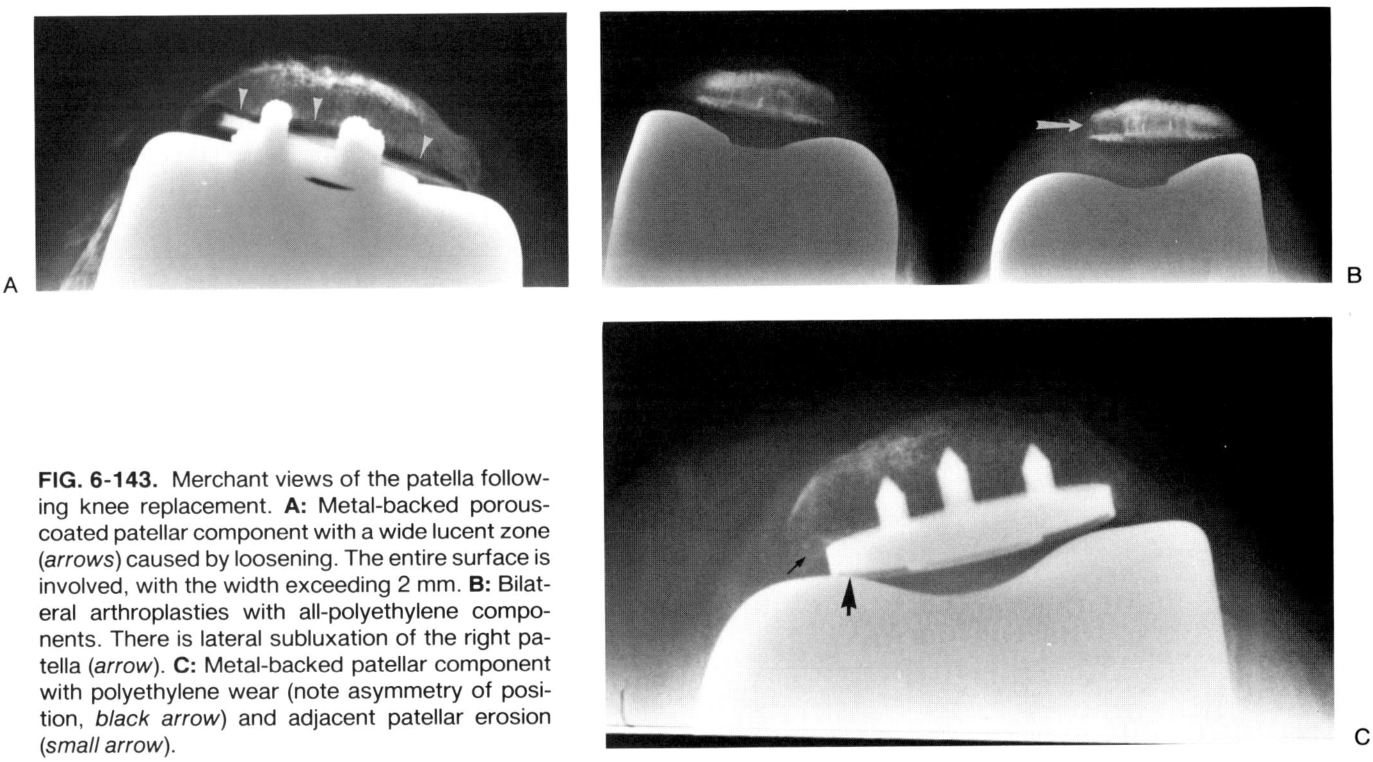

FIG. 6-143. Merchant views of the patella following knee replacement. **A:** Metal-backed porous-coated patellar component with a wide lucent zone (*arrows*) caused by loosening. The entire surface is involved, with the width exceeding 2 mm. **B:** Bilateral arthroplasties with all-polyethylene components. There is lateral subluxation of the right patella (*arrow*). **C:** Metal-backed patellar component with polyethylene wear (note asymmetry of position, *black arrow*) and adjacent patellar erosion (*small arrow*).

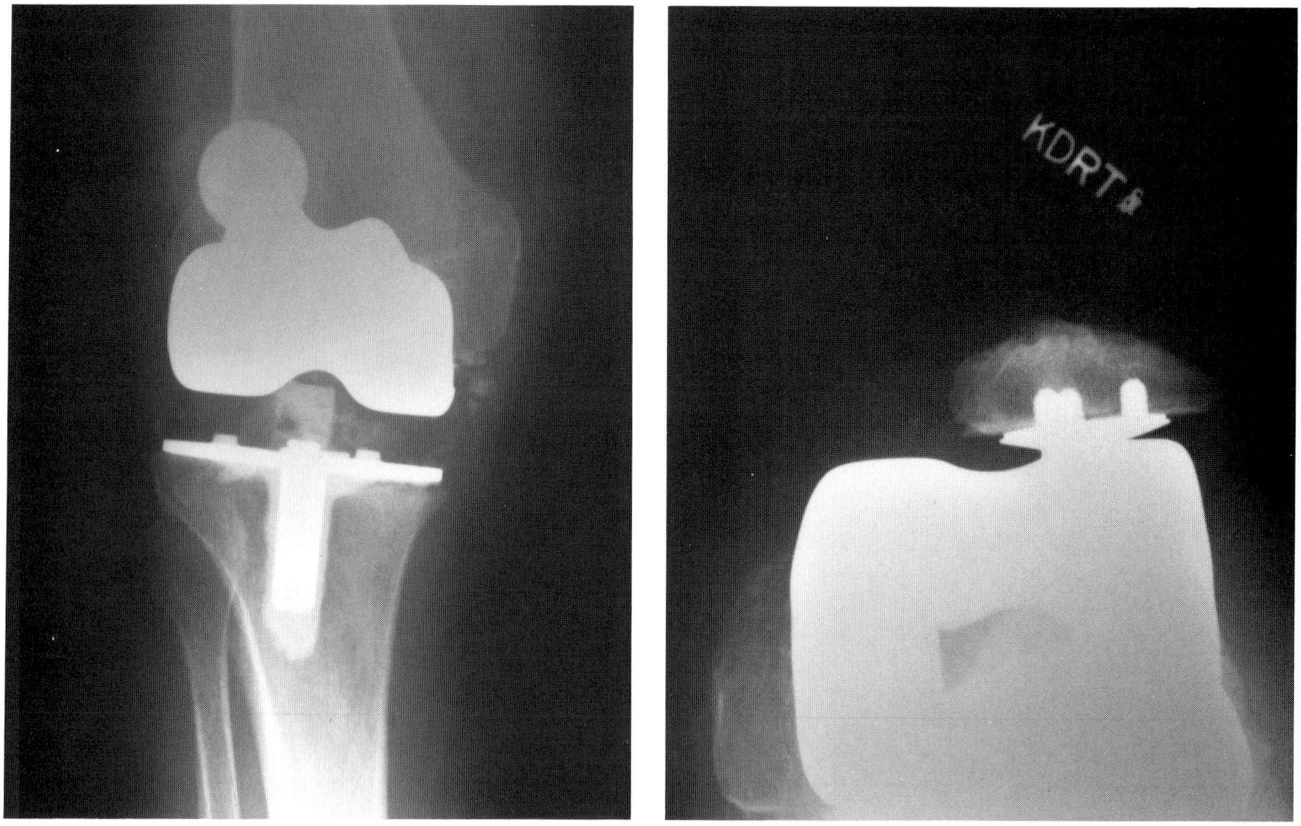

A

B

FIG. 6-144. The AP **(A)** and Merchant **(B)** views demonstrating lateral subluxation of the patella with a metal-backed patellar component. The component is in good position and does not appear loose (Fig. 6-106A).

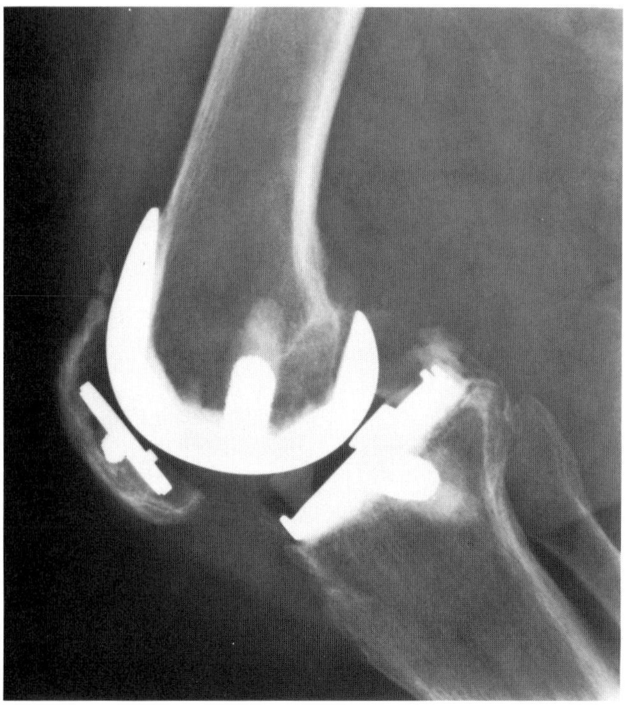

FIG. 6-145. Lateral view of a cemented PCA arthroplasty with gross loosening of the patellar component.

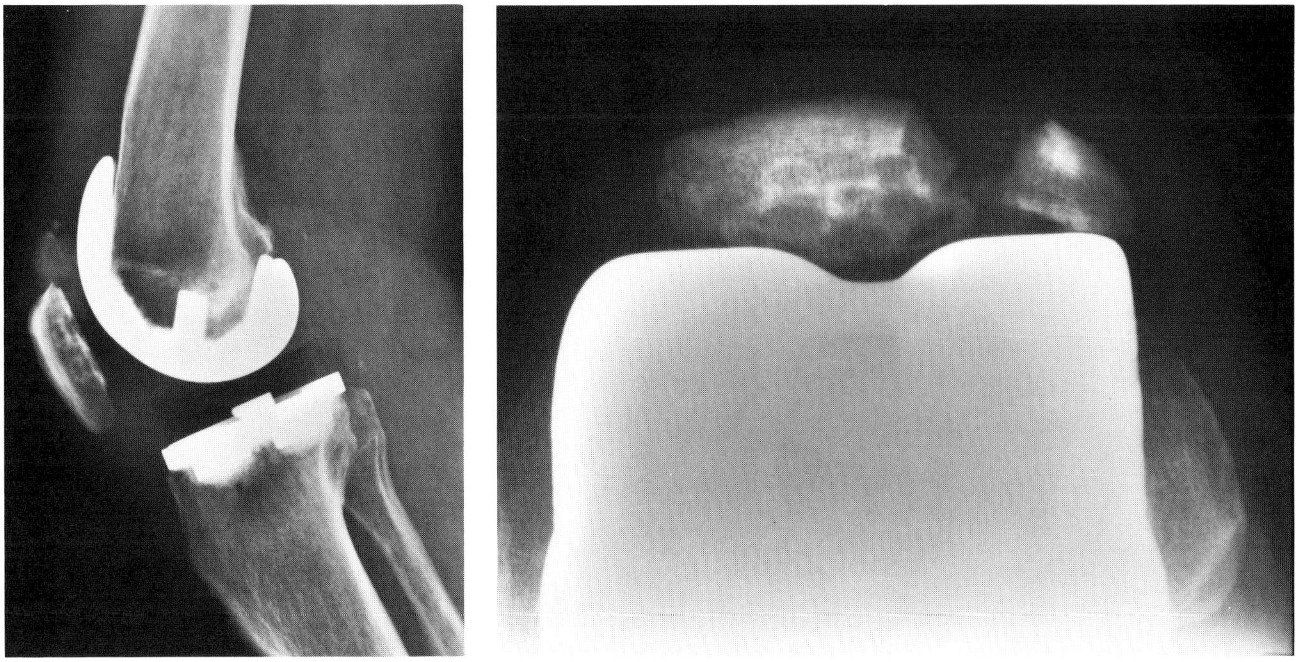

A B

FIG. 6-146. Lateral **(A)** and Merchant **(B)** views of a Miller-Galante II (tibial component option with four short pegs) demonstrating a patellar fracture.

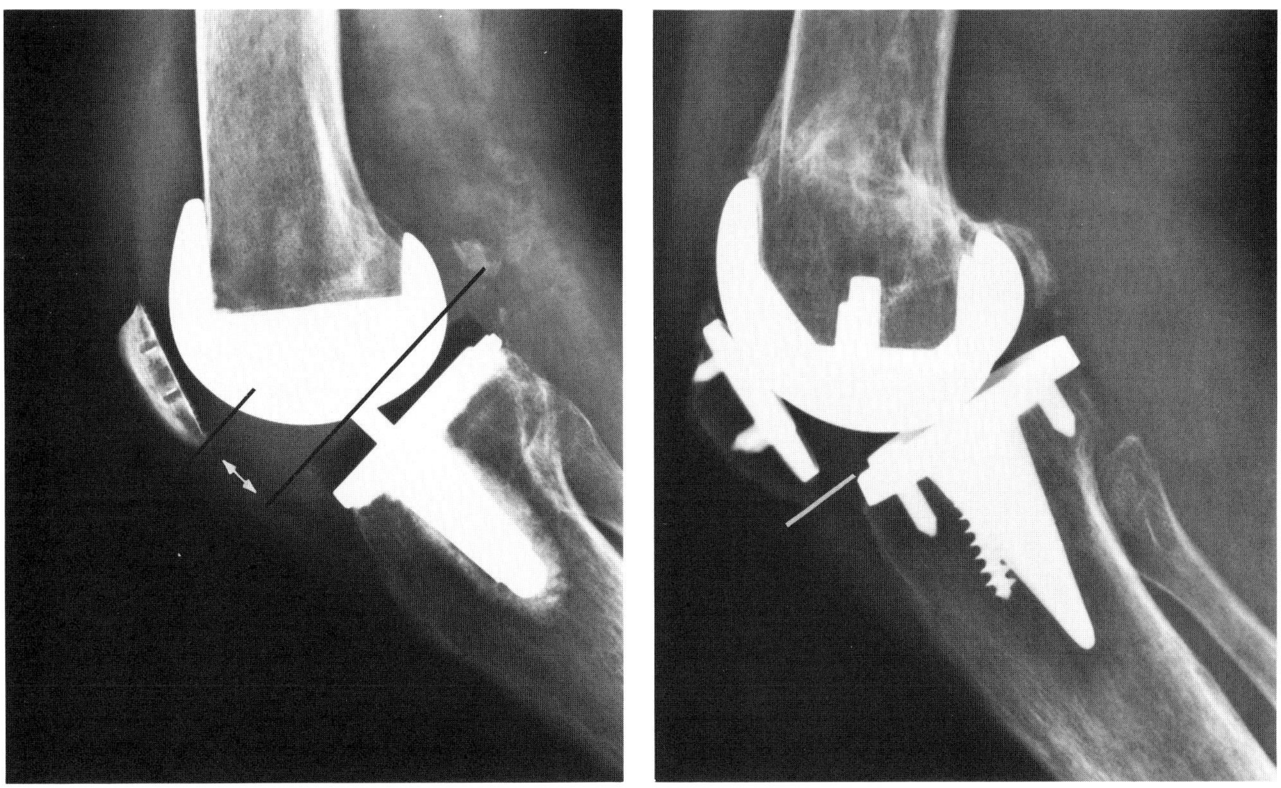

A B

FIG. 6-147. Lateral views of the knee. **A:** Normal patellar position (> 10 mm). **B:** Patella infra. There is no distance (*white line*) between the patellar component and the anterior margin of the tibial component.

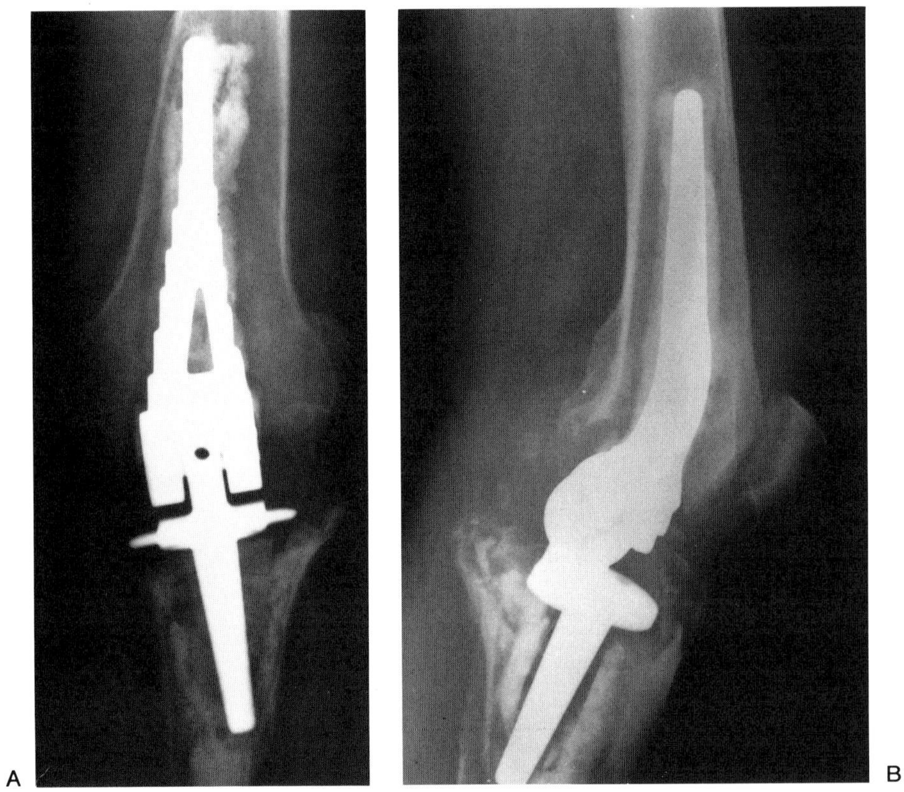

FIG. 6-148. The AP **(A)** and lateral **(B)** radiographs of a grossly loose Noiles hinge prosthesis (Fig. 6-110).

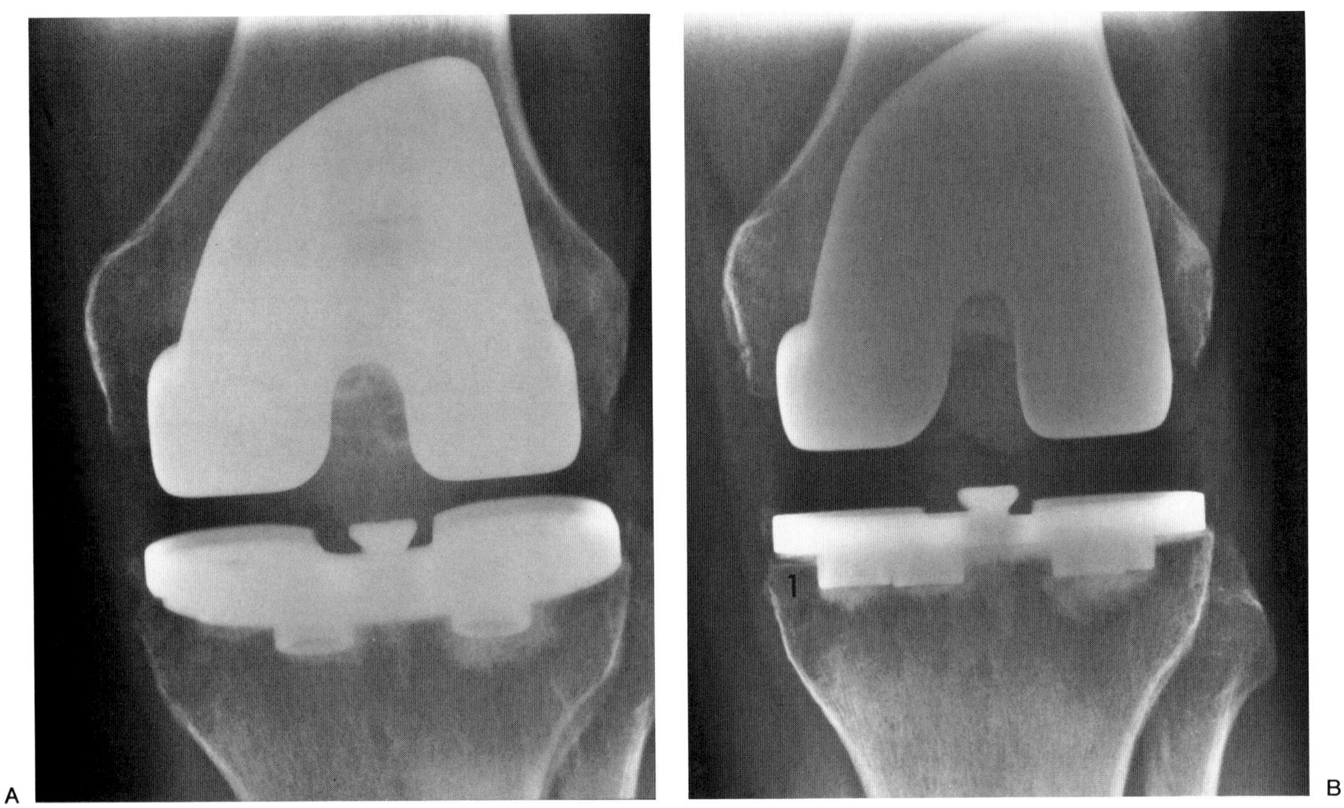

FIG. 6-149. Routine radiograph **(A)** and fluoroscopically positioned tibial component **(B)**. The component interface can only be effectively studied when the interface is clearly seen (B). Incomplete thin lucent line in zone 1 (B).

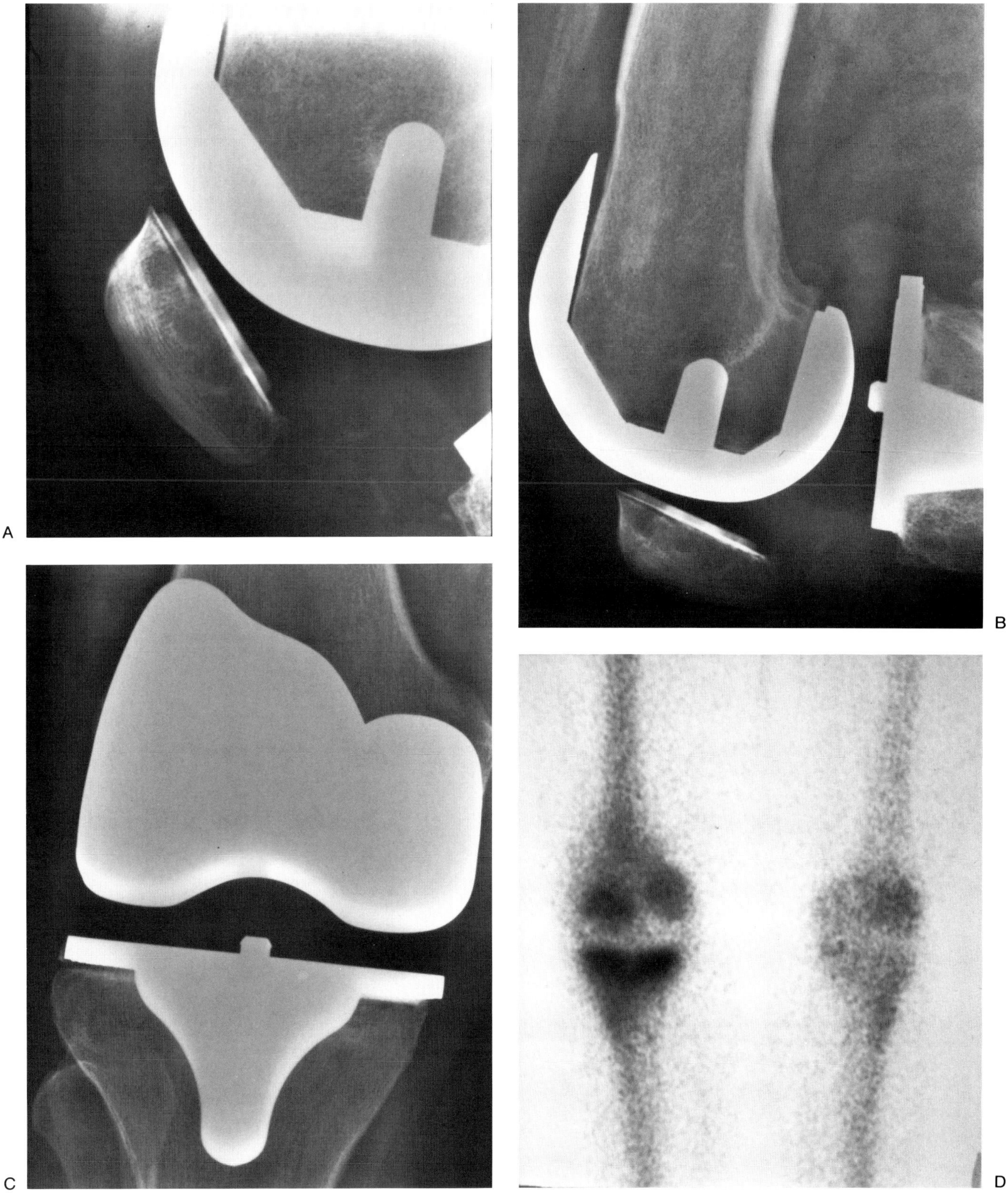

FIG. 6-150. Fluoroscopically positioned spot views of the patella **(A)**, femoral component **(B)**, and tibial component **(C)** demonstrating incomplete lucent lines in a patient with knee pain. **D:** Technetium-99m bone scan shows intense uptake in the tibia, which is more indicative of loosening.

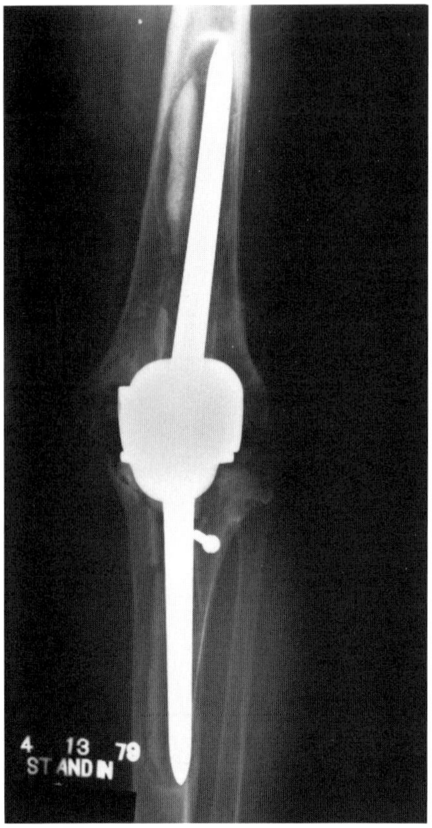

FIG. 6-151. An AP view of the knee with a Guepar hinged prosthesis. There are large lucent zones and cement fractures caused by loosening.

A 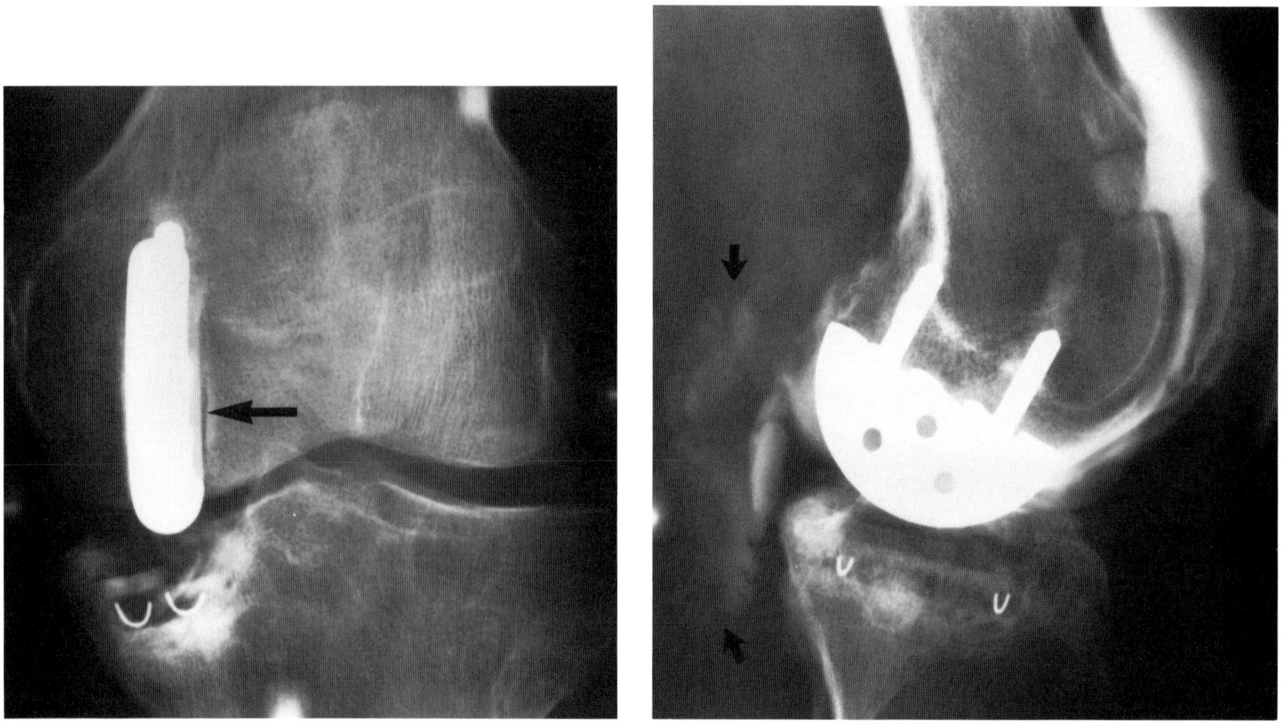 B

FIG. 6-152. A: An AP view of the knee with polycentric medial compartmental arthroplasty. There is a lucent line (*arrow*) along the femoral component. **B:** Lateral view (unsubtracted) shows a popliteal cyst (*arrows*).

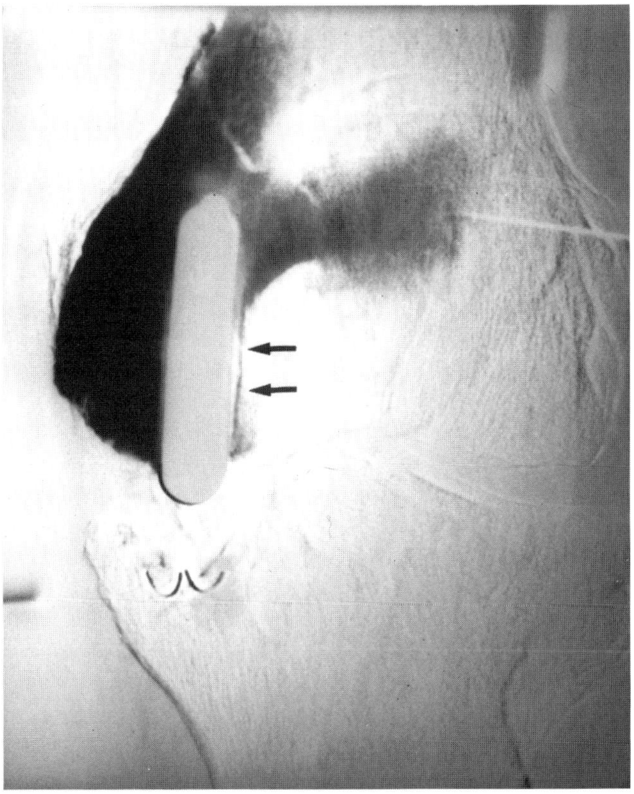

C

FIG. 6-152. (*Continued.*) **C:** The AP subtraction view shows contrast along the component (*arrows*) caused by loosening.

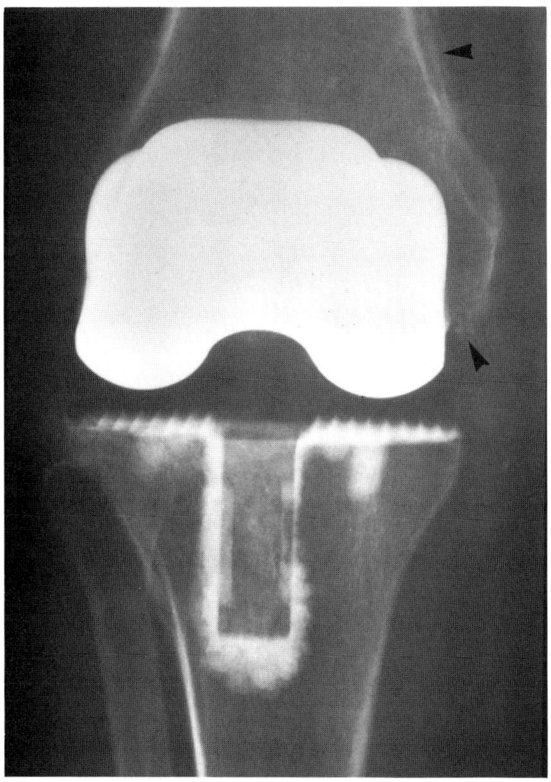

FIG. 6-153. An AP view of a total condylar knee with a cemented all-polyethylene tibial component. There is bone loss in the medial femoral condyle (*lower arrow*) and periosteal reaction (*upper arrow*) caused by infection.

meticulous postoperative care can prevent or reduce the incidence of wound infections.[129,131]

Deep infection is a more significant problem. Patients often present with persistent pain for 6 months or longer postoperatively. Large series have reported the incidence of deep infection to range from 1% to 19%.[62,180] The Mayo clinic incidence was 1.2%.[129] A large series by Wilson et al.[179] reported an incidence of 1.6% in 4,171 patients. A large series in Sweden (12,118 patients) reported an incidence of deep infection of 1.7%.[62] The incidence of infection varies with the type of prosthesis. Hinged prostheses became infected in 19%; stabilized components, in 5.1%; resurfacing designs, in 2.8%; and unicompartmental components, in only 0.8% of cases.[62,139] The incidence of infection with revision arthroplasty is also higher (9%).[130]

Routine laboratory studies, including the erythrocyte sedimentation rate, white blood cell counts, and cultures should be obtained. Joint aspiration, which is performed with arthrography or alone, is also useful. The accuracy of joint aspiration in the identification of infection varies from 70% to 98%. A sensitivity of 67%, a specificity of 92%, and an accuracy of 83%, which were reported by Cuckler et al.,[82] were comparable to the results we found.[63]

The imaging of patients with suspected infection is often complex. Routine radiographs can be useful to demonstrate swelling, effusion, and bone changes. Serial radiographs are useful for abrupt changes in lucent lines and poorly defined lucent areas, and periosteal new bone may be identified (Figs. 6-153 to 6-155).[63,159] Unfortunately, routine radiographs are often normal. Sinus tracts can be studied with fine catheters to determine if they are superficial or communicate with the joint space.[63]

Radionuclide imaging is commonly used in patients with suspected infections. Most prefer technetium-99m methylene diphosphonate (MDP) or sulfur colloid scans in combination with indium-111-labeled leukocytes or gallium-67 (Fig. 6-156).[82,133] The accuracy of technetium-gallium scans is reported to be 60% to 80%, and technetium-99m MDP combined with indium-111-labeled leukocyte scans improve the accuracy to 85% to 93%. Technetium-sulfur colloid combined with indium-111-labeled leukocytes provides an accuracy of 96% to 97%.[123,133,146]

Infections are most commonly due to *Staphylococcus aureus* (64%), *Pseudomonas aeruginosa* (12%), *Escherichia coli* (5%), and anaerobic organisms (6%); various other organisms account for the remaining 13%.[129] Depending on the virulence of the organism and other clinical factors, Rand[139] and others[180] described basic approaches to the patient with deep infection as follows:

Antibiotic therapy is used if the (1) surgical risk is too high, (2) there is a low-virulence organism, (3) the organism is susceptible to oral antibiotics, (4) the patient can tolerate antibiotics, and (5) the components are not loose.

Débridement is indicated for early infection with no component loosening. Antibiotic therapy is given with the débridement.

Resection arthroplasty includes the removal of components with no attempt at revision. For example, patients with polyarticular rheumatoid arthritis and little physical demand may be treated in this manner.

Arthrodesis is used to relieve pain, but motion is lost (Fig. 6-157). This is best suited to patients with greater mobility, younger individuals, or those with highly virulent organisms.

Two-stage revision includes the removal of the implant and all cement in the first stage. The infected tissues undergo débridement. The second stage is 6 weeks of intravenous antibiotics through a in dwelling catheter. The final stage is revision arthroplasty.[162,180]

Fractures

Fractures occur more frequently with osteopenia; loose components; components, such as hinged prostheses, that require more bone removal; and technical problems during surgery.[124,129,159] Fractures in the supracondylar region (Fig. 6-158) occur most frequently, but patellar fractures (Fig. 6-146) and femoral and tibial condyles also occur.[80,120] Stress or insufficiency fractures also occur, especially in patients with underlying osteopenia (Fig. 6-159). The incidence of fractures following knee arthroplasty is 1.2% to 3.0%.[80,120,159] Treatment may be accomplished without component removal (Fig. 6-158), depending on the location and extent of the fractures. Component fracture is unusual but can occur, especially with hinged components (Fig. 6-160).

Cordeiro et al.[80] described a specially designed revision system with long intramedullary femoral and tibial stems. This system provided improved treatment results in patients with periprosthetic fractures compared with conservative methods. Five patients were treated conservatively, and five had the tibial component modeled after a Freeman revision prosthesis (Fig. 6-161). The femoral component was an ICLH prosthesis with a long stem to follow valgus and anterior femoral curves (Fig. 6-161).[80]

Instability

Ligament instability also occurs following joint arthroplasty. This complication varies with the type of components but can occur in up to 13% of cases.[118] Preoperative deformities are often corrected by releasing the ligaments on the concave side of the joint and using an appropriate polyethylene spacer to make the articular surface uniform (Fig. 6-162).[156,159] Postoperative insta-

(*text continues on page 524*)

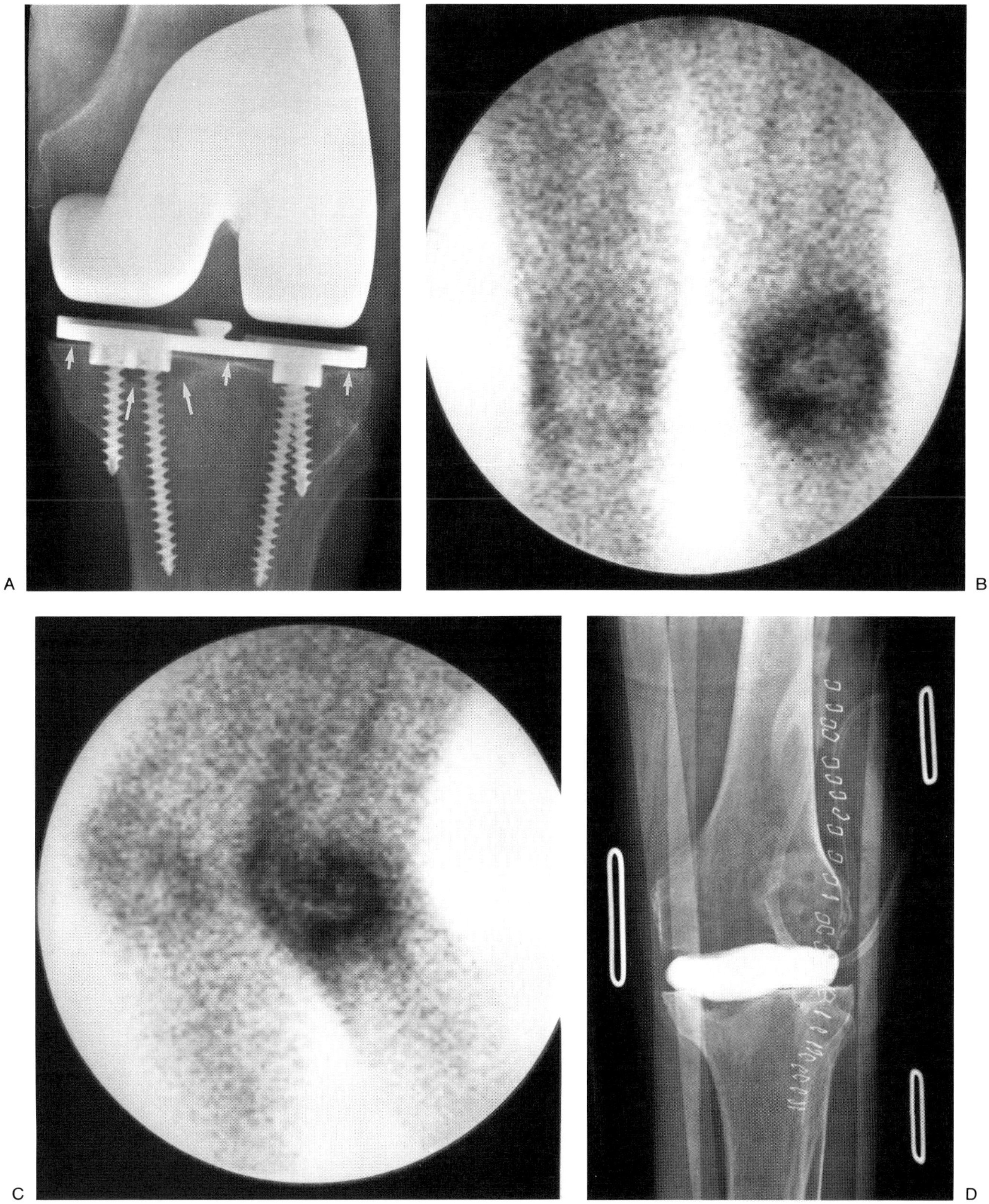

FIG. 6-154. A: An AP view of an uncemented Miller-Galante with screws. There is a lucent line along the entire undersurface of the metal tray (*small arrows*) with an irregular zone (*large arrows*) medially caused by infection. The AP **(B)** and lateral **(C)** views of the indium-111-labeled leukocyte scan show marked increased uptake. **D:** The components were removed, and an antibiotic-impregnated spacer was left in place.

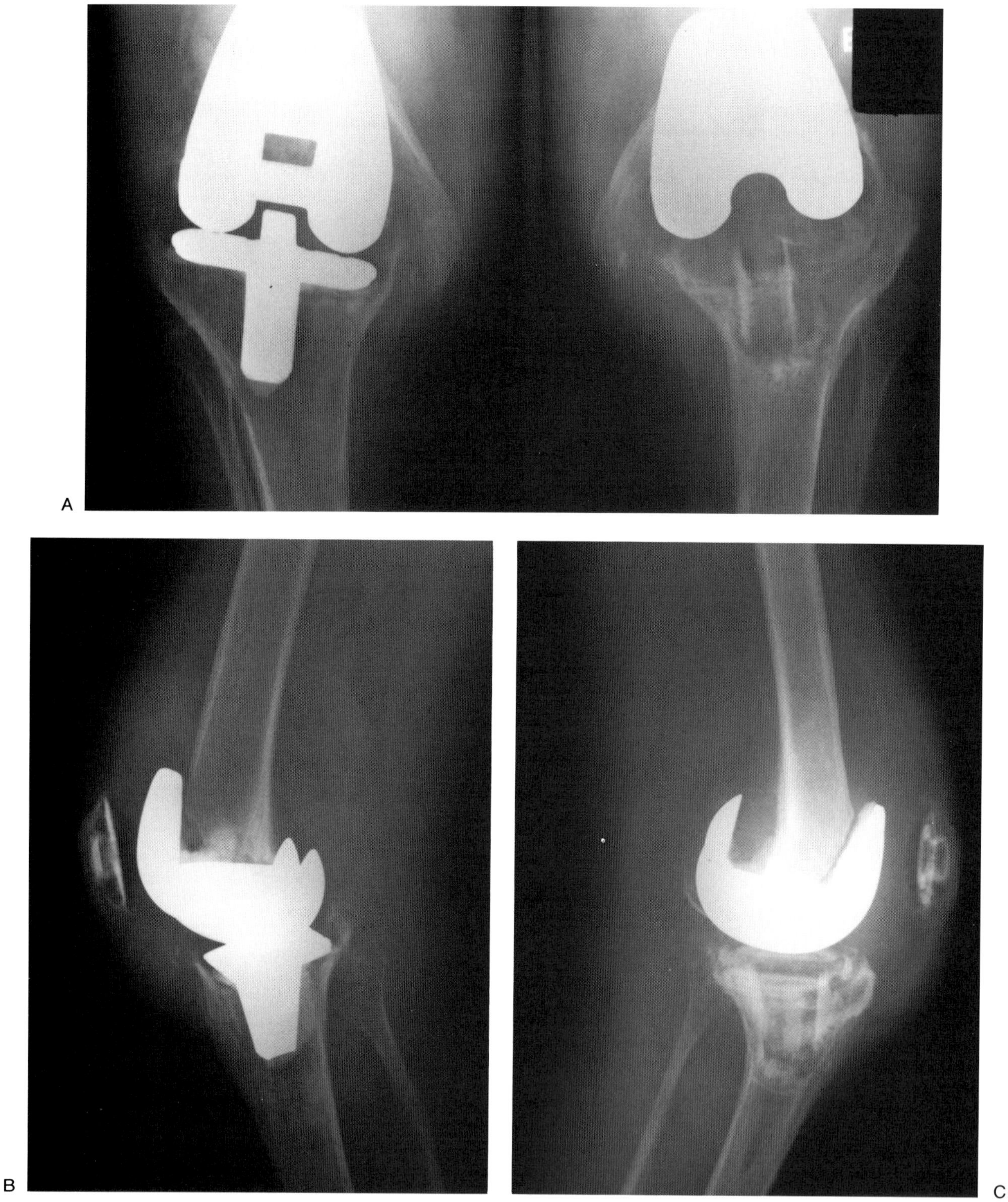

FIG. 6-155. The AP standing (A) and lateral (B,C) views demonstrate irregular lucency at the component interfaces, soft tissue swelling, and effusions in a patient with infections bilaterally.

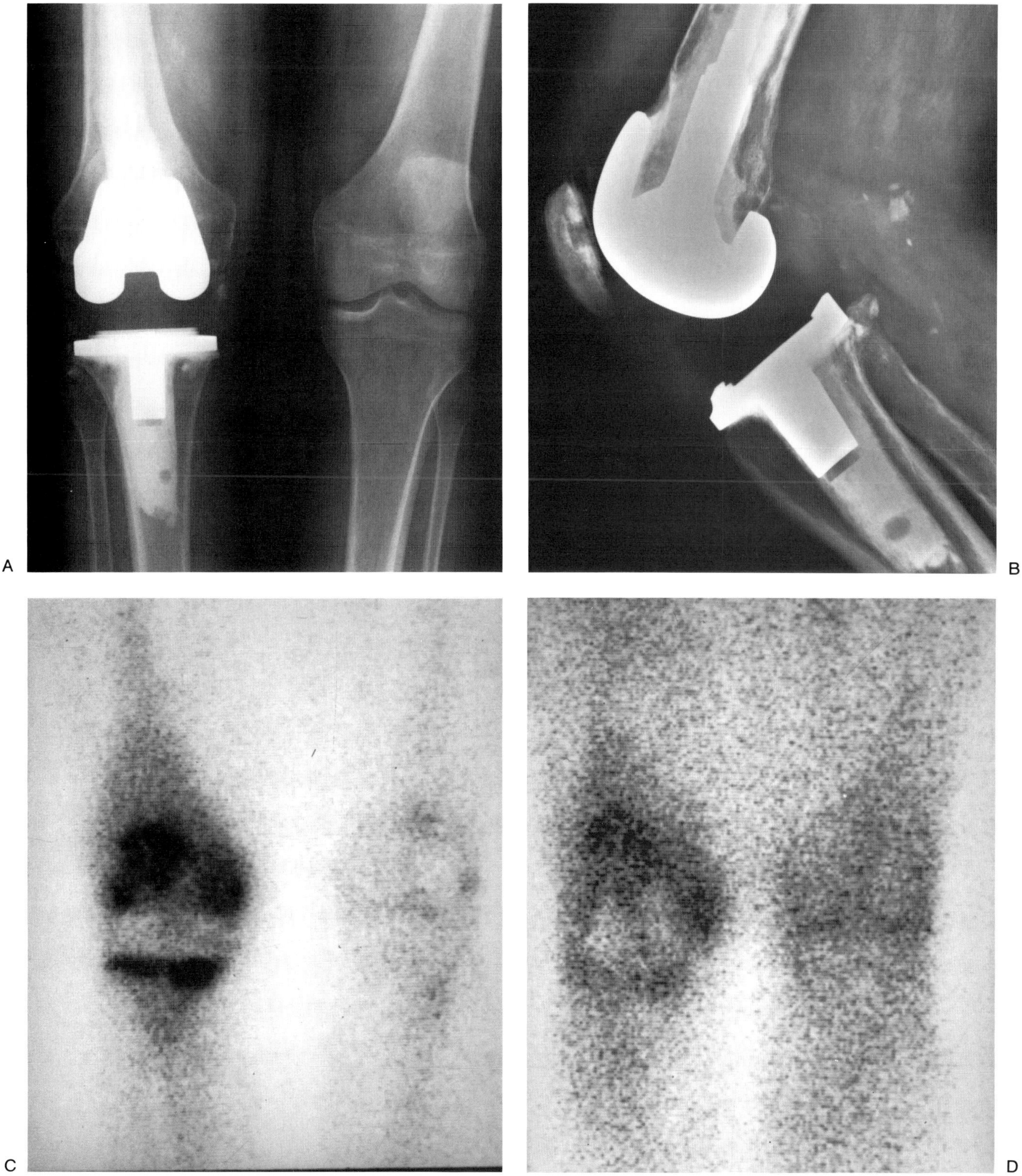

FIG. 6-156. The AP (A) and lateral (B) views of the knee demonstrating a right knee replacement with cemented components and an augmented femoral stem. Technetium-99m MDP (C) and indium-111-labeled leukocyte scans (D) show increased uptake caused by infection.

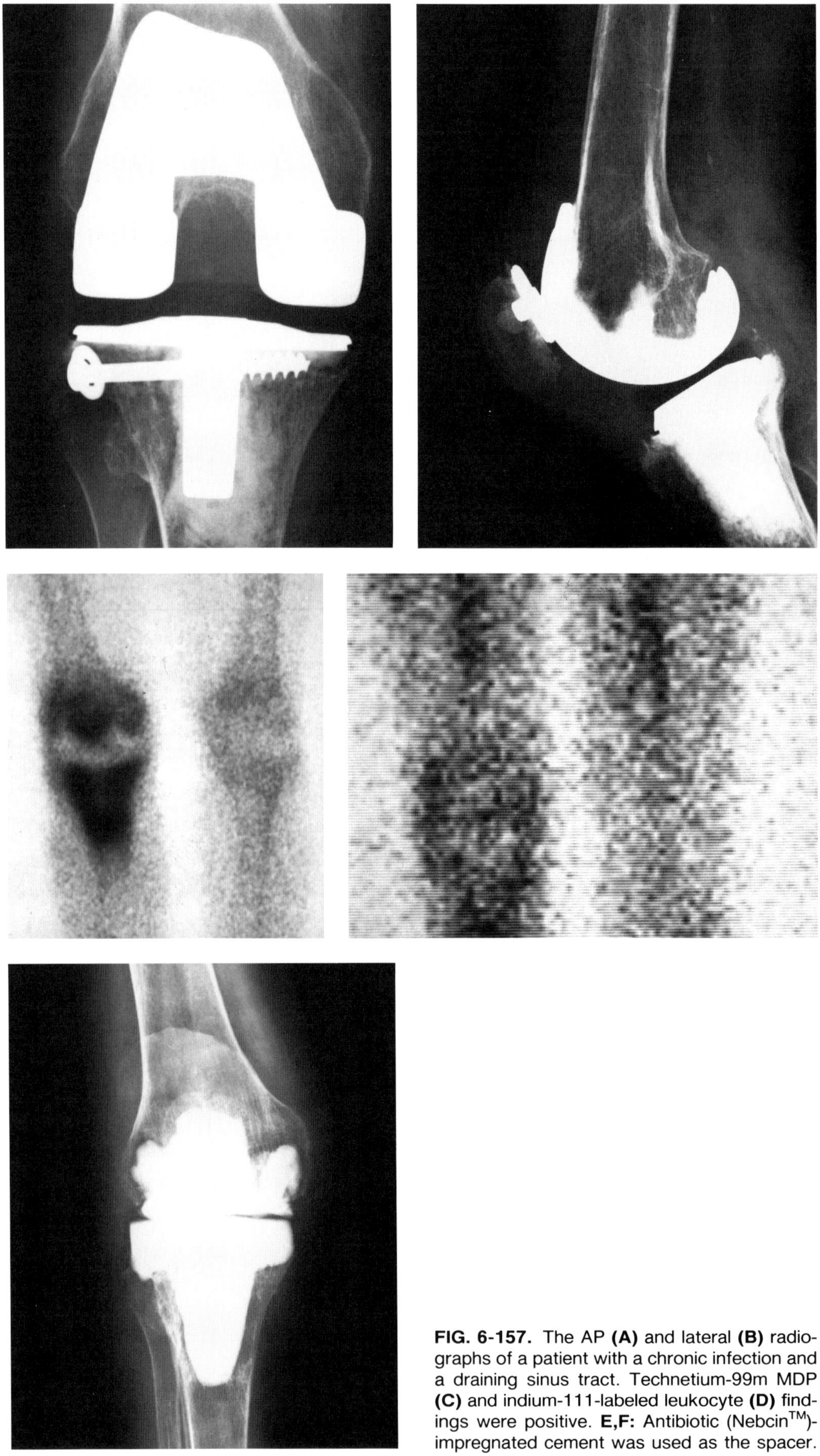

FIG. 6-157. The AP **(A)** and lateral **(B)** radiographs of a patient with a chronic infection and a draining sinus tract. Technetium-99m MDP **(C)** and indium-111-labeled leukocyte **(D)** findings were positive. **E,F:** Antibiotic (Nebcin^{TM})-impregnated cement was used as the spacer.

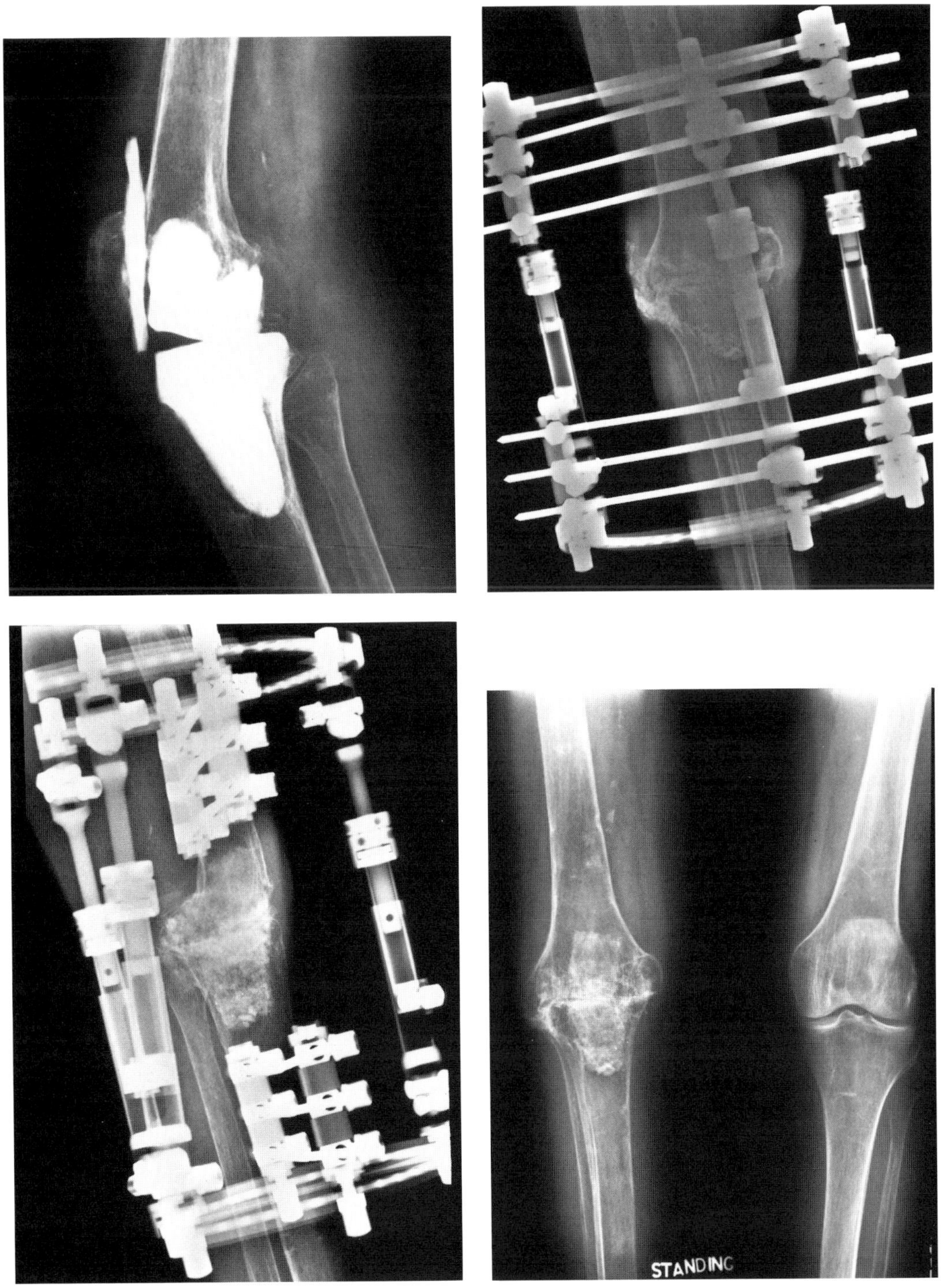

F G H I

FIG. 6-157. (*Continued.*) **G,H:** Weeks later, the cement was removed and an arthrodesis performed using an Ace-Fischer external fixator. **I:** The arthrodesis healed with fusion present 5 months later.

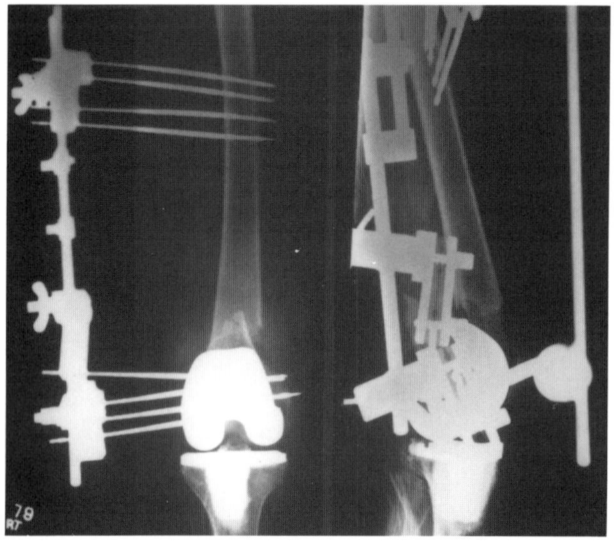

A B

FIG. 6-158. The AP **(A)** and lateral **(B)** views of a supracondylar fracture treated with external Hoffman fixation. (From Rand JA, Berquist TH. The knee. In: Berquist TH, ed. *Imaging of orthopedic trauma and surgery.* Philadelphia: WB Saunders, 1986;293–391.)

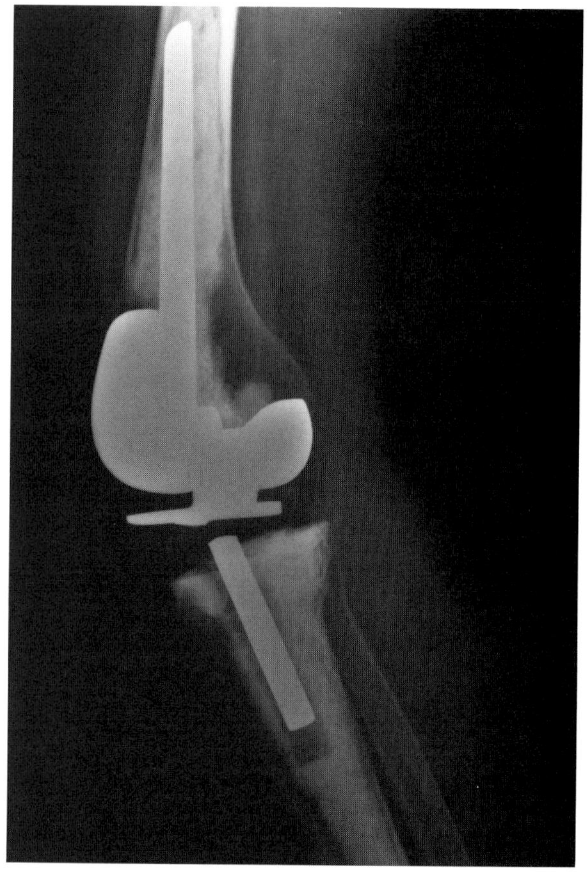

FIG. 6-160. Oblique view of the knee demonstrating a fracture of the tibial stem of a Kinematic™ rotating hinge prosthesis.

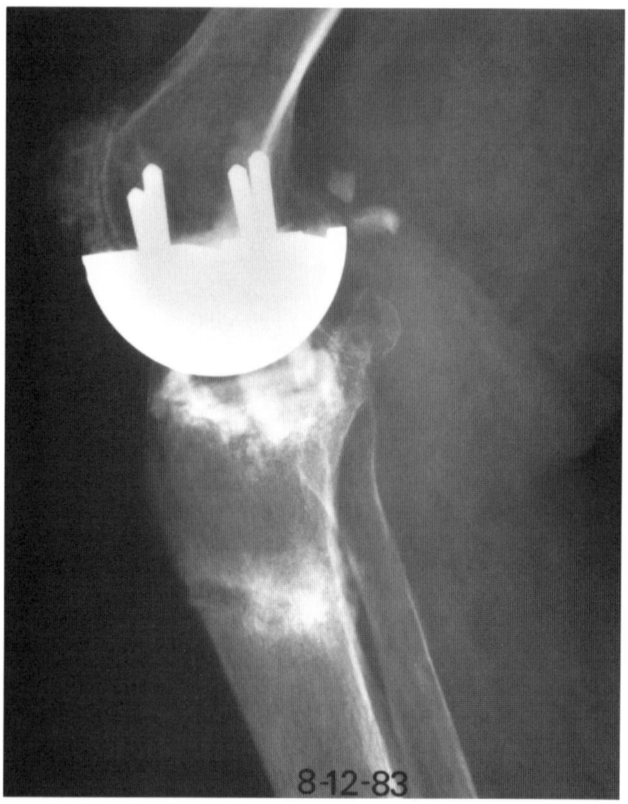

FIG. 6-159. Lateral view of the knee with polycentric components. There is a proximal tibial stress fracture. (From Rand JA, Berquist TH. The knee. In: Berquist TH, ed. *Imaging of orthopedic trauma and surgery.* Philadelphia: WB Saunders, 1986;293–391.)

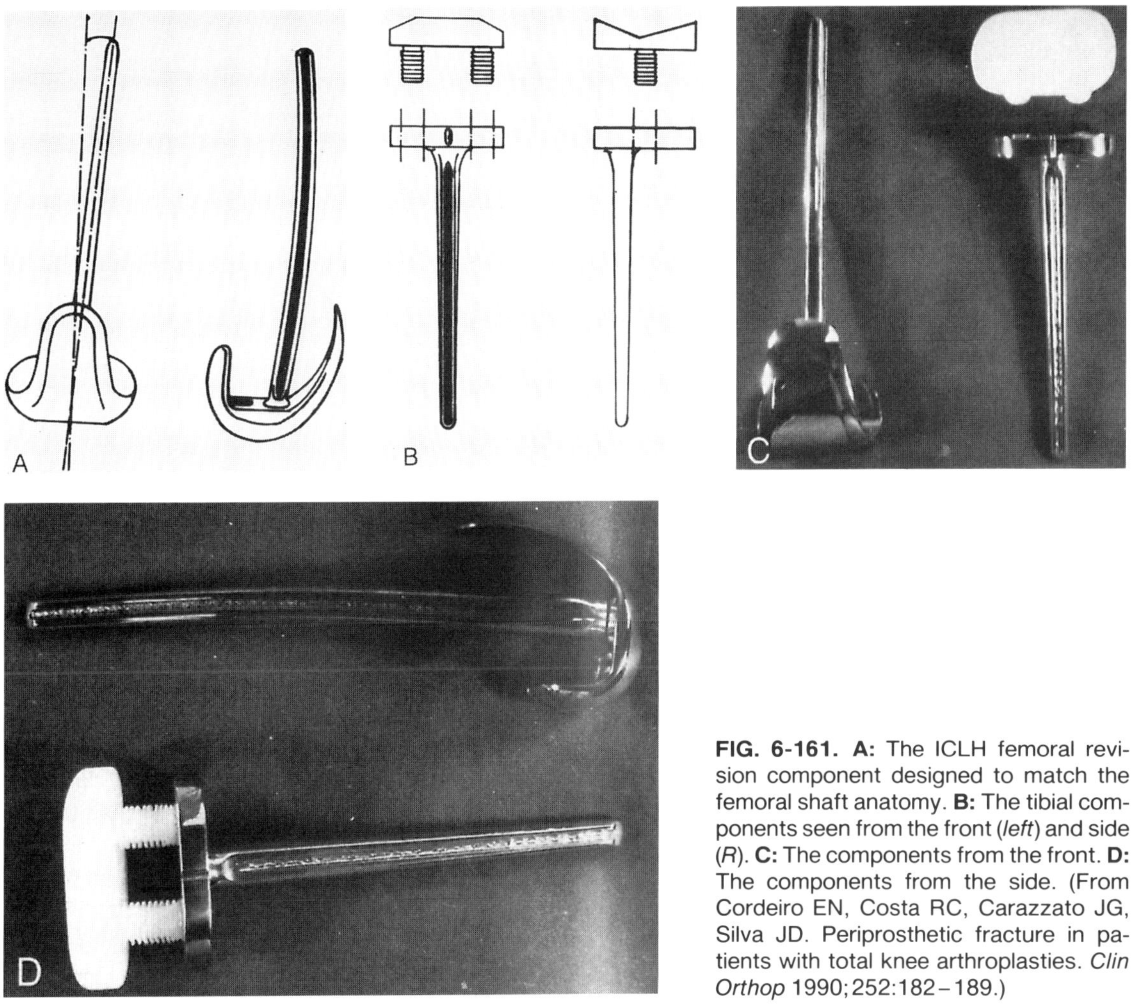

FIG. 6-161. **A:** The ICLH femoral revision component designed to match the femoral shaft anatomy. **B:** The tibial components seen from the front (*left*) and side (*R*). **C:** The components from the front. **D:** The components from the side. (From Cordeiro EN, Costa RC, Carazzato JG, Silva JD. Periprosthetic fracture in patients with total knee arthroplasties. *Clin Orthop* 1990;252:182–189.)

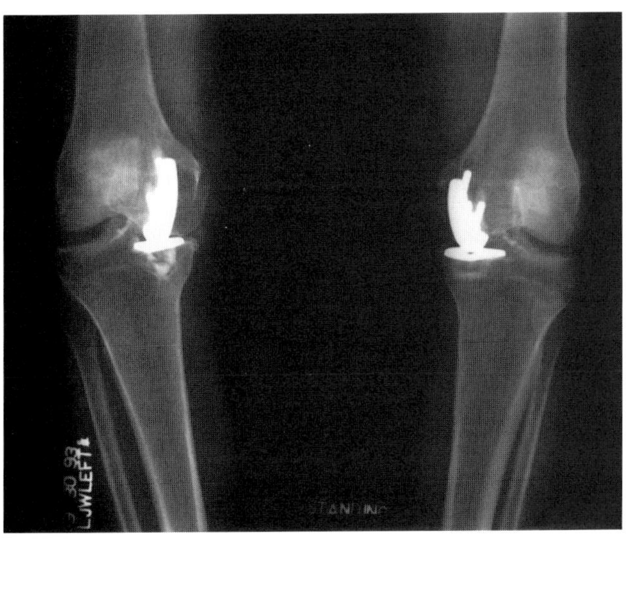

FIG. 6-162. Standing AP views of the knees after bilateral medial compartmental arthroplasty. There is obvious lateral laxity and impingement on the tibial spine on the right. Changes on the left are more subtle.

bility may occur in the AP plane, or be varus, valgus, or rotary in nature.[159]

The clinical evaluation of instability is part of the knee scoring system. A total of 25 points is awarded if there is no instability (< 5 mm of movement), in the AP direction (10 points), or less than 5° in the mediolateral direction (15 points).[103] Measurements can be made clinically, or usual radiographic stress views may be used.[63]

Stress views should be performed fluoroscopically to ensure proper alignment. The AP, varus, and valgus stress views are obtained.[63]

Other Complications

Additional complications include polyethylene wear, synovitis related to metal or polyethylene, myositis ossificans, osteolysis, and peroneal nerve palsy.[59,61,74,93,126,136,158] Pes anserinus bursitis is seen more often with unicompartmental procedures and with medial overhang of the tibial component.

Dissociation of the polyethylene from tibial and patellar components can occur in addition to wear, which results in wear particles in the joint space (Fig. 6-163).[59,74,83,110,119] Thin polyethylene surfaces tend to show more wear problems. Noncongruent surfaces also tend to show more wear.[77] Seven percent of cases reported by Tsao et al.[174] failed because of polyethylene wear. Wear particles result in giant cell reactions in the synovial tissues, and synovitis and osteolysis (Figs. 6-164 and 6-165) can occur.[61,119,177] An effusion seen on the lateral view may be the earliest radiographic feature. Juxtaarticular osteopenia has also been described with osteolysis.[177]

Metal-induced synovitis also occurs.[79] Cobalt-chromium alloys are more locally toxic. Titanium-aluminum-vanadium alloys are less toxic locally but appear to create more systemic inflammatory responses by inducing prostaglandin E_2, interleukin-1 and -6, and tumor necrosis factor.[177]

Deep Venous Thrombosis and Pulmonary Emboli

Certain factors appear to increase the incidence of deep venous thrombosis. Obesity, prolonged immobilization, previous venous disease, and hyperlipidemia have been implicated.[111,130] There does not seem to be a significant difference whether one knee is operated on or both are done at the same time.[130] The incidence of deep venous thrombosis ranges from 0.4% to 3%.[88,120,130] Pulmonary emboli occur in about 1% of patients who undergo knee replacement surgery. The incidence of both complications is lower than that with hip arthroplasty.[88,130]

The imaging of deep venous thrombosis can be accomplished with ultrasonography (compression and color-flow techniques, Fig. 6-166) or venography.

The thigh and popliteal regions are easily examined with ultrasound. The calf is more accurately studied with contrast venography. However, in our practice, sonography is the screening technique of choice. In patients with suspected pulmonary emboli, a ventilation-perfusion scan is performed.[63]

MISCELLANEOUS PROCEDURES

There are other procedures about the knee that require some form of fixation and/or instrumentation. Pre- and postoperative imaging plays a significant role in the selection and follow-up of patients for osteotomy, arthrodesis (discussed earlier), and other orthopedic procedures.[63,183]

Osteotomy

Unilateral or unicompartmental osteoarthritis may be treated with proximal tibial or supracondylar femoral osteotomies. The rationale for these procedures is to reduce the load to the involved compartment and transfer the load to the uninvolved side of the femorotibial articulation.[183,187]

Osteotomy is indicated in patients who are younger (< 65 years old) with unicompartmental pain (medial or lateral compartment), which correlates with the radiographic involvement (Fig. 6-167).[183] Supracondylar femoral osteotomies are reserved for disorders originating in the femur with valgus deformity (Fig. 6-168).[129]

The contraindications for tibial osteotomy include severe vascular disease, reduced range of motion, flexion contracture, significant bone loss, and ligament instability.[183,184]

The preoperative imaging should include a knee series (lateral, notch, Merchant, and standing AP views) to evaluate the degree of arthrosis and tibiofemoral angles. Full-length standing views (Fig. 6-169) are best for measuring the mechanical axis and tibiofemoral angle. Subtle joint space narrowing may be more easily assessed using the PA flexion standing technique.[154] In patients with more generalized symptoms, a radionuclide scan should be considered to exclude the involvement of both compartments.[183,184]

Routine radiographs are used to calculate the angle desired and the amount of bone to remove (Fig. 6-169A). Coventry[183] supports overcorrecting a varus deformity into valgus by 10°. Fixation is achieved using staples (Figs. 6-170 and 6-171), condylar plates and screws (Fig. 6-172), or modifications of the plate and screw technique. Miniaci et al.[187] used a prebent half-tubular plate and screws (Figs. 6-173 and 6-174) to prevent the loss of correction postoperatively. Giebel et al.[185] devised a blade plate and screw technique to ensure compression of the fragments at the osteotomy site (Fig. 6-175).

(*text continues on page 536*)

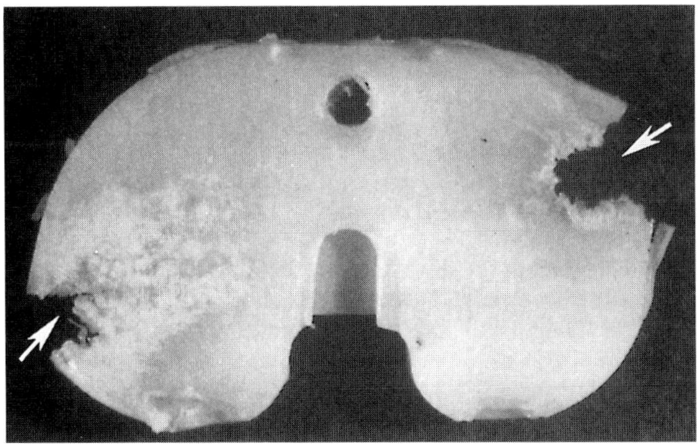

FIG. 6-163. Tibial component with irregular polyethylene wear, leaving large areas of fragmentation (*white arrows*). The posterior portion is cut out for the PCL.

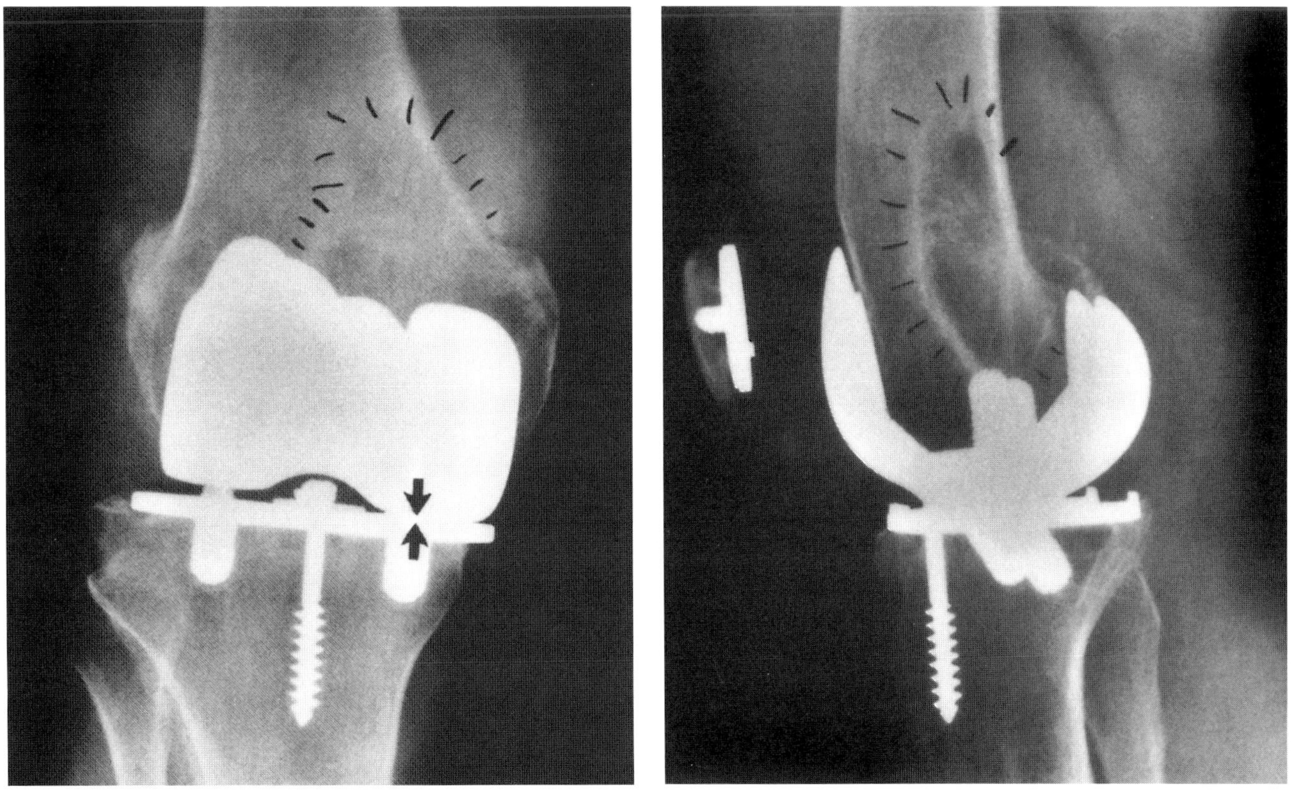

A B

FIG. 6-164. The AP **(A)** and lateral **(B)** views of the knee in a patient with a PCA knee. There is massive osteolysis caused by a foreign-body response to polyethylene particles. Early recognition allows revision before bone loss becomes this extensive. (From Kilgus DJ, Funahaski AM, Campbell PA. Massive femoral osteolysis and early disintegration of a polyethylene-bearing surface of a total knee replacement. *J Bone Joint Surg* [*Am*] 1992;74A:770–774.)

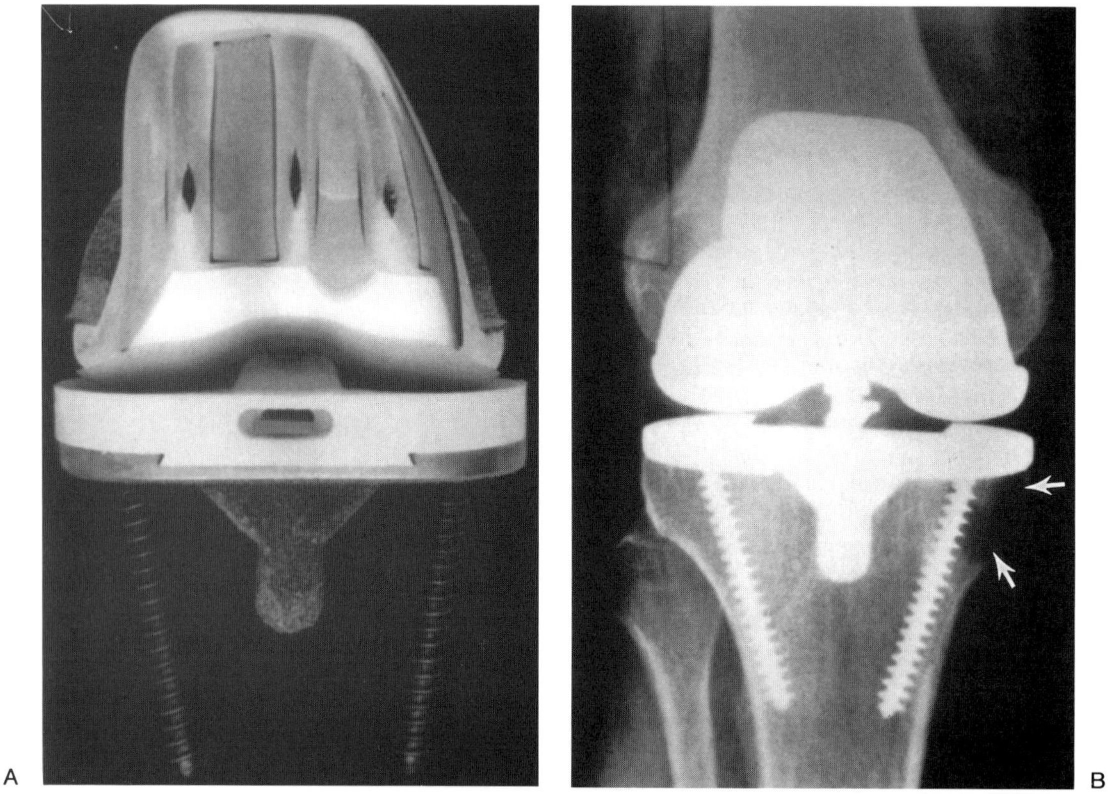

Fig. 6-165. **A:** Synatomic total knee with porous-coated cobalt-chromium femoral, tibial, and metal-backed patellar component. **B:** An AP view of the knee demonstrating medial tibial osteolysis (*arrows*). (From Peters DC et al. Osteolysis after total knee arthroplasty without cement. *J Bone Joint Surg* [*Am*] 1992;74A:864–876.)

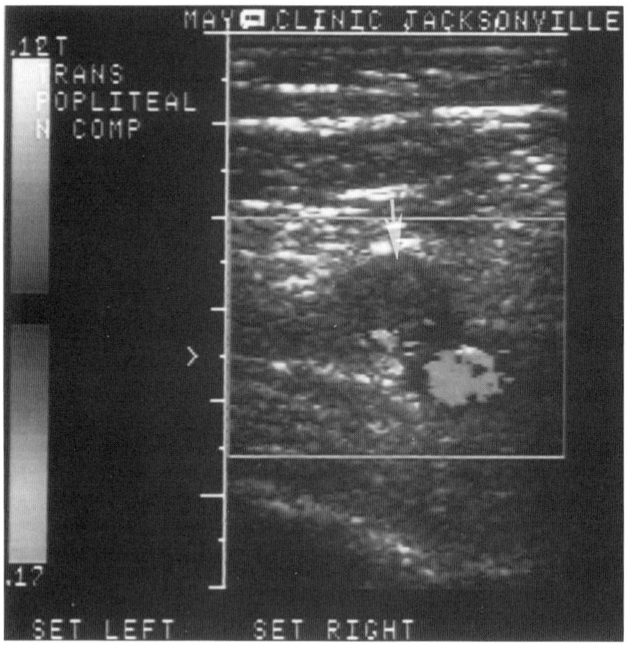

FIG. 6-166. Ultrasonographic scan of the popliteal vein (*arrow*) with compression shows failure of the vein to compress and increased echoes caused by deep venous thrombosis.

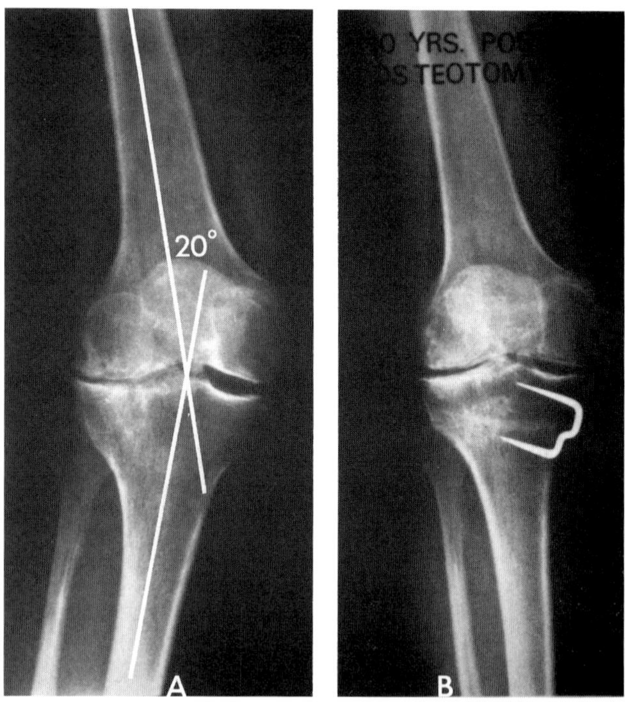

FIG. 6-167. Varus osteotomy. **A:** An AP standing view of the right knee preoperatively demonstrates degenerative changes in the lateral compartment with a 20° valgus tibiofemoral angle. **B:** Postoperative standing AP view 10 years later shows the lateral joint space is still open, and the tibiofemoral angle is 7° valgus. (From Coventry MB. Proximal tibial varus osteotomy for osteoarthritis of the lateral compartment of the knee. *J Bone Joint Surg* [*Am*] 1987;69A:32–38.)

A 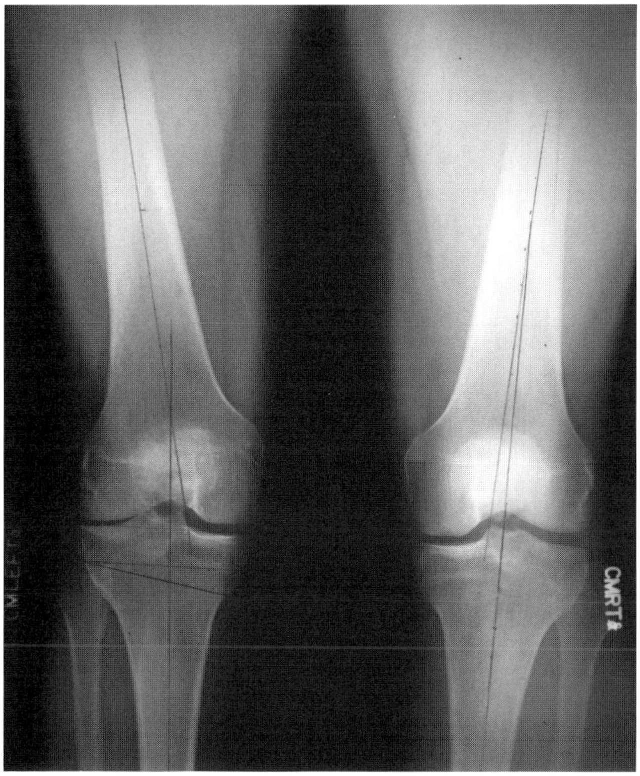

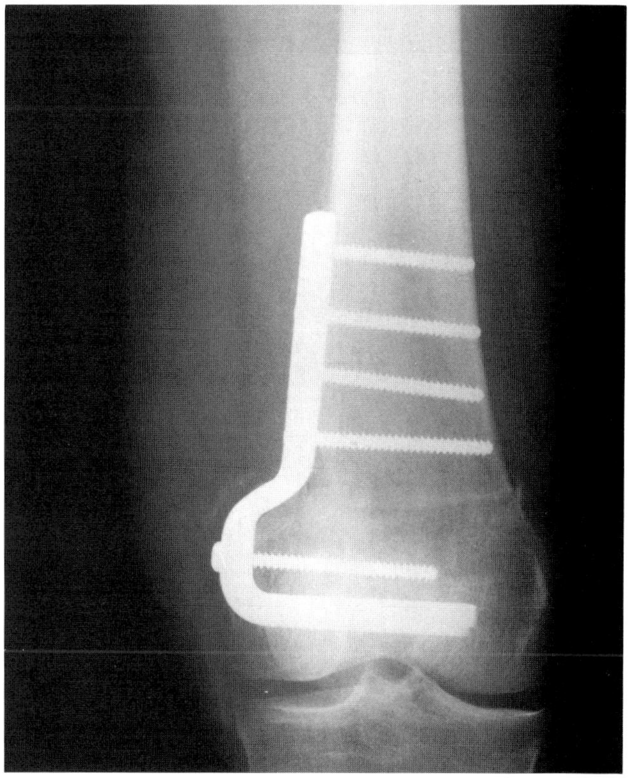 B

C 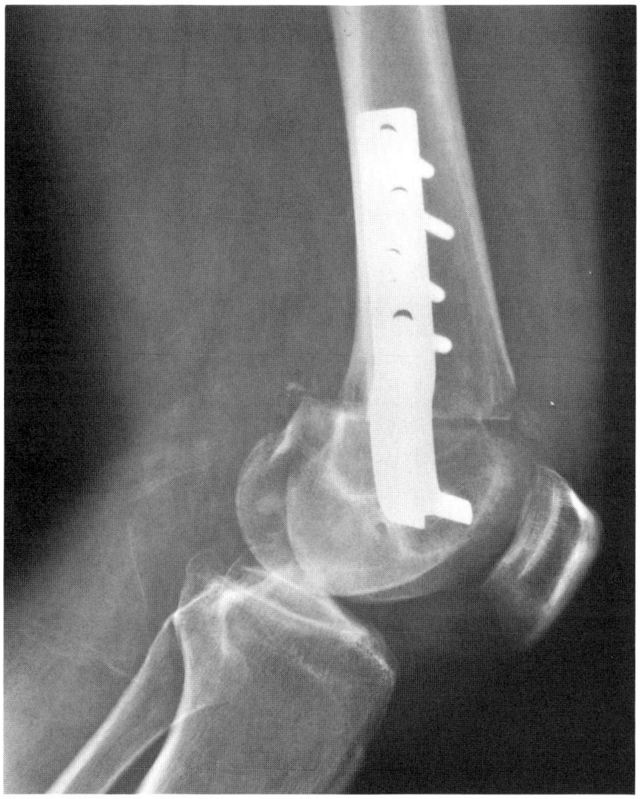

FIG. 6-168. A: Osteoarthritis with valgus deformity in the right knee. Distal femoral osteotomy with a condylar blade plate and five cortical screws demonstrated on AP **(B)** and lateral **(C)** radiographs.

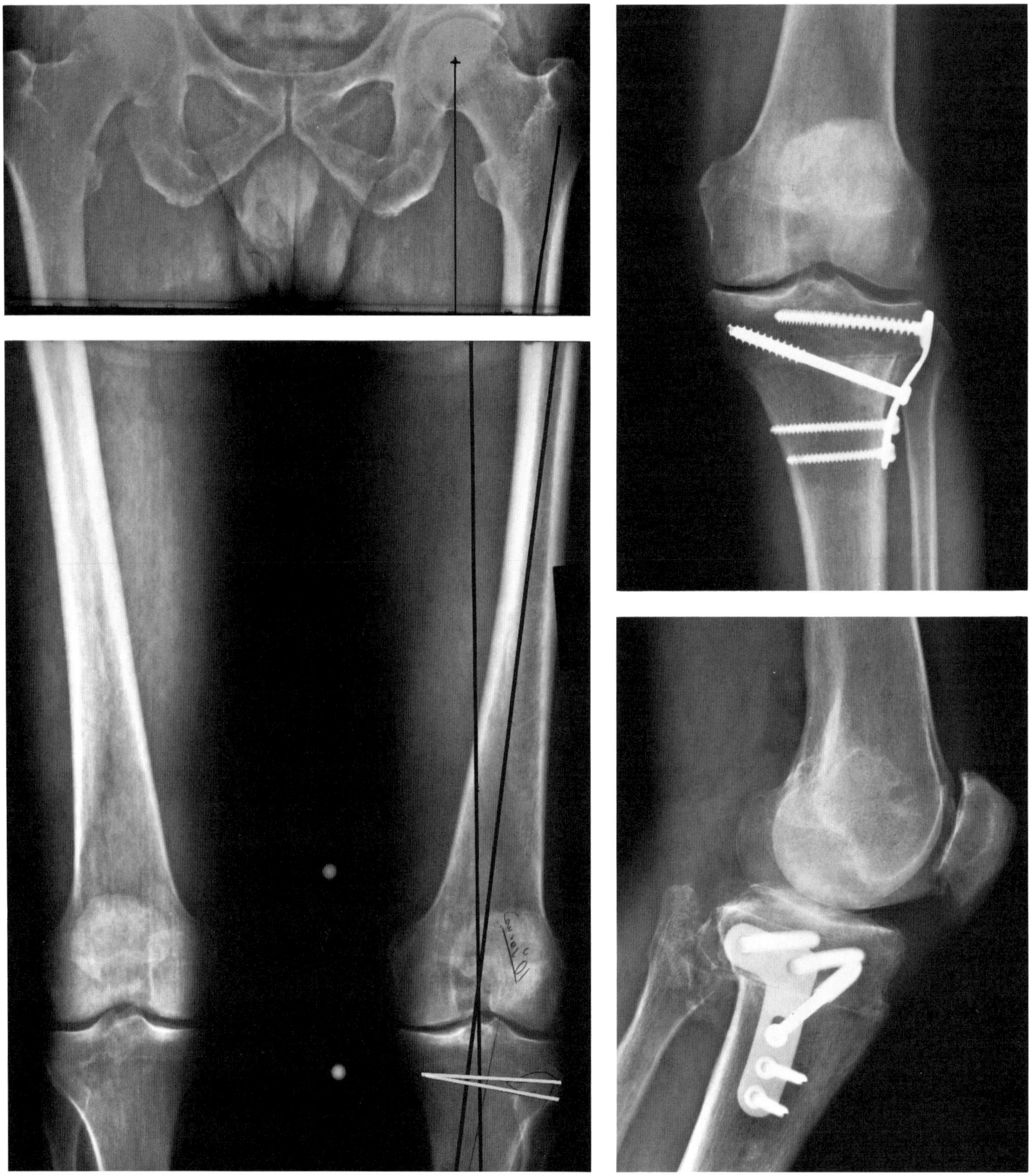

A B C

FIG. 6-169. A: Standing full-length view of the lower extremities. The mechanical axis, tibiofemoral angles, and planned wedge cuts are demonstrated. **B,C:** The AP and lateral valgus osteotomies with the "L" condylar plate, two cortical and two cancellous screws, and a lag screw for fixation.

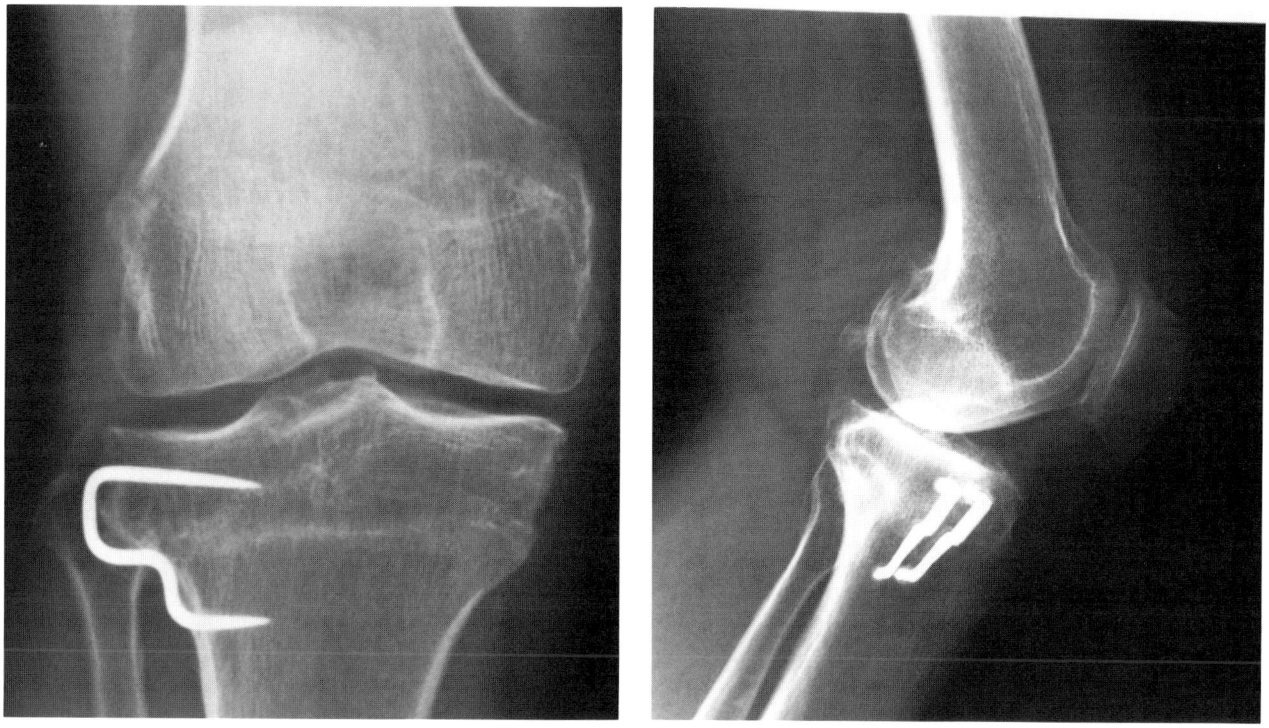

A B

FIG. 6-170. The AP **(A)** and lateral **(B)** radiographs of a healed upper tibial osteotomy with fixation using two Coventry osteotomy staples.

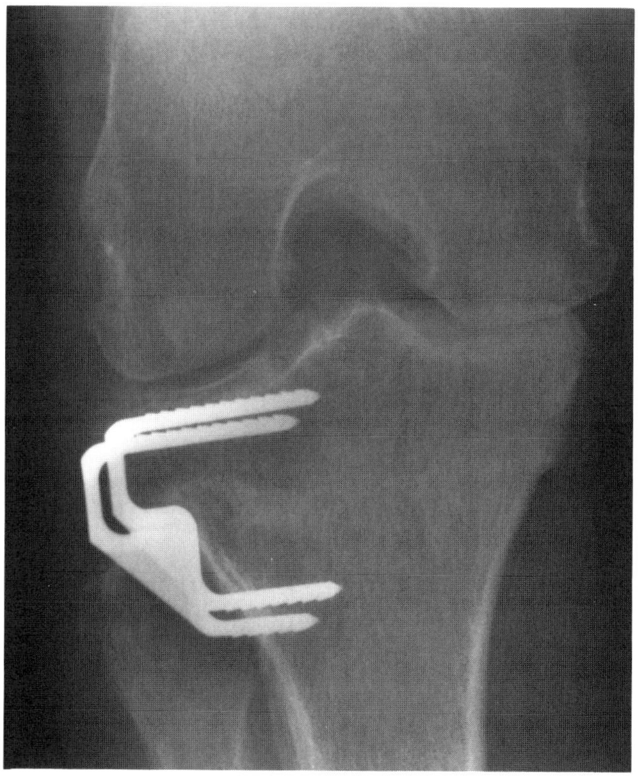

FIG. 6-171. An AP radiograph of a healed upper tibial osteotomy using barbed staples.

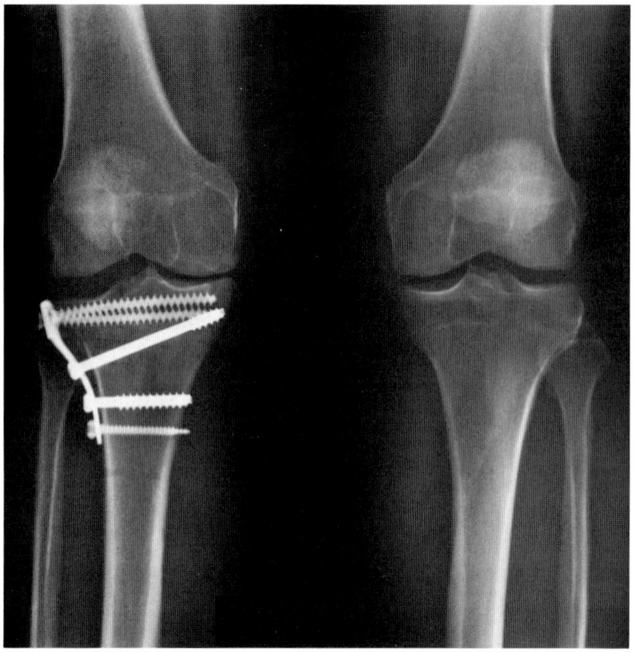
A

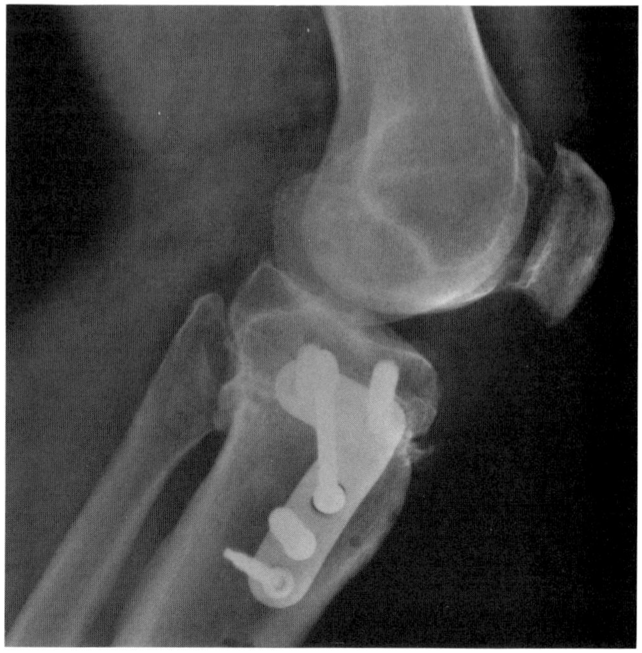
B

FIG. 6-172. Standing AP **(A)** and lateral **(B)** radiographs after right upper tibial osteotomy. Fixation achieved with the L buttress plate. There are two cancellous screws in the upper plate, a central angled short-threaded screw, and distal cancellous and cortical screws.

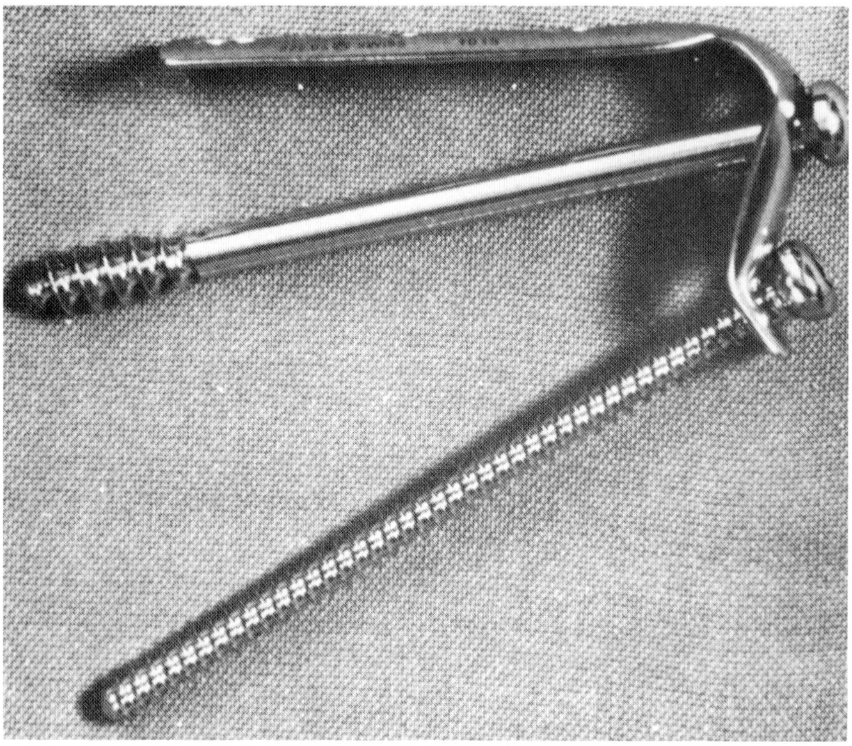
A

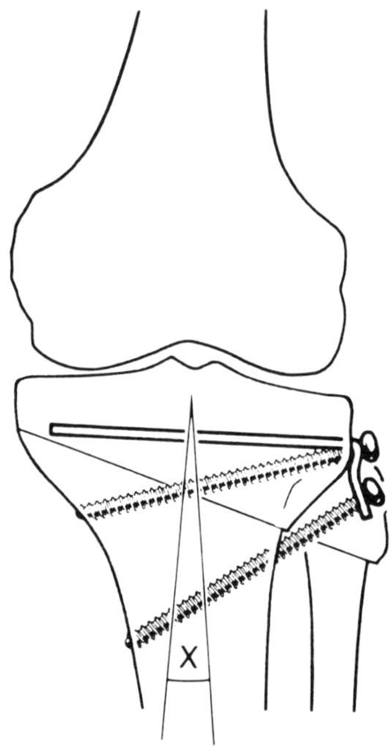

B

FIG. 6-173. A: Five-hole one-half tubular plate prebent between the third and fourth and fourth and fifth holes. Two screws are inserted, with the upper partially threaded screw crossing the osteotomy site and the lower screw entering the tibia below the osteotomy. **B:** The modified plate and screws for fixation after osteotomy corrected by X degrees. (From Miniaci A, Ballmer FT, Ballmer PM, Jakob RP. Proximal tibial osteotomy: a new fixation device. *Clin Orthop* 1989;246:250–259.)

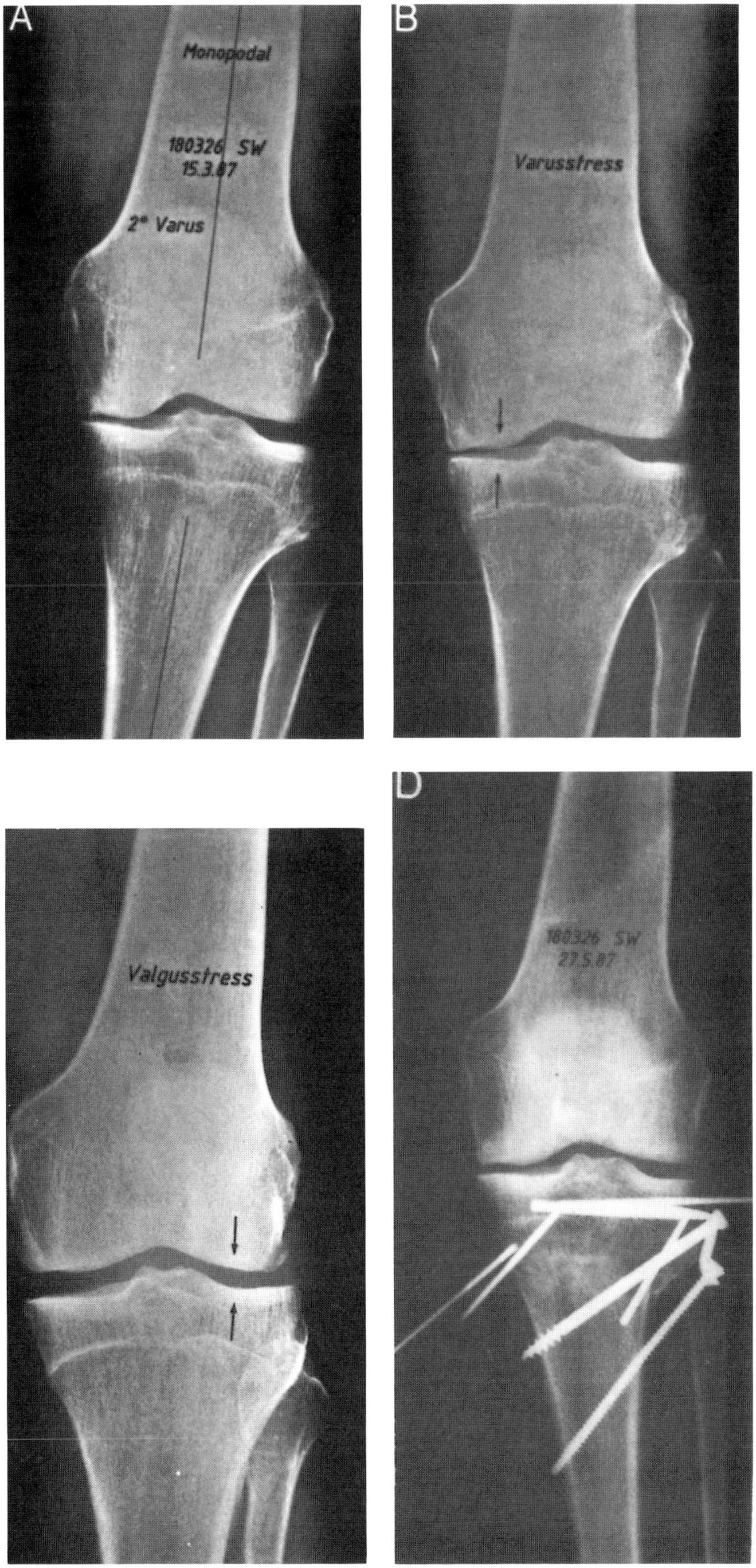

FIG. 6-174. A 61-year-old man with medial joint line pain. **A:** Standing view demonstrating 2° varus deformity and medial compartment narrowing. **B:** Varus stress view demonstrating progressive medial narrowing (*arrows*). **C:** Valgus stress view demonstrating maintenance of the lateral joint space (*arrows*). **D:** Intraoperative radiograph taken to ensure the proper positioning of plate and screws. (See **E** and **F** on next page.)

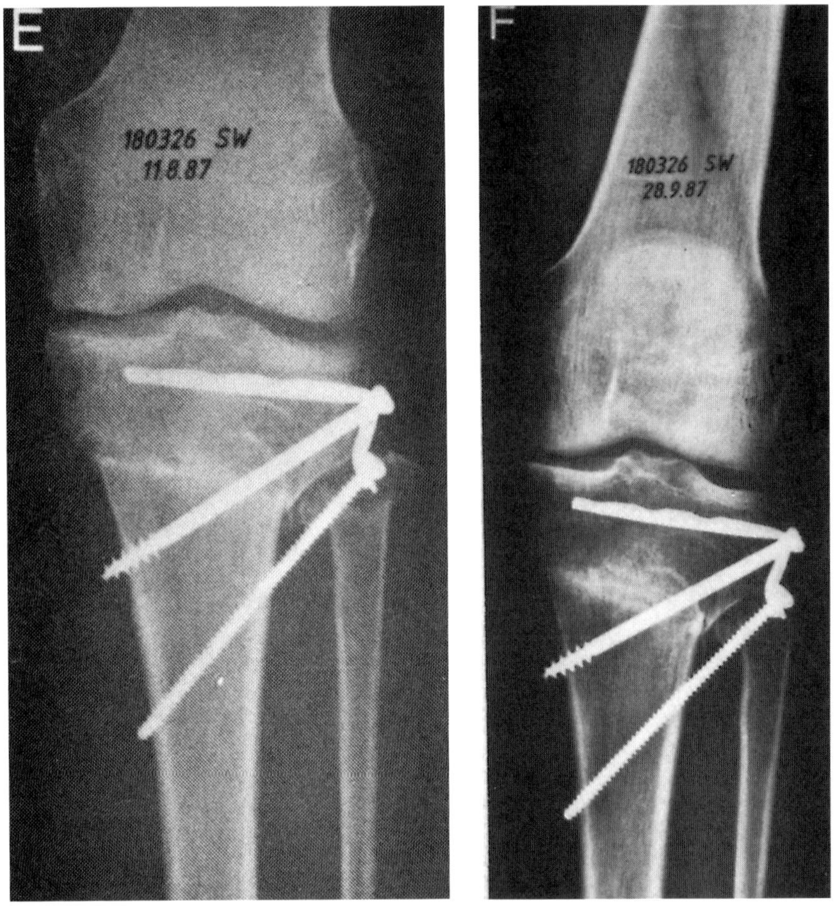

FIG. 6-174. (*Continued.*) **E:** An AP radiograph at 10 weeks postoperatively. **F:** An AP radiograph at 16 weeks. The patient was ambulating and pain free. (From Miniaci A, Ballmer FT, Ballmer PM, Jakob RP. Proximal tibial osteotomy: a new fixation device. *Clin Orthop* 1989;246:250–259.)

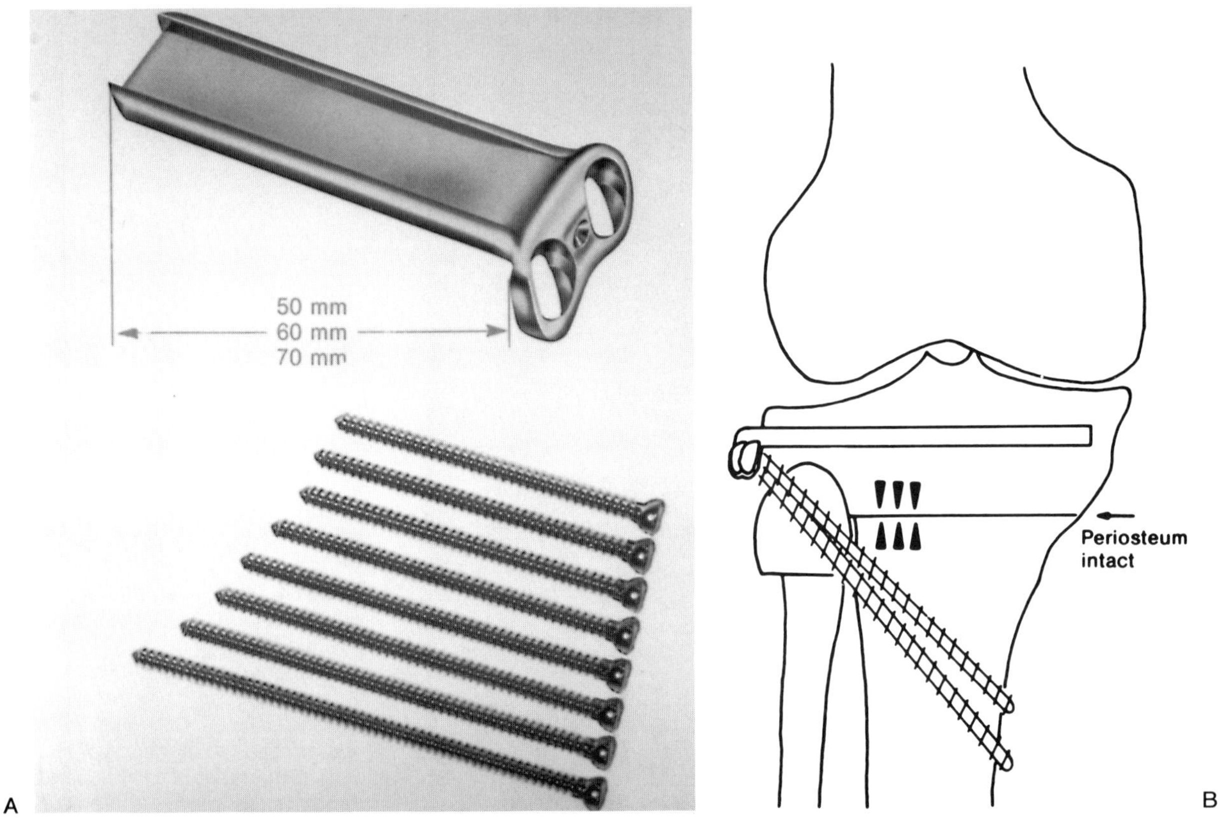

FIG. 6-175. A: The Giebel blade plate and stainless steel screws for osteotomy. **B:** Osteotomy. The periosteum is left intact medially. (Courtesy of Link America, Denville, NJ, and G. Giebel.)[185]

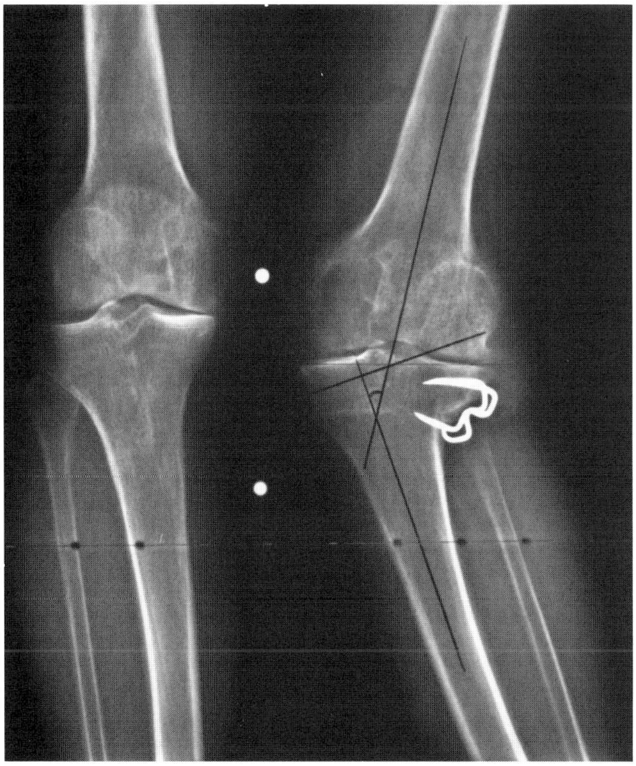

FIG. 6-176. Standing AP views of the knees with an old osteotomy on the left. The correction has been lost, the staples have buckled, and one has partially pulled out.

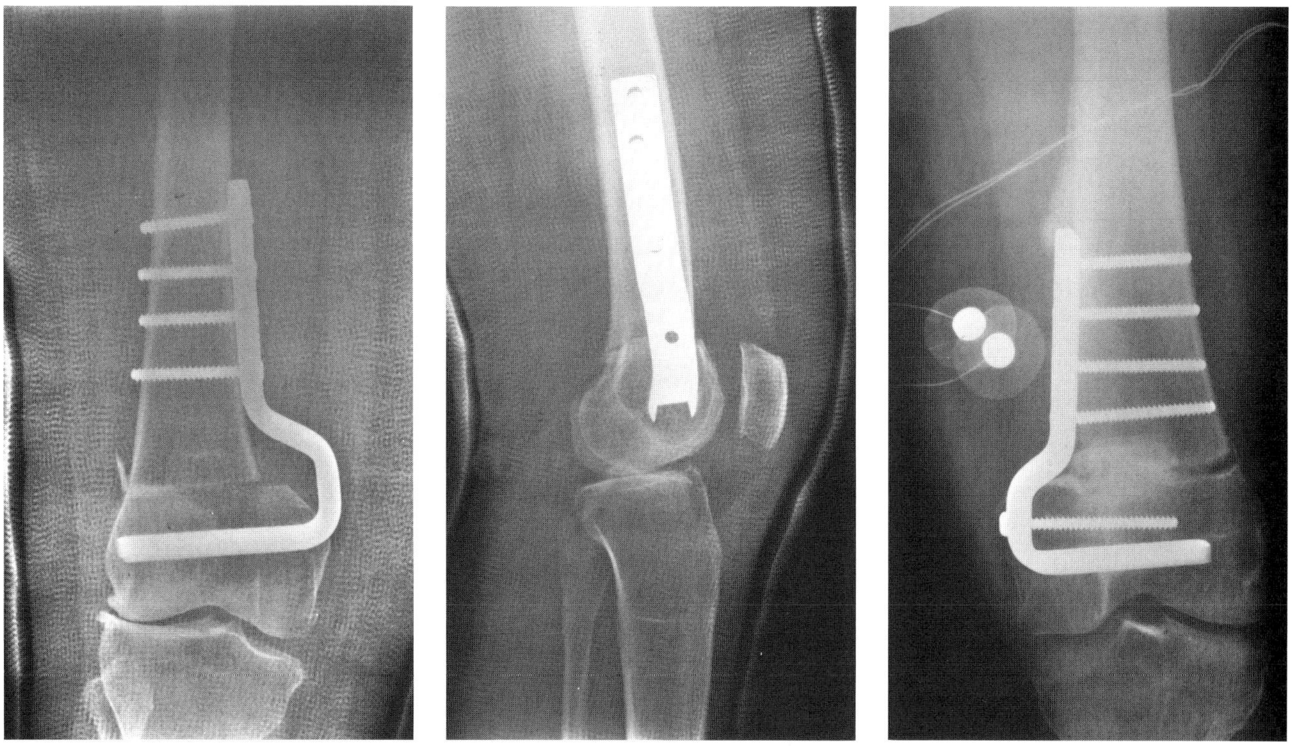

B C

FIG. 6-177. Distal femoral osteotomy with condylar blade plate and four cortical screws for fixation. The AP **(A)** and lateral **(B)** views postoperatively demonstrate the sharply defined osteotomy line. **C,D:** Four months later, the osteotomy fracture is still not healed, and there is widening medially. (See **D** and **E** on next page.)

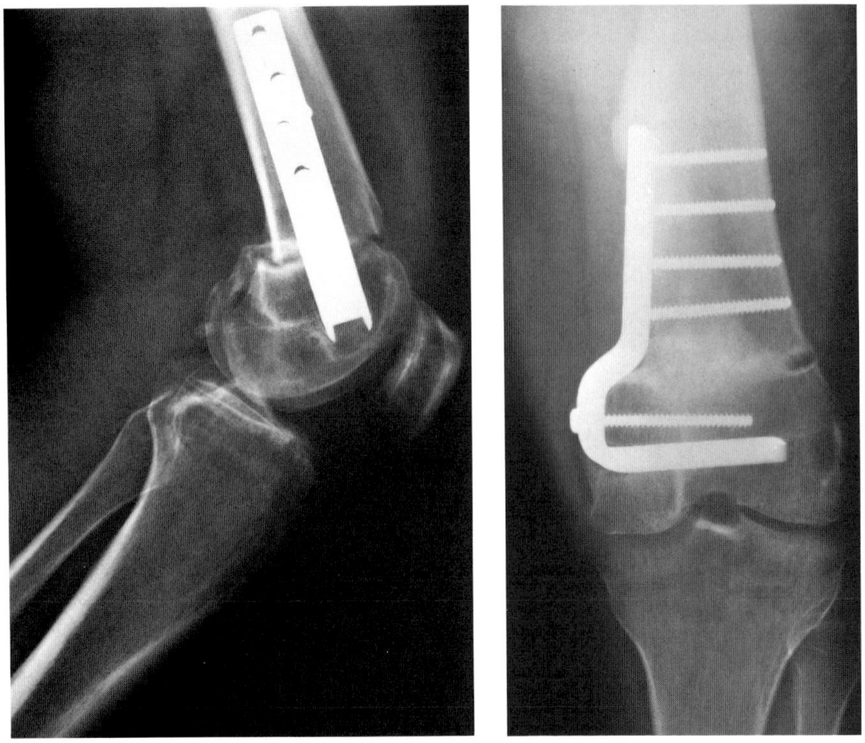

D,E

FIG. 6-177. (*Continued.*) **E:** An AP radiograph at 7 months shows bony union, except at the medial margin.

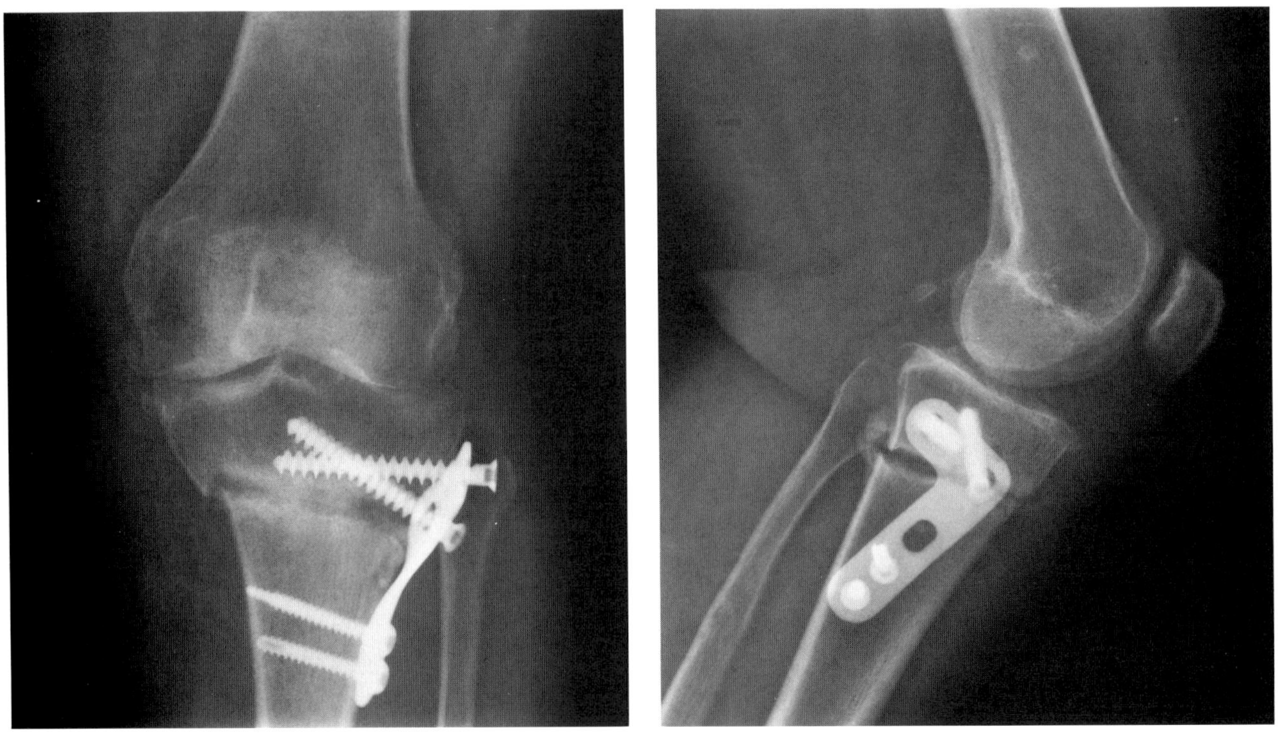

A B

FIG. 6-178. The AP **(A)** and lateral **(B)** radiographs of a nonunion with pull out of the proximal screws. Note the tilted position of the L buttress plate on the lateral view.

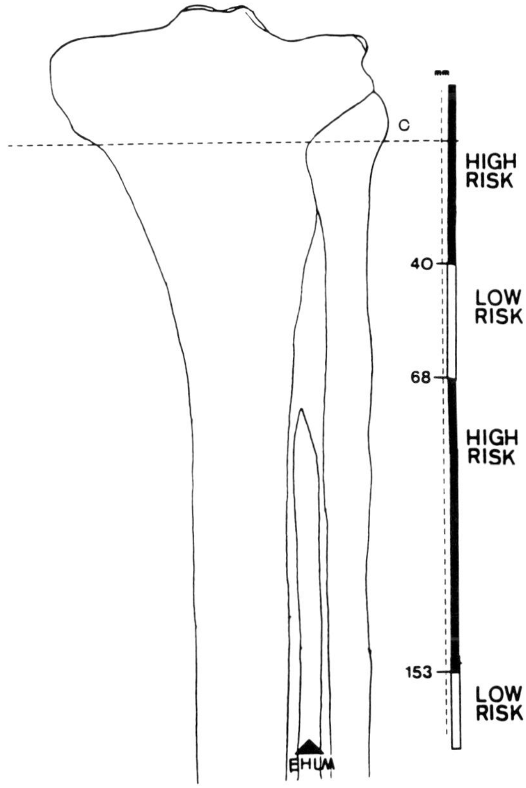

FIG. 6-179. The high-risk zones for intraoperative injury to the peroneal nerve. (From Kirgis A, Albrecht S. Palsy of the deep peroneal nerve after proximal tibial osteotomy. *J Bone Joint Surg* [*Am*] 1992;74A:1180–1185.)

Osteotomy Complications

Osteotomy has been used for years to treat unicompartmental knee arthritis.[183,187] Although most studies demonstrate good results in more than 85% of patients, it is not unusual for the joint to continue to deteriorate.[187] Other complications include a loss of correction (Fig. 6-176), nonunion or delayed union (Figs. 6-177 and/or Fig. 6-178), infection, deep venous thrombosis, and deep peroneal nerve palsy (Fig. 6-179).[183,185,187]

Imaging of most complications can be identified with serial radiographs. Standing AP views, either full-length (hip to ankle) (Fig. 6-176) or standard views, are the most useful for evaluating the loss of correction. Venous complications can be evaluated with sonography or venography. Peroneal nerve injury may be most easily identified.

REFERENCES

Trauma

1. Apple JS, Martinez S, Allen NB, Caldwell DS, Rice JR. Occult fractures of the knee: tomographic evaluation. *Radiology* 1985;148:383–387.
2. Balkfors B. The course of knee-ligament injuries. *Acta Orthop Scand Suppl* 1982;198:1–99.
3. Ballmer PM, Ballmer FT, Jacob RP. Reconstruction of the anterior cruciate ligament alone in the treatment of combined instability with complete rupture of the medial collateral ligament. *Arch Orthop Trauma Surg* 1991;110:139–141.

3a. Barquet A, Massaferro J, Dubra A, Nun F. Ipsilateral open fracture of the femur and tibia treated using the dynamic ASIF-BM tubular external fixation: case reports. *J Trauma* 1991;31:1312–1315.

4. Bernau A, Berquist TH. *Orthopedic positioning in diagnostic radiology.* Baltimore: Urvan and Schwartzenberg; 1983.
5. Berquist TH. *MRI of the musculoskeletal system.* 2nd ed. New York: Raven Press; 1990.
6. Berquist TH. *Imaging of orthopedic trauma.* 2nd ed. New York: Raven Press; 1992.
7. Berquist TH. *Imaging in sports injuries.* Rockville, MD: Aspen Press; 1992.
8. Biyani A, Mathers NC, Sharma JC. Percutaneous tension band wiring for minimally displaced fractures of the patella. *Int Orthop* 1990;14:281–283.
9. Blake R, McBride A. The floating knee: ipsilateral fractures of the tibia and femur. *South Med J* 1975;68:13–16.
10. Boström A. Fractures of the patella. *Acta Orthop Scand Suppl* 1972;143:1–80.
11. Burkhart SS, Peterson HA. Fractures of the proximal tibial epiphysis. *J Bone Joint Surg [Am]* 1979;61A:996–1002.
12. Burri C, Bartzke G, Coldewey J, Muggter E. Fractures of the tibial plateau. *Clin Orthop* 1979;138:84–93.
13. Butler MS, Brumback RJ, Ellison T, Poka A, Bathon GH, Burgess AR. Interlocking nailing for ipsilateral fractures of the femoral shaft and distal part of the femur. *J Bone Joint Surg [Am]* 1991;73A:1492–1502.
14. Cohen SH, Ehrlich GE, Kaufman MS, Cope C. Thrombophlebitis following knee surgery. *J Bone Joint Surg [Am]* 1973;55A:106–112.
15. Curtis MJ. Internal fixation for fractures of the patella. A comparison of two methods. *J Bone Joint Surg [Br]* 1990;72B:280–282.
16. Daffner RH, Tabas JH. Trauma oblique radiographs of the knee. *J Bone Joint Surg [Am]* 1987;69A:568–572.
17. Dahlstedt L, Dalen N, Jonsson U. Goretex prosthetic ligament vs. Kennedy ligament augmentation device in anterior cruciate ligament reconstruction. *Acta Orthop Scand* 1990;61:217–224.
18. Drennan DB, Locher FG, Maylahn DJ. Fractures of the tibial plateau. Treatment by closed reduction and spica cast. *J Bone Joint Surg [Am]* 1979;61A:989–995.
19. Eqund N. The axial view of the patellofemoral joint. *Acta Radiol* 1986;27:101–104.
20. Fairclough JA, Graham GP, Dent CM. Radiologic sign of chronic anterior cruciate ligament deficiency. *Injury* 1990;21:401–402.
21. Fraser RD, Hunter GA, Waddel JP. Ipsilateral fracture of the femur and tibia. *J Bone Joint Surg [Br]* 1978;60B:510–515.
22. Giles JB, DeLee DC, Heckman JD, Keever JE. Supracondylar-intercondylar fractures of the femur treated with a supracondylar plate and lag screw. *J Bone Joint Surg [Am]* 1982;64A:864–870.
23. Hall EM. Radiographic diagnosis and accuracy of knee joint effusions. *Radiology* 1975;115:49–54.
24. Healy WL, Brooker AF. Distal femoral fractures: comparison of open and closed methods of treatment. *Clin Orthop* 1983;174:166–171.
25. Hohl M. Tibial condylar fractures. *J Bone Joint Surg [Am]* 1967;49A:144–1467.
26. Hohl M, Larson RL, Jones DC. Fractures and dislocations of the knee. In: Rockwood CA, Green DP, eds. *Fractures in adults.* 3rd ed. Philadelphia: JB Lippincott; 1992:1429–1591.
27. Hohl M, Luck LV. Fractures of the tibial condyle. A clinical experimental study. *J Bone Joint Surg [Am]* 1956;38A:1001–1018.
28. Holmblad EC. Posteroanterior x-rays of the knee in flexion. *JAMA* 1937;109:1196–1197.
29. Hooper GJ. Radiological assessment of anterior cruciate ligament deficiency. *J Bone Joint Surg [Br]* 1986;68B:292–296.
30. Howell SM, Taylor MA. Failure of reconstruction of the anterior cruciate ligament due to impingement by the intercondylar roof. *J Bone Joint Surg [Am]* 1993;75A:1044–1055.
31. Hughston JC. Subluxation of the patella. *J Bone Joint Surg [Am]* 1968;50A:1003.
32. Inoue M, Shino K, Hirose H, Horibe S, Ono K. Subluxation of the patella: computed tomography analysis of patellofemoral congruence. *J Bone Joint Surg [Am]* 1988;70A:1331–1337.
33. Jacobsen K. Stress radiographic assessment of anteroposterior, medial and lateral stability of the knee joint. *Acta Orthop Scand* 1976;47:335–344.
34. Kaufman SL, Martin LG. Arterial injuries associated with complete dislocation of the knee. *Radiology* 1992;184:153–155.
35. Kumberlin GE. Radiologic assessment of the patellofemoral articulation and subluxation of the patella. *Radiol Technol* 1975;45:129–137.
36. Lachiewicz PF, Funcik T. Factors influencing the results of open reduction and internal fixation of tibial plateau fractures. *Clin Orthop* 1990;259:210–215.
37. Lansinger O, Bergman B, Korner L, Andersson GBJ. Tibial condylar fractures: a twenty year follow-up. *J Bone Joint Surg [Am]* 1986;68A:13–18.
38. Malghem J, Maldaque B. Patellofemoral joint: 30° axial radiograph with lateral rotation of the leg. *Radiology* 1989;170:566–567.
39. Manaster BJ, Remley K, Newman AP, Mann FA. Knee ligament reconstruction: plain film analysis. *AJR Am J Roentgenol* 1988;150:337–342.
40. Merchant AC, Mercark L, Jacobsen RH, Coal CR. Roentgenographic analysis of the patellofemoral congruence. *J Bone Joint Surg* 1974;56:1391–1396.
41. Mooney V, Nickel VL, Harvey JP, Snelson R. Cast-brace treatment for fracture of the distal part of the femur. *J Bone Joint Surg [Am]* 1970;52A:1563–1578.
42. Moore TM. Fracture-dislocation of the knee. *Clin Orthop* 1981;156:128–140.
43. Neer CS, Granthan A, Sheldon ML. Supracondylar fracture of the adult femur. A study of one hundred and ten cases. *J Bone Joint Surg [Am]* 1967;49A:591–613.
44. Polakoff DR, Bucholz RW, Ogden JA. Tension band wiring of displaced tibial tuberosity fractures in adolescents. *Clin Orthop* 1986;209:161–165.
45. Quan-Yi L, Jia-Wen W. Fracture of the patella treated by open reduction and external compressive skeletal fixation. *J Bone Joint Surg [Am]* 1987;69A:83–89.
46. Rand JA, Berquist TH. The knee. In: Berquist TH, ed. *Imaging*

of orthopedic trauma. 2nd ed. New York: Raven Press; 1992:333–432.
47. Rasmussen PS. Tibial condylar fractures. Impairment of knee joint stability as an indication for surgical treatment. *J Bone Joint Surg [Am]* 1973;55A:1331–1350.
48. Ries MD, Meinhard BP. Medial external fixation with lateral plate internal fixation in metaphyseal tibial fractures. *Clin Orthop* 1990;256:215–223.
49. Scapinelli R. Blood supply to the human patella. Its relation to ischemic necrosis after fracture. *J Bone Joint Surg [Br]* 1967;48B:563–570.
50. Schatzker J, Lambert DC. Supracondylar fractures of the femur. *Clin Orthop* 1979;138:77–83.
51. Schatzker J, McBroom R, Bruce D. The tibial plateau fracture. The Toronto experience: 1968–1975. *Clin Orthop* 1979;138:94–104.
52. Seinsheimer F. Fractures of the distal femur. *Clin Orthop* 1980;153:169–180.
53. Shino K, Inoue M, Horibe S, Hamada M, Ono K. Reconstruction of the anterior cruciate ligament using allogenic tendon: long term followup. *Am J Sports Med* 1990;18:457–465.
54. Stewart MJ, Sisk, TD, Wallace SL Jr. Fractures of the distal third of the femur. A comparison treatment method. *J Bone Joint Surg [Am]* 1966;48A:784–807.
55. Stokel EA, Sadasivan KK. Tibial plateau fractures: standardized evaluation of operative results. *Orthopedics* 1991;14:263–270.
56. VanRoay JJAM, Roaymaters ELPD, Daydee HW. Knee ligament injuries combined with ipsilateral tibial and femoral diaphyseal fractures: the "floating knee." *Arch Orthop Trauma Surg* 1991;110:75–77.
57. Waisor RE, Insall JN. Bone-block iliotibial band reconstruction for anterior cruciate insufficiency. *Clin Orthop* 1990;250:197–206.
58. Zickel RE, Fietti VG, Lawsing JF, Cochran GVB. A new intramedullary fixation device for the distal third of the femur. *Clin Orthop* 1977;125:185–191.

Total Knee Arthroplasty

59. Anderson HN, Ernest C, Franndsen PA. Polyethylene failure of metal backed patellar components. *Acta Orthop Scand* 1991;62:1–3.
60. Apel DM, Tozzi JM, Dorr LD. Clinical comparison of all polyethylene and metal-backed tibial components in total knee arthroplasty. *Clin Orthop* 1991;273:243–252.
61. Bauer TW, Saltarelli M, McMahon JT, Wilde AH. Regional dissemination of wear debris from total knee prosthesis. *J Bone Joint Surg [Am]* 1993;75A:106–111.
62. Bengtson S, Knutson K. The infected knee arthroplasty. A 6 year follow-up of 357 cases. *Acta Orthop Scand* 1991;62:301–311.
63. Berquist TH. *Imaging of orthopedic trauma and surgery*. Philadelphia: WB Saunders; 1986.
64. Berquist TH. *MRI of the musculoskeletal system*. 2nd ed. New York: Raven Press; 1990.
65. Bloebaum RD, Rhodes DM, Rubman MH, Hofmann AA. Bilateral tibial components of different cementless designs and materials. *Clin Orthop* 1991;268:179–187.
66. Boyd AD, Ewald FC, Thomas WH, Poss R, Sledge CB. Long-term complications after total knee arthroplasty with or without patellar resurfacing. *J Bone Joint Surg [Am]* 1993;75A:674–681.
67. Brandt KD, Fife RS, Brainstein EM, Katz B. Radiographic grading of the severity of knee osteoarthritis: relation of the Kellgren and Lawrence grade to a grade based on joint space narrowing and correlation with arthroscopic evidence of articular cartilage degeneration. *Arthritis Rheum* 1991;34:1381–1386.
68. Brunker MR, Haddad RJ, Cook SD, Cash JD, James PT, Tan EH. Four year average followup on cemented PCA total knees: clinical and roentgenographic analysis. *Orthopedics* 1990;13:831–837.
69. Bryan RS, Peterson LFA. Polycentric total knee arthroplasty. *Orthop Clin North Am* 1973;4:575–585.
70. Buechel FF, Pappas MJ, Makris G. Evaluation of contact stress on metal-backed patellar replacements. *Clin Orthop* 1991;273:190–197.
71. Burger RR, Basch T, Hopson CN. Implant salvage in infected total knee arthroplasty. *Clin Orthop* 1991;273:105–112.
72. Chan WP, Lang P, Steven MP, Sack K, Majunder S, Stoller DW, Basch C, Genant HK. Osteoarthritis of the knee—comparison of radiography, CT and MR imaging to assess extent and severity. *AJR Am J Roentgenol* 1991;157:799–806.
73. Chestnut WJ. Preoperative diagnostic protocol to predict candidates for unicompartmental arthroplasty. *Clin Orthop* 1991;273:146–150.
74. Christensen OM, Christiansen TJ, Johansen T. Polyethylene failure in a PCA unicompartmental knee prosthesis. *Acta Orthop Scand* 1990;61:578–579.
75. Clayton ML, Thirupathi R. Patellar complications after total condylar arthroplasty. *Clin Orthop* 1982;170:152–155.
76. Cloutier J. Long term results after non-constrained total knee arthroplasty. *Clin Orthop* 1991;273:63–65.
77. Collier JP, Mayor MB, McNamara JL, Surprenant VA, Jensen RE. Analysis of the failure of 122 polyethylene inserts from uncemented tibia components. *Clin Orthop* 1991;273:232–242.
78. Collins DN, Heim SA, Nelson CL, Smith P III. Porous coated anatomic total knee arthroplasty. *Clin Orthop* 1991;267:128–136.
79. Cooke DTV, Collins A, Wevers HW. Failure of a knee prosthesis accelerated by shedding of beads from the porous metal surface. *Clin Orthop* 1990;258:204–208.
80. Cordeiro EN, Costa RC, Carazzato JG, Silva JD. Periprosthetic fracture in patients with total knee arthroplasties. *Clin Orthop* 1990;252:182–189.
81. Coventry MB. Upper tibial osteotomy. *Clin Orthop* 1984;182:46–52.
82. Cuckler JM, Star AM, Alavi A, Noto RB. Diagnosis and management of infected total joint arthroplasty. *Orthop Clin North Am* 1991;22:523–530.
83. Davis PF, Bocell JR, Tullos HS. Dissociation of the tibial component in total knee arthroplasty. *Clin Orthop* 1991;272:199–204.
84. Dood CAF, Hungerford DS, Krackow KA. Total knee arthroplasty fixator: comparison of early results of paired cemented versus uncemented porous coated anatomic knee prosthesis. *Clin Orthop* 1990;260:66–70.
85. Elia EA, Lotke PA. Results of revision total knee arthroplasty associated with significant bone loss. *Clin Orthop* 1991;271:114–121.
86. Ewald FC, Jacobs MA, Miegel RE, et al. Kinematic total knee replacement. *J Bone Joint Surg [Am]* 1984;66A:1032–1040.
87. Friedman RJ, Block J, Galante JO, Jacobs JJ, Skinner HB. The current concepts in orthopedics biomaterials and implant fixation. *J Bone Joint Surg [Am]* 1993;75A:1086–1109.
88. Gill ES, Mills DM. Long-term follow-up evaluation of 1,000 consecutive cemented total knee arthroplasties. *Clin Orthop* 1991;273:66–76.
89. Gilula LA, Staple TW. Radiology of recently developed total knee prosthesis. *Radiol Clin North Am* 1975;13:57–66.
90. Grace JN, Rand JA. Patellar instability after total knee arthroplasty. *Clin Orthop* 1988;230:168.
91. Grace JN, Sun FH. Fracture of the patella after total knee arthroplasty. *Clin Orthop* 1988;230:168–175.
92. Groh GI, Porter J, Elliott J, Pear AJ. Results of total knee arthroplasty using the posterior stabilized condylar prosthesis. *Clin Orthop* 1991;269:58–62.
93. Gross TP, Lennon DW. Osteolytic cyst-like area associated with polyethylene and metallic debris after total knee replacement with an uncemented Vitallium prosthesis. *J Bone Joint Surg [Am]* 1992;74A:1096–1102.
94. Haynes DR, Rogers SD, Hay S, Pearcy MJ, Howie DW. The differences in toxicity and release of bone resorbing mediators induced by titanium and cobalt-chromium alloy wear particles. *J Bone Joint Surg [Am]* 1993;75A:825–834.
95. Hodge A, Chandler HP. Unicompartmental knee replacement: a comparison of constrained and unconstrained designs. *J Bone Joint Surg [Am]* 1992;74A:877–882.
96. Hofmann AA, Murdock LE, Wyatt RWB, Alpert JP. Total knee arthroplasty: two-four year experience using an asymmetric tibial

tray and a deep trochlear-grooved femoral component. *Clin Orthop* 1991;269:78–88.

97. Hofmann AA, Wyatt RWB, Beck SW, Alpert J. Cementless total knee arthroplasty in patients over 65 years old. *Clin Orthop* 1991;271:28–34.
98. Hohl WM, Crawfurd E, Zelicof SB, Ewald FC. The total condylar knee prosthesis in complex knee reconstruction. *Clin Orthop* 1991;273:91–97.
99. Hue FC, Fitzgerald RH Jr. Hinged total knee arthroplasty. *J Bone Joint Surg [Am]* 1990;65A:513–519.
100. Hungerford DS, Krackow KA. Total joint arthroplasty of the knee. *Clin Orthop* 1985;192:23–33.
101. Hungerford DS, Krackow KA, Kenna RV. Two to five year experience with cementless porous-coated total knee prosthesis. In: Rand JA, Dorr LD, eds. *Proceedings of the Knee Society*. Rockville, MD: Aspen Publishing; 1986:215–235.
102. Insall JN, Dorr LD, Scott RD, Scott WN. Rationale of the Knee Society clinical grading system. *Clin Orthop* 1989;248:13–14.
103. Insall JN, Kelly M. The total condylar prosthesis. *Clin Orthop* 1986;205:43–48.
104. Insall JN, Lachiewicz PF, Barstein AH. The posterior stabilized condylar prosthesis. A modification of the total condylar design. *J Bone Joint Surg [Am]* 1982;64A:1317–1323.
105. Insall JN, Scott WN, Ranawat CS. The total condylar knee prosthesis. *J Bone Joint Surg [Am]* 1979;61A:173–180.
106. Insall JN, Tria AJ, Scott, WN. The total condylar knee prosthesis. The first five years. *Clin Orthop* 1979;145:68–77.
107. Kaiser AD, Whileside LA. The effect of screws and pegs on the initial fixation stability of an uncemented unicondylar knee replacement. *Clin Orthop* 1990;259:169–178.
108. Kantor SG, Schneider R, Insall JN, Becker MW. Radionuclide imaging of asymptomatic versus symptomatic total knee arthroplasties. *Clin Orthop* 1990;260:118–123.
109. Kershaw CJ, Therman AEG. The Attenborough knee. A four to ten year review. *J Bone Joint Surg [Br]* 1988;70B:89–93.
110. Kilgus DJ, Funahaski AM, Campbell PA. Massive femoral osteolysis and early disintegration of a polyethylene-bearing surface of a total knee replacement. *J Bone Joint Surg [Am]* 1992;74A:770–774.
111. Kim Y. Incidence of deep vein thrombosis after cementless and cemented knee replacement. *J Bone Joint Surg [Br]* 1990;72B:779–783.
112. Koshino T, Morii T, Wada J, Takahaski S. Unicompartmental replacement with the Marmor modular knee operative procedure and results. *Bull Hosp Jt Dis Orthop Inst* 1991;51:119–131.
113. Kraay MJ, Meyers SA, Goldberg VM, Figgie HE, Conroy PA. "Hybrid" total knee arthroplasty with the Miller-Galante prosthesis. *Clin Orthop* 1991;273:32–41.
114. Krugluger J, Zenz P, Parzer R, Jantsch S, Hackel H. Long term analysis of Sheehan total knee arthroplasty. *Int Orthop* 1991;15:149–154.
115. Larson KR, Cracchiolo A III, Dorey FJ, Finerman GAM. Total knee arthroplasty in patients after patellectomy. *Clin Orthop* 1991;264:243–254.
116. Lee JG, Keating EM, Ritter MA, Faris PM. Review of the all polyethylene tibial component in total knee arthroplasty. *Clin Orthop* 1990;260:87–92.
117. Lettin AWF, Kavanagh TG, Grary D, Scales JT. Assessment of survival and clinical results of Stanmore total knee replacement. *J Bone Joint Surg [Br]* 1984;66B:355–361.
118. Lewallen DG, Bryan RS, Peterson LFA. Polycentric total knee arthroplasty. A 10 year follow-up study. *J Bone Joint Surg [Am]* 1984;66A:1211–1218.
119. Lundstrand A, Ryd L, Stenström A. Polyethylene failure in two total knees. *Acta Orthop Scand* 1990;61:575–577.
120. Lovelock JE, Griffiths HJ, Silverstein AM, Anson PS. Complications of total knee replacement. *AJR Am J Roentgenol* 1984;141:985–992.
121. Mazas FB. The GUEPAR Group: Guepar total knee prosthesis. *Clin Orthop* 1973;94:211–221.
122. Melhoff MA, Sledge CB, Bender CE. Comparison of cemented and cementless hip and knee replacements. *Arthritis Rheum* 1990;33:293–297.
123. Merkel KD, Brown ML, Decranjee MK, Fitzgerald RH. Comparison of indium labeled leukocyte imaging with sequential technetium gallium scanning in the diagnosis of low grade musculoskeletal sepsis. *J Bone Joint Surg [Am]* 1985;67A:465–476.
124. Merkel KD, Johnson EW. Supracondylar fracture of the femur after total knee arthroplasty. *J Bone Joint Surg [Am]* 1986;68A:29–43.
125. Merkow RL, Soundry M, Insall JN. Patellar dislocation following total knee replacement. *J Bone Joint Surg [Am]* 1985;67A:1321–1327.
126. Milliano MT, Whiteside L. Articular surface material effect on metal-backed patellar components. *Clin Orthop* 1991;273:204–214.
127. Moran CG, Purdei IM, Lees TA, Midwinter MJ. Survivorship of the uncemented porous-coated anatomic knee replacement. *J Bone Joint Surg [Am]* 1991;73A:848–857.
128. Moreland JR, Hanker GJ. Lower extremity axial alignment in males. In: Dorr LD, ed. *The knee. Papers of the first scientific meeting of the Knee Society*. 1985.
129. Morrey BF. *Joint replacement arthroplasty*. New York: Churchill Livingstone; 1991.
130. Morrey BF, Adams RA, Ilstrup DM, Bryan RS. Complications and mortality associated with bilateral and unilateral total knee arthroplasty. *J Bone Joint Surg [Am]* 1987;69A:484–488.
131. Nichols SJ, Landon GG, Tullos HS. Arthrodesis with dual plates after failed total knee arthroplasty. *J Bone Joint Surg [Am]* 1991;73A:1020–1024.
132. Outerbridge RE. Etiology of chondromalacia patella. *J Bone Joint Surg [Br]* 1961;43B:752–757.
133. Palestro CJ, Swyer AJ, Kim CK, Goldsmith SJ. Infected knee prosthesis: diagnosis with In-111 leukocyte, Tc-99m sulfur colloid and Tc-99m MDP imaging. *Radiology* 1991;179:645–648.
134. Patel DV, Aichroth PM, Wand JS. Posteriorly stabilized (Insall-Burstein) total condylar knee arthroplasty. *Int Orthop* 1991;15:211–218.
135. Patel DV, Ferris BD, Aichroth PM. Radiologic study of alignment after total knee replacement. *Int Orthop* 1991;15:209–210.
136. Peters PC, Engh GA, Dwyer KA, Vink TN. Osteolysis after total knee arthroplasty without cement. *J Bone Joint Surg [Am]* 1992;74A:864–876.
137. Peterson LFA. Current status of total knee arthroplasty. *Arch Surg* 1977;112:1099–1104.
138. Piraino D, Richmond D, Freed H, Belhobehl G, Schils J, Stulberg B. Total knee replacement: radiologic findings in failure of porous-coated metal backed patellar component. *AJR Am J Roentgenol* 1990;155:555–558.
139. Rand JA. Alternatives to reimplantation for salvage of total knee arthroplasty complicated by infection. *J Bone Joint Surg [Am]* 1993;75A:282–288.
140. Rand JA. Bone deficiency in total knee arthroplasty. Use of metal augmentation wedge. *Clin Orthop* 1991;271:63–71.
141. Rand JA. Selection of the prosthesis. In: Morrey BF, ed. *Joint replacement arthroplasty*. New York: Churchill Livingstone; 1991:981–988.
142. Rand JA. Unicemented TKA: results. In: Berquist TH, ed. *Imaging of orthopedic trauma and surgery*. Philadelphia: WB Saunders; 1986:1021–1027.
143. Rand JA. Revision total knee arthroplasty. In: Berquist TH, ed. *Imaging of orthopedic trauma and surgery*. Philadelphia: WB Saunders; 1986:1093–1112.
144. Rand JA, Bergman NR. Cemented total knee arthroplasty: results. In: Berquist TH, ed. *Imaging of orthopedic trauma and surgery*. Philadelphia: WB Saunders; 1986:1007–1019.
145. Rand JA, Berquist TH. The knee. In: Berquist TH, ed. *Imaging of orthopedic trauma and surgery*. Philadelphia: WB Saunders; 1986:293–391.
146. Rand JA, Brown ML. The value of indium 111 leukocyte scanning in the evaluation of painful or infected total knee arthroplasties. *Clin Orthop* 1990;259:179–182.
147. Rand JA, Chao EYS, Stauffer RN. Kinematic rotating-hinge total knee arthroplasty. *J Bone Joint Surg [Am]* 1987;69A:489–497.
148. Rand JA, Coventry MB. Ten year evaluation of geometric total knee arthroplasty. *Clin Orthop* 1988;232:168–173.
149. Rand JA, Ilustrup DM. Survivorship analysis of total knee arthroplasty. Cumulative rates of survival for 9,200 total knee arthroplasties. *J Bone Joint Surg [Am]* 1991;73A:397–409.
150. Rorabeck CH, Bourne RB, Lewis PL, Nott L. The Miller-Galante

knee prosthesis for treatment of osteoarthritis. *J Bone Joint Surg [Am]* 1993;75A:402–408.
151. Rosenberg AG, Barden RM, Galante JO. Cemented and ingrowth fixation of the Miller-Galante prosthesis. Clinical and roentgenographic comparison after 3-6 year follow-up studies. *Clin Orthop* 1990;260:71–79.
152. Rosenberg AG, Verner JJ, Galante JO. Clinical results of total knee revision using the total condylar III prosthesis. *Clin Orthop* 1991;273:89–90.
153. Rosenberg AG, Paulos LE, Parker RD, Coward DB, Scott SM. The forty-five degree posteroanterior flexion weight bearing radiograph of the knee. *J Bone Joint Surg [Am]* 1988;70A:1479–1482.
154. Rosenquist R, Bylander B, Knutson K, Rydholm U, Rööser B, Eqund N, Lidgren L. Loosening of porous coating of bicompartmental prostheses in patients with rheumatoid arthritis. *J Bone Joint Surg [Am]* 1986;68A:538–542.
155. Ryd L, Lindstrand A, Stenström A, Selvick G. Porous coated anatomic tricompartmental tibial components. *Clin Orthop* 1991;251:189–197.
156. Sambatakakis A, Wilton TJ, Newton G. Radiographic signs of persistent soft tissue imbalance after knee replacement. *J Bone Joint Surg [Br]* 1991;73B:751–756.
157. Samuelson K, Nelson L. An all-polyethylene cementless tibial component. A 5 to 9 year follow-up study. *Clin Orthop* 1990;260: 93–97.
158. Schneider R, Abenovoli AM, Soundry M, Insall J. Failure of total condylar knee replacement. Correlation of radiographic clinical and surgical findings. *Radiology* 1984;152:309–315.
159. Schneider R, Goldman AB, Insall JN. Knee prosthesis. *Semin Roentgenol* 1986;21:29–46.
160. Scott RD, Cobb AG, McQueary FG, Thornhill TS. Unicompartmental knee arthroplasty. Eight to twelve year follow-up evaluation with survivorship analysis. *Clin Orthop* 1991;271:96–100.
161. Scott RD, Santore RF. Unicondylar unicompartmental replacement for osteoarthritis of the knee. *J Bone Joint Surg* 1981;63: 536–544.
162. Seligson D, Popharn GJ, Voos K, Henry SL, Faghri M. Antibiotic-leaking from polymethyl methacrylate beads. *J Bone Joint Surg [Am]* 1993;75A:714–720.
163. Shemagaki H, Bechtold JE, Sherman RE, Gustilo RB. Stability of initial fixation of the tibial component in cementless total knee arthroplasty. *J Orthop Res* 1990;8:64–71.
164. Shiers L. Arthroplasty of the knee. Preliminary report of a new method. *J Bone Joint Surg [Br]* 1954;36B:553–560.
165. Shindell R, Neumann R, Connolly JF, Jordon OM. Evaluation of the Noiles hinged knee prosthesis. A 5 year study of 17 knees. *J Bone Joint Surg [Am]* 1986;68A:579–586.
166. Staehli JW, Cass JR, Morrey BF. Condylar total knee arthroplasty after failed proximal tibial osteotomy. *J Bone Joint Surg [Am]* 1987;69A:28–31.
167. Stern SH, Insall JN. Posterior stabilized prosthesis. Results after follow-up of nine to 12 years. *J Bone Joint Surg [Am]* 1992;74A: 980–986.
168. Stockley L, Douglas DL, Elson RA. Bicondylar St. Georg Sledge knee arthroplasty. *Clin Orthop* 1990;225:228–234.
169. Stuart MJ. Indications and patient selection. In: Morrey BF, ed. *Joint replacement arthroplasty.* New York: Churchill Livingstone; 1991:971–979.
170. Stuart MJ, Rand JA. Total knee arthroplasty in young adults who have rheumatoid arthritis. *J Bone Joint Surg [Am]* 1988;70A:84–87.
171. Stuckin SA, Ruoff M, Matarese W. Cementless total knee arthroplasty in patients with inflammatory arthritis and compromised bone. *Clin Orthop* 1991;273:42–51.
172. Tateishi H, Maraoka T, Yoh K, Iwata Y, Futani H, Yamada H, Maruo S. A long term follow-up study in unicompartmental replacement with a Marmor knee prosthesis and the introduction of a new ceramic prosthesis. *Bull Hosp Jt Dis Orthop Inst* 1991;51:132–139.
173. Teewy SM, Krackow KA, Hungerford DS, Jones M. Primary total knee arthroplasty in patients with severe varus deformity. *Clin Orthop* 1991;273:19–31.
174. Tsao A, Mintz L, McRae CR, Stulberg D, Wright T. Failure of the porous-coated anatomic prosthesis in total knee arthroplasty due to severe polyethylene wear. *J Bone Joint Surg [Am]* 1993;75A:19–26.
175. Tooms RE, Harkness JW. Arthroplasty: introduction and overview. In: Crenshaw AH, ed. *Campbell's operative orthopedics.* 8th ed. Vol. 1. St. Louis: CV Mosby; 1992:371–387.
176. Walldius B. Arthroplasty of the knee using an endoprosthesis. *Acta Orthop Scand* 1960;30:137–148.
177. Weissman BN, Scott RD, Brick GW, Carson JM. Radiographic detection of metal-induced synovitis as a complication of arthroplasty of the knee. *J Bone Joint Surg [Am]* 1991;73A:1002–1007.
178. Whiteside LA. The effect of patient age, gender, and tibial component fixation or pain relief after cementless total knee arthroplasty. *Clin Orthop* 1991;271:21–27.
179. Wilson MG, Kelley K, Thornhill TS. Infection as a complication of total knee-replacement arthroplasty. *J Bone Joint Surg [Am]* 1990;72A:878–883.
180. Windsor RE. Management of total knee arthroplasty infection. *Orthop Clin North Am* 1991;22:531–537.
181. Wright J, Ewald FC, Walter PS, Thomas WH, Poso R, Sledge CB. Total knee arthroplasty with the Kinematic prosthesis. *J Bone Joint Surg [Am]* 1990;72A:1003–1009.
182. Young HH. Use of a hinged Vitallium prosthesis for arthroplasty of the knee: a preliminary report. *J Bone Joint Surg [Am]* 1963;45A:1627–1642.

Miscellaneous Procedures

183. Coventry MB. Upper tibial osteotomy. *Clin Orthop* 1984;182: 46–52.
184. Coventry MB. Proximal tibial varus osteotomy for osteoarthritis of the lateral compartment of the knee. *J Bone Joint Surg [Am]* 1987;69A:32–38.
185. Giebel G, Tscherne H, Daiber M. Tibial head osteotomy in the treatment of arthrosis of the knee. *Orthopade* 1985;14:144–153.
186. Kirgis A, Albrecht S. Palsy of the deep peroneal nerve after proximal tibial osteotomy. *J Bone Joint Surg [Am]* 1992;74A:1180–1185.
187. Miniaci A, Ballmer FT, Ballmer PM, Jakob RP. Proximal tibial osteotomy: a new fixation device. *Clin Orthop* 1989;246:250–259.

Imaging Atlas of Orthopedic Appliances and Prostheses,
edited by T.H. Berquist.
Mayo Clinic Foundation © 1995.
Published by Raven Press, Ltd., New York.

CHAPTER 7

The Tibial Shaft

Jerald H. Pietan, Mark P. Brodersen, and Thomas H. Berquist

Fractures and fixation for the knee and upper tibia were discussed in Chapter 6, and fractures of the distal tibia and plafond are discussed in Chapter 8. This section concentrates on fixation devices for the tibial and fibular shafts.

FRACTURES

Fractures of the shafts of the tibia and fibula are common long bone fractures. These injuries account for more days lost from school or work annually in the United States than do any other long bone fractures.[40] The treatment of tibial and fibular fractures is similar; therefore, we refer primarily to the tibia.

The lower leg is the most common site of combined bone and soft tissue injury.[29] The relatively exposed subcutaneous location of the tibial shaft makes it vulnerable to direct high-energy forces, such as those associated with motor vehicle accidents or gunshot wounds, which frequently result in severe soft tissue damage with tibial and fibular comminution that produce difficult orthopedic challenges. The complexity of these fractures has fostered advocates for a variety of treatment methods.[46,47,51,56,57,65] Direct trauma fractures can be transverse, segmental, or comminuted; indirect injuries are usually oblique or spiral. These indirect injuries usually result from falls or injuries in which the foot is fixed. The fibula can remain intact; however, the greater the injury force is, the greater is the likelihood that both the tibia and fibula will be fractured.[7,11,51] Fractures should be described according to the (1) precise anatomic location, (2) pattern of the fracture line, (3) position of the fragments, (4) degree of comminution, and (5) open or closed nature of the fracture.[7]

Fractures are more common in the middle and distal third of the tibial shaft.[7,51] Distal tibial fractures may extend into the tibial plafond and are discussed in Chapter 8.

Classification

The current treatment of tibial fractures includes both operative and nonoperative methods. The treatment choice is based on the type of fracture, the medical condition of the patient, and the experience of the orthopedic surgeon.[7,10,16,39,56,65] Many classification methods have been developed that aid the orthopedic surgeon in management decisions and fracture prognosis.

Soft tissue injuries may be associated with open and closed tibial fractures. The degree of soft tissue injury influences the selection of fixation devices for management.[3,32,33,39,51,56,61] The classifications based on the severity of soft tissue damage include the following.

1. In the Muller[56] classification, grade I fractures are compounded from within, with minimal soft tissue damage. Grade II fractures are compounded from without; the soft tissue injury is much less severe than the degree of bone injury. Grade III fractures are comminuted, with extensive skin and muscle damage.
2. The Gustilo and Anderson[32] classification is similar but further subdivides grade III injuries because of the significant differences in prognosis.[14] Grade IIIA injuries have adequate residual soft tissue coverage. Grade IIIB injuries are more severe with periosteal stripping, bone exposure, and extensive contamination. With grade IIIC, there is arterial injury requiring repair. The incidence of nonunion increases from 27% to 43% when the injuries increase from grade

J. H. Pietan and T. H. Berquist: Mayo Medical School and Department of Diagnostic Radiology, Mayo Clinic Jacksonville, Jacksonville, Florida 32224.

M. P. Brodersen: Mayo Medical School and Department of Orthopedic Surgery, Mayo Clinic Jacksonville, Jacksonville, Florida 32224.

IIIA to grade IIIB. Amputations may be indicated in up to 25% of grade IIIB open fractures. Nonunion is the rule, and infection rates reach 57%. Amputations are eventually required in 78% of grade IIIC open fractures.[14,15]
3. Tscherne and Gotzen[69] classified soft tissue injuries associated with closed fractures. This classification progresses from grade 0 (absent or negligible soft tissue damage) to grade III (extensively contused or crushed soft tissue, including major vascular rupture) and is helpful in treatment decisions in regard to closed fractures.[61]

There are other osseous classifications that aid in the management decisions and in determining the prognosis.

Ellis[25] classified tibial fractures based on severity (Fig. 7-1). A fracture of minor severity is undisplaced and not angulated and involves only a minor degree of comminution or a minor open wound. One of moderate severity is complete displacement or angulation, with a small degree of comminution or a minor open wound. One of major severity involves a major comminution or a major open, wound with total displacement of the fracture. Ellis found that bony union occurred at approximately 10 weeks in a fracture of minor severity; 15 weeks, in moderate; and 23 weeks, in major severity, with delayed union rate rising from 2% in minor and 11% in moderate to 60% in the major severity group.[26]

The Nicoll[58] classification, based on the most significant factors affecting union, is helpful to determine the prognosis in the closed treatment of tibial fractures. The factors are (1) initial displacement; (2) comminution; and (3) associated soft tissue wounds, infection, and distraction. These parameters are graded from moderate to severe or nil to slight. With this system, the outcome of any type of tibial fracture could be reasonably predicted. In his series of 705 patients (674 treated conservatively), the incidence of delayed union or nonunion varied from 9% in the most favorable type to 39% in the least favorable.

Johner and Wruhs[44] developed a classification based on the morphology of the fracture (Fig. 7-2). The factors that influence the treatment, prognosis, and outcome are the (1) mechanics of the accident, (2) degree of comminution, (3) displacement of the fracture, and (4) open or closed nature of the fracture. They found that displacement was not a reliable criterion and that the fracture pattern was the most important factor in the prognosis. The classification by fracture morphology has approximately the same prognostic importance as the classification into open or closed fractures. Spiral fractures, regardless of the degree of comminution, have less local complications and no poor final results; bending nonspiral fractures have the worst prognosis. Spiral fractures are caused by indirect forces; nonspiral bending fractures involve crush injuries, with varying degrees of soft tissue injury.

Preoperative Imaging

Standard routine views of the tibia and fibula include anteroposterior (AP) and lateral projections (Fig. 7-3). Soft tissues of the leg, knee, and ankle must be included on the films to evaluate possible associated injuries. Oblique projections can give additional information about the fracture's rotation and alignment.[7]

Additional imaging techniques are usually not required. Computed tomography (CT) may be helpful in certain spiral fractures.[28,49] Magnetic resonance imaging (MRI) may be indicated to evaluate soft tissue interposition or injury.[8] Angiography or MRI may be helpful to evaluate vascular injury.[7,35]

Treatment Options

The basic principles of fracture management include the (1) maintenance or restoration of functional length, (2) restoration of normal weight-bearing alignment, (3) preservation of soft tissue, and (4) adjustment of the treatment to fit the fracture.[14]

The goal of fracture management is acceptable reduction.[51] This means good alignment and rotation as nearly perfect as possible. The ankle and knee joints must be parallel. Russell et al.[63] sets goals of 5% for varus or valgus angulation (Fig. 7-4), 10% for anterior and posterior angulation, 10% or less for rotation, and 1 cm or less for length discrepancy.

Tibial fractures can be managed by a variety of reduction methods.[51,63,70] With any fracture, orthopedic surgeons use the method of reduction and immobilization that has proved satisfactory in their experience.[10,17,21,39,67] The treatment choices are (1) closed reduction with cast or brace immobilization, (2) external fixation, (3) intramedullary nailing techniques, and (4) open reduction with internal fixation.

Closed Reduction with Cast or Brace Immobilization

Most tibial shaft fractures are managed by closed reduction and cast application.[63] There are various casting techniques; long leg casts with 0% to 5% knee flexion are frequently used. Patellar-tendon-bearing (PTB) below-the-knee casts, as described by Sarmiento,[65] are also commonly used (Fig. 7-5). Early weight bearing is important in the treatment of these fractures.[65]

Advantages[63,65]

- Early weight bearing, which is important to minimize hospitalization and stimulate bone healing
- Avoids exposure to the risk of infection by surgery or pin insertion
- Avoids the need for sophisticated equipment or implants

(*text continues on page 547*)

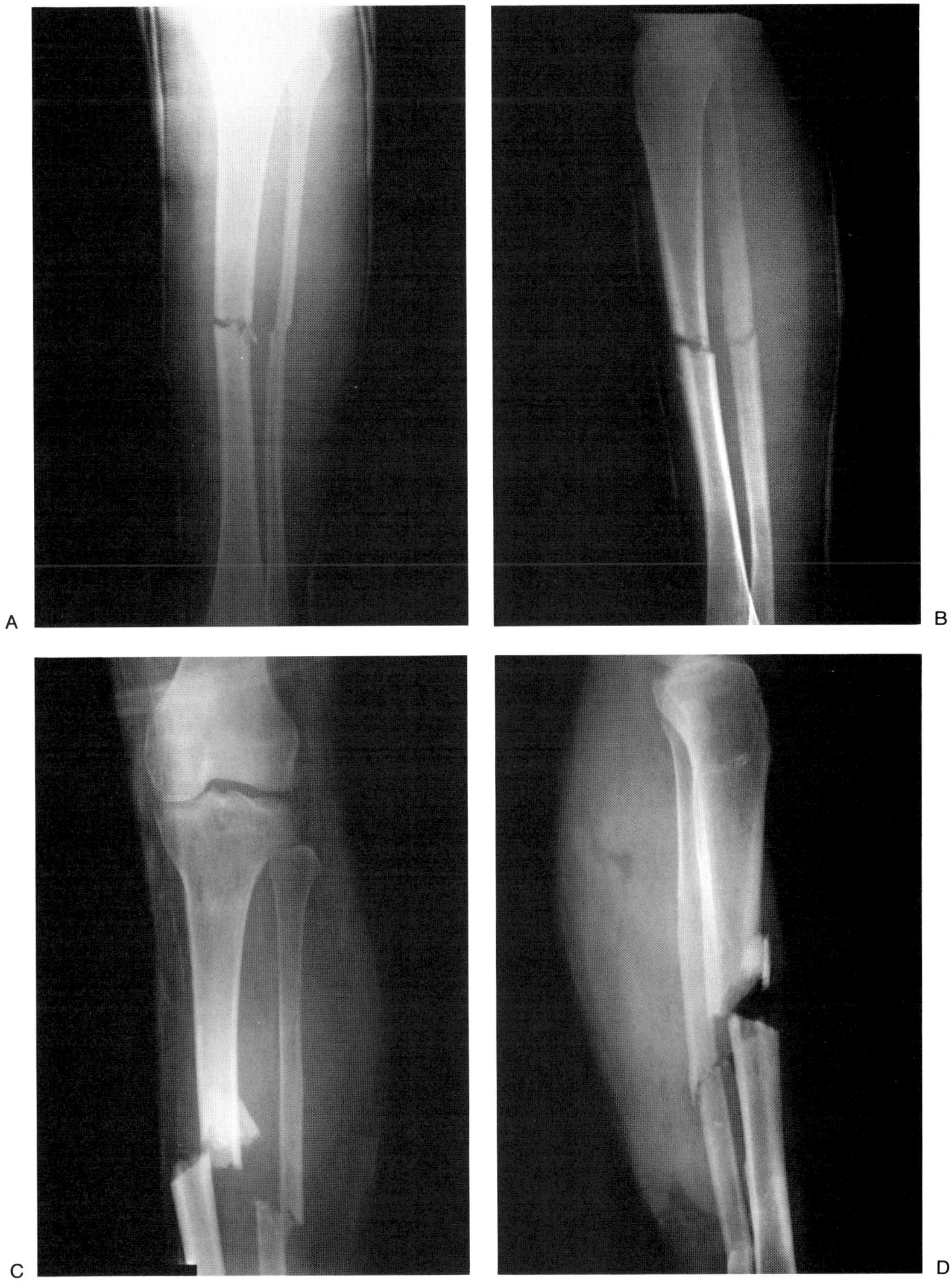

FIG. 7-1. Ellis classification based on severity. In fractures of minor severity, the AP **(A)** and lateral **(B)** views of the tibia and fibula demonstrate midshaft fractures with good apposition and no significant angulation. In those of major severity, the AP **(C)** and lateral **(D)** radiographs demonstrate comminuted displaced midshaft fractures with bone loss and angulation.

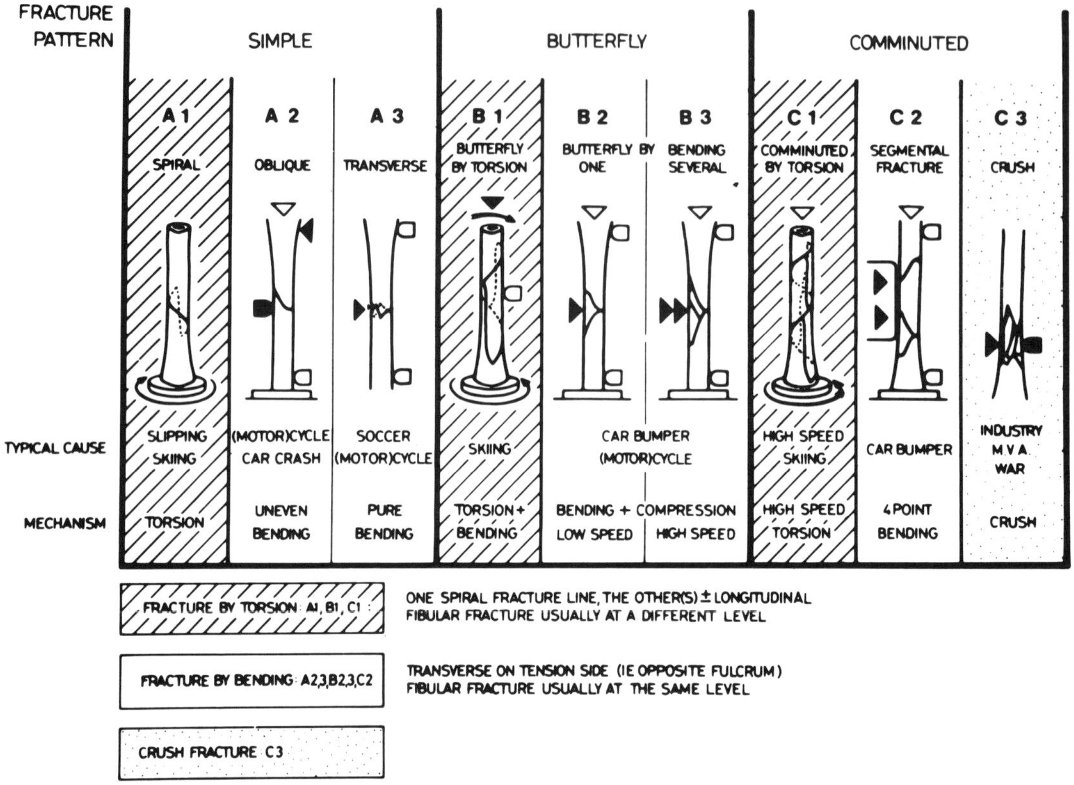

A

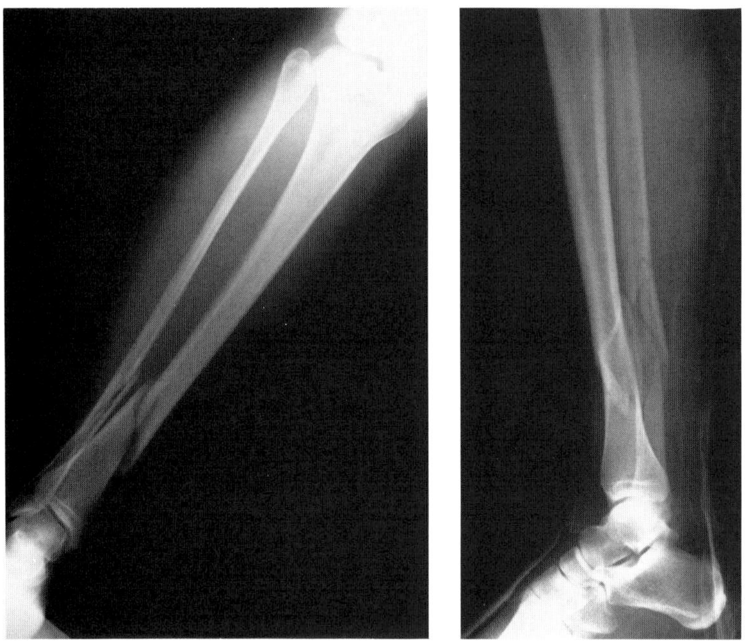

B,C

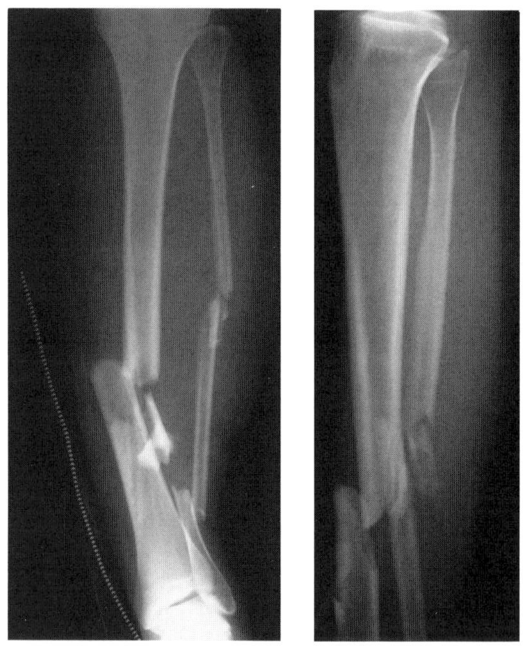

D,E

FIG. 7-2. A: Johner and Wruhs classification based on fracture morphology. This figure demonstrates the pattern and mechanism of injury. (From Johner R, Wruhs O. Classification of tibial shaft fractures and correlation with results after rigid internal fixation. *Clin Orthop* 1983;178:7–25.) The AP **(B)** and lateral **(C)** radiographs demonstrate spiral fractures caused by indirect forces. In nonspiral bending fractures, the AP **(D)** and lateral **(E)** radiographs demonstrate crush injuries with varying degrees of soft tissue injury.

A 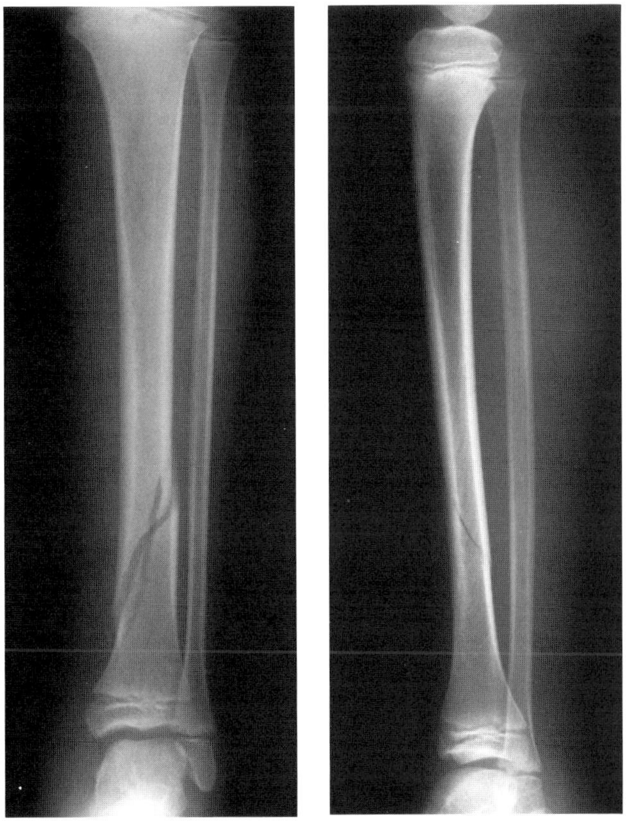 B

FIG. 7-3. Standard AP **(A)** and lateral **(B)** views of the tibia and fibula should include the soft tissue of the leg, knee, and ankle. Note the distal tibial spiral fracture, which is minimally displaced and seen best on the AP (A) view.

A,B 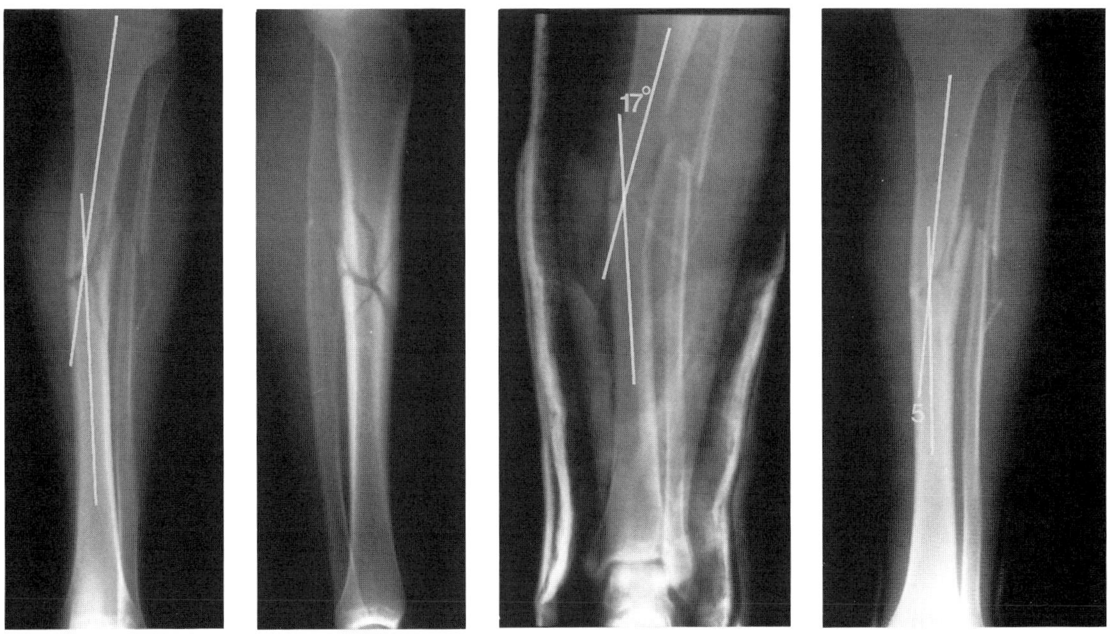 C,D

FIG. 7-4. Comminuted fractures of the midtibia and fibula. There is slight medial angulation on the AP view **(A)** and minimal displacement on the lateral view **(B)**. **C:** The AP view immediately following reduction shows increased angulation (17°). **D:** Following remanipulation, the angulation is reduced to 5°. (See **E** and **F** on next page.)

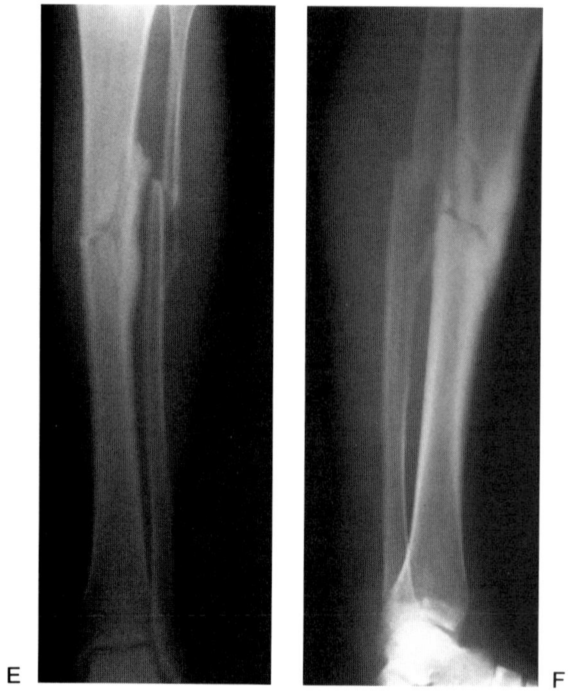

FIG. 7-4. (*Continued.*) The AP **(E)** and lateral **(F)** views 3 months after reduction show healing with good callus. There is no significant angulation. (From Berquist TH. *Imaging of orthopedic trauma,* 2nd ed. New York: Raven Press, 1992.)

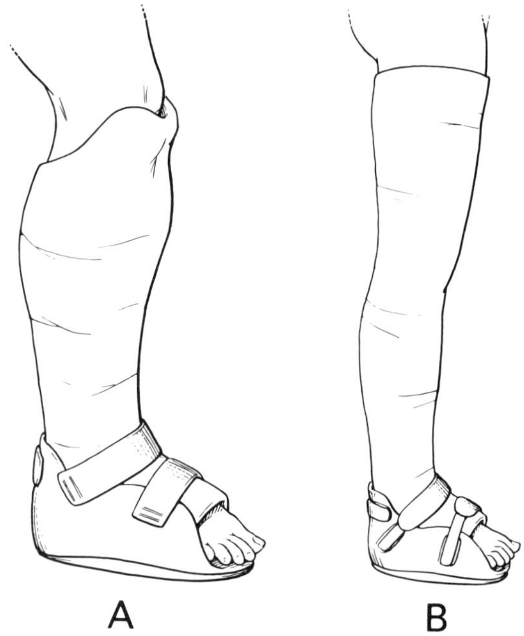

FIG. 7-5. Examples of PTB **(A)** and long leg **(B)** casts.

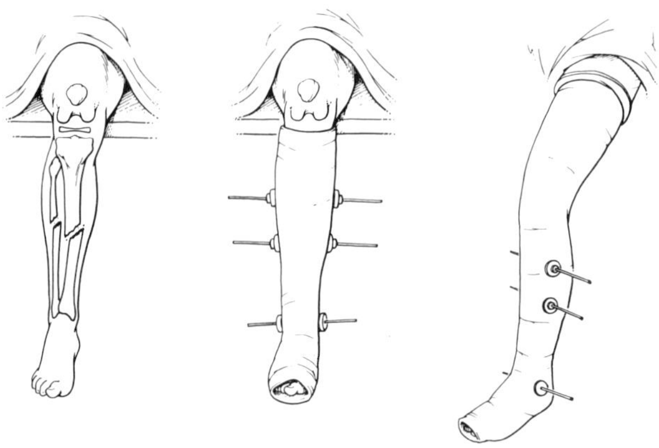

FIG. 7-6. Pin and plaster technique for fracture fixation.

TABLE 7-1. *Indications for external fixation*[4-6]

Open fractures with soft tissue injuries
Management of fractures with bone loss
Closed severely unstable fractures
Closed fractures in patients with
Burns
Head injuries
Neurosensory deficits
Compartment syndromes
Bone-lengthening procedures
Treatment of
Nonunion
Infected nonunion
Malunion

Disadvantages[63,65]
- Compliant patient needed, i.e., one who is receptive to treatment advice and willing to accept the risk of some residual fracture deformity
- Loss of subtalar motion and malunion more frequent after closed treatment than after an operative approach[63]

Traction

This is rarely used in tibial shaft fractures today.[63]

External Fixation

External fixators are commonly used for tibial shaft fractures because of the relatively high frequency of open fractures with significant soft tissue injury. External fixation is usually reserved for fractures that cannot be treated by other means.[7,63] The proponents of modern improved fixators suggest widening the indications for external fixation.[4-6,29,30,68] The general indications for external fixation are shown in Table 7-1.

External fixation devices stabilize fractures by holding the bone fragments in place with percutaneous pins, screws, or wires attached to an external frame. Steinmann pins, Schanz screws, or threaded half screws are frequently used.

One simple form of external fixation is pin and plaster (Fig. 7-6). Two Kirschner wires (K wires) or Steinmann pins are placed above and one below the fracture and are incorporated into the plaster.[2] This method can be used to treat closed or grade 1 fractures and to maintain reduction in some oblique or comminuted closed tibial shaft fractures.[23]

External fixators have been developed by using a multitude of different frame materials and designs.[2,4,6,22,42,63] Usually, they are classified by the type of pin and frame configuration.

Behrens classified two main types of external fixators: (1) pin and (2) ring. Pin fixators are subdivided into simple and clamp types. There are four standard frames that can be built with these devices, i.e., either unilateral or bilateral frames that can be in one or two planes.[4] The choice of fixator and frame depends on the mechanical needs for fracture management and the needs for wound access (Table 7-2).

If a fracture permits, axial compression should be applied.[66]

Advantages[5]
- Stabilization away from the fracture site
- Wound access
- Wide variety of management options
- Adjustable during treatment
- Addition of other means of internal fixation permitted
- Minimal adjacent joint interference
- Mobilization of patient to weight bearing

Disadvantages[6,63]
- Contractures possible
- Pin tract infections and osteomyelitis
- Pain

TABLE 7-2. *External fixators: general advantages and disadvantages*[38]

Simple pin	Clamp	Ring
Advantages		
Variable pin placement	Final reduction possible after application	Angulation and rotational deformities may be gradually corrected
Tremendous number of configuration possibilities	Good wound access	Smaller wires may cause less skin irritation and reduce the incidence of pin tract infections
Versatile good wound access		
Disadvantages[a]		
Fracture must be reduced before application	Pin placement dictated by clamp configuration	Wound access limited
Little adjustment possible after application	Limited variety of frame configurations	Bulky frame
	Gradual adjustment not possible	
	Reduction may be lost with release of articulation	

[a] Some of the newer fixators designs have eliminated these problems.

Fracture through pin tracts
Bulky so may not be accepted by patient

Examples of External Fixators

Simple Pin Fixators. Independent articulations connect each pin with a longitudinal rod (Fig. 7-7).[4,38]

Roger Anderson. Multiple pins are inserted as either transfixion pins or half pins. Each pin attaches to a clamp that has a connection to an aluminum rod (Fig. 7-8).[38]

Orthofix™. This is a lightweight unilateral external fixator (dynamic axial fixator, Fig. 7-9). The body is made of anodized aluminum light alloy with stainless steel linings at bearing surfaces.[20] It has a single telescoping bar with a ball and socket articulation at each end, which clamps with self-tapping screws. It can be locked at an angle for axial alignment, and the telescoping ability allows conversion from a rigid to dynamic fixation.

The Orthofix™ half pin is unique, with a 6-mm shank and a conical threaded portion. Choa et al.[17] state that this larger pin gives improved mechanical properties. The unilateral Orthofix™ with half pins compares in rigidity to quadrilateral fixators with transfixing full pins.

Its main advantages are its ease of application and versatility, the ability to reduce and adjust a fracture after its application, and the acceptance by patients of the lightweight smooth single bar.[17,20]

AO/ASIF fixator. This device is built of four components: Steinmann pins, Schanz screws, 11-mm diameter tubes, and several adjustable clamps (Fig. 7-10). This fixator can be arranged in many configurations. AO/ASIF recommends three particular configurations: unilateral frame, bilateral frame, and three-dimensional triangular. All of these may be used in tibial fractures.[6,66]

Wagner apparatus. This is a large telescoping rectangular column that holds two Schanz screws placed above and below the fracture (Fig. 7-11). Absolute rigid immobilization is possible with this system.[18,19,68]

Clamp fixators. Pins are held by clamps that are then attached the longitudinal rod by an articulation (Fig. 7-12).[38]

Hoffmann system. This apparatus consists of heavily threaded pins placed above and below the fracture, with an adjustable frame that has four vertical supports (Fig. 7-13).[7] Hoffmann developed the fixator in 1938.[45,50]

Triple-frame Vidal system. In 1968, Vidal modified the Hoffmann frame from a single-half-pin unit to a quadrilateral bicortical system.[47] This improves the rigidity of the quadrangular frame by (1) increasing the pin's diameter from 4 to 6 mm, (2) adding transverse coupling, and (3) adding half pins at an angle to the transfixion pins (Fig. 7-14).[38,71]

Hammer system. This unilateral frame consists of a square connecting rod with two universal ball and socket joints that hold two Schanz screws above and below the fracture. The mechanical characteristics of the ball joint provide adequate rigidity for unilateral application no matter what the type or location of the injury, and its versatility permits a large number of possible pin-insertion planes (Fig. 7-15).[36,37]

Behrens[4,5] believes unilateral frames are more desirable because of better wound access, less joint stiffness, and less chance of neurovascular damage.[6,38]

Carbon-Fiber Fixators. Radiolucent frames cause less interference with the radiographic evaluation of fractures than do metal frames. Several of these frames are available; one example is the Carbon Monotube™ (Fig. 7-16).

Ring Fixators. Frames are built of rings or partial rings connected to rods. Transfixion pins or wires above and below the fracture are connected to the rings to stabilize the fracture.[38]

Ilizarov frame. This frame was developed by Dr. Gauriil Ilizarov in Kurgan, Siberia, in 1951. Reportedly used in more than 1 million cases worldwide, it was first used in the West in 1981.[43] Although used in acute-fracture treatment by Ilizarov, the primary use in the United States is for the treatment of pseudarthrosis, bone defects, and deformities (Fig. 7-17).[38,55]

It can be assembled in more than 600 different ways to match the specific orthopedic need. Preplanning is necessary because only minor adjustments are possible after the application is complete.[43]

Monticelli-Spinelli fixator. A modified Ilizarov frame was designed primarily for leg-lengthening procedures (Fig. 7-18).[18,38]

Ace-Fischer fixator. This is a ring fixator in which the rings are connected by rods with universal joints at each end (Fig. 7-19). It has the ability to compress or distract.[19,38]

Hex-Fix™ fixator. This has features of simple, clamp, and ring fixators (Fig. 7-20).[38] It has a single hexagonal bar and spools with locking rings and 4.0-, 5.0-, and 6.0-mm diameter pins that allow uniplanar or multiplanar configurations. It also has an adapter that allows coupling with an Ilizarov ring.

Complications of External Fixation

The complications of external fixation can be reduced by proper pin placement in "safe soft tissue corridors," as described by Behrens[5] and Behrens and Searles[6] (Fig. 7-21).

Pin Tract Infection. Pin placement through fleshy areas increases the incidence of infection. Smaller wires in ring fixators have a lower incidence of infection.[38]

Pin Loosening and Breakage. The loosening rate increases over time, and loosening is inevitable if the pin is left in long enough.[63] Loosening decreases stability and increases the opportunity for infection.[5,38] Proper pin insertion and selection is critical.[5]

(*text continues on page 560*)

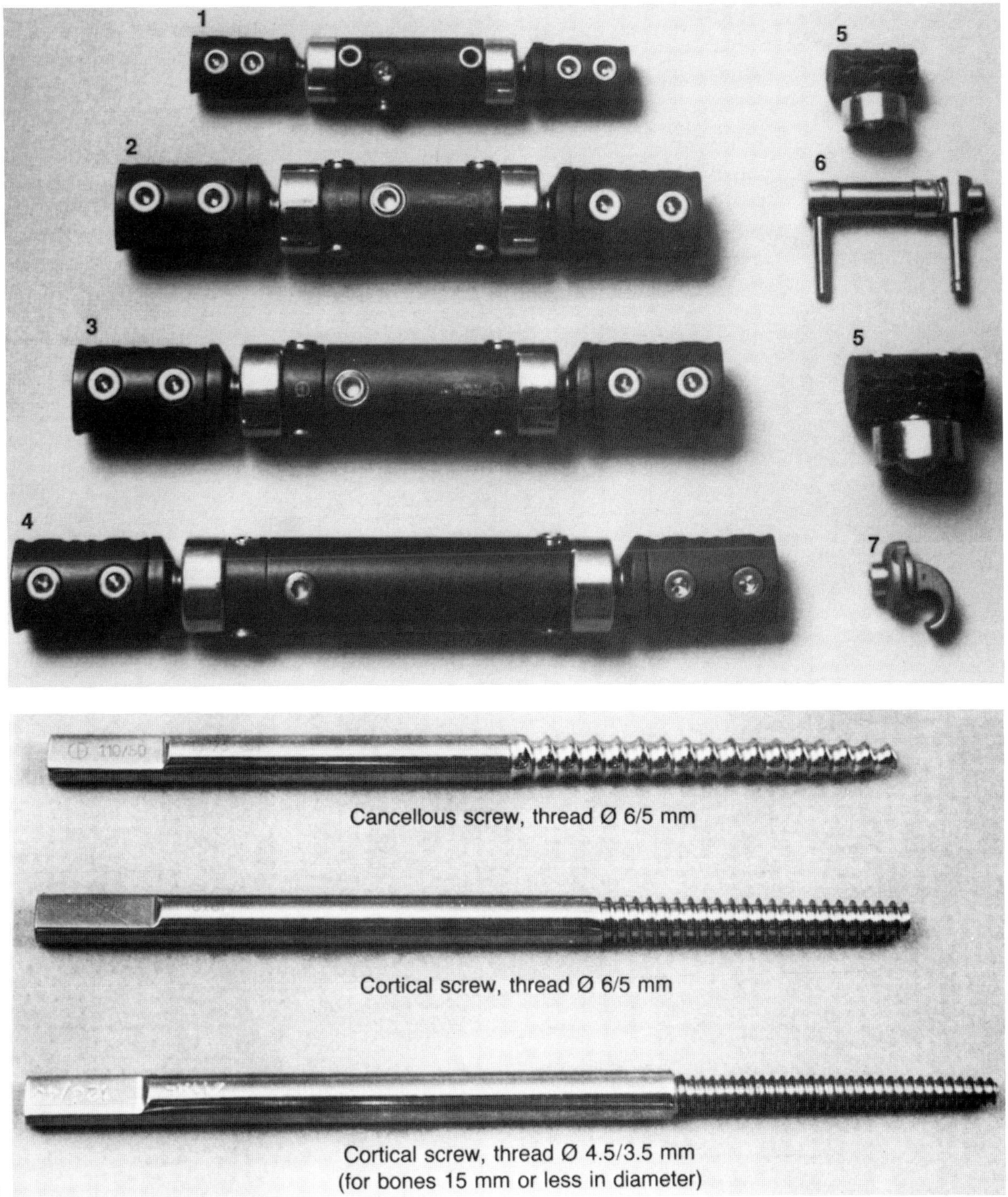

FIG. 7-7. Simple pin fixator. Independent articulations connect each pin with a longitudinal rod. Different-sized Orthofix™ fixators **(A)** and different screws attach to the end of mounted universal articulations **(B)**. (Courtesy of EBI Medical Systems, Parsippany, NJ.)

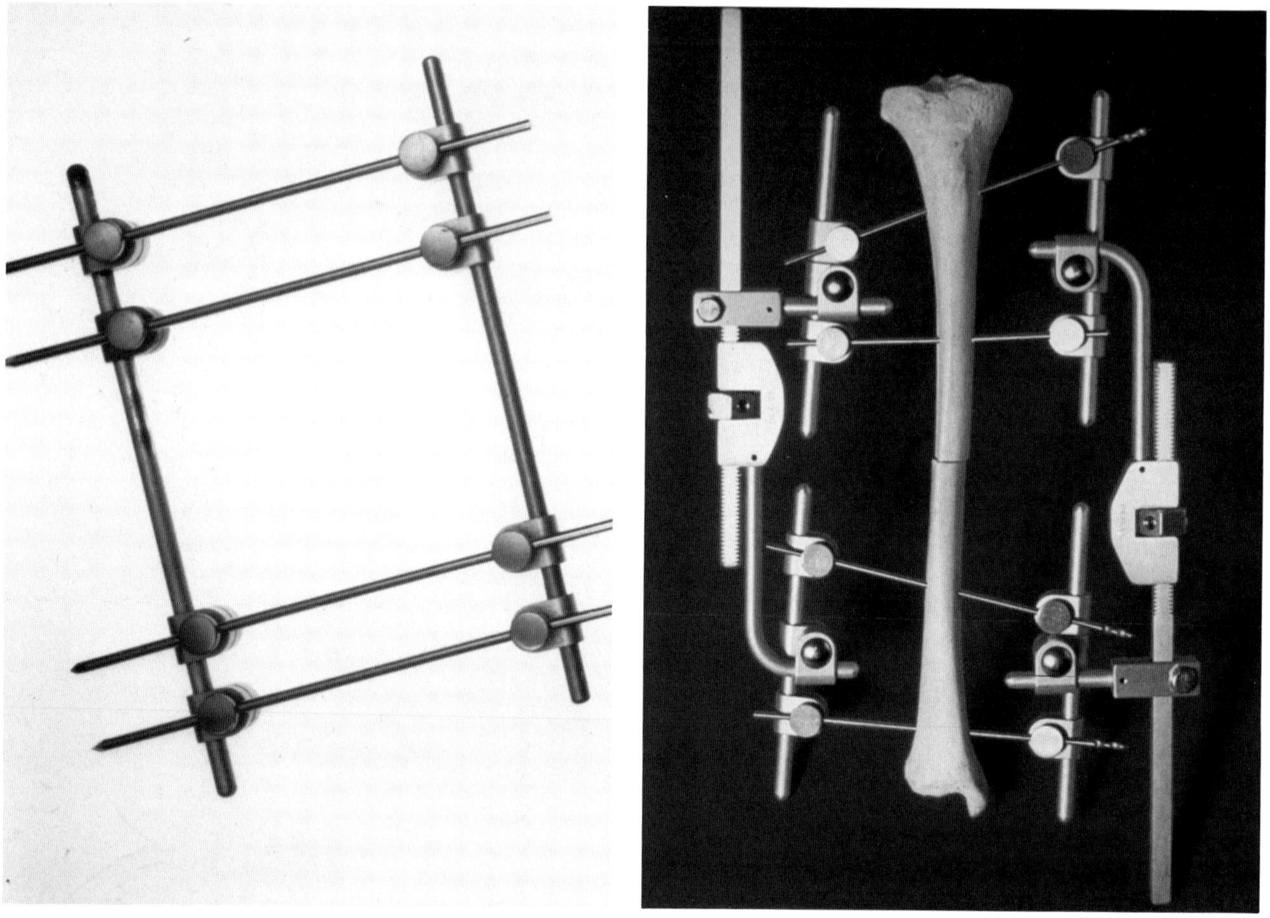

A B

FIG. 7-8. Original Roger Anderson fixator **(A)** and new Roger Anderson fixator with a device to allow compression of the fracture surfaces **(B)**. (From Berquist TH. *Imaging of orthopedic trauma,* 2nd ed. New York: Raven Press, 1992.)

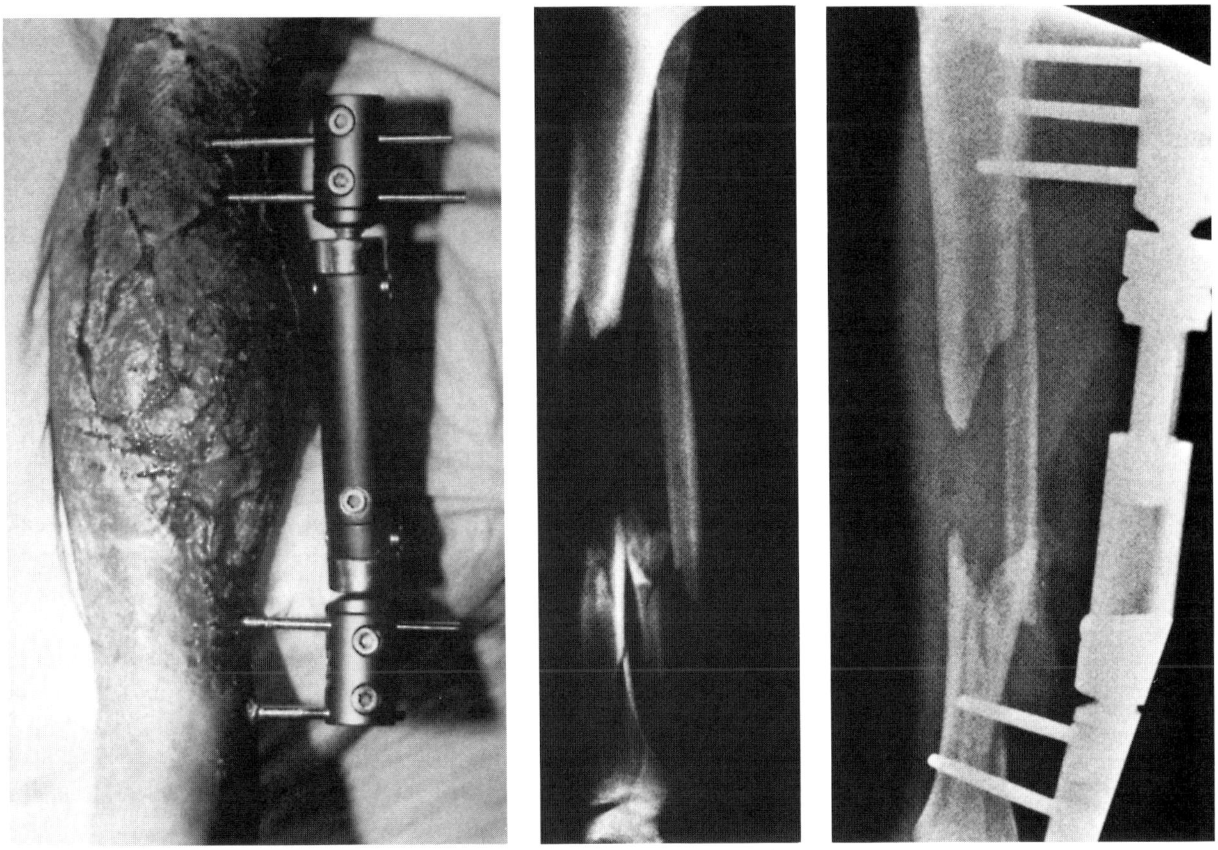

A B,C

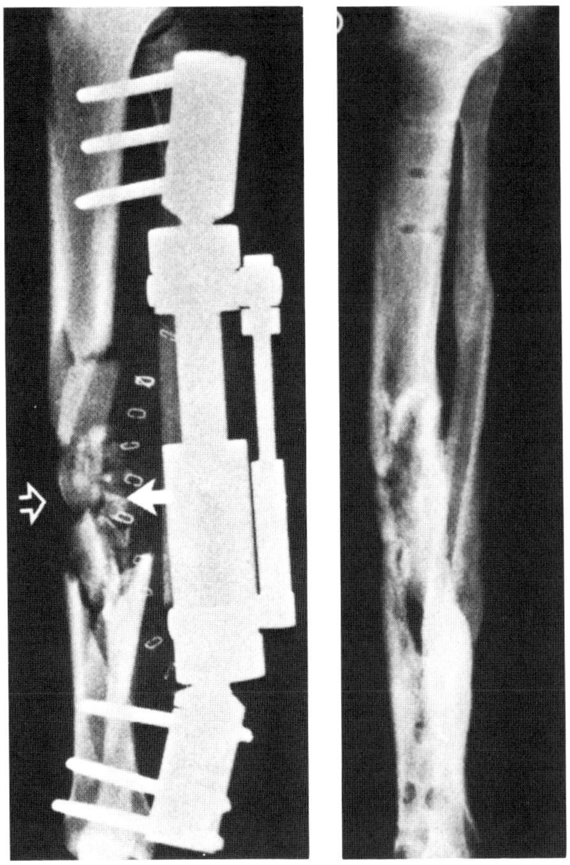

D,E

FIG. 7-9. Orthofix™ fixator (dynamic axial fixator). **A:** unilateral fixator allows easy access to a soleus skin flap for treatment of this open tibial fracture. The fixation of a type III unstable open tibial fracture with segmental bone loss **(B)**, the fracture postfixation **(C)** and after bone grafts **(D)**, and the healed fracture **(E)**. (From Melendez EM, Colon C. Treatment of open tibial fractures with the OrthoFix™ fixator. *Clin Orthop* 1989;241:224–230.)

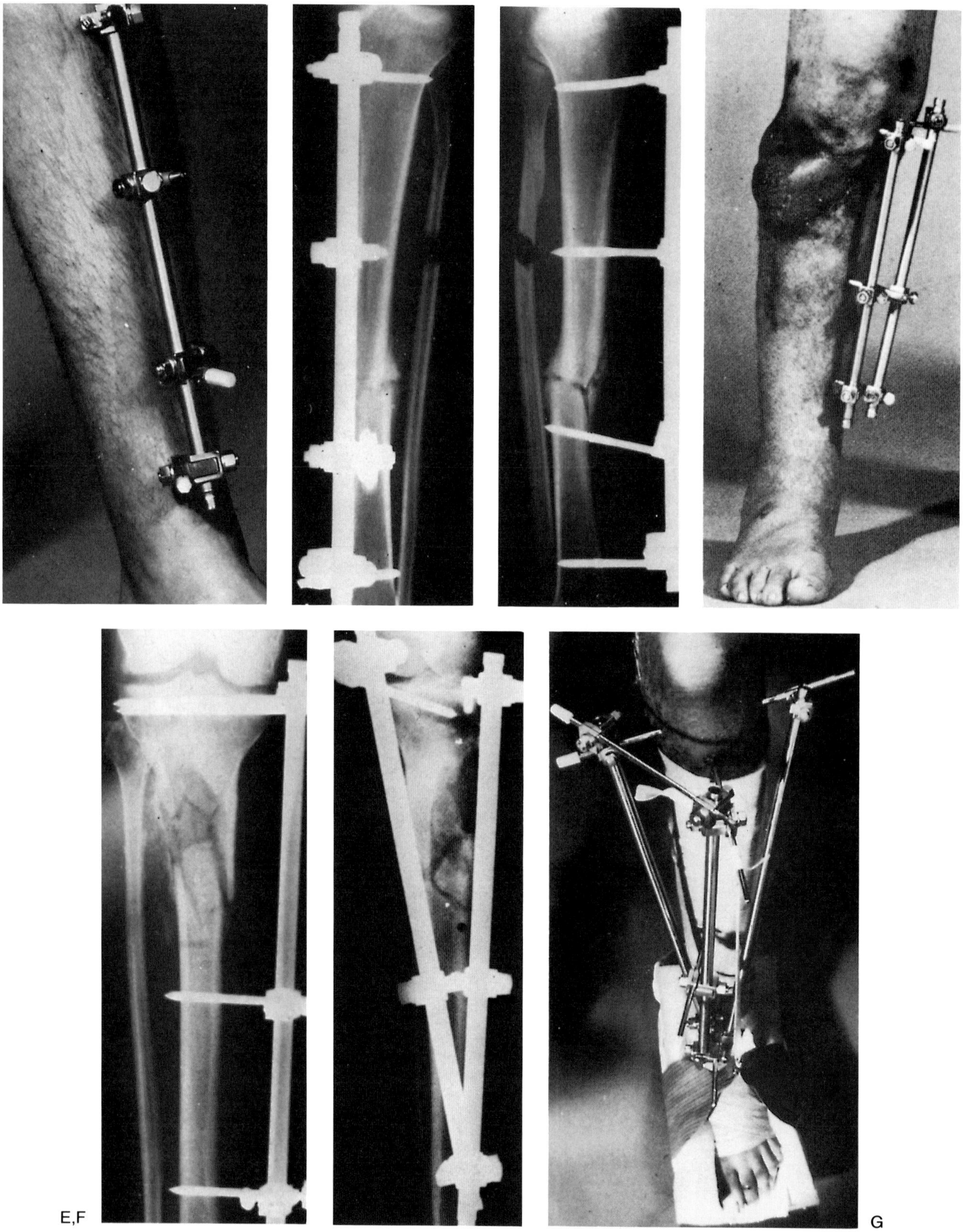

A,B C,D E,F G

FIG. 7-10. The AO/ASIF fixator. Hypertrophic nonunion of a tibial fracture treated with a unilateral frame in one plane **(A)**, as shown by AP **(B)** and lateral **(C)** radiographs. Major severity fractures treated by a unilateral fixator in two planes **(D)**, as shown by AP **(E)** and lateral **(F)** radiographs and three-dimensional fixation for greater stability **(G)**. (From Behrens F, Searles K. External fixation of the tibia. Basic concepts and prospective evaluation. *J Bone Joint Surg* [*Br*] 1986;68:246–254.)

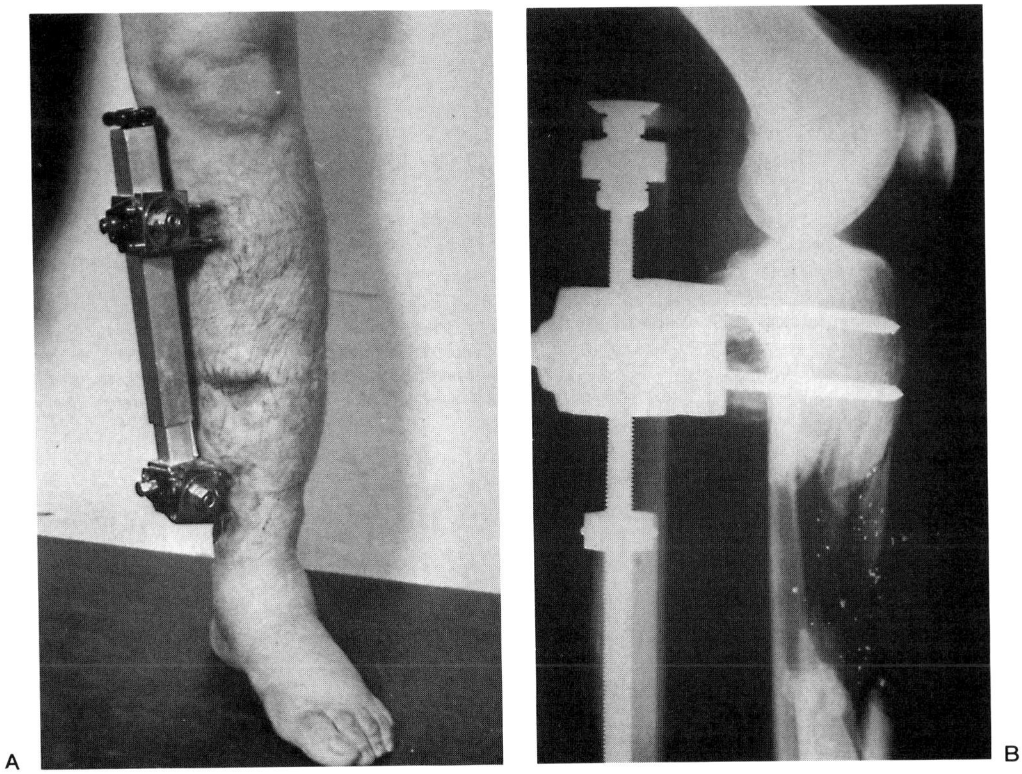

FIG. 7-11. Wagner apparatus. **A:** Open tibial fracture treated with Wagner external fixator. **B:** Lateral radiograph of open tibial fracture after gunshot wound. There is good alignment with Wagner fixation. (From Stein H, Makin M. Use of the Wagner apparatus in fractures of lower limb. *Orthop Rev* 1980; 9.)

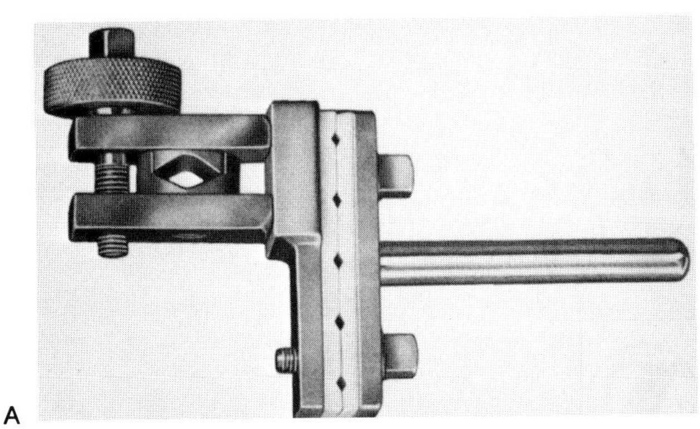

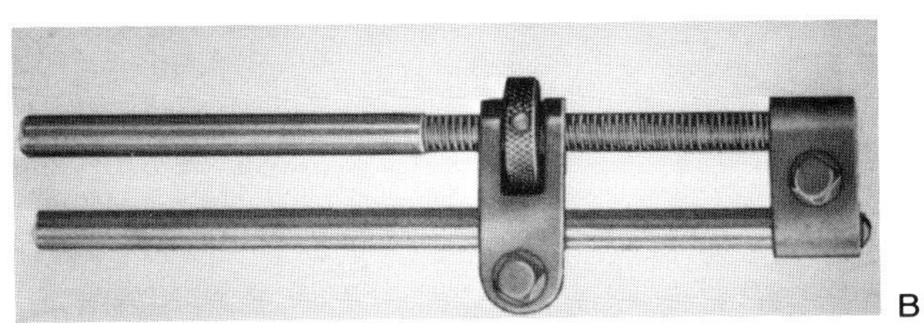

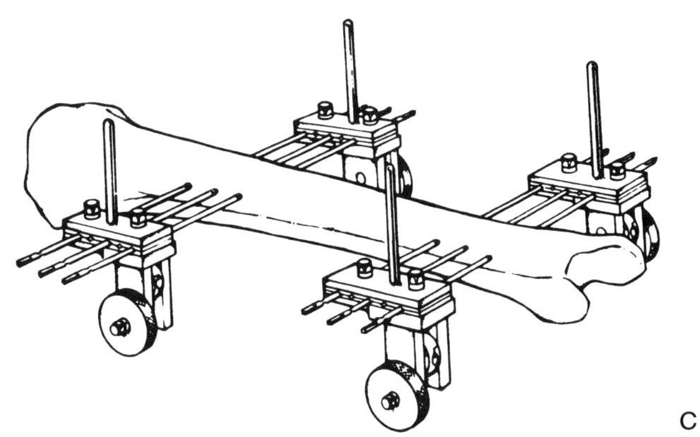

FIG. 7-12. Clamp fixator. Hoffman pin clamp for fixation to a connecting rod and a five-slot clamp for fixation pins or half pins **(A)**, adjustable connecting rod **(B)**, and four clamps with six transfixation pins **(C)**. Two adjustable rods are clamped on each side of (C) for the biplanar configuration. (Courtesy of Zimmer, Warsaw, IN.)

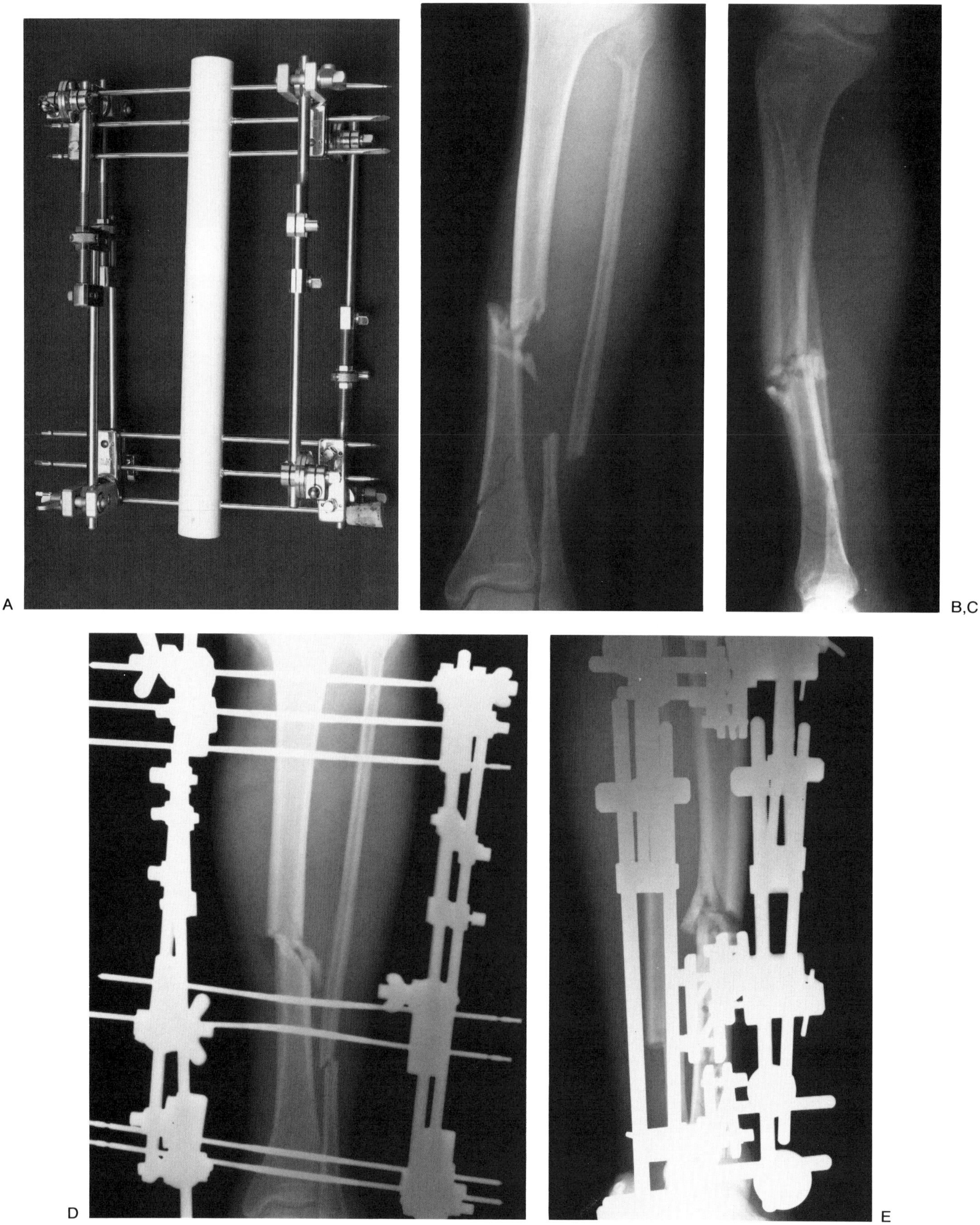

FIG. 7-13. A: Hoffmann fixator. Type III displaced comminuted tibial fracture, as shown by AP **(B)** and lateral **(C)** radiographs. Postreduction AP **(D)** and lateral **(E)** radiographs with Hoffman frame.

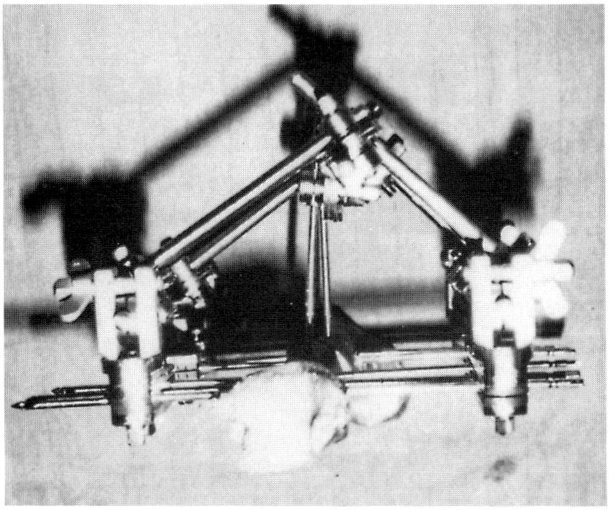

FIG. 7-14. "Chalet" configuration of triangular triple frame fixator. (From Vidal J, Nakach G, Orst G. New biomechanical study of Hoffmann external fixation. *Orthopedics* 1984;7: 654–670.)

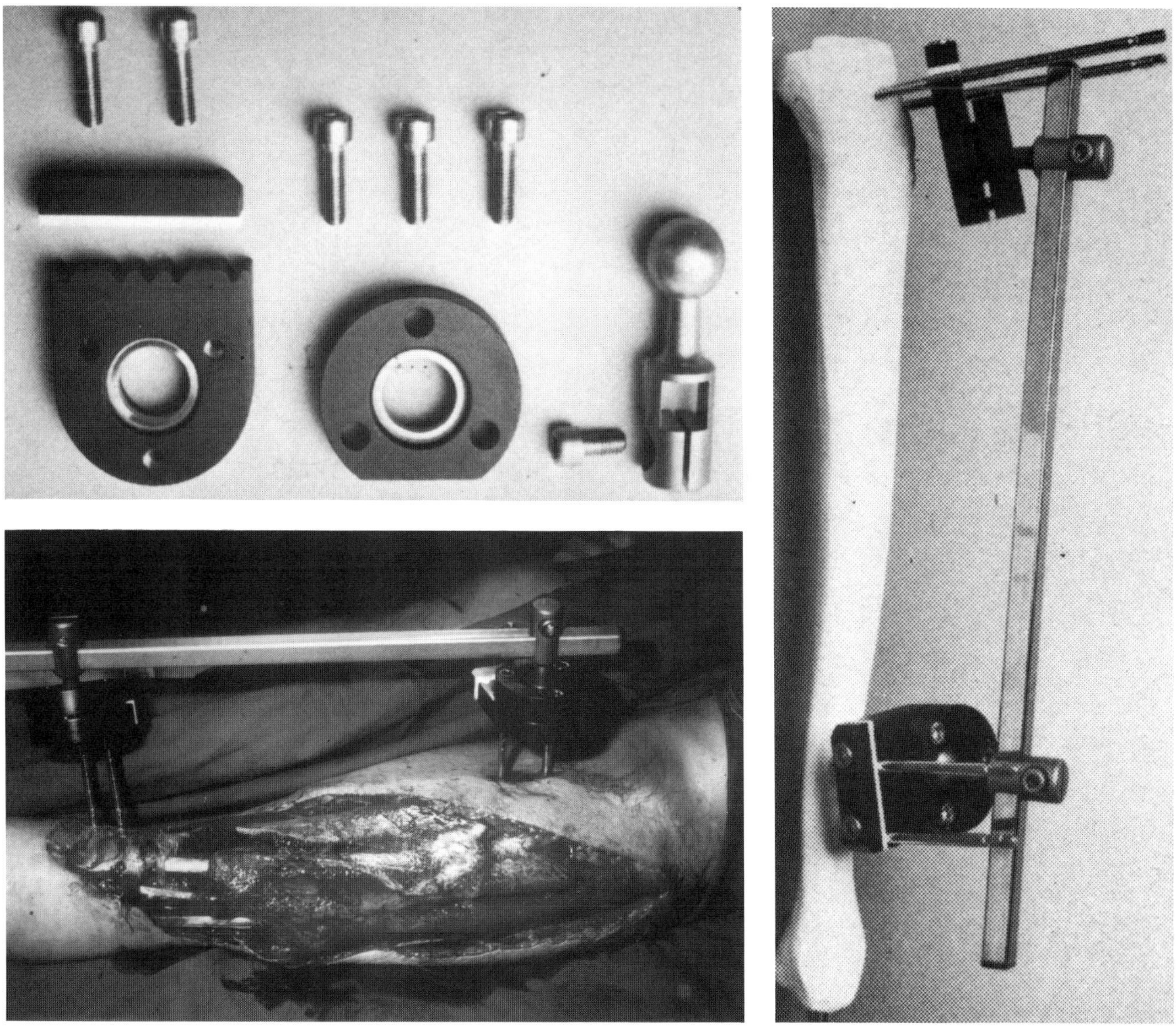

A

C

B

FIG. 7-15. Hammer system. **A:** Components of a disassembled universal ball joint. Unilateral frame mounted on a tibial model **(B)** and used in the treatment of a type IIIB tibial fracture on first postoperative day after débridement **(C)**. (From Hammer R. A new device for external fixation. *Acta Orthop Scand* 1988;59:708–711.)

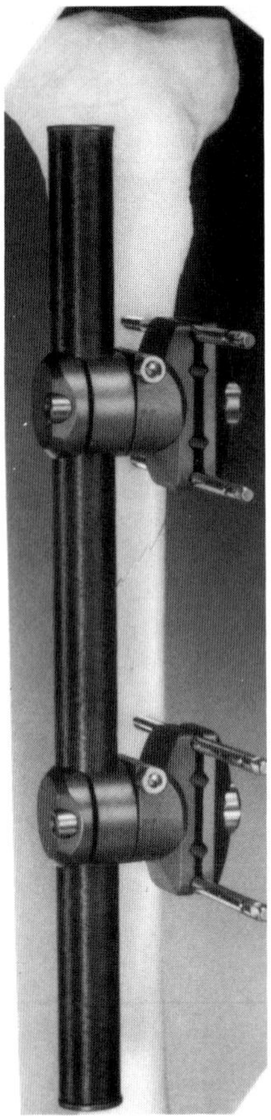

FIG. 7-16. Carbon fiber fixator. A Carbon Monotube™ fixator. (Courtesy of Howmedica, Rutherford, NJ.)

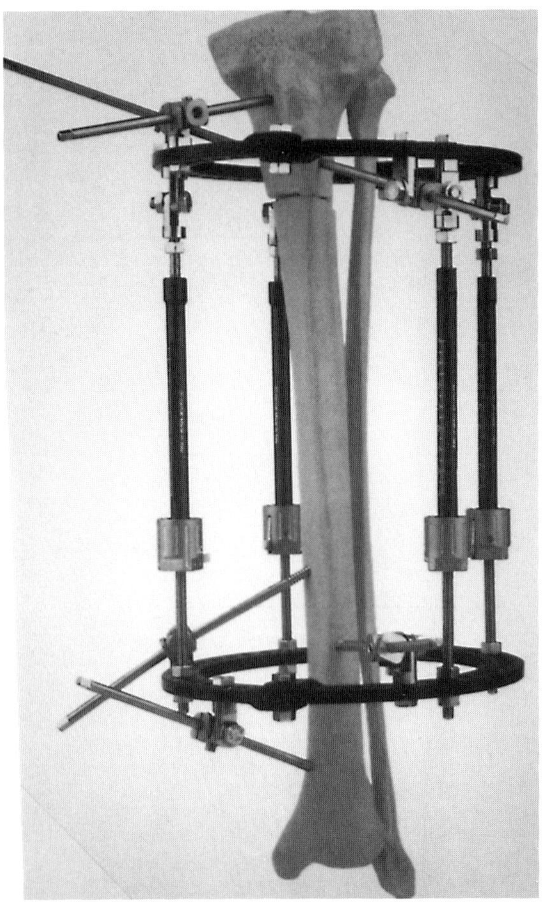

A

FIG. 7-17. A: The Ilizarov fixator on a bone model. (Courtesy of Smith and Nephew Richards, Memphis, TN.)

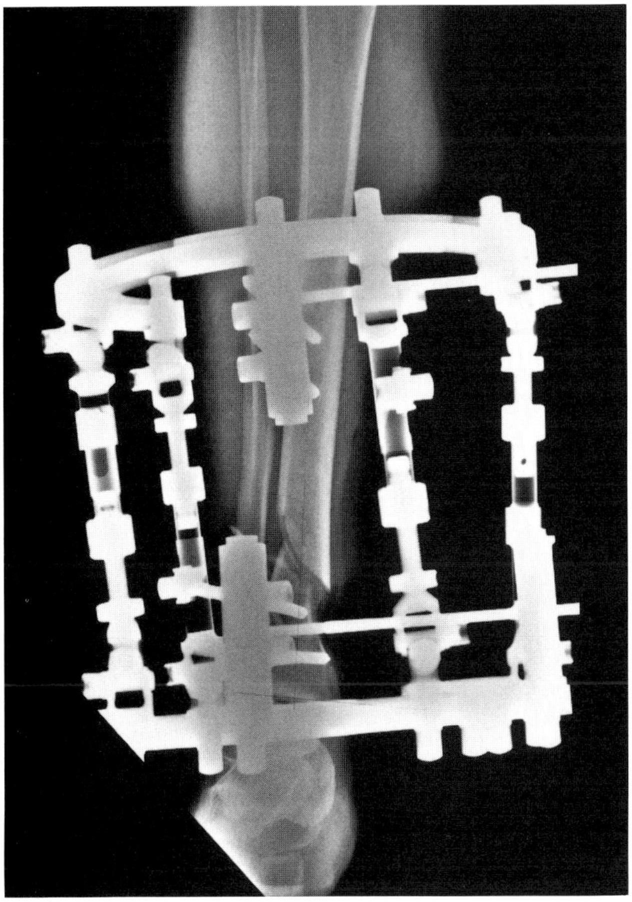

B

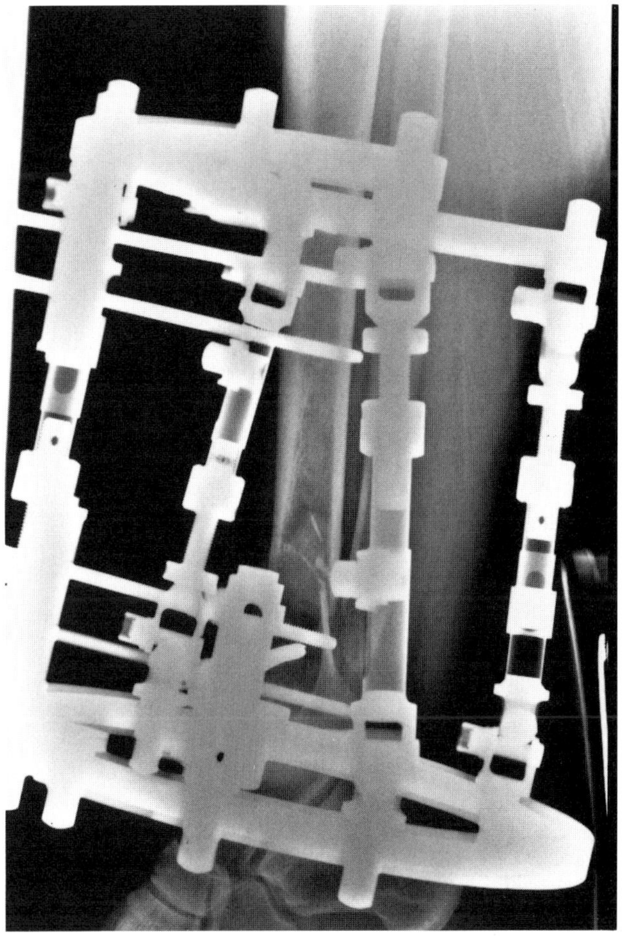

C

FIG. 7-17. (*Continued.*) The AP **(B)** and lateral **(C)** radiographs of fixation of a distal tibial fracture using an Ilizarov frame.

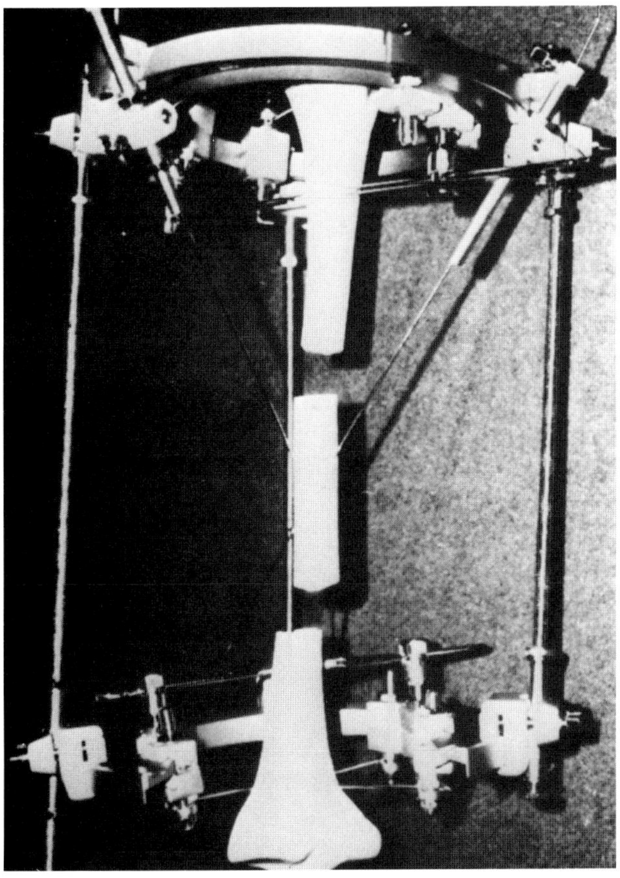

FIG. 7-18. A Monticelli-Spinelli fixator setup for bone transport with oblique directional wires. (From Green SA. The Ilizarov method: Rancho technique. *Orthop Clin North Am* 1991;22.)

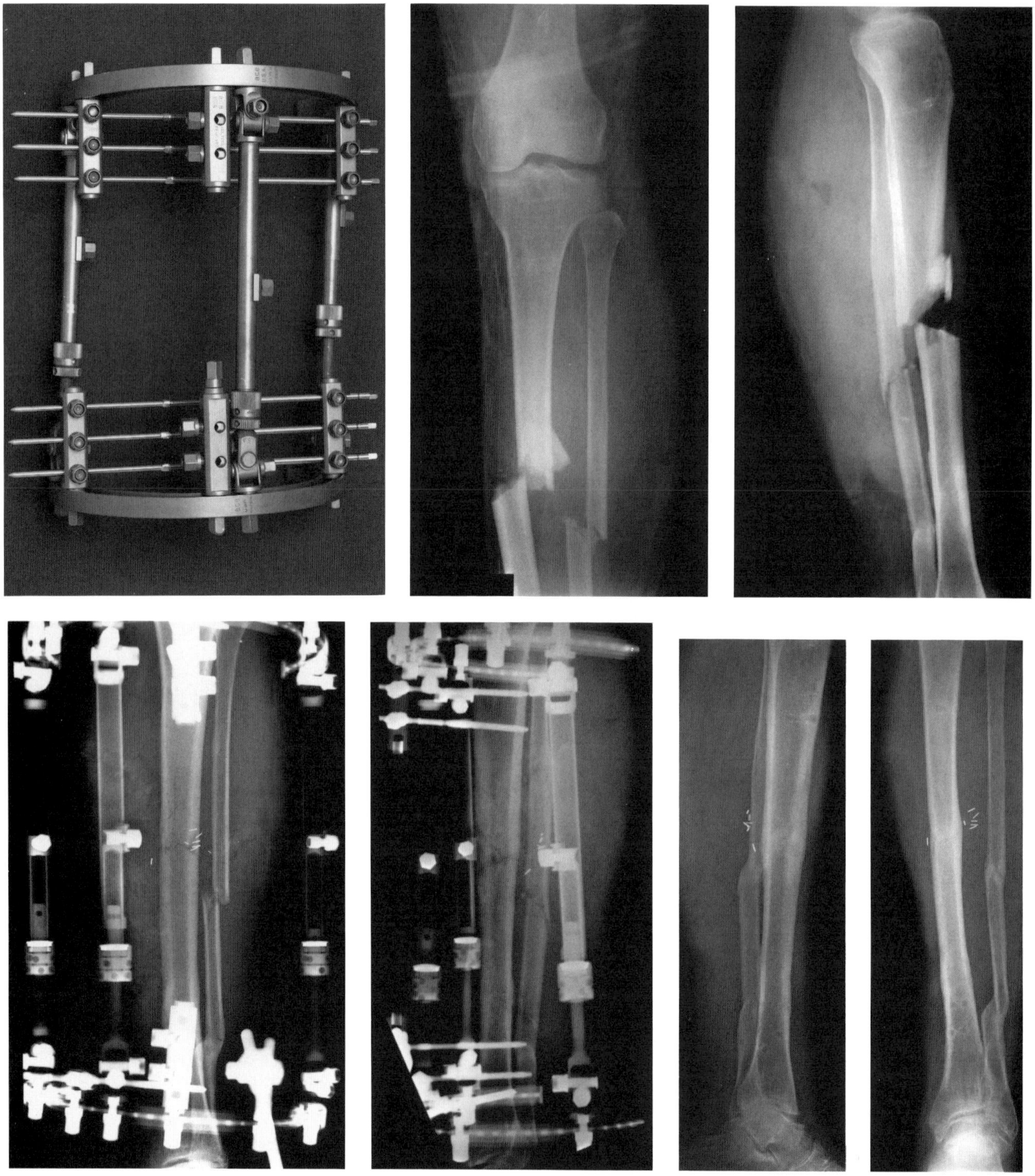

A,B C D,E F,G

FIG. 7-19. A: A Fischer fixator. The AP **(B)** and lateral **(C)** radiographs of an open type IIIA fracture. The fracture was reduced with a Fischer frame **(D,E)**. Lateral **(F)** and AP **(G)** radiographs 6 months later with the fractures healed. (From Berquist TH. *Imaging of orthopedic trauma,* 2nd ed. New York: Raven Press, 1992.)

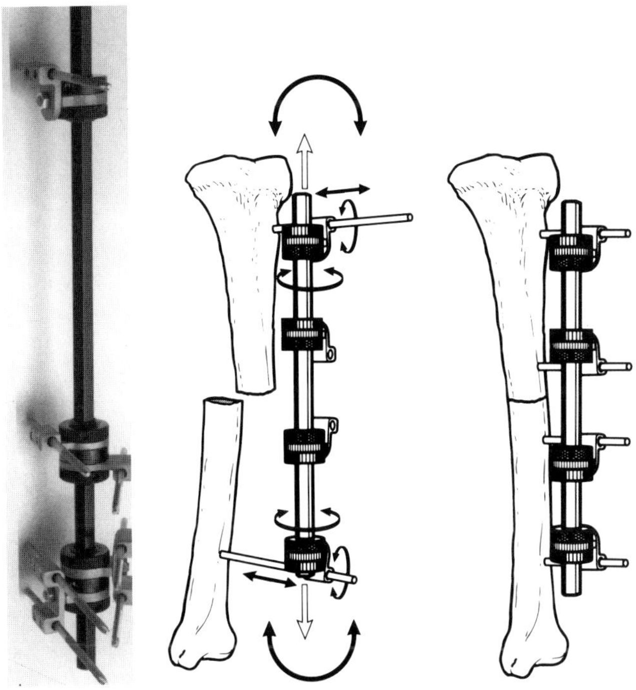

A B,C

FIG. 7-20. A: Hex-Fix™ fixator. External fixator during reduction of a diaphyseal tibial fracture **(B)** and after reduction **(C)**. (Courtesy of Smith and Nephew Richards, Memphis, TN.)

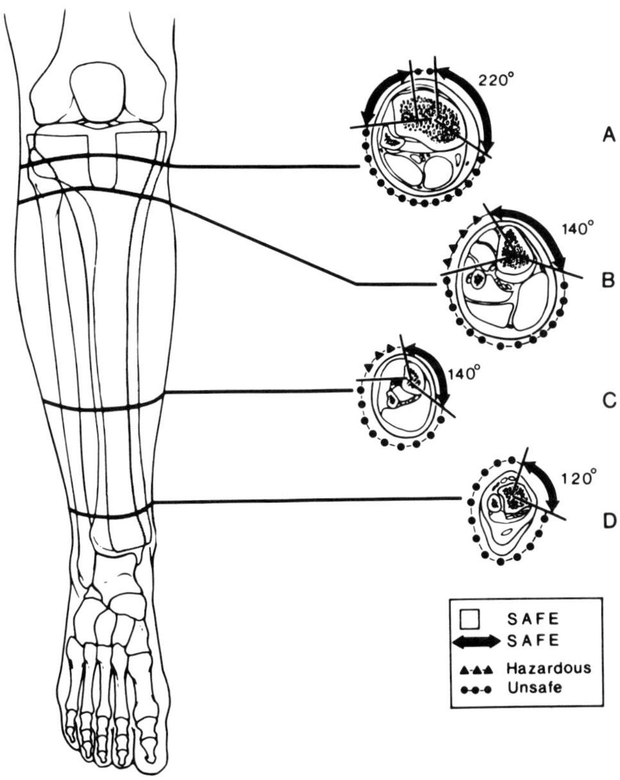

FIG. 7-21. Behrens's[5] "safe, hazardous and unsafe corridors for placement of transfixation pins and/or wires." **A:** In the proximal to tibial tuberosity, safe insertion zones are shown (*arrows*); the posterior region and the area under the patellar tendon are unsafe. **B:** In the area just below the tibial tuberosity, the anterior zone is safe (*arrows*), with the hazardous area indicated (triangular). **C:** In the distal third of leg, the safe zone is identified (*arrows*). **D:** Two inches above the ankle is a safe zone (*arrow*), with the danger zone indicated (*dots*) and no hazardous area at this level. (From Behrens F. General theory and principles of external fixation. *Clin Orthop* 1989;241:15–23.)

Limitation of Joint Motion. Transfixion of the foot dorsiflexors may lead to permanent ankle stiffness.[6,38]

Neurovascular Damage and Compartment Syndrome. The placement of half pins is safer than is that of transfixion pins.[38] Placement through the anterolateral compartment may produce compartment syndrome if bleeding increases the intracompartmental pressure.

Malalignment and Malunion. It is important to match the involved leg to the uninvolved normal leg. Even if perfect alignment is obtained initially, any pin loosening or weight bearing can lead to deformities.[38]

Delayed Union or Nonunion. With this form of treatment, problems with union occur. This is most likely due more to the severity of the injury for which the device is used than to the device itself (Fig. 7-22).[38]

Dynamization and Build Down

In the later stages of fracture healing, gradual frame modification or build down improves the opportunity for union.[6]

Intramedullary Nailing

Intramedullary nails can be placed by either an open or closed technique, with or without reaming. Lottes[52] was an early proponent of closed intramedullary nailing. Compared with external fixation, the advantage of internal fixation is a lower infection rate, especially with the closed technique, and no soft tissue impingement.[63]

Ender Nails

Multiple flexible pins are placed in medial and lateral entrance sites in the proximal tibia (Fig. 7-23). Angulation and rotation are resisted by the spring force of the pins.[63] They are useful in certain fractures, such as type 1 or 2 open fractures, short oblique distal tibial fractures,[7,51] and middle third shaft fractures.[63]

The placement of Ender nails without reaming produces less damage to the medullary endosteal circulation,[63] but reaming allows the placement of larger stronger nails.[38]

Intramedullary nails are useful in short oblique or transverse fractures of the middle third that are angulated or displaced, segmental tibial fractures, and nonunions.[7]

Lottes's[52] closed technique required a short incision at the tibial tuberosity, and the nail was placed without the modern image intensifiers that are now used to guide both the reaming and placement. Closed techniques have less chance of infection or disturbances of the soft tissue's vascularity, but open techniques are needed if a closed approach fails.[63]

If rotation occurs with intramedullary devices, external supports, such as a cast or brace, may be necessary initially during management.[6,13,17]

Interlocking Intramedullary Nails

Bone screws can be placed transversely through the nail and bone at either or both ends of the nail to increase the stability and prevent rotation or displacement of the fracture. These devices allow intramedullary nailing of more comminuted and more distal or proximal shaft fractures than was previously possible.[7,48,72]

A static configuration is achieved by placing screws at both ends of the nail; a dynamic configuration results when the screws are placed at the proximal or distal end of the nail with compression of the fracture by weight bearing. Generally, the dynamic configuration is used in more stable fractures; the static configuration is indicated when stability is required (Fig. 7-24).[7,10,24,63]

Several types of interlocking intermedullary nails are available. There are reamed and nonreamed types.

AO/ASIF Nail. This is a thin-walled open nail with a cloverleaf cross-section and anterior longitudinal slitting (Fig. 7-25). There are two proximal holes for cortical screws and two holes distally for the placement of antirotational wires inserted down through the nail. The newer design AO/ASIF nail allows proximal and distal interlocking. Proximal round and oval holes allow dynamic or static interlocking. Distally, there are two transverse locking holes and an anterior hole for use in difficult fractures.[66]

Russell-Taylor™ Nail. This nail has a cloverleaf and is designed to be used as an unreamed interlocking nail (Fig. 7-26). It is not slotted like the AO/ASIF and Grosse-Kempf nails. The nonslotted closed design increases the torsional rigidity of the nail. The increased wall thickness in the smaller-diameter Delta™ nails maintains the strength for unreamed placement in smaller medullary canals. There are two proximal and two distal holes that allow either dynamic or static interlocking configurations.[63,64]

Grosse-Kempf Nail. This is a modification of the Küntscher nail that is slotted posteriorly (Fig. 7-27). It also has two proximal and distal holes. Bone and Johnson[10] were the authors to first describe the use of an interlocking intermedullary nail in this country.[63]

Brooker-Wills Nail. This differs from the other nails because distal stability is achieved by blades (Fig. 7-28). Proximal holes are present for screw fixation.[12]

Percutaneous Cerclage Fixation

Certain torsional fractures can be fixed by percutaneous cerclage (Fig. 7-29). Habernek et al.[34] state that "this method should be used only for torsional fractures

(*text continues on page 567*)

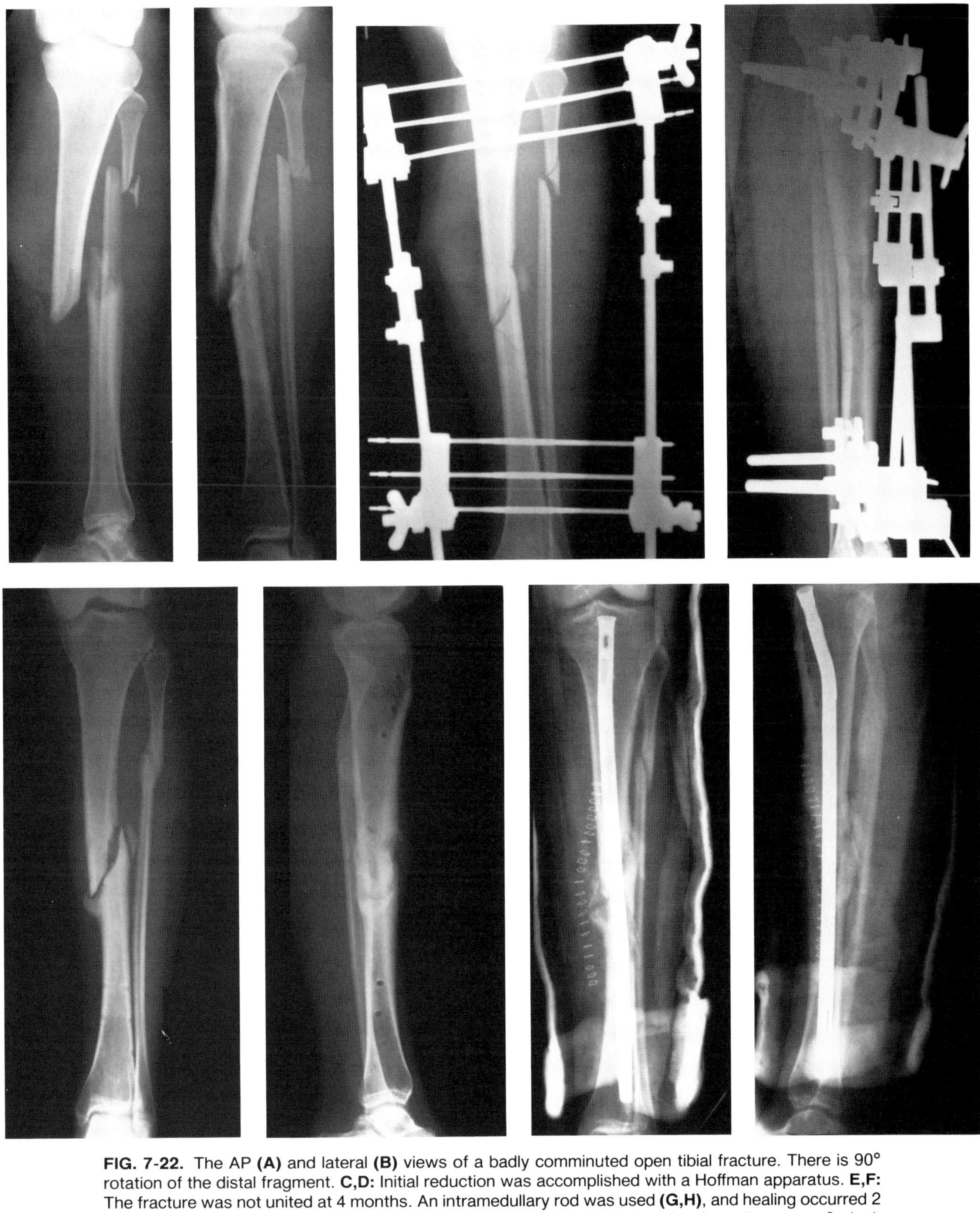

A,B C,D E,F G,H

FIG. 7-22. The AP **(A)** and lateral **(B)** views of a badly comminuted open tibial fracture. There is 90° rotation of the distal fragment. **C,D:** Initial reduction was accomplished with a Hoffman apparatus. **E,F:** The fracture was not united at 4 months. An intramedullary rod was used **(G,H)**, and healing occurred 2 months later **(I,J)**. (See **I** and **J** on next page.) (From Berquist TH. *Imaging of orthopedic trauma,* 2nd ed. New York: Raven Press, 1992.)

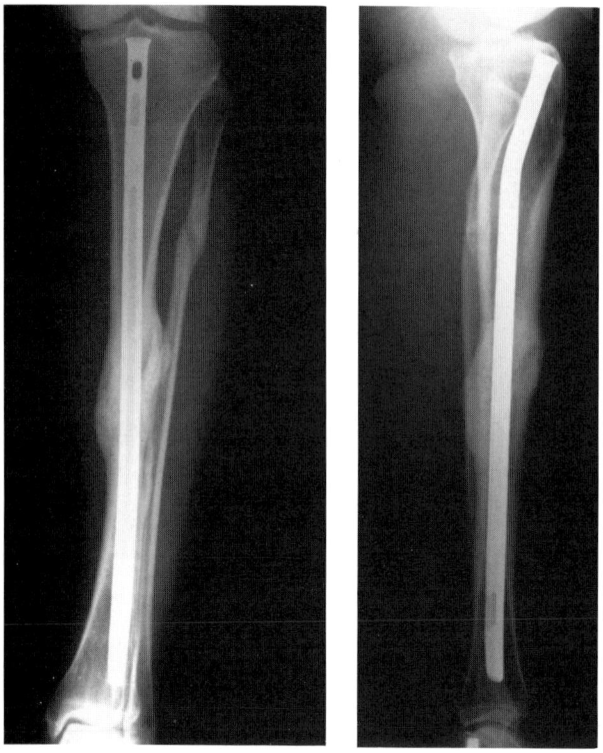

I J **FIG. 7-22.** *Continued.*

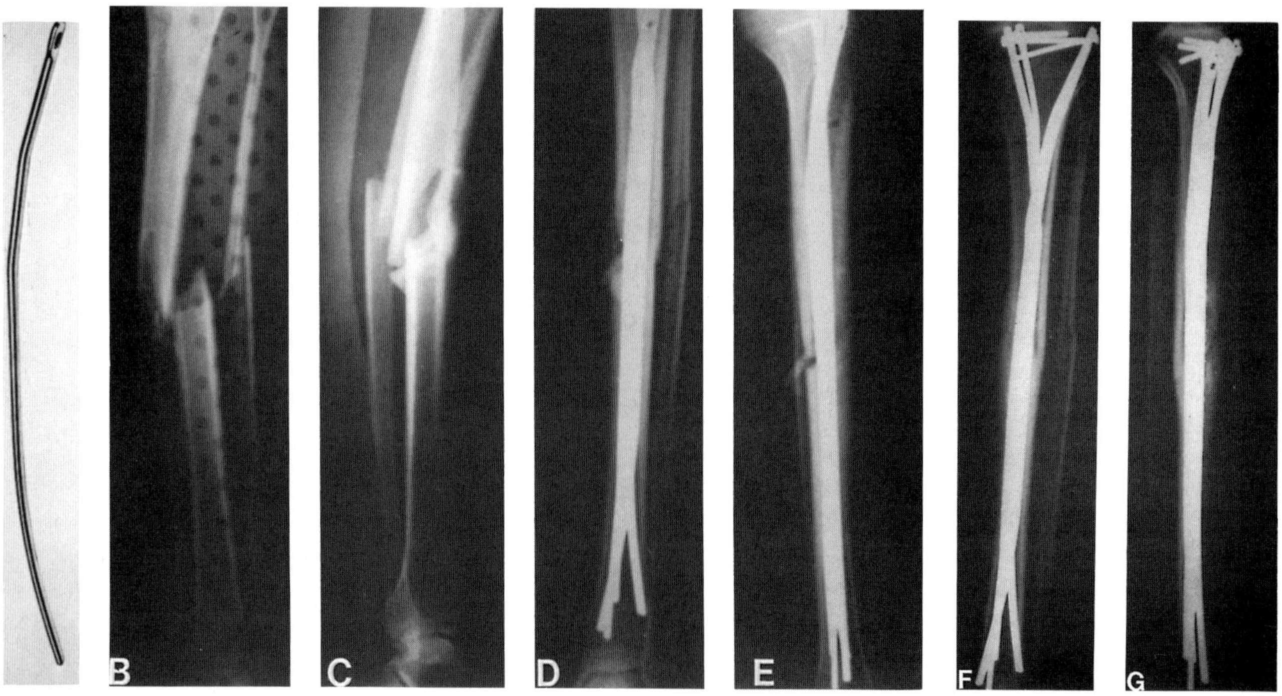

FIG. 7-23. A: Ender nail. (Courtesy of Zimmer, Warsaw, IN.) The AP **(B)** and lateral **(C)** radiographs of a grade II open tibial fracture. The AP **(D)** and lateral **(E)** radiographs showing reduction with 4.0-mm Ender nails. **F,G:** Radiographs show healing at 5 months. (From Holbrook JL, Swiontkowski MF, Sanders R. Treatment of open fractures of the tibial shaft: Ender nailing versus external fixation. *J Bone Joint Surg* [*Am*] 1989;71A:1231–1238.)

A,B 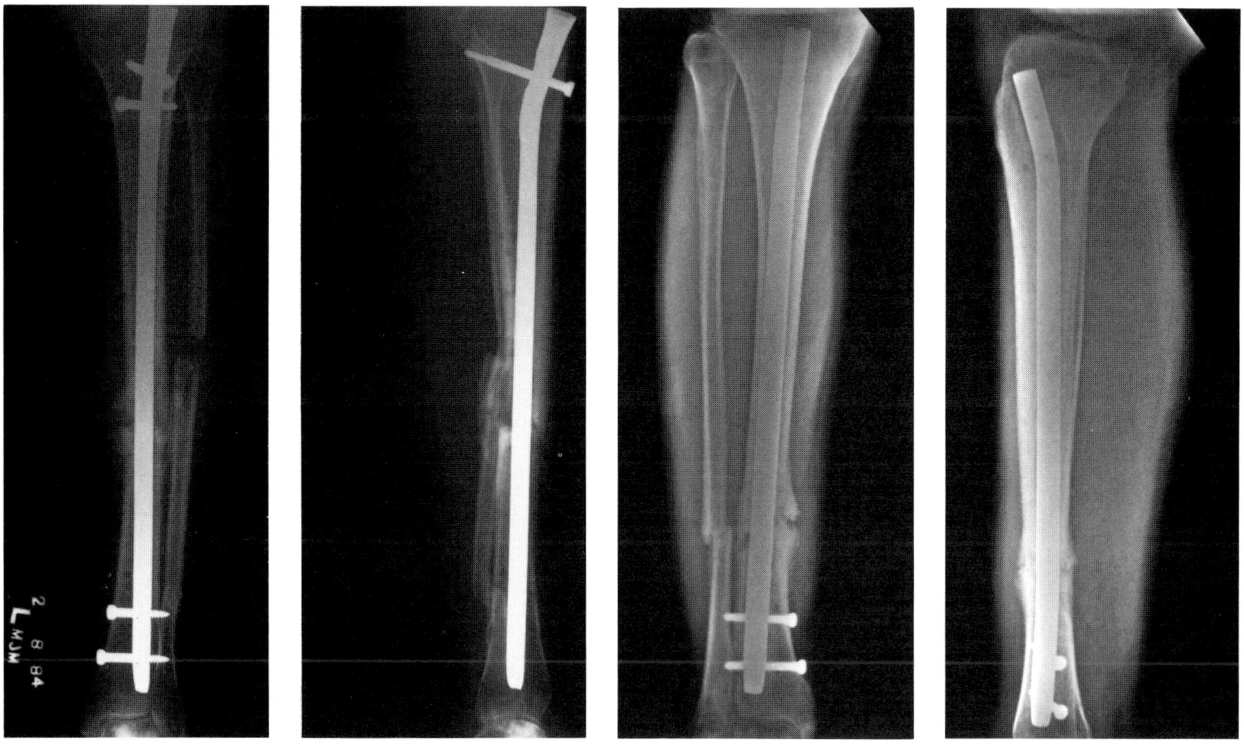 C,D

FIG. 7-24. The AP **(A)** and lateral **(B)** radiographs of the static intramedullary nail technique. The AP **(C)** and lateral **(D)** radiographs of distal tibial and fibular fractures treated with a dynamic (screws distally) technique using a Russell-Taylor™ nail.

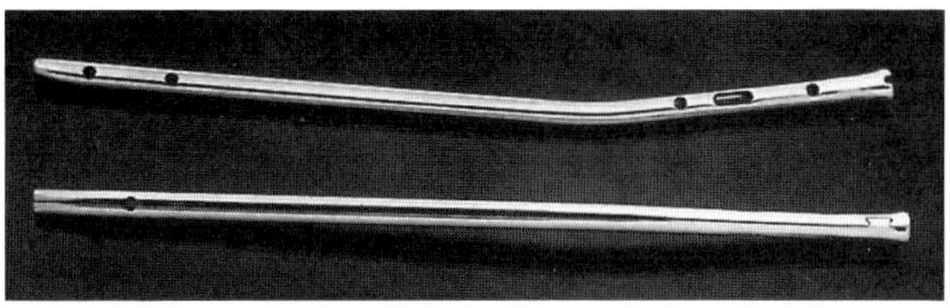

FIG. 7-25. AO/ASIF interlocking intramedullary nail. (From Ruedi T. Intramedullary nailing with interlocking. *Arch Orthop Trauma Surg* 1990;103:317–320.)

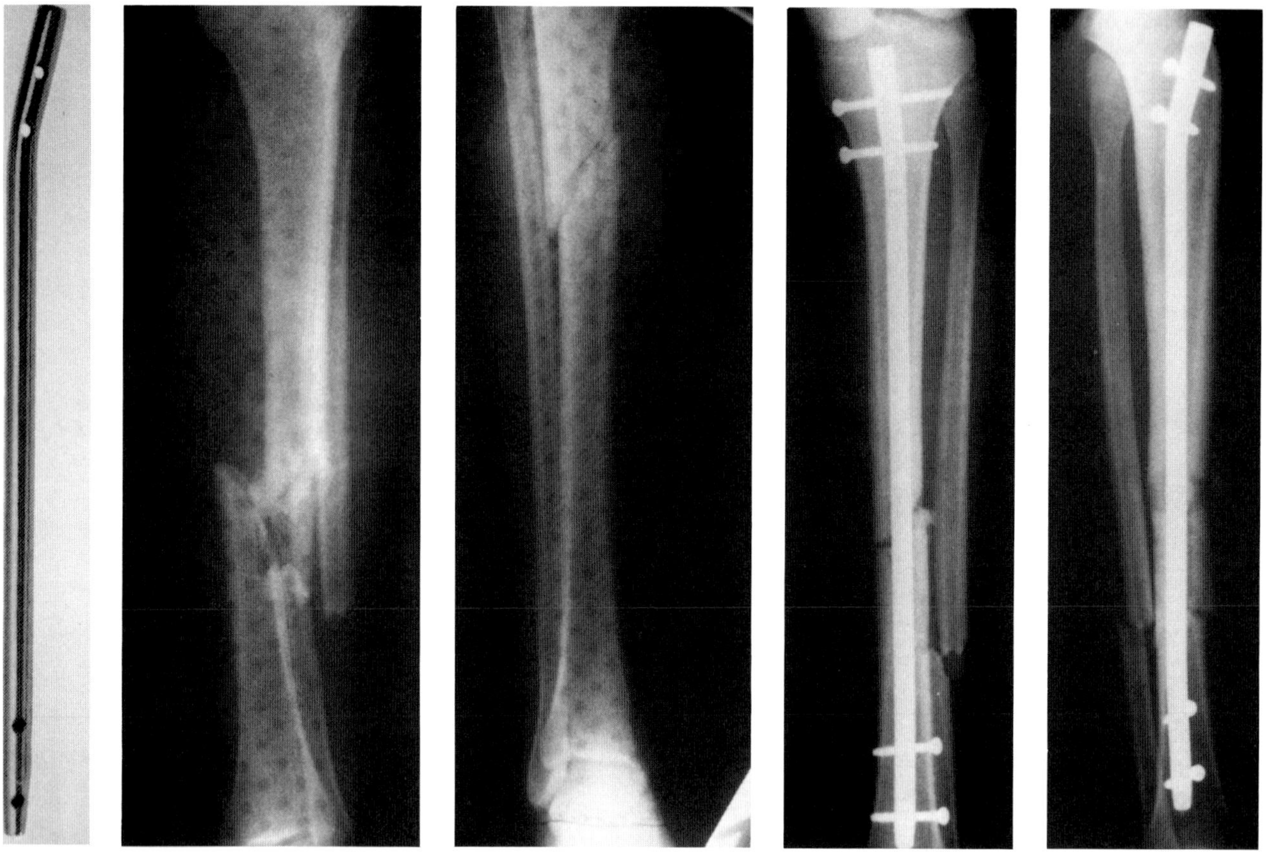

A,B,C

D,E

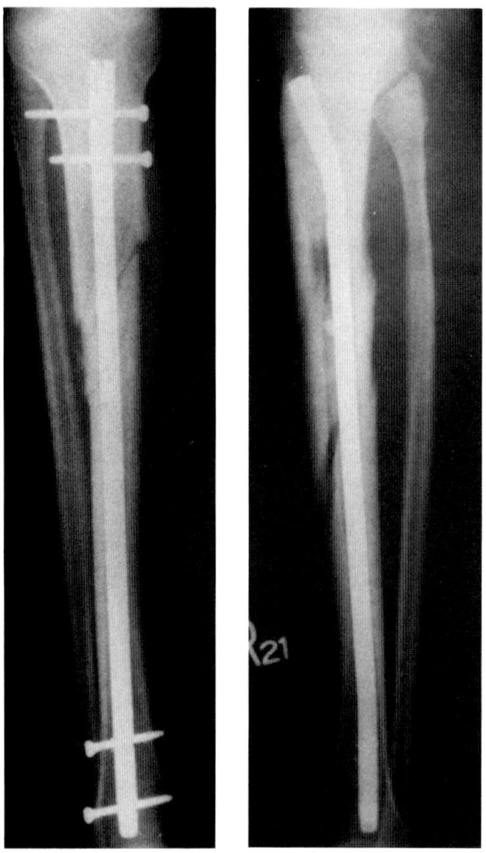

F,G

FIG. 7-26. A: Russell-Taylor™ nail. (Courtesy of Smith and Nephew Richards, Memphis, TN.) Intramedullary nailing in a static configuration of a grade II open fracture of the left tibia **(B)** and grade III open fracture of the right tibia **(C)**. Postnailing radiographs show AP **(D)** and lateral **(E)** views of the left tibia and AP **(F)** and lateral **(G)** views of the right tibia. (From Whittle AP, Russell TA, Taylor JC, LaVelle DG. Treatment of open fractures of the tibial shaft with the use of interlocking nailing without reaming. *J Bone Joint Surg* [*Am*] 1992;74A.)

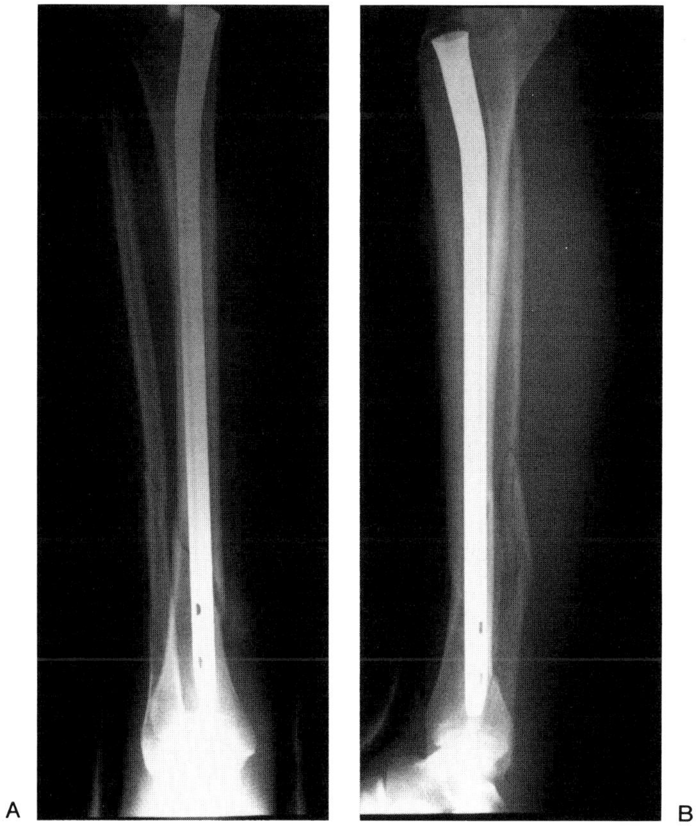

FIG. 7-27. Grosse-Kempf nail. The AP **(A)** and lateral **(B)** radiographs of a tibial fracture with a Grosse-Kempf intramedullary nail.

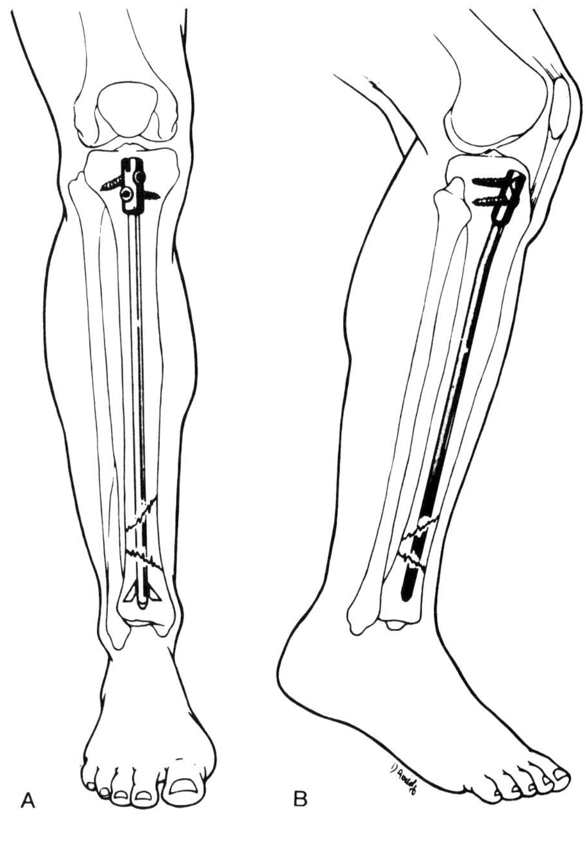

FIG. 7-28. Brooker-Wills nail. The Brooker-Wills seen from the front **(A)** and side **(B)**. (From Brooker AF Jr, Epps H, Constable D. New tibial interlocking nail system. *J Orthop Trauma* 1987;1:257–259.)

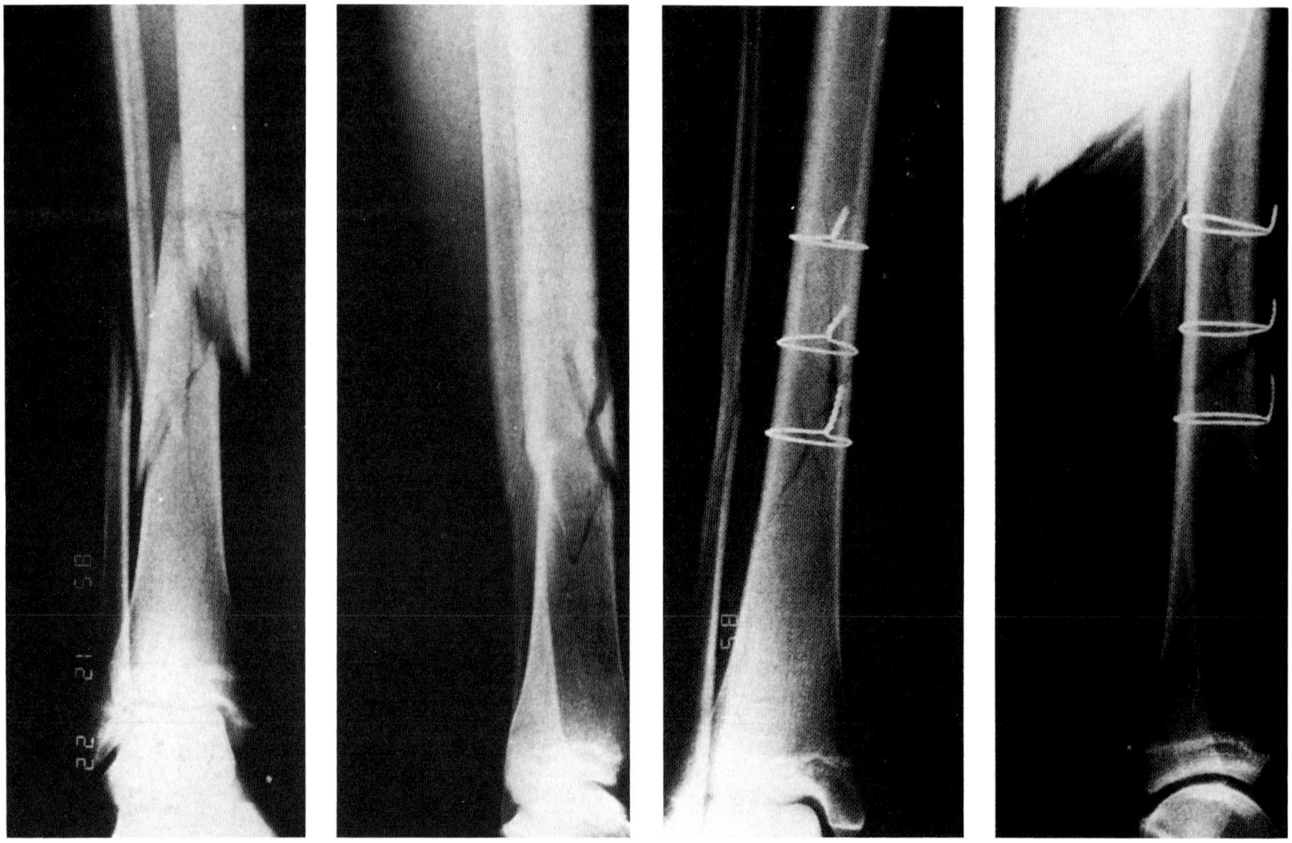

A,B C,D

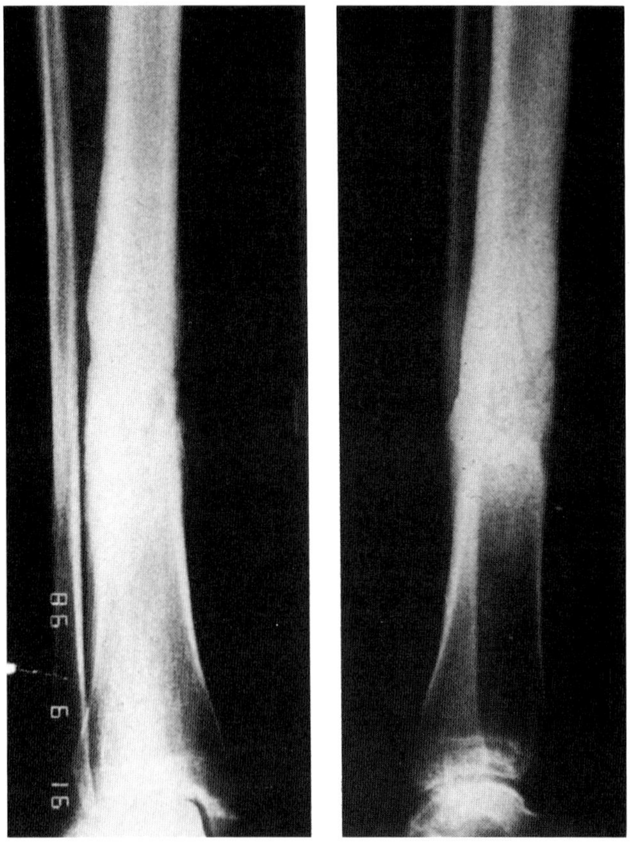

E,F

FIG. 7-29. Percutaneous cerclage wire fixation. The AP **(A)** and lateral **(B)** radiographs of a comminuted torsional tibial fracture, after percutaneous cerclage wire fixation **(C,D)**, and follow-up radiographs after healing and wire removal **(E,F)**. (From Habernek H, Walch G, Dengg C. Cerclage for torsional fractures of the tibia. *J Bone Joint Surg* [*Br*] 1989;71:311–313.)

(Johner and Wruhs classification type A1, B1 and sometimes C1) in which the length of the fracture line exceeds twice the diameter of the tibia and full reduction has been achieved by manipulation under radiographic control."

Open Reduction and Internal Fixation

Certain oblique tibial fractures can be fixed with multiple screws to achieve anatomic reduction with minimal soft tissue dissection.[7] Casting or bracing is necessary with this method. Some cases of delayed union can be treated with bone grafts and multiple screws (Fig. 7-30).[7,51,63]

Compression Plate and Screws

This type of fixation is useful in certain situations but has largely been replaced by other treatment methods, such as intramedullary nailing.[7,29,32,63]

Indications
- Tibial shaft fractures with interarticular extension at the knee or ankle
- Malunions or nonunions (Fig. 7-31)[63,73]

Careful attention to maintaining the vascular integrity of the bone is necessary for good healing.[7]

Advantages[7,70]
- Better anatomic results
- Shorter mean healing time

Disadvantages[7,63,70]
- Increased risk of infection
- Increased duration of hospital stay
- Fixation or implant failure
- Increased rate of delayed union or nonunion
- Refractures through screw holes

The AO/ASIF group has recommended the techniques and indications for this method.[66]

LEG-LENGTH DISCREPANCY

Leg-length discrepancies are common problems with multiple causes.[18,27,31]

The need for surgical intervention for leg-length discrepancy of the tibia and/or the femur is determined by multiple factors. Differences of 2 cm or less can be managed with shoe lifts.[18,31] Epiphysodesis of the uninvolved extremity can be used for discrepancies of 5 cm or less.[19] A greater deformity may require lengthening procedures.[18,27,31]

Bone-lengthening concepts were initially introduced by Codivilla in 1905.[55] Modern bone-lengthening procedures, as developed by Ilizarov,[41] use a corticotomy, with resection of the cortex and preservation of the medullary canal. The fibula is transsected at a different level than is the tibial corticotomy (Fig. 7-32).[43,55]

Distraction can be achieved immediately with fixation or by gradual distraction. A two-level corticotomy can speed the bone-lengthening process with less chance of fracture or soft tissue problems, but it is technically more difficult.[43]

Rezaian and Abtahi[60] used a closed tibial osteotomy and indirect fibular epiphyseal distraction with a bilateral-frame external fixator (Fig. 7-33).

The frequency and distance of gradual distraction is variable. Some surgeons use 1 to 2 mm once a day; others used 0.25 mm four times a day.[18,19,43]

The process is followed radiographically. If no calcification is present at the site, the distraction is reversed to compression for several days, and then, the distraction is reinstituted.[43]

The Rancho technique modified Ilizarov's method by substituting titanium half pins for transfixion wires and added hinges and clamps that were attached to the rings.[30] Orthofix™ and Wagner unilateral half frame external fixators are now frequently used for leg lengthening. Also, a corticotomy and progressive distraction are used (Fig. 7-34).[18,19,31,55] After the desired length is obtained, internal fixation with a bone graft is inserted.[18]

The surgical procedures involving the epiphyseal plate include stapling and distraction.

Epiphysodesis

The proximal tibial and fibular or the distal femoral epiphysis are stapled to arrest growth. The opposite extremity continues to grow, reducing the length discrepancy between the legs.[18]

Epiphyseal Distraction and Chondrodiastasis

This method involves slow symmetric epiphyseal distraction to correct short or angulated limbs (Fig. 7-35).[1,18,54]

Preoperative Imaging

The imaging for leg-length procedures includes routine radiographs, scanograms, or CT.[59]

COMPLICATIONS AND POSTOPERATIVE IMAGING

Delayed union is a common complication of tibial fractures and occurs in up to 15% of all patients.[7,51,65] Nonunion can occur with any type of fracture but is more frequent in high-energy displaced comminuted

(text continues on page 572)

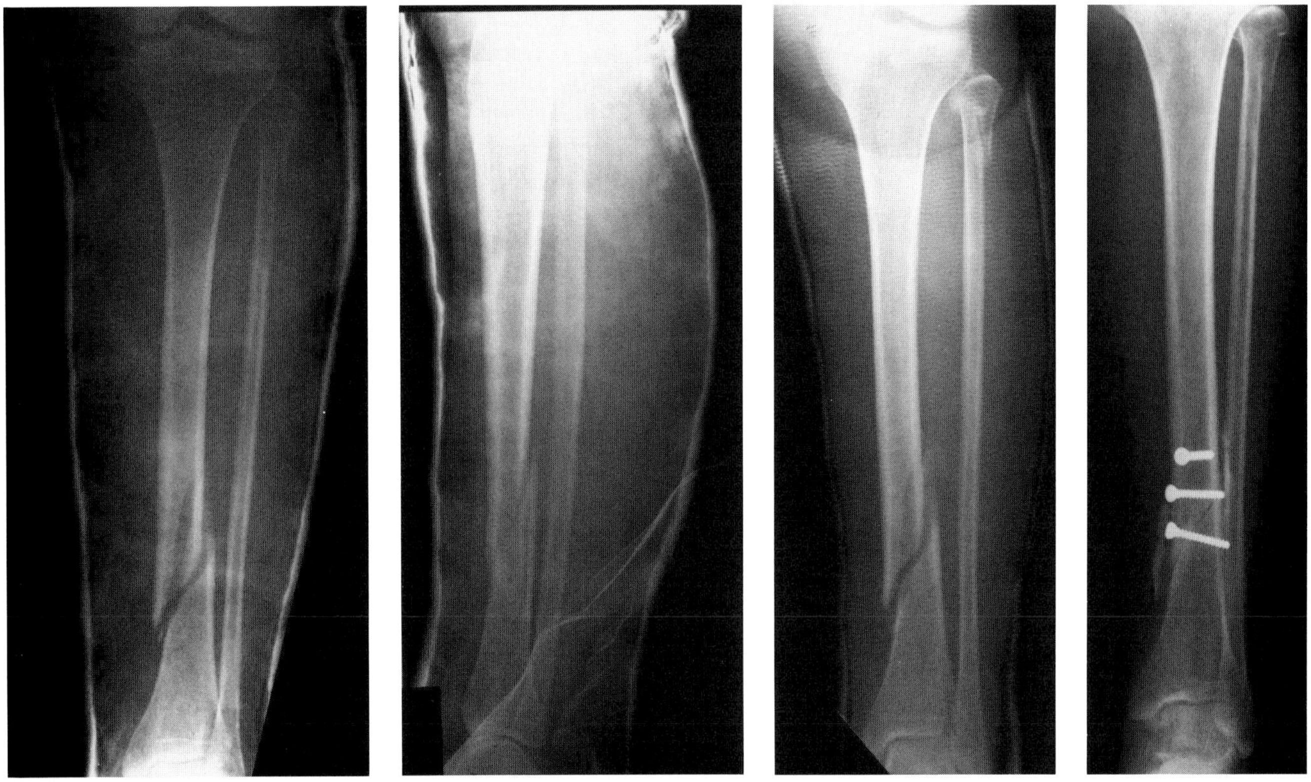

A,B C,D

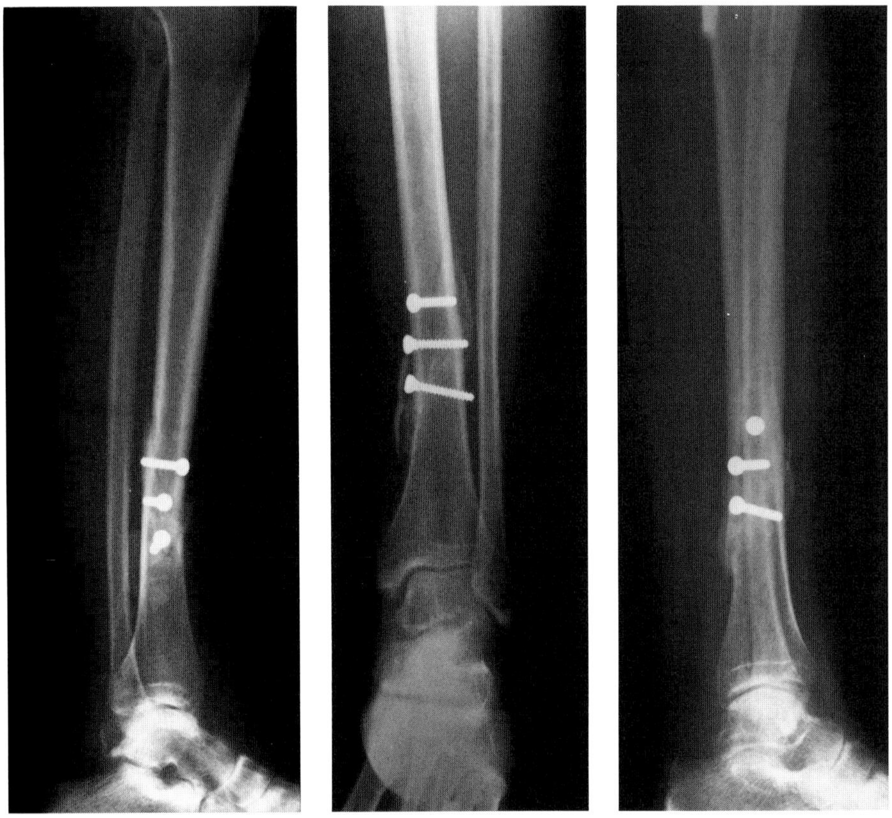

E,F,G

FIG. 7-30. The AP **(A)** and lateral **(B)** views of the tibia showing a distal spiral fracture of the tibia and proximal fibular fracture. **C:** Follow-up radiographs with fracture in PTB cast at 3 months shows minimal callus. Bone grafts and leg screws were used **(D,E)**, and healing occurred at 5 months **(F,G)**. (From Berquist TH. *Imaging of orthopedic trauma,* 2nd ed. New York: Raven Press, 1992.)

A,B

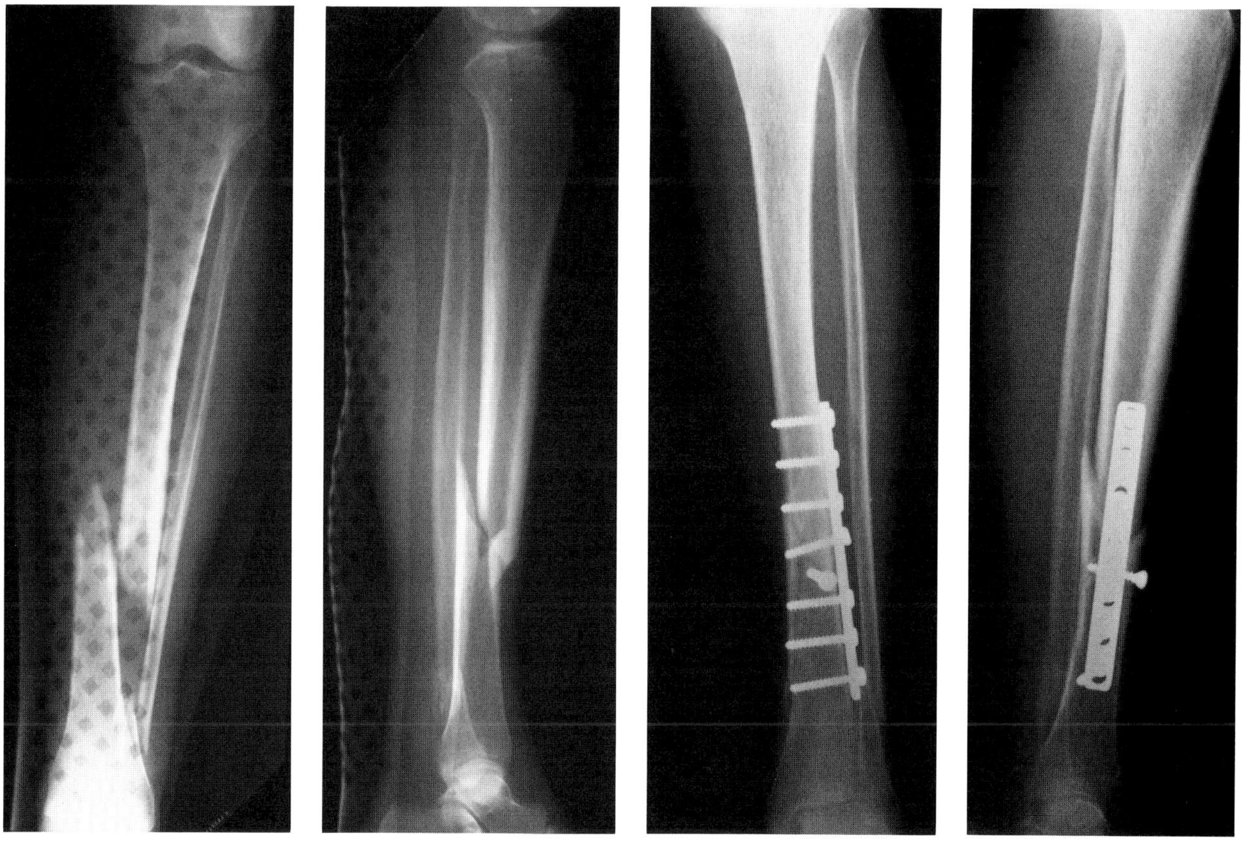

C,D

FIG. 7-31. The AP **(A)** and lateral **(B)** views of overriding fracture of the distal tibia and fibula with several centimeters of shortening. **C,D:** Reduction was accomplished with a seven-hole AO plate and screws. (From Berquist TH. *Imaging of orthopedic trauma,* 2nd ed. New York: Raven Press, 1992.)

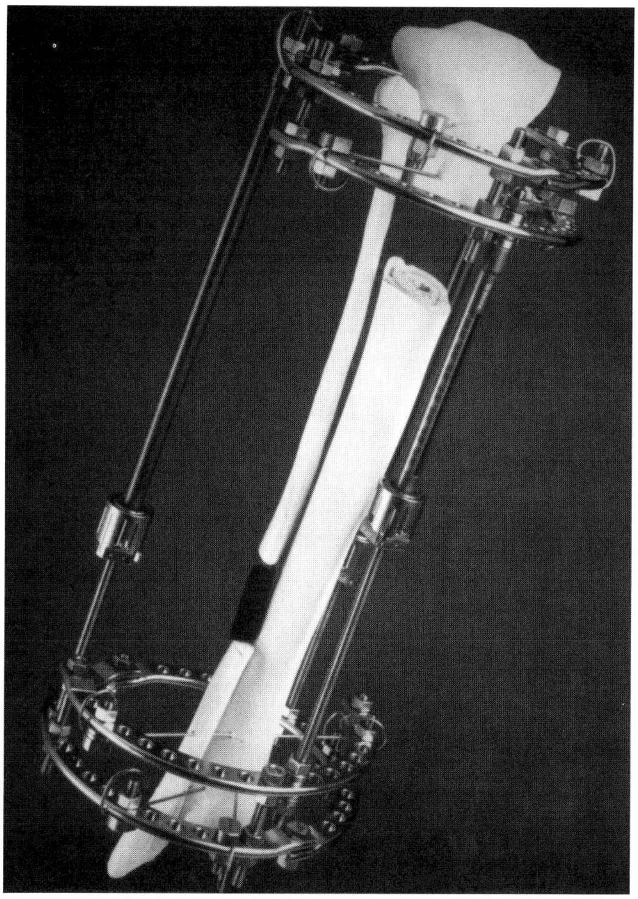

FIG. 7-32. Ilizarov bone-lengthening frame with tibial corticotomy and a distally transsected fibula. (Courtesy of Smith and Nephew Richards, Memphis, TN.)

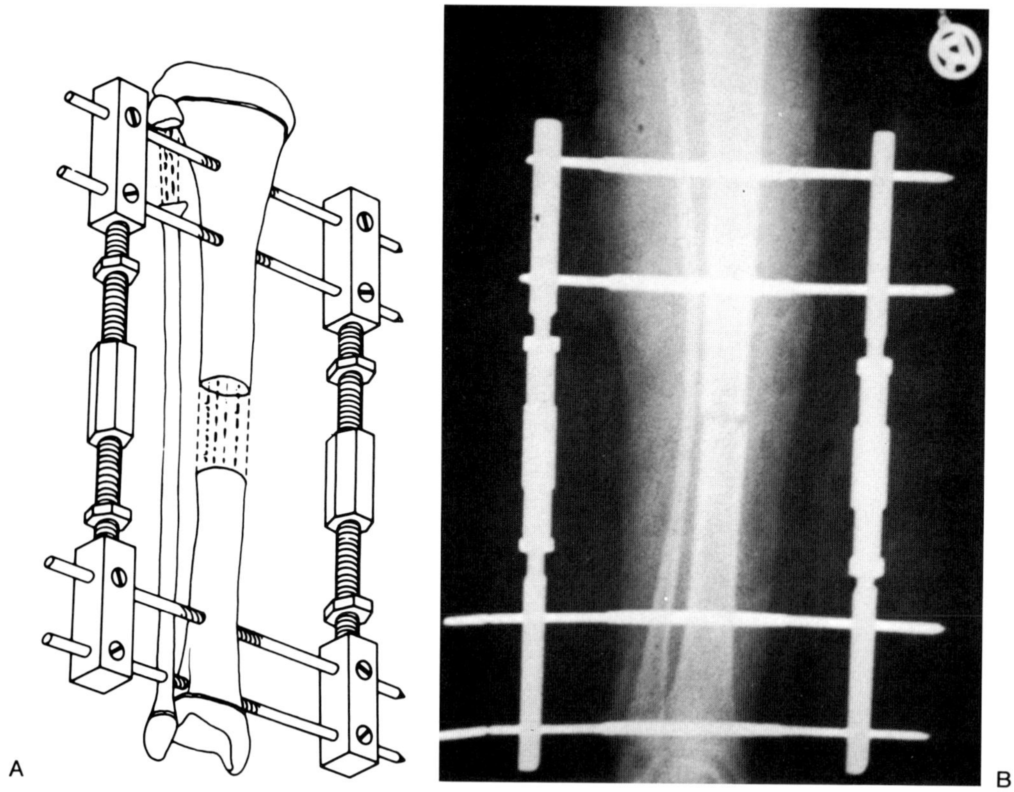

FIG. 7-33. Rezaian technique uses a closed tibial osteotomy, direct tibial distraction, and indirect fibular epiphyseal distraction with a bilateral frame **(A)** and radiograph **(B)**. (From Rezaian SM, Abtahi M. A simple and safe technique for tibial lengthening. *Clin Orthop* 1986;207.)

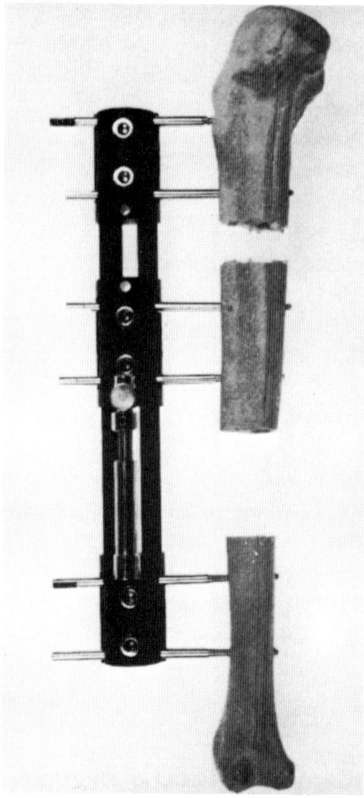

FIG. 7-34. Orthofix™ unilateral fixator modified for leg lengthening. (From Green SA. The Ilizarov method: Rancho technique. *Orthop Clin North Am* 1991;22.)

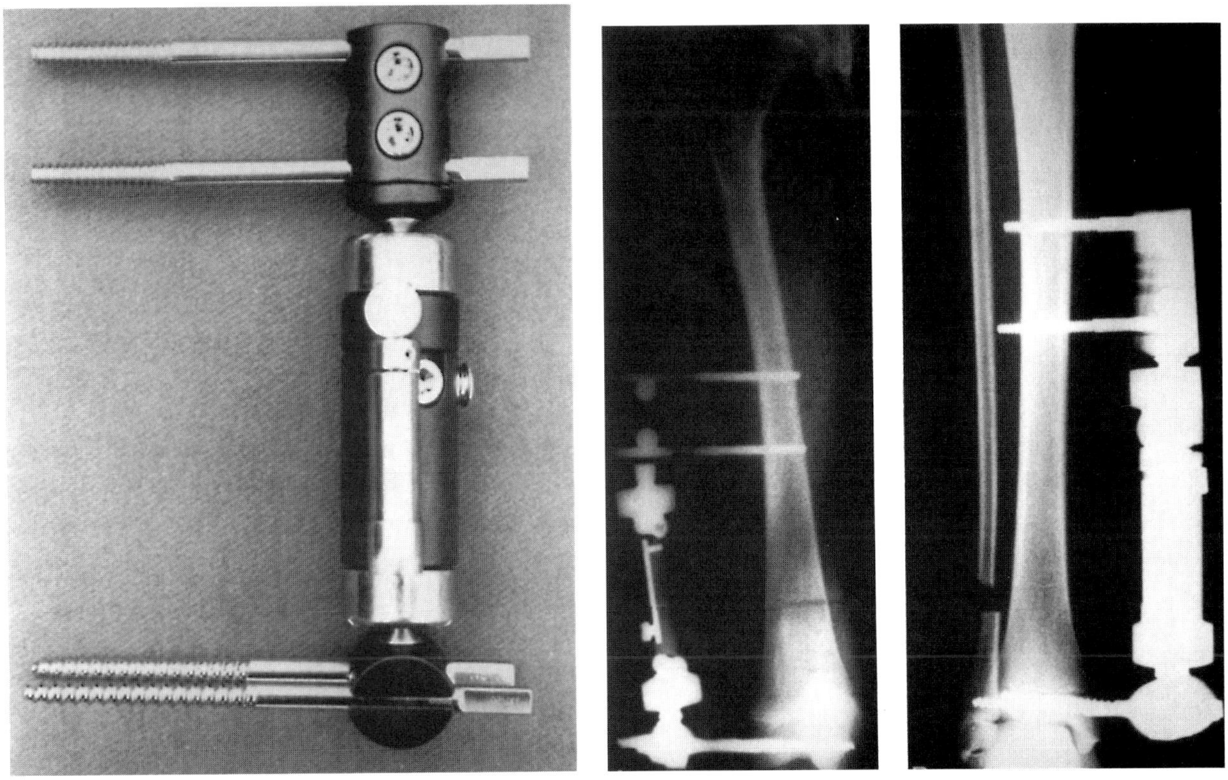

A B

FIG. 7-35. Epiphyseal distraction. Orthofix™ modified for chondrodiastasis **(A)**, with radiographs of fixator in place for femoral and tibial lengthening **(B)**. (From Aldegheri R, Trevella G, Lavini F. Epiphyseal distraction: chondrodiastasis. *Clin Orthop* 1989;241.)

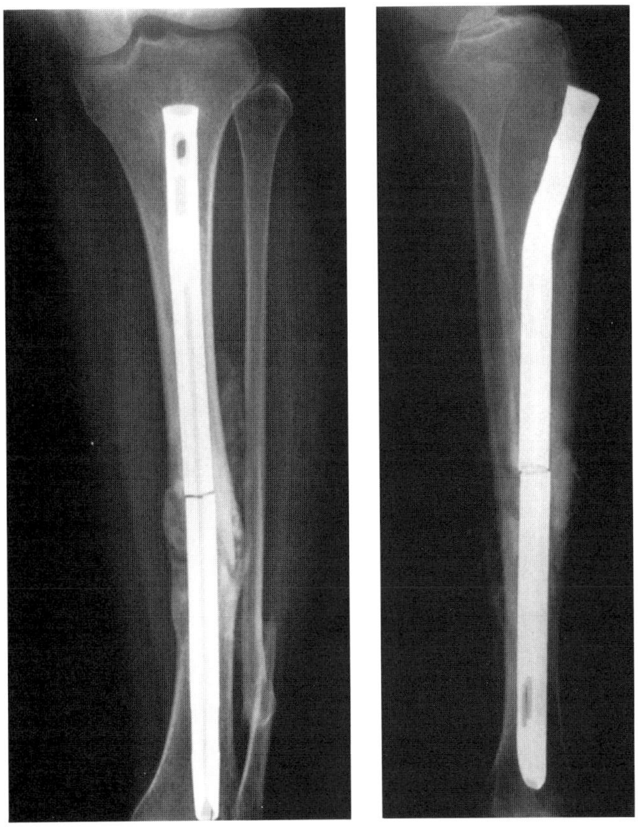

FIG. 7-36. Fixation failure. Midtibial shaft nonunion with fractured intramedullary nail.

open fractures.[7] Treatment includes bone grafts, fibular osteotomy, intramedullary nailing, compression plating, and electrical stimulation.[7,9]

The healing time of the fracture is approximately the same for proximal, middle, and distal third tibial shaft fractures. The presence or absence of an associated fibular fracture does affect tibial healing. The intact fibula adds structural support but can also contribute to an angular deformity of the tibia, delayed union, or nonunion. The resection of a small segment of fibula may be necessary for appropriate tibial healing.[7,21]

Delayed union, malunion, and nonunion can be evaluated with serial routine radiographs, which are obtained in at least two projections. Conventional tomography can be helpful in evaluating fractures with internal metallic fixation that could cause artifacts that would interfere with the CT or MRI results.[7,8]

Infections are most frequently seen after high-energy open fractures that have skin loss or necrosis and after open reduction with internal fixation of fractures with skin coverage failure.[63] Infection also occurs in pin tracts and other open techniques.[7,63] The techniques of MRI and radionuclide studies can be more effective in the early detection of infection than are routine radiographs.[7,8]

Instrument failure can occur with any fixation device. If the time for healing exceeds the structural life of the device, it may fail (Fig. 7-36). Therefore, if delayed healing or a deformity in the device occurs, a revision should be considered.[63]

Soft tissue complications are seen because the lower leg is the most common site of combined bone and soft tissue injury.[29] Neurovascular injuries, skin loss, and/or necrosis are common in high-energy injuries.[15,33] Compartment syndromes result from increased pressure as a result of edema and hemorrhage following fracture.[63]

Soft tissue injuries may also be related to the hardware used. Soft tissue impingements with wire or screw fixation and with protruding screws, plates, or nails are examples.[5,6] Soft tissue injuries may be evaluated by MRI, venography, and arteriography. Compartment syndromes are best evaluated by clinical findings and conventional intracompartmental measurement techniques.[7,8]

REFERENCES

1. Aldegheri R, Trevella G. Lavini F. Epiphyseal distraction: chondrodiastasis. *Clin Orthop* 1989;241.
2. Anderson R. An automatic method of treatment for fractures of the tibia and fibula. *Surg Gynecol Obstet* 1934;58:639–646.
3. Bach AW, Hansen ST Jr. Plates versus external fixation in severe open tibial shaft fractures: a randomized trial. *Clin Orthop* 1989;241:89–94.
4. Behrens F. A primer of fixator devices and configurations. *Clin Orthop* 1989;241:5–14.
5. Behrens F. General theory and principles of external fixation. *Clin Orthop* 1989;241:15–23.
6. Behrens F, Searles K. External fixation of the tibia. Basic concepts and prospective evaluation. *J Bone Joint Surg [Br]* 1986;68:246–254.
7. Bender CE, Campbell DC II, Berquist TH. The tibia, fibula, and calf. In: Berquist TH, ed. *Imaging of orthopedic trauma.* 2nd ed. New York: Raven Press; 1992.
8. Berquist TH. *Magnetic resonance of the musculoskeletal system.* New York: Raven Press; 1990.
9. Bohler L. *The treatment of fractures.* 5th ed. New York: Grune and Stratton; 1958.
10. Bone LB, Johnson KD. Treatment of tibial fractures by reaming and intramedullary nailing. *J Bone Joint Surg [Am]* 1989;68A:877–886.
11. Boyer RS, Jaffee RB, Nixon GW, Condon VR. Trampoline fracture of the proximal tibia in children. *AJR Am J Roentgenol* 1986;146:83–85.
12. Brooker AF Jr, Epps H, Constable D. New tibial interlocking nail system. *J Orthop Trauma* 1987;1:257–259.
13. Caplin RD, Veith RG, Hansen ST. Treatment of failures after plating of tibial fractures. *J Bone Joint Surg [Am]* 1986;68A:1231–1236.
14. Carpenter EB. Management of fractures of the shaft of the tibia and fibula. *J Bone Joint Surg [Am]* 1966:48A:1640–1646.
15. Caudle RJ, Stern PJ. Severe open fractures of the tibia. *J Bone Joint Surg [Am]* 1987;69:801–807.
16. Chapman MW. Immediate internal fixation in open fractures. *Orthop Clin North Am* 1980;11:579–591.
17. Choa EYS, Hein TJ. Mechanical performance of the standard Orthofix external fixator. *Orthopedics* 1988;11:1057–1069.
18. Coleman SS. Lower limb length discrepancy. In: Lovell WW, Winter RB, ed. *Pediatric orthopedics.* Vol. 2. Philadelphia: JB Lippincott; 1986:281–865.
19. Dahl MT, Fischer DA. Lower extremity lengthening by Wagner's method and by callous distraction. *Orthop Clin North Am* 1991;22:643–649.
20. De Bastiani G, Aldeghiri R, Brivio LR. The treatment of fractures with a dynamic axial fixator. *J Bone Joint Surg [Br]* 1984;66B:538–545.
21. DeLee JC, Hickman JD, Lewis AG. Partial fibulectomy for ununited fractures of the tibia. *J Bone Joint Surg [Am]* 1981;63A:1390–1395.
22. Edge AJ, Denham RA. External fixation for complication tibial fractures. *J Bone Joint Surg [Br]* 1981;63:92–97.
23. Edwards CC. *Current concepts of external fixation of fractures.* Berlin: Springer-Verlag; 1982.
24. Ekeland A, Thoresen BO, Alho A, Stromsoe K, Folleras G, Haukebo A. Interlocking intramedullary nailing in the treatment of tibial fractures. A report of 45 cases. *Clin Orthop* 1988;231:205–215.
25. Ellis H. Disabilities after tibial shaft fractures. *J Bone Joint Surg [Br]* 1958;40:190–197.
26. Ellis H. The speed of healing after fracture of the tibial shaft. *J Bone Joint Surg [Br]* 1958;40:42–46.
27. Faber FWM, Keessen W, van Roermund PM. Complications of leg lengthening. *Acta Orthop Scand* 1991;62:327–332.
28. Gershuni DH, Shyhar MJ, Thompson B, Resnick D, Donald G, Akeson WH. A comparison of conventional radiography and computed tomography in the evaluation of spiral fractures of the tibia. *J Bone Joint Surg [Am]* 1985;67A:1388–1395.
29. Gotzen L, Haas N. The operative treatment of tibial shaft fractures with soft tissue injuries. In: Tscherne H, Gotzen L, eds. *Fractures with soft tissue injuries.* Berlin: Springer-Verlag; 1984.
30. Green SA. The Ilizarov method: Rancho technique. *Orthop Clin North Am* 1991;22.
31. Guichet JM, Spivak JM, Trouilloud P, Grammont PM. Lower limb-length discrepancy. An epidemiologic study. *Clin Orthop* 1991;272:235–241.
32. Gustilo RB, Anderson JT. Prevention of infection in the treatment of 1025 open fractures of long bones. *J Bone Joint Surg [Am]* 1976;58:453–458.
33. Gustilo RB, Mendoza RM, Williams DN. Problems in the management of type III (severe) open fractures: a new classification of type III open fractures. *J Trauma* 1984;24:742–746.

34. Habernek H, Walch G, Dengg C. Cerclage for torsional fractures of the tibia. *J Bone Joint Surg [Br]* 1989;71:311–313.
35. Hall RF, Gonzales M. Fracture of the proximal part of the tibia and fibula associated with an entrapped popliteal artery. *J Bone Joint Surg [Am]* 1986;68A:941–944.
36. Hammer R. A new device for external fixation. *Acta Orthop Scand* 1988;59:708–711.
37. Hammer R, Lidman D, Nettelblad H, Ostrup L. Team approach to tibial fracture. 37 consecutive type III cases reviewed after 2–10 years. *Acta Orthop Scand* 1992;63:471–476.
38. Harkess JW, Ramsey WC, Harkess J. Principles of fractures and dislocations. In: Rockwood CA Jr, Green DP, Bucholz RW. *Rockwood and Green's fractures in adults.* 3rd ed. New York: JB Lippincott; 1991.
39. Holbrook JL, Swiontkowski MF, Sanders R. Treatment of open fractures of the tibial shaft: Ender nailing versus external fixation. *J Bone Joint Surg [Am]* 1989;71A:1231–1238.
40. Holbrook TL, Grazier K, Kelsey JL, Stauffer RN. *The frequency of occurrence, impact and cost of musculoskeletal conditions in the United States.* A.A.O.S., 1984.
41. Ilizarov GA. Clinical application of the tension-stress effect for limb lengthening. *Clin Orthop* 1990;250:8–26.
42. Ilizarov GA. The tension-stress effect on the genesis and growth of tissues. *Clin Orthop* 1989;239:264–285.
43. *The original Ilizarov system: general surgical technique brochure.* Memphis, TN: Smith & Richards, 1990.
44. Johner R, Wruhs O. Classification of tibial shaft fractures and correlation with results after rigid internal fixation. *Clin Orthop* 1983;178:7–25.
45. Karlstrom G, Olerud S. External fixation of severe open tibial fractures with Hoffmann frame. *Clin Orthop* 1983;180:68–77.
46. Kempf I, Grosse A, Rigaut P. The treatment of noninfected pseudoarthrosis of the femur and tibia with locked intramedullary nailing. *Clin Orthop* 1986;212:142–154.
47. Kimmel RB. Results of treatment using the Hoffmann external fixator for fractures of the tibial diaphysis. *J Trauma* 1982;22:960–965.
48. Klemm KW, Borner M. Interlocking nailing of complex fractures of the femur and tibia. *Clin Orthop* 1986;212:89–100.
49. Laasonen EM, Jokio P, Lindholm TS. Tibial torsion measured by computed tomography. *Acta Radiol* 1984;25:325–329.
50. Lawyer RB, Lubbers LM. Use of the Hoffman apparatus in the treatment of unstable tibial fractures. *J Bone Joint Surg [Am]* 1980;62:1264–1273.
51. Leach RE. Fractures of the tibia and fibula. In: Rockwood CA, Green DP. *Fractures in adults.* 2nd ed. Vol. 2. Philadelphia: JB Lippincott; 1984:1593–1663.
52. Lottes JO. Intramedullary fixation for fracture of shaft of tibia. *South Med J* 1952;45:407–414.
53. Melendez EM, Colon C. Treatment of open tibial fractures with the OrthoFix™ fixator. *Clin Orthop* 1989;241:224–230.
54. Monticelli G, Spinelli R. Distraction epiphysiolysis as a method of limb lengthening: I. experimental study: II. morphological investigation: III. clinical applications. Clin Orthop 1981;154:254.
55. Mosely CF. Leg lengthening: a historical perspective. *Orthop Clin North Am* 1991;22:555–561.
56. Muller ME, Allgower M, Schneider R, Willenegger H. *Manual of internal fixation; techniques recommended by the AO group.* Berlin: Springer-Verlag; 1979.
57. Nicoll EA. Closed and open management of tibial fractures. *Clin Orthop* 1974;105:144–153.
58. Nicoll EA. Fractures of the tibial shaft. A survey of 705 cases. *J Bone Joint Surg [Br]* 1964;46:373–387.
59. Pugh DG, Winkler NT. Scanography for leg length measurement: an easy satisfactory method. *Radiology* 1966;87:130–133.
60. Rezaian SM, Abtahi M. A simple and safe technique for tibial lengthening. *Clin Orthop* 1986;207.
61. Rommens P, Schmit-Neuerburg KP. Ten years of experience with the operative management of tibial shaft fractures. *J Trauma* 1987;27:917–927.
62. Ruedi T. Intramedullary nailing with interlocking. *Arch Orthop Trauma Surg* 1990;109:317–320.
63. Russell TA, Taylor JC, Lavelle DG. Fractures of the tibia and fibula. In: Rockwood CA, Green DP. *Fractures in adults.* 3rd ed. Vol. 2. Philadelphia: JB Lippincott; 1991:1915–1982.
64. Russell TA, Taylor JC, LaVelle DG. Russell-Taylor tibial nail system. Memphis, TN: Smith and Nephew Richards, 1993.
65. Sarmiento A. A functional below-the-knee cast for tibial fracture. *J Bone Joint Surg [Am]* 1967;49A:855–875.
66. Sequin F, Texhammar R. *AO/ASIF instrumentation.* Berlin: Springer-Verlag; 1981.
67. Sledge SL, Johnson KD, Henley MB, Watson JT. Intramedullary nailing with reaming to treat non-union of the tibia. *J Bone Joint Surg [Am]* 1989;71A:2004–2029.
68. Stein H, Makin M. Use of the Wagner apparatus in fractures of lower limb. *Orthop Rev* 1980;9.
69. Tscherne H, Gotzen L. *Fractures with soft tissue injuries.* Berlin: Springer-Verlag; 1984.
70. van der Linden W, Larsson K. Plate fixation versus conservative treatment of tibial shaft fractures. *J Bone Joint Surg [Am]* 1979;61A:873–878.
71. Vidal J, Nakach G, Orst G. New biomechanical study of Hoffmann external fixation. *Orthopedics* 1984;7:654–670.
72. Whittle AP, Russell TA, Taylor JC, LaVelle DG. Treatment of open fractures of the tibial shaft with the use of interlocking nailing without reaming. *J Bone Joint Surg [Am]* 1992;74A.
73. Wiss DA, Johnson DL, Miao M. Compression plating for nonunion after failed external fixation of open tibial fractures. *J Bone Joint Surg [Am]* 1992;74A:1279–1285.

Imaging Atlas of Orthopedic Appliances and Prostheses,
edited by T.H. Berquist.

Published by Raven Press, Ltd., New York.

CHAPTER 8

Foot and Ankle

Thomas H. Berquist and Harold B. Kitaoka

There are numerous imaging techniques for evaluating the foot and ankle. The array of surgical procedures for traumatic conditions and reconstructive procedures (arthropathies and neuromuscular disorders) is also extensive. As in the other chapters, this chapter outlines the preoperative imaging techniques required to evaluate foot and ankle disorders and reviews the mechanisms of injury and classifications, when appropriate, for traumatic injuries in specific areas. Operative procedures that use fixation devices for either trauma or reconstructive purposes are also reviewed.

PREOPERATIVE IMAGING EVALUATION

There are numerous imaging techniques that may be used in the preoperative assessment of patients with foot and ankle disorders. This section reviews the general techniques with specific variations referred to in later sections as they apply to specific anatomic areas or clinical disorders.

Routine Radiography

Ankle

The radiographic evaluation of the ankle should include anteroposterior (AP), lateral, and mortise views.[2,3,29] Following trauma, an external oblique projection is also routinely obtained in our practice (Fig. 8-1).[3] Standing AP and lateral views are obtained when there is no history of acute trauma. The mortise view is particularly important to assess the symmetry of the talus within the boundaries of the tibia and fibula. The lateral view should be carefully evaluated for the presence of an effusion, and the pre-Achilles fat triangle should be studied to be certain there is no posterior soft tissue injury.[39] The presence of an effusion suggests an intact capsule and ligaments, which may be useful in the immediate postinjury evaluation. However, small tears may close, reducing the reliability of this sign after 48 hours. The presence of an effusion should also raise the suspicion of subtle fractures, such as a talar dome fracture, which may require conventional or computed tomography (CT) for further evaluation.[3]

Stress Views

Stress views of the ankle may be helpful for evaluating suspected ligament injuries and differentiating them from minor sprains.[3,19] In the acute setting, stress views may be difficult to perform because of pain and swelling of the involved area. To obtain accurate results, injection of local anesthetic may be useful prior to performing the stress views. Views should be obtained using varus and valgus stress. It is important that the varus and valgus stress views be performed in neutral and plantar flexed positions to ensure accuracy. Because normal talar tilt may approach 25° in a hypermobile ankle, it is essential to compare both ankles for an accurate assessment. On varus-valgus stress views, a difference of 3 mm between the injured and uninjured side may indicate ligament injury. If the injured ankle exceeds that of the normal ankle by 5°, using a slightly different technique, a ligament injury is also most likely to be present. A difference of 10° allows the diagnosis of a ligament injury with more certainty (Fig. 8-2).[5,13,15,26,28,33,38]

The AP stress views (Fig. 8-3) can be obtained by placing the patient's heel on a support so that the ankle and

(text continues on page 578)

T. H. Berquist: Mayo Medical School and Department of Diagnostic Radiology, Mayo Clinic Jacksonville, Jacksonville, Florida 32224.
H. B. Kitaoka: Mayo Medical School and Department of Orthopedic Surgery, Mayo Clinic, Rochester, Minnesota 55903.

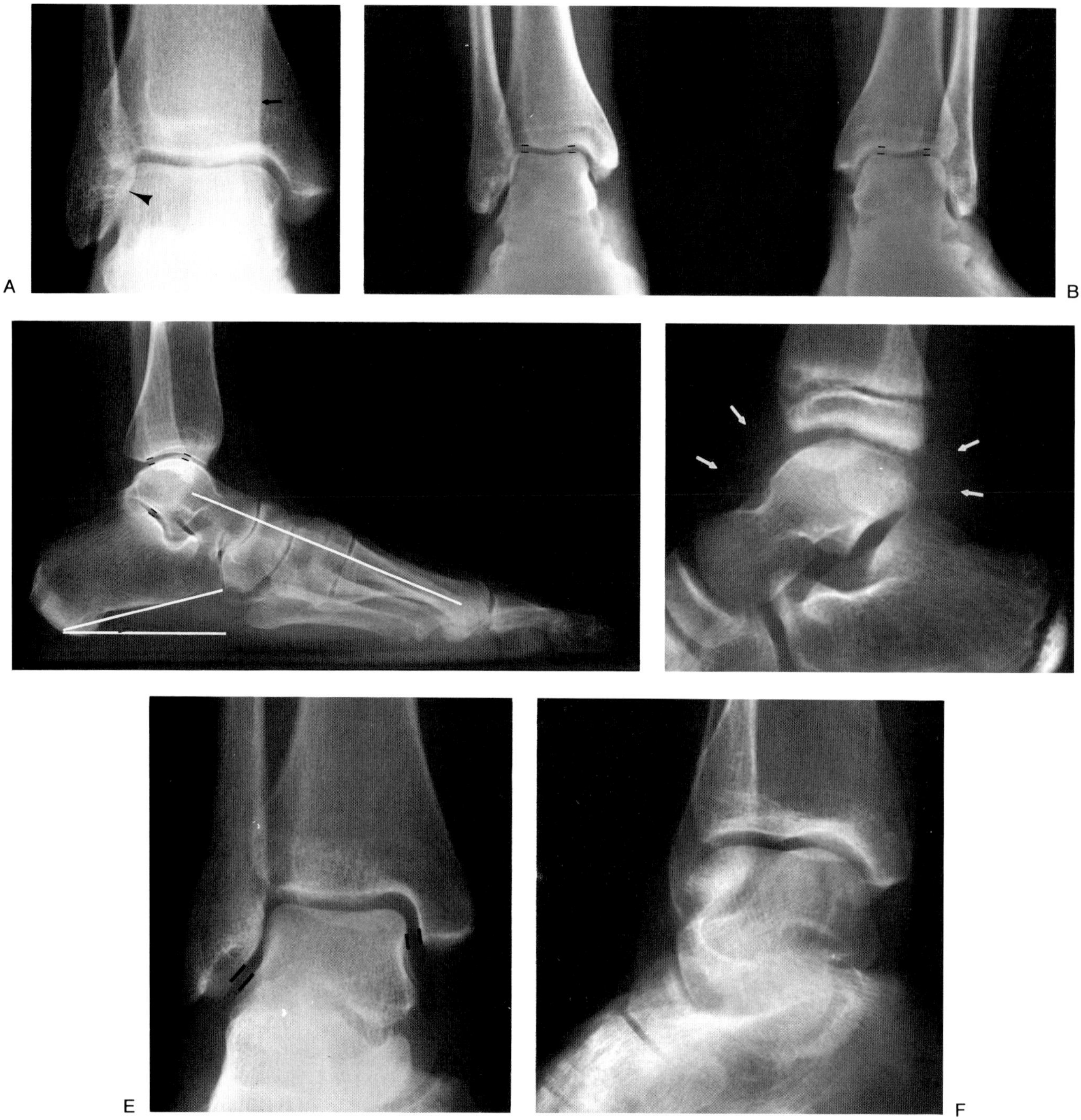

FIG. 8-1. Routine views of the ankle. **A:** An AP view of the ankle. The fibula overlaps the lateral talus (*arrowhead*). The Achilles tendon shadow projects over the tibia (*black arrow*) and should not be confused with a pathologic condition. **B:** Standing AP views for assessment of joint-space width and congruency. There is slight symmetric narrowing of both ankles (*lines*). **C:** Normal standing lateral view of the foot and ankle. The ankle and subtalar joints (*lines*) are clearly seen. The normal talus, tarsal, and first metatarsal alignment (*white line*) and normal calcaneal inclination (20° to 30°) are demonstrated. **D:** Lateral view of the ankle demonstrating an effusion (*arrows*) with anterior "teardrop." **E:** Mortise view with joint space clearly defined and no overlap of the fibula and talus. **F:** External oblique view that provides an additional view of the medial talar dome and medial malleolus.

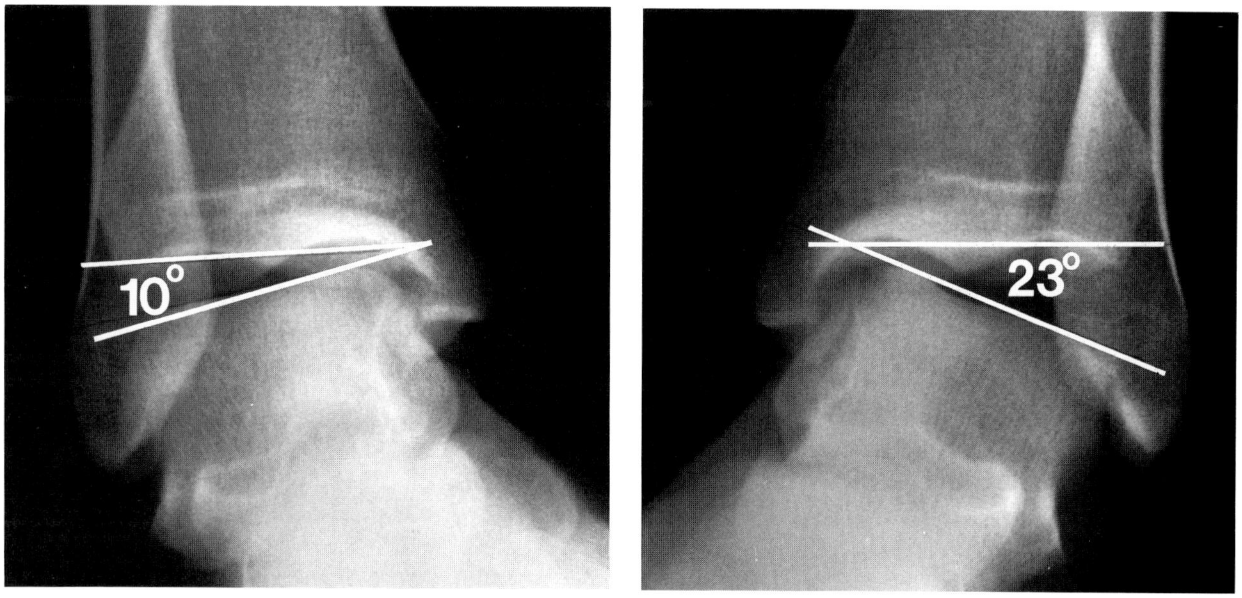

FIG. 8-2. Varus and valgus stress views. Valgus stress views of the normal right **(A)** and abnormal left **(B)** ankle. The normal ankle opens 10°, but the injured side opens 23° because of anterior talofibular and calcaneofibular ligament disruption.

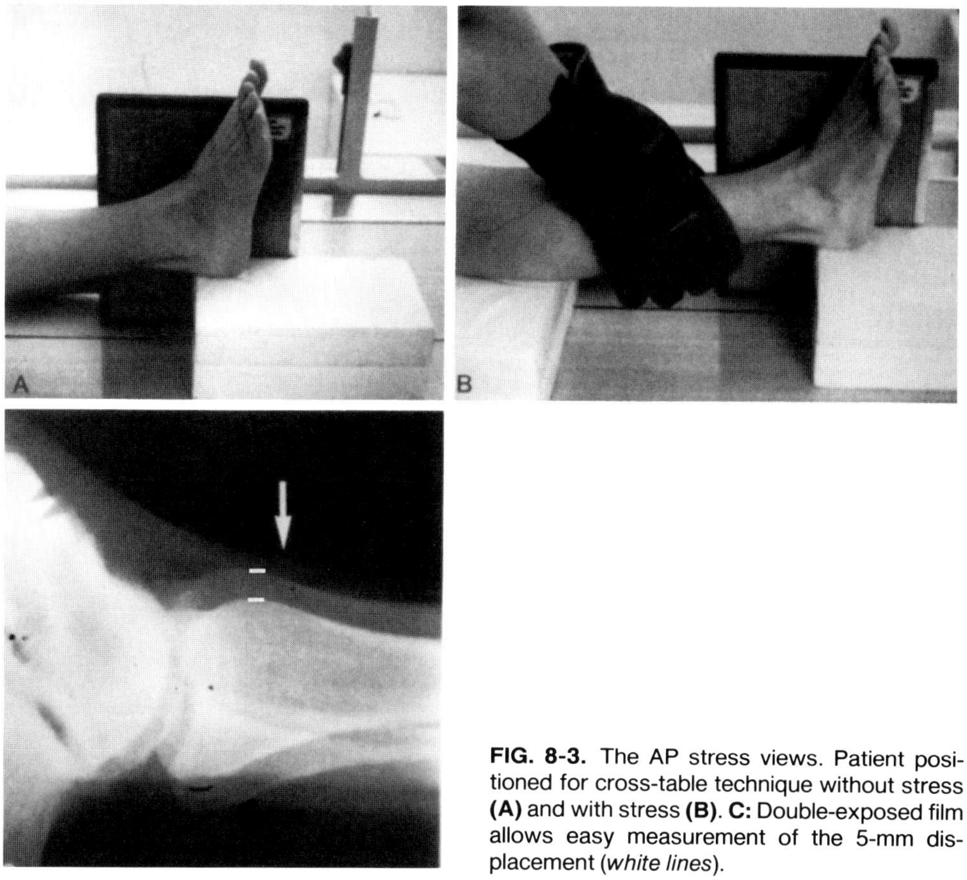

FIG. 8-3. The AP stress views. Patient positioned for cross-table technique without stress **(A)** and with stress **(B)**. **C:** Double-exposed film allows easy measurement of the 5-mm displacement (*white lines*).

knee are level. This removes stress from the ankle. An initial radiograph is obtained, and a second one is double exposed after stress is applied to the anterior tibia. This technique allows the measurement of the degree of displacement of the talus in relation to the tibia. Talar shift > 2.5 mm should be considered abnormal.[3,28]

Foot

Routine radiographs of the foot should be obtained in the AP, lateral, and oblique views (Figs. 8-1C and 8-4).[2,3] In the nonacute trauma setting, standing AP and lateral views of the foot and ankle are also essential to evaluate the anatomy properly and obtain accurate measurements, which are used to evaluate deformities. These measurements are discussed later with appropriate reconstructive procedures.

Isolated views of the phalanges are also important when the anatomy of an individual toe needs to be defined better. The AP, lateral, and oblique views are routinely obtained.[2,3]

Special Views

The complex anatomy of the hindfoot may require further views for a more complete evaluation. The axial calcaneal view is obtained in addition to the lateral view (Fig. 8-5) and provides important information regarding the width of the calcaneus following trauma and the talocalcaneal articulations.[35] Subtalar views may also be obtained in different positions; however, because of difficulty in the technique, fluoroscopic positioning is preferred.[3,27] The sesamoid view (Fig. 8-6) is useful in patients with medial forefoot symptoms to assess the position and condition of the sesamoids for suspected diagnoses, such as fracture or avascular necrosis.[11]

CT and Conventional Tomography

The complex osseous anatomy of the foot and ankle may make it necessary to evaluate the articular relationships or the position of the fracture fragments further with conventional (Fig. 8-7) or CT (Fig. 8-8).[3,16,23–25,31] Also, CT is useful in selected patients with suspected soft tissue abnormalities.[36,37] These techniques are particularly useful in evaluating subtle suspected trauma or for preoperative planning purposes. The three-dimensional reconstruction of CT images may be useful for planning the surgical repair of complex fractures.[42]

Ultrasonography

The most severe limitation of diagnostic ultrasonography is the inability to penetrate gas or bone. In our practice, ultrasonography is used in the lower extremity for the evaluation of suspected muscle, tendon, and ligament injuries and vascular abnormalities.[3,6,8]

Real-time ultrasonography has gained acceptance in the evaluation of Achilles tendon and other superficial soft tissue structures of the foot and ankle (Fig. 8-9). Ultrasonography is particularly suited for these structures because of its low cost and ability to study tendon motion.[3,17,32]

Radionuclide Studies

Radionuclide bone scans can provide important information in patients with numerous suspected injuries.[3,10] They are also occasionally useful preoperatively in assessing the extent of articular involvement prior to operations such as arthrodesis. Routine radiographs easily demonstrate the site of fracture in most patients with a clinical history of trauma. In subtle cases, radionuclide studies may demonstrate areas of increased uptake, which should be visible in 80% of patients within 24 hours of injury and 95% within 72 hours of injury (Fig. 8-10).[9,20]

Magnetic Resonance Imaging (MRI)

For the detection of musculoskeletal abnormalities in the foot and ankle, MRI is a valuable technique.[4,30] Soft tissue injuries can be detected and classified (Fig. 8-11). Subtle osseous injuries and ischemic changes can also be detected (Fig. 8-12).[3,4,14] An evaluation of the response to treatment is also possible.

Patients should be positioned in the most comfortable and effective position to evaluate the specific clinical problem. Surface or head coils, which allow a comparison of both feet and ankles, are commonly used. Spin-echo (SE) sequences using a T2-weighted double-echo technique (SE 2,000, 80/20) are effective for the detection of both soft tissue and articular abnormalities. New fast-scan gradient-echo techniques are also useful (T2*-weighted images) for reducing the examination time and allowing cine-looped motion studies.

Interventional Techniques

Interventional techniques in the foot and ankle are used for diagnostic and therapeutic purposes. The techniques include arthrography (Fig. 8-13), tenography (Fig. 8-14), and diagnostic and therapeutic injections (Fig. 8-15).[1,5,7,12,18,34,40,41] Proper use of these techniques permits us to obtain additional information regarding ligament and tendon disorders and to localize symptomatic articular regions, which may be useful for planning procedures, such as arthrodesis.[7,21,22] These techniques

(text continues on page 585)

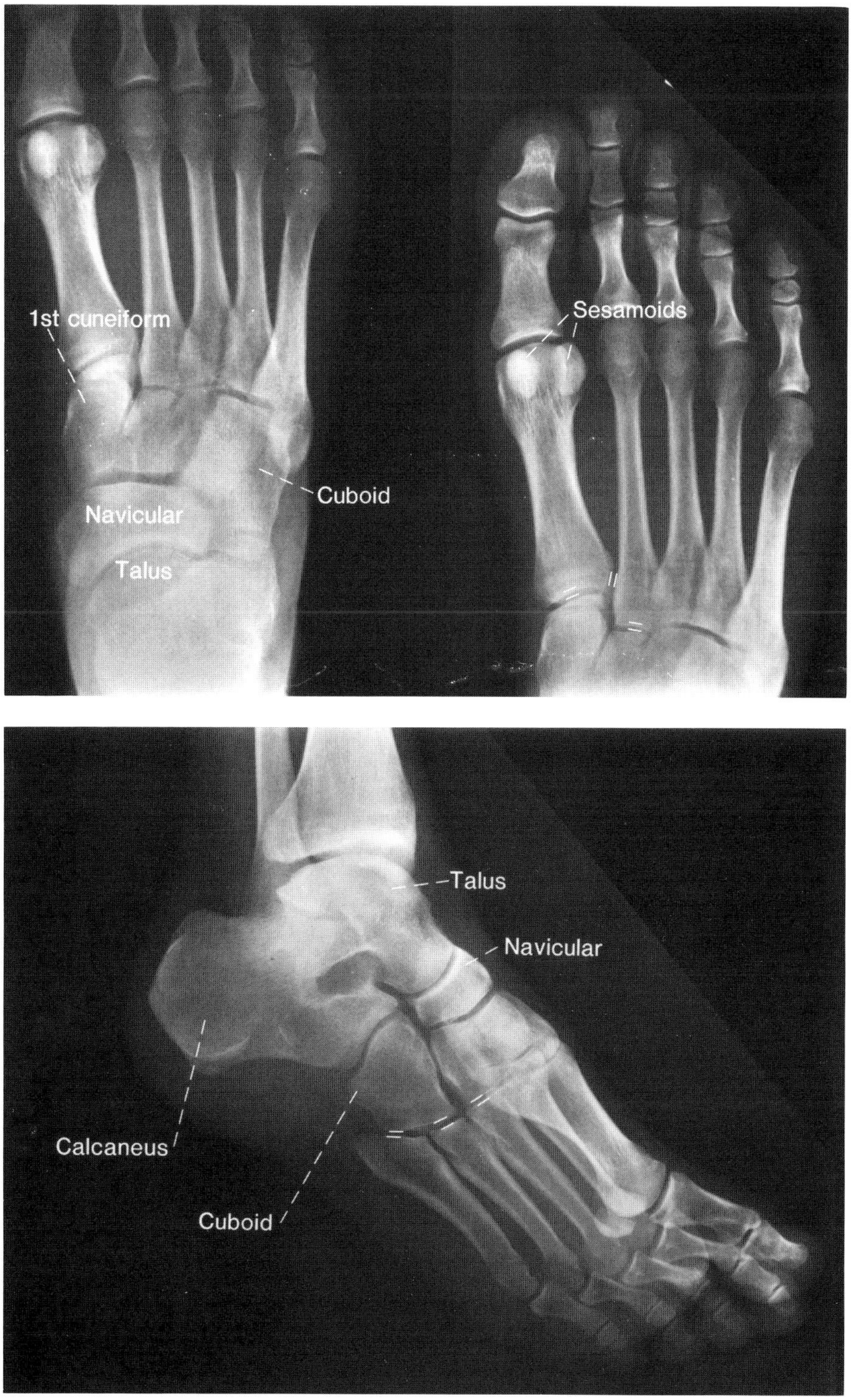

A

B

FIG. 8-4. The AP **(A)** and oblique **(B)** views of the foot. (From Berquist TH. *Radiology of the foot and ankle.* New York: Raven Press, 1989.)

A 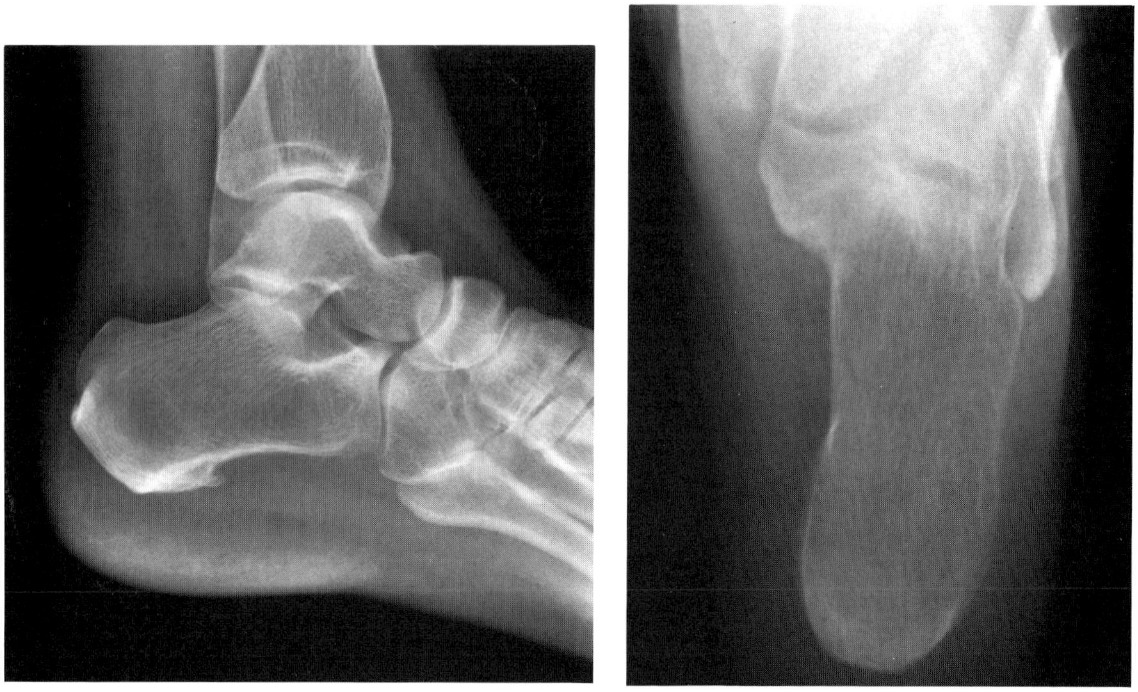 B

FIG. 8-5. Normal lateral **(A)** and axial **(B)** views of the calcaneus provide improved geometry and better definition of the subtalar joints.

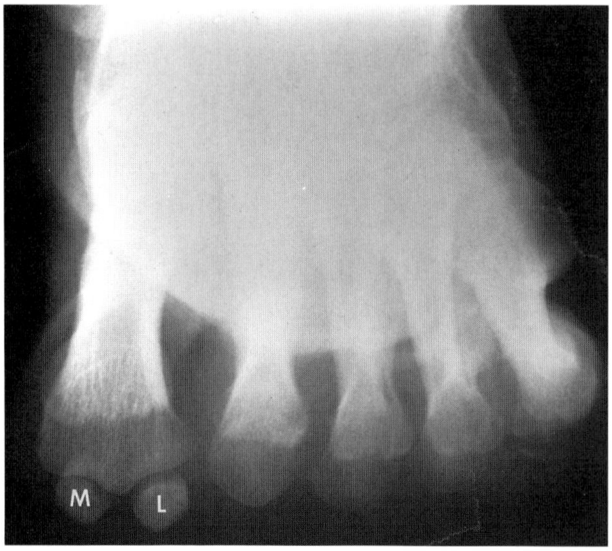

FIG. 8-6. Normal sesamoid view showing the normal relationships of the medial (*M*) and lateral (*L*) sesamoids to the first metatarsal.

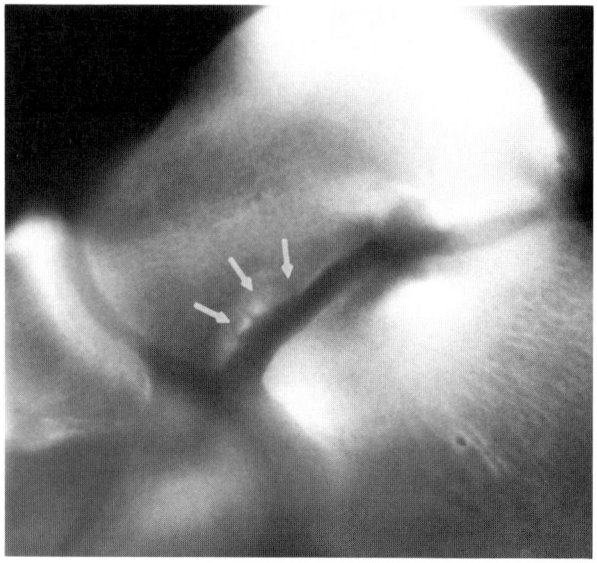

FIG. 8-7. Lateral tomogram demonstrating a subtle talar articular fracture (*arrows*), which was not evident on routine radiographs.

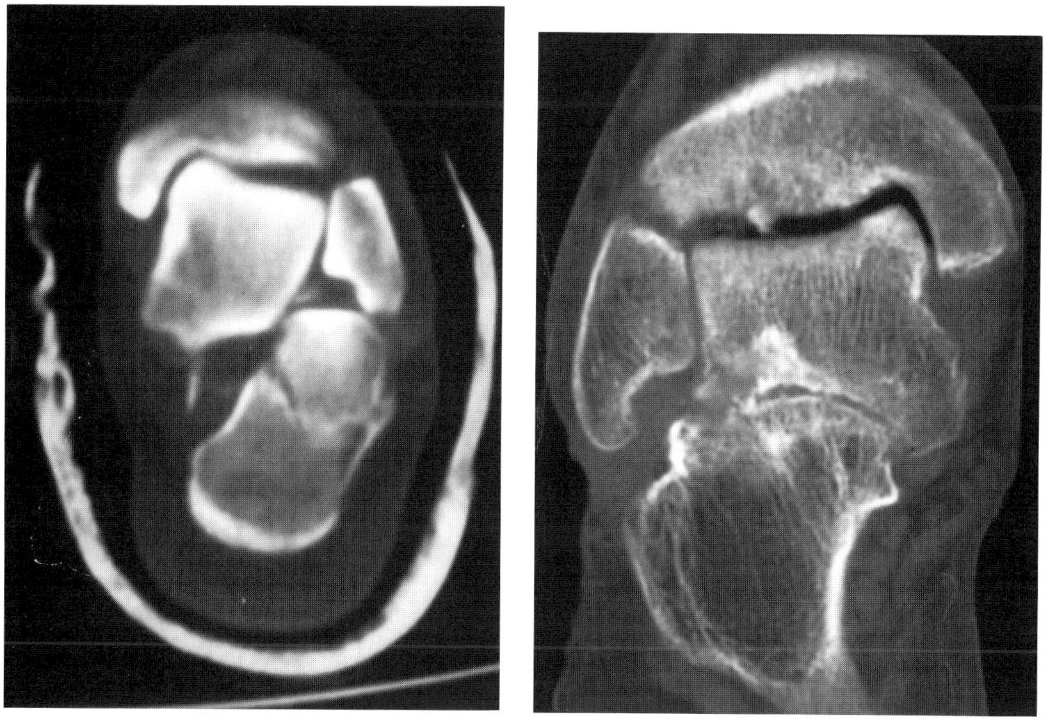

A B

FIG. 8-8. The CT images. **A:** Complex calcaneal fracture-dislocation. **B:** Posttraumatic arthrosis of the subtalar and tibiotalar joints seen in the coronal plane.

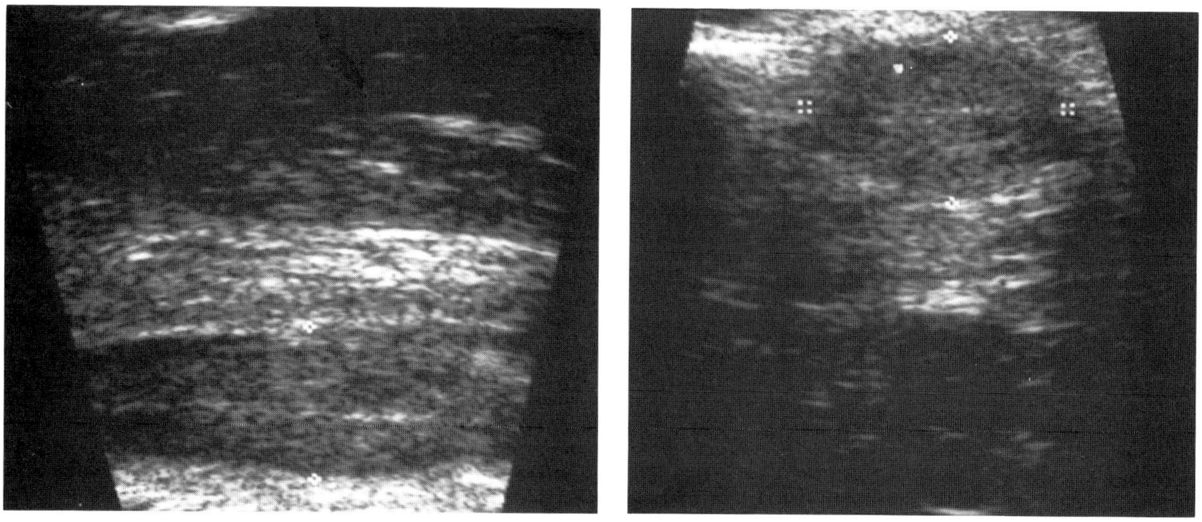

A B

FIG. 8-9. Longitudinal **(A)** and transverse **(B)** sonogram demonstrating thickening and slight increase in internal echoes as a result of a low-grade Achilles tendon tear.

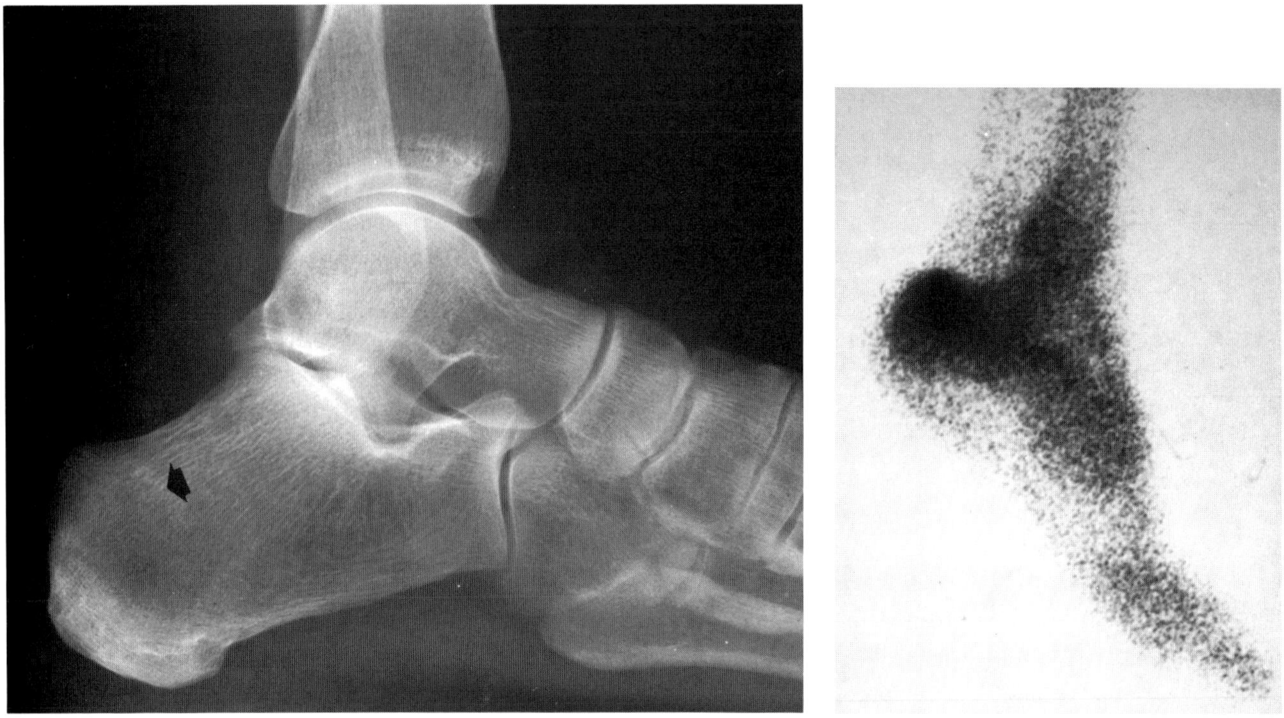

A B

FIG. 8-10. **A:** Routine lateral radiograph with subtle linear condensation (*arrow*). **B:** Radionuclide scan shows intense uptake caused by a stress fracture.

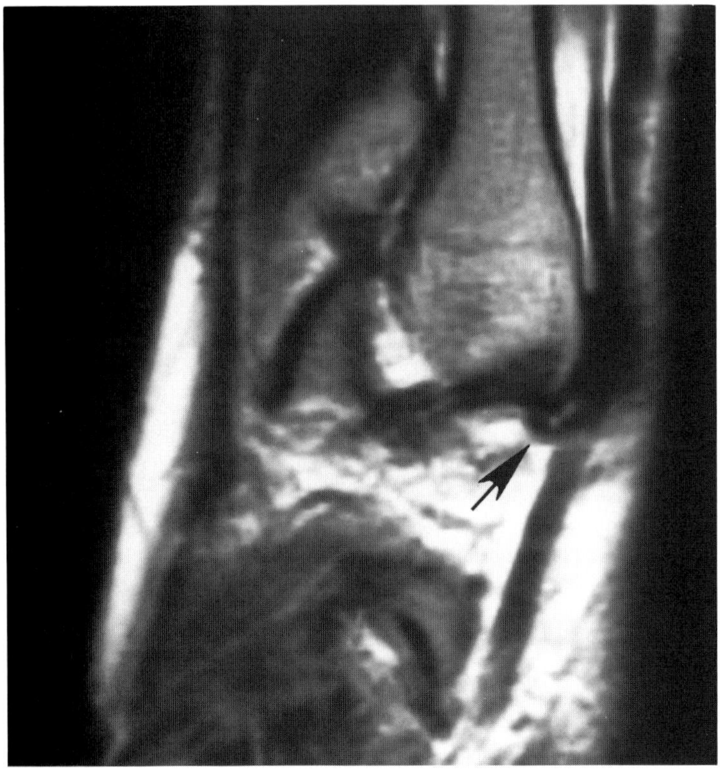

FIG. 8-11. Sagittal SE 500/20 image demonstrating a peroneal tendon tear. The proximal portion (*arrow*) is buckled at the malleolar tip.

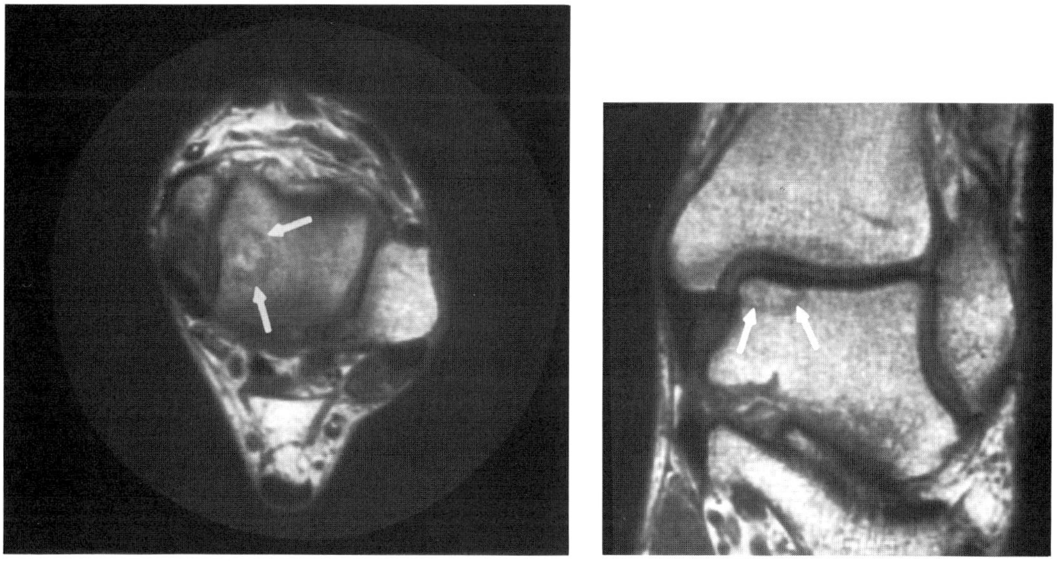

A B

FIG. 8-12. Axial **(A)** and coronal **(B)** SE 500/20 images demonstrate a talar dome fracture (*arrows*) in a patient with suspected soft tissue injury.

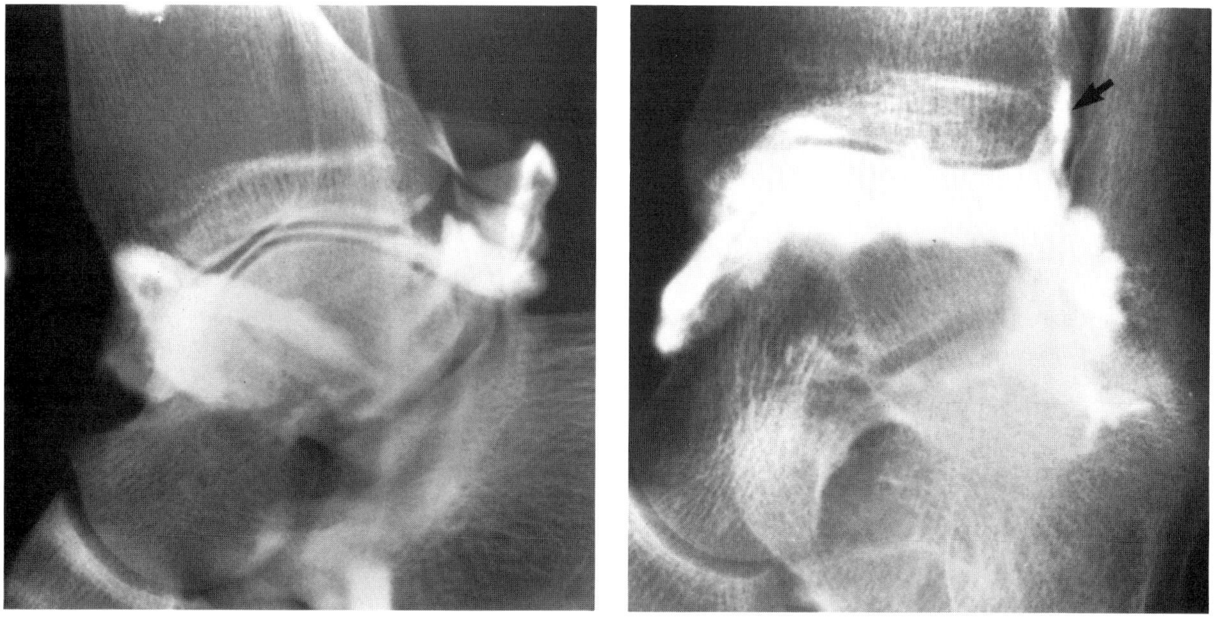

A B

FIG. 8-13. Normal lateral view **(A)** and mortise view **(B)** after contrast injection in the tibiotalar joint. Note the normal syndesmotic recess (*arrow*) in B.

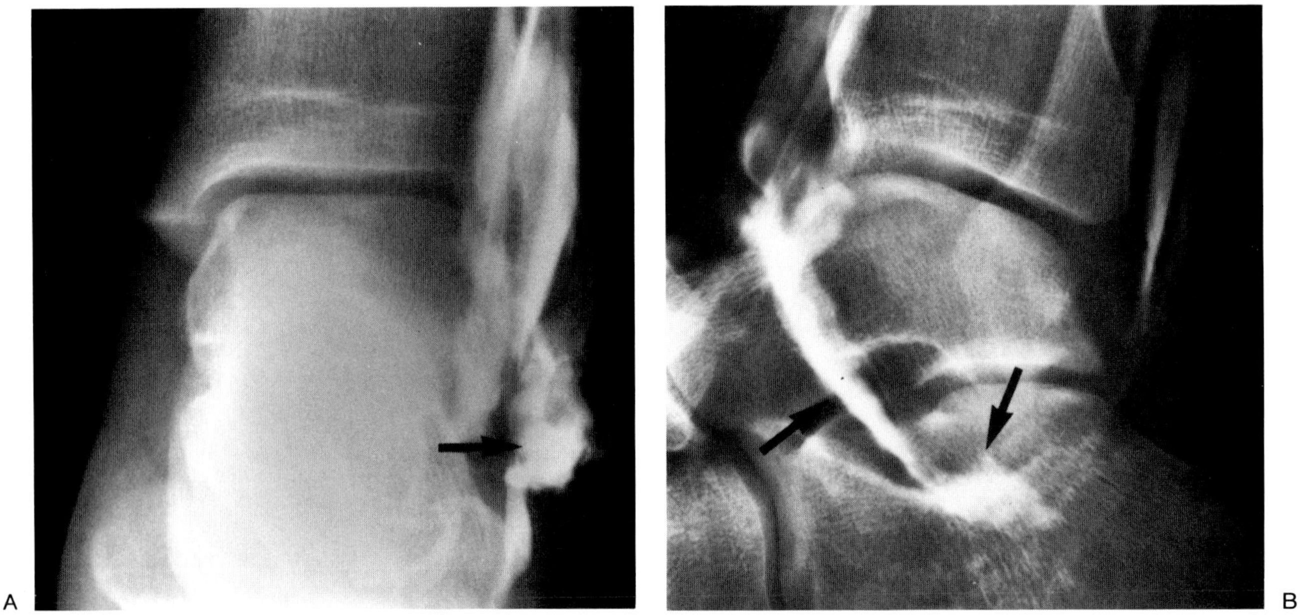

FIG. 8-14. The AP (A) and lateral (B) views of a peroneal tenogram. There is extravasation (*arrows*) but no filling of the ankle joint to indicate ligament tear.

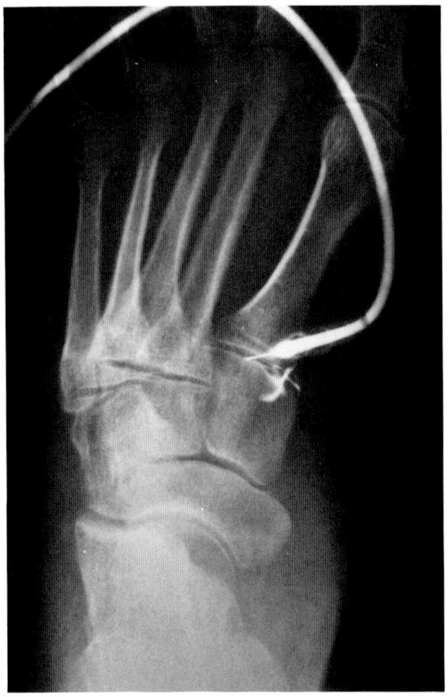

FIG. 8-15. Fluoroscopically monitored injection of the first tarsometatarsal joint. A contrast agent is injected to confirm the needle's position prior to injection of anesthetic and/or steroid for diagnostic or therapeutic purposes.

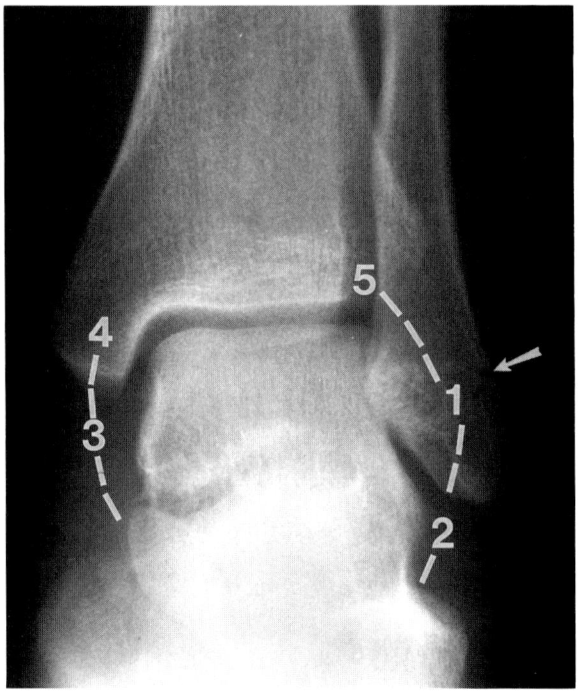

FIG. 8-16. An AP radiograph demonstrating the ring concept created by bones and ligaments of the ankle. Common breaks in the ring are (*1*) lateral malleolus, (*2*) lateral ligaments, (*3*) medial ligaments, (*4*) medial malleolus, and (*5*) syndesmosis. Subtle lateral malleolar fracture (*arrow*).

are easily accomplished using fluoroscopic guidance (see Chapter 1).[3]

TRAUMA

The management of foot and ankle fractures is a common problem for orthopedic surgeons, emergency room physicians, family practice physicians, and radiologists. Imaging plays an important role in assessing the degree of bone and soft tissue injury and in following the healing process.

The discussion of specific foot and ankle fractures and fracture dislocations is most easily accomplished using anatomic regions. Therefore, ankle, hindfoot, midfoot, and forefoot injuries are discussed separately.

Ankle Fractures

Adult and childhood fractures are managed somewhat differently and are discussed separately.

The evaluation of adult ankle fractures includes an assessment of the fracture fragments and an accurate description of associated ligament injuries. Determining the extent of bone and soft tissue involvement is important in predicting the mechanism of injury, which in turn, has significant treatment implications.[43,44,47,59,68,70]

When evaluating ankle fractures, we commonly consider the bones and ligaments as a ring-like structure in the coronal plane (Fig. 8-16). This concept was popularized by Neer[71] and other authors.[61,64] The ring is made up of the medial malleolus, tibial plafond, distal tibiofibular ligaments and syndesmosis, the lateral malleolus, lateral ligament complex, talus, and medial ligaments. Breaks in the ring commonly occur at five sites, either alone or in combination. A shift of the talus indicates a disruption of the ring in at least two locations (Fig. 8-17). The five common sites of injury include (1) lateral malleolus, (2) lateral ligaments, (3) deltoid ligaments, (4) medial malleolus, and (5) syndesmosis. Other injuries, such as fractures of the tibial plafond, occur with axial loading and various degrees of plantar flexion and, frequently, result in comminution of the distal tibia.[47,68,73]

Classification

Most ankle injuries occur as a result of inversion or eversion forces. The mechanism is, however, rarely pure; frequently, abduction, adduction, lateral rotation, or axial loading occur in addition to eversion and inversion.[43,44,60,61,65,70,72,82–86] Two common adult classifications for ankle fractures are the Lauge-Hansen[64] and the Weber classifications.[68,70,81]

The Lauge-Hansen[64] classification is summarized in Table 8-1.[43,47] This classification system is based on the position of the foot and direction of the force at the time of injury. Four basic categories of injury are described with several levels of injuries in each category. From a radiographic standpoint, the appearance of the talus within the ankle mortise and the appearance of the fibular fracture are key features in defining the mechanism of injury (Figs. 8-18 to 8-21).[43,47,64]

Some find the previous classification too difficult and cumbersome; therefore, the Weber classification is more frequently used, especially by orthopedic surgeons.[68,80] This classification is based on the level of the fibular fracture in predicting the degree of syndesmotic injury and mortise displacement. The AO group modified the Weber classification into subgroups.[70] Table 8-2 summarizes the Weber classification system (Figs. 8-22 to 8-24).

Certain fractures, such as the tibial plafond fracture, do not fit neatly into these classifications. These injuries typically occur in patients younger than 50 years of age

(text continues on page 590)

TABLE 8-1. *Lauge-Hansen classification*[43,64]

Stage	Characteristics
Pronation-abduction	
I	Ruptured deltoid ligament or transverse medial malleolar fracture
II	Disruption of the distal tibiofibular ligaments (anterior and posterior)
III	Oblique fibular fracture at the joint level (best seen on AP view)
Pronation-lateral rotation	
I	Rupture of the deltoid ligament or transverse medial malleolar fracture
II	Disruption of the anterior tibiofibular ligament and interosseous membrane
III	Fibular fracture above the joint space (usually 6 cm or more above the joint line)
IV	Posterior tibial chip fracture or rupture of posterior tibiofibular ligament
Supination-adduction	
I	Lateral ligament injury or transverse lateral malleolar fracture below the ankle joint
II	Steep oblique fracture of the medial malleolus
Supination-lateral rotation	
I	Disruption of the anterior tibiofibular ligament
II	Spiral fracture of the distal fibula near the joint (best seen on the lateral view)
III	Rupture of the posterior tibiofibular ligament
IV	Transverse fracture of the medial malleolus

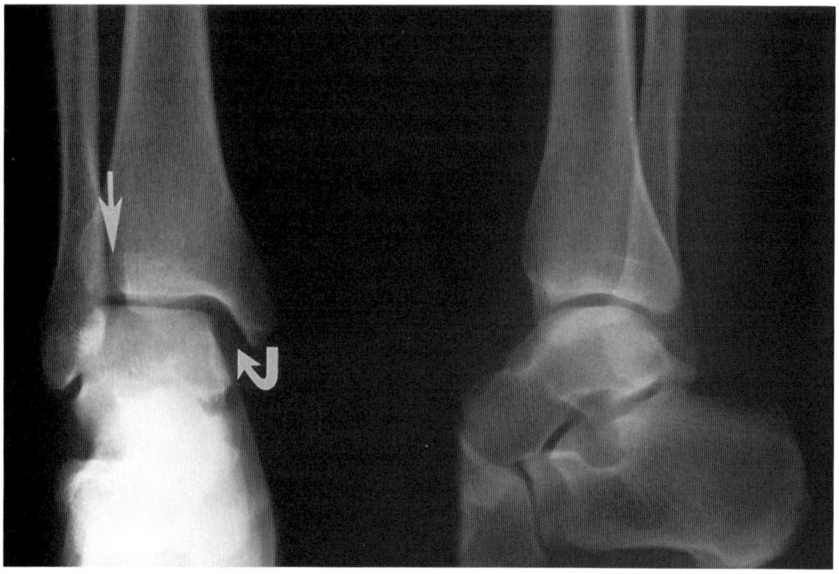

FIG. 8-17. The AP and lateral views of the ankle. The talus is shifted laterally with widening of the ankle mortise medially (*curved arrow*), which was caused by a pronation-lateral rotation injury with disruption of the medial ligaments, anterior distal tibiofibular ligament, and distal syndesmosis (*vertical arrow*).

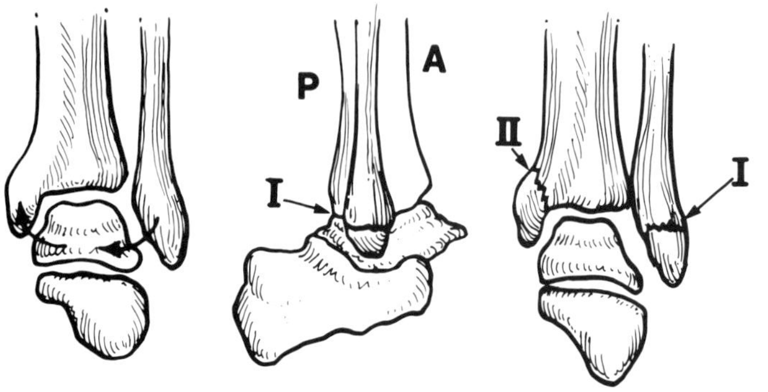

A

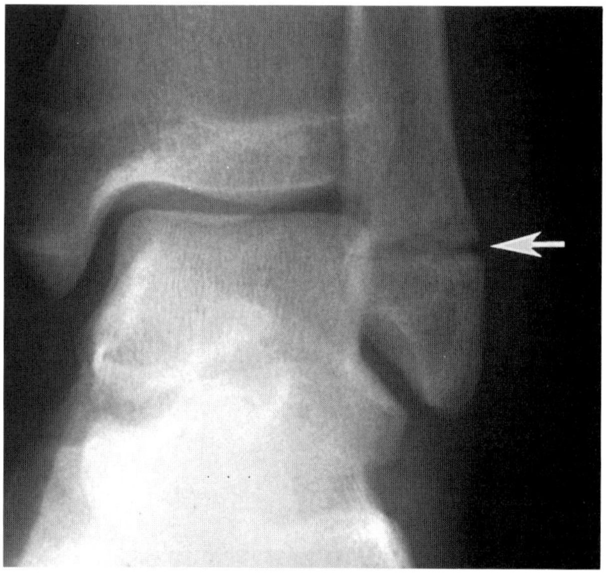

B

FIG. 8-18. A: Supination-adduction injury. Stage I, transverse fracture of the lateral malleolus at or below the joint line or lateral ligament rupture; stage II, oblique medial malleolar fracture. (From Berquist TH. *Imaging of orthopedic trauma and surgery.* Philadelphia: WB Saunders, 1986.) **B:** Supination-adduction stage I with a transverse lateral malleolar fracture (*arrow*).

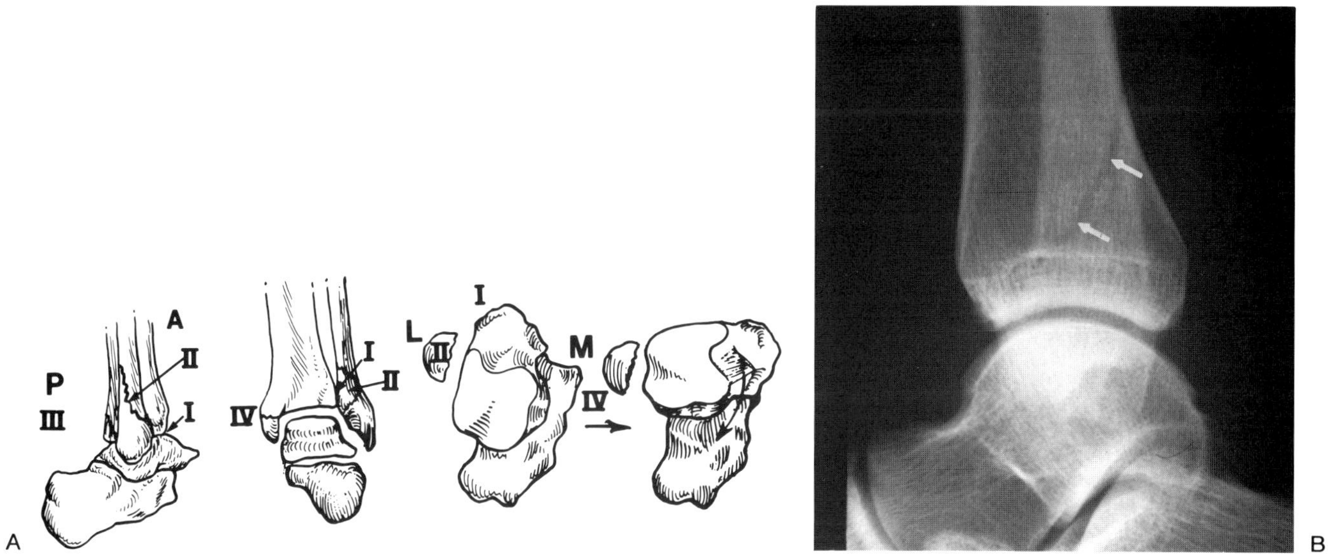

FIG. 8-19. A: Supination-lateral rotation injury. Stage I, disruption of the anterior distal tibiofibular ligament; stage II, spiral fibular fracture extending above the joint line and best seen on the lateral view; stage III, posterior tibial fracture; stage IV, transverse fracture of the medial malleolus. (From Berquist,[47A] with permission.) **B:** Lateral view of the ankle demonstrating a stage II supination-lateral rotation injury. Note the oblique fibular fracture (*arrows*).

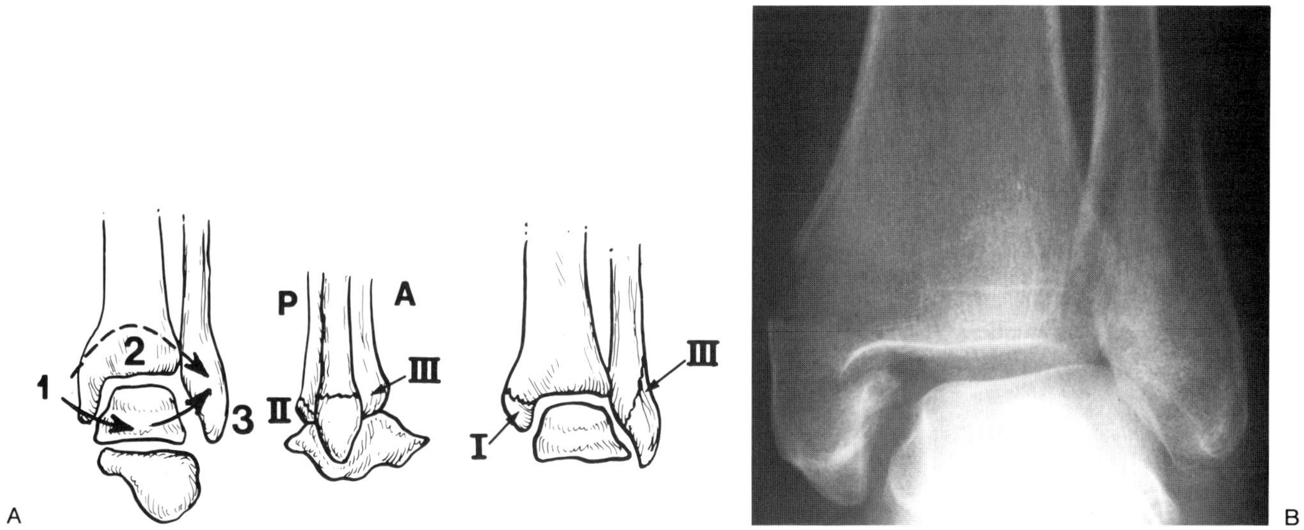

FIG. 8-20. A: Pronation-abduction injury. Stage I, transverse fracture of the medial malleolus or medial ligament disruption; stage II, posterior tibial fracture or distal tibiofibular ligament injury; stage III, oblique fibular fracture seen best on the AP view. (From Berquist TH. *Imaging of orthopedic trauma and surgery.* Philadelphia: WB Saunders, 1986.) **B:** An AP radiograph demonstrating a stage III injury with medial malleolar fracture and an oblique fibular fracture.

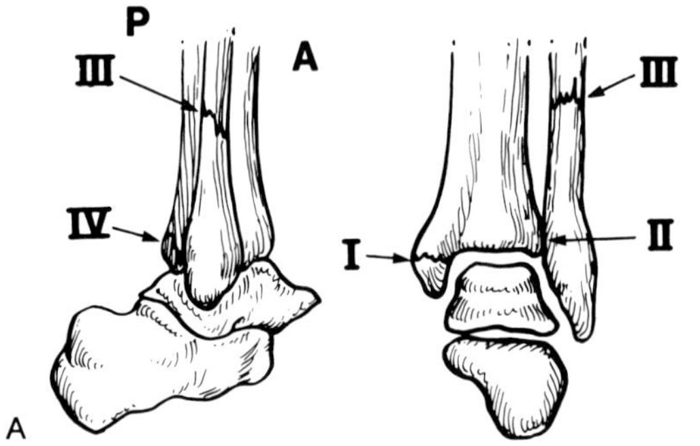

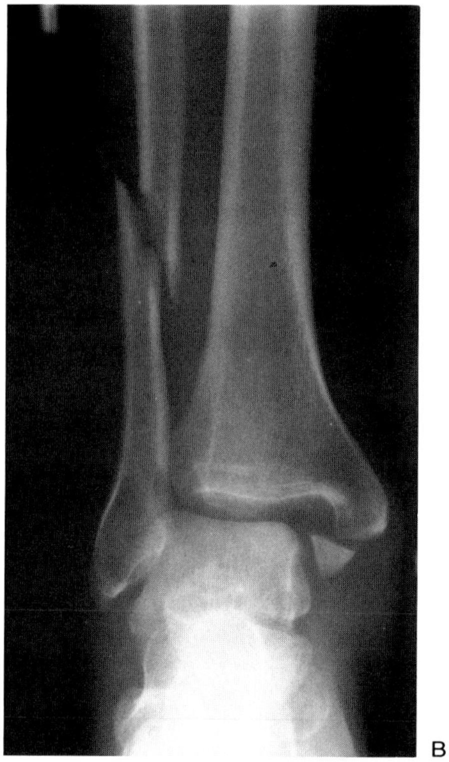

FIG. 8-21. **A:** Pronation-lateral rotation injury. Stage I, transverse fracture of the medial malleolus or medial ligament injury; stage II, rupture of the distal tibiofibular ligament and syndesmosis; stage III, fibular fracture well above the joint (usually >6 cm); stage IV, posterior tibial fracture. (From Berquist TH. *Imaging of orthopedic trauma and surgery.* Philadelphia: WB Saunders, 1986.) **B:** An AP view of a stage III pronation-lateral rotation injury with medial malleolar fracture, widened syndesmosis, and a high fibular fracture.

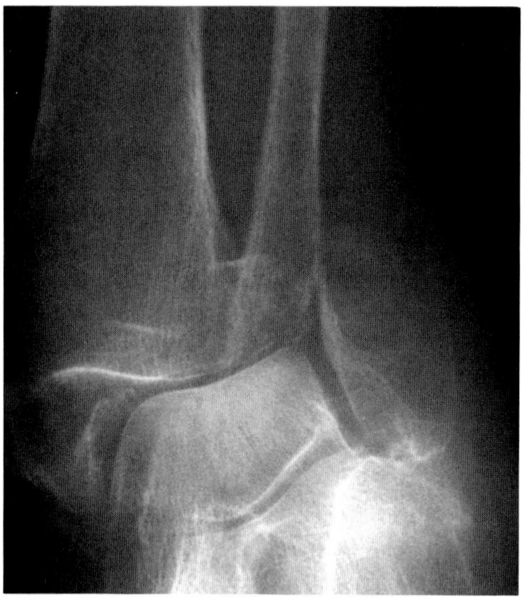

FIG. 8-22. An AP radiograph of a Weber type A2 fracture. There is a medial malleolar fracture with fibular fracture below the syndesmosis. This is similar to a pronation-abduction stage III Lauge-Hansen injury.

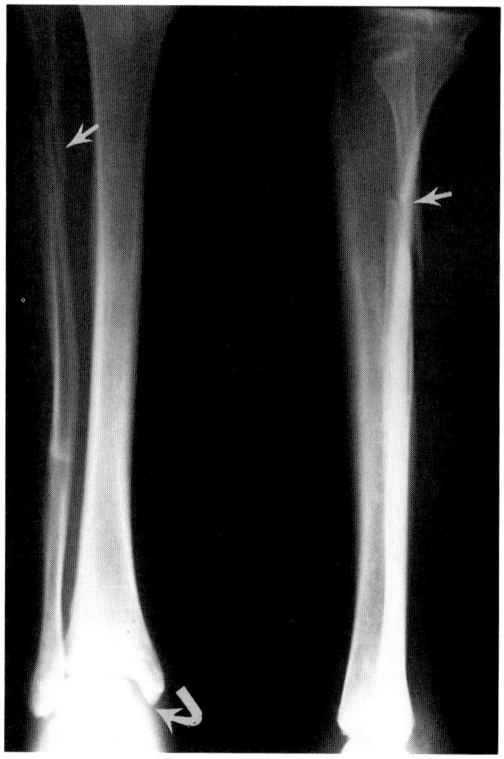

FIG. 8-23. The AP and lateral views of the leg demonstrating a Weber type C3 fracture (*arrows*). There is also a medial ligament tear (*lower curved arrow*).

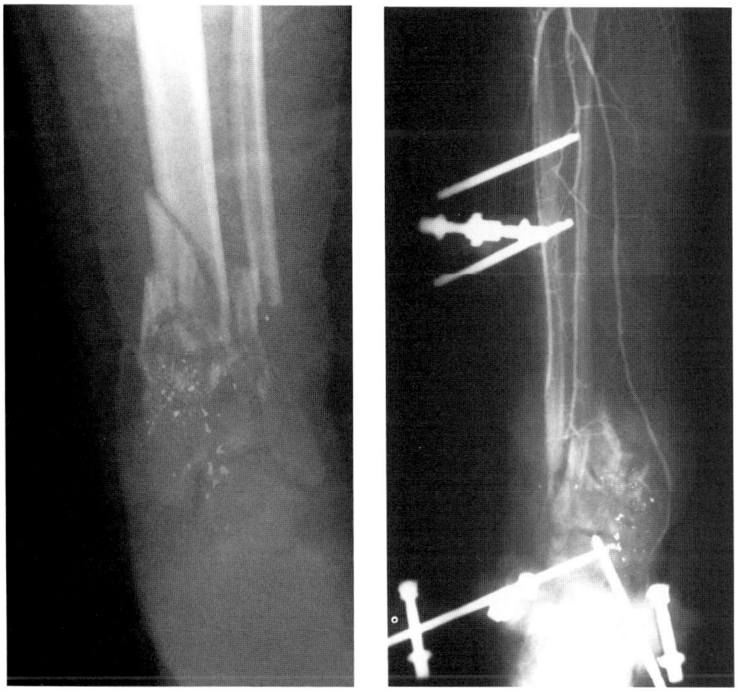

A,B

FIG. 8-25. A: Comminuted plafond fracture and multifragment fibular fracture caused by a gunshot wound. **B:** Angiogram obtained after external fixation shows distal vascular occlusions.

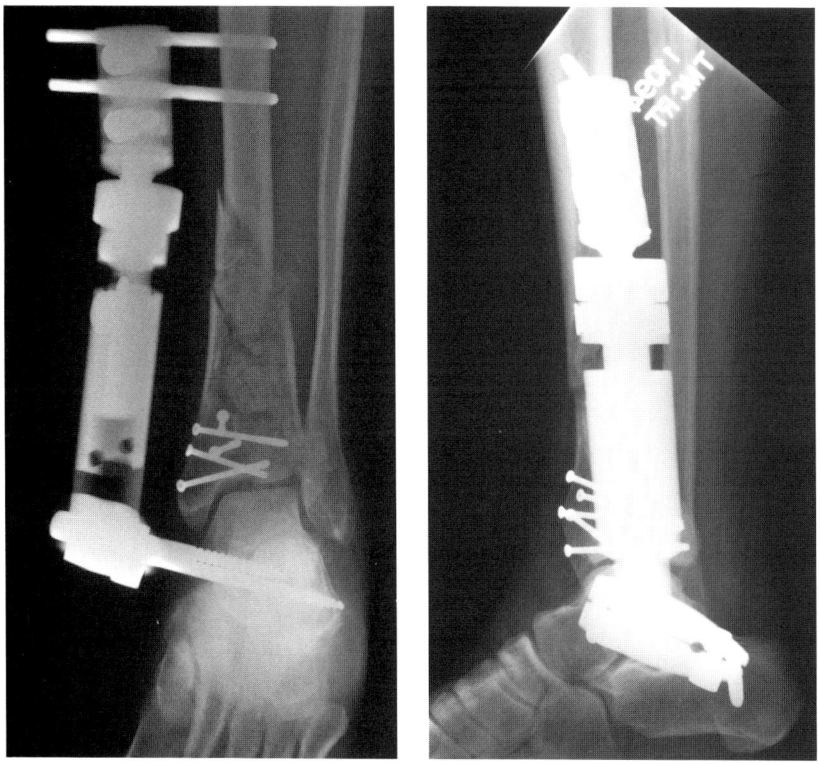

A,B

FIG. 8-26. The AP **(A)** and lateral **(B)** radiographs of a comminuted pilon fracture with five interfragmentary screws and an Orthofix™ unilateral fixator for fixation.

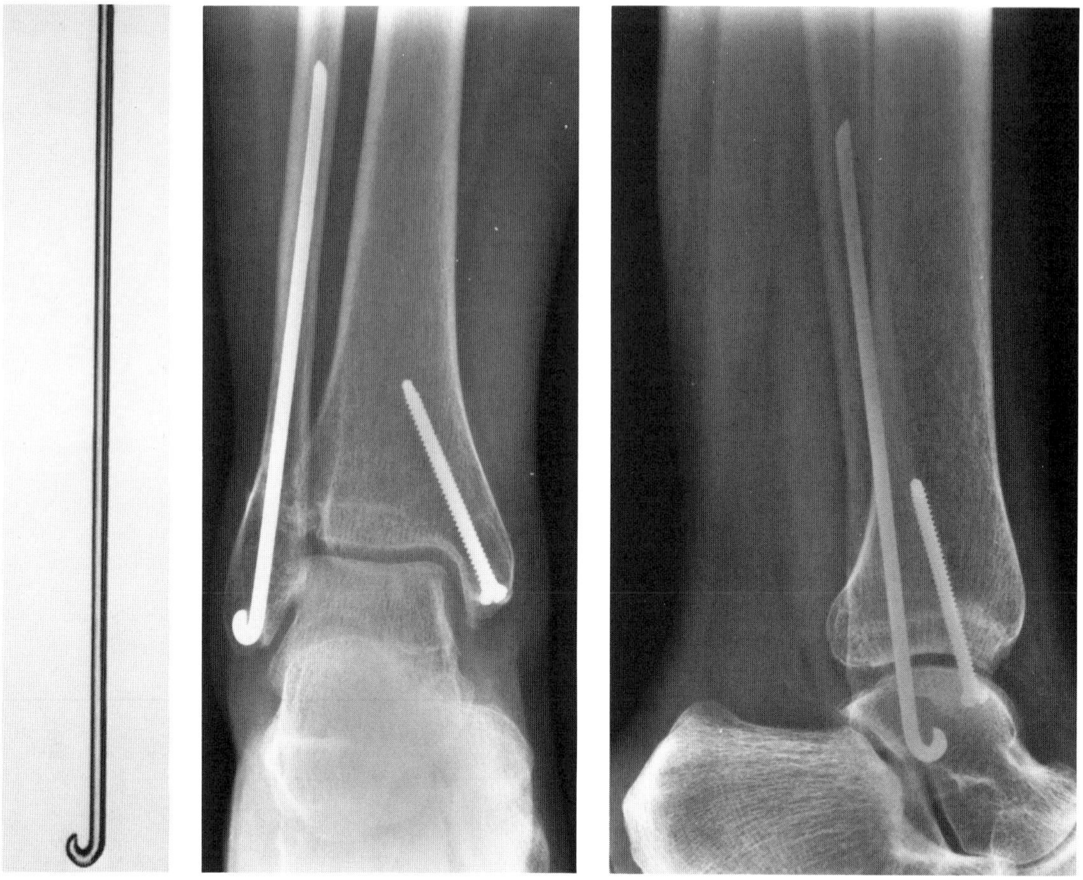

A,B C

FIG. 8-27. **A:** A Rush pin. (Courtesy of Zimmer, Warsaw, IN.) The AP **(B)** and lateral **(C)** radiographs of the ankle demonstrating internal fixation of the fibula fracture with a Rush pin. There is a single cortical screw in the medial malleolus. The fractures are healed.

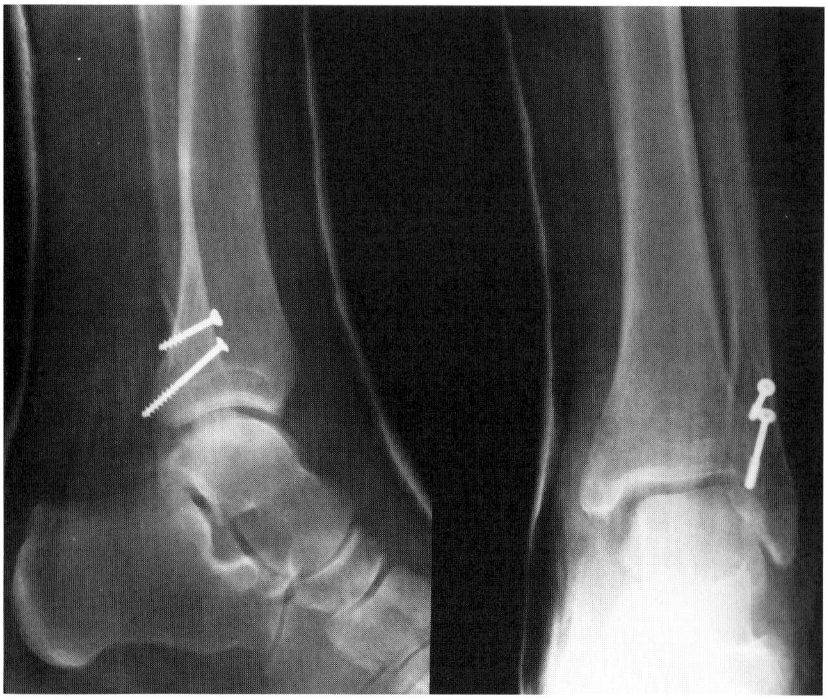

A,B

FIG. 8-28. Lateral **(A)** and AP **(B)** radiographs with two cancellous screws for fixation of an oblique fibular fracture. Note the ankle mortise is not anatomically reduced as medial widening is seen.

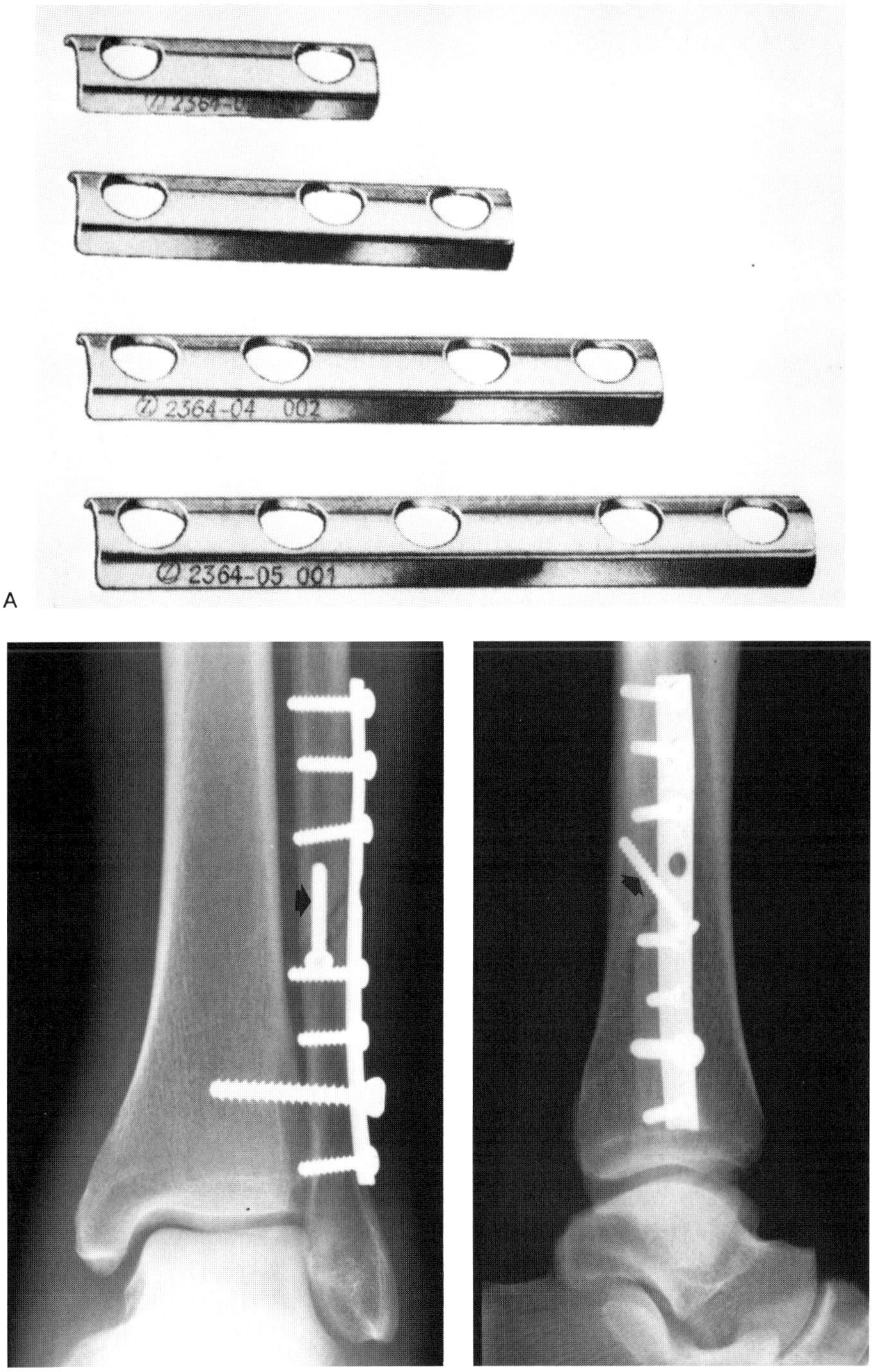

A

B

C

FIG. 8-29. A: Two- to five-hole semitubular plates. (Courtesy of Zimmer, Warsaw, IN.) The AP **(B)** and lateral **(C)** radiographs of a high fibular fracture treated with an eight-hole plate, six cortical screws, a larger syndesmosis screw, and a single interfragmentary screw (*arrow*).

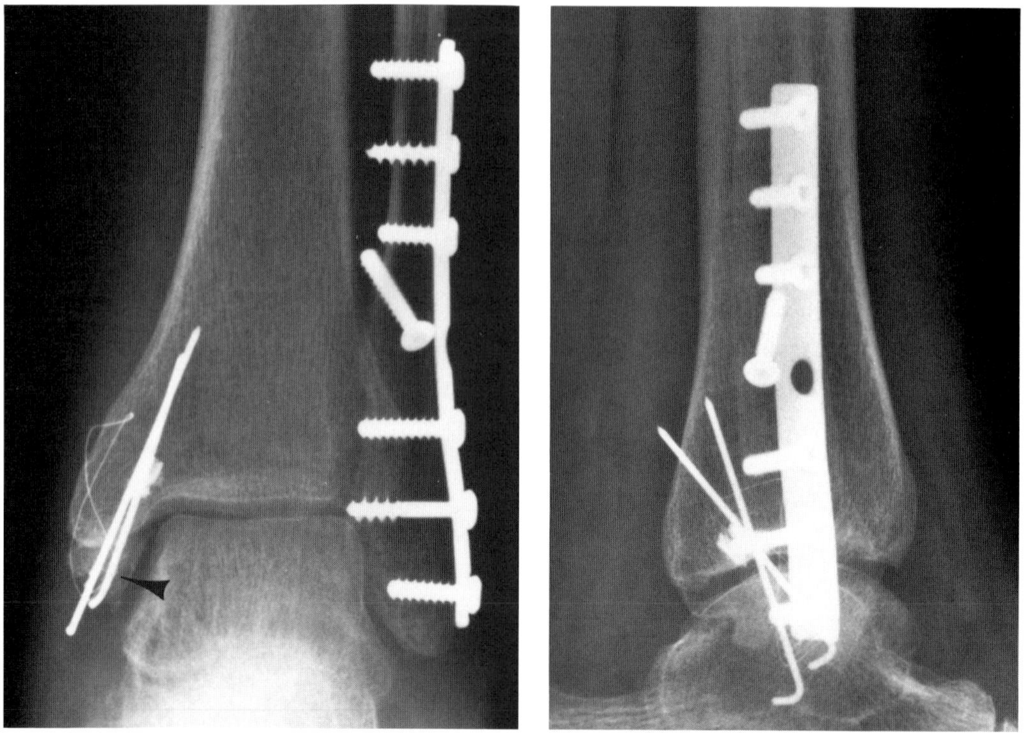

A B

FIG. 8-30. Bimalleolar fracture of the left ankle with K-wire and tension-band fixation of the medial malleolus and plate and screw fixation of the fibular fracture. The AP **(A)** and lateral **(B)** radiographs show a healed fibular fracture. There is questionable pin migration or loss of reduction of the medial malleolar tip (*arrow*).

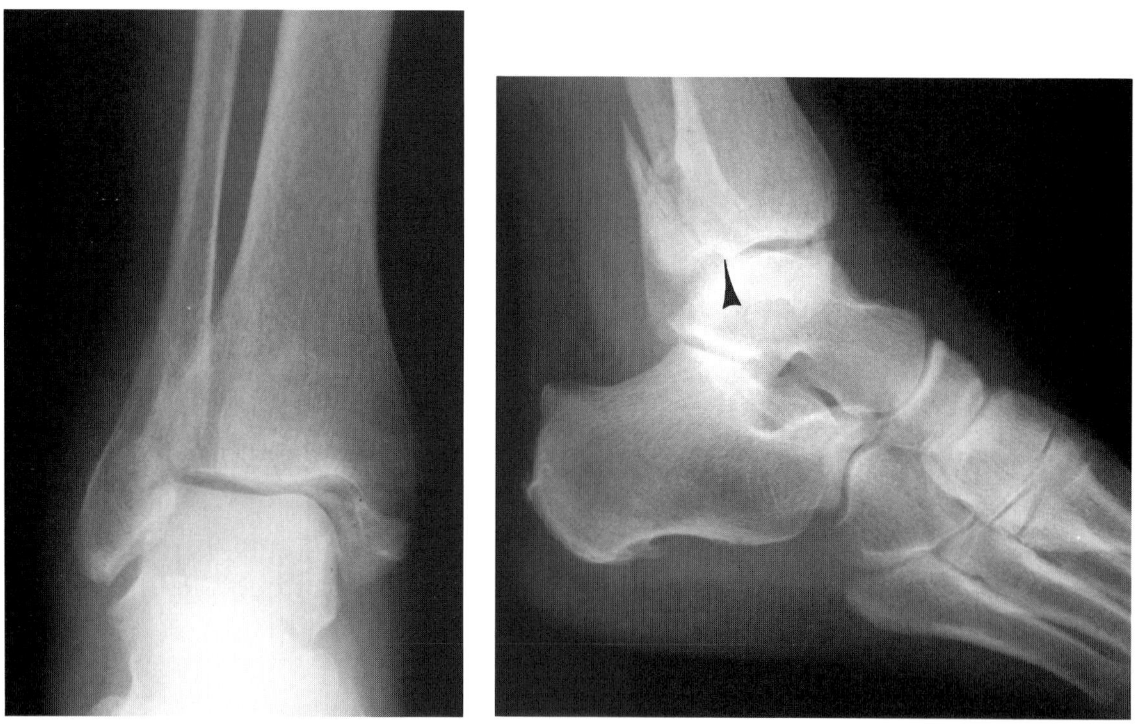

A B

FIG. 8-31. The AP **(A)** and lateral **(B)** views of a Weber type B fibular fracture with a medial malleolar fracture. The posterior tibial fragment involves approximately 25% of the articular surface (*arrow*) in B. Internal fixation with tension band and K wires with a fully threaded cancellous screw for the medial malleolus, two cancellous screws to fix the posterior tibial fragment, and a six-hole plate for the fibular fracture.

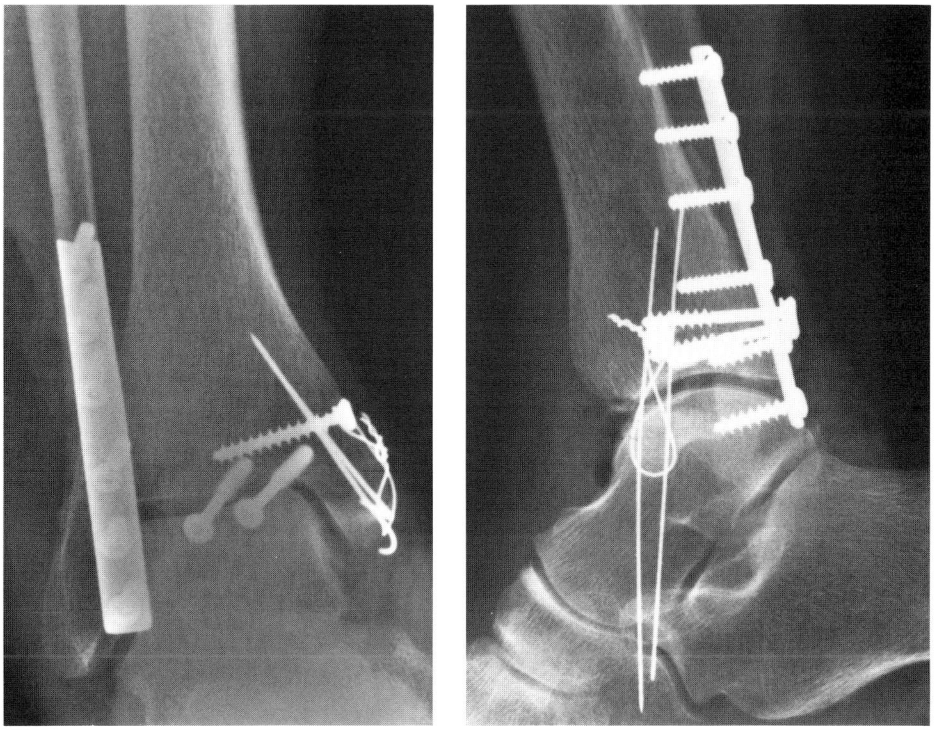

C D

FIG. 8-31. (*Continued.*) The AP postoperative **(C)** and lateral intraoperative **(D)** films show excellent reduction. There is no tibial articular defect.

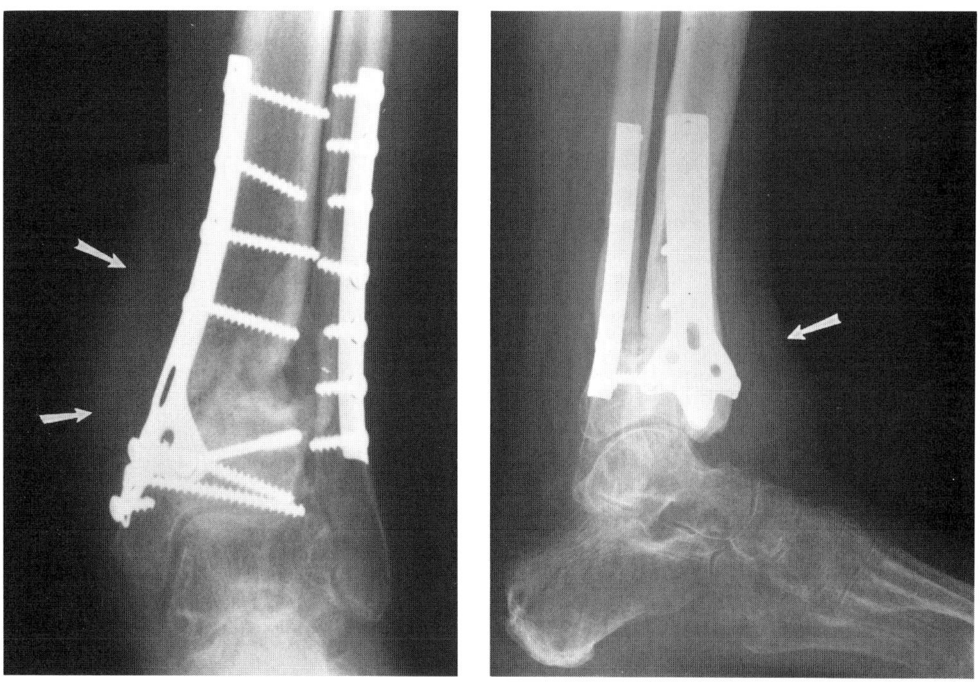

A B

FIG. 8-32. The AP **(A)** and lateral **(B)** radiographs of an old plafond fracture with a fibular fracture. A one-third tubular plate was used for the fibular fracture and a cloverleaf plate, for the tibial fracture. The tibial fracture line is open laterally because of local bone loss. Soft tissue prominence anteriorly and medially (*arrows*) caused by muscle flap.

diaphyseal and metaphyseal fractures are frequently incomplete, and in most cases, there is a posterior cortical break with buckling or a torus-type fracture. Ankle fractures in children most commonly involve the growth plate, and ligament injuries are more uncommon than they are in adults. The distal tibial epiphysis is the second most common site for growth plate fracture. In Rogers's[75] series, 25% of 118 physeal injuries involved the distal tibia or fibula. These fractures can result in growth articular deformity if the proper diagnosis and treatment are not implemented.

The same forces that cause fracture and/or ligament disruption in adults also cause similar fractures in children. In children, the growth plates are two- to five fold weaker than the ligaments; therefore, fractures of the physis occur more commonly than do ligament injuries. The fracture patterns that evolve are thus related to age, the ligament of attachment, and the type of force applied.[47,75,77]

The most commonly used classification of physeal injuries was described by Salter and Harris.[77] This classification is used because of its prognostic significance and the easy use of radiographic patterns. Salter-Harris classifications are summarized in Figure 8-33.

More recently, the Lauge-Hansen[64] system has been combined with the Salter-Harris[77] system. The former is an accurate method commonly applied to adult injuries. Dias and Giegerich[54] and Dias and Tachdjian[55] combined these classifications (Fig. 8-34), which are summarized in Table 8-4.

Several ankle fractures do not clearly fit this classification scheme.[47,67,79] Triplane fractures are usually caused by external rotation forces, with or without associated plantar flexion.[50,62,67] The fractures consist of three fragments instead of two. The first fragment involves the anterolateral portion of the tibia and has the appearance of a Salter-Harris type III fracture radiographically. The second fragment is the remainder of the tibial epiphysis with the metaphyseal attachment. The third fragment is the tibial diaphysis (Figs. 8-35 and 8-36).[50,67] About 6% of epiphyseal fractures are triplane injuries.[51,52] The prognosis is similar to that in the Salter-Harris type IV fracture.[47,50,67,74]

The juvenile Tillaux fracture (Fig. 8-37) is a Salter-Harris type III fracture of the lateral tibial epiphysis. The fragment is displaced by the distal tibiofibular ligaments when the foot is externally rotated.[47,63]

Treatment

The mechanism of injury may often be determined by a careful evaluation of ankle radiographs and a knowledge of ankle injury classification systems.

Fractures involving the growth plate should be reduced gently to avoid increasing damage to the growth plate. In most cases, treatment can be accomplished using closed techniques.[48,49,51,55] Internal fixation and open reduction may be required with significantly displaced fractures, as noted earlier for adult fractures. In pediatric ankle fractures, it is generally preferable to avoid fixation across the growth plate. In some instances, it is useful to fix fractures with small-caliber K wires across the growth plate. Other fixation devices, such as large compression screws, may lead to malalignment because of their effects on the growth plate (Fig. 8-38).

Follow-up examination of these patients with radiography, or in some cases, tomography or MRI may be helpful to be sure that the growth plate is not adversely affected.[47]

Talar Fractures

Talar fractures account for only 6% of all foot and ankle injuries (Table 8-5).[92–94,97,98,104] The talar neck fracture is the second most common type of talar injury after avulsion fractures.[101] These injuries usually occur during abrupt dorsiflexion of the foot, which is most often associated with motor vehicle accidents or following a significant fall.[88,91,92,96,107] The most used classification for

(text continues on page 600)

TABLE 8-4. *Ankle growth plate fractures in children: Dias-Tachdjian classification*[54,55]

Stage	Characteristics
Supination-inversion	
I	Traction on lateral ligaments leads to Salter-Harris I or II fracture of fibula. Rarely, ligament tear or avulsion fracture of the fibula occurs (Fig. 8-34A–C)
II	Greater inversion force leads to Salter-Harris III or IV fracture of the medial tibia in addition to grade I changes (Fig. 8-34A–C)
Supination-plantar flexion	Salter-Harris I or II of distal tibia. The metaphyseal fragment is best seen on the lateral view (Fig. 8-34D)
Supination-external rotation	
I	Salter-Harris II of distal tibia with spiral component similar to supination-plantar flexion (Fig. 8-34E)
II	Grade I plus spiral fibular fracture above the growth plate
Pronation-eversion-external rotation	Tibial and fibular physes fracture simultaneously; Salter-Harris II of the tibia with fibular fracture above the growth plate (5–6 cm, Fig. 8-34F)

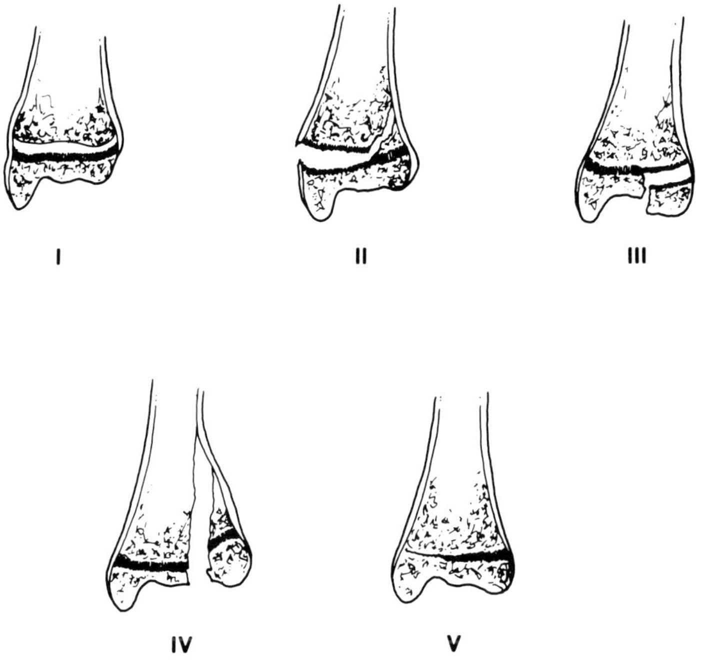

FIG. 8-33. Salter-Harris physeal fractures.[75,77] Type I, growth plate fracture with no diaphyseal or epiphyseal involvement (6%); type II, physeal fracture existing through the metaphysis (75%); type III, physeal fracture extending through the epiphysis (8%); type IV, fracture through the epiphysis and metaphysis (10%); type V, compression of the physis (1%).

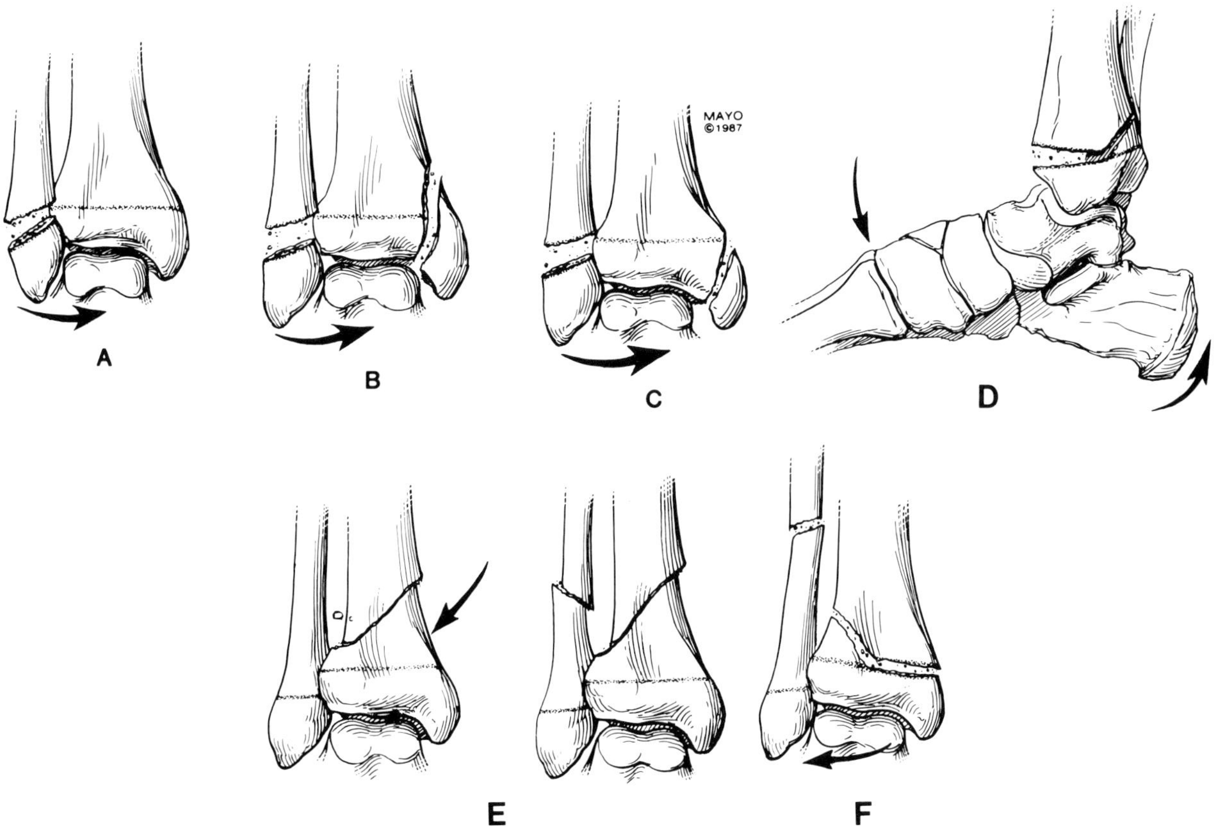

FIG. 8-34. Injuries in the Dias-Tachdjian classification combining the Lauge-Hansen and Salter-Harris classifications. **A–C:** Supination-inversion: stage I (Salter-Harris I or II fibular fracture); stage II, Salter-Harris I or II fibular fracture with medial malleolar fracture. **D:** Supination-plantar flexion: Salter-Harris I or II of the distal tibia. Metaphyseal fragment best seen on the lateral view. **E:** Supination-external rotation: stage I (Salter-Harris II or oblique distal tibial fracture); stage II, tibial fracture plus fibular fracture well above the growth plate. **F:** Pronation-eversion external rotation: fractures of the fibula above the growth plate with a Salter-Harris II of the tibia. (From Berquist TH. *Radiology of the foot and ankle.* New York: Raven Press, 1989.)

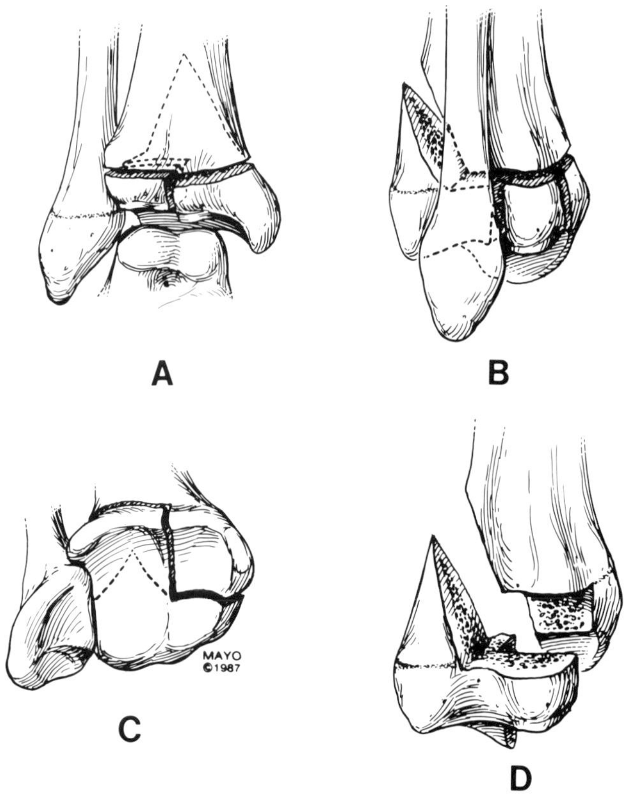

FIG. 8-35. Triplane fracture. **A:** Seen anteriorly. **B:** Seen laterally. **C:** Seen from below. **D:** Fragments separated. (From Berquist TH. *Radiology of the foot and ankle.* New York: Raven Press, 1989.)

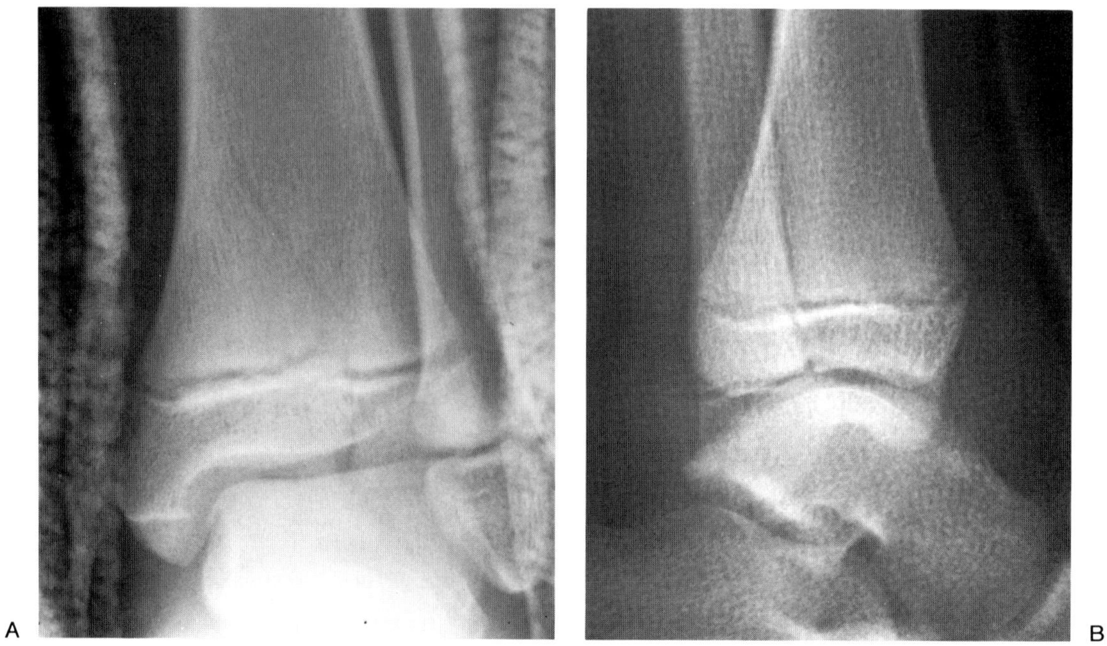

FIG. 8-36. The AP **(A)** and lateral **(B)** radiographs of a triplane fracture. This looks like a Salter-Harris II on the AP and a Salter-Harris III or IV on the lateral view.

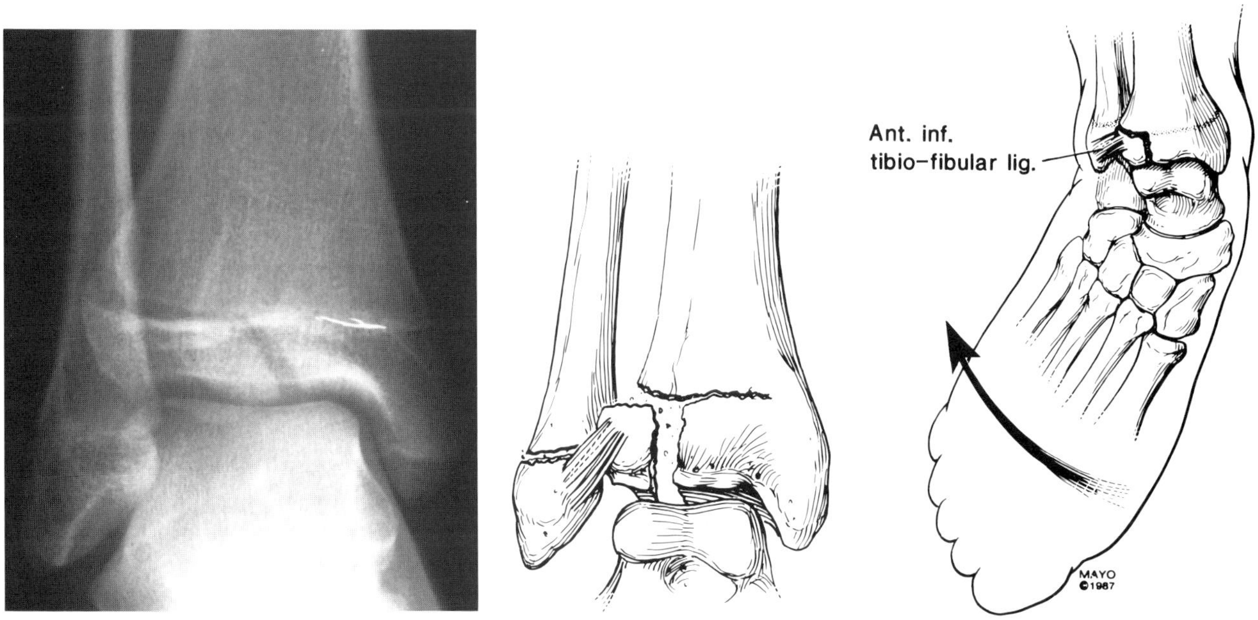

A,B

C

FIG. 8-37. **A:** An AP view of the ankle demonstrating a lateral Salter-Harris III of the distal tibia, a juvenile Tillaux fracture. **B:** Illustration of a juvenile Tillaux fracture. **C:** Mechanism of injury.

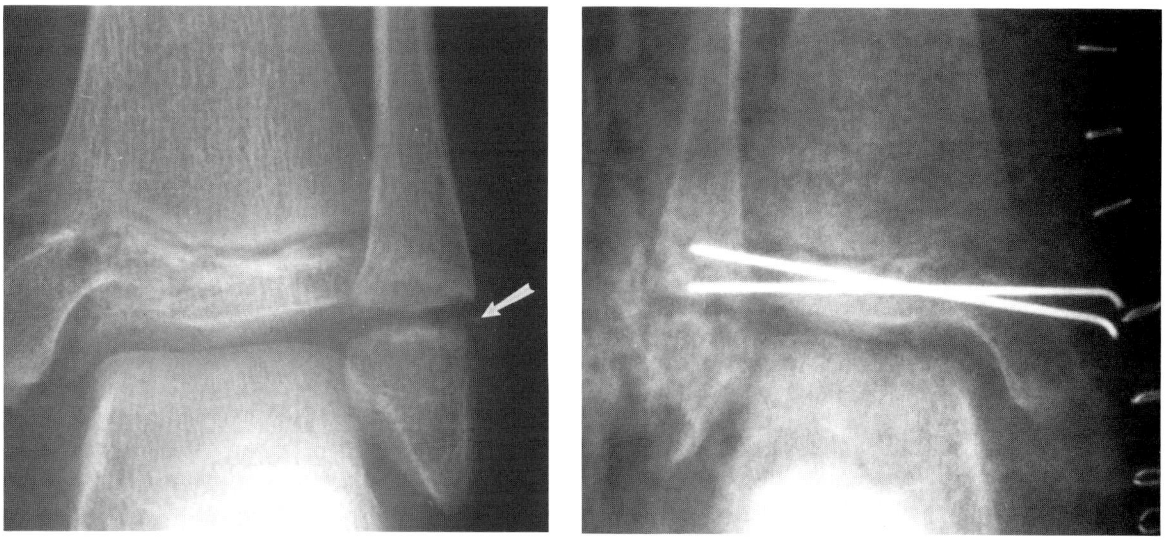

A

B

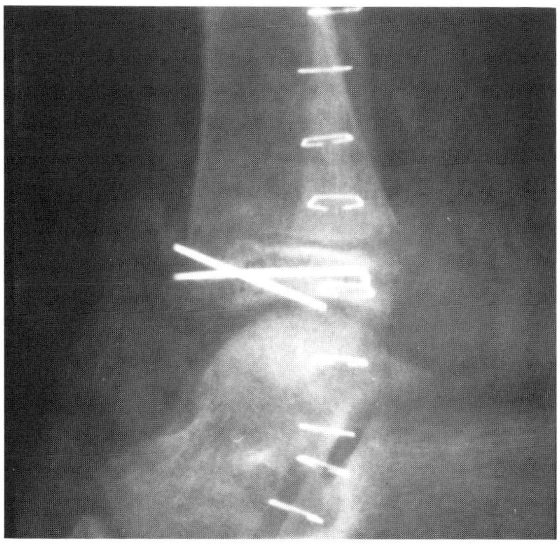

C

FIG. 8-38. **A:** An AP radiograph of a displaced medial epiphyseal fracture. There is a slightly displaced Salter-Harris II (*arrow*) of the fibula. The AP **(B)** and lateral **(C)** radiographs after K-wire fixation. The K wires do not cross the physis.

TABLE 8-5. *Talar fractures*[87,88,91,96,103]

Fracture type	Incidence rates[a] (%)
Fractures	
Chip or avulsion	40–49
Neck	28–32
Body	11–14
Compression	5–10
Fracture-dislocations	
Neck fracture with subtalar dislocation	45–50
Neck fracture with posterior body dislocation	30–40
Body fracture with subtalar dislocation	9–12
Total dislocation	3–12

[a] Variable, owing to multiple series.

talar neck injuries was devised by Hawkins[98] and modified by Canale and Kelly[91] to include four categories of injury (Table 8-6). Routine radiographs are usually adequate for the diagnosis of talar fractures (Fig. 8-39). Keep in mind that up to 20% of patients have associated medial malleolar fractures, which may be more obvious.[89,98] Sixteen percent of patients have fractures in other bones of the ipsilateral foot. Tomography or CT may be required to detect subtle undisplaced fractures.[88,90,95,102]

Treatment

Treatment should be instituted as soon as possible after the radiographs have been assessed and the fracture is properly classified.[87,99,100,102,105,106,108] Undisplaced Hawkins type I fractures can be treated with a below-the-knee cast for 8 to 12 weeks. Fractures that are minimally displaced may be reduced with closed techniques and immobilized in a cast. Open reduction and internal fixation with compression screws or K wires is often needed to maintain reduction in types II through IV. The prognosis is improved with these injuries if adequate open reduction can be obtained.[99,100,102]

Because of the vascular anatomy to the body of the talus, significant complications can occur.[103] The complications are summarized later.[88,102]

Calcaneal Fractures

The calcaneus is the largest tarsal bone; because of its complex anatomy, it can be difficult to image with routine radiographic techniques. It is also the most commonly fractured bone in the adult foot, accounting for 60% of foot fractures and 2% of all skeletal fractures.[109,116,119,123] Calcaneal fractures in children are much less common and tend to be less extensive. Also, unlike those in adults, calcaneal fractures in children are generally extraarticular.[109,126] In adults, 70% to 75% of calcaneal fractures are intraarticular, and 25% to 30% are extraarticular.[119,123]

The most severe adult calcaneal fractures are due to falls or motor vehicle accidents, which result in axial loading of the calcaneus (Fig. 8-40). Less severe avulsion and extraarticular fractures occur with twisting injuries or muscle pulls.[114,119] Classifications of calcaneal injuries were proposed by Rowe et al.[125] and Essex-Lopresti.[112] The Rowe classification is less commonly used. The Essex-Lopresti classification divides fractures into two major categories: intraarticular and extraarticular (Table 8-7).

Schmidt and Weiner[126] combined these classifications to provide a system that could be used for adults and children (Table 8-8). A type 6 category was added because of the significant soft tissue injury seen with posterior calcaneal fractures in children (Fig. 8-41).[126]

Paley and Hall[121] devised a classification system based on findings on the lateral radiograph. The system is a modification of the Essex-Lopresti and Soeur-Remy classifications (Fig. 8-42).[112,121]

Treatment

The treatment of simple or extraarticular calcaneal fractures is much less controversial than is the management of complex intraarticular fractures.[120] The goal of treatment is to reestablish the articular alignment, particularly the posterior facet (Böhler's angle), and maintain a normal calcaneal width. Furthermore, motion is also important to maintain normal function.[112,118,119,125]

If recognized, type 1 (Schmidt and Weiner) fractures

(text continues on page 605)

TABLE 8-6. *Talar neck fractures and fracture dislocations*[88,91,97,98,101]

Type	Definition	Incidence rates[a] (%)
I	Undisplaced vertical neck fracture	11–21
II	Displaced vertical neck fracture with subtalar subluxation or dislocation	40–42
III	Displaced vertical neck fracture with subluxation or dislocation of both tibiotalar and subtalar joints	23–47
IV	Displaced vertical fracture of the talus with subtalar or tibiotalar dislocation and subluxation or dislocation of the talonavicular joint	5

[a] Incidence rate >100% due to multiple series.

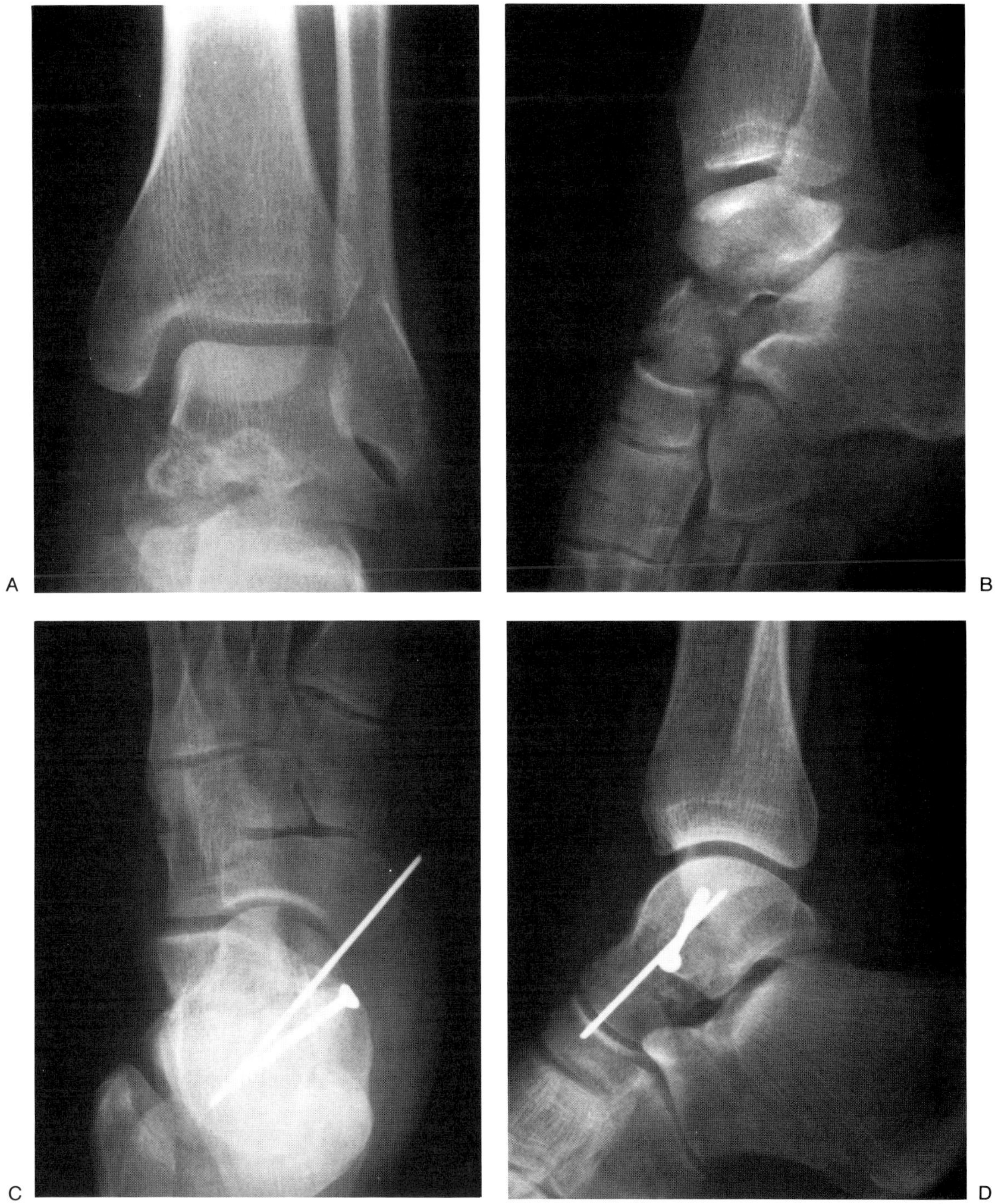

FIG. 8-39. The AP (A) and lateral (B) radiographs demonstrating a talar neck fracture. The AP (C) and lateral (D) radiographs after K-wire and cancellous screw fixation.

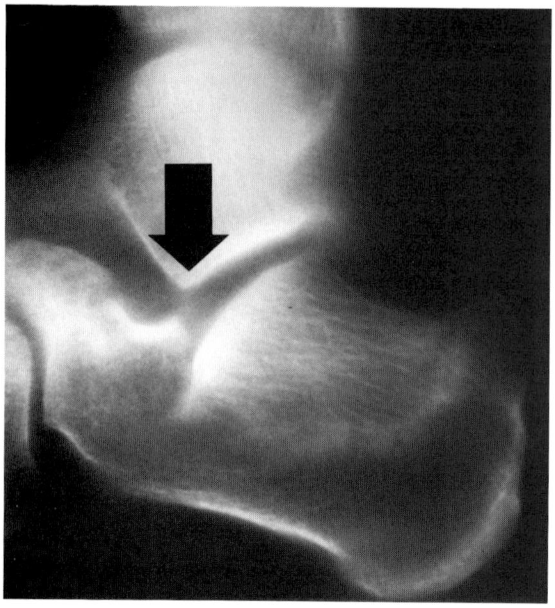

FIG. 8-40. Lateral tomogram demonstrating axial loading force, resulting in a calcaneal fracture.

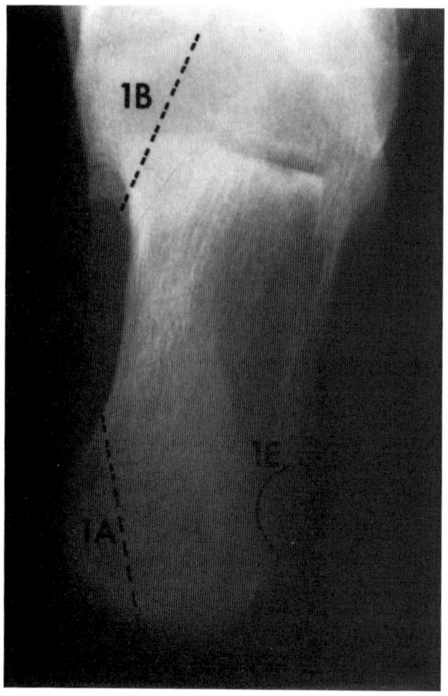

A

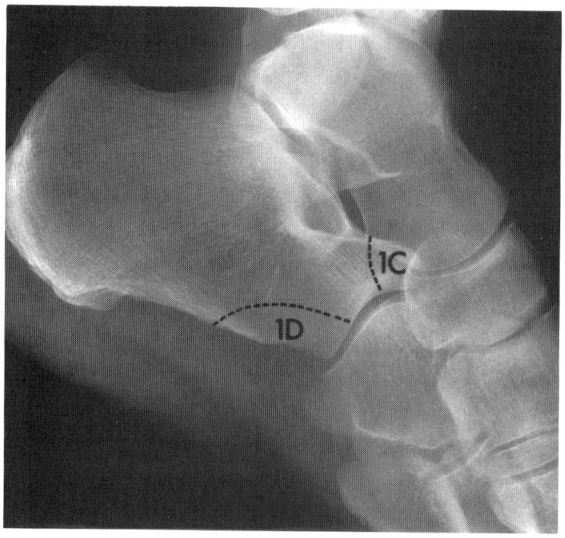

B

FIG. 8-41. Schmidt and Weiner[124] modification of the Rowe and Essex-Lopresti classifications for calcaneal fractures. **A:** Axial calcaneal view demonstrating type 1A, tuberosity or apophysis fracture; type 1B, sustentacular fracture; type 1E, avulsion fracture. **B:** Lateral view of the calcaneus demonstrating a type 1C, anterior process fracture; type 1D, inferolateral fracture.

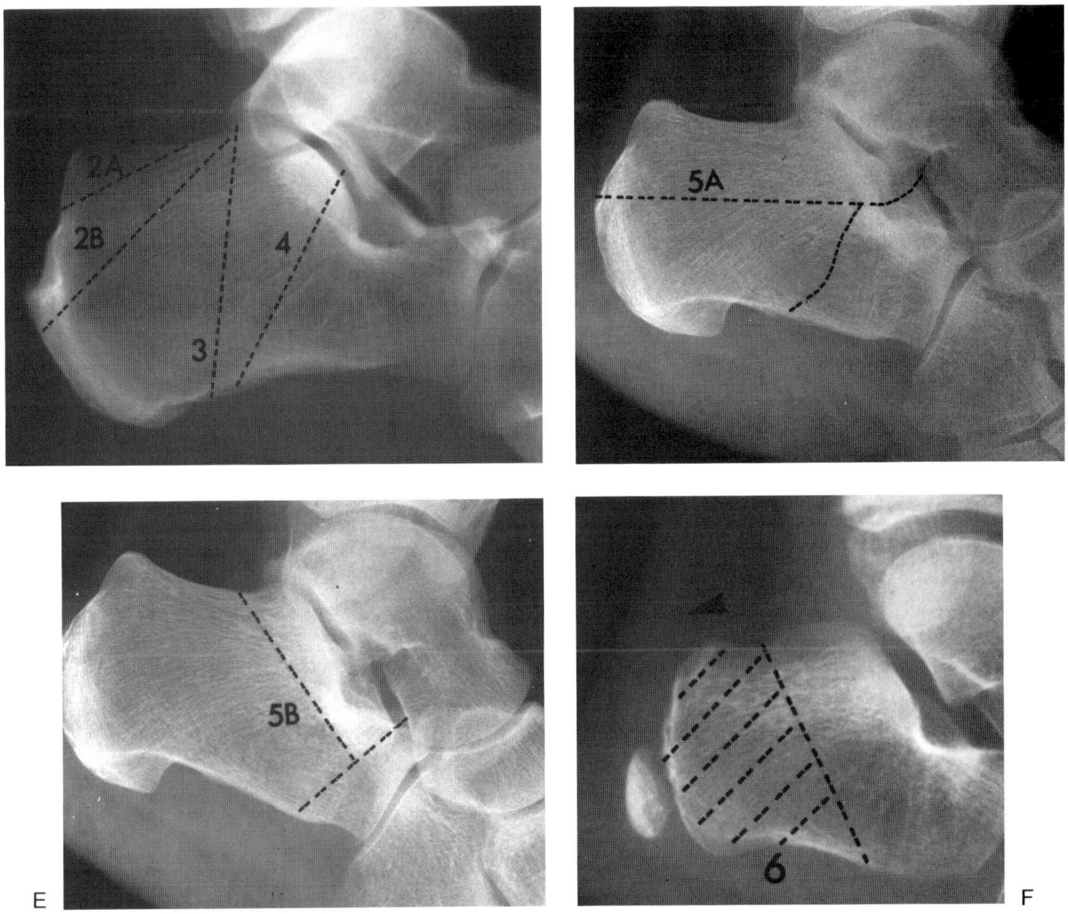

FIG. 8-41. (*Continued.*) **C:** Lateral view of the calcaneus demonstrating type 2A, beak fracture; type 2B, Achilles avulsion fracture; type 3, undisplaced fracture without subtalar joint involvement; type 4, linear fracture involving the subtalar joint. **D:** Lateral calcaneal radiograph demonstrating type 5A, tongue-type, compression fracture of the subtalar joint. **E:** Lateral calcaneal radiograph demonstrating type 5B, joint depression type of fracture. **F:** Lateral view of the calcaneus in a child demonstrating a type 6 fracture with loss of the Achilles insertion (*arrow*). (From Berquist TH. *Radiology of the foot and ankle.* New York: Raven Press, 1989.)

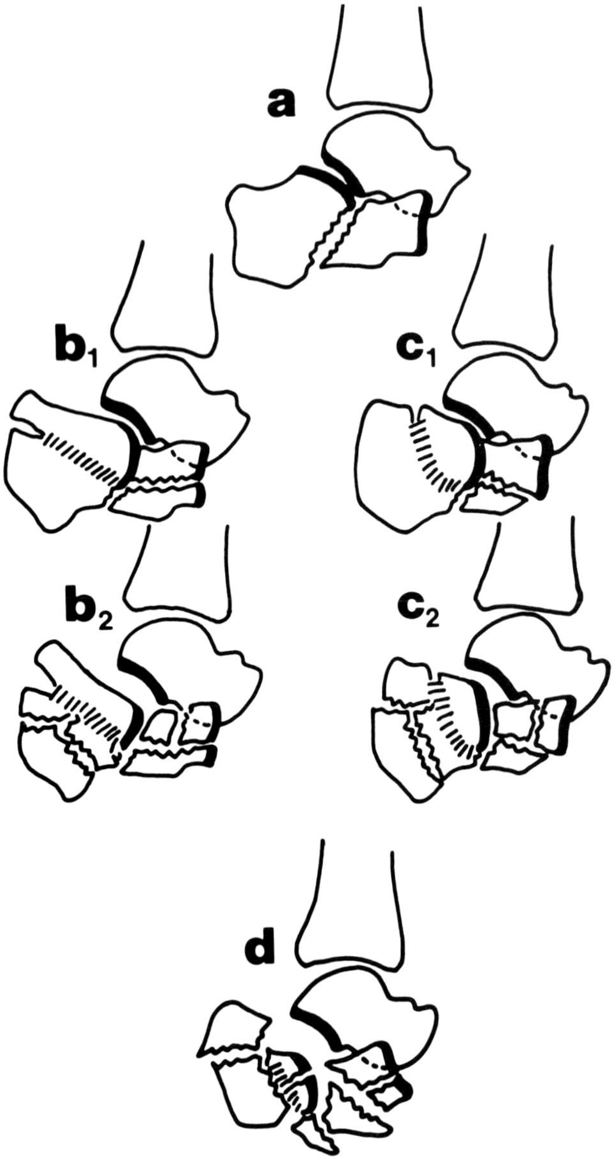

FIG. 8-42. Paley and Hall modification of Essex-Lopresti and Soeur-Remy classifications for calcaneal fractures. The classification is based on lateral radiographic features. Type a, two-part injury; type b1, tongue fracture with anterior and posterior secondary fracture lines; type b2, tongue fracture with comminution; type c1, central depression with anterior and posterior secondary fractures; type c2, central depression with comminution; type d, complex comminuted fracture. (From Paley D, Hall H. Intra-articular fractures of the calcaneus. A critical analysis of results and prognostic factors. *J Bone Joint Surg* [*Am*] 1993;75A:342–354.)

TABLE 8-7. *Essex-Lopresti classification of calcaneal fractures*[111,118]

I. No subtalar joint involvement
  A. Tuberosity fractures
    1. Break type
    2. Medial avulsion
    3. Vertical
    4. Horizontal
  B. Calcaneocuboid joint involvement
II. Involving subtalar joint
  A. Undisplaced
  B. Displaced
  C. Gross comminution

are generally not difficult to treat. The detection of these injuries may be particularly difficult in children in whom 81% of extraarticular fractures are missed on routine radiographs.[126] Types 1A and 1E (Fig. 8-41) can be treated with closed reduction and cast immobilization for 6 weeks.[118] Fractures of the sustentaculum (type 1B) and the calcaneocuboid articulation (types 1C and 1D, Fig. 8-41) may require more aggressive therapy.[112,118,119,125] Internal fixation or excision may be required for displaced fractures.[119,124]

The treatment of types 4 and 5 fractures (Fig. 8-41) is more controversial. Lateral radiographs to evaluate Böhler's angle and axial views or CT to evaluate calcaneal width and fragmentation are essential (Fig. 8-43).[109,110,113,115,122,123]

Multiple approaches to the treatment of these fractures have been proposed. Subtalar arthrodesis and triple arthrodesis were considered appropriate at one time; however, open reduction with accurate fixation have become more popular recently (Fig. 8-44). If comminution is too severe and adequate reduction cannot be achieved, closed treatment with early motion or arthrodesis may be appropriate in selected cases.[117,119,124,125,127,128]

Associated fractures with calcaneal injuries are common. Bilateral calcaneal fractures occur in 10% of patients because of the mechanism of injury, which may be a fall and landing on both feet. Lower-extremity fractures on the ipsilateral side occur in 24% to 26% of patients, and spine injury, usually lumbar compression fractures, are associated with calcaneal fractures in 10% to 30% of adults.[109,111,126,128]

Mid- and Forefoot Fractures

The midfoot is made up of the lesser tarsal bones (navicular, cuboid, and three cuneiforms). Joint stability is provided by numerous static and dynamic elements, such as the ligaments and tendons.[141]

Injuries of the bones of the midtarsal joints have been classified by Main and Jowett.[145] Their classification is based on the deformity force and the resulting displacement. Five categories of injury were established as follows: (1) medial, 30% of injuries; (2) longitudinal, 41% of injuries; (3) lateral, 17% of injuries; (4) plantar, 7% of injuries; and (5) crush injury, 5% of total injuries.

Medial forces cause inversion, resulting in dorsal avulsion fractures of the talus or navicular and lateral margins of the calcaneus or cuboid, medial subluxation of the forefoot, and rotation dislocation of the talonavicular joint.[145]

Longitudinal forces cause compression of the metatarsals with forces transmitted to the cuneiforms, causing compression of the navicular between the cuneiforms and talar head.

Lateral forces are usually due to falls causing medial distraction, which may lead to avulsion fractures of the navicular or talus and lateral impaction, causing compression of the calcaneus and/or cuboid. Lateral subluxation of the talonavicular joint may also occur.[141,145]

Plantar forces result in talonavicular or calcaneonavicular subluxation or dislocation with associated periarticular avulsions.

There are no consistent patterns of injury with crush injuries.[141,145]

Isolated tarsal fractures without associated joint involvement are uncommon (Fig. 8-45), especially in children.[134,141,145] For example, navicular fractures are avulsion injuries in 47% of patients, 29% involve the body, and 24% involve the tuberosity.[134] Isolated fractures of

(text continues on page 609)

TABLE 8-8. *Calcaneal fractures: classification and incidence*[112,115,119,125,126]

Type	(Schmidt and Weiner modification of Rowe and Essex-Lopresti)	Incidence rates (%)
1C	(Anterior process)	15
1A	(Tuberosity)	6
1B	(Sustentaculum tali)	3
1D and 1E		1
2	(A beak or B Achilles avulsion)	3–4
3	(Linear extraarticular)	19
4	(Intraarticular, linear)	10–24
5A	(Tongue type)	5
B	(Joint depression or comminution)	43–60

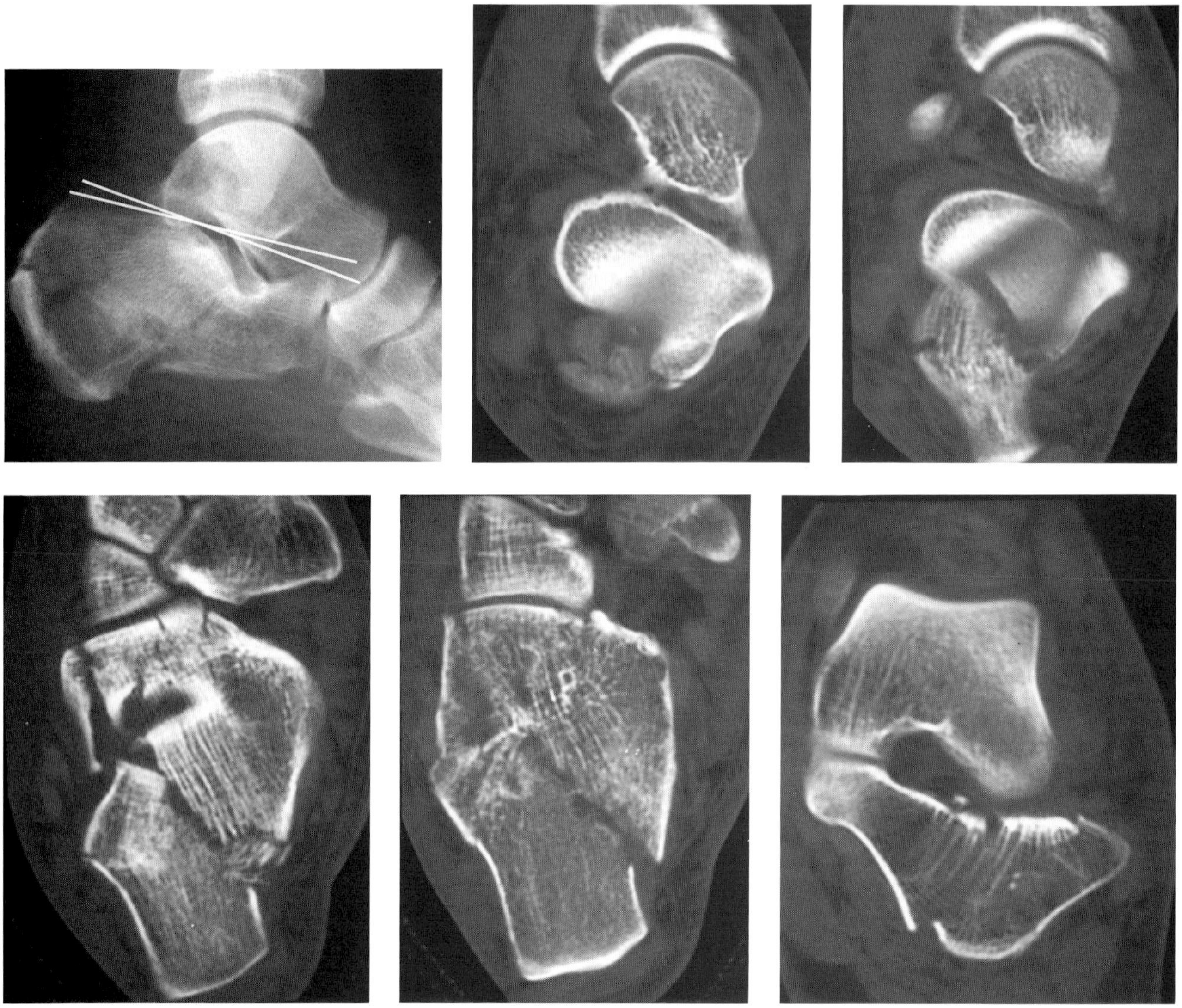

A,B

C

D,E

F

FIG. 8-43. Type 5 calcaneal fracture. **A:** Lateral view of the calcaneus demonstrates compression with reduction of Böhler's angle (normal, 20° to 40°). **B–E:** Axial CT images demonstrate the position of the fragments, calcaneal widening, and involvement of the calcaneocuboid and posterior subtalar joint. **F–H:** Coronal CT images demonstrating subtalar joint involvement.

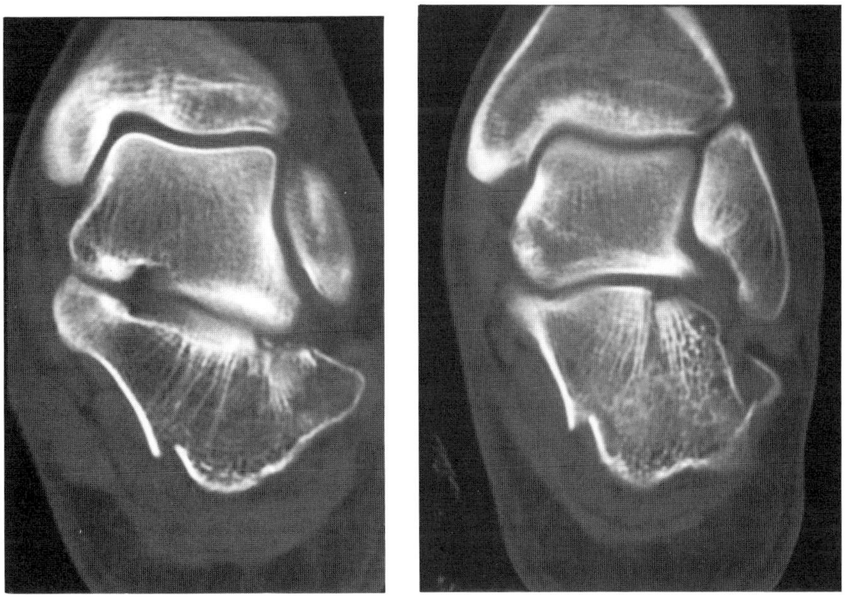

G H

FIG. 8-43. *Continued.*

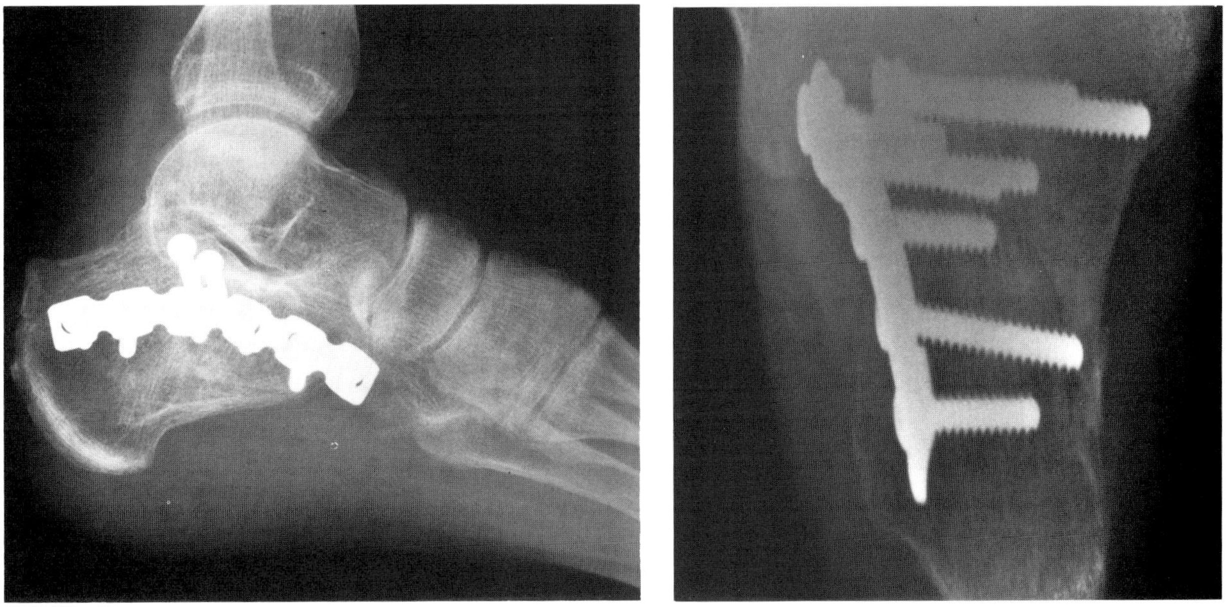

A B

FIG. 8-44. Lateral **(A)** and axial **(B)** images after internal fixation with two compression screws in the posterior facet and a pelvic reconstruction plate shaped to follow the bony contour and six screws. Calcaneal width is restored and Böhler's angle, improved.

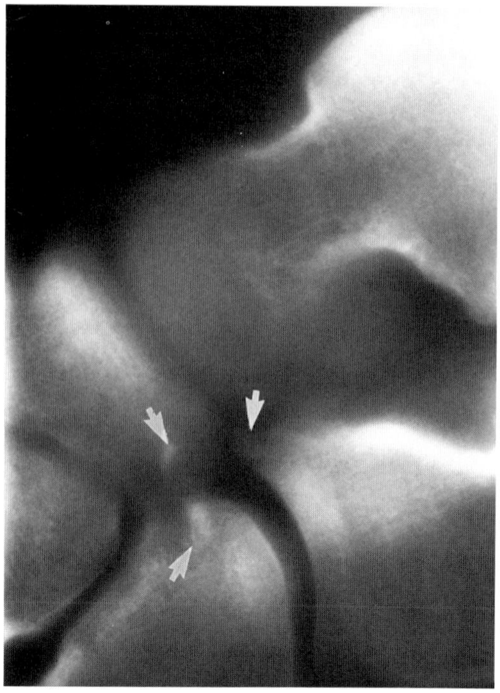

FIG. 8-45. Lateral tomogram demonstrating avulsion fractures (*arrows*) of the calcaneocuboid articulation.

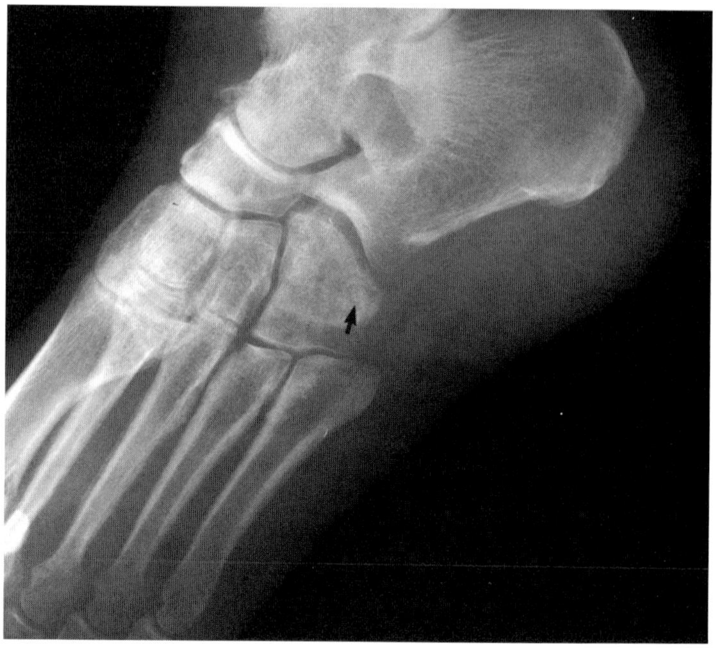

FIG. 8-46. Oblique view of the foot demonstrating a compression injury (*arrow*) of the cuboid.

A

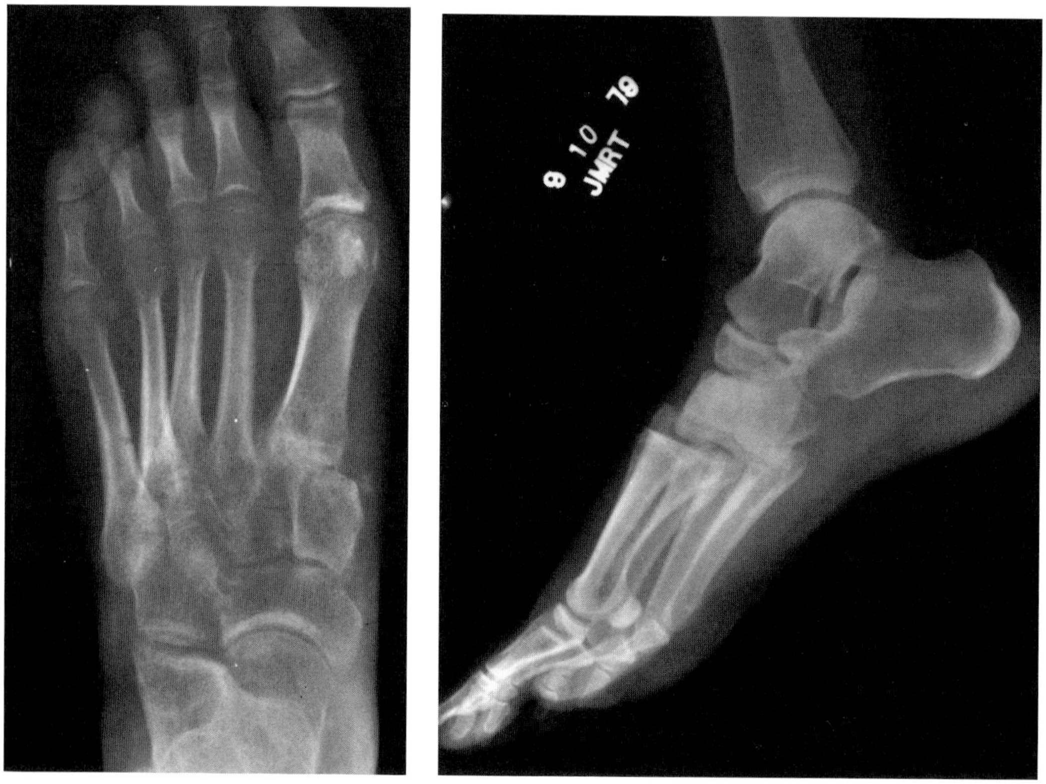

B

FIG. 8-47. The AP **(A)** view and lateral views in a different patient **(B)** demonstrating tarsometatarsal dislocations.

the cuneiforms and cuboid (Fig. 8-46) are uncommon in children and adults.[139–141]

Tarsometatarsal fracture dislocations are commonly referred to as Lisfranc injuries (Fig. 8-47) Typically, the injury occurs with forced plantar flexion of the foot, with or without associated rotation. This can occur during a fall or landing on the toes, which forces the forefoot into plantar flexion. Other mechanisms include falls with the forefoot fixed or compression of the foot caused by a heavy object striking the heel when the patient is in the kneeling position.[129–131,133,146,148]

Metatarsal fractures are common. These injuries are usually a result of direct trauma caused by a heavy object striking the foot. However, twisting or shearing injuries may also lead to fracture. The neck of the metatarsal is weaker than the shaft, which explains the higher incidence of fracture in this location.

Fractures at the base of the fifth metatarsal are common in children and adults. Two basic fracture patterns with different prognoses can be distinguished. Avulsion of the proximal tuberosity of the fifth metatarsal is common. This is due to an abrupt pull of the peroneus brevis. This fracture must be distinguished from a growth plate injury in the younger child. The second type of fifth metatarsal base fracture is referred to as the Jones fracture. This fracture involves the proximal diaphysis and metaphysis and should be treated differently. Internal fixation is frequently required.[130,132,142,143]

Treatment

Most forefoot injuries can be identified and classified on routine radiographs. Midfoot injuries can be subtle and easily overlooked or complex, requiring conventional tomography or CT to define the injury prior to therapy.[135,138] Today, many prefer CT.[146,147]

Midfoot Fracture-Dislocations

Most subluxations or minimally displaced fractures ($\leq$2 mm) are treated nonoperatively. Treatment failures or more significant injuries can be managed with arthrodesis operations and screw fixation.[136,137,145]

Metatarsal and Phalangeal Fractures

Most phalangeal and metatarsal fractures can be treated nonoperatively. Significantly displaced fractures may require open reduction with screws or pin fixation (Fig. 8-48).[130,141,144]

Jones fractures (Fig. 8-49) can be difficult to manage. Plates or cancellous screws (Fig. 8-50) may be required for union.[142,144,147]

Postoperative Imaging and Complications

Routine radiographic evaluation following treatment is essential to ensure proper healing and to be certain that reduction is maintained. In some cases, more sophisticated techniques, such as CT or MRI, may be required.[149,150] These techniques may be adversely affected by metal implants (Fig. 8-51). In addition, MRI is particularly useful for evaluating problems in the soft tissues, either with neurovascular structures or tendon interposition or deformity. For purposes of this discussion and because of certain differences in complications, it is best to discuss the evaluation of complications anatomically.

Ankle

The complications following ankle fracture differ somewhat in children and adults. Table 8-9 lists common ankle complications. In adults, arthritis is the most common long-term complication, occurring in 30% to 40% of patients, regardless of the type of treatment used (Fig. 8-52). The incidence is higher with displaced plafond fractures and when a syndesmosis is poorly reduced, leading to chronic instability.[149,157]

Malunion and nonunion may occur even when adequate reduction is obtained (Fig. 8-53). Nonunion occurs most commonly after avulsion of the medial malleolus. The incidence is 10% to 15% higher after closed than after open reduction.[149,163,166] The evaluation of nonunion can be accomplished with routine radiographs, but in many cases, CT or conventional tomography is helpful to define the region of interest better. If there is no significant metal in the area of interest, T2-weighted MRI sequences are also useful to differentiate union from nonunion or fibrous union. In children, MRI is also useful to evaluate the viability of the growth plate following ankle fractures.[150] A loss of reduction and instrument failure are uncommon with ankle injuries, but they do occur (Fig. 8-54).

(text continues on page 614)

TABLE 8-9. *Complications of ankle fractures*[149,152,154–156,158,160,163,166–169]

Osteoarthritis
Chronic instability
Nonunion
Malunion
Physeal deformity
Leg-length discrepancy
Reflex sympathetic dystrophy
Infection
Adhesive capsulitis
Tendon rupture or dislocation
Synovial chondromatosis
Tarsal tunnel syndrome
Neurovascular injury
Pes cavovarus deformity

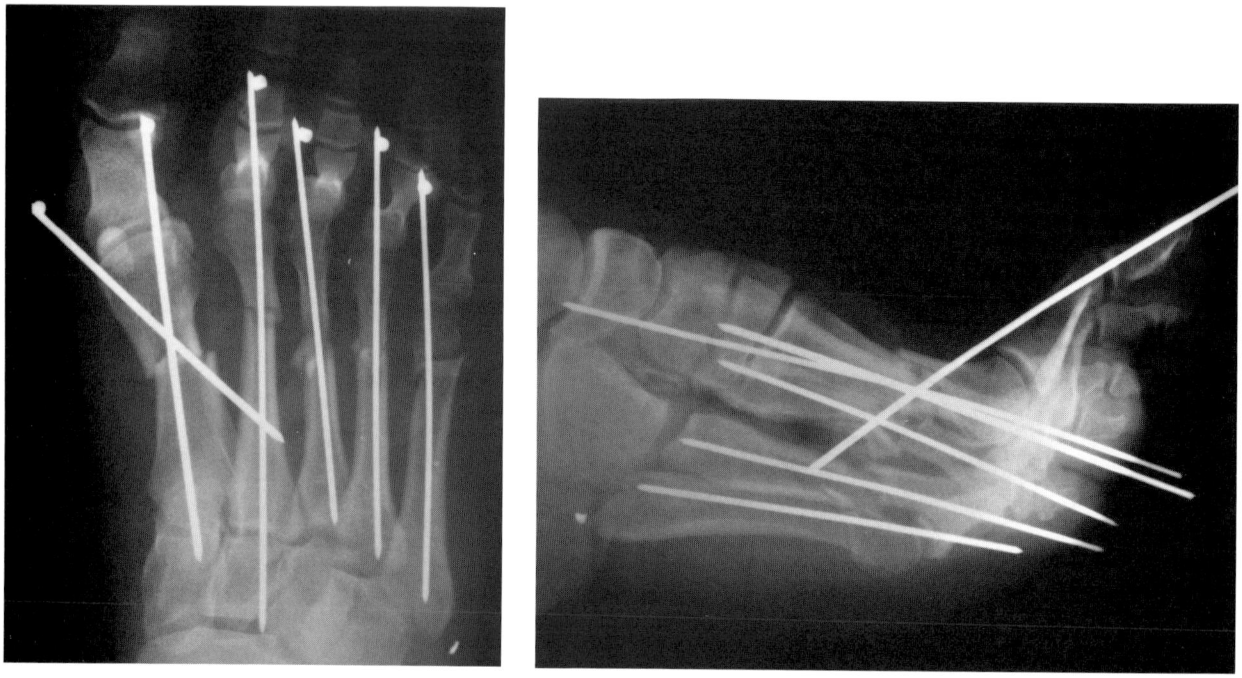

A B

FIG. 8-48. The AP **(A)** and lateral **(B)** radiographs of comminuted displaced distal metatarsal fractures after K-wire fixation.

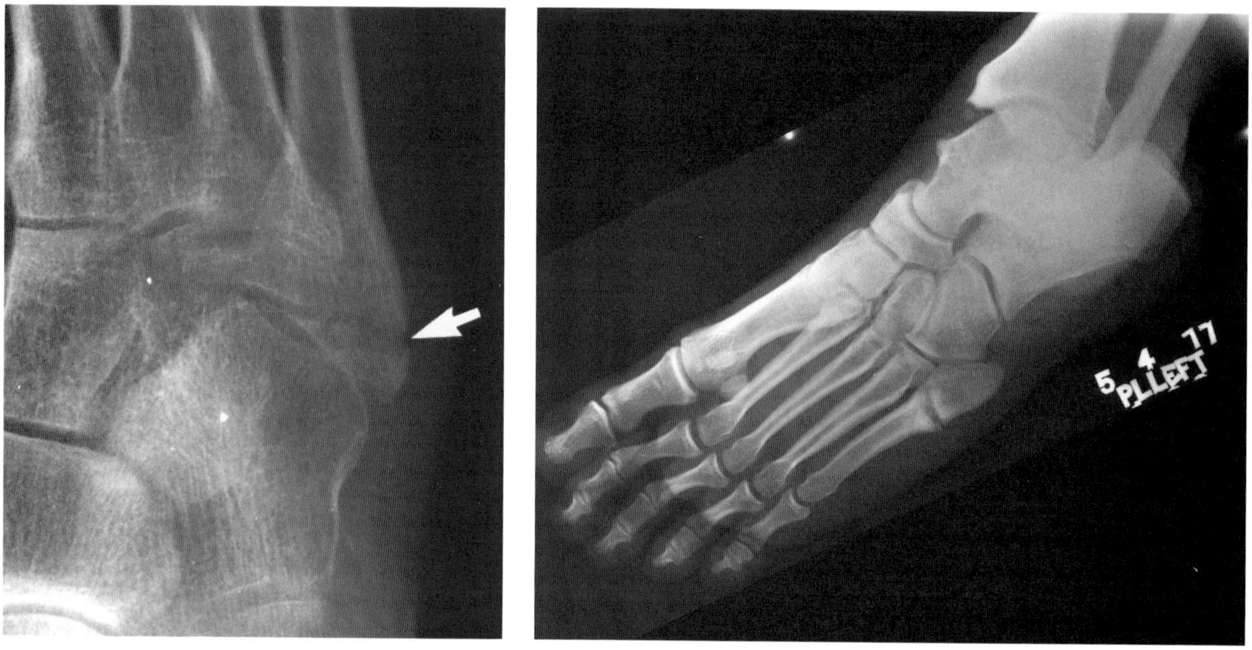

A B

FIG. 8-49. Radiographs of the typical transverse fracture of the fifth metatarsal base **(A)** and oblique radiograph of the foot demonstrating a nonunited Jones fracture **(B)**.

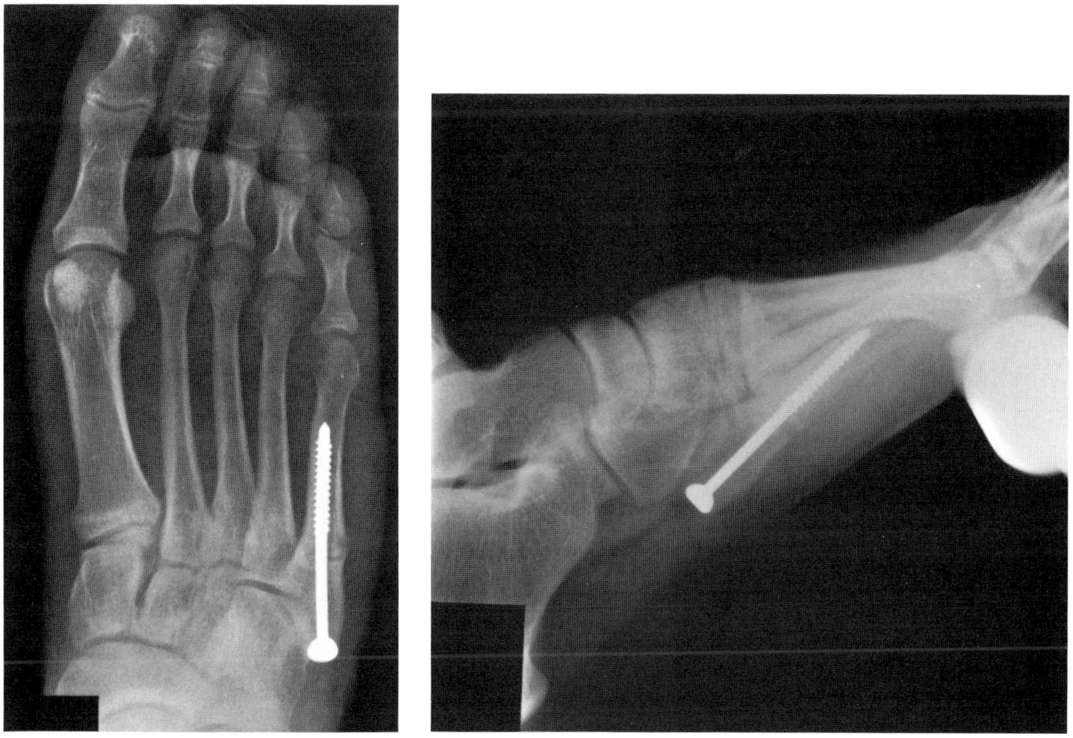

A B

FIG. 8-50. The AP **(A)** and lateral **(B)** radiographs of a proximal diaphyseal fracture of the fifth metatarsal with a long cancellous screw for fixation.

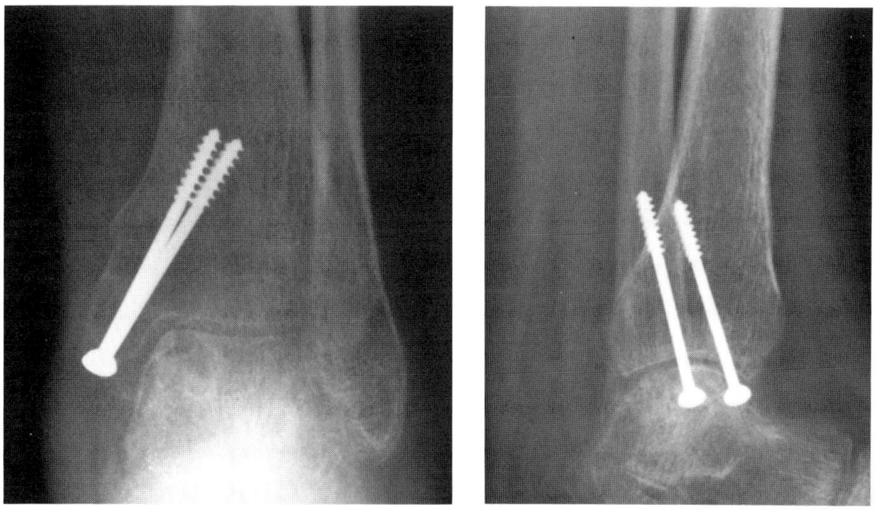

A B

FIG. 8-51. The AP **(A)** and lateral **(B)** radiographs in a patient with persistent ankle pain and swelling after healing of a medial malleolar fracture with two malleolar screws in place. (See **C-G** on next page.)

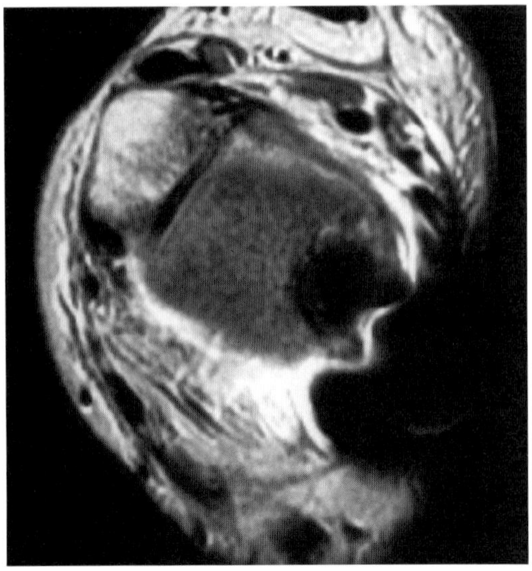

C

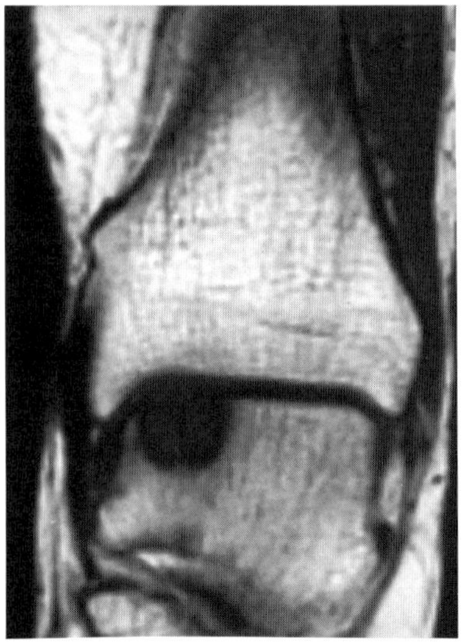

D

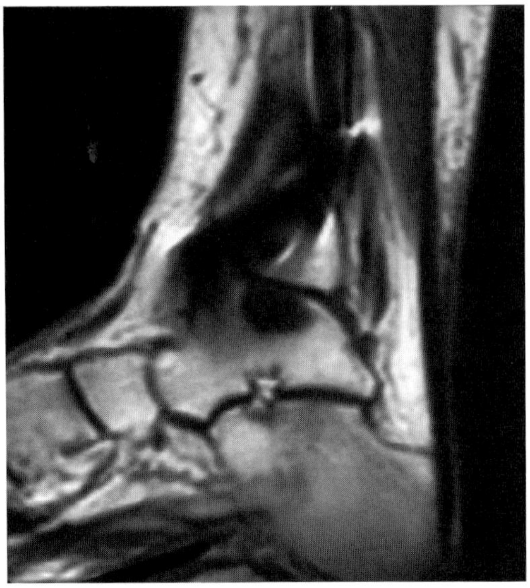

E

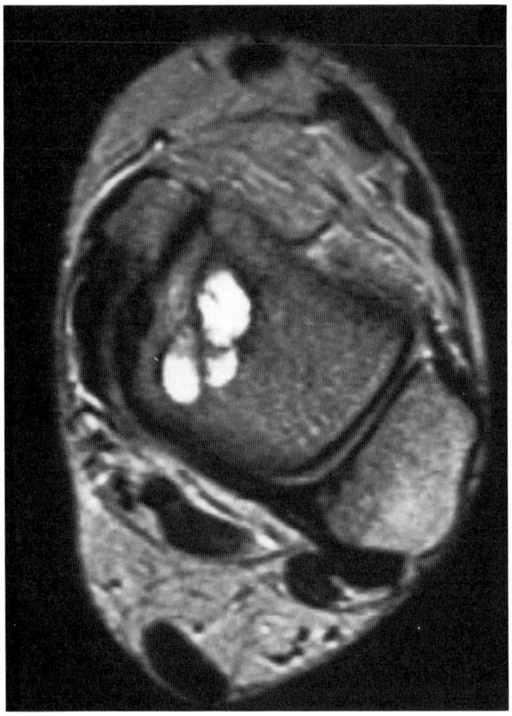

F

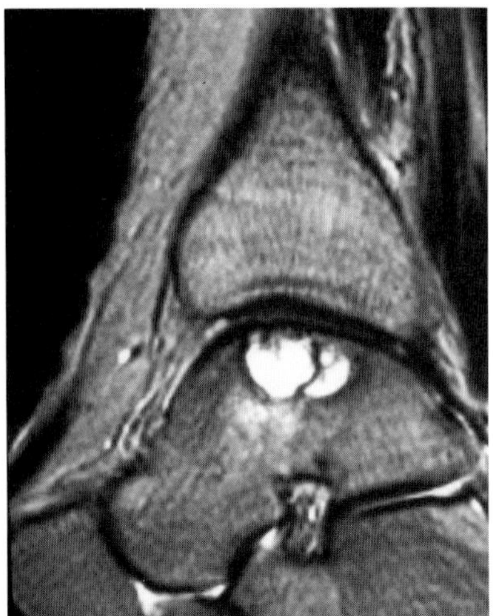

G

FIG. 8-51. (*Continued.*) Axial **(C)**, coronal **(D)**, and sagittal **(E)** SE 500/20 images show metal artifact with a low-intensity abnormality in the medial talar dome. Axial **(F)** and sagittal **(G)** SE 2,000/60 images show an old well-defined talar dome defect with no bone fragment in the defect.

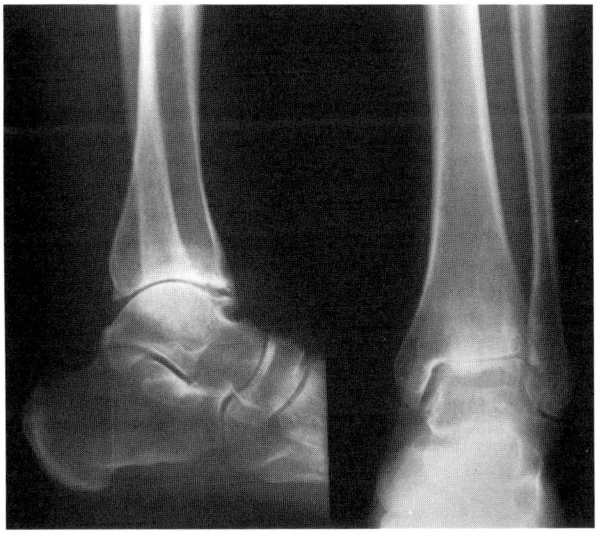

FIG. 8-52. Lateral and AP views of the ankle 2 years after fracture demonstrating degenerative arthritis with marked joint space narrowing.

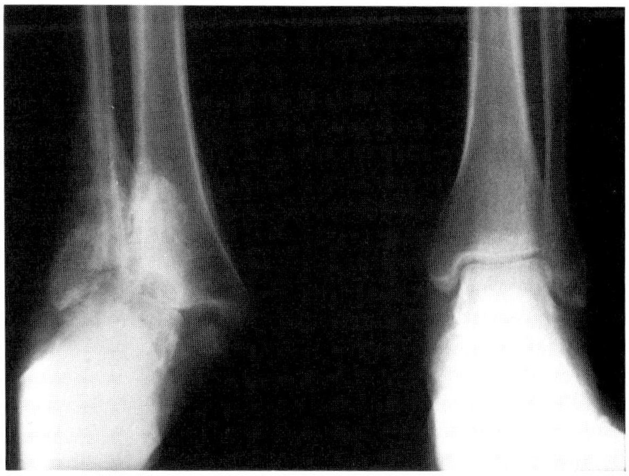

FIG. 8-53. Standing AP view of the ankles demonstrating a nonunited medial malleolar fracture, fibular malunion, and subluxation with talar tilt on the right.

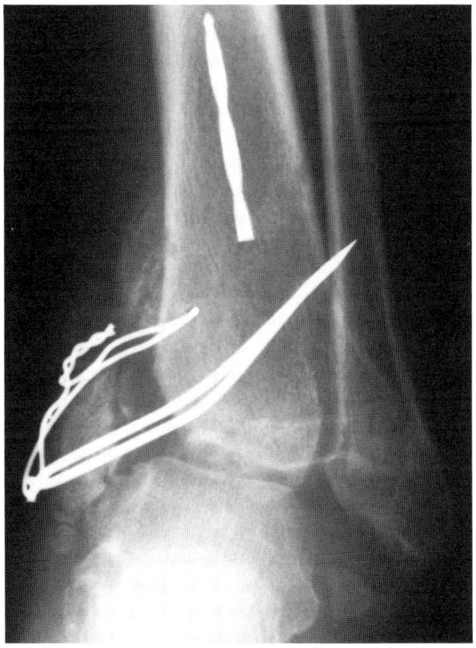

FIG. 8-54. An AP view of the ankle demonstrating failed K-wire and tension-band wire technique for a medial malleolar fracture. The fracture is not united, and the ankle is unstable.

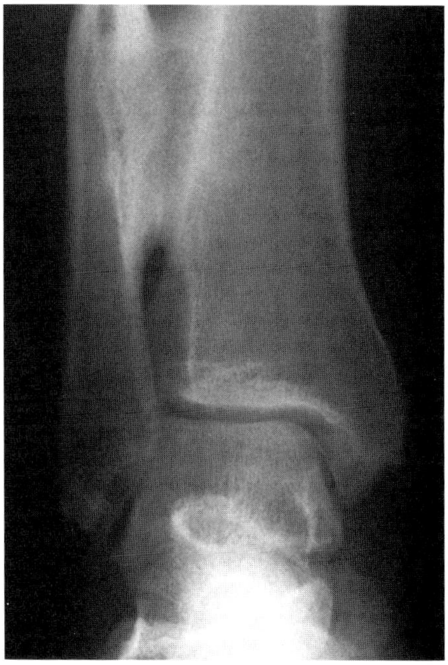

FIG. 8-55. An AP view of the ankle after fracture. There is a large area of ossification (synostosis) in the syndesmosis.

Ossification of the syndesmosis can occur after ankle fractures (Fig. 8-55). Most often, it is incomplete. However, complete bone fusion can occur, usually when a syndesmosis screw has been used. These changes are usually obvious on routine radiographs. However, the scarring and stenosis may be truly fibrotic in nature, in which case MRI or CT is more helpful.[150]

Infection, although uncommon, occurs more frequently with open techniques (Fig. 8-56). The incidence is higher with open or contaminated injuries.[149,163]

In children, the most common problem encountered is premature or asymmetric closure of the physis. This may be related to the type of growth plate injury. Salter-Harris types III to V and triplane fractures tend to have a guarded prognosis. There is also a potential for problems if fixation devices cross the growth plate.[149,156]

The deformity caused by a growth plate fracture may lead to a leg-length discrepancy or angular deformity. Excision of the osseous bar can be performed if less than 50% of the growth plate is involved. If greater than 50% of the growth plate is affected, contralateral epiphysiodesis is generally performed. These procedures are generally preferred for younger patients who have at least 1 year of growth remaining. When angular deformities are greater than 10°, surgeons may consider performing a wedge osteotomy at the same time that the bar is resected. Prior to planning the surgical procedure, tomograms or MRI scans of the affected growth plate are used to define the degree of closure better (Fig. 8-57).[149,152,154,156]

Leg-length discrepancy occurs in 10% to 30% of pediatric patients. If the leg-length difference is less than 2 cm, it may not require surgery.[152,154]

Other complications include rotational malalignment, delayed or nonunion, and avascular necrosis. Rotational deformities are more common with triplane injuries. The deformity may be significant, requiring derotational osteotomy. The assessment of the degree of deformity is most easily accomplished by using CT or MRI, which allow the degree of rotation to be more easily documented.[149,150]

Talar Fractures and Dislocations

Complications are particularly common after displaced talar neck fractures (Hawkins types II to IV).[151,159] Avascular necrosis, if untreated, progresses through stages. Early identification and evaluation of the extent of involvement is most easily accomplished with MRI if there is no significant metal in the area of interest (Fig. 8-58).[150] Radiographic changes may be apparent in 6 to 8 weeks. Disuse leads to subchondral lucency if the vascular supply is intact. If this feature is not evident (Fig. 8-59), avascular necrosis should be considered.[159,161,162]

Posttraumatic arthritis is common after talar neck fractures. The incidence increases with the severity of injury. Delayed healing is fairly common with talar neck fractures, occurring in 15% of patients. Nonunion is considered if the fractures have not healed by 6 months. It occurs in approximately 4% of cases overall. However, the incidence is higher with Hawkins types II and III fractures.[149,159,163]

Malunion is more common in complex injuries, occurring in up to 15% of cases. Other complications include infection.[149,164,168]

Calcaneal Fractures

Chronic pain may occur after calcaneal fractures. The prognosis is more guarded with central depression than with tongue-type fractures (Figs. 8-41 and 8-42).[165] Pain may be related to arthrosis, nerve entrapment, or tendon impingement.[164] Even in the presence of metal implants, CT is probably the best way to evaluate bone and articular changes (Fig. 8-60).[149] Routine radiographs should also be carefully evaluated. The standing lateral foot, oblique foot, and standing AP ankle views are most useful. Böhler's angle, heel width, joint incongruity or arthrosis, and the lateral foot angles can be evaluated and followed. Calcaneal width and Böhler's angle tend to be the most useful in predicting the prognosis.[165] Diagnostic subtalar or tarsal joint injections along with CT are useful prior to considering arthrodesis.[149]

Mid- and Forefoot Injuries

Delayed union, malunion, and nonunion are complications that may occur regardless of the fracture site.[149,153,170] Persistent pain following midfoot fractures is not uncommon, and it is usually due to arthritis. In this case, arthrodesis of the involved joints may be required.[163] In particular, CT and selected joint injections with anesthetic are useful prior to planning surgery.

JOINT RECONSTRUCTION

Ankle

The ankle is among the most frequently injured joints. Arthrosis is common following injury. Rheumatoid arthritis also frequently involves the ankle. Ankle arthroplasty was developed to provide a functional, pain-free joint and avoid arthrodesis.[171,177,181,183,184,187,197,205]

Newton[200] reported on 50 patients who used a prosthesis he designed in 1973 (Fig. 8-61). There were failures in 38% and loosening in 24% of patients.

Several types of ankle joint replacements were devel-

(text continues on page 620)

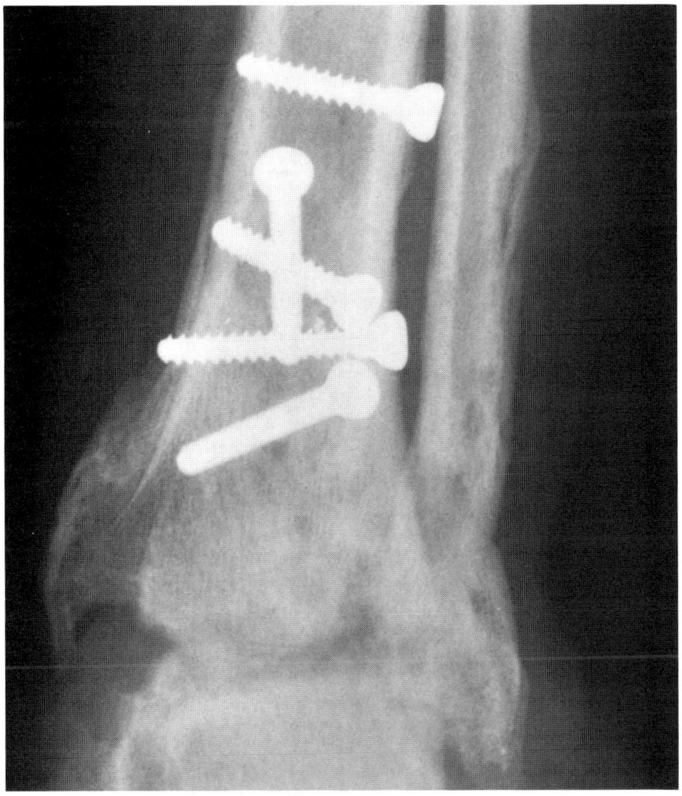

FIG. 8-56. The AP radiographs after internal fixation of a complex open plafond fracture. There is marked articular destruction and sclerosis caused by chronic osteomyelitis with septic arthritis.

A

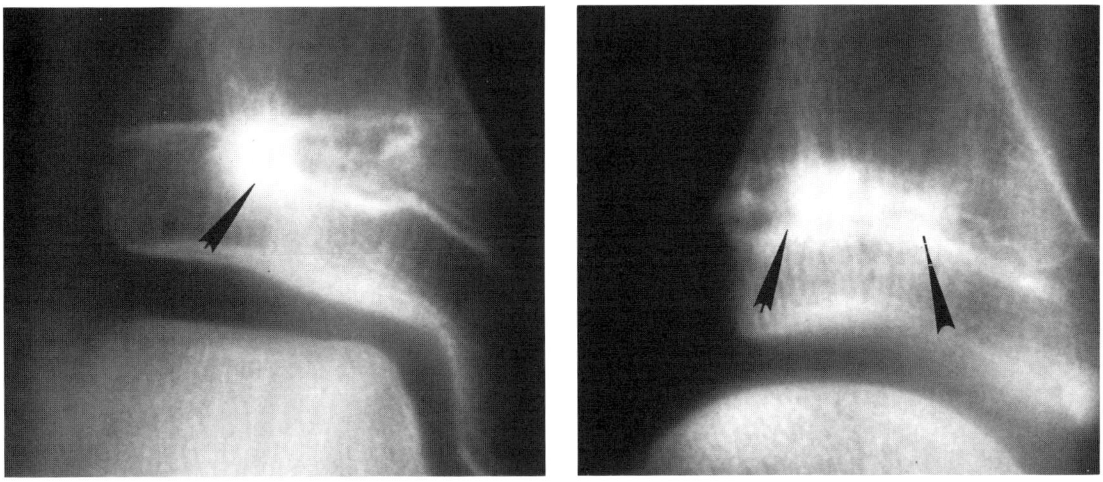

B

FIG. 8-57. Previous fracture through the distal tibial physis. The AP **(A)** and lateral **(B)** tomograms demonstrate a bony bar (*arrows*) involving < 50% of the growth plate. There is articular incongruency (*lines*). (See **C-E** on next page.)

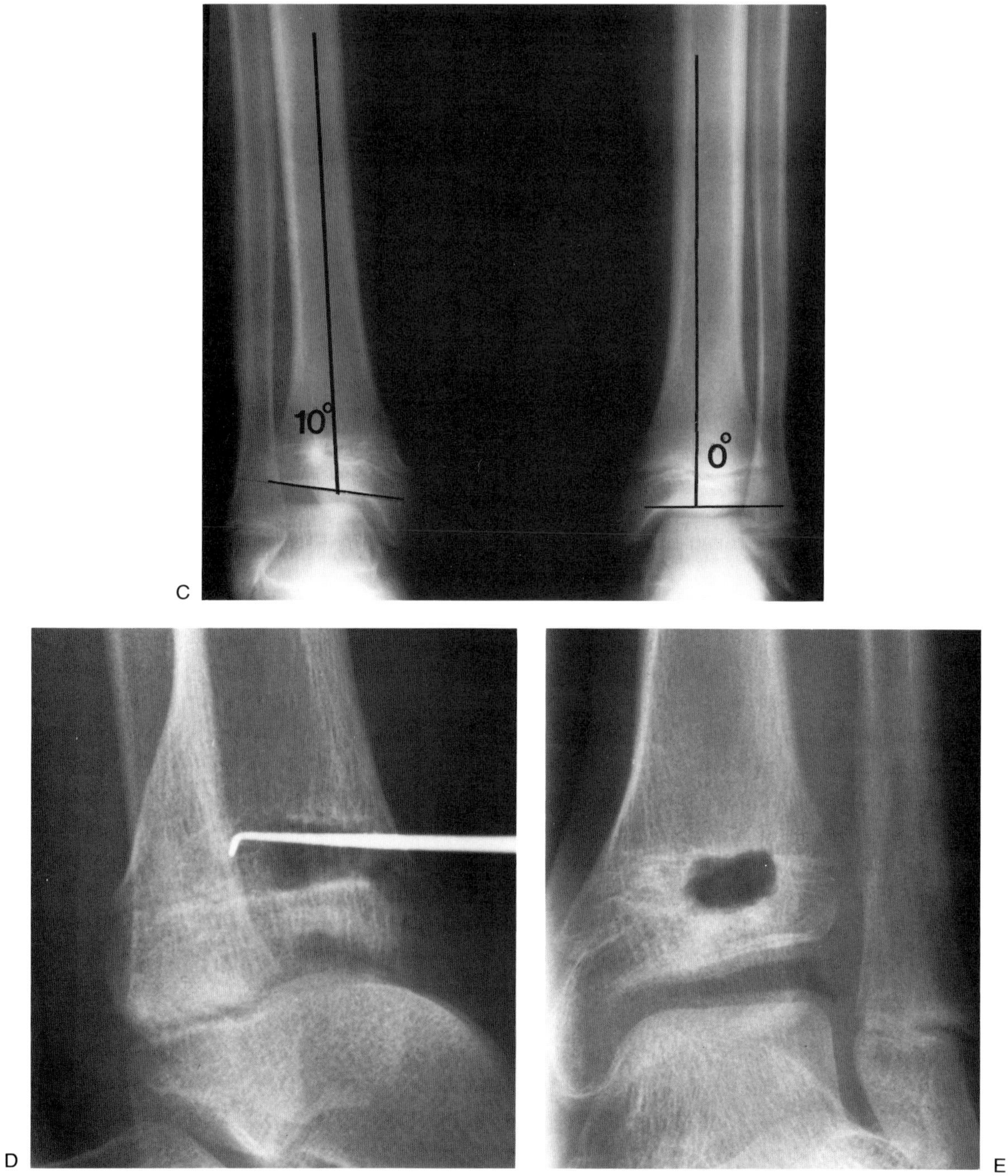

FIG. 8-57. (*Continued.*) **C:** Standing AP views show 10° of incongruency and slight leg-length discrepancy. Operative **(D)** and postoperative **(E)** radiographs showing resection of the bony bar.

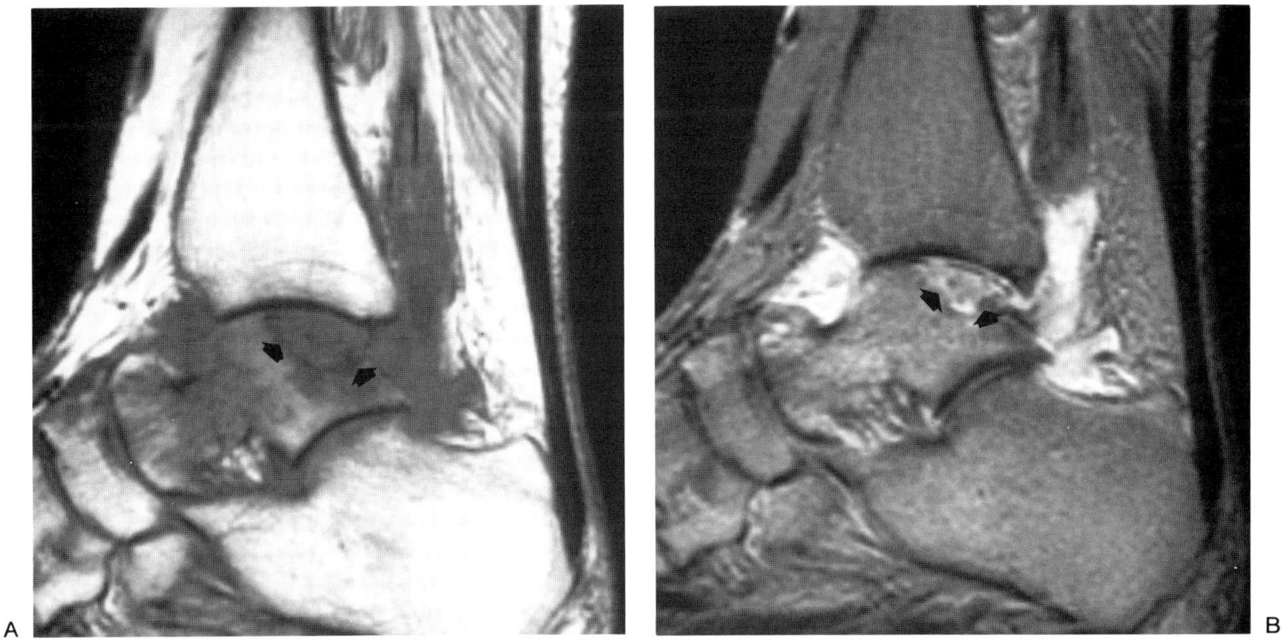

FIG. 8-58. Sagittal T1 (SE 500/20) **(A)** and T2 (SE 2,000/60) **(B)** images after talar neck fracture. There is an ankle effusion and avascular necrosis (*arrows*).

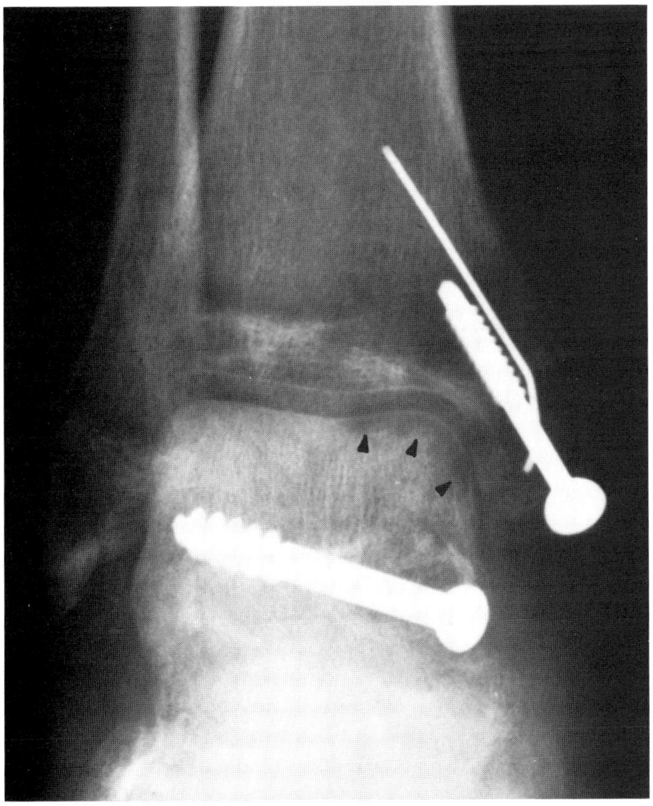

FIG. 8-59. An AP view of the ankle after internal fixation of the medial malleolus and talar neck. There is subchondral lucency medially, indicating vascular supply to this region is intact (*arrows*). There is sclerosis of the lateral talar dome as a result of avascular necrosis.

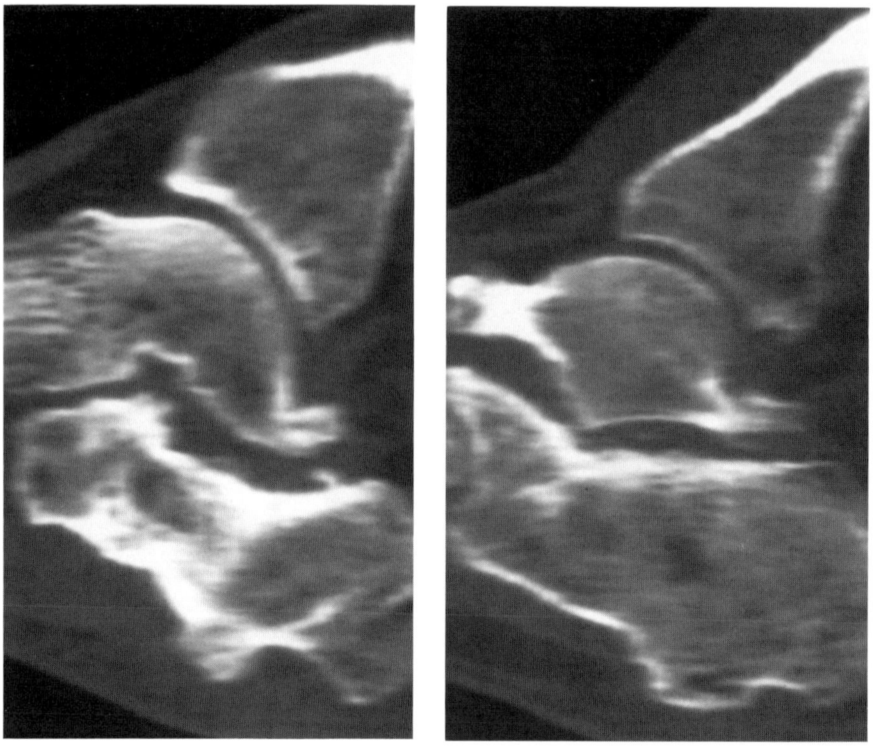

A B

FIG. 8-60. A, B: Sagittal reformatted CT images after calcaneal fracture with deformity and marked subtalar arthrosis.

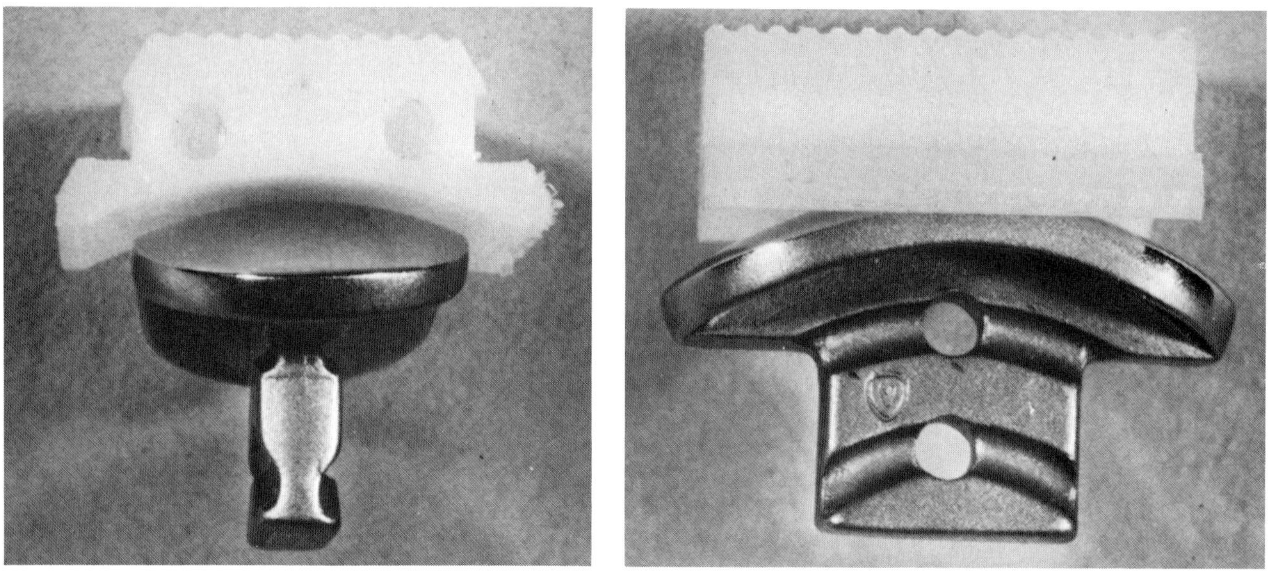

A B

FIG. 8-61. Newton ankle prosthesis seen from the front **(A)** and side **(B)**. The tibial component is high-density polyethylene with a flat upper surface and curved articulating surface. The talar component is cobalt-chromium alloy. Both components were cemented.

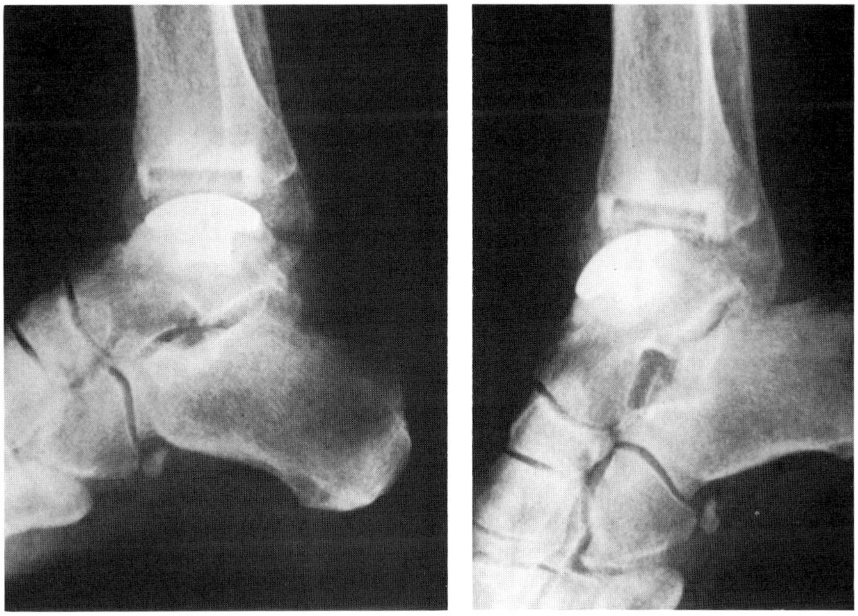

C D

FIG. 8-61. (*Continued.*) Lateral radiographs in extension **(C)** and flexion **(D)** demonstrate the appearance and motion allowed. (From Newton SE. Total ankle arthroplasty. *J Bone Joint Surg [Am]* 1982;64A: 104.)

A,B

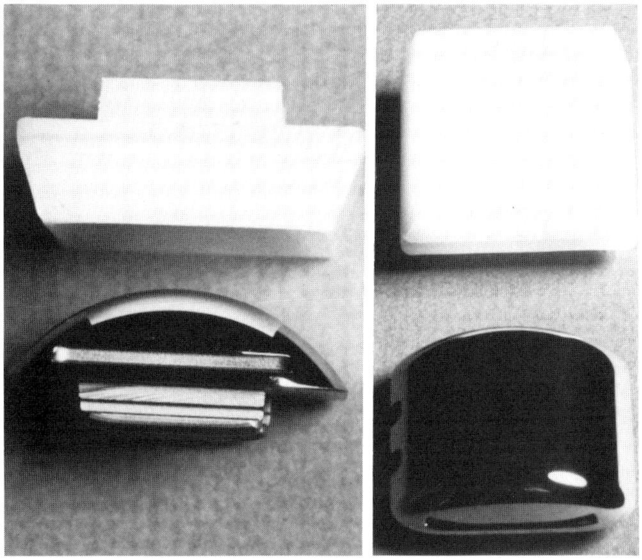

FIG. 8-62. The Mayo ankle arthroplasty components seen from the side **(A)** and top **(B)**. Metal talar and polyethylene tibial components. The AP **(C)** and lateral **(D)** radiographs of cemented components in good position. (From Johnson KA. Total ankle arthroplasty. In: Berquist TH, ed. *Imaging of orthopedic trauma and surgery.* Philadelphia: WB Saunders, 1986;491–494.)

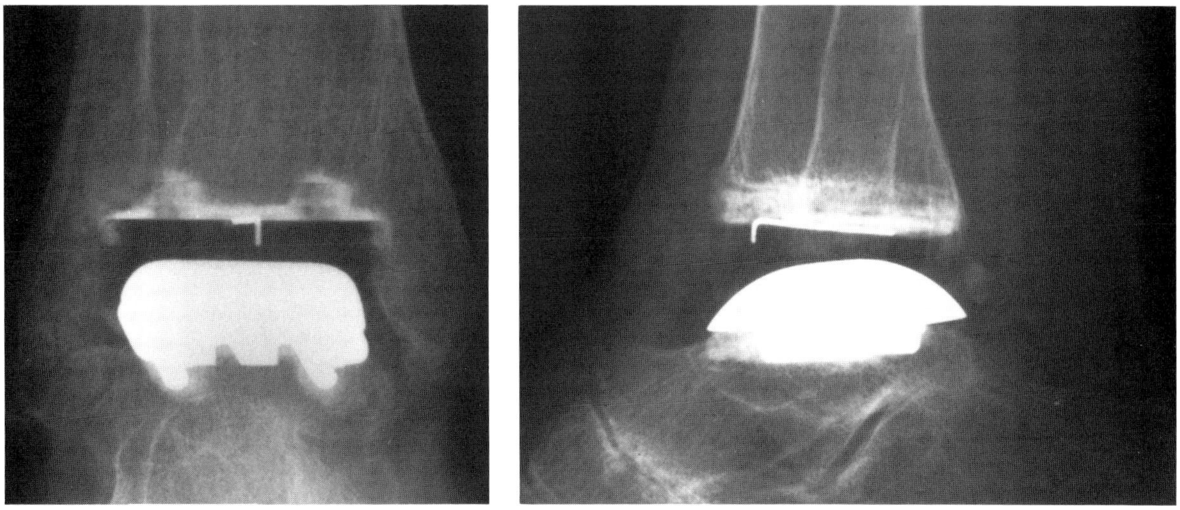

C D

oped. Satisfactory early results were achieved in most cases. The implants are divided according to their design philosophy, similar to those of the hip and knee. One group of implants essentially allows motion in flexion and extension (constrained); the other group allows some motion in multiple directions (nonconstrained).[185,186,209,210] The materials used in each are largely metal-polyethylene combinations. Ceramic implants are also available.[208] None of the components designed thus far appears to show significant superiority over any other. Figures 8-61 to 8-67 show examples of different types of ankle arthroplasties.[173,178,179] Our experience at the Mayo Clinic reflects the general experience of others with ankle-replacement procedures.[185–191,195,200,209] In a report from this institution of 102 arthroplasties of the ankle, the best results were obtained in patients with rheumatoid arthritis and those with posttraumatic osteoarthritis who were older than 60 years of age. A survivorship analysis of 204 primary Mayo total ankle arthroplasties studied by Kitaoka et al.[194] demonstrated survival rates of 79%, 65%, and 61% at 5, 10, and 15 years, respectively. Significantly higher risks of failure were observed in patients who had undergone previous operative procedures or who were 57 years of age or younger.

The use of ankle arthroplasty in other diagnostic categories of ankle disease has been less successful. The contraindications include previous arthrodesis, failed arthroplasty, and avascular necrosis of the talus.[185]

Metatarsophalangeal Joint Replacement

Resection arthroplasty, cheilectomy, and arthrodesis have been used for years to deal with diseases of the first metatarsophalangeal joint.[192] The Mayo procedure (resection of the metatarsal head) and Keller procedure (resection of the base of the proximal phalanx of the first toe) were popular in the past, but problems have been recognized with both operations, such as recurrent hallux valgus, hallux extensus, loss of flexor strength, and weight transfer to the lateral metatarsal heads. Other procedures, such as arthrodesis, occasionally have problems with union or interphalangeal arthrosis, and osteotomy procedures can be associated with recurrent deformity, malunion, nonunion, and avascular necrosis.[206,207]

Joint-replacement arthroplasty was developed as an alternative to these techniques in an effort to relieve pain and improve function.[182,192,196] The indications for great toe arthroplasty include hallux valgus, hallux rigidus, degenerative joint disease, rheumatoid arthritis, and failed surgical procedures. Although this discussion emphasizes first metatarsophalangeal joint replacement, the lesser metatarsophalangeal joints have also been replaced in patients with Frieberg's disease, subluxation, rheumatoid arthritis, and bunionette deformities.[172,175,176,188,190,192,193,199,206,207]

Arthroplasty designs have changed significantly since the 1950s. The early designs included a metal stemmed metatarsal head resurfacing implant and acrylic implants for the first metatarsal head and proximal phalanx.[192,207] In 1965, Swanson designed a silicone single-stemmed resurfacing implant for the proximal phalanx (Fig. 8-68).[207] Other designs have also been developed (Figs. 8-69 to 8-71).[172,188,198] Double-stemmed Silastic™ implants were subsequently introduced (Figs. 8-72 and 8-73).The clinical evaluation considers the patient's age and activity level, radiographic features of severe arthrosis, and the underlying disease process.[192,198] A scoring system similar to that used for arthroplasty in other regions can be used to evaluate symptoms and postoperative function.[199]

Preoperative radiographs should include standing AP and lateral views of the foot (Fig. 8-74). The AP view is used to evaluate the first to second metatarsal angles (intermetatarsal angle), joint congruence, and the angles of the great toe (metatarsophalangeal angle, Fig. 8-74). The CT images can be used to evaluate bone stock in patients with rheumatoid arthritis.

Postoperative Imaging and Complications

As in other arthroplasties, loosening and infection are worrisome complications. For ankle replacement, the incidence of deep infection ranges from 2.7% to 3.5%.[185,186,209] Infection appears to be more common in patients with rheumatoid arthritis (Fig. 8-75).[203] Patients may experience persistent pain, which is often related to loosening (Fig. 8-76).[185] Impingement of the talar components beneath the fibula is also a cause of pain (Fig. 8-77). This usually occurs from component subsidence into the talus and tibia over time. Other complications include instability (Fig. 8-78) and fracture during implant insertion.[174,185,186,192,194,201–202,204,209] Table 8-10 lists complications of ankle arthroplasty. The results of ankle arthroplasty with longer follow-up have been a concern because of loosening, component migration, and impingement.

Imaging of ankle arthroplasties postoperatively requires serial routine radiographs. Standing AP and lateral ankle images are required for an accurate evaluation of ankle implants. Stress views may occasionally be useful in patients with suspected instability.

(text continues on page 634)

TABLE 8-10. *Ankle replacement arthroplasty: complications*[185–187, 197]

Delayed wound healing
Loosening
Deep infection
Talofibular impingement
Instability
Pain, implant removed

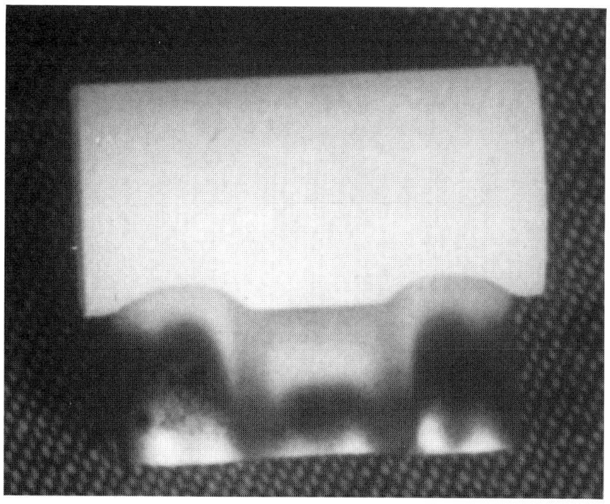

A

FIG. 8-63. Conaxial (Beck-Steffee) ankle arthroplasty. (DePuy, Warsaw, IN.) **A:** Seen from the front. **B:** Lateral view of the tibial polyethylene component and metal talar dome. **C:** An AP radiograph demonstrating the double-dome configuration seen on the AP view. There is a medial malleolar stress fracture (*arrow*). Lateral **(D)** and AP **(E)** radiographs later show the medial malleolar fracture healed; a fibular stress fracture has also healed. The tibial component is loose. (From Wynn AH, Wilde AH. Long-term follow-up of the conaxial (Beck-Steffee) total ankle arthroplasty. *Foot Ankle* 1992;13:303–306.)

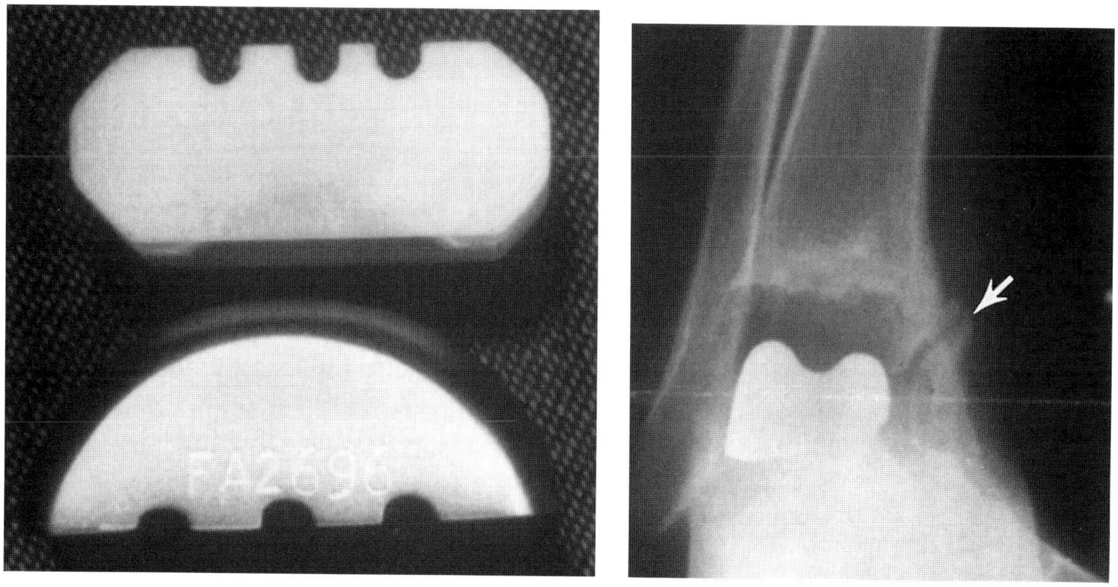

B C

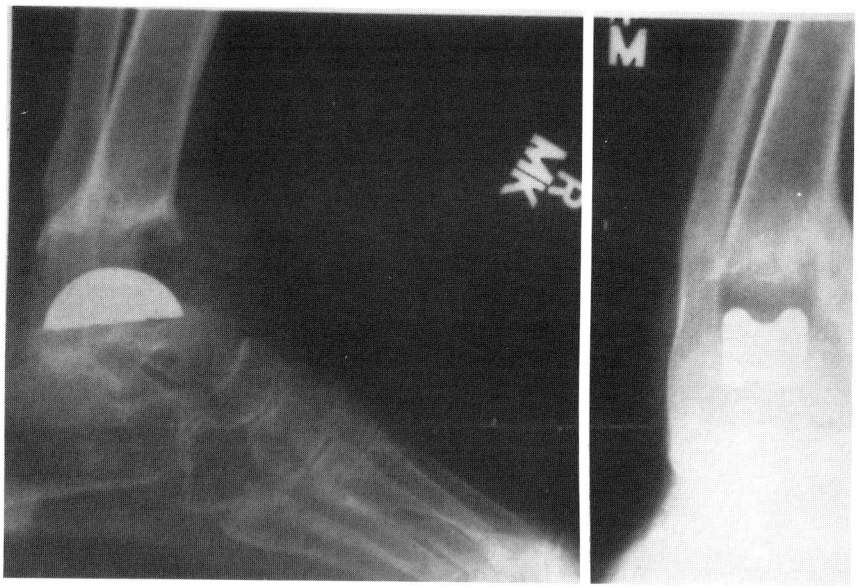

D E

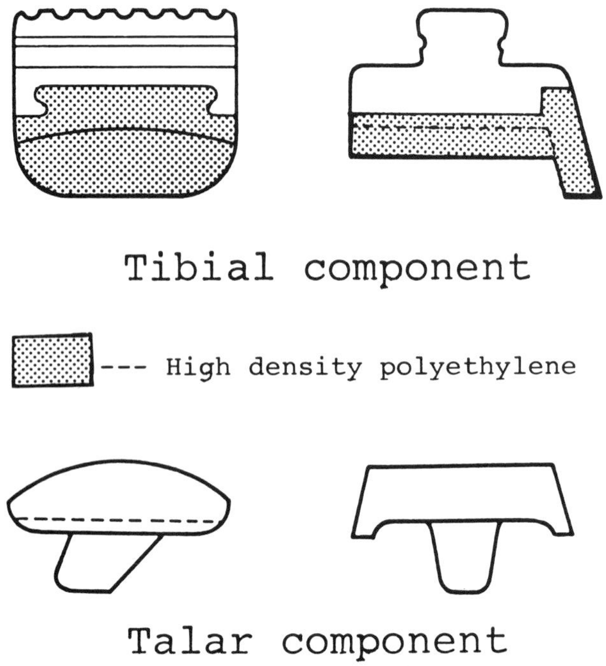

A

FIG. 8-64. A: A ceramic-polyethylene prosthesis with a medial facet on the tibial component. B: Uncemented ceramic prosthesis 6 months after insertion. There is minimal callus anterior to the tibial component (*arrow*). C: Lateral radiograph taken in dorsiflexed position at 6 years shows a good result with anterior callus (*arrows*). (From Takakura Y, Tanaka Y, Sugimoto K, Tamai S, Masuhara K. Ankle arthroplasty: a comparative study of cemented metal and uncemented ceramic prosthesis. *Clin Orthop* 1990;252:209–216.)

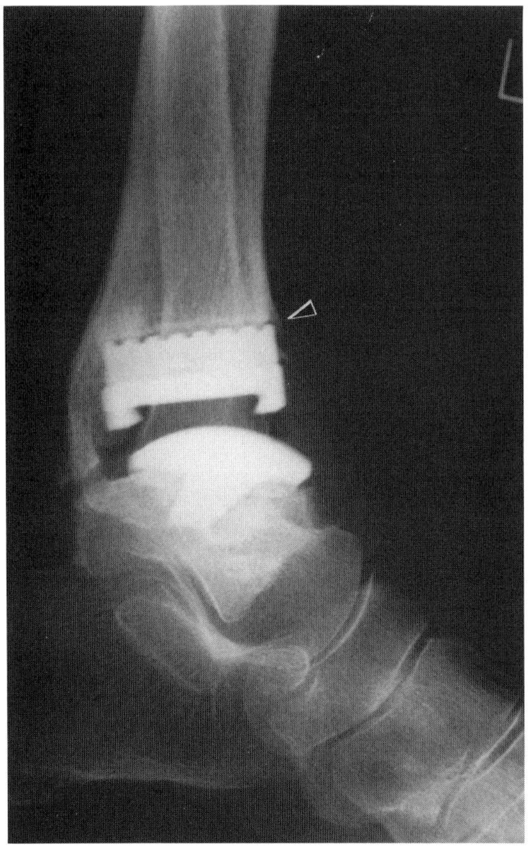

B

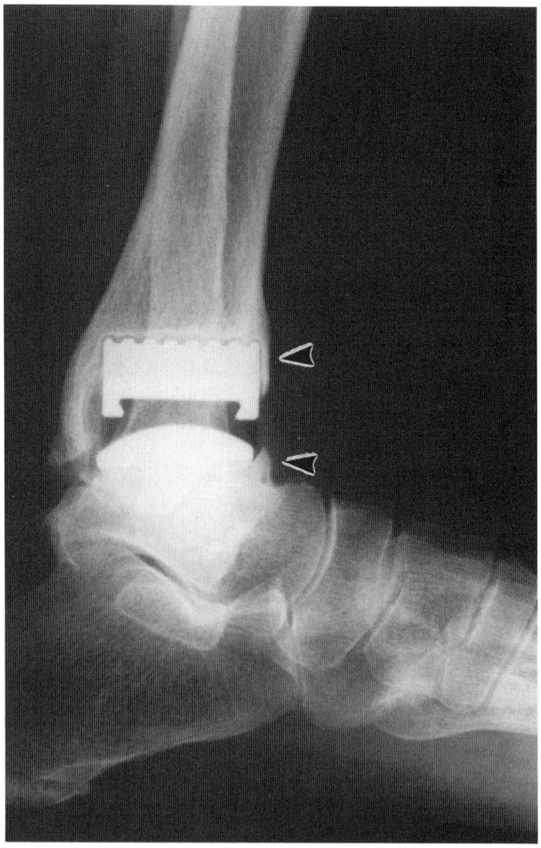

C

A,B

C

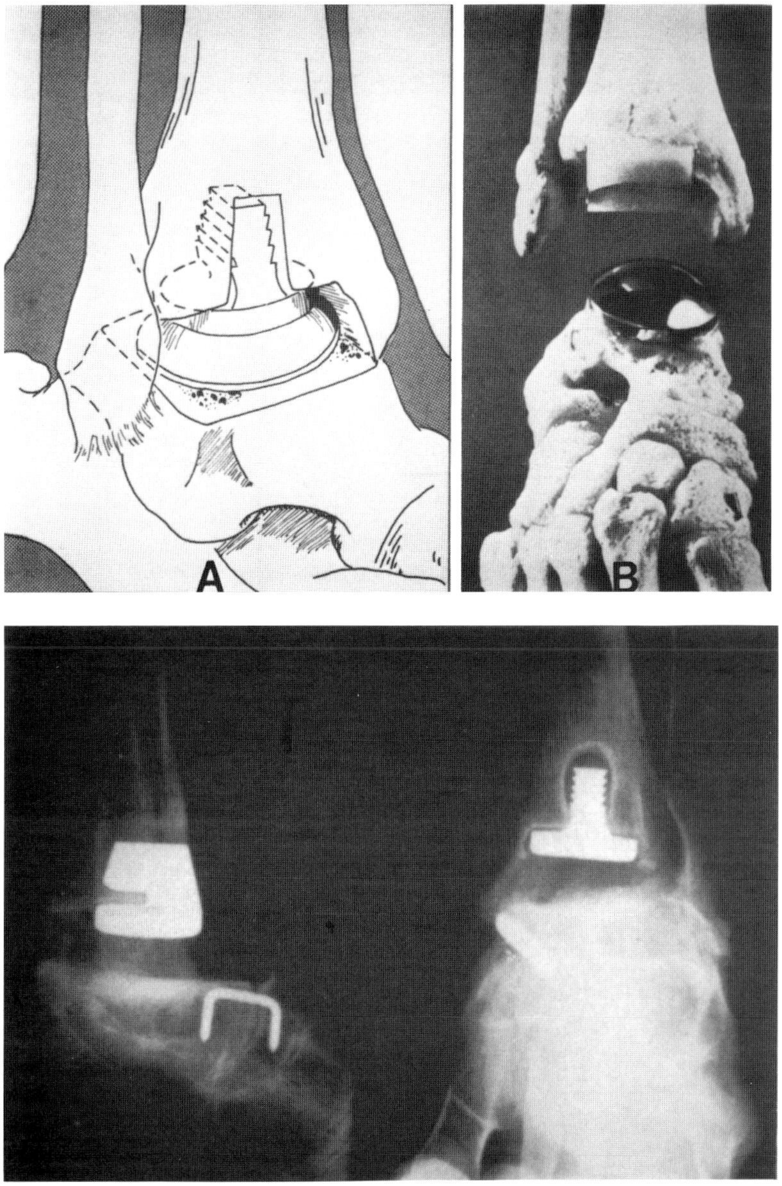

FIG. 8-65. Unconstrained ankle arthroplasties. **A:** Richard Smith ankle with steel tibial and polyethylene talar implant. **B:** Bath and Wessex implants with steel talar dome and polyethylene tibial components. **C:** The AP and lateral radiographs of a Smith prosthesis. (From Kirkup J. Rheumatoid arthritis and ankle surgery. *R Natl Hosp Rheum Dis* 1990;49:837–844.)

A,B

C,D

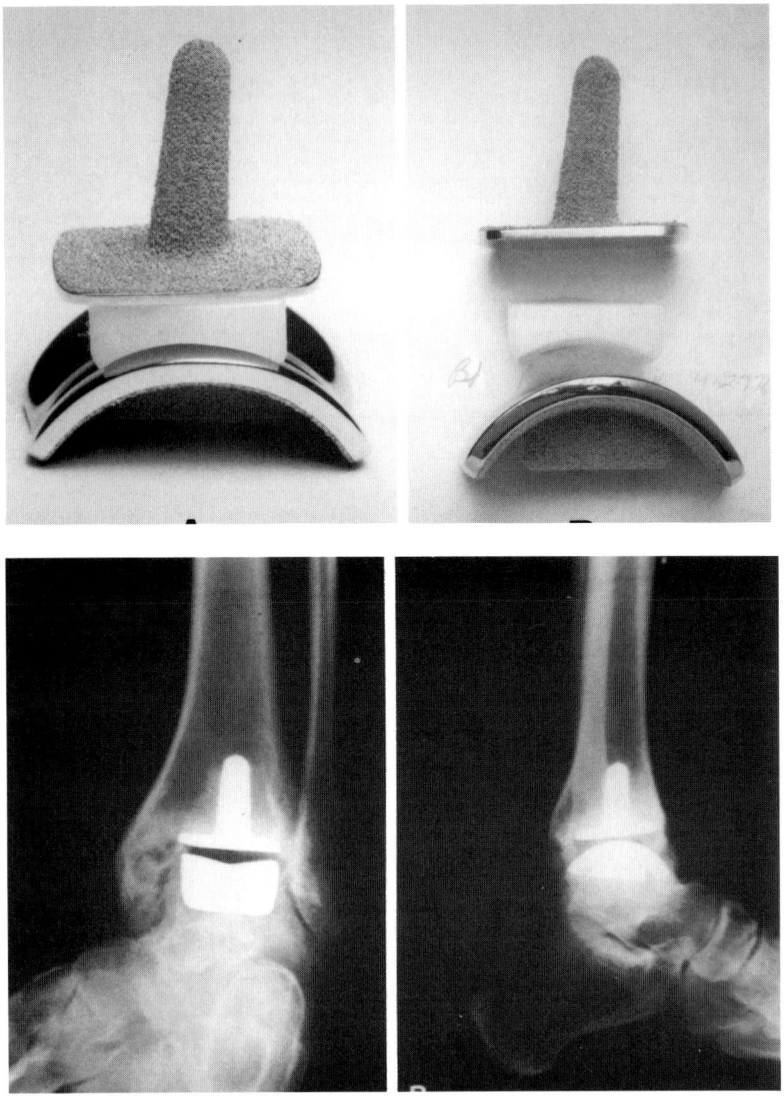

FIG. 8-66. New Jersey porous-coated unconstrained ankle system. (DePuy, Warsaw, IN.) Sintered-bead porous-coated tibial and talar components of cobalt-chromium-molybdenum alloy with an ultrahigh molecular weight polyethylene bearing seen from the side **(A)** and separated **(B)**. The AP **(C)** and lateral **(D)** radiographs demonstrate solid fixation. (From Buechel FF, Pappas MJ, Iorio LJ. New Jersey low contact stress total ankle replacement: biomechanical rationale and review of 23 cementless cases. *Foot Ankle* 1988;8:279–290.)

A

B

C,D

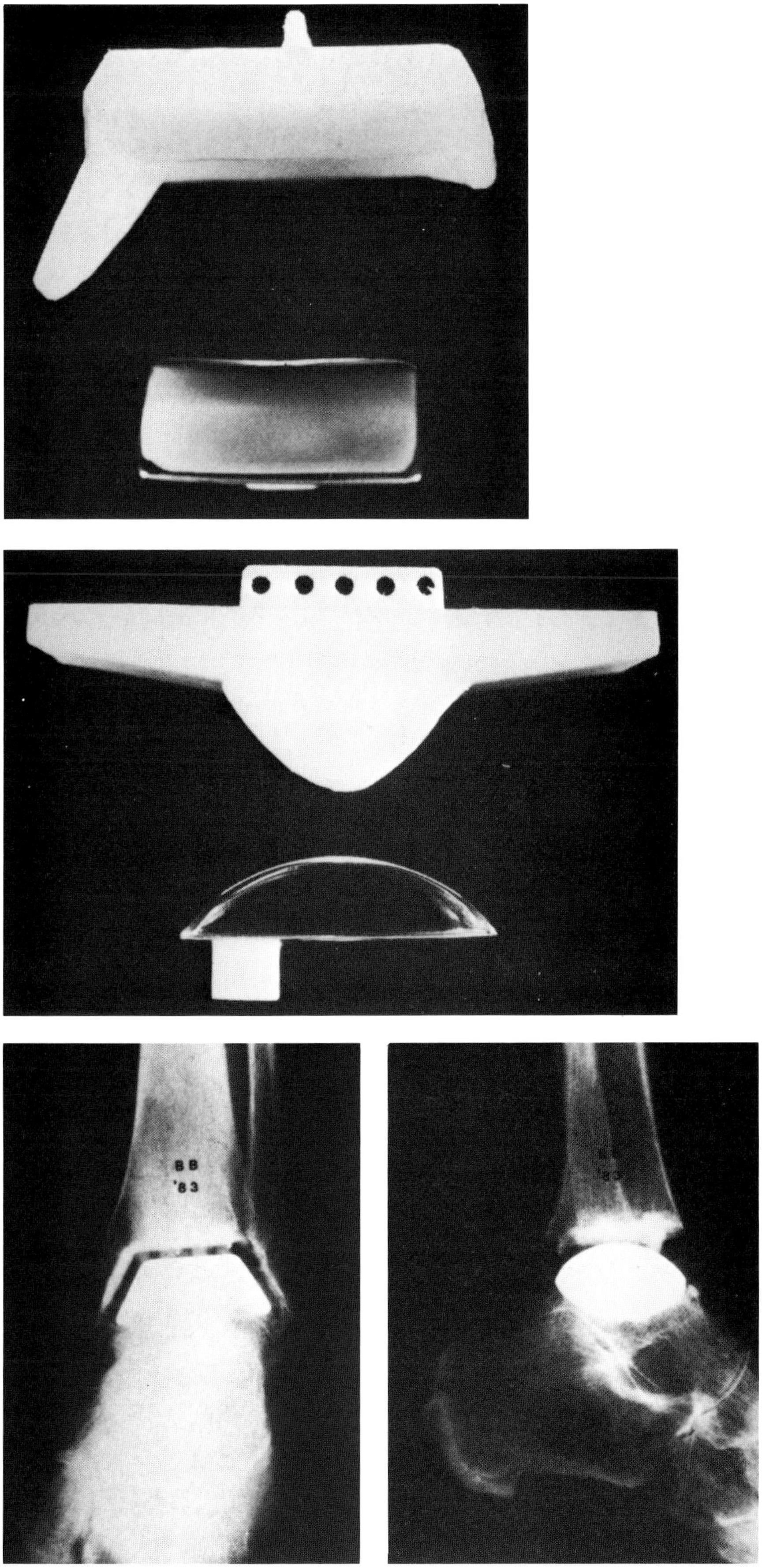

FIG. 8-67. The Imperial College London Hospital Mark VII prosthesis seen from the front **(A)** and side **(B)**. The polyethylene tibial component has a flange for fibular articulation. The AP **(C)** and lateral **(D)** radiographs 4 years later with no loosening or infection. (From Bolton-Maggs BG, Sudlow RA, Freeman MAR. Total ankle arthroplasty: a long-term review of the London Hospital experience. *J Bone Joint Surg* [*Br*] 1985; 67B:785–790.)

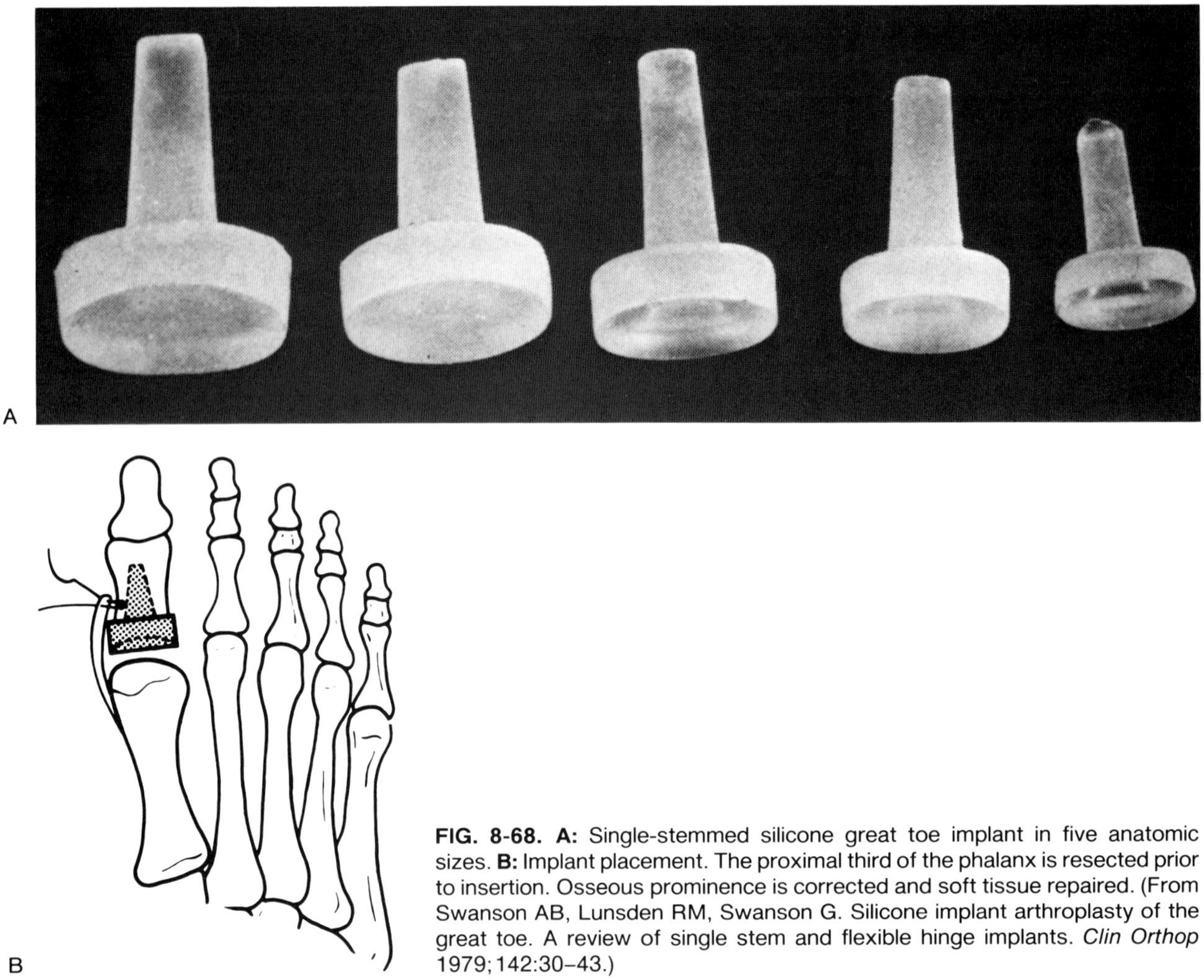

FIG. 8-68. **A:** Single-stemmed silicone great toe implant in five anatomic sizes. **B:** Implant placement. The proximal third of the phalanx is resected prior to insertion. Osseous prominence is corrected and soft tissue repaired. (From Swanson AB, Lunsden RM, Swanson G. Silicone implant arthroplasty of the great toe. A review of single stem and flexible hinge implants. *Clin Orthop* 1979;142:30–43.)

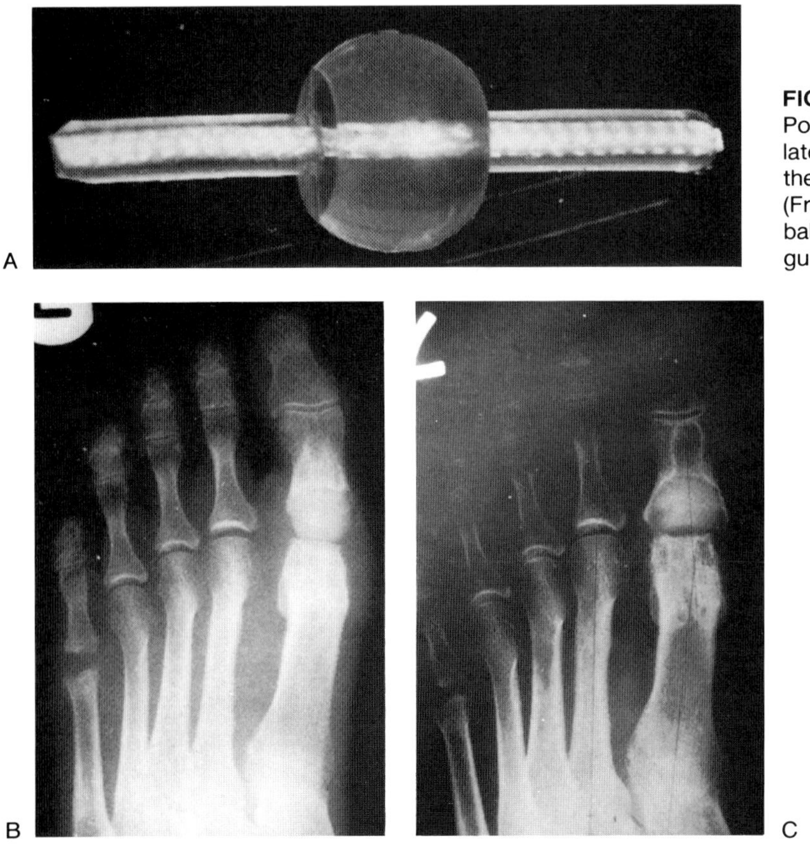

FIG. 8-69. A: Silicone ball spacer with double stems. Postoperative **(B)** radiograph and follow-up 4 years later **(C)** demonstrating settling of the prosthesis into the metatarsal and proximal migration of sesamoids. (From Broughton NS, Doran A, Meggitt BF. Silastic ball spacer arthroplasty in management of hallux valgus and hallus rigidus. *Foot Ankle* 1990;10:61–64.)

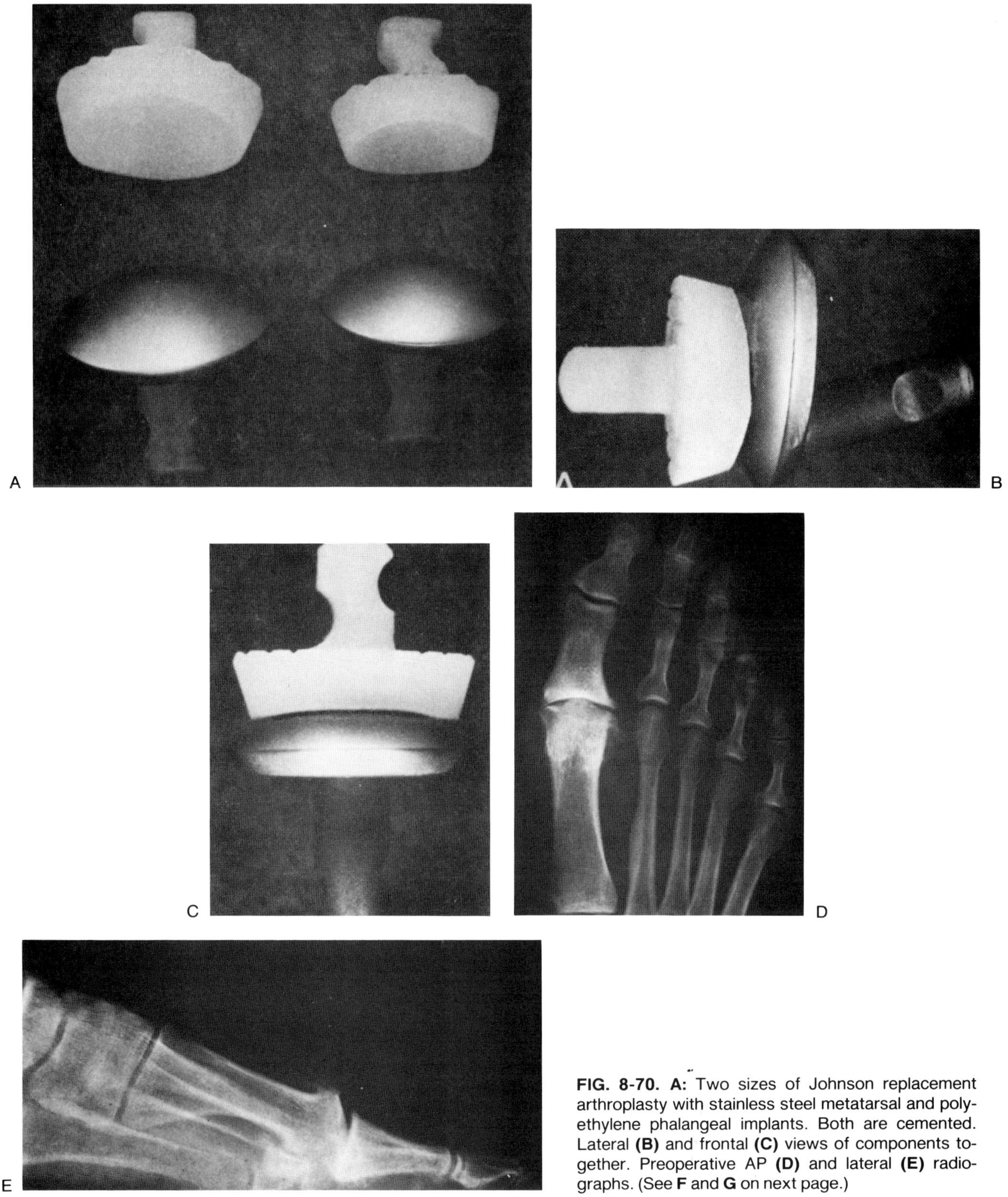

FIG. 8-70. A: Two sizes of Johnson replacement arthroplasty with stainless steel metatarsal and polyethylene phalangeal implants. Both are cemented. Lateral **(B)** and frontal **(C)** views of components together. Preoperative AP **(D)** and lateral **(E)** radiographs. (See **F** and **G** on next page.)

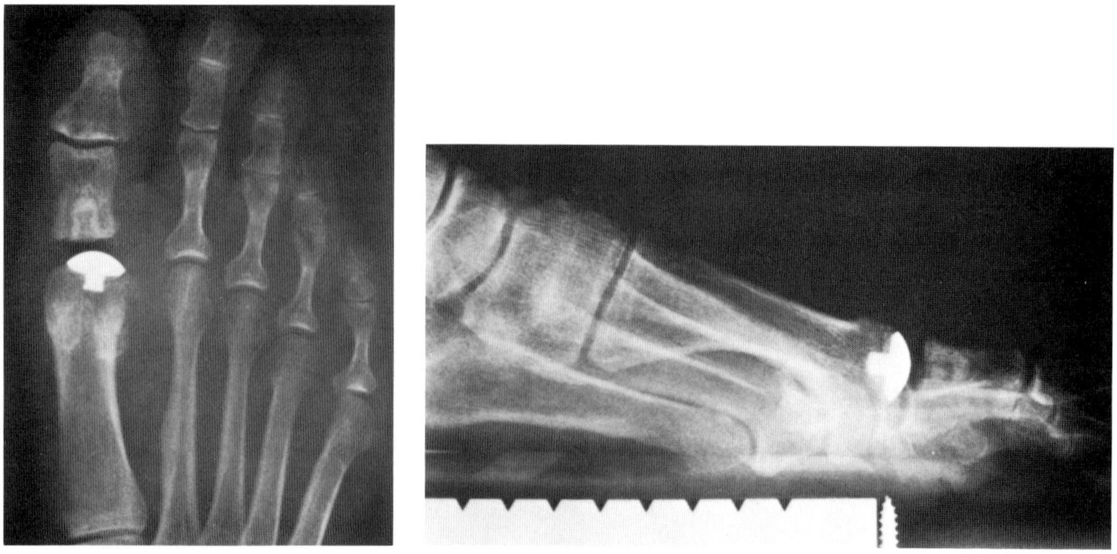

F G

FIG. 8-70. (*Continued.*) Postoperative AP **(F)** and lateral **(G)** radiographs with components in place. (From Johnson KA, Buck PG. Total replacement arthroplasty of the first metatarsophalangeal joint. *Foot Ankle* 1981;1:307–314.)

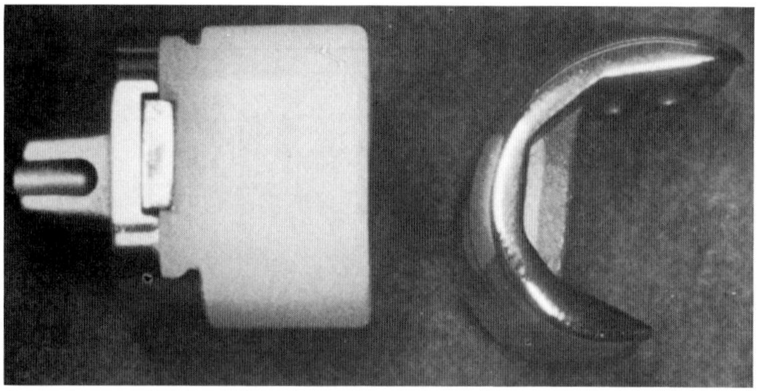

A

FIG. 8-71. A: Semiconstrained system with titanium metatarsal head and phalangeal tray with polyethylene insert. Radiographs in the AP **(B)** and lateral **(C)** projections with components in place. (From Merkle PF, Sculco TP. Prosthetic replacement of the first metatarsophalangeal joint. *Foot Ankle* 1989;9:267–271.)

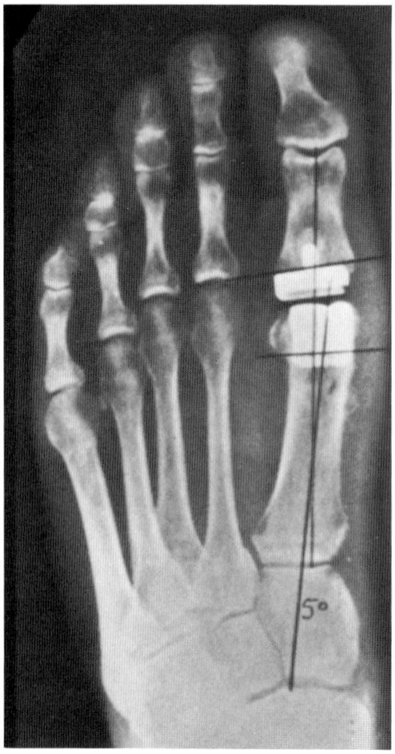

B

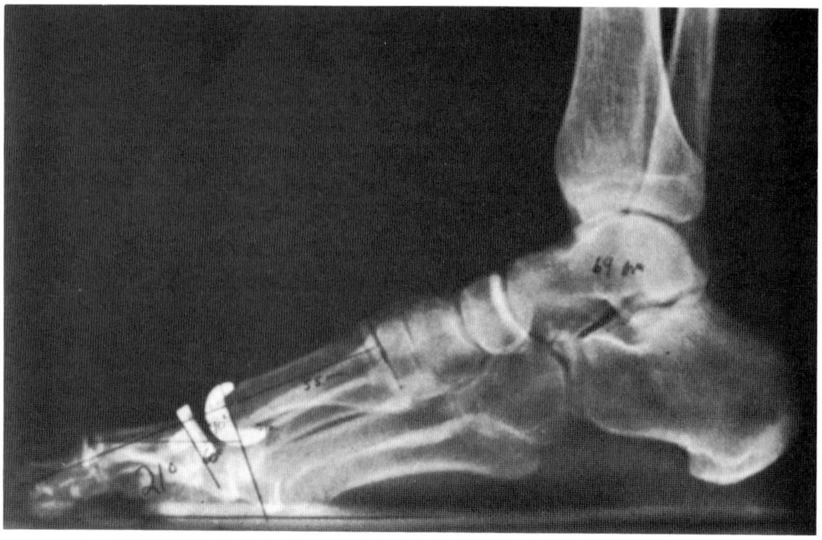

C

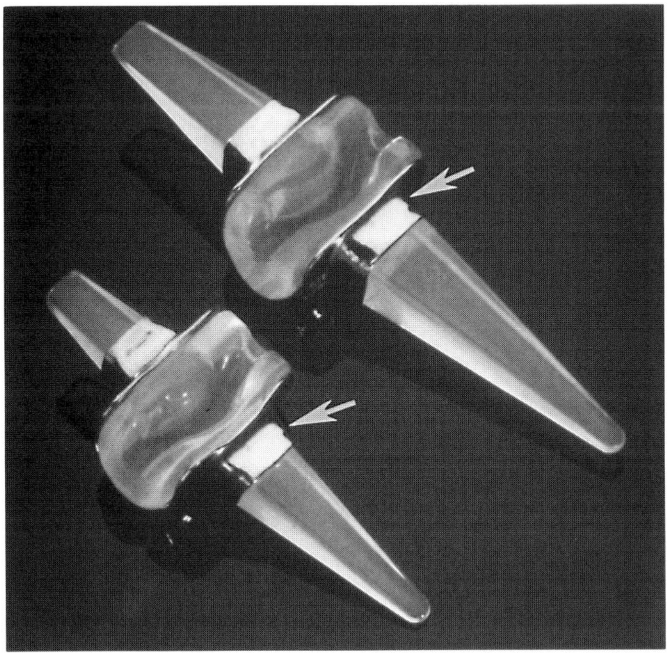

A

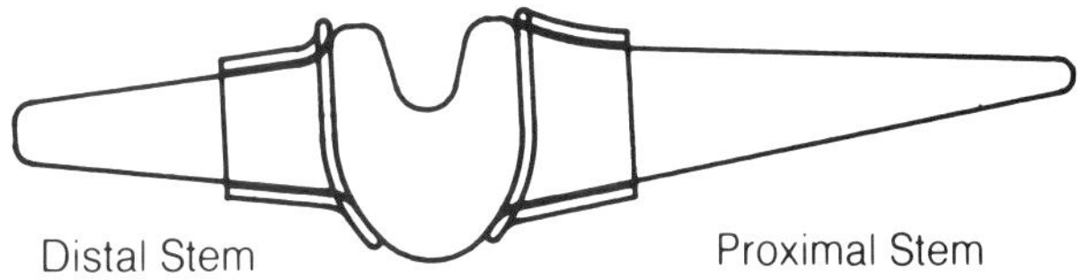

B

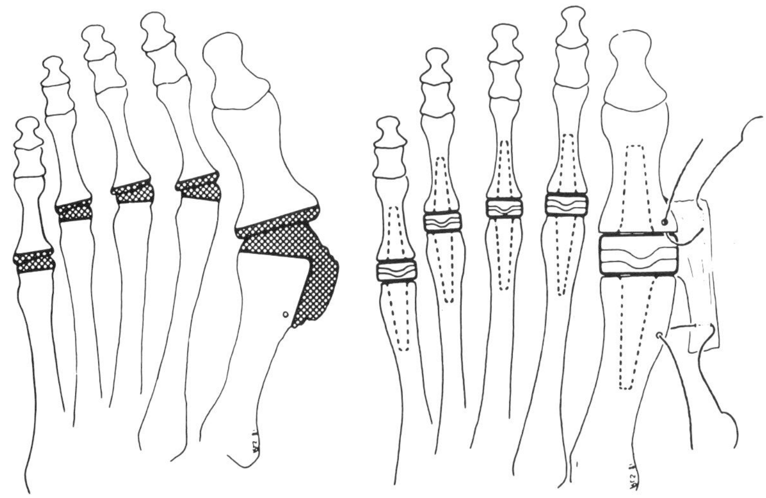

C D

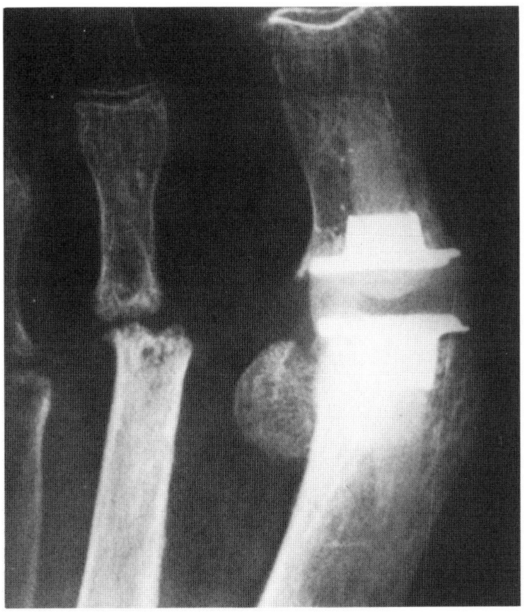

E

FIG. 8-72. Swanson Silastic™ H.P. 100 flexible hinge toe implant with flexible hinge grommet. **A:** Implants. The titanium grommet (*arrows*) is designed to provide a shield between the bone and silicone portion of the implant. **B:** Lateral illustration of the distal and proximal stem and grommets. Bone resections **(C)** for lesser toes and great toe with hallux valgus prior to implants **(D)**. **E:** An AP radiograph of the foot demonstrating a great toe implant in place. (Courtesy of Wright Medical Technology, Arlington, TN, and Dr. A. B. Swanson.[206,207])

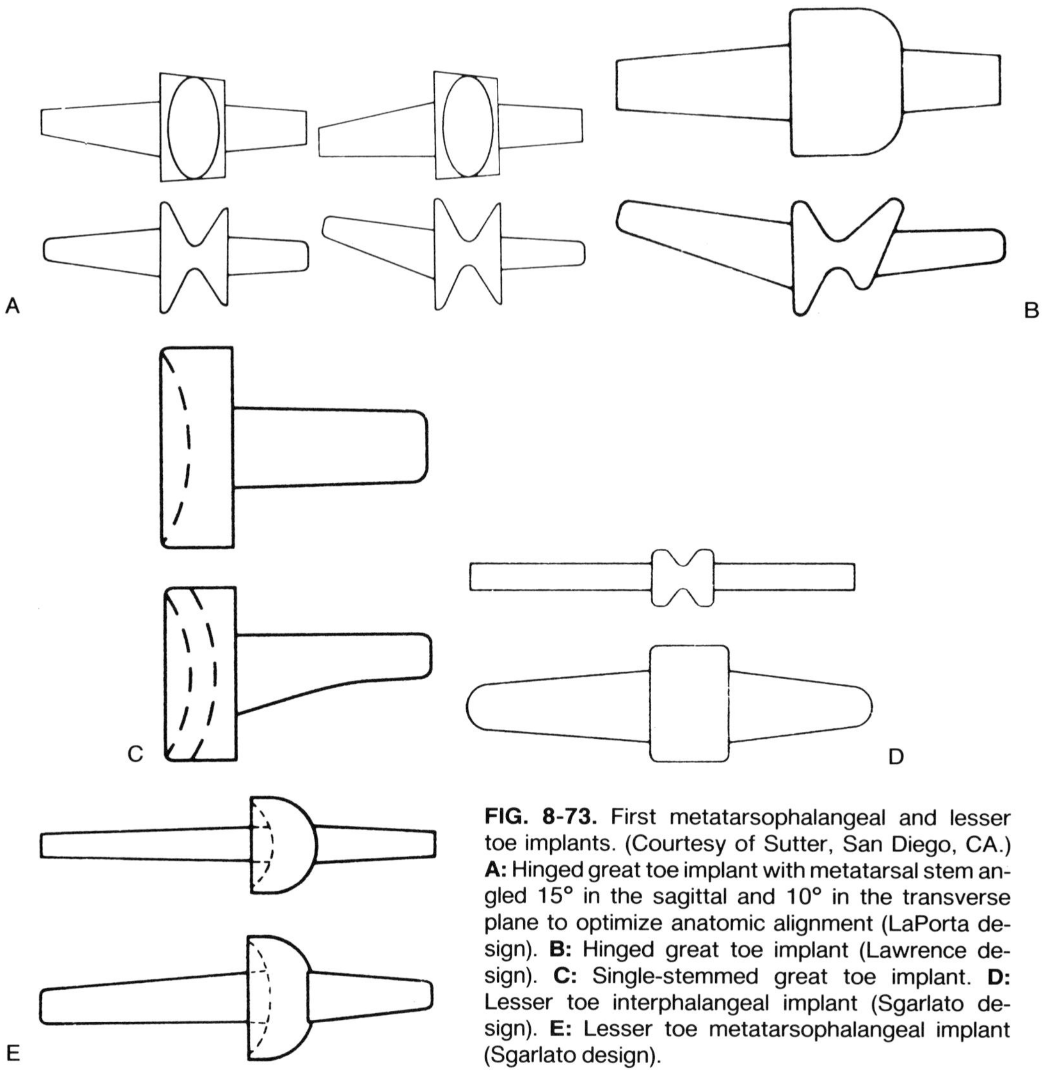

FIG. 8-73. First metatarsophalangeal and lesser toe implants. (Courtesy of Sutter, San Diego, CA.) **A:** Hinged great toe implant with metatarsal stem angled 15° in the sagittal and 10° in the transverse plane to optimize anatomic alignment (LaPorta design). **B:** Hinged great toe implant (Lawrence design). **C:** Single-stemmed great toe implant. **D:** Lesser toe interphalangeal implant (Sgarlato design). **E:** Lesser toe metatarsophalangeal implant (Sgarlato design).

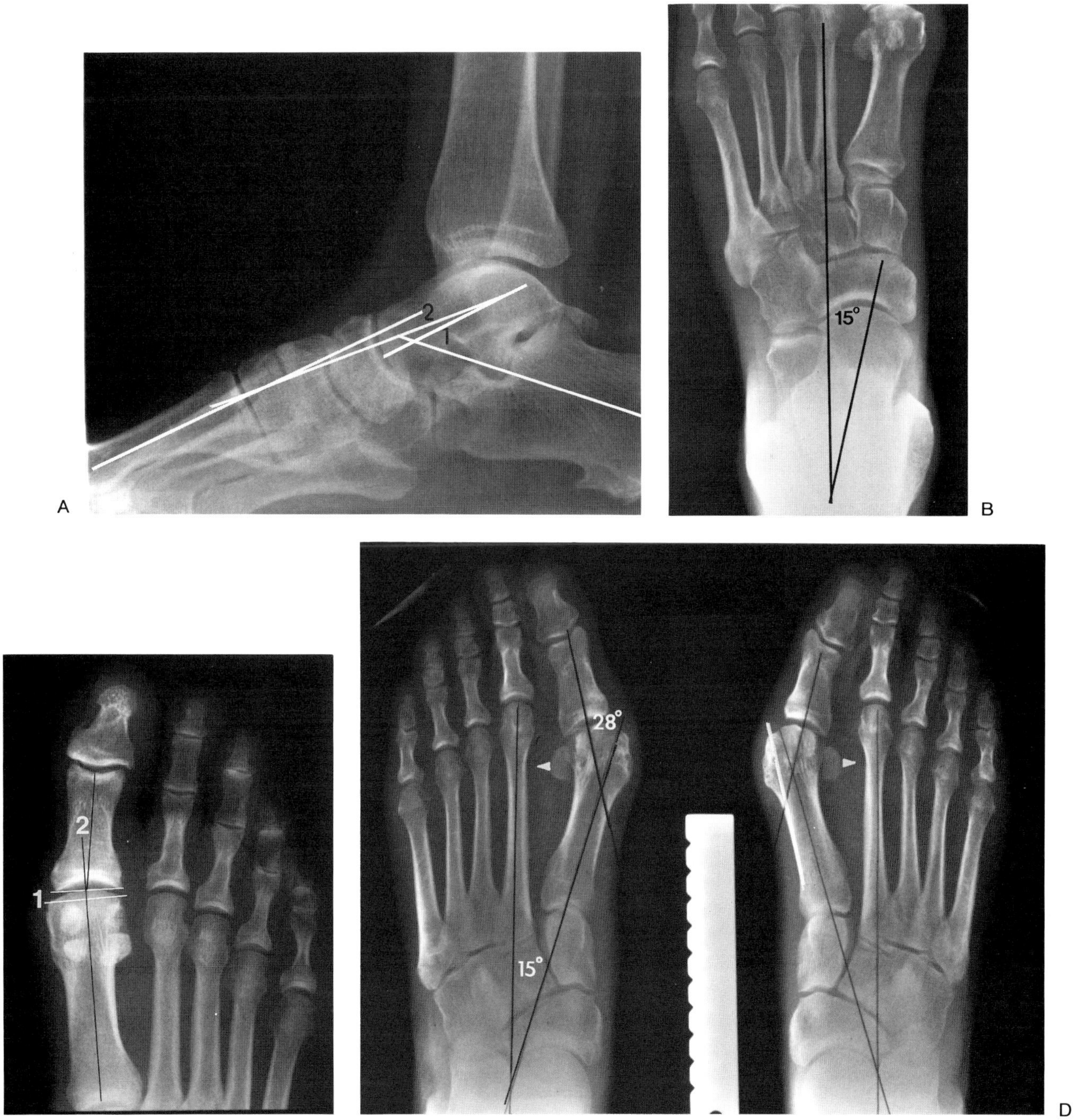

FIG. 8-74. **A:** Standing lateral view of the foot and ankle demonstrating the talocalcaneal (*1*; normal, 25° to 30°) and talar first metatarsal angle (*2*; normal, 4° to +4°). **B:** An AP view of the foot demonstrating the talar second metatarsal angle (normal, 6° to 42°). **C:** Normal AP view of the forefoot. *1,* The first metatarsal phalangeal joint is almost perfectly congruent (*lines* along articular margins); *2,* normal metatarsal phalangeal angle should be < 15°. **D:** Standing AP views of both feet with bilateral metatarsus varus and hallux valgus deformities. Both great toes are pronated. The intermetatarsal angles are both 15° (normal, < 9°). This angle is formed by lines bisecting the first and second metatarsals. The metatarsal phalangeal angle formed by lines through the first metatarsal and proximal phalanx should be < 15°. In this patient, the angle is 28°. There is also apparent lateral dislocation of the sesamoids caused by medial rotation of the first metatarsal (*arrows*). A *white line* drawn along the first metatarsal shaft on the right defines the size of the medial eminence. (See **E** on next page.)

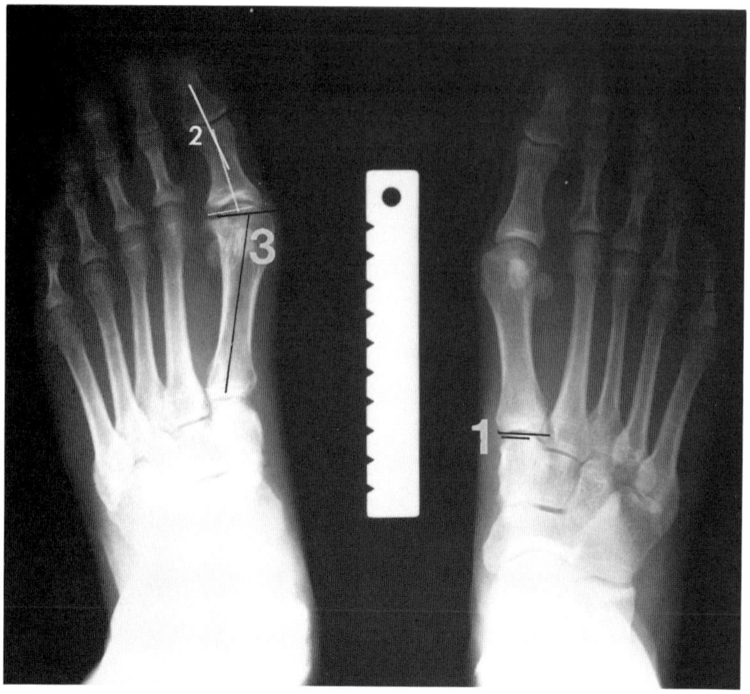

E

FIG. 8-74. (*Continued.*) **E:** Bilateral standing AP views with mild deformity on the right and more marked changes on the left with arthrosis. *1*, The cuneiform-metatarsal angle is flat and congruent; *2*, the normal interphalangeal angle is < 10°. The angle formed by a line bisecting the articular surface in this patient is increased. *3*, Distal metatarsal articular surface angle (normal, < 10° lateral deviation) is formed by a line bisecting the shaft and metatarsal head.

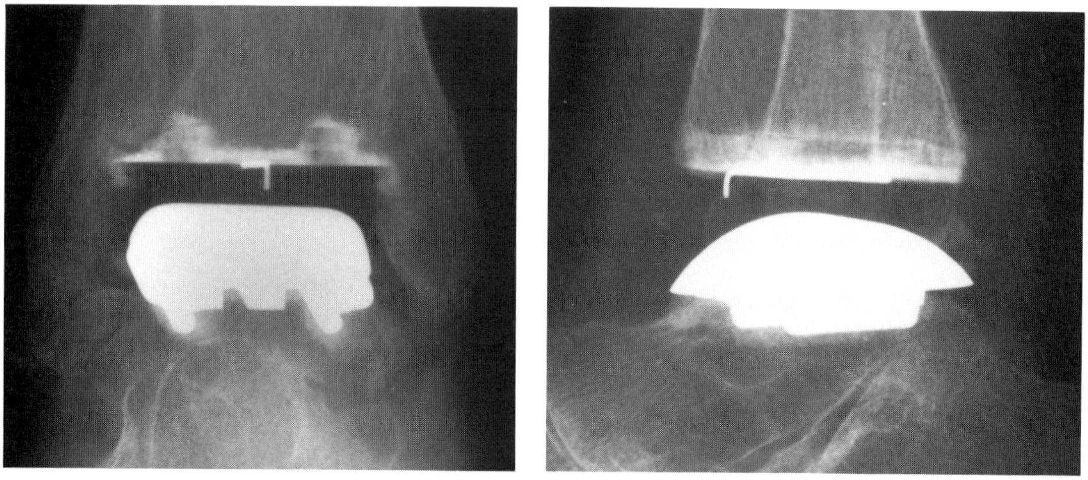

A B

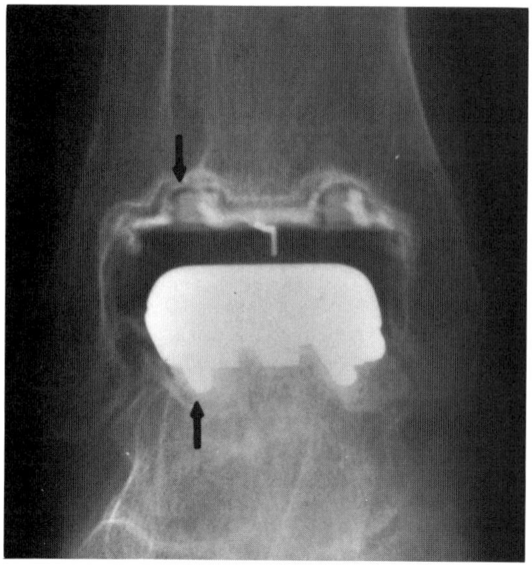

C

FIG. 8-75. Mayo ankle system. The AP **(A)** and lateral **(B)** radiographs after surgery are normal. **C:** The AP view 3 years after surgery demonstrates lucency at the bone-cement interface (*arrows*) more obvious laterally due to infection. (From Johnson KA. Total ankle arthroplasty. In: Berquist TH, ed. *Imaging of orthopedic trauma and surgery.* Philadelphia: WB Saunders, 1986;491–494.)

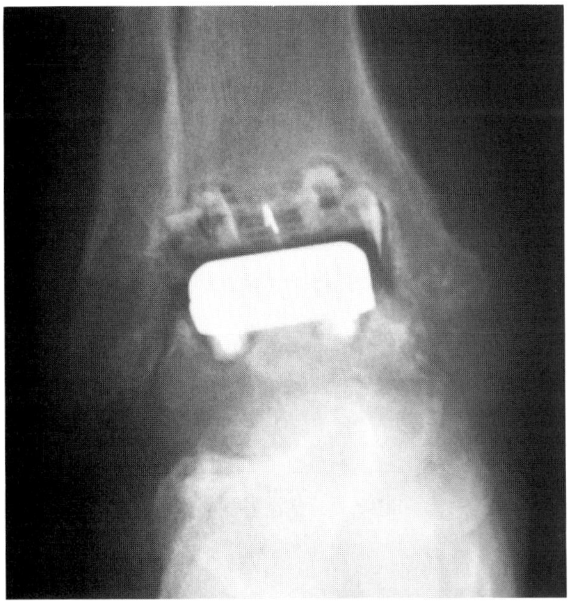

FIG. 8-76. An AP view following ankle arthroplasty with loosening of both components and malleolar impingement on the talus.

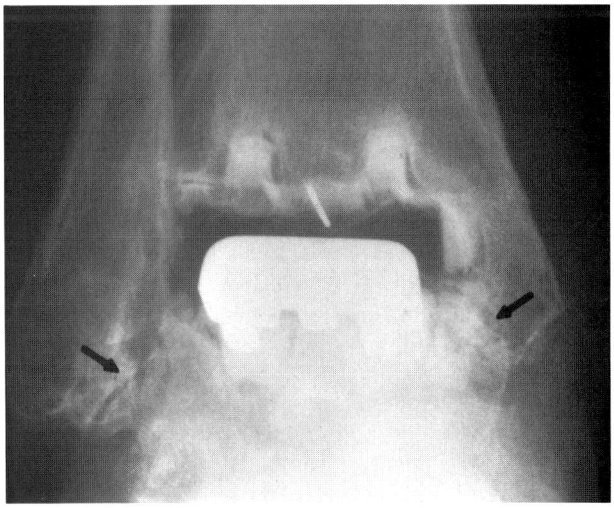

FIG. 8-77. An AP view demonstrating medial and lateral talar impingement (*arrows*). (From Johnson KA. Total ankle arthroplasty. In: Berquist TH, ed. *Imaging of orthopedic trauma and surgery*. Philadelphia: WB Saunders, 1986;491–494.)

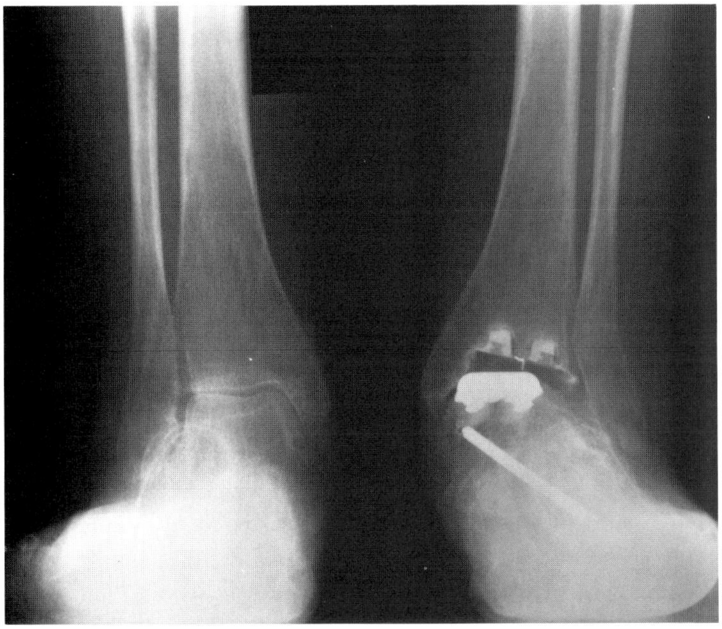

FIG. 8-78. Standing AP views show joint space narrowing in the right ankle and subluxation of the arthroplasty on the left. Threaded Steinmann pin for subtalar arthrodesis.

TABLE 8-11. *Metatarsophalangeal arthroplasty: complications*[176,180,193,206,207]

Painful plantar keratosis
Osteophytes around implants
Implant fracture (double-stem silicone)
Restricted motion
Deep infection
Recurrent deformity
Stress fractures

Oblique views and standing AP and lateral foot radiographs are also used to assess metatarsophalangeal arthroplasty. Lucency at the prosthesis-bone interface is usually obvious on serial radiographs (Figs. 8-79 and 8-80). Joint aspiration is useful in patients who have undergone arthroplasty who have suspected infections. Routine radiographs may not be able to differentiate loosening from infection. Other imaging studies, specifically combined technetium-99m and indium-111-labeled leukocyte scans or technetium-99m and gallium-67 studies may be useful.

The correlation with clinical results and radiography is poor (Fig. 8-79). Granberry et al.[180] categorized radiographic features based on the deformity of the implants (Fig. 8-81 and Table 8-11). Implants in the foot and ankle have, in general, not achieved the success reported in other joints (Figs. 8-80 and 8-81).[180,186,189]

ARTHRODESIS AND MISCELLANEOUS PROCEDURES

Arthrodesis

Numerous techniques are available for arthrodesis of the ankle, hindfoot, midfoot, and forefoot.[217,219,221,222,229,230,233,235] The techniques are similar in that soft tissue dissections should be minimized; joint surfaces, optimally prepared; and some type of internal or external fixation, used.[222] Some type of bone graft is used with some arthrodesis techniques.[217,228,233]

Ankle Arthrodesis

Ankle arthrodesis is performed to restore activity and relieve pain. The procedure is most commonly performed in adults for the conditions listed as follows:[219,222,223,227,232,234,235]

1. Arthrosis
   - Osteoarthritis
   - Rheumatoid arthritis
   - Posttraumatic arthritis
   - Infection
2. Selected cases of severe acute trauma
3. Failed ankle arthroplasty
4. Tumors

In children, the indications include painful posttraumatic or septic arthritis, paralytic disorders, and congenital deformities.[230]

The preoperative clinical evaluation is performed using an ankle scoring system, which assists in patient selection and the postoperative evaluation.[226,231] The scoring system proposed by Mazur et al.[231] is based on pain level, function, and alignment of the foot and ankle.

The preoperative imaging should include routine standing AP and lateral ankle radiographs (Fig. 8-74). Mortise and oblique views should also be evaluated.[212,215]

The talocalcaneal and talar-first metatarsal angles are evaluated on the lateral view. Osteoarthritis can also be graded to assist in evaluating progression on postoperative radiographs. Grade 1 arthrosis consists of joint space narrowing without secondary changes. Grade 2 osteoarthritis includes moderate sclerosis and osteophyte formation along with joint space narrowing. Grade 3 changes have severe sclerosis and osteophyte formation.[221]

Preoperative CT (Fig. 8-82) may be useful to evaluate bone loss fully in patients with erosive arthritis or severe trauma.[229] In addition, MRI is useful in patients with suspected avascular necrosis of the talus.[214] Diagnostic injections are also useful to confirm joint involvement prior to surgery.[213]

At least 30 techniques have been described for performing ankle arthrodesis.[216,226,229,232,235] Internal and external fixation techniques have been advocated, depending on the clinical setting.[226,229,233,235]

External Fixation

External fixation techniques are preferred by some authors for ankle arthrodesis. This technique may be particularly useful following failed arthrodesis or failed total ankle arthroplasty.[226,229] Also, patients with osteopenia or those who require large bone grafts should be treated with external fixation.[217,226] External fixation may be accomplished with several different systems. Figures 8-83 to 8-86 demonstrate commonly used external fixators for ankle arthrodesis.[217,225]

Internal Fixation Techniques

Internal fixation techniques may use several types of internal fixation plates and cancellous screws with or without bone graft.[215,224,226,230] Internal fixation can be used in most patients with adequate bone stock to hold the screws.[217]

Compression arthrodesis is a technique originally used by Wagner and Pock[229,234] and modified by Gschivend

(text continues on page 641)

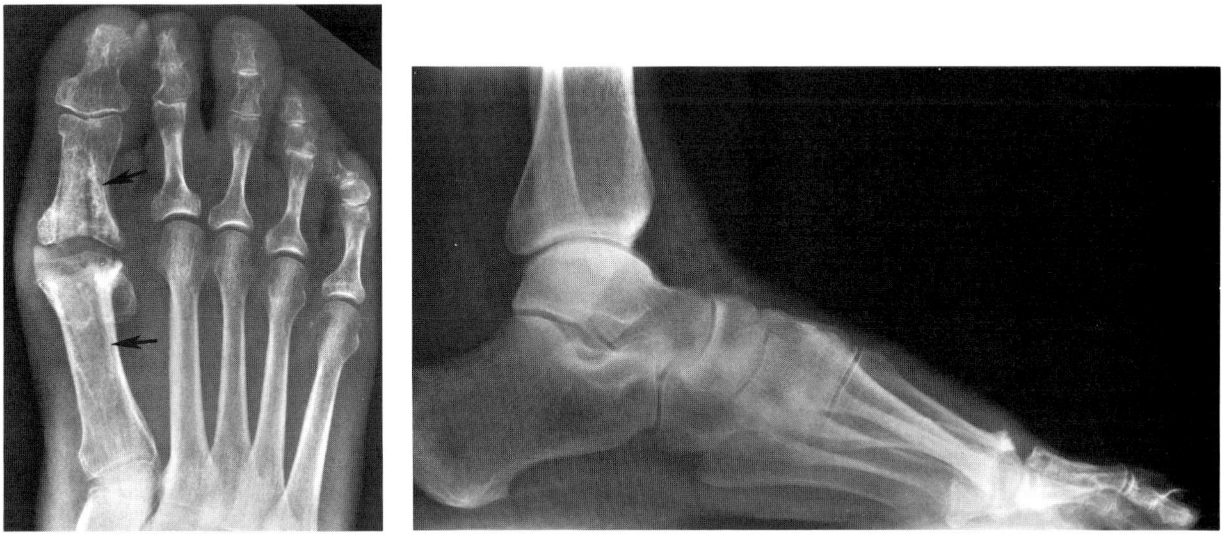

A B

FIG. 8-79. The AP **(A)** and lateral **(B)** standing radiographs of a double-stemmed (*arrows*) silicone arthroplasty. There is lucency around the component stems (*arrows*). Clinically, the patient was doing well.

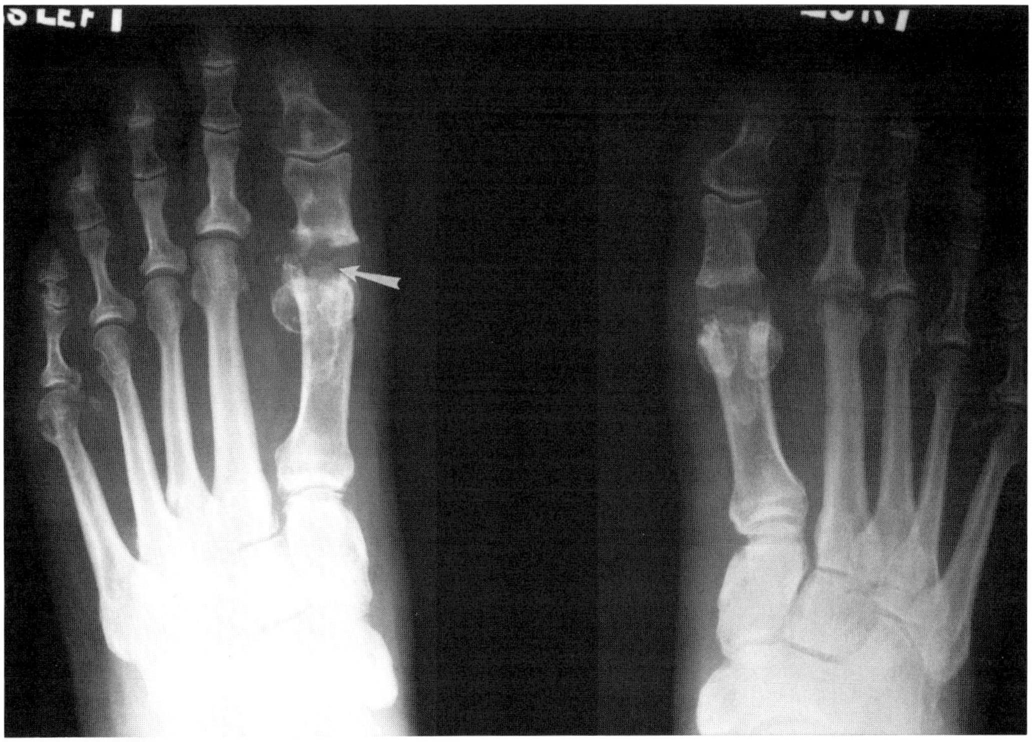

FIG. 8-80. Standing AP views of the feet in a patient with bilateral first metatarsophalangeal implants with double stems. The implant on the right is normal. There is deformity and a fracture at the stem-hinge junction on the left (*arrow*). There are erosive changes of rheumatoid arthritis bilaterally.

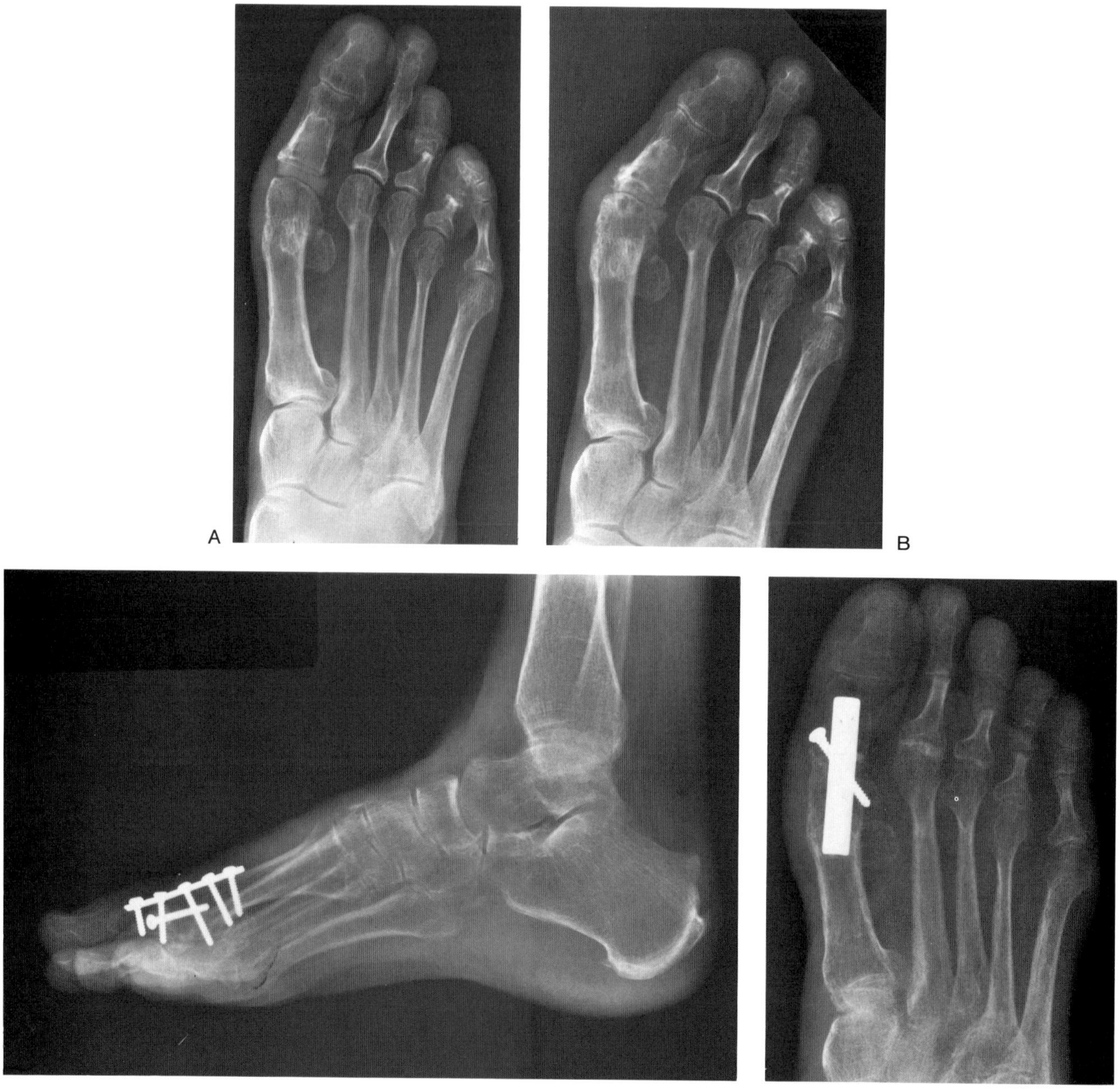

FIG. 8-81. Progressive fracture and failure of a single-stemmed silicone implant over a period of 5 years. **A:** Postoperative AP. **B:** Five years later, with implant fracture and recurrent deformity. Lateral **(C)** and AP **(D)** views after removal of the implant and arthrodesis.

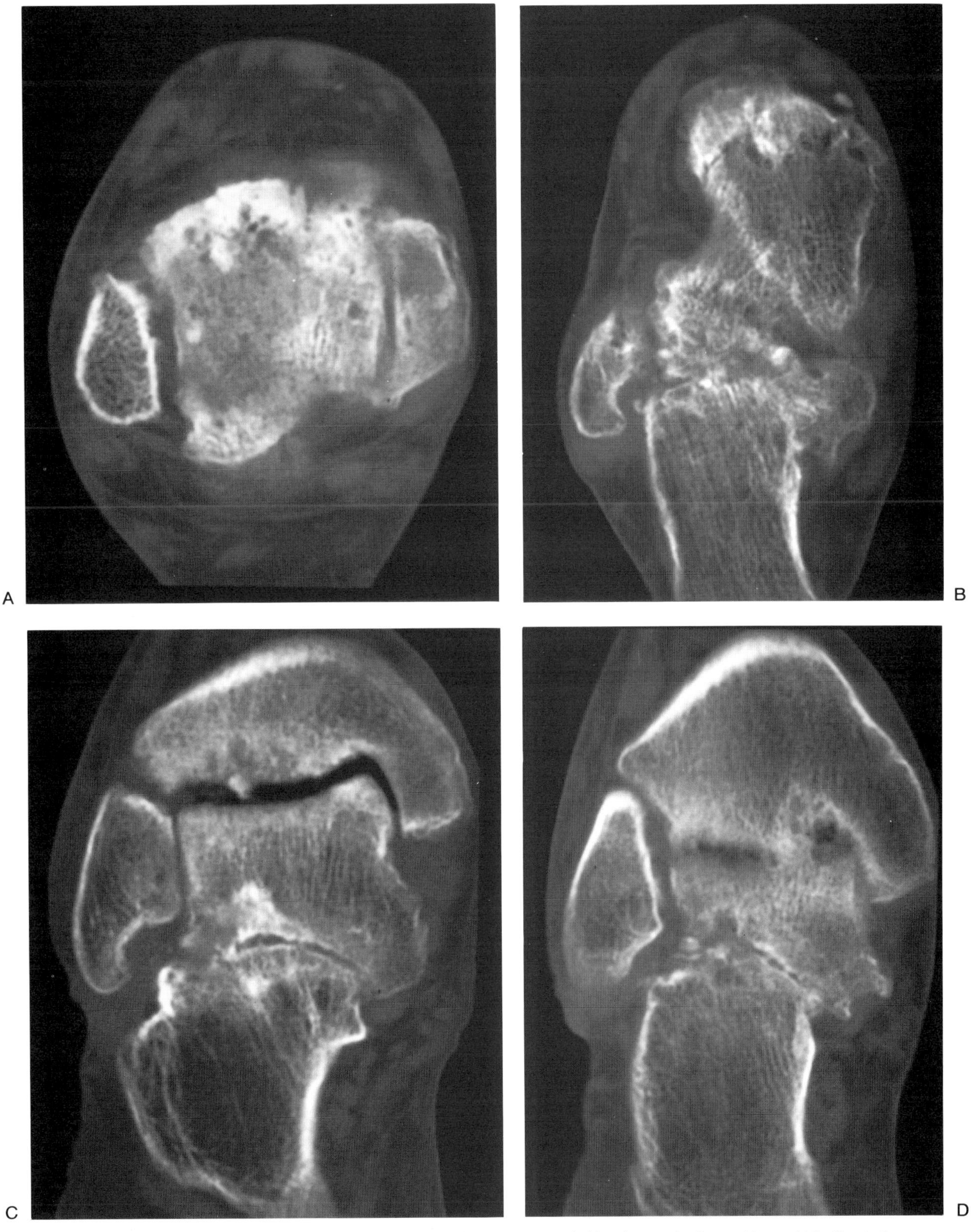

FIG. 8-82. Preoperative CT images demonstrating severe arthritic change in the ankle and hindfoot. **A, B:** Axial images. **C, D:** Coronal images.

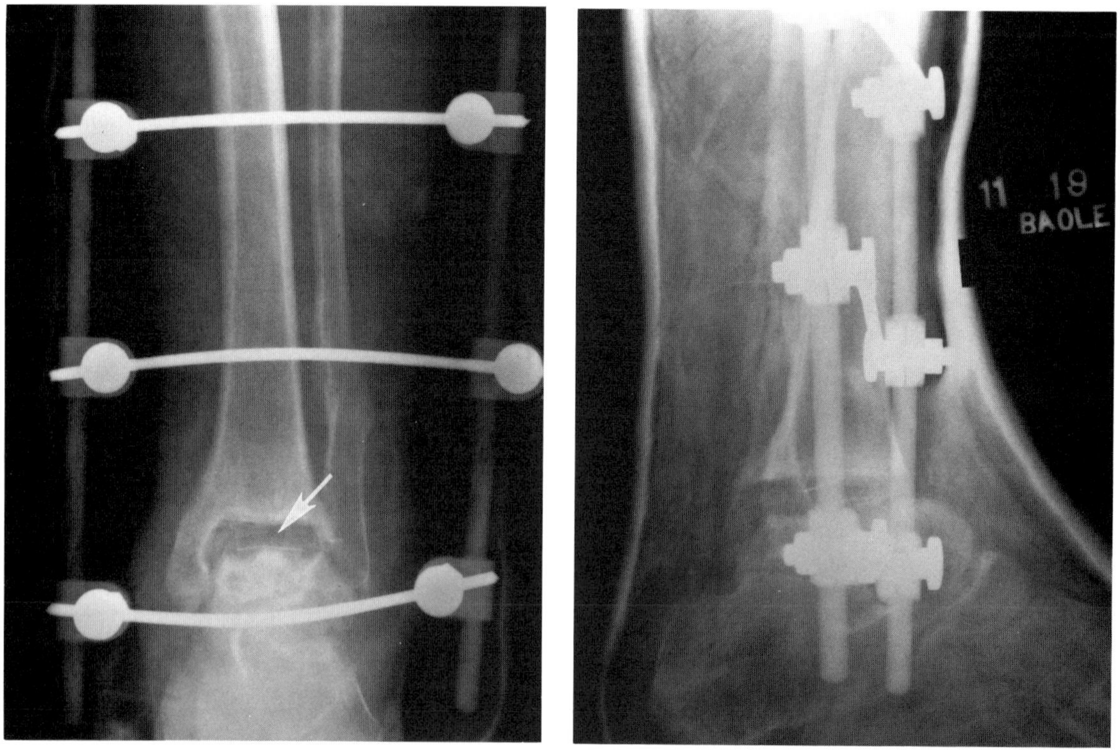

A B

FIG. 8-83. The AP **(A)** and lateral **(B)** radiographs of an ankle arthrodesis with iliac bone graft (*arrow*) and external fixation with a Roger-Anderson apparatus for failed total ankle replacement with large bony deficit.

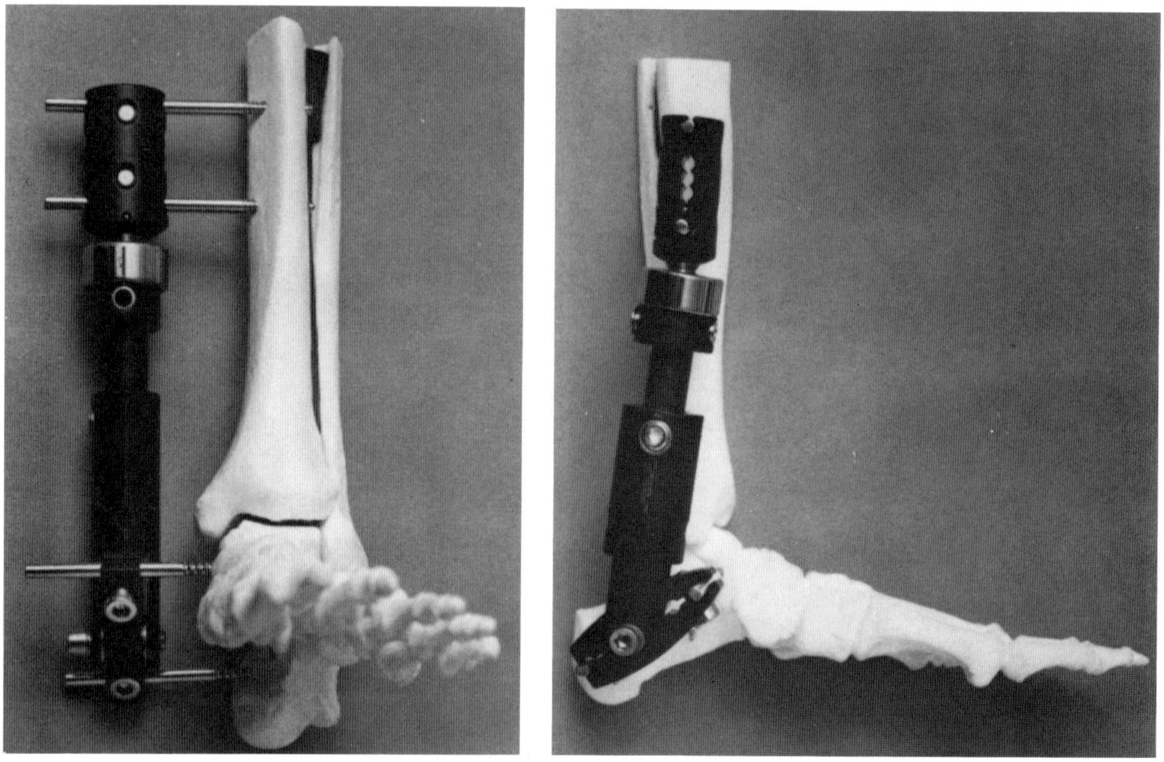

A B

FIG. 8-84. Frontal **(A)** and lateral **(B)** photos of the Orthofix™ uniaxial external fixator with the foot maintained in neutral position. (Courtesy of EBI Medical Products, Parsippany, NJ). Extending fixation across subtalar level occasionally, but not routinely, desirable.

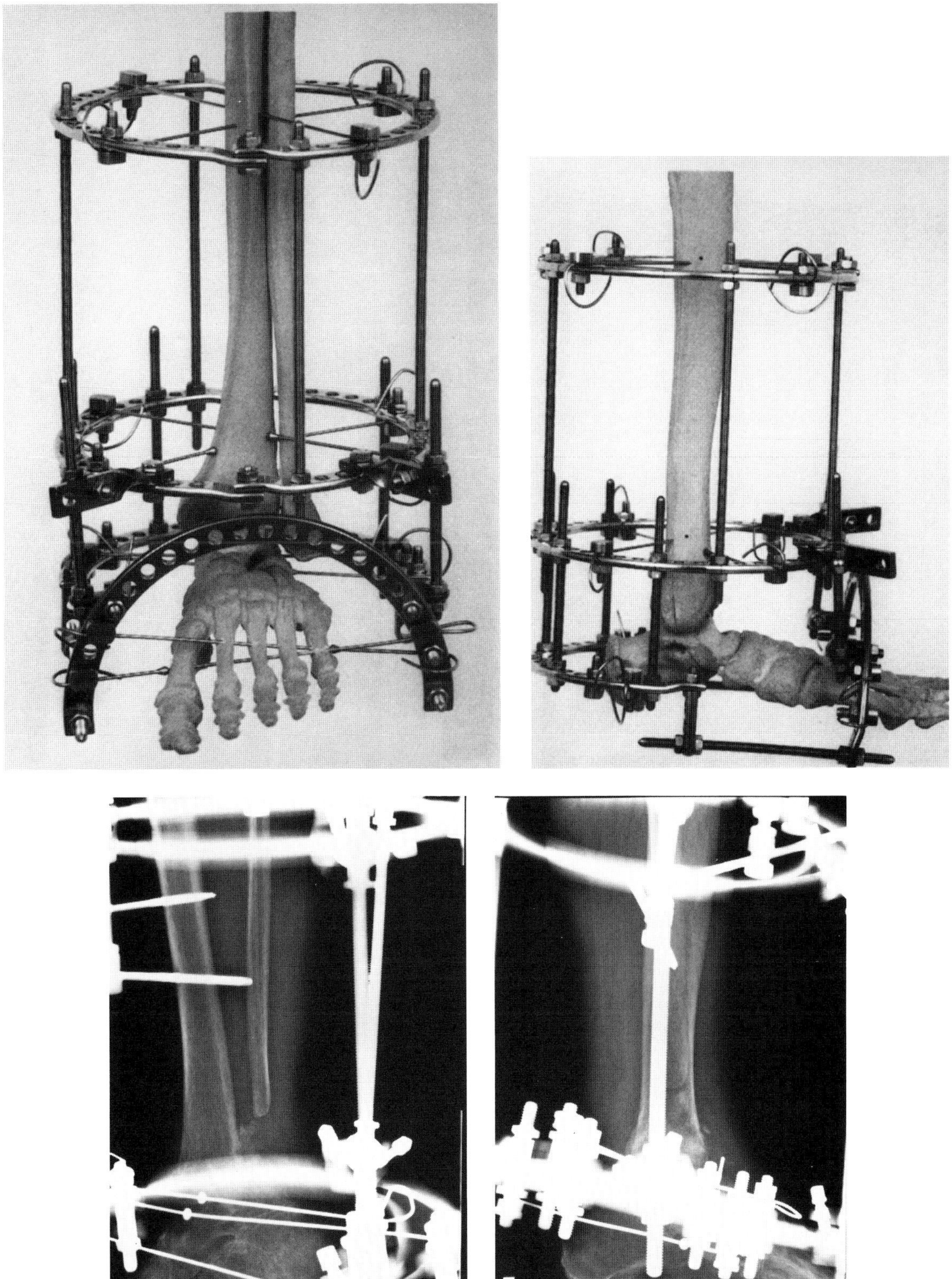

A B C D

FIG. 8-85. A plastic bone model with the Ilizarov external fixator seen from the front **(A)** and side **(B)**. There are two full rings applied to the tibia and two half-rings to the foot. Both threaded pins and wires are used. The AP **(C)** and lateral **(D)** radiographs with Ilizarov external fixator and distal fibula for bone graft. (From Johnson JE, Clanton TO, Baxter DE, et al. Ilizarov ankle arthrodesis. *Clin Orthop* 1992;280: 160–169.)

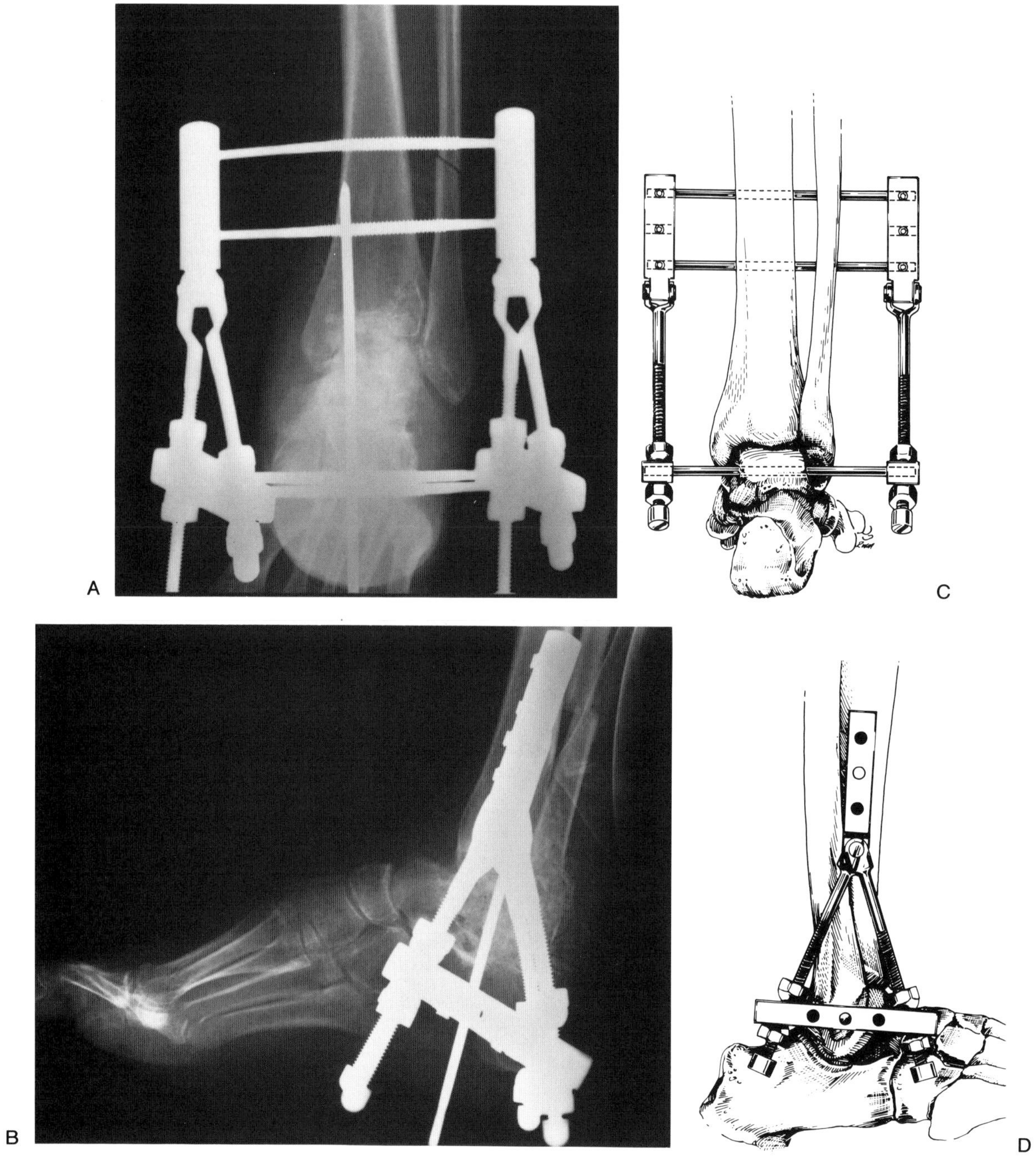

FIG. 8-86. Tibiotalocalcaneal arthrodesis with Calandruccio triangular compression frame. The AP **(A)** and lateral **(B)** radiographs of combined Steinmann pin and Calandruccio compression device. Note pins in the calcaneus. The Calandruccio triangular compression device seen from behind **(C)** and the side **(D)** with more conventional pin placement in talus and tibia for ankle arthrodesis. (C, D : Courtesy Smith and Nephew Richards, Memphis, TN.)

and Steiger.[222,229] This technique uses a lateral approach and fibular osteotomy. The fibula can be used for the bone graft. The outer half of the fibula is used as an onlay graft with screw fixation. Oblique screws are placed across the prepared articular surfaces of the tibia and talus. The foot is maintained in neutral to slight plantar flexed position (Fig. 8-87).[219,229]

Plate techniques have also been described, both as primary and revision procedures (Fig. 8-88). Gruen and Mears[222] described the use of a 95° blade plate with a posterior approach. This technique was advocated for salvage in patients with significant soft tissue compromise by previous injury, surgery, or infection. The Achilles tendon is separated from the calcaneus with a bone block (Fig. 8-89A) and reattached after the blade plate is positioned (Fig. 8-89B).[222] The Wolf blade-plate technique has also been used (Fig. 8-90).[235] Anterior tension-plate techniques were described by Mears et al.[232] A solid arthrodesis was obtained in 82% of 17 patients (Fig. 8-91). This technique is usually used in patients with mild deformity and no significant bone loss.[235]

Hindfoot Arthrodesis

Triple arthrodesis (talonavicular, talocalcaneal, and calcaneocuboid) was initially performed in children or polio patients with failed foot.[222,223] Today, selective arthrodesis of one or more joints is commonly performed. The indications include rheumatoid arthritis, traumatic arthritis, congenital deformities, neurologic deformities, posterior tibialis tendon dysfunction, or other conditions leading to pain and instability.[222]

The patients are evaluated clinically using a grading scale similar to that described for ankle function.[218,231] The talocalcaneal and talar-first metatarsal angles (Fig. 8-74) are measured as described earlier. The talar height (most superior aspect of the talar dome to the weight-bearing surface), calcaneal pitch angle, and tibial-calcaneal angle should all be evaluated on the standing lateral view (Fig. 8-92). The talocalcaneal angle (normal, 30° to 50° in infants and young children and 15° to 30° in those > 5 years old) and other tarsometatarsal angles (Fig. 8-92) are measured on the AP standing view.[218,229] In addition, CT may be useful for assessing bone stock and articular abnormalities. In selected cases, joint injections are performed using a local anesthetic to confirm which joints are causing the symptoms. This technique is useful when there is a question about the source(s) of symptoms.[212,213]

Although percutaneous pin fixation techniques can be used, many surgeons prefer internal fixation, with or without bone grafting.[211,221,222,229] Staples or cancellous screws are most often used (Figs. 8-93 to 8-95). Dowel grafts are round 12-to 14-mm bone plugs obtained from the iliac crest, which may be useful in selected cases. A similar round hole is drilled through the articular portion of the opposing bones in the joint to be fused. The joint with the dowel is maintained with staples, pins, or screws (Fig. 8-96).[217,218]

Mid- and Forefoot Arthrodesis

The indications for mid- and forefoot fusions are similar to those described previously. Preoperative radiographs in the standing AP, standing lateral, and oblique positions are required. Isolated lateral views of individual digits should be obtained when isolated digital deformities are being considered for repair.[212] Preoperative CT and diagnostic midfoot injections may be useful in potentially complex cases.[212,213]

Surgical techniques are designed to prepare the articular surface and apply fixation, typically, using screws, staples, or plate and screw combinations (Figs. 8-97 to 8-99).[217,229]

Complications

Complications of foot and ankle arthrodesis occasionally occur.[221,223,229] Nonunion has been reported in up to 40% of ankle arthrodesis (Fig. 8-99), although new techniques have improved these figures significantly.[232,235]

Wound, pin tract, and deep bone or soft tissue infections can occur in up to 19% of patients.[223,226] External fixators and internal fixation hardware can interfere with imaging (Fig. 8-99). Conventional tomography, CT, and MRI may be useful in a given clinical setting. Combined radionuclide imaging using technetium-99m with gallium-67 or labeled white cells can also be used in patients with suspected infections.[213,215] Aspiration of areas of suspected infection, such as pseudarthrosis sites, can be performed easily using fluoroscopic guidance.[212,213]

The position of the fused ankle, hindfoot, or forefoot can be measured using routine radiographs and by comparing pre- and postoperative angles.[226] Postoperative arthrosis of adjacent nonfused joints may occur. This can be assessed and graded using serial radiographs (Fig. 8-100).[212,221]

Other complications, including soft tissue injury and fracture through pin tracts (Fig. 8-101), may also occur.[221,223,226,229] Amputation rates as a result of treatment failure have been reported in up to 6.4% of patients with failed ankle fusions.[223]

Epiphysiodesis

Epiphysiodesis is not an uncommon treatment for leg-length discrepancy in the tibia and femur. This procedure is performed less frequently in the foot and ankle (Figs. 8-102 and 8-103). In the foot, first metatarsal

(text continues on page 656)

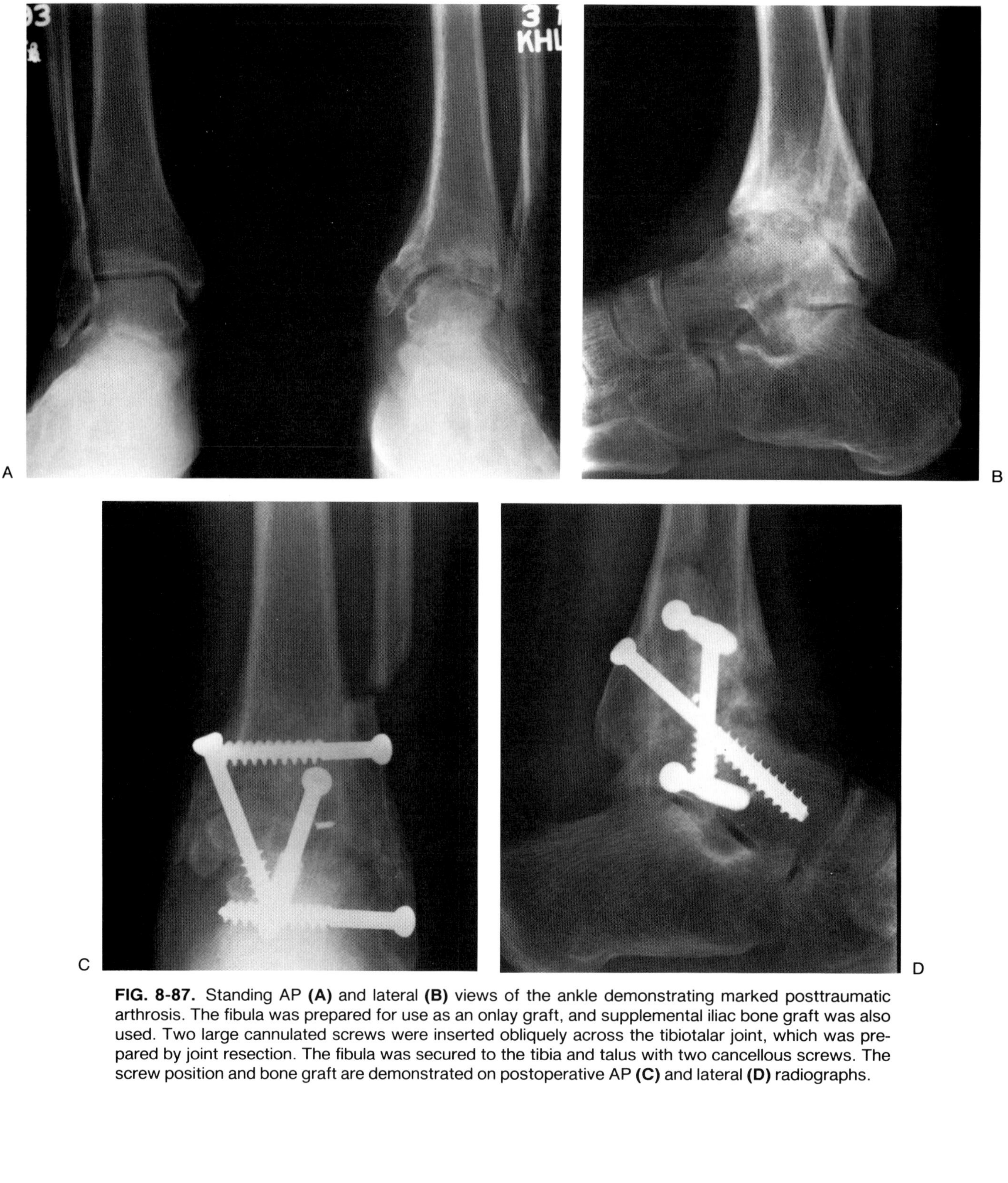

FIG. 8-87. Standing AP **(A)** and lateral **(B)** views of the ankle demonstrating marked posttraumatic arthrosis. The fibula was prepared for use as an onlay graft, and supplemental iliac bone graft was also used. Two large cannulated screws were inserted obliquely across the tibiotalar joint, which was prepared by joint resection. The fibula was secured to the tibia and talus with two cancellous screws. The screw position and bone graft are demonstrated on postoperative AP **(C)** and lateral **(D)** radiographs.

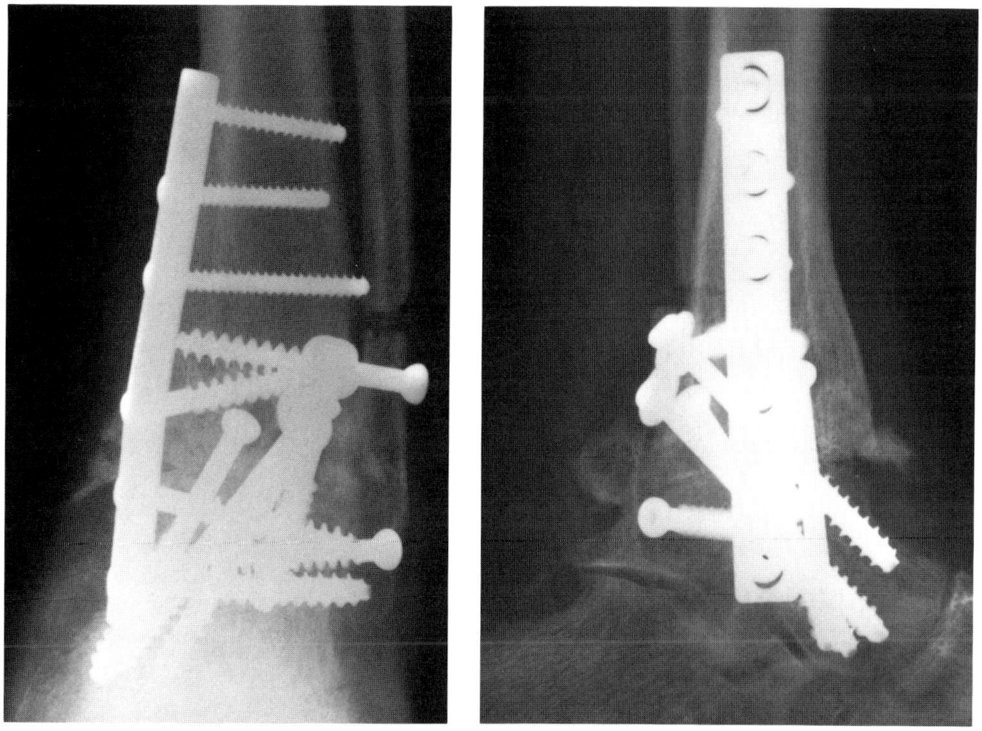

A B

FIG. 8-88. The AP **(A)** and lateral **(B)** radiographs of a nonunion using bone graft and internal fixation screws across the ankle joint; a plate and screws were added medially; and a fibular onlay graft, laterally.

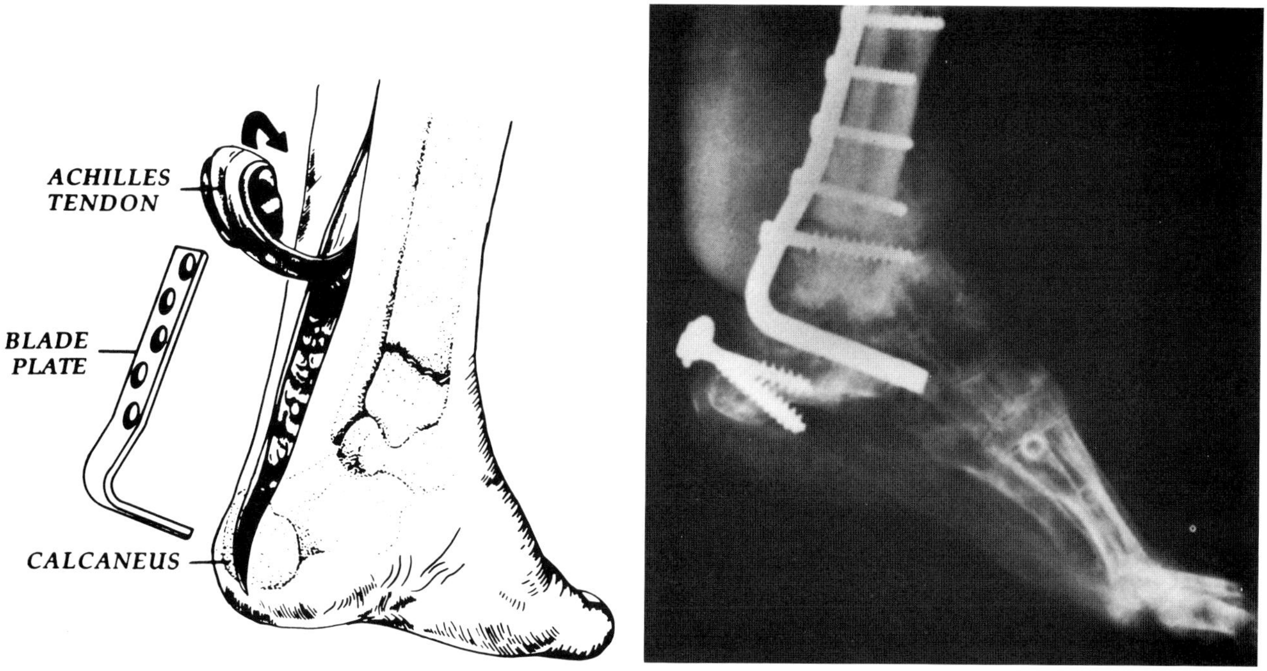

A B

FIG. 8-89. A: Positioning of the five-hole 95° blade plate into the posterior calcaneus for tibiotalocalcaneal arthrodesis. The Achilles tendon and bone block have been elevated. **B:** Lateral radiograph demonstrating the five-hole blade plate in place and two 6.5-mm cancellous screws with ligament washers to reattach the Achilles tendon and bone block. (From Gruen GS, Mears DC. Arthrodesis of the ankle and subtalar joints. *Clin Orthop* 1991;268:15–20.)

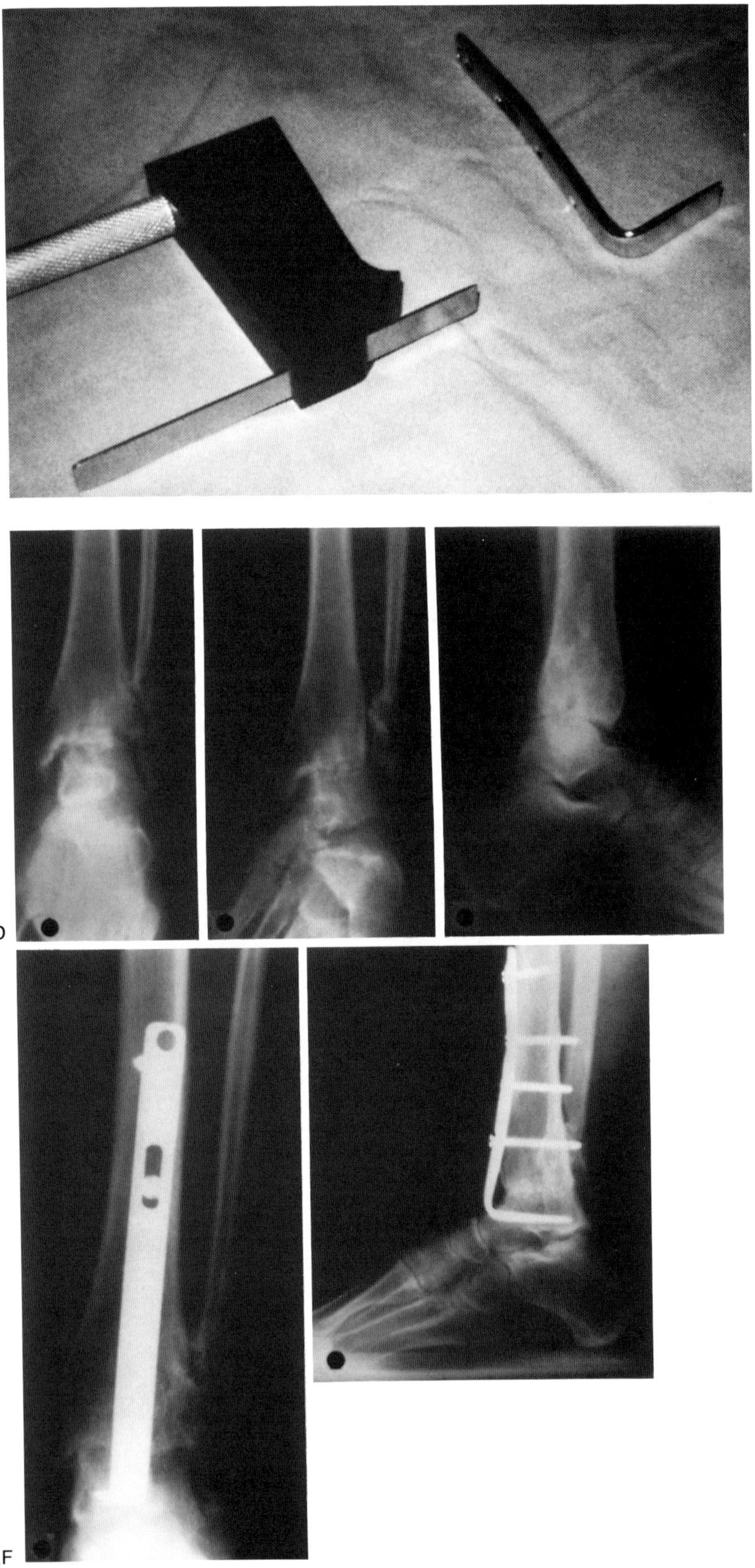

FIG. 8-90. A: The Wolf blade plate with osteotome. **B–D:** The AP, oblique, and lateral views of the ankle after open fracture dislocation. The AP **(E)** and lateral **(F)** radiographs after arthrodesis with Wolf blade plate and cortical screws. (From Weltmer JB, Choi SH, Shenoy A, Schwartsman V. Wolfe blade plate ankle arthrodesis. *Clin Orthop* 1991;268:107–111.)

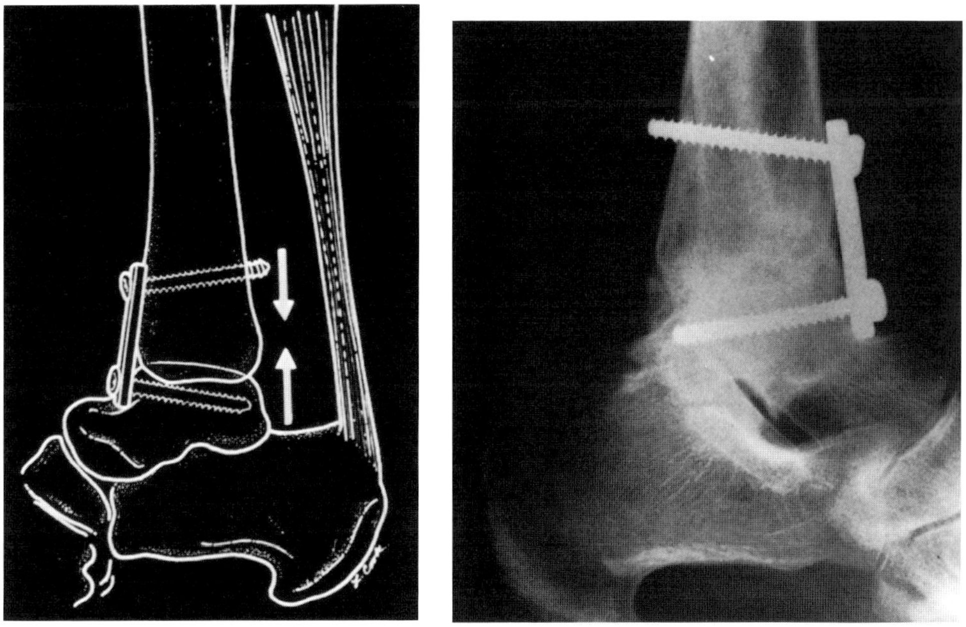

A B

FIG. 8-91. **A:** Anterior tension-plate technique with screws in the tibia and talus. The Achilles tendon is converted to a compressive force (*arrows*). **B:** Lateral radiograph demonstrating solid fusion with anterior plate and two cortical screws. (From Mears DC, Gordon RG, Kann SE, Kann JN. Ankle arthrodesis with an anterior tension plate. *Clin Orthop* 1991;268:70–77.)

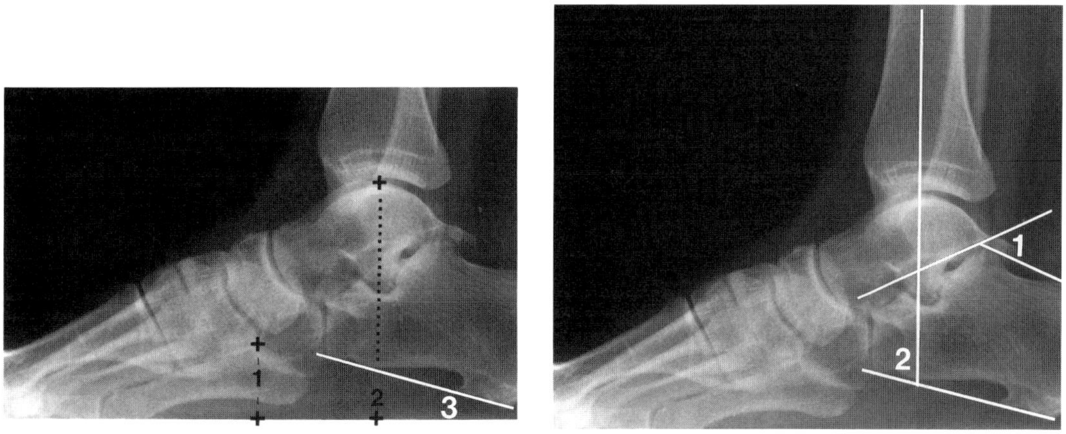

A B

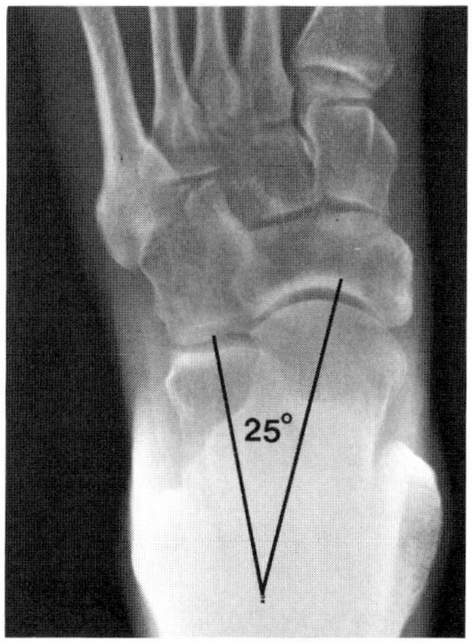

C

FIG. 8-92. **A:** Standing lateral view of the foot and ankle. *1,* Fifth metatarsal height, i.e., distance from the upper articular surface (+) to the weight-bearing surface (normal, 2.3 to 3.8 cm); *2,* talar height, i.e., distance from the most superior aspect of the talar articular surface to the weight-bearing surface; *3,* calcaneal pitch angle, angle formed by weight-bearing surface and a line along the inferior calcaneus (normal, 10° to 30°). **B:** Standing lateral view of the foot and ankle. *1,* Böhler's angle, i.e., angle formed by lines along the posterior calcaneus and posterior articular margin and the posterior articular margin and anterior superior calcaneal margin (normal, 22° to 48°); *2,* tibiocalcaneal angle, i.e., vertical line through the center of the tibia and a line along the inferior calcaneus (normal, 60° to 90°). **C:** Standing AP view of the foot. (see Fig. 8-74 for talar-second metatarsal angle). Talocalcaneal angle (normal, 30° to 50° in patients < 5 years old and 15° to 30° in patients > 5 years old.)

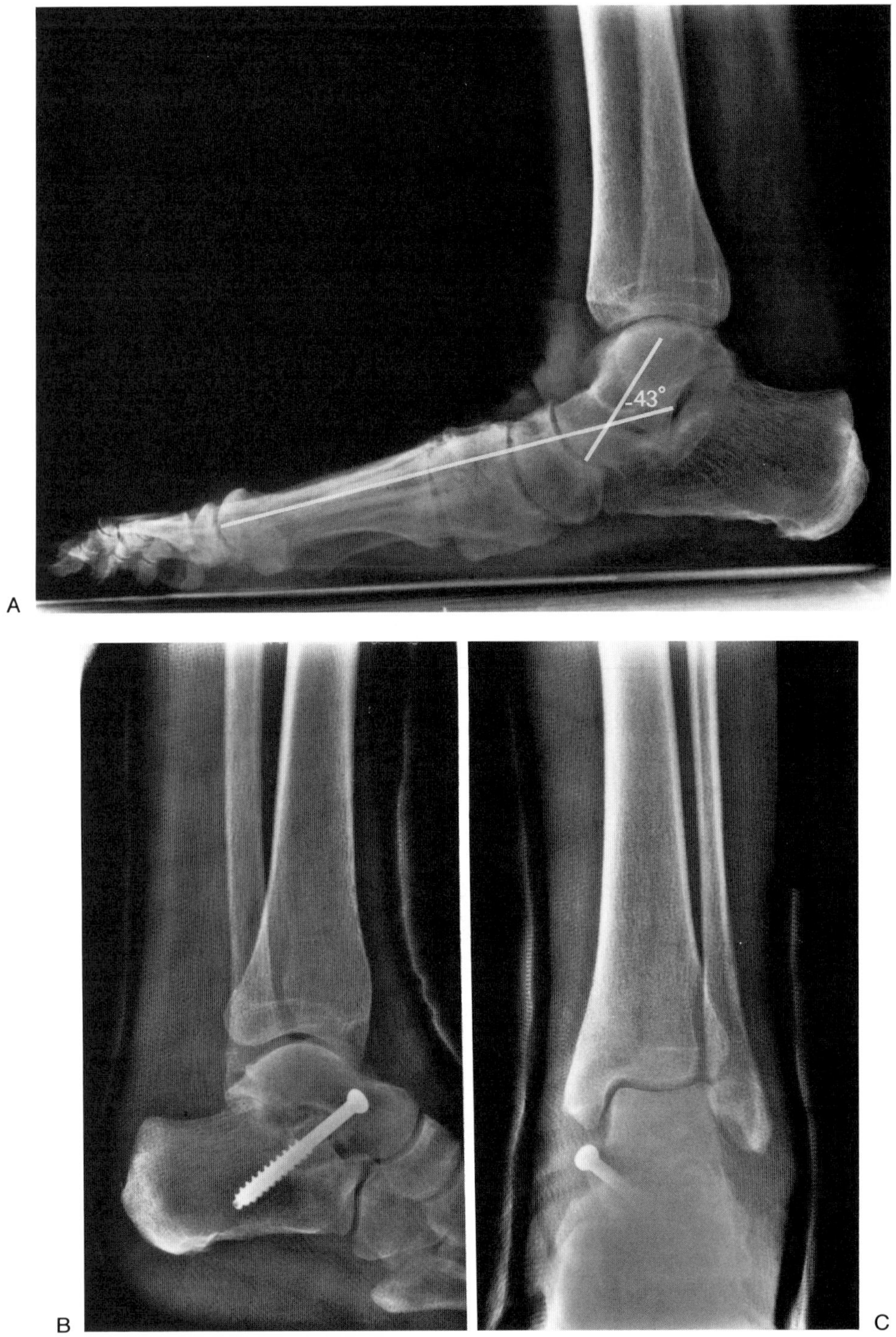

FIG. 8-93. **A:** Standing lateral view of the foot in a patient with posterior tibial tendon dysfunction. Note the marked flatfoot deformity with talar-first metatarsal angle of −43°. **B, C:** Lateral and AP views after arthrodesis with iliac bone graft and a single cancellous screw.

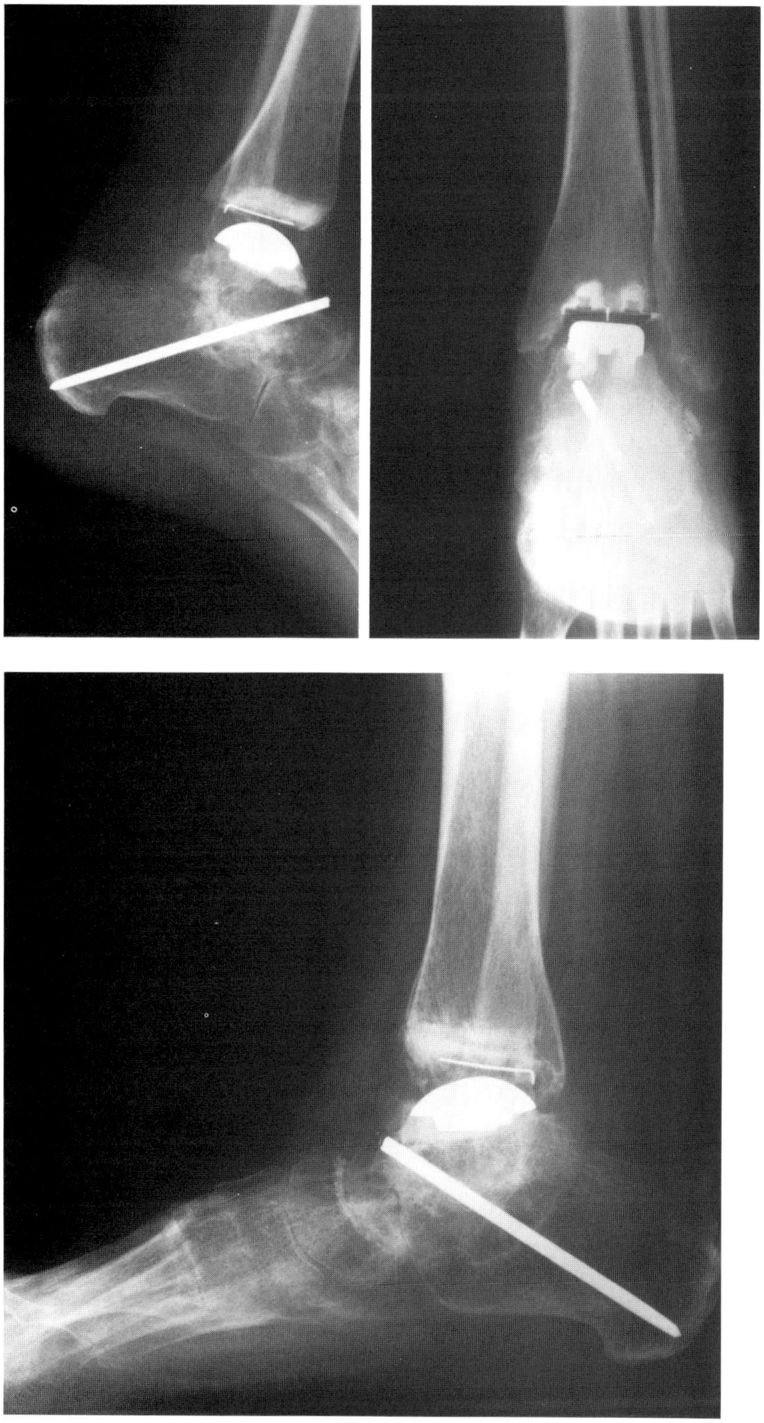

FIG. 8-94. Lateral **(A)**, AP **(B)**, and standing lateral **(C)** views of the foot with a threaded Steinmann pin and bone graft for subtalar arthrodesis. Ankle arthroplasty.

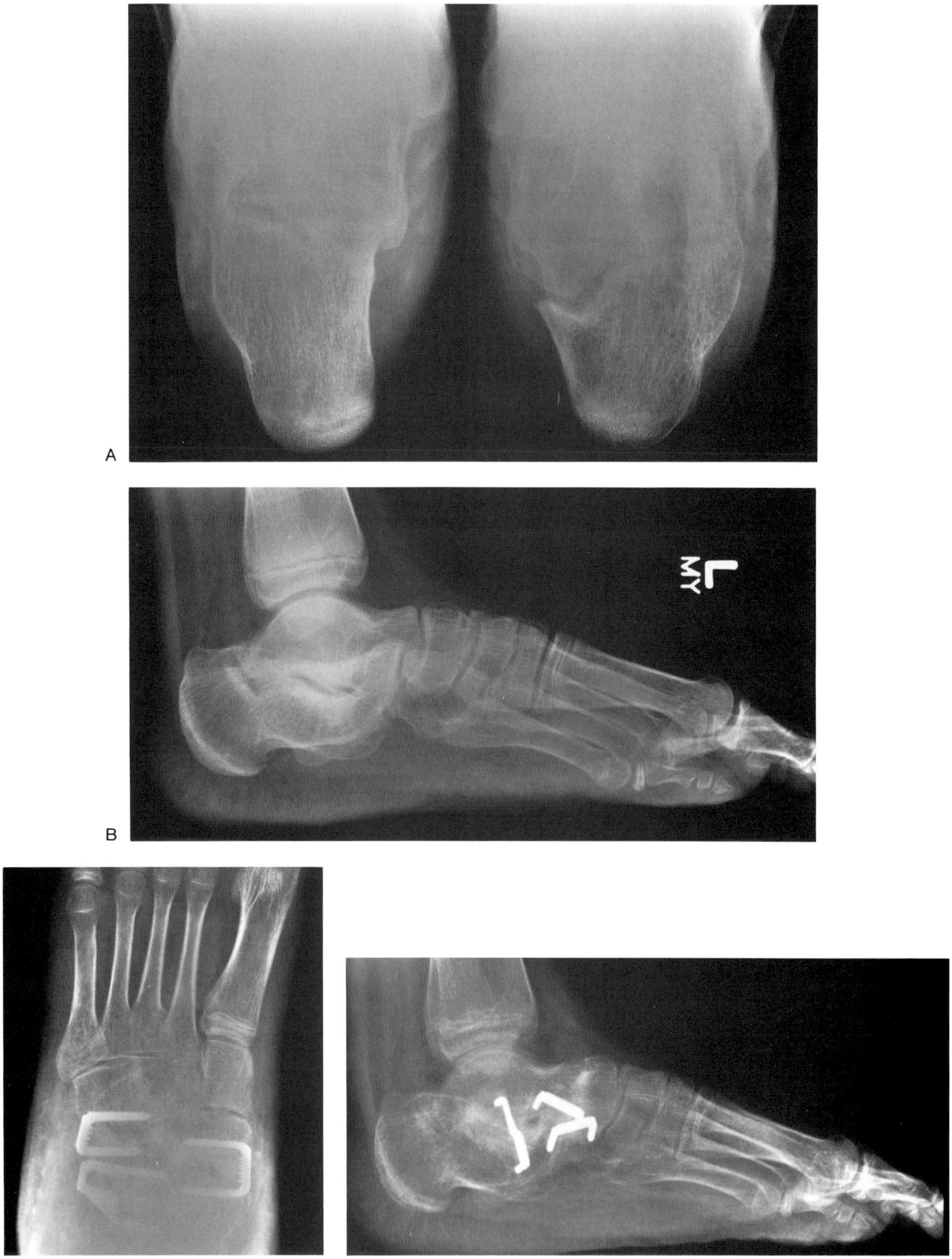

A

B

C

D

FIG. 8-95. Axial **(A)** and standing lateral view **(B)** of the left foot in a child with pes planus and neutrophic hindfoot deformity. The AP **(C)** and lateral **(D)** radiographs after triple arthrodesis with staple fixation. (Courtesy of Dr. John Mazur, Nemours Children's Clinic, Jacksonville, FL.)

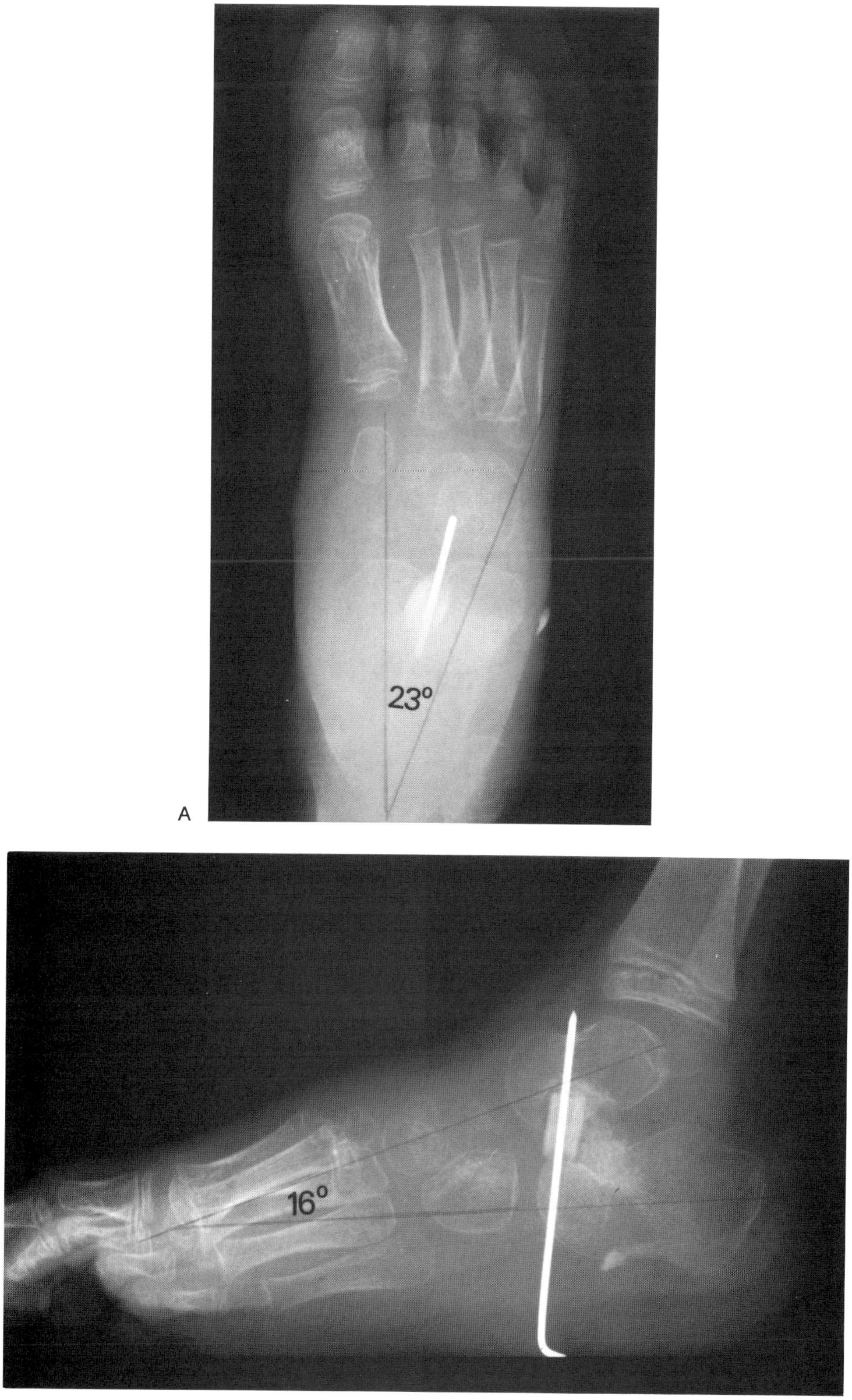

A

B

FIG. 8-96. The AP **(A)** and lateral **(B)** radiographs after Grice procedure with bone dowel and pin fixation.

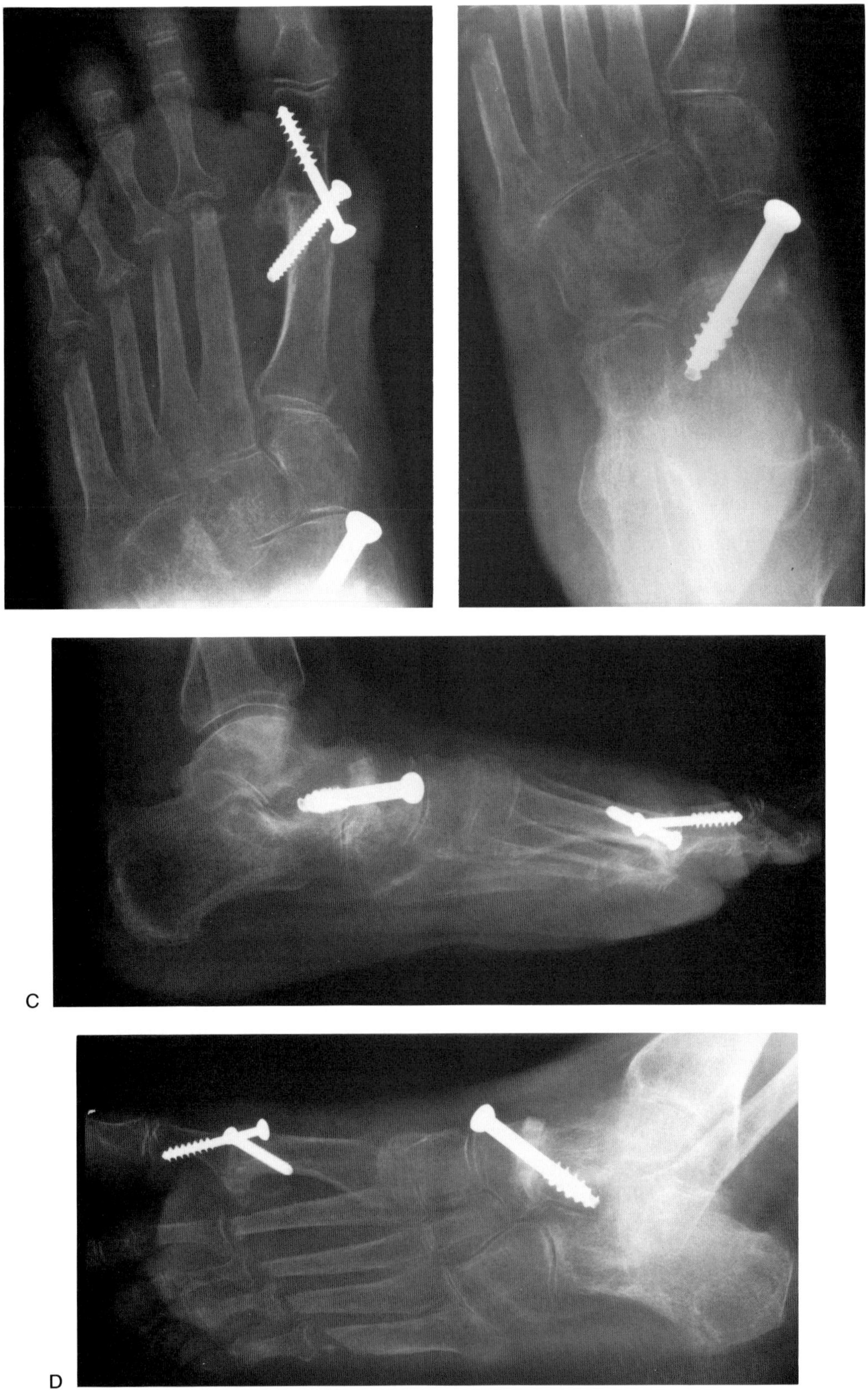

A B C D

FIG. 8-97. A 58-year-old woman with rheumatoid arthritis. The AP **(A, B)**, lateral **(C)**, and oblique **(D)** radiographs after forefoot arthroplasty, including first metatarsophalangeal arthrodesis with screws. Fusion in slight valgus and dorsiflexion is preferable. Talonavicular arthrodesis was performed using iliac crest graft (not always required) and a cannulated cancellous screw.

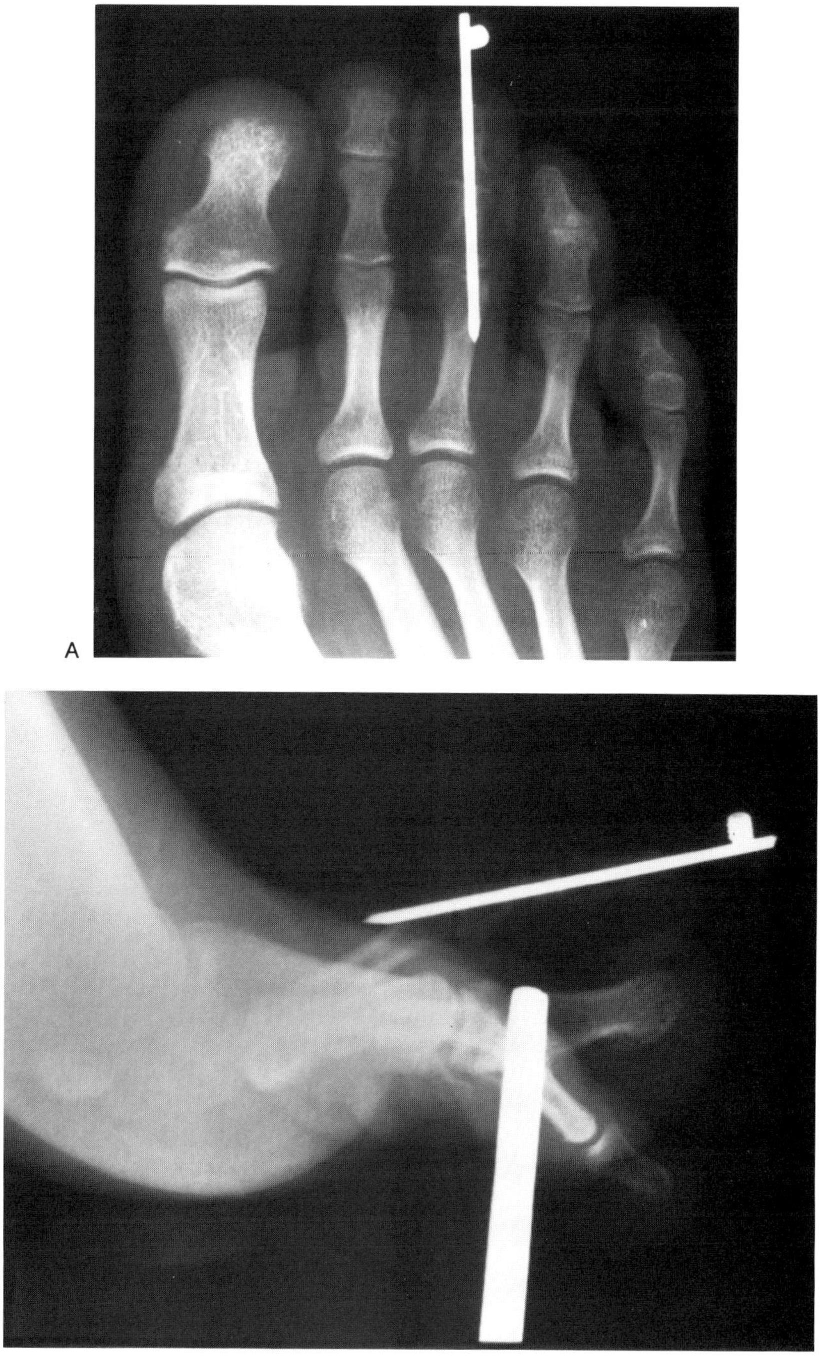

A

B

FIG. 8-98. The AP **(A)** and lateral **(B)** radiographs after distal interphalangeal resection arthroplasty and K-wire fixation.

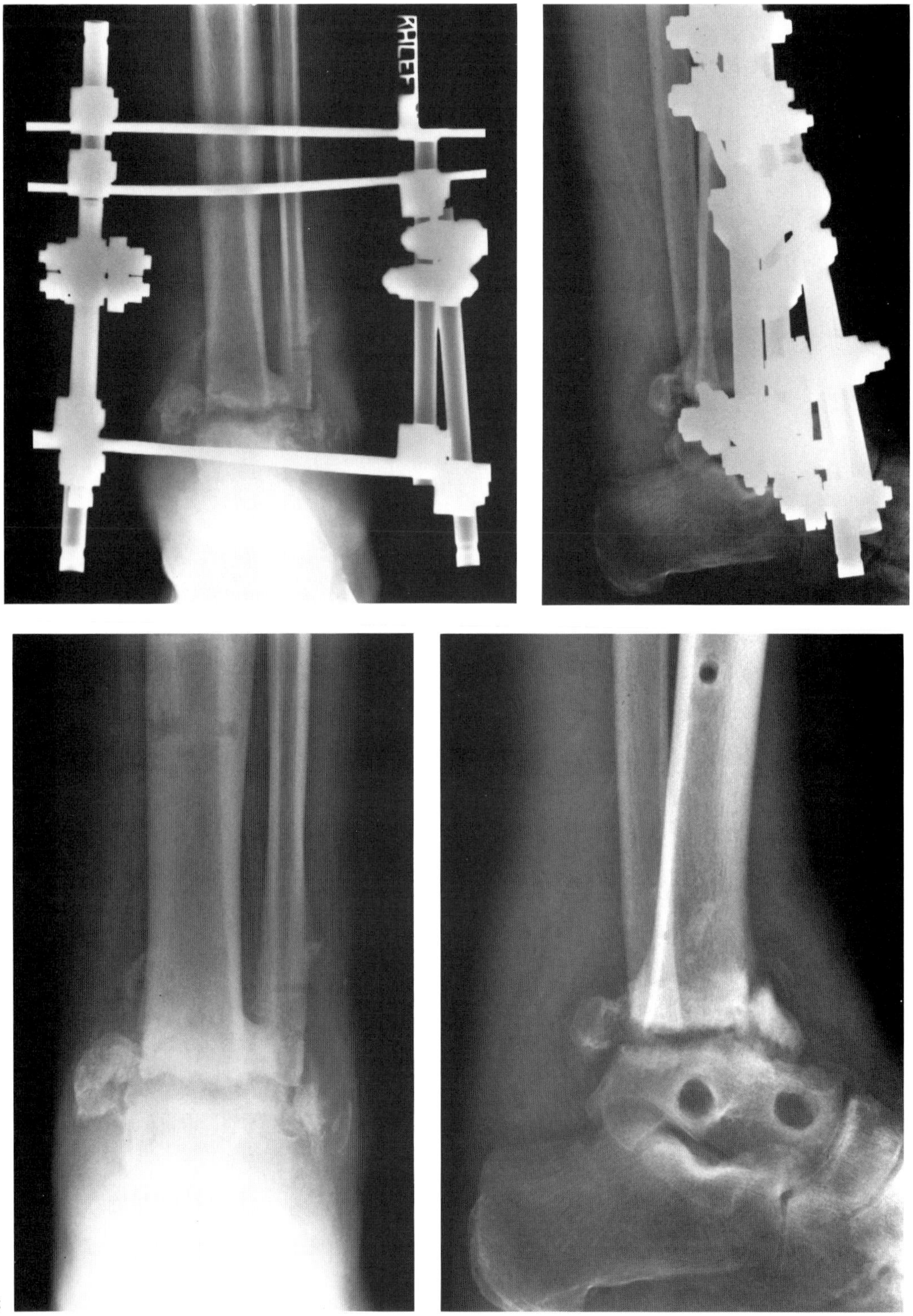

FIG. 8-99. The AP **(A)** and lateral **(B)** views of the ankle with attempted arthrodesis using an AO frame. There is irregularity and sclerosis at the fusion site as a result of nonunion and fragmentation of the tibial margin. Following frame removal, the AP **(C)** and lateral **(D)** radiographs show marked enlargement of the talar pin tracts caused by motion. This can also be seen with chronic infection. Sequestra in pin tracts are a useful finding for the diagnosis of infection.

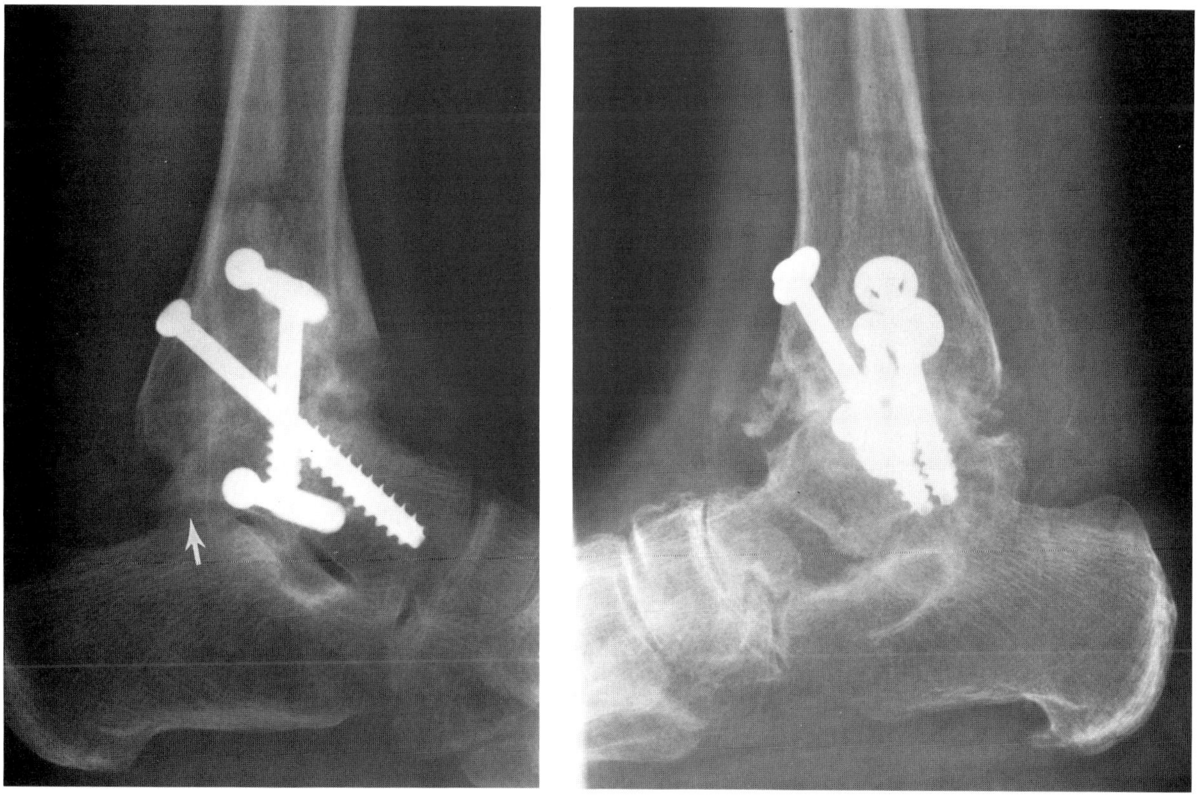

A B

FIG. 8-100. Lateral views of the ankle and hindfoot after ankle arthrodesis. **A:** Lateral radiograph suggests early grade 1 changes with joint-space narrowing in the posterior subtalar joint (*arrow*). **B:** Advanced osteoarthritis in the subtalar joint in a patient who underwent an ankle fusion operation.

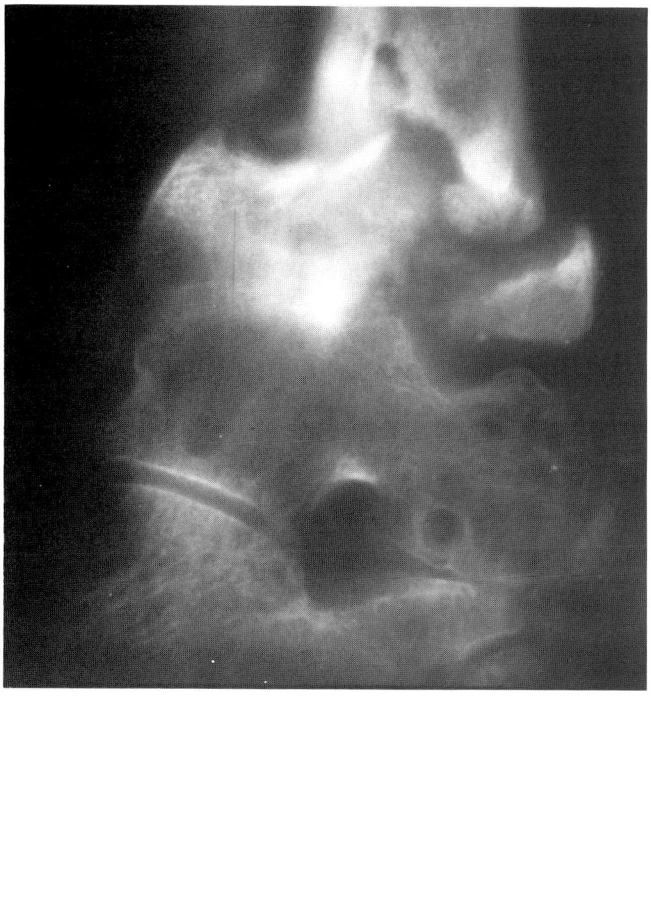

FIG. 8-101. Lateral tomogram after ankle fusion. There is a displaced fracture through an external fixator pin tract just above the fusion site.

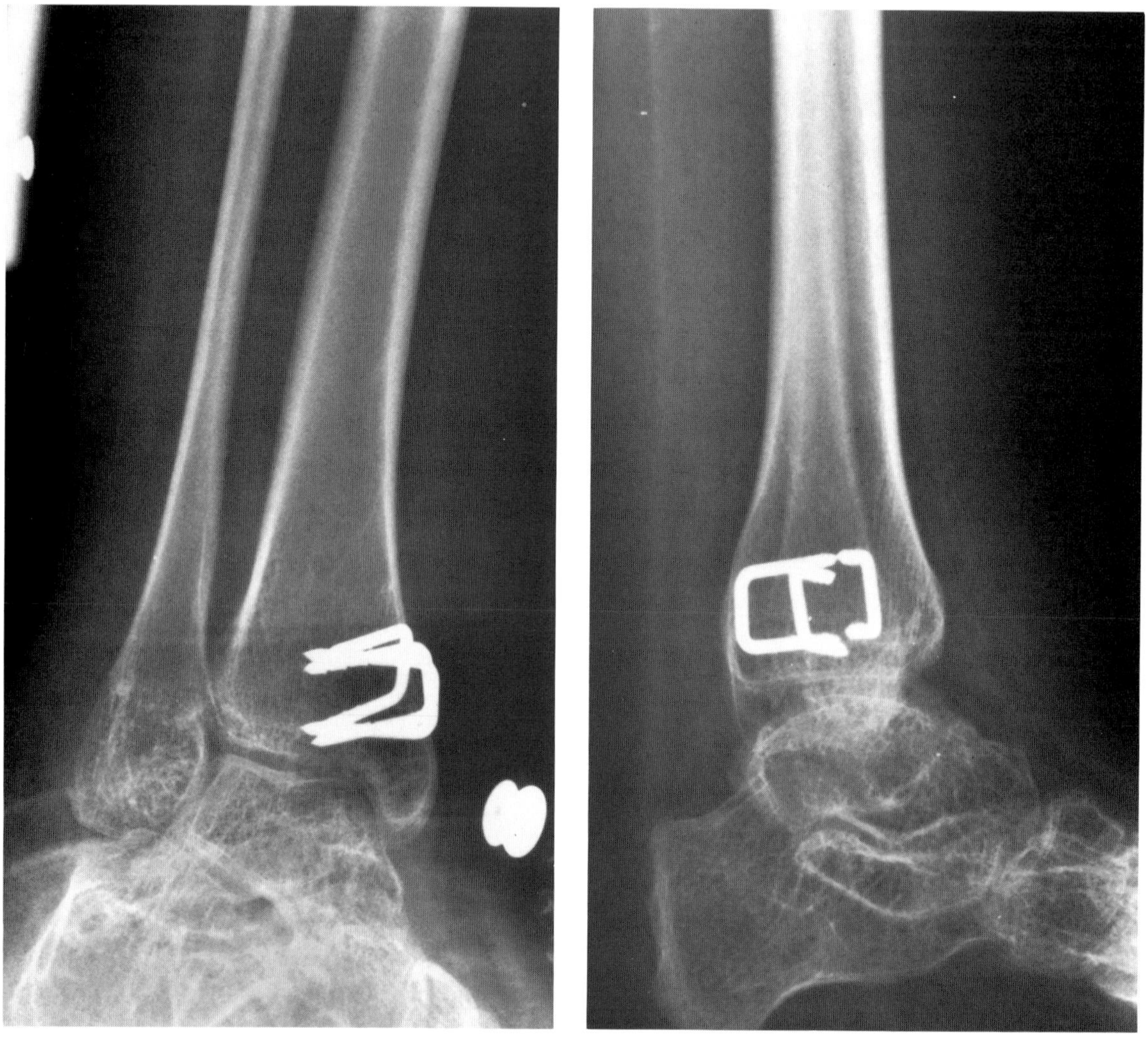

A B

FIG. 8-102. The AP **(A)** and lateral **(B)** radiographs of an old healed distal tibial epiphysodesis using barbed staples. (Courtesy of Dr. John Mazur, Nemours Children's Clinic, Jacksonville, FL.)

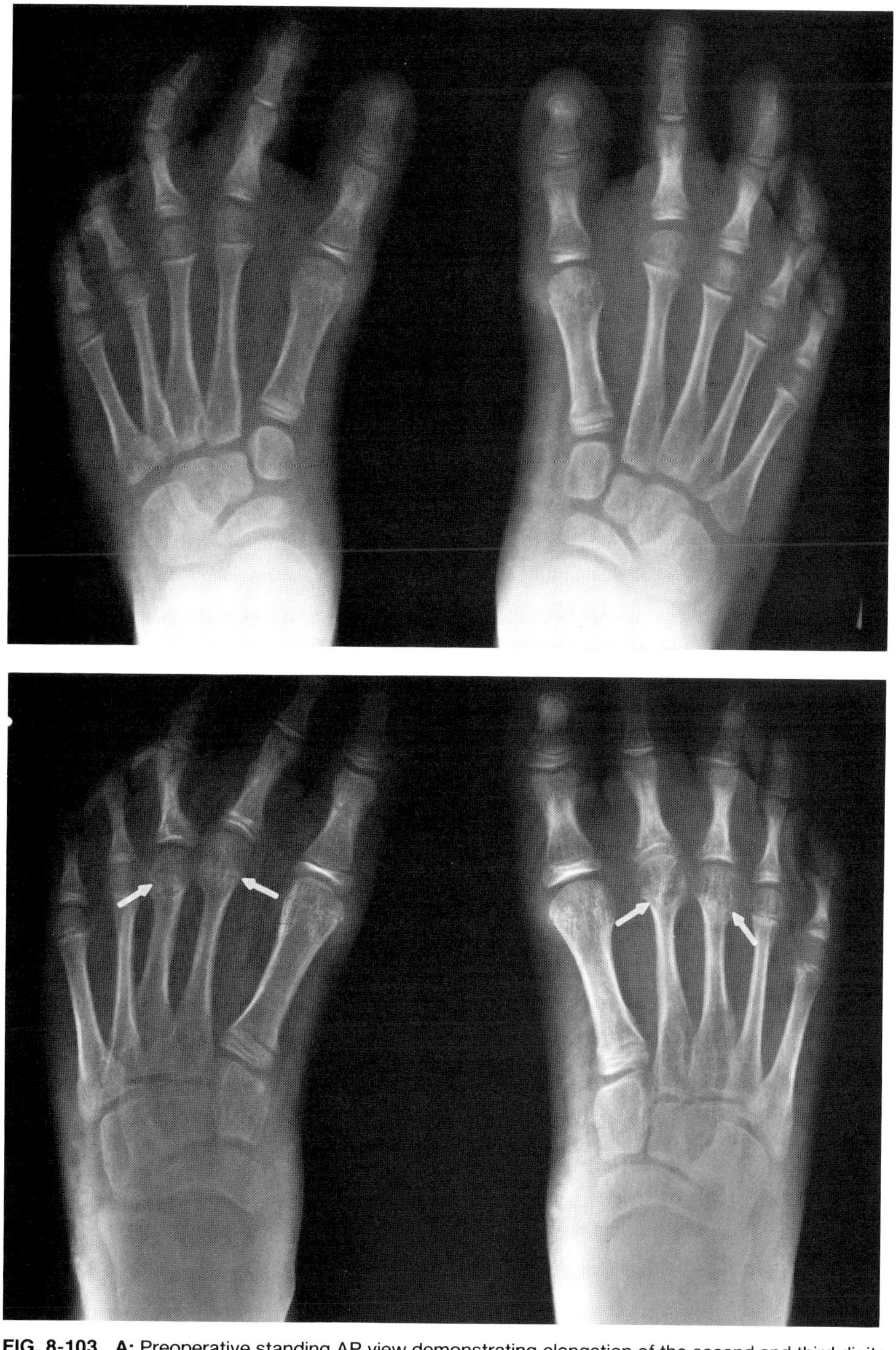

A

B

FIG. 8-103. A: Preoperative standing AP view demonstrating elongation of the second and third digits bilaterally. **B:** After healed epiphysodeses (*arrows*) of the distal second and third metatarsals, the discrepancy in length was improved. (Courtesy of Dr. John Mazur, Nemours Children's Clinic, Jacksonville, FL.)

growth ceases at 15 to 16 years in boys and 13 to 14 years in girls.[236]

The applications of this technique in the foot and ankle could be for metatarsus primus adductus and ankle valgus. Some authors have managed the former by stapling the lateral aspect of the first metatarsal epiphysis when the patient was about age 8 years. The lateral 25% of the growth plate should be closed. Others have managed ankle valgus by stapling 30% to 40% of the distal tibial physis.[216,236]

REFERENCES

Imaging Techniques

1. Ala-Ketola L, Puronen J, Koivisto E, Purepera M. Arthrography in the diagnosis of ligament injuries and classification of ankle injuries. *Radiology* 1977;125:63–68.
2. Ballinger WR. *Merrill's atlas of roentgenographic positions and standard radiographic procedures.* 5th ed. St. Louis: CV Mosby; 1982.
3. Berquist TH. *Radiology of the foot and ankle.* New York: Raven Press; 1989.
4. Berquist TH. *MRI of the musculoskeletal system.* 2nd ed. New York: Raven Press; 1990.
5. Black HM, Brand RL, Eichelberger MR. An improved technique for the evaluation of ligamentous injury in severe ankle sprains. *Am J Sports Med* 1978;6:276–282.
6. Blei CL, Nirschl RP, Grant EG. Achilles tendon: US diagnosis of pathologic conditions. *Radiology* 1986;159:765–767.
7. Bleikrodt RP, Kingma LM, Binnendijk B, Klein JP. Injuries of the lateral ankle ligaments. Classification with tenography and arthrography. *Radiology* 1989;173:347–349.
8. Bluth EI, Merritt CR, Sullivan MA. Grey scale ultrasound evaluation of the lower extremities. *JAMA* 1982;247:3127–3129.
9. Brown ML, Swee RG, Johnson KA. Bone scintigraphy of the calcaneus. *Clin Nucl Med* 1986;11:530–536.
10. Burkus JK, Sella EJ, Southwick WO. Occult injuries of the talus diagnosed by bone scan and tomography. *Foot Ankle* 1984;4:316–324.
11. Causton J. Projection of the sesamoid bones in the region of the first metatarsophalangeal joints. *Radiology* 1943;9:39–40.
12. Dory MA. Arthrography of the ankle joint in chronic instability. *Skeletal Radiol* 1986;15:291–294.
13. Edeiken J, Colter JM. Ankle injury. The need for stress views. *JAMA* 1978;240:1183–1184.
14. Erickson SJ, Quinn SF, Kneeland JB, et al. MR imaging of the tarsal tunnel and related spaces. *AJR Am J Roentgenol* 1990;155:323–328.
15. Evans GA, Frenyo SD. The stress-tenogram in the diagnosis of ruptures of the lateral ligament of the ankle. *J Bone Joint Surg [Br]* 1979;61B:347–351.
16. Floyd EJ, Ransom RA, Dailey JM. Computed tomography scanning of the subtalar joint. *J Am Podiatry Assoc* 1984;74:533–537.
17. Fornage BD. Achilles tendon: US examination. *Radiology* 1986;159:759–764.
18. Freiberger RH, Kaye J. *Arthrography.* New York: Appleton-Century-Crofts; 1979.
19. Frolich H, Gotzen L, Adam D. Evaluation of stress roentgenogram of the upper ankle joint. *Unfallchirurg* 1980;83:457–461.
20. Geslian JE, Thrall JH, Espenosa JL, Older RA. Early detection of stress fractures using Tc-99m polyphosphate. *Radiology* 1976;121:683–687.
21. Gilula LA, Oloff L, Caputi R, Destouet JM, Jacobs A, Solomon MA. Ankle tenography: a key to unexplained symptomatology. *Radiology* 1984;151:581–587.
22. Goergen TG, Resnick D. Arthrography of the ankle. In: Dalinka M, ed. *Arthrography.* New York: Springer-Verlag; 1981.
23. Goiney RC, Connell DG, Nichols DM. CT evaluation of tarsometatarsal fracture dislocation injuries. *AJR Am J Roentgenol* 1985;144:985–990.
24. Heger L, Wulff K. Computer tomography of the calcaneus: normal anatomy. *AJR Am J Roentgenol* 1985;75:123–129.
25. Heger L, Wulff K, Seddigi MSA. Computed tomography of calcaneal fractures. *AJR Am J Roentgenol* 1985;145:131–137.
26. Horsfield D, Murphy G. Stress views of the ankle joint in lateral ligament injury. *Radiography* 1985;51:7–11.
27. Isherwood I. A radiologic approach to the subtalar joint. *J Bone Joint Surg [Br]* 1961;43B:566–574.
28. Johannsen A. Radiologic diagnosis of lateral ligament lesion of the ankle. A comparison between talar tilt and anterior drawer sign. *Acta Orthop Scand* 1978;49:259–301.
29. Jonsson K, Fredin HO, Cederlund CG. Width of the normal ankle joint. *Acta Radiol* 1984;25:147–149.
30. Kneeland JB, Macrandor S, Middleton WD, Cates CD, Jesmanowicz A, Hyde JS. MR imaging of the normal ankle: correlation with anatomic sections. *AJR Am J Roentgenol* 1988;151:117–123.
31. Martinez S, Herzenberg JE, Apple JS. Computed tomography of the hindfoot. *Orthop Clin North Am* 1985;16:481–496.
32. Mathieson JR, Connell DG, Cooperberg PL, Lloyd-Smith DR. Sonography of the Achilles tendon and adjacent bursae. *AJR Am J Roentgenol* 1988;151:127–131.
33. Morrey BF, Cass JF, Johnson KA, Berquist TH. The foot and ankle. In: Berquist TH, ed. *Imaging of orthopedic trauma and surgery.* Philadelphia: WB Saunders; 1986:407–498.
34. Olson RW. Ankle arthrography. *Radiol Clin North Am* 1981;19:255–268.
35. Pritsch M, Heim M, Horoszowski H, Farine I. The significance of the axial foot projection in diagnosis of metatarsal pathology. *Arch Orthop Trauma Surg* 1981;98:139–141.
36. Rosenberg ZS, Feldman F, Singson RD. Intra-articular calcaneal fractures: computed tomographic analysis. *Skeletal Radiol* 1987;16:105–113.
37. Rosenberg ZS, Johss MH, Noto AM, et al. Rupture of the posterior tibial tendon: CT and surgical findings. *Radiology* 1988;176:489–493.
38. Sauser DD, Nelson RC, Lavine MH, Wa CW. Acute injuries of the lateral ligaments of the ankle: comparison of stress radiography and arthrography. *Radiology* 1983;148:643–657.
39. Towbin R, Dimbar JS, Towbin J. Teardrop sign: plain film recognition of ankle effusion. *AJR Am J Roentgenol* 1980;134:985–990.
40. Vuust M. Arthrographic diagnosis of ruptured calcaneofibular ligament: a new projection tested on experimental post mortem. *Acta Radiol* 1980;21:123–128.
41. Vuust M, Niedermann B. Arthrographic diagnosis of ruptured calcaneofibular ligament. II. Clinical evaluation of a new method. *Acta Radiol* 1980;21:231–234.
42. Woolson ST, Porvati D, Fillingham LL, Vassiliodis A. Three-dimensional imaging of the ankle from computed tomography. *Foot Ankle* 1985;6:2–6.

Trauma: Ankle Fractures

43. Arimoto HR, Forrester DM. Classification of ankle fractures: an algorithm. *AJR Am J Roentgenol* 1980;135:1057–1063.
44. Ashhurst APC, Bromer RS. Classification and mechanism of fractures of the leg bones involving the ankle. *Arch Surg* 1922;4:51–129.
45. Behrens F. A primer of fixation devices and configurations. *Clin Orthop* 1989;251:5–14.
46. Behrens F. General theories and principles of external fixation. *Clin Orthop* 1980;241:15–23.
47. Berquist TH. *Radiology of the foot and ankle.* New York: Raven Press; 1989.
48. Bishop PA. Fractures and epiphyseal separations of the ankle. *AJR Am J Roentgenol* 1932;67:28–49.
49. Carothers CO, Crenshaw AH. Clinical significance of a classifi-

cation of epiphyseal injuries at the ankle. *Am J Surg* 1955;89: 879–889.
50. Cone RO III, Nguyen V, Flournoy JG, Guerra J. Triplane fracture of the distal tibia epiphysis: radiologic and CT studies. *Radiology* 1984;153:763–767.
51. Cooperman DR, Spiegel PG, Laros GS. Tibial fractures involving the ankle in children. *J Bone Joint Surg [Am]* 1978;60A:1040–1045.
52. Crenshaw AH. Injuries of the distal tibial epiphysis. *Clin Orthop* 1965;41:98–107.
53. DeCosta T, Alvarey R, Trevino S. External fixation of the foot and ankle. *Foot Ankle* 1986;7:40–48.
54. Dias LS, Giegerich CR. Fractures of the distal tibia epiphysis in adolescence. *J Bone Joint Surg [Am]* 1983;56A:438–444.
55. Dias LS, Tachdjian MO. Physeal injuries of the ankle in children. *Clin Orthop* 1956;136:230–233.
56. Edeiken J, Cotler JM. Ankle trauma. *Semin Roentgenol* 1978;13: 145–155.
57. Etter C, Ganz R. Long-term results of tibial plafond fractures treated with open reduction and internal fixation. *Arch Orthop Trauma Surg* 1991;110:277–283.
58. Eventon I, Salama R, Goodwin DRA, Weissman SL. An evaluation of surgical and conservative treatment of fractures of the ankle in 200 patients. *J Trauma* 1978;18:271–274.
59. Griffiths HJ. Trauma to the ankle and foot. *Crit Rev Diagn Imaging* 1979;26:45–105.
60. Hall H. A simplified workable classification of ankle fractures. *Foot Ankle* 1980;1:5–10.
61. Kelikian H, Kelikian AS. *Disorders of the ankle.* Philadelphia: WB Saunders; 1985.
62. King TF, Bright RW, Hensinger RN. Distal tibial physeal fractures in children that may require open reduction. *J Bone Joint Surg [Am]* 1984;66A:647–657.
63. Kleiger B, Mankin JJ. Fracture of the lateral portion of the distal tibial epiphysis. *J Bone Joint Surg [Am]* 1964;46A:25.
64. Lauge-Hansen N. Fractures of the ankle. II. Combined experimental-surgical and experimental-radiological investigations. *Arch Surg* 1950;60:957–985.
65. Leach RE. Fractures of the tibial plafond. *Instr Course Lect* 1979;28:88–93.
66. Leeds HC, Erlich MG. Instability of the distal tibiofibular syndesmosis after bimalleolar and trimalleolar fractures. *J Bone Joint Surg [Am]* 1984;66A:490–503.
67. Lynn MD. The triplane distal tibial epiphyseal fracture. *Clin Orthop* 1972;86:187–190.
68. Morrey BF, Cass JR, Johnson KA, Berquist TH. Imaging of orthopedic trauma and surgery. In: Berquist TH, ed. *Foot and ankle.* Philadelphia: WB Saunders; 1986:407–498.
69. Müller ME, Allgower M, Willenegger H. *Manual of internal fixation. Techniques recommended by AO-ASIF group.* Berlin: Springer-Verlag; 1991.
70. Müller ME, Nazarian S, Koch P. *The AO classification of fractures.* New York: Springer-Verlag; 1988.
71. Neer CS II. Injuries of the ankle joint: evaluation. *Conn Med* 1953;17:580–583.
72. Olerud C. Supination-eversion ankle fractures sustained during downhill skiing. *Acta Orthop Trauma Surg* 1985;104:129–131.
73. Ovadia DN, Beals RK. Fractures of the tibial plafond. *J Bone Joint Surg [Am]* 1986;68A:543–551.
74. Peiró A, Araal J, Mortos F, Mut T. Triplane distal tibial epiphyseal fracture. *Clin Orthop* 1981;160:196–200.
75. Rogers LF. Radiology of epiphyseal injuries. *Radiology* 1970;96: 289–299.
76. Ruedi T. Fractures of the lower end of the tibia into the ankle joint: results of 9 years after open reduction and internal fixation. *Injury* 1973;5:130–134.
77. Salter RB, Harris WR. Injuries involving the epiphyseal plate. *J Bone Joint Surg [Am]* 1963;45A:587–622.
78. Slone RM, Heare MM, VanderGrund RA, Montgomery WJ. Orthopedic fixation devices. *Radiographics* 1991;11:823–847.
79. Spiegel PG, Cooperman DR, Laros GS. Epiphyseal fractures of the distal ends of the tibia and fibula. *J Bone Joint Surg [Am]* 1978;60A:1046–1050.
80. VanderGreind RA, Savoie FH, Hughes JL. Fractures of the ankle. In: Rockwood CA, Green DP, Bucholz RW, eds. *Rockwood and Green's fractures in adults.* 3rd ed. Vol. 2. Philadelphia: JB Lippincott; 1991:1983–2039.
81. Winkler B, Weber BG, Simpson LA. The dorsal antiglide plate in the treatment of Danis-Weber type B fractures of the distal fibula. *Clin Orthop* 1990;259:204–209.
82. Yablon IG, Heller FG, Shouse L. The key role of the lateral malleolus in displaced fractures of the ankle. *J Bone Joint Surg [Am]* 1977;59A:169–173.
83. Yablon IG, Wasilewski S. Management of unstable ankle fractures. *Foot Ankle* 1980;1:11–19.
84. Yde J. The Lauge-Hansen classification of malleolar fractures. *Acta Orthop Scand* 1980;51:181–192.
85. Yde J, Kristensen KD. Ankle fractures: supination eversion fractures of stage IV. *Acta Orthop Scand* 1980;51:981–990.
86. Yde J, Kristensen KD. Ankle fractures: supination eversion fractures stage II. Primary and late operative and nonoperative treatment. *Acta Orthop Scand* 1980;51:695–702.

Talar Fractures and Dislocations

87. Alexander AH, Lichtman DM. Surgical treatment of transchondral talar dome fractures. *J Bone Joint Surg [Am]* 1980;62A:646–652.
88. Berquist TH. *Radiology of the foot and ankle.* New York: Raven Press; 1989.
89. Blair HC. Comminuted fractures and fracture dislocations of the body of the talus. *Am J Surg* 1943;59:37–43.
90. Burkus JK, Sella FJ, Southwick WO. Occult injuries of the talus diagnosed by bone scan and tomography. *Foot Ankle* 1984;4: 316–324.
91. Canale ST, Kelly FB. Fractures of the neck and the talus. *J Bone Joint Surg [Am]* 1978;60A:143–156.
92. Coltart WD. Aviator's astragalus. *J Bone Joint Surg [Br]* 1952;34B:545–566.
93. Detenbeck LC, Kelly PJ. Total dislocation of the talus. *J Bone Joint Surg [Am]* 1969;51A:283–288.
94. Flick AB, Gould N. Osteochondritis dessicans of the talus: review of the literature and a new surgical approach for medial dome lesions. *Foot Ankle* 1985;5:165–185.
95. Floyd FJ, Ransom RA, Dailey JM. Computed tomography scanning of the subtalar joint. *J Am Podiatry Assoc* 1984;14:533–537.
96. Gross RH. Fractures and dislocations of the foot. In: Rockwood CA, Winkins KE, Kuig RE, eds. *Fractures in children.* Vol. 3. Philadelphia: JB Lippincott; 1984:1043–1103.
97. Hawkins LG. Fractures of the lateral process of the talus. *J Bone Joint Surg [Am]* 1965;47A:1170–1175.
98. Hawkins LG. Fractures of the neck of the talus. *J Bone Joint Surg [Am]* 1970;52A:991–1002.
99. Kelikian H, Kelikian AS. *Disorders of the ankle.* Philadelphia: WB Saunders; 1985.
100. Kleiger B, Ahmed M. Injuries of the talus and its joints. *Clin Orthop* 1976;121:243–262.
101. Lorentzen JE, Christensen SB, Krogsoe O, Snepper O. Fractures of the neck of the talus. *Acta Orthop Scand* 1977;48:115–120.
102. Morrey BF, Cass JR, Johnson KA, Berquist TH. Foot and ankle. In: Berquist TH, ed. *Imaging of orthopedic trauma and surgery.* Philadelphia: WB Saunders; 1986:407–498.
103. Mulfinger GL, Trueta JC. The blood supply of the talus. *J Bone Joint Surg [Br]* 1970;52B:160–167.
104. Pennal GF. Fractures of the talus. *Clin Orthop* 1963;30:53–63.
105. Segal D, Waselewski S. Total dislocation of the talus. *J Bone Joint Surg [Am]* 1980;62A:1370–1372.
106. Seltzer SE, Weissman BN, Braunstein EM, Adams DF, Thomas WH. Computed tomography of the hind foot. *J Comput Assist Tomogr* 1094;8:488–497.
107. Snepper O, Christensen SB, Krogsoe O, Lorentzen J. Fracture of the body of the talus. *Acta Orthop Scand* 1977;48:317–324.
108. Swanson TV, Bray TJ, Holmes GB. Fractures of the talar neck. A mechanical study of fixation. *J Bone Joint Surg [Am]* 1992;74A: 544–551.

Calcaneal Fractures

109. Berquist TH. *Radiology of the foot and ankle.* New York: Raven Press; 1989.
110. Böhler L. Diagnosis, pathology, and treatment of fractures of the os calcis. *J Bone Joint Surg* [*Am*] 1931;13A:75–89.
111. Cave EF. Fracture of the os calcis—the problem in general. *Clin Orthop* 1963;30:64–66.
112. Essex-Lopresti P. The mechanism, reduction technique, and results in fractures of the os calcis. *Br J Surg* 1952;39:395–419.
113. Gellman M. Fractures of the anterior process of the calcaneus. *J Bone Joint Surg* 1931;13:877–879.
114. Gilmer PW, Herzenberg J, Frank JL, Silverman P, Morteney S, Goldner JL. Computerized tomographic analysis of acute calcaneal fractures. *Foot Ankle* 1986;6:184–193.
115. Gross RH. Fractures and dislocations of the foot. In: Rockwood CA, Wilkins KE, King RE, eds. *Fractures in children.* Vol. 3. Philadelphia: JB Lippincott; 1991:1043–1103.
116. Guyer BH, Levinsuhn EM, Fredrickson BE, Bailey GL, Formikell M. Computed tomography of calcaneal fractures: anatomy, pathology, dosimetry and clinical relevance. *AJR Am J Roentgenol* 1985;145:911–919.
117. Hall MC, Pennal GF. Primary subtalar arthrodesis in treatment of severe fractures of the calcaneus. *J Bone Joint Surg* [*Br*] 1960;42B:336–343.
118. Lance EM, Corey EJ, Wade PA. Fractures of the os calcis. *J Trauma* 1964;4:15–56.
119. Morrey BF, Cass JF, Johnson KA, Berquist TH. Foot and ankle. In: Berquist TH, ed. *Imaging of orthopedic trauma and surgery.* Philadelphia: WB Saunders; 1986:407–498.
120. Norfay JF, Rogers LF, Adams GP, Graves HC, Herser WJ. Common calcaneal avulsion fracture. *AJR Am J Roentgenol* 1980;134:119–123.
121. Paley D, Hall H. Intra-articular fractures of the calcaneus. A critical analysis of results and prognostic factors. *J Bone Joint Surg* [*Am*] 1993;75A:342–354.
122. Renfrew DL, El-Khoury GY. Anterior process fractures of the calcaneus. *Skeletal Radiol* 1985;14:121–125.
123. Rosenberg ZS, Feldman F, Surgson RD. Intra-articular calcaneal fractures: computed tomographic analysis. *Skeletal Radiol* 1987;16:105–113.
124. Ross SDK, Sowerby RR. The operative treatment of fractures of the os calcis. *Clin Orthop* 1985;199:132–143.
125. Rowe CR, Sakillarides HT, Freeman PA. Fractures of the os calcis. A long term follow-up study in 146 patients. *JAMA* 1963;184:920–924.
126. Schmidt TL, Weiner DS. Calcaneal fractures in children. An evaluation of the nature of injury in 56 children. *Clin Orthop* 1982;171:150–155.
127. Slatis P, Kroduoto O, Santavista S, Laasonen EM. Fractures of the calcaneus. *J Trauma* 1979;19:939–943.
128. Stephenson JR. Displaced fractures of the os calcis involving the subtalar joint: the key role of the superomedial fragment. *Foot Ankle* 1983;4:91–101.

Midfoot and Forefoot Fractures

129. Aitken AP, Paulsen D. Dislocation of the tarsometatarsal joints. *J Bone Joint Surg* [*Am*] 1963;45A:246–260.
130. Anderson LD. Injuries of the forefoot. *Clin Orthop* 1977;122:18–27.
131. Cain PR, Seligson D. Lisfranc's fracture-dislocation with intercuneiform dislocation. *Foot Ankle* 1981;2:156–160.
132. Carp L. Fracture of the fifth metatarsal bone with special reference to delayed union. *Ann Surg* 1927;86:308–320.
133. Cassebaum WH. Lisfranc fracture dislocations. *Clin Orthop* 1963;30:116–129.
134. Eichenholtz SN, Levene DB. Fracture of the tarsal navicular bone. *Clin Orthop* 1964;34:142–157.
135. English TA. Dislocation of the metatarsal bone and adjacent bone. *J Bone Joint Surg* [*Br*] 1964;46B:700–704.
136. Foster SC, Foster RR. Lisfranc's tarsometatarsal fracture dislocation. *Radiology* 1976;120:79–83.
137. Gissane W. A dangerous type of fracture of the foot. *J Bone Joint Surg* [*Br*] 1951;33B:535–538.
138. Goiney RC, Connell DG, Nichols DM. CT evaluation of tarsometatarsal fracture-dislocation injuries. *AJR Am J Roentgenol* 1985;144:985–990.
139. Gross RH. Fractures and dislocation of the foot. In: Rockwood CA, Wilkins KE, King RE, eds. *Fractures in children.* Vol. 3. Philadelphia: JB Lippincott; 1984:1043–1103.
140. Hardcastle PH, Reschauer R, Kutscha-Lissberg E, Schoffman W. Injuries of the tarsometatarsal joint: incidence, classification and treatment. *J Bone Joint Surg* [*Br*] 1982;64B:349–356.
141. Heckman JD. Fractures of the foot and ankle. In: Rockwood CA, Green DP, eds. *Fractures in adults.* Philadelphia: JB Lippincott: 1991:2041–2182.
142. Jones R. Fracture of the base of the fifth metatarsal bone by indirect violence. *Ann Surg* 1902;35:697–700.
143. Kavanaugh JH, Borower TD, Mann RV. The Jones' fracture revisited. *J Bone Joint Surg* [*Am*] 1978;60A:776–782.
144. Lewis AG, DeLee JC. Type I complex dislocation of the 1st metatarsophalangeal joint—open reduction through a dorsal approach. *J Bone Joint Surg* [*Am*] 1984;66A:1120–1123.
145. Main BJ, Jowett RL. Injuries of the mid-tarsal joint. *J Bone Joint Surg* [*Br*] 1975;57B:89–97.
146. Norfray JF, Feline RA, Steinberg RI, Galinski AW, Gilula LA. Subtleties of Lisfranc fractures-dislocation. *AJR Am J Roentgenol* 1981;137:1151–1156.
147. Slone RM, Heare MM, VanderGriend RA, Montgomery WJ. Orthopedic fixation devices. *Radiographics* 1991;11:823–847.
148. Wiley JJ. The mechanism of tarsometatarsal joint injuries. *J Bone Joint Surg* [*Br*] 1971;53B:474–482.

Trauma: Postoperative Imaging and Complications

149. Berquist TH. *Radiology of the foot and ankle.* New York: Raven Press; 1989.
150. Berquist TH. *MRI of the musculoskeletal system.* 2nd ed. New York: Raven Press; 1990.
151. Canale ST, Kelly FB. Fractures of the neck of the talus. *J Bone Joint Surg* [*Am*] 1978;60A:143–156.
152. Carothers CO, Crenshaw AH. Clinical significance of classification of epiphyseal injuries of the ankle. *Am J Surg* 1955;89:879–889.
153. Cassebaum WH. Lisfranc fracture dislocations. *Clin Orthop* 1963;30:116–129.
154. Cooperman DR, Spiegel PG, Laros GS. Tibial fractures of the ankle in children. *J Bone Joint Surg* [*Am*] 1978;60A:1040–1045.
155. DeZwart DF, Davidson JSA. Rupture of the posterior tibial tendon associated with fractures of the ankle. *J Bone Joint Surg* [*Am*] 1983;65A:260–262.
156. Dias LS, Giegerich CR. Fractures of the distal tibial epiphysis in adolescence. *J Bone Joint Surg* [*Am*] 1983;65A:438–444.
157. Etter C, Ganz R. Long-term results of tibial plafond fractures treated with open reduction and internal fixation. *Arch Orthop Trauma Surg* 1991;110:277–283.
158. Griffiths HJ, Utz R, Burke J, Bonfiglio T. Adhesive capsulitis of the hip and ankle. *AJR Am J Roentgenol* 1985;144:101–105.
159. Hawkins LG. Fractures of the neck of the talus. *J Bone Joint Surg* [*Am*] 1970;52A:991–1002.
160. Jenkins D, Campbell LG. Synovial chondromatosis of the ankle. *J Am Podiatry Assoc* 1981;71:666–670.
161. Lorentzen JE, Christiansen SB, Krogsoe O, Snepper O. Fractures of the neck of the talus. *Acta Orthop Scand* 1977;48:115–120.
162. Mindell EB, Cisek EE, Kartalian G, Dziab JM. Late results of injuries of the talus. *J Bone Joint Surg* [*Am*] 1963;45A:221–245.
163. Morrey BF, Cass JR, Johnson KA, Berquist TH. Foot and ankle. In: Berquist TH, ed. *Imaging of orthopedic trauma.* 2nd ed. New York: Raven Press; 1992:453–578.
164. Myerson M, Quill E. Late complications of fractures of the calcaneus. *J Bone Joint Surg* [*Am*] 1993;85A:331–341.

165. Paley D, Hall H. Intra-articular fractures of the calcaneus. A critical analysis of results and prognostic factors. *J Bone Joint Surg [Am]* 1993;75A:342–354.
166. Pettrone FA, Gail M, Pu D, Fitzpatrick T, VanHerpe LB. Quantitative criteria for prediction of results of displaced fracture of the ankle. *J Bone Joint Surg [Am]* 1983;65A:667–677.
167. Salter RB, Harris WR. Injuries involving the physeal plate. *J Bone Joint Surg [Am]* 1963;45A:587–622.
168. Slone RM, Heare MM, VanderGriend RA, Montgomery WJ. Orthopedic fixation devices. *Radiographics* 1991;11:823–847.
169. Spiegel PG, Cooperman DR, Laros GS. Epiphyseal fractures of the distal ends of the tibia and fibula. *J Bone Joint Surg [Am]* 1978;60A:1046–1050.
170. Wiley JJ. Tarsometatarsal joint injuries in children. *J Pediatr Orthop* 1981;1:255–260.

Joint Reconstruction

171. Bolton-Maggs BG, Sudlow RA, Freeman MAR. Total ankle arthroplasty: a long-term review of the London Hospital experience. *J Bone Joint Surg [Br]* 1985;67B:785–790.
172. Broughton NS, Doran A, Meggitt BF. Silastic ball spacer arthroplasty in management of hallux valgus and hallus rigidus. *Foot Ankle* 1990;10:61–64.
173. Buechel FF, Pappas MJ, Iorio LJ. New Jersey low contact stress total ankle replacement: biomechanical rationale and review of 23 cementless cases. *Foot Ankle* 1988;8:279–290.
174. Burge P, Evans M. Effect of surface replacement arthroplasty or stability of the ankle. *Foot Ankle* 1986;7:10–17.
175. Cracchiolo A III, Kitaoka HB, Leventen EO. Silicone implant arthroplasty for second metatarsophalangeal joint disorders with and without hallux valgus deformities. *Foot Ankle* 1988;9:10–18.
176. Cracchiolo A III, Weltmer JB, Lian G, Dalseth T, Dorey F. Arthroplasty of the first metatarsophalangeal joint. *J Bone Joint Surg [Am]* 1992;74A:552–563.
177. Cuckler JM, Rhoad RC. Alternatives to hip, knee and ankle arthroplasty. *Curr Opin Rheumatol* 1991;3:81–87.
178. Demottaz JB, Mazur JM, Thomas WH, Sledge CB, Simon SR. Clinical study of total ankle replacement with gait analysis. A preliminary report. *J Bone Joint Surg* 1979;61:976.
179. Dini AA, Bassett FH III. Evaluation of the early results of Smith total ankle replacement. *Clin Orthop* 1980;146:228–230.
180. Granberry WM, Noble PC, Bishop JO, Tullos HS. Use of a hinged silicone prosthesis for replacement arthroplasty of the first metatarsophalangeal joint. *J Bone Joint Surg [Am]* 1991;73A: 1453–1459.
181. Grumbue NA, Santoro JP, Chinn ES. Continuous passive motion following partial ankle joint arthroplasty. *J Foot Surg* 1990;29:557–566.
182. Helal B, Chen SC. Arthroplastik dis grosszehen Grundgelenks mit einer neuen Silastik-Endoprostheses. *Orthopade* 1982;11: 200–206.
183. Hensley JP. Anterior ankle arthroplasty. *Clin Podiatr Med Surg* 1991;8:625–635.
184. Hensley JP, Saltrick K, Le T. Anterior ankle arthroplasty. A retrospective study. *J Foot Surg* 1990;29:169–172.
185. Johnson KA. Total ankle arthroplasty. In: Berquist TH, ed. *Imaging of orthopedic trauma and surgery.* Philadelphia: WB Saunders; 1986:491–494.
186. Johnson KA. Total joint arthroplasty. The foot. *Mayo Clin Proc* 1979;54:576–578.
187. Johnson KA. Ankle replacement arthroplasty. In: Morrey BF, ed. *Joint replacement arthroplasty.* New York: Churchill Livingstone; 1991:1173–1182.
188. Johnson KA, Buck PG. Total replacement arthroplasty of the first metatarsophalangeal joint. *Foot Ankle* 1981;1:307–314.
189. Kabra SG. Articulated cadaveric bones as a structural endoskeleton in an ankle-foot prosthesis: a preliminary report. *J Rehabil Res Dev* 1990;27:43–52.
190. Kampner SL. Long-term experience with total joint prosthetic replacement for the arthritic great toe. *Bull Hosp Jt Dis Orthop Inst* 1987;47:153–177.
191. Kirkup J. Rheumatoid arthritis and ankle surgery. *R Natl Hosp Rheum Dis* 1990;49:837–844.
192. Kitaoka HB. Historical perspective of foot and ankle arthroplasty. In: Morrey BF, ed. *Joint replacement arthroplasty.* New York: Churchill Livingstone; 1991:1157–1171.
193. Kitaoka HB, Cracchiolo A III. Stress fracture of the lateral metatarsal following double-stemmed silicone implant arthroplasty of the hallux metatarsophalangeal joint. *Clin Orthop* 1989;239:211–215.
194. Kitaoka HB, Patzer GL, Ilstrup DM, Mallricks SL. Survivorship analysis of Mayo total ankle arthroplasties. *J Bone Joint Surg [in press]*.
195. Kitaoka HB, Romness DW. Arthrodesis for failed ankle arthroplasty. *J Arthroplasty* 1992;7:277–284.
196. Laird L. Silastic joint arthroplasty of the great toe. A review of 228 implants using double stemmed implant. *Clin Orthop* 1990;255: 268–272.
197. McMaster WC. Total ankle arthroplasty. *Adv Orthop Surg* 1986;9:264–272.
198. Merkel PF, Sculco TP. Prosthetic replacement of the first metatarsophalangeal joint. *Foot Ankle* 1989;9:267–271.
199. Moeckel BH, Sculco TP, Alexiades MM, Dossick PA, Inglis AE, Ranawat CS. The double stemmed silicone-rubber implant for rheumatoid arthritis of the first metatarsophalangeal joint. *J Bone Joint Surg [Am]* 1992;74A:564–570.
200. Newton SE. Total ankle arthroplasty. *J Bone Joint Surg [Am]* 1982;64A:104.
201. Pappas M, Buechel F, DePalma AF. Cylindrical total ankle joint replacement. *Clin Orthop* 1976;118:82.
202. Scholz KC. Total ankle arthroplasty using biological fixation components compared to ankle arthrodesis. *Orthopedics* 1987;10:125–131.
203. Smith EJ, Wood PLR. Ankle arthrodesis in rheumatoid patient. *J Bone Joint Surg [Br]* 1990;72B:530.
204. Smith SR, Morgan CG, Pinder IM. Results and complications of ankle arthrodesis. *J Bone Joint Surg [Br]* 1990;72B:530.
205. Stauffer RN. Total joint arthroplasty. The ankle. *Mayo Clin Proc* 1979;54:570–757.
206. Stockley I, Betts RP, Getty CJ, Rowley DI, Duckworth T. A prospective study of forefoot arthroplasty. *Clin Orthop* 1989;248: 213–218.
207. Swanson AB, Lunsden RM, Swanson G. Silicone implant arthroplasty of the great toe. A review of single stem and flexible hinge implants. *Clin Orthop* 1979;142:30–43.
208. Takakura Y, Tanaka Y, Sugimoto K, Tamai S, Masuhara K. Ankle arthroplasty: a comparative study of cemented metal and uncemented ceramic prosthesis. *Clin Orthop* 1990;252:209–216.
209. Weissman BN, Sledge CB. *Orthopedic radiology.* Philadelphia: WB Saunders; 1986.
210. Wynn AH, Wilde AH. Long-term follow-up of the conaxial (Beck-Steffee) total ankle arthroplasty. *Foot Ankle* 1992;13:303–306.

Arthrodesis and Miscellaneous Procedures

211. Alexander IJ, Kotschi H. Redirecting K-wires and Steinmann pins. *Foot Ankle* 1990;10:243.
212. Berquist TH. *Radiology of the foot and ankle.* New York: Raven Press; 1989.
213. Berquist TH. Diagnostic and therapeutic injections as an aid to musculoskeletal diagnosis. *Semin Intervent Radiol* 1993;10:326–343.
214. Berquist TH. *MRI of the musculoskeletal system.* New York: Raven Press; 1990.
215. Carrier DA, Harris CM. Ankle arthrodesis with Steinmann pins in rheumatoid arthritis. *Clin Orthop* 1991;268:10–14.
216. Coughlin MJ. Juvenile bunions. In: Mann RA, Coughlin MJ, eds. *Surgery of the foot and ankle.* 6th ed. St. Louis: CV Mosby-Year Book; 1993:297–340.
217. Cracchiolo A III. Surgical arthrodesis techniques for foot and ankle pathology. *Instr Course Lect* 1990;39:49–63.

218. Cracchiolo A III. Hindfoot arthrodesis in adults utilizing a dowel graft technique. *Clin Orthop* 1990;251:193–203.
219. Dennis DA, Clayton ML, Wong DA, Mack RP, Susiman MH. Internal fixation compression arthrodesis of the ankle. *Clin Orthop* 1990;253:212–220.
220. Grace DL, Cracchiolo A. A method of evaluating results of forefoot surgery. *Clin Orthop* 1985;198:208.
221. Graves SC, Mann RA, Graves KO. Triple arthrodesis in older adults. *J Bone Joint Surg [Am]* 1993;75A:355–362.
222. Gruen GS, Mears DC. Arthrodesis of the ankle and subtalar joints. *Clin Orthop* 1991;268:15–20.
223. Helm R. The results of ankle arthrodesis. *J Bone Joint Surg [Br]* 1990;72B:141–143.
224. Holt ES, Hansen ST, Mayo KA, Sangeorzan BJ. Ankle arthrodesis using internal screw fixation. *Clin Orthop* 1991;268:21–28.
225. Johnsson EE, Weltmen J, Lian GJ, Cracchiolo A. Ilizarov ankle arthrodesis. *Clin Orthop* 1992;280:160–169.
226. Kitaoka HB, Anderson PJ, Morrey BF. Revision of ankle arthrodesis with external fixation for nonunion. *J Bone Joint Surg [Am]* 1992;74A:1191–1200.
227. Kitaoka HB, Romness DW. Arthrodesis for failed ankle arthroplasty. *J Arthroplasty* 1992;7:277–284.
228. Malarkey RF, Binski JC. Ankle arthrodesis with Calandruccio frame and bimalleolar only grafting. *Clin Orthop* 1991;268:44–48.
229. Mann RA, Coughlin MJ. *Surgery of the foot and ankle.* 6th ed. St. Louis: CV Mosby-Year Book; 1993.
230. Mann RA, VanMonen JW, Wapner KL, et al. Ankle fusion. *Clin Orthop* 1991;268:49–55.
231. Mazur JM, Schwartz E, Simon SR. Ankle arthrodesis. Long term follow-up with quit analysis. *J Bone Joint Surg [Am]* 1979;61A:964–975.
232. Mears DC, Gordon RG, Kann SE, Kann JN. Ankle arthrodesis with an anterior tension plate. *Clin Orthop* 1991;268:70–77.
233. Moeckel BH, Patterson BM, Inglis AE, Sculco TP. Ankle arthrodesis: a comparison of internal and external fixation. *Clin Orthop* 1991;268:78–83.
234. Morrey BF, Wiedeman GP Jr. Complications and long-term results of ankle arthrodesis following trauma. *J Bone Joint Surg [Am]* 1980;62A:777–784.
235. Weltmer JB, Choi SH, Shenoy A, Schwartsman V. Wolfe blade plate ankle arthrodesis. *Clin Orthop* 1991;268:107–111.
236. Wertheimer SJ. Role of epiphysiodesis in the management of deformities of the foot and ankle. *J Foot Surg* 1990;29:459–462.

Imaging Atlas of Orthopedic Appliances and Prostheses,
edited by T.H. Berquist.
Mayo Clinic Foundation © 1995.
Published by Raven Press, Ltd., New York.

CHAPTER 9

The Shoulder

Thomas H. Berquist and James K. DeOrio

Imaging of shoulder disorders has been facilitated by computed tomography (CT), arthrography, and magnetic resonance imaging (MRI). This section stresses pre- and postoperative imaging techniques for shoulder trauma, arthroplasty, and arthrodesis and other surgical procedures. Techniques using instrumentation are emphasized. The indications for specific modalities are discussed with each category of procedure.

IMAGING TECHNIQUES

There are numerous invasive and noninvasive imaging techniques for the evaluation of shoulder disorders.[4,27,32,47] Routine radiography remains the primary screening technique.[6] Selection of the appropriate projections is essential to document the anatomy and pathologic condition.[2,4,12,17,26,29,55]

Routine Radiography

Standard and, when appropriate, special radiographic views provide most of the information required to evaluate osseous pathologic disorders in the shoulder. A demonstration of shoulder anatomy requires a minimum of two to three radiographic projections. We prefer the anteroposterior (AP), axillary, and scapular "Y" views for trauma or screening of shoulder pathologic conditions (Fig. 9-1).[3,4,16,22,37,38,46,61,64,66] We frequently add the supraspinatus outlet view to our standard series to see the anterior acromion in profile. This is obtained in a manner similar to the scapular Y view, but the tube is angled 15° to the feet (Fig. 9-2).

The AP view should be obtained with the patient rotated 40° to 45° posteriorly to assess the glenohumeral joint more accurately. These two structures overlap on the standard nonrotated AP view (Fig. 9-3).[3,4,29]

The transthoracic view is an alternative to the scapular Y view, and it can be combined with the AP view to achieve the obligatory minimal two views at 90° (Fig. 9-4).[4,11]

Special views of the shoulder may be indicated in some clinical situations or when the lesion is not clearly identified on standard views.[4,12,64,66,70] These views are designed to visualize more subtle glenoid lesions, Hill-Sachs deformities, calcifications, or other subtle fractures.[4,38,49] Hill-Sachs lesions may be more easily identified on internal rotation views or special views, such as the West Point view or Stryker notch view.[4,60,65] The West Point view is a prone axillary view with the arm abducted 90° and the forearm hanging off the radiographic table. The x-ray tube is positioned with the central ray projecting 25° medially and 25° off the horizontal.[60] This view is especially useful for the identification of anterior glenoid rim abnormalities in patients with instability.[4]

The Stryker notch view is most useful for identifying Hill-Sachs lesions. The patient is supine with the hand adjacent to or on top of the head and the elbow directly vertically. The central beam is angled 10° cephalad and centered on the coracoid. This technique detects nearly 90% of Hill-Sachs lesions.[4]

Other oblique views have been introduced more recently.[26,42] The apical oblique view[26] is obtained with the patient sitting or supine with the involved shoulder rotated posteriorly 45°, which is similar to the true AP view. The central beam is centered on the shoulder and

(text continues on page 665)

T. H. Berquist: Mayo Medical School and Department of Diagnostic Radiology, Mayo Clinic Jacksonville, Jacksonville, Florida 32224.

J. K. DeOrio: Mayo Medical School and Department of Orthopedics, Mayo Clinic Jacksonville, Jacksonville, Florida 32224.

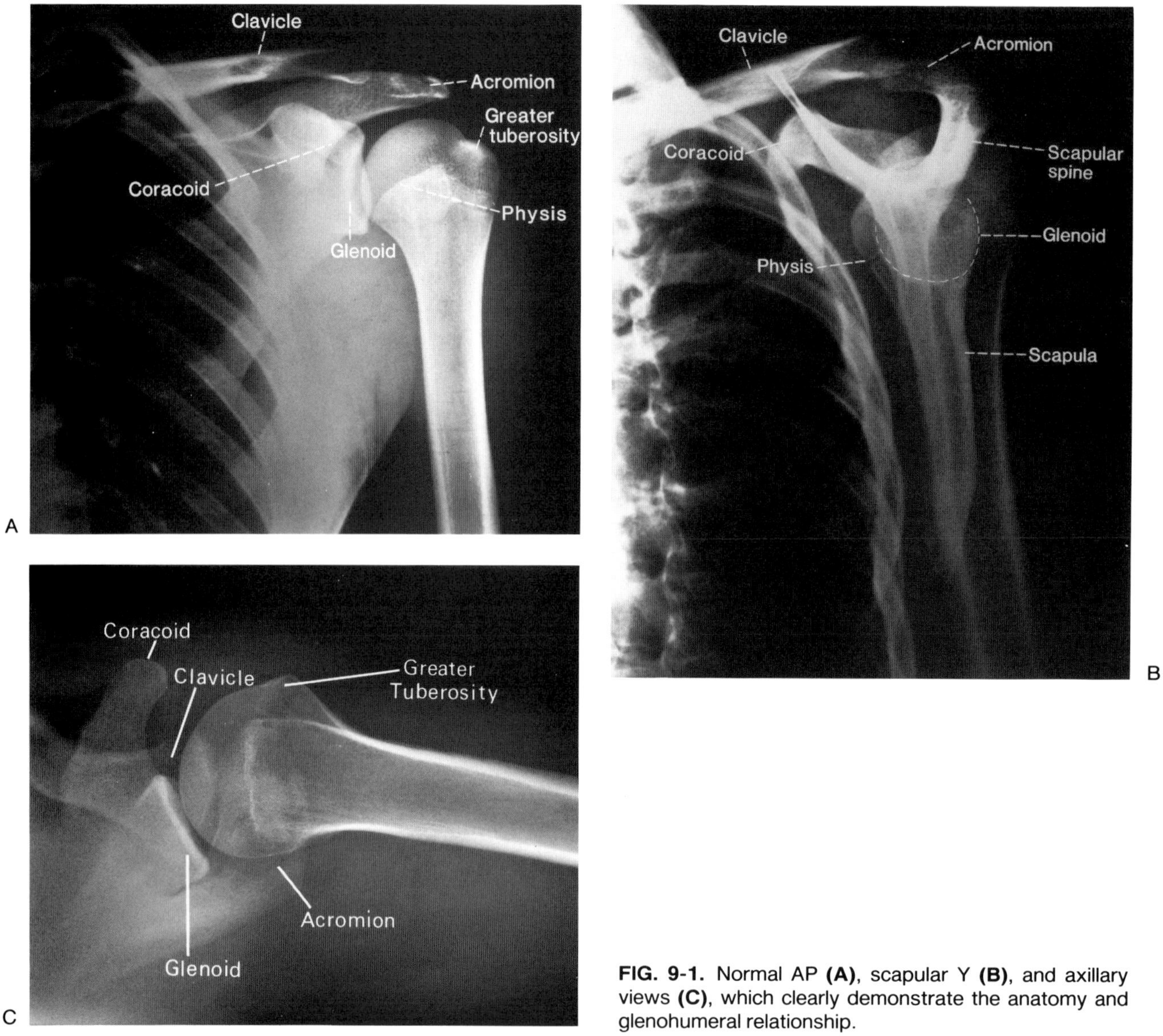

FIG. 9-1. Normal AP **(A)**, scapular Y **(B)**, and axillary views **(C)**, which clearly demonstrate the anatomy and glenohumeral relationship.

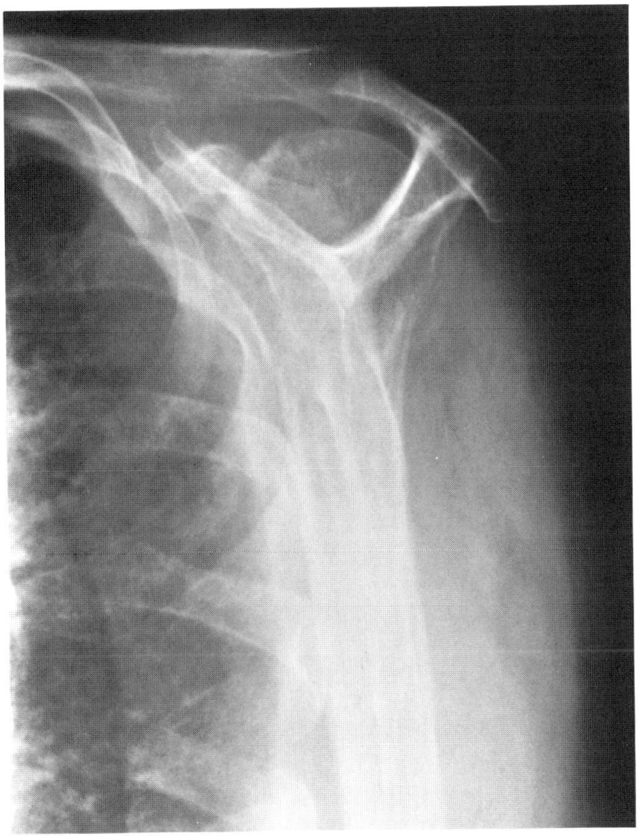

FIG. 9-2. Supraspinatus outlet view demonstrating the acromial configuration (curved type 2), distal clavicle, and humeroacromial relationship.

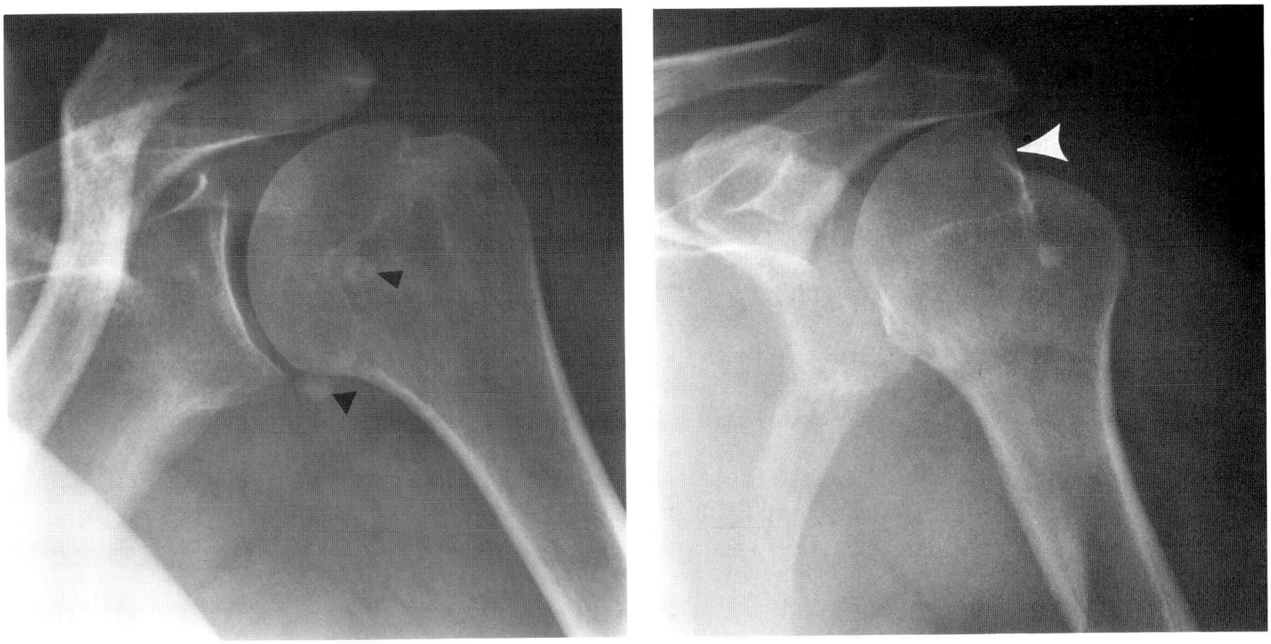

A B

FIG. 9-3. A: True AP view (rotated posteriorly 45°) of the left shoulder demonstrating the glenohumeral joint. There are two loose bodies (*arrow*). **B:** Standard AP in internal rotation demonstrates the Hill-Sachs deformity (*arrow*), but the glenohumeral joint is not seen *en face*.

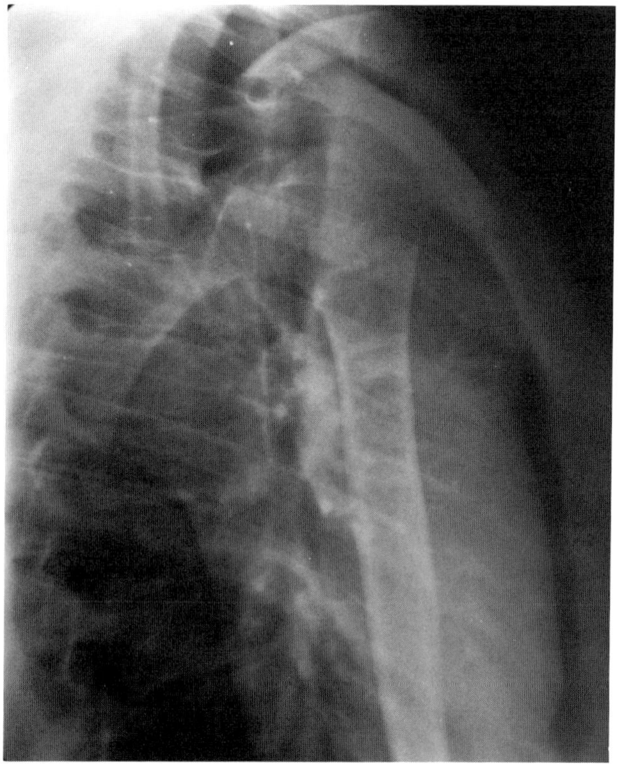

FIG. 9-4. Normal transthoracic view of the shoulder and upper humerus.

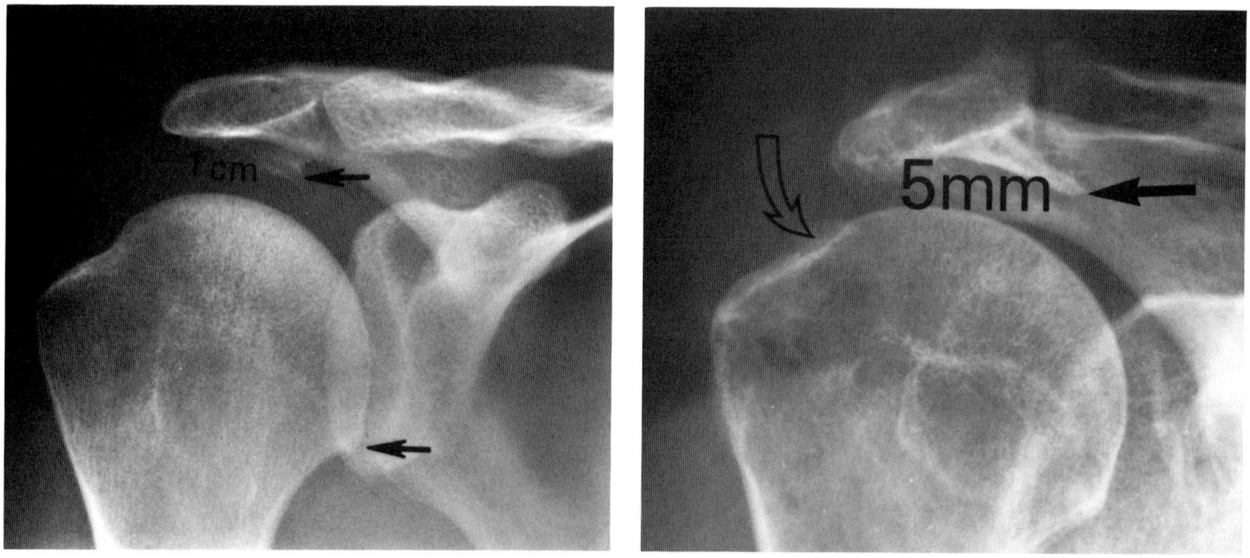

A B

FIG. 9-5. A: An AP view of the shoulder using standard (not angled 45°) technique. The humeroacromial space is 1 cm (normal, ≥0.7 cm). However, there are subacromial spurs (*upper arrow*) and early inferior eburnation at the inferior margin of the humeral head (*lower arrow*). **B:** An AP view of the shoulder in a patient with a chronic rotator cuff tear. The humeroacromial space is reduced to 5 mm, and there are acromioclavicular joint spurs (*black arrow*) and greater tuberosity new bone formation (*open curved arrow*).

angled 45° inferiorly. This view provides a coronal profile of the glenohumeral joint for more accurate detection of intraarticular fractures, Hill-Sachs lesions, and glenoid injuries.[26] Acromial changes may be more easily assessed using an AP oblique view, with the tube angled 30° caudad. This technique is useful for detecting subtle subacromial abnormalities in patients with suspected impingement.[17,41]

Routine radiographic projections are useful in the detection of numerous abnormalities, including rotator cuff tears.[4,67] A simple evaluation of the secondary bone changes and humeroacromial space can provide valuable information (Fig. 9-5).[4,13,18,21] Fluoroscopy can be used for positioning in difficult cases.[4,53]

Localized views of the clavicle, scapula, and sternoclavicular joints are also obtained when necessary. These views are described in the trauma section as they apply to specific injuries and orthopedic procedures.[7,36,37]

Conventional Tomography or CT

Currently, CT has largely replaced conventional linear or complex-motion tomography in the assessment of the shoulder.[4,14,33] Alone or combined with arthrography, CT is useful for the detection of subtle osseous or articular pathologic conditions,[4,10,19,20,43,47] and it provides excellent bone and soft tissue detail to assess trauma (Fig. 9-6), labral pathologic disorders (Fig. 9-7), and bone stock, which needs to be evaluated prior to orthopedic implant positioning or selection.[4,14,51,63]

Ultrasonography

The role of ultrasonography in the evaluation of shoulder disorders is evolving. Early studies demonstrated features associated with rotator cuff tears, including motion patterns of the supraspinatus and echo patterns within the tendon substance. Rotator cuff tears typically have four patterns: (1) focal cuff thinning, (2) nonvisualization of the cuff, (3) discontinuity of echo patterns, and (4) a central echogenic band in the substance of the tendon.[8,32,49] As experience with this technique has increased, the applications have expanded to include biceps tendon disorders.

The accuracy reports for rotator cuff tears range from 63% to 94%, depending on the author; the results are superior at those institutions that use this modality daily and when done by operators who have sound anatomic knowledge and consistent technique.[8,9,49]

MRI

In particular, MRI is useful in the shoulder because of its ability to detect lesions in the rotator cuff and abnormalities in the glenohumeral joint, acromioclavicular joint, osseous lesions, and periarticular soft tissue abnormalities.[5,40,56] Small or partial cuff tears may not be as accurately detected without some type of intraarticular contrast agent (normal saline, iodinated contrast, or gadolinium). Also motion and/or stress studies are not as easy to perform with MRI techniques.[4]

The techniques and pulse sequences used for shoulder examinations vary to some degree, depending on the suspected abnormality. For screening purposes, we typically obtain axial and oblique coronal T2-weighted images (spin-echo [SE] 2,000/80, 20) with or without fat suppression. New fast T2-weighted sequences or T2* gradient-echo sequences can also be used. Sagittal images are useful to evaluate impingement, acromial configuration, and marrow abnormalities in the humeral head (Figs. 9-8 and 9-9).[5,40,56,71,72]

On T2- or T2*-weighted images, the signal intensity is increased in the areas of abnormality (Fig. 9-9), providing excellent contrast between tendon and cuff tears.[5,71,72] Increasing the signal intensity between the first and second echoes of a T2-weighted sequence is helpful in differentiating granulation tissue from a true tear (which increases on the second echo).[5]

Marrow abnormalities are easily appreciated on T1-weighted SE or short TI-inversion recovery sequences.

The accuracy of MRI in the detection of full-thickness rotator cuff tears is > 90%. Compared with double-contrast arthrography, both MRI and the arthrographic technique demonstrated sensitivities of 92% and specificities of 100% for normal rotator cuffs.[9,71,72]

Arthrography, Bursography, and Diagnostic and Therapeutic Injections

Arthrography is still a useful technique pre- and postoperatively.[4,6,10,24,30,34] Capsular abnormalities, loose bodies, subtle synovial changes, and complete and partial rotator cuff tears can be evaluated (Fig. 9-10).[4,30,52,54,60] Postoperatively, arthrography with a subtraction technique (see Chapter 1, Fig. 9-11) is useful for the detection of subtle loosening and to obtain fluid for culture in patients with suspected infections. In patients without a joint prosthesis, we routinely obtain internal and external rotation AP views, both prone and supine axillary views, and stress or weight-bearing views to assess instability (Fig. 9-12).[4,25] When the subtraction technique is used, we usually position the patient with the shoulder in a neutral position or in external rotation. The patient must not move until the injection is completed and the postinjection film is obtained. Routine and stress views can then be obtained as appropriate.[4,15,25,43] Arthrography can also be combined with CT in patients with suspected instability (Fig. 9-7).[35,48]

Distention arthrography can be used to assist with the treatment of patients with mild to moderate adhesive

(text continues on page 671)

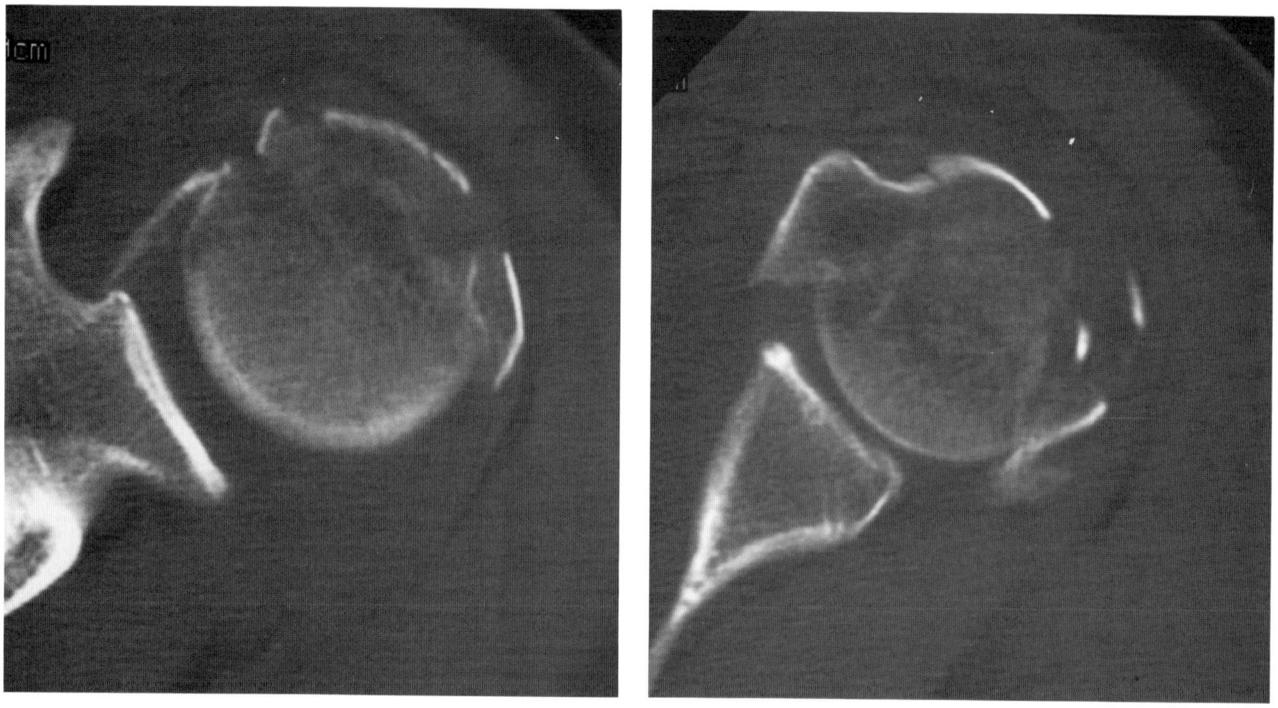

A B

FIG. 9-6. A,B: Axial CT images of a complex humeral head and neck fracture. There is no glenoid involvement; CT is particularly useful to evaluate the glenoid and scapula.

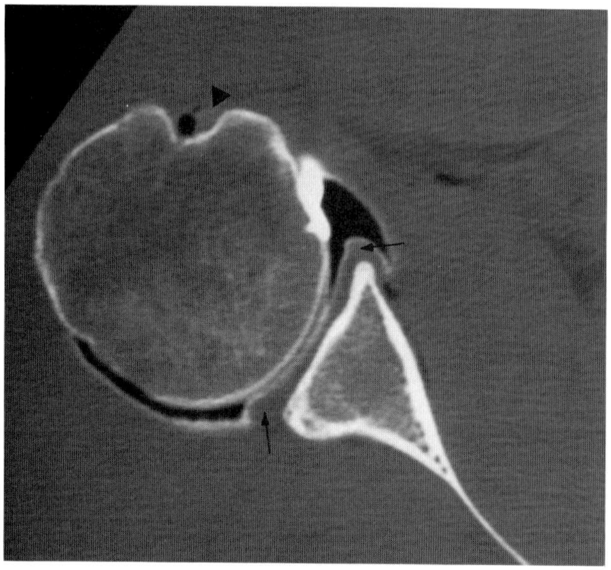

FIG. 9-7. Double-contrast CT arthrogram demonstrating the normal glenoid labrum (*arrows*) and biceps tendon (*arrowhead*).

A

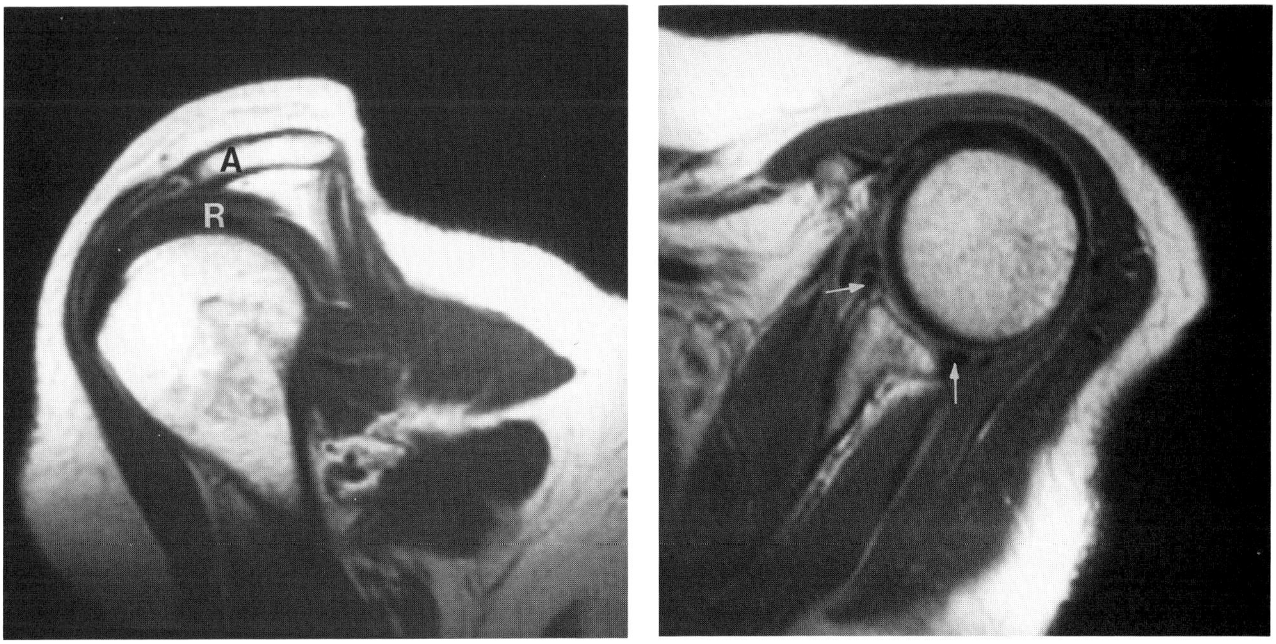

B

FIG. 9-8. Sagittal **(A)** and axial **(B)** SE 500/15 images of the shoulder demonstrating the rotator cuff (*R*) and anterior angulated acromion (*A*) in A. The normal appearance of the glenoid labrum is demonstrated (*arrows*) on the axial image (B).

A

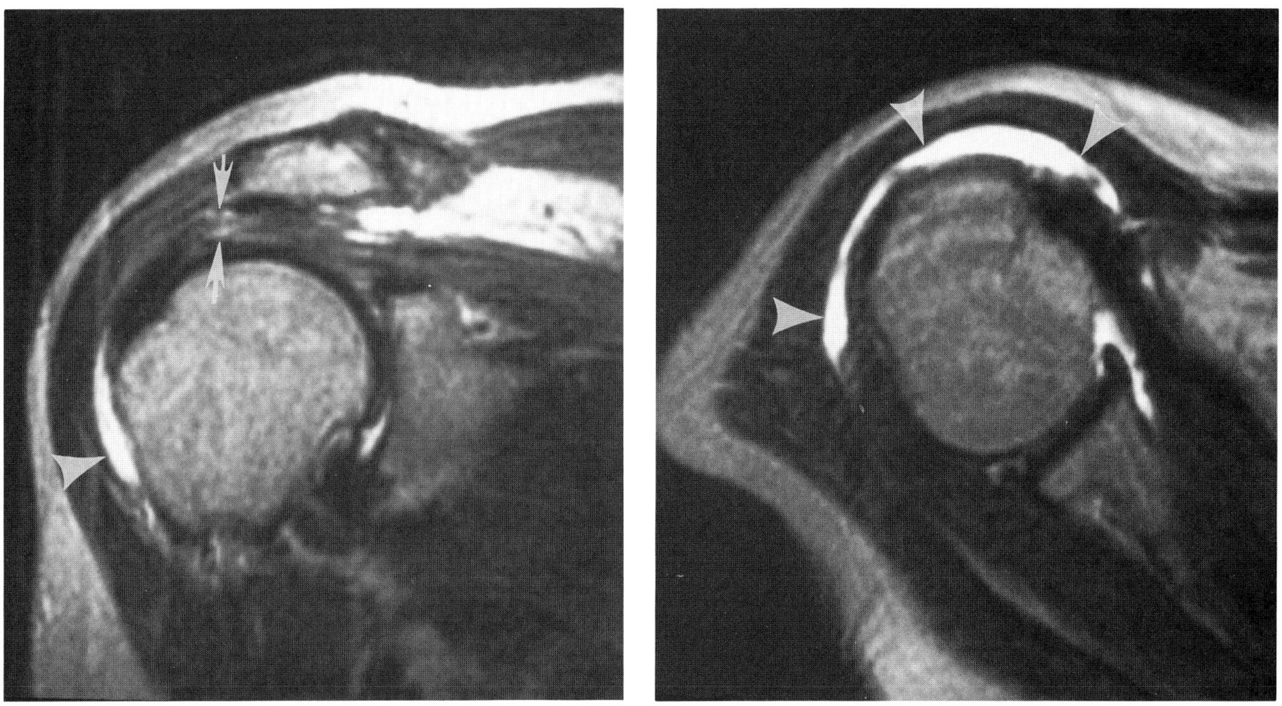

B

FIG. 9-9. Coronal **(A)** and axial **(B)** T2-weighted SE 2,000/80 images demonstrating a small irregular rotator cuff tear (*arrows*) with increased signal caused by fluid in the subdeltoid bursa (*arrowheads*).

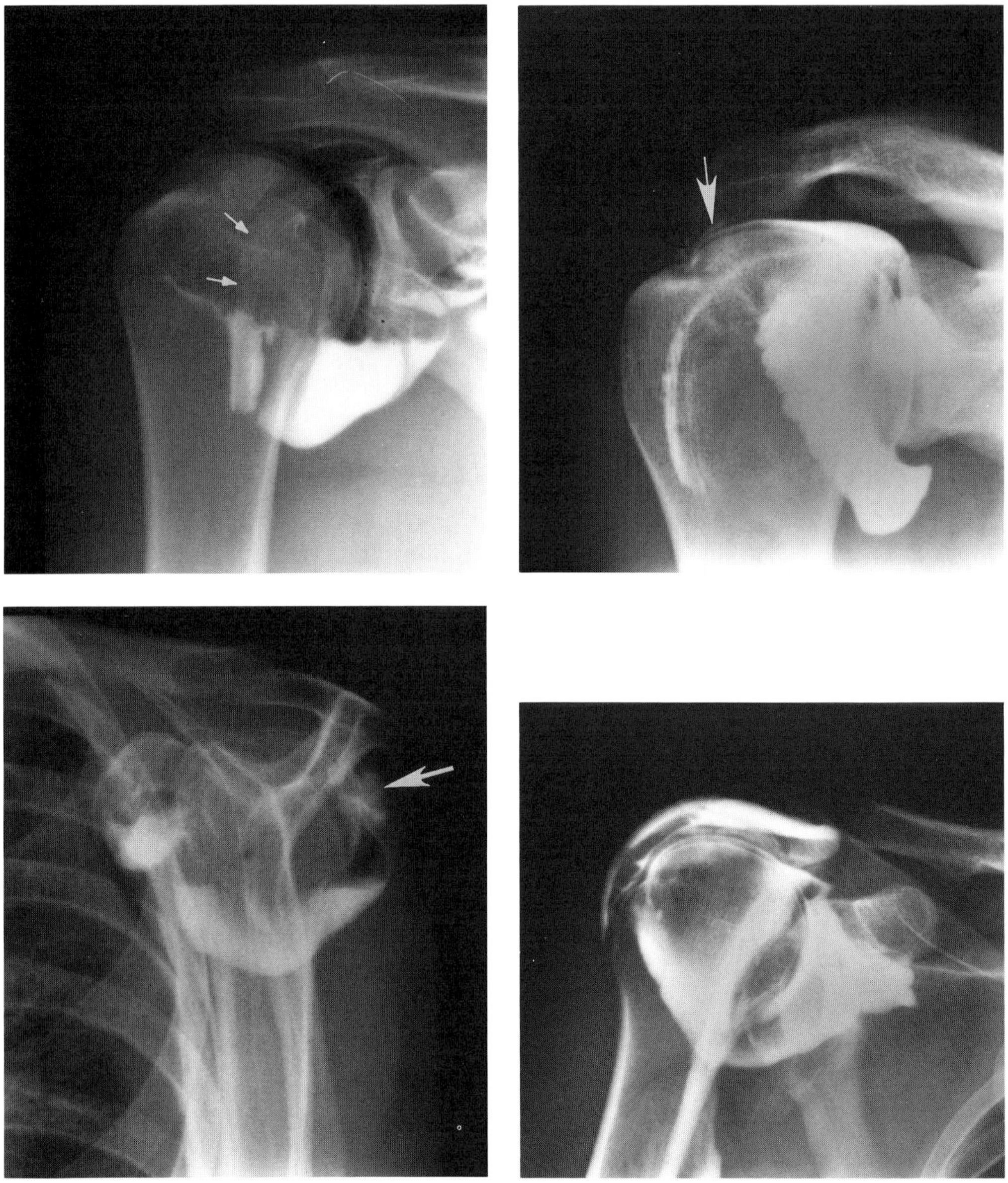

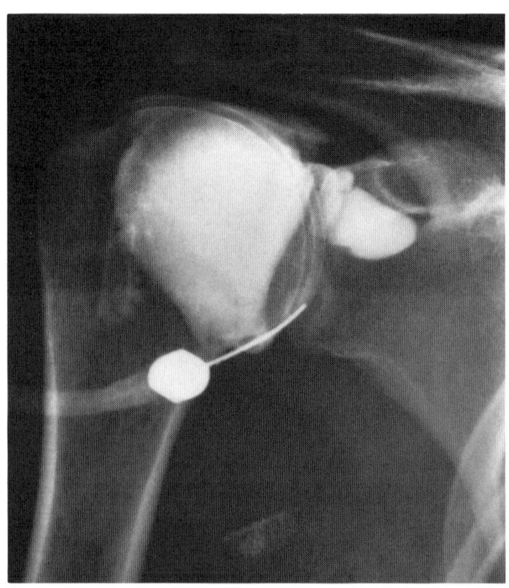

FIG. 9-10. Arthrography. **A:** Normal double-contrast arthrogram with internal rotation. Note the biceps tendon (*arrows*) and normal capsular volume. **B:** External rotation view with a small peripheral partial tear (*arrow*). **C:** Scapular Y view with a partial tear more posteriorly (*arrow*). **D:** Complete rotator cuff tear with contrast in the subacromial and subdeltoid bursae. **E:** Single-contrast arthrogram demonstrating moderate adhesive capsulitis with decreased capsular volume.

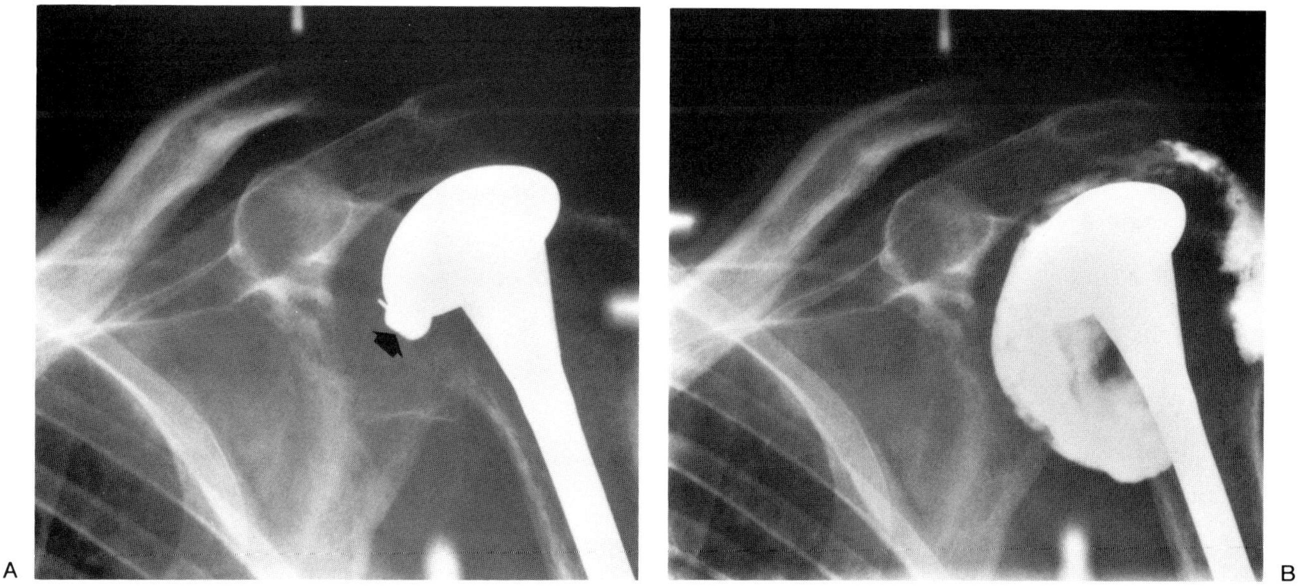

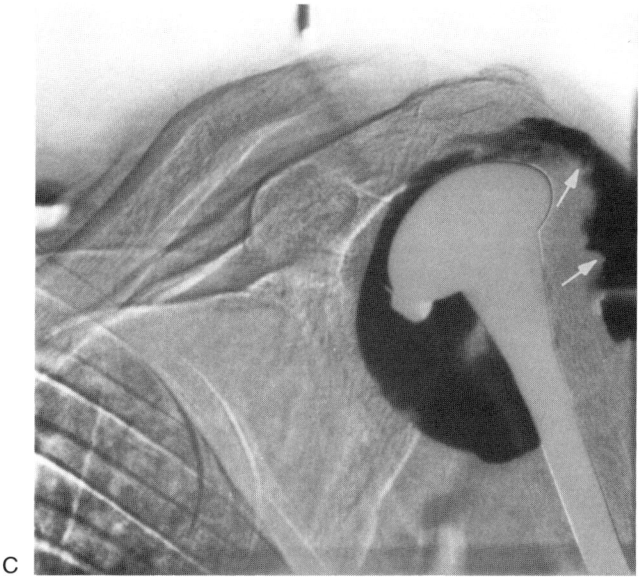

FIG. 9-11. Subtraction arthrogram and fluid aspiration after shoulder endoprosthesis in a patient with a low-grade infection. **A:** Preinjection film (mask) with needle (*arrow*) in place. **B:** Postinjection film taken with patient motionless between A and B. **C:** Subtraction film demonstrating a large capsule with synovial proliferation (*arrows*) but no evidence of loosening.

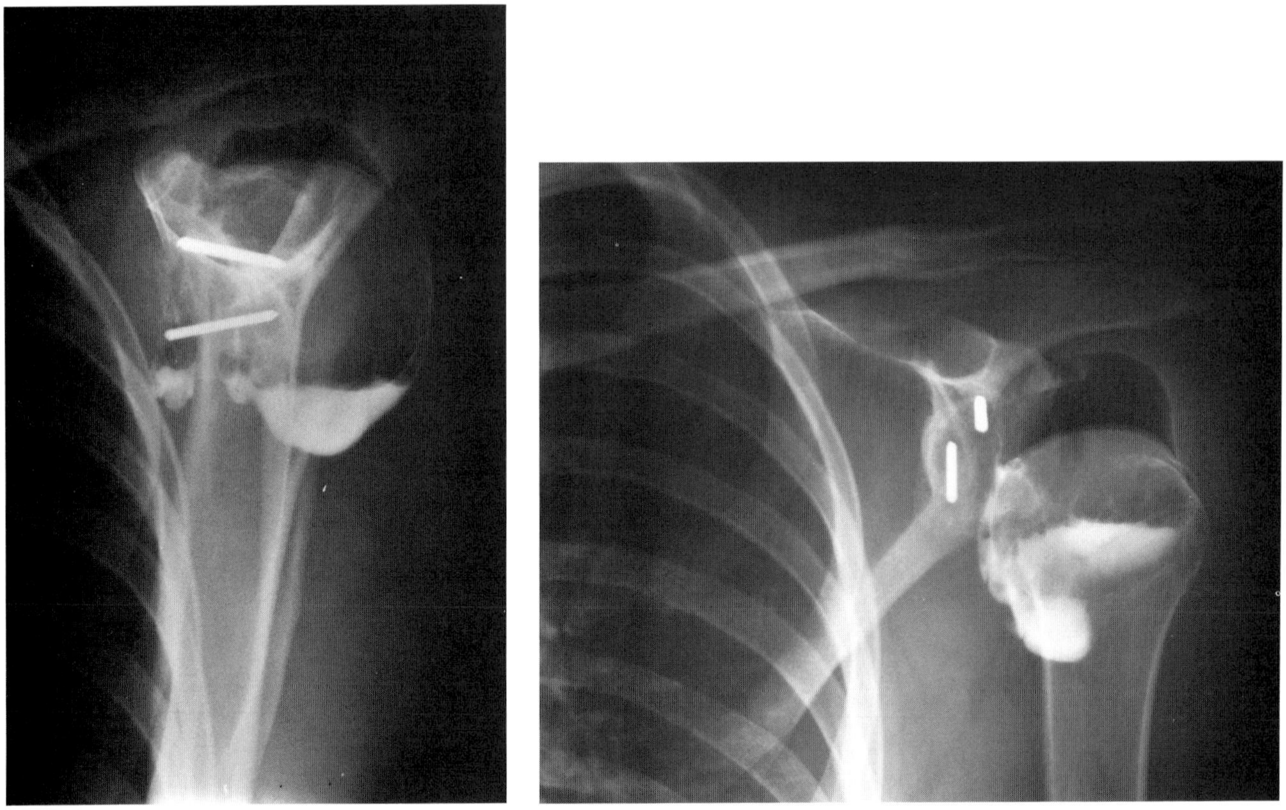

A B

FIG. 9-12. Postoperative anterior repair with two pins anteriorly, continued pain, and questionable instability. Scapular Y view **(A)** and stress view **(B)** demonstrate anterior capsular deformity and subluxation (B).

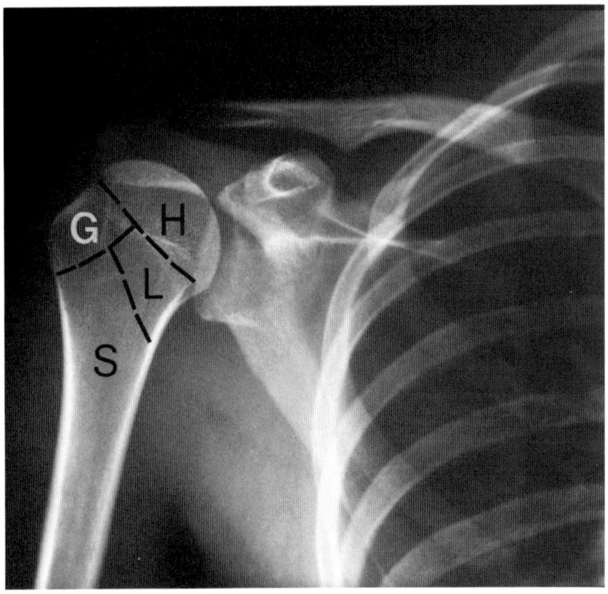

FIG. 9-13. Radiograph of the shoulder demonstrating the typical lines of fracture and segments in proximal humeral injuries. *H,* head; *G,* greater tuberosity; *L,* lesser tuberosity; *S,* shaft.

capsulitis (Fig. 9-10E).[1] The joint is gradually distended with Marcaine™ (Sanofi Winthrop, New York, NY) or Xylocaine™ (Astra, Westborough, MA) and contrast medium to evaluate the progress of the technique. The procedure is terminated when the capsule begins to extravasate the contrast agent. Celestone™ (Schering, Kenilworth, NJ) can be added if necessary.[1,6,28,52,57–59]

Arthrography does not evaluate the upper surface of the rotator cuff. Therefore, some authors advocate performing bursography in patients with normal arthrograms to define the bursa and upper aspect of the rotator cuff.[6,23,45,50,59,65,69] Diagnostic injections of the bursa or acromioclavicular joint can also be performed to localize the site of symptoms prior to instituting therapy.[7,48,68]

Arthrograms and diagnostic and therapeutic injections are invasive but safe techniques with low complication rates.[4,6,31]

Other diagnostic techniques, such as venography and angiography, are most frequently used in acute trauma with suspected vascular injury or to evaluate postoperative complications.[4]

TRAUMA

Some fractures and fracture-dislocations can be treated conservatively with closed reduction. Surgical intervention with implants that must be evaluated radiographically is stressed in this section. The classification categories are also important to understand because they apply to the selection of treatment methods.

Proximal Humeral Fractures

Fractures of the proximal humerus are common in elderly patients and account for about 5% of all fractures. The injury is usually due to a minor fall.[84,95,108,150] Fractures tend to follow the physeal lines that divide the humerus into four parts: the head, shaft, greater tuberosity, and lesser tuberosity (Fig. 9-13).[81,93] Neer[137] proposed the most commonly used classification, which is based on the number of segments and angular deformities.[118,119] The fragments are considered displaced if there is 1 cm or more of displacement or greater than 45° of angular deformity. Most (80% to 85%) fractures are undisplaced. A summary of the Neer classification and the incidence of injuries follows.[81,137]

One-part fracture, undisplaced or no segment displaced, 80%

Two-part fracture, one segment displaced in relation to other three (Fig. 9-14), 13%

Three-part fracture, two segments displaced in relation to the other two, 3%

Four-part fracture, all fragments displaced (Fig. 9-15), 4%

The AO classification is a modification of the Neer classification. This system is based on the vascular supply and likelihood of avascular necrosis (AVN).[84,113,134,150]

Type A, no vascular isolation of humeral head and AVN unlikely; extracapsular with two to four segments

Type B, partial isolation of the humeral head with a low probability for AVN

Type C, total isolation of the humeral head with a high risk for AVN

Both systems can be complex, with a high interobserver error.[161,162] We prefer the Neer classification used with only four categories described earlier.

Treatment

One- and two-part fractures can usually be treated with closed reduction.[109] The arm is immobilized with a sling or Velpeau immobilizer, followed by early mobilization to avoid adhesive capsulitis.[81,95,105,137]

Internal fixation is generally required to reduce and stabilize three-part fractures (Figs. 9-16 to 9-18).[105,133] Certain three-part fractures and most four-part fractures are treated with endoprostheses because of the high incidence of AVN (Fig. 9-19).[137]

The choice of fixation devices depends on the type of injury, patient's age, bone stock, and degree of soft tissue injury.[137,150] Kirschner wires (K wires, Fig. 9-18), screws (Fig. 9-17), or screw-plate systems (Fig. 9-20) may be used.[113,137,150] Medullary rods, such as Rush rods (Fig. 9-16), can be used, but rotation is a problem without proximal locking screws; impingement may also create symptoms necessitating removal.[133,150]

Clavicle Fractures

Clavicle fractures occur commonly, especially in children (Fig. 9-21). The injury is usually due to a fall with the hand outstretched or a direct blow transmitted through the shoulder.[81,138]

Most fractures occur in the midclavicle (80%). Allman[73] classified clavicle fractures by location. Group I fractures (80%) involve the middle third (Fig. 9-21), group II fractures involve the distal clavicle (lateral to the coracoclavicular ligament, 15%), and group III fractures involve the medial clavicle. The sternocleidomastoid muscle tends to elevate the proximal fragment, and the weight of the arm lowers the distal fragment.[73,138,177]

Radiographic evaluation of the middle and distal clavicle can be easily accomplished with AP and angled AP (15°, with 40° cephalad for subtle injuries) views (Fig. 9-22).[81] The medial clavicle is more difficult to evaluate because of overlying bone and soft tissue structures. Centering on the medial clavicle with the tube angled 40°

(text continues on page 678)

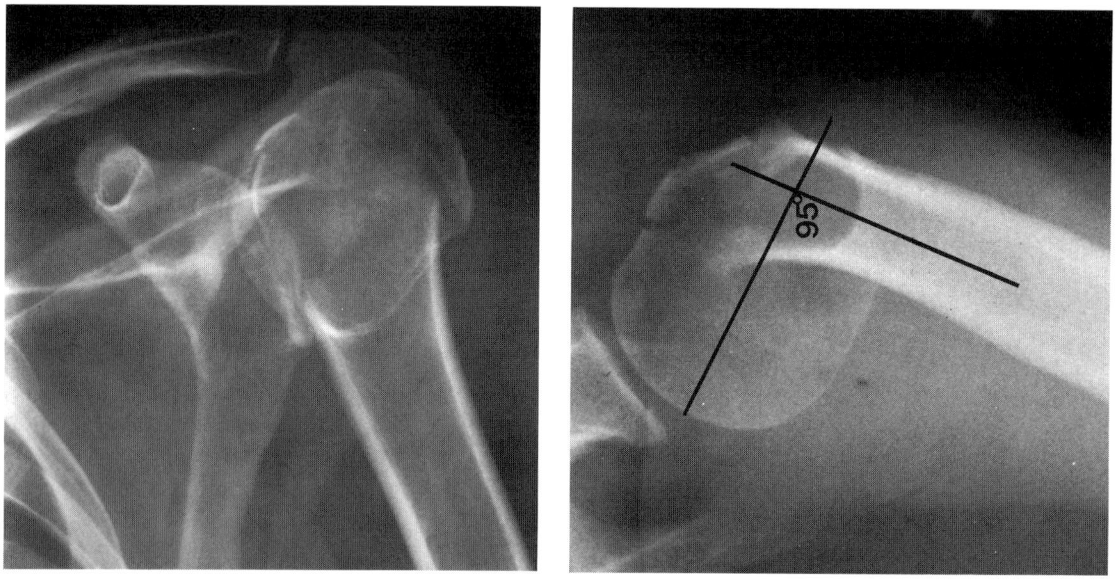

A B

FIG. 9-14. A: An AP view shows comminuted fracture of the proximal humerus. Is there a fragment angled > 45° or displaced 1 cm? **B:** Axillary view shows the head is rotated and angulated > 45°, a two-part fracture.

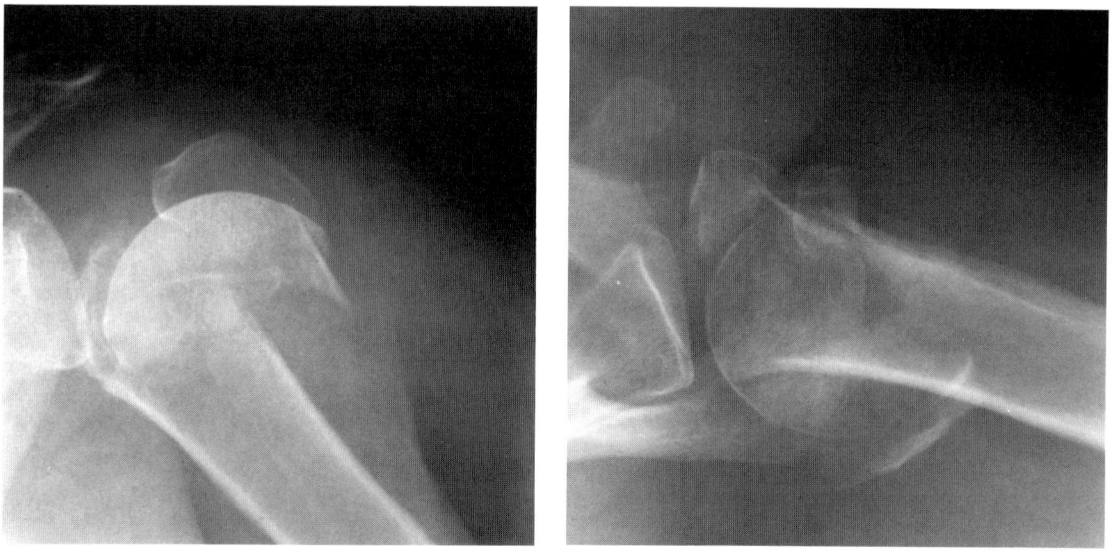

A B

FIG. 9-15. The AP **(A)** and axillary **(B)** views of a four-part fracture with all fragments displaced.

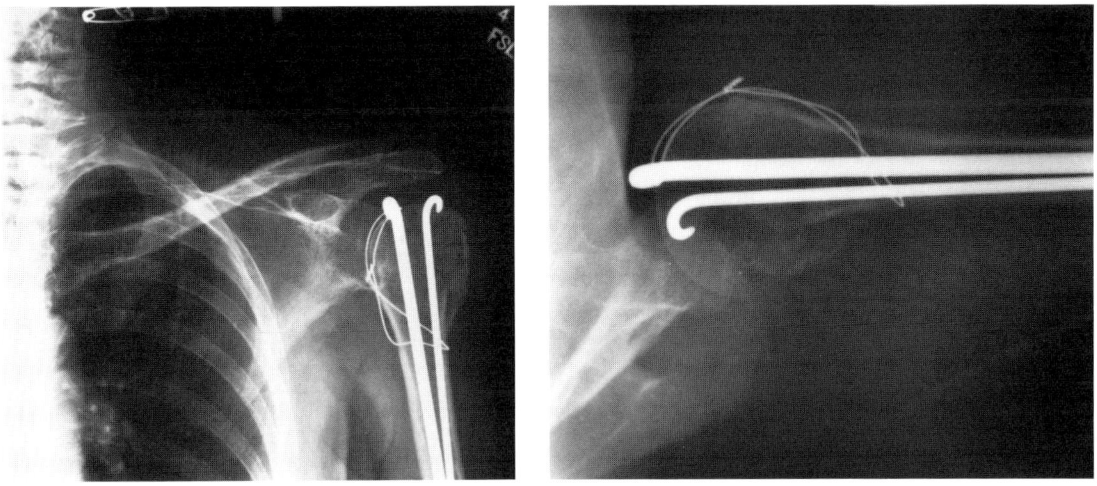

A B

FIG. 9-16. Three-part fracture of the proximal humerus reduced with two Rush rods and tension-band wiring. The AP **(A)** and axillary **(B)** radiographs.

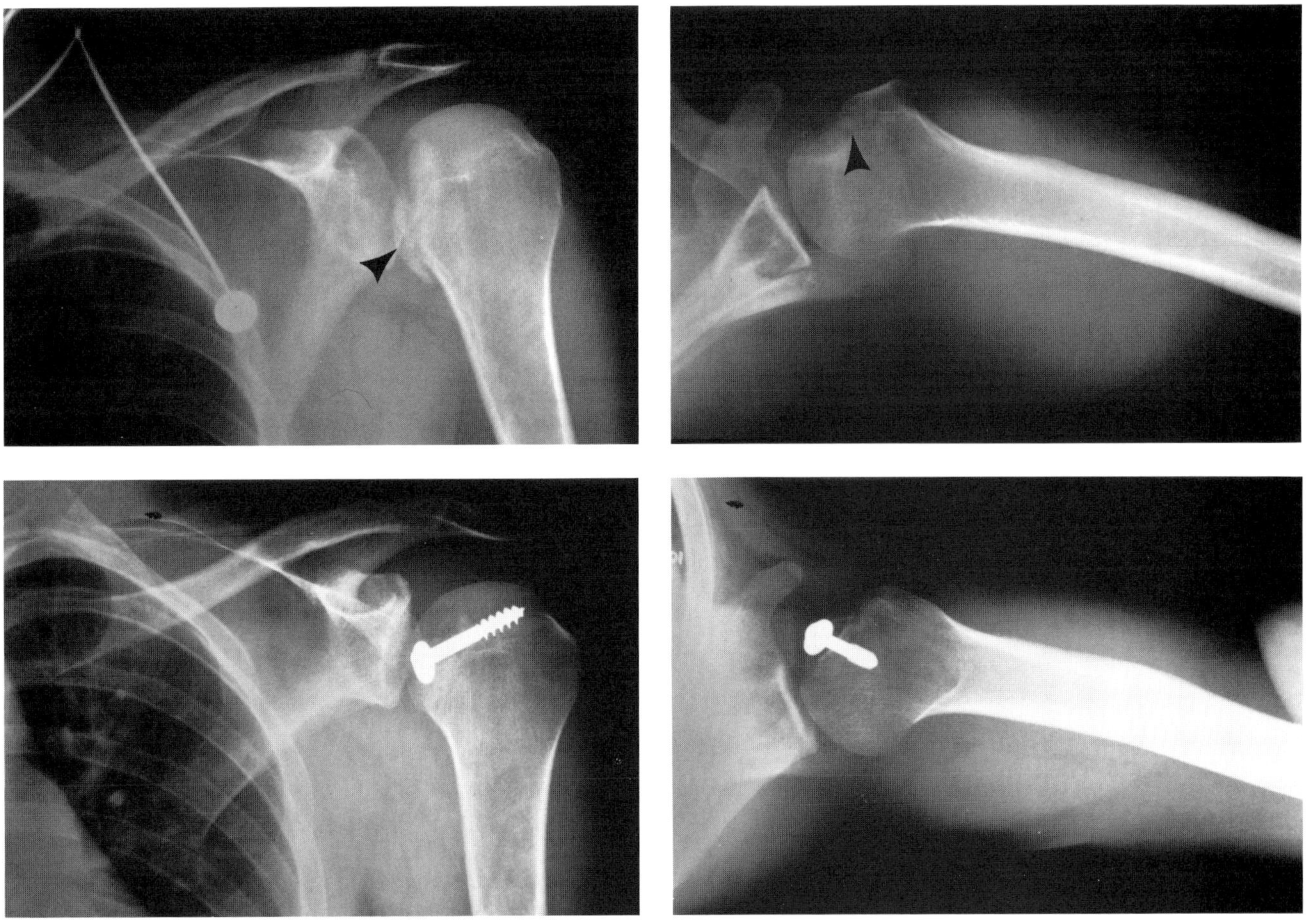

A B C D

FIG. 9-17. The AP **(A)** and axillary **(B)** radiographs demonstrating a fracture of the humeral head and lesser tuberosity (*arrow*). The AP **(C)** and axillary **(D)** radiographs after reduction and internal fixation with a single cancellous screw and washer.

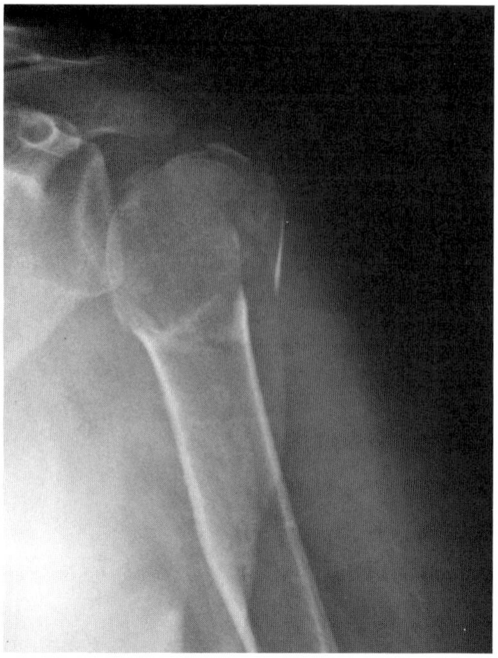

A

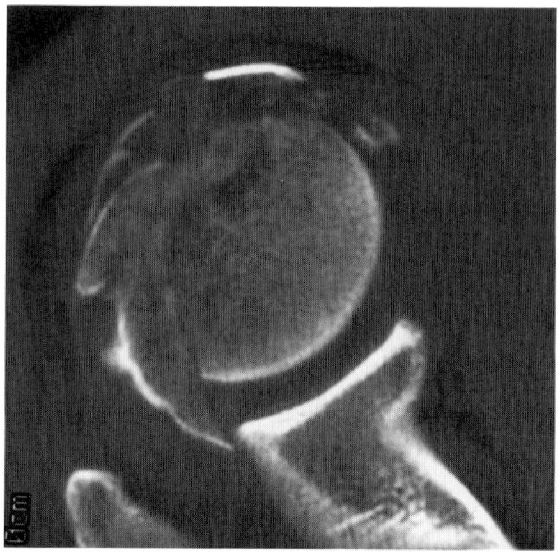

B

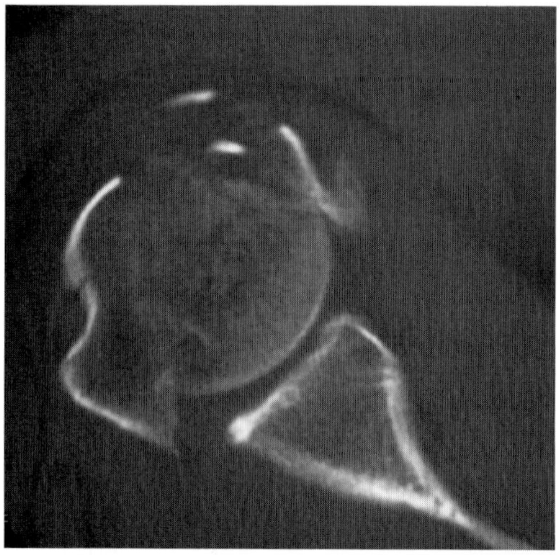

C

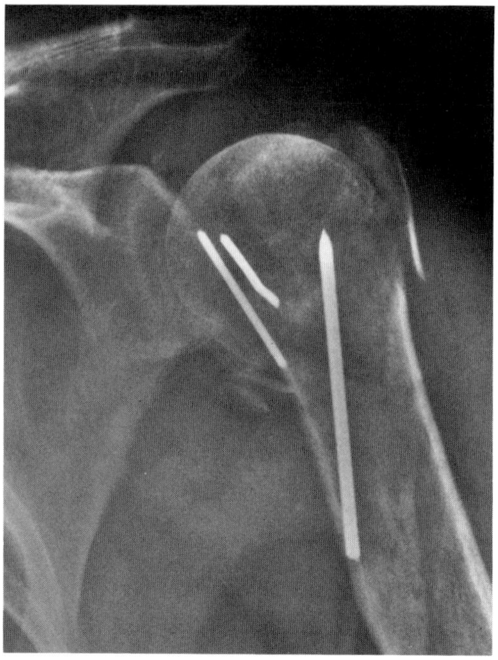

D

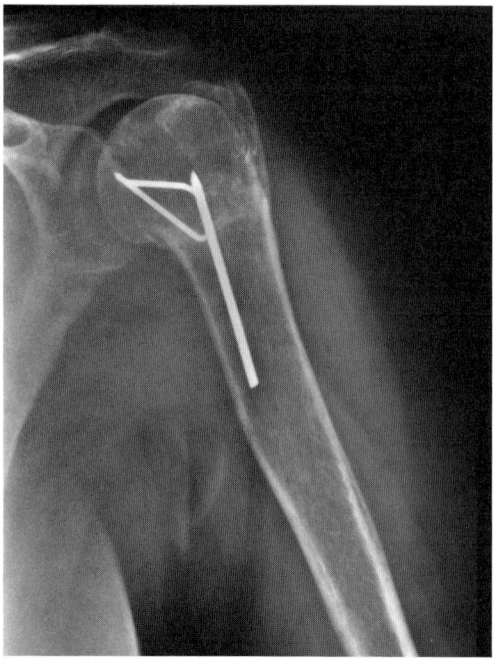

E

FIG. 9-18. An AP radiograph **(A)** and CT images **(B,C)** of a four-part fracture with inferior subluxation caused by a hemarthrosis. **D:** Open reduction and internal fixation with K wires from the lesser tuberosity into the head and a Steinmann pin to secure the head fragments. The greater tuberosity is still slightly displaced. **E:** Radiograph after healing 4 months later.

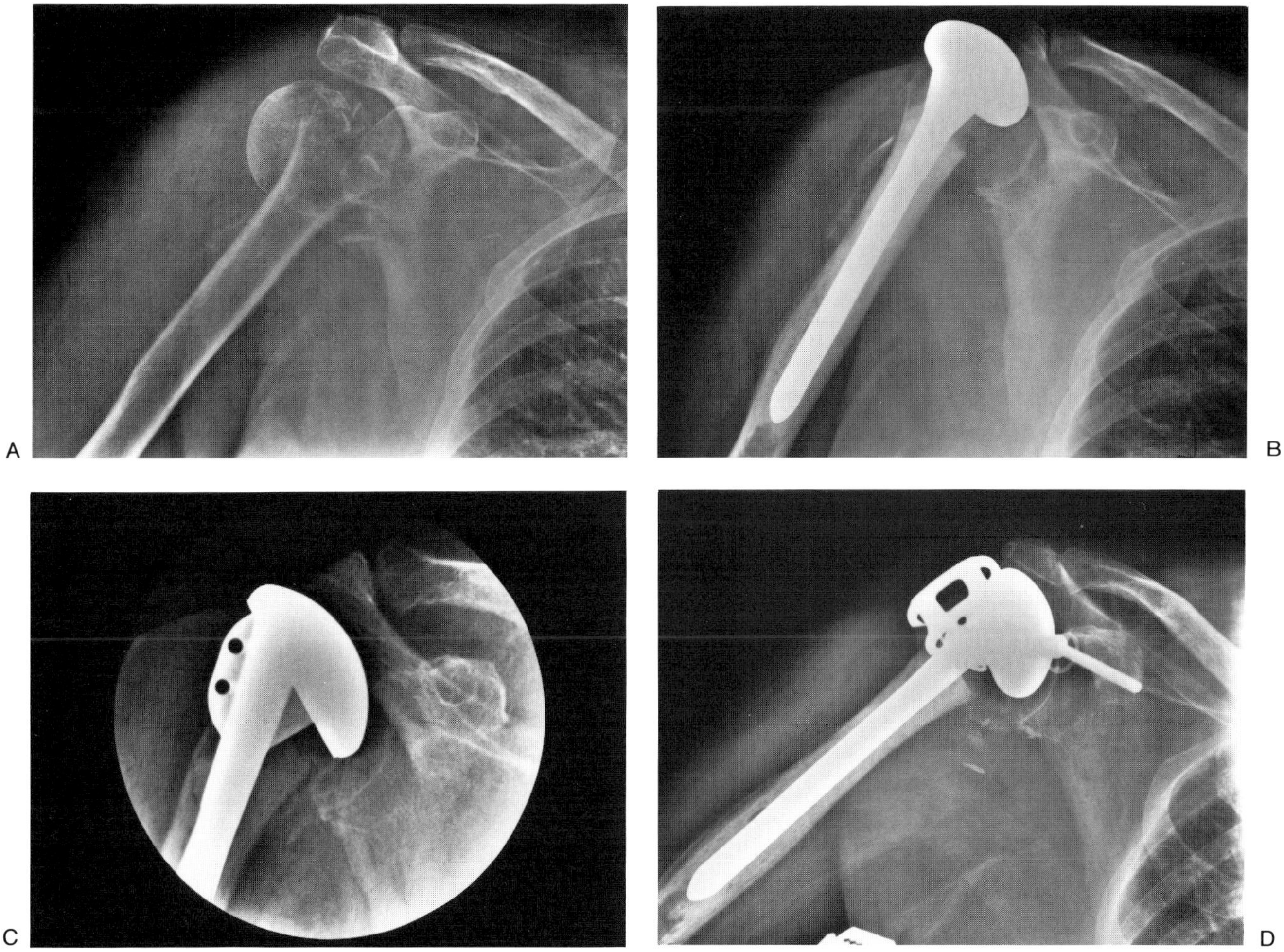

FIG. 9-19. A: Comminuted four-part fracture of the proximal humerus with marked displacement of the humeral head. **B:** Postoperative view with a cemented Neer endoprosthesis. **C:** Fluoroscopically positioned view taken during stress maneuvers because of continued pain and instability. **D:** Revision surgery with addition of Dall-Miles cable system and anterior screw with soft tissue washer to repair the capsule and soft tissues.

A 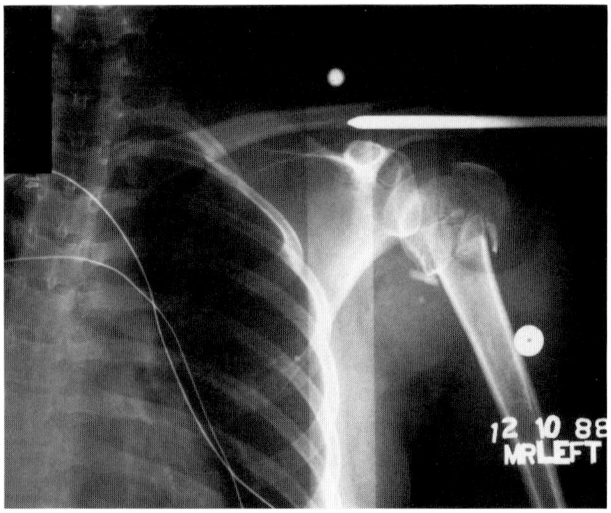

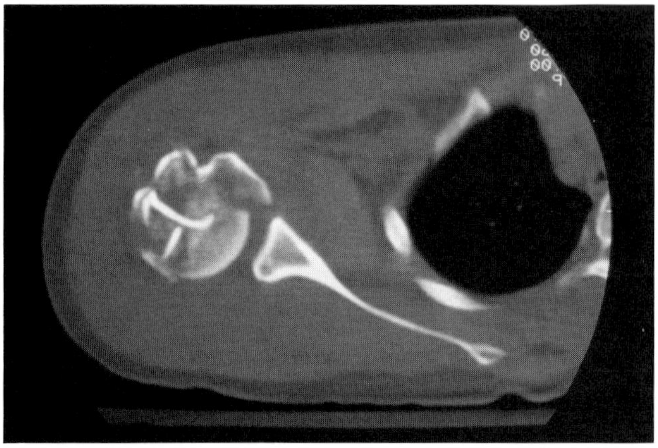 B

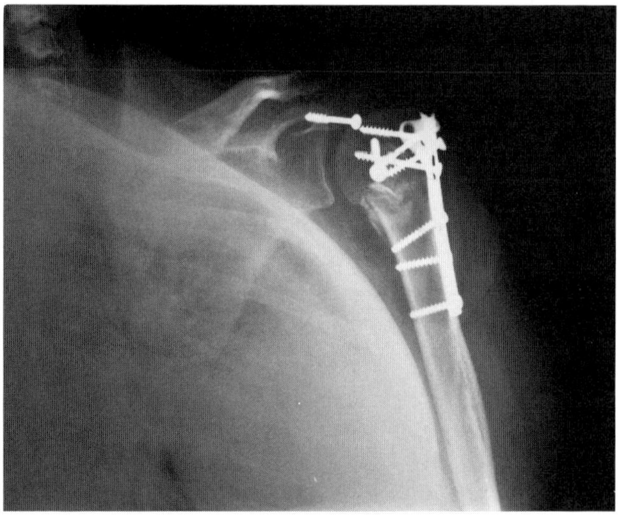 C

FIG. 9-20. A: Comminuted fracture of the left humeral head and neck. A Steinmann pin was used to stabilize the distal clavicle fracture. **B:** A CT image demonstrating the position of the fragments. **C:** Postoperative radiograph demonstrating reduction with a cloverleaf plate with the end cut off and proximal cancellous and distal cortical screws. The coracoid was removed for exposure and was resecured with a single cancellous screw.

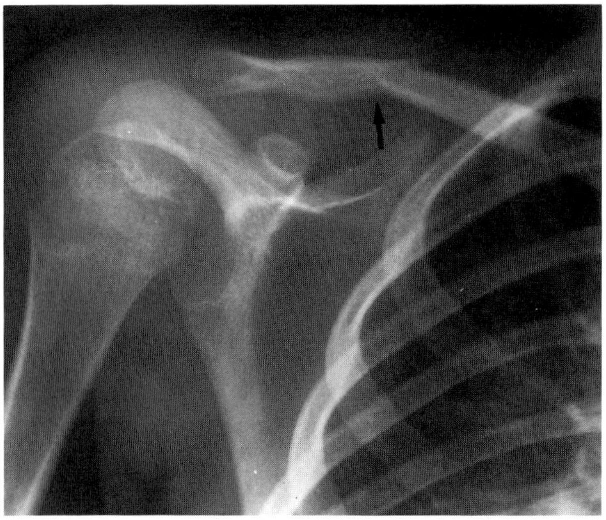

FIG. 9-21. Slightly angulated fracture of the right midclavicle (*arrow*).

A
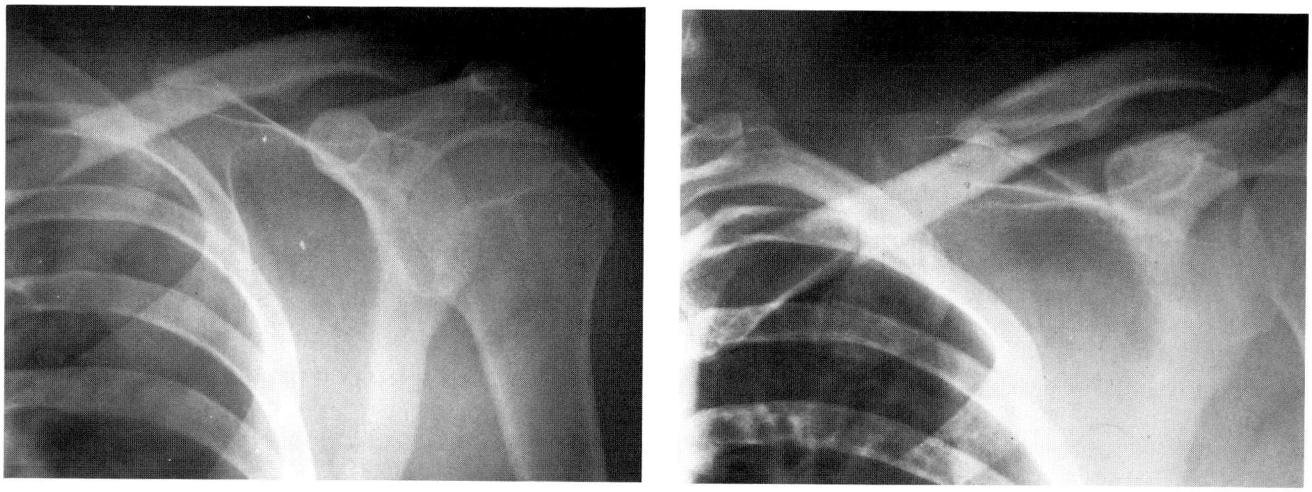
B

FIG. 9-22. A: An AP view of the clavicle. The medial clavicle is not completely shown. No fracture is evident. **B:** Angled view clearly demonstrates the fracture of the midclavicle proximal to the coracoclavicular ligament.

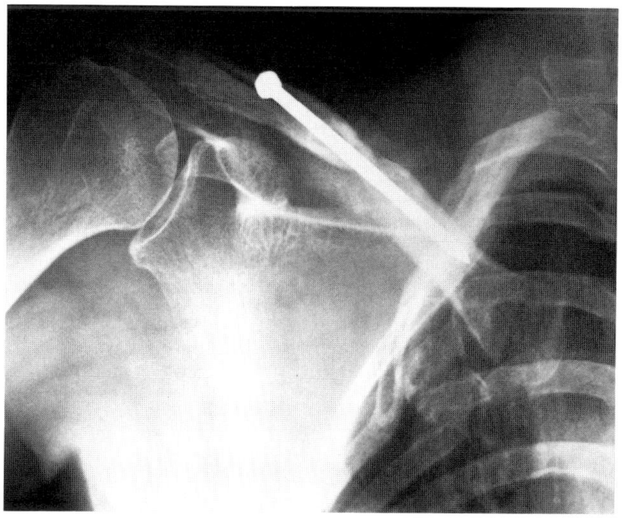

FIG. 9-23. Badly displaced midclavicle fracture internally fixed with a Knowles pin.

A
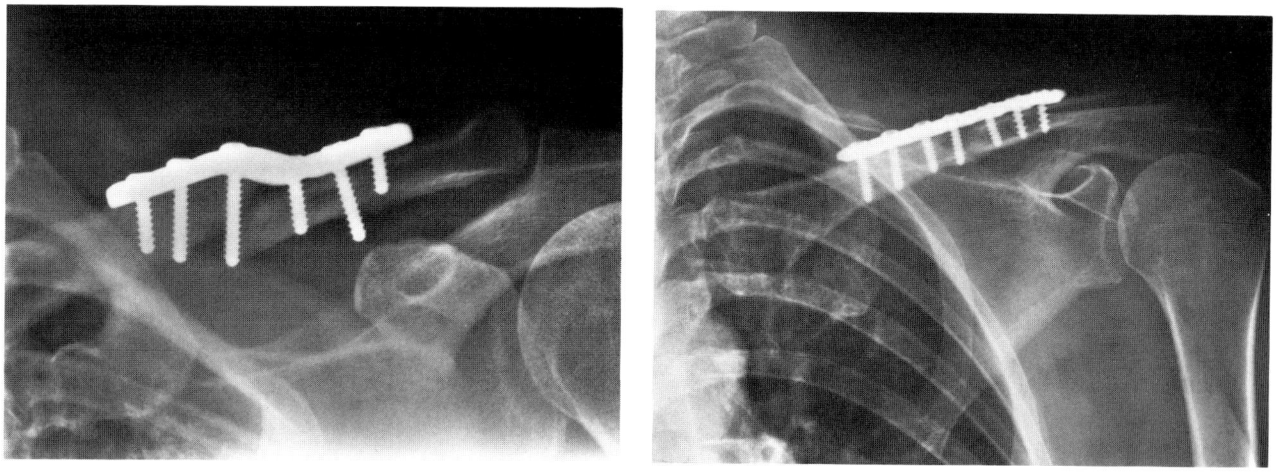
B

FIG. 9-24. A: Fracture of the midclavicle with a prebent DC plate and six cortical screws for fixation. **B:** Fracture of the midclavicle internally fixed with a seven-hole reconstruction plate and five cortical and two cancellous screws distally.

cephalad may be useful. However, in difficult or subtle cases, CT is most effective.

Treatment

Most clavicle fractures can be treated conservatively by using shoulder support (e.g., a "figure-eight" dressing).[127,138,139,141]

Open reduction and internal fixation is used in the following situations.[121,127,173,177]

1. Neurovascular compromise or entrapment
2. Distal clavicle fractures with coracoclavicular ligament rupture
3. Fractures with severe angulation or comminution
4. Patient who cannot tolerate closed treatment techniques
5. Symptomatic nonunion of previous closed reduction

Internal fixation can be accomplished with pins (Fig. 9-23) or plate and screw techniques (Fig. 9-24).[121,173,177] Reconstruction plates, dynamic compression plates (Fig. 9-24), or semitubular plates can be used (see Chapter 2).[121]

Scapular Fractures

Scapular fractures are uncommon and account for only 1% of all fractures and 3% to 5% of shoulder injuries.[84,150] Major trauma, typically motor vehicle accidents, is the usual mechanism of injury. There is a high incidence of associated injuries, which may require treatment prior to dealing with the scapular fracture (Table 9-1).[152,168]

There are several classification schemes that have been used. Anatomically, the injuries can be described by the structure involved: spine, acromion, glenoid neck, articular, or coracoid. Scapular neck and body fractures occur most commonly.[84,150]

Zdravkovic and Damholt[176] classified body fractures as type I, apophyseal fractures (including the coracoid and acromion) as type II, and fractures of the glenoid neck and articular surface as type III. The latter are the most difficult to treat. Thompson et al.[168] classified small body fractures and coracoid and acromial fractures as type I, glenoid and glenoid neck fractures as type II, and major body fractures as type III.

TABLE 9-1. *Scapular fractures: associated injuries*[150,152,168,176]

Injury	Percent of cases
Pneumothorax	53
Pulmonary contusion	11–54
Rib fractures	27–54
Clavicular fractures	23–39
Brachial plexus injury	5–13

The use of the anatomic description is the simplest. However, because of the significance of glenoid fractures, the Ideberg classification (Fig. 9-25) has been commonly used.[101,111,112] Type I fractures (Fig. 9-25) involve the anterior (type IA) or posterior (type IB) glenoid rim. Type II fractures (Fig. 9-25B) occur with force directed through the humeral head inferiorly. Type III fractures (Fig. 9-25C) involve the superior glenoid and occur with force directed superiorly through the humeral head. Type IV fractures (Fig. 9-25D) occur with force directed centrally leading to a split of the glenoid and scapula. Type V fractures (Fig. 9-25E) are combinations of types II to IV injuries.

Imaging of the scapula typically includes AP (Fig. 9-26) and lateral views. Axillary or scapular Y views may be required to evaluate the coracoid, glenoid, and spine more accurately (Fig. 9-27).[81] Subtle and complex injuries should be evaluated with CT.[81,90,104,156,176]

Treatment

Nonoperative treatment is recommended for most scapular fractures.[117,169,176] Open reduction has been recommended for articular fractures or fractures involving the scapular neck and clavicle (Fig. 9-28).[117,121] Internal fixation may specifically be required if greater than 25% of the articular surface is involved and the fragment is displaced. Secondary instability is common if left untreated (Figs. 9-29 and 9-30).[111,112] Multiple techniques can be used including K wires, interfragmentary screws (Fig. 9-29), and staples (Fig. 9-31).[101,117,121] Postoperatively, true AP and axillary views should be obtained to evaluate the glenoid articular surface. Fluoroscopic positioning may be required.[81]

Glenohumeral Dislocations

Glenohumeral dislocations are the most frequent, accounting for 50% of all dislocations.[81,84,109] Ninety-seven to 98% are anterior, about 2% are posterior, and rarely, inferior or superior dislocations occur.[77,78,97,107,129,152]

Most anterior dislocations result from a fall with the arm abducted and externally rotated. Rarely, dislocations occur after direct posterior trauma.[81,84,109,153] As the humeral head is displaced anteriorly, injury to the subscapularis tendon, anterior capsule, and glenohumeral ligaments occur to varying degrees. Osseous or glenoid labral injuries (Bankart, Fig. 9-32) occur in up to 50% of cases, and posterolateral humeral head (Hill-Sachs, Fig. 9-33) lesions occur in 67% to 76% of anterior dislocations.[78,81,107] Fractures of the greater tuberosity occur in 15% of cases (Fig. 9-34). The biceps tendon can become trapped between the humeral head and tuberosity fragment.[81,103]

Posterior dislocations occur during falls with the arm internally rotated and adducted, with electroconvulsive

(text continues on page 685)

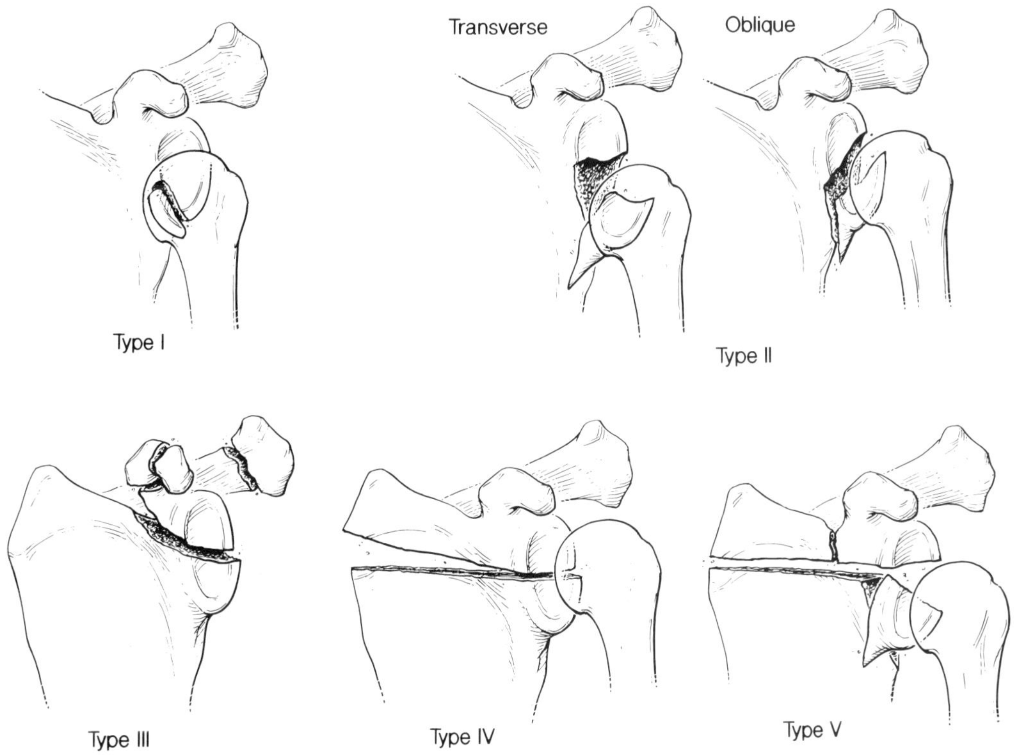

FIG. 9-25. The Ideberg classification. Type I, fracture of the glenoid rim (IA, anterior; IB, posterior). Subluxation or dislocation may be associated (type IA illustrated). Type II, larger transverse or oblique fragment caused by force directed through the humeral head inferiorly. Type III, force from humeral head directed superiorly, leading to superior glenoid fracture. The coracoid and acromion may be involved. Type IV, humeral head driven centrally leading to a split of the glenoid and scapular body. Type V, combinations of types II, III, and IV.

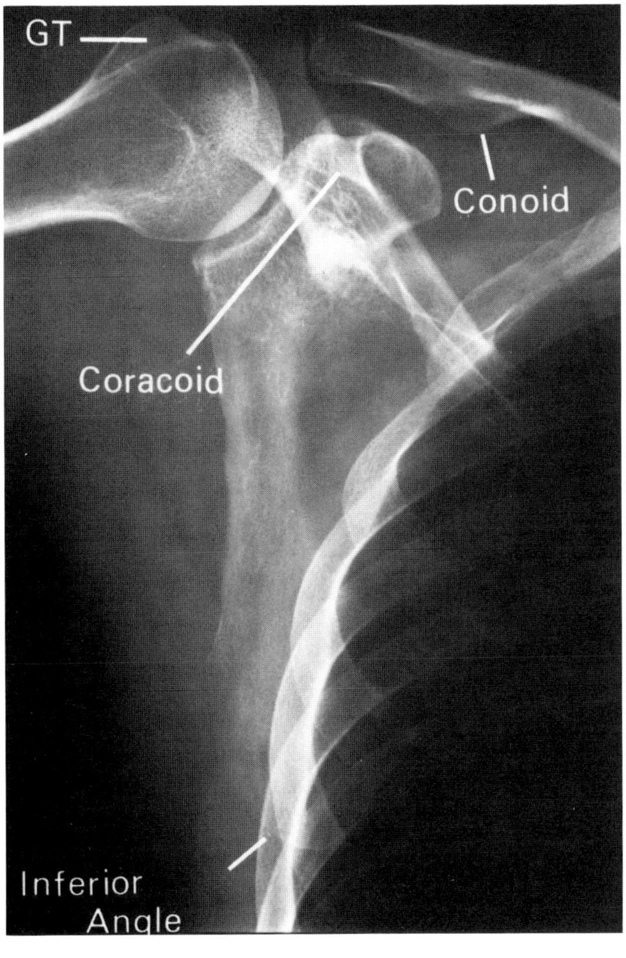

FIG. 9-26. Normal AP view of the scapula.

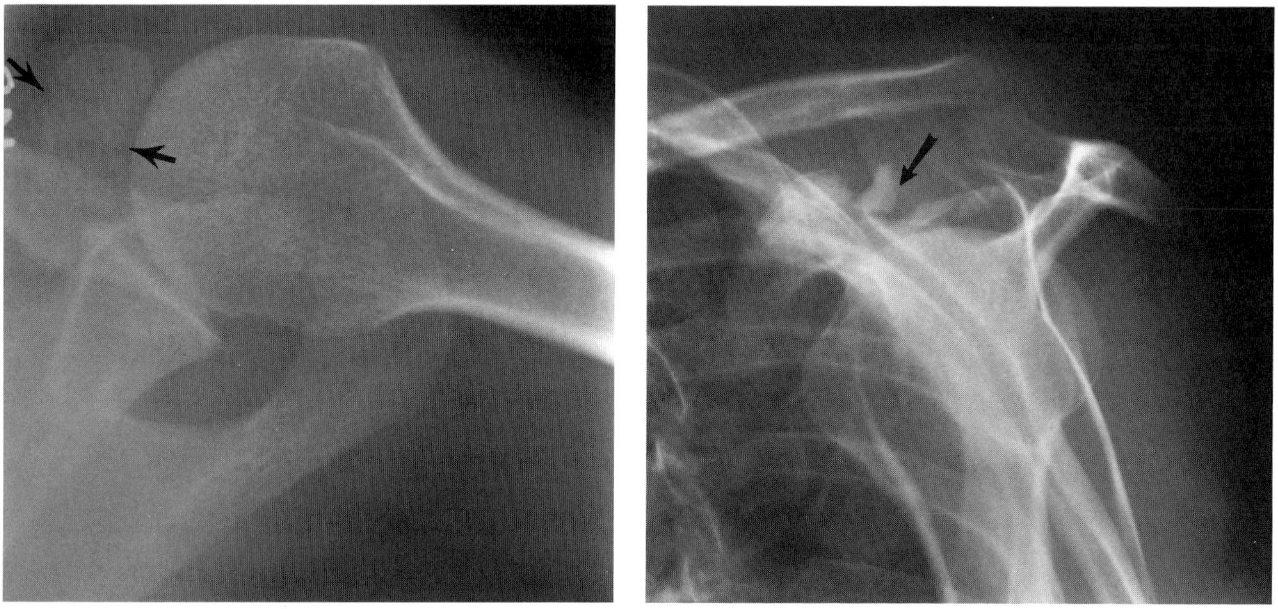

A B

FIG. 9-27. Axillary **(A)** and scapular Y **(B)** views demonstrating coracoid fractures (*arrows*).

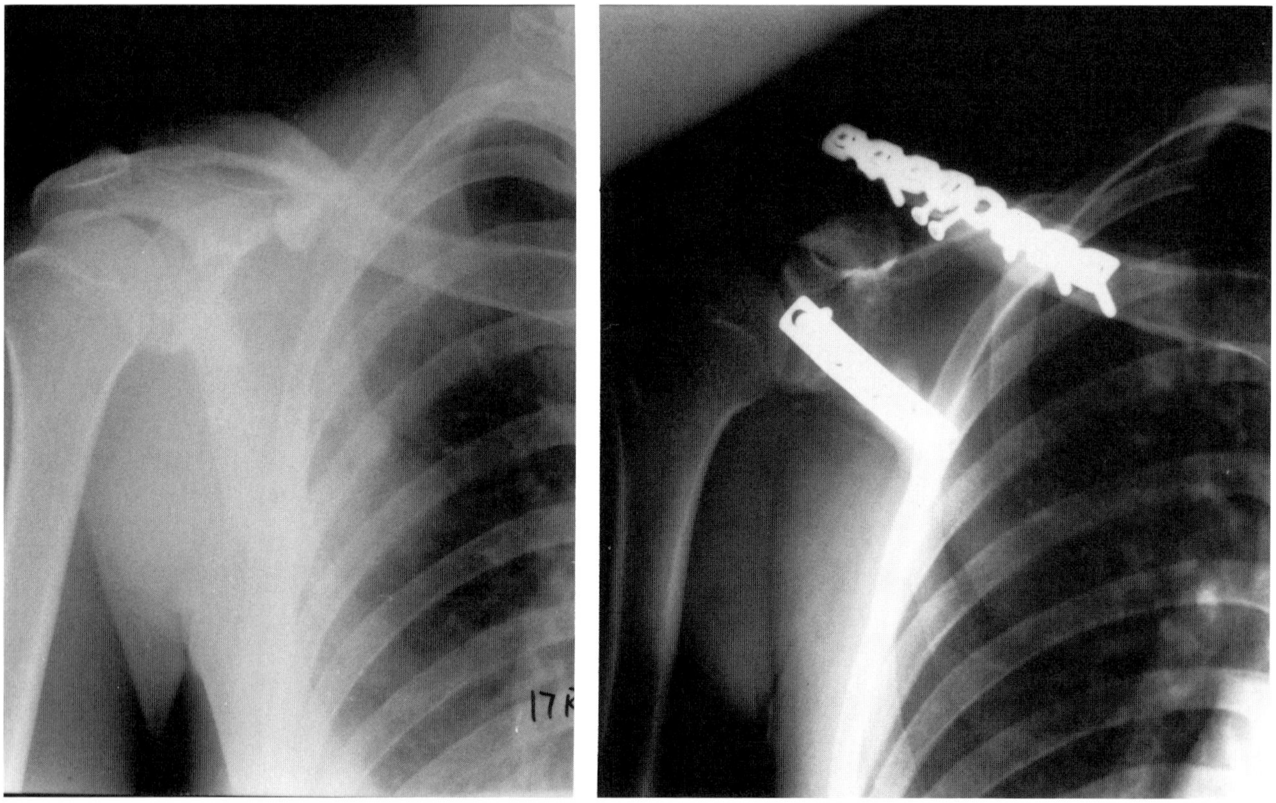

A B

FIG. 9-28. **A:** An AP radiograph demonstrating a displaced glenoid neck fracture and comminuted mid-clavicle fracture. **B:** Operative reduction of the glenoid neck with plate and screws. The clavicle fracture is reduced with a reconstruction plate and screws. The glenoid is reduced with a DC plate and screws. (From Leung KS, Lans TP. Open reduction and internal fixation of ipsilateral fractures of the scapular neck and clavicle. *J Bone Joint Surg* [*Am*] 1993;75A:1015–1018.)

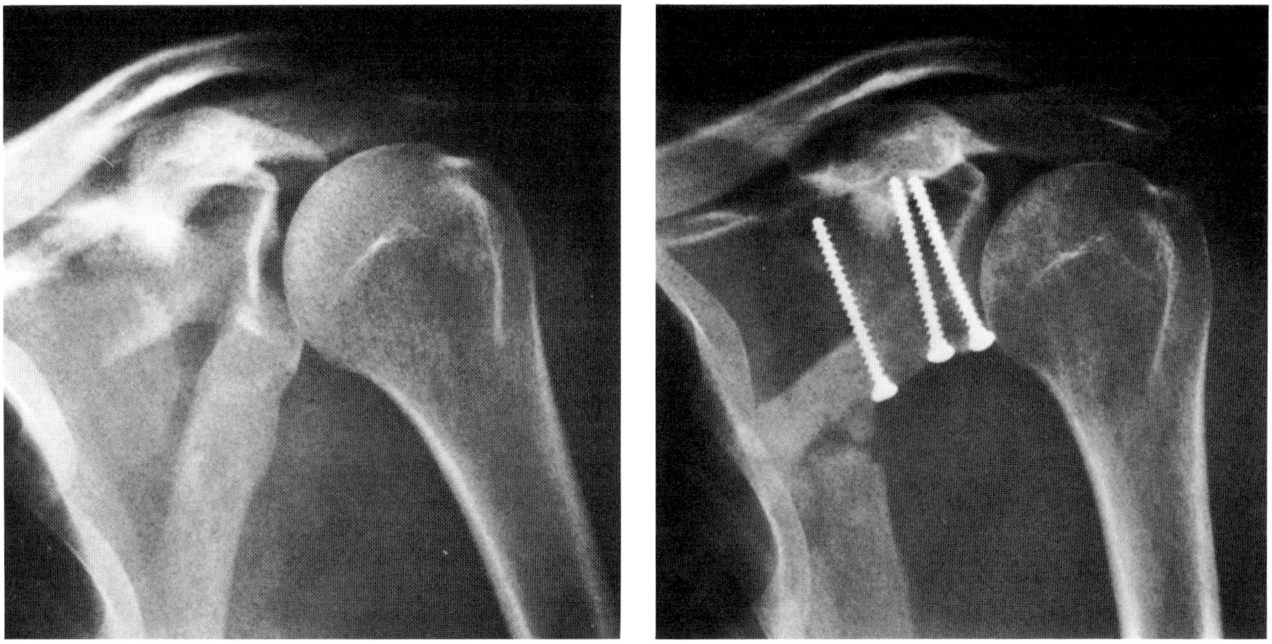

A B

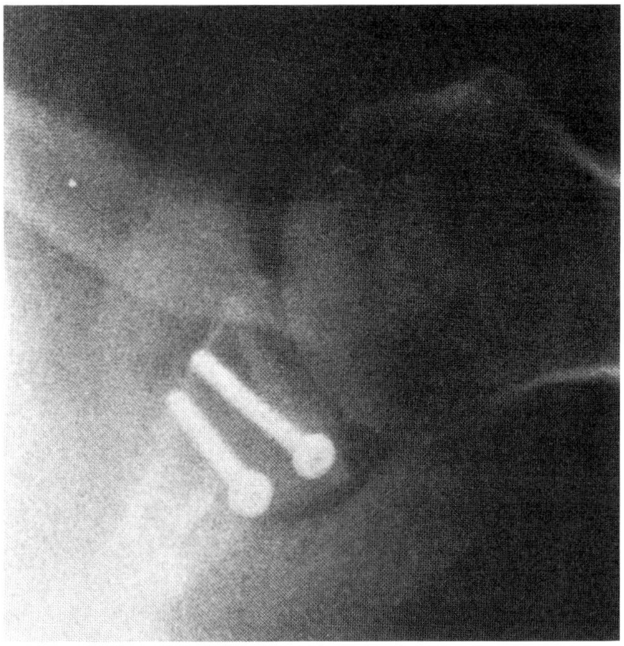

C

FIG. 9-29. A: Split (type IV) fracture of the glenoid and scapular body. The AP **(B)** and axillary **(C)** views after reduction with three interfragmentary screws. (From Kavanagh BF, Bradway JK, Cofield RH. Open reduction and internal fixation of displaced intra-articular fractures of the glenoid fossa. *J Bone Joint Surg* [*Am*] 1993;75A:479–484.)

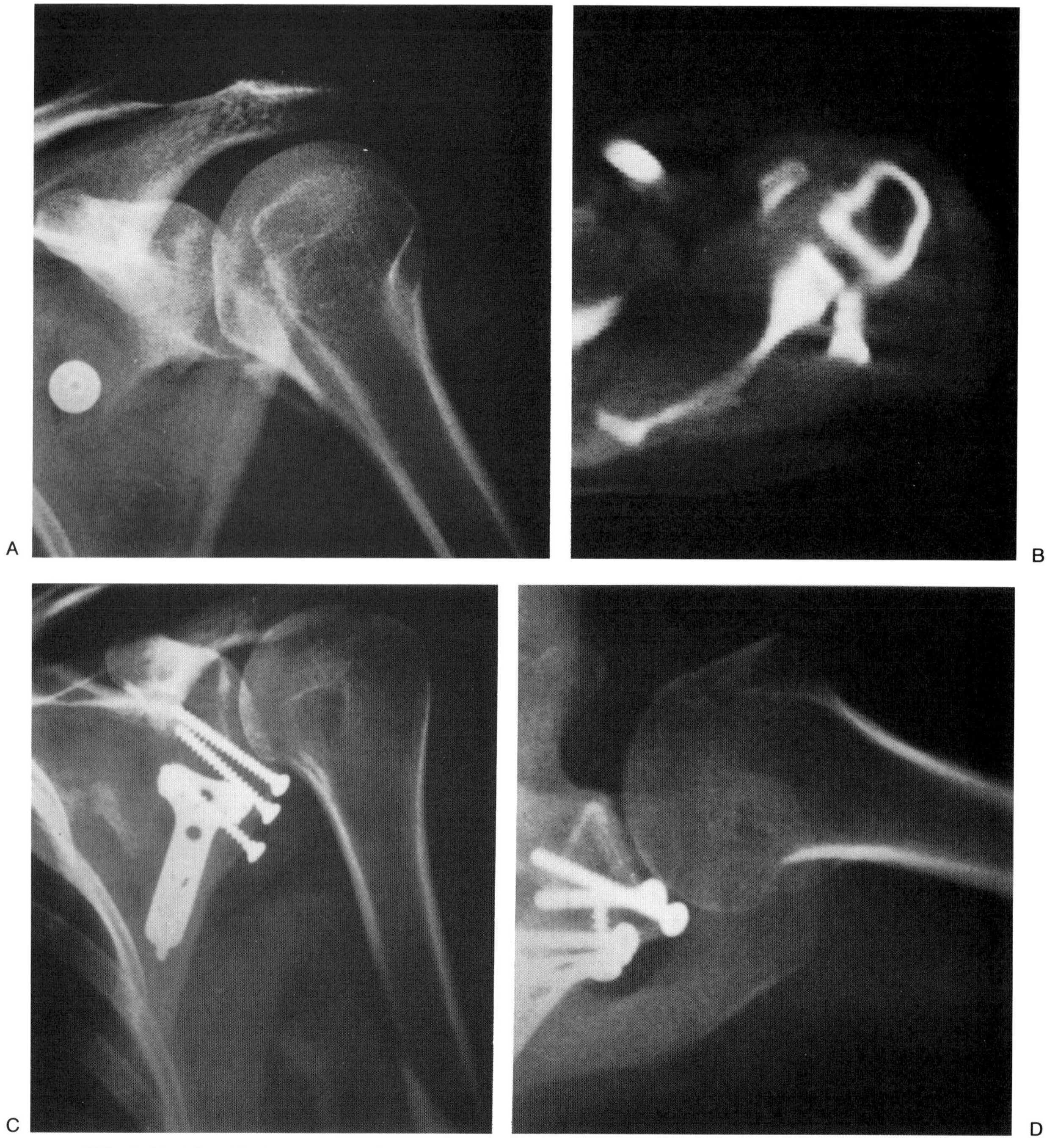

FIG. 9-30. The AP view (A) and CT (B) of a glenoid fossa fracture. The AP (C) and axillary (D) views after reduction with a T buttress plate and interfragmentary screws. (From Kavanagh BF, Bradway JK, Cofield RH. Open reduction and internal fixation of displaced intra-articular fractures of the glenoid fossa. *J Bone Joint Surg* [*Am*] 1993;75A:479–484.)

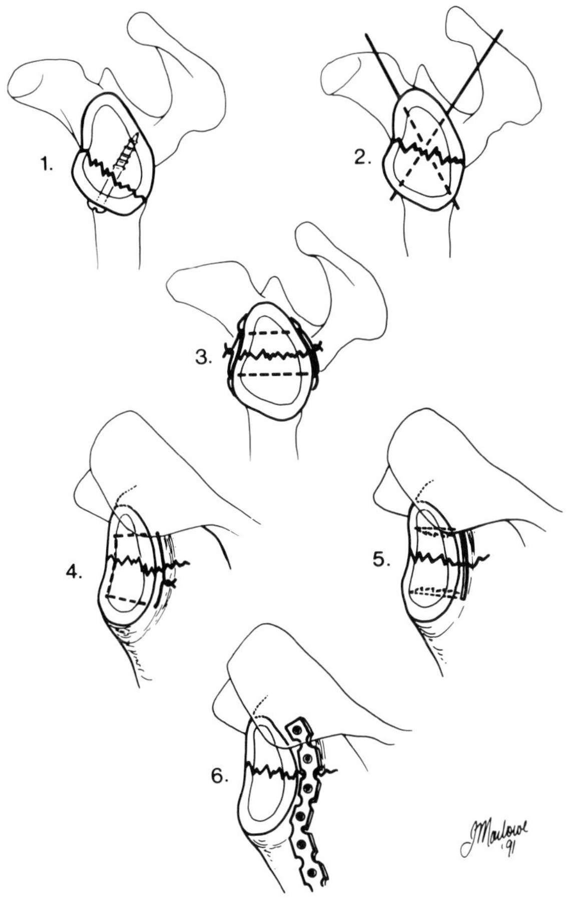

FIG. 9-31. Techniques for the reduction of glenoid fossa fractures. *1,* Lag screw; *2,* K wires; *3,* K wires and cerclage wires; *4,* cerclage wire or suture; *5,* staples; *6,* buttress or reconstruction plate. (From Goss TP. Fractures of the glenoid cavity. *J Bone Joint Surg* [*Am*] 1992;74A:299–305.)

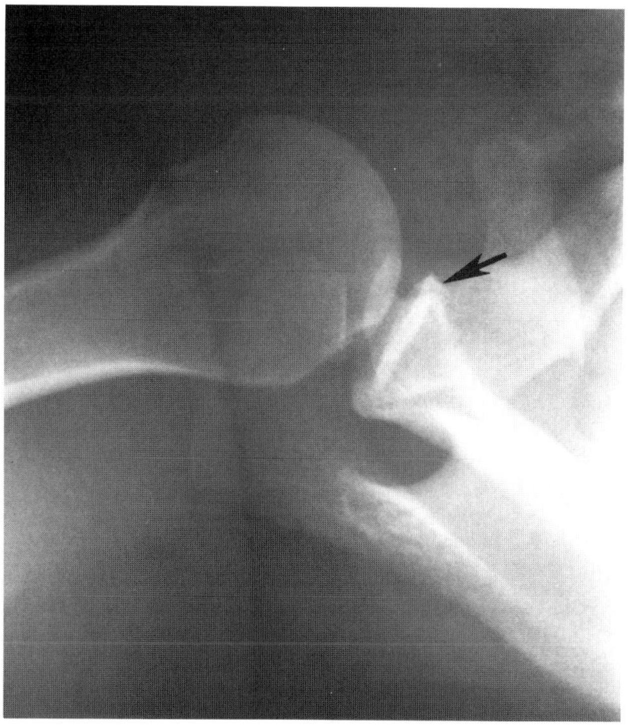

FIG. 9-32. Axillary view after anterior dislocation demonstrating an anterior labral fracture (*arrow*).

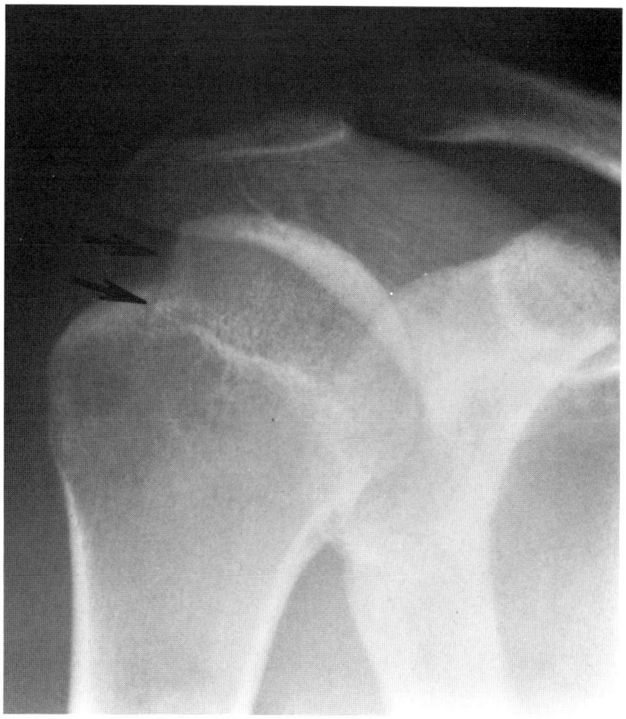

FIG. 9-33. An AP view of the shoulder demonstrating a Hill-Sachs lesion (*arrows*).

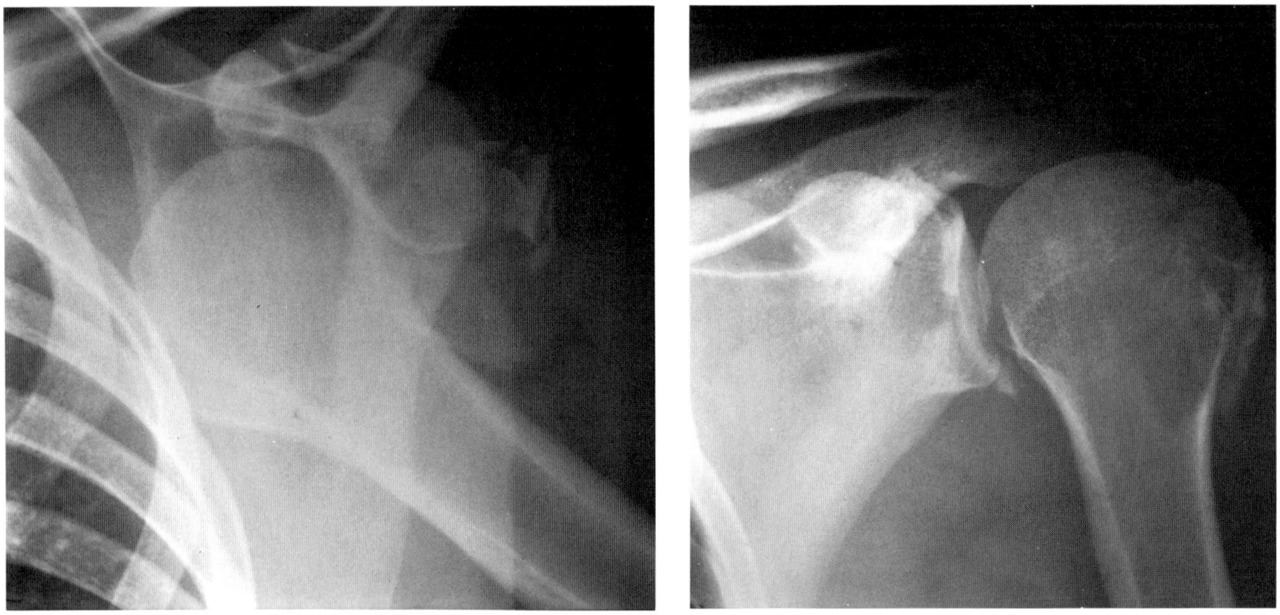

A B

FIG. 9-34. Prereduction AP **(A)** and postreduction AP **(B)** views of an anterior dislocation with associated glenoid and greater tuberosity fractures.

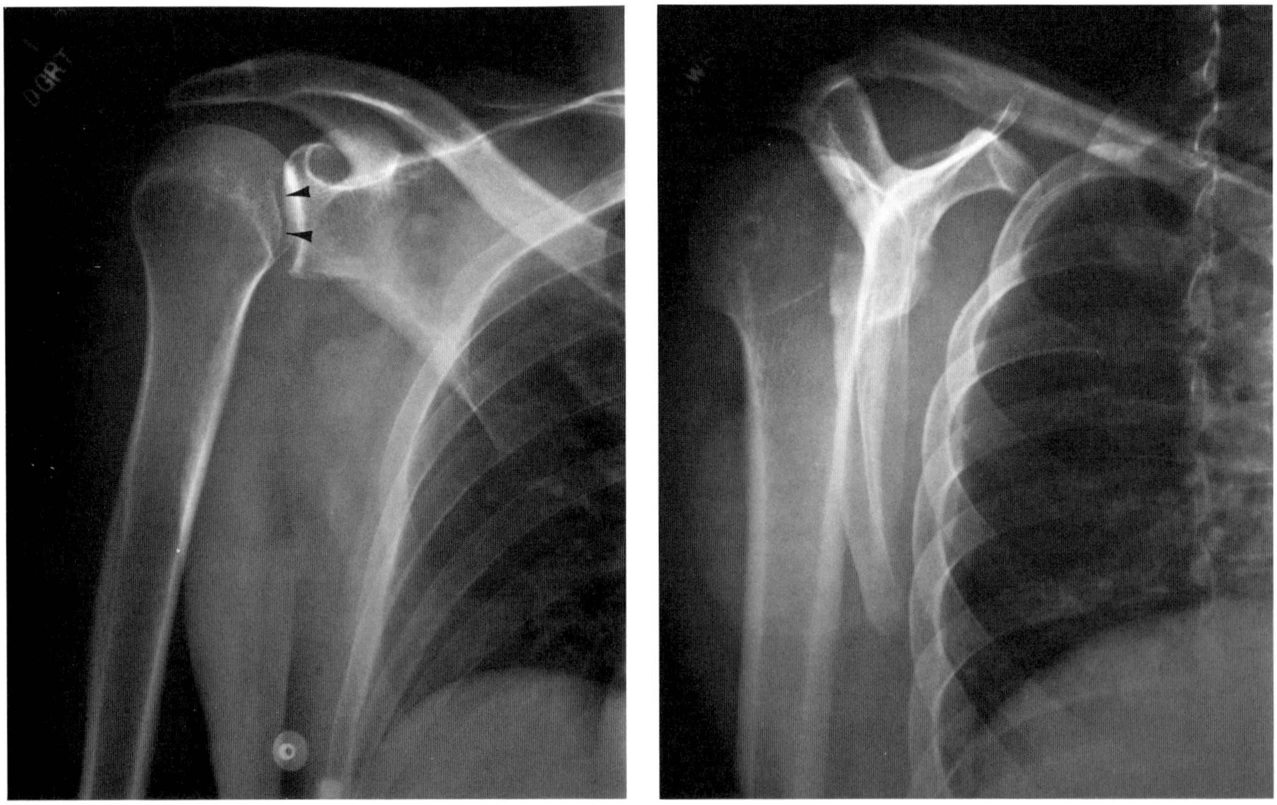

A B

FIG. 9-35. Posterior dislocation. **A:** An AP view demonstrating the arm in internal rotation with a trough sign (*arrowheads*) medially. **B:** Scapular Y view clearly demonstrates the posterior position of the humeral head.

therapy, and following direct anterior trauma.[74,91,129] Posterior capsule, glenoid run, and anteromedial humeral head (75% of cases) injury may be associated. Lesser tuberosity fractures occur with about 25% of posterior dislocations.[81,92]

Routine radiography, using AP, scapular Y, and axillary views, should ensure the diagnosis of all types of dislocation or subluxations (Fig. 9-35). After reduction, many of the osseous injuries (Fig. 9-34) may be more easily appreciated.[81]

Treatment

The treatment of acute dislocation is generally closed manipulation and reduction. We will concentrate on operative procedures designed to deal with the problem of recurrent dislocations.

Recurrent dislocation is the most frequent complication of shoulder dislocations.[96,110,150,155,159,163,164,170,171] Recurrence is most common after anterior dislocations and more common in younger patients (55% < 22 years old). Associated Bankart (84%), Hill-Sachs (76%), and capsular laxity (83%) are common in patients with recurrent dislocation and instability.[155] Recurrent dislocation occurs less frequently with posterior dislocations.[74,81,92,129]

Conventional arthrography with fluoroscopic stress views is useful for evaluating stability and capsular deformity. The proper demonstration of the direction of instability (anterior, posterior, inferior, or multidirectional) is important for selecting the best technique for repair. Both CT and MRI can be used to evaluate the glenoid, glenoid labrum, and pericapsular soft tissues (MRI superior) preoperatively.[81,83,136]

There are numerous procedures for the treatment of patients with recurrent dislocation or instability. The orthopedic fixation technique may not be apparent radiographically in all procedures. Thus, the type of procedure performed may not be definable on radiographic images. Most procedures have been designed for anterior instability. The repairs may be primarily soft tissue reconstructions or involve coracoid transfers or bone blocks.[100,116,145,147,150] The procedures used and a brief description are summarized in the next section.

Anterior Repairs

Bankart Repair.[78,150,154,155] The anterior capsule is reattached to the glenoid. Soft tissue anchors may be used (Fig. 9-36). There is an approximately 2% redislocation incidence.

Staple Capsulorrhaphy.[96,142,165] The detached glenoid is secured to the capsule with staples. The recurrence rate is 28%, with 11% staple loosening. Staple migration and cartilage penetration are the major complications.

Putti-Platt Procedure.[110,144,148] The subscapularis is divided 2.5 cm from its insertion, and the capsule is opened. The lateral end is reattached to the "most convenient soft tissue structure along the anterior rim of the glenoid cavity."[150] The medial end is brought over the lateral segment to insert on the greater tuberosity. This can be combined with a Bankart procedure. There is 30% decreased range of motion and 14% recurrent instability.

Magnuson-Stack Procedure.[116,125,126,131] The subscapularis tendon is transferred from the lesser tuberosity to the greater tuberosity. There is a 2% recurrence rate.

McLaughlin Procedure.[129,150] This procedure is for use with large anteromedial humeral head defects. The subscapularis is transferred from the lesser tuberosity into the defect (Fig. 9-37A). Neer modified this technique by including the lesser tuberosity with the tendon and securing it to the defect (Fig. 9-37B) with a bone screw.

Trillat Procedure.[85,147,150] This is a coracoid osteotomy. The coracoid and tendon attachments are moved inferiorly and laterally and reattached with a bone screw.

Bristow-Helfet Procedure.[76,147,150,151,175] The subscapularis muscle and tendon are split, and the coracoid is resected and reattached to the anterior glenoid neck with a bone screw (Fig. 9-38B).

Latarjet Procedure.[146,150,153,167] This technique transfers a larger segment of coracoid than does the Bristow procedure with the conjoined tendon. The bone is laid flat on the anterior glenoid (Fig. 9-38C) and held with one or two screws.

Eden-Hybbinette Procedure.[120,150] This procedure extends the coracoid (Fig. 9-39) by using an iliac bone graft. The subscapularis is also shortened.

Boytchev Procedure.[147,150] The coracoid and conjoined tendons are moved deep to the subscapularis and reattached to the coracoid base.

Connally Procedure.[147,150] This is a mirror image of the McLaughlin procedure. The infraspinatus is transferred into a large posterolateral humeral head defect.

Saha Procedure.[150] The latissimus dorsi is transferred onto the greater tuberosity to reinforce the subscapularis.

Nicola Procedure.[147,150] The long head of the biceps is transferred across the anterior humerus to serve as a check rain.

Gallie Procedure.[100,150] Autogenous fascia is used to create new ligaments between the anterior inferior capsule and humeral neck.

Humeral Osteotomy.[150,171] A proximal humeral osteotomy is done with rotation of the humeral head and plate and screw fixation. The results are good in 90%, but most require plate removal.

Arthroscopic anterior repairs can also be performed to reattach the labrum or capsule to the glenoid.[115,132]

Posterior instability can be corrected using the reverse Putti-Platt procedure, a posterior glenoid osteotomy, posterior bone blocks, or a transfer of the long head of the biceps behind the humeral head (Boyd-Sisk procedure).[150] Patients with multidirectional instability may

(text continues on page 688)

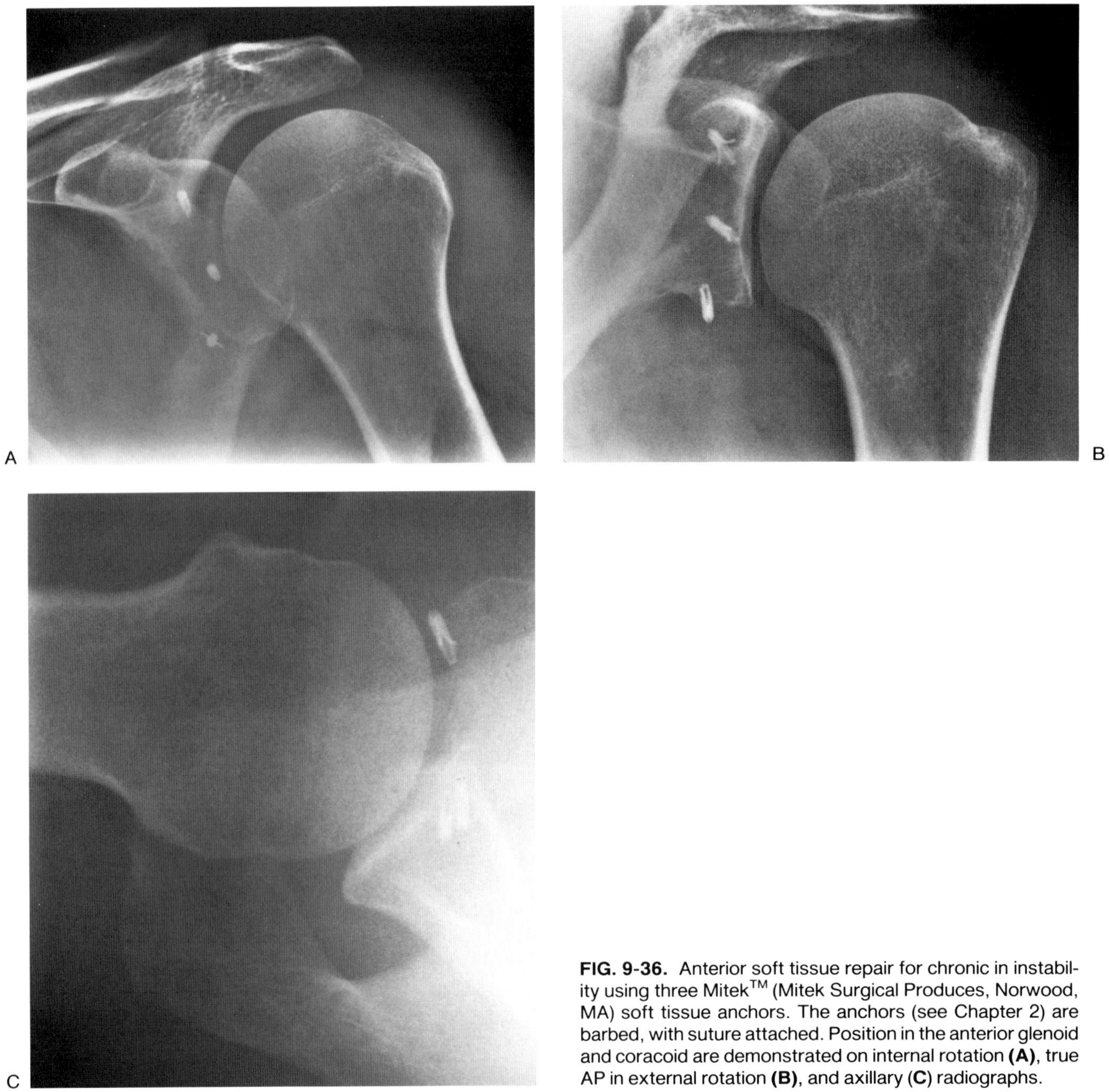

FIG. 9-36. Anterior soft tissue repair for chronic in instability using three Mitek™ (Mitek Surgical Produces, Norwood, MA) soft tissue anchors. The anchors (see Chapter 2) are barbed, with suture attached. Position in the anterior glenoid and coracoid are demonstrated on internal rotation **(A)**, true AP in external rotation **(B)**, and axillary **(C)** radiographs.

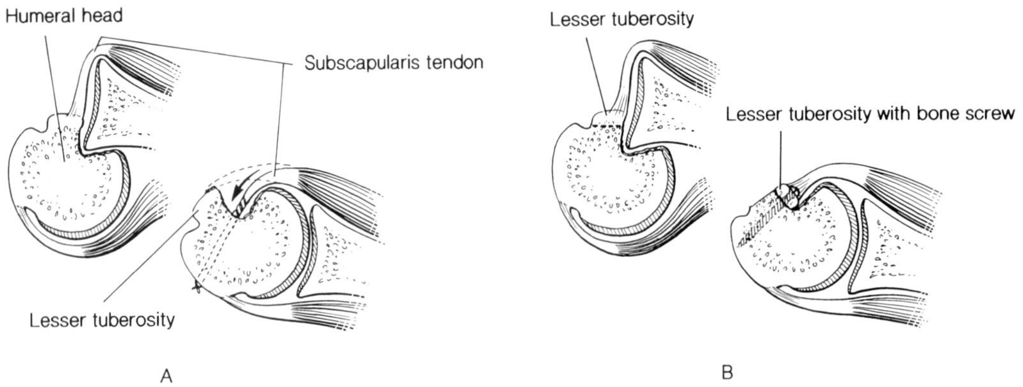

FIG. 9-37. A: The McLaughlin procedure with transfer of the subscapularis tendon into the large anteromedial humeral head defect. **B:** Neer modified this technique by including the lesser tuberosity with the tendon.

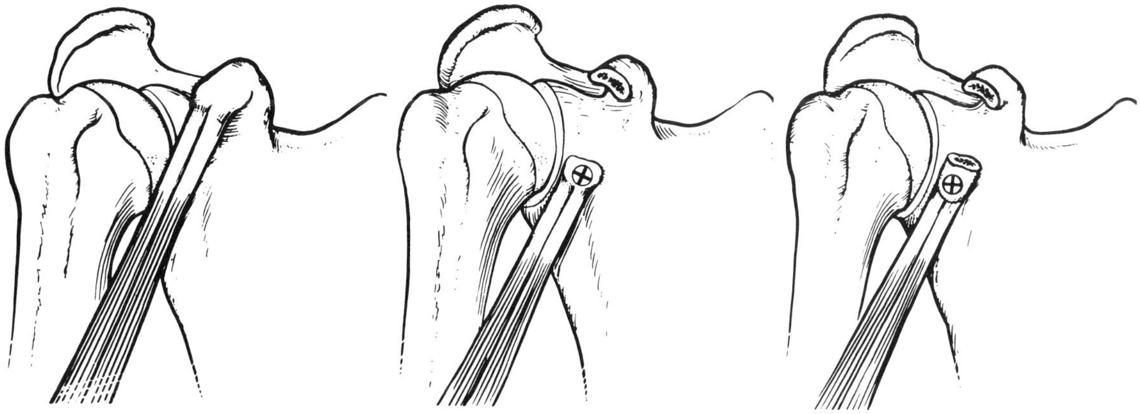

A,B C

FIG. 9-38. The normal coracoid and conjoined tendon **(A)**, coracoid transfer described by Bristow **(B)**, and transfer of coracoid to the glenoid neck, as described by Latarjet **(C)**. (From Young DC, Rockwood CA. Complications of a failed Bristow procedure and their management. *J Bone Joint Surg* [*Am*] 1991;73A:969–981.)

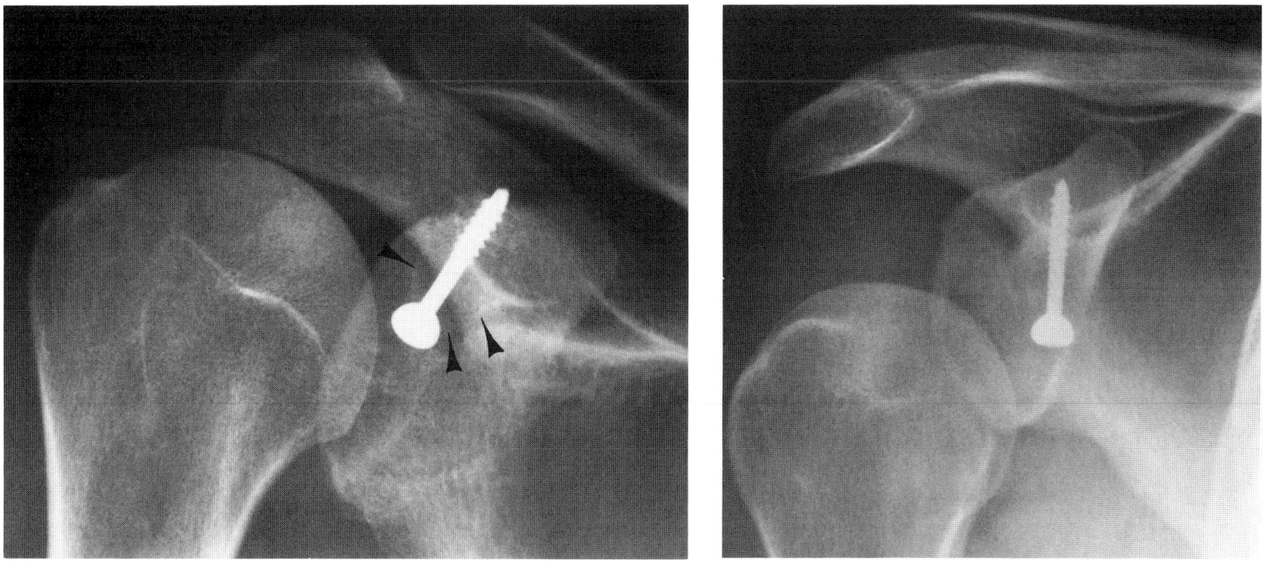

A B

FIG. 9-39. Radiographs of coracoid extension using iliac bone graft and screw fixation, the Oudard procedure. **A:** An AP radiograph after healing (note the coracoid extension, *arrows*). **B:** Recurrent instability 7 months later.

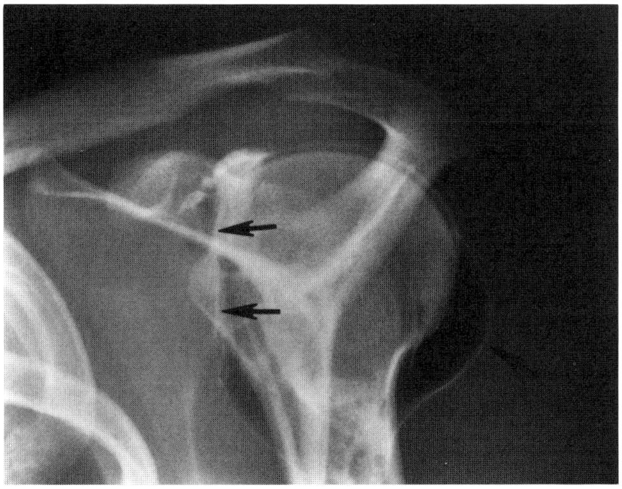

FIG. 9-40. Scapular Y view after a double-contrast arthrogram showing a tight (*arrows*) anterior capsule in a patient with previous anterior repair and decreased range of motion.

require more aggressive surgery, combined procedures, or arthrodesis.

Depending on the symptoms and type of fixation, follow-up imaging can be accomplished with routine radiography (Fig. 9-39) or arthrography with or without CT and fluoroscopically positioned stress views. This allows an assessment of the bone, soft tissue, metal implant, capsule size, and recurrent instability (Figs. 9-12 and 9-40).[81]

Acromioclavicular Dislocation

Dislocations of the acromioclavicular joint account for about 12% of all dislocations. The injury usually occurs after a fall with the force directed at the point of the shoulder. Less commonly, indirect force from superior displacement of the humeral head creates the dislocation.[73,75,81,150]

Allman[73] described acromioclavicular injuries based on the extent of ligament disruption. Type I injuries have a few fibers torn. Type II injuries have rupture of the acromioclavicular ligaments and capsule, and type III injuries involve rupture of the acromioclavicular and coracoclavicular ligaments (Table 9-2 and Fig. 9-41).[73,150] Rockwood[150] added three additional categories (types IV to VI, Fig. 9-41).

Routine radiographs of the shoulder or clavicle are normal with type I injuries. The AP views of the clavicle and acromioclavicular joint with the tube angled 10° to 15° to the head reduce bony overlap. In addition, lateral views are important to assess the position (anterior, superior, and posterior) of the distal clavicular articular surface. Axillary views are also useful for joint assessment.[81,150] Type II or III injuries require weight-bearing views for the diagnosis. We prefer to use a transverse 14 × 17 film to allow a comparison of both shoulders with and without weight bearing (Fig. 9-42). A weight of 8 to 10 pounds is attached to each wrist for weight-bearing views. If patients are allowed to hold the weights, they may involuntarily splint the shoulder, reducing the accuracy of the study.[81] Types IV to VI injuries may be evident without stressing the acromioclavicular joint (Fig. 9-43).[81] Arthrography of the acromioclavicular joint is useful in type II injuries to exclude meniscal and capsular entrapment.[81]

Treatment

Most injuries can be managed conservatively using adhesive straps, figure-eight bandage, slings, or braces.[150] Certain type II injuries have persistent pain, which may be due to clavicular osteolysis or derangement of the acromioclavicular joint.[79] Resection arthroplasty or débridement of the joint may be required.[102,135]

Surgical treatment for type III injuries may concentrate on the acromioclavicular joint, coracoclavicular repair, or both. Resection of the distal clavicle and dynamic muscle transfers may also be used.[80,86–88,99,135,150]

Intraarticular repairs can be accomplished with smooth or threaded Steinmann pins.[99] Most authors do not use K wires because of their small size and tendency to migrate or fracture.[99,150] Cortical screws can also be used, although the incidence of osteolysis of the clavicle is somewhat higher (8 of 13 cases reported by Esckola et al.[99]). This may be prevented by resection of the distal clavicle during repair.[166]

Extraarticular repairs concentrate on the repair of the coracoclavicular disruption. Bosworth[86,87] described the use of a cancellous screw (Fig. 9-44). Tsou[169] described the use of a cannulated screw in 1989. Other modifications include wire or mersilene suture fixation of the coracoid to the clavicle, fixation with the repair of the ligaments, and combined repair of the coracoclavicular ligament with reattachment of the deltoid and trapezius to the clavicle (Fig. 9-45).[80,150]

Dynamic muscle transfers can be accomplished by coracoid osteotomy with transfer of the coracoid and biceps tendon or tendon alone to the clavicle using a screw for fixation.[98,150]

Combined intra- and extraarticular techniques may be required for type IV to VI injuries because of the significant clavicular displacement and soft tissue injury.[150]

Sternoclavicular Dislocations

Dislocations of the sternoclavicular joints are uncommon, accounting for only about 3% of shoulder dislocations.[81,89,150,160] These strong support structures require significant trauma, generally applied through the shoulder before dislocation can occur.[81,150] Posterolateral forces transmitted medially cause anterior dislocation.

(text continues on page 691)

TABLE 9-2. *Acromioclavicular dislocation: classification, radiographic features, and prognosis*[73,81,150]

Classification	Radiographic features	Prognosis
Type I: acromioclavicular ligament strain	Normal	No instability, excellent
Type II: rupture of the capsule and coracoclavicular ligaments	Joint wide; clavicle may be slightly elevated	90% recovery with closed therapy, 10% require surgery
Type III: rupture of the acromioclavicular and coracoclavicular ligaments	Elevated clavicle; increased coracoclavicular distance	Closed or open therapy; internal fixation, 80% good results, 20% require reoperation

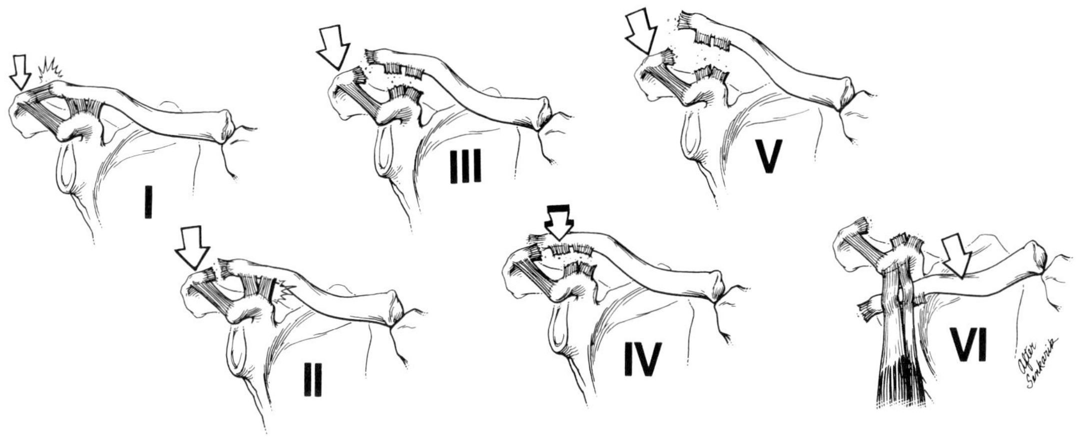

FIG. 9-41. Acromioclavicular ligament injury.[73,150] Type I, sprain of acromioclavicular ligaments; type II, disruption of acromioclavicular ligaments with intact coracoclavicular ligaments; type III, disruption of both acromioclavicular and coracoclavicular ligaments; type IV, disruption of both ligament complexes with posterior clavicular displacement; type V, disruption of both ligament complexes with superior elevation of the distal clavicle; type VI, disruption of the ligament complexes with anterior entrapment.

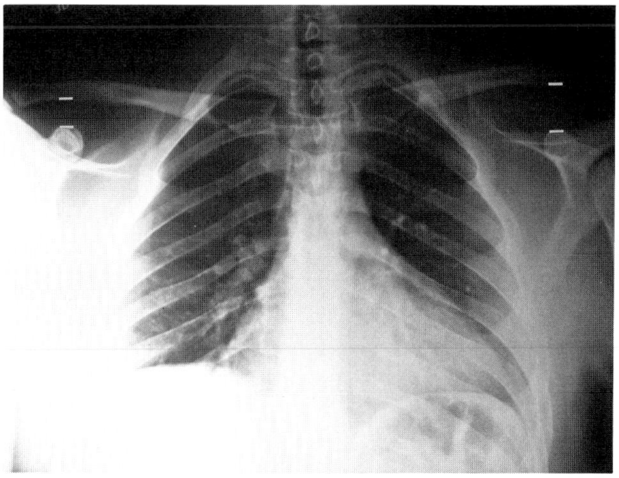

FIG. 9-42. Weight-bearing views demonstrate increased coracoclavicular distance on the left (*white lines*) as a result of a type III injury. The coracoclavicular ligaments are disrupted when the difference in coracoclavicular distance between the normal and abnormal side exceeds 5 mm.

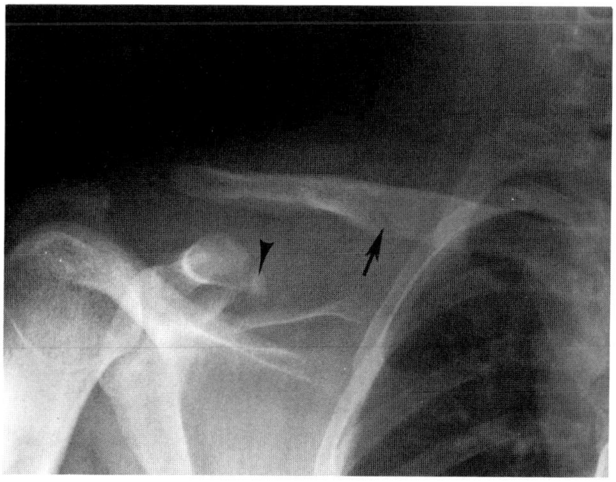

FIG. 9-43. Routine AP view of the clavicle demonstrating a type IV injury with associated fractures of the clavicle (*arrow*) and coracoid (*arrowhead*).

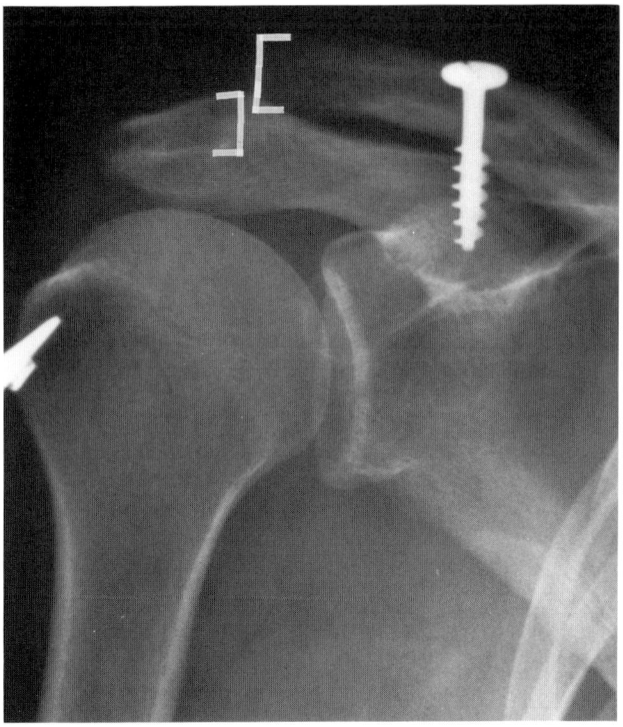

FIG. 9-44. Bosworth-type repair with a cancellous screw and washer. The threads partially penetrate the coracoid. Note the persistent subluxation of the acromioclavicular joint (*white lines*).

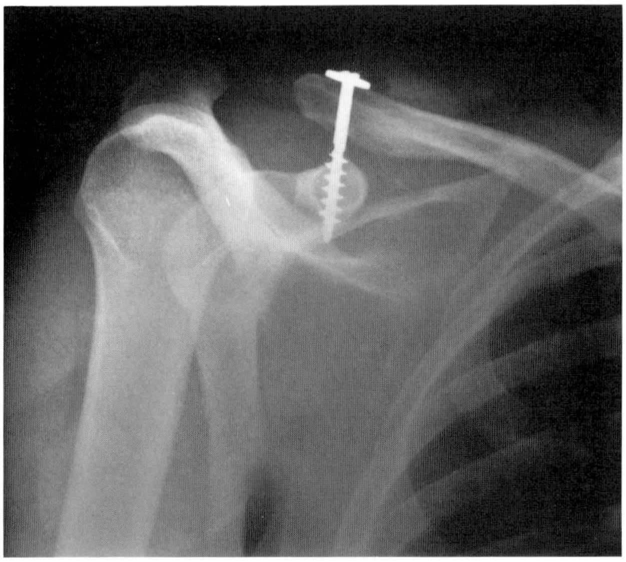

FIG. 9-45. An AP view of the shoulder after type IV dislocation with resection of the distal clavicle and a lag screw well positioned in the coracoid.

Direct anterior trauma causes posterior dislocation. Posterior dislocations are much more uncommon, accounting for 3 of 60 sternoclavicular dislocations in Nettles and Linscheid's[140] series. Bilateral dislocations are rare.[150] Anterior dislocations may be palpable, but posterior dislocations may be subtle and difficult to diagnose radiographically. Posterior dislocations must be diagnosed early because of the potential tracheal and great vessel injury.[89,94,160]

Allman[73] classified sternoclavicular dislocations similarly to acromioclavicular dislocations. Type I injuries are sprains with slight tearing of the sternoclavicular ligament. Type II injuries have disruption of the sternoclavicular ligaments. The sternoclavicular and costoclavicular ligaments are both torn in type III dislocations.

Imaging of the sternoclavicular joint is difficult with routine radiographs because of overlapping bony structures.[81] Angled and oblique techniques have been described (Fig. 9-46).[81,124] Tomography may be useful. However, CT is preferred for its ease of interpretation and its ability to detect associated soft tissue, vascular, or tracheal injury (Fig. 9-47).[81,89,160,174]

Treatment

Most sprains or moderate subluxations are treated conservatively. When reduction cannot be maintained, some prefer open ligament repair with temporary pin fixation. Complications related to the use of pins in this region are significant; many surgeons do not choose to use them.[150] Therefore, even complete dislocations are most often reduced without metallic fixation devices.[143,150,157,158]

Complications and Postoperative Imaging

Postreduction imaging of fractures and dislocations of the shoulder requires an understanding of the complications that are related to the initial injury and treatment.

Malunion of displaced clavicular fractures is not unusual. However, nonunion of clavicle fractures (1% to 2%) is rare and also infrequent with proximal humeral fractures (Fig. 9-48).[71,78,143] Routine radiography is usually sufficient for the detection of these complications. Subtle changes are more easily appreciated with conventional tomography or CT.[81] When nonunion of the greater tuberosity is suspected, CT or arthrography may be required to exclude interposition of the biceps tendon.[81,114]

Articular complications are not uncommon following intraarticular fractures or dislocations.[81,149] Osteoarthritis is a common complication, regardless of the joint involved (glenohumeral, acromioclavicular, or sternoclavicular). Fixation devices (Fig. 9-16), such as Rush rods used for fixation of proximal humeral fractures, can cause impingement.[81,150] Adhesive capsulitis is also a problem following glenohumeral fracture-dislocation.[82] Recurrent instability following trauma or surgical procedures for glenohumeral instability is most easily assessed with conventional techniques instead of MRI. In fact, conventional or CT arthrography provides the necessary information regarding the capsular volume, postoperative capsular deformity, and capsulitis, and stress views can define the extent of instability (Figs. 9-7, 9-10, and 9-12).[81,82,95]

Neurovascular complications (Fig. 9-49) can occur with glenohumeral, clavicular, and sternoclavicular injuries.[81,106,123,130,172,178] Either MRI or angiographic techniques may be required in this setting.

Implant complications include pin migration, screw or staple pull out, and implant fracture (Figs. 9-50 to 9-54).[81,122,125,128,150,178] Routine radiographs or fluoroscopically positioned spot views may be adequate to define these problems. However, in some cases, CT may be required to evaluate bone blocks and other subtle osseous complications.[81]

Other complications include AVN of the humeral head (most common with four-part fractures) and myositis ossificans; MRI is most effective for the detection of AVN unless there is too much metal in the region of interest. In addition, CT is preferred for evaluating myositis ossificans.[81,82]

SHOULDER ARTHROPLASTY

Glenohumeral joint replacement arthroplasty has become the technique of choice for patients with articular damage and pain that does not respond to more conservative measures.[181,182,185,194,195,205]

Indications and Preoperative Evaluation

Shoulder arthroplasty is most commonly performed because of pain and decreased function caused by rheumatoid arthritis, osteoarthritis, AVN, or trauma.[194,205,210,211,224] Table 9-3 lists the indications in order of decreasing frequency.

(text continues on page 696)

TABLE 9-3. *Shoulder replacement: arthroplasty indications*[183,193–195,205,206,218,220–222]

Indications
Osteoarthritis
Rheumatoid arthritis
Traumatic arthritis
Rotator cuff arthropathy
Avascular necrosis
Old infection
Systemic lupus erythematosus
Ankylosing spondylitis
Radiation necrosis
Hemophilia

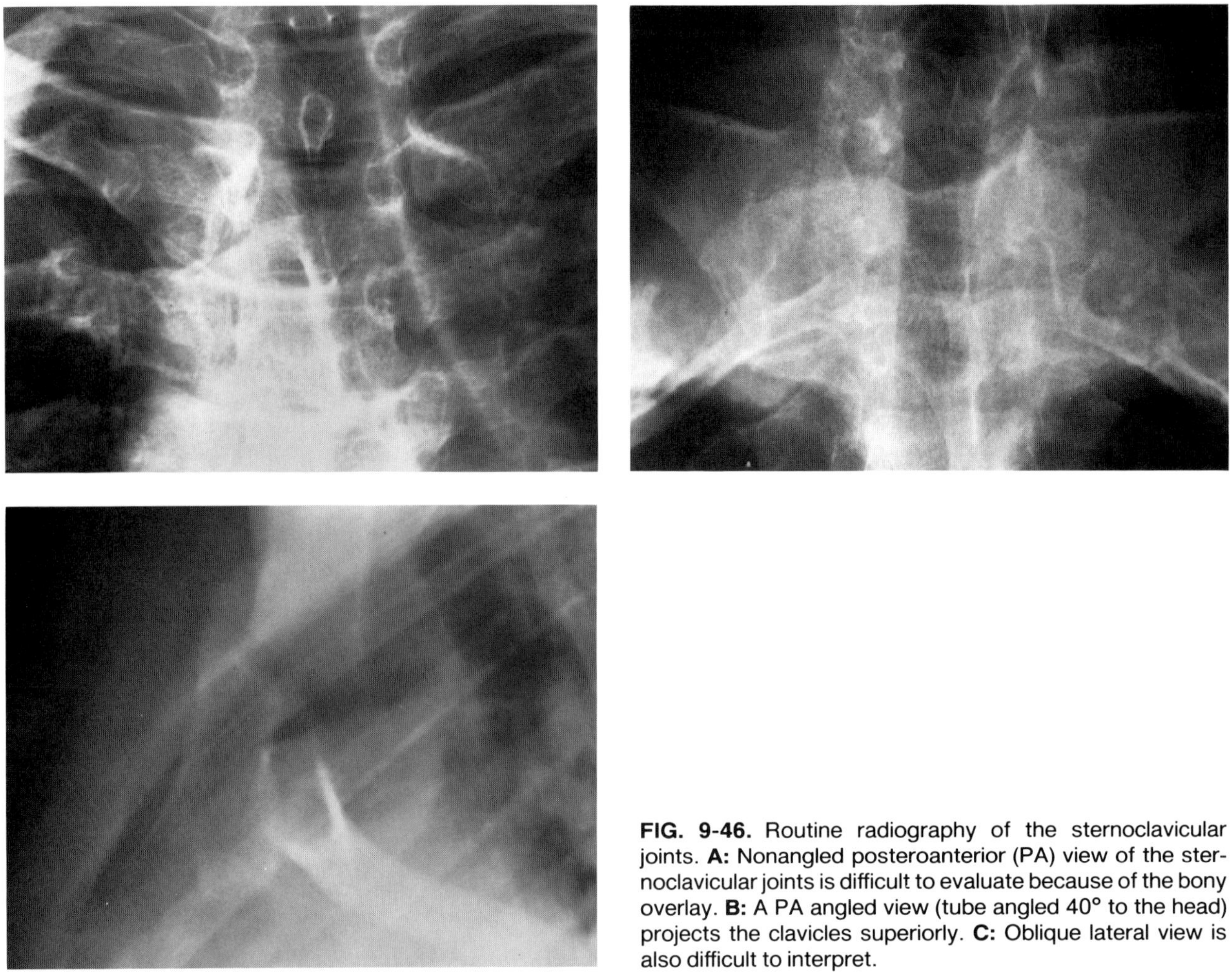

A

B

C

FIG. 9-46. Routine radiography of the sternoclavicular joints. **A:** Nonangled posteroanterior (PA) view of the sternoclavicular joints is difficult to evaluate because of the bony overlay. **B:** A PA angled view (tube angled 40° to the head) projects the clavicles superiorly. **C:** Oblique lateral view is also difficult to interpret.

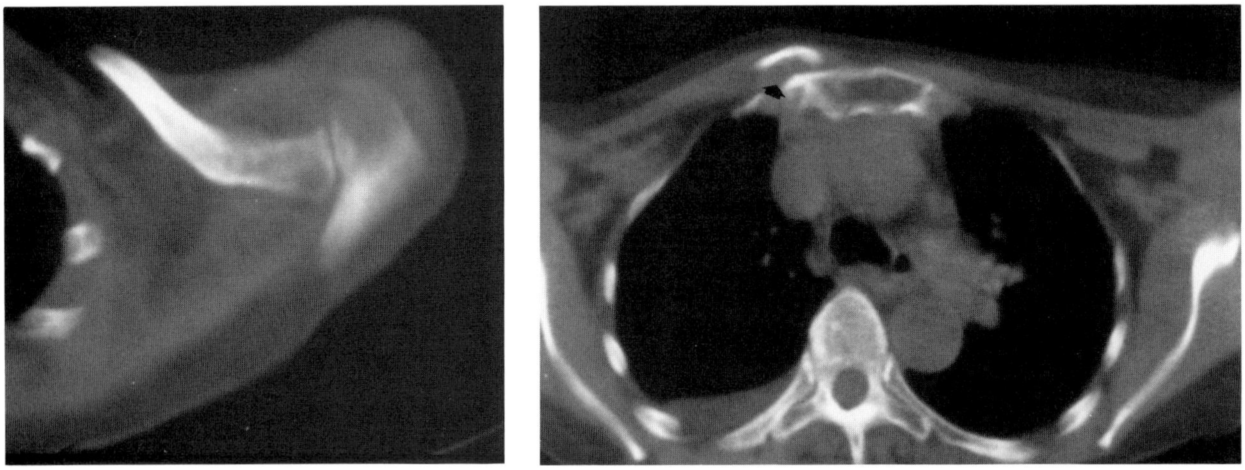

A

B

FIG. 9-47. The CT images after sternoclavicular trauma. **A:** Normal clavicle and acromioclavicular joint. **B:** Fracture dislocation (*arrow*) on the right.

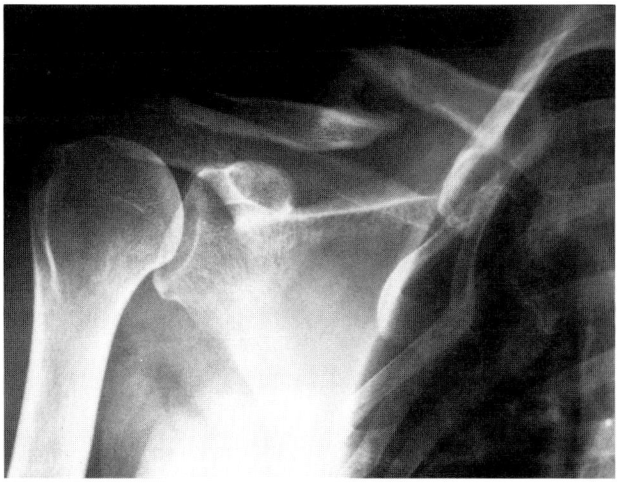

FIG. 9-48. An AP view of the clavicle with a nonunited overriding fracture.

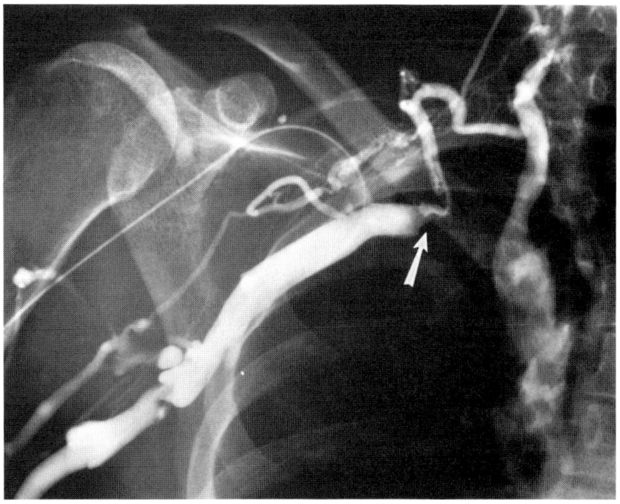

FIG. 9-49. Right arm venogram after sternoclavicular subluxation with venous occlusion (*arrow*).

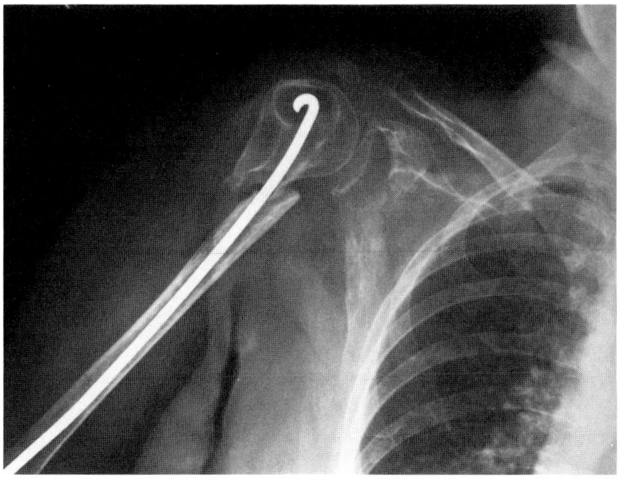

FIG. 9-50. Old proximal humeral fracture treated with a single Rush rod. The rod is loose, and the fracture is not united.

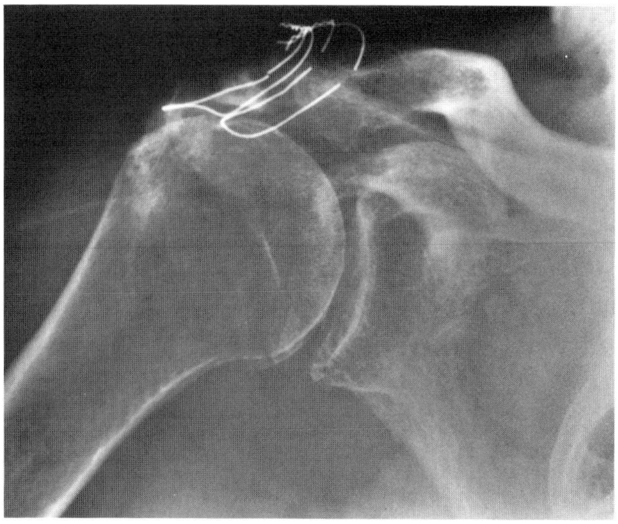

FIG. 9-51. An AP radiograph of the shoulder demonstrating wire fracture after acromioclavicular repair. There is advanced rotator cuff arthropathy.

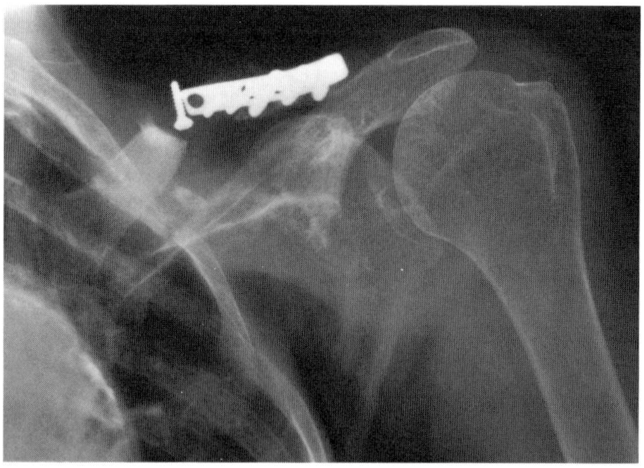

FIG. 9-52. Nonunited clavicle fracture, which is internally fixed with a six-hole one-third tubular plate. One of the screws has pulled out and migrated.

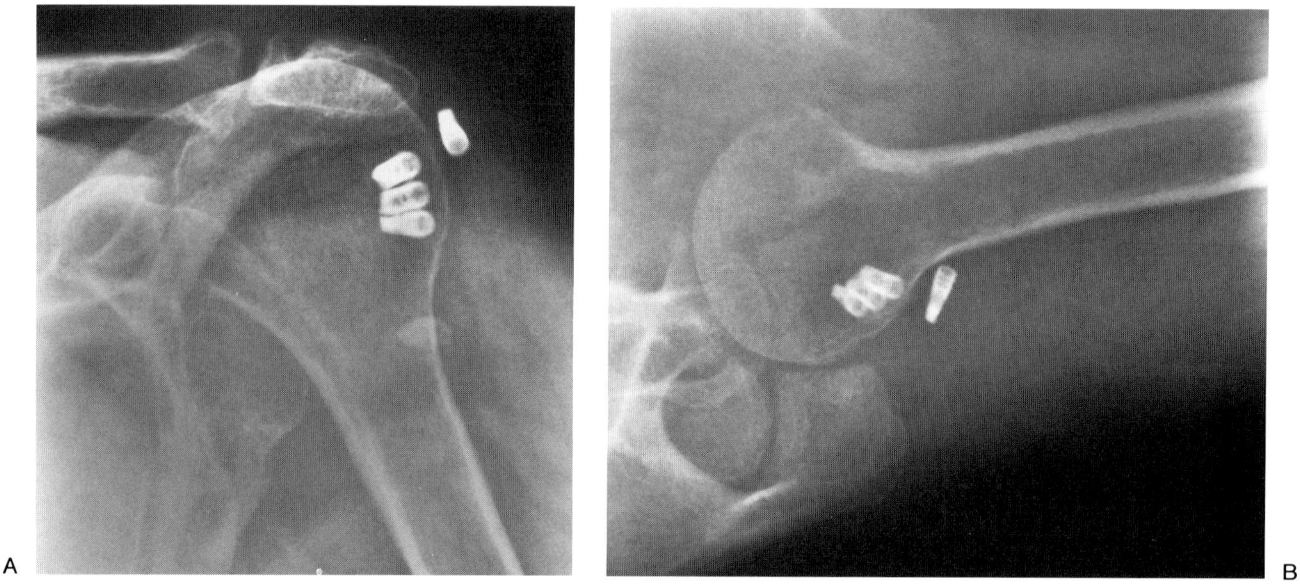

FIG. 9-53. The AP **(A)** and axillary **(B)** views after posterior repair using four Statek™ (Zimmer, Warsaw, IN) soft tissue anchors. One of the anchors has pulled out (see Chapter 2).

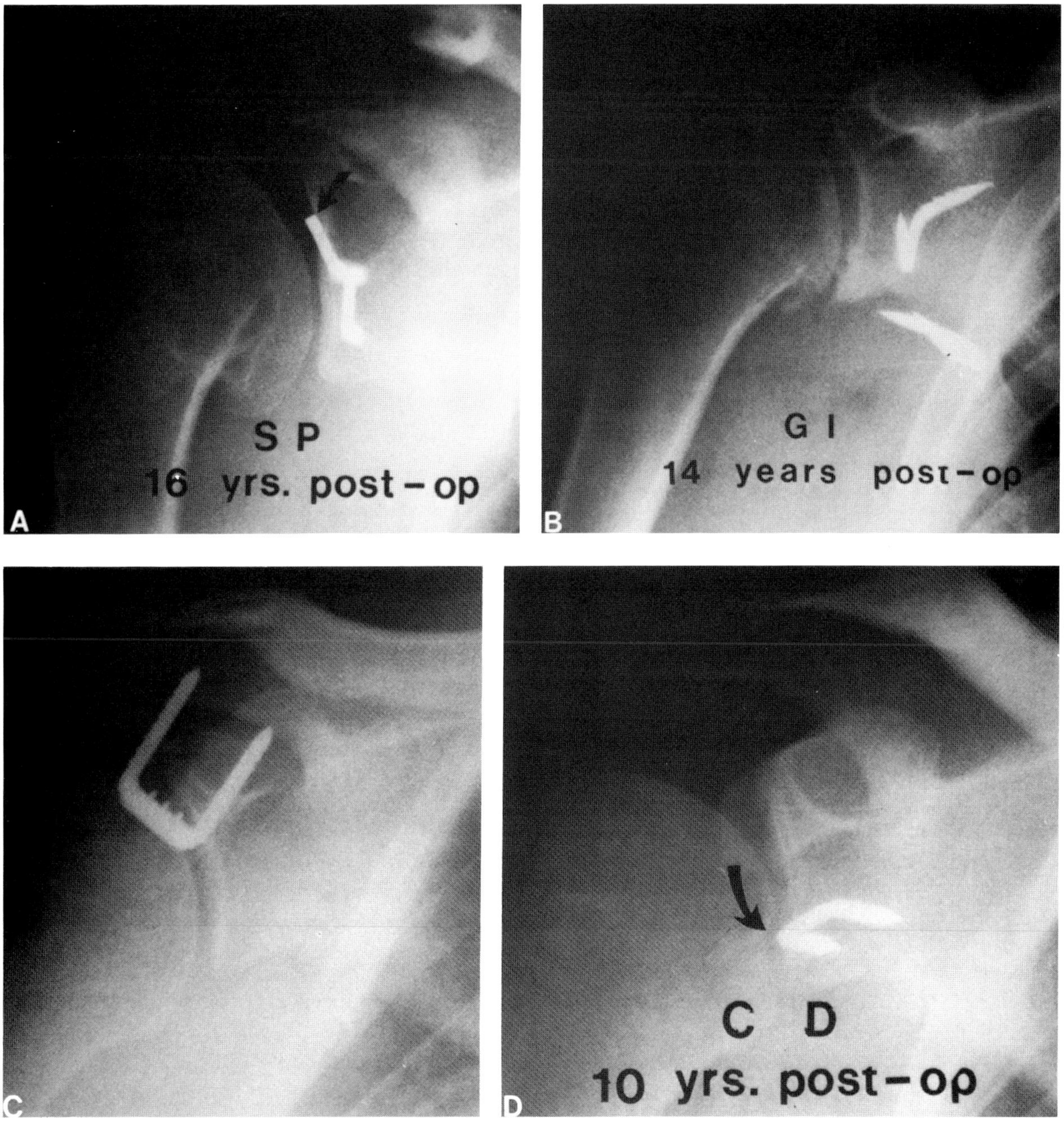

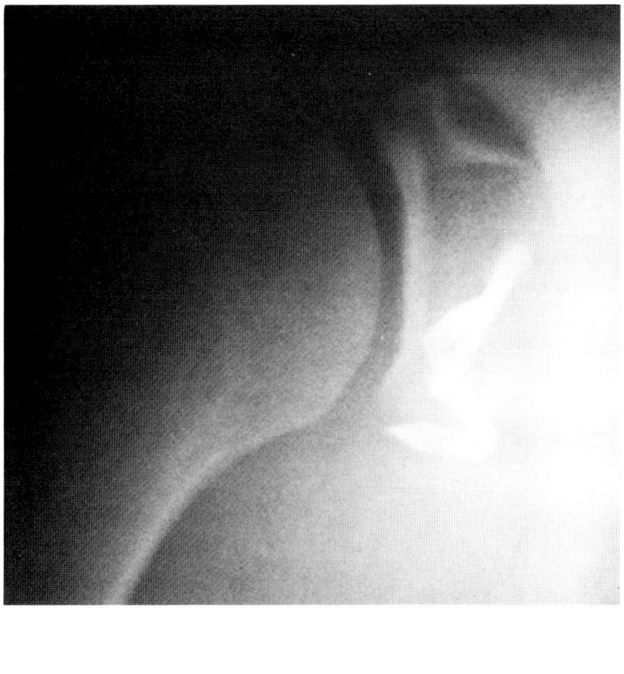

FIG. 9-54. Staple complications. **A:** Staple (*arrow*) penetrating the articular cartilage at time of placement. **B:** Migration of the inferior staple. **C:** Staple is too superior, and the upper prong is not in bone. **D:** Staple impinging on the humeral head. **E:** Bent staple with one prong under the glenoid. (From O'Driscoll SW, Evans DC. Long-term results of staple capsulorrhaphy for anterior instability of the shoulder. *J Bone Joint Surg* [*Am*] 1993;75A:249–258.)

Whatever the underlying condition, the prognosis and selection of repair technique varies with the extent of joint, bone, and soft tissue involvement. The extent of synovial disease, capsular and rotator cuff involvement, and bone structural changes are important. Bone loss may be caused by trauma, erosive arthritis, AVN, or osteopenia.[193–196,205]

As with other joints discussed in previous chapters, a scoring system has been devised for shoulder evaluation.[180,205] The University of California at Los Angeles scoring system is commonly used to grade the pain, function, and strength pre- and postoperatively.[180] The system uses a ten-point scale for pain, function, and range of motion. The scores in each category are graded as excellent (nine to ten points), good (six to eight points), fair (four to five points), or poor (one to three points). Patients with severe pain preoperatively (one to three points) may have significant improvement. However, patients with advanced rheumatoid arthritis and poor function and range of motion should not expect as much improvement in these categories postoperatively as can those patients with less severe disease.[205]

Preoperative imaging may require multiple modalities, depending on the physical examination and other clinical data. True AP, axillary, and scapular Y views should be available to evaluate the joint spaces and osseous abnormalities (Fig. 9-55).[179,186,202] The evaluation of bone stock, especially in the glenoid, is most easily accomplished with CT, the use of which should be considered in patients with trauma (Fig. 9-56), osteopenia, or erosive arthritis with bone loss to plan the operative procedure and determine the extent of bone grafting that may be necessary.[186,221,234] Soft tissue structures are most easily evaluated with MRI. When instability is suspected, we prefer arthrography with fluoroscopically positioned stress views and CT when necessary to define the extent of instability.[186] Templates (Fig. 9-57) can be used preoperatively to serve as a guide to component selection and sizing.

Component Selection and Configurations

Although there are alternative techniques to implant arthroplasty (Fig. 9-58), this discussion concentrates on joint replacement techniques.[216]

Design choices for shoulder arthroplasty include constrained, semiconstrained, and anatomic or nonconstrained systems (Figs. 9-59 to 9-66).[179,180,184,193–195,212,226] Constrained components are intended for patients with a loss of rotator cuff mechanism or when there is inadequate soft tissue strength and support.[225] Constrained prosthesis have limited indications and an unacceptably high incidence of loosening (25% for cemented). They are not commonly used today (Figs. 9-67 and 9-68).[212,215,226] Therefore, this review concentrates on commonly used current nonconstrained designs.

Humeral Components

The first prosthetic arthroplasty of the shoulder was performed by Pein in 1893.[183] Prior to the 1950s, arthrodesis or resection arthroplasty (Fig. 9-58) were the only effective surgical techniques for glenohumeral arthritis.[231] Several humeral designs, including metal cup arthroplasty (Fig. 9-69) and Silastic™ and plastic implants were attempted with limited success.[198]

In 1952, Neer replaced the humeral head with a Vitallium prosthesis. This was followed by reports of further success in pain relief and function using humeral implants in 1955.[219] Today, the Neer prosthesis has multiple head sizes and 14 varieties of stems (Fig. 9-70).[231]

Bipolar components (Fig. 9-71) were designed by Swanson in 1975.[233] Swanson et al.[233] reported results with this system, which is recommended for patients with cuff arthroplasty or superior subluxation of the humeral head in patients with rheumatoid arthritis. In a series of 35 patients, this group reported 89% pain relief with 79° of flexion and 28° of external rotation postoperatively. When vertical or superior subluxation occurs with a bipolar system, the larger unfixed cup helps distribute the deltoid muscle forces over a larger area of the acromion (Fig. 9-72).

Modular humeral components have become popular today. These systems provide increased flexibility with regard to head and stem interchange and selection. Biomodular™ (Biomet, Warsaw, IN; Fig. 9-73), Fenlin™ (Zimmer, Warsaw, IN; Fig. 9-74), Global™ (DePuy, Warsaw, IN; Figs. 9-75 and 9-76), and Select™ (Intermedics, Austin, TX) have modular heads. With some variation, all humeral components have proximal holes for suturing soft tissue or bone fragments and stabilization fins.

Glenoid Components

Both metal-backed and all-polyethylene glenoid components are available (Figs. 9-75C,D; 9-76D; and 9-77 to 9-80). Fixation is accomplished using pegs, fins, a keel, or cancellous screws. The pegs or screws tend to have less problem with pull out. Neer et al.[222] suggested using metal-backed glenoid components in younger, more active patients. Occasionally, the thicker metal-backed designs make closure of the capsule difficult, and instead, an all-polyethylene component is cemented in position. Hooded glenoid components are designed to improve stability in patients with rotator cuff deficiency (Fig. 9-79).[180]

Hemiarthroplasty Versus Total Shoulder Arthroplasty

Numerous humeral component designs have been developed for hemiarthroplasty.[206,208,218,221] The metal cup

(text continues on page 717)

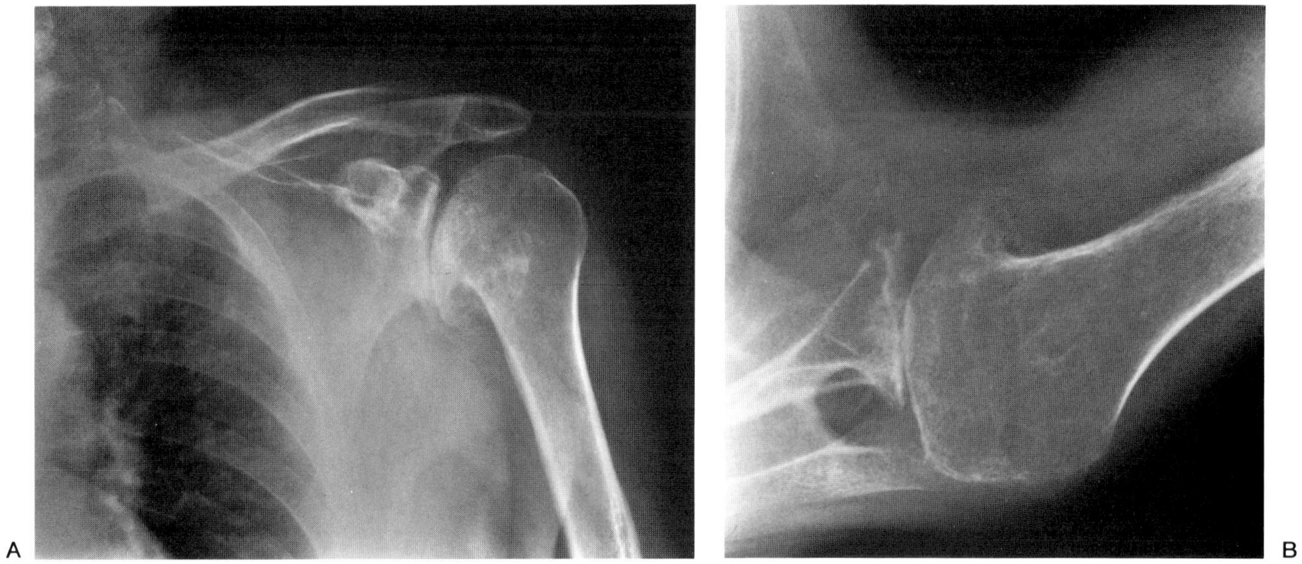

FIG. 9-55. Preoperative radiographs. A: True AP of the left shoulder demonstrating joint space narrowing and deformity with new bone formation of the inferomedial humeral head. The lower glenoid is flattened and deformed. B: Axillary view demonstrating joint space narrowing and flattening of the humeral head and glenoid with posterior subluxation.

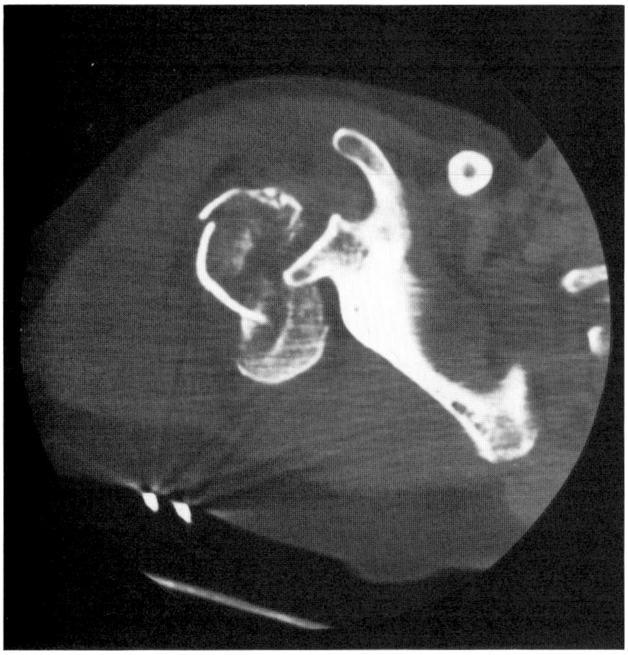

FIG. 9-56. A CT scan after a four-part humeral fracture with posterior dislocation and impaction. The glenoid is normal; CT imaging is useful to exclude glenoid injury or evaluate osteopenia or erosive arthropathy.

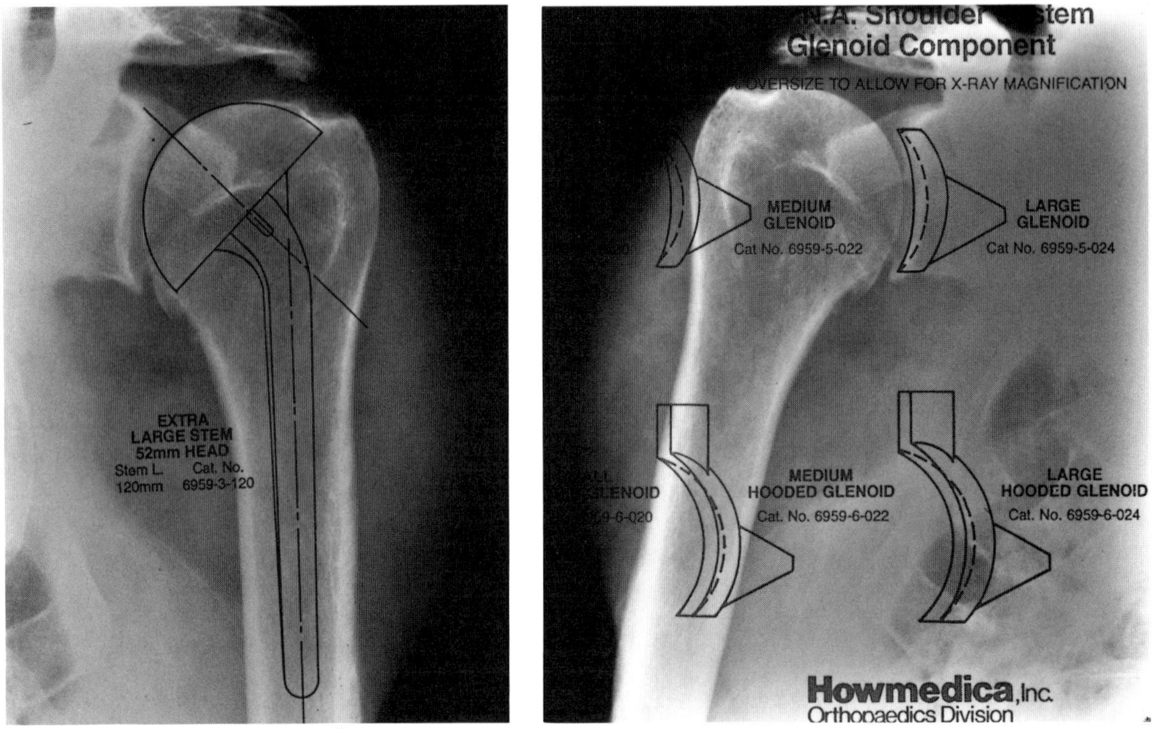

A B

FIG. 9-57. Preoperative templates. **A:** An AP view of the left shoulder with template aligned over the humerus for humeral component selection. **B:** The AP view of the right shoulder with glenoid component template sheet aligned to evaluate the larger glenoid component. (templates, D.A.N.A.™ shoulder. Courtesy of Howmedica, Rutherford, NJ.)

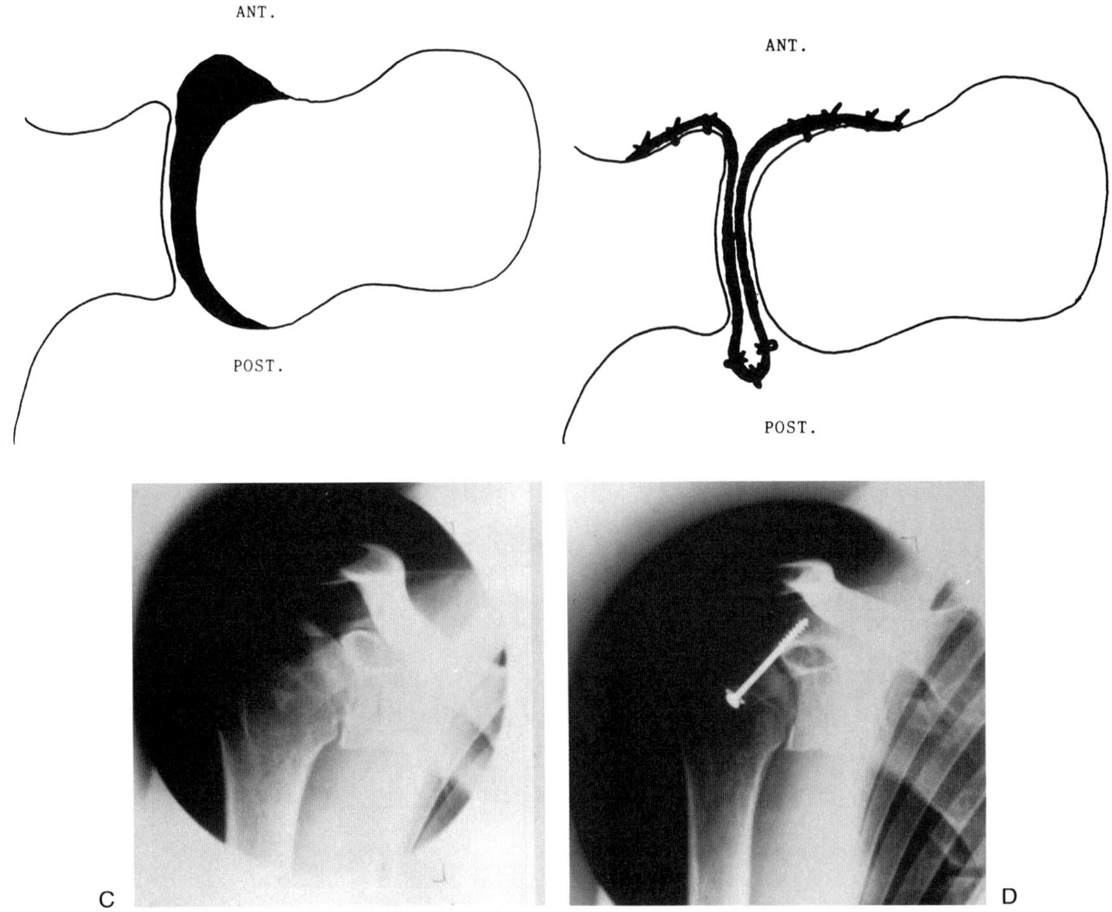

FIG. 9-58. Resection interpositioning arthroplasty (RIAP). **A:** Bone resection. **B:** Interposed dura mater membrane at RIAP. Pre- **(C)** and postoperative **(D)** radiographs after resection interpositioning arthroplasty. A coracoid osteotomy was also performed with a single cancellous screw and washer for fixation. (From Milbrink J, Wigren A. Resection arthroplasty of the shoulder. *Scand J Rheumatol* 1990; 19: 432–436.)

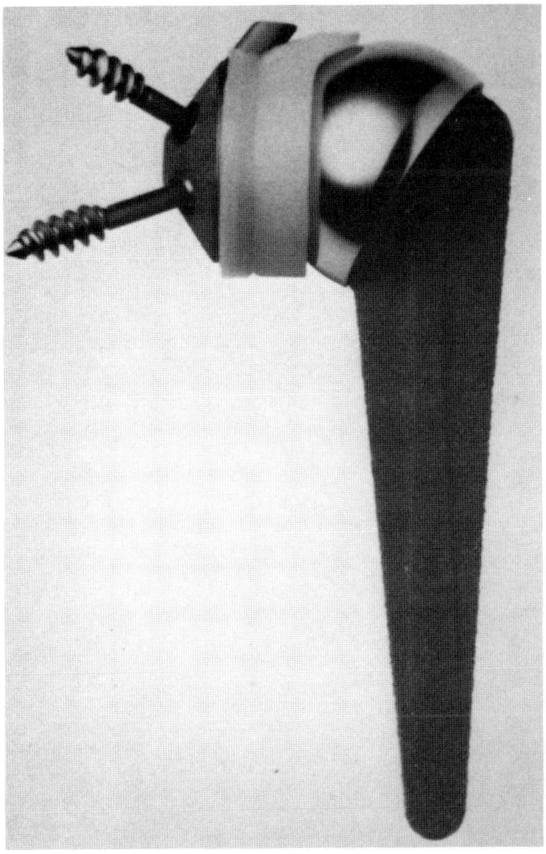

A

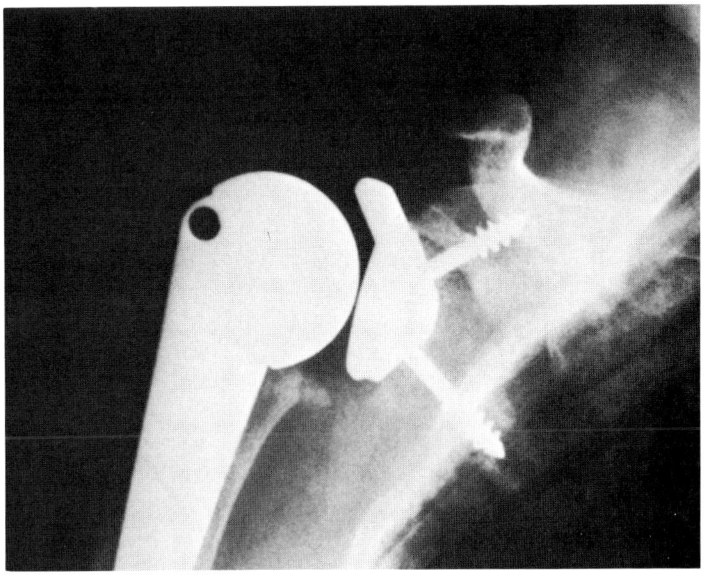

B

FIG. 9-59. A: The English-McNab porous-coated shoulder prosthesis.[199] (From Faludi and Weiland,[199] with permission.) **B:** An AP radiograph of the English-McNab shoulder prosthesis, i.e., metal-backed porous-coated glenoid component with screws for fixation, porous-coated humeral component, and semiconstrained.[184] The authors describe this prosthesis as essentially nonconstrained in their original article.[215] (From McElwain JP, English E. The early results of porous-coated total shoulder arthroplasty. *Clin Orthop* 1987;218:217–224.)

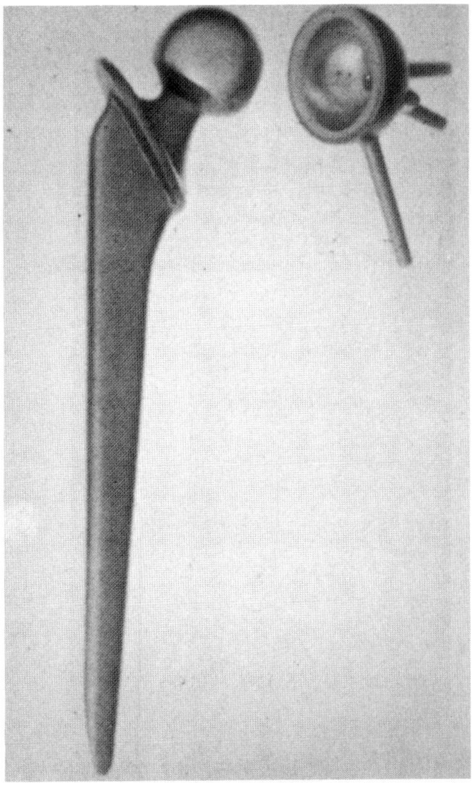

A

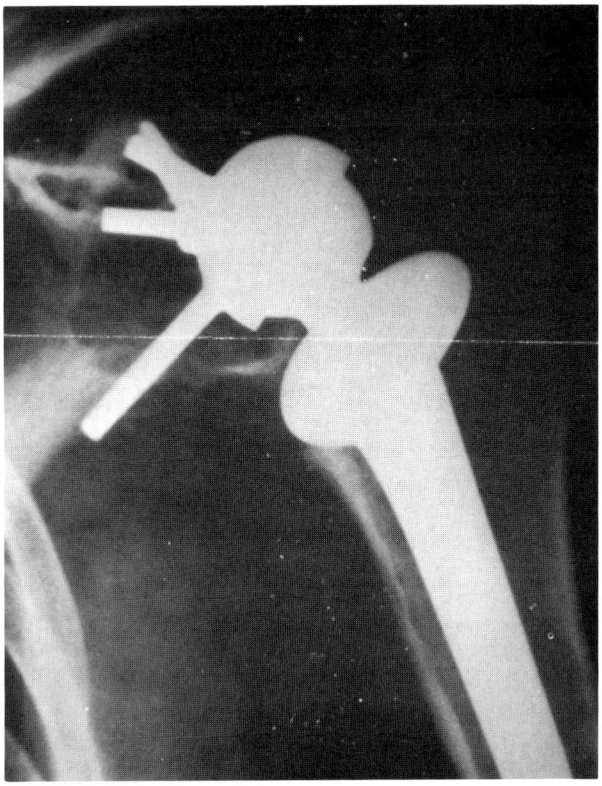

B

FIG. 9-60. A: The semiconstrained Mark II Stanmore prosthesis. Cobalt-chrome ball and socket design.[212] (From Lettin et al.,[212] with permission.) **B:** An AP radiograph of the semiconstrained Stanmore prosthesis.[196] (From Coughlin MJ, Morris JM, West WF. The semiconstrained total shoulder arthroplasty. *J Bone Joint Surg [Am]* 1979;61A:574–581.)

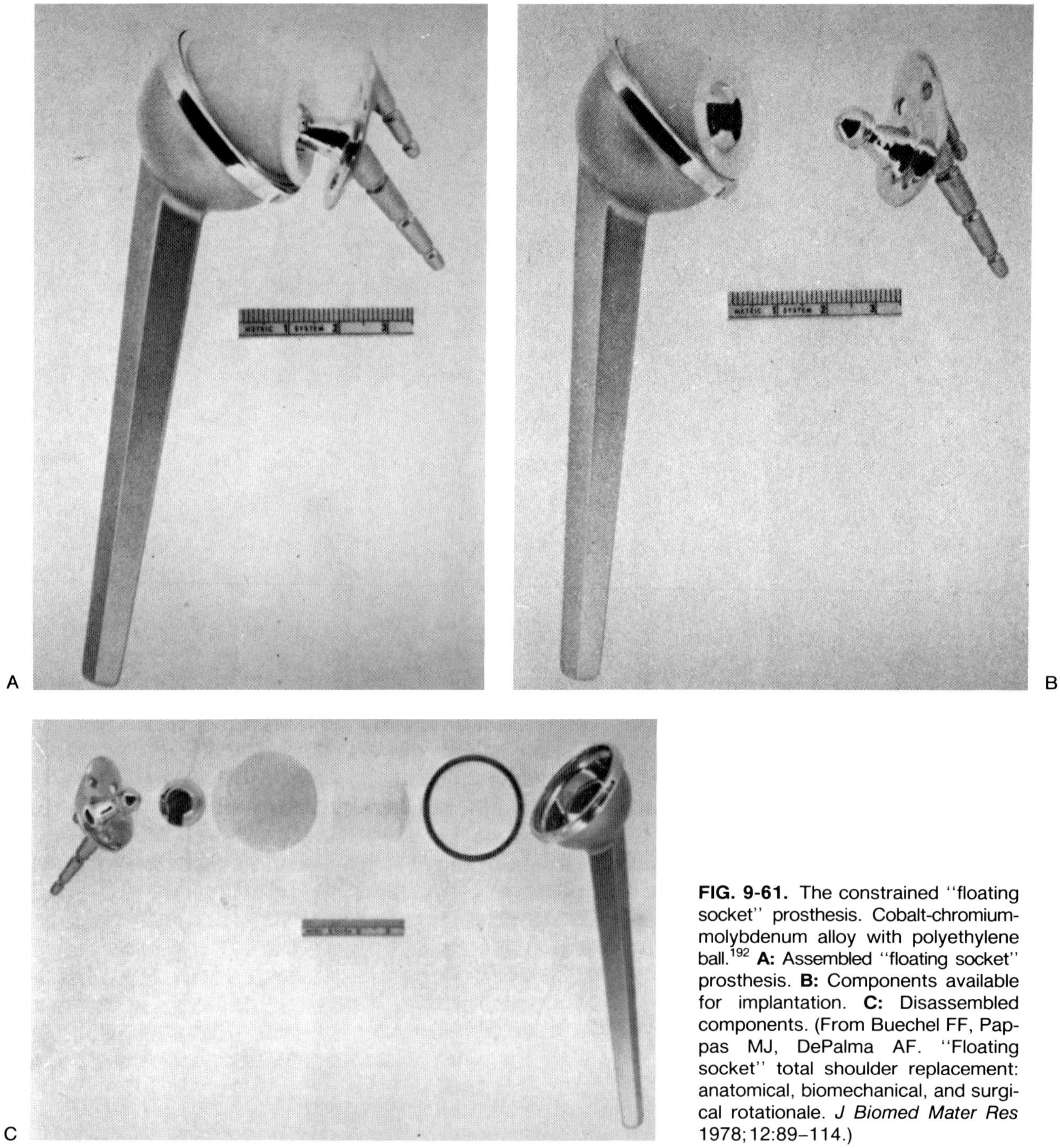

FIG. 9-61. The constrained "floating socket" prosthesis. Cobalt-chromium-molybdenum alloy with polyethylene ball.[192] **A:** Assembled "floating socket" prosthesis. **B:** Components available for implantation. **C:** Disassembled components. (From Buechel FF, Pappas MJ, DePalma AF. "Floating socket" total shoulder replacement: anatomical, biomechanical, and surgical rotationale. *J Biomed Mater Res* 1978;12:89–114.)

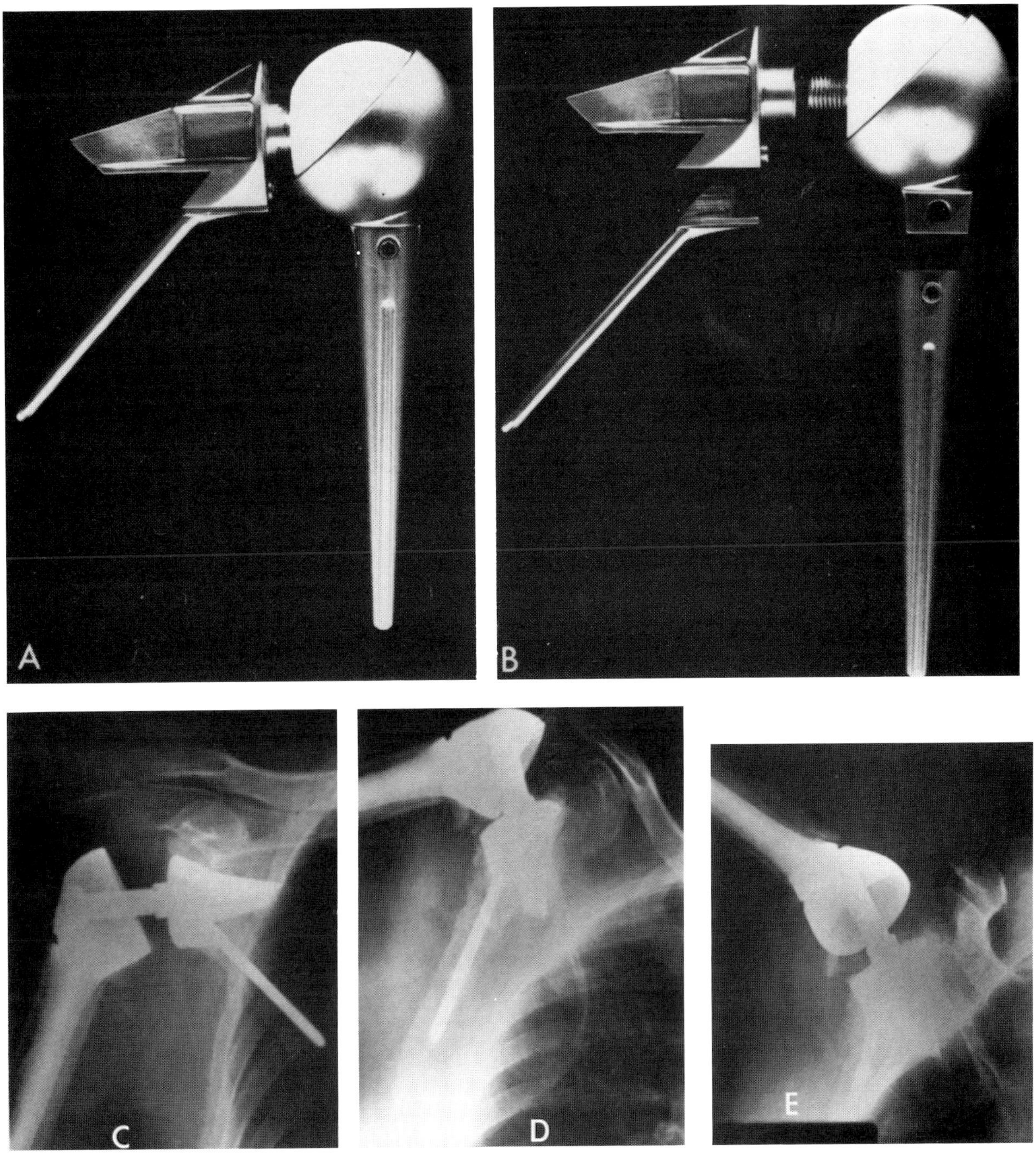

FIG. 9-62. The Fenlin™ reverse ball and socket constrained shoulder arthroplasty with components assembled **(A)** and disassembled **(B)**. Polyethylene ball and metal cup. Metal components, titanium-aluminum-vanadium alloy.[201] Radiographs with prosthesis in place **(C)**, elevated to 70° mainly by scapulothoracic motion **(D)**, and elevated greater than 70° **(E)** as a result of prosthetic motion. (From Fenlin JM. Total glenohumeral joint replacement. *Orthop Clin North Am* 1975;6:565–583.)

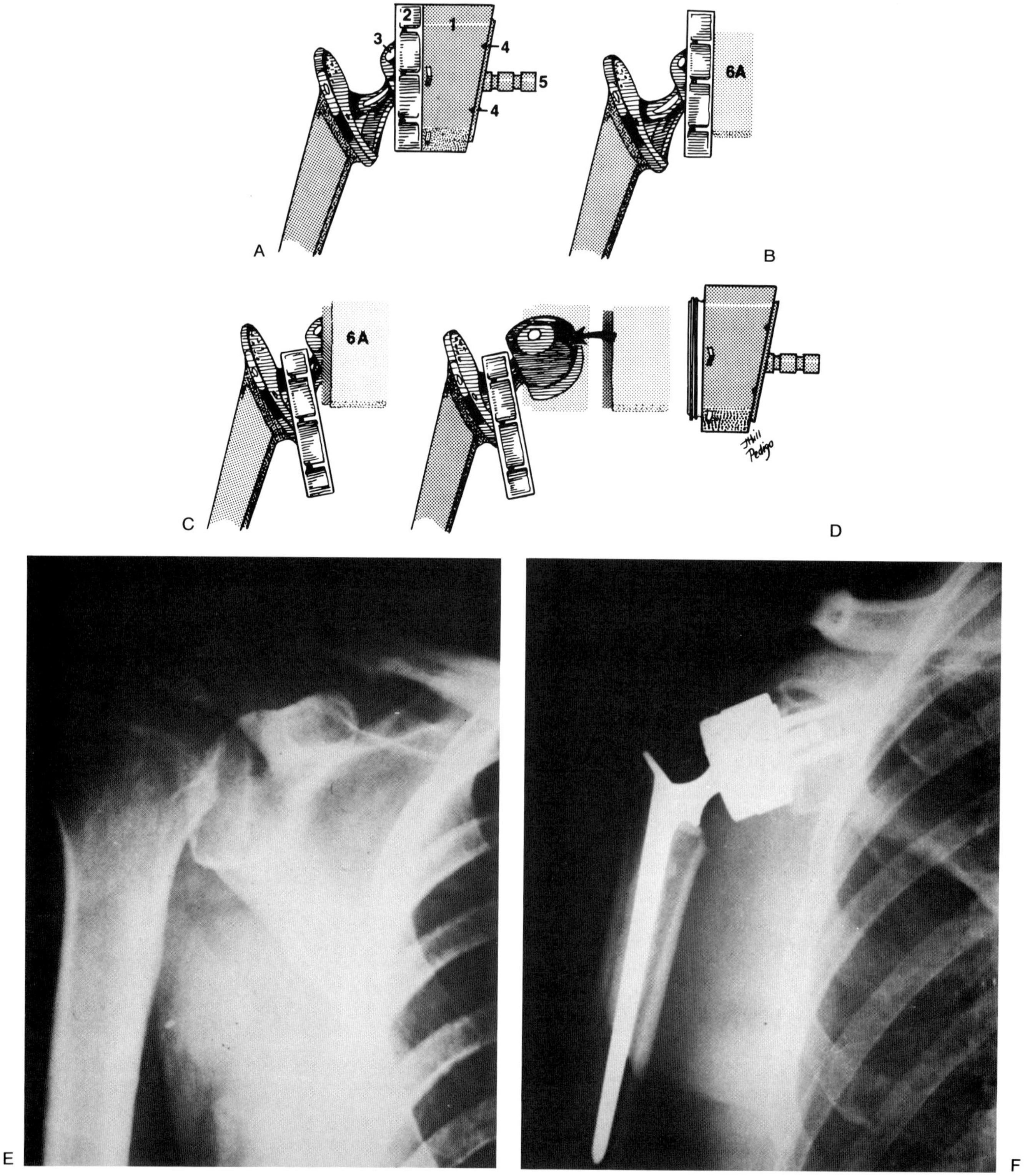

FIG. 9-63. The constrained Michael Reese total shoulder (MRTS). **A:** Assembled: *1,* metal glenoid cup; *2,* tightened metal locking ring; *3,* series II humeral head; *4,* position of eccentric screw holes; *5,* metal stem. **B:** Prosthesis with metal cup removed. **C:** Metal ring pulled over neck demonstrating polyethylene peripheral lip (*6,* in A). **D:** Disassembled shows metal ring fits over neck and polyethylene inserts placed over head before attaching metal cup. **E:** Preoperative radiograph in a patient with superior humeral migration caused by rotator cuff disease. **F:** An AP radiograph after implantation of the MRTS. (From Post M, Haskell SS, Jablon M. Total shoulder replacement with a constrained prosthesis. *J Bone Joint Surg* [*Am*] 1980;62A:327–335.)

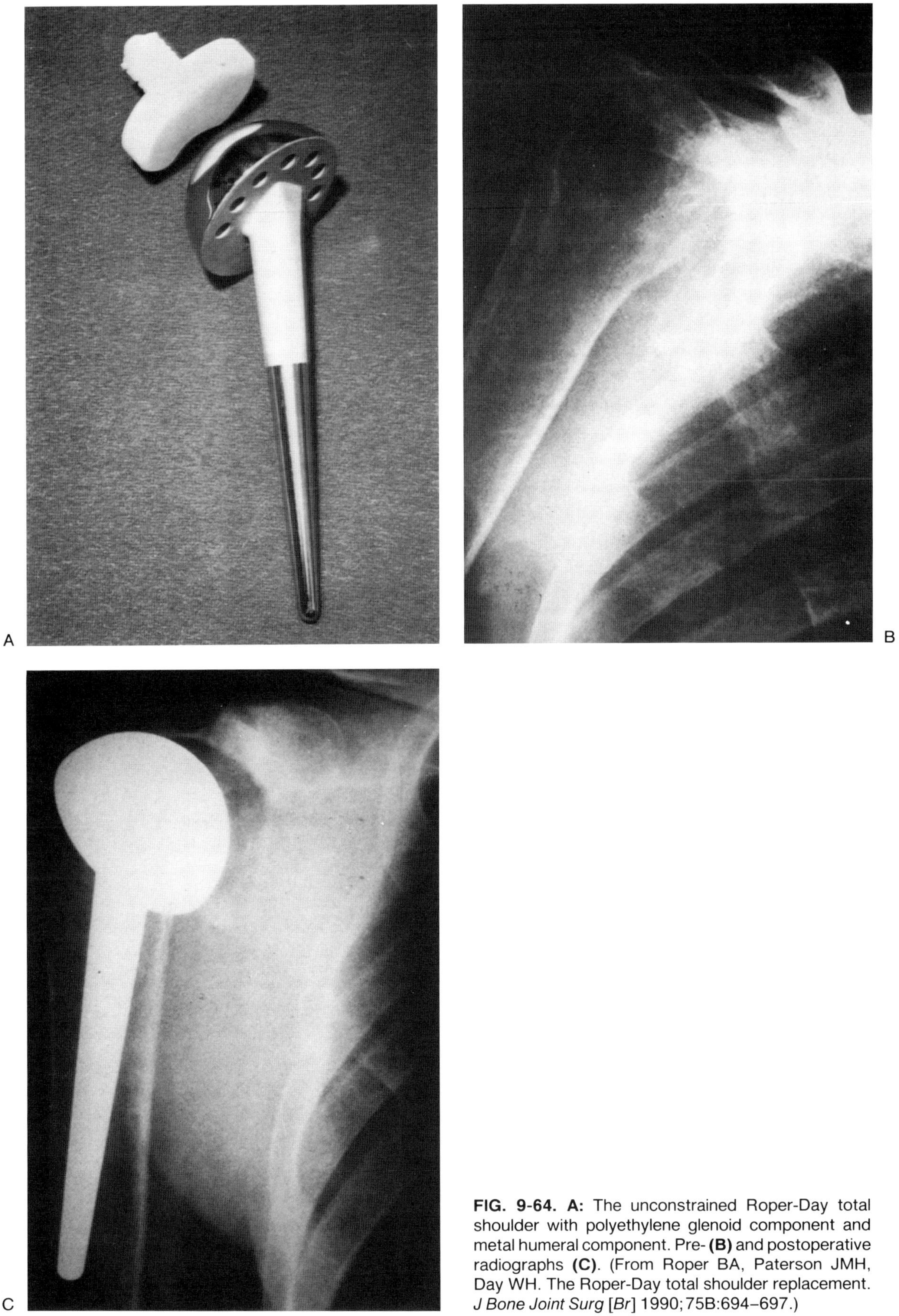

FIG. 9-64. **A:** The unconstrained Roper-Day total shoulder with polyethylene glenoid component and metal humeral component. Pre- **(B)** and postoperative radiographs **(C)**. (From Roper BA, Paterson JMH, Day WH. The Roper-Day total shoulder replacement. *J Bone Joint Surg* [*Br*] 1990;75B:694–697.)

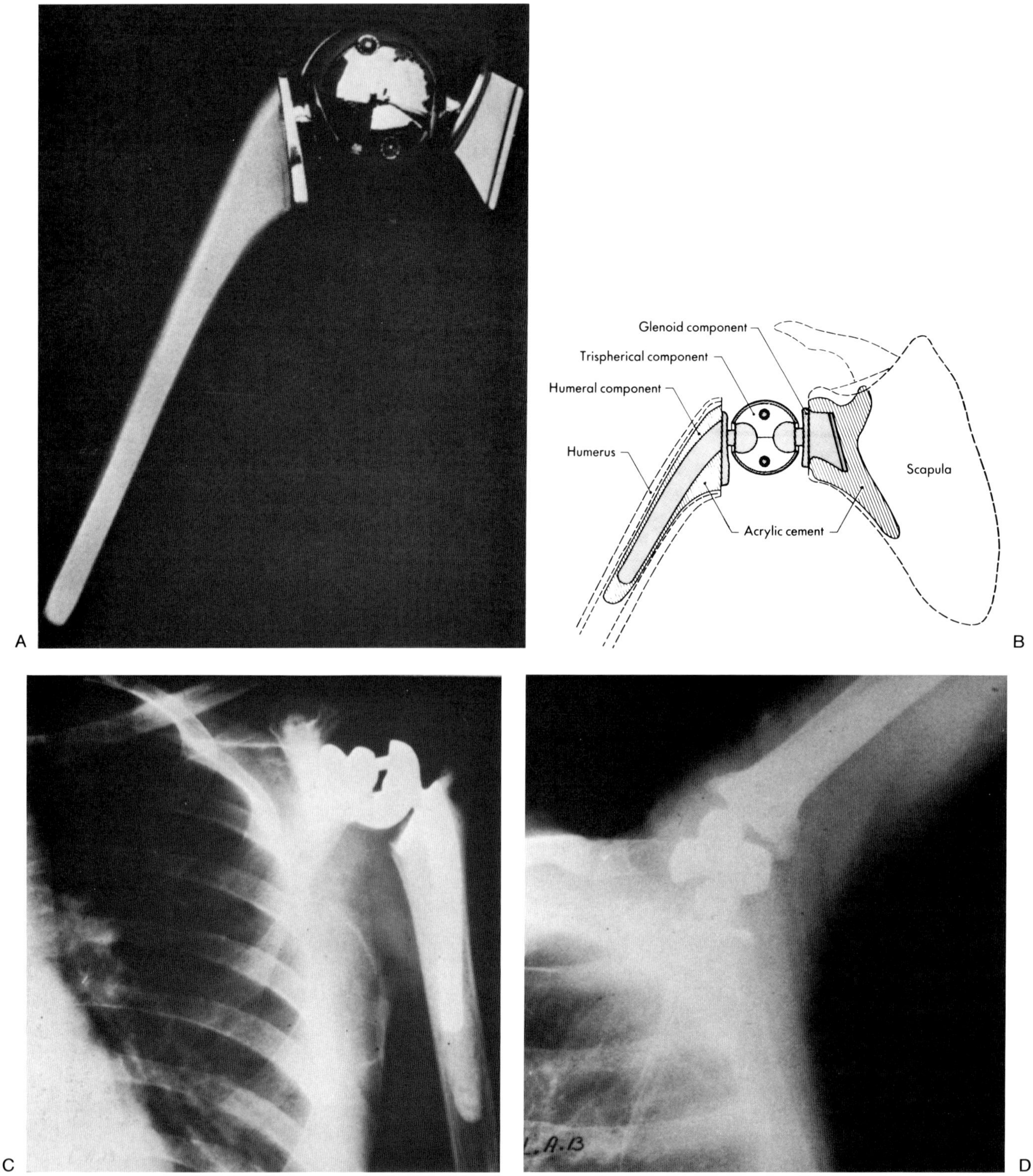

FIG. 9-65. Photograph **(A)** and illustration of components in place **(B)**. Trispheric total shoulder prosthesis composed of scapular, humeral, and central polyethylene spheres. Radiographs of the shoulder at the side **(C)** and with arm raised **(D)** 1 year after surgery. (From Gristura AG, Webb L. The trispherical total shoulder. In: Inglis AE, ed. *American Academy of Orthopedic Surgeons Symposium on Total Joint Replacement of the Upper Extremity*. St. Louis: CV Mosby, 1982; 50.)

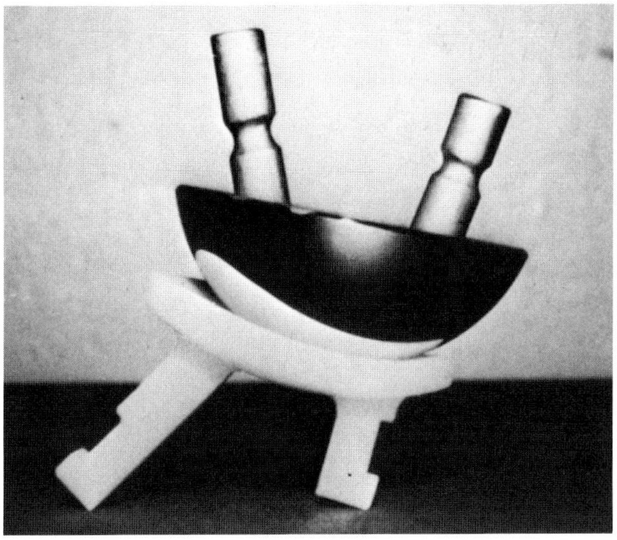

FIG. 9-66. The unconstrained resurfacing O'Leary-Walker total shoulder. (From Warren RF, Ranawat CS, Inglis AE. Total shoulder replacement indications and results of the Neer nonconstrained prosthesis. In: Inglis AE, ed. *American Academy of Orthopedic Surgeons Symposium on Total Joint Replacement of the Upper Extremity*. St. Louis: CV Mosby, 1982;56.)

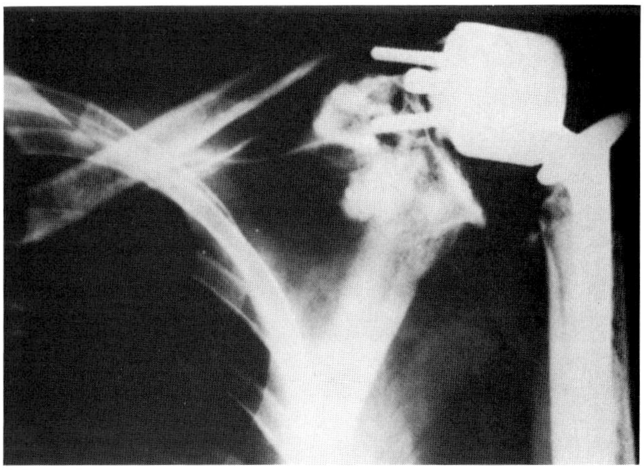

FIG. 9-67. An AP radiograph of the left shoulder after MRTS (constrained). The glenoid component has pulled out and displaced superiorly. (From Post M. Constrained arthroplasty of the shoulder. *Orthop Clin North Am* 1987;18:455.)

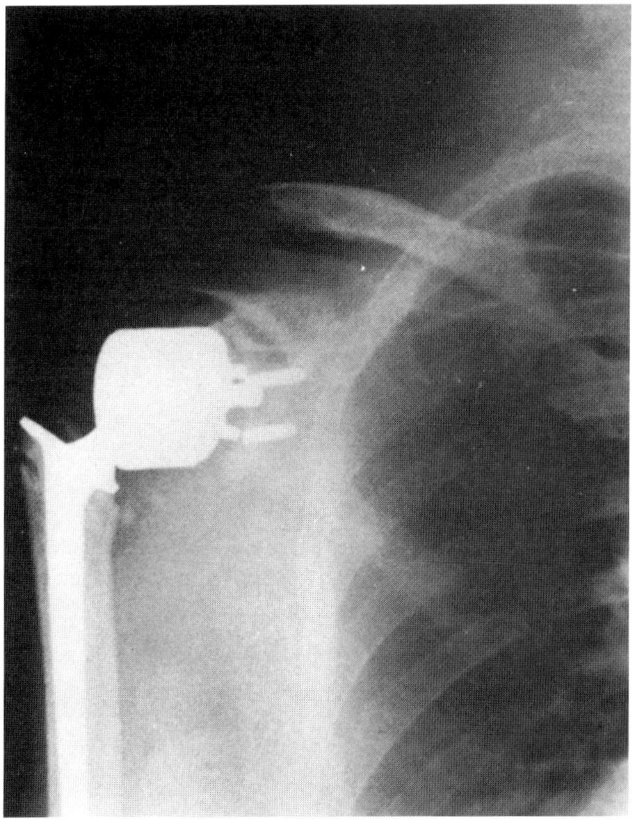

FIG. 9-68. An AP view of the right shoulder with a series II MRTS (constrained) with fracture of the glenoid screws. (From Post M. Constrained arthroplasty of the shoulder. *Orthop Clin North Am* 1987;18:455.)

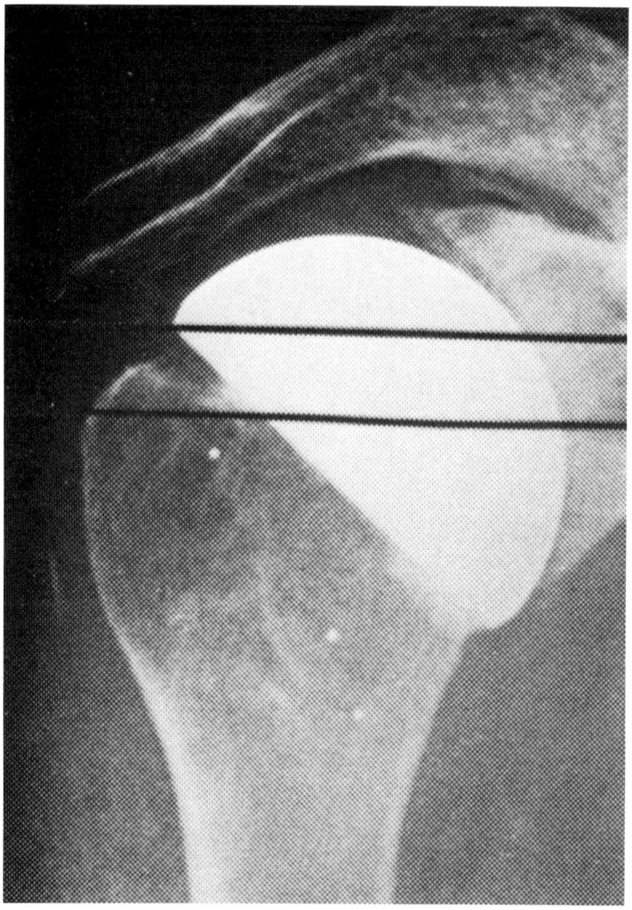

A

FIG. 9-69. **A:** Radiograph of metal cup arthroplasty with lines for CT image selection. **B,C:** CT images (window width, 4,800; window level, 400). Cement (*arrows*) and osseous anatomy are well demonstrated inside the cup. (From Eqund N, Jonsson E, Lidgren L, Kelly I, Pettersson H. Computed tomography of humeral head cup arthroplasties. *Acta Radiol* 1987;28:71.)

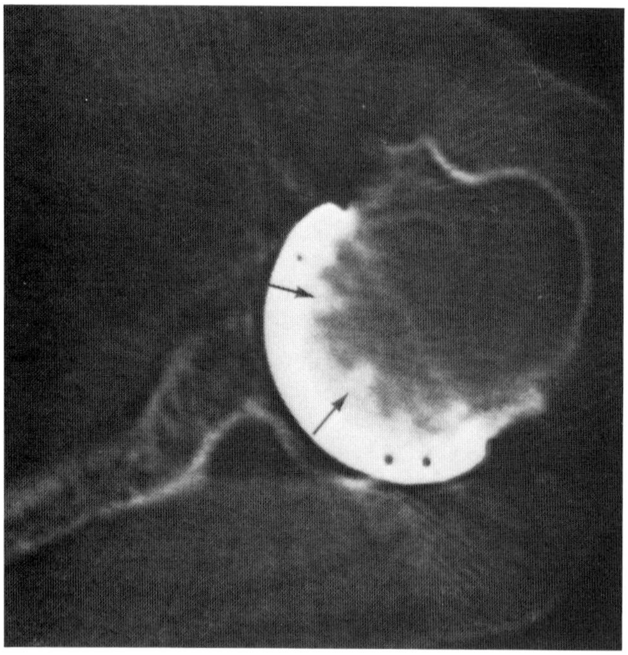

B

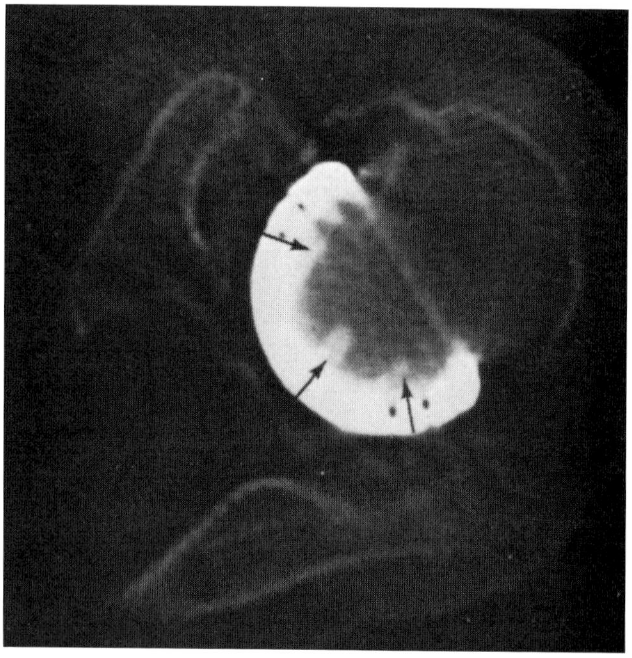

C

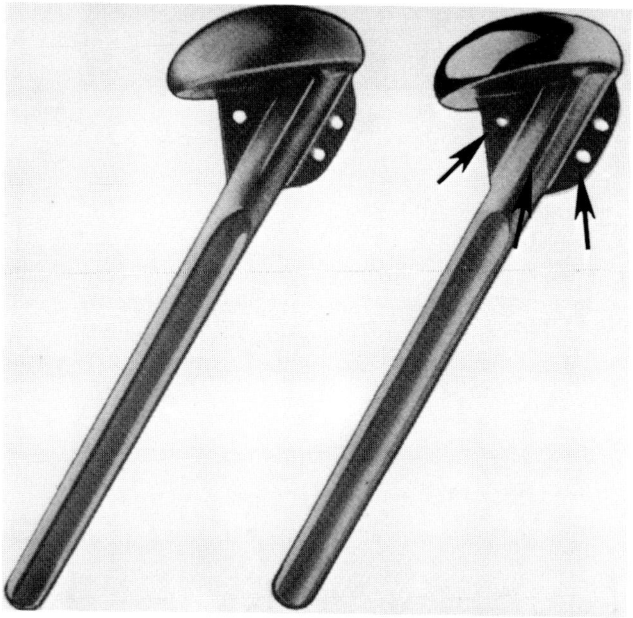

FIG. 9-70. Total Shoulder II™ humeral components constructed of cobalt-chromium-molybdenum alloy. There are four fins (*arrows*) directly under the head to assist with fit and reduce rotation. Stems are grooved to improve cement fixation. **Left:** 23-mm head, 6.3-mm diameter shaft, 125-cm length; provisional. **Right:** implant. (Courtesy of Zimmer, Warsaw, IN.)

A

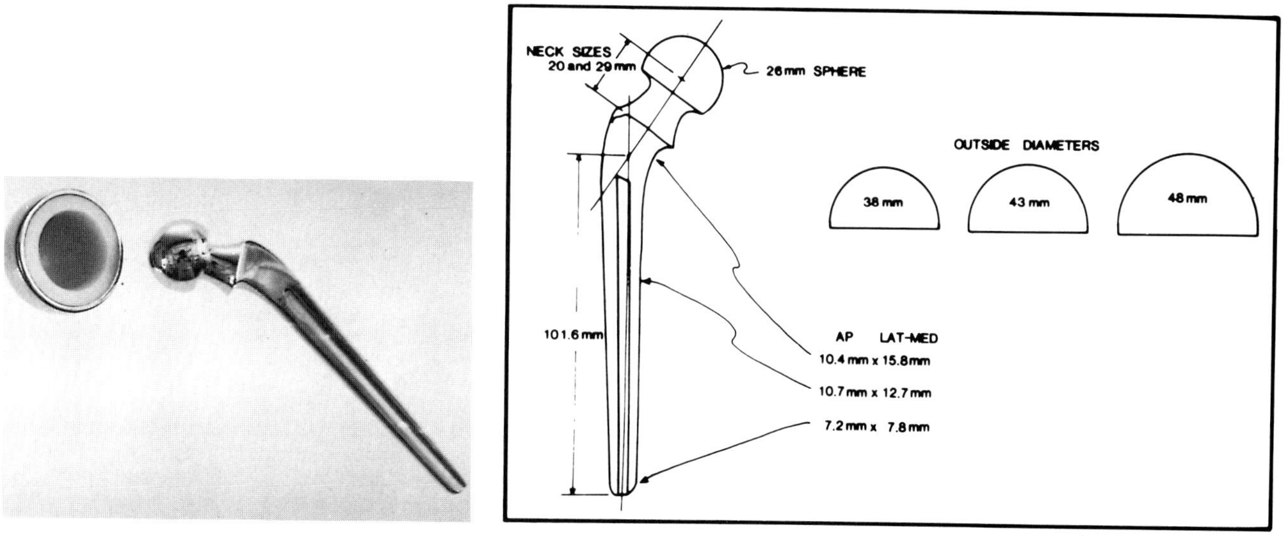

B

FIG. 9-71. A: The metal cup with polyethylene bearing and the humeral component. The glenoid component is not fixed to bone. **B:** Cup sizes are available in 14 diameters (36 to 50 mm). The humeral component has neck lengths of 20 and 29 mm, with stem lengths as illustrated. (From Swanson AB, Swanson GD, Sattel AB, Cendo RD, Hynes D, Jarning W. Bipolar implant shoulder arthroplasty. *Clin Orthop* 1989;249:227–247.)

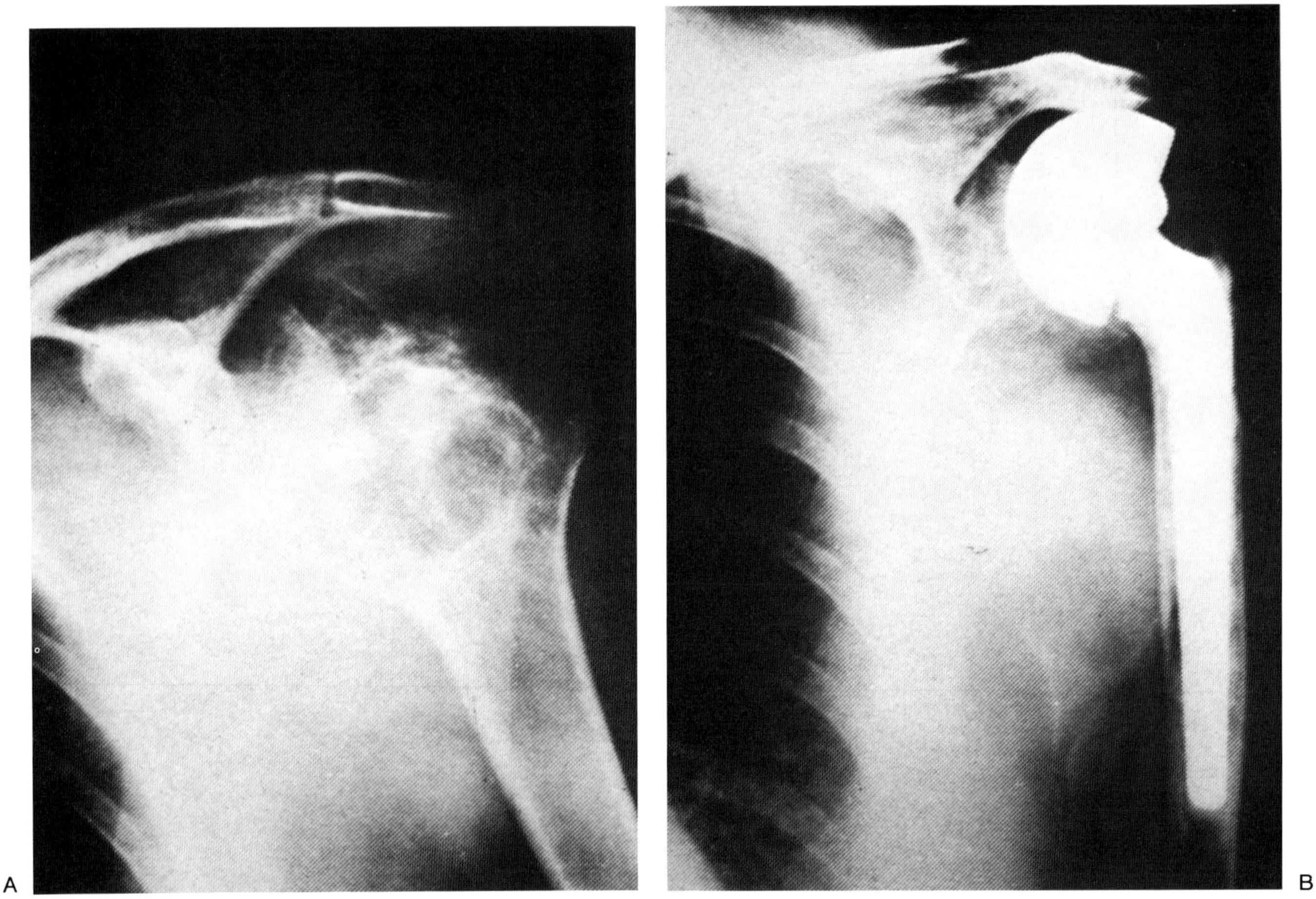

FIG. 9-72. **A:** Preoperative radiograph 7 years posthumeral head fracture. **B:** Bipolar implant 8 years after insertion. (From Swanson AB, Swanson GD, Sattel AB, Cendo RD, Hynes D, Jarning W. Bipolar implant shoulder arthroplasty. *Clin Orthop* 1989;249:227–247.)

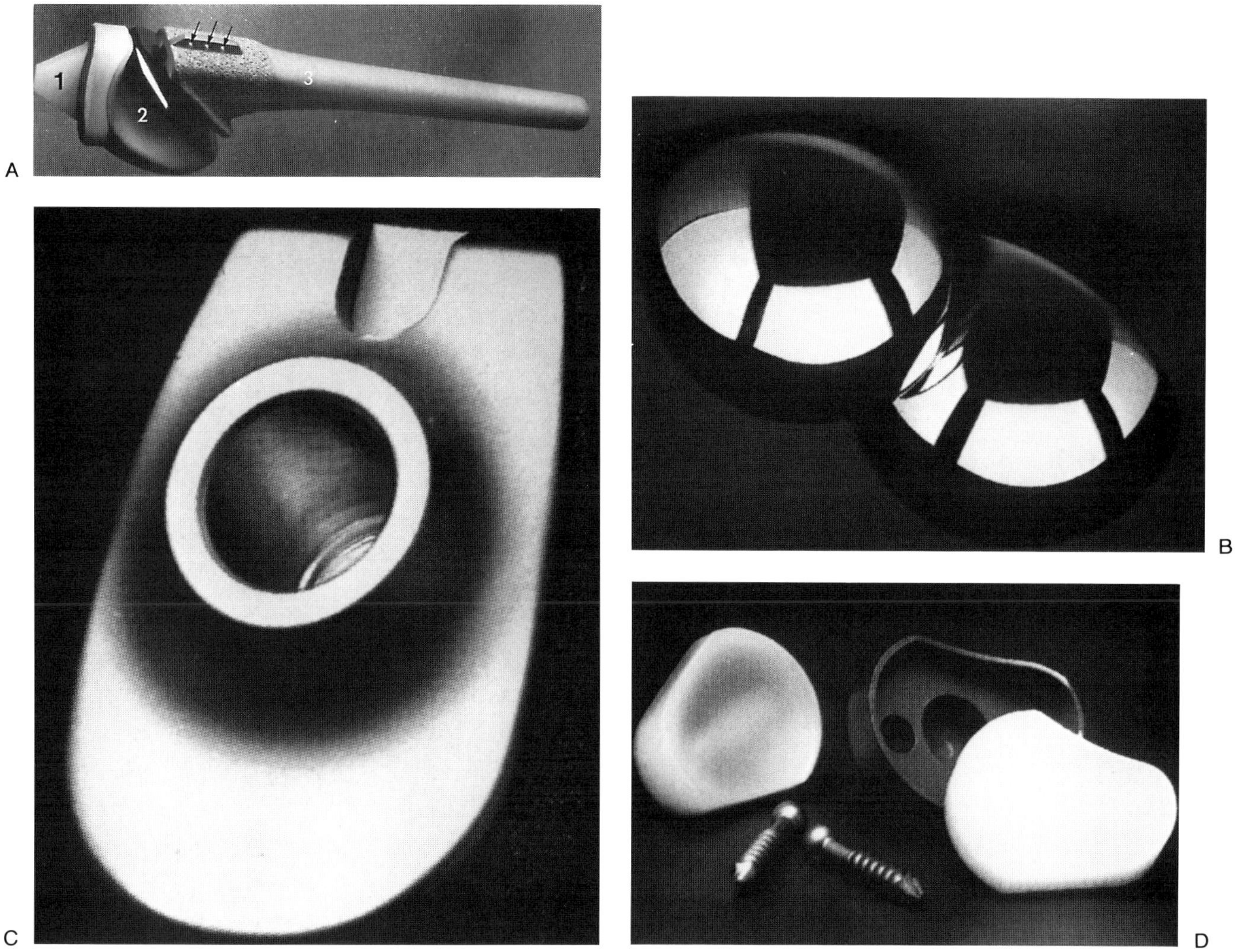

FIG. 9-73. Biomodular™ shoulder system. (Courtesy of Biomet, Warsaw, IN.) **A:** The glenoid component (*1*), modular head (*2*), and humeral stem (*3*). The humeral stem is porous coated proximally with three lateral suture holes (*arrows*) placed for tuberosity fixation. The stem has a Morse-type taper proximally. **B:** Modular heads. **C:** Neck insert. **D:** Porous-coated metal-backed glenoid component with two cancellous screws and two thicknesses of glenoid polyethylene inserts.

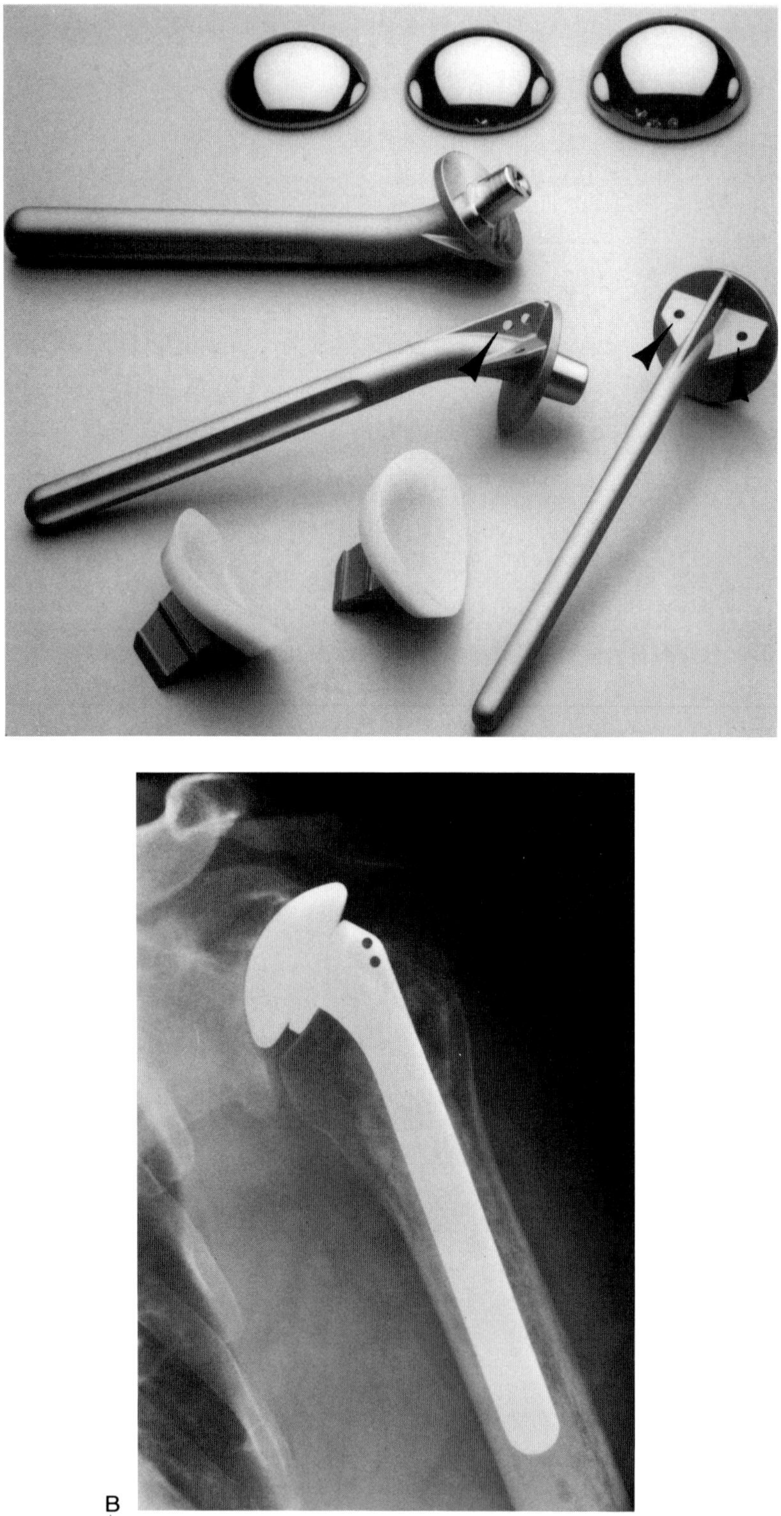

A

B

FIG. 9-74. Fenlin™ total shoulder system (A: Courtesy of Zimmer, Warsaw, IN.) **A:** Cobalt-chromium-molybdenum alloy humeral components. There are three proximal fins (*arrows*) with holes in each fin for bone and soft tissue reattachment. Morse-type taper proximally. The stem is grooved to facilitate cement fixation. Modular heads top. Glenoid implants (*below*) with barbed keel of cobalt-chromium-molybdenum and ultrahigh molecular weight polyethylene articular surface. **B:** Radiograph of a cemented modular Fenlin™ humeral component.

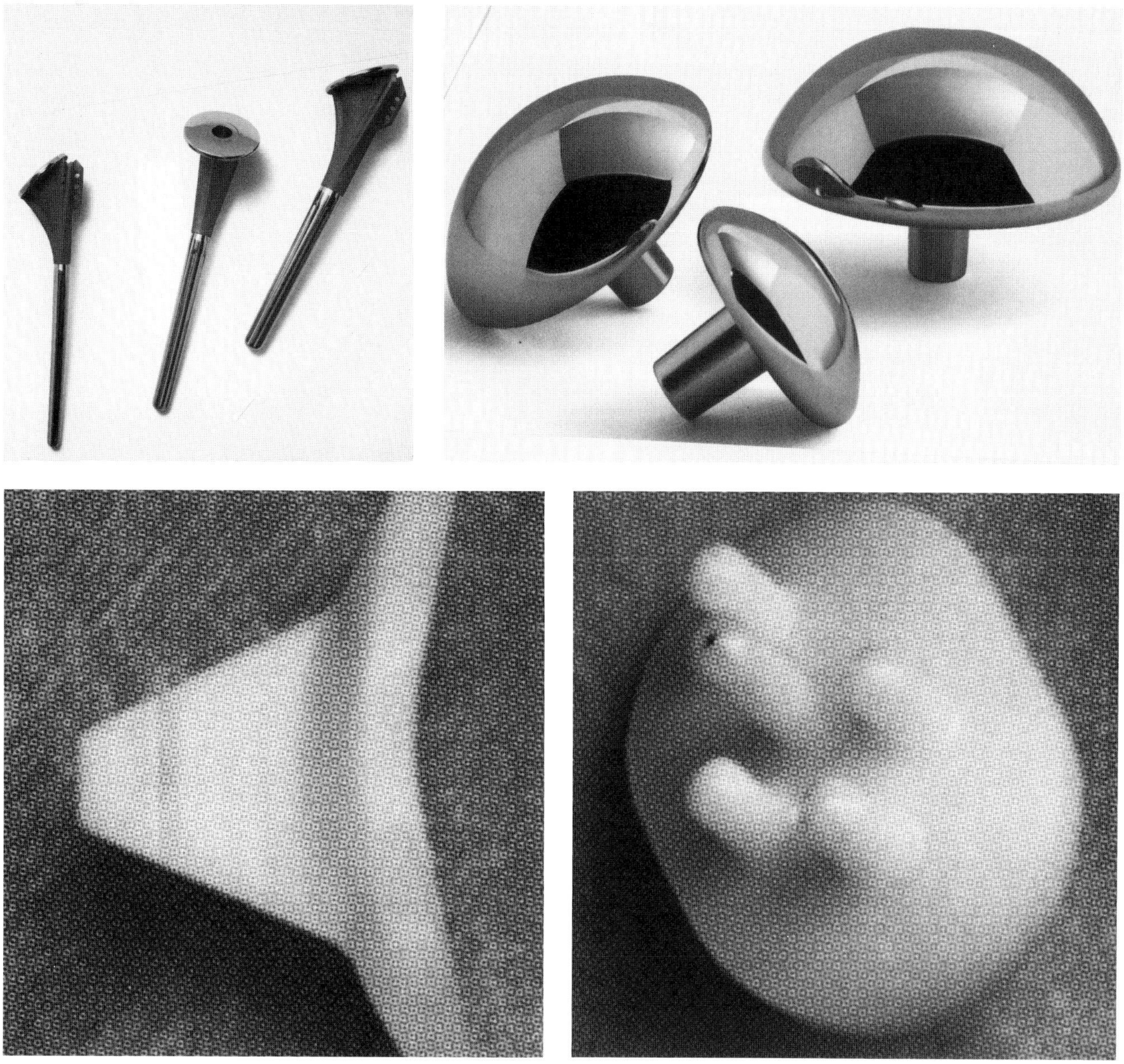

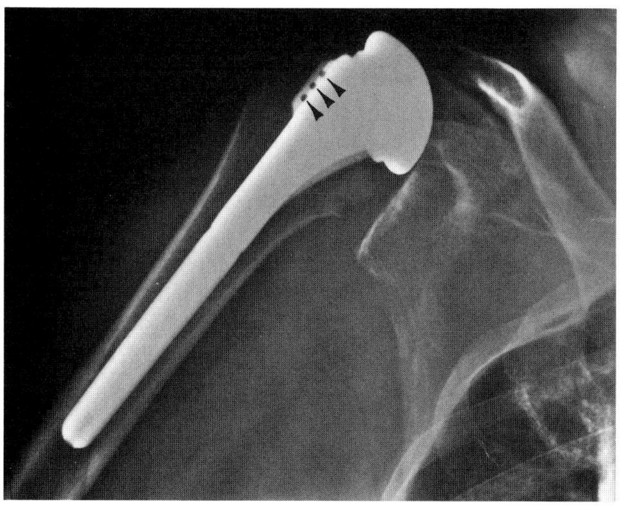

FIG. 9-75. Global™ total shoulder arthroplasty. (A–D: Courtesy of DePuy, Warsaw, IN.) **A:** Humeral stem with three lateral holes and porous-coated neck. The distal stem is grooved to enhance cement fixation. **B:** Three of 19 humeral head options. Keeled **(C)** and five-pegged **(D)** polyethylene glenoid components. **E:** An AP radiograph of a Global™ modular humeral component. Note the stem design and three lateral holes (*arrowheads*).

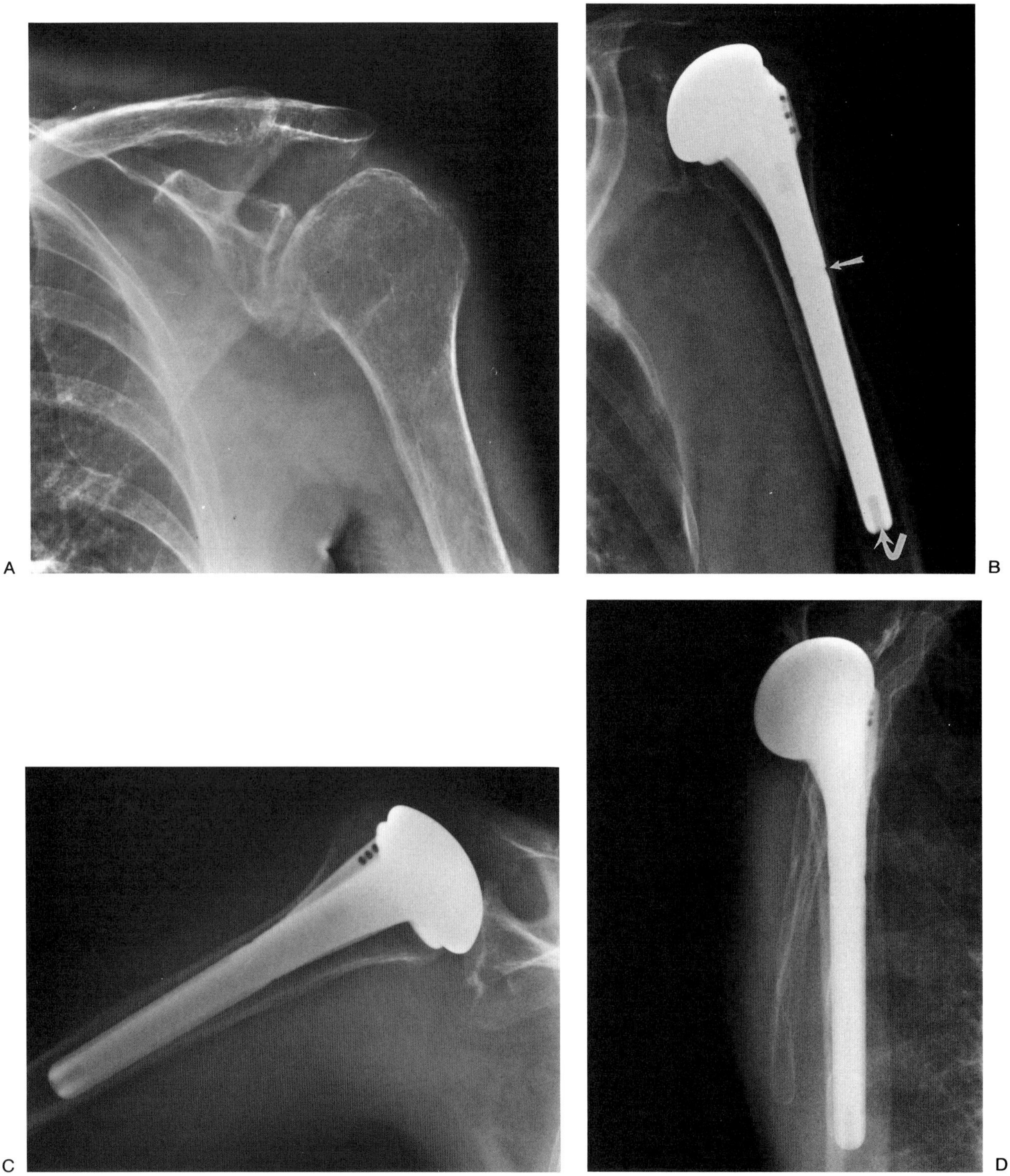

FIG. 9-76. A: An AP radiograph demonstrating osteoarthritis. The AP **(B)**, axillary **(C)**, and scapular Y **(D)** views after placement of a Global™ modular humeral component. Note the three lateral suture holes in the neck, the sectioned appearance of the midstem (*arrow*), and lucency in the tip (*curved arrow*), which is intended for a centralizer when cement is used.

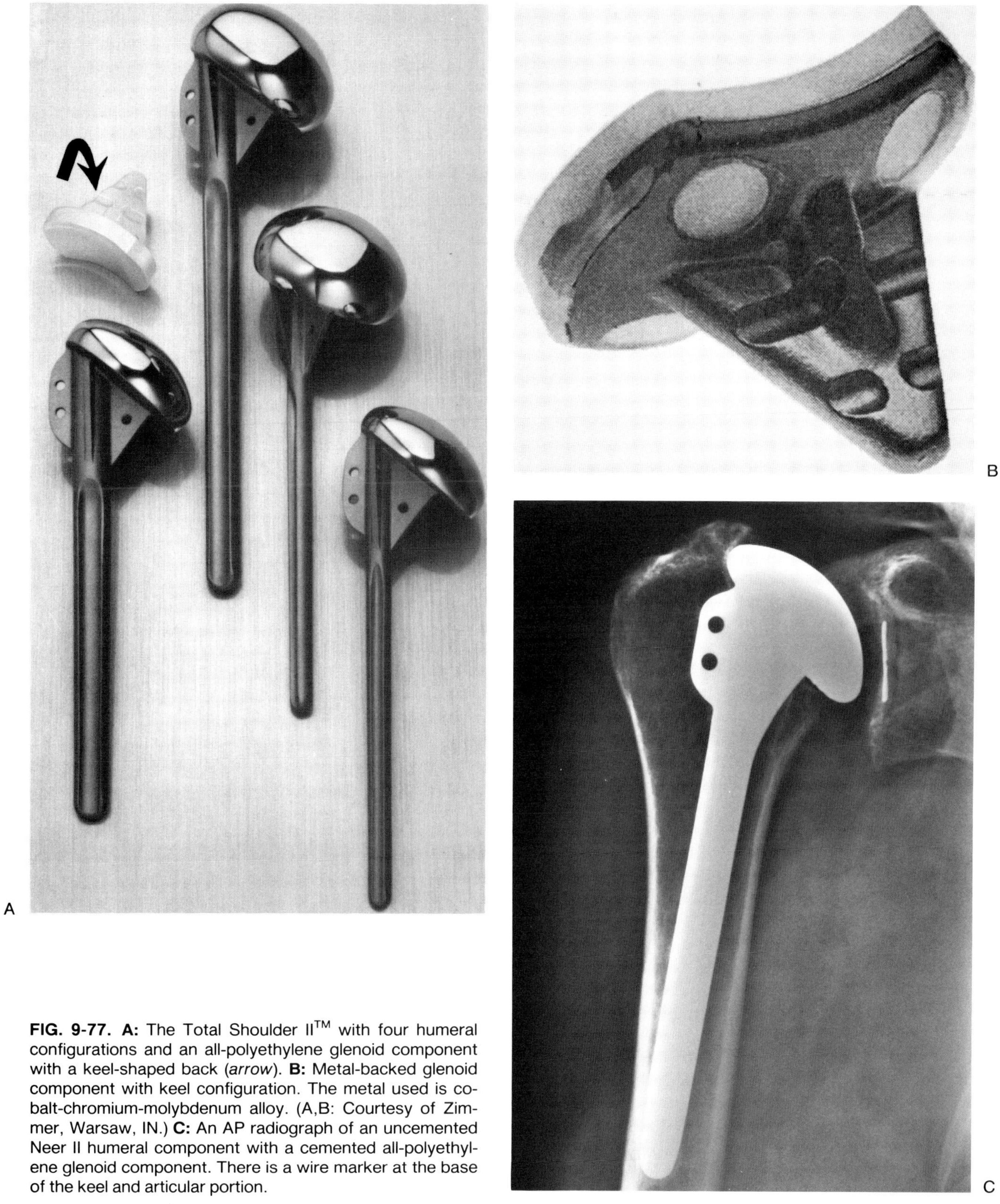

FIG. 9-77. A: The Total Shoulder II™ with four humeral configurations and an all-polyethylene glenoid component with a keel-shaped back (*arrow*). **B:** Metal-backed glenoid component with keel configuration. The metal used is cobalt-chromium-molybdenum alloy. (A,B: Courtesy of Zimmer, Warsaw, IN.) **C:** An AP radiograph of an uncemented Neer II humeral component with a cemented all-polyethylene glenoid component. There is a wire marker at the base of the keel and articular portion.

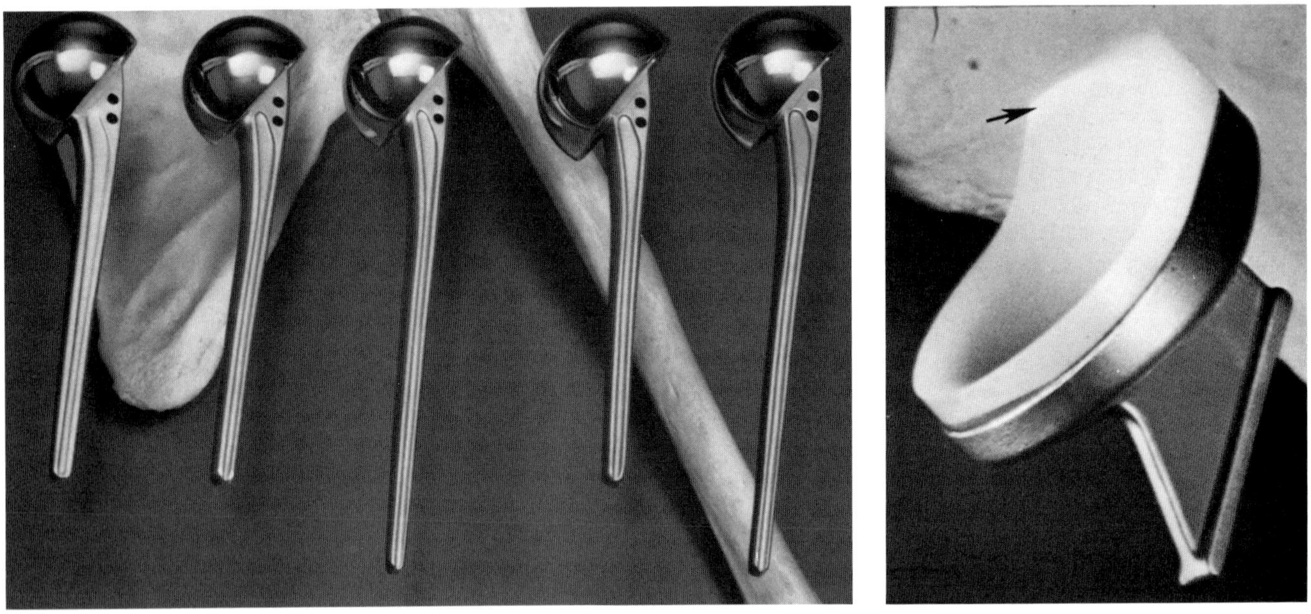

A B

FIG. 9-78. Monospherical™ shoulder system. (Courtesy of Howmedica, Rutherford, NJ.) **A:** Humeral components with two upper holes and variable stem lengths and diameters. **B:** The metal-backed glenoid component. There is an upper glenoid lip (*arrow*) on the polyethylene surface.

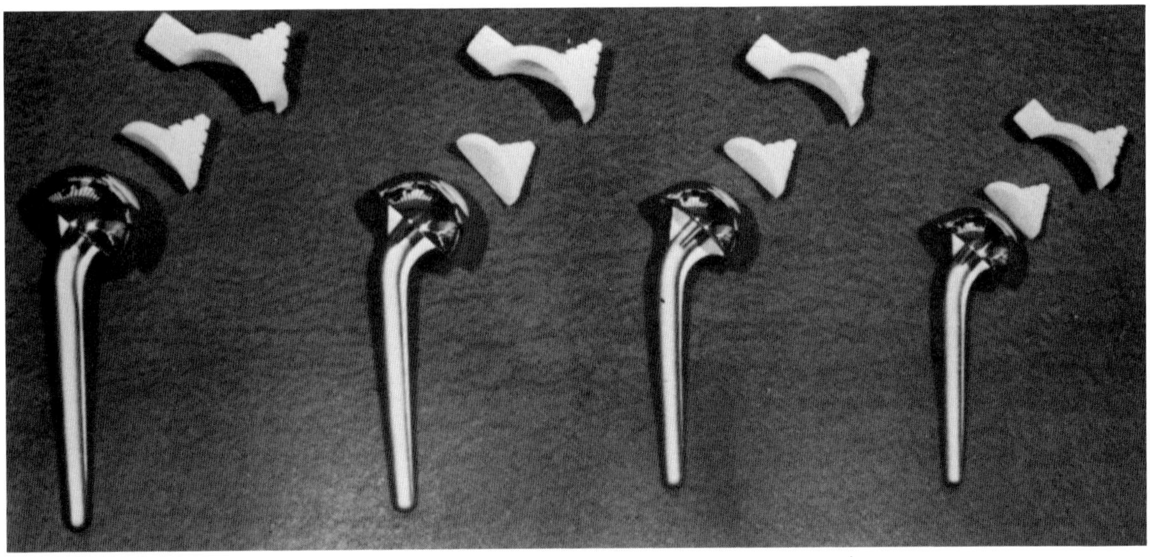

A

FIG. 9-79. D.A.N.A.™ (*d*esigned *a*fter *n*atural *a*natomy) total shoulder. **A:** Photograph of the four humeral component sizes and regular or hooded polyethylene glenoid components.

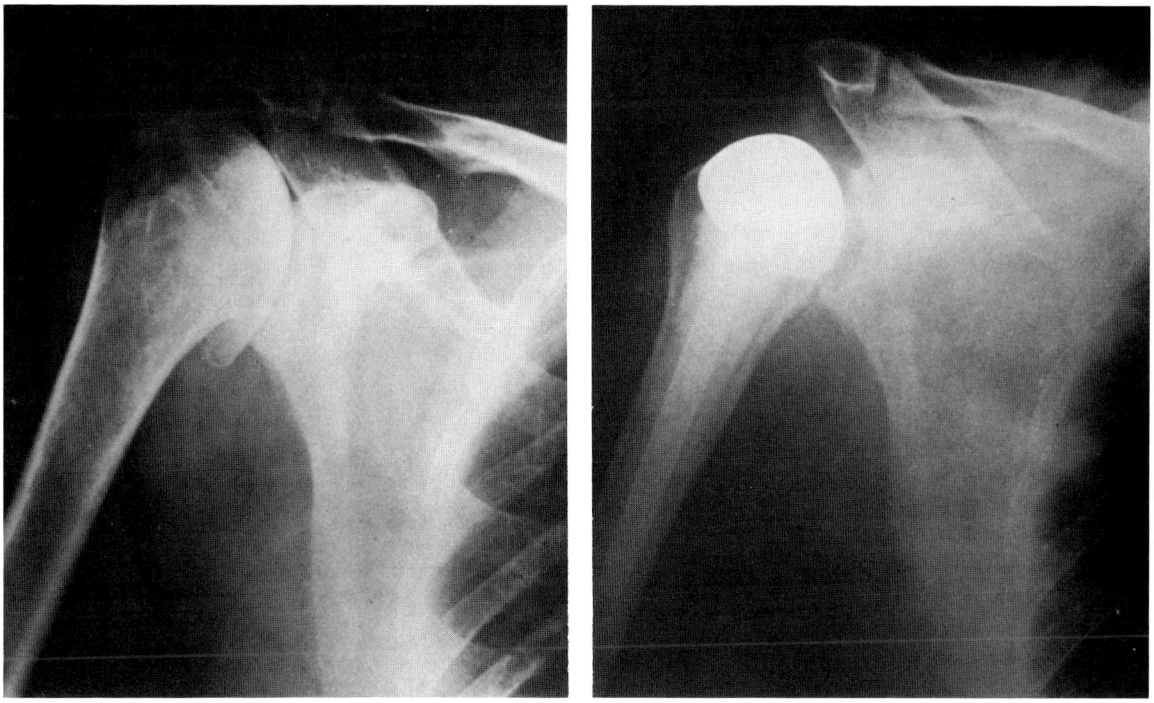

B C

FIG. 9-79. (*Continued.*) Pre- **(B)** and postoperative **(C)** radiographs. (From Amstutz HC, Thomas BJ, Kabo JM, Jinnah RH, Dorey FJ. The Dana total shoulder arthroplasty. *J Bone Joint Surg* [*Am*] 1988; 70A: 1174–1182.)

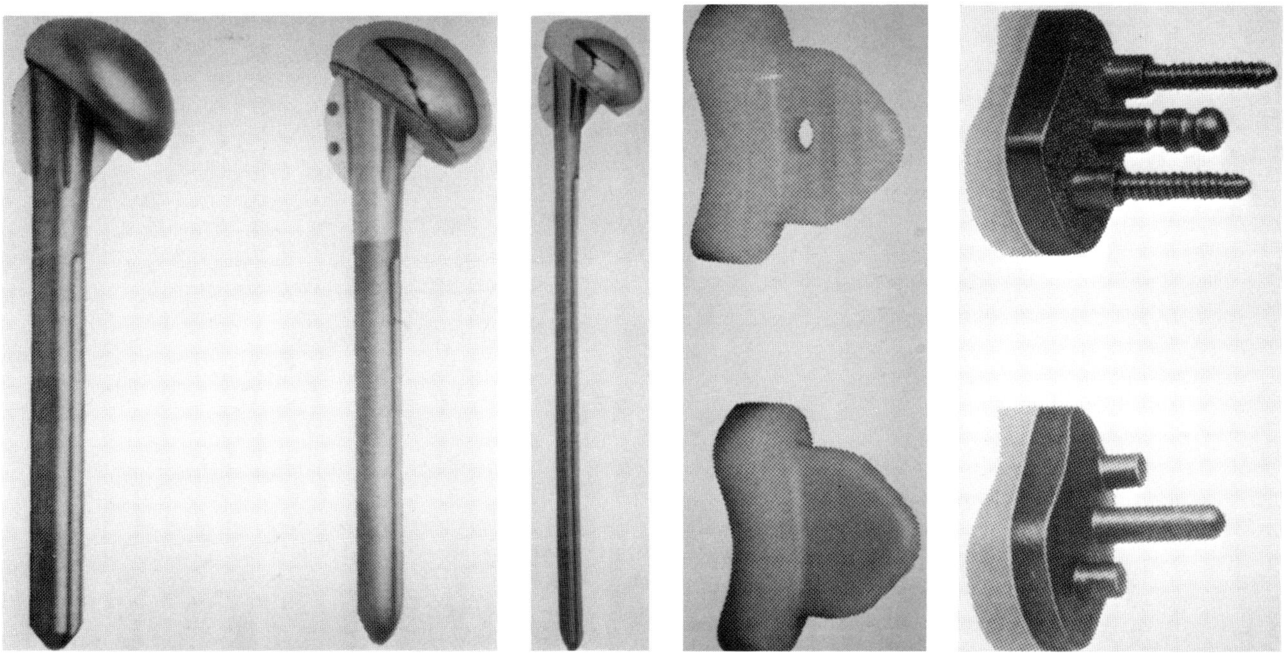

A,B C,D

FIG. 9-80. The Cofield shoulder. (A,B: Courtesy of Smith and Nephew Richards, Memphis, TN.) **A:** Standard-stem humeral component (chromium-cobalt), 143 mm. **B:** Long stem, 241 mm. **C:** Polyethylene glenoid component. **D:** Metal-backed glenoid component. (See **E** on next page.)

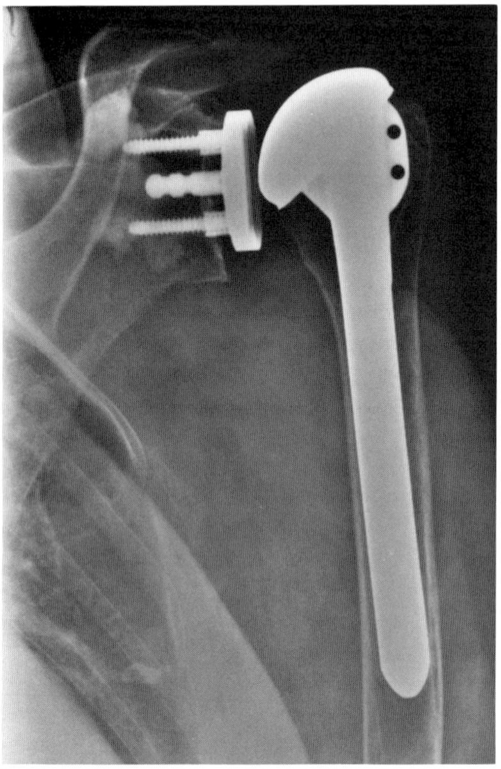

E

FIG. 9-80. (*Continued.*) **E:** An AP radiograph demonstrating a Cofield shoulder. The humeral component is similar to the Neer prosthesis.

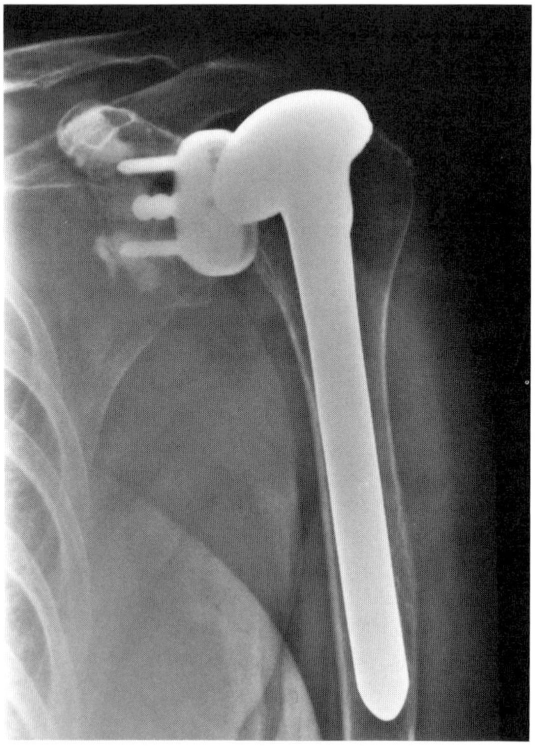

A

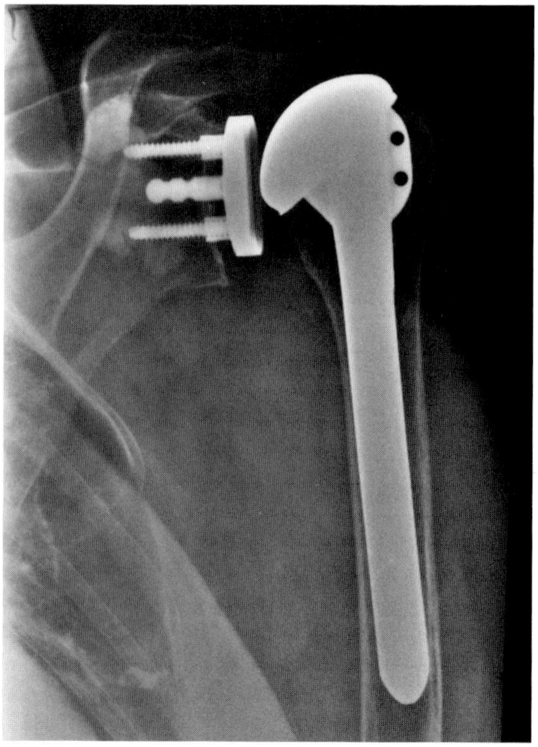

B

FIG. 9-81. A: An AP view of the shoulder (Cofield shoulder), which does not adequately demonstrate the glenoid component or the head-neck region of the humeral component. **B:** Fluoroscopically positioned AP view clearly demonstrates the glenoid component and bone interfaces and the humeral component.

arthroplasty (Fig. 9-69) provided significant pain relief with varied success in improved function or range of motion.[231] Swanson et al.[233] developed a bipolar prosthesis (Figs. 9-71 and 9-72), which was primarily used for patients with rotator cuff deficiency or superior subluxation secondary to rheumatoid arthritis.[232,233]

Today, Neer or modular humeral components are frequently used (Figs. 9-73 to 9-81).[185,206,218] The latter allow more flexibility in head selection, and soft tissue tension and greater tuberosity repair are facilitated.[218] The utility of hemiarthroplasty varies with the indication.[185,189,202,204,234] Zuckerman and Cofield[239] reported pain relief in 83% of patients with osteoarthritis and 89% of patients with rheumatoid arthritis. The range of motion was more improved in patients with osteoarthritis. Although most authors report good to excellent results for pain relief and improved function, the range of motion is only consistently improved when the indication for hemiarthroplasty is fracture or AVN.[209,221] Some authors perform glenoid osteotomy in conjunction with hemiarthroplasty.[185]

Total shoulder arthroplasty provides the most consistent results for pain relief and improved range of motion. Pain relief is noted in about 90% of patients. Range of motion improves more consistently in patients with osteoarthritis than in patients with rotator cuff arthropathy or rheumatoid arthritis. Unconstrained systems are more commonly used than semiconstrained. Constrained systems are rarely used today because of their high failure rate.[185,191,203,207,222,227,235,237,238]

Most components are cemented, although porous-coated implants are available.[237] Weiss et al.[237] reported no difference in the results obtained using cemented Neer and uncemented English-McNab glenoid components (Fig. 9-59).

Postoperative Imaging and Complications

The complications related to shoulder arthroplasty vary with the type of prosthesis (unconstrained, semiconstrained, unconstrained, and hemiarthroplasty) and underlying pathologic condition (soft tissue integrity and bone stock).[183,187,188,195,203,221,222] Table 9-4 summarizes the complications noted with shoulder arthroplasty. The total reported complications range from 9% to 38%.[237]

Glenoid component loosening is the most common complication with total shoulder replacement.[179,180,195,203] The average incidence with unconstrained components is 4.7% (range, 3% to 15%). Semiconstrained components have an average incidence of around 12%.[185,195,203,222]

Humeral component loosening occurs less frequently. The average incidence is less than 1% (range, 1% to 7%) with a slightly higher incidence with constrained shoulder arthroplasties.[193,194,212] Subsidence of the humeral component (sinking of the humeral implant into the shaft) occurs in about 7% of patients.[179]

TABLE 9-4. *Shoulder arthroplasty: Complications*[179,180,195,203,207,218,222]

Complication	Incidence rates (%)
Glenoid loosening	3–15
Humeral component loosening	5
Humeral component subsidence	7
Subluxation-dislocation	6
Superior migration (rotator cuff tear in 24%)	22
Nerve injury	1–2
Infection	<1–3
Humeral fracture	1.6

Superior migration, subluxation, and dislocation of the humeral head have all been reported.[179,188,222] Subluxation or dislocation occur in 1% to 3% of patients (range, 1% to 18%).[179,193,194] Superior migration has been reported in 22% to 53%.[203,235] Migration does not correlate with pain. It is believed to be related to rotator cuff tears, inadequate cuff repair, or failed cuff repair.[183,188] This finding has also been associated with glenoid loosening.[188,203] Rotator cuff tears were confirmed in 24% of the patients with superior migration reported on by Boyd et al.[188] Most of these patients had rheumatoid arthritis (79%). Rotator cuff tears were detected postoperatively in 10% of patients with osteoarthritis.

Infection does not occur often with shoulder arthroplasty. Deep infection occurs in less than 1% of unconstrained and 2% to 3% of patients with constrained prostheses.[193,194] However, infection rates with constrained components as high as 15% have been reported. Infection with hemiarthroplasty is rare.[179,193,194]

Nerve injury occurs more frequently in patients with previous surgery or trauma in whom scar tissue compromises surgical dissection.[197] The incidence of nerve injury is still only about 1% to 2%.[193]

Fractures of the humeral shaft are uncommon indeed.[187,190] Seven fractures in 436 patients (1.6%) were reported by Boyd et al.[190] Most fractures can be treated conservatively. However, fixation with plastic bands or Dall-Miles cables may be indicated. The complications of humeral fractures include radial nerve injury (6% to 25%) and nonunion (0% to 13%).[187,190]

Revision surgery with component replacement or removal or soft tissue repair may be indicated.[193,194]

Imaging of patients after shoulder arthroplasty plays a significant role in their evaluation. Routine radiographs should be obtained at 2, 6, and 12 months and then yearly, assuming there are no indications for implant failure.[180,186,200,202] Most authors suggest true AP, axillary, and scapular Y views for implant evaluation. This would be adequate for most patients who have undergone hemiarthroplasty. However, the evaluations of glenoid components and some humeral components are

(text continues on page 722)

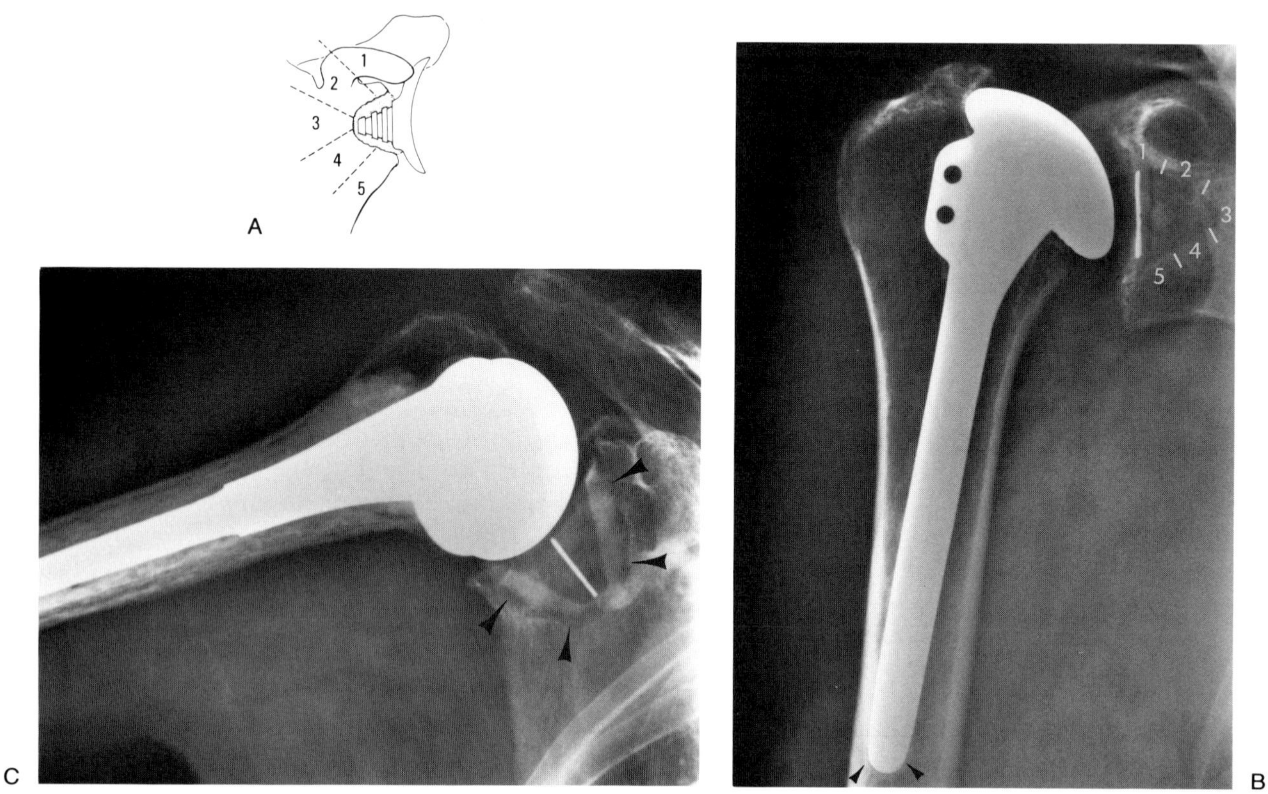

FIG. 9-82. **A:** The zones to evaluate lucent lines about the glenoid component. (From Amstutz HC, Thomas BJ, Kabo JM, Jinnah RH, Dorey FJ. The Dana total shoulder arthroplasty. *J Bone Joint Surg* [*Am*] 1988;70A:1174–1182.) **B:** Uncemented humeral component (Neer) and polyethylene keel type of glenoid component. The zones for evaluating the glenoid keel type of component are numbered. Lucent lines in zones 1 and 5 are common. There are thin lucent zones at the humeral tip (*arrows*) and in zone 1, which are of no significance. Note the superior position of the humeral head compared with that of the glenoid. Perfect interface position is unusual because of preoperative soft tissue deficiencies. **C:** Cemented modular shoulder arthroplasty with a wide irregular lucent zone (*arrows*) around the entire glenoid component, suggesting loosening. Lucency in zones 2 to 4 (the deeper zones) is usually more significant. Slight lucency in zones 1 and 5 is almost always evident.

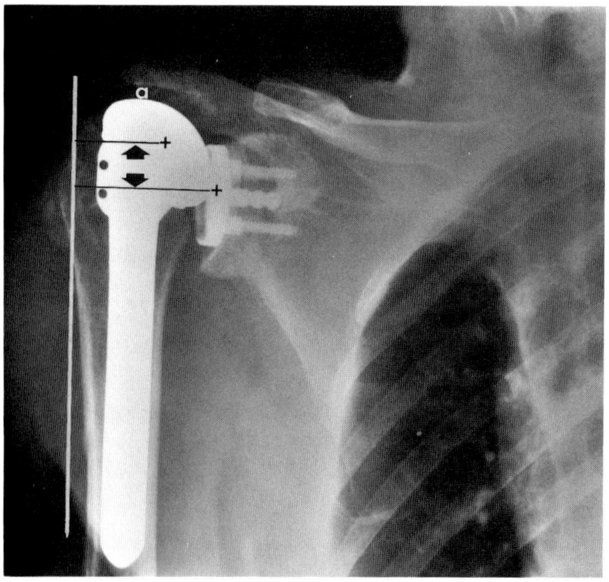

FIG. 9-83. Shoulder arthroplasty with superior migration and reduced subacromial space (*a*). Follow-up evaluation can be more consistent by selecting the center of the glenoid (+) and humeral head (+) and drawing lines (*black*) to a line (*white*) perpendicular to the humeral component.[203]

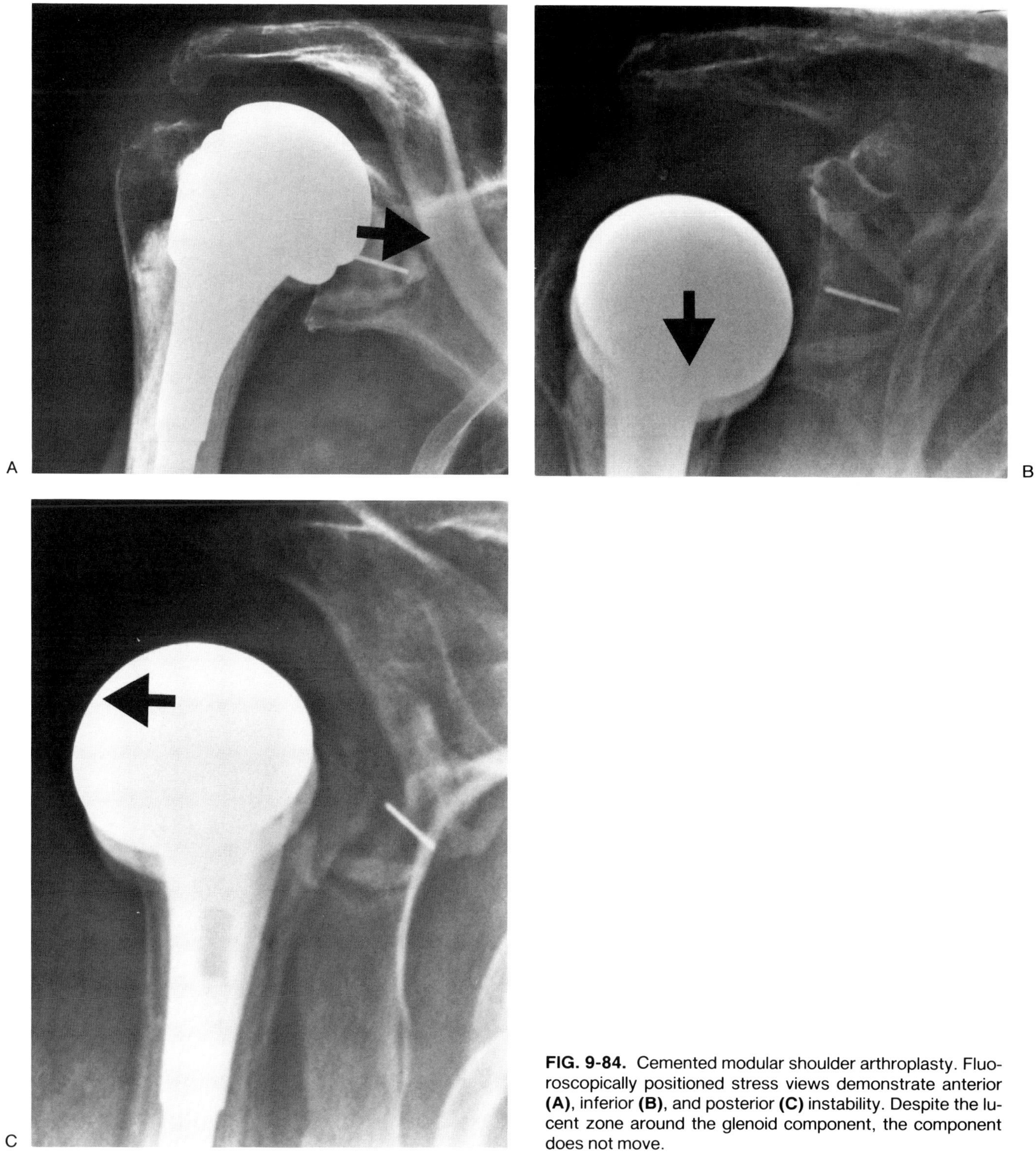

FIG. 9-84. Cemented modular shoulder arthroplasty. Fluoroscopically positioned stress views demonstrate anterior (A), inferior (B), and posterior (C) instability. Despite the lucent zone around the glenoid component, the component does not move.

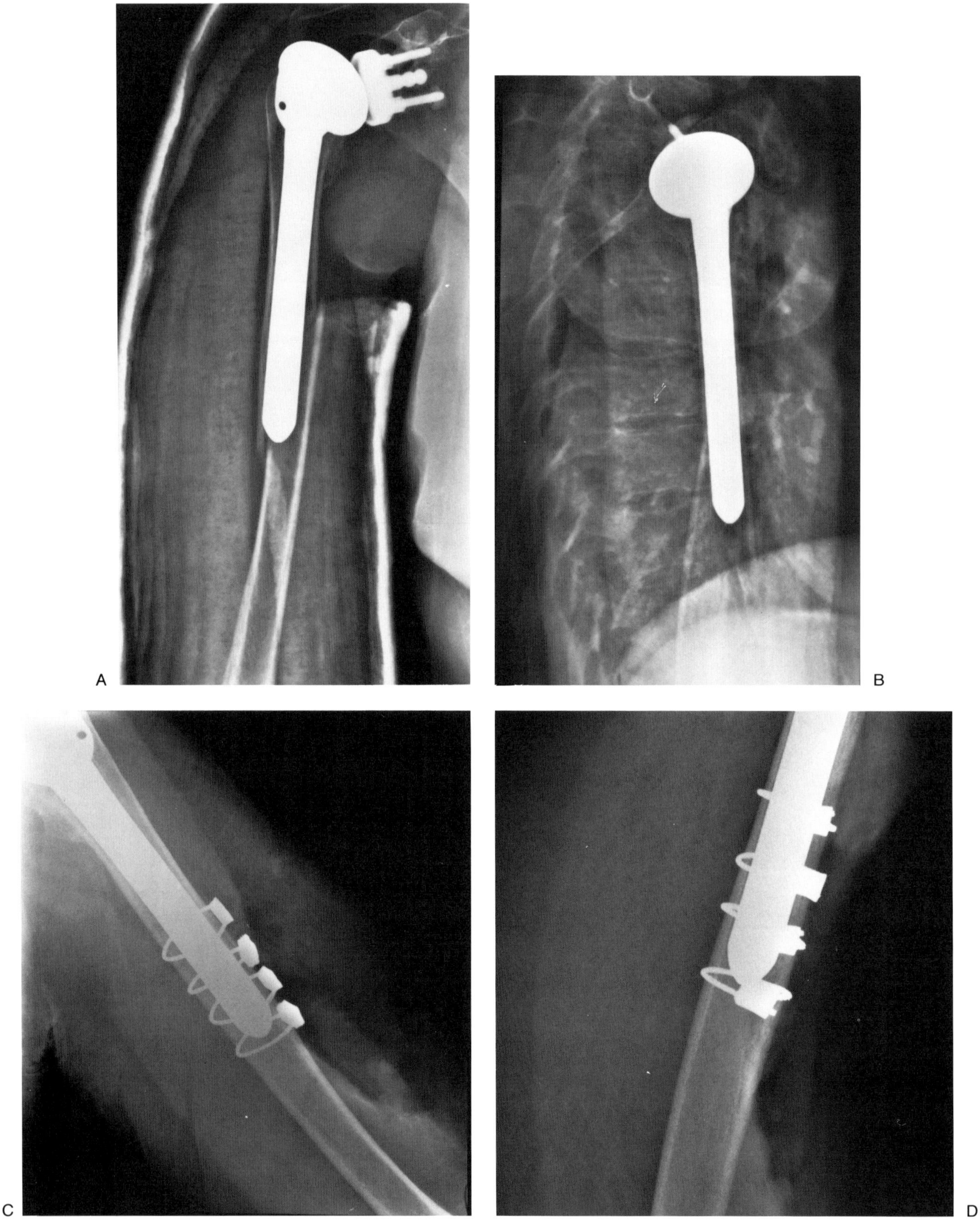

FIG. 9-85. The AP **(A)** and transthoracic **(B)** radiographs of a patient with a shoulder arthroplasty and a fracture at the tip of the humeral component treated initially with a closed-cast technique. The AP **(C)** and lateral **(D)** views after open reduction and fixation with four Dall-Miles cables.

A,B

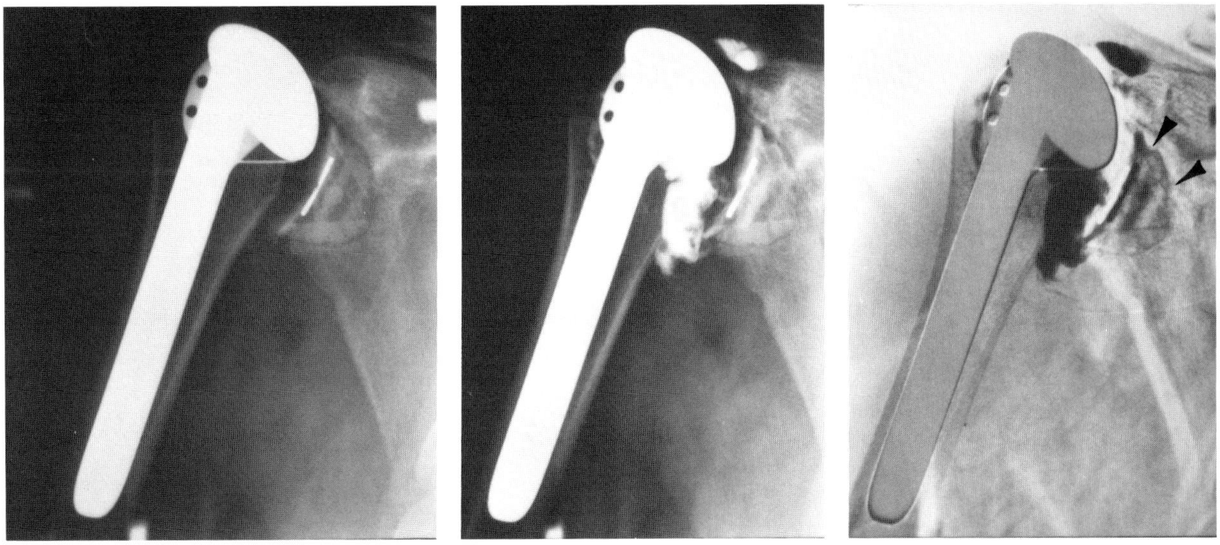

C

FIG. 9-86. Mask **(A)**, postinjection film **(B)**, and subtracted result **(C)** demonstrating loosening (*arrows*) of the glenoid component.

A

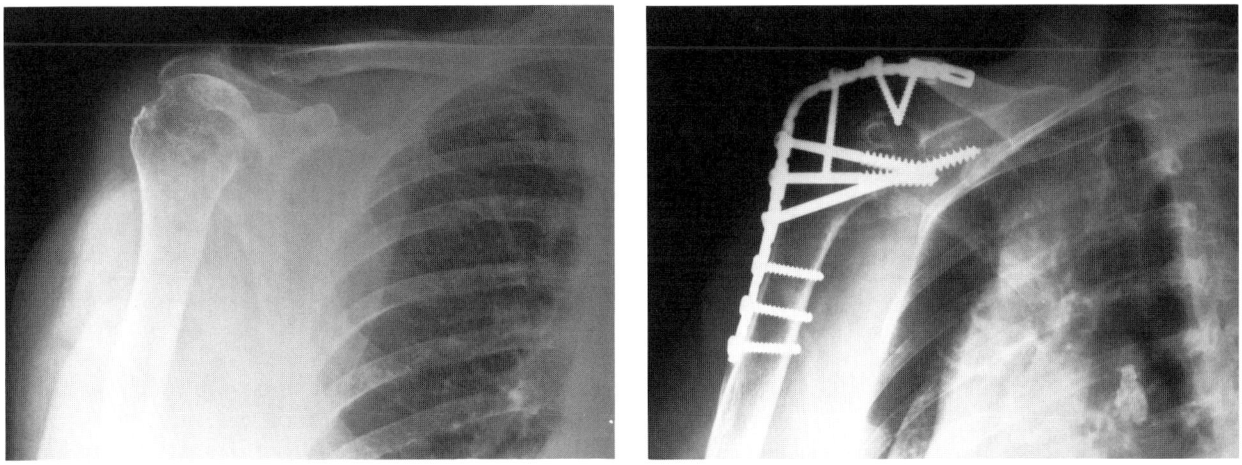

B

FIG. 9-87. A: An AP view of the shoulder with erosive arthritis, rotator cuff deficiency, and clavicular erosion caused by rheumatoid arthritis. **B:** Arthrodesis was performed using a reconstruction plate and cortical and cancellous screws. There is solid union at 6 months.

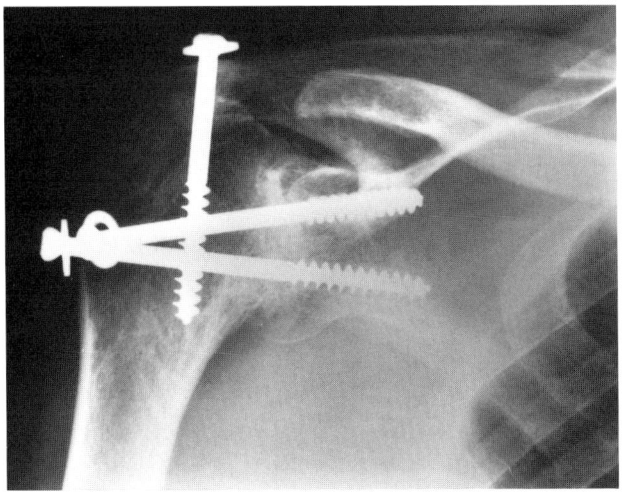

FIG. 9-88. An AP view of the shoulder after arthrodesis with three cancellous screws and washers.

inconsistent unless the images are obtained after fluoroscopic alignment (Fig. 9-81).[186] Consistency in positioning is essential to evaluate the component's position and lucent lines.[186,197]

Routine radiographic features, especially on serial films, can provide valuable information concerning loosening, infection, and component migration.[186,197]

Lucent lines are a common finding. This finding is particularly common around the glenoid component (≥80%).[186,193,194] Loosening is also more common with the glenoid than with the humeral component. Loosening rates of up to 30% have been reported for the glenoid component.[197] Lucent lines may be caused by numerous factors, e.g., (1) surgical trauma; (2) incomplete removal of cartilage, blood, or soft tissues; (3) faulty cement technique; (4) local thermal changes. They do not necessarily indicate loosening. Progressive widening of lucent zones, especially if irregular and greater than 2 mm, is a more accurate indicator of loosening (Fig. 9-82).[186,197,237] Progressive migration (Fig. 9-83) has also been associated with an increased incidence of glenoid loosening, along with cuff deficiency.[203]

Motion or stress studies can be performed to evaluate component loosening. The motion of the component can be more easily assessed in this fashion. Also, instability is more easily evaluated in this manner (Fig. 9-84).[186]

Routine radiographic features of infection include areas of bone destruction, endosteal scalloping, and periosteal new bone formation. Features of loosening (irregular lucent lines > 2 mm) are commonly noted in patients with infected arthroplasties.[186,197]

Routine radiographs are also generally effective for the detection of fractures complicating shoulder arthroplasty (Fig. 9-85).[187,190]

Arthrography (conventional or subtraction) is useful for joint aspiration in patients with suspected infection. When contrast media fills a cavity, a bone defect or sinus tract infection is the likely cause.[186] Also the injection of anesthetic can confirm the site of pain as intraarticular. Arthrograms can be useful to evaluate loosening, but they are not as effective as when they are performed in the hip (Fig. 9-86). Rotator cuff tears, instability, and superior migration are more effectively evaluated.[186,197]

Radionuclide studies are commonly used in the hip and knee to evaluate loosening and potential infection.[186,197,214,223,229,236] These techniques are not as frequently used in the shoulder. Classically, technetium-99m phosphate complexes have been used. Focal areas of uptake have been associated with loosening and more diffuse changes, with infection.[197] However, increased tracer may be evident around components for more than 1 year following surgery.[186] The compared results of scans with technetium-99m and gallium-67 or indium-111-labeled white blood cells are commonly more accurate in patients with suspected infections.[213,230] More recently, intraarticular injection of technetium-99m sulfur colloid has been used in conjunction with arthrography. Early reports suggest these techniques are complementary.[214,229,236]

ARTHRODESIS AND MISCELLANEOUS PROCEDURES

The procedures used to treat instability were discussed previously. The treatment options for shoulder arthropathies (in addition to joint replacement) include synovectomy, humeral, and/or glenoid osteotomy, resection arthroplasty, and arthrodesis.[240–249]

Synovectomy and osteotomy have been described for inflammatory arthropathy, primarily, rheumatoid arthritis.[242] Limited joint débridement to remove osteophytes, loose bodies, and synovial abnormalities is accomplished arthroscopically today.[242]

Shoulder arthrodesis was used historically for the treatment of conditions that are now more frequently treated with shoulder arthroplasty. Today, this technique is most commonly used for failed arthroplasty that cannot be revised, neuromuscular paralysis, or chronic infection.[240,242–244,248,250]

Preoperative imaging should include routine radiographs (true AP, axillary, and scapular Y views) and, if necessary, CT to evaluate bone loss and glenoid anatomy.

Both internal and external fixation techniques have been used (Figs. 9-87 and 9-88). External fixation was suggested by Kocialkowski and Wallace[247] because of the incidence of nonunion and the long protective period required when internal fixation was used alone. A Hoffmann external fixator system was used in conjunction with a dynamic compression plate and screw.[247] Several screw and plate combinations or screws alone have been used for internal fixation (Figs. 9-87 and 9-88).[242,247–251]

Postoperative imaging is done with routine radiographs in AP and lateral positions to confirm the position of the humerus in relation to the glenoid and to evaluate the position of the hardware.[248] Fluoroscopic stress views may be useful in patients with suspected nonunion.

The most common complications are nonunion, stress fractures, and infection.

REFERENCES

Imaging Techniques

1. Andren L, Lundberg BJ. Treatment of rigid shoulders by joint distention arthrography. *Acta Orthop Scand* 1965;36:45–53.
2. Bateman JE. *The shoulder and neck.* 2nd ed. Philadelphia: WB Saunders; 1978.
3. Bernau A, Berquist TH. *Orthopedic positioning in diagnostic radiology.* Baltimore: Urban and Schwarzenberg; 1983.
4. Berquist TH. *Imaging of orthopedic trauma.* New York: Raven Press; 1992.

5. Berquist TH. *MRI of the musculoskeletal system*. New York: Raven Press; 1990.
6. Berquist TH. Diagnostic and therapeutic injections as an aid to musculoskeletal diagnosis. *Semin Intervent Radiol* 1993;10:326–343.
7. Bosworth BM. Complete acromioclavicular dislocation. *N Engl J Med* 1949;241:221–225.
8. Brandt TD, Cardone BW, Grant TH, Post M, Weiss CA. Rotator cuff sonography: a reassessment. *Radiology* 1989;173:323–327.
9. Burk LD, Karasick D, Kurtz AB. Rotator cuff tears: prospective comparison of MR imaging with arthrography, sonography, and surgery. *AJR Am J Roentgenol* 1989;153:87–92.
10. Callaghan JJ, McNiesch LM, Dehaven JP, Savory CG, Polly DW. A prospective comparison of double contrast computed tomography, arthrography and arthroscopy of the shoulder. *Am J Sports Med* 1988;16:13–20.
11. Clements RW. Adaptation of the technique for radiology of the glenohumeral joint in the lateral position. *Radiol Technol* 1979;51:305.
12. Cone RO, Danzig L, Resnick D, Goldman AB. The bicipital groove. Radiographic, anatomic, and pathologic study. *AJR Am J Roentgenol* 1983;141:781–788.
13. Cone RO III, Resnick D, Danzig L. Shoulder impingement syndrome: radiographic evaluation. *Radiology* 1984;150:29–33.
14. Danzig L, Resnick D, Greenway G. Evaluation of unstable shoulders by computed tomography. *Am J Sports Med* 1982;10:138–141.
15. DePalma AF. Loss of scapulohumeral motion. *Ann Surg* 1952;135:193–204.
16. DeSmet AA. Axillary projection in radiography of the nontraumatized shoulder. *AJR Am J Roentgenol* 1980;143:511–518.
17. DeSmet AA. Anterior oblique projection in radiography of the traumatized shoulder. *AJR Am J Roentgenol* 1980;134:515–518.
18. DeSmet AA, Ting YM. Diagnosis of rotator cuff tear on routine radiographs. *Can Assoc Radiol J* 1977;28:54–57.
19. Deutsch AL, Resnick D, Mink JH, et al. Computed and conventional arthrotomography of the glenohumeral joint: normal anatomy and clinical experience. *Radiology* 1984;153:603–609.
20. El-Koury GY, Albright JB, Yousef MA, Montgomery WJ, Tuck SL. Arthrotomography of the glenoid labrum. *Radiology* 1979;131:333–337.
21. Ellis VH. The diagnosis of shoulder lesions due to injuries to the rotator cuff. *J Bone Joint Surg [Br]* 1953;35B:72–74.
22. Flinn RM, MacMillan CL, Campbell DR, et al. Optimal radiography of the acutely injured shoulder. *Can Assoc Radiol J* 1983;34:128.
23. Fulenda H, Mikasa M, Yamanaka K. Incomplete thickness rotator cuff tears diagnosed by subacromial bursography. *Clin Orthop* 1987;223:51–58.
24. Garcia JF. Arthrography. *Curr Probl Diagn Radiol* 1980;9:1.
25. Garcia JF. Arthrographic visualization of rotator cuff tears. Optimal application of stress to the shoulder. *Radiology* 1984;150:595.
26. Garth WP, Slappey CE, Ochs CW. Roentgen demonstration of instability of the shoulder: the apical oblique projection. *J Bone Joint Surg [Am]* 1984;66A:1450–1453.
27. Genoe GA, Moeller JA. Normal shoulder variations in the technetium-99m polyphosphate bone scan. *South Med J* 1974;67:659.
28. Gilula LA, Schoenecker PL, Murphy WA. Shoulder arthrography as a treatment modality. *AJR Am J Roentgenol* 1978;131:1047–1048.
29. Golding FC. The shoulder: the forgotten joint. *Br J Radiol* 1962;35:149–158.
30. Goldman AB, Dines DM, Warren RF. *Shoulder arthrography: technique, diagnosis and clinical correlation*. Boston: Little, Brown; 1982.
31. Hall FM. Morbidity from shoulder arthrography. Etiology, evidence, and prevention. *AJR Am J Roentgenol* 1981;136:56–62.
32. Harke AT, Grissom LE, Finkelstein MS. Evaluation of the musculoskeletal system with sonography. *AJR Am J Roentgenol* 1988;150:1253–1261.
33. Hatfield MK, Gross BH, Glazer GM, Martel W. Computed tomography of the sternum at its articulation. *Skeletal Radiol* 1984;11:197–203.
34. Hattrup SJ, Cofield RH, Berquist TH, McGough PF, Hoffmeyer DJ. Shoulder arthrography for determination of size of rotator cuff tear. *J Shoulder Elbow Surg* 1992;1:98–105.
35. Haynor DR, Shuman WP. Double contrast CT arthrography of the glenoid labrum and shoulder girdle. *Radiographics* 1984;4:411–421.
36. Heinig CF. Retrosternal dislocation of the clavicle: early recognition, x-ray diagnosis, and management. *J Bone Joint Surg [Am]* 1968;50A:830.
37. Hermodsson I. Roentgenologische Studien über die traumatischen and habituellen Schultergelenkverrenkungen nach vorn and nach unten. *Acta Radiol* 1934;20[Suppl]:1.
38. Hill NH, Sachs MD. The grooved defect of the humeral head. A frequently unrecognized complication of dislocations of the shoulder joint. *Radiology* 1940;35:690–701.
39. Holt PD, Keats TE. Calcific tendinitis: a review of the usual and unusual. *Skeletal Radiol* 1993;22:1–9.
40. Holt RG, Helms CA, Steinbach L, Neumann C, Mink PL, Genant HK. Magnetic resonance imaging of the shoulder: rotationale and current applications. *Skeletal Radiol* 1990;19:5–14.
41. Kilcoyne RF, Reddy PK, Lyons F, Rockwood CA. Optimal plain film imaging of the shoulder impingement syndrome. *AJR Am J Roentgenol* 1989;153:795–797.
42. Korngerth PJ, Salazar AM. The apical oblique view of the shoulder: its usefulness in acute trauma. *AJR Am J Roentgenol* 1987;149:113–116.
43. Kotzen LM. Roentgen diagnosis of rotator cuff tears. *AJR Am J Roentgenol* 1971;112:507–511.
44. Lee FA, Gwinn JL. Retrosternal dislocation of the clavicle. *Radiology* 1974;110:631–634.
45. Lie S, Mast WA. Subacromial bursography. *Radiology* 1982;144:626–630.
46. Mazuijian M. Lateral profile view of the scapula. *Radiol Technol* 1953;25:24.
47. McGlynn FJ, El-Koury G, Albright JP. Arthrotomography of the glenoid labrum in shoulder instability. *J Bone Joint Surg [Am]* 1982;64A:506–518.
48. McNiesh LM, Callaghan JJ. CT arthrotomography of the shoulder: variations of the glenoid labrum. *AJR Am J Roentgenol* 1987;149:963–966.
49. Middleton WD, Reinus WR, Totty WG, Madson CL, Murphy WA. Ultrasonographic evaluation of the rotator cuff and biceps tendon. *J Bone Joint Surg [Am]* 1986;68A:440–450.
50. Mikasa M. Subacromial bursography. *J Jpn Orthop Assoc* 1979;53:225.
51. Neer CS II. Displaced proximal humeral fractures. Part I. Classification and evaluation. *J Bone Joint Surg [Am]* 1970;52A:1077–1089.
52. Neviasser JS. Adhesive capsulitis of the shoulder. *J Bone Joint Surg* 1953;27:211–222.
53. Newhouse KE, El-Khoury GY, Nepala JV, Montgomery WJ. The shoulder impingement view: a fluoroscopic technique for detection of subacromial spurs. *AJR Am J Roentgenol* 1988;151:539–541.
54. Older MWJ, McIntyre JL, Lloyd GJ. Distention arthrography of the shoulder. *Can J Surg* 1976;19:203.
55. Quesada F. Technique for the roentgen diagnosis of fractures of the clavicle. *Surg General* 1926;42:4261–4281.
56. Rafii M, Finoznia H, Sherman O, et al. Rotator cuff lesions: signal patterns at MR imaging. *Radiology* 1990;177:817–823.
57. Rathburn JB, McNab I. Microvascular pattern of the rotator cuff. *J Bone Joint Surg [Br]* 1970;52B:540–553.
58. Reeves B. The natural history of frozen shoulder syndrome. *Scand J Rheum* 1975;4:193–196.
59. Resnick D. Arthrography, tenography, and bursography. In: Resnick D, Niwayama G, eds. *Diagnosis of bone and joint disorders*. Philadelphia: WB Saunders; 1988.
60. Rokous JR, Feagin JA, Abbott HG. Modified axillary roentgenogram. A useful adjunct in the diagnosis of recurrent instability of the shoulder. *Clin Orthop* 1972;82:84–86.
61. Rubin SA, Gray RL, Green WR. The scapular "Y": a diagnostic aid in shoulder trauma. *Radiology* 1974;110:725–726.
62. Simmonds FA. Shoulder pain with particular reference of "frozen" shoulder. *J Bone Joint Surg [Br]* 1949;31B:834–838.

63. Singson RD, Feldman F, Bigliani L. CT arthrographic patterns in recurrent glenohumeral instability. *AJR Am J Roentgenol* 1987;149:749–753.
64. Slivka J, Resnick D. An improved radiographic view of the glenohumeral joint. *Can Assoc Radiol J* 1979;30:83–85.
65. Strizak AM, Torrance CD, Jackson W, et al. Subacromial bursography: an anatomical and clinical study. *J Bone Joint Surg [Am]* 1982;64A:196–201.
66. Wallace WA, Hellier M. Improving radiographics of the injured shoulder. *Radiography* 1983;49:229.
67. Weiner DS, MacNab I. Superior migration of the humeral head: a radiographic aid to diagnosis of rotator cuff tear. *J Bone Joint Surg [Br]* 1970;52B:524–527.
68. Weston WJ. Arthrography of the acromioclavicular joint. *Australas Radiol* 1974;18:213–214.
69. Weston WJ. The subdeltoid bursa. *Australas Radiol* 1973;17:214.
70. Zanca P. Shoulder pain: involvement of the acromioclavicular joint. Analysis of 1000 cases. *AJR Am J Roentgenol* 1971;112:493–506.
71. Zlatkin MB, Dalinka MK. The glenohumeral joint. *Top Magn Reson Imaging* 1989;1:1–13.
72. Zlatkin MB, Iannotti JP, Roberts MC, et al. Rotator cuff disease: diagnostic performance of MR imaging. *Radiology* 1989;172:223–229.

Trauma

73. Allman FL. Fractures and ligamentous injuries of the clavicle and its articulations. *J Bone Joint Surg [Am]* 1967;49A:774–784.
74. Arndt JH, Sears AD. Posterior dislocation of the shoulder. *AJR Am J Roentgenol* 1965;94:639–645.
75. Arner O, Sandahl U, Ohrling H. Dislocation of the acromioclavicular joint: a review of the literature and report of 56 cases. *Acta Chir Scand* 1957;113:140–152.
76. Artz T, Huffer JM. A major complication of the modified Bristow procedure for recurrent dislocation of the shoulder. *J Bone Joint Surg [Am]* 1972;54A:1293–1296.
77. Aston JW Jr, Gregory CF. Dislocation of the shoulder with significant fracture of the glenoid. *J Bone Joint Surg [Am]* 1973;55A:1531–1533.
78. Baukart ASB. Recurrent or habitual dislocation of the shoulder joint. *BMJ* 1923;2:1132–1133.
79. Bateman FE. Athletic injuries about the shoulder in throwing and body-contact sports. *Clin Orthop* 1962;23:75–83.
80. Bearden JM, Hughston JC, Whatley GS. Acromioclavicular dislocation: method of treatment. *Am J Sports Med* 1973;4:5–17.
81. Berquist TH. *Imaging of orthopedic trauma.* 2nd ed. New York: Raven Press; 1992.
82. Berquist TH. Diagnostic and therapeutic injections as an aid to musculoskeletal diagnosis. *Semin Intervent Radiol* 1993;10:326–343.
83. Berquist TH. *MRI of the musculoskeletal system.* 2nd ed. New York: Raven Press; 1990.
84. Bigliani LU, Craig EU, Butters KP. Fractures of the shoulder. In: Rockwood CA, Green DP, Bucholz RW, eds. *Rockwood and Green's fractures in adults.* 3rd ed. Vol. 1. Philadelphia: JB Lippincott; 1991:871–1020.
85. Bodey WN, Denham RA. A free bone block operation for recurrent anterior dislocation of the shoulder. *Injury* 1983;15:184–188.
86. Bosworth BM. Complete acromioclavicular dislocation. *N Engl J Med* 1949;241:221–225.
87. Bosworth BM. AC separation: a new repair method. *Surg Gynecol Obstet* 1941;73:866–871.
88. Brunelli G, Brunvilli F. The treatment of A/C dislocation by transsection of the short biceps head. *Int Orthop* 1988;12:105–108.
89. Buckerfield CT, Castle ME. Acute retrosternal dislocation of the clavicle. *J Bone Joint Surg [Am]* 1984;66A:379–384.
90. Castagno AA, Shuman AA, Kilcoyne RF, Haynor DR, Morris ME, Matson FA. Complex fractures of the proximal humerus: role of CT in treatment. *Radiology* 1987;165:759–762.
91. Cave EF, Burke FE, Boyd RJ. *Posterior dislocation in trauma management.* Chicago: Year Book; 1974:437.
92. Cisternino SJ, Rogers LF, Stuffleban BC, Kruglik GD. The trough line: a radiographic sign of posterior dislocation. *AJR Am J Roentgenol* 1978;130:951–954.
93. Codman EA. *The shoulder: rupture of the supraspinatus tendon and other lesions in or about the subacromial bursa.* Boston: Thomas Todd; 1934.
94. Cope R, Riddervald HO. Posterior dislocation of the sternoclavicular joint. Report of two cases with emphasis on the radiographic management and early diagnosis. *Skeletal Radiol* 1988;17:247–258.
95. DePalma AF, Contilli RA. Fractures of the upper end of the humerus. *Clin Orthop* 1961;20:73–93.
96. Detoit GT, Roux D. Recurrent dislocation of the shoulder. A 24 year study of Johannesburg stapling operation. *J Bone Joint Surg [Am]* 1956;38A:1–12.
97. Downey EF Jr, Cartes DJ, Bower AC. Unusual dislocations of the shoulder. *AJR Am J Roentgenol* 1983;140:1207–1210.
98. Earwaker J. Isolated avulsion of the lesser tuberosity of the humerus. *Skeletal Radiol* 1990;19:121–125.
99. Esckola A, Vainionpaa S, Korkola O, Rokkonen P. Acute complete acromioclavicular dislocation: a prospective randomized trial with smooth and threaded Kirschner wires and cortical screws. *Ann Chir Gynecol* 1987;76:323–326.
100. Gallie WE, LeMesurier AB. Recurrent dislocation of the shoulder. *J Bone Joint Surg [Br]* 1948;30B:9–18.
101. Goss TP. Fractures of the glenoid cavity. *J Bone Joint Surg [Am]* 1992;74A:299–305.
102. Gurd FB. Treatment of complete dislocation of the outer end of the clavicle. A hitcher to undescribed operation. *Ann Surg* 1941;113:1094–1098.
103. Hall RH, Isaac E, Booth CR. Dislocation of the shoulder with special reference to accompanying small fractures. *J Bone Joint Surg [Am]* 1959;41A:489–494.
104. Harris RD, Harris HJ. The prevalence and significance of missed scapular fractures in blunt chest trauma. *AJR Am J Roentgenol* 1988;151:747–750.
105. Hawkins RJ, Bell RH, Gurr K. The three-part fracture of the proximal part of the humerus. *J Bone Joint Surg [Am]* 1986;68A:1410–1414.
106. Hayes JM, VanWinkle GN. Axillary artery injury with minimally displaced fracture of the neck of the humerus. *J Trauma* 1983;23:431–433.
107. Hill AA, Sachs MD. The grooved defect of the humeral head—a frequently unrecognized complication of dislocations of the shoulder joint. *Radiology* 1940;35:690–701.
108. Horak J, Nilsson BE. Epidemiology of fractures of the upper end of the humerus. *Clin Orthop* 1975;112:250–253.
109. Hovelius L. Anterior dislocation of the shoulder in teen-agers and young adults. *J Bone Joint Surg [Am]* 1987;69A:393–399.
110. Hovelius L, Thorling J, Freden H. Recurrent anterior dislocation of the shoulder. Results after Bankart and Putti-Platt operations. *J Bone Joint Surg [Am]* 1979;61A:566–569.
111. Ideberg R. Unusual glenoid fractures: a report of 92 cases. *Acta Orthop Scand* 1987;58:191–192.
112. Ideberg R. Fractures of the scapula involving the glenoid fossa. In: Bateman JE, Welsh RP, eds. *Surgery of the shoulder.* Toronto: BC Decker; 1984:63–66.
113. Jakoli RP, Kristiansen T, Mayo K, Ganz R, Miller RE. Classification and aspects of treatment in fractures of the proximal humerus. In: Bateman JE, Welsh RP, eds. *Surgery of the shoulder.* Toronto: BC Decker; 1984.
114. Janeiki CJ, Barnett DC. Fracture-dislocation of the shoulder with biceps tendon interposition. *J Bone Joint Surg [Am]* 1979;61A:141–143.
115. Johnson LL. Arthroscopy of the shoulder. *Orthop Clin North Am* 1980;11:197–204.
116. Karadumas J, Reutis G, Varouchas W. Repair of recurrent anterior dislocation of the shoulder using transfer of the subscapularis tendon. *J Bone Joint Surg [Am]* 1980;62A:1147–1149.
117. Kavanagh BF, Bradway JK, Cofield RH. Open reduction and in-

ternal fixation of displaced intra-articular fractures of the glenoid fossa. *J Bone Joint Surg [Am]* 1993;75A:479–484.
118. Kilcoyne RF, Shuman WP, Matson FA III, Rockwood CA. The Neer classification of displaced humeral fractures. Spectrum of findings on plain radiographs and CT scans. *AJR Am J Roentgenol* 1990;154:1029–1033.
119. Kristiansen B, Andersen WLS, Olsen CV, VanMarken J. The Neer classification of fractures of the proximal humerus. An assessment of interobserver variation. *Skeletal Radiol* 1988;17:420–422.
120. Lavic K. Habitual shoulder dislocation. *Acta Orthop Scand* 1961;30:252–264.
121. Leung KS, Lans TP. Open reduction and internal fixation of ipsilateral fractures of the scapular neck and clavicle. *J Bone Joint Surg [Am]* 1993;75A:1015–1018.
122. Lindsey RW, Gutowski WT. The migration of a broken pin after fracture of the AC joint. A case report and review of the literature. *Orthopedics* 1986;9:413–416.
123. Linson MA. Axillary artery thrombosis after fracture of the humerus. *J Bone Joint Surg [Am]* 1980;62A:1214–1215.
124. Lourie JA. Tomography in diagnosis of posterior dislocation of the sternoclavicular joint. *Acta Orthop Scand* 1980;51:579–580.
125. Lyons FA, Rockwood CA. Migration of pins in operations on the shoulder. *J Bone Joint Surg [Am]* 1990;72A:1262–1267.
126. Magnuson PB, Donaghue JR, Good RP, Stack AJ. The Magnuson-Starck procedure for treatment of recurrent glenohumeral dislocation. *Am J Sports Med* 1984;12:133–137.
127. Manshe DJ, Szabo RM. The operative treatment of mid shaft clavicular non-unions. *J Bone Joint Surg [Am]* 1985;67A:1367–1371.
128. Mazet RJ. Migration of K-wire from shoulder region into the lung. A report of 2 cases. *J Bone Joint Surg [Am]* 1943;25A:477–483.
129. McLaughling HL. Posterior dislocations of the shoulder. *J Bone Joint Surg [Am]* 1952;34A:584–590.
130. Miller DS, Boswich JA. Lesions of the brachial plexus associated with fractures of the clavicle. *Clin Orthop* 1969;64:144–149.
131. Miller LS, Donaghue JR, Good RP, Starck AJ. The Magnuson Stack procedure for treatment of recurrent glenohumeral dislocation. *Am J Sports Med* 1984;12:133–137.
132. Morgan CD, Bodenstat AB. Arthroscopic Bankart suture repair: early technique and results. *Arthroscopy* 1987;3:111–122.
133. Mouradian WA. Displaced proximal humeral fractures: 7 year experience with a modified Zickel supracondylar device. *Clin Orthop* 1986;212:209–218.
134. Müller ME, Nazarian S, Koch P, Schatzker J. *The comprehensive classification of fractures of long bones.* New York: Springer-Verlag; 1990:54–63.
135. Mumford EB. Acromioclavicular dislocation. *J Bone Joint Surg* 1941;23:799–802.
136. Neer CS II. Anterior acromioplasty for chronic impingement syndrome in the shoulder. A preliminary report. *J Bone Joint Surg [Am]* 1972;54A:41–50.
137. Neer CS II. Displaced proximal humeral fractures. Part I: classification and evaluation. *J Bone Joint Surg [Am]* 1970;52A:1077–1089.
138. Neer CS II. Fractures of the distal clavicle with detachment of the coracoclavicular ligament in adults. *J Trauma* 1963;3:99–110.
139. Neer CS II. Fractures of the distal third of the clavicle. *Clin Orthop* 1968;58:43–50.
140. Nettles JL, Linscheid R. Sternoclavicular dislocations. *J Trauma* 1968;8:158–164.
141. Neviaser JS. The treatment of fractures of the clavicle. *Surg Clin North Am* 1963;43:1555–1563.
142. O'Driscoll SW, Evans DC. The DuToit staple capsulorrhaphy for recurrent dislocation of the shoulder. Twenty year experience in six Toronto hospitals. *Orthop Trans* 1988;12:731.
142A. O'Driscoll SW, Evans DC. Long-term results of staple capsulorrhaphy for anterior instability of the shoulder. *J Bone Joint Surg [Am]* 1993;75A:249–258.
143. Omer GE. Osteotomy of the clavicle in surgical reduction of anterior sternoclavicular dislocation. *J Trauma* 1967;7:584–590.
144. Osmund-Clarke H. Habitual dislocation of the shoulder: the Putti-Platt operation. *J Bone Joint Surg [Br]* 1948;30B:19–25.
145. Oudard P. La luxation recidivante de l'épaule (varieté antero-interne) procède opération. *J Chir* 1924;23:13–25.
146. Pascoet G, Jung F, Foucher G, Kehr P. Treatment of recurrent dislocation of the shoulder by preglenoid artificial ridge using the Latarjet-Vittori technique. *J Med Strasburg* 1975;6:501–504.
147. Post M, Morrey BF, Hawkins RJ. *Surgery of the shoulder.* St. Louis: Mosby-Year Book; 1990.
148. Quigley TB, Freedman PA. Recurrent dislocation of the shoulder: preliminary report of personal experience with seven Bankart and 92 Putti-Platt operations in 99 cases over 25 years. *Am J Surg* 1974;128:595–599.
149. Quinn SF, Glass TA. Post-traumatic osteolysis of the clavicle. *South Med J* 1983;76:307.
150. Rockwood CA, Green DP, Bucholz RW. *Rockwood and Green's fractures in adults.* 3rd ed. Vol. 1. Philadelphia: JB Lippincott; 1991.
151. Rockwood CA Jr, Young DC. Complications and manifestations of Bristow shoulder reconstruction. *Orthop Trans* 1989;13:232.
152. Rowe CR. Fractures of the scapula. *Surg Clin North Am* 1972;43:1565–1571.
153. Rowe CR. Prognosis in dislocation of the shoulder. *J Bone Joint Surg [Am]* 1956;38A:957–977.
154. Rowe CR, Zarins B. Recurrent transient dislocation of the shoulder. *J Bone Joint Surg [Am]* 1981;63A:863–872.
155. Rowe CR, Zarins B, Ciullo JV. Recurrent anterior dislocation of the shoulder after surgical repair: apparent causes of treatment failure. *J Bone Joint Surg [Am]* 1984;66A:159–168.
156. Rubenstein JD, Ebraheim NA, Kellam JF. Traumatic scapulothoracic dislocation. *Radiology* 1985;157:297–298.
157. Salvatore J. Sternoclavicular joint dislocation. *Clin Orthop* 1968;58:51–55.
158. Sanders JO, Lyons FA, Rockwood CA. Management of dislocation of both ends of the clavicle. *J Bone Joint Surg [Am]* 1990;72A:399–402.
159. Schultz TJ, Jacobs B, Patterson RL. Unrecognized chronic dislocation of the shoulder. *J Trauma* 1969;9:1009–1023.
160. Selesnick FH, Jablow M, Frank C, Post W. Retrosternal dislocation of the clavicle. A report of 4 cases. *J Bone Joint Surg [Am]* 1984;66A:287–291.
161. Sidor ML, Zucherman JD, Lyon T, Koval K, Cuomo F, Schoenberg N. The Neer classification system for proximal humeral fractures. *J Bone Joint Surg [Am]* 1993;75A:1745–1750.
162. Siebenrock KA, Gerber C. The reproducibility of classification of fractures of the proximal end of the humerus. *J Bone Joint Surg [Am]* 1993;75A:1751–1755.
163. Simeone FA. Neurological complications of closed shoulder injuries. *Orthop Clin North Am* 1975;6:499.
164. Simonet WT, Cofield RH. Prognosis in anterior shoulder dislocation. *Am J Sports Med* 1984;12:19–23.
165. Sisk TD, Boyd HB. Management of recurrent anterior dislocation of the shoulder: deTort type of stapling capsulorrhaphy. *Clin Orthop* 1974;103:150–156.
166. Smith MJ, Stewart MJ. Acute acromioclavicular separations. *Am J Sports Med* 1979;7:62–71.
167. Tagliahue D, Esposito A. Latarjet's operation in recurrent dislocation of the shoulder in athletes. *Ital J Sports Traumatol* 1980;2:91–100.
168. Thompson DA, Flynn TC, Miller PW, Fischer RP. Significance of scapular fractures. *J Trauma* 1985;25:974–977.
169. Tsou PM. Percutaneous cancellous screw coracoid fixation for acute acromioclavicular dislocation. *Clin Orthop* 1989;243:112–121.
170. Turkel SJ, Pinto MW, Marshall JL, Girgis FG. Stabilizing mechanism preventing anterior dislocation of the glenohumeral joint. *J Bone Joint Surg [Am]* 1981;63A:1208–1217.
171. Weber BG, Simpson LA, Hardegger F. Rotational humeral osteotomy for recurrent anterior dislocation of the shoulder associated with a large Hill-Sachs lesion. *J Bone Joint Surg [Am]* 1984;66A:1443–1450.
172. White EM, Kattapuram SV, Jupiter JB. Case report 241. Post-traumatic pseudoaneurysm. *Skeletal Radiol* 1983;10:178.
173. Wilkin RM, Johnson RM. Ununited fractures of the clavicle. *J Bone Joint Surg [Am]* 1983;65A:773–778.

174. Worman LW, Leagus C. Intrathoracic injury following retrosternal dislocation of the clavicle. *J Trauma* 1967;7:416–423.
175. Young DC, Rockwood CA. Complications of a failed Bristow procedure and their management. *J Bone Joint Surg [Am]* 1991;73A:969–981.
176. Zdravkovic D, Damholt VV. Comminuted and severely displaced fractures of the scapula. *Acta Orthop Scand* 1974;45:60–65.
177. Zenni EJ, Krieg JK, Rosen MJ. Open reduction and internal fixation of clavicle fractures. *J Bone Joint Surg [Am]* 1981;63A:147–151.
178. Zucherman JD, Matsen FA. Complications about the glenohumeral joint related to the use of screws and staples. *J Bone Joint Surg [Am]* 1984;66A:175–180.

Arthroplasty

179. Alibradi P, Weissman BN, Thornhell T, Nippoor N, Sosman JL. Evaluation of a nonconstrained total shoulder prosthesis. *AJR Am J Roentgenol* 1988;151:1169–1172.
180. Amstatz HC, Thomas BJ, Kabo JM, Jinnah RH, Dorey FJ. The Dana total shoulder arthroplasty. *J Bone Joint Surg [Am]* 1988;70A:1174–1182.
181. An KN, Morrey BF. The shoulder: biomechanics. In: Morrey BF, ed. *Joint replacement arthroplasty.* New York: Churchill Livingstone; 1991:397.
182. Arntz CT, Jackins S, Matsen FA III. Prosthetic replacement of the shoulder for treatment of defects in the rotator cuff and the surface of the glenohumeral joint. *J Bone Joint Surg [Am]* 1993;75A:485–491.
183. Barrett WP, Franklin JL, Jackins SE, Wyss CR, Matsen FA III. Total shoulder arthroplasty. *J Bone Joint Surg [Am]* 1987;69A:865–872.
184. Becker DA. Prosthetic design, surgical technique and rehabilitation. In: Morrey BF, ed. *Joint replacement arthroplasty.* New York: Churchill Livingstone, 1991.
185. Bell SN, Geschwend N. Clinical experience with total arthroplasty and hemiarthroplasty of the shoulder using a Neer prosthesis. *Int Orthop* 1986;10:217–222.
186. Berquist TH. *Imaging of orthopedic trauma and surgery.* Philadelphia: WB Saunders; 1985.
187. Bonutto PM, Hawkins RJ. Fracture of the humeral shaft associated with total replacement of the shoulder. *J Bone Joint Surg [Am]* 1992;74A:617–618.
188. Boyd AD Jr, Alibadi P, Thornhill TS. Postoperative proximal migration in total shoulder arthroplasty. *J Arthroplasty* 1991;6:31–37.
189. Boyd AD, Thomas WH, Scott RD, Sledge CB, Thornhill TS. Total shoulder arthroplasty vs. hemiarthroplasty. *J Arthroplasty* 1990;5:329–336.
190. Boyd AD, Thornhill TS, Barnes CL. Fractures adjacent to humeral prosthesis. *J Bone Joint Surg [Am]* 1992;74A:1498–1504.
191. Brenner BC, Ferlic DC, Clayton ML, Dennis DA. Survivorship of unconstrained total shoulder arthroplasty. *J Bone Joint Surg [Am]* 1989;71A:1289–1296.
192. Buechel FF, Pappas MJ, DePalma AF. "Floating socket" total shoulder replacement: anatomical, biomechanical and surgical rotationale. *J Biomed Mater Res* 1978;12:89–114.
193. Cofield RH. Results and complications. In: Morrey BF, ed. *Joint replacement arthroplasty.* New York: Churchill Livingstone; 1991:437.
194. Cofield RH. Unconstrained total shoulder prosthesis. *Clin Orthop* 1983;173:97–108.
195. Cofield RH. Total shoulder arthroplasty with the Neer prosthesis. *J Bone Joint Surg [Am]* 1984;66A:899–906.
196. Coughlin MJ, Morris JM, West WF. The semiconstrained total shoulder arthroplasty. *J Bone Joint Surg [Am]* 1979;61A:574–581.
197. Craig EV. Total shoulder replacement. *Orthopedics* 1988;11:125–136.
198. Eqund N, Jonsson E, Lidgren L, Kelly I, Pettersson H. Computed tomography of humeral head cup arthroplasties. *Acta Radiol* 1987;28:71.
199. Faludi DD, Weiland AJ. Cementless total shoulder arthroplasty: preliminary experience with 13 cases. *Orthopedics* 1983;6:431–437.
200. Feldman F. The radiology of total shoulder prosthesis. *Semin Roentgenol* 1986;1:47–65.
201. Fenlin JM. Total glenohumeral joint replacement. *Orthop Clin North Am* 1975;6:565–583.
202. Figgie HE, Inglis AE, Goldberg VM, Ranawat CS, Figgie MP, Wile JM. Analysis of factors affecting the long term results of total shoulder arthroplasty in inflammatory arthritis. *J Arthroplasty* 1988;3:123–130.
203. Franklin JL, Barrett WP, Jackins SE, Matsen FA III. Glenoid loosening in total shoulder arthroplasty. *J Arthroplasty* 1988;3:39–46.
204. Frich LH, Sojbjerg JO, Sneppen O. Shoulder arthroplasty in complex and chronic proximal humeral fractures. *Orthopedics* 1991;14:949–954.
205. Friedman RJ, Thornhill TS, Thomas WH, Sledge CB. Non-constrained total shoulder replacement in patients who have rheumatoid arthritis and class IV function. *J Bone Joint Surg [Am]* 1989;71A:494–498.
206. Gristina AG, Romano RL, Mannire GC, Webb LX. Total shoulder replacement. *Orthop Clin North Am* 1987;18:445–453.
206A. Gristura AG, Webb L. The trispherical total shoulder. In: Inglis AE, ed. *American Academy of Orthopedic Surgeons Symposium on Total Joint Replacement of the Upper Extremity.* St. Louis: CV Mosby; 1982:50.
207. Hawkins RJ, Bell RH, Jallay B. Total shoulder arthroplasty. *Clin Orthop* 1989;242:188–194.
208. Kay SP, Amstatz HC. Shoulder hemiarthroplasty at UCLA. *Clin Orthop* 1988;228:42–48.
209. Inglis AE. Advances in implant arthroplasty. *Clin Exp Rheumatol* 1989;7:141–144.
210. Kelly IG, Foster RS, Fisher WD. Neer shoulder replacement in rheumatoid arthritis. *J Bone Joint Surg [Br]* 1987;69B:723–726.
211. Laurence M. Replacement arthroplasty of the rotator cuff deficient shoulder. *J Bone Joint Surg [Br]* 1991;73B:916–919.
212. Lettin AW, Copeland SA, Scales JT. The Stanmore total shoulder arthroplasty. *J Bone Joint Surg [Br]* 1982;64B:47–51.
213. Magnuson JE, Brown ML, Hauser MF, Berquist TH, Fitzgerald RH, Klee GG. In-111-labeled leukocyte scintigraphy in suspected orthopedic prosthesis infection: comparison with other imaging modalities. *Radiology* 1988;168:235–239.
214. Maxon HR, Schneider HJ, Hopson CN, Miller EH, VonStein DE, Kereuakes JG, Cummings DD, McDevitt RM. A comparative study of indium-111 DTPA radionuclide and iotholamate meglumine roentgenographic arthrography in the evaluation of painful hip arthroplasty. *Clin Orthop* 1989;245:156–159.
215. McElwain JP, English E. The early results of porous-coated total shoulder arthroplasty. *Clin Orthop* 1987;218:217–224.
216. Milbrink J, Wigren A. Resection arthroplasty of the shoulder. *Scand J Rheumatol* 1990;19:432–436.
217. Moeckel BH, Altchek DW, Warren RF, Wickiewicz TL, Dines DM. Instability of the shoulder after arthroplasty. *J Bone Joint Surg [Am]* 1993;75A:492–499.
218. Moeckel BH, Dines DM, Warren RF, Altchek DW. Modular hemiarthroplasty for fractures of the proximal part of the humerus. *J Bone Joint Surg [Am]* 1992;74A:884–889.
219. Neer CS II. Articular replacement of the humeral head. *J Bone Joint Surg [Am]* 1955;31A:215–228.
220. Neer CS II. Replacement arthroplasty for glenohumeral osteoarthritis. *J Bone Joint Surg [Am]* 1974;56A:1–13.
221. Neer CS II, Morrison DS. Glenoid bone grafting in total shoulder arthroplasty. *J Bone Joint Surg [Am]* 1988;70A:1154–1162.
222. Neer CS II, Watson KC, Stanton FJ. Recent experience in total shoulder replacement. *J Bone Joint Surg [Am]* 1982;64A:319–337.
223. Oates E. Scintigraphic diagnosis of infection and inflammation. *Appl Radiol* 1992;21:48–53.
224. Pahle JA, Kvarmes L. Shoulder replacement arthroplasty. *Ann Chir Gynaecol* 1985;74:85–89.
225. Post M. Constrained arthroplasty of the shoulder. *Orthop Clin North Am* 1987;18:455.
225A. Post M, Haskell SS, Jablon M. Total shoulder replacement with

a constrained prosthesis. *J Bone Joint Surg* [*Am*] 1980;62A:327–335.
226. Post M, Jablon M. Constrained total shoulder arthroplasty. A critical review. *Clin Orthop* 1979;144:130–150.
227. Rietveld ABM, Daanen HAM, Rozing PM, Obermann WR. The lever arm in glenohumeral abduction after hemiarthroplasty. *J Bone Joint Surg* [*Br*] 1988;70B:561–565.
228. Roper BA, Paterson JMH, Day WH. The Roper-Day total shoulder replacement. *J Bone Joint Surg* [*Br*] 1990;75B:694–697.
229. Rosenthall L, Aldis AE, Hill RO. Combined radionuclide and radiocontrast arthrography for evaluating hip arthroplasty. *Eur J Nucl Med* 1985;10:531–534.
230. Schauwecken DS. The scintigraphic diagnosis of osteomyelitis. *AJR Am J Roentgenol* 1992;158:9–18.
231. Schutts JP, Hawkins RJ. Advances in shoulder surgery. *Int Orthop* 1989;13:57–60.
232. Swanson AB. Bipolar implant shoulder arthroplasty. In: Bateman JE, Welsh RP, eds. *Surgery of the shoulder.* St. Louis: CV Mosby; 1984:211–223.
233. Swanson AB, Swanson GD, Sattel AB, Cendo RD, Hynes D, Jarning W. Bipolar implant shoulder arthroplasty. *Clin Orthop* 1989;249:227–247.
234. Thomas BJ, Amstutz HC, Cracchiolo A. Shoulder arthroplasty for rheumatoid arthritis. *Clin Orthop* 1991;265:125–128.
235. Vahvanen V, Hämälainen M, Paavolainen P. The Neer II replacement for rheumatoid arthritis of the shoulder. *Int Orthop* 1989;13:57–60.
236. Uri G, Wellman H, Capello W, Robb J, Greenman G. Scintigraphic and x-ray arthrographic diagnosis of femoral prosthesis loosening. *J Nucl Med* 1984;25:661–663.
236A. Warren RF, Ranawat CS, Inglis AE. Total shoulder replacement indications and results of the Neer nonconstrained prosthesis. In: Inglis AE, ed. *American Academy of Orthopedic Surgeons Symposium on Total Joint Replacement of the Upper Extremity.* St. Louis: CV Mosby; 1982:56.
237. Weiss A-PC, Adams MA, Moore JR, Weiland AJ. Unconstrained shoulder arthroplasty. *Clin Orthop* 1990;257:86–90.
238. Wilde AH, Bonden LS, Brews JJ. Experience with the Neer total shoulder replacement. In: Bateman JE, Welsh RP, eds. *Surgeries of the shoulder.* St. Louis: CV Mosby; 1984:224–228.
239. Zuckerman JD, Cofield RH. Proximal humeral prosthesis replacement in glenohumeral arthritis. Presented at American Shoulder and Elbow Surgeons, New Orleans, February, 1986 (abst).

Arthrodesis and Miscellaneous Procedures

240. Beltran JE, Trilla JC, Barjau R. Simplified compression arthrodesis of the shoulder. *J Bone Joint Surg* [*Am*] 1975;57A:538.
241. Benjamin A, Herschowitz D, Arden GP. The treatment of arthritis of the shoulder joint by double osteotomy. *Int Orthop* 1979;3:21.
242. Boyd AD, Thornhill TS. Surgical treatment of osteoarthritis of the shoulder. *Rheum Dis Clin North Am* 1988;14:591–611.
243. Cofield RH. Shoulder arthrodesis and resection arthroplasty. In: Inglis AE, ed. *AAOS Instruction Course Lectures.* St. Louis: CV Mosby; 1985.
244. Cofield RH. Shoulder arthrodesis and resection arthroplasty. In: Evarts CM, ed. *Surgery of the musculoskeletal system.* 2nd ed. New York: Churchill Livingstone; 1990.
245. Cofield RH, Briggs BT. Glenohumeral arthrodesis: operative and long term functional results. *J Bone Joint Surg* [*Am*] 1979;61A:668–677.
246. Hawkins RJ, Neer CS II. A functional analysis of shoulder fusion. *Clin Orthop* 1987;223:65.
247. Kocialkowski A, Wallace WA. Shoulder arthrodesis using an external fixator. *J Bone Joint Surg* [*Br*] 1991;73B:180–181.
248. Mak JY, Hall JE. Arthrodesis of the shoulder in children. *J Bone Joint Surg* [*Am*] 1990;72A:582–586.
249. Neer CS II, Kirby RM. Revision of humeral head and total shoulder arthroplasties. *Clin Orthop* 1982;170:189.
250. Richards RR, Sherman RM, Hudson AR, Waddell JP. Shoulder arthrodesis using a pelvic-reconstruction plate. *J Bone Joint Surg* [*Am*] 1988;70A:416–421.
251. Rowe CR. Arthrodesis of the shoulder used in treating painful conditions. *Clin Orthop* 1983;173:92–96.

Imaging Atlas of Orthopedic Appliances and Prostheses,
edited by T.H. Berquist.
Mayo Clinic Foundation © 1995.
Published by Raven Press, Ltd., New York.

CHAPTER 10

Humeral Shaft

Thomas H. Berquist and Mark P. Brodersen

Humeral shaft fractures account for 1% of all fractures. Most can be treated using closed techniques; however, internal and external fixation techniques are also frequently used, depending on the type and location of the fracture.[1,5,8,29]

MECHANISM OF INJURY

There are several unique features of the humerus that present special problems in the treatment of fractures. First, the humerus is the most freely movable bone. Scapulohumeral motion can amplify this. Second, the humerus functions as a lever; therefore, nearly all stress to the bone is in tension from or is at an angle to the long axis of the bone. Weight bearing and compression forces are not problems in fracture management. Finally, when the patient is upright, the bone hangs vertically and thus is influenced by gravity alone, allowing realignment of fracture fragments.[4,16,17]

The location of the fracture in relationship to the muscle attachments affects the direction of the displacement of the bone fragments. Fractures of the proximal third (between the pectoralis major and deltoid insertions) result in the medial displacement of the proximal fragment that goes to the pole of the musculus pectoralis. Fractures distal to the deltoid tuberosity result in the abduction of the proximal fragment from the pull exerted by the deltoid and the proximal displacement of the fragment from pull exerted by the brachialis and biceps (Fig. 10-1).[8,16]

Direct force from either blunt or penetrating injuries is the most frequent cause of fractures of the humeral shaft. Transverse fractures are usually the result of a bending force. Spiral fractures occur from a combination of bending and rotational forces. Compression forces acting on the humerus tend to affect either end but not the diaphysis. Indirect forces, such as falling directly on the elbow or on the outstretched hand, vigorous throwing of objects, or even violent muscle contraction can also result in fracture of the humeral shaft. The level of fracture is described as being upper, middle, or lower third (Fig. 10-2). Sixty-nine percent of fractures occur at the midshaft level. Of these fractures, 61% are transverse; 18%, oblique; 17%, spiral; and 4%, comminuted or segmental.[1,8,11,13,19]

Fractures at the junction of the middle and distal thirds of the humeral shaft are particularly difficult to manage. Injury to the main nutrient artery may contribute to the delayed union or nonunion. The radial nerve is also at risk in fractures at this level. Closed reduction may damage the nerve in this setting. For this reason, open reduction and internal fixation of these fractures is recommended, especially if there is any evidence of chronic radial nerve involvement.[8,18]

PREOPERATIVE IMAGING

Standard recumbent views include anteroposterior (AP) and lateral projections. The transthoracic view is also useful in evaluating the position of fragments and determining the extent of angulation of the fractures.

With severe trauma, additional injury to the radius and ulna or shoulder may occur. Therefore, evaluation of the forearm and shoulder may also be required.[1]

TREATMENT

The treatment options for humeral shaft fractures depend on the patient's age, the type and level of fracture,

(text continues on page 731)

T. H. Berquist: Mayo Medical School and Department of Diagnostic Radiology, Mayo Clinic Jacksonville, Jacksonville, Florida 32224.

M. P. Brodersen: Mayo Medical School and Department of Orthopedic Surgery, Mayo Clinic Jacksonville, Jacksonville, Florida 32224.

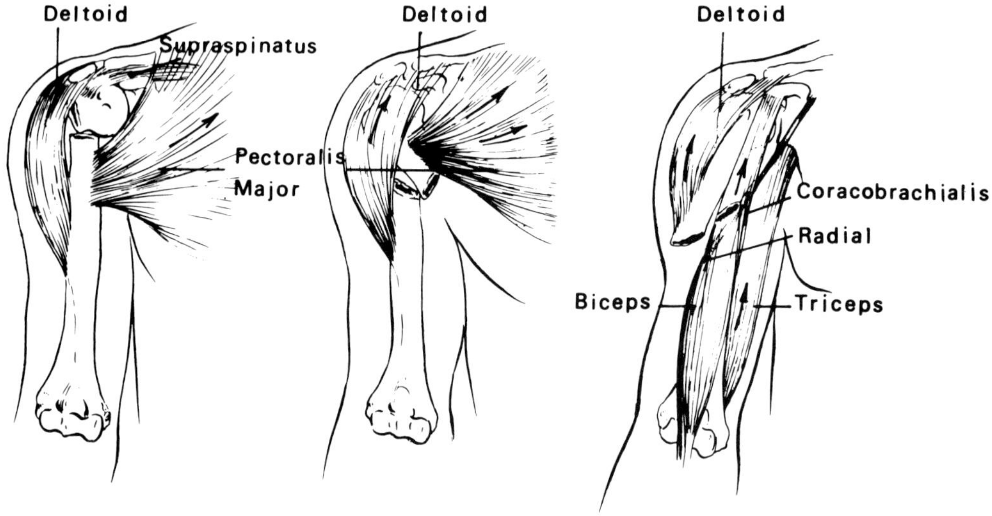

FIG. 10-1. Muscle forces on humeral fractures. (From Epps CH, Grant RE. Fractures of the shaft of the humerus. In: Rockwood CA, Green DP, Bucholz KW, eds. *Rockwood and Green's fractures in adults,* 3rd ed. Vol. 1. Philadelphia: JB Lippincott 1991;843–869.)

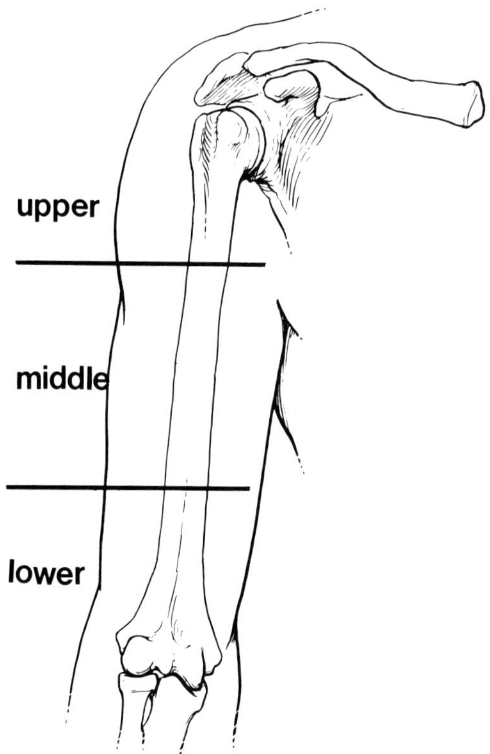

FIG. 10-2. Fractures of the humeral shaft are described according to their location as upper, middle, or lower third.

the degree of fracture displacement, muscle development, and associated injuries. Closed primary treatment may include dependent traction (long arm hanging cast, Fig. 10-3), thoracobrachial immobilization (open Velpeau-type cast) or various other casts and splints.[1,4,8,17,18,25,29]

Perfect alignment and apposition of the fracture fragment is not as essential as it would be with the weight-bearing structures in the lower extremity. Anterior angulation of up to 20° and varus angulation of up to 30° can usually be accepted without compromising function or appearance. Fractures of the distal third of the humerus are more significant, and as the involvement approaches the elbow, alignment is more critical.[8,19]

The indications for primary operative treatment include (1) displaced transverse fractures or short oblique fractures (Fig. 10-4), (2) long spiral fractures with displacement that suggest soft tissue interposition (Fig. 10-5), and (3) compound or open fractures with vascular or neural complications.

External Fixation

External fixators are commonly used with complex open wounds (Table 10-1) to provide a method for realignment and stabilization while maintaining access to the wound (see Chapter 2, Figs. 2-71 and 2-72). Unilateral frame fixators are commonly used for the humerus in this setting (Figs. 10-6 to 10-8).[1,8]

Internal Fixation

Internal fixation of the humeral shaft can be accomplished with closed intramedullary nailing, open intramedullary nailing, or plate and screw techniques.[3,8,23–28]

Plate and Screw Fixation

Plate and screw fixation techniques provide rigid fixation and control of fracture fragments and the fracture gap. The regenerating blood supply is protected, allowing primary bone healing across the fracture site. The major disadvantages are increased bone exposure, with the risk to the local vascular supply and infection. Also, stress protection by the rigid implants decreases bone strength.[1] Bone grafting (Fig. 10-4) is commonly used in conjunction with plate and screw fixation. Methyl methacrylate is also used in osteopenic patients to improve screw purchase (Fig. 10-9).[1,27] Union rates of up to 97% can be achieved with plate and screw techniques.[27]

TABLE 10-1. *External fixation of humeral shaft fractures: indications*[1,6,8,9,13,14]

Marked comminution
Infected nonunion
Bone loss
Severe open wounds
Elderly patients who cannot be immobilized
Associated forearm fractures

Intramedullary Nailing

Intramedullary nailing of humeral fractures can be accomplished using open or closed techniques. Multiple nail configurations are available for humeral intramedullary nailing. Intramedullary nails maintain alignment, and newer interlocking designs prevent the rotation of the fracture fragments.[3,6,8] The operative procedure is less extensive than that with plate and screw techniques; therefore, the local blood supply is less likely to be affected. The fixation is less rigid than that with plate and screw fixation. Healing generally occurs in 7 to 8 weeks with uncomplicated intramedullary nailing.[3,6,7,8]

Hackethal Stacked Nailing[7]

This technique uses smooth Steinmann pins of 3.2 mm and smaller diameters to pack the medullary canal (Fig. 10-10). The pins are inserted 5 cm above the olecranon and cut or bent at the cortical margin after insertion. From 3 to 11 pins may be used, depending on the size of the medullary canal. Durbin et al.[7] reported 92% union with this technique.

Rush Rods and Ender Nailing[3,8,15,20]

Ender nails can be used for humeral shaft fractures. The nails (usually two) can be inserted into the greater tuberosity below the level of the rotator cuff (Fig. 10-11) or above the olecranon (Fig. 10-12) and flared in the proximal metaphysis.[15] Epicondylar entry ports have also been used but with poor results. If the superior entry point is too high (above the rotator cuff), impingement can be a problem postoperatively.

These closed procedures are usually performed within 24 hours of injury and are best suited for the severely injured multiple trauma patient. Union rates of 94% have been reported using these techniques (Figs. 10-13 through 10-15).[3,15]

True/Flex™ Humeral Rod

This solid rod has five flutes giving it a "star"-shaped cross-sectional diameter. The rods are available in 6-, 8-, and 10-mm diameters and five lengths (23 to 31 cm); they are constructed of titanium alloy. A cobalt-chromium screw cap secures the rod and provides axial locking (Fig. 10-16).

(text continues on page 749)

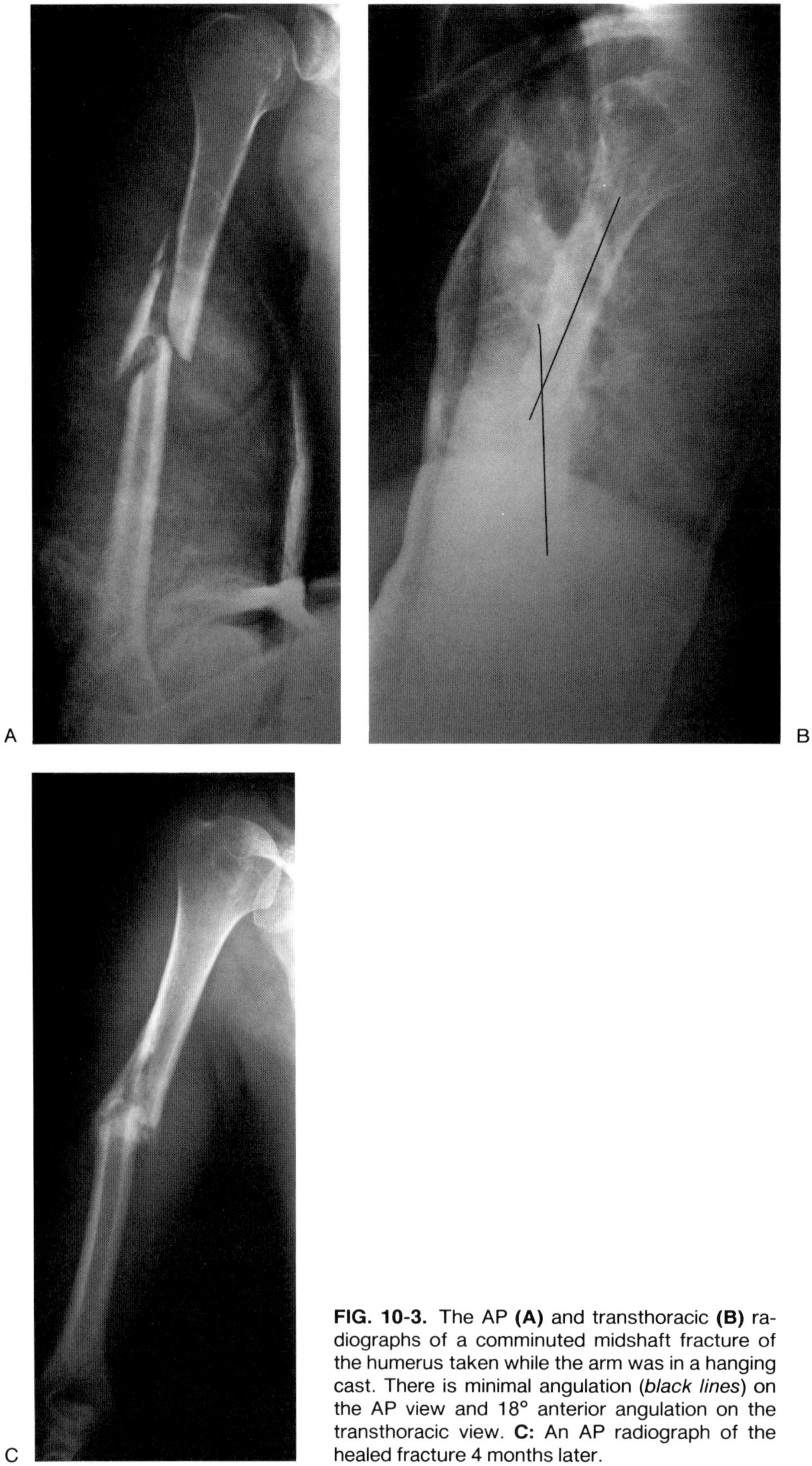

FIG. 10-3. The AP **(A)** and transthoracic **(B)** radiographs of a comminuted midshaft fracture of the humerus taken while the arm was in a hanging cast. There is minimal angulation (*black lines*) on the AP view and 18° anterior angulation on the transthoracic view. **C:** An AP radiograph of the healed fracture 4 months later.

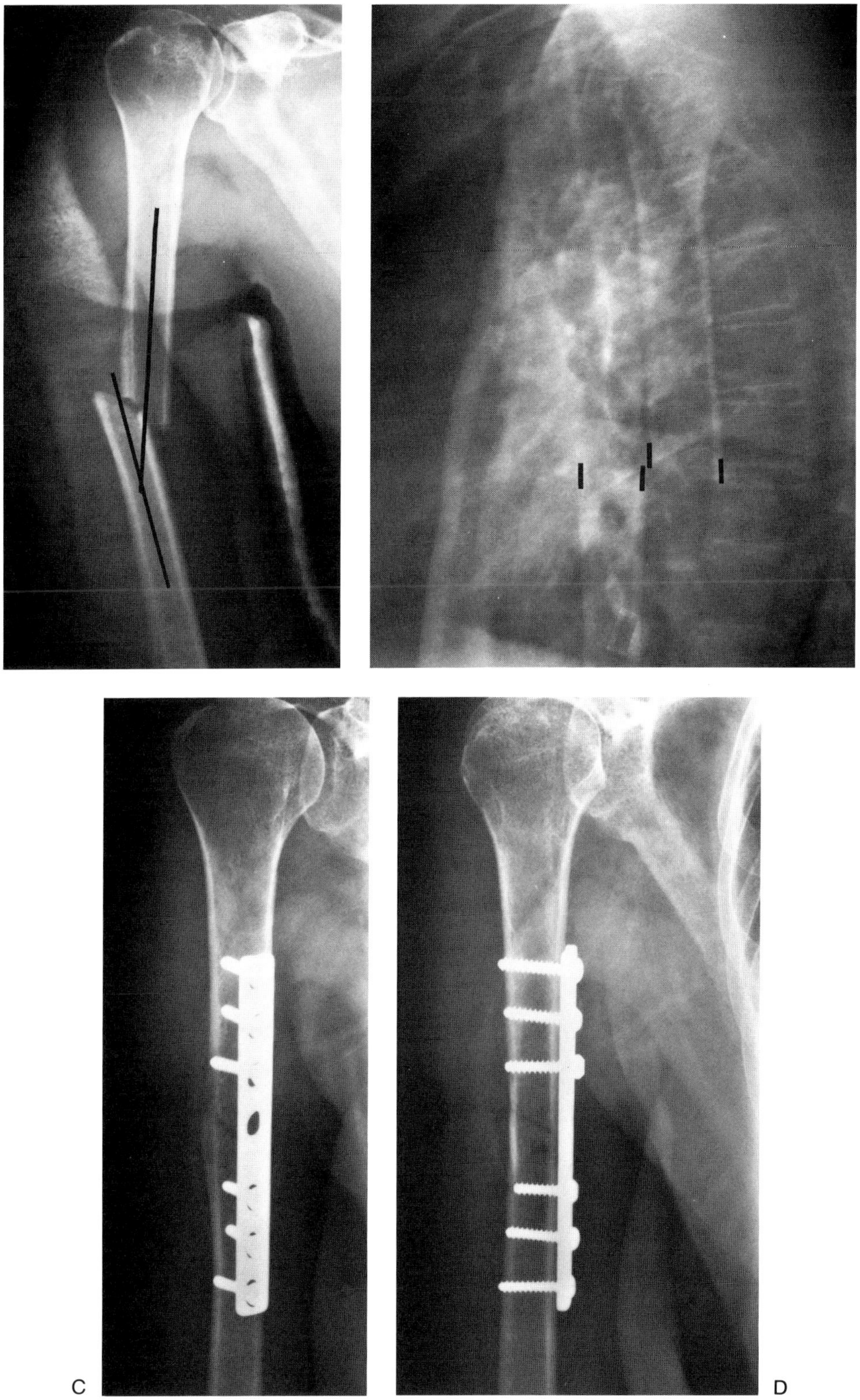

A B C D

FIG. 10-4. The AP **(A)** and transthoracic **(B)** views of a short oblique fracture of the midhumeral shaft with 25° angulation on the AP view (A) and no bony apposition (*lines* mark cortex) on the lateral view (B). Radiographs taken while the arm was in a hanging cast. **C,D:** The fracture did not unite and required dynamic compression (DC) plate and screw fixation with bone grafting 6 months later.

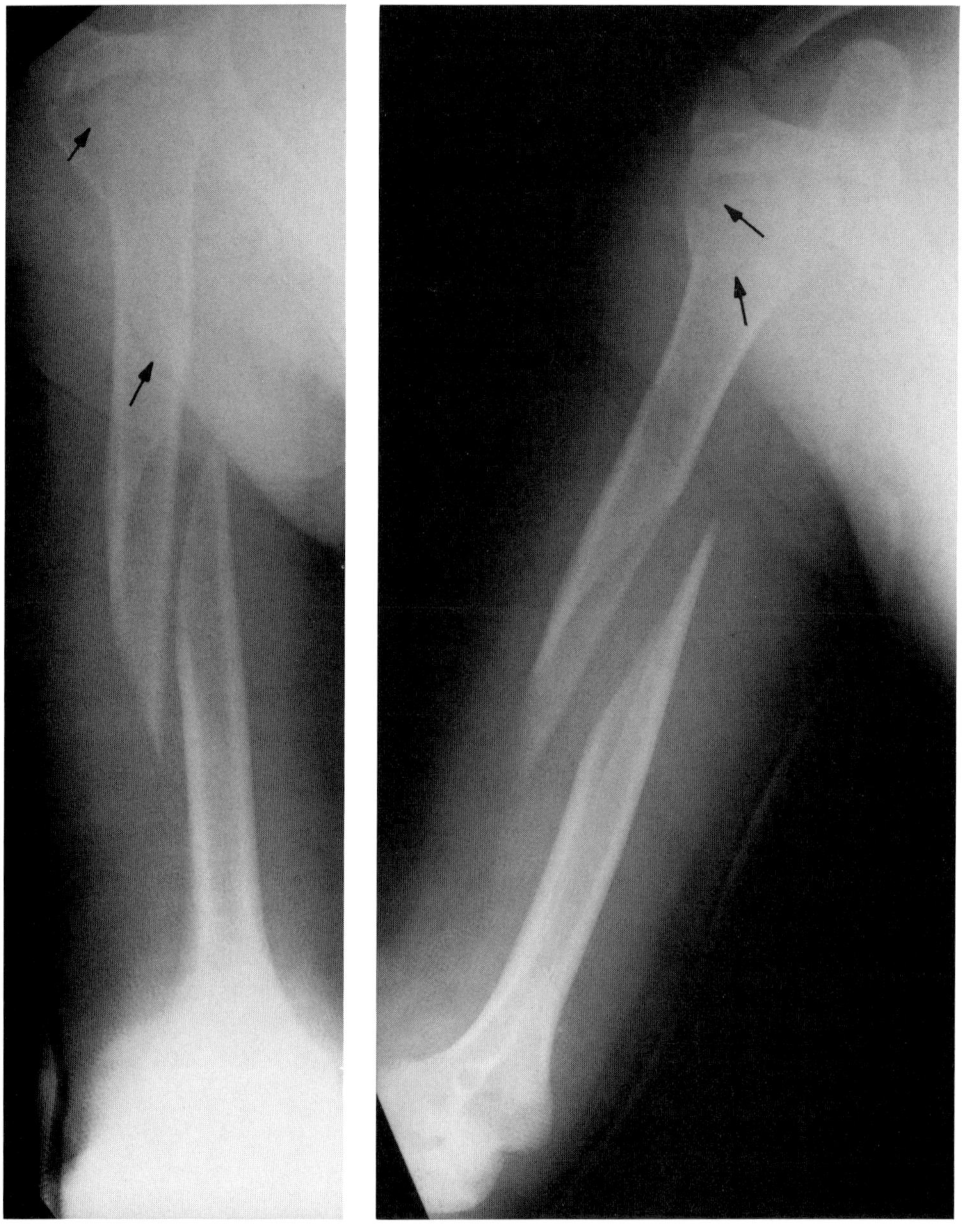

A B

FIG. 10-5. A,B: Long spiral fracture of the midhumeral shaft with separation of the fragments as a result of soft tissue interposition. There is also an undisplaced fracture of the proximal humerus and greater tuberosity (*arrows*).

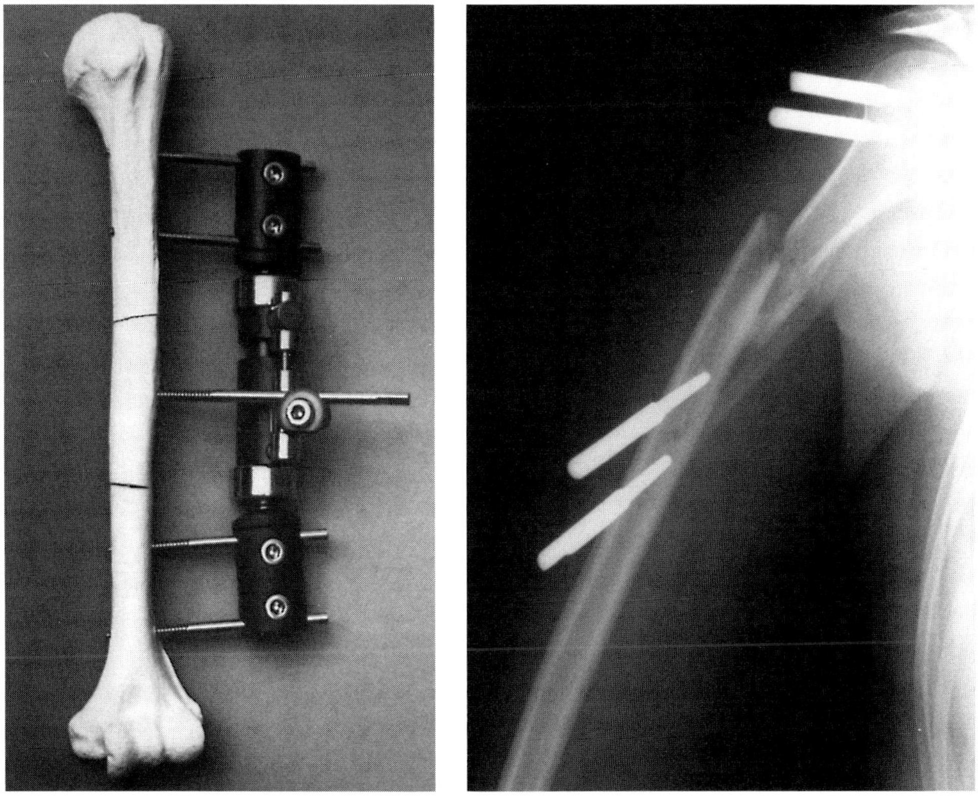

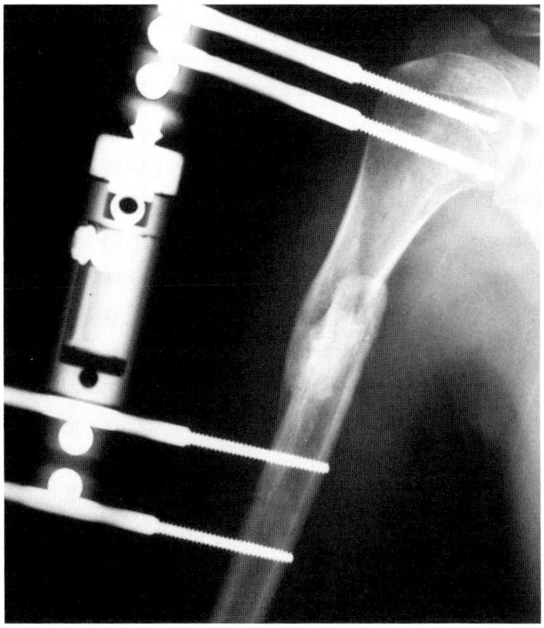

FIG. 10-6. A: The Orthofix™ fixator in a bone model. (Courtesy of EBI Medical Systems, Parsippany, NJ.) **B:** Comminuted upper humeral fracture at the junction of the proximal and middle thirds of the shaft with fixation pins above and below the fracture. **C:** Postreduction radiographs with Orthofix™ (EBI Medical Systems, Parsippany, NJ) fixation and healing fracture.

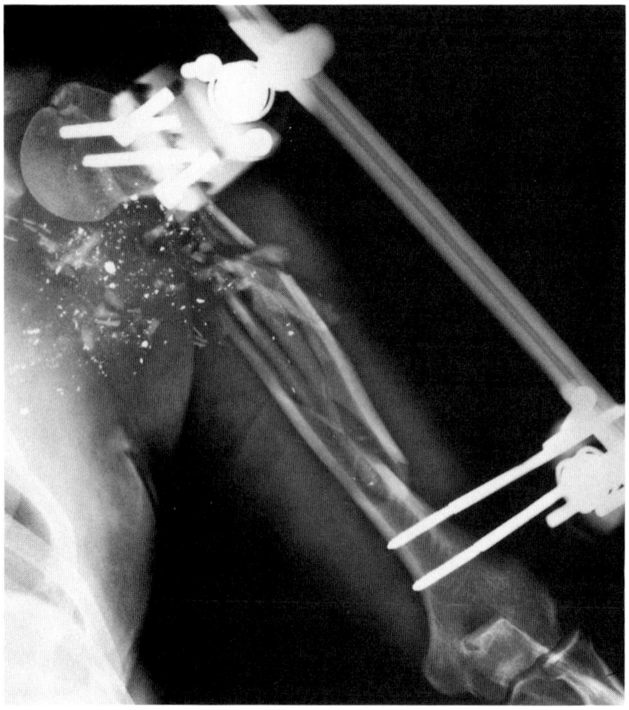

FIG. 10-7. Gunshot wound to the left humerus, resulting in extensive soft tissue injury and humeral fragmentation. External fixation with a unilateral Hex-Fix™ (Smith and Nephew Richards, Memphis, TN) fixator.

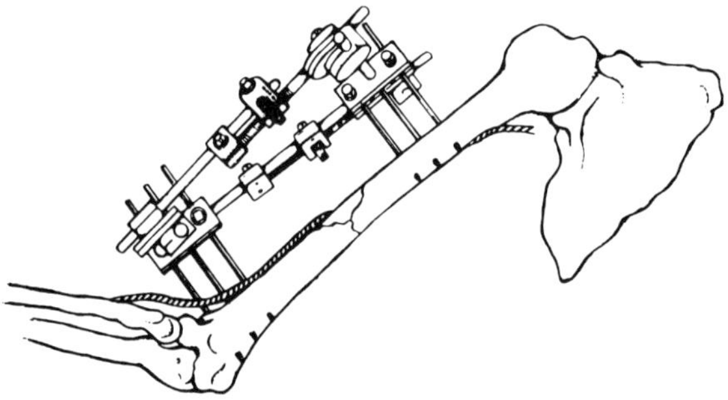

A

FIG. 10-8. A: Hoffmann fixator for a comminuted midhumeral fracture. (Courtesy of Zimmer, Warsaw, IN.) **B:** Angulated overriding left midhumeral fracture. **C:** Reduction and healing achieved with Hoffmann external fixator.

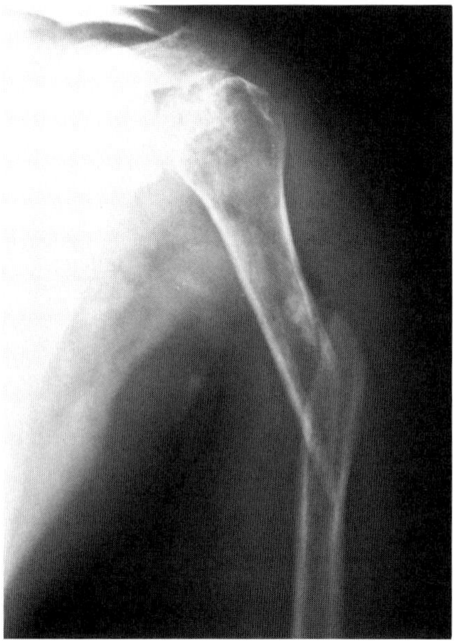

B

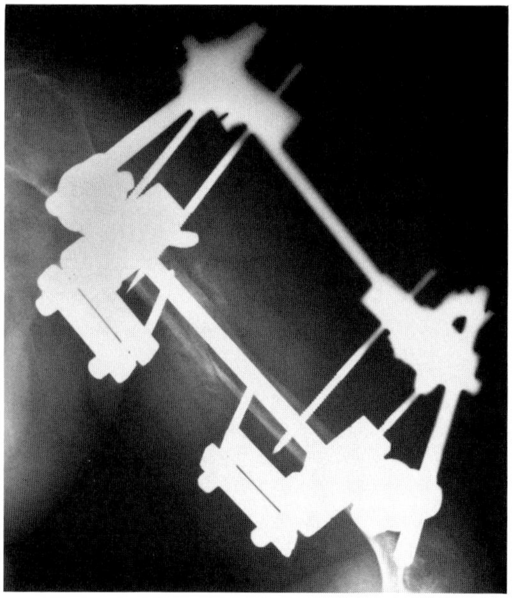

C

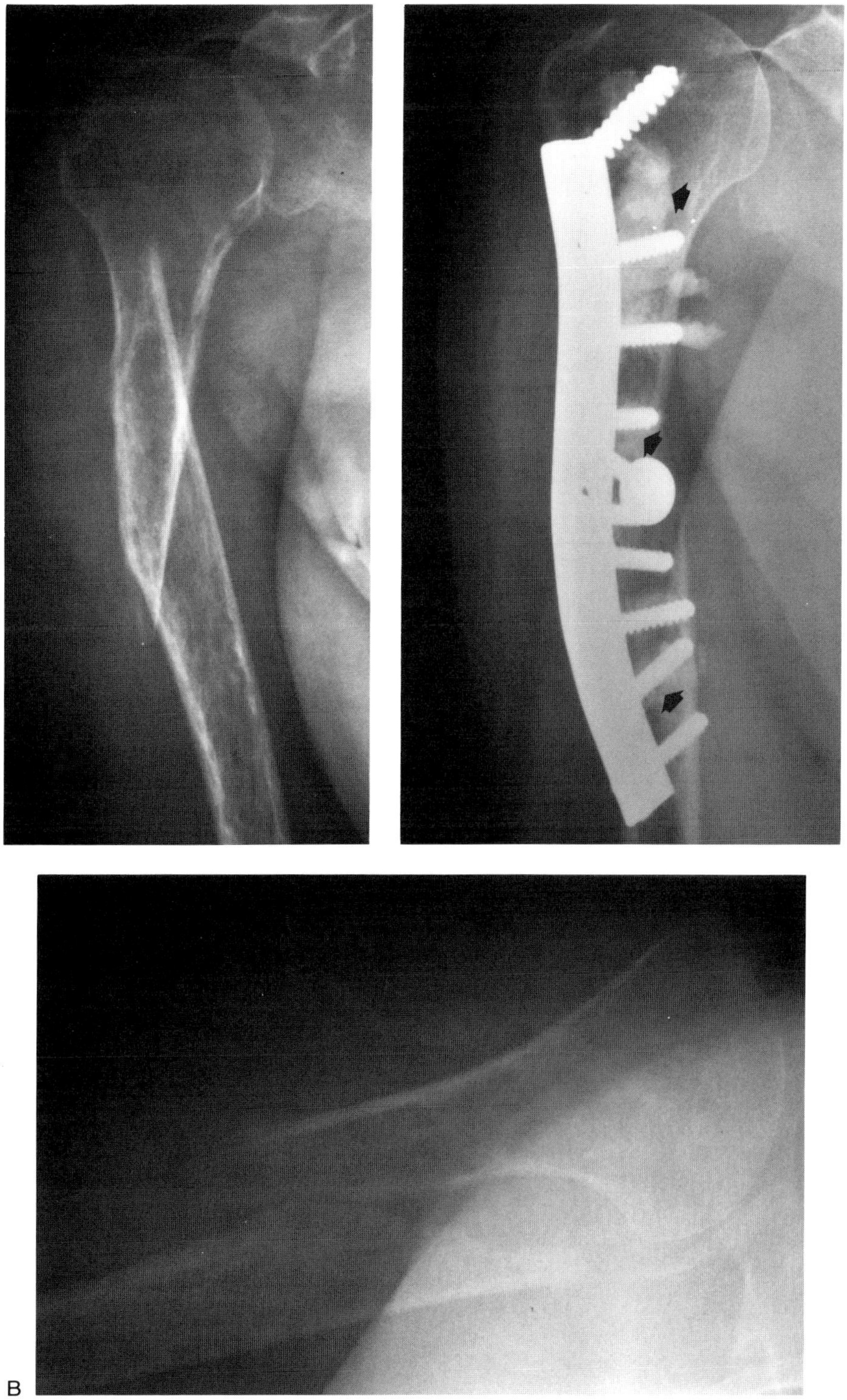

A C

B

FIG. 10-9. The AP **(A)** and axillary **(B)** radiographs of an overriding fracture of the humerus at the junction of the proximal and middle thirds. The bone is osteopenic. **C:** The DC plate and screws with methyl methacrylate (*arrows*) used to enhance screw purchase.

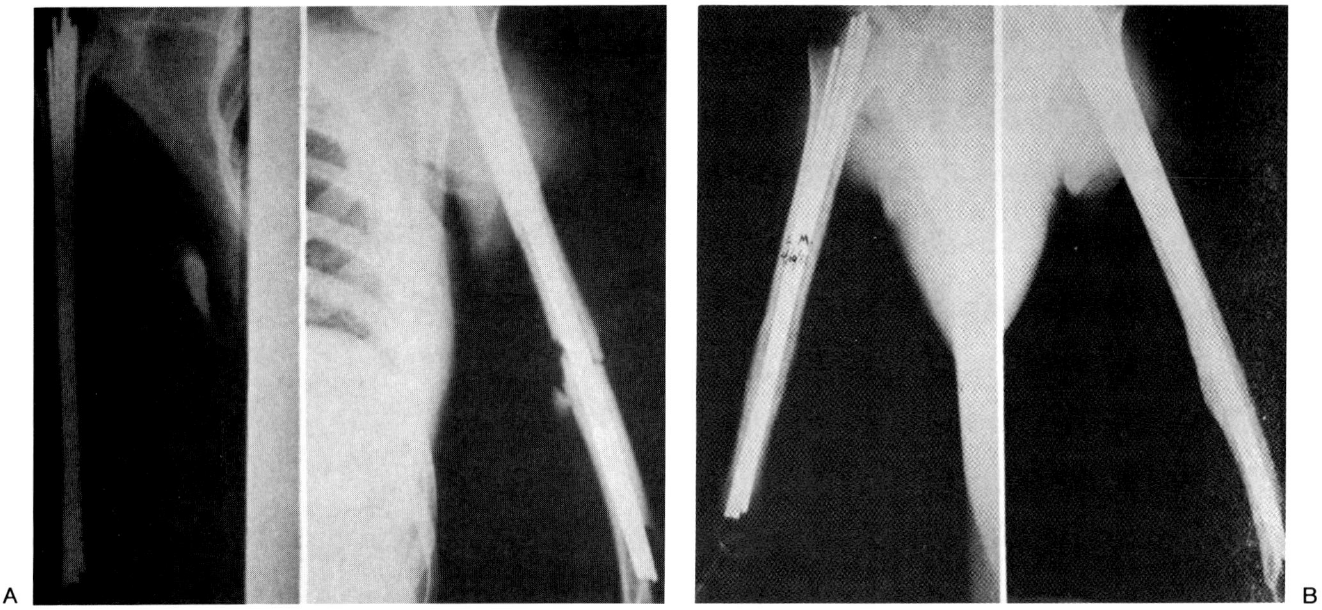

FIG. 10-10. Hackethal stacked nailing. The AP and lateral **(A)** radiographs postoperatively and **(B)** after healing. (From Durbin RA, Gottesman MJ, Saunders KC. Hackethal stacked nailing of humeral shaft fractures. *Clin Orthop* 1983;179:168–174.)

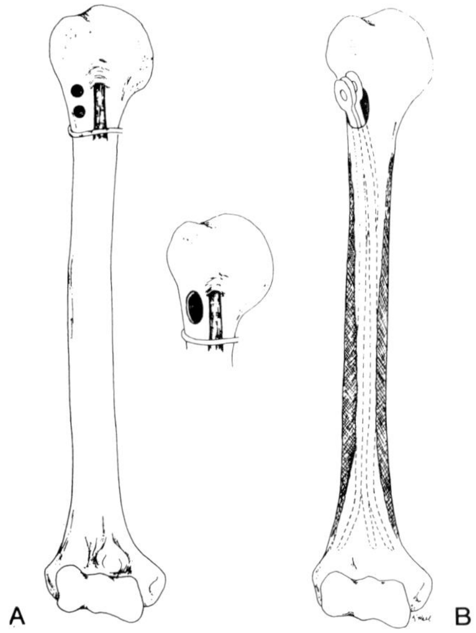

FIG. 10-11. A: Proximal portal and preparation for Ender nails or Rush rods. **B:** The implants should enter anterolaterally below the level of the rotator cuff. (From Hall RF, Pankovich AM. Ender nailing of acute fractures of the humerus. A study of closed fixation by intramedullary nails without reaming. *J Bone Joint Surg* [*Am*] 1987;69A:558–567.)

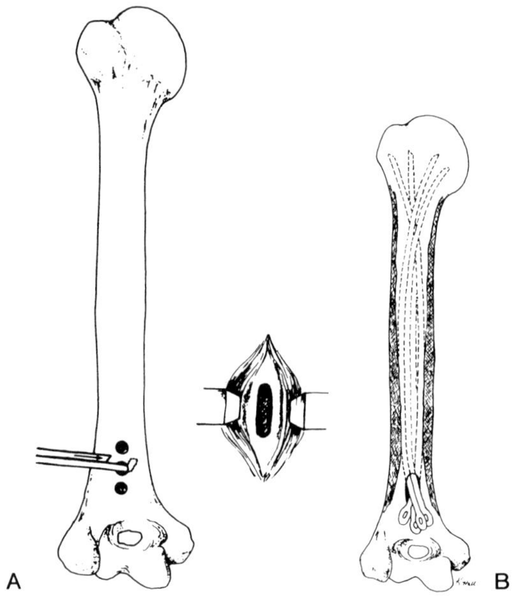

FIG. 10-12. A: Distal entry port preparation for Ender nails or Rush rods. Three holes are made, and a rongeur is used to create an elliptic entry port (*right*). **B:** There are four Ender nails in place. (From Hall RF, Pankovich AM. Ender nailing of acute fractures of the humerus. A study of closed fixation by intramedullary nails without reaming. *J Bone Joint Surg* [*Am*] 1987;69A:558–567.)

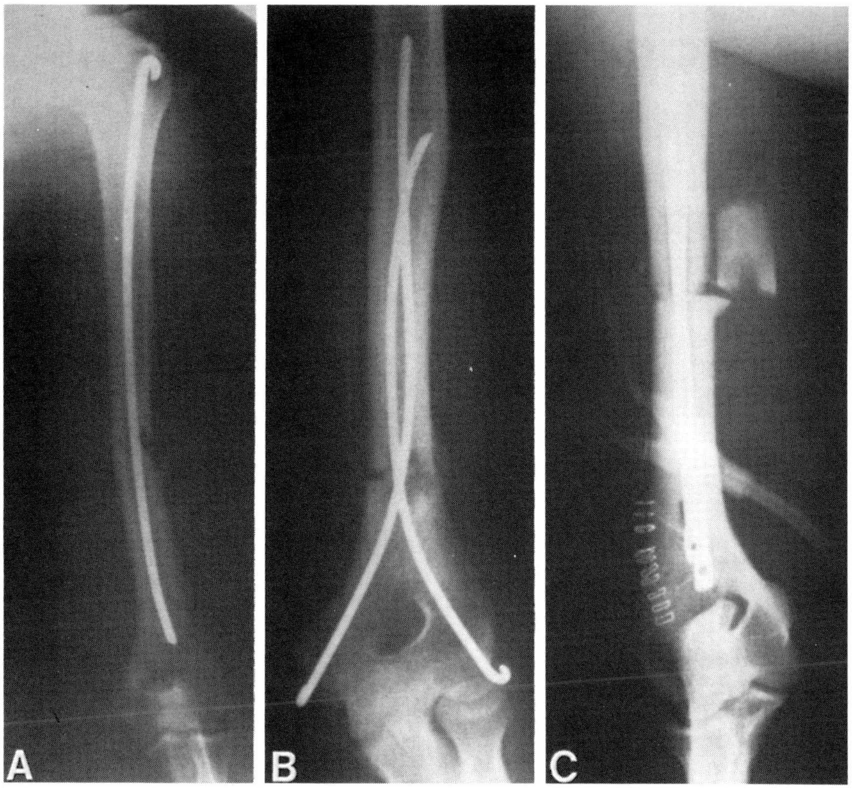

FIG. 10-13. **A:** Antegrade insertion of a Rush rod into the greater tuberosity for a fracture of the humerus at the junction of the mid and distal thirds. **B:** Rush rods inserted through epicondylar portals for a distal humeral fracture. **C:** Retrograde insertion of Rush rods through the preferred portal above the olecranon. (From Brumback RH, Bosse MJ, Poka A, Burgess AR. Intramedullary stabilization of humeral shaft fractures in patients with multiple myeloma. *J Bone Joint Surg [AM]* 1986;68A:910–970.)

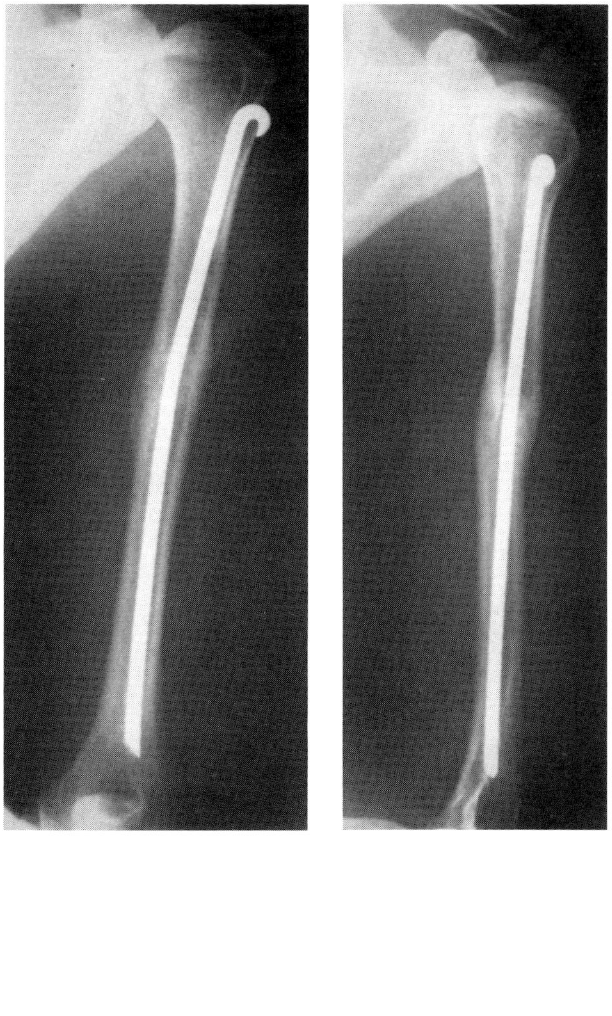

A,B

FIG. 10-14. The AP **(A)** and lateral **(B)** radiographs of a healed midshaft fracture with Rush rod fixation. Note the entry portal is lower and more optimal than in Fig. 10-13A. (From Brumback RH, Bosse MJ, Poka A, Burgess AR. Intramedullary stabilization of humeral shaft fractures in patients with multiple myeloma. *J Bone Joint Surg [AM]* 1986;68A:910–970.)

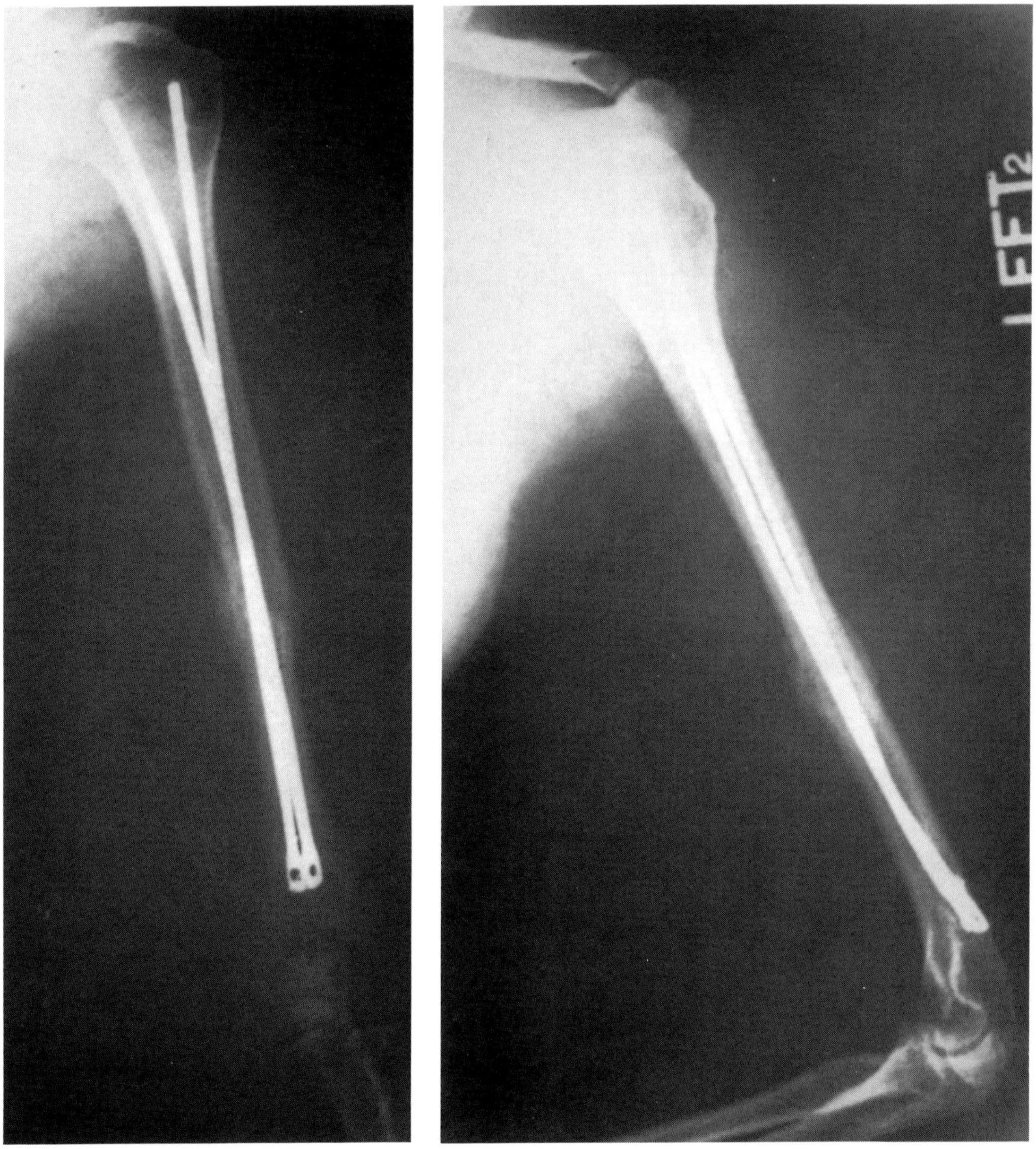

A B

FIG. 10-15. The AP **(A)** and lateral **(B)** radiographs of Ender nails inserted in the preferred supraolecranon portal. The nails are flared in the upper humeral metaphysis. The distal fracture is healed. (From Brumback RH, Bosse MJ, Poka A, Burgess AR. Intramedullary stabilization of humeral shaft fractures in patients with multiple myeloma. *J Bone Joint Surg* [*Am*] 1986; 68A:910–970.)

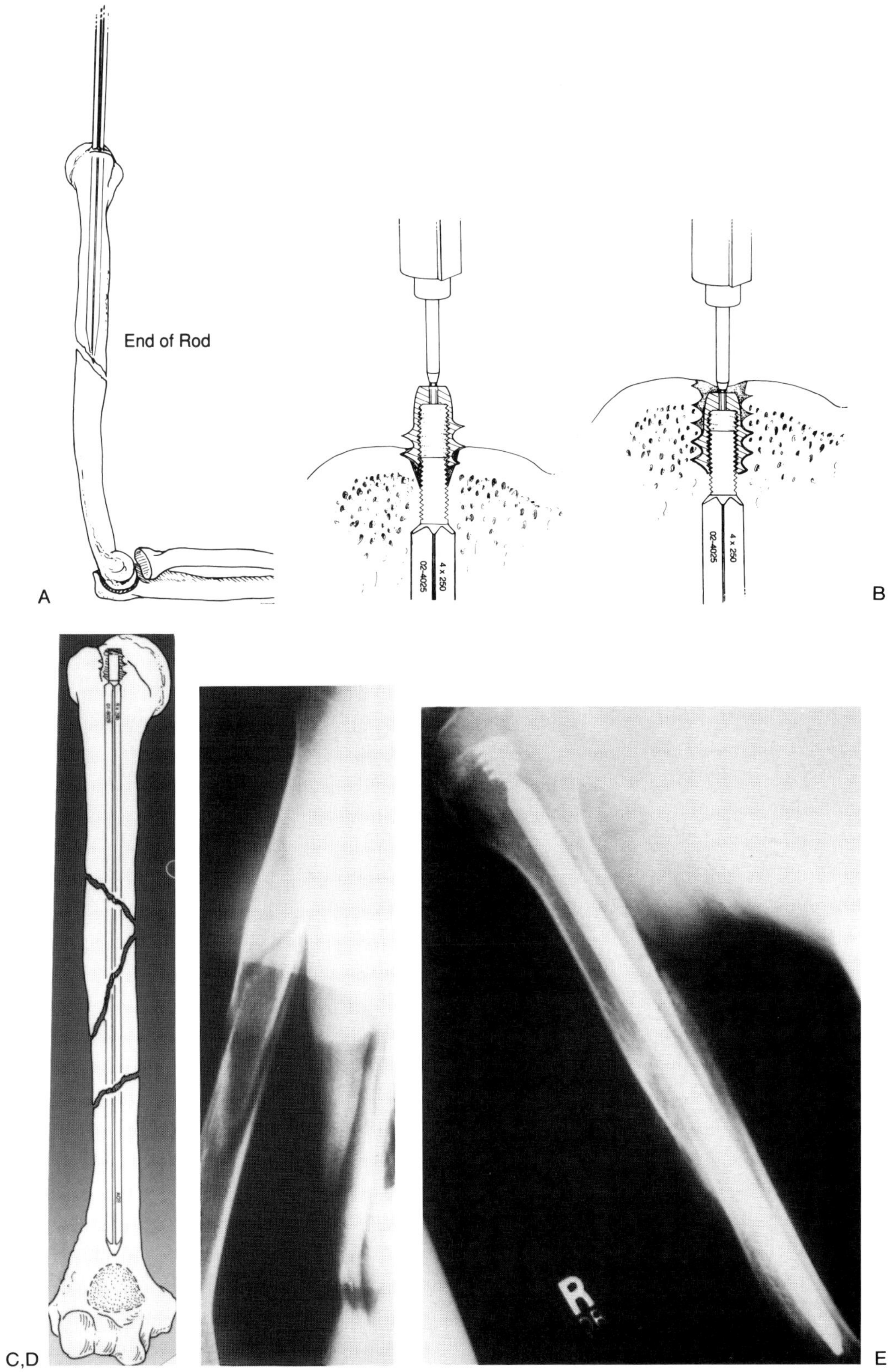

FIG. 10-16. A: Insertion of a True/Flex™ rod (nonreamed) for a midhumeral fracture. **B:** Locking cap is inserted after rod is positioned. **C:** True/Flex™ rod for reduction of a comminuted midhumeral fracture. The AP radiograph **(D)** preoperatively and **(E)** after reduction with a True/Flex™ rod. (Courtesy of Applied OsteoSystems, Walnut Creek, CA. Radiographs courtesy of Dr. Jeffrey Carter, Dallas/Fort Worth Medical Center, Grand Prairie, TX.)

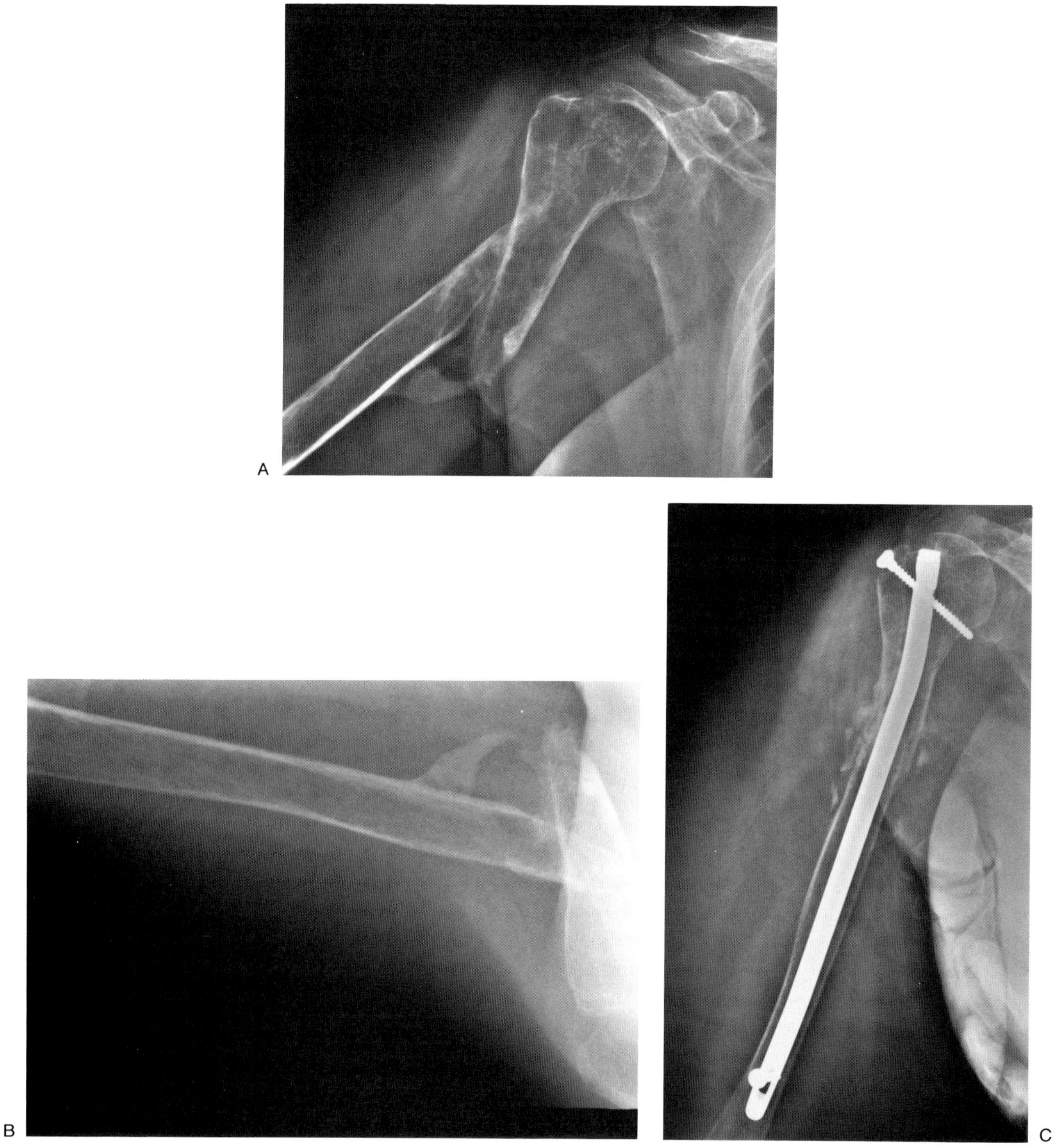

FIG. 10-17. The AP (A) and lateral (B) radiographs of a proximal humeral nonunion. Reduction and fixation achieved using an interlocking intramedullary AO nail with single locking screws proximally and distally. There is iliac bone graft in addition. Note the reamed area in the proximal humerus.

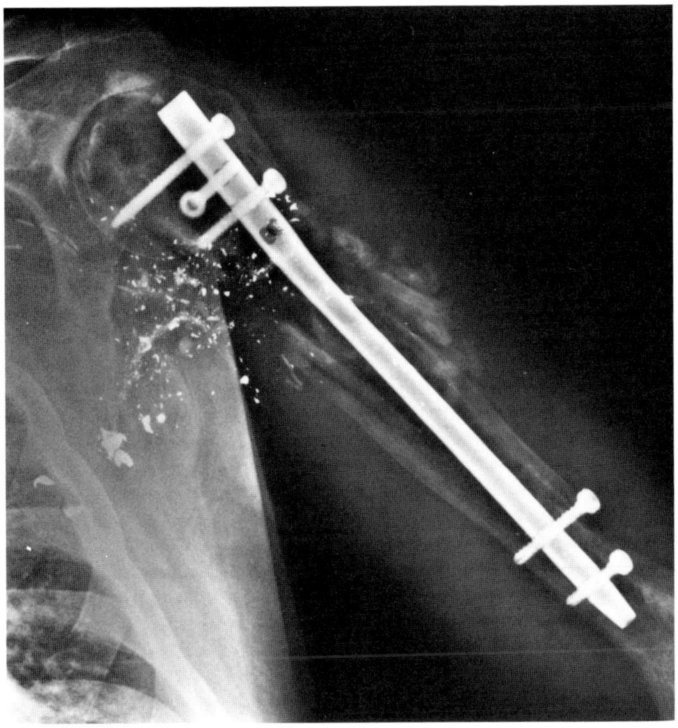

FIG. 10-18. Badly comminuted fracture of the humerus after a gunshot wound. Internal fixation with a hollow interlocking medullary nail and three proximal and two distal locking screws. The canal is reamed prior to placement of this type of nail (Biomet Uniflex^{TM} nail, Biomet, Warsaw, IN).

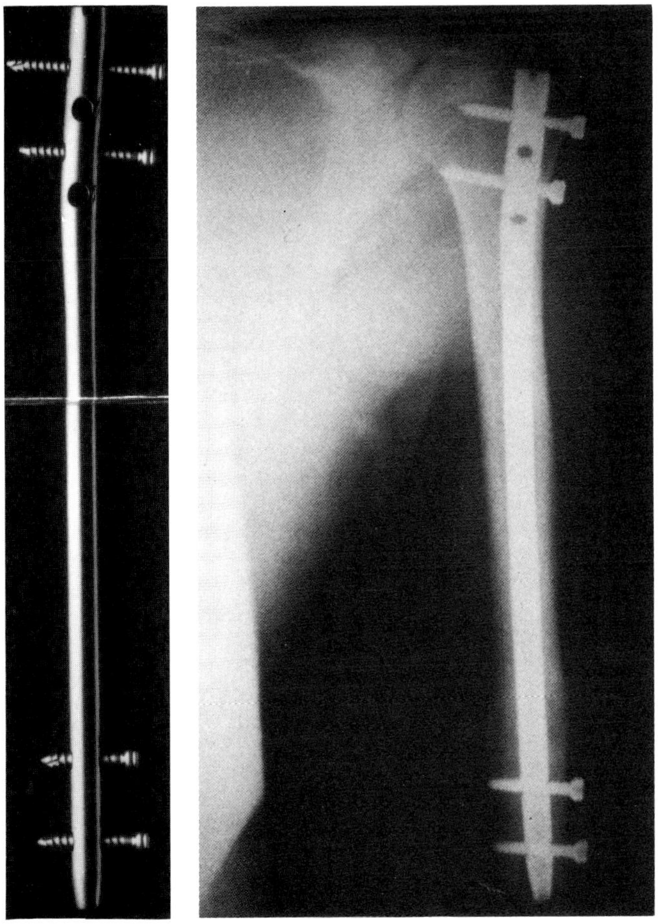

A,B

FIG. 10-19. A: The Biomet Uniflex^{TM} nail with proximal and distal locking screws. **B:** An AP radiograph of a healed distal humeral fracture with the Uniflex^{TM} nail and two proximal and distal locking screws in place. (Courtesy of Biomet, Warsaw, IN.)

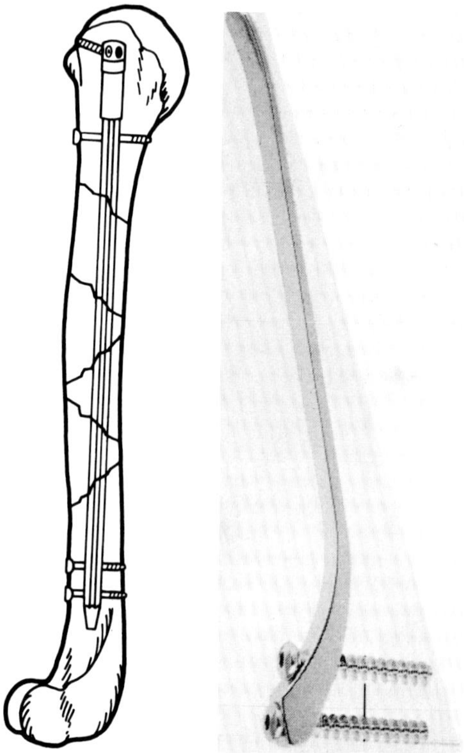

A,B

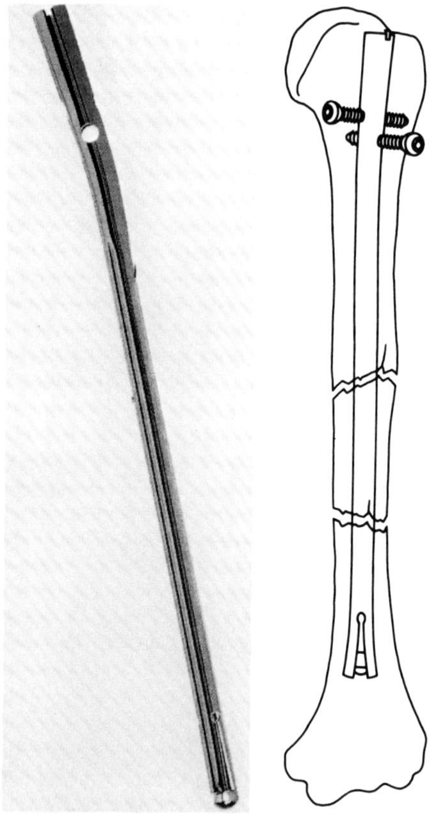

C,D

FIG. 10-20. A: The Alta^{TM} modular trauma humeral intramedullary nail, which is solid and fluted. **B:** The Mouradian^{TM} humeral fixation device. Photograph **(C)** and illustration **(D)** of the Seidel^{TM} locking humeral nail. The distal end can be expanded to prevent rotation of the distal fragment. (Courtesy of Howmedica, Rutherford, NJ.)

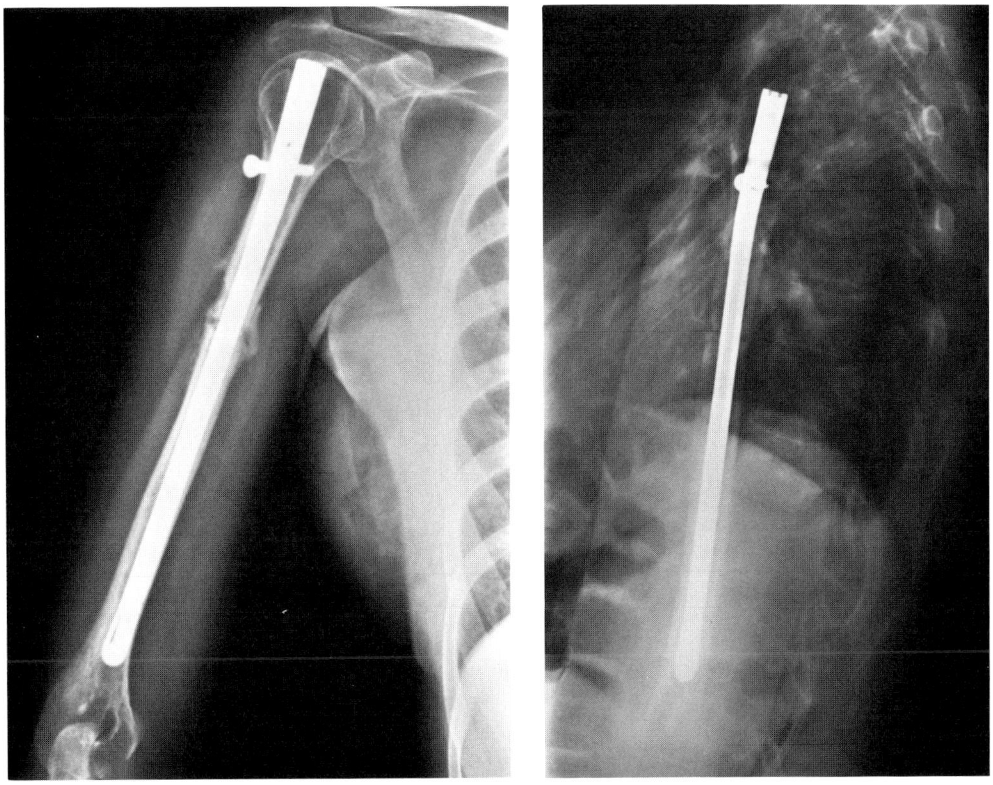

FIG. 10-21. The AP **(A)** and transthoracic **(B)** radiographs of a healing upper humeral fracture with a Seidel™ locking nail in place.

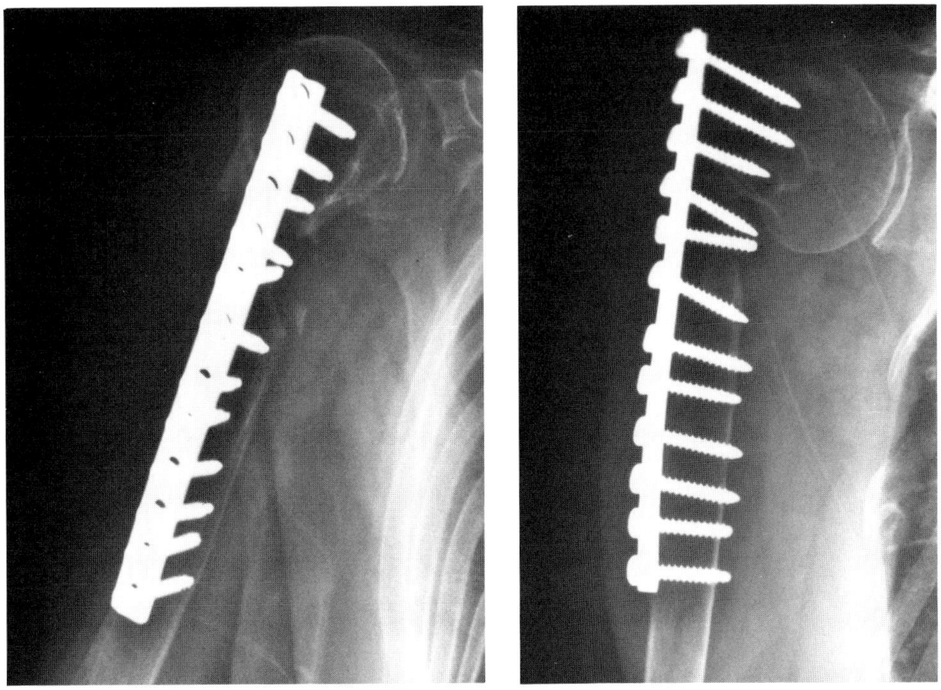

FIG. 10-22. A,B: Radiographs of the right humerus after plate and screw fixation of a proximal humeral fracture. The bone is osteopenic. The proximal fragment has pulled free (B), and there is atrophic non-union.

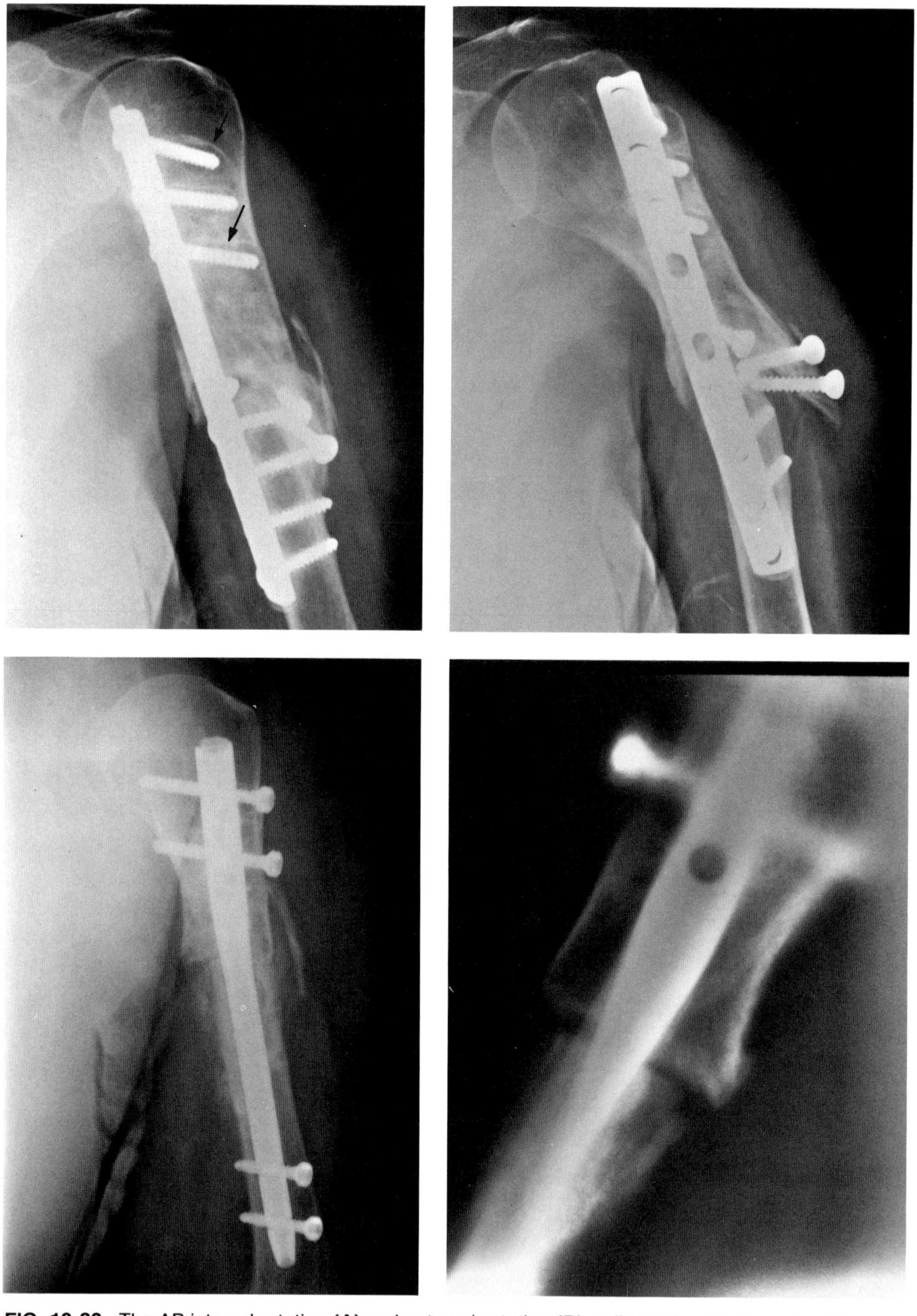

A B C D

FIG. 10-23. The AP internal rotation **(A)** and external rotation **(B)** radiographs of a hypertrophic nonunion caused by failed plate and screw fixation. Note the lucency around the upper screws (*arrows*). **C:** The fracture was undergone débridement, and the plate and screws were replaced with an interlocking medullary nail. **D:** Tomogram shows sclerosis of the osteotomy margins as a result of persistent nonunion.

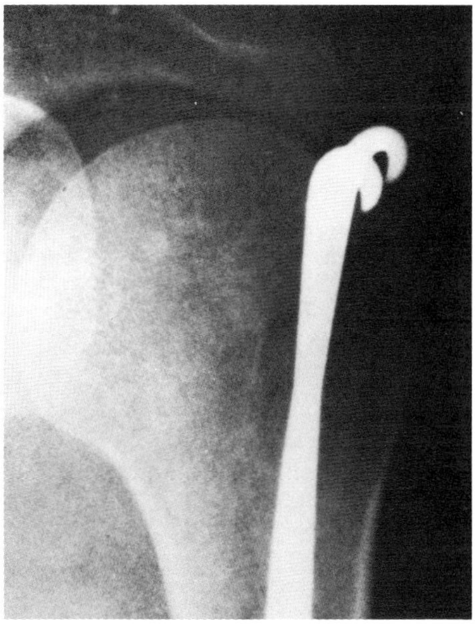

FIG. 10-24. Radiograph of the humerus with two Rush rods inserted proximally. The ends are above the normal insertion point, causing impingement. (From Brumback RH, Bosse MJ, Poka A, Burgess AR. Intramedullary stabilization of humeral shaft fractures in patients with multiple myeloma. *J Bone Joint Surg* [*Am*] 1986;68A:910–970.)

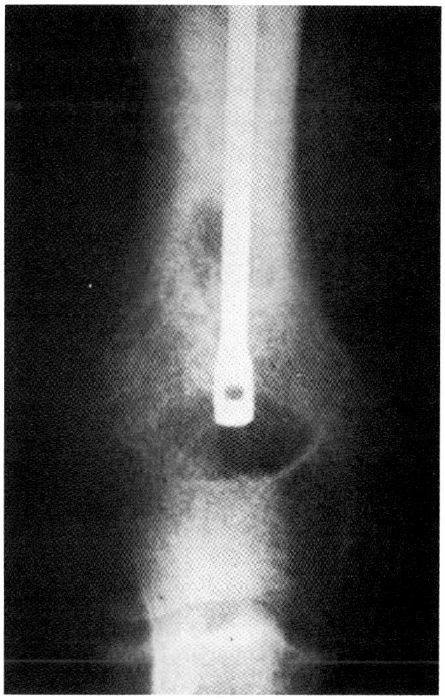

FIG. 10-25. Radiograph of the distal humerus showing an Ender nail projecting into the olecranon fossa, which leads to reduced elbow extension. (From Brumback RH, Bosse MJ, Poka A, Burgess AR. Intramedullary stabilization of humeral shaft fractures in patients with multiple myeloma. *J Bone Joint Surg* [*Am*] 1986;68A:910–970.)

A

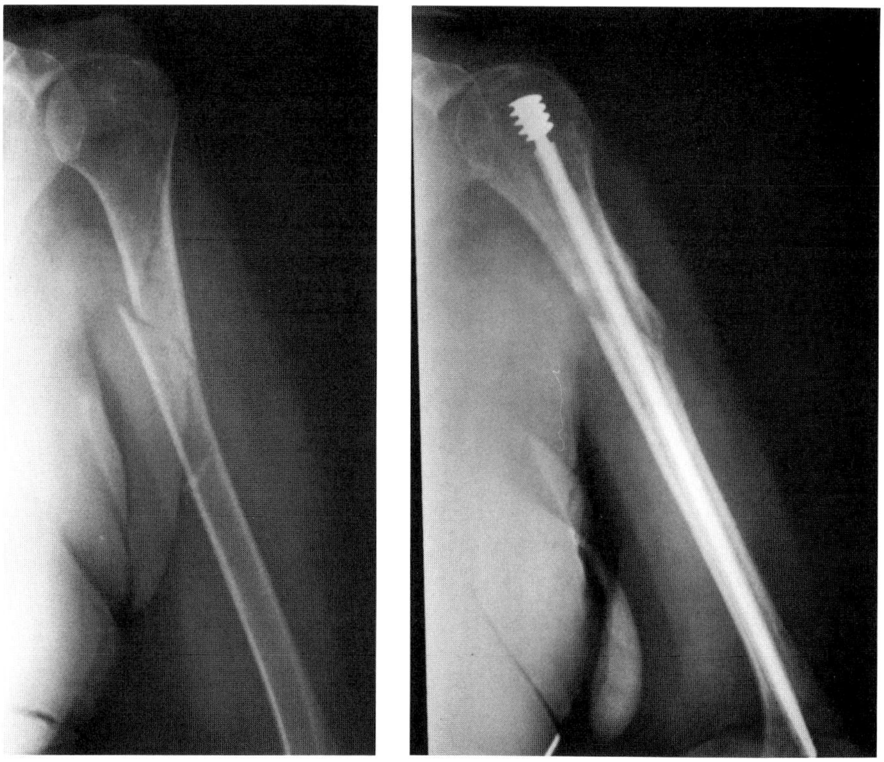

B

FIG. 10-26. A: An AP radiograph of the left humerus demonstrates a comminuted fracture at the junction of the proximal and distal thirds of the humerus. Internal **(B)** and external **(C)** rotation views after reduction with a True/Flex™ nail. (See **C-E** on next page.)

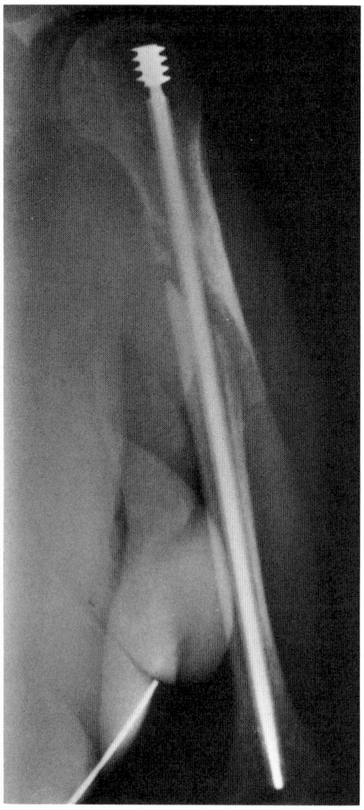

C

FIG. 10-26. (*Continued.*) The tip projected into the olecranon fossa, which caused some limitation of extension. Internal **(D)** and external **(E)** rotation views 4 months later demonstrate nonunion with dissociation of the screw cap (*arrow*).

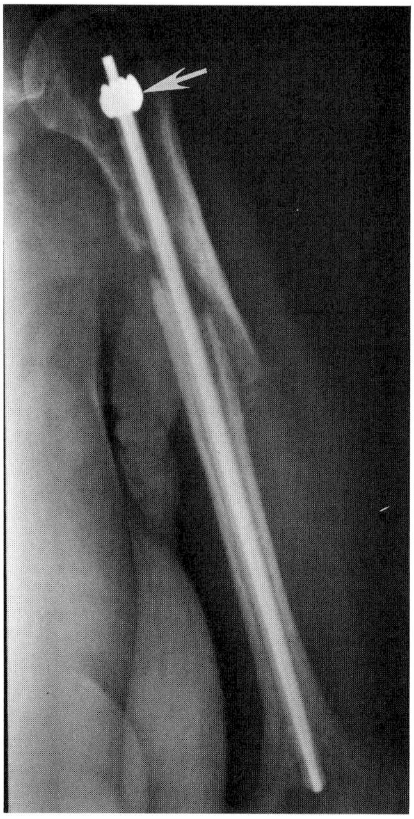

D

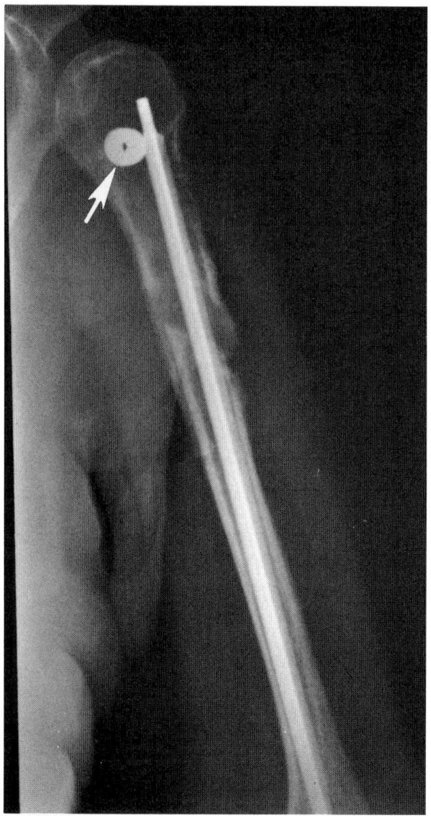

E

The indications are similar to those for other intramedullary nails. Rods such as these are not usually used if there is infection, osteopenia, or a risk of crossing a growth plate.

Interlocking Intramedullary Nails

Interlocking intramedullary nails similar to those described in Chapters 2, 5, and 7 are also available for humeral fracture fixation. The interlocking nail systems provide excellent fixation, with superior reduction and diminished problems with rotation. These techniques offer superior load sharing compared with plate and screw fixation, and less soft tissue damage occurs during surgery.[28] These systems are particularly useful for nonunions (Fig. 10-17), pathologic fractures, severely comminuted fractures (Fig. 10-18), or failed initial instrumentation techniques.[8,28]

Open or solid interlocking nails are available (Figs. 10-19 to 10-22). The nail length can be measured using a radiograph of the unaffected humerus or using fluoroscopy and a guide wire during the procedure.[27]

POSTOPERATIVE IMAGING AND COMPLICATIONS

Delayed union, nonunion, and malunion are fairly common. Delayed union is defined as the absence of union at 8 weeks. Both delayed union and nonunion are associated with poor apposition or distraction of the fracture fragments, interference of blood supply, open injury with infection, or soft tissue interposition. In unstable fractures with osteoporotic bone (Fig. 10-9), it is difficult to maintain fixation with internal techniques (Figs. 10-22 and 10-23).[1,22]

Instrument failure (screw pull out) and rod migration can also create problems after internal fixation (Figs. 10-23 through 10-26).[10,23]

Deep infection is a potential problem with internal fixation; pin tract infection can occur with external fixation.[14,17,25,27,29]

Soft tissue complications include neurovascular injury and myositis ossificans. The latter is far more common with elbow fracture-dislocations. Radial nerve injury occurs in 5% to 10% of humeral fractures. The injury may be the result of direct trauma or bruising, stretching, or entrapment between fracture fragments. Operative intervention is required if spontaneous recovery does not occur.[2,25]

Postoperative imaging can usually be accomplished with routine radiographic techniques. In the presence of internal fixation, conventional tomography may be useful to evaluate fracture healing (Fig. 10-23D). In this setting, computed tomography and magnetic resonance imaging (MRI) are less effective.

Pin tract infections can be evaluated with fluoroscopic positioning and radiographic spot views.[2] Deep infections can be difficult to detect in the presence of orthopedic implants.[1,2,21] Combined imaging with indium-111-labeled white blood cells and technetium-99m methylene diphosphate is an excellent imaging technique. Neopola et al.[21] reported a sensitivity of 86%, an accuracy of 82%, and a negative predictive value of 94% when diagnosing infection in nonunited fractures.

The technique of MRI is particularly suited for the evaluation of neurovascular complications. In the presence of intramedullary nailing, the artifact is minimal compared with that seen with compression plate and screw fixation. In the presence of significant metal, which would create problems with MRI, other techniques should be considered. Vascular abnormalities may be further evaluated with angiography. There may be no adequate imaging technique for neural injury in this setting.[1,2,12]

REFERENCES

1. Berquist TH. *Imaging of orthopedic trauma.* 2nd ed. New York: Raven Press; 1991.
2. Berquist TH. *MRI of the musculoskeletal system.* 2nd ed. New York: Raven Press; 1990.
3. Brumback RH, Bosse MJ, Poka A, Burgess AR. Intramedullary stabilization of humeral shaft fractures in patients with multiple myeloma. *J Bone Joint Surg* [*Am*] 1986;68A:910–970.
4. Caldwell JA. Treatment of fractures of the humeral shaft by hanging cast. *Surg Gynecol Obstet* 1940;70:421–425.
5. Christensen NO. Kirster intramedullary seaming and nail fixation for nonunion of the humerus. *Clin Orthop* 1976;116:222–226.
6. Debastiani G, Aldegheri R, Briviol R. The treatment of fractures with a dynamic axial fixation. *J Bone Joint Surg* [*Br*] 1984;66B: 538–545.
7. Durbin RA, Gottesman MJ, Saunders KC. Hackethal stacked nailing of humeral shaft fractures. *Clin Orthop* 1983;179:168–174.
8. Epps CH, Grant RE. Fractures of the shaft of the humerus. In: Rockwood CA, Green DP, Bucholz KW, eds. *Rockwood and Green's fractures in adults.* 3rd ed. Vol. 1. Philadelphia: JB Lippincott; 1991:843–869.
9. Fenyo G. O-fractures of the shaft of the humerus. *Acta Chir Scand* 1971;137:221–226.
10. Foster RJ, Dixon GL, Back AW, Appleyard RW, Green TM. Internal fixation of fractures and non-unions of the humeral shaft. *J Bone Joint Surg* [*Am*] 1985;67A:857–864.
11. Garth WP, Leberte MA, Cool TA. Recurrent fractures of the humerus in a baseball pitcher. *J Bone Joint Surg* [*Am*] 1988;70A: 305–306.
12. Greene TL, Louis DS. Compartment syndrome in the arm: a complication of the pneumatic tourniquet. *J Bone Joint Surg* [*Am*] 1983;65A:270–272.
13. Gregersen HN. Fractures of the humerus from muscle violence. *Acta Orthop Scand* 1971;42:506–512.
14. Gustilo RB, Andersen JT. Prevention of infection in the treatment of one thousand and twenty-five fractures of the long bones. *J Bone Joint Surg* [*Am*] 1976;58A:453–458.
15. Hall RF, Pankovich AM. Ender nailing of acute fractures of the humerus. A study of closed fixation by intramedullary nails without reaming. *J Bone Joint Surg* [*Am*] 1987;69A:558–567.
16. Hollinshead WH. The back and limbs. In: *Anatomy for surgeons.* 3rd ed. Vol. 3. New York: Harper and Row; 1982.
17. Holm CL. Management of humeral shaft fractures. *Clin Orthop* 1970;71:132–139.
18. Holstein A, Lewis GB. Fractures of the humerus with radial nerve paralysis. *J Bone Joint Surg* [*Am*] 1963;45A:1382–1388.

19. Kleinerman L. Fractures of the shaft of the humerus. *J Bone Joint Surg* [*Br*] 1966;48B:105–111.
20. Mann RJ, Neal FG. Fractures of the humeral shaft in adults. *South Med J* 1964;58:264–268.
21. Neopola JV, Seabold JE, Marsh JL, Kirchner PT, El-Khoury GY. Diagnosis of infection in ununited fractures: combined imaging with indium-111-labeled leukocytes and technetium-99m methylene diphosphonate. *J Bone Joint Surg* [*Am*] 1993;75A:1816–1822.
22. Rooney PJ, Cockshott WP. Pseudarthrosis following proximal humeral fractures. A possible mechanism. *Skeletal Radiol* 1986;15: 21–24.
23. Rosen H. The treatment of nonunions and pseudarthroses of the humeral shaft. *Orthop Clin North Am* 1990;21:725–742.
24. Seidel H. Humeral locking nail: a preliminary report. *Orthopedics* 1989;12:219–226.
25. Shaw JL, Sakellorides H. Radial nerve paralysis associated with fractures of the humerus. *J Bone Joint Surg* [*Am*] 1967;49A:889.
26. Stern PJ, Mattingly DA, Pomeroy DL, Zenni EJ, Kreig JK. Intramedullary fixation of humeral shaft fractures. *J Bone Joint Surg* [*Am*] 1984;66A:639–646.
27. VanderGriend R, Tomasin J, Ward EF. Open reduction and internal fixation of humeral shaft fractures. *J Bone Joint Surg* 1986;68A:430–433.
28. Ward EF, White JL. Interlocked intramedullary nailing of the humerus. *Orthopedics* 1989;12:135–141.
29. Zagorski JB, Latta LL, Zych GA, Furneton AR. Diaphyseal fractures of the humerus. Treatment with prefabricated braces. *J Bone Joint Surg* [*Am*] 1988;70A:607–610.

Imaging Atlas of Orthopedic Appliances and Prostheses,
edited by T.H. Berquist.
Mayo Clinic Foundation © 1995.
Published by Raven Press, Ltd., New York.

CHAPTER 11

The Elbow

Thomas H. Berquist and Stephen D. Trigg

The imaging of elbow disorders can be a complex problem. Routine radiographs can be obtained easily. However, because of the anatomy and positioning problems, examination of the elbow with other techniques, specifically, magnetic resonance imaging (MRI) can be difficult. In this chapter, we emphasize pre- and postoperative imaging of trauma and joint-replacement arthroplasty along with other common orthopedic disorders in which implants are used.

IMAGING

Routine Radiography

Routine radiographs remain the initial screening technique for screening suspected elbow pathologic disorders. A minimum of two views is required. Anteroposterior (AP) and lateral views may be sufficient in some cases. We routinely obtain both oblique views in addition to the AP and lateral views in patients with trauma (Fig. 11-1). Oblique views are particularly important in skeletally immature patients.[3,5]

The relationship of the radial head to the capitellum should be constant on all projections (Fig. 11-2).[5] The radius is normally bowed at the level of the tubercle. However, a line through the midradial articular surface should intersect the center of the capitellum on all radiographic projections.[6]

T. H. Berquist: Mayo Medical School and Department of Diagnostic Radiology, Mayo Clinic Jacksonville, Jacksonville, Florida 32224.

S. D. Trigg: Mayo Medical School and Department of Orthopedic Surgery, Mayo Clinic Jacksonville, Jacksonville, Florida 32224.

Careful evaluation of fat pads is essential. The anterior and posterior fat pads are intracapsular but extrasynovial. The posterior fat pad is normally obscured because of its location within the olecranon fossa. The anterior fat pad is generally visible on the lateral view (Fig. 11-1B). The lateral view should be carefully studied to detect any elevation of the anterior fat pad. The posterior fat pad becomes visible in the presence of an effusion or hemarthrosis (Fig. 11-3).[1,9,10] Cross-table lateral views may be more specific after trauma for the identification of lipohemarthroses.[1,5]

The supinator fat stripe lies ventral to the radial head and neck on the surface of the supinator muscle. Fractures of the radial head or neck nearly always displace or obliterate this structure. Other elbow injuries affect the supinator fat stripe in 82% of cases (Fig. 11-4).[5,20]

The anterior humeral line is useful in children. A line along the anterior humerus should pass through the middle third of the capitellum (Fig. 11-5). The position of the capitellum and the presence of changes in the fat pads is important for detecting subtle supra- or intracondylar fractures of the humerus in children.[3,5] Should there be any question of subtle injury, the opposite side should be radiographed for comparison.[6]

Additional views are sometimes useful in patients with subtle abnormalities (Fig. 11-6). The radial head-capitellar view is obtained in a manner similar to the lateral view except the tube is angled 45°. This projects the radial head and capitellum away from overlying structures, which allows subtle fractures to be more easily appreciated.[5,13,14] Axial views can be obtained to provide further information regarding the epicondyles, olecranon, and medial and lateral supracondylar columns (Figs. 11-7 and 11-8).[5,16]

Fluoroscopically positioned stress views are useful for evaluating instability. Varus and valgus stress views

(text continues on page 757)

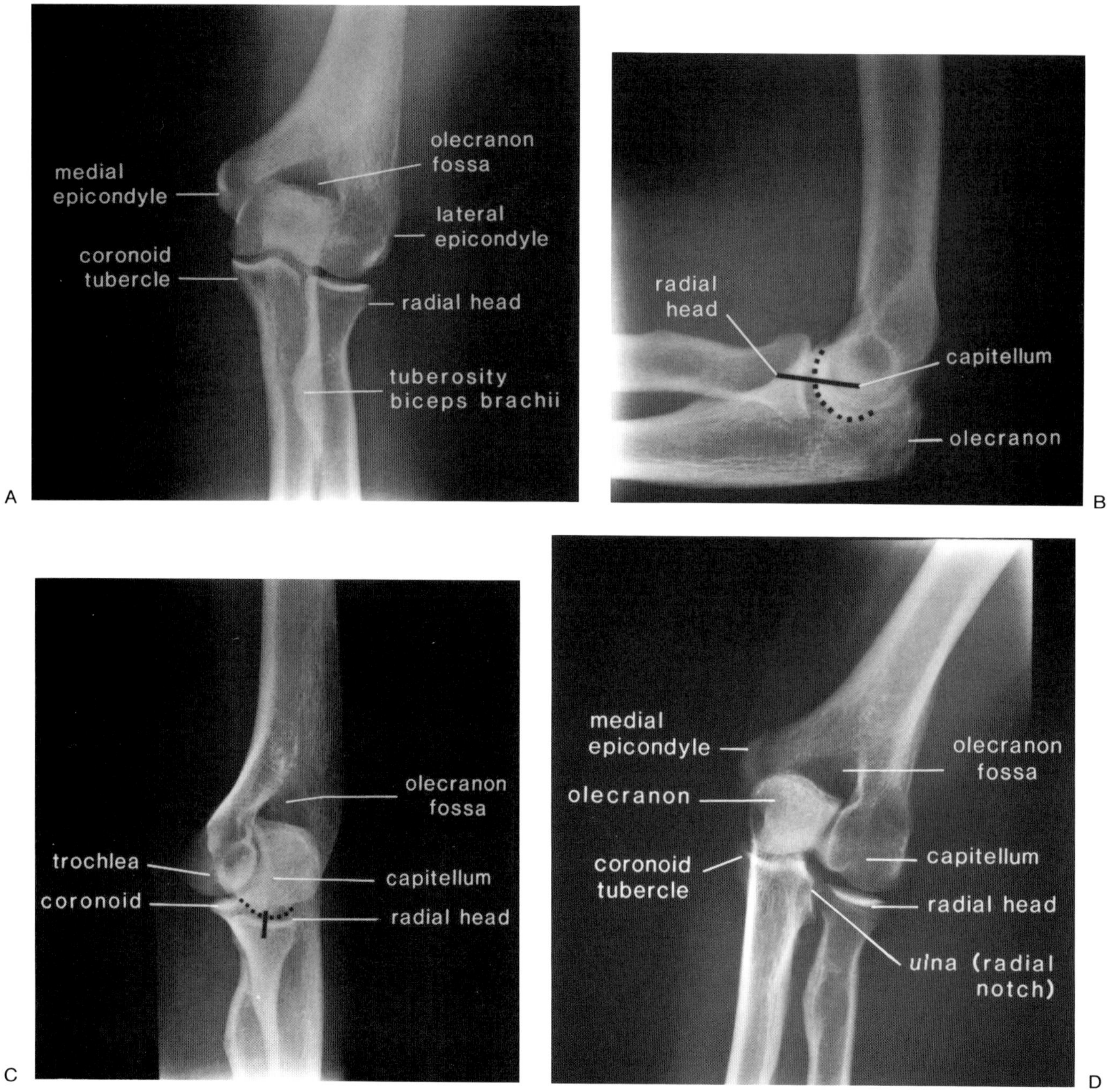

FIG. 11-1. Routine radiographs with anatomy labeled. The AP **(A)**, lateral **(B)**, oblique views **(C,D)**. (From Berquist TH. *Imaging of orthopedic trauma,* 2nd ed. New York: Raven Press, 1992.)

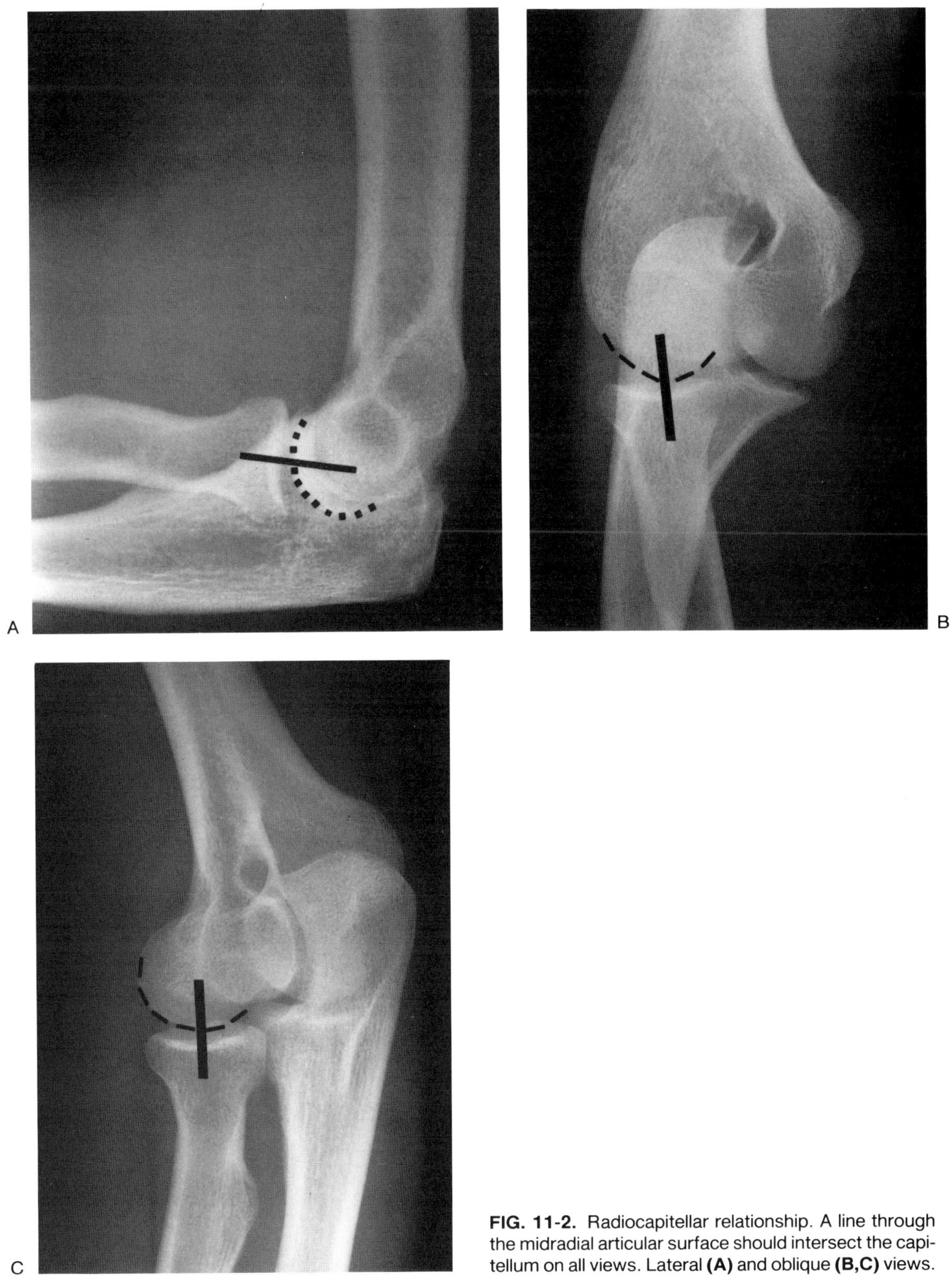

FIG. 11-2. Radiocapitellar relationship. A line through the midradial articular surface should intersect the capitellum on all views. Lateral **(A)** and oblique **(B,C)** views.

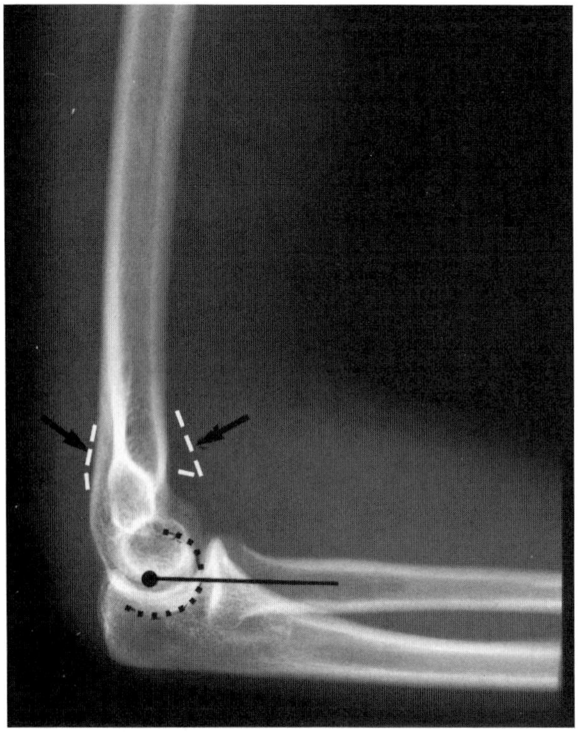

FIG. 11-3. A lateral view of the elbow demonstrating displaced anterior and posterior (*white broken lines*) fat pads in a patient with a subtle radial head fracture.

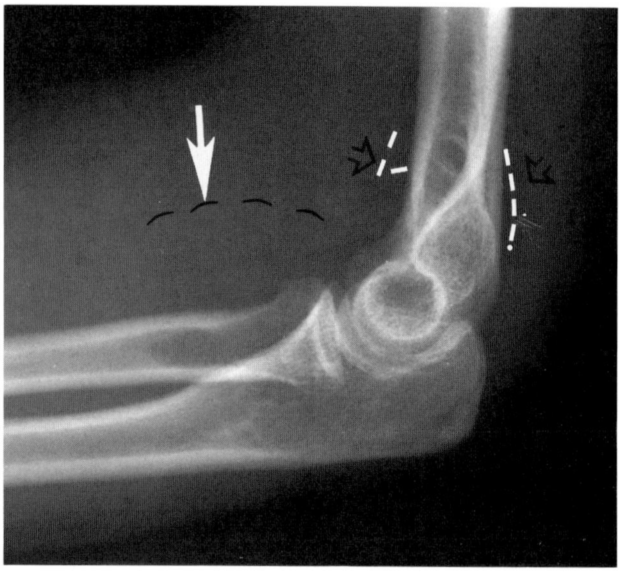

FIG. 11-4. Subtle radial head fracture. The lateral view shows a displaced supinator fat stripe (*white arrow, broken black line*) and elevated fat pads (*open arrows, white broken lines*).

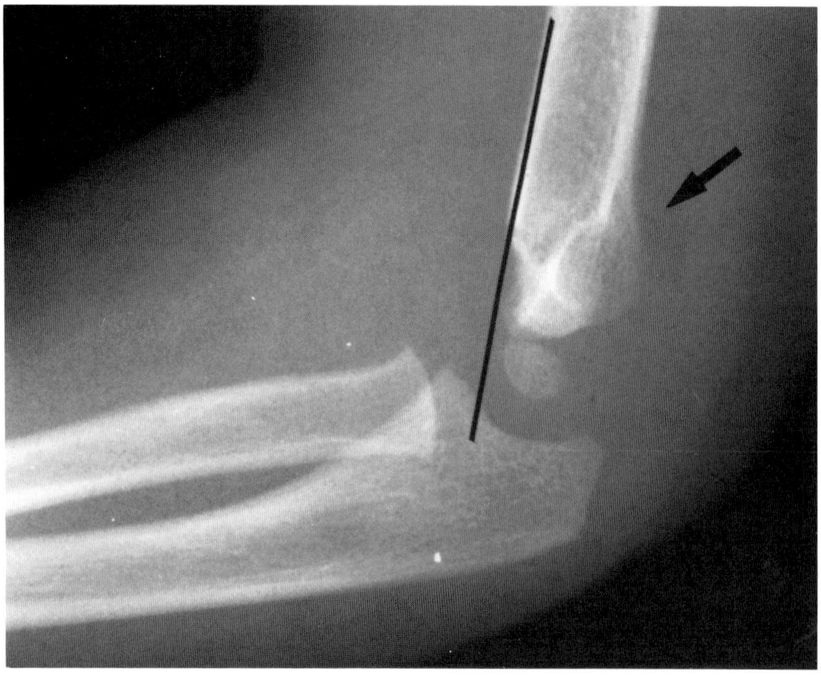

FIG. 11-5. Lateral view of the elbow in a child with a supracondylar fracture. The anterior humeral line passes anterior to the capitellum. Note the displaced posterior fat pad (*arrow*).

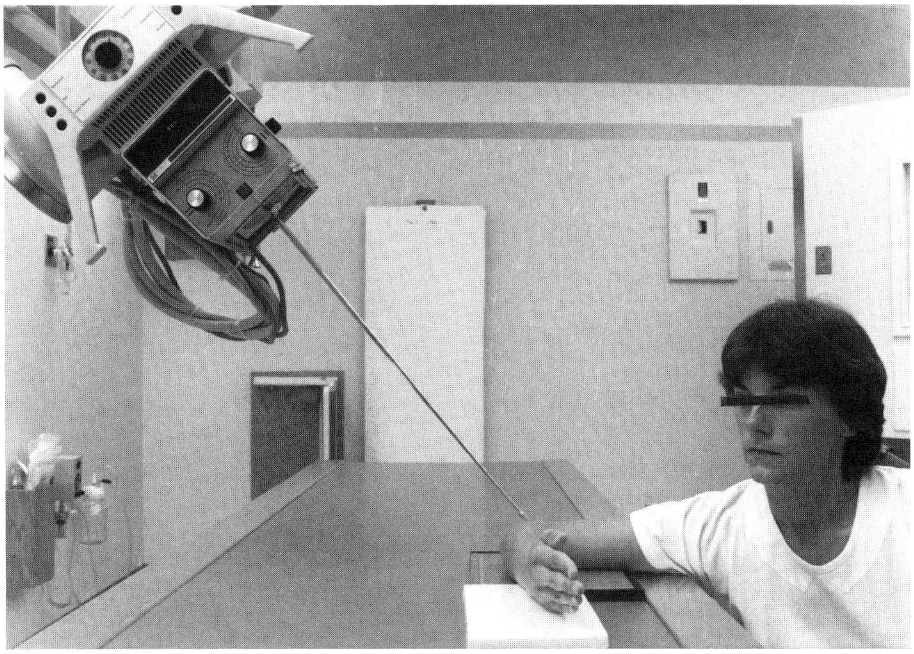

A

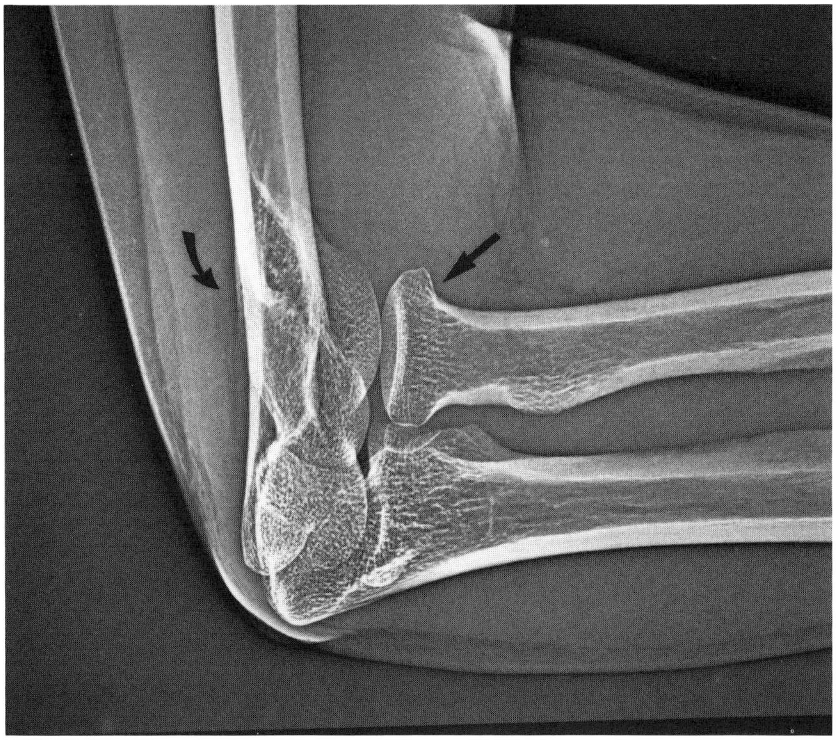

B

FIG. 11-6. A: A patient positioned for a radial head capitellar view. The tube is angled 45°. **B:** Xerograph demonstrates a subtle radial head fracture (*straight arrow*) and a posterior fat pad (*curved arrow*). (From Berquist TH. Diagnostic radiographic techniques in the elbow. In: Morrey BF, ed. *The elbow and its disorders,* 2nd ed. Philadelphia: WB Saunders, 1993; 98–119.)

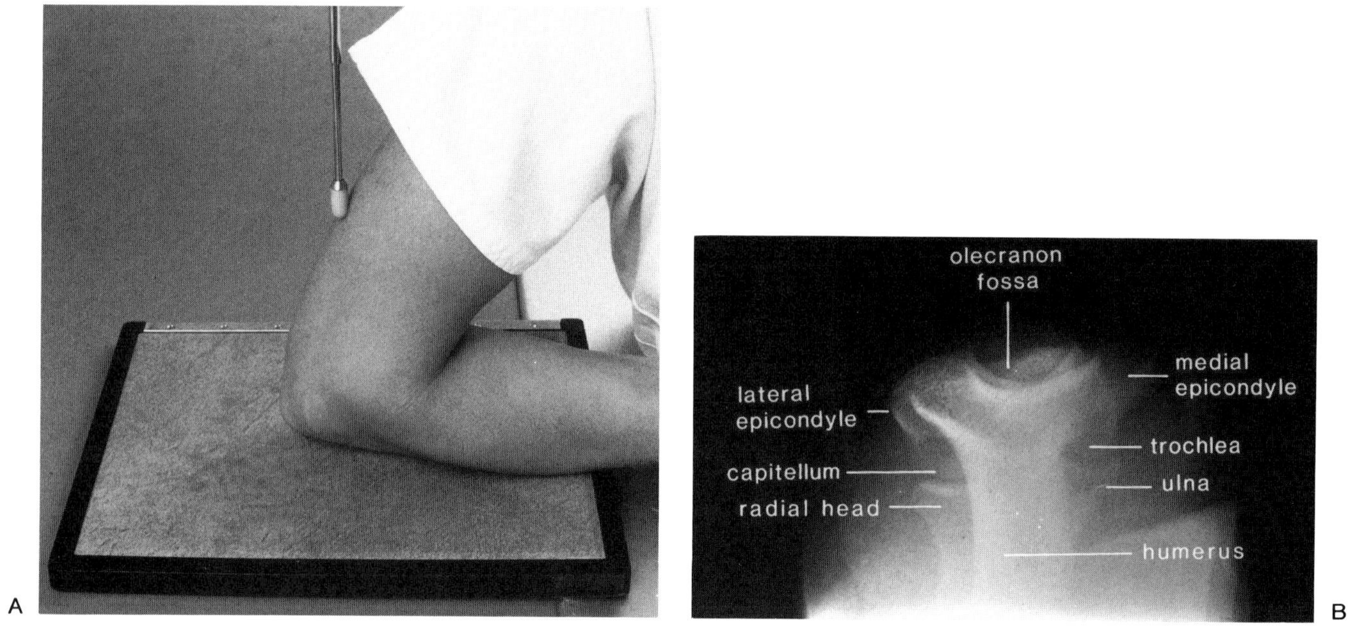

FIG. 11-7. Patient positioned **(A)** and radiograph **(B)** of an axial view of the distal humerus. (From Berquist TH. Diagnostic radiographic techniques in the elbow. In: Morrey BF, ed. *The elbow and its disorders,* 2nd ed. Philadelphia: WB Saunders, 1993; 98–119.)

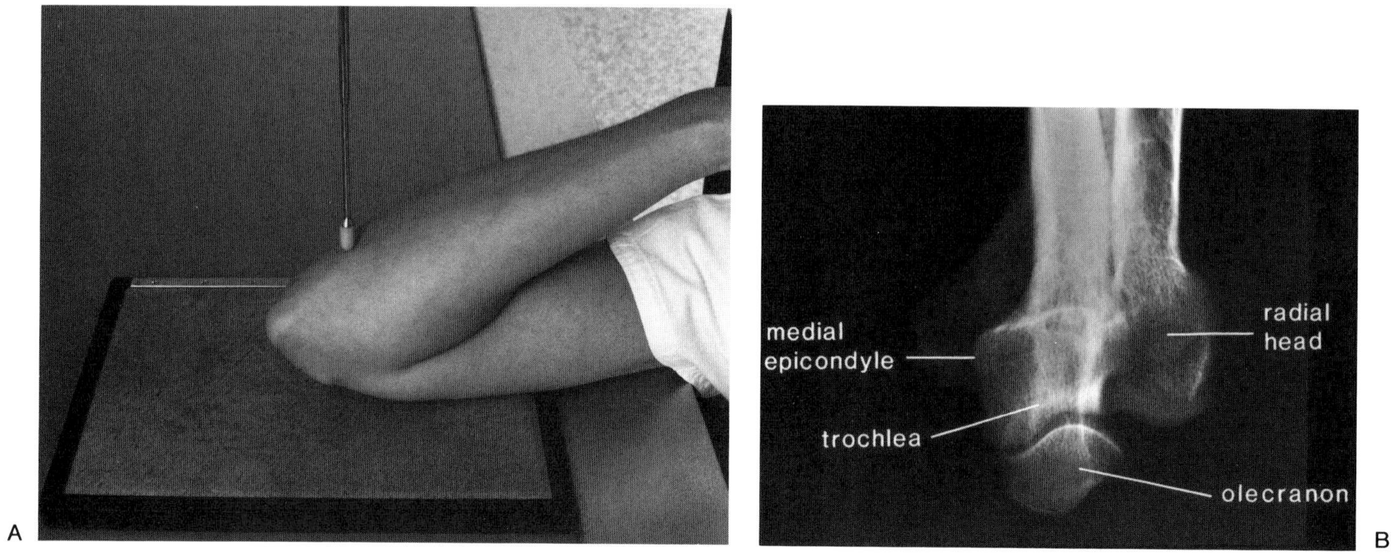

FIG. 11-8. Patient positioned **(A)** and radiograph **(B)** of the axial view in the reverse position, which demonstrates the olecranon, trochlea, and medial epicondyle. (From Berquist TH. Diagnostic radiographic techniques in the elbow. In: Morrey BF, ed. *The elbow and its disorders,* 2nd ed. Philadelphia: WB Saunders, 1993; 98–119.)

should be performed on the normal and involved side for comparison. An increase in the joint space of 2 mm greater on the involved side than on the uninvolved side is abnormal (Fig. 11-9).[5,17,18]

Arthrography and Injections

Elbow arthrography and diagnostic and therapeutic injections of articular and periarticular structures are useful techniques in selected patients with elbow disorders (Fig. 11-10).[5,8,12,16] Arthrography provides valuable information regarding the synovial lining, capsular volume, articular deformities, and loose bodies (Fig. 11-11).[2,5,12,16] Routine fluoroscopically positioned spot views and stress views are obtained after injection. In many patients, we use a double-contrast technique and also obtain computed tomographic (CT) or conventional tomographic images after injection (Fig. 11-12).[5,11,15,19,21] Joint aspiration for fluid analysis can be performed prior to the contrast agent injection for the arthrogram. This may be especially useful in patients with suspected infections after arthroplasties.[7]

The injections are also useful for the localization of symptoms. Xylocaine™ (Astra, Westborough, MA) or a longer acting anesthetic, such as Marcaine™ (Sanofi Winthrop, New York, NY) can be injected alone or with Celestone™ (Schering, Kenilworth, NJ) to diagnose and treat chronic pain syndromes.[7,8]

MRI, CT, and Ultrasound

The technique of CT is commonly used for the evaluation of complex fractures. Reconstructions in multiple planes or three-dimensional reconstructions may be required with severe injuries.[5,15] Ultrasound techniques can be used for periarticular soft tissue masses or superficial tendon abnormalities. We prefer MRI to evaluate subtle soft tissue injury, nerve compression syndromes, or suspected physeal injuries and their complications in children.[4,6] These techniques are discussed more fully as they apply to specific conditions later in this chapter.

TRAUMA

Fractures and fracture dislocations of the elbow can be complex and difficult to treat.[34,40] This section reviews injuries and classification schemes with an emphasis on those injuries that may require fixation by either the internal or percutaneous routes.

Distal Humeral Fractures

Supracondylar fractures are extraarticular. If the joint is involved, these injuries are considered intercondylar or transcondylar with extension.[52] Most supracondylar fractures occur in children (80%).[70,71] The second most common group involves insufficiency fractures through osteoporotic bone in elderly patients. These fractures generally occur after a fall on the outstretched hand, which causes extension at the elbow and a shearing fracture of the distal humerus. Flexion-type injuries caused by direct trauma to the posterior aspect of a fully flexed elbow occur less commonly.

In children, intercondylar extension and physeal injuries are unusual.[59,76] Peterson[76] reported that only 20 of 330 physeal fractures involved the distal humerus.

Different classification systems are used for adult and pediatric supracondylar fractures. The El-Ahwany[45] system correlates radiographic features with management, complications, and prognosis (Fig. 11-13).[59] The AP, axial flexed (Fig. 11-8), and lateral views are useful in the pediatric age group. The axial view demonstrates tilt of the distal fragment, and the lateral view rotary changes because most supracondylar fractures result in some rotation of the distal fragment.[45,59] Short oblique fractures are unstable and may cause neurovascular compromise (Fig. 11-13). Transcondylar fractures (Fig. 11-13B) are distal to the olecranon fossa, occur after age 6 years, and are often angled anteriorly.[70] The Salter-Harris classification is used for physeal fractures. Unfortunately, unossified epiphyses are difficult to evaluate on routine radiographs (Fig. 11-14).[76] MRI can be used to evaluate the physes and unossified ossification centers if indicated.

In adults, injuries are most often due to extension, but flexion injuries do occur.[70,71] On lateral radiographs, supracondylar fractures typically demonstrate posterior displacement of the distal fragment if the mechanism of injury was extension (Fig. 11-15A) and anterior displacement (Fig. 11-15B) with flexion injuries.[5,71]

Until recently, adult fractures were classified as supracondylar, intercondylar, epicondylar, and condylar, with numerous classification systems for each.[24,36,49,71,82] Today, a more simplified approach to the distal humerus is commonly used, which considers all this information but views the distal humerus as two diverging columns that hold the trochlea between them (Fig. 11-16).[57,67]

The AO classification is a much more comprehensive system with multiple subgroups. Type A fractures (Figs. 11-15 to 11-17) are extraarticular. Type B fractures (Figs. 11-18 and 11-19) are extraarticular with intraarticular extension, and type C fractures are intraarticular. Each type is further divided into three groups, with each group containing three subgroups (i.e., A → A1, A2, and A3 → A1.1, A1.2, and A1.3), thus covering almost any fracture of the distal humerus previously described (Fig. 11-18).[72] Table 11-1 describes the AO classification system.[57,58,72]

T and Y supracondylar fractures were also classified by Riseborough and Radin[82] in 1969. This classification is also useful in treatment planning. This classification corresponds to AO type C injuries (Fig. 11-20).[72]

(text continues on page 765)

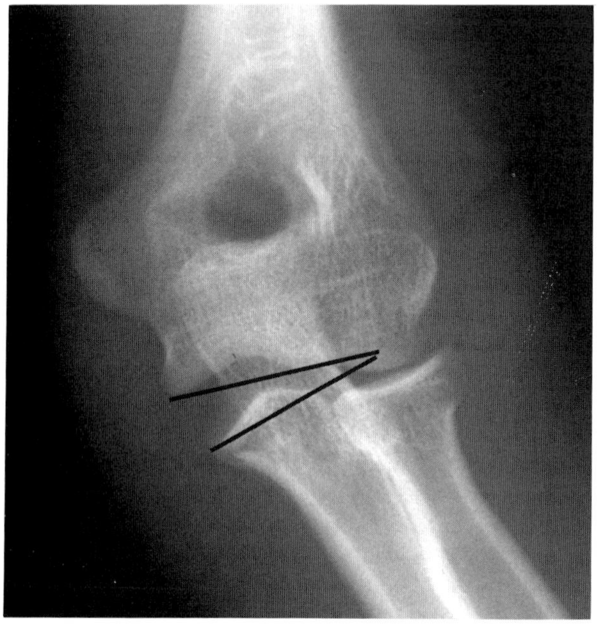

FIG. 11-9. Stress view of the elbow demonstrating medial instability.

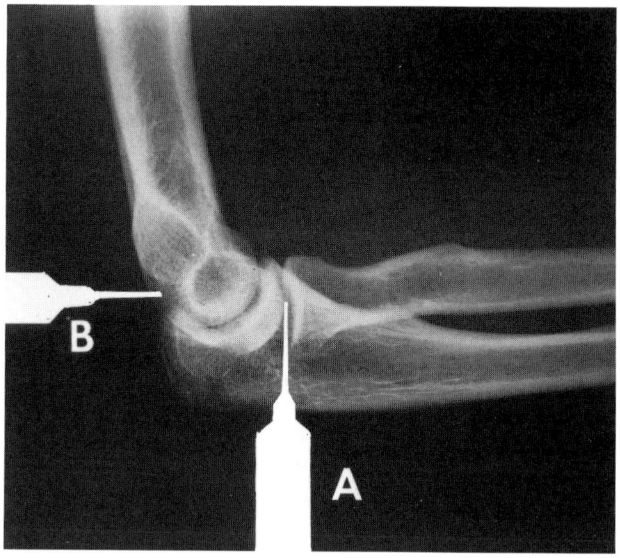

FIG. 11-10. Injection sites for elbow arthrography. **A:** Radiocapitellar joint entered laterally. **B:** Posterior entry above the olecranon. (From Berquist TH. *Imaging of orthopedic trauma,* 2nd ed. New York: Raven Press, 1992.)

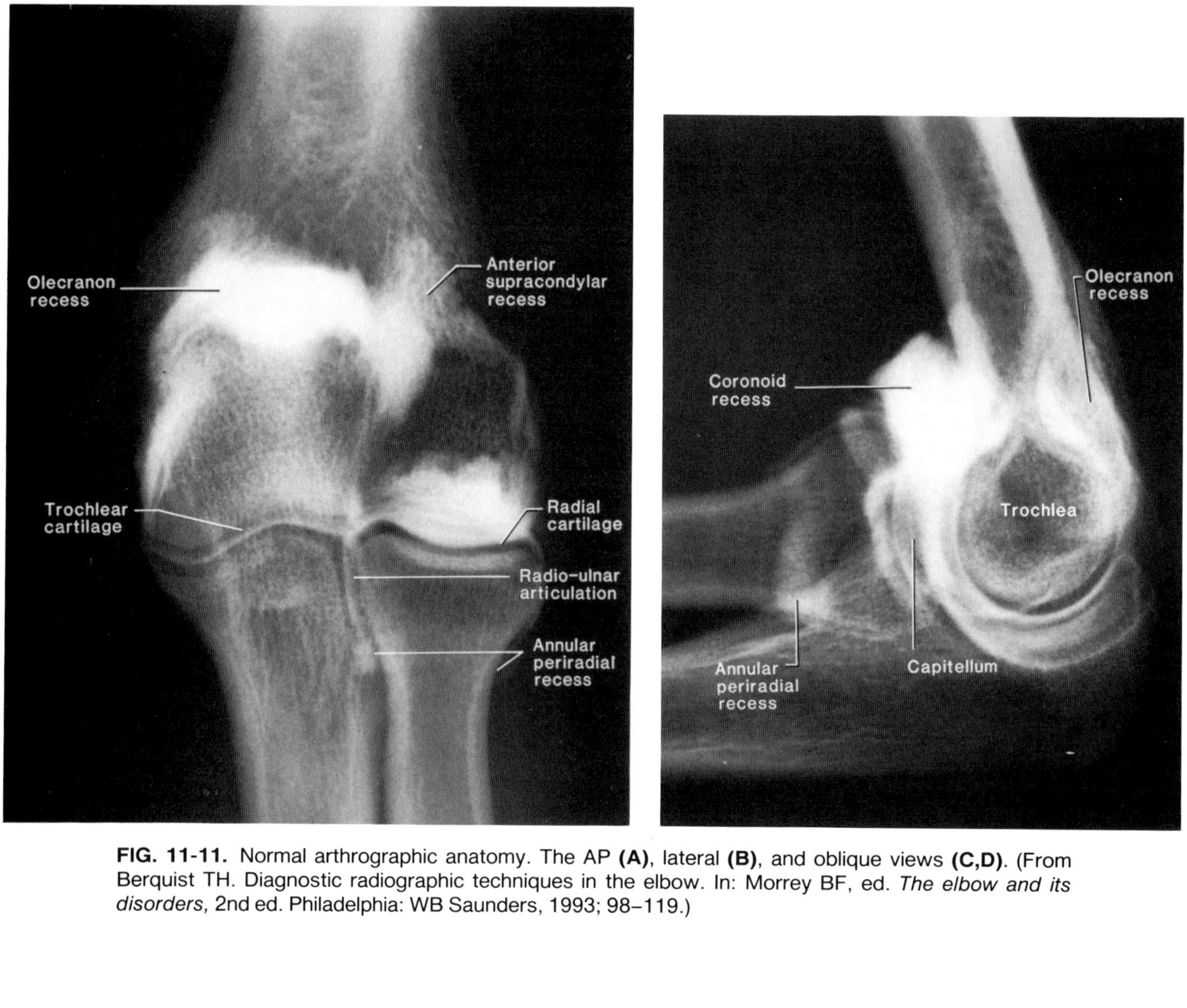

A B

FIG. 11-11. Normal arthrographic anatomy. The AP **(A)**, lateral **(B)**, and oblique views **(C,D)**. (From Berquist TH. Diagnostic radiographic techniques in the elbow. In: Morrey BF, ed. *The elbow and its disorders,* 2nd ed. Philadelphia: WB Saunders, 1993; 98–119.)

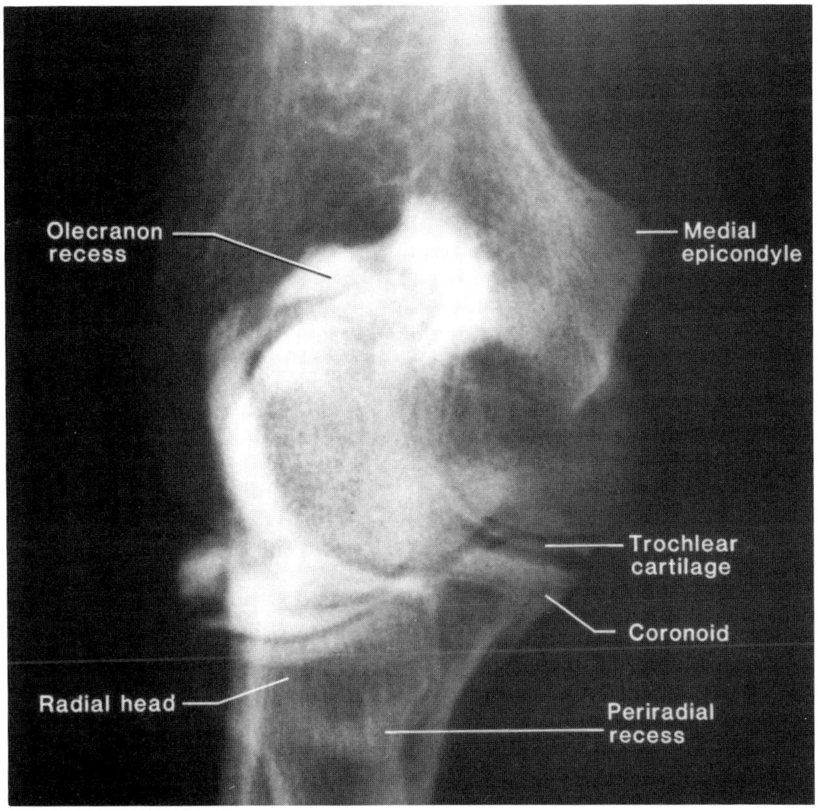

C

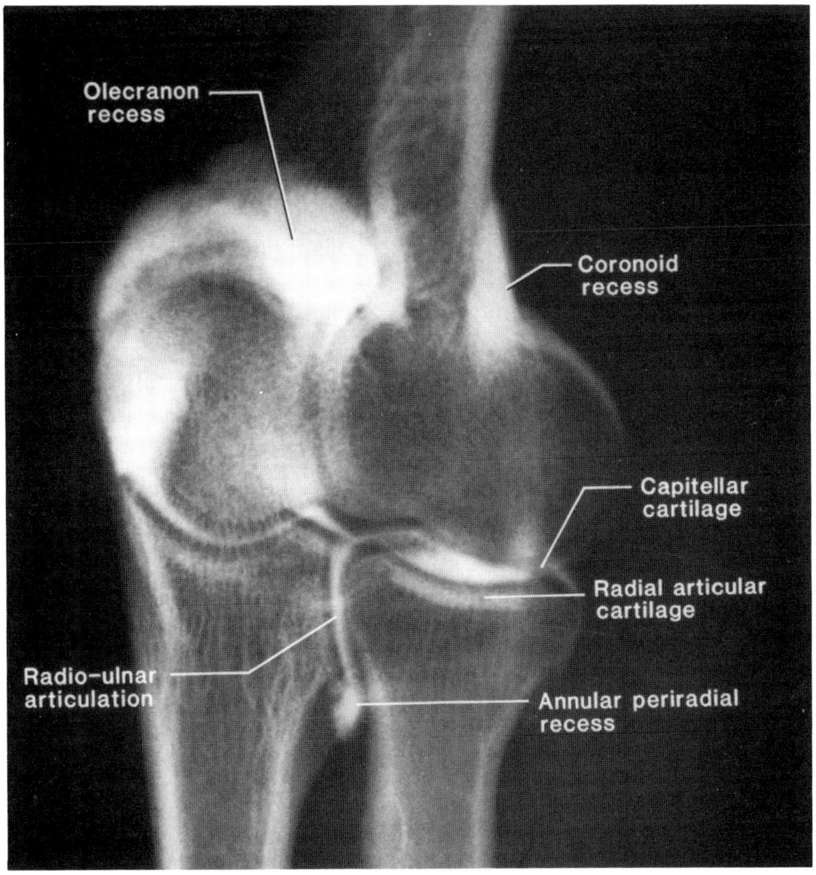

D

FIG. 11-11. *Continued.*

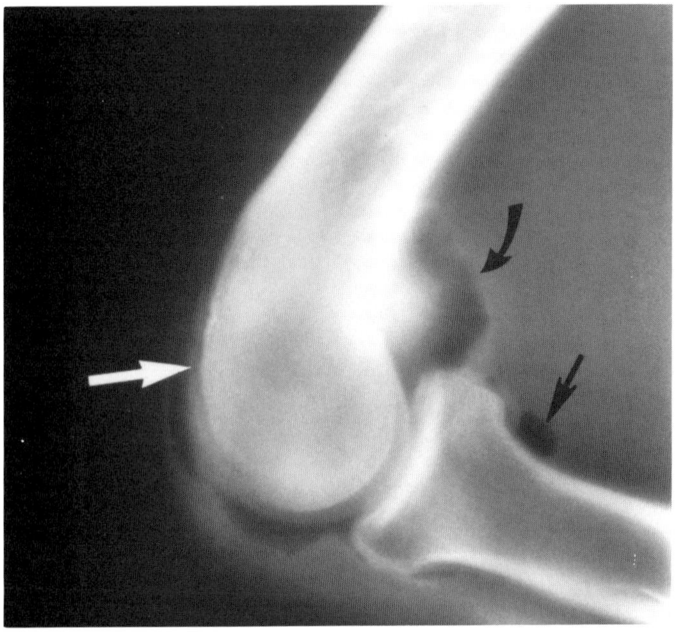

FIG. 11-12. Lateral view of a double-contrast arthrotomogram demonstrating the capsular volume (*arrows*).

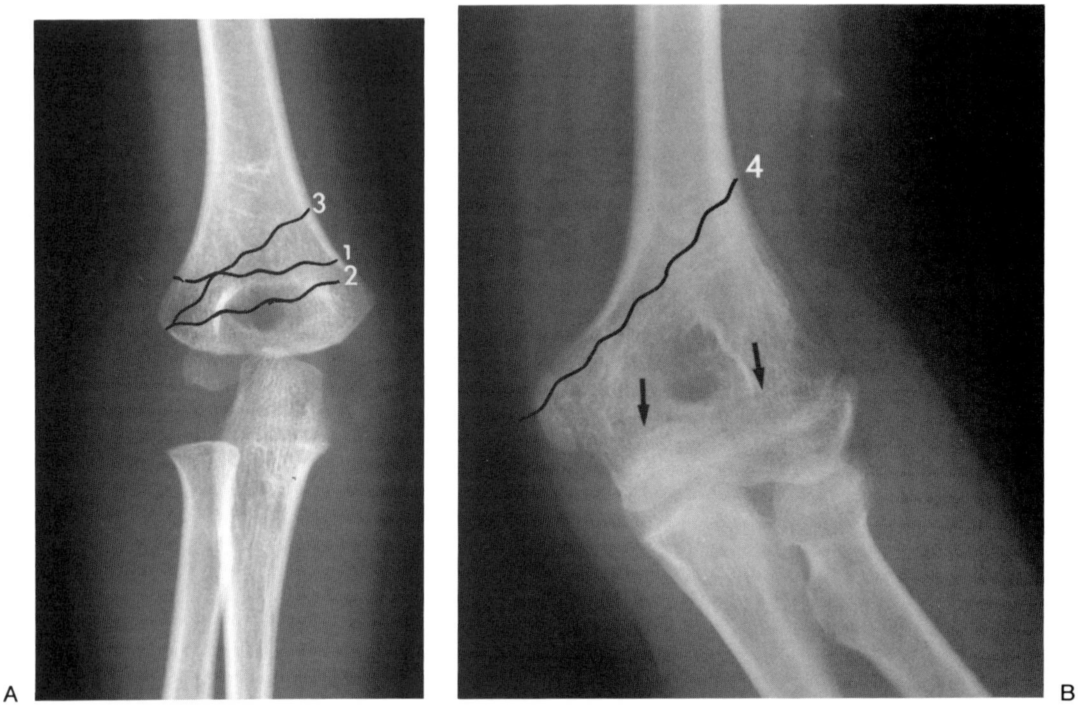

FIG. 11-13. The El-Ahwany[45] classification. **A,1:** Supracondylar type 1, a high transverse fracture; **2:** supracondylar type 2, short oblique fracture; **3:** supracondylar type 3, steep oblique fracture, which is unstable and likely to cause neurovascular compromise; **B,4:** supracondylar type 4, steep oblique fracture liable to immediate neurovascular compromise. A low transverse-transcondylar fracture. Forward displacement is common (*arrows*).

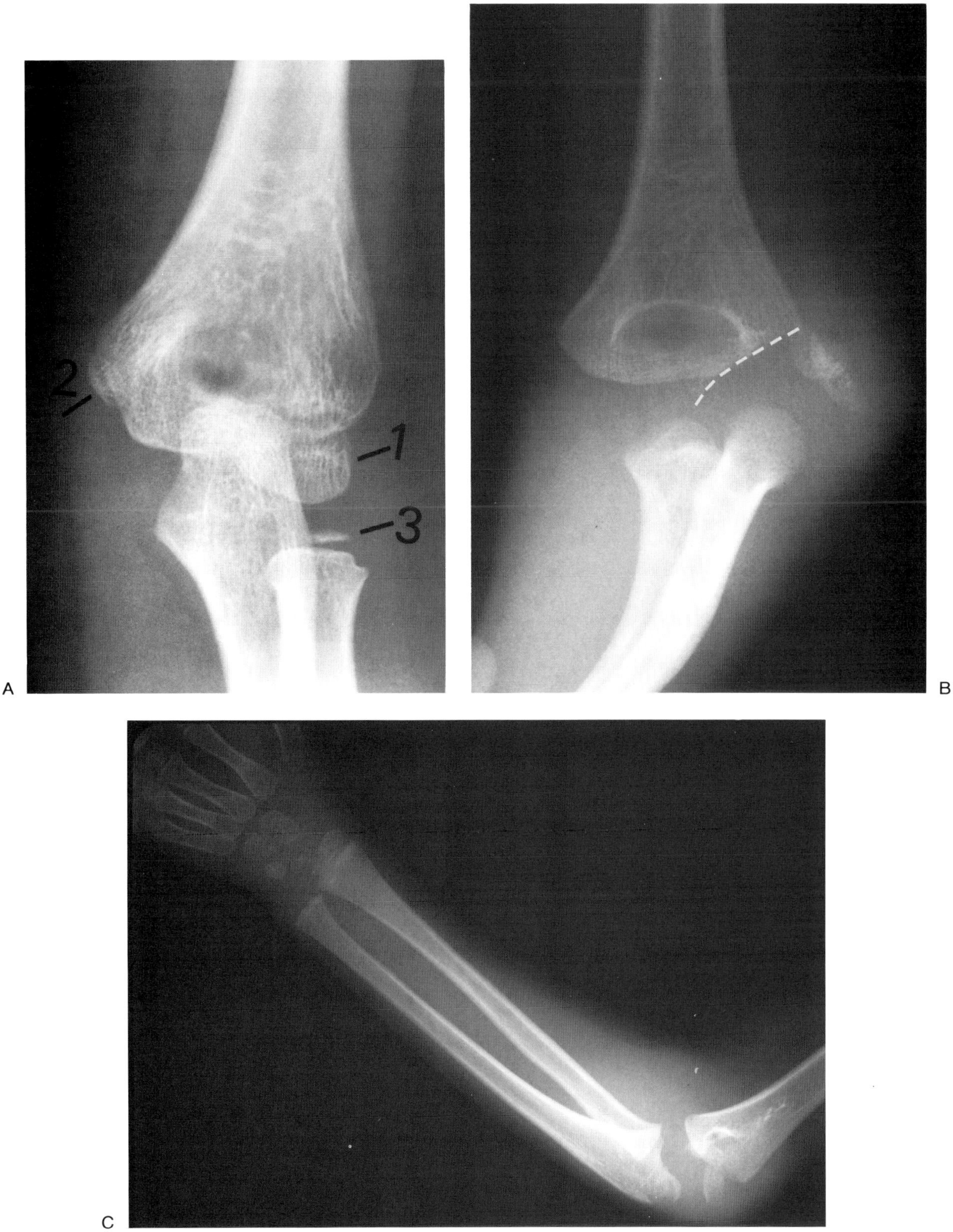

FIG. 11-14. A: Ossification of the distal humeral growth centers. Capitellum (*1*) appears by age 2 years, medial epicondyle (*2*) by age 4 years, and radial head (*3*) by age 5 years. The trochlea (not ossified here) ossifies by age 8 years; the olecranon, by age 9 years; and the lateral epicondyle, by ≥ age 10 years.[30,31] The AP **(B)** and lateral **(C)** views of the elbow in a 3-year-old child with a Salter-Harris type IV fracture (*white dotted line* in B) with displacement of a portion of the metaphysis and ossification center of the capitellum. Proper positioning is restricted by swelling and displacement.

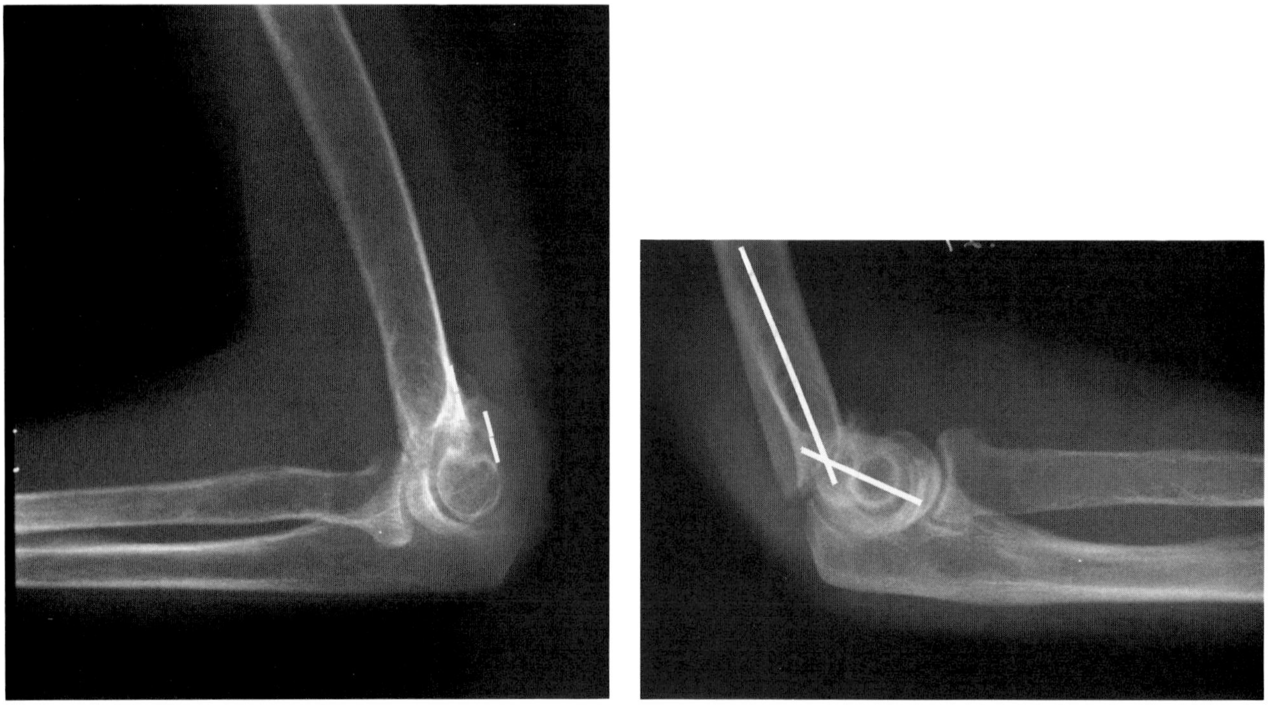

A B

FIG. 11-15. **A:** Lateral view of the elbow demonstrating a supracondylar fracture with posterior displacement (*lines*) of the distal fragment. **B:** Lateral view of a flexion injury with anterior displacement (*lines*) of the distal fragment.

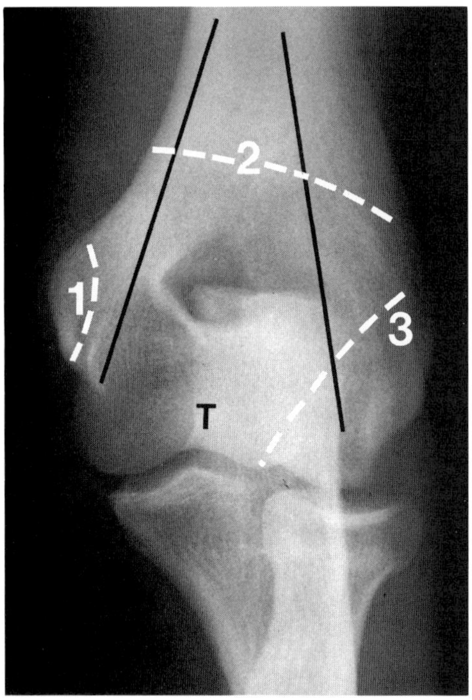

FIG. 11-16. An AP radiograph demonstrating the two-column (*black lines*) concept with the trochlea (*T*) held between the two columns.[57] Fractures (*white broken lines*) can be extraarticular (*1*), cross both columns (*2*, supracondylar), or intraarticular involving one (*3*) or both columns.[67]

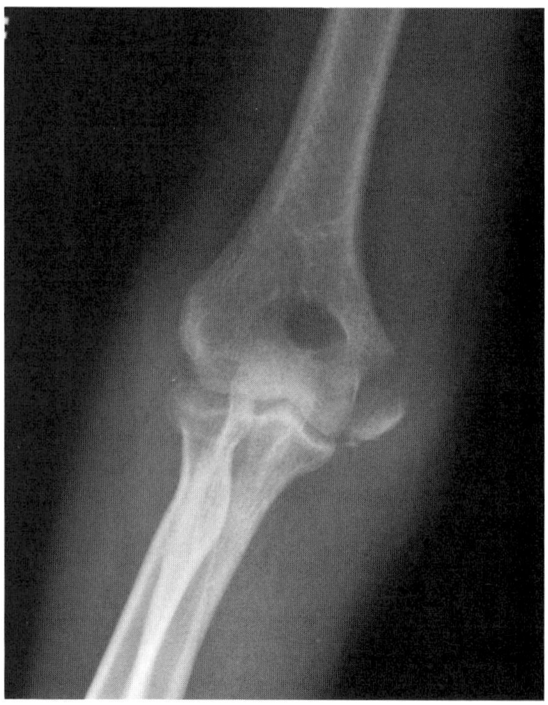

FIG. 11-17. An AP view of the elbow demonstrating a displaced avulsion fracture (AO type A1.3) of the medial epicondyle.

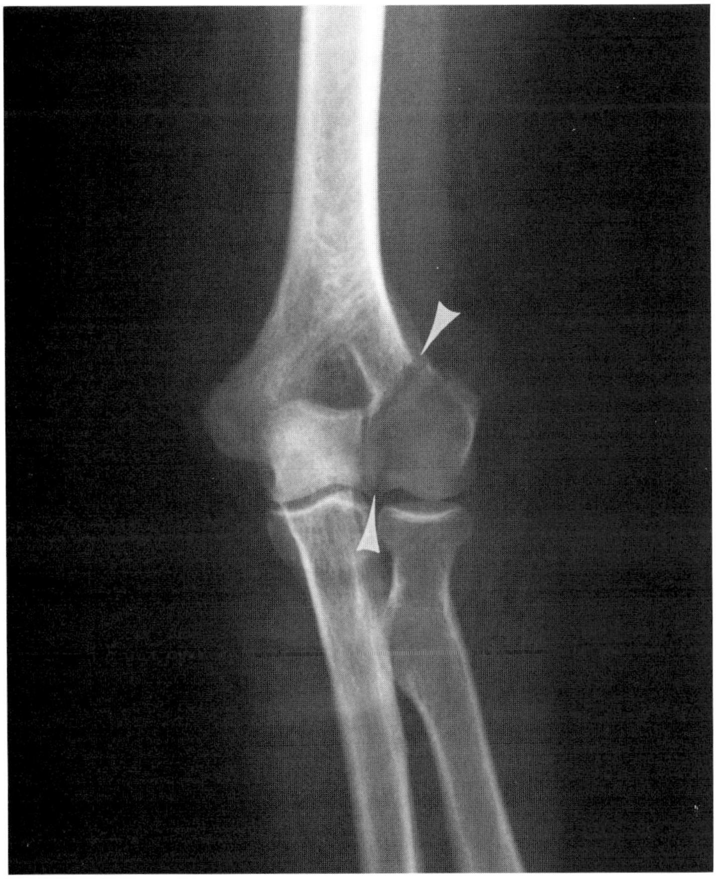

FIG. 11-18. An AP view of the elbow with a lateral column fracture (*arrows*) entering the margin of the trochlea (AO type B1.2).

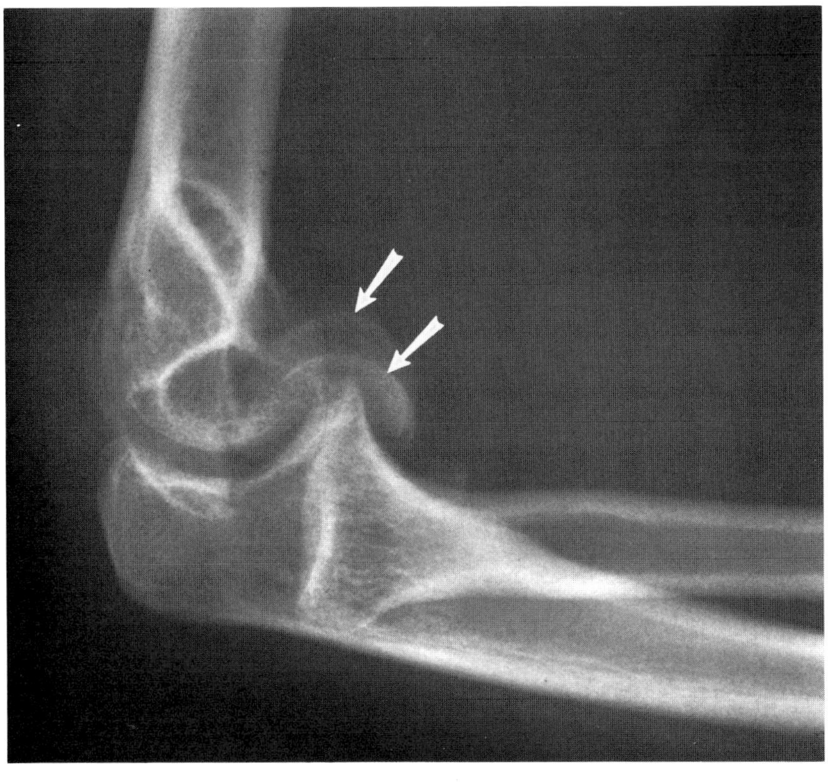

FIG. 11-19. Lateral view of the elbow demonstrating displaced coronal fracture involving the trochlea and capitellum (*arrows*). Note the double density, confirming involvement of both structures.

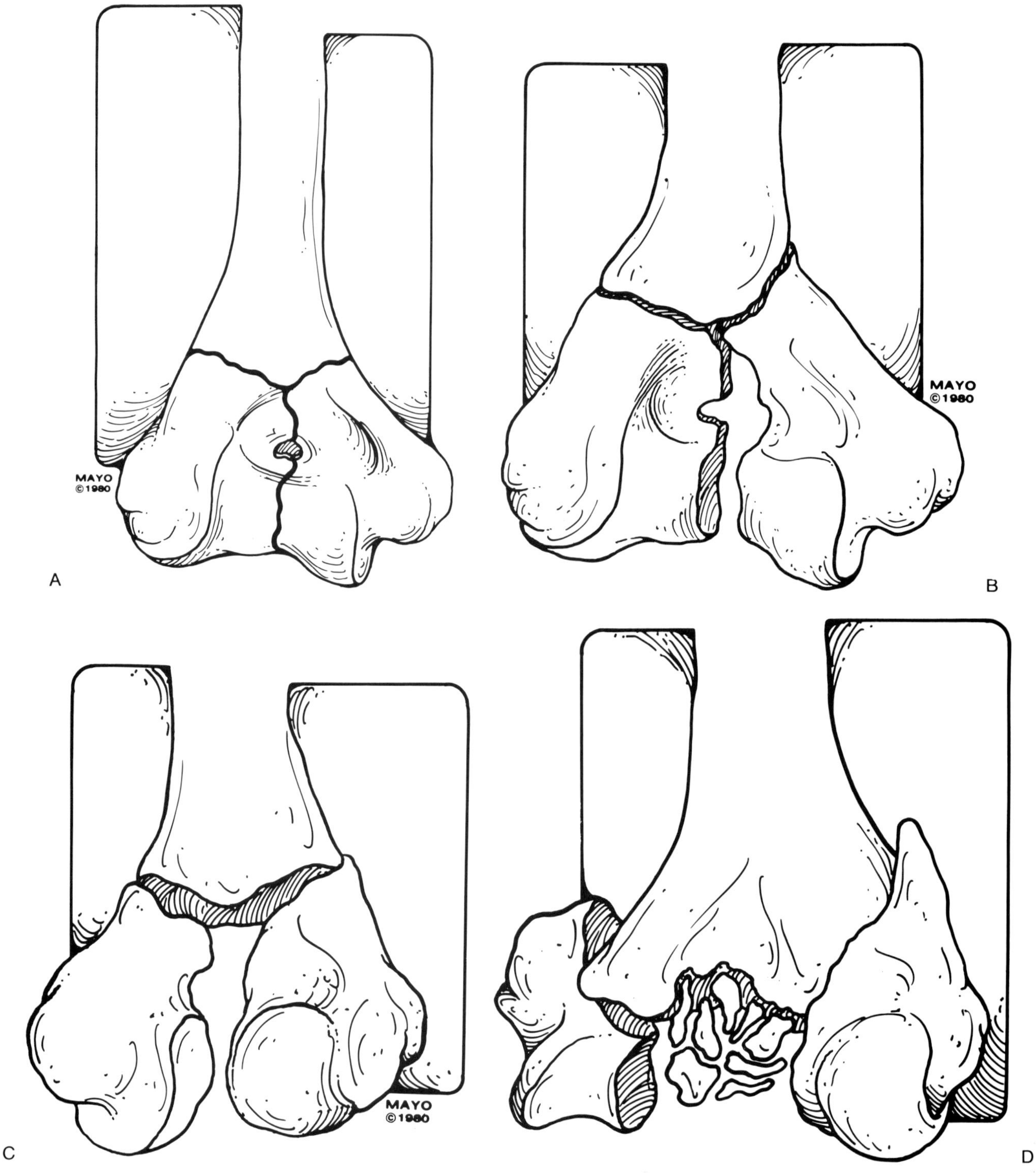

FIG. 11-20. The Riseborough and Radin classification of Y and T fractures. **A:** Type I, undisplaced fracture. **B:** Type II, displaced without significant rotation. **C:** Type III, displaced with condylar rotation. **D:** Type IV, displaced and comminuted. (From Bryan RS. Fractures about the elbow in adults. *Instr Course Lect* 1981;30:200–223.)

TABLE 11-1. *AO classification of distal humeral fractures*[57,58,72]

Type			Description
A			Extraarticular
	A1		Extraarticular avulsion fracture
		A1.1	Lateral epicondyle avulsion
		A1.2	Medial epicondyle avulsion with minimal displacement
		A1.3	Medial epicondyle avulsion with >3 mm displacement or medial joint space entrapment (Fig. 11-17)
	A2		Extraarticular involving both columns (Fig. 11-16, part 2) without articular extension
		A2.1	Abduction injury with an oblique fracture extending laterally to medially
		A2.2	Adduction injury with oblique fracture extending inferiorly medially to laterally
		A2.3	Transverse low fracture with posterior or anterior displacement (Fig. 11-15)
	A3		Comminuted extraarticular fracture
		A3.1	Transverse two-column fracture with intact wedge
		A3.2	Transverse two-column with comminution of one column
		A3.3	Transverse with comminution of both columns
B			Single-column fracture extending to the articular surface
	B1		Lateral fracture involving the articular surface
		B1.1	Lateral fracture entering the capitellum
		B1.2	Lateral fracture entering the trochlea
		B1.3	Lateral-column fracture with comminution of the articular surface
	B2		Medial fracture involving the articular surface
		B2.1	Medial fracture entering the margin of the joint surface
		B2.2	Medial fracture entering the trochlear groove
		B2.3	Medial fracture with articular comminution
	B3		Coronal articular fracture (best seen on lateral radiograph)
		B3.1	Coronal fracture involving the capitellum
		B3.2	Coronal fracture involving the trochlea
		B3.3	Coronal fracture involving both the trochlea and capitellum (Fig. 11-19)
C			Intraarticular fractures involving both columns
	C1		T- or Y-shaped intraarticular with no fragmentation
		C1.1	Supracondylar fracture entering the midjoint space or trochlea with minimal displacement
		C1.2	Supracondylar fracture as described in C1
		C1.3	T-shaped epiphyseal fracture
	C2		T- or Y-shaped fracture with metaphyseal comminution (Fig. 11-25)
		C2.1	Intact wedge laterally
		C2.2	Comminuted lateral column and wedge
		C2.3	Comminution of both columns
	C3		Comminuted articular surface
		C3.1	Articular surface fragmented with simple T- or Y-shaped metaphyseal fracture
		C3.2	Metaphyseal wedge
		C3.3	Fragmentation of the metaphysis and articular surface

Treatment

The treatment of distal humeral fractures should be designed to restore anatomy, particularly articular surfaces, and maintain distal humeral anteversion and the normal valgus carrying angle of the elbow (range, 5° to 20°; average, 15°).[33,52,54,70,71] Undisplaced or minimally displaced fractures may be treated conservatively with closed reduction and casting in adults and children.[51,52,58,59,61,76]

Traction

Traction can be used in children or adults (Fig. 11-21), but this technique is less frequently used in adults, who tolerate long-term bed rest more poorly than do children. Overhead traction with the elbow flexed 90° using a percutaneous olecranon Kirschner wire (K wire) or screw in the olecranon (Fig. 11-21) is commonly used. The screw technique is simpler, and nerve injury is less likely to occur than with through-and-through pinning.[44,53,59,76,80]

Percutaneous Pinning

Percutaneous pin fixation using K wires (typically 0.062-inch smooth K wires) is useful in unstable fractures in adults and children.[37,58,59] The advantages of percutaneous pinning include (1) reduced incidence of lost reduction compared with closed cast immobilization, (2) the elbow does not have to be maintained in flexion (children should be casted in 120° flexion, and (3) improved flexibility for clinical and radiographic evaluation (Figs. 11-22 and 11-23).[59]

(*text continues on page 768*)

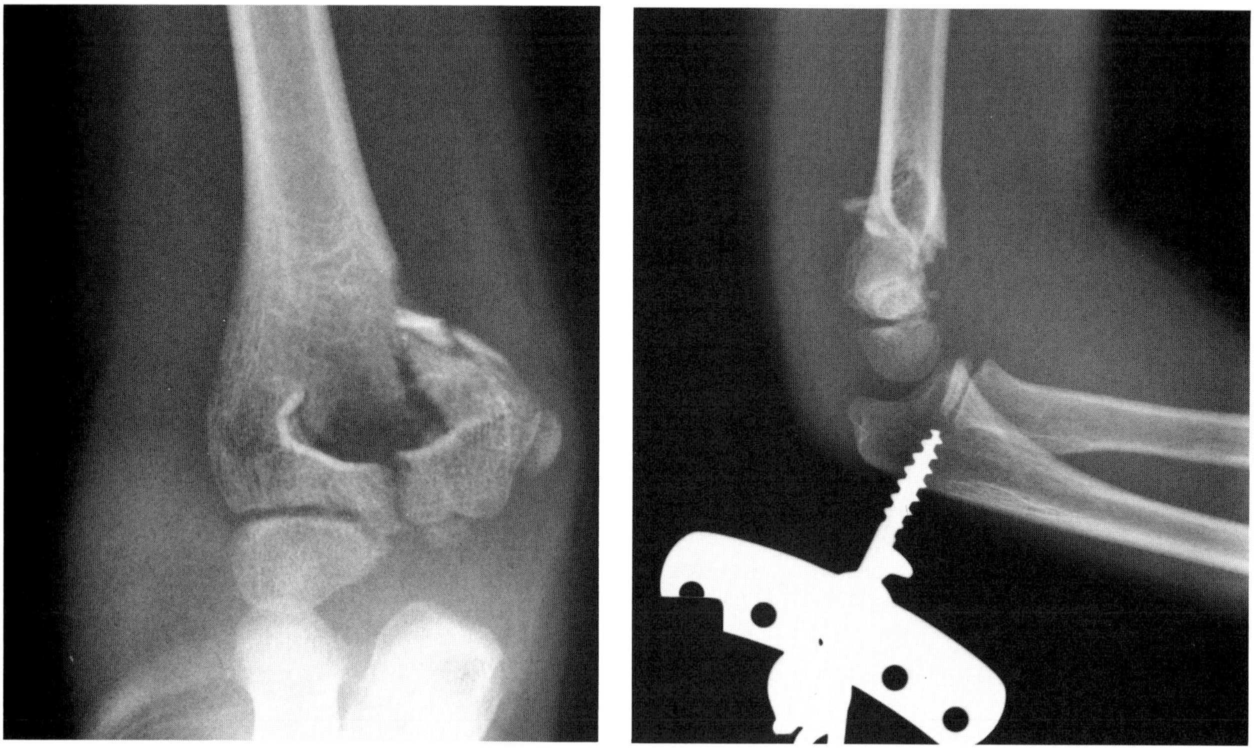

A B

FIG. 11-21. The AP **(A)** and lateral **(B)** views of the elbow in a child with a comminuted intraarticular fracture. The medial column is fragmented and the lateral column, minimally displaced. The medial portion of the fracture extends through the metaphysis and epiphysis (Salter-Harris type IV). The distal fragment is still posteriorly displaced slightly. Traction accomplished with 90° flexion using an olecranon screw.

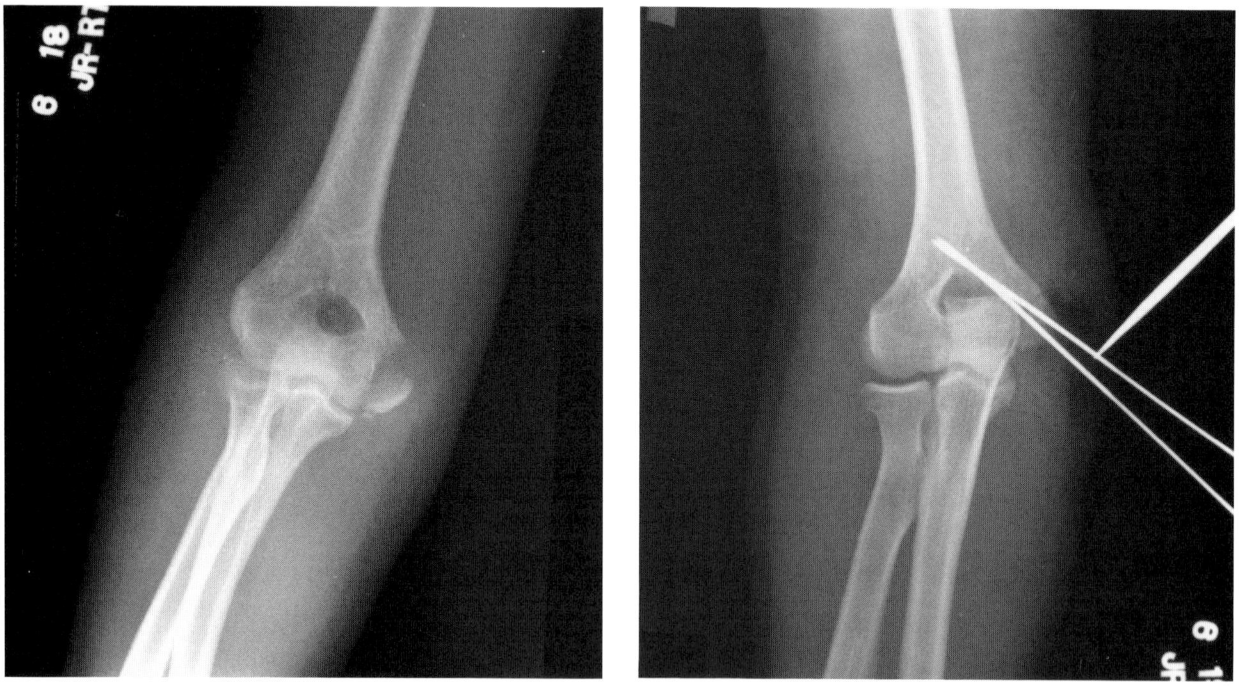

A B

FIG. 11-22. A: An AP radiograph of the elbow demonstrating a displaced medial epicondylar fracture. **B:** The anatomic position was restored with two percutaneous K wires, which were placed with fluoroscopic guidance.

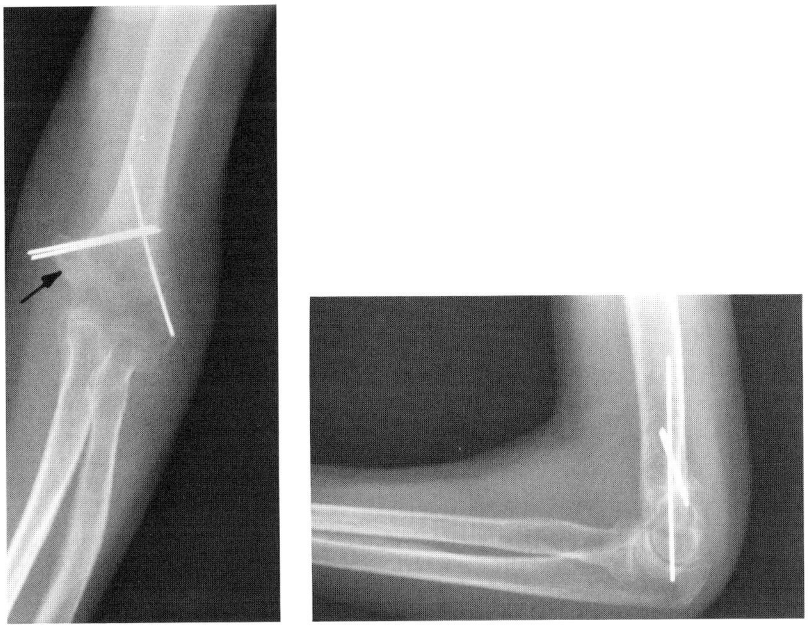

A,B

FIG. 11-23. The AP **(A)** and lateral **(B)** views of bilateral epicondyle fractures reduced with K-wires. The medial epicondyle is rotated slightly and more proximally than normal (*arrow*).

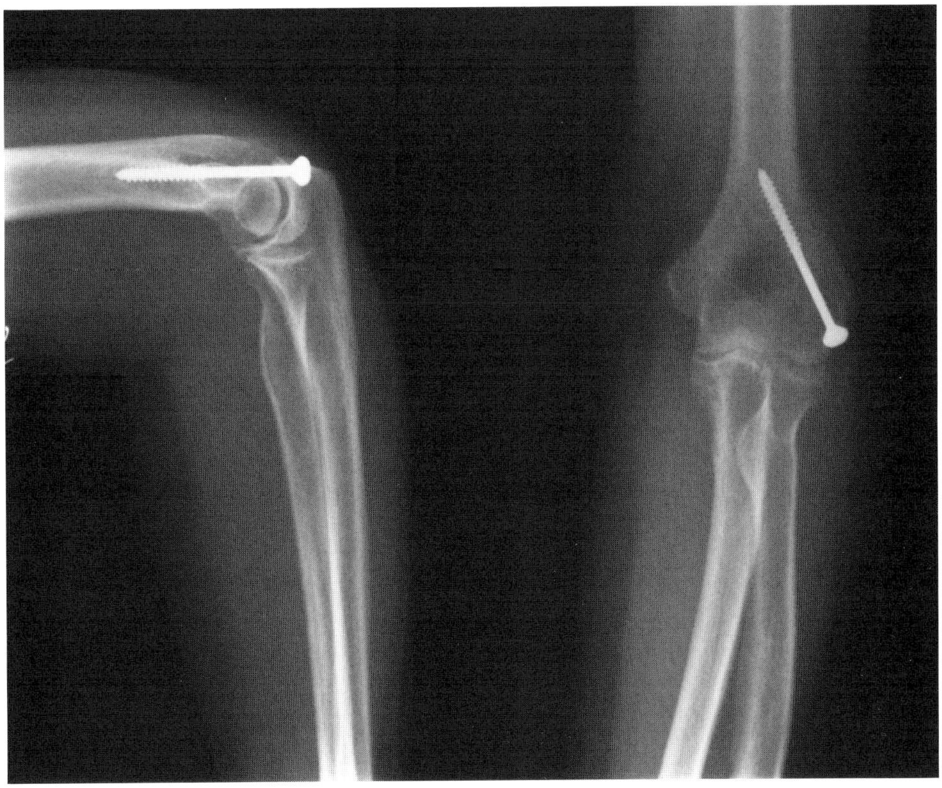

FIG. 11-24. Fracture of the lateral condyle reduced using a single cancellous screw.

Open Reduction and Internal Fixation

Surgical reduction is important for unstable, displaced, or rotated column fractures, such as AO type C or Riseborough and Radin types III and IV fractures.[52,71] The indications for open reduction include (1) an open fracture that requires débridement, (2) displaced unstable fractures, (3) neurovascular compromise, (4) recognized neurovascular compromise after reduction, and (5) fractures that cannot be reduced because of soft tissue interposition.[58]

Articular fragments can be reduced with K wires under fluoroscopic guidance. Cancellous screws, one-third semitubular plates, or reconstruction plates can be used, as necessary, to restore the medial and lateral columns. Areas with significant bone loss may require grafting. When the posterior approach is used, an olecranon osteotomy is performed.[32,36,46,51,52,58] This is reduced and internally fixed at the time of surgery and should not be confused for a more complex fracture by the uninformed imager.[71] Figures 11-24 to 11-29 demonstrate various surgical implants for distal humeral fractures.

Radial Head Fractures

Radial head fractures account for 2% to 5% of all fractures.[26,29,52,70,71] Nearly one third of elbow fractures involve the radial head.[34,70] Most radial head fractures occur in adults (85%). Radial neck fractures are more common in children.[70,71]

The mechanism of injury is usually a fall on the outstretched arm with the forearm pronated (Fig. 11-30).[70,71] A direct blow is an uncommon cause of radial head fractures.[52,70,71]

The most commonly used classification system was proposed by Mason.[66] Type I fractures are undisplaced or minimally displaced fractures that involve less than one third of the head or neck (Figs. 11-31A and 11-32). Type II fractures of the radial head involve one third of the articular surface and are displaced or impacted > 2 mm (Figs. 11-31B and 11-33) or result in angulation of the radial neck (Figs. 11-31B and 11-33B). Type III radial head fractures are comminuted (Fig. 11-31C), and type IV fractures include any radial head fracture associated with ulnohumeral dislocation (Figs. 11-31D and 11-34).[66,70,71] Associated ligament and neurovascular injuries are fairly common. Fractures of the olecranon or coronoid also occur with radial head fractures.[70] Up to 50% of capitellar fractures occur with radial head injuries. These fractures often involve the articular surface, and they are easily overlooked on routine radiographs.[70,71]

Imaging of the elbow in patients with suspected radial head injuries can usually be accomplished with AP, lateral, 45° lateral oblique, and in some cases, radial head capitellar views. Attention to soft tissue changes, specifically the fat pads and supinator fat stripe (Figs. 11-3, 11-6, and 11-35), is important to avoid overlooking type I injuries.[29,71] In patients with more complex injuries, further evaluation with CT (reformatted images or three-dimensional reconstruction may be required) or thin-section trispiral tomography should be considered to enhance treatment planning.[29,60]

Treatment

Type I injuries are managed conservatively.[70–72] The management of type II injuries (Figs. 11-31B and 11-33) is more controversial.[23,34,52,71] Early resection of the radial head is most commonly performed if excision is considered (Fig. 11-36).[23,67,70] This treatment remains controversial compared with conservative therapy. Resection of the radial head is generally reserved for injuries involving > 30% of the articular surface and in which the displacement is > 2 to 3 mm with a loss of elbow motion or when crepitus of the fragments is noted at the radiocapitellar surface.[23,34,70] Type III fractures are treated with early excision of the radial head. Type IV fractures are frequently complex injuries. The elbow should be reduced immediately.[30,70,71] Large single head fractures can be reduced with small compression screws (Figs. 11-37 and 11-38).[30,73,74] Comminuted fractures may require radial head resection.[70,71]

Prosthetic replacement of the radial head is generally reserved for injuries with resulting instability.[70,84] Instability is commonly seen with type IV injuries (Fig. 11-31D). Monteggia fractures with radial head fracture in addition to dislocation, radial head fractures with medial ligament tears, and radial head fractures with associated coronoid fractures are included in this group of injuries.[50,65,77,78]

Various prosthetic designs have been used, but the Silastic™ prosthesis designed by Swanson is most commonly used today (Fig. 11-39).[70,84] The results are good in most cases. However, most authors still recommend reserving implants for patients with posttraumatic instability.[50,70,84]

Fractures of the Proximal Ulna

The ulnar olecranon is particularly susceptible to fracture because of its subcutaneous position. Most fractures are intraarticular, which can alter joint function in addition to compromising stability.[29] Fractures with disruption of the triceps fascial expansions tend to be more displaced.[29,35]

Olecranon fractures occur from direct blows or falls on the flexed elbow. There are several classification schemes with which radiologists should be familiar.[29,35]

The Colton[39] classification is commonly used for olecranon fractures. Type I fractures are undisplaced (Fig.

(*text continues on page 778*)

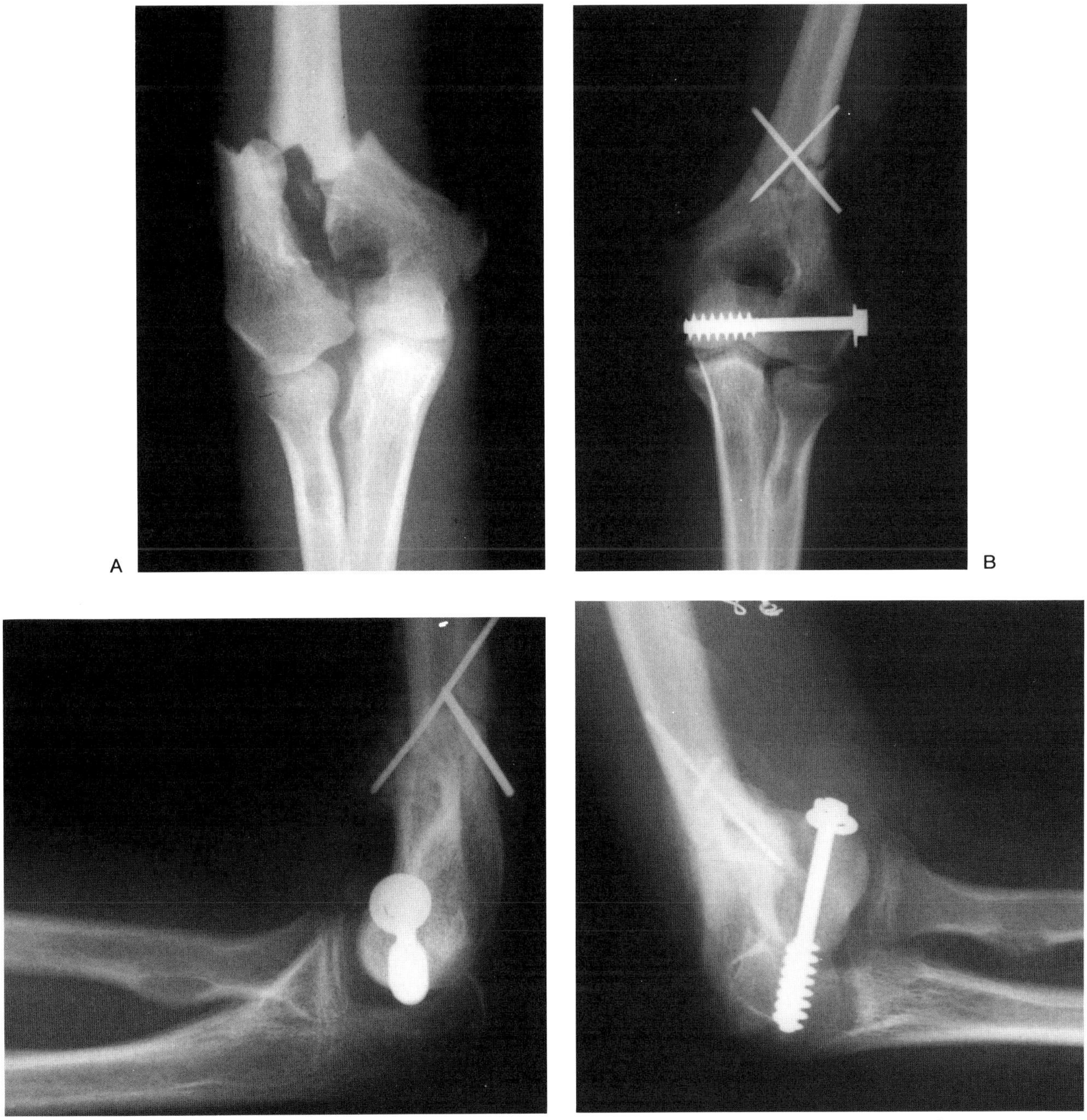

FIG. 11-25. A: An AP radiograph of a comminuted Y fracture with rotation of the medial and lateral fragments. Riseborough and Radin type III and AO type C2. **B:** The AP view after reduction and internal fixation using two crossed K wires proximally and a cancellous screw and washer to reduce the articular fragments (medial and lateral columns). **C,D:** Lateral and oblique views demonstrate healing with little articular deformity.

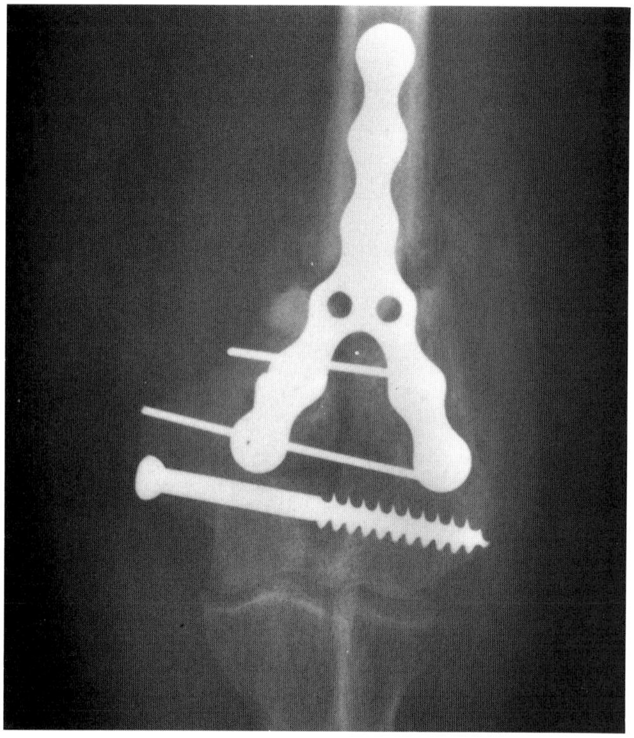

FIG. 11-26. An AP view of a healing Y supracondylar fracture reduced with two K wires, a Y reconstruction plate (see Chapter 2), and a distal cancellous screw.

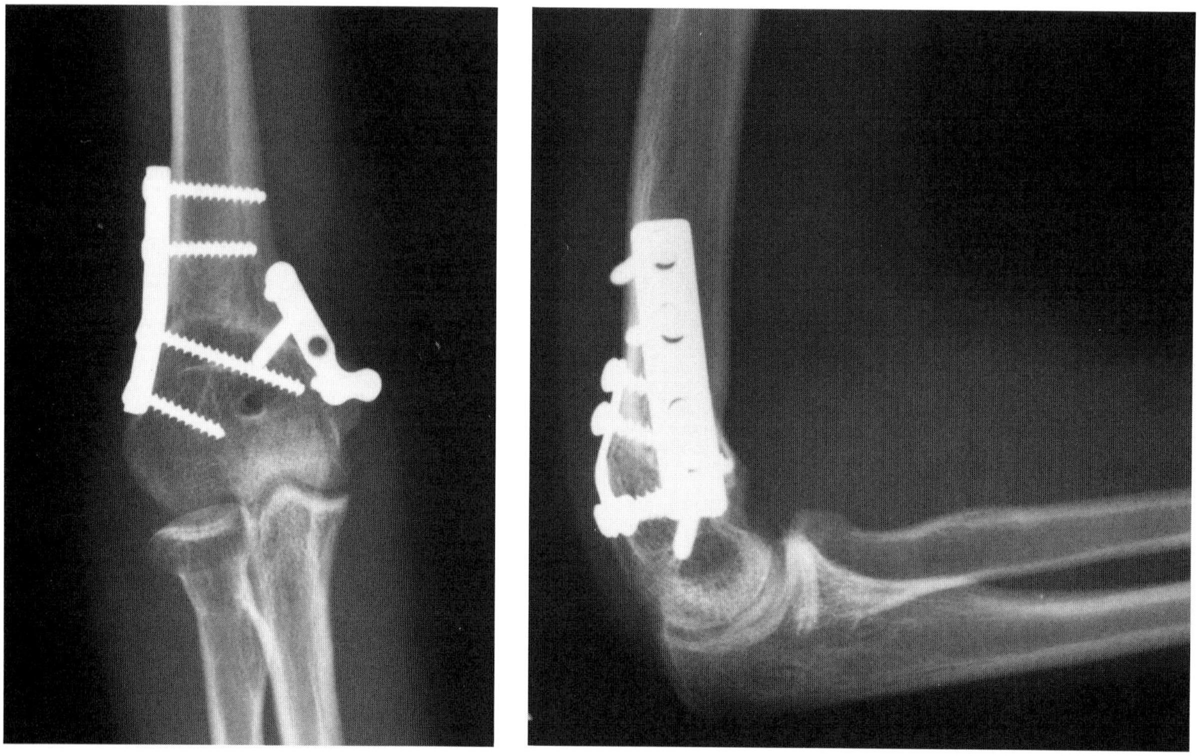

A

B

FIG. 11-27. The AP **(A)** and lateral **(B)** radiographs of a healed fracture. The lateral column was restored with a dynamic compression (DC) plate and four cortical screws. The medial column was reduced with an oblique miniplate and screws.

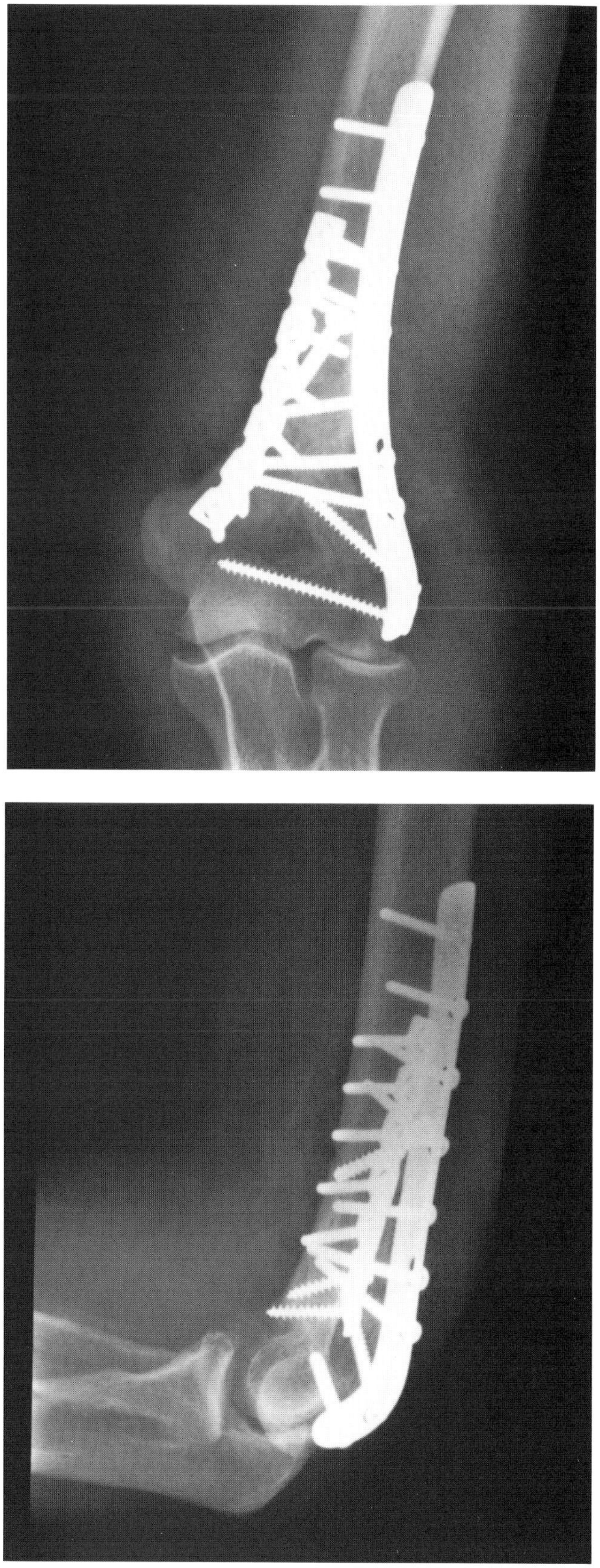

A

B

FIG. 11-28. The AP **(A)** and lateral **(B)** radiographs of a healed AO type C2.3 fracture with medial column reconstruction using a straight reconstruction plate (note notches in plate) and a semitubular plate laterally.

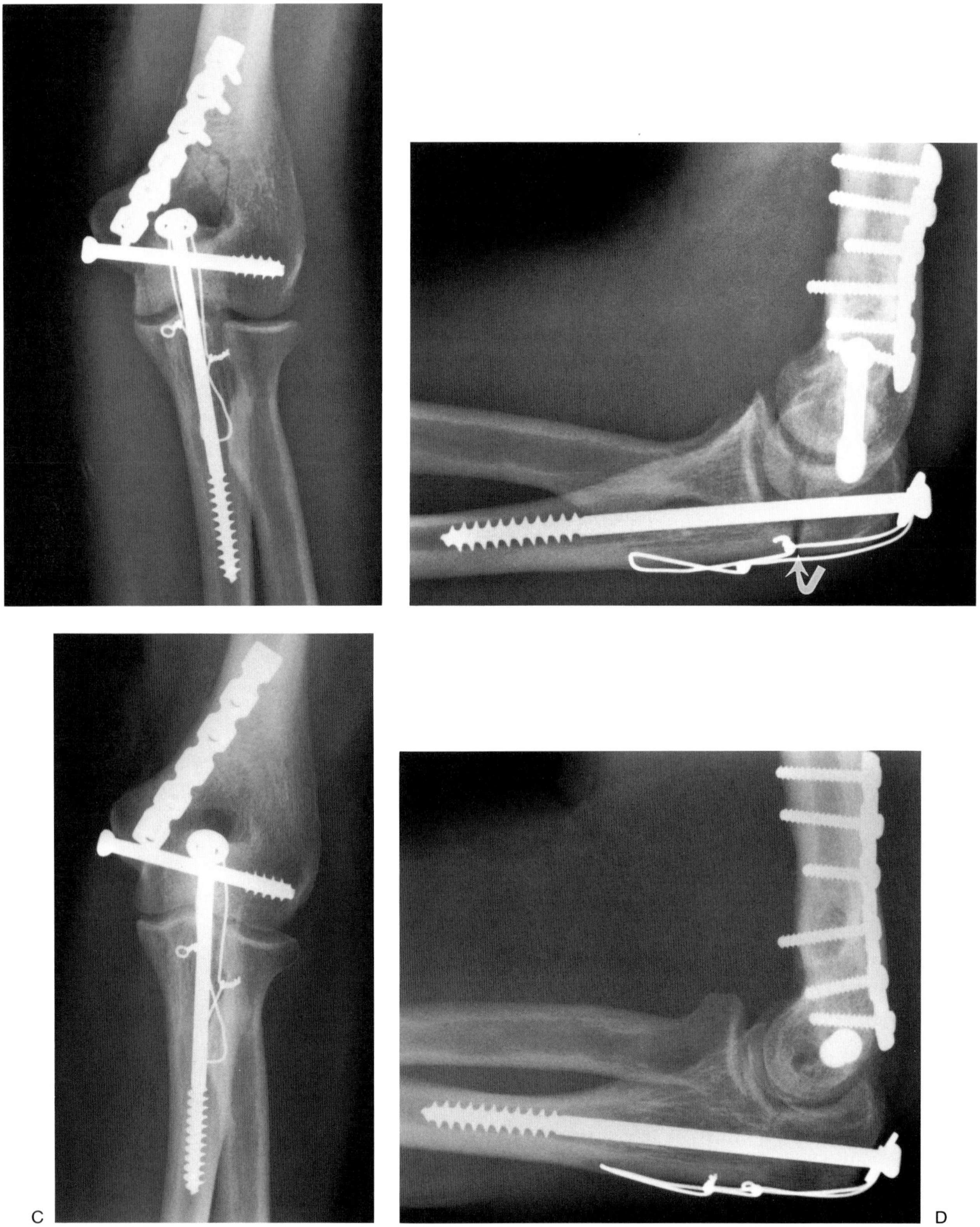

FIG. 11-29. The AP **(A)** and lateral **(B)** radiographs after reduction of a comminuted medial column fracture with intraarticular extension (AO type B2.3). Reduction was performed with an olecranon osteotomy (*curved arrow*). The medial column is reduced with a reconstruction plate and six cortical screws. There is a single transcondylar cancellous screw. The osteotomy is reduced with a long cancellous screw with a washer and tension-band wire. The AP **(C)** and lateral **(D)** views show the fracture and osteotomy are healed 9 months later.

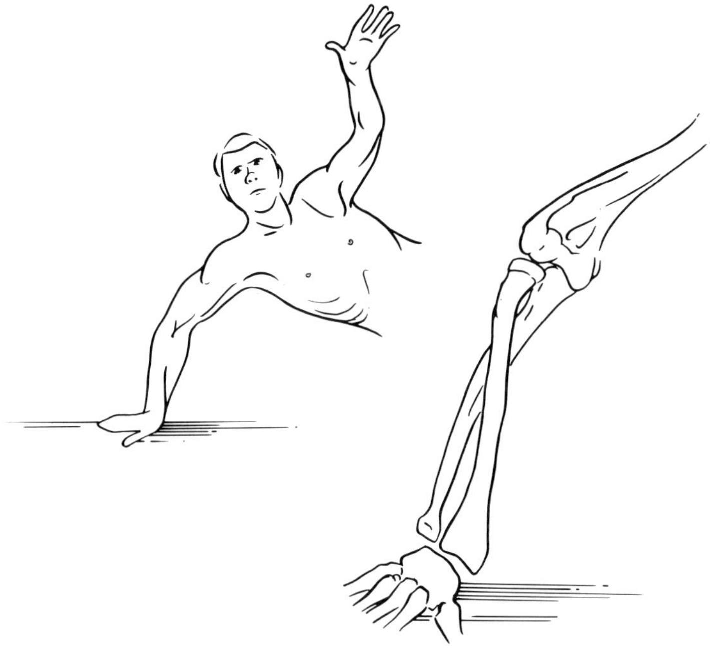

FIG. 11-30. Mechanism of injury of radial head fractures is most often a fall on the outstretched arm with the elbow partially flexed and the forearm pronated. (From Morrey BF, Berquist TH. The elbow. In: Berquist TH, ed. *Imaging of orthopedic trauma,* 2nd ed. New York: Raven Press, 1992;675–730.)

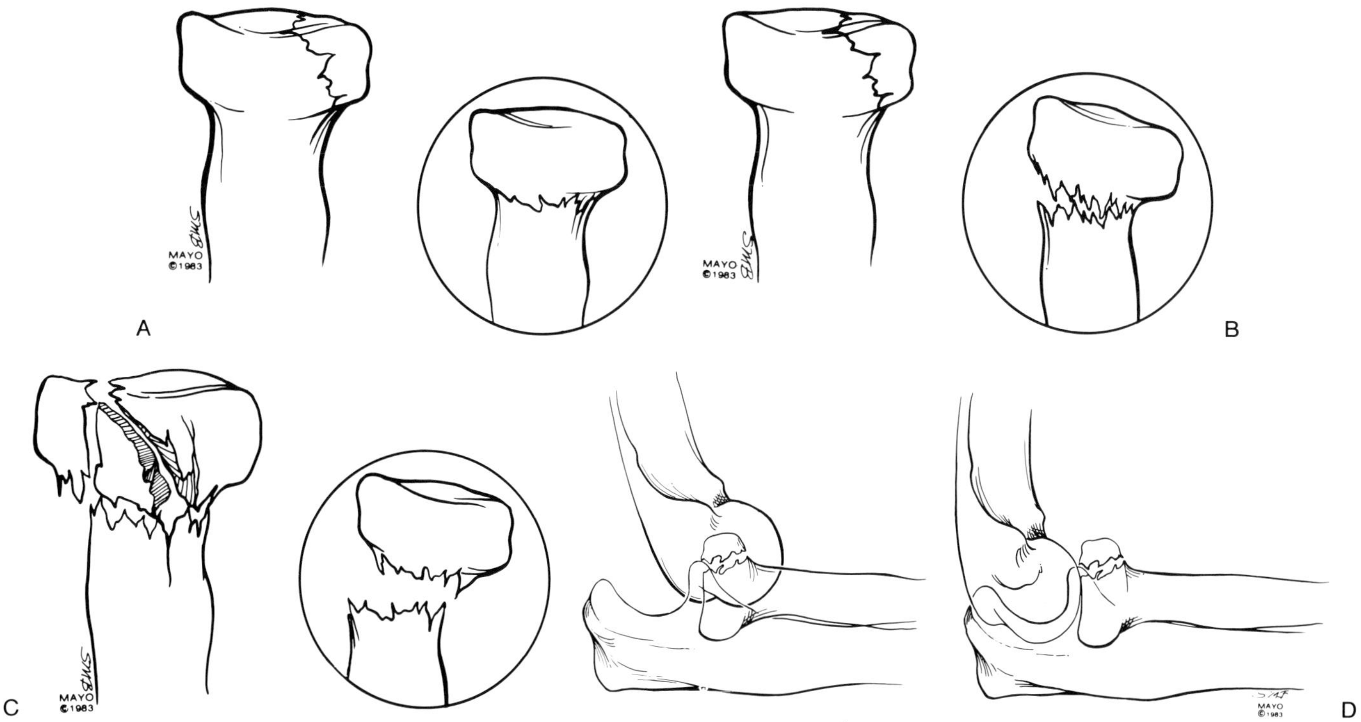

FIG. 11-31. Mason classification of radial head and neck fractures. **A:** Type I, minimally displaced or undisplaced. **B:** Type II, fracture involves one third of the radial head with > 2 mm of displacement or a neck fracture with 20° to 30° angulation. **C:** Type III, comminuted fracture of the radial head. **D:** Type IV, any radial head fracture with associated ulnohumeral dislocation. (From Morrey BF, Berquist TH. The elbow. In: Berquist TH, ed. *Imaging of orthopedic trauma,* 2nd ed. New York: Raven Press, 1992;675–730.)

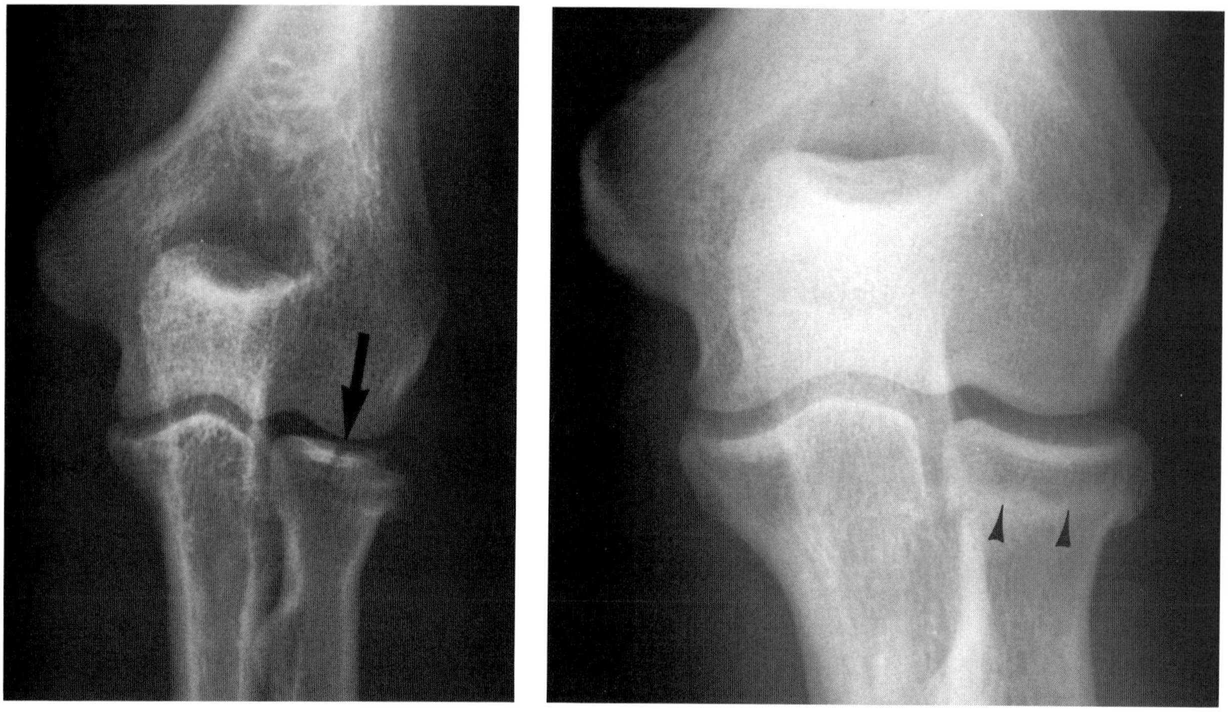

A B

FIG. 11-32. Type I radial fractures. **A:** Undisplaced radial head fracture (*arrow*). **B:** Slightly impacted radial neck fracture (*arrows*).

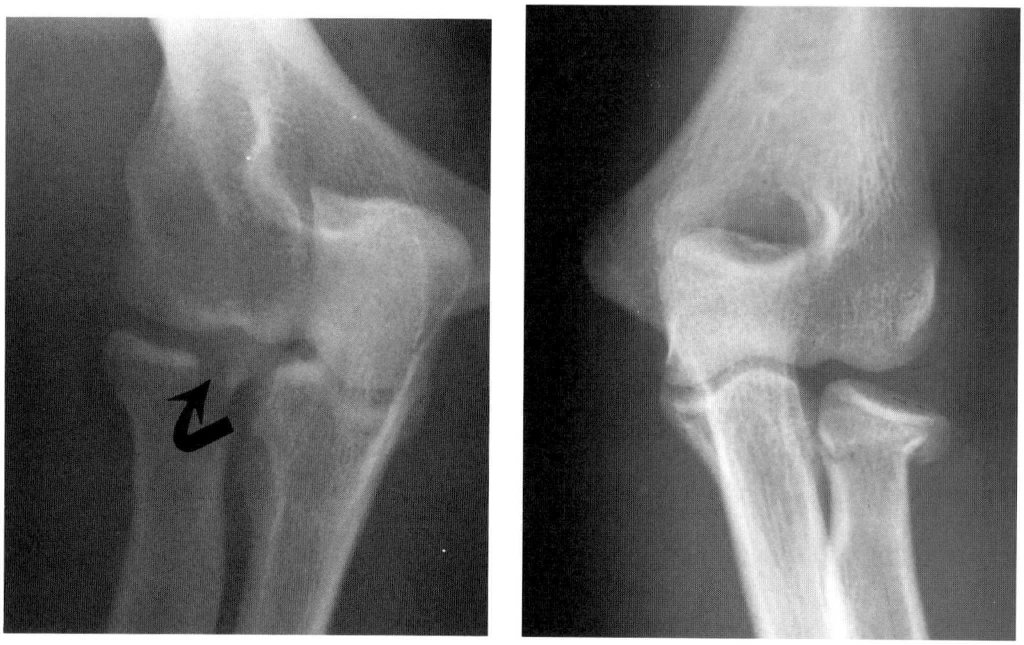

A B

FIG. 11-33. Type II radial fractures. **A:** Displaced radial head fracture (*arrow*). **B:** Displaced angulated radial neck fracture.

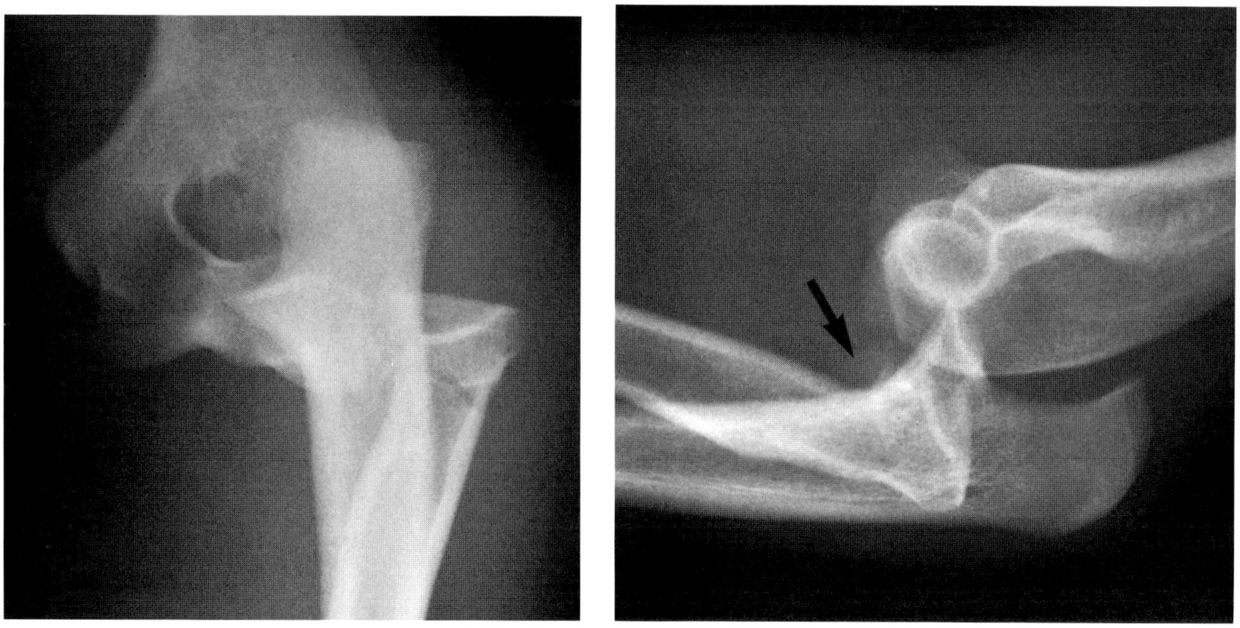

A B

FIG. 11-34. Type IV radial fracture (*arrow*) with posterolateral dislocation demonstrated on AP **(A)** and lateral **(B)** radiographs.

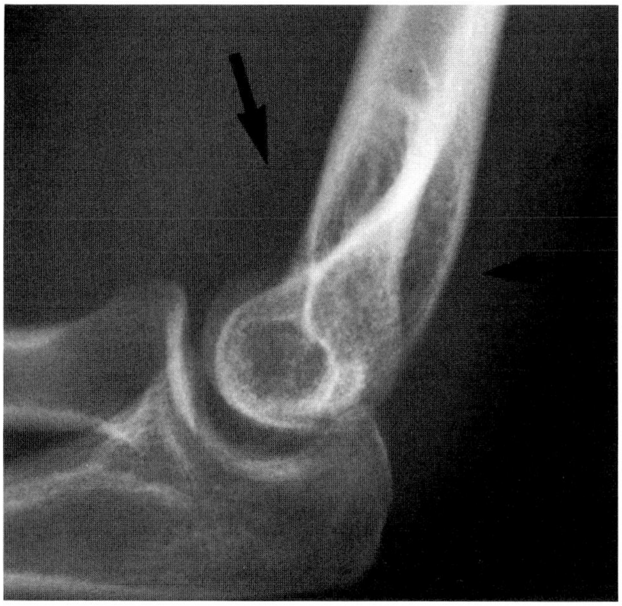

FIG. 11-35. Type I radial head fracture. Lateral radiograph of the elbow following trauma. No fracture is evident, but both the anterior and posterior fat pads are displaced (*arrows*).

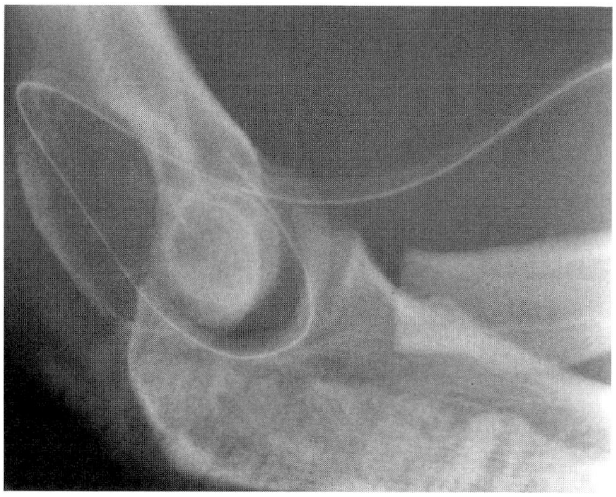

FIG. 11-36. Type II radial head fracture treated with radial head resection. The Kocher excision is most commonly used. The incision is made between the anconeus and extensor carpi ulnaris with care taken not to disrupt the ulnar humeral ligament.[70]

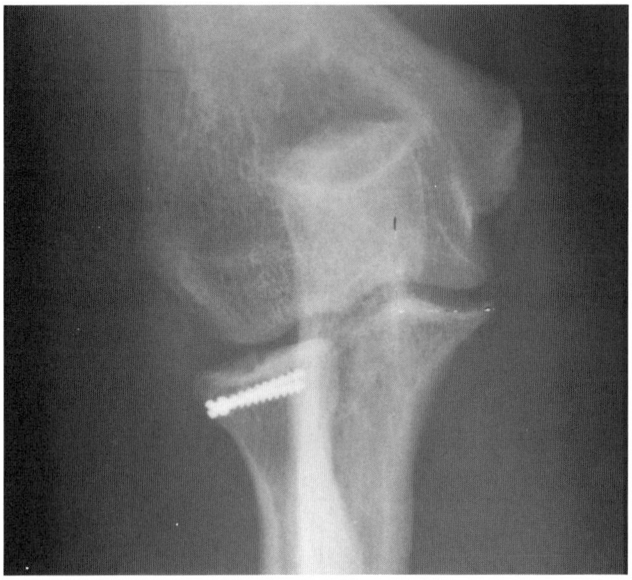

FIG. 11-37. An AP view of the elbow after fracture of the radial head with ulnohumeral dislocation. The single fragment was reduced with two small compression screws. There is slight residual articular deformity.

A

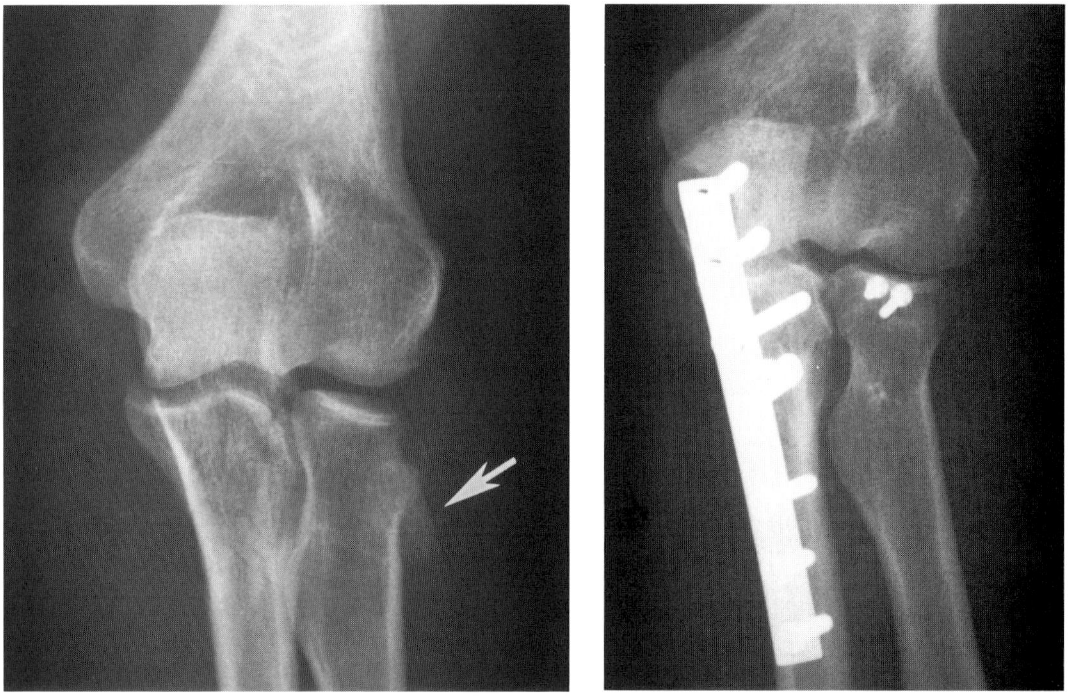

B

C

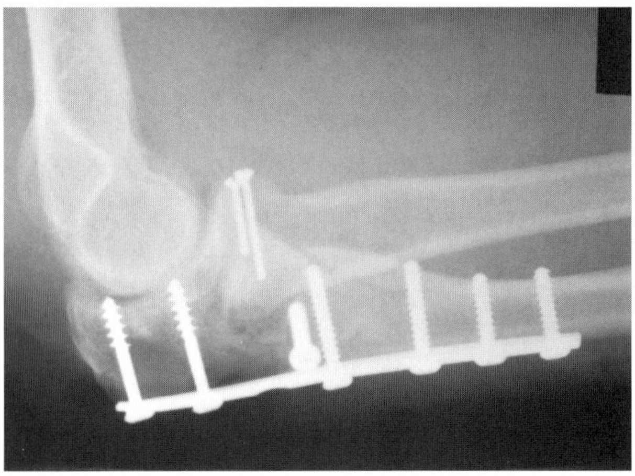

FIG. 11-38. A: An AP view of the elbow with a displaced radial head fracture (*arrow*) and associated proximal ulnar fracture. Oblique **(B)** and lateral **(C)** radiographs after reduction of the radial head fracture with two compression screws. The ulnar fracture was reduced using a semitubular plate and four cortical screws, two proximal cancellous screws, and a single lag screw.

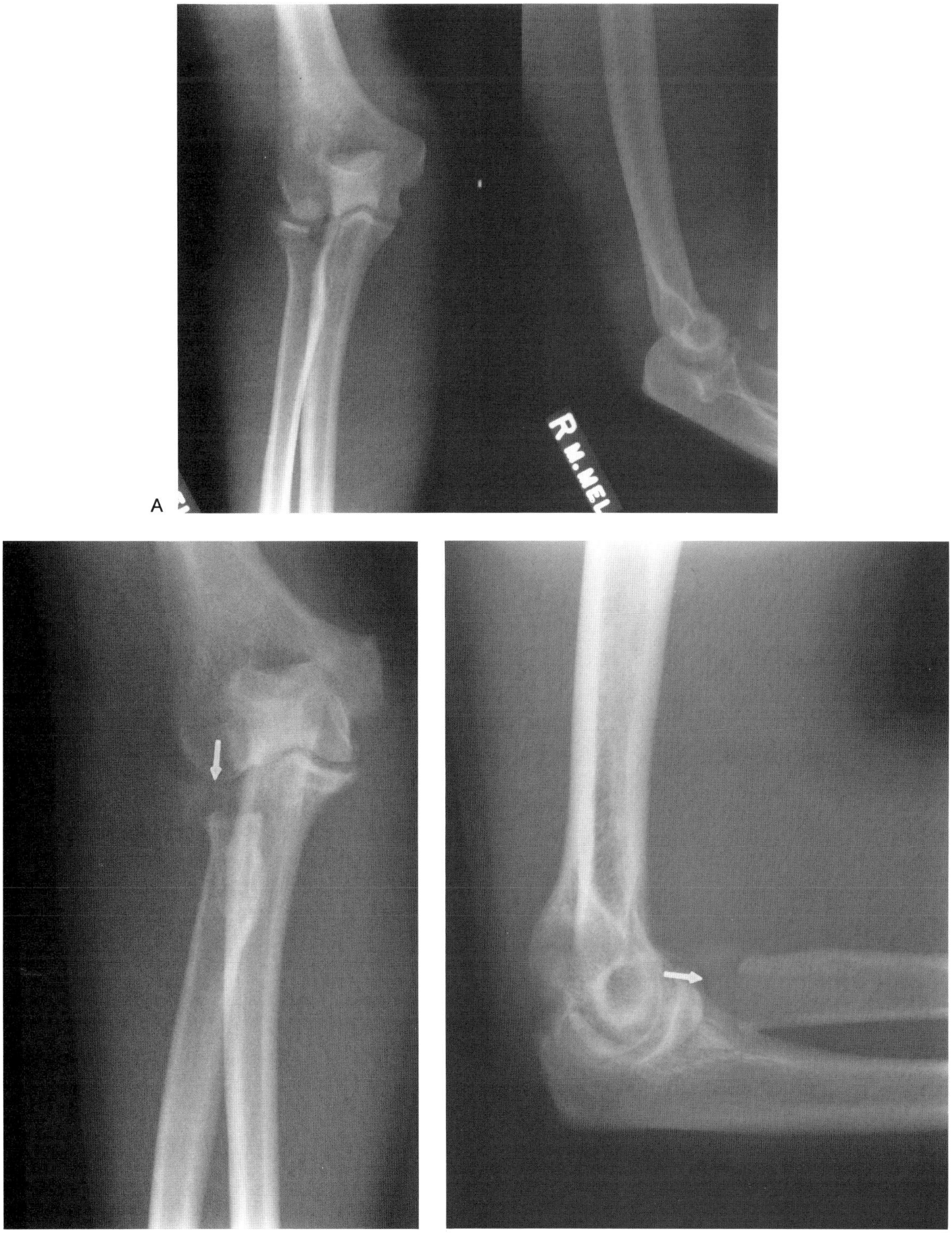

A B C

FIG. 11-39. A: The AP and lateral views of the elbow demonstrating a comminuted radial head fracture. The AP **(B)** and lateral **(C)** radiographs 2 years after a Silastic^{TM} radial head implant. The articular surface (*small arrows*) has fractured.

11-40). Type II fractures are avulsion injuries with transverse or oblique configurations (Fig. 11-40). Type III fractures are oblique or transverse and involve the articular surface, and type IV fractures are comminuted (Figs. 11-40 and 11-41). Type V fractures are associated with dislocation (Figs. 11-40 and 11-42).[39,70,71] The AO classification is based on the location and radial involvement (type A), joint involvement (type B), or degree of comminution (type C).[72] Mayo Clinic authors devised a simpler scheme based on displacement, stability, and comminution.[35,70] Type I fractures are undisplaced (fragment separation < 2 mm) with minimal comminution (5% of olecranon fractures). Type II fractures are displaced but stable. These injuries may be comminuted and account for 85% of proximal ulnar fractures. Type III fractures are displaced and unstable and may be comminuted (Fig. 11-41).[35]

The radiographic evaluation is usually complete with routine views. The lateral view is most important to determine the degree of comminution and fracture displacement (Figs. 11-41 and 11-42).[29]

Treatment

The treatment goals include restoring the articular surface and maintaining stability and range of motion.[34,35,52] Undisplaced fractures are uncommon, but these injuries are usually managed conservatively with cast or splint immobilization.[35,70] Unstable or displaced fractures (types II and III) may be managed with internal fixation or excision with triceps mechanism repair.[35,48,64,81,85]

Several approaches can be used for open reduction and internal fixation. Rigid fixation should be achieved to allow early motion.[35,41,70]

Wiring

Tension-band wiring (see Chapter 2) is used to transform distraction forces into compression forces with a figure-eight wire technique and K wires. This technique is usually reserved for noncomminuted injuries with moderate displacement (Fig. 11-43).

Intramedullary Fixation

Intramedullary fixation is typically achieved using Steinmann pins, Rush rods, or long cancellous screws (Fig. 11-44). Tension-band wiring may be used in conjunction with cancellous screws (see Chapter 12).[35,64,70]

Bicortical Screw Fixation

An oblique olecranon may be reduced using a lag screw that extends from cortex to cortex (Fig. 11-45).[35]

Plate and Screw Fixation

Semitubular or one-third tubular plates, cloverleaf plates (Figs. 11-46 and 11-47), or other configurations can be used. Skin irritation is a common postoperative complication with this technique because of the subcutaneous location of the olecranon, and it may necessitate later hardware removal.[35,70]

Coronoid Fractures

Isolated coronoid fractures are uncommon. Most are associated with other fractures or dislocation of the elbow.[35,79] The incidence is 2% to 10% with posterior elbow dislocations (Fig. 11-48). Instability after a coronoid fracture is common.[29]

Regan and Morrey[79] classified these fractures into three categories (Fig. 11-49). Type I fractures involve only the coronoid tip (Fig. 11-48). Type II fractures involved 50% or less of the coronoid and type III injuries, $>50\%$ of the coronoid. The fractures were further classified as A (no associated dislocation) or B (associated elbow dislocation).

Most displaced fractures can be identified on the lateral view. Subtle injuries may not be detected without CT or conventional tomography. The coronoid is frequently partially obscured on routine radiographs.[29]

Treatment

Types I and II fractures can be immobilized with a sling or cast for less than 3 weeks. Type III fractures are immobilized longer (≥ 4 weeks). Satisfactory results are reported in 72% of patients who do not have associated dislocations.[79]

Monteggia Fracture

Monteggia fractures involve the proximal ulna, with associated dislocation of the radial head (Fig. 11-50).[29] This injury comprises only 7% of ulnar fractures.[68,70,75]

Monteggia fractures were classified by Bado[28] into four categories. Type I lesions are ulnar fractures associated with anterior dislocation of the radial head. This is the most common category (50% to 75%), especially in children (Fig. 11-51). The radial head is dislocated posteriorly or posterolaterally in type II injuries. This injury is more common in adults, and the ulnar fracture is usually more proximal.[28,29] Type III injuries have lateral or anterolateral radial head dislocations (Fig. 11-50). This injury is also more common in children. Type IV lesions have an anteriorly dislocated radial head with fractures of the proximal radius and ulna.[28]

Usually, AP, lateral, and oblique radiographs are adequate for the diagnosis and classification of Monteggia

(*text continues on page 785*)

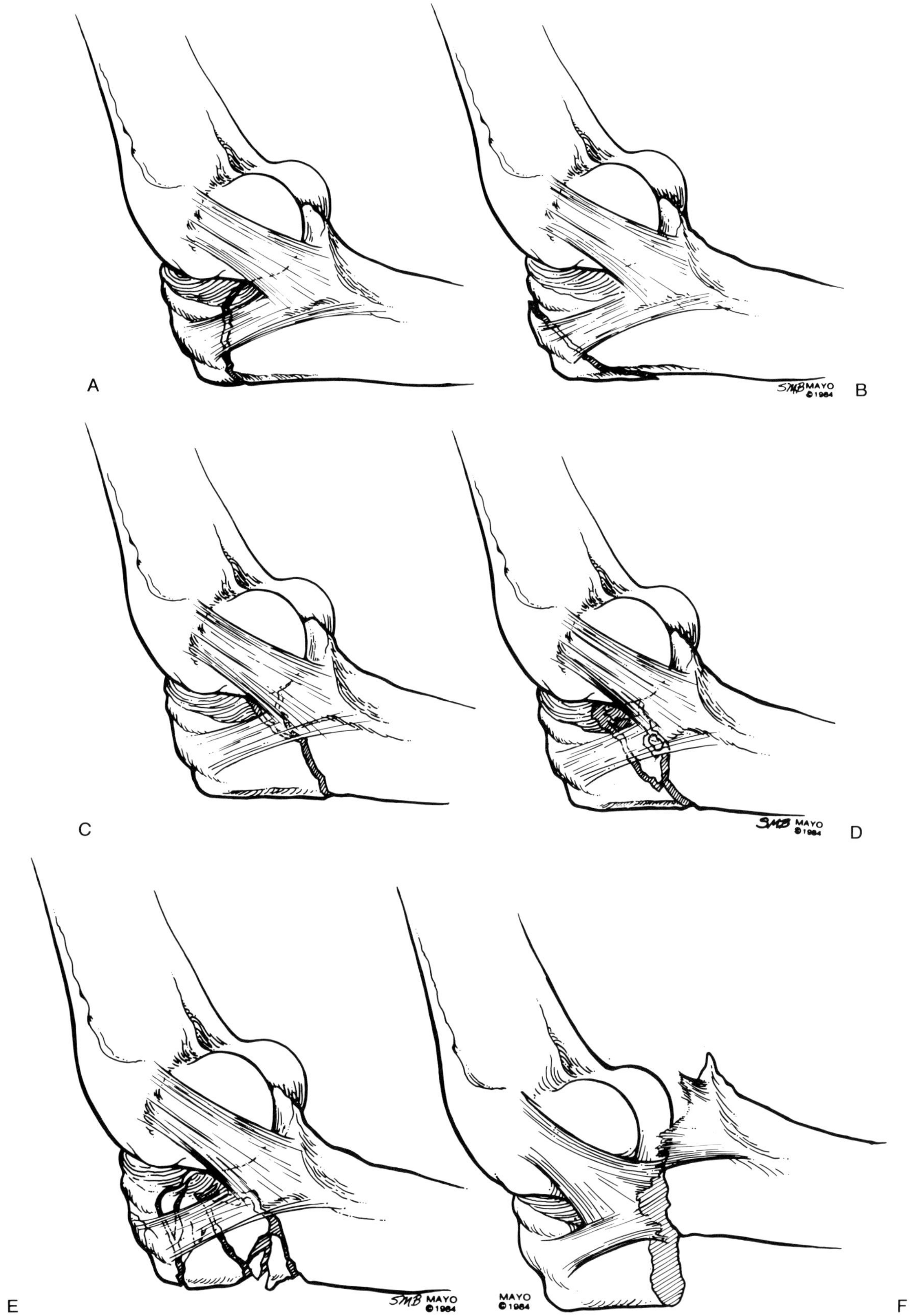

FIG. 11-40. Classification of olecranon fractures.[35,39,70] **A,B:** Avulsion fractures. **C,D:** Oblique fractures with joint involvement. **E:** Comminuted olecranon fracture. **F:** Fracture dislocation. (From Morrey BF, Berquist TH. The elbow. In: Berquist TH, ed. *Imaging of orthopedic trauma,* 2nd ed. New York: Raven Press, 1992;675–730.)

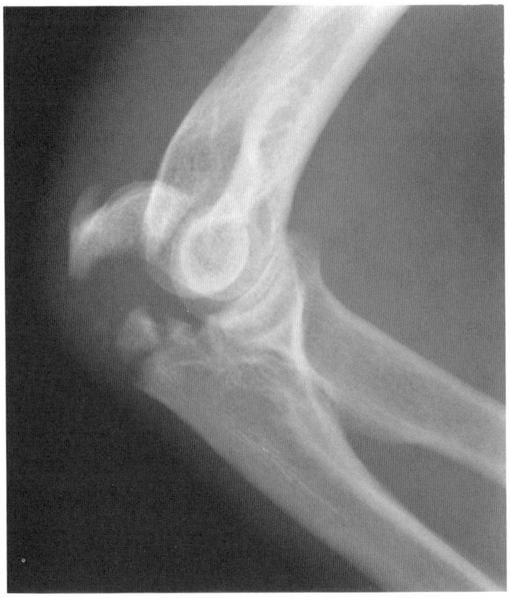

FIG. 11-41. Lateral radiograph demonstrating a comminuted displaced olecranon fracture.

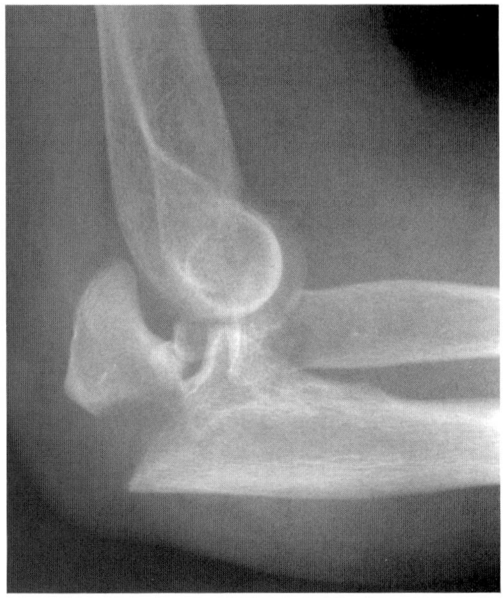

FIG. 11-42. Lateral radiograph demonstrating an olecranon fracture dislocation with radial head involvement.

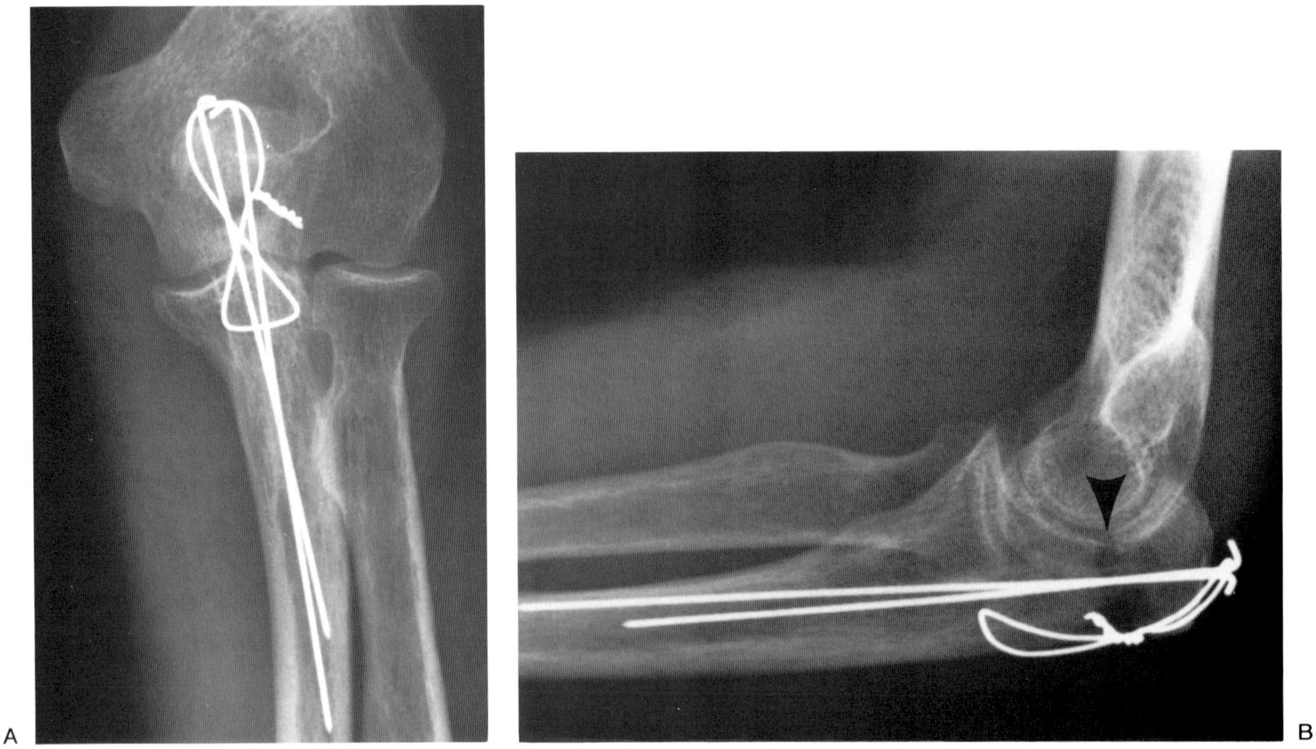

FIG. 11-43. The AP **(A)** and lateral **(B)** radiographs of an intraarticular olecranon fracture reduced with a tension-band and K-wire technique. There is slight (*arrow*) residual articular deformity.

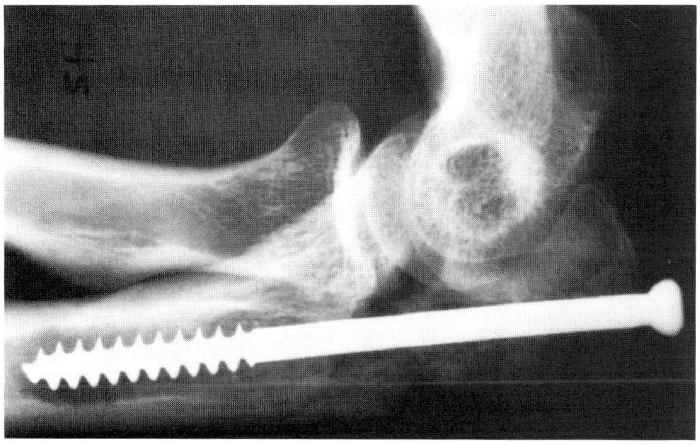

FIG. 11-44. Lateral radiograph demonstrating a displaced olecranon fracture internally fixed with a long cancellous screw. There is nonunion with a large lucent zone around the screw threads caused by loosening.

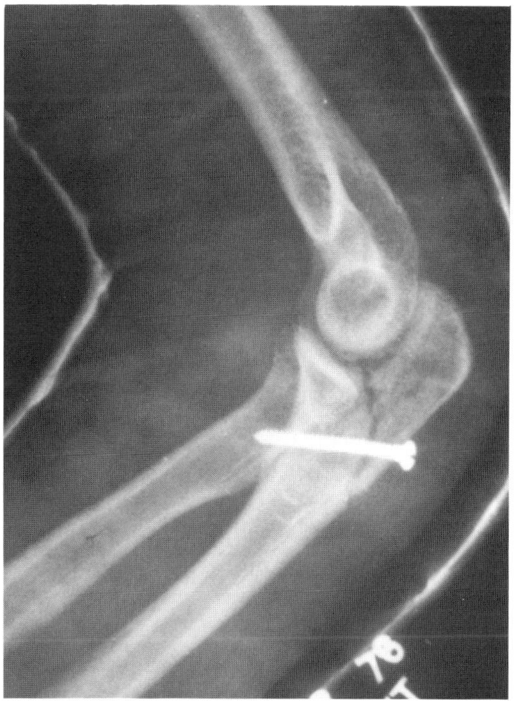

FIG. 11-45. Oblique olecranon fracture reduced with bicortical screw technique.

A 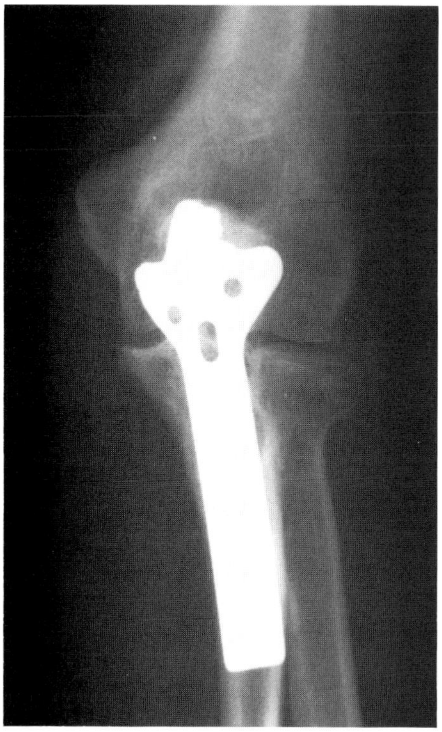

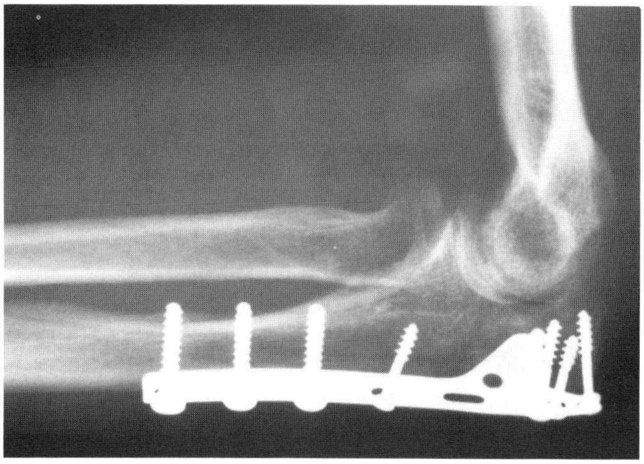 B

FIG. 11-46. The AP (A) and lateral (B) radiographs of an olecranon fracture with internal fixation using a cloverleaf plate and three distal cortical screws, with minicancellous screws proximally.

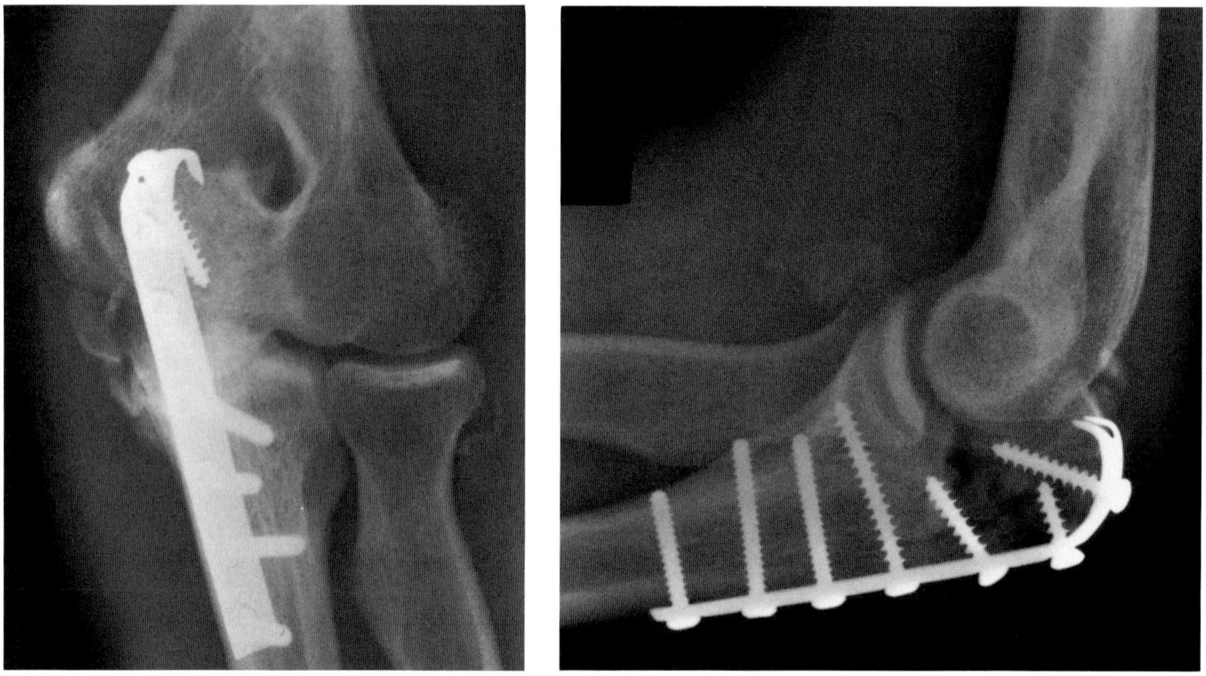

A B

FIG. 11-47. Comminuted olecranon fracture. The AP **(A)** and lateral **(B)** internally fixed with a shaped one-third tubular plate with a cut proximal end crimped into the bone. There are three distal cortical and four proximal cancellous screws.

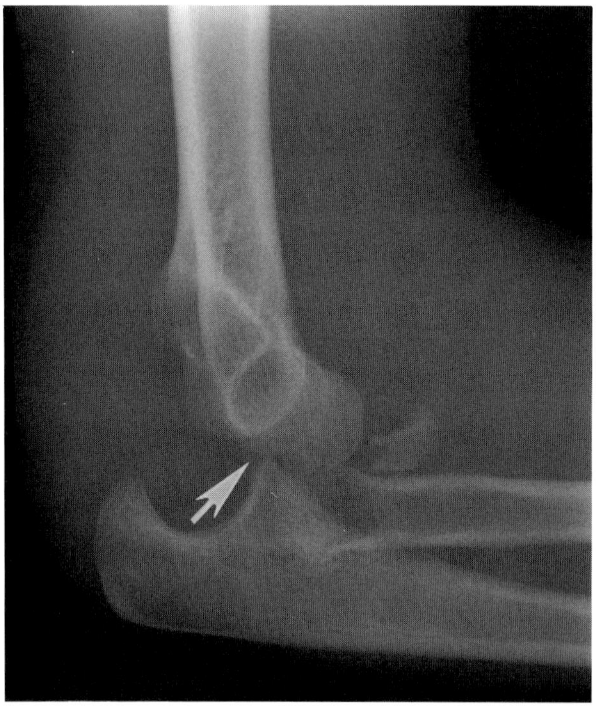

FIG. 11-48. Lateral view of the elbow with a posterior dislocation. There is an associated radial head fracture and a small type I (*arrow*) coronoid fracture.

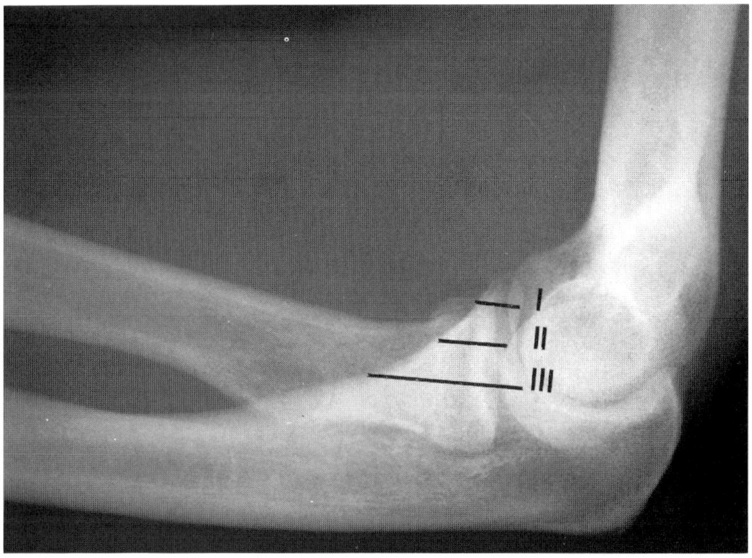

FIG. 11-49. Regan-Morrey classification of coronoid fractures. Type I, avulsion of the coronoid tip; type II, fracture involving 50% or less of the coronoid; type III, fractures involving greater than 50% of the coronoid. (From Berquist TH. *Imaging of orthopedic trauma*. New York: Raven Press, 1992.)

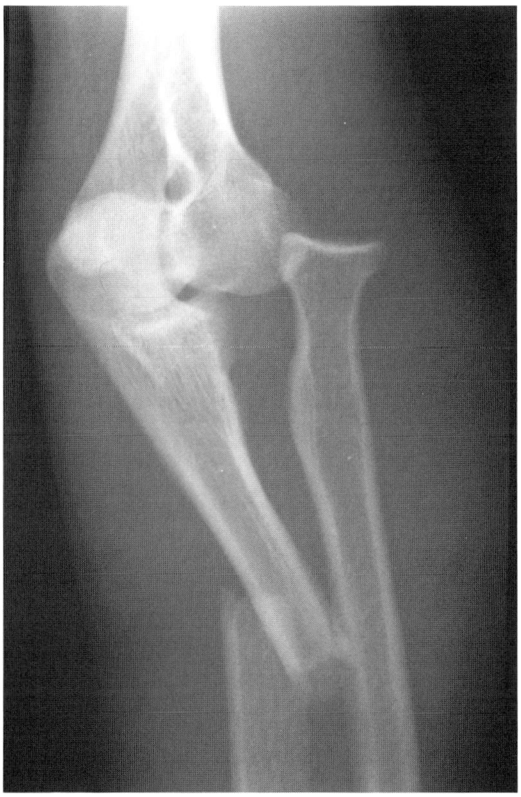

FIG. 11-50. An AP view of the elbow demonstrating an obvious Monteggia lesion with fracture of the ulna and dislocation of the radial head.

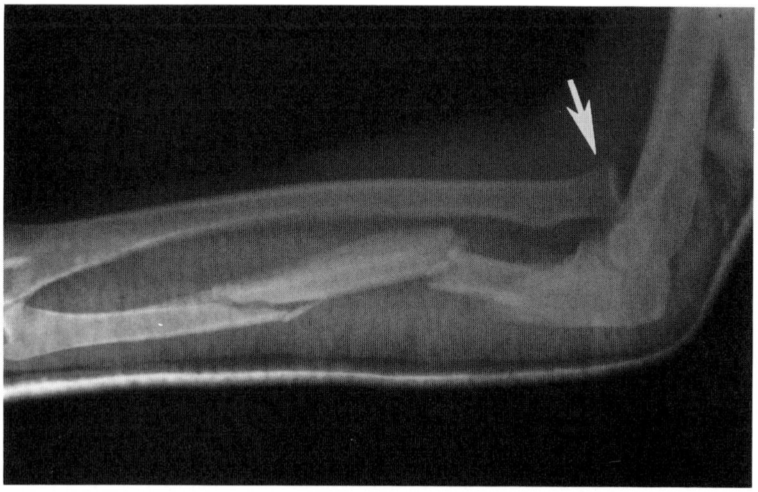

A

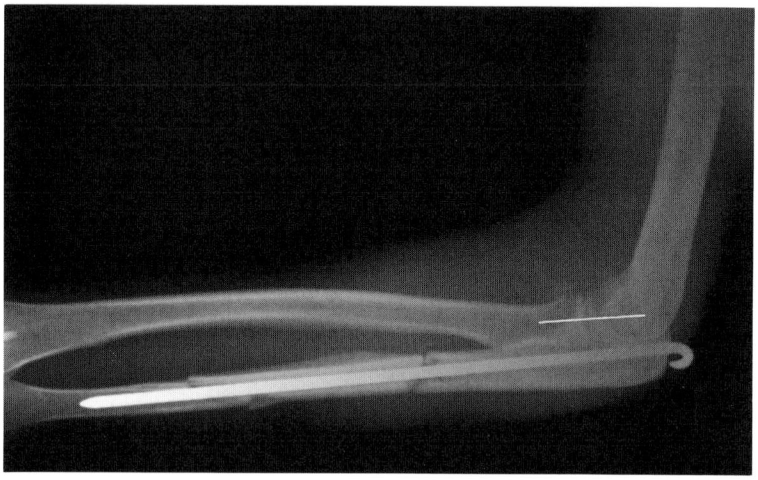

B

FIG. 11-51. Type I Monteggia lesion. **A:** Lateral radiograph with a comminuted ulnar fracture and anterior dislocation of the radial head (*arrow*). **B:** Internal fixation of the ulna was achieved with a Rush rod, and the radial head (*line* to capitellum) is reduced.

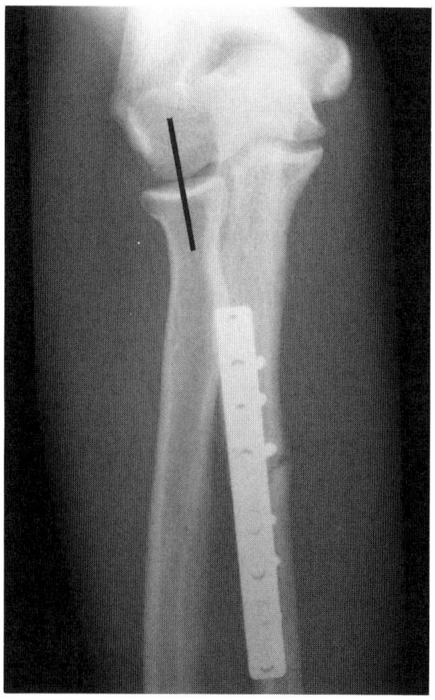

A

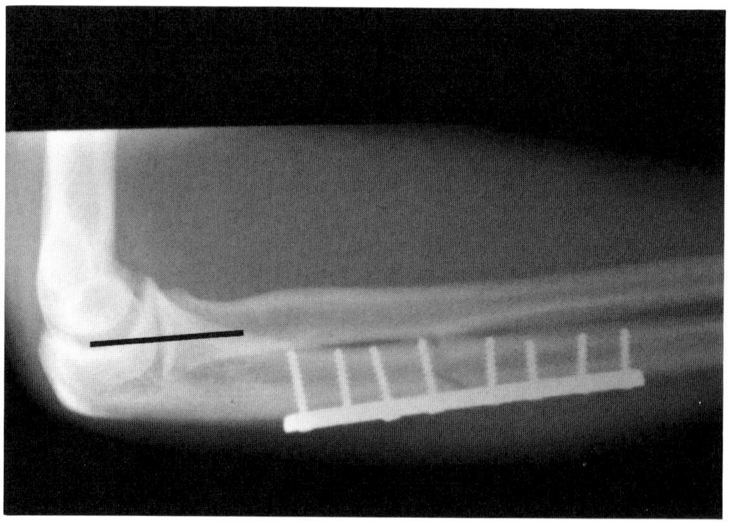

B

FIG. 11-52. Monteggia lesion with radial head (*line*) in normal position. The AP **(A)** and lateral **(B)** radiographs demonstrate DC plate fixation of the ulnar fracture.

injuries.[29] A dislocation may be inadvertently reduced prior to imaging, which results in an improper assessment of the severity of the injury. This occurs in about 16% of cases.[78]

Treatment

Closed treatment can be used for children and type I injuries.[28] Most authors prefer internal fixation of the ulnar fracture, using a compression plate and screw technique (Fig. 11-52).[28,34,35,78] Intramedullary nailing (Fig. 11-51) can also be used (see Chapter 12). Resection of the radial head may be required when radial head fracture is associated with the dislocation.[36]

Dislocations

Elbow dislocations are the most common dislocations in children and the second most common major joint dislocation in adults.[56,62] Most dislocations are caused by a fall on the outstretched upper extremity.[29,70,83] Posterior dislocations occur most frequently (Fig. 11-48). Anterior dislocations are rare and usually occur in children. The radius and ulna may also separate (divergent dislocation) with disruption of the interosseous membrane. This injury requires more significant trauma and is even rarer than an anterior dislocation.[42,62] Associated fractures are common.[38,72] Radial head and neck fractures occur in 5% to 10%; epicondylar avulsions, in 12%; and coronoid fractures, in 10% of elbow dislocations.[34,47,62,70,71,78] The fractures are treated based on the criteria described earlier. Most isolated dislocations are reduced by using closed techniques.

Postoperative Imaging and Complications

Routine radiographs should be obtained after closed or open reduction with internal fixation, using the same projections as the prereduction examination when possible.[29] This facilitates comparisons of the reduction and prereduction fragment positions and is useful to identify injuries overlooked on prereduction images (Fig. 11-53).

In children, the position of the distal fragment should be reviewed in supracondylar fractures. This can be accomplished on the lateral view. The AP view is used to evaluate the growth centers and Bauman's angle (Figs. 11-54 and 11-55).[59,70]

Routine radiographs are also used to evaluate arthrosis, heterotopic bone or calcification, myositis ossificans, cross-union, nonunion, and malunion.[22,29,35,43,69,70,71] Implant failures (Figs. 11-45 and 11-56) are also detected with routine views. In some cases, fluoroscopic positioning may be required.[29,62] In addition, CT is useful for evaluating early myositis ossificans and suspected nonunions.[29,60]

Stress views with or without arthrography are useful to evaluate postreduction instability (Figs. 11-57 and 11-58).[29]

Compartment syndrome, which is caused by hemorrhage and edema, neurovascular injury, avascular necrosis, physeal status, and certain other complications, requires additional studies.[25,27,29,70,71]

Neural injuries can occur with dislocation, Monteggia lesions, and distal humeral fractures.[25,27,58,62] Radial, ulnar, or medial nerves may be injured as a result of direct trauma or stretching. The median nerve may be trapped intraarticularly with dislocation.[62] When imaging is indicated, MRI is superior for evaluating neural, physeal, and periarticular soft tissue abnormalities. It is also most useful for the diagnosis of early avascular necrosis.[29]

Vascular injuries include intimal tears, thrombosis, and disruptions.[25,63,64] Angiography may be required to evaluate these injuries fully. Magnetic resonance angiography shows great promise and may provide a noninvasive means for evaluating vascular integrity.[29]

ELBOW ARTHROPLASTY

Elbow-replacement arthroplasty has evolved over many years with continued modification of implants and improving surgical techniques. Resection and interposition techniques were performed as early as 1885 primarily for tuberculosis.[91] Beginning in 1947, constrained or hinged implants began to be developed. From 1970 to 1975, cemented metal hinged replacement implants, similar in function to those developed for the knee (see Chapter 6), were used. Less constrained implants (semiconstrained and resurfacing systems) have been evolving since the mid-1970s, which has decreased the rate of implant failure and loosening.[91,104,114,123,124] Alternative procedures, such as resection arthroplasty and arthrodesis, are infrequently selected today if elbow-replacement arthroplasty can be accomplished.[90,114]

The choice of the implant and patient selection depends on clinical features (including age, activity level, and expectations) and the radiographic evaluation of bone and soft tissue disease.[90] The degree of pain, instability, and loss of motion are major determining factors.[90,95,97–98,122]

Patient Selection

In considering patient selection, we should remember that the goals of elbow-replacement arthroplasty are pain relief, improved stability, and mobility.[101,103] An arc of 30° to 130° of motion will provide the necessary function.[90,123]

The primary indications for replacement arthroplasty are rheumatoid arthritis, osteoarthritis, and posttraumatic arthritis.[90,103,114] The contraindications include

(*text continues on page 789*)

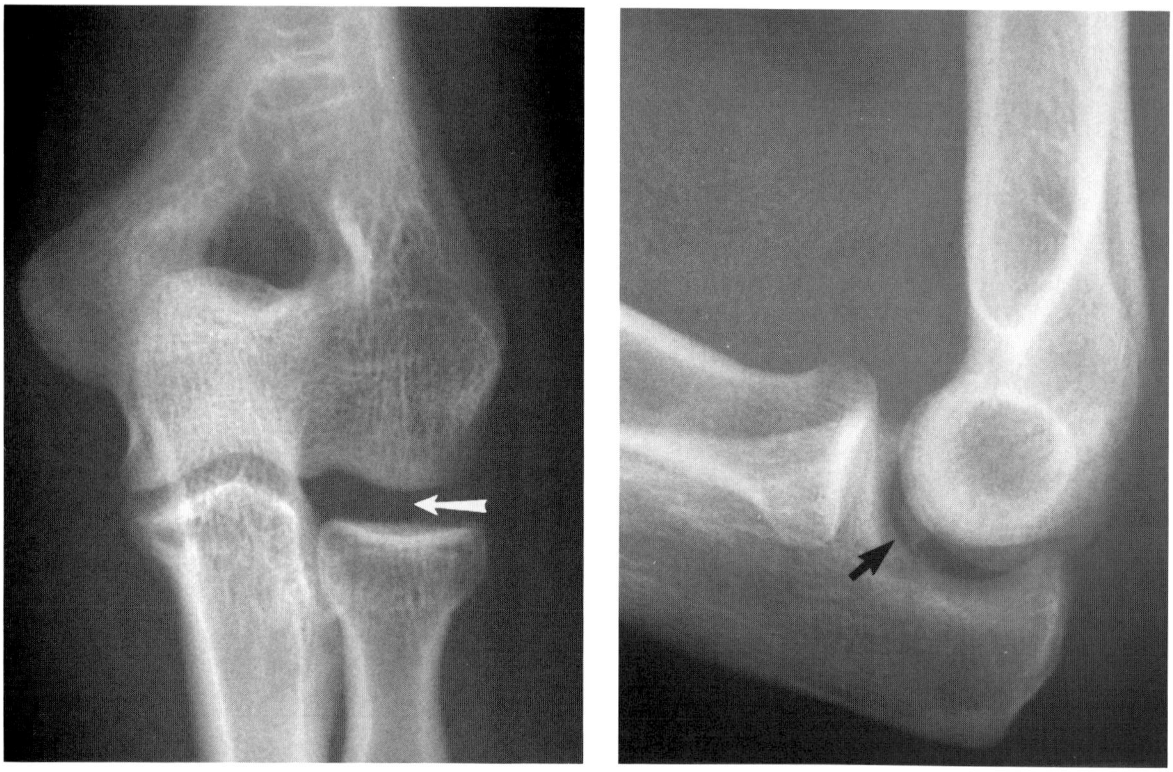

A B

FIG. 11-53. Postreduction views. **A:** An AP view in a patient with postreduction pain. Note the widened radiocapitellar joint caused by a subtle (*arrow*) osteochondrial fragment. **B:** Lateral view in a patient with persistent pain and snapping after reduction of a fracture dislocation. There is a bone fragment (*arrow*) in the joint space. In these situations, CT or CT arthrography would be useful to define the anatomy better.

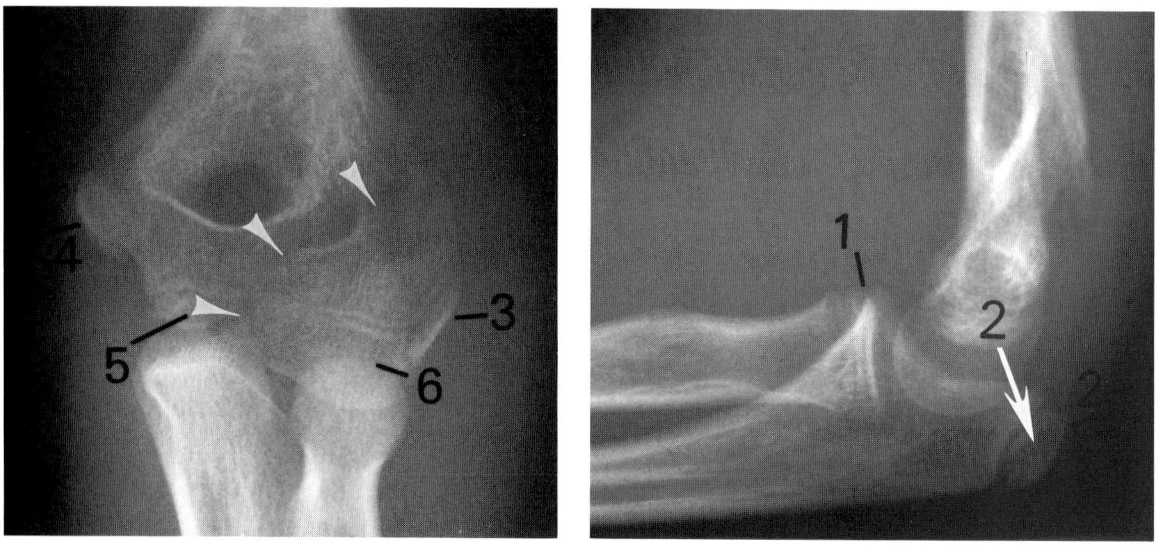

A B

FIG. 11-54. The AP **(A)** and lateral **(B)** radiographs after a Salter-Harris type IV fracture (*arrows*) of the lateral condyle. There is overgrowth of the distal lateral humerus, which neutralizes the carrying angle. Ossification centers: *1,* radial; *2,* olecranon; *3,* lateral epicondyle; *4,* medial epicondyle; *5,* trochlea; *6,* capitellum. Normal carrying angles:[59] in adults, 5° to 20°; average, 15°; in children aged 3 to 11 years, 0° to 11°; average, 5° to 6°.

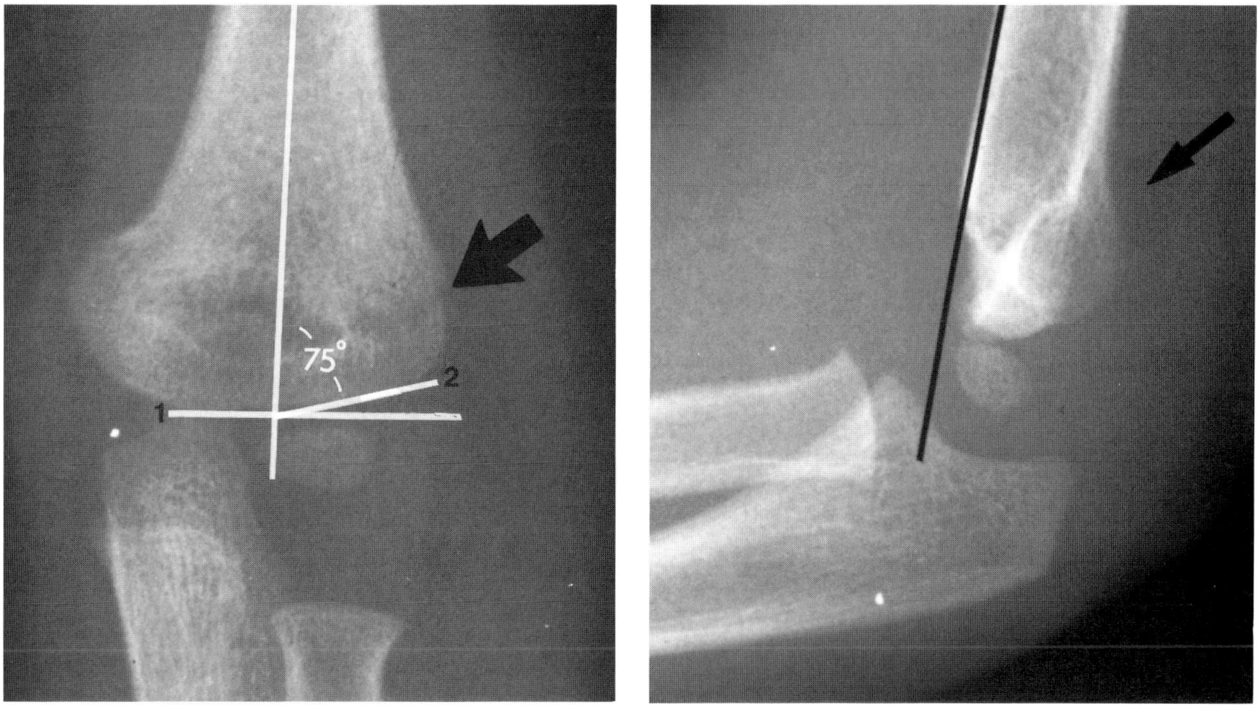

A B

FIG. 11-55. The AP **(A)** and lateral **(B)** postreduction views of a transcondylar fracture (*arrow*). The anterior humeral line (B) and Bauman's angle are demonstrated. Bauman's angle is formed by a line perpendicular to the humeral axis (*1*) and a line (*2*) tangential to the lateral humeral metaphysis. (Normal, 70° to 75°; both normal and injured side should be measured for comparison.)

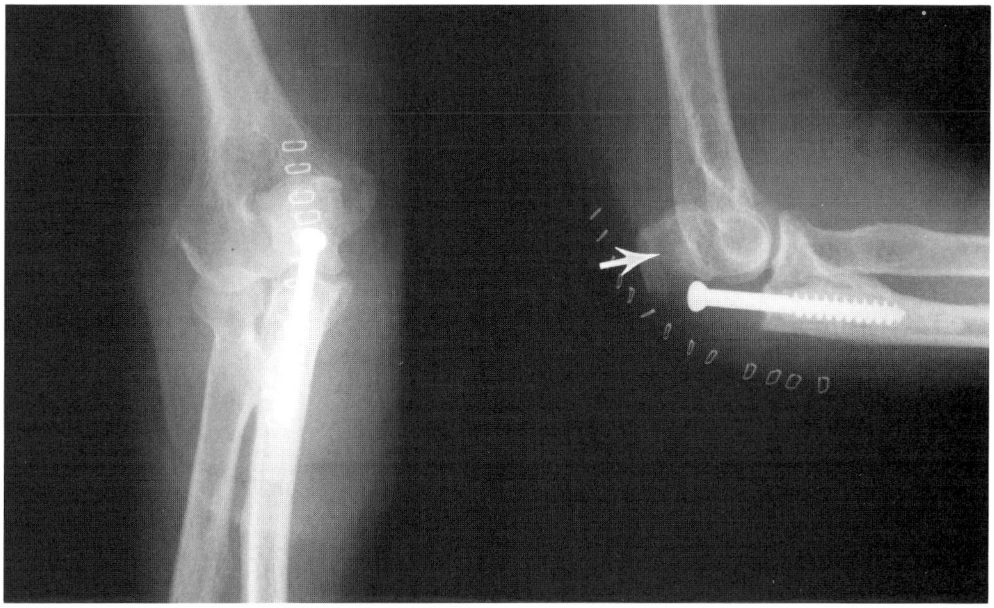

A B

FIG. 11-56. The AP **(A)** and lateral **(B)** views of a cancellous screw for fixation of an olecranon fracture. The olecranon has pulled free (*arrow*).

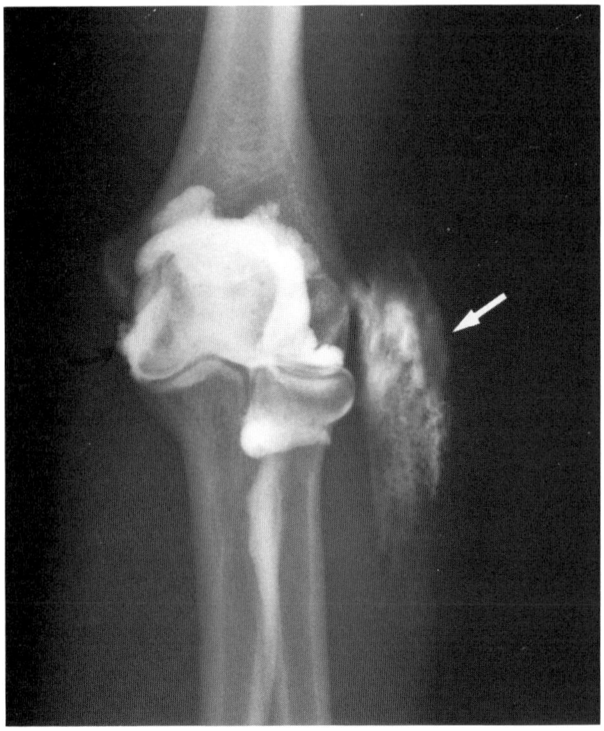

FIG. 11-57. An AP arthrographic view in a patient with a lateral capsular injury and instability. There is extravasation of contrast agent (*arrow*).

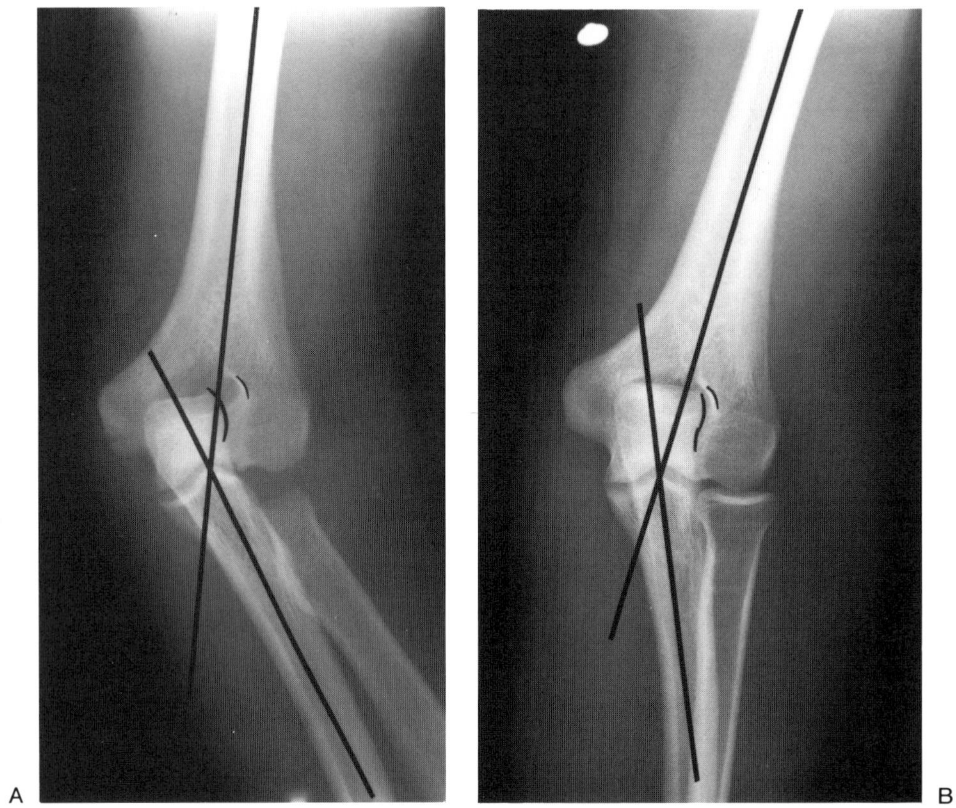

FIG. 11-58. Radial head resection following a type III fracture. Stress **(A)** view shows instability compared with a normal stress view **(B)**.

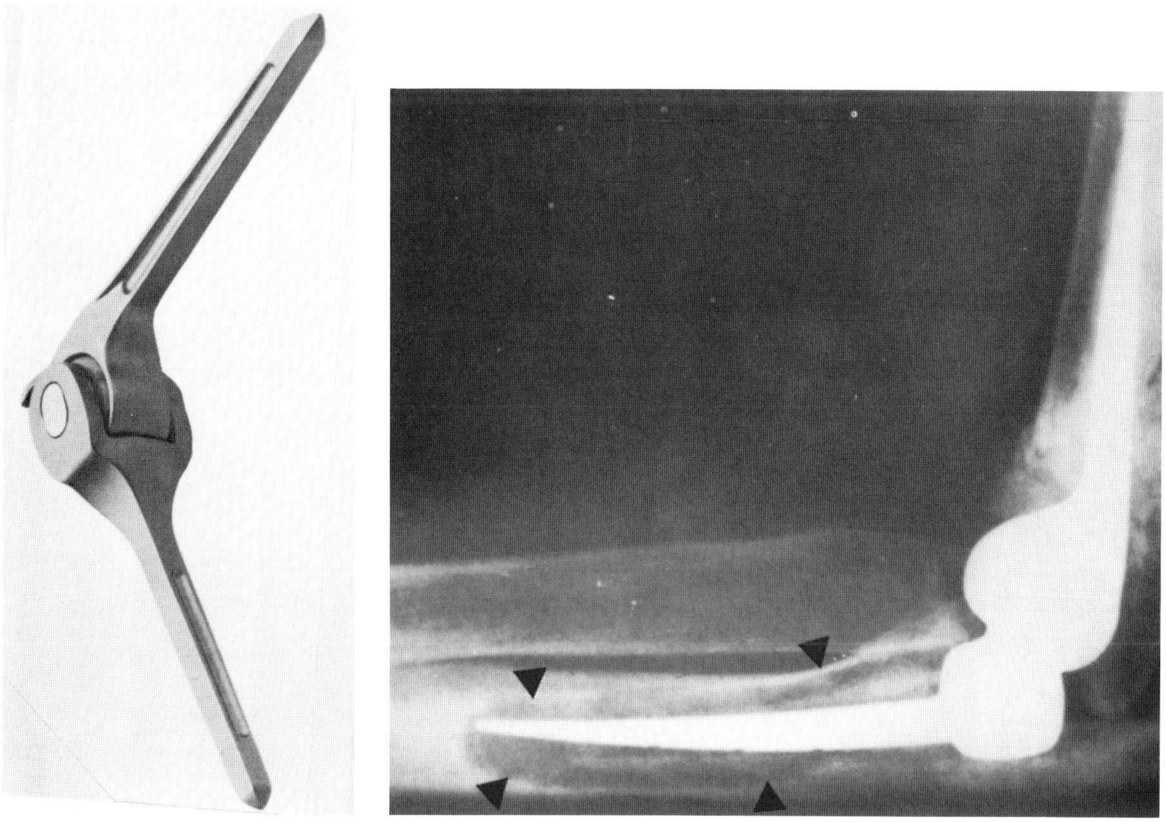

A B

FIG. 11-59. A: The Schlein hinged prosthesis. (Courtesy of Howmedica, Rutherford, NJ.) **B:** Lateral radiograph of a GSB hinged elbow system demonstrating a wide lucent zone at the bone-cement interface (*arrows*) caused by loosening. (From Garrett JC et al. Loosening associated with GSB hinge total elbow replacement in patients with rheumatoid arthritis. *Clin Orthop* 1977;127:170–174.)

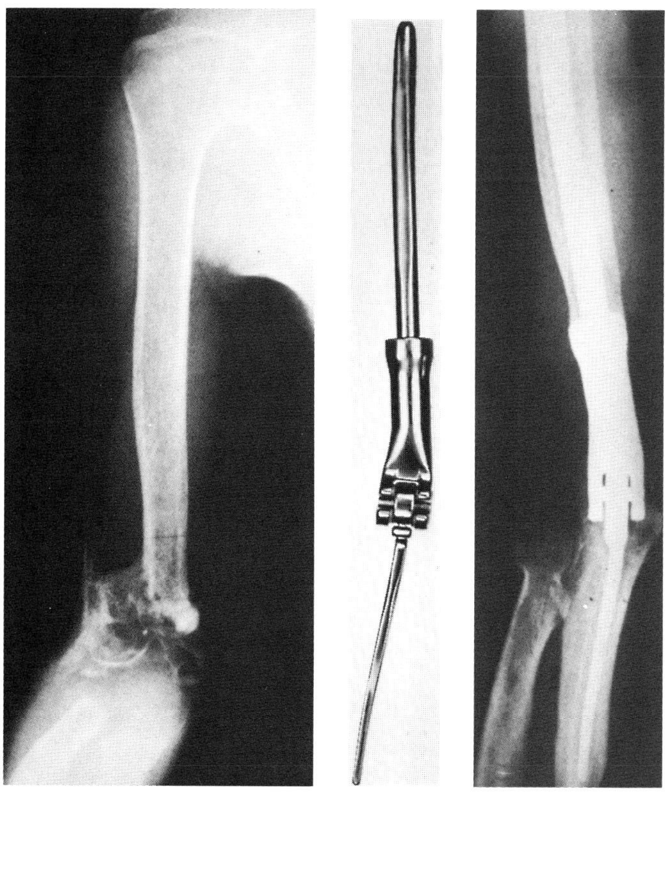

A,B,C

FIG. 11-60. Preoperative AP radiograph **(A)**, humeral replacement prosthesis with hinged articulation **(B)**, and postoperative radiograph with the system in place **(C)**. (From Ross AC, Sneath RS, Scales JT. Endoprosthetic replacement of the humerus and elbow joint. *J Bone Joint Surg* [*Br*] 1987;69B:652–655.)

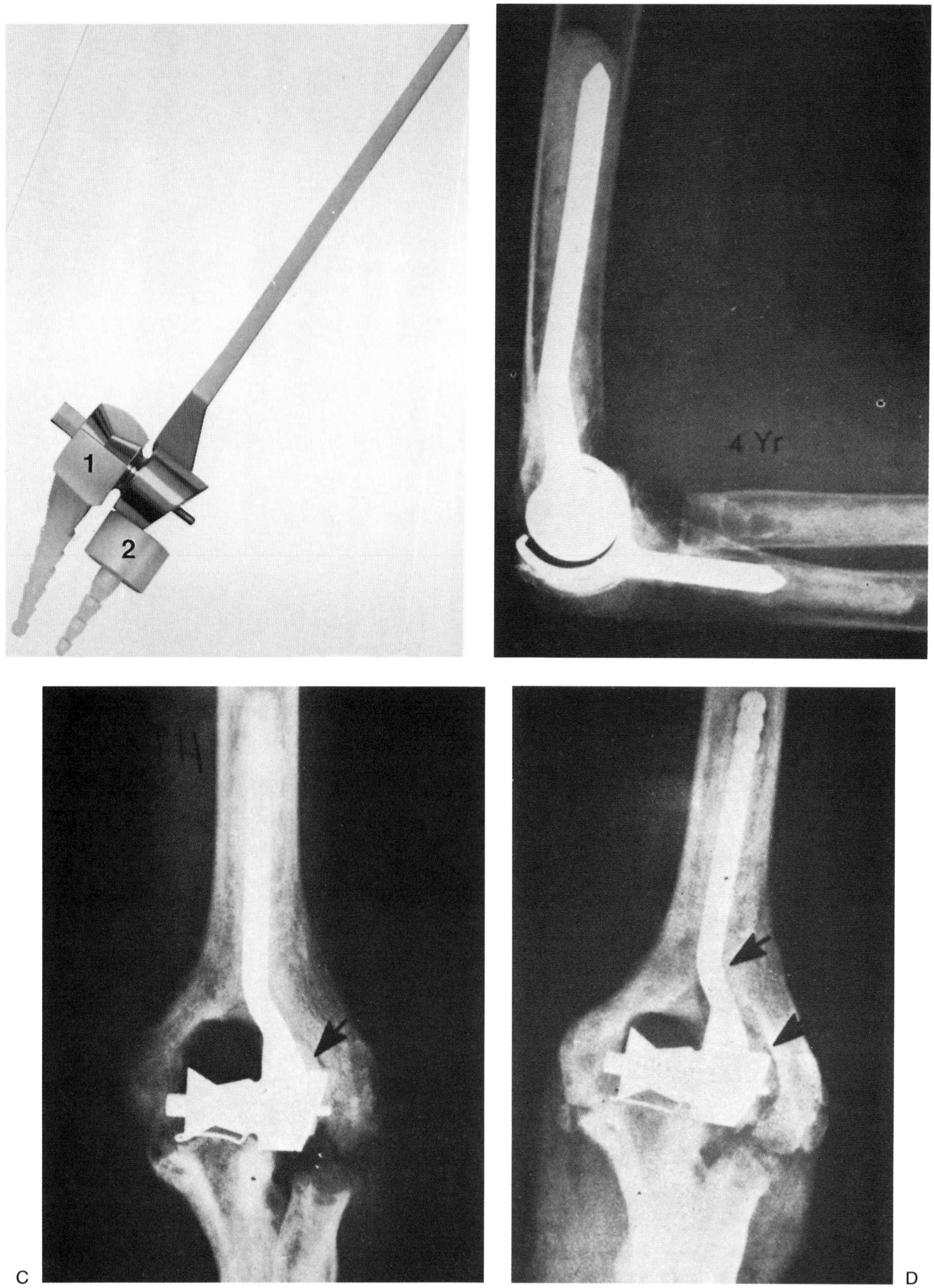

FIG. 11-61. Mayo elbow. **A:** The Mayo elbow with long humeral stem and snap-fit ulnar (*1*) and polyethylene (*2*) radial head component. The components are cemented. (Courtesy of Howmedica, Rutherford, NJ.) **B:** Lateral radiograph after Mayo implants. Cement extends beyond the component tips, with no loosening. An AP **(C)** view 1 year after surgery shows a lucent zone at the bone-cement interface (*arrow*). An AP radiograph **(D)** at 5 years shows progression of the lucent zone (*arrows*). No loosening clinically. (B–D: From Morrey BF, Bryan RS, Dobyns HJ, Linscheid RL. Total elbow arthroplasty. *J Bone Joint Surg* [*Am*] 1981;3A:1050–1063.)

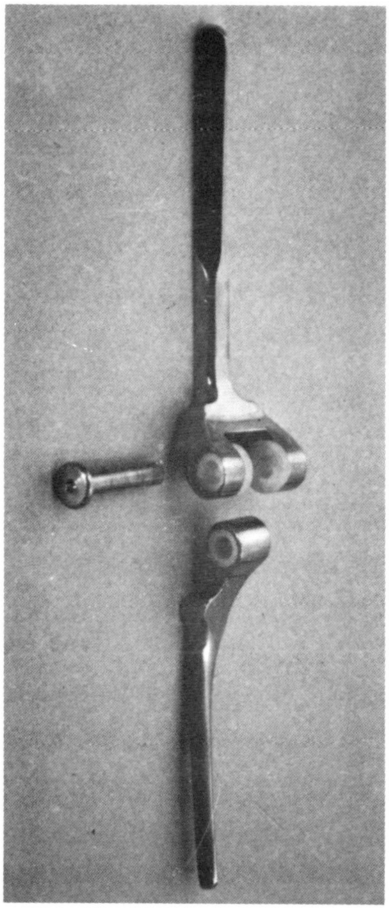

FIG. 11-62. The Coonrad hinged prosthesis with titanium stems and polyethylene bushings. (From Morrey BF, Bryan RS, Dobyns HJ, Linscheid RL. Total elbow arthroplasty. *J Bone Joint Surg* [*Am*] 1981;3A:1050–1063.)

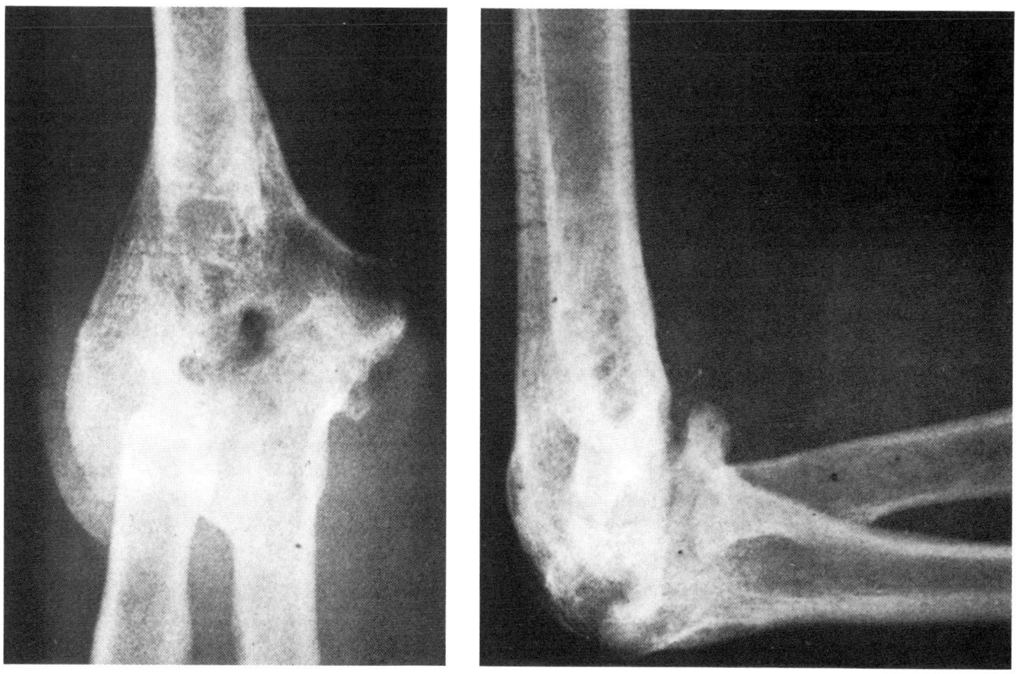

A B

FIG. 11-63. The AP **(A)** and lateral **(B)** radiographs in a 25-year-old man with advanced posttraumatic arthritis.

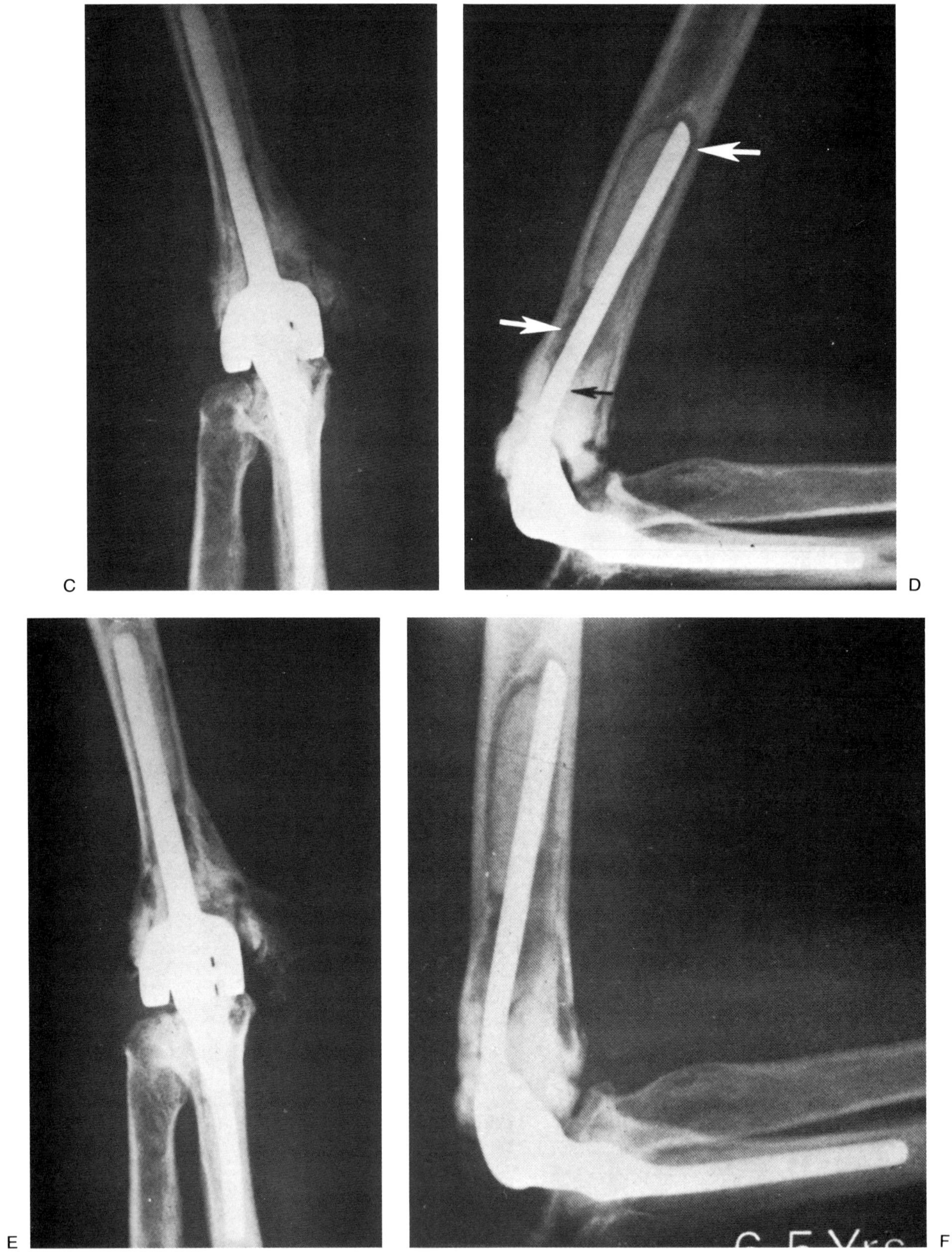

FIG. 11-63. (*Continued.*) The AP **(C)** and lateral **(D)** radiographs 2 years after insertion of a Coonrad prosthesis show lucency at the bone-cement (*white arrows*) and metal-cement interfaces (*black arrow*). The AP **(E)** and lateral **(F)** radiographs 5 years later show minimal progression. (From Morrey BF, Bryan RS, Dobyns HJ, Linscheid RL. Total elbow arthroplasty. *J Bone Joint Surg* [*Am*] 1981;3A:1050–1063.)

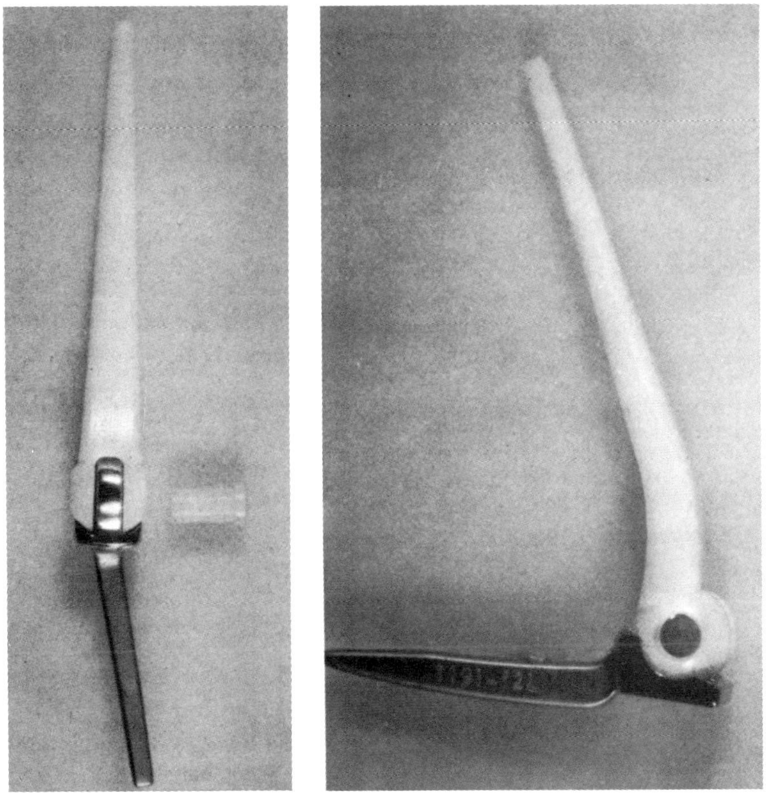

A,B

FIG. 11-64. Frontal **(A)** and side **(B)** photographs of the Pritchard-Walker prosthesis. (From Inglis AE. Tri-axial total elbow replacement: indications, surgical technique, and results. In: Inglis AE, ed. *American Academy of Orthopedic Surgery total joint replacement in the upper extremity*. St. Louis: CV Mosby, 1980;100–112.)

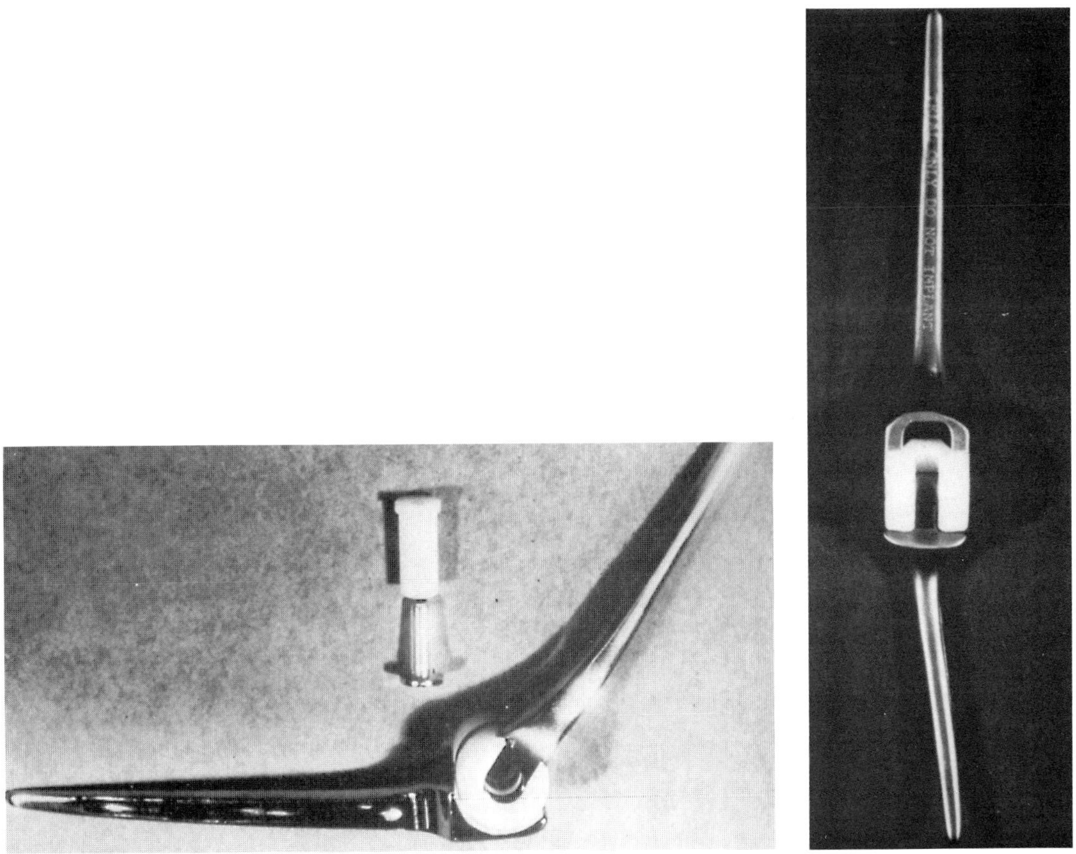

A B

FIG. 11-65. Triaxial elbow system. **A:** First generation: chromium-cobalt humeral and ulnar components articulate with a polyethylene axle; 10° to 12° of varus-valgus and 4° to 6° of rotational motion are possible. **B,C:** Second generation: a polyethylene bearing replaced the first-generation axle. (From Inglis AE. Tri-axial total elbow replacement: indications, surgical technique, and results. In: Inglis AE, ed. *American Academy of Orthopedic Surgery total joint replacement in the upper extremity*. St. Louis: CV Mosby, 1980;100–112.)

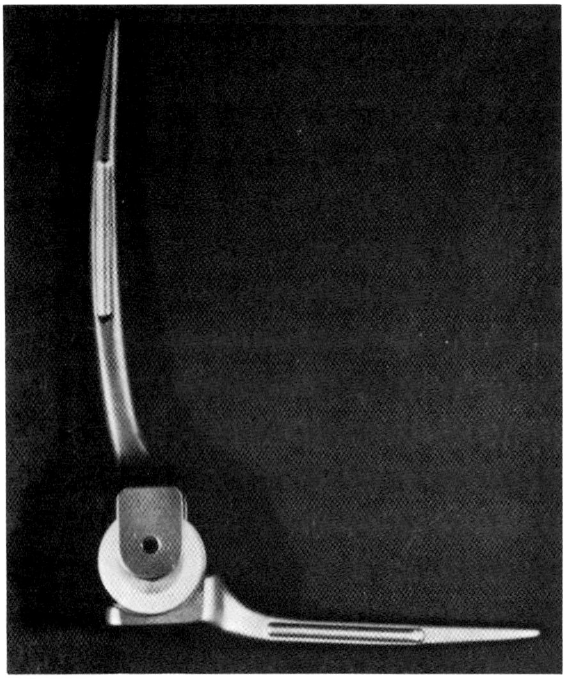

C

FIG. 11-65. *Continued.*

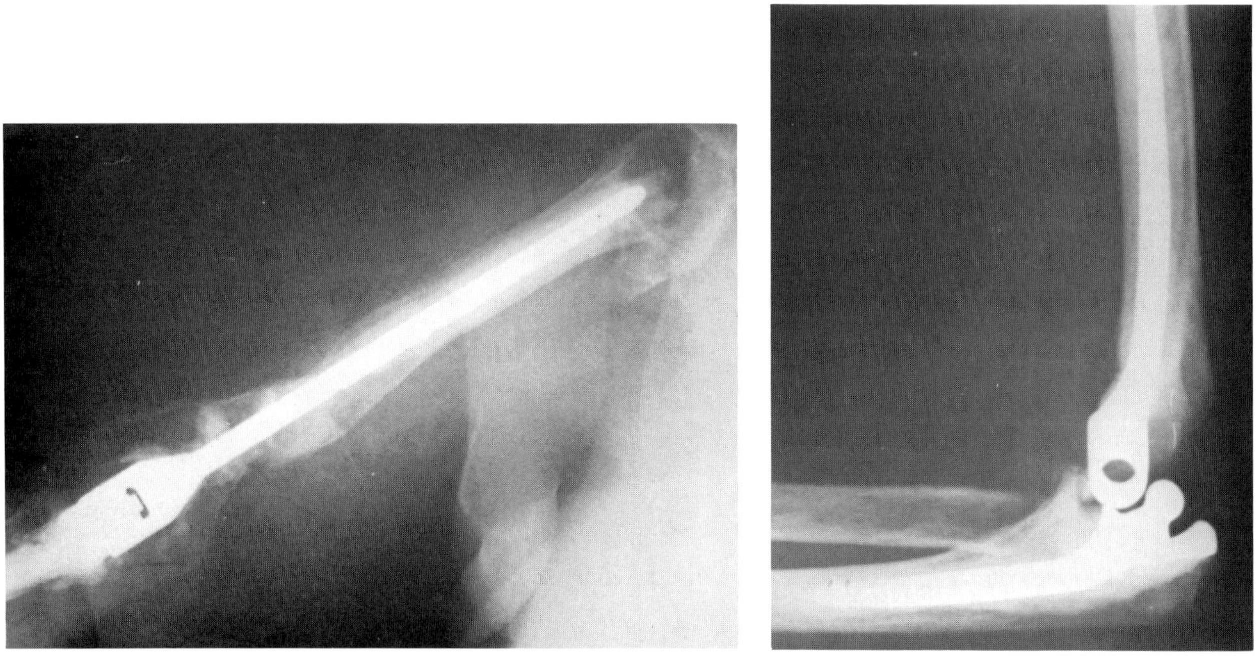

A B

FIG. 11-66. A: An AP radiograph of the long stemmed triaxial prosthesis. The humeral fracture is healed. **B:** Lateral radiograph of a failed triaxial implant as a result of a broken axle. (From Inglis AE. Tri-axial total elbow replacement: indications, surgical technique, and results. In: Inglis AE, ed. *American Academy of Orthopedic Surgery total joint replacement in the upper extremity.* St. Louis: CV Mosby, 1980;100–112.)

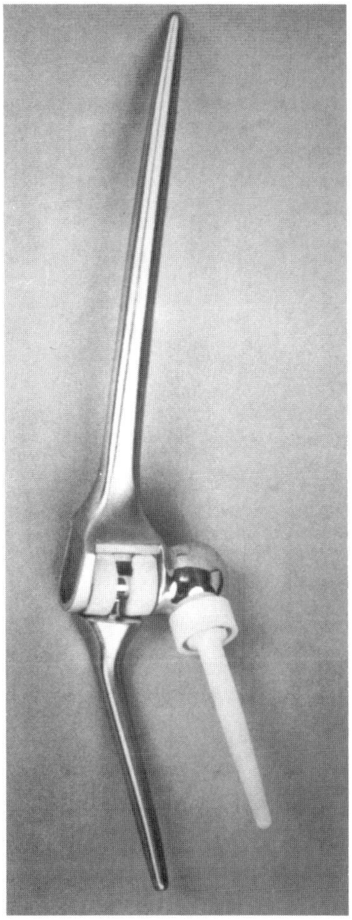

FIG. 11-67. The AHSC (Volz) elbow prosthesis. Cobalt-chromium ulnar and humeral components, a polyethylene snap-fit interface, and polyethylene radial component. (From Brumfield RH, Volz RG, Green JF. Total elbow arthroplasty: a clinical review of 30 cases employing the Mayo and AHSC prosthesis. *Clin Orthop* 1981;158:137–141.)

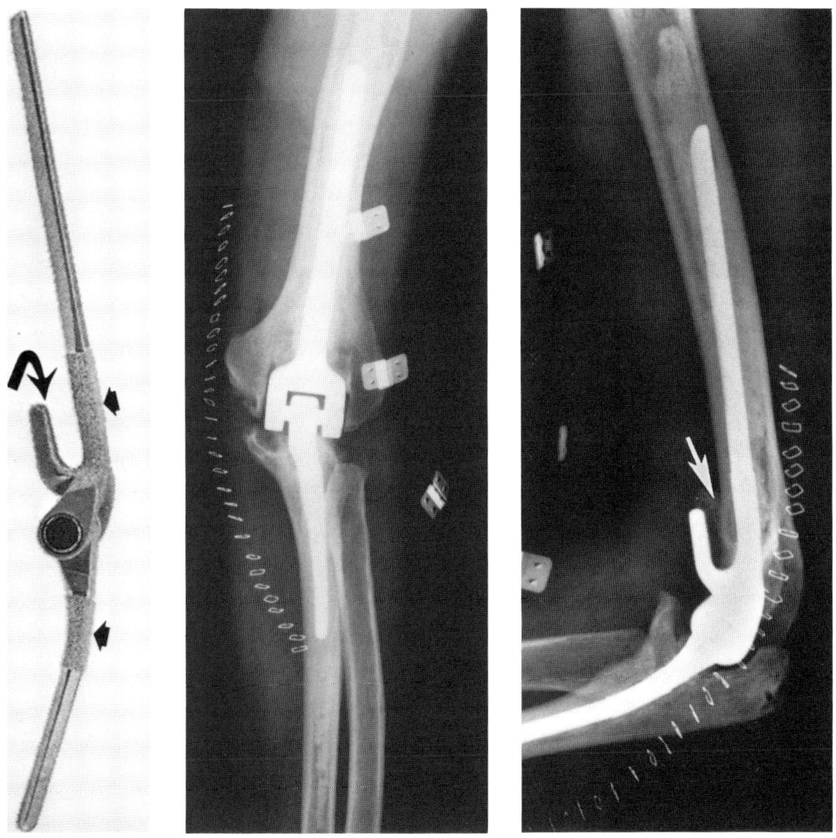

A,B,C

FIG. 11-68. A: The Coonrad-Morrey elbow system. Loose polyethylene hinge, beaded stems segments (*arrows*), and anterior extension (*curved arrow*) differ from the original Coonrad design. (Courtesy of Zimmer, Warsaw, IN.) The AP **(B)** and lateral **(C)** radiographs of the Coonrad-Morrey elbow. Note the bone graft (*arrow*) between the humerus and anterior extension.

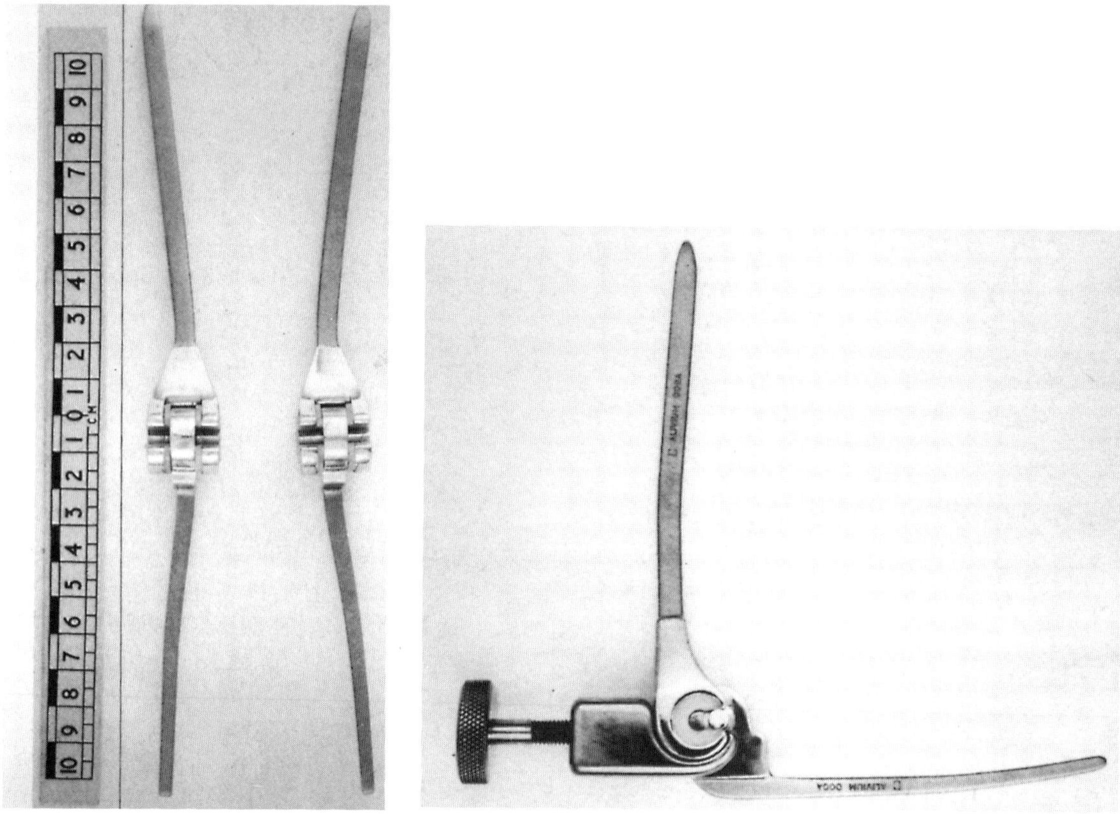

A B

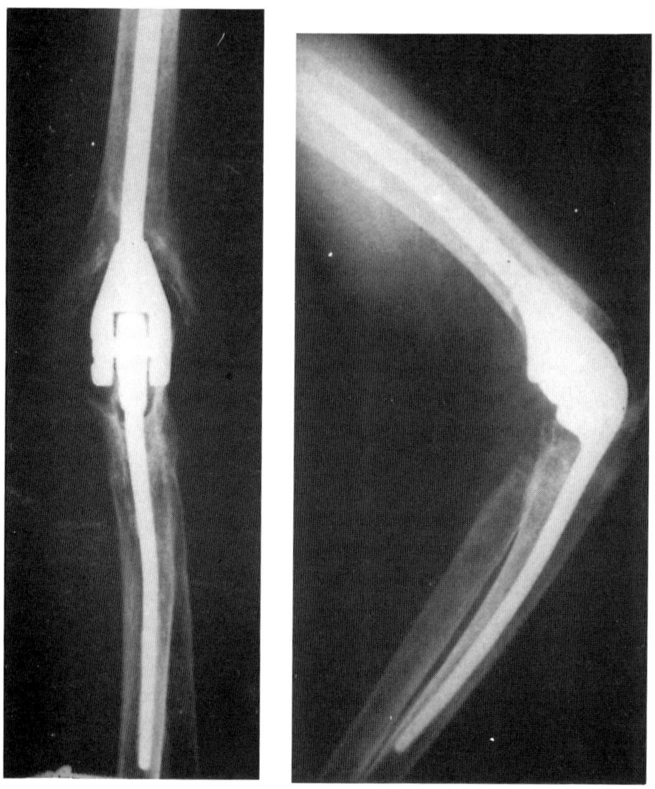

C,D

FIG. 11-69. Stanmore total elbow system. **A:** Components for the right and left elbow assembled with offsets for the normal carrying angles of the elbow. **B:** Components seen from the side with disarticulating tool in place. The AP **(C)** and lateral **(D)** radiographs with components in place. The system resembles the Morrey elbow on the AP radiograph. However, the anterior extension seen on the lateral radiograph (Fig. 11-68C) allows easy identification of the Morrey system. (From Johnson JR, Getty CJM, Lettin AWF, Glasgow MMS. The Stanmore total elbow replacement for rheumatoid arthritis. *J Bone Joint Surg [Br]* 1984;66B:732–736.)

This design was used primarily for patients with rheumatoid arthritis. Good results were achieved in 77% of patients.[105]

Unconstrained (Resurfacing) Systems

Unconstrained or resurfacing implants are designed to reproduce the anatomy of the normal sigmoid notch and condylar surface.[101,110] The original designs were stemless (Fig. 11-70), but today most have stems to improve fixation. This type of system is not usually effective in patients with poor bone stock or ligament instability.[96,101,108,109]

Capitellocondylar (Ewald) Elbow System[95–99]

The original Ewald system (1973) shown in Figure 11-70A did not have stems. The most recent design (Fig. 11-70B) has stems on both components.[98] Initial experience demonstrated satisfactory results in 87% of patients.[95] Newer stem designs provide greater implant stability.[110]

Souter-Strathclyde™ (Howmedica, Rutherford, NJ)[89,95,106,117,121]

The ulnar component is constructed of ultrahigh molecular weight polyethylene. The humeral component is Vitallium™ with medial and lateral epicondylar projections (Fig. 11-71). The ulnar component is designed so there is 8° of valgus angulation when the elbow is extended and 6° with flexion to maintain the normal carrying angle. As with other unconstrained components, pain relief and improved motion were achieved. Instability and dislocation can be as high as 14%. Pöll and Rozing[117] reported dislocations in 9% of their patients.

ERS™ (DePuy, Warsaw, IN)[110,118,119]

This system designed by Pritchard and consists of three components (Fig. 11-72). The humeral component is cobalt-chromium with a stem aligned in 8° of valgus.[118,119] The ulnar and radial components have partially porous surfaces with snap-fit polyethylene inserts. The radial and ulna inserts comes in various thicknesses to improve stability and flexibility at surgery.[118] Linscheid[110] reported improved motion (39° to 123°) and pain relief in patients postimplant.

Kudo Hingeless Prosthesis[95,108,109]

The original prosthesis was designed and used in the early 1970s (type I). The humeral component was stainless steel and fit the condylar configuration. The ulnar component was polyethylene with a short stem. A later modification (Fig. 11-73) has a saddle-shaped condylar component with an all-polyethylene ulnar component and a heel-type stem. Kudo et al.[108,109] have used this system primarily in patients with rheumatoid arthritis (Fig. 11-74). The results were excellent in 53% of patients and fair in 36% of the initial series.[95]

Guildford Elbow[107]

The Guildford elbow has dual components to replace the humeroulnar joint. The radial head is resected. The humeral component (Fig. 11-75) is chromium-cobalt-molybdenum and the ulnar, polyethylene. The components have a narrow appearance on the AP radiograph (Fig. 11-76). Pain relief was reported in 82% and improved function, in 73% of 44 cases. However, revision was necessary in 12%.[107]

Other metal-to-polyethylene unconstrained designs (Table 11-3) include the London, Liverpool nonblocked (West Germany), and Isizaki (Japan) designs.[95]

Postoperative Imaging and Complications

The complications that occur with elbow-replacement arthroplasty do not affect the eventual outcome in most cases. They may be related to the disease process, type of implant (unconstrained, semiconstrained, or constrained), surgical technique (Fig. 11-77), and of course, patient compliance.[101,107,112,114] Table 11-4 summarizes the complications of total elbow arthroplasty.

Loosening is a more common problem in the humeral than in the ulnar component. However, the incidence is still low (1% to 2%) for semiconstrained components. Loosening is common with constrained metal hinge components (23% to 31%).[92,99,114,115] Progressive lucency at the bone-cement interface to > 2 mm is indicative of loosening. However, lucent areas, especially at the artic-

TABLE 11-4. *Elbow arthroplasty: complications*[92,94–98,101,109,112–116]

Complication	Incidence rate (%)
Loosening	
Semiconstrained	1–2
Constrained	23–31
Instability	5–18
Implant failure	
Component fracture	1
Linkage failure	3
Infection (deep)	1–5
Ulnar nerve injury	
Permanent	2
Transient	22–26
Cortex penetration (30% for revision systems)	5–30
Triceps deficiency	5

(*text continues on page 807*)

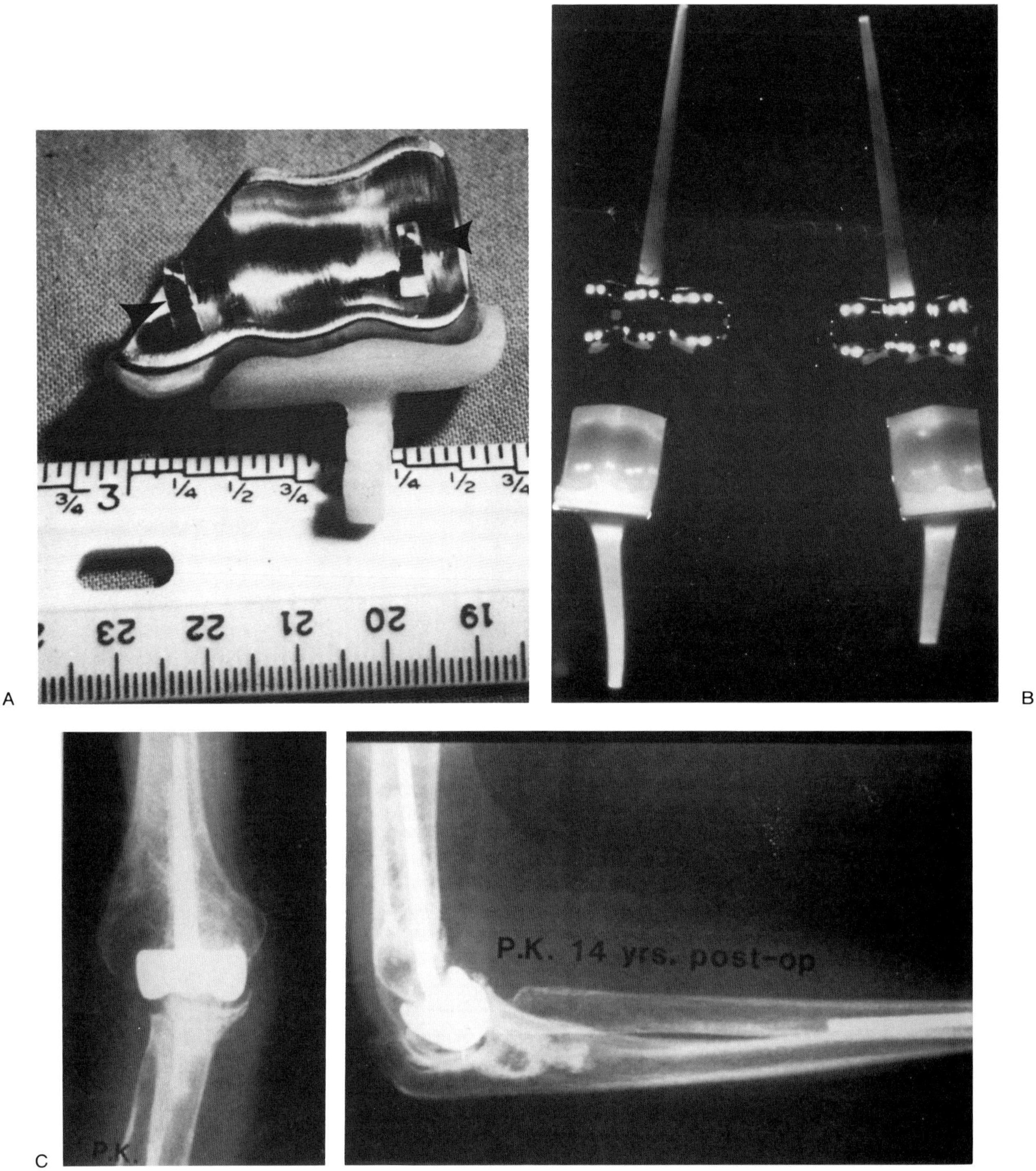

FIG. 11-70. **A:** Prototype resurfacing arthroplasty developed in 1973. There are two short pegs on the condylar resurfacing component (*arrows*) but no stem. There is a short stem on the polyethylene ulnar component. **B:** Latest generation capitellocondylar design with humeral and ulnar stems. The ulnar stem on the left is longer. Both are angled to maintain the normal carrying angle of the elbow. **C:** The AP and lateral radiographs 14 years after a capitellocondylar implant with a polyethylene ulnar component. There is no evidence of loosening. (From Ewald FC, Simmons ED, Sullivan JA, et al. Capitellocondylar total elbow replacement in rheumatoid arthritis. *J Bone Joint Surg* [*Am*] 1993;75A:498–507.)

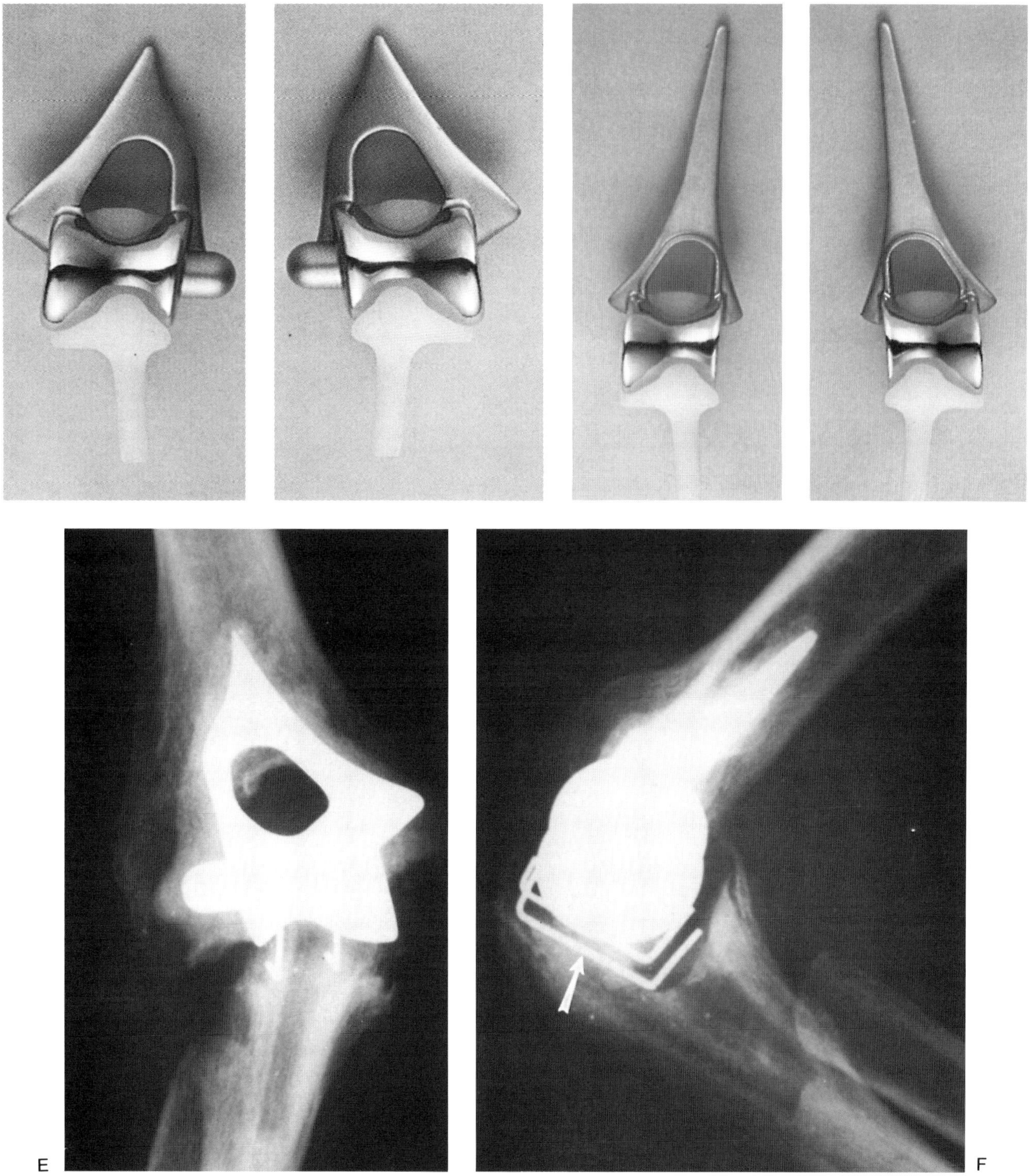

A,B C,D

E F

FIG. 11-71. Souter-Strathclyde^{TM} elbow. (Courtesy of Howmedica, Rutherford, NJ.) The large left **(A)** and right **(B)** components. Long stem, medium sized left **(C)** and right **(D)**. The AP **(E)** and lateral **(F)** radiographs of a Souter-Strathclyde^{TM} elbow at 10 years. The heel portion of the olecranon component has wire markers (*arrow*). Both components are cemented.

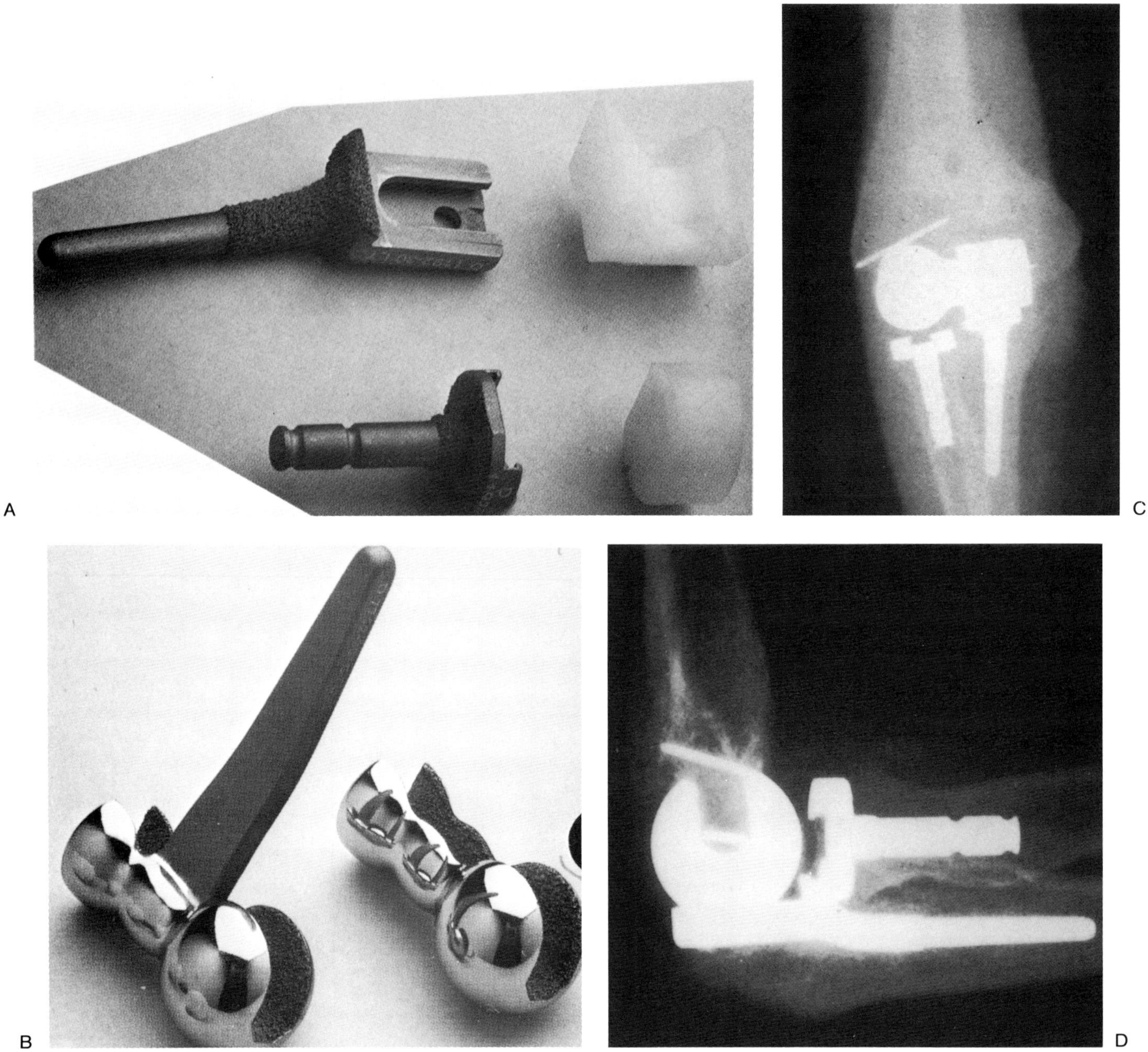

FIG. 11-72. ERS™ (Pritchard). (Courtesy of DePuy, Warsaw, IN.) **A:** Ulnar and radial components with snap-fit polyethylene bearings. The proximal ulnar stem is porous coated. Polyethylene bearings come in several thicknesses. **B:** Universal (*right*) and stemmed (*left*) humeral components with anatomic trochlear and capitellar surfaces. The AP **(C)** and lateral **(D)** radiographs demonstrating a universal nonstemmed humeral component.

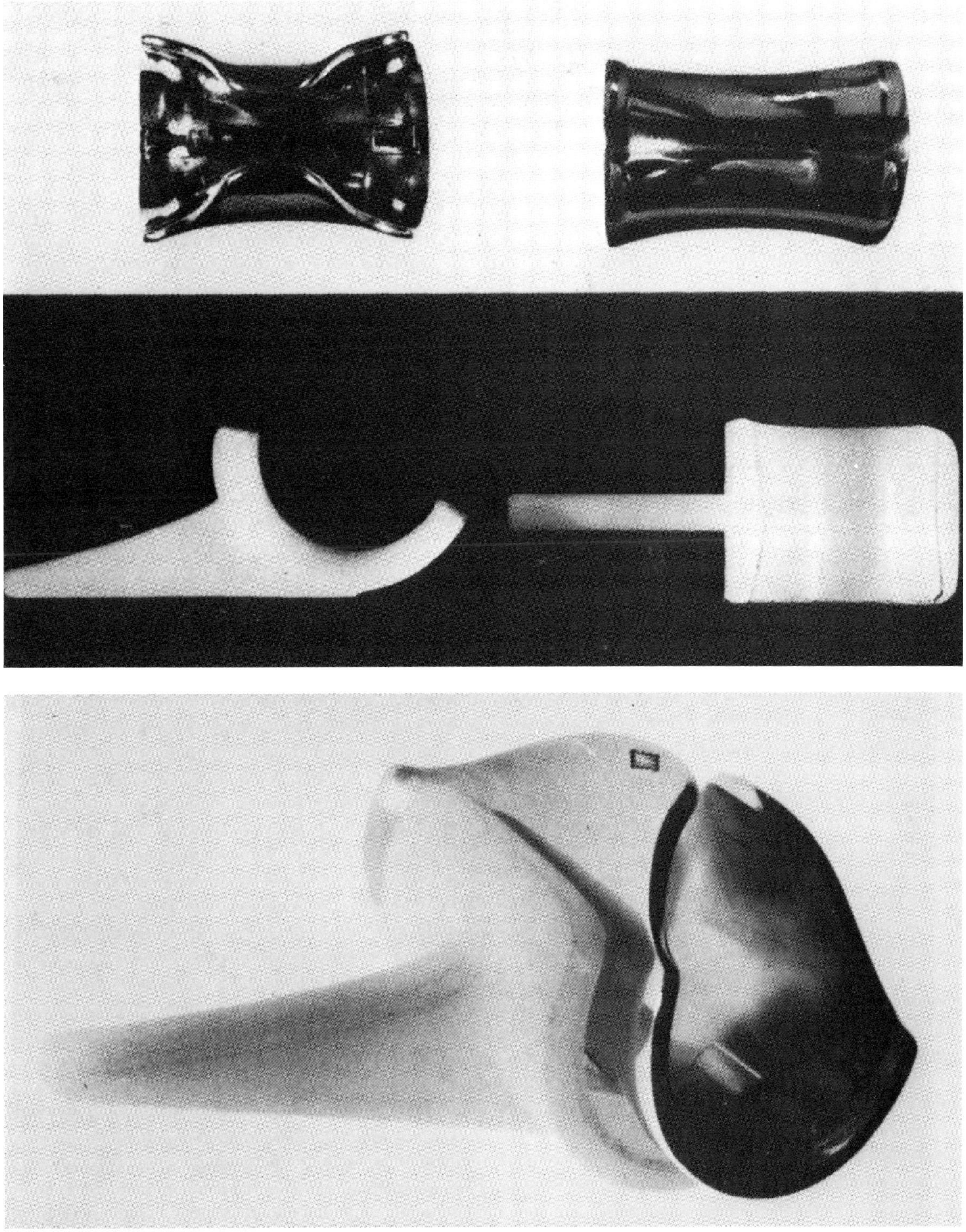

A

B

FIG. 11-73. Kudo hingeless prosthesis type 2. **(A)** The humeral and ulnar components disarticulated. **(B)** Components articulated. (From Kudo H, Iwano K, Watanobe S. Total replacement of the rheumatoid elbow with a hingeless prosthesis. *J Bone Joint Surg* [*Am*] 1980;62A:277–285.)

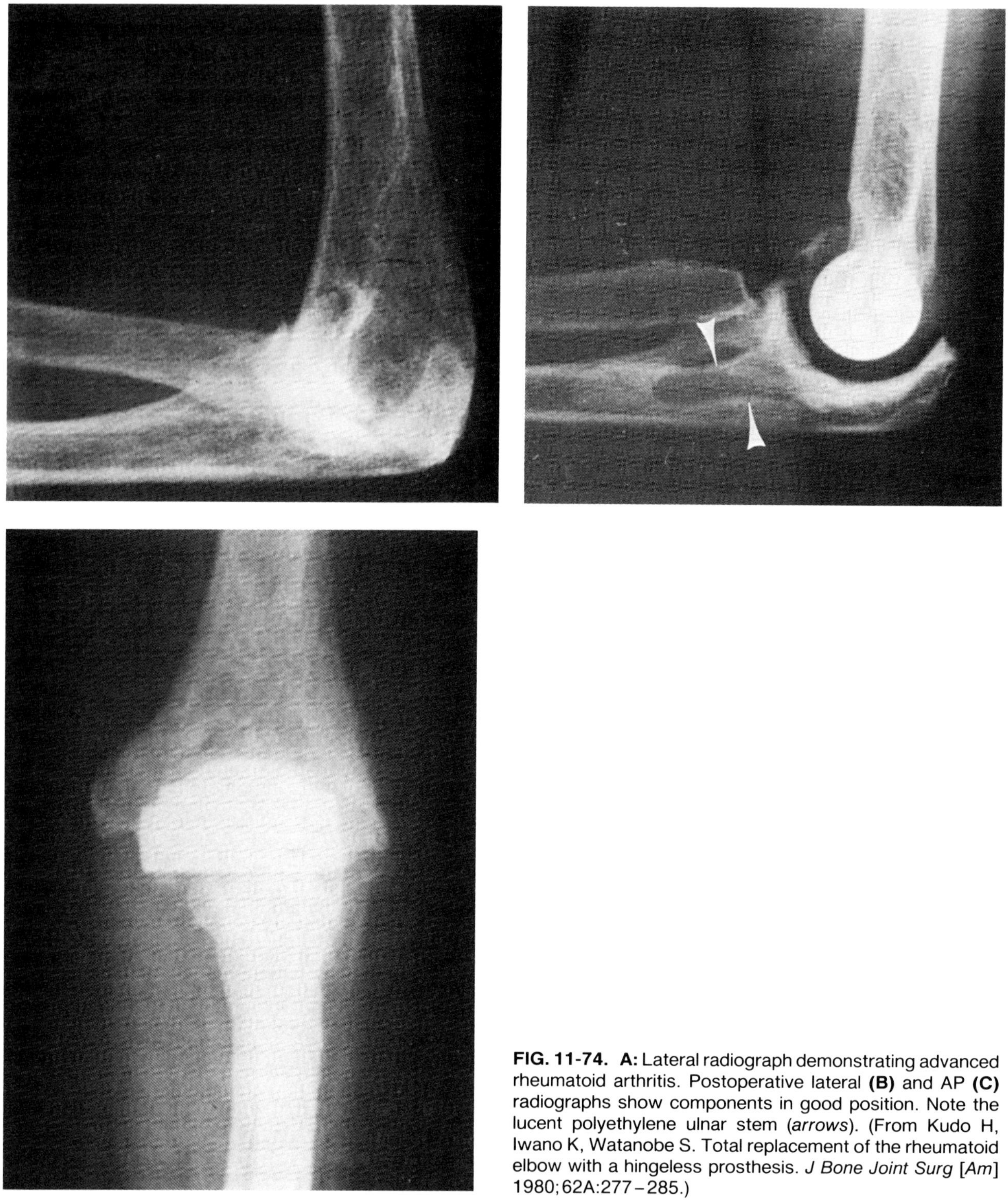

A B C

FIG. 11-74. A: Lateral radiograph demonstrating advanced rheumatoid arthritis. Postoperative lateral **(B)** and AP **(C)** radiographs show components in good position. Note the lucent polyethylene ulnar stem (*arrows*). (From Kudo H, Iwano K, Watanobe S. Total replacement of the rheumatoid elbow with a hingeless prosthesis. *J Bone Joint Surg* [*Am*] 1980;62A:277–285.)

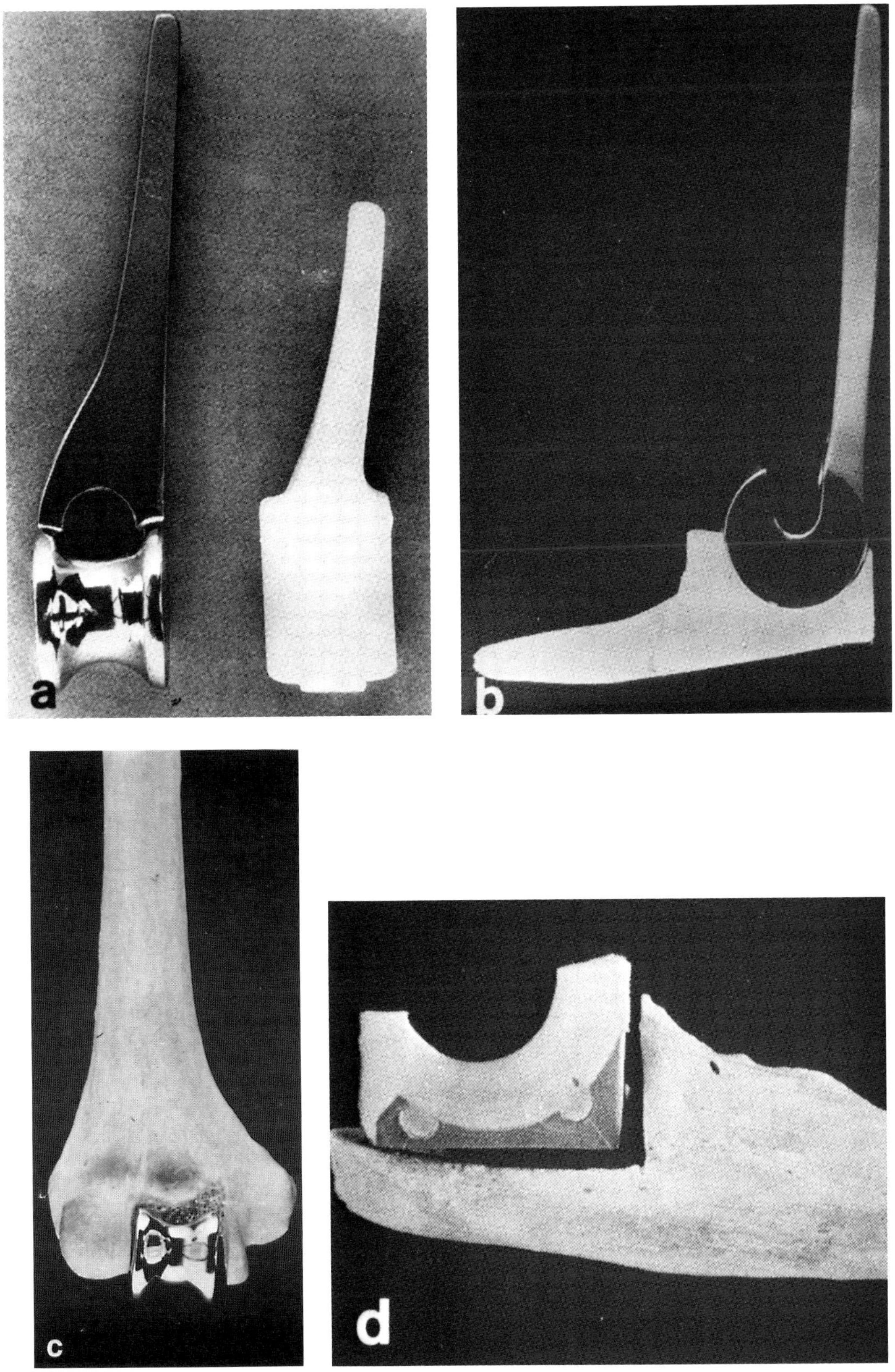

FIG. 11-75. Guildford elbow. **A:** Humeral and ulnar components seen from the front. **B:** Articulated components seen from the side. **C:** Humeral component in a bone model seen from the front. **D:** Ulnar component in a bone model seen from the side. (From Karanjia ND, Stiles PJ. The Guildford elbow. *Int Orthop* 1990;14:315–319.)

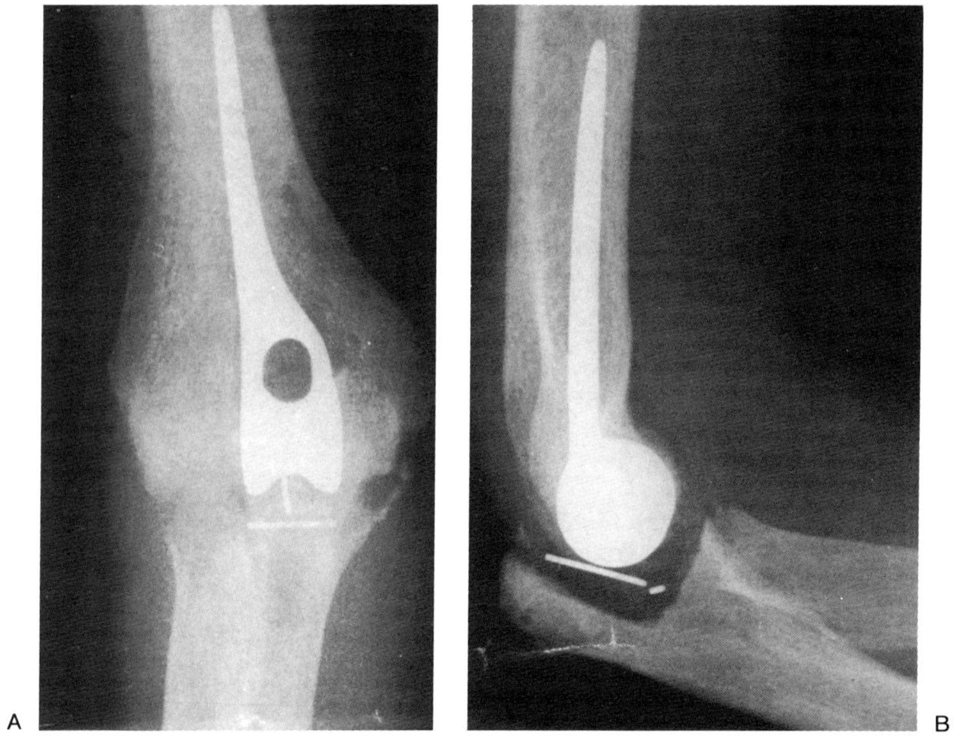

FIG. 11-76. The AP **(A)** and lateral **(B)** radiographs of the Guildford elbow. (From Karanjia ND, Stiles PJ. The Guildford elbow. *Int Orthop* 1990;14:315–319.)

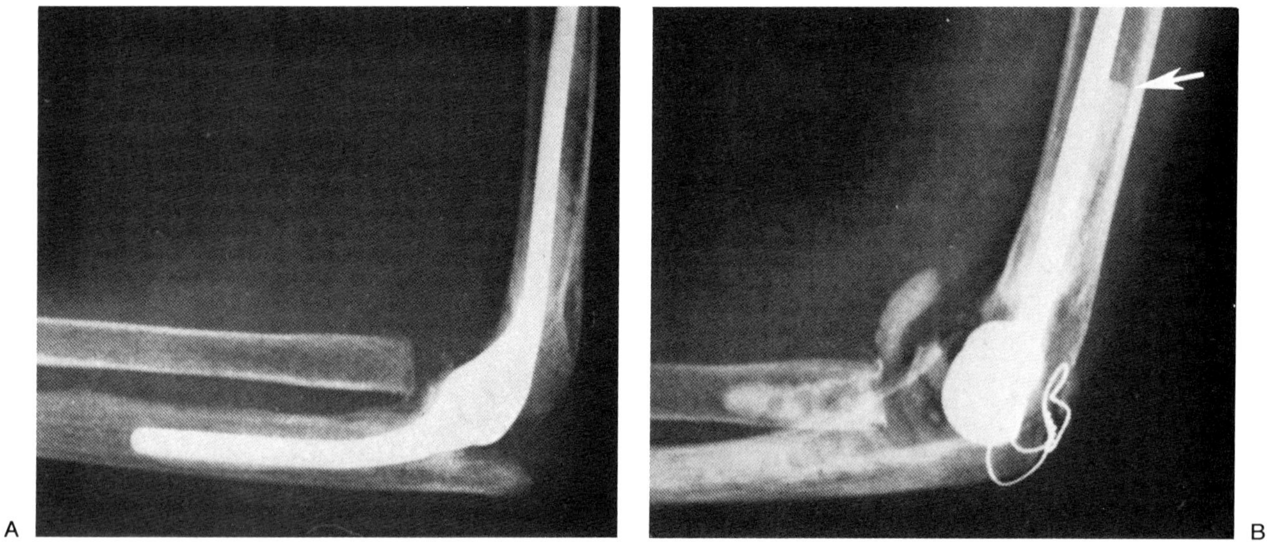

FIG. 11-77. Lateral radiographs of the elbow after total elbow replacement. **A:** Coonrad prosthesis with resection of the radial head. The cement is not evenly distributed around the components and beyond the component tips. The radiograph is also inadequate because the entire humeral component and cement beyond the stem are not included on the radiograph. **B:** Mayo prosthesis with adequate cement technique around the ulnar and radial components. The cement is not extended to include the entire humeral component (*arrow*). There is also a large cement collection in the antecubital region. (From Morrey BF, Bryan RS, Dobyns HJ, Linscheid RL. Total elbow arthroplasty. *J Bone Joint Surg* [*Am*] 1981;3A:1050–1063.)

ular margins of the humeral component are fairly common and not necessarily symptomatic. Lucent zones about the radial component have been reported in up to 50% of patients.[97] Humeral subsidence is also common in patients with rheumatoid arthritis. This finding does not necessarily indicate a poor prognosis.[108]

Subluxation and dislocation are most common with unconstrained components. The incidence is 5% to 18% (Fig. 11-78).[95–99,107,117]

Implant failure (e.g., fracture or linkage failure; Fig. 11-66B) is not a common problem. Implant fractures (Fig. 11-79) are easily detected with routine radiography.[114] Fracture of the component stem through the cortex occurs most commonly with constrained prostheses (30%). Unconstrained and semiconstrained implants penetrate the cortex in about 5% of cases.[115]

Deep infection occurs with an incidence of 1% to 5%.[92,115] Implant removal is often required. The corrective alternatives include simple resection arthroplasty, revision, or arthrodesis.[93,94,101] Reimplantation or revision can be considered if there is no bacterial growth after 6 weeks of antibiotic therapy.[101] Joint aspiration is a simple technique to obtain fluid for cultures.[87]

Other soft tissue abnormalities include instability, triceps deficiency, and transient or permanent nerve injury. The ulnar nerve is most commonly affected. Permanent injury is reported in only 2% of cases.[92,96,106]

The implant revision may be partial (Fig. 11-80C) (i.e., radial head implant added) or total. The indications include implant fracture or failure, sepsis, instability (e.g., unconstrained revised to semiconstrained), or loosening.[93,94,113] Arthrodesis is an option but not a popular method of treating arthroplasty failures.[101,113] Resection arthroplasty or the insertion of new components with longer stems and bone grafting (Fig. 11-80) is more commonly performed. Morrey[113] prefers reimplantation, especially for loosening. It is important to have adequate bone stock if implant revision is to be used.

Postoperative imaging can be difficult because of the elbow's mobility. Full extension is necessary for a normally positioned AP radiograph. This may be difficult in the immediate postoperative period or even later in patients with reduced motion. When true AP and lateral radiographs cannot be obtained (Fig. 11-80), fluoroscopic positioning should be considered to obtain optimal data on component position and metal-cement and bone-cement interfaces. The cement normally extends several centimeters beyond the component tips. The entire area must be included on the radiographs (Fig. 11-81).

Serial radiographs, optimally positioned, are useful for evaluating loosening, subsidence, component failure, and gross instability (Figs. 11-81 to 11-85). Subtle instability may require fluoroscopically positioned spot views. Progressive lucent lines that exceed 2 mm in width indicate loosening (Fig. 11-85). Endosteal scalloping or more irregular lucent lines suggest infection.[115] Aspiration with fluoroscopic guidance is useful to obtain fluid for culture in patients with suspected infection.[86,87]

CT can be used to evaluate bone stock prior to primary or revision arthroplasty; MRI is not frequently used postoperatively because of the metal artifact and difficulties with positioning.[86,87]

ARTHRODESIS

The elbow is the link between the hand and the shoulder. Fusion of this joint should not be entertained lightly in the presence of shoulder abnormalities, specifically reduced internal and external rotation. The position of the elbow after fusion is also important, depending on patient needs and activity level. If the shoulder and hand are normal, most authors fuse the elbow at or near 90° of flexion.[126,130]

Indications

Arthrodesis of the elbow is performed for pain, instability, arthroplasty failure, marked traumatic deformity, and sepsis.[125–130] This technique is not commonly used today.[126,129]

Surgical Techniques

There are numerous approaches to elbow arthrodesis. The underlying disease process and bone stock are important in the selection of a technique. When minimal bone removal is required, internal fixation with bone grafting and bone screws (Fig. 11-86) or external fixation techniques may be adequate.[126,128,130] In patients with sepsis, external fixation may be preferred.[126] Plate and screw techniques (Fig. 11-87) are preferred by some authors.

Imaging and Complications

The failure rate of arthrodesis may be as high as 53%.[128] Nonunion or pseudarthrosis, implant failure, fracture adjacent to fusion, and deep infection are the most common complications.[126]

Routine radiography and even conventional tomography may be the most useful methods to evaluate fusion in the presence of significant metal implant material. Also, CT can be used with bone algorithms to reduce metal artifact; MRI is difficult to use because of the flexed elbow and metal artifact. Fluoroscopic positioning, stress views, or guidance for injection or aspiration may be useful to evaluate motion and exclude infected fluid.

(text continues on page 814)

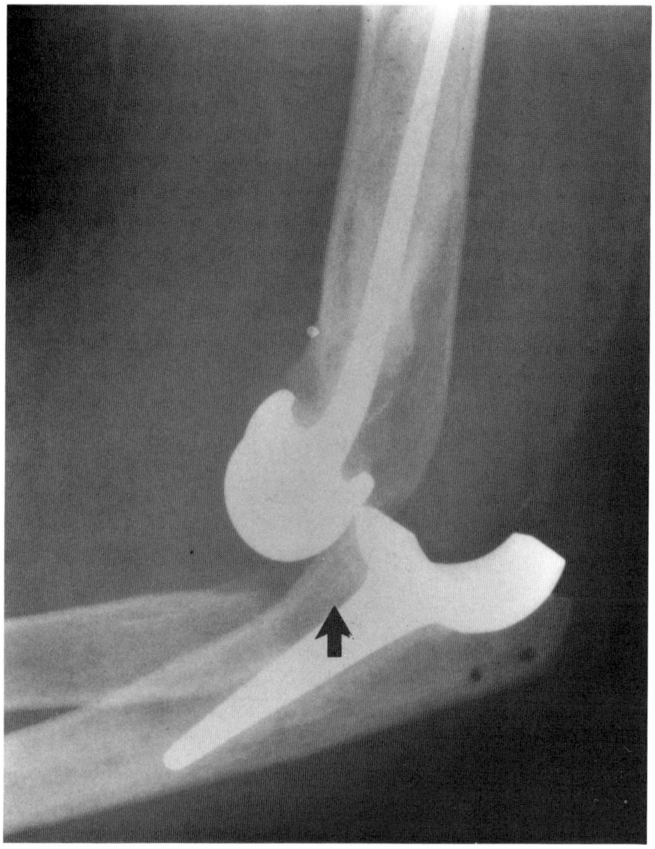

FIG. 11-78. Lateral radiograph of a capitellocondylar arthroplasty with a metal-backed ulnar component. The radial head (*arrow*) has been resected. There is posterior dislocation.

A,B

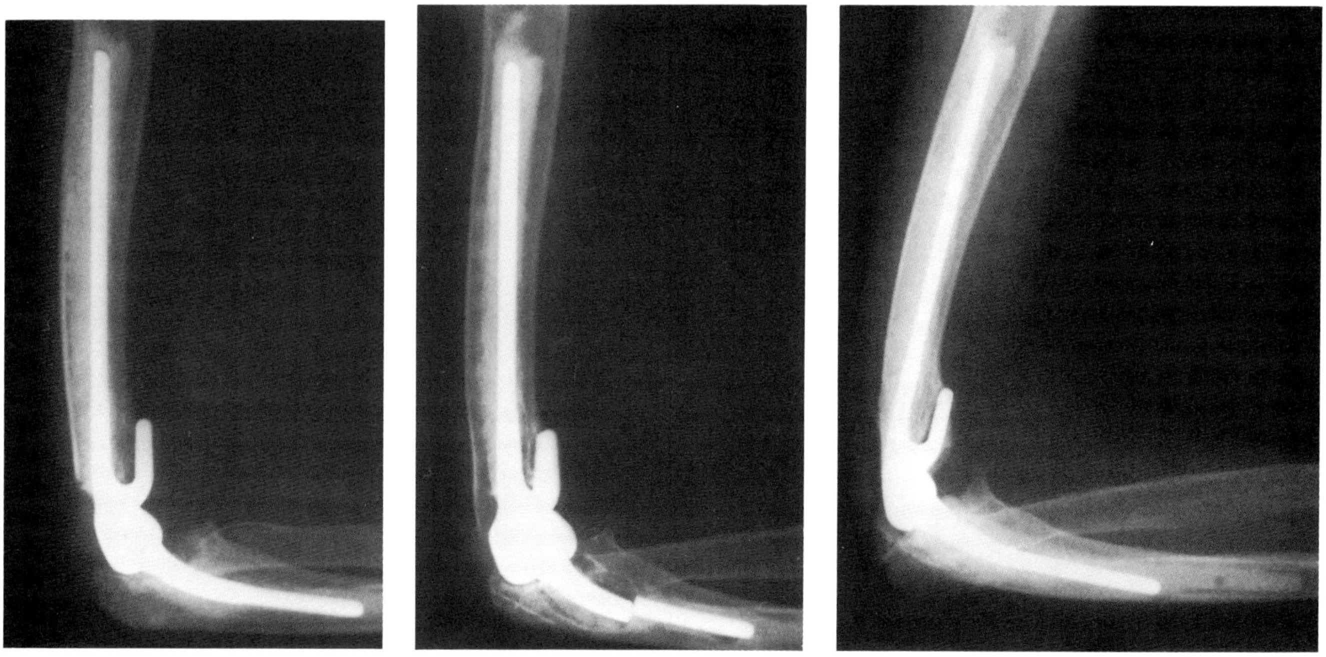

C

FIG. 11-79. Lateral radiographs of a Coonrad-Morrey implant at 3 months **(A)** and at 3 years with a fracture of the ulnar stem **(B)**. The component was successfully revised **(C)**. (From Morrey BF, Adams RA. Semiconstrained arthroplasty for the treatment of rheumatoid arthritis of the elbow. *J Bone Joint Surg* [*Am*] 1992;74A:479–490.)

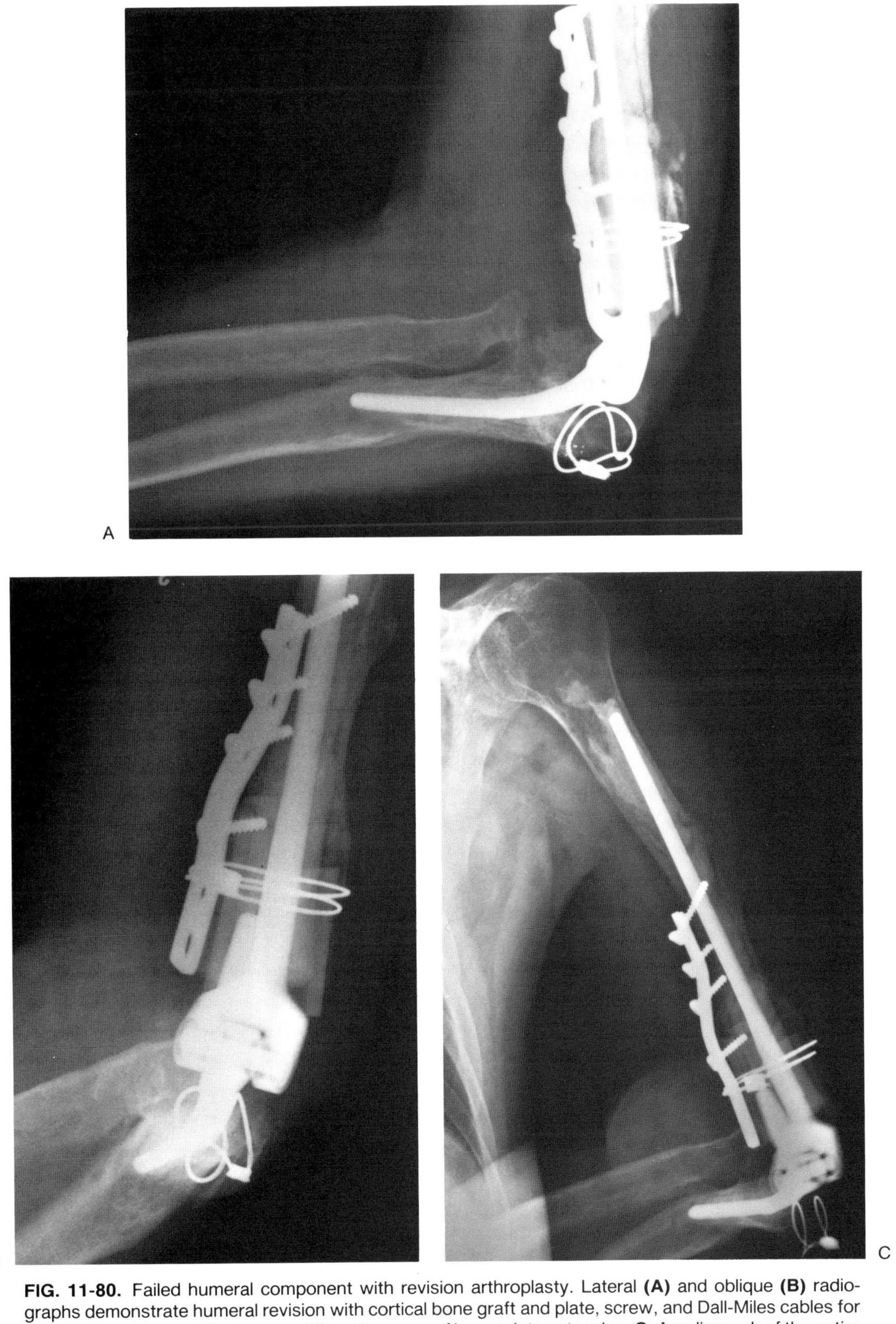

FIG. 11-80. Failed humeral component with revision arthroplasty. Lateral **(A)** and oblique **(B)** radiographs demonstrate humeral revision with cortical bone graft and plate, screw, and Dall-Miles cables for graft fixation. The positioning was difficult because of incomplete extension. **C:** A radiograph of the entire humerus was required to evaluate the long stem humeral component.

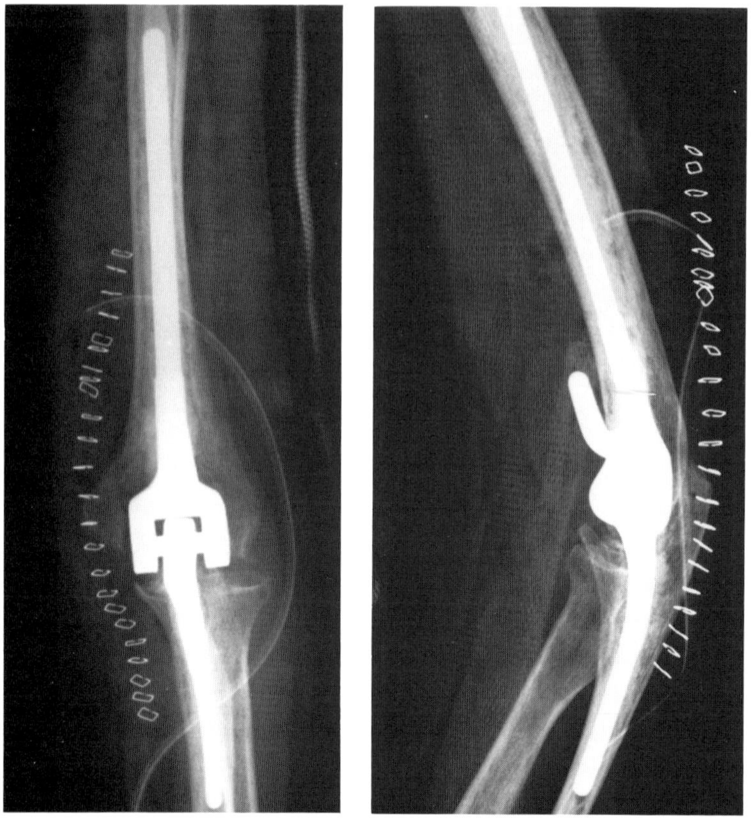

A,B

FIG. 11-81. The AP **(A)** and lateral **(B)** radiographs taken after placement of a long-stem (humeral) Coonrad-Morrey prosthesis. The components are entirely included on the AP view, and the component-cement and cement-bone interfaces are easily evaluated. The lateral view is poorly positioned, and the humeral component not completely included on the film.

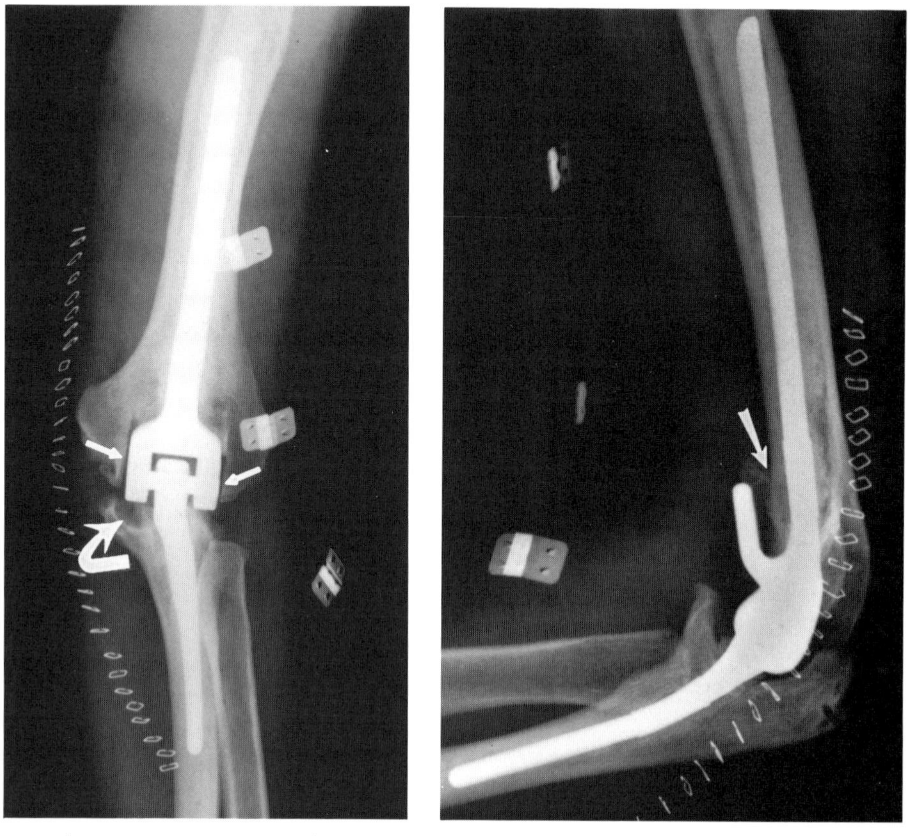

A B

FIG. 11-82. The AP **(A)** and lateral **(B)** radiographs of a Coonrad-Morrey implant. The lucent area adjacent to the humeral component (*arrows*) immediately after surgery is of no importance. There is also a small area of marrow with no cement (*curved arrow*) in the proximal ulna. Note the anterior bone graft (*arrow*) placed around the proximal ulnar component, which should not be confused with loosening.

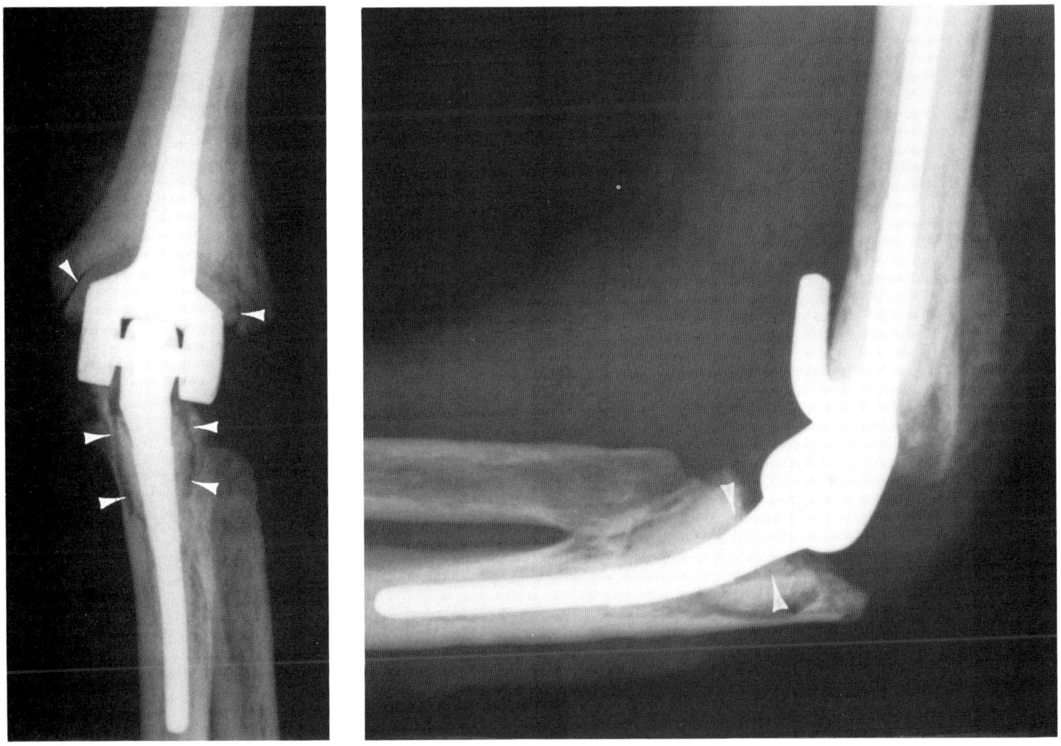

A B

FIG. 11-83. The AP **(A)** and lateral **(B)** radiographs demonstrate lucent zones (*arrowheads*) about both components. There was no clinical loosening. The patient was asymptomatic. There is also lucency at the metal-cement interface on the lateral view (*arrowheads*).

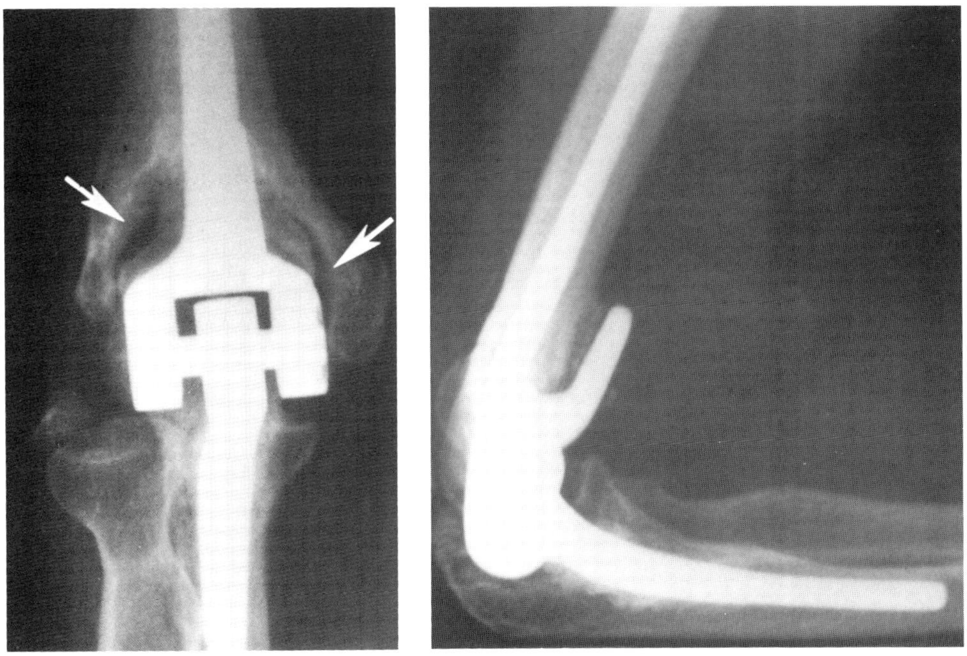

A B

FIG. 11-84. The AP **(A)** and lateral **(B)** radiographs 5 years after placement of a Coonrad-Morrey prosthesis. There is bone resorption along the distal humeral component (*arrows*) which, to date, has not been clinically significant. (From Morrey BF, Adams RA. Semiconstrained arthroplasty for the treatment of rheumatoid arthritis of the elbow. *J Bone Joint Surg* [*Am*] 1992;74A:479–490.)

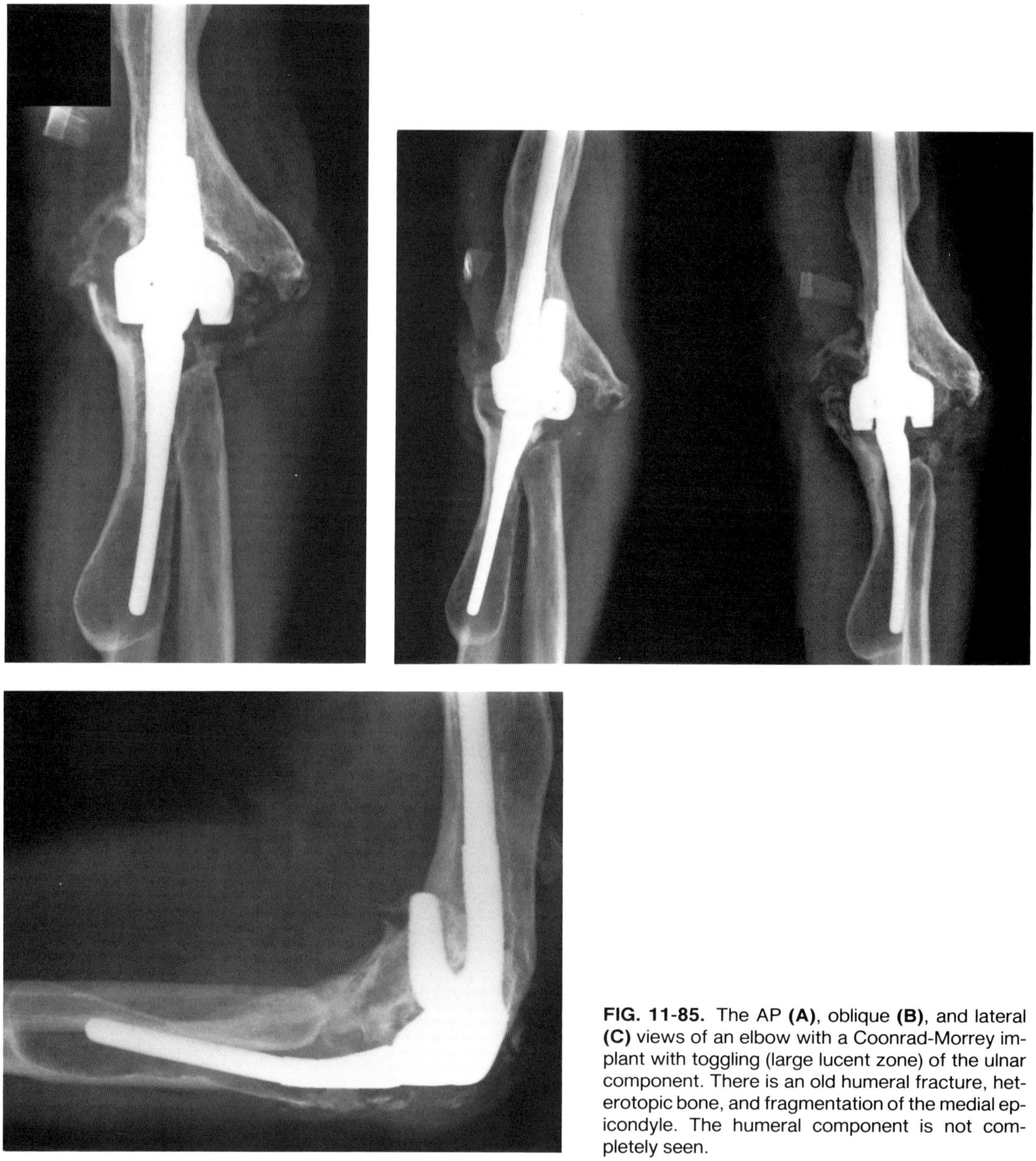

A

B

C

FIG. 11-85. The AP **(A)**, oblique **(B)**, and lateral **(C)** views of an elbow with a Coonrad-Morrey implant with toggling (large lucent zone) of the ulnar component. There is an old humeral fracture, heterotopic bone, and fragmentation of the medial epicondyle. The humeral component is not completely seen.

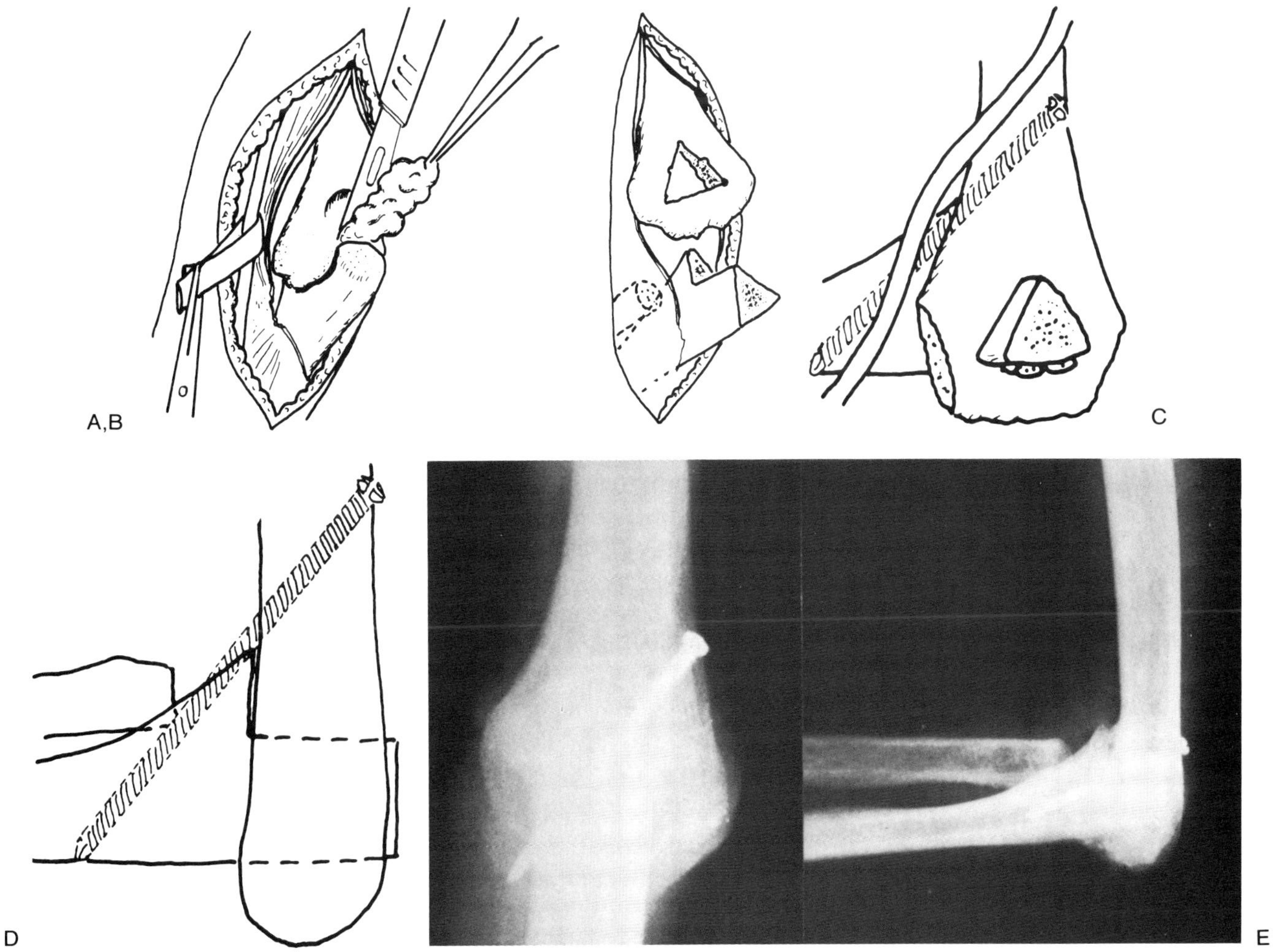

FIG. 11-86. Technique of joint débridement, synovectomy, and radial head excision.[124] **A:** Ulnar nerve isolated and triceps attachment released and posterior synovectomy done. **B:** Radial head excision, anterior synovectomy, olecranon, and humerus configured. **C:** Medial and lateral epicondyles removed, olecranon inserted into humerus, screw inserted. **D:** Completed procedure seen from the side. **E:** The AP and lateral views demonstrating fusion with 90° of flexion. (From Arafiles RP. A new technique of fusion for tuberculosis of the elbow. *J Bone Joint Surg* [*Am*] 1981;63A:1396–1400.)

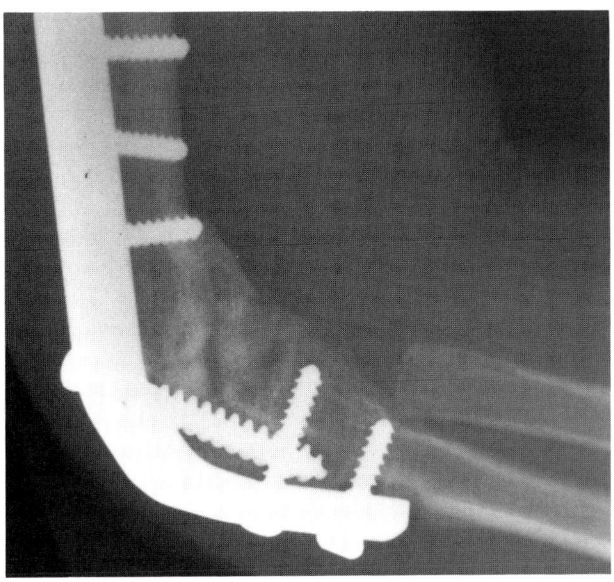

FIG. 11-87. Lateral radiograph after arthrodesis using a preshaped DC plate and cortical screws with a single longer cancellous screw for the olecranon. The elbow is fused at near 90° of flexion. The radial head had been resected.

REFERENCES

Imaging

1. Arger PH, Oberhircher PE, Miller WT. Lipohemarthrosis. *AJR Am J Roentgenol* 1974;121:97–100.
2. Bassett LW, Mirra JM, Forrester DM, Gold RH, Berstein ML, Rollins JS. Post-traumatic osteochondral "loose body" of the olecranon fossa. *Radiology* 1981;141:635–638.
3. Bernau A, Berquist TH. *Positioning techniques in orthopedic radiology.* Baltimore: Urban and Schwarzenberg; 1983.
4. Berquist TH. The elbow and wrist. *Top Magn Reson Imaging* 1989;3:15–27.
5. Berquist TH. *Imaging of orthopedic trauma.* 2nd ed. New York: Raven Press; 1992.
6. Berquist TH. *MRI of the musculoskeletal system.* 2nd ed. New York: Raven Press; 1990.
7. Berquist TH. Diagnostic and therapeutic injections as an aid to musculoskeletal diagnosis. *Semin Intervent Radiol* 1993;10:326–343.
8. Berquist TH. Diagnostic radiographic techniques in the elbow. In: Morrey BF, ed. *The elbow and its disorders.* 2nd ed. Philadelphia: WB Saunders; 1993:98–119.
9. Bledsoe RC, Izenstark JL. Displacements of fat pads in disease and injury to the elbow. A new radiographic sign. *Radiology* 1959;73:717–724.
10. Bohrers P. The fat pad sign following elbow trauma. *Clin Radiol* 1970;21:90–94.
11. Eto RT, Anderson PW, Harley JD. Elbow arthrography with the application of tomography. *Radiology* 1975;115:283–288.
12. Freiberger RH, Kaye JJ. *Arthrography.* New York: Appleton-Century-Crofts; 1979.
13. Greenspan A, Norman A. Radial-head-capitellar view: an expanded imaging approach to elbow injury. *Radiology* 1987;164:272–274.
14. Hall-Craggs MA, Showon PJ, Chapman M. Assessment of the radial head capitellar view and dorsal fat pad sign in acute elbow trauma. *AJR Am J Roentgenol* 1985;145:607–609.
15. Hindman BW, Schreiber RR, Wiss DA, Ghilorducci MJ, Avolio RE. Supracondylar fractures of the humerus. Prediction of cubitus varus deformity with CT. *Radiology* 1988;168:513–515.
16. Hudson TM. Elbow arthrography. *Radiol Clin North Am* 1981;19:227.
17. Kohn AM. Soft tissue alterations in elbow trauma. *AJR Am J Roentgenol* 1959;82:867–874.
18. London JT. Kinematics of the elbow. *J Bone Joint Surg [Am]* 1981;63A:529–535.
19. Pavlov H, Ghilman B, Warren RF. Double contrast arthrography of the elbow. *Radiology* 1979;130:87–95.
20. Rogers SL, MacEwan DW. Changes due to trauma in the fat plane overlying the supinator muscle. A radiographic sign. *Radiology* 1969;92:954.
21. Surgson RD, Feldman F, Rosenberg ZS. Elbow joint: assessment with double-contrast CT arthrography. *Radiology* 1986;160:167–173.

Trauma

22. Ackerman G, Jupiter JB. Non-union of fractures of the distal end of the humerus. *J Bone Joint Surg [Am]* 1988;70A:75–83.
23. Adler JB, Shaftan GW. Radial head fractures. Is excision necessary. *J Trauma* 1964;4:115–136.
24. Alvarez E, Paetl M, Winburg G, Pearlman HS. Fracture of the capitellum humeri. *J Bone Joint Surg [Am]* 1975;57A:1093–1096.
25. Amsallum JL, Blankstein A, Bass A, Horozowski H. Brachial artery injury: a complication of posterior dislocation of the elbow. *Orthop Rev* 1986;15:379–382.
26. Arner O, Ehengren K, VonSchrieb T. Fractures of the head and neck of the radius. A clinical and roentgenographic study of 310 cases. *Acta Chir Scand* 1957;112:115–134.
27. Ashbell TS, Kleinert HE, Kutz JE. Vascular injuries about the elbow. *Clin Orthop* 1967;50:107–127.
28. Bado JL. The Monteggia lesion. *Clin Orthop* 1967;50:71–86.
29. Berquist TH. *Imaging of orthopedic trauma.* New York: Raven Press; 1992.
30. Broberg MA, Morrey BF. Results of treatment of fracture-dislocations of the elbow. *Clin Orthop* 1987;216:109.
31. Brodeur AE, Silkerstein MJ, Graviss ER. *Radiology of the pediatric elbow.* Boston: GK Hall Publishers; 1981.
32. Brown AO, O'Riordan M, Quinlan W. Supracondylar fractures of the humerus in adults. *Injury* 1986;17:184–186.
33. Brown RF, Morgan RG. Intercondylar T-shaped fractures of the humerus. *J Bone Joint Surg [Br]* 1971;53B:425–428.
34. Bryan RS. Fractures about the elbow in adults. *Instr Course Lect* 1981;30:200–223.
35. Cabanela ME, Morrey BF. Fractures of the proximal ulna and olecranon. In: Morrey BF, ed. *Disorders of the elbow.* Philadelphia: WB Saunders; 1993:405–440.
36. Cassebaum WH. Open reduction of "T" and Y-fractures of the lower end of the humerus. *J Trauma* 1969;9:915–925.
37. Childress HM. Transarticular pin fixation in supracondylar fractures of the elbow in children. *J Bone Joint Surg [Am]* 1972;54A:1548–1552.
38. Colbert S. Surgical management of fractures of the capitellum humeri. *Acta Orthop Scand* 1977;48:603–606.
39. Colton CL. Fractures of the olecranon in adults. Classification and management. *Injury* 1973;5:121–127.
40. Conn J, Wade PA. Injuries of the elbow. A ten year review. *J Trauma* 1961;1:248–268.
41. Coonran RW. Nonunion of the olecranon and proximal ulna. In: Morrey BF, ed. *The elbow and its disorders.* Philadelphia: WB Saunders; 1993:429–440.
42. DeLee JC. Transverse divergent dislocation of the elbow in a child. *J Bone Joint Surg [Am]* 1981;63A:322.
43. Earwaker J. Post-traumatic calcification of the annular ligament of the radius. *Skeletal Radiol* 1992;21:149–154.
44. Edman P, Lohr G. Supracondylar fractures of the humerus treated with olecranon traction. *Acta Chir Scand* 1963;126:505–516.
45. El-Ahwany MD. Supracondylar fractures of the humerus in children with a note on surgical correction of late cubitus varus. *Injury* 1973;6:46.
46. Figgie MP, Inglis AE, Mow CS, Figgie HE. Salvage of non-union of the supracondylar fracture of the humerus by total elbow arthroplasty. *J Bone Joint Surg [Am]* 1989;71A:1058–1065.
47. Fowles JV, Kassab MT. Fracture of the capitellum humeri. Treatment of excision. *J Bone Joint Surg [Am]* 1974;56A:794–798.
48. Gartsman GM, Sculco TP, Otis JC. Operative treatment of olecranon fractures. *J Bone Joint Surg [Am]* 1981;63A:718–721.
49. Grantham SA, Norris TR, Bush DC. Isolated fracture of the humeral capitellum. *Clin Orthop* 1981;161:262–269.
50. Harrington IJ, Torentas AA. Replacement of the radial head in the treatment of unstable elbow fractures. *Injury* 1981;12:405–412.
51. Horne G. Supracondylar fracture of the humerus in adults. *J Trauma* 1980;20:71–74.
52. Hotchkiss RN, Green DP. Fractures and dislocations of the elbow. In: Rockwood CA, Green DP, Bucholz RW, eds. *Rockwood and Green's fractures in adults.* 3rd ed. Vol. 1. Philadelphia: JB Lippincott; 1991:739–841.
53. Hoyer A. Treatment of supracondylar fractures of the humerus by skeletal traction in an abduction splint. *J Bone Joint Surg [Am]* 1952;34A:623–637.
54. Jessing P. Monteggia lesions and their complicating nerve damage. *Acta Orthop Scand* 1975;46:601–609.
55. Johansson H, Olerud S. Operative treatment of intercondylar fractures of the humerus. *J Trauma* 1971;11:836–843.
56. Johnsson O. Capsular and ligament injuries of the elbow joint. *Acta Chir Scand* 1982;287:50–65.
57. Jupiter JB. Fractures of the distal humerus. In: Browner B, Jupiter JB, Levine A, Trafton P, eds. *Skeletal trauma.* Vol. II. Philadelphia: WB Saunders; 1991:1151.
58. Jupiter JB, Morrey BF. Fractures of the distal humerus in the

adult. In: Morrey BF, ed. *The elbow and its disorders.* 2nd ed. Philadelphia: WB Saunders; 1993:328–366.
59. Klassen RA. Supracondylar fractures of the elbow in children. In: Morrey BF, ed. *The elbow and its disorders.* 2nd ed. Philadelphia: WB Saunders; 1993:206–247.
60. Kuhlman JE, Fishman EK, Magid D, Scott WW, Brooker AF, Siegelman SS. Fracture nonunion: CT assessment with multiplanar reconstruction. *Radiology* 1988;167:483–488.
61. Lansinger O, More K. Intracondylar T-fractures of the humerus in adults. *Arch Orthop Trauma Surg* 1982;100:37–42.
62. Linscheid RL, O'Driscoll SW. Elbow dislocations. In: Morrey BF, ed. *The elbow and its disorders.* 2nd ed. Philadelphia: WB Saunders; 1993.
63. Lipscomb PR, Burleson RJ. Vascular and neural complications of the humerus in children. *J Bone Joint Surg [Am]* 1955;37A: 487–492.
64. MacAusland WR Jr, Wyman ET. Treatment of fractures of the olecranon by screw or nail fixation. *Ann Surg* 1942;116:293–296.
65. MacKay I, Fitzgerald B, Miller JH. Silastic replacement of the head of the radius in trauma. *J Bone Joint Surg [Br]* 1979;61B: 494–497.
66. Mason MB. Some observations on the fractures of the head of the radius with a review of 100 cases. *Br J Surg* 1954;42:123–132.
67. Mehne DK, Jupiter JB. Fractures of the distal humerus. In: Browner B, Jupiter J, Levine A, Trafton P, eds. *Skeletal trauma.* Vol. 2. Philadelphia: WB Saunders; 1991:1146.
68. Mobley JE, Jones JM. Monteggia fractures. *Mayo Clinic Proc* 1955;30:497–504.
69. Mohan K. Myositis ossificans traumatica of the elbow. *Int Surg* 1972;57:475–478.
70. Morrey BF. *The elbow and its disorders.* Philadelphia: WB Saunders; 1993.
71. Morrey BF, Berquist TH. The elbow. In: Berquist TH, ed. *Imaging of orthopedic trauma.* 2nd ed. New York: Raven Press; 1992:675–730.
72. Müller ME, Nazarian S, Koch P, Schaftzher J. *Comprehensive classification of fractures of the long bones.* Berlin: Springer-Verlag; 1990.
73. Odenheimer K, Harvey JP Jr. Internal fixation of fracture of the head of the radius. *J Bone Joint Surg [Am]* 1979;61A:785–787.
74. Paulson JO, Tophoj K. Fracture of the head and neck of the radius. *Acta Orthop Scand* 1974;45:66–75.
75. Penrose JH. The Monteggia fracture with posterior dislocation of the radial head. *J Bone Joint Surg [Br]* 1951;33B:65–73.
76. Peterson HA. Physeal fractures of the elbow. In: Morrey BF, ed. *The elbow and its disorders.* 2nd ed. Philadelphia: WB Saunders; 1993:248–265.
77. Radin EL, Riseborough EJ. Fractures of the radial head. *J Bone Joint Surg [Am]* 1966;48A:1055–1061.
78. Reckling FW, Cordell LB. Unstable fracture-dislocations of the forearm. The Monteggia and Galeazzi lesions. *Arch Surg* 1968;96:999–1007.
79. Regan W, Morrey BF. Fractures of the coronoid process of the ulna. *J Bone Joint Surg [Am]* 1989;71A:1348–1354.
80. Reich RS. Treatment of the intracondylar fractures of the elbow by means of traction. *J Bone Joint Surg* 1936;18:997–1004.
81. Rettig AC, Waugh TR, Evanski PM. Fracture of the olecranon: a problem of management. *J Trauma* 1979;19:23–28.
82. Riseborough EJ, Radin EL. Intercondylar T fractures of the humerus in the adult. Comparison of operative and nonoperative treatment in 29 cases. *J Bone Joint Surg [Am]* 1969;51A:130–141.
83. Scharplat D, Allgower M. Fractures-dislocations of the elbow. *Injury* 1976;7:143–159.
84. Swanson AB, Jaegar SH, LaRochelle D. Comminuted fractures of the radial head. The role of silicone implant replacement arthroplasty. *J Bone Joint Surg [Am]* 1981;63A:1039–1049.
85. Wainwright D. Fractures of the olecranon process. *Br J Surg* 1942;29:403–406.

Arthroplasty

86. Berquist TH. *Imaging of orthopedic trauma.* New York: Raven Press; 1992.
87. Berquist TH. Diagnostic and therapeutic injections as an aid to musculoskeletal diagnosis. *Semin Intervent Radiol* 1993;10:326–343.
88. Brumfield RH, Volz RG, Green JF. Total elbow arthroplasty: a clinical review of 30 cases employing the Mayo and AHSC prosthesis. *Clin Orthop* 1981;158:137–141.
89. Burnett R, Fyfe IS. Souter-Strathclyde arthroplasty of the rheumatoid elbow. *Acta Orthop Scand* 1991;62:52–54.
90. Cooney WP. Elbow arthroplasty: indications and implant selection. In: Morrey BF, ed. *The elbow and its disorders.* 2nd ed. Philadelphia: WB Saunders; 1993:629–637.
91. Coonrad RW. History of elbow arthroplasty. In: Inglis AE, ed. *American Academy of Orthopedic Surgery total joint replacement in the upper extremity.* St. Louis: CV Mosby; 1980:75–90.
92. Coonrad RW. Seven year follow-up of Coonrad total elbow replacement. In: Inglis AE, ed. *American Academy of Orthopedic Surgery total joint replacement in the upper extremity.* St. Louis: CV Mosby; 1980:91–99.
93. Dee R. Revision surgery after failed elbow endoprosthesis. In: Inglis AE, ed. *American Academy of Orthopedic Surgery total joint replacement in the upper extremity.* St. Louis: CV Mosby; 1980: 126–140.
94. Dee R. Nonimplantation salvage in failed reconstructive procedures of the elbow. In: Morrey BF, ed. *The elbow and its disorders.* 2nd ed. Philadelphia: WB Saunders; 1993:690–695.
95. Ewald FC. Nonconstrained metal-to-plastic total elbow replacement. In: Inglis AE, ed. *American Academy of Orthopedic Surgery total joint replacement in the upper extremity.* St. Louis: CV Mosby; 1980:141–149.
96. Ewald FC, Jacobs MA. Total elbow arthroplasty. *Clin Orthop* 1984;182:137–142.
97. Ewald FC, Scheinberg RD, Poss R, Thomas WH, Scott RD, Sledge CB. Capitellocondylar total elbow arthroplasty. *J Bone Joint Surg [Am]* 1980;62A:1259–1263.
98. Ewald FC, Simmons ED, Sullivan JA, Thomas WH, Scott RD, Poss S, Thornhill TS, Sledge CB. Capitellocondylar total elbow replacement in rheumatoid arthritis. *J Bone Joint Surg [Am]* 1993;75A:498–507.
99. Friedman RJ, Lee DE, Ewald FC. Nonconstrained total elbow arthroplasty. *J Arthroplasty* 1989;4:31–37.
100. Garrett JC, Ewald FC, Thomas WH, Sledge CB. Loosening associated with G.S.B hinge total elbow replacement in patients with rheumatoid arthritis. *Clin Orthop* 1977;127:170–174.
101. Goldberg VM, Figgie HE III, Inglis AF, Figgie MP. Total elbow arthroplasty. *J Bone Joint Surg [Am]* 1988;70A:778–783.
102. Inglis AE. Tri-axial total elbow replacement: indications, surgical technique, and results. In: Inglis AE, ed. *American Academy of Orthopedic Surgery total joint replacement in the upper extremity.* St. Louis: CV Mosby; 1980:100–112.
103. Inglis AE, Pellicci PM. Total elbow replacement. *J Bone Joint Surg [Am]* 1980;62A:1252–1258.
104. Johnson EW, Schlein AP. Vitallium prosthesis for the olecranon and proximal part of the ulna. *J Bone Joint Surg [Am]* 1970;52A: 721–724.
105. Johnson JR, Getty CJM, Lettin AWF, Glasgow MMS. The Stanmore total elbow replacement for rheumatoid arthritis. *J Bone Joint Surg [Br]* 1984;66B:732–736.
106. Jonsson B, Larsson S. Elbow arthroplasty in rheumatoid arthritis. *Acta Orthop Scand* 1990;61:344–347.
107. Karanjia ND, Stiles PJ. The Guildford elbow. *Int Orthop* 1990;14:315–319.
108. Kudo H, Iwano K. Total elbow arthroplasty with a nonconstrained surface-replacement prosthesis in patients with rheumatoid arthritis. *J Bone Joint Surg [Am]* 1990;72A:355–362.
109. Kudo H, Iwano K, Watanobe S. Total replacement of the rheumatoid elbow with a hingeless prosthesis. *J Bone Joint Surg [Am]* 1980;62A:277–285.
110. Linscheid RL. Resurfacing elbow replacement arthroplasty rationale, technique and results. In: Morrey BF, ed. *The elbow and its disorders.* 2nd ed. Philadelphia: WB Saunders; 1993:638–647.
111. Lowe LW, Miller AJ, Allum RL, Higginson DW. The development of an unconstrained elbow arthroplasty. *J Bone Joint Surg [Br]* 1984;66B:243–247.
112. Morrey BF. Complications of elbow replacement surgery. In:

Morrey BF, ed. *The elbow and its disorders.* 2nd ed. Philadelphia: WB Saunders; 1993:665–675.
113. Morrey BF. Revision of failed elbow arthroplasty. In: Morrey BF, ed. *The elbow and its disorders.* 2nd ed. Philadelphia: WB Saunders; 1993:676–689.
114. Morrey BF, Adams RA. Semiconstrained arthroplasty for the treatment of rheumatoid arthritis of the elbow. *J Bone Joint Surg* [*Am*] 1992;74A:479–490.
115. Morrey BF, Adams RA. Semiconstrained elbow replacement arthroplasty: rationale, technique and results. In: Morrey BF, ed. *The elbow and its disorders.* 2nd ed. Philadelphia: WB Saunders; 1993:648–664.
116. Morrey BF, Bryan RS, Dobyns HJ, Linscheid RL. Total elbow arthroplasty. *J Bone Joint Surg* [*Am*] 1981;3A:1050–1063.
117. Pöll RG, Rozing PM. Use of the Souter-Strathclyde total elbow prosthesis in patients who have rheumatoid arthritis. *J Bone Joint Surg* [*Am*] 1991;73A:1227–1233.
118. Pritchard RW. Long-term follow-up study: semiconstrained elbow prosthesis. *Orthopedics* 1981;4:151–155.
119. Pritchard RW. Anatomic surface elbow arthroplasty. *Clin Orthop* 1983;179:223–230.
120. Ross AC, Sneath RS, Scales JT. Endoprosthetic replacement of the humerus and elbow joint. *J Bone Joint Surg* [*Br*] 1987;69B:652–655.
121. Souter WA. Total replacement of the elbow joint. In: *Proceedings of the Combined Meeting of the Orthopedic Association of the English-Speaking World.* 1977;59B:99–100.
122. Street DM, Stevens PS. A humeral replacement prosthesis for the elbow. *J Bone Joint Surg* [*Am*] 1974;6A:1147–1158.
123. Torzilli PA. Biomechanics of the elbow. In: Inglis AE, ed. *American Academy of Orthopedic Surgery total joint replacement in the upper extremity.* St. Louis: CV Mosby; 1980:150–168.
124. Volz RG. Development and clinical analysis of new semiconstrained total elbow prosthesis. In: Inglis AE, ed. *American Academy of Orthopedic Surgery total joint replacement in the upper extremity.* St. Louis: CV Mosby; 1980:111–124.

Arthrodesis

125. Arafiles RP. A new technique of fusion for tuberculosis of the elbow. *J Bone Joint Surg* [*Am*] 1981;63A:1396–1400.
126. Beckenbaugh RD. Arthrodesis. In: Morrey BF, ed. *The elbow and its disorders.* 2nd ed. Philadelphia: WB Saunders; 1993:696–703.
127. Figgie MP, Inglis AE, Mow CS, Wolfe SW, Suilo TP, Figgie HE III. Results of reconstruction for failed total elbow arthroplasty. *Clin Orthop* 1990;253:123.
128. Koch M, Lipscomb PR. Arthrodesis of the elbow. *Clin Orthop* 1967;50:151.
129. Rashkoff E, Burkhalter WE. Arthrodesis of the salvaged elbow. *Orthopedics* 1986;9:733.
130. Snider WJ, DeWitt HJ. Functional study for optimum position of the elbow for arthrodesis or ankylosis. *J Bone Joint Surg* [*Am*] 1973;55A:1305.

Imaging Atlas of Orthopedic Appliances and Prostheses,
edited by T.H. Berquist.
Mayo Clinic Foundation © 1995.
Published by Raven Press, Ltd., New York.

CHAPTER 12

The Radius and Ulna

Thomas H. Berquist and Mark P. Brodersen

Orthopedic appliances are primarily used for fracture treatment in the radius and ulna. A discussion of distal ulna osteotomy or lengthening procedures is included in Chapter 13. Therefore, this chapter emphasizes the imaging and management of fractures of the radial and ulnar shafts.

FOREARM FRACTURES

Mechanism of Injury

Fractures of the radius and ulna may occur separately or together. The mechanism of injury is usually a direct blow to the forearm during a motor vehicle accident or a severe fall on the outstretched hand. Associated injuries of the elbow or wrist are fairly common.[1,7,26,29]

Classification

Fractures of either or both forearm bones are classified according to the level of fracture, degree of displacement and angulation, degree of comminution, and whether they are open or closed. Each feature has a significant impact on the treatment considerations and prognosis. Figure 12-1 illustrates the classification system developed by the Orthopedic Trauma Association.[9] Comminuted fractures (groups 4 to 7) are more frequently open injuries.[1,7,9,16]

T. H. Berquist: Mayo Medical School and Department of Diagnostic Radiology, Mayo Clinic Jacksonville, Jacksonville, Florida 32224.

M. P. Brodersen: Mayo Medical School and Department of Orthopedic Surgery, Mayo Clinic Jacksonville, Jacksonville, Florida 32224.

In Smith and Sage's[29] series of 555 forearm fractures in 330 adult patients, approximately 75% involved both bones, 15% involved the ulna alone, and 10% involved the radius alone. About three fifths of the fractures involved adjacent proximal and distal thirds of the radial and ulnar shafts. Figure 12-2 illustrates the incidence of forearm fractures in the proximal, mid and distal thirds of the radius and ulna.

Two additional fractures are associated with accompanying articular injuries. The Monteggia fracture is associated with dislocation of the radial head. This injury was originally described in 1814 as a "fracture of the proximal third of the ulna and an anterior dislocation of the proximal epiphysis of the radius."[3] Type I injuries (60% of Monteggia fractures, Fig. 12-3) present with anterior dislocation of the radial head and a fracture of the ulnar shaft, which is typically angulated anteriorly. Type II injuries (15% of cases) differ in that the radial head is dislocated posteriorly or posterolaterally and the ulnar fracture is more often angulated posteriorly. Type III Monteggia lesions (20% of cases) have anterolateral or lateral dislocation of the radial head and fracture of the ulnar metaphysis. Type IV injuries (5% of cases) present with anterior dislocation of the radial head with fractures of the proximal thirds of the radius and ulna.[1,4,16,24]

In 1929, Valande[31] described the reverse Monteggia lesion or a fracture of the distal radius. Galeazzi described the associated subluxation or dislocation of the distal radioulnar joint (Fig. 12-4) in 1934.[1,7,17,20,24]

Preoperative Imaging Evaluation

Although the clinical presentation of fracture of the forearm bones is usually obvious, radiographic evaluation is essential to evaluate the position of the fracture fragments and to exclude associated wrist and elbow in-

(*text continues on page 820*)

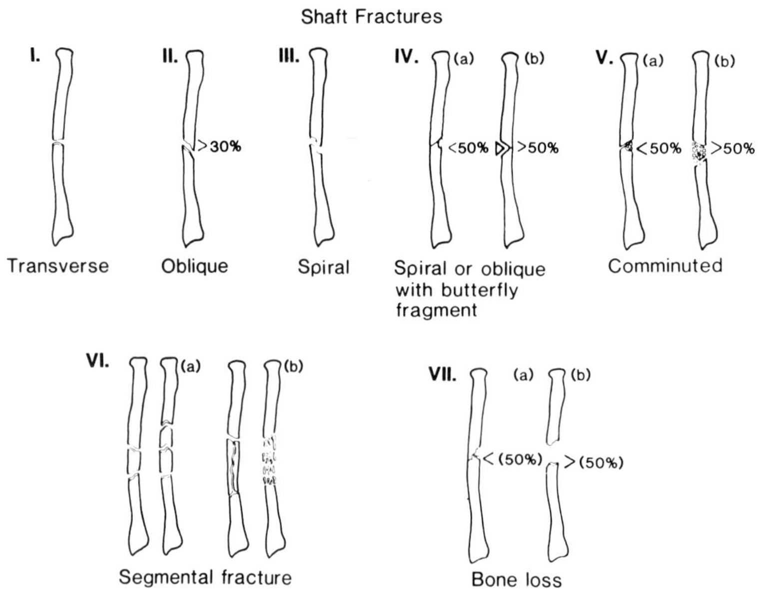

FIG. 12-1. Forearm fracture classification of the Orthopedic Trauma Association. (From Chapman MW, Gordon JE, Zissimos AG. Compression plate fixation of acute fractures of the diaphysis of the radius and ulna. *J Bone Joint Surg* [*Am*] 1989;71A:159–169.)

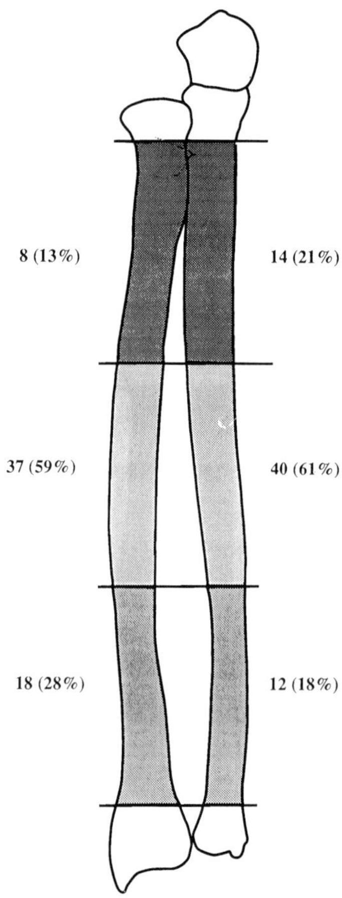

FIG. 12-2. Location of radial and ulnar fractures. (From Chapman MW, Gordon JE, Zissimos AG. Compression plate fixation of acute fractures of the diaphysis of the radius and ulna. *J Bone Joint Surg* [*Am*] 1989;71A:159–169.)

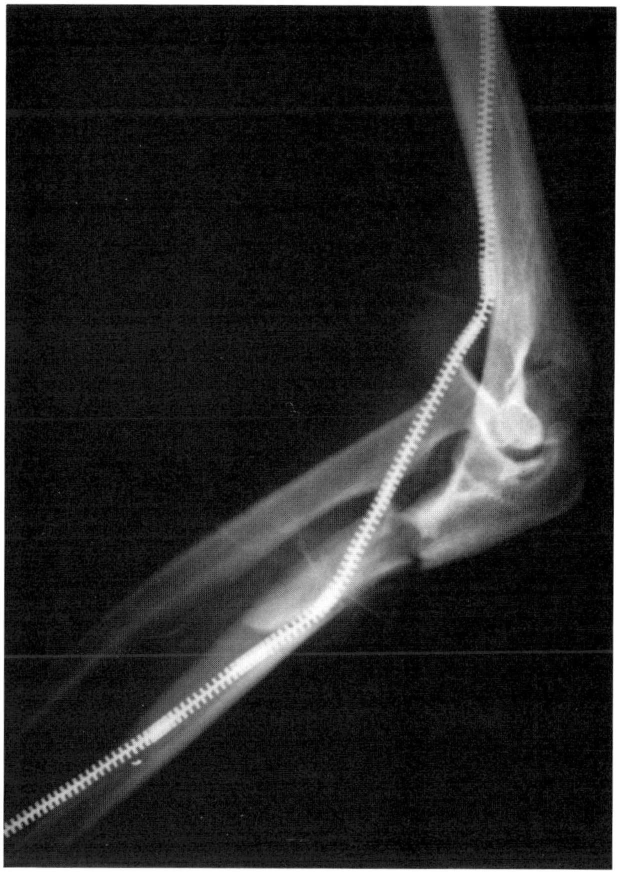

A

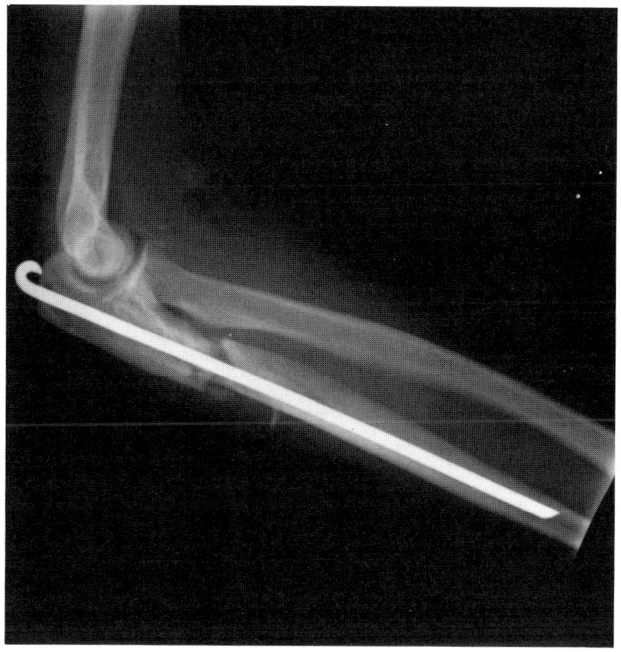

B

FIG. 12-3. A: Lateral view of the forearm and elbow demonstrating a type I Monteggia injury with anterior dislocation of the radial head and a fracture of the proximal ulna. **B:** Postoperative lateral radiograph after reduction with a Rush rod.

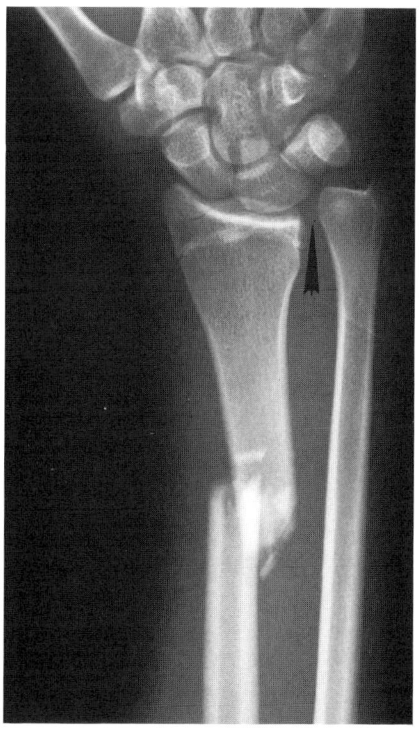

A

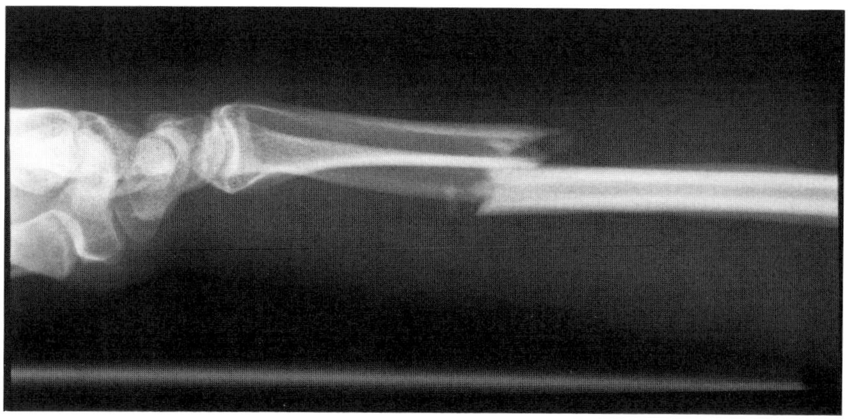

B

FIG. 12-4. Galeazzi fracture. The AP **(A)** and lateral **(B)** views of the wrist and distal forearm demonstrating a comminuted overriding radial fracture with dislocation of the distal radioulnar joint, which is more easily appreciated on the AP (A) view.

juries. Routinely, anteroposterior (AP) and lateral views of the forearm are obtained. Using 7 × 17-inch extremity cassettes allows the elbow and wrist to be included also. Separate series of elbow and wrist images may be required in certain cases.[4,5,7] More detailed examinations with conventional or computed tomography are usually not necessary.[7,20]

The use of the radiocapitellar line is helpful to avoid overlooking subluxation or dislocation of the radial head (Fig. 12-5).[15]

Treatment Options

The goals of treatment are to restore and maintain the length of the arm, achieve anatomic alignment, prevent rotational deformity, and maintain normal function (pronation and supination).[2] Treatment with internal fixation is frequently required. However, certain fractures can be managed conservatively.[2,8,19,20,30]

Conservative Therapy

Undisplaced fractures of the shaft about the radius and ulna (type I) are rare. The treatment usually consists of immobilization and a well-molded long arm cast with the elbow flexed 90° and the hand in neutral position.[7,20,28]

The undisplaced fracture of the ulna alone, also called the nightstick fracture because of the mechanism of injury, is usually caused by a direct blow and is fairly common. These too can be treated with conservative techniques.[1,7,20]

Isolated undisplaced fractures of the proximal radius alone are rare. The forearm muscles support and protect this region. Therefore, severe injuries to this area are more likely to injure both the radius and ulna.

Because these fractures can become displaced easily, weekly films are taken initially to be certain that the position of the fracture is maintained. Each new series of films must be compared with the original films to exclude even slight displacements or rotation.

Operative Therapy

Most authors report poor results when closed treatment is used for forearm fracture management. The indications for operative intervention are as follows:[1,20]

1. All displaced diaphyseal fractures
2. Displaced radial fractures with > 10° angulation or involvement of the proximal or distal articulations
3. Ulnar fractures with > 10° angulation
4. Monteggia fractures
5. Galeazzi fractures
6. Open fractures
7. Fracture with compartment syndrome

Surgical intervention should be performed within 24 hours of the injury when possible.[20,25,27]

Displaced fractures of the shafts of the radius and ulna present a difficult challenge and treatment problem. The fracture fragments are frequently rotated, and satisfactory results are difficult to obtain using conservative techniques. If the fragments are not properly aligned, rotational function is diminished with healing. Generally, fractures proximal to the pronator teres insertion on the radius result in supination of the proximal radial fragments. In fractures distal to the insertion of the pronator teres, the major forces of the biceps and supinator muscles are neutralized; therefore, the fragments are minimally displaced. Because the proximal ulnar fragment remains stable, the position for immobilization must be governed by the position of this fragment. Thus, for satisfactory reduction, the distal radial fragment must be rotated to align with the proximal fragment.[7,13]

Evans[13] described a method that allows the correct rotational position of the forearm during reduction. He emphasized a standardized technique by obtaining AP views of both the involved elbow and the normal side. The elbow is flexed 90°, and the tube is angled 20° toward the joint space. By locating the position of the radial tuberosity on the radiograph, the rotational position of the proximal radial fragment can be determined, and thus, the radial fragment can be properly reduced (Figs. 12-6 and 12-7).

Open reduction with some form of internal fixation offers the best chance for successful alignment and functional results. Various devices, including medullary nails, such as Rush rods; Kirschner wires (K wires); Steinmann pins; Lottes nails; and Sage triangular nails, have been used. Plate and screw fixation with or without bone grafting has also been used.[1,2,9,19,20,21]

Intramedullary Nailing

Intramedullary nailing of forearm fractures actually preceded the use of this technique for the treatment of femoral fractures.[30]

The anatomy of the ulna is better suited to intramedullary fixation.[18,23] The medullary canal is straight and large enough to allow a pin or nail of adequate strength to be inserted (Fig. 12-3).[29] The radius is curved, and the canal narrows (Fig. 12-8). Therefore, the nail selected is limited by the narrowest diameter of the canal.[18,29] This configuration limits reaming of the entire canal. Also, the configuration of the nail must be shaped prior to insertion to ensure that the radial configuration is main-

(text continues on page 829)

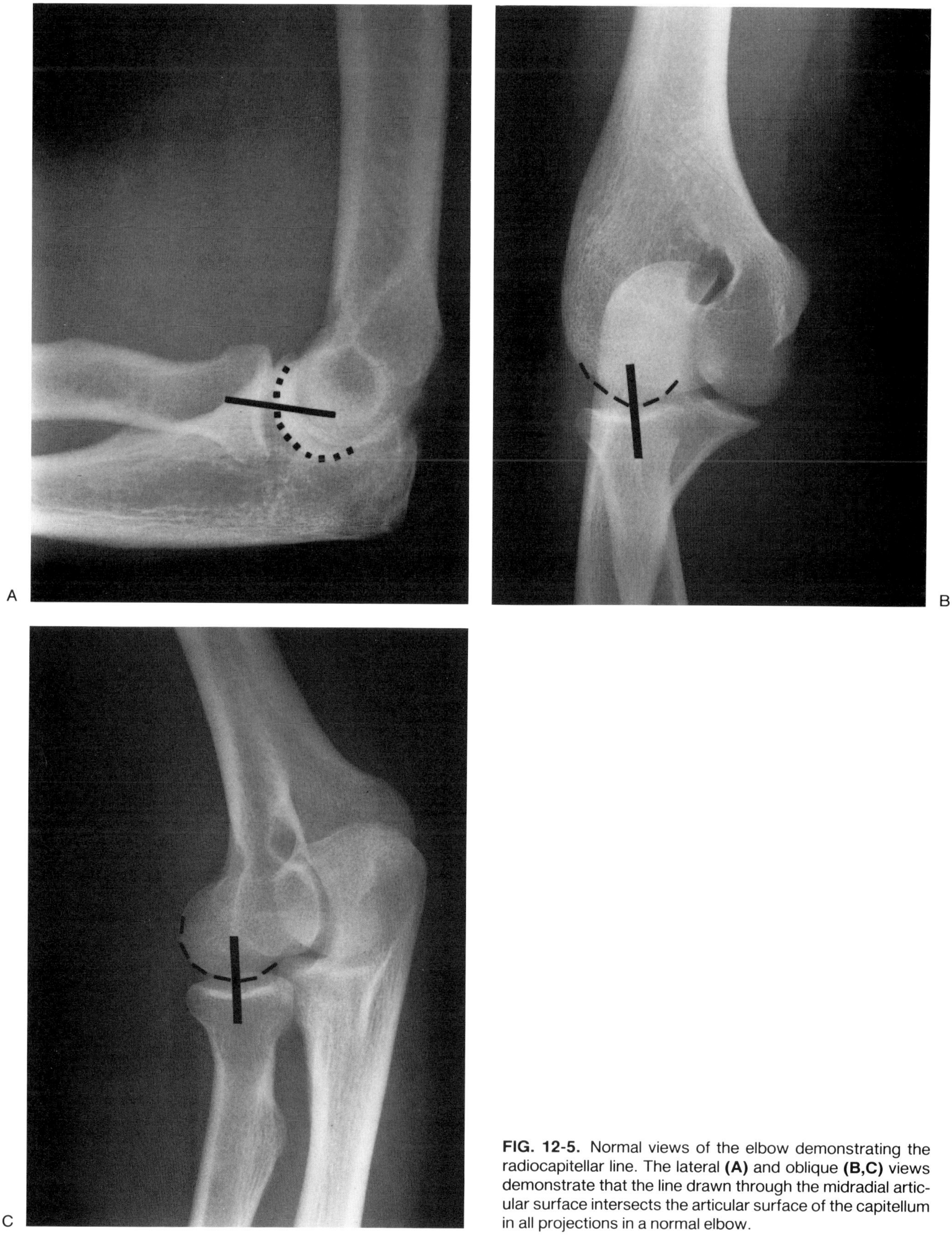

FIG. 12-5. Normal views of the elbow demonstrating the radiocapitellar line. The lateral **(A)** and oblique **(B,C)** views demonstrate that the line drawn through the midradial articular surface intersects the articular surface of the capitellum in all projections in a normal elbow.

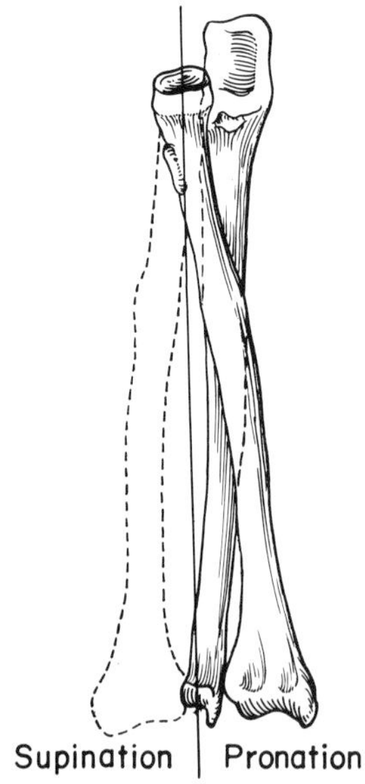

FIG. 12-6. Positional relationships of the radius and ulna with pronation and supination.

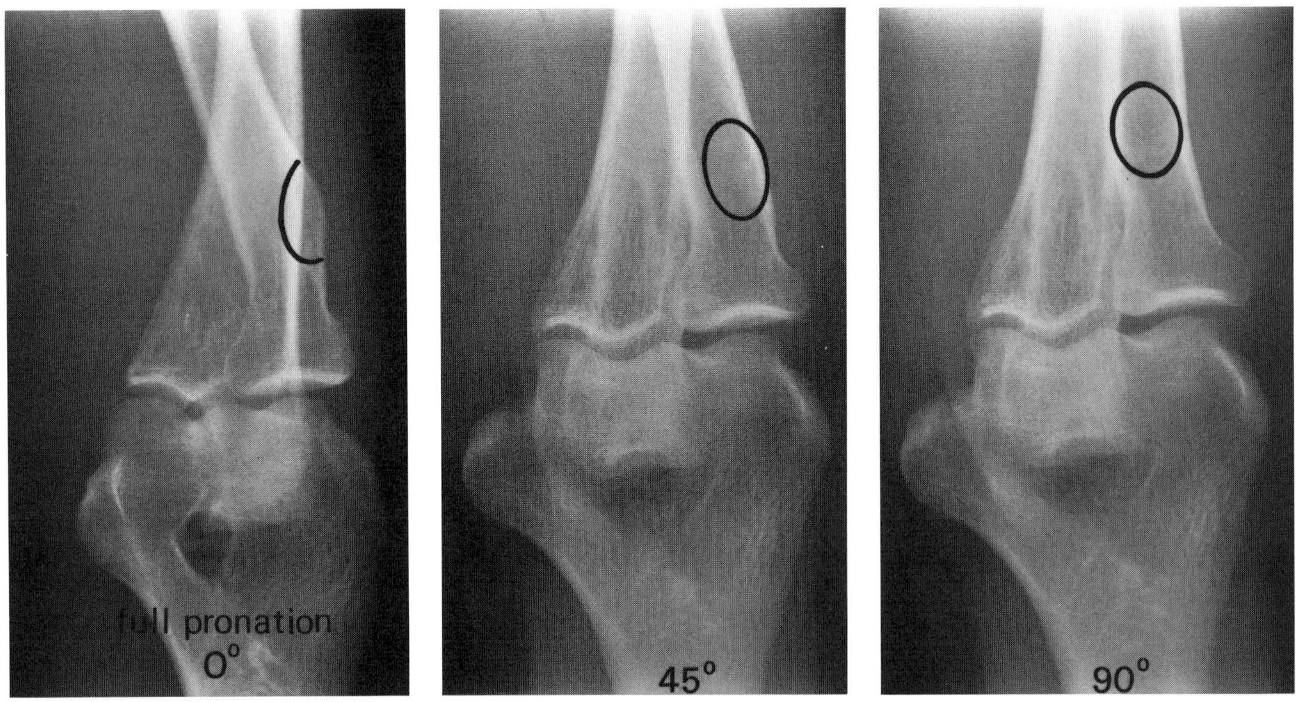

A B,C

FIG. 12-7. Radiographs of the elbow demonstrating the position of the radial tuberosity in different degrees of pronation and supination. Full pronation **(A)**, 45° **(B)**, 90° **(C)**, 135° **(D)**, and 180° full supination **(E)**.

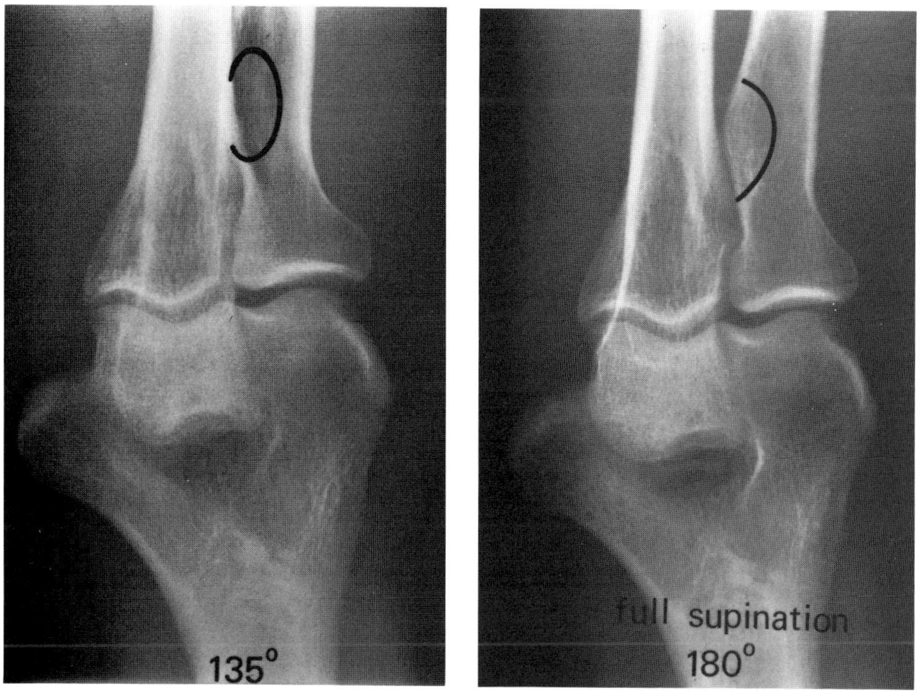

D E

FIG. 12-7. *Continued.*

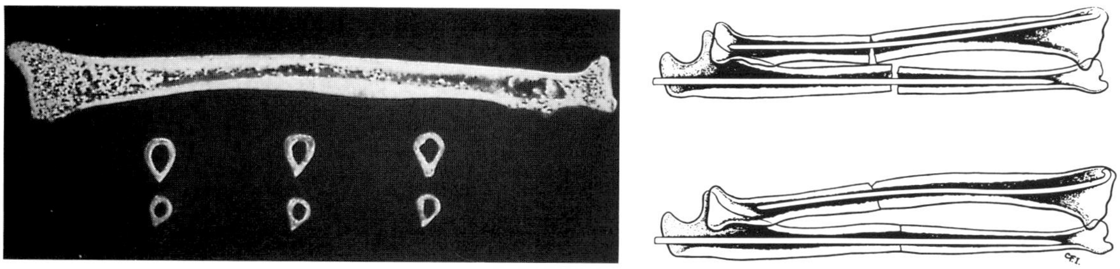

A B

FIG. 12-8. A: Anatomy of the radius with cross-sections demonstrating the variations in the size of the medullary canal. **B:** The radius and ulna with intramedullary nailing of radial and ulnar fractures. Loss of the normal radial curve (*upper drawing*) results in a loss of apposition of the ulnar fragments. (From Sage FB. Medullary fixation of fractures of the forearm: a study of the medullary canal of the radius and a report of 50 fractures of the radius treated with a prebent triangular nail. *J Bone Joint Surg* [*Am*] 1959;41A:1489–1516.)

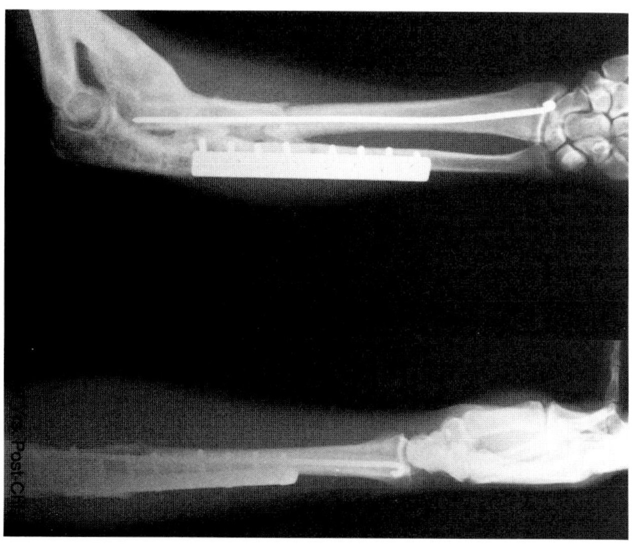

FIG. 12-9. The AP and lateral views of the forearm with an old ulnar fracture, which was plated. A more recent radial fracture was treated with a Rush pin inserted near Lister's tubercle in the distal radius. Note fixation of the elbow in flexion by the anterior heterotopic ossification.

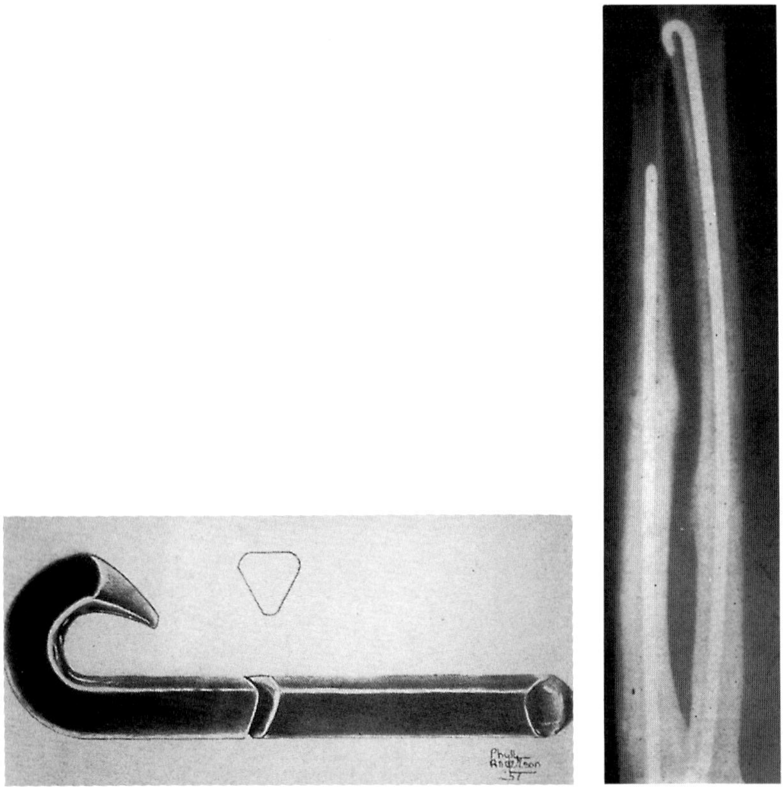

A,B

FIG. 12-10. A: Triangular solid intramedullary forearm rod. Available in 3-, 4-, and 5-mm diameters. **B:** Radiograph with triangular stainless steel rod, which looks radiographically similar to a Rush pin. (From Ritchey JJ, Richardson JP, Thompson MS. Rigid medullary fixation of forearm fractures. *South Med J* 1958;51:852–856.)

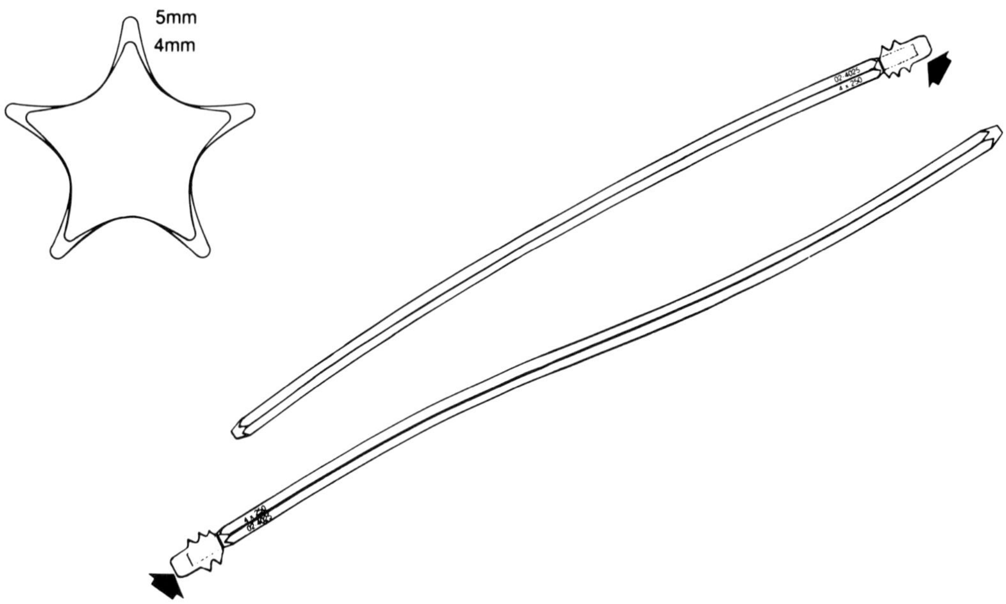

FIG. 12-11. Fluted locking True/Flex™ intramedullary nail with cross-section (*upper left*) of the configuration. The rod is titanium, and the locking cap (*arrow*) is cobalt-chromium alloy. (Courtesy of Applied Osteo Systems, Walnut Creek, CA.)

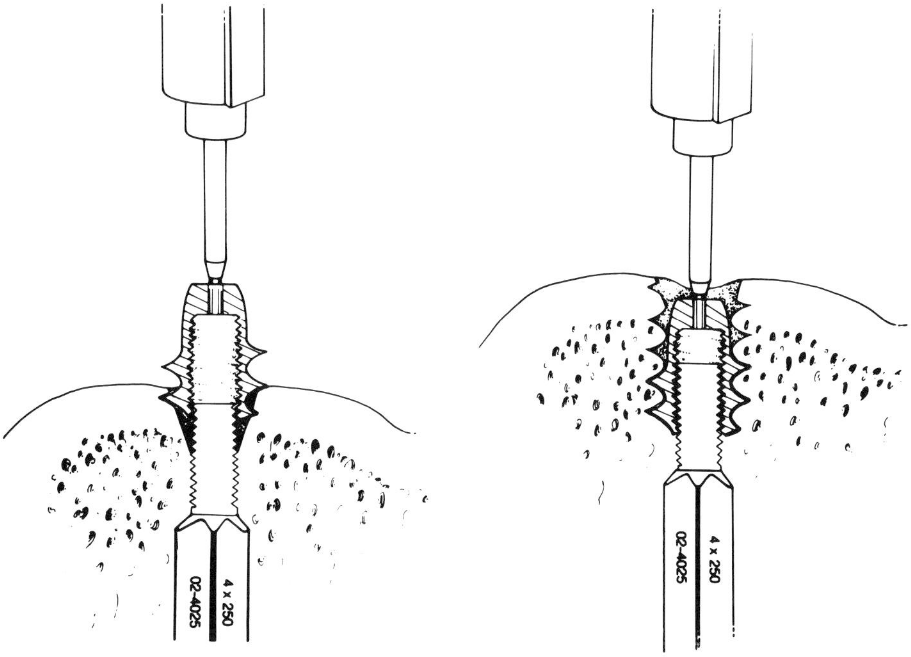

FIG. 12-12. Insertion of the locking cap. (Courtesy of Applied Osteo Systems, Walnut Creek, CA.)

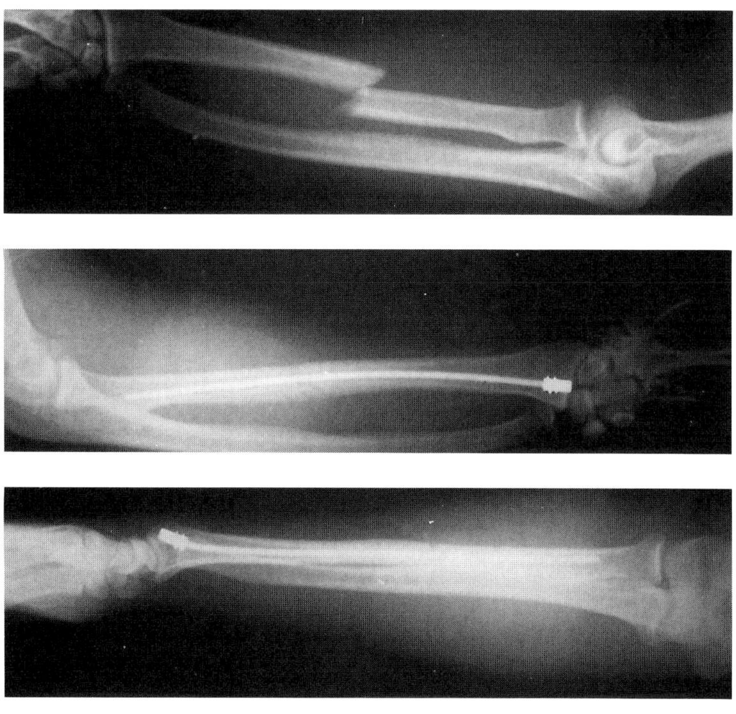

A

B

C

FIG. 12-13. A: Radiograph of a midradial fracture with displacement. The AP **(B)** and lateral **(C)** radiographs after reduction with a True/Flex™ radial rod. The locking cap is in the distal radius. (Courtesy of Dr. J. Dan Carter, Woodland Heights Medical Center, Lufkin, TX, and Applied Osteo Systems, Walnut Creek, CA.)

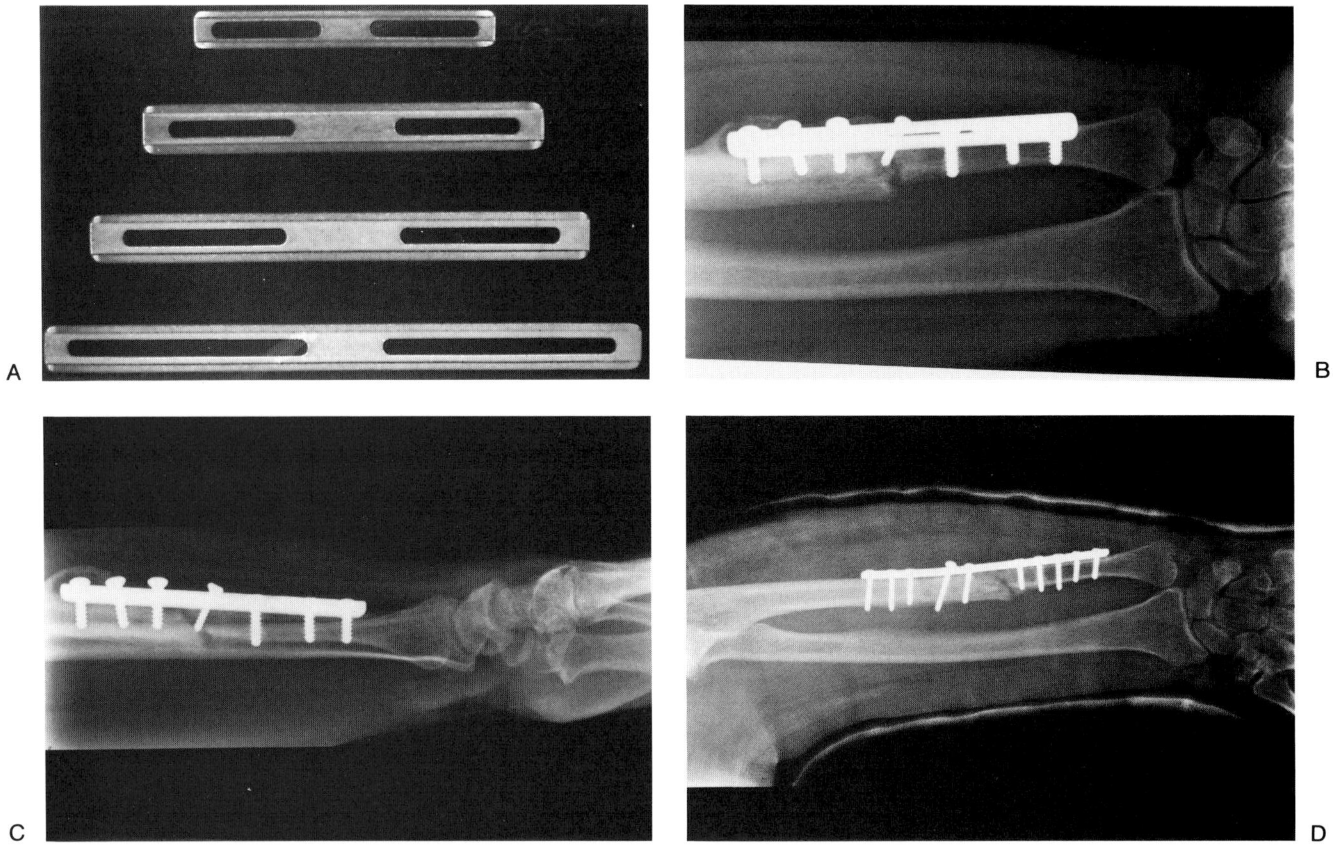

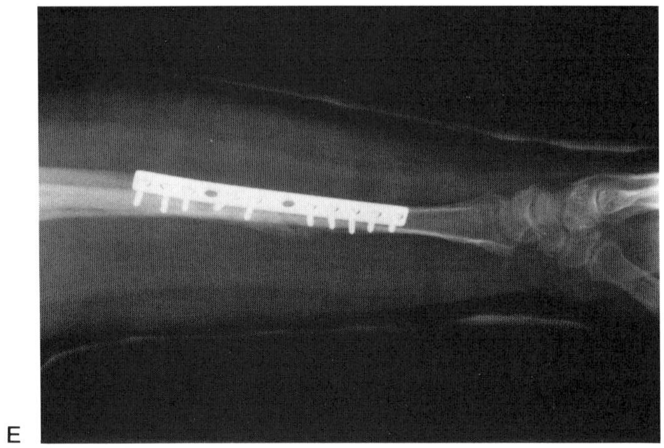

FIG. 12-14. A: Slotted Eggers plates. (From Eggers et al.,[12] with permission.) The AP **(B)** and lateral **(C)** views of the distal forearm demonstrating a distal ulnar fracture with slotted plate and screw fixation. The plate and proximal screws are loose, and the fracture has not healed. The AP **(D)** and lateral **(E)** radiographs after revision with a 12-hole compression plate.

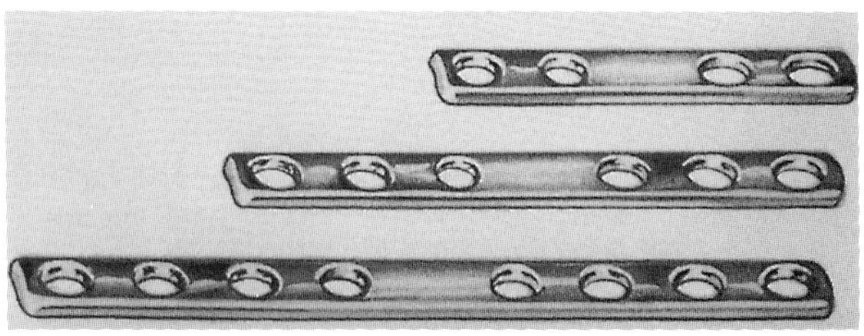

FIG. 12-15. Forearm compression plates with four, six, and eight holes. (Courtesy of Zimmer, Warsaw, IN.)

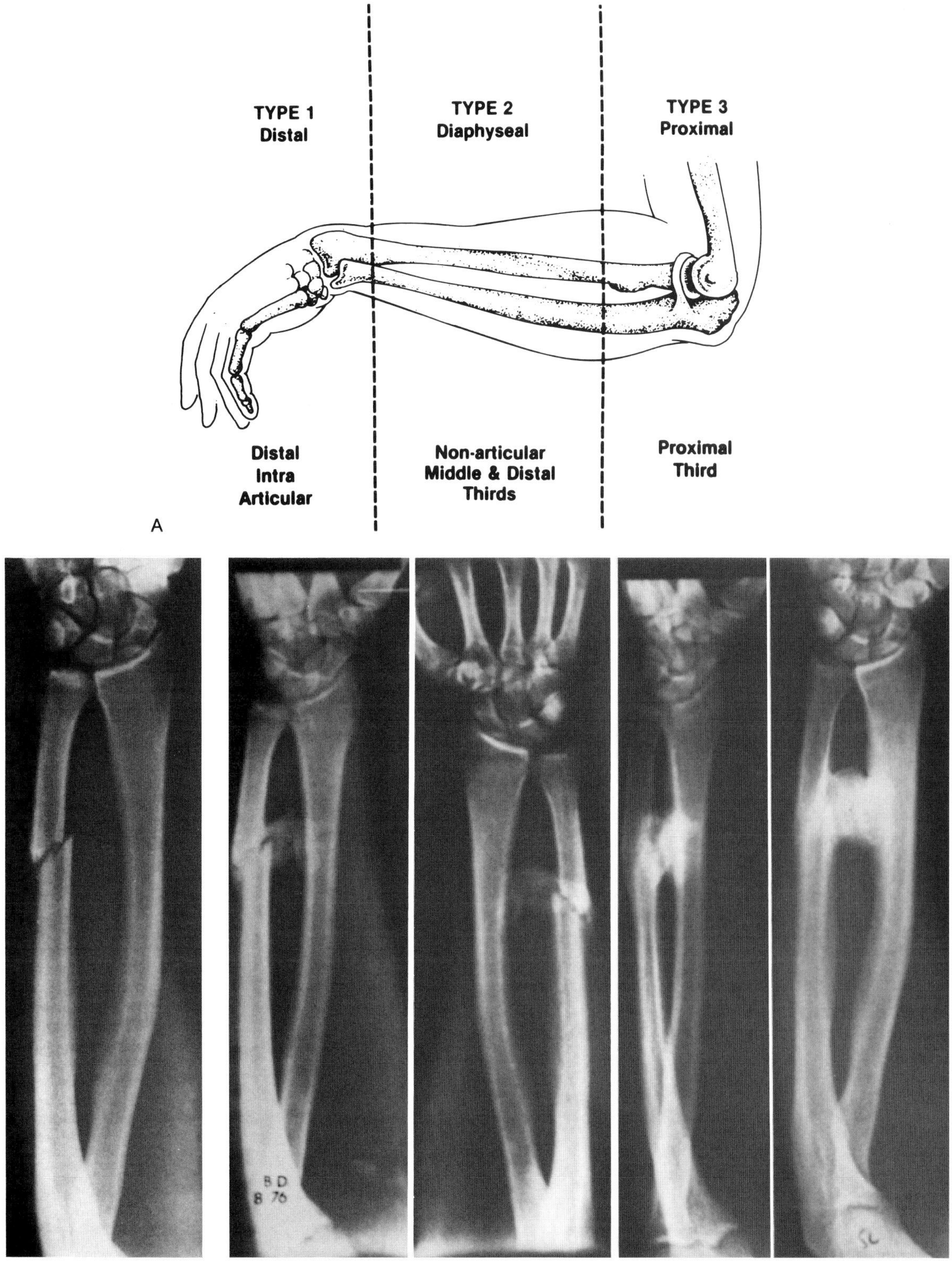

B,C,D

E, F

FIG. 12-16. Cross-union. **A:** Classification of cross-unions. Type 1, distal articular portion of the forearm; type 2, midforearm; type 3, proximal third of forearm. **B:** Isolated fracture of the distal ulna. **C–F:** Evolving bridging callus with cross-union (F) 14 months after injury. (From Vince KG, Miller JE. Cross-union complicating fracture of the forearm. Part I: adults. *J Bone Joint Surg* [*Am*] 1987;69A:640–660.)

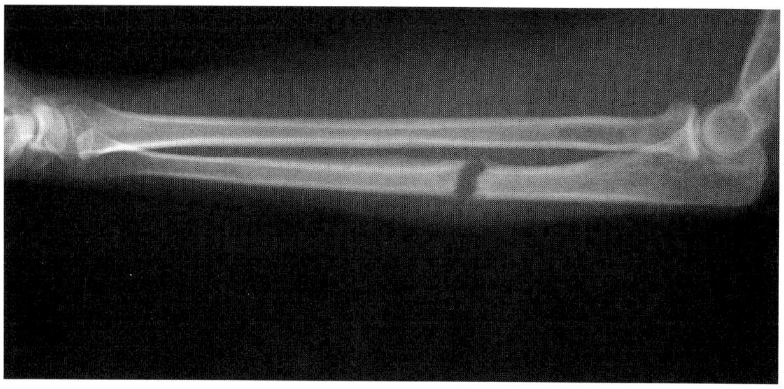

A

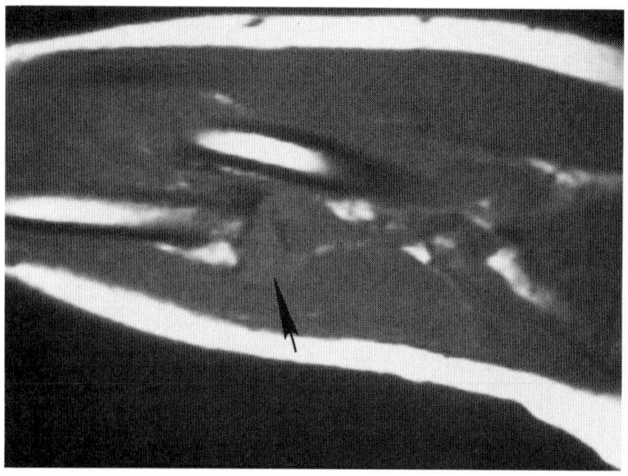

B

FIG. 12-17. Nonunion. **A:** Lateral radiograph of a well-aligned fracture of the ulna with widening and irregularity at the fracture site. **B:** The MRI scan shows soft tissue interposition (*arrow*).

tained. The use of a rigid nail may lead to loss of the radial curve. If the nail or pin is too flexible, the muscle forces will deform the radius at the fracture site.[29]

The nail's length can be measured using radiographs of the uninvolved forearm preoperatively. The nail should be about 1 cm shorter than the radius or ulna to avoid penetration of the distal articulation.[30] Open and closed techniques can be used. The radius is typically entered at Lister's tubercle.[29,30] The ulna is usually entered at the olecranon.[20,29,30]

Types of Medullary Nails
- Rush pins (Fig. 12-9)
- K-wires
- Küncher V nails
- Lottes nails
- Ritchey stainless steel rod (Fig. 12-10)
- Street nail-square
- Fluted locking nails (Figs. 12-11 to 12-13)

Both K-wires and Rush pins are round and do not prevent rotation of the fragments. Square, triangular, or fluted configurations (Fig. 12-10) are more effective at reducing rotation. Sage and Ritchey nails are triangular.[25,27,30] VonSaal, Schneider (miniature of femoral nail, see Chapters 2 and 5), Tibone, and Street nails have a square cross-sectional configuration.[30] The True/Flex™ nail has a fluted cross-sectional configuration and locking cap to provide a system similar to locking femoral and tibial nails. The fluted configuration (Fig. 12-11) reduces rotational problems.

The most popular method of treatment of displaced fractures of the radius and ulna is compression plate fixation. Autogenous bone grafts are used if a significant degree of comminution is present (types V through VII).[9] Anderson et al.[1] reported satisfactory results with compression plate fixation in 240 patients with acute diaphyseal fractures of the radius and ulna. Union occurred in 97.9% of radius fractures and 96.3% of ulnar fractures. Satisfactory or excellent results were obtained in more than 90% of patients.

Slotted Eggers plates were used early on (Fig. 12-14), but compression plates (Fig. 12-15) or semitubular plates are used more commonly today.[1,9] In most cases, the radius and ulna are exposed with separate incisions, and only the area to be plated is exposed by subperiosteal dissection. Interfragmentary screws may be used with the plate or independently for comminuted fractures.

The follow-up radiographic evaluation for open reduction is similar to that for closed. The difference is that the loss of reduction in the early posttreatment phase is less likely with internal fixation. Because rigid fixation is achieved, especially with plate and screw fixation, the healing callus is reduced, and radiographic evidence of healing may be less apparent.

COMPLICATIONS

The complications of fracture and treatment include nonunion (Fig. 12-14), malunion, infection, neurovascular injury, compartment syndrome, and cross-union.[1,7,9,10,14,17A,27,30,32] The latter results in complete loss of pronation and supination. Vince and Miller[32] classified cross-union based on the anatomic location. Type 1 cross-unions occur in the distal intraarticular region; type 2, in the diaphyseal; and type 3, in the proximal radius and ulna. Cross-unions can occur more frequently in patients with fractures at the same level (Fig. 12-16).[32]

Nonunion has been reported in up to 12% of patients treated with closed reduction, 7% of patients treated with intramedullary nailing, and 2% to 3% of patients treated with compression plates.[1,2,29,30] The normal average time for fracture healing is 7 to 8 weeks (Fig. 12-17).[2]

Refracture after plate removal is an additional complication of forearm fractures. This may occur in up to 11% of cases. The fracture typically occurs within the first 4 months after plate removal. If the plates require removal, the radiographs should be carefully evaluated or tomography should be considered prior to plate removal. Fracture sites with residual lucent areas are more prone to fracture after plate removal. This complication can be diminished by keeping plates in position for 12 to 18 months and then protecting the forearm for 4 to 6 weeks after removal. Some authors do not recommend removal. Implant fracture is unusual.[1,2,8,11,17A,27,29]

Neural injuries have been reported in one sixth of forearm fractures. The radial nerve is involved in 60% of the injuries with the remainder involving the ulnar and median nerves.[1,7,22]

The imaging of complications is usually possible with routine radiographs. Fluoroscopic positioning may be required to evaluate pin tracts and other abnormalities better, which may be a concern for refracture. On occasion, conventional tomography is useful. Conventional tomograms are less affected by the presence of metal than are computed tomograms.[6]

Soft tissue complications, such as neural injury, are most easily evaluated with magnetic resonance imaging (MRI). However, the success of this technique varies, depending on the type and amount of metal present. Plate and screw fixation causes considerably more local distortion in image quality than does a medullary nail.[6]

REFERENCES

1. Anderson LD, Meyer FN. Fractures of the shafts of the radius and ulna. In: Rockwood CA, Green DE, Buchols RW, eds. *Fractures in adults*. Vol. 1. Philadelphia: JB Lippincott; 1991:697–737.
2. Anderson LD, Sisk TD, Tooms RE, Park WI III. Compression plate fixation in acute diaphyseal fractures of the radius and ulna. *J Bone Joint Surg* [*Am*] 1975;57A:287–297.

3. Bado JL. The Monteggia lesion. *Clin Orthop* 1967;50:71–86.
4. Ballinger PW. *Merrill's atlas to roentgenographic positioning and standard radiologic procedures.* 5th ed. St. Louis: CV Mosby; 1982.
5. Bernau A, Berquist TH. *Orthopedic positioning in diagnostic radiology.* Baltimore: Urban and Schwarzenberg; 1983.
6. Berquist TH. *MRI of the musculoskeletal system.* New York: Raven Press; 1990.
7. Berquist TH. *Imaging of orthopedic trauma.* 2nd ed. New York: Raven Press; 1992.
8. Caden JG. Internal fixation of fractures of the forearm. *J Bone Joint Surg [Am]* 1961;43A:1115–1121.
9. Chapman MW, Gordon JE, Zissimos AG. Compression plate fixation of acute fractures of the diaphysis of the radius and ulna. *J Bone Joint Surg [Am]* 1989;71A:159–169.
10. DeLee JC. External fixation of the forearm and wrist. *Orthop Rev* 1981;6:43–48.
11. DeLuca PA, Lindsey RW, Rowe PA. Refracture of bones in the forearm after removal of compression plates. *J Bone Joint Surg [Am]* 1988;70A:1372–1376.
12. Eggers GWN, Ainsworth WH, Shindler TO, Pomerat CM. Clinical significance of the contact-compression factor in bone surgery. *Arch Surg* 1951;62:467–474.
13. Evans EM. Rotational deformity in the treatment of fractures of both bones of the forearm. *J Bone Joint Surg [Am]* 1945;27A:373–379.
14. Failla JM, Amadio PC, Morrey BF. Post traumatic proximal radioulnar synostosis. *J Bone Joint Surg [Am]* 1989;71A:1208–1213.
15. Giustra PE, Killoran PJ, Fierman RS, Root JA. The missed Monteggia fracture. *Radiology* 1974;110:45–47.
16. Grace TG, Eversmann WW. Forearm fractures. *J Bone Joint Surg [Am]* 1980;62A:433–438.
17. Gustilo RB, Anderson JT. Prevention of infection in the treatment of 1025 open fractures of the long bones: retrospective and prospective analysis. *J Bone Joint Surg [Am]* 1976;58A:453–458.
17A. Hidaka S, Gustilo RB. Refracture of bones of the forearm after plate removal. *J Bone Joint Surg [Am]* 1984;66A:1241–1243.
18. Hollinshead WH. *Anatomy for surgeons.* 3rd ed. Vol. 3. New York: Harper and Row; 1982.
19. Jinkins WJ, Lockhart LD, Eggers GWN. Fractures of the forearm in adults. *South Med J* 1960;53:669–679.
20. Mallin BA. Principles of management of forearm fractures. In: Chapman MW, Madison M, eds. *Operative orthopedics.* Vol. 1. Philadelphia: JB Lippincott; 1988:263–271.
21. Patrick J. Study of supination and pronation with special reference to the treatment of forearm fractures. *J Bone Joint Surg [Am]* 1946;28A:737–748.
22. Poppi M. Fracture of the distal radius with ulnar nerve palsy. *J Trauma* 1978;18:278–279.
23. Rang M. *Anatomy of orthopaedics.* Baltimore: Williams and Wilkins; 1966.
24. Reckling FW, Cordell LD. Unstable fracture-dislocation of the forearm (Monteggia and Galeazzi lesions). *J Bone Joint Surg [Am]* 1982;64A:999–1007.
25. Ritchey JJ, Richardson JP, Thompson MS. Rigid medullary fixation of forearm fractures. *South Med J* 1958;51:852–856.
26. Rogers LF. *Radiology of skeletal trauma.* New York: Churchill Livingstone; 1993.
27. Sage FB. Medullary fixation of fractures of the forearm: a study of the medullary canal of the radius and a report of 50 fractures of the radius treated with a prebent triangular nail. *J Bone Joint Surg [Am]* 1959;41A:1489–1516.
28. Sarmiento A, Cooper JS, Sinclair WF. Forearm fractures. Early functional bracing—a preliminary report. *J Bone Joint Surg [Am]* 1975;57A:297–304.
29. Smith H, Sage FP. Medullary fixation of forearm fractures. *J Bone Joint Surg [Am]* 1957;39A:91–98.
30. Street DM. Intramedullary forearm nailing. *Clin Orthop* 1986;212:219–230.
31. Valande M. Luxation en arrière du aibitus avec fracture de la diaphyse radiale. *Bull Mem Soc Natl Chir* 1929;55:435–437.
32. Vince KG, Miller JE. Cross-union complicating fracture of the forearm. Part I: adults. *J Bone Joint Surg [Am]* 1987;69A:640–660.

Imaging Atlas of Orthopedic Appliances and Prostheses,
edited by T.H. Berquist.
Mayo Clinic Foundation © 1995.
Published by Raven Press, Ltd., New York.

CHAPTER 13

Hand and Wrist

Thomas H. Berquist and Stephen D. Trigg

The complex bone and soft tissue anatomy of the hand and wrist present a continuing challenge to radiologists. We must deal with the detection of lesions and their characterization or classification on a daily basis. Interpreting postoperative images and defining the nature of our patients' symptoms in this setting can be even more difficult.

This chapter concentrates on the pre- and postoperative imaging of trauma, arthroplasty, and other common orthopedic procedures. Emphasis is placed on conditions treated with implants or fixation devices.

IMAGING TECHNIQUES

Routine radiography, including fluoroscopically positioned spot views, remains the first step for imaging hand and wrist disorders.[7,9,24,26]

Hand

Posterolateral (PA), lateral, and oblique views are essential for the evaluation of the hand. When a specific finger is involved, it should be isolated, and PA, oblique, and lateral views should be obtained (Fig. 13-1).[2,4,7]

Special views designed to demonstrate the metacarpal heads (Brewerton view) and navicular-trapezium-first metacarpal articulations (Burman view) can also be obtained. However, unless technologists perform these views frequently, the quality may be inconsistent.[2,12,14,36] Fluoroscopic positioning is a simple alternative.[7,26,28]

Stress views of the thumb or fingers may be indicated to evaluate soft tissue injuries. Generally, a local anesthetic injection is required to improve accuracy in the acutely injured or painful joint. Contrast media can be injected at the same time to provide a more specific diagnosis.[7,10,54]

Wrist

Routinely, PA, lateral, and oblique views are obtained. The PA view provides significant bone and soft tissue information to assist in evaluating the other routine views and selecting additional imaging studies. Subtle fractures, specifically involving the scaphoid, can be easily overlooked. The navicular fat stripe is useful in this regard. This fat plane (Fig. 13-2) lies between the radial collateral ligament and the tendon sheaths of the abductor pollicis longus and extensor pollicis brevis. This structure is inconsistently seen in children but easily identified in 96% of adults. Terry and Ramin[58] noted the absence or displacement of the navicular fat stripe in 88% of fractures on the radial side of the wrist and 87% of scaphoid fractures.

The articular surfaces of the bones of the wrist should be parallel with 1- to 2-mm joint spaces. A change in the joint spaces or arcs formed by the carpal bones (Fig. 13-3) may indicate subluxation or dislocation.[7,17,26,28]

There are multiple measurements that can be determined on the PA view. Several commonly used ratios are the carpal height (Fig. 13-4) and carpal ulnar distance (Fig. 13-5).[7,47] The normal carpal height ratio should be 0.54 ± 0.03 compared with the third metacarpal. However, because the third metacarpal may not be completely included on PA views of the wrist, an alternative

(*text continues on page 836*)

T. H. Berquist: Mayo Medical School and Department of Diagnostic Radiology, Mayo Clinic Jacksonville, Jacksonville, Florida 32224.

S. D. Trigg: Mayo Medical School and Department of Orthopedic Surgery, Mayo Clinic Jacksonville, Jacksonville, Florida 32224.

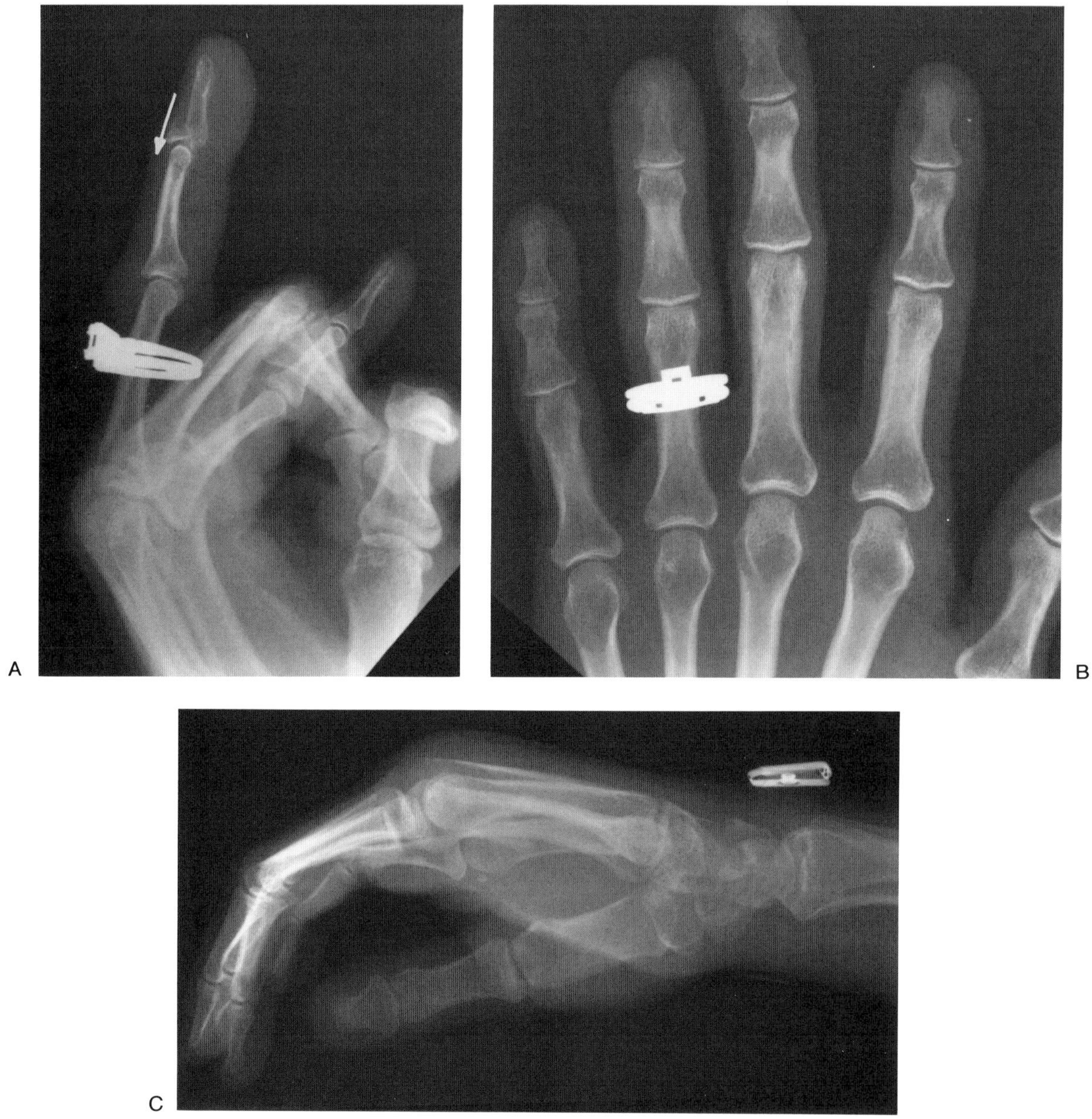

FIG. 13-1. Lateral **(A)** and PA **(B)** radiographs of the left hand demonstrating a dorsal plate fracture of the distal phalanx of the fourth finger. The fragment is pulled proximally (*arrow*) by the extensor attachment. Radiographs of individual fingers prevent the overlap problems seen on lateral views of the entire hand **(C)**, which make it difficult to exclude fractures or identify fracture sites.

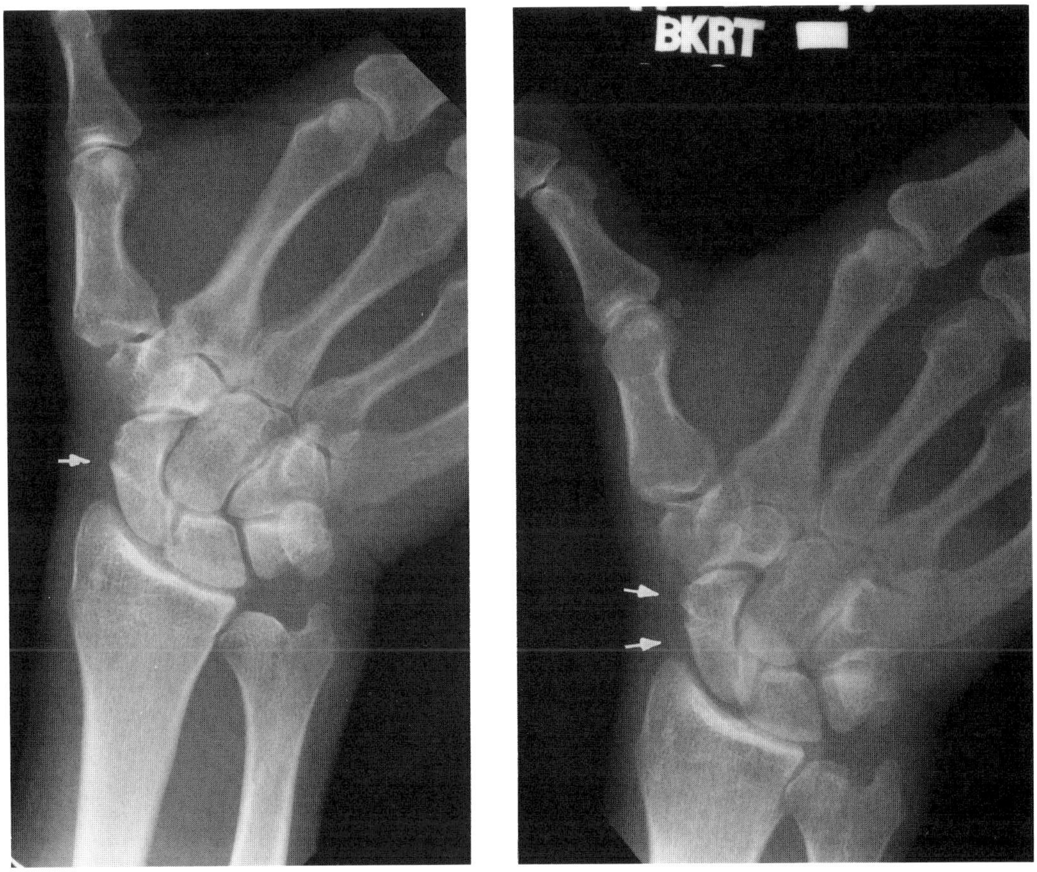

FIG. 13-2. Scaphoid views of the wrist demonstrating the normal navicular fat stripe (*arrows*).

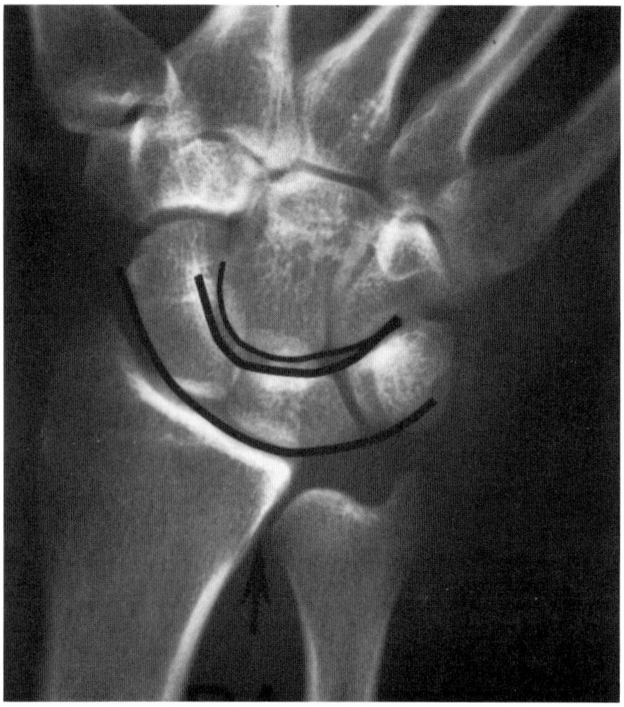

A

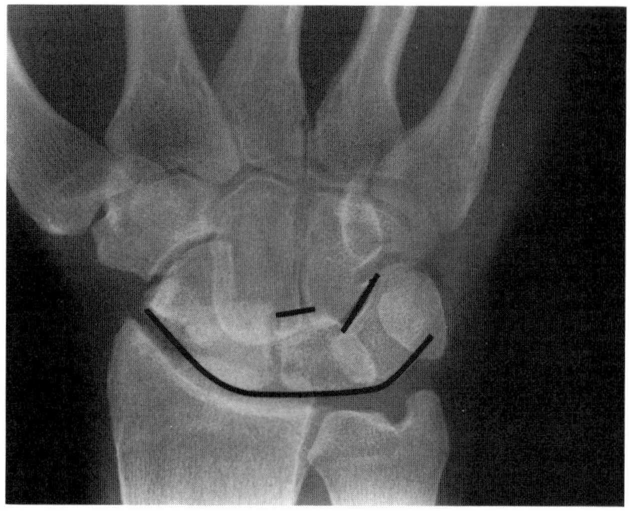

B

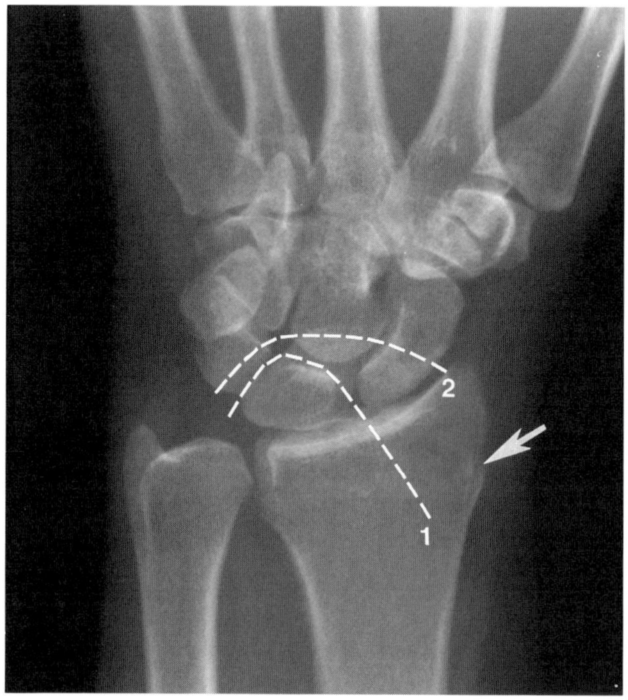

C

FIG. 13-3. Normal joint spaces and arcs of the wrist on the PA view. **A:** A PA radiograph of the wrist demonstrating the normal arcs formed by the carpal bones. The distal radioulnar joint is shown in profile (*arrow*). **B:** A PA view of the wrist demonstrating interrupted arcs in a patient with a transscaphoid perilunate dislocation. **C:** Arcs formed by the vulnerable zones of the wrist are aligned in the opposite direction of the articular arcs. *1,* Lesser arc follows the radial styloid midcarpal joint and lunotriquetral joint; *2,* greater arc passes through the scaphoid, capitate, and triquetrum. These arcs are considered in fracture and instability patterns in the wrist.[17] Note the radial fracture (*arrow*) and scapholunate space widening along the lesser arc (1), which was caused by ligament injury.

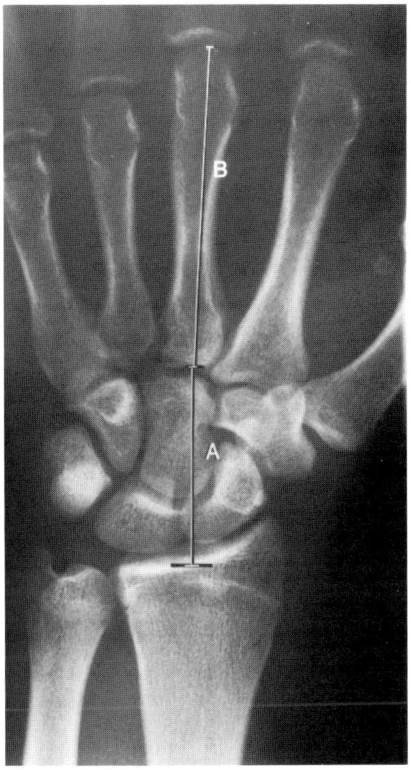

A

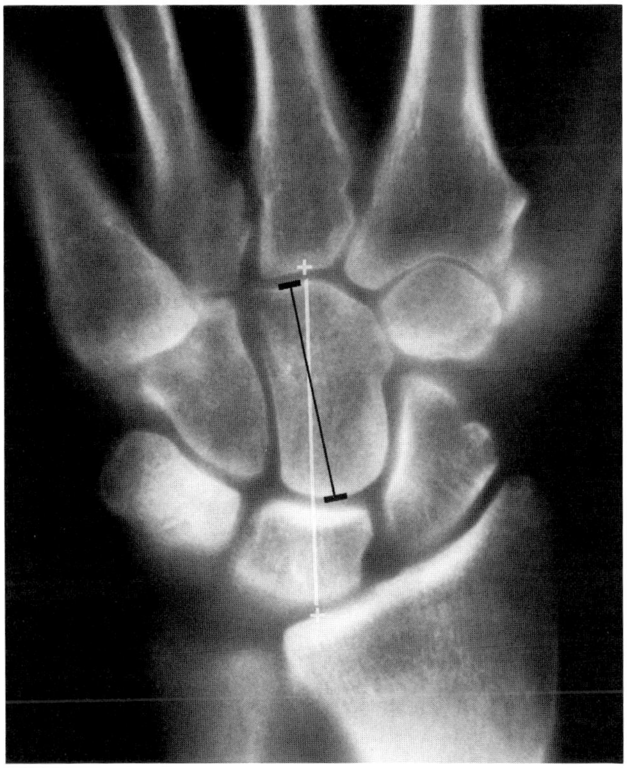

B

FIG. 13-4. Carpal height ratio. **A:** The conventional technique is the ratio of the carpal height (distal radial articular surface to the base of the third metacarpal) to the length of the third metacarpal (normal, 0.54 ± 0.03).[7] **B:** The modified carpal height ratio described by Nattrass et al.[47] The carpal height is measured along the third metacarpal axis from the third metacarpal base to the radial articular surface (+) divided by the capitate length (*black lines*; normal, 1.57 ± 0.06).

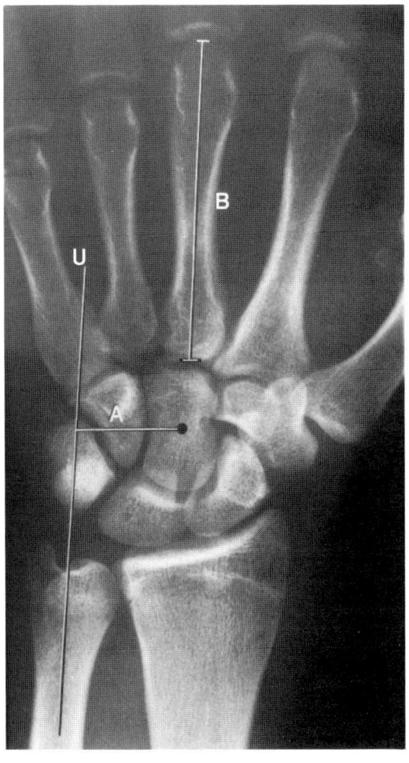

FIG. 13-5. The carpal ulnar distance forms a ratio of 0.30 ± 0.03 with the length of the third metacarpal. A line is constructed parallel to the ulnar shaft (*u*). The measurement of a perpendicular from ulnar line to the center of the capitate **(A)** over the third metacarpal height **(B)** forms the carpal ulnar ratio.[7]

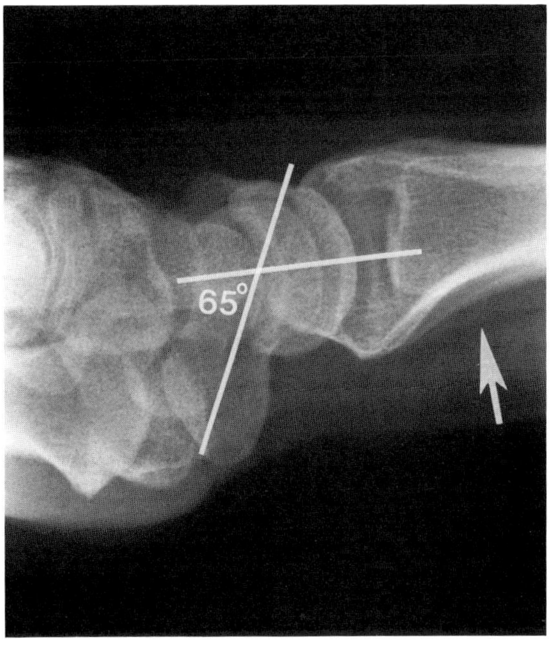

FIG. 13-6. Lateral radiographs of the wrist demonstrating the normal pronator fat strip (*arrow*). The scapholunate angle is normally 47° with the wrist in neutral position. With radial or ulnar deviation, this angle can decrease to 30° or increase to 60°, providing the range of normal. In this case, the angle is increased to 65°.

method can be used. Nattrass et al.[47] described using the carpal height divided by the capitate length (Fig. 13-4B). This new method was found to be consistent bilaterally but reduced in patients with carpal collapse, as expected. The carpal ulnar ratio is calculated by dividing a line perpendicular to the ulnar shaft to the center of the capitate by the third metacarpal height (Fig. 13-5).[7,48]

The lateral view of the wrist also provides significant information with subtle soft tissue signs and important carpal measurements.[7,26,28] The pronator fat stripe passes along the volar aspect of the distal radius approximately 1 cm from the diaphyseal-metaphyseal junction (Fig. 13-6). Subtle displacement or obliteration of the fat plane is common with distal radial fractures.[7]

Each carpal bone can be identified on the lateral view—an interesting and rewarding exercise. In the neutral position (not often seen radiographically), the radius, lunate, capitate, and third metacarpal should be aligned. Slight radial or ulnar deviation or mild flexed or extended projections cause disruption of this straight line pattern.[7]

There are two obvious carpal collapse patterns that can be identified on the lateral radiograph. The most common is the dorsal intercalated segment instability (DISI, Fig. 13-6). This is characterized by dorsiflexion of the lunate and palmar flexion of the scaphoid, which results in an increased scapholunate angle. This pattern is most often associated with scaphoid fractures or scapholunate ligament injuries.[7,17] The volar intercalated segment instability pattern is characterized by a palmar flexed lunate and a decrease in the scapholunate angle. This pattern is most commonly seen with lunotriquetral ligament injuries, midcarpal sprains, and rheumatoid arthritis.[7,17]

Special views, such as the carpal tunnel view, pisiform view, dorsal tangential views, and fluoroscopically positioned spot views or motion studies may also be required.[1,7,10–14,18,21,22,34–36,62] Motion studies include PA views with radial and ulnar deviation, lateral views with the wrist flexed and extended, and the clenched-fist view.[1,7,26,28,49,62] Noting the relationships of the carpal bones in different positions is useful for evaluating the articulations and instability patterns (Fig. 13-7).[18,22,33,49,63]

Conventional and Computed Tomography (CT)

Thin-section (1 to 3 mm) conventional tomography or CT is useful for detecting subtle fractures and other bony pathologic disorders. We typically use PA and lateral projections for complex motion tomography. However, in certain cases, oblique positions are preferred to improve the position of specific carpal bones.[7,56] When CT is used, several positions or reformatted images may be necessary to evaluate the positions of fragments. This is especially important for scaphoid fractures.[7,15,40,51,56,57]

In addition, CT is preferred for evaluating the distal radioulnar joints (DRUJ). Neutral, pronation, and supination positions should be considered for patients with suspected subluxation. Arthrography can be combined with either conventional tomography or CT to enhance the diagnosis of articular disorders.[3,7,16,50,60] Three-dimensional CT reconstructions are possible, but they are not frequently obtained.[59,61]

Radionuclide Imaging

Three-phase radionuclide studies of the hand and wrist are useful for evaluating acute and chronic trauma related disorders. Technetium-99mm coupled with phosphate compounds, such as methylene diphosphonate, is commonly used. Three-phase imaging provides additional advantages over the usual delayed (2 to 3 hours) bone images (phase III).[23,26,29] The first phase (I) provides flow information as rapid sequence images are obtained during the first 1 to 2 minutes after bolus injection. Soft tissue distribution can be evaluated 5 to 10 minutes after the injection (phase II). Diffusely increased or abnormal uptake is not unusual during the first two phases. The lack of focal uptake on the delayed images is useful for excluding osseous pathologic conditions.[7,28,29,44] Focal uptake localizes the osseous abnormality so that additional studies, such as CT, can further define the cause of the lesion.[24]

Radionuclide scintigraphy is most commonly used for subtle osseous pathologic conditions (Fig. 13-8), reflex sympathetic dystrophy, bone ischemia, and early infection.[7,23,32,44]

Magnetic Resonance Imaging (MRI)

An effective technique for demonstrating soft tissue and osseous pathologic conditions, MRI provides superior soft tissue contrast and multiple image plane capabilities with excellent anatomic detail and superior contrast between pathologic and normal tissues.[5,6,7,31,55,64] It has been used for the detection of soft tissue injury, including ligament injuries of the wrist, osseous trauma, avascular necrosis, and neoplasms. As a preoperative tool for patients requiring orthopedic implants (fixation devices or arthroplasty), the technique is not commonly required.[5,7] Therefore, an in-depth discussion of techniques is not indicated here.

In the postoperative setting, we rarely use MRI because the metal artifact in generally too significant to permit adequate evaluation of the region of interest.[7] However, evaluating fracture healing or early avascular necrosis is easily accomplished in patients treated with closed reduction and cast or splint immobilization. (Fig. 13-9).[5,7] Both T1- and T2-weighted sequences should be obtained. Two image planes (typically axial and coronal) are usually necessary for a complete evaluation of patients with suspected posttraumatic complications.[5]

Arthrography, Tenography, and Diagnostic Injections

Arthrograms, tenograms, and diagnostic injections (soft tissue, tendon sheath, and articular) are commonly performed in our practice to evaluate and localize patient symptoms.[7,8] Although they are invasive, these techniques have a low complication rate and provide valuable information to assist with preoperative planning and to evaluate postoperative complications.[7,8,41,50]

At some institutions, MRI has replaced arthrography to evaluate the triangular fibrocartilage complex (TFC) and scapholunate ligament.[30,64] However, the ability to perform diagnostic injections in conjunction with arthrography provides valuable information concerning the localization of a symptom.[8] Therefore, we still prefer arthrography in difficult orthopedic cases.[7,8]

The findings on wrist arthrograms must be correlated with clinical symptoms. Three-compartment injections are often required, although this is somewhat controversial.[38,39,41,42] We initially start in the most symptomatic region and continue with other compartments as indicated, depending on the radiographic findings (Fig. 13-10).[7] It is important to perform stress studies and document abnormalities fluoroscopically (video tape) during the procedure.[7,19,20,27,37] A correlation of arthrographic findings with clinical symptoms is not always possible.[45,46] Normal communications between the radiocarpal and lunotriquetral ligament have been reported in 36% and the radioulnar joint and radiocarpal joint in 7% to 35% of patients.[7,25,27] Other communications are also seen in normal individuals. In some cases, diagnostic injection of an anesthetic agent can be helpful.[8] In the presence of a normal arthrogram and no pain relief from such an injection, the clinician may proceed to tenography or MRI.[7,52,53]

The joints of the hand, wrist, and tendon sheaths are easily entered using fluoroscopic guidance. Contrast and anesthetic agent injections are useful in detecting articular or tendon sheath abnormalities.[7,8]

TRAUMA

Fractures and fracture-dislocations of the hand and wrist occur commonly. The common injury patterns, classifications, and methods of fixation are reviewed according to the anatomic region. Complications and postoperative imaging are discussed together at the end of this section.

Distal Radius and Ulna

Fractures of the distal radius account for 17% of all fractures seen in the emergency room.[72] These fractures also most frequently require manipulation for reduction, which necessitates radiographic monitoring.[72,85]

There are five basic fracture patterns that have eponyms. These include Colles's fracture, the Smith fracture, Barton's fracture, the chauffeur's fracture, and the Galeazzi fracture.[72] The fracture patterns and classifications are outlined separately. The treatment and postoperative imaging of complications are discussed together to avoid redundancy.

Colles's Fracture

The Colles's fracture was initially described in 1813 prior to the development of the x-ray machine.[121] The term is well known and frequently used incorrectly. The term should be restricted to fractures of the radial metaphysis or epiphysis with dorsal displacement of the distal fragment. There may be involvement of the radiocarpal or distal radial ulnar joint, and an associated ulnar styloid or distal ulnar fracture is frequently present (Fig. 13-11).[72,85,121]

This fracture most commonly results from a fall on the outstretched hand. Elderly patients with osteopenia are particularly susceptible.[72,121] Several classification systems have been proposed for Colles's fractures. The AO classification is the most complex. There are three major categories of fracture with three subcategories in each group. Type A fractures are extraarticular. Type B fractures are partially articular. Type C fractures are completely articular. We prefer to use the Frykman[103] classification because it is simpler to use and correlation with the prognosis is possible. This system is based on articular involvement of the radiocarpal joints or DRUJ and the presence or absence of an associated ulnar styloid fracture (Table 13-1 and Fig. 13-12).[72,103]

Cooney et al.[85] also recommend the "universal" classification, which is a modification of the Garland and Wesley[106] method. Distal radial fractures are classified as extraarticular (type I, undisplaced; type II, displaced) or intraarticular. The type I fractures are similar to Frykman type I injuries (Fig. 13-12A). Type III intraarticular fractures are undisplaced, and type IV are displaced (see Fig. 13-20). Type IV fractures are subdivided into A, reducible, stable; B, reducible, unstable; and C, irreducible.[85,106]

Smith Fracture

The Smith fracture was originally described in 1847 by Robert Smith.[144] This is basically a reverse Colles's

TABLE 13-1. *Frykman classification of Colles-type fractures*[103]

Type	Fracture location	Distal ulnar fracture
I	Extraarticular	Absent
II	Extraarticular	Present
III	Intraarticular involving radiocarpal joint	Absent
IV	Intraarticular involving radiocarpal joint	Present
V	Intraarticular involving distal radioulnar joint	Absent
VI	Intraarticular involving distal radioulnar joint	Present
VII	Intraarticular involving both radiocarpal and distal radioulnar joints	Absent
VIII	Intraarticular involving both radiocarpal and distal radioulnar joints	Present

fracture, and the term should be restricted to fractures of the distal radial metaphysis or epiphysis that are displaced or angulated in a volar or palmar direction (Fig. 13-13).[72,144] Smith fractures can occur during a fall on the flexed wrist or from dorsal trauma.[72,85] These fractures have been classified by Thomas.[163] Type I fractures are extraarticular. The type II fracture is a typical Barton's volar fracture, and type III fractures are oblique juxtaarticular fractures with increased instability (Fig. 13-14).[72,163]

Barton's Fracture

Barton's fracture is credited to John Rhea Barton who described the injury in 1838.[91,96,143,164] The injury, by definition, is a marginal rim fracture of the radius that displaces along with the carpal bones, producing a fracture subluxation (Fig. 13-15). The injury typically involves the volar or dorsal lip of the radius. The dorsal radius is more commonly involved. The volar injury is the injury described by Thomas as a type II fracture.[163]

Chauffeur's Fracture (Radial Styloid Fracture)

The chauffeur's fracture is an intraarticular radial styloid fracture. The fracture line typically extends from the junction of the scaphoid and lunate fossae on the radial articular surface obliquely to below the radial styloid (Fig. 13-16). The injury usually occurs with axial trauma and was originally ascribed to the backfire of the original automobiles, causing the starting crank to turn and break the wrist of the chauffeur.[95]

Galeazzi Fracture

The Galeazzi fracture is usually a distal radial diaphysis fracture with associated subluxation or dislocation of the DRUJ.[72,85,134] The radial fracture may occur more distally near the metaphysis or more proximally near the elbow. Unfortunately, the radioulnar joint injury is easily overlooked radiographically. Both injuries should be treated at the same time (Fig. 13-17).

Treatment

The prereduction images should include PA, lateral, and oblique views of the wrist. The forearm, including the elbow, should be imaged in patients with shaft fractures or suspected articular involvement. The wrist must be carefully studied to identify the following features in fractures of the distal radius and ulna.

1. Number of fragments
2. Degree of angulation or displacement
3. Articular involvement
4. Loss of radial length
5. Signs of ligament injury (joint-space incongruity)

In some cases, fluoroscopic spot views or prereduction CT or conventional tomography are required to define the position of the fragments more accurately.[72,129]

The treatment options include closed reduction with cast immobilization, external fixation, and open reduction with internal fixation. The treatment goals for distal radial fractures should include anatomic reduction as soon as possible with maintenance of radial length or neutral ulnar variance. The radial angle should be 0° to 10° palmar on the lateral radiograph, and there should be 14° of ulnar inclination of the PA view. Articular congruity is important. There is some variability in fracture reduction parameters, depending on the patient's age and activity and the priority of other injuries that may have occurred during the same event.[72,85]

Seventy-five to 80% of undisplaced fractures can be treated with closed reduction and cast immobilization. Radiographs should be obtained weekly for 3 weeks to confirm that reduction is maintained.[86,99,104,121]

For purposes of this atlas, we concentrate on reduction techniques using orthopedic fixation devices. Fixation may be achieved using external, internal, or combined techniques, depending on the extent of injury.[81,84,86,121]

External Fixation

External fixation is achieved by using finger traction with 8 to 10 pounds of counterweight for 5 to 10 minutes. An axillary block is typically used to facilitate the procedure. External fixation devices are generally left in place for 8 weeks followed by 2 to 3 weeks of splint immobilization.[86] Pin and plaster techniques were used early in the treatment of distal radial fractures.[80] However, stiffness and decreased motion resulted after immobilization for 6 to 8 weeks.[80,86] External fixators can cause

(*text continues on page 844*)

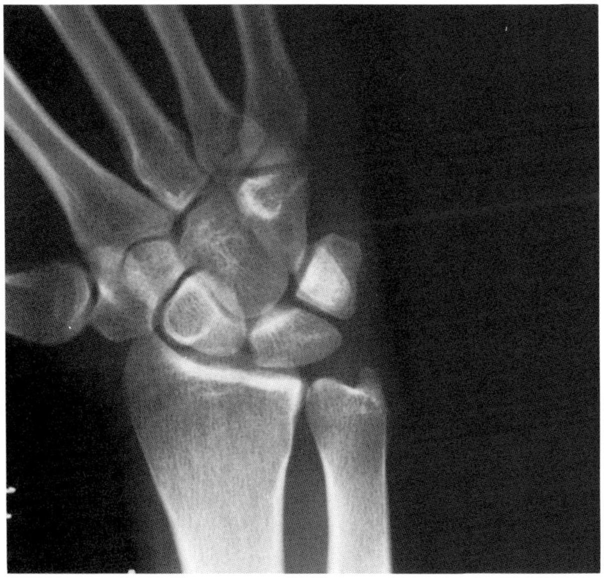

A

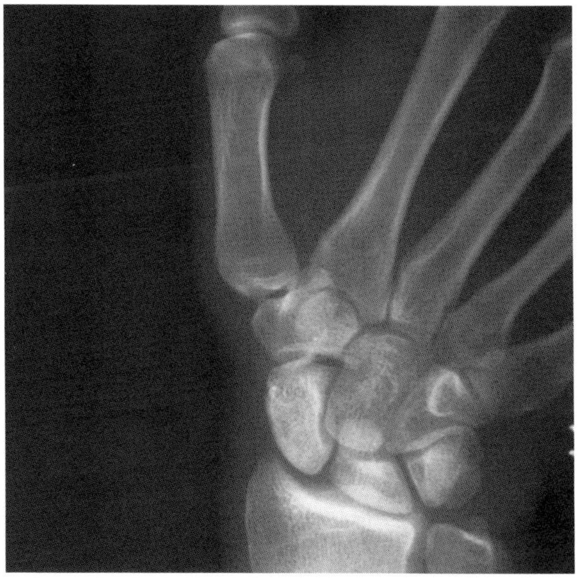

B

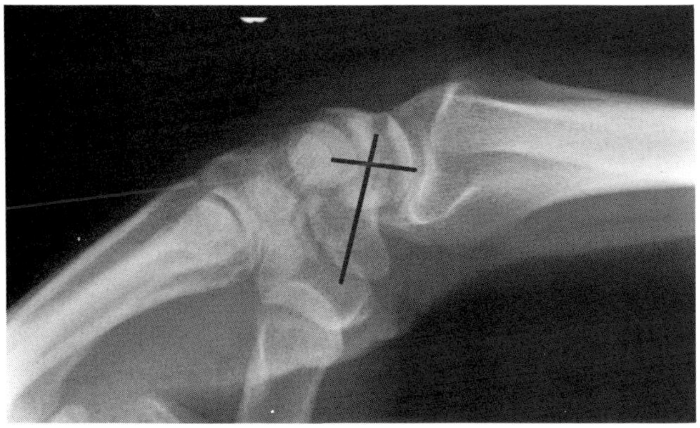

C

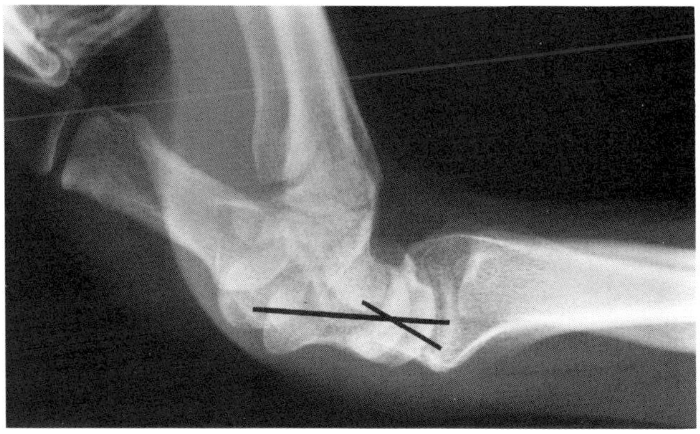

D

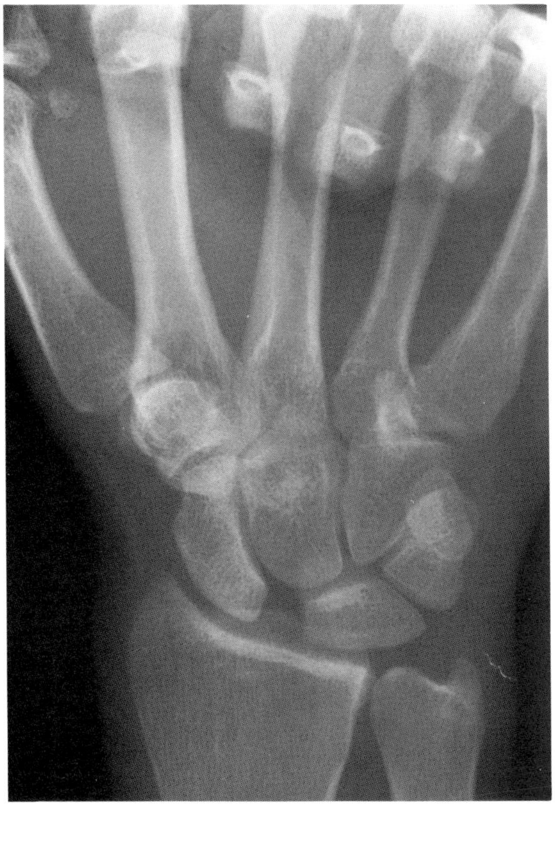

E

FIG. 13-7. Motion series. **A:** A PA radiograph with radial deviation. **B:** A PA radiograph with ulnar deviation. **C:** Lateral with wrist flexed. **D:** Lateral with wrist extended (note changes in scapholunate angles in C and D). **E:** Clenched-fist PA radiograph demonstrating obvious separation of the scapholunate space as a result of ligament injury.

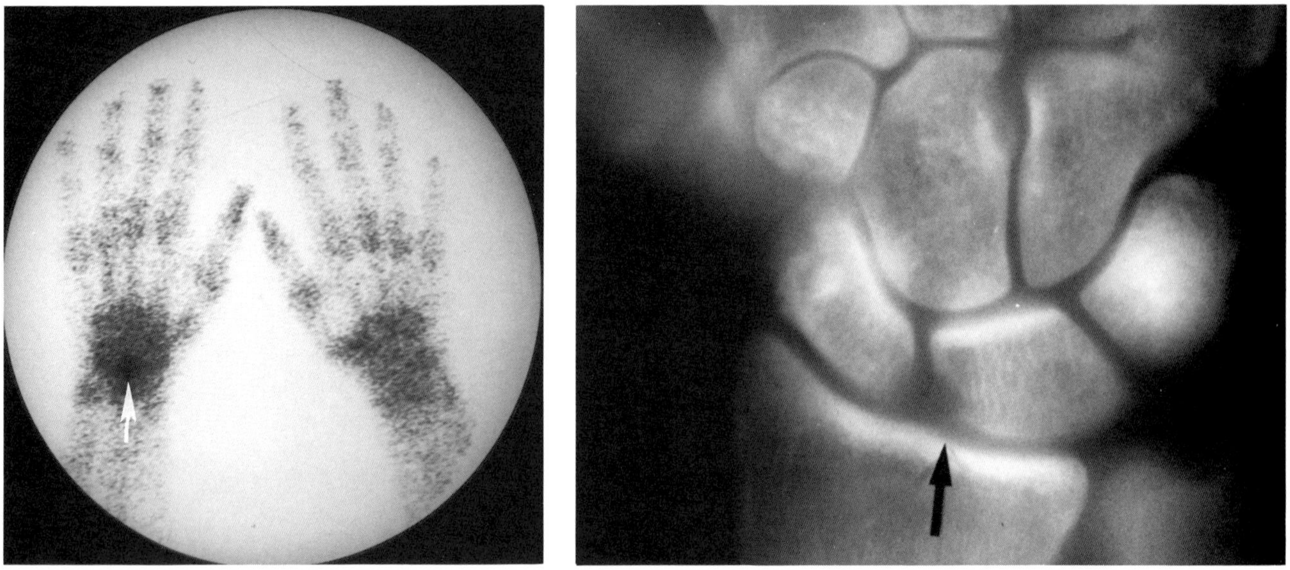

A B

FIG. 13-8. Chronic posttraumatic wrist pain. **A:** The PA delayed radionuclide images demonstrate a focal area of increased tracer (*arrow*) in the midproximal carpal row. **B:** The anteroposterior (AP) tomogram demonstrates a small posttraumatic osteochondral defect in the lunate (*arrow*).

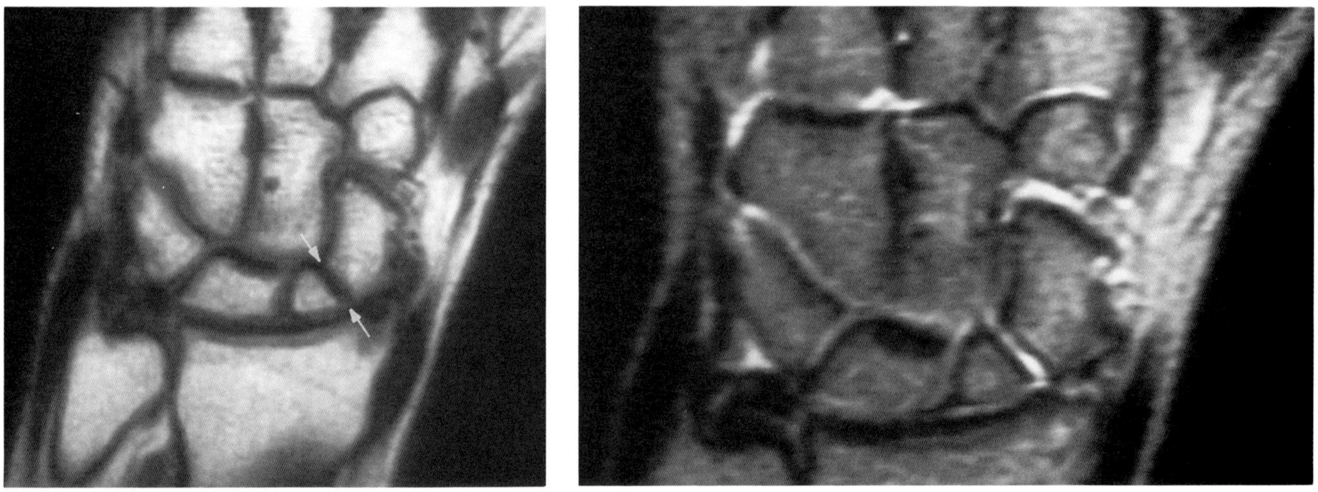

A B

FIG. 13-9. A patient with wrist pain after scaphoid fracture treated with cast immobilization. **A:** Coronal spin-echo (SE) 500/20 (TR 500 msec, TE 20 msec) (T1-weighted) image shows a linear dark area of low signal intensity through the proximal scaphoid (*arrows*). The signal intensity in the proximal fragment is normal. There is no avascular necrosis. **B:** Coronal SE 2,000/80 (TR 2000 msec, TE 80 msec) image shows a high signal intensity in the fracture region as a result of fluid and nonunion. (From Berquist TH. *MRI of the musculoskeletal system,* 2nd ed. New York: Raven Press, 1990.)

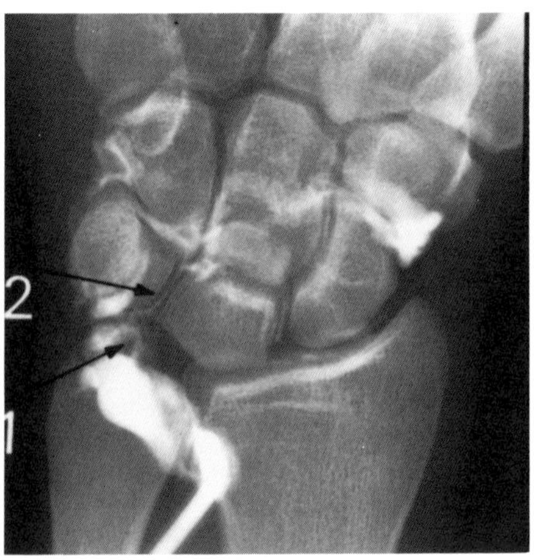

FIG. 13-10. A patient with ulnar wrist pain. The DRUJ was injected, and the injection and arthrogram were video taped and fluoroscopically monitored. There is communication with the radiocarpal joint through a TFC defect (*1*) and also communication with the midcarpal compartment (*2*) as a result of a lunotriquetral ligament injury.

A 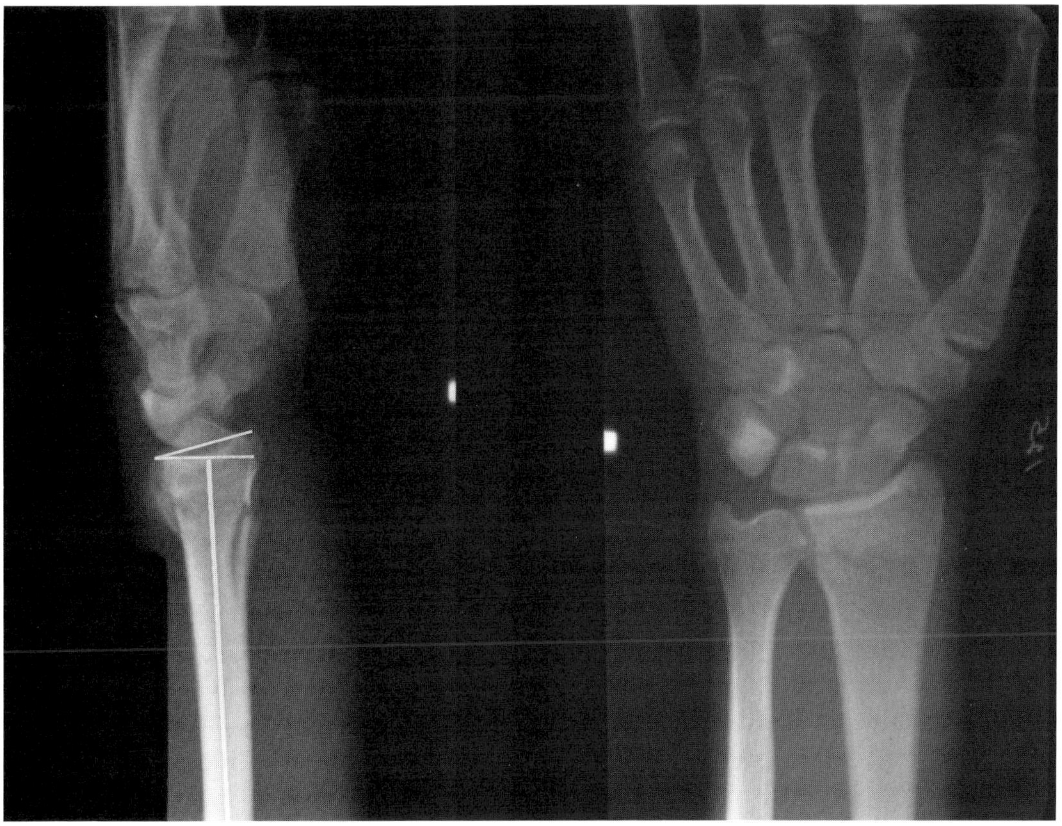 B

FIG. 13-11. Lateral **(A)** and PA **(B)** radiographs of the wrist demonstrating a typical Colles's fracture with dorsal displacement of the distal fragment. The fracture is minimally displaced, but the distal radial angle (normal, volar 12°) is dorsally directed 10° from the vertical (*lines*).

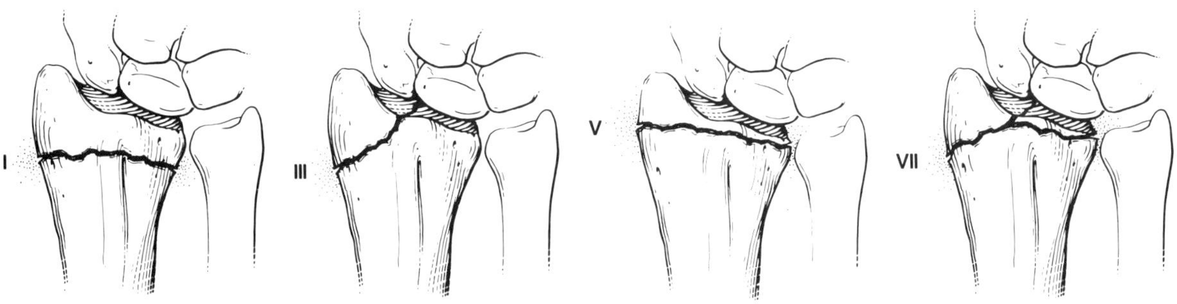

A,B C,D

FIG. 13-12. Frykman Classification for distal radial fractures.[103] **A:** Type I, extraarticular fracture of the distal radius without ulnar styloid involvement; type II, with ulnar styloid involvement. **B:** Type III, fracture involving the radio carpal joint without ulnar styloid fracture; type IV, with associated ulnar styloid fracture. **C:** Type V, fractures involving the DRUJ; type VI, with associated ulnar styloid fracture. **D:** Type VII, fractures involving the radiocarpal joint and DRUJ; type VIII, with associated ulnar styloid fracture. (From Berquist TH. *Imaging of orthopedic trauma,* 2nd ed. New York: Raven Press, 1992.)

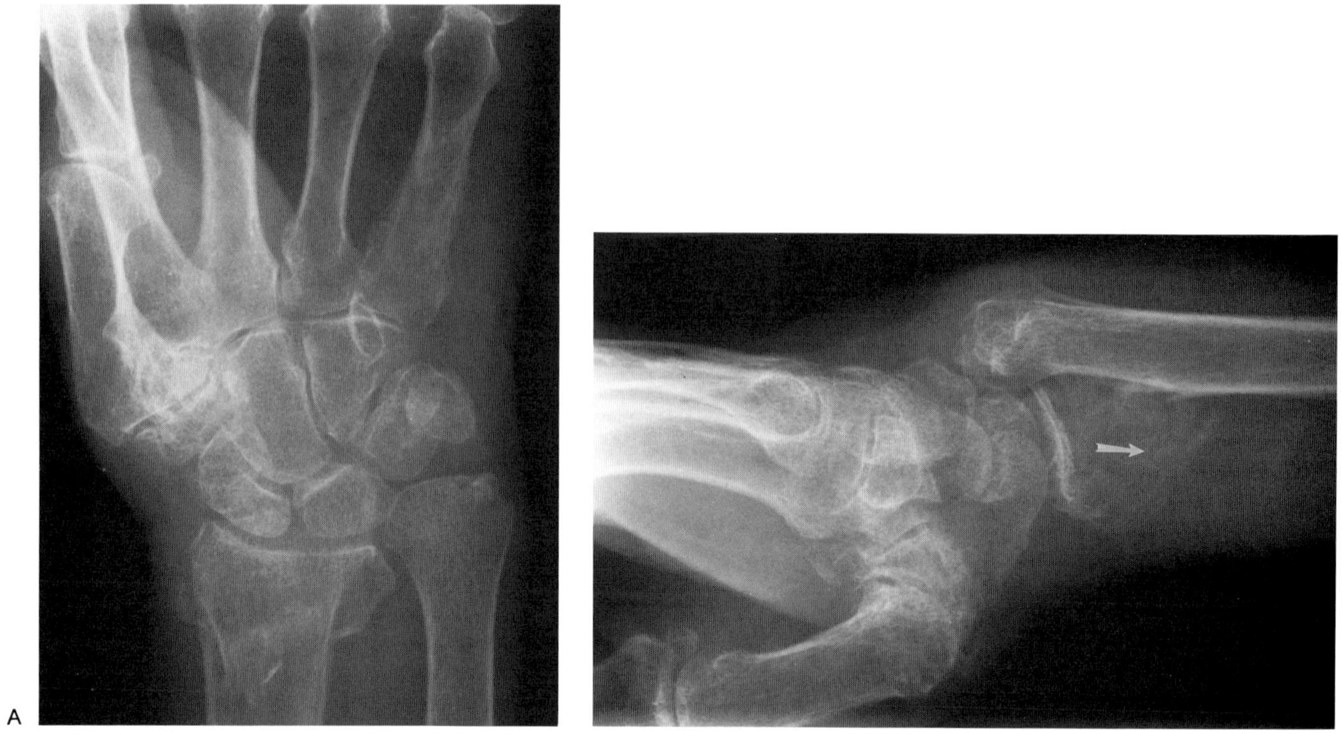

FIG. 13-13. The PA **(A)** and lateral **(B)** radiographs demonstrating a type II Smith fracture. The large volar fragment is displaced proximally (*arrow*). The classification is most easily assessed on the lateral view.

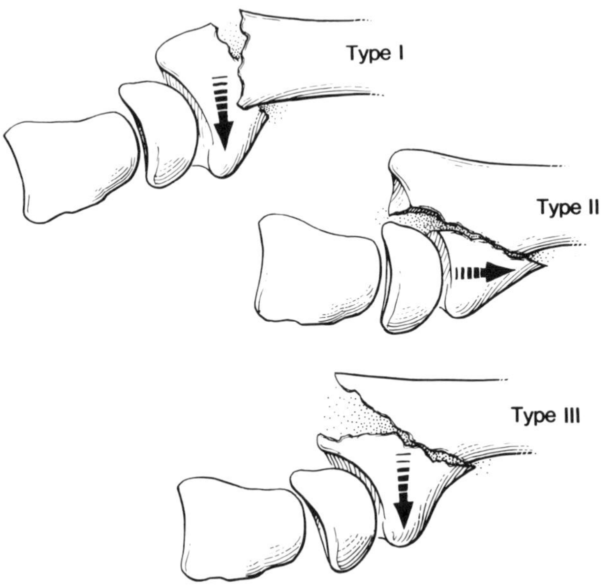

FIG. 13-14. Thomas[163] classification of Smith fractures. Type I, extraarticular; type II, volar intraarticular; type III, oblique juxtaarticular. (From Berquist TH. *Imaging of orthopedic trauma,* 2nd ed. New York: Raven Press, 1992.)

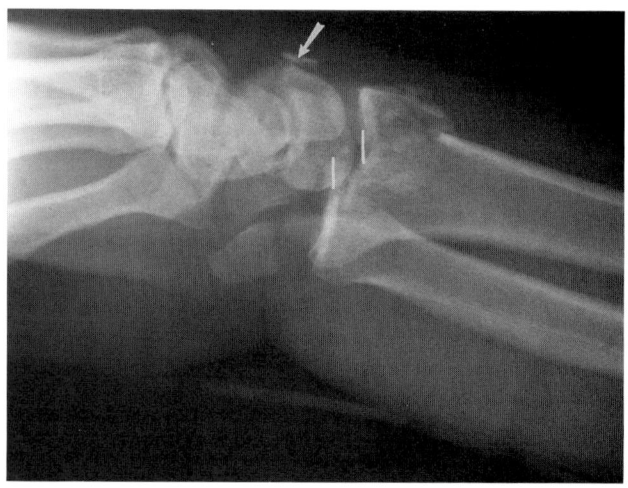

FIG. 13-15. Poorly positioned lateral view of the wrist demonstrating a dorsal Barton's fracture with subluxation of the wrist dorsally and a dorsal triquetral fracture (*arrow*). There is 5 mm of articular deformity (*lines*) as a result of proximal displacement of the distal fragment.

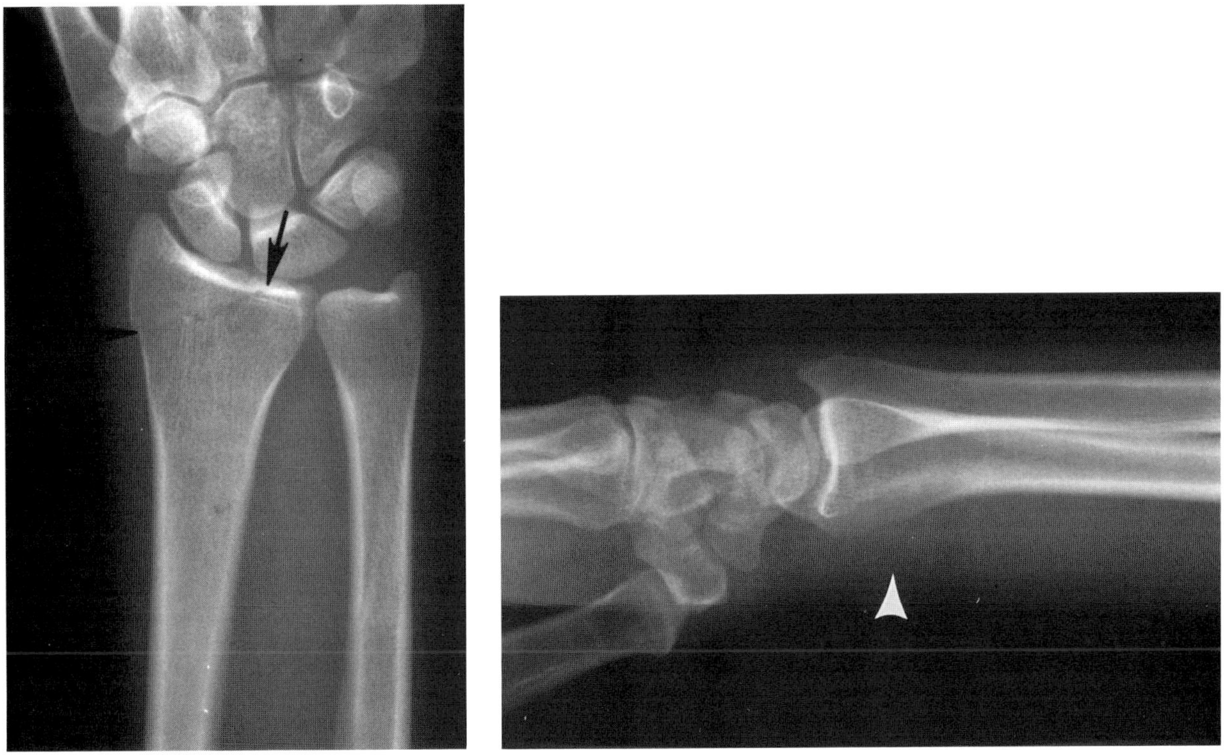

A B

FIG. 13-16. **A:** A PA radiograph of the wrist demonstrating a chauffeur's fracture. The fracture line (*arrows*) extends obliquely from the lunate fossa to below the radial styloid. **B:** The fracture is not evident on the lateral view. However, the pronator fat stripe is obliterated (*arrow*).

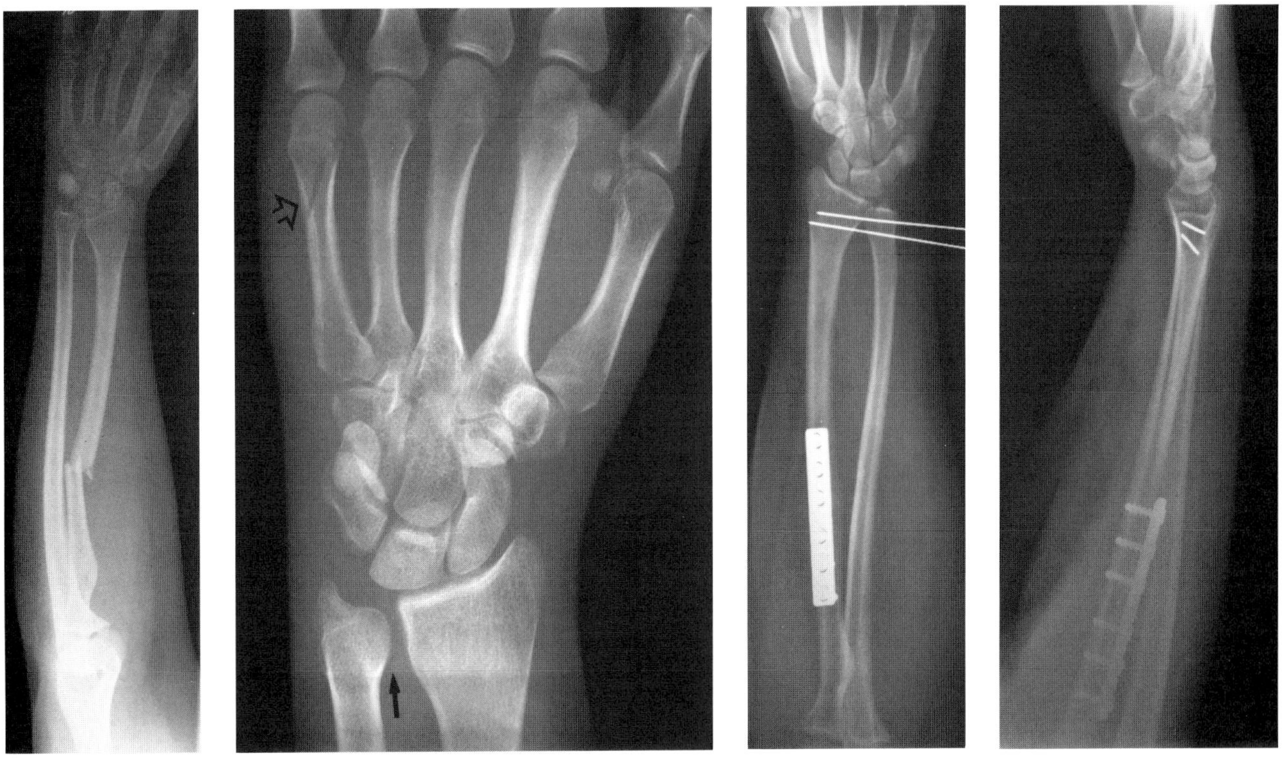

A,B C,D

FIG. 13-17. Radiographs of the forearm **(A)** and PA view of the wrist **(B)** demonstrating a proximal radial diaphysis fracture (A) and widening (*arrow*) of the distal radioulnar joint. Note also the oblique fracture of the fifth metacarpal (*open arrow*). **C,D:** The radial injury was treated with a semitubular plate and six cortical screws. There are two temporary K-wires to secure the DRUJ.

similar problems. However, in recent years, the fixators have been adapted to allow motion without loss of reduction. Clyburn[80] designed an external fixator with a ball joint at the center of wrist rotation (proximal capitate or capitolunate articulation). Other fixators are now available that offer similar features. Both 3- and 4-mm half pins can be used for external fixation, but the pullout strength is superior with 4-mm half pins.[150] Figures 13-18 to 13-24 demonstrate examples of external fixation devices.

Percutaneous pins can be used alone (Fig. 13-25) or with external fixation devices (Fig. 13-24) for displaced (universal type II), articular (universal type III), or reducible displaced intraarticular fractures (universal type IVA).[85]

Internal Fixation

Open reduction and internal fixation may be indicated for displaced articular fractures, especially if the articular deformity is greater than 2 mm or cannot be maintained with percutaneous pins or external fixators. Volar Barton's fractures or Smith fractures may be difficult to reduce and stabilize without a buttress plate. Plates used for the hand and wrist are demonstrated in Figs. 13-26 to 13-29.[67,76,169]

Carpal Fractures

Carpal fractures commonly involve multiple bones or associated ligaments. This must be kept in mind when evaluating images after trauma.[72]

Scaphoid Fractures

The scaphoid is the most frequently fractured carpal bone.[72,85,93,102,175] These fractures account for 70% of carpal fractures and more than one half of all carpal injuries. Transscaphoid perilunate dislocation must be excluded.[72,77,85]

Scaphoid fractures are classified by their location (Fig. 13-30) and the direction of the fracture line.[72,147] The prognosis is the most guarded for proximal fractures because of the increased incidence of nonunion and avascular necrosis of the proximal fragment.[85,90] Russe[147] classified scaphoid fractures according to the direction of the fracture line (Fig. 13-31). Type I fractures are oblique to the long axis of the scaphoid and perpendicular to the long axis of the wrist (Fig. 13-31A). These fractures tend to compress with minimal shearing forces. Type II fractures are perpendicular to the long axis of the scaphoid and oblique to the plane of the wrist (Fig. 13-31B). Shearing forces are slightly more significant in this setting. Type III fractures (Fig. 13-31C) have the worst prognosis because of their parallel nature compared with the longitudinal axis of the wrist, leading to significant shearing forces, which cause displacement and increased risk of nonunion.[72,147]

The imaging of suspected scaphoid fractures should begin with radiographs in the PA and lateral projection with a scaphoid view (Fig. 13-32).[72] Displacement or obliteration of the navicular fat stripe is a useful sign. In the presence of this sign or a strong clinical suspicion of a subtle fracture, the patient's wrist can be splinted or immobilized with a cast and restudied in 10 to 14 days. A radionuclide scan can be obtained 24 to 48 hours after the injury as an alternative.[139,142] If the scan results are positive, thin-section complex motion tomography or CT should be performed to confirm the fracture and define its position.[72,153,162]

The treatment of undisplaced scaphoid fractures is usually cast immobilization (long arm or short thumb spica) for 4 to 6 weeks.[82,85,107] Fractures of the waist or proximal pole may require longer periods of immobilization.[82,85] Conventional tomography or CT in the PA and sagittal planes are used to be certain that the proper alignment is achieved and maintained.[72,153]

Displaced scaphoid fractures are treated more aggressively.[85,170] A fracture is considered displaced if the fragments have a ≥ 1-mm step off or there is more than 60° of scapholunate or 15° of lunocapitate angulation. Following reduction, the interscaphoid angle should be less than 25° in the lateral view or sagittal plane and less than 30° to 35° on PA images.[85,152–154] If reduction can be maintained, the fracture can be immobilized, as described earlier. If not, percutaneous Kirschner wires (K-wires) or open reduction and internal fixation with K-wires or a compression screw (Herbert screw) are indicated (Fig. 13-33).[82,85,130,133,145]

Other Carpal Fractures

Fractures of the other carpal bones occur less frequently than do scaphoid fractures.[65,69,72,85,93,102,175] The triquetrum is the second most commonly fractured carpal bone.[77] Injuries are usually the result of a direct blow or dorsal shearing or avulsion forces. The latter are more common, occurring at the site of ulnotriquetral ligament attachment. Therefore, fractures are usually most easily identified on the lateral view (Fig. 13-34).[72]

Fractures of the remaining carpal bones are also usually due to direct blows, compression, or shearing forces directed from the distal radius or metacarpals and ligament avulsion.[72,74,85,115,140] Detection of these injuries may be difficult on routine radiographs. Fluoroscopically positioned spot views or CT may be required (Fig. 13-35).[72,108]

The treatment of these carpal fractures is almost accomplished with cast immobilization.[85,87,90] Displaced fractures may require open reduction with K-wire or screw fixation (Fig. 13-36) if the position cannot be

(*text continues on page 857*)

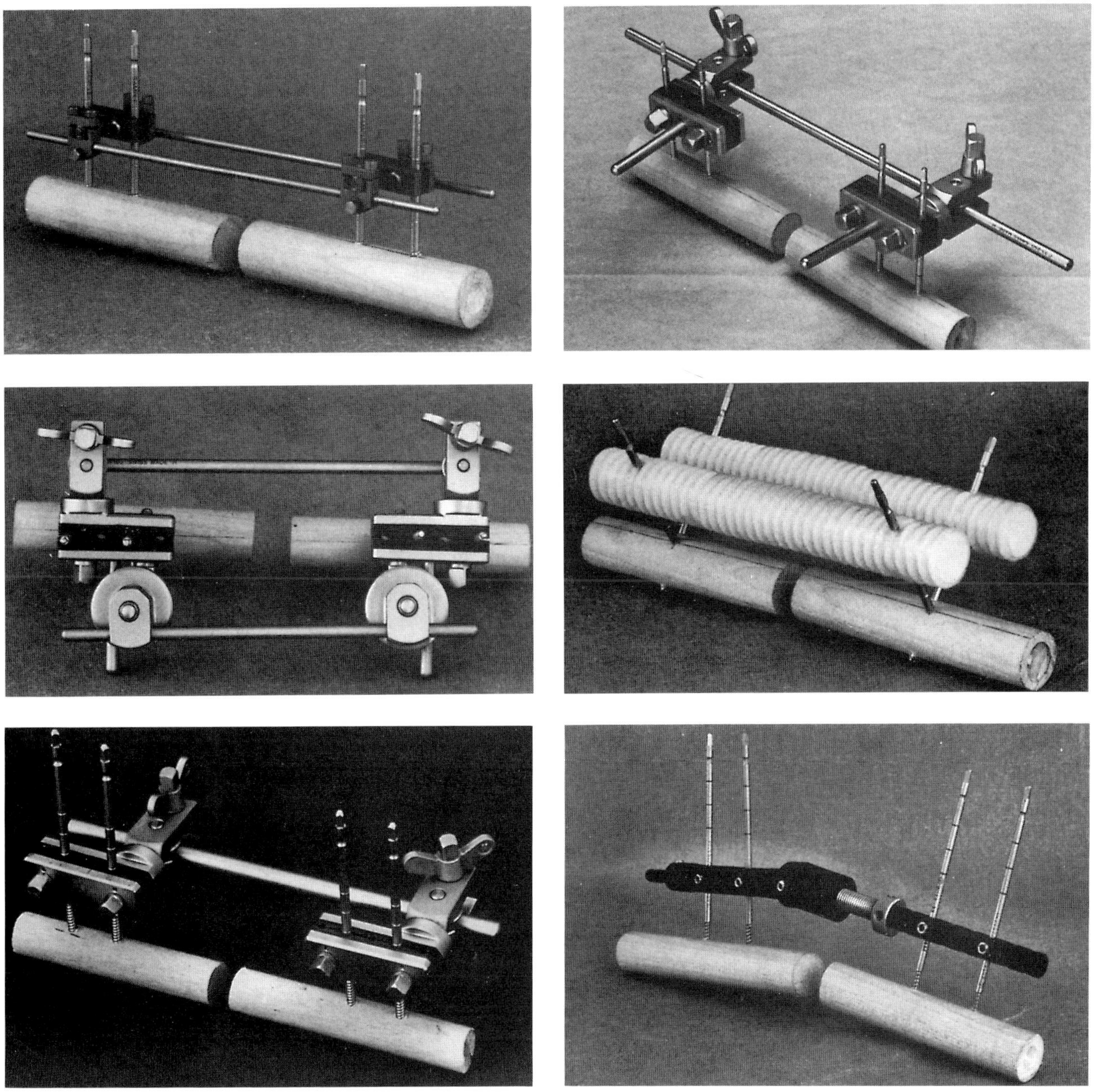

A B C D E F

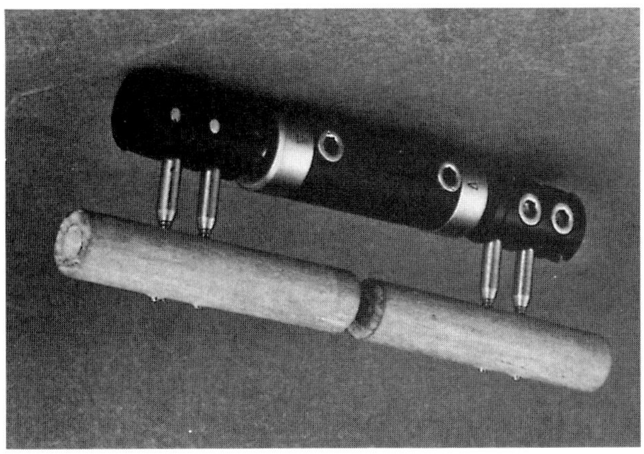

G

FIG. 13-18. External fixators used for unstable wrist fractures. **A:** The Hanson Baylor Mini Hoffman fixator is lightweight with low rigidity and contains four pins, two proximal and two distal, with two rods and clamps (Howmedica, Rutherford, NJ). **B:** The C series unilateral Hoffman fixator has a single rod, two proximal and two distal pins, and intermediate rigidity (Howmedica, Rutherford, NJ). **C:** The C series Hoffman bilateral frame fixator has central rod connectors with bilateral rods and rigid fixation (Howmedica, Rutherford, NJ). **D:** The methyl methacrylate external fixator has rigid fixation with two methyl methacrylate tubes and four angled half pins. **E:** The standard Hoffman external fixator has rigid fixation and a heavier fixator (Howmedica, Rutherford, NJ). **F:** The Clyburn external fixator with a ball joint to allow wrist motion is lightweight and a rigid fixator (Zimmer, Warsaw, IN). **G:** The Orthofix™ fixator is a rigid fixator, more rigid than the others shown here, with a moderate weight (EBI, Parsippany, NJ). (From Frykman GK et al. Comparison of eleven external fixators for treatment of unstable wrist fractures. *J Hand Surg* [*Am*] 1989;14A:247–254.)

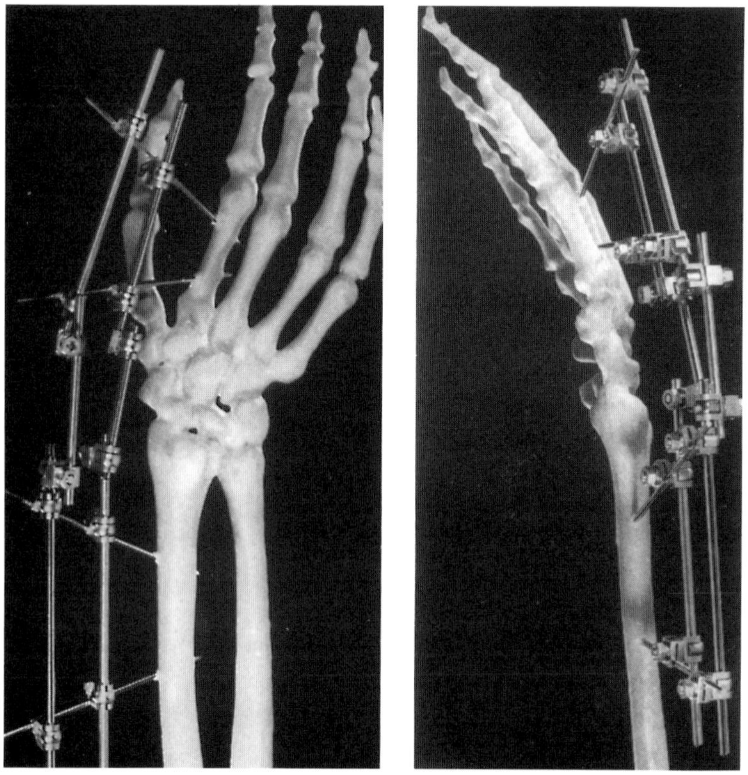

A,B

FIG. 13-19. The AO small external fixator seen from above **(A)** and the side **(B)**. (From Prince H, Worlock P. The small AO external fixator in treatment of distal forearm fractures. *J Hand Surg* 1988;13B:294–297.)

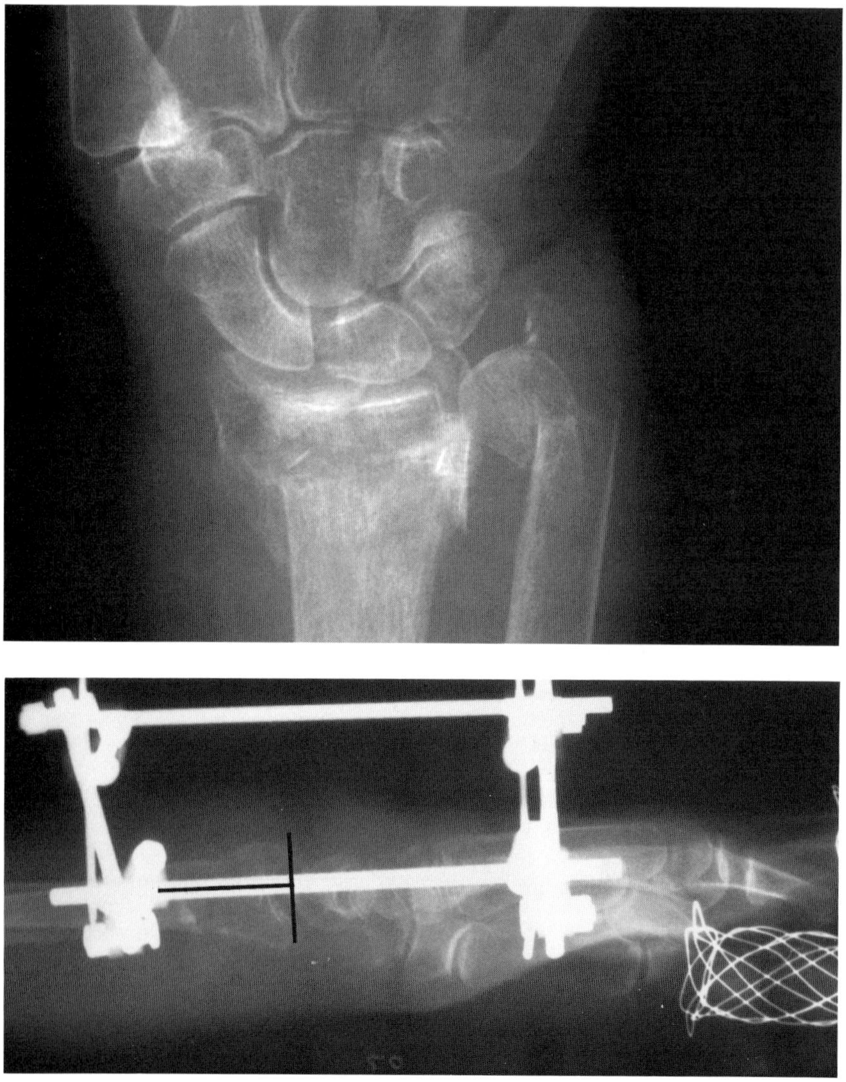

A

C

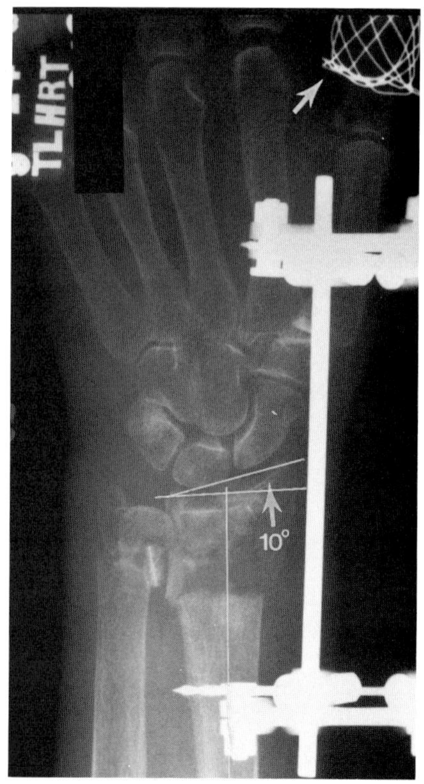

B

FIG. 13-20. Complex distal radial and ulnar fractures treated with external fixation. **A:** A PA radiograph demonstrating a Frykman type VIII fracture with radial shortening and angulation of the ulna. **B:** Reduction with finger traction (*arrow*) and external fixation. The angle of radial inclination is 10°, and there is ulnar minus variance. **C:** Lateral view with quadrilateral frame fixator. The distal radial angle is neutral.

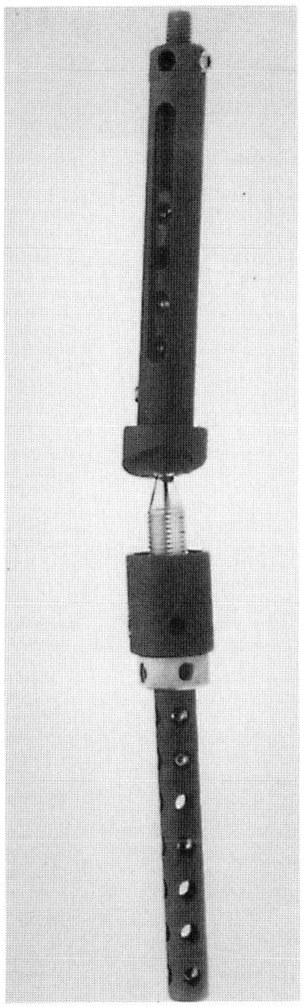

FIG. 13-21. Clyburn external fixation. (Courtesy of Zimmer, Warsaw, IN.)

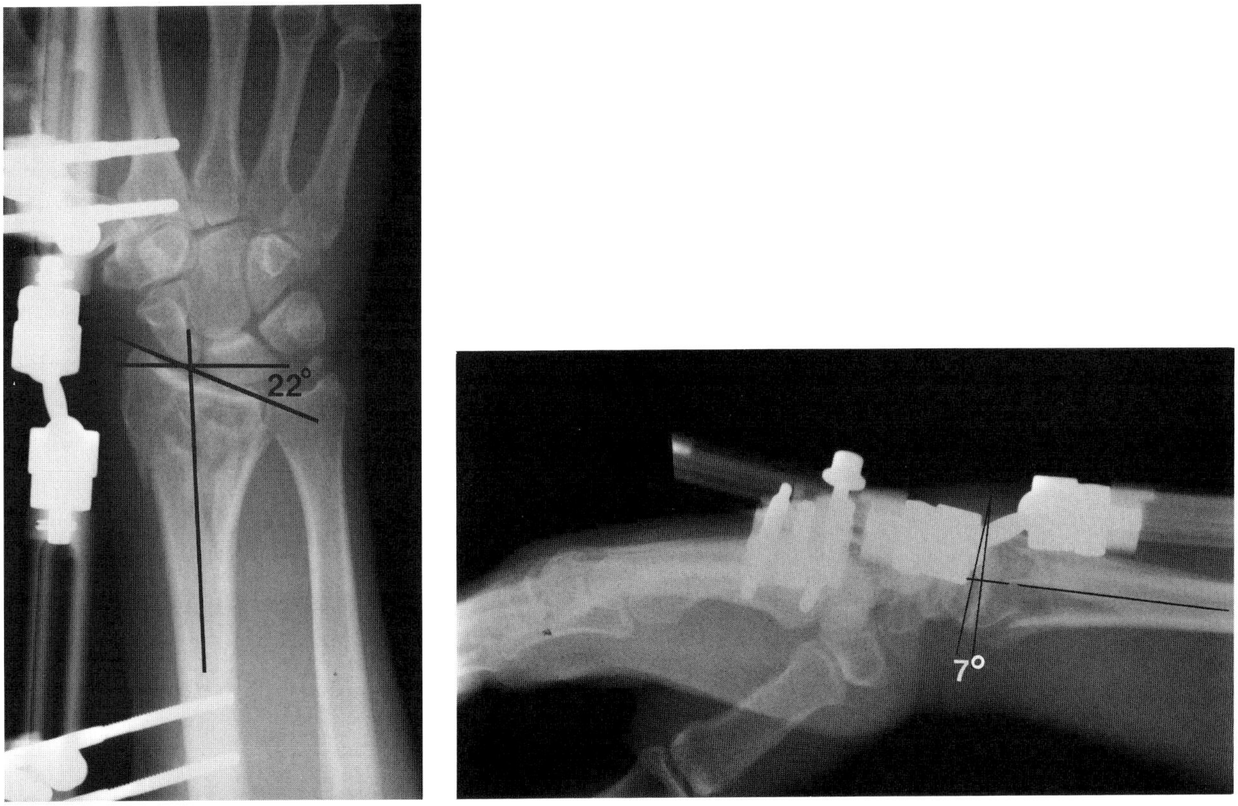

FIG. 13-22. A: A PA radiograph with an Orthofix™ external fixator. This is of Frykman type VIII fracture. The radial length is restored, and there is no ulnar positive variance. The radial inclination (normal, 16° to 28°, with angular distal radial articular surface in the coronal plane) is 22°. Less than 5° indicates a poor prognosis.[129] B: Lateral radiograph shows a distal radial angle or palmar tilt (normal, 0° to 22°) of [minus]7° or 7° of dorsal tilt.

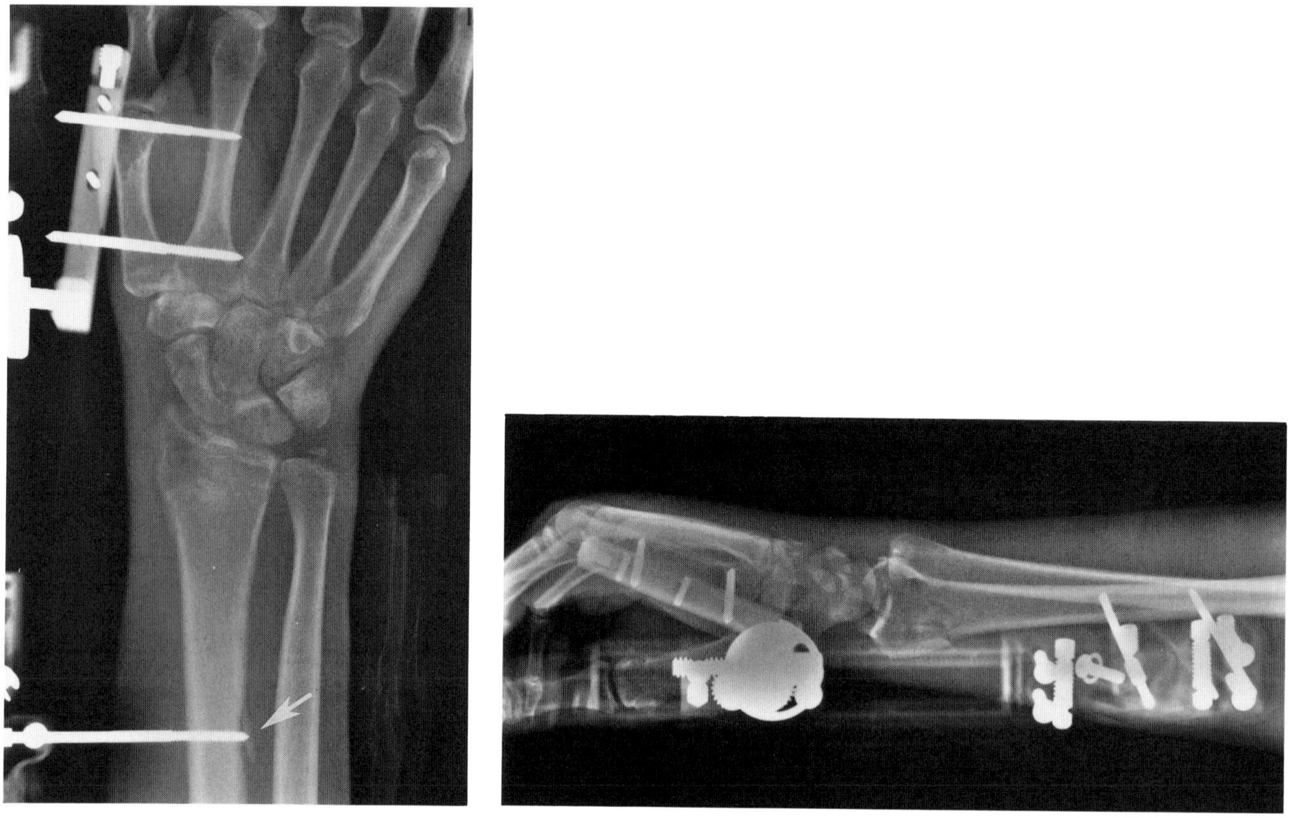

A B

FIG. 13-23. The PA **(A)** and lateral **(B)** radiographs of a Frykman type VIII fracture with external fixator (Agee wrist jack). The position of the fragment appears good on the PA view. One of the proximal pins has fractured through the distal cortex (*arrow*). This may be of no clinical consequence. Two distal pins in the second metacarpal.

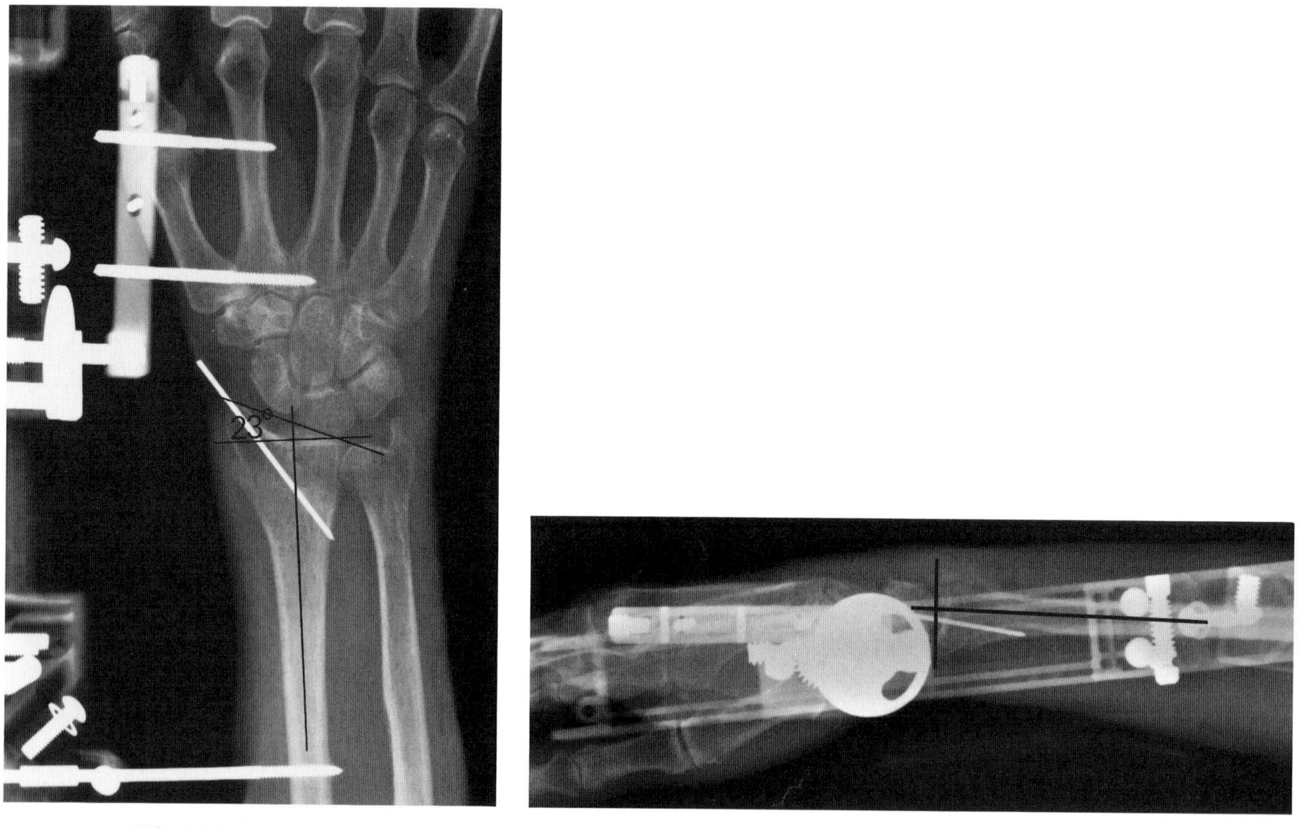

A B

FIG. 13-24. The PA **(A)** and lateral **(B)** radiographs of a comminuted intraarticular fracture of the distal radius with a percutaneous K wire across the radial styloid and an external fixator in place (Agee wrist jack). The radial inclination on the PA view (A) is 23°, and there is slight ulnar minus variance. On the lateral view, the distal radial angle is neutral.

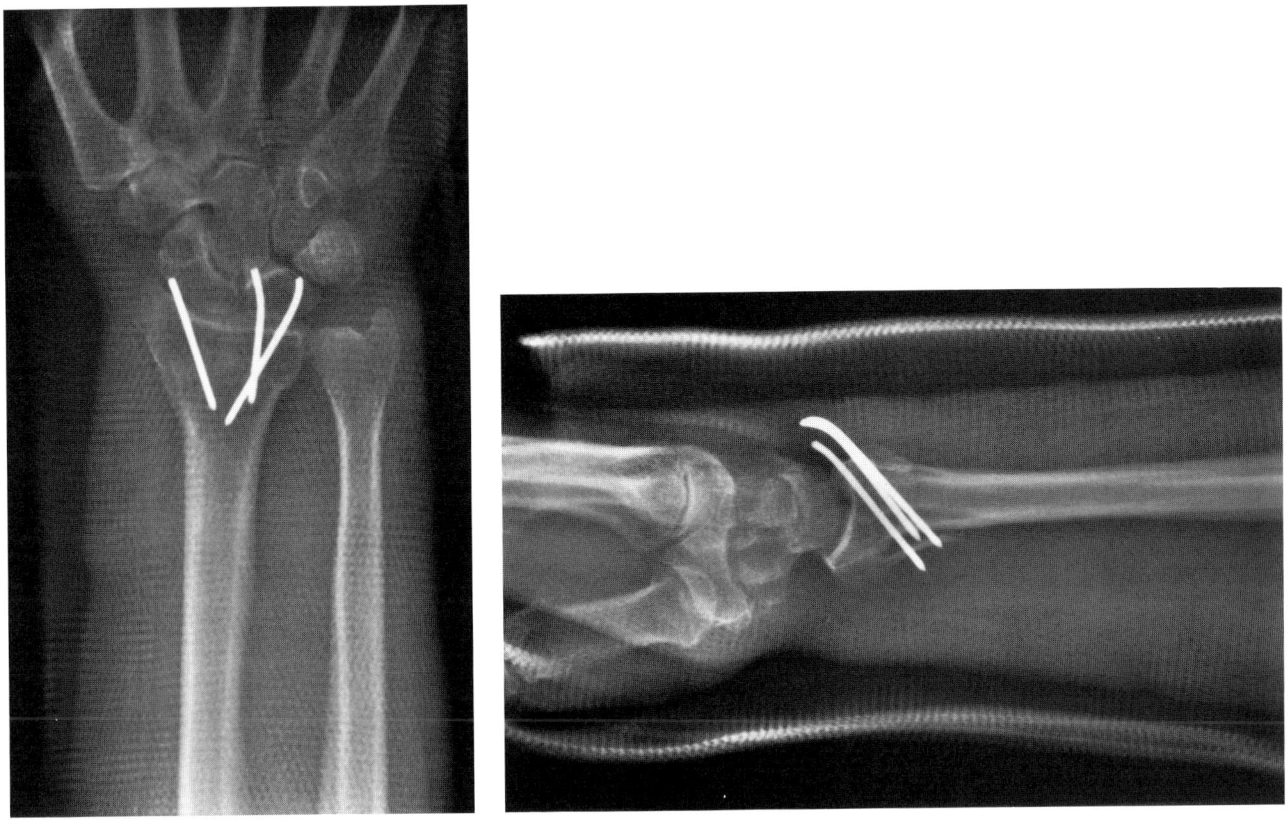

A B

FIG. 13-25. The PA **(A)** and lateral **(B)** radiographs of a minimally displaced distal radial articular fracture reduced with three percutaneous K-wires inserted dorsally and cast immobilization.

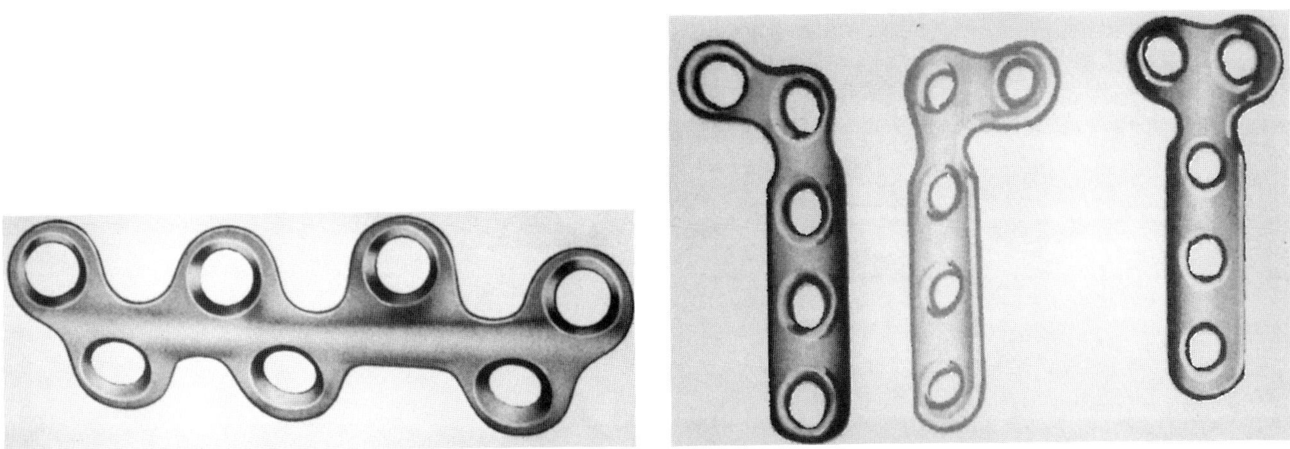

A B

FIG. 13-26. Fixation devices for the hand and wrist. (Courtesy of Zimmer, Warsaw, IN.) **A:** Small fragment plate with staggered screw holes. **B:** Small left, right, and T epiphyseal plates. (See **C-G** on next page.)

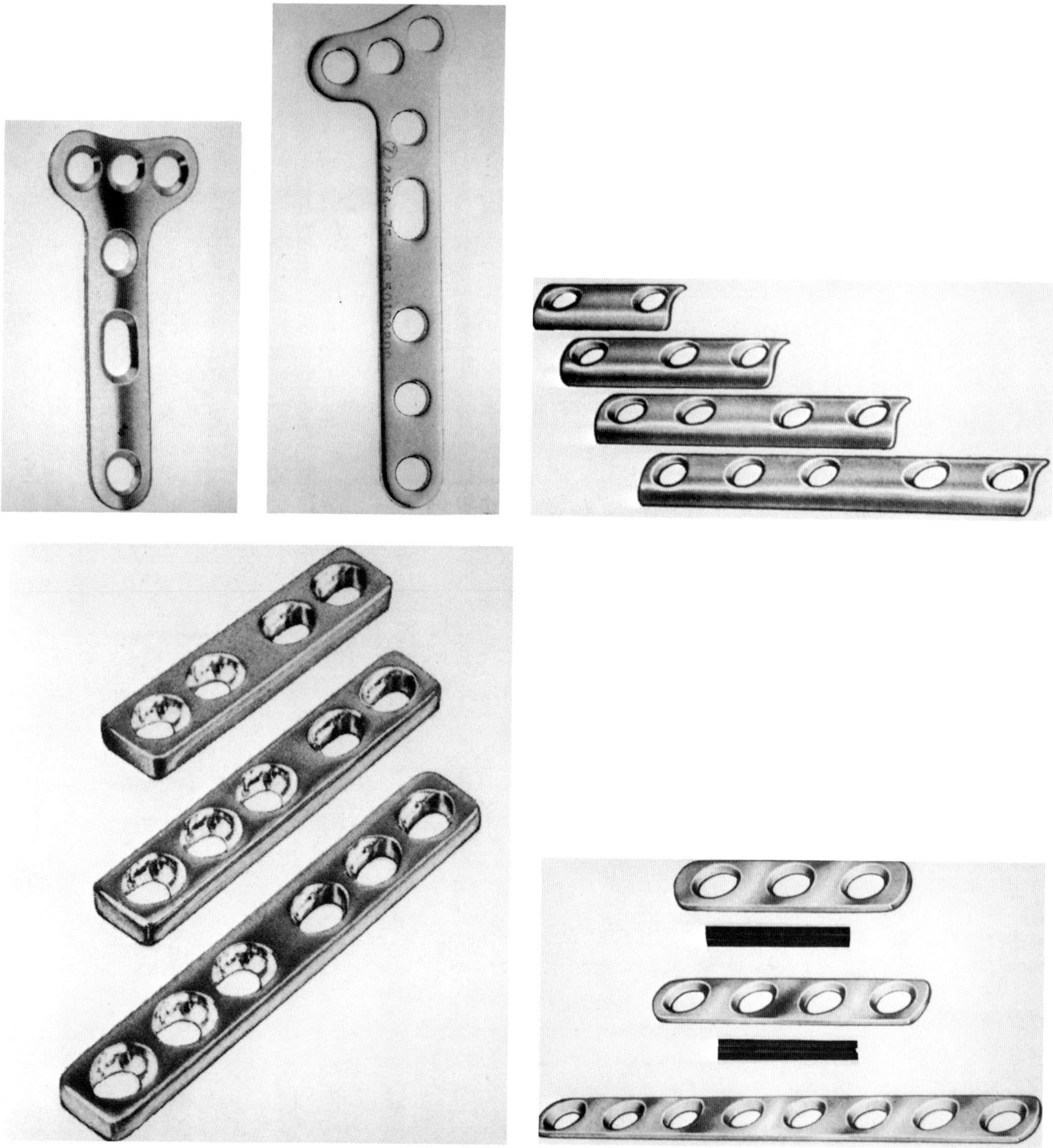

C,D E F G

FIG. 13-26. (*Continued.*) **C:** Small T buttress plate for the distal radius. **D:** Oblique T plate for the distal radius. **E:** Small one-third tubular plates with two to five holes. **F:** Small self-compressing plates with four, five, and six holes. **G:** Small thin miniplates with three, four, and eight holes.

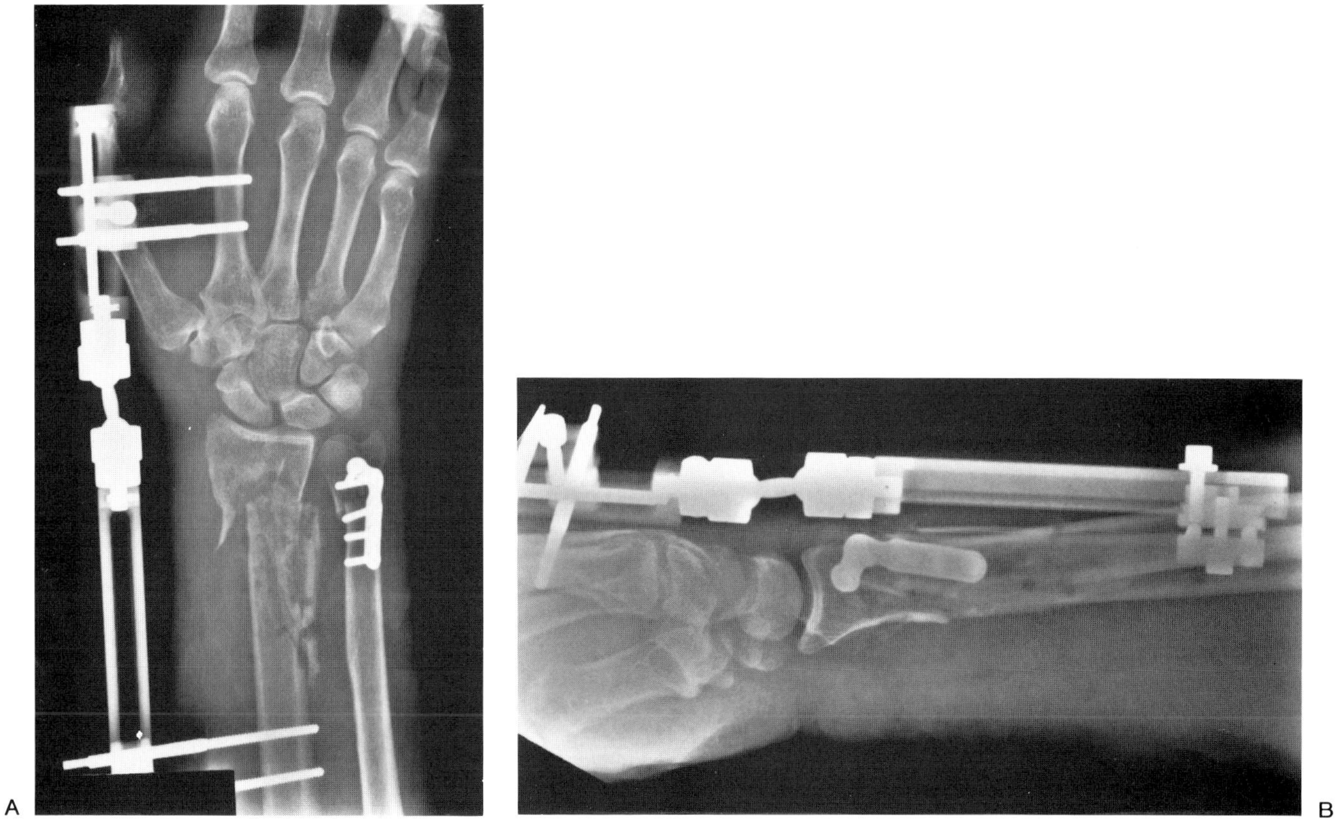

FIG. 13-27. Combined external and internal fixation for a comminuted distal radial fracture that spared the articular surface and a displaced distal ulnar fracture. The PA **(A)** and lateral **(B)** radiographs demonstrate a Orthofix™ external fixator for radial fracture fixation and a small epiphyseal plate and five small cortical screws for fixation of the ulna. The radial length is maintained.

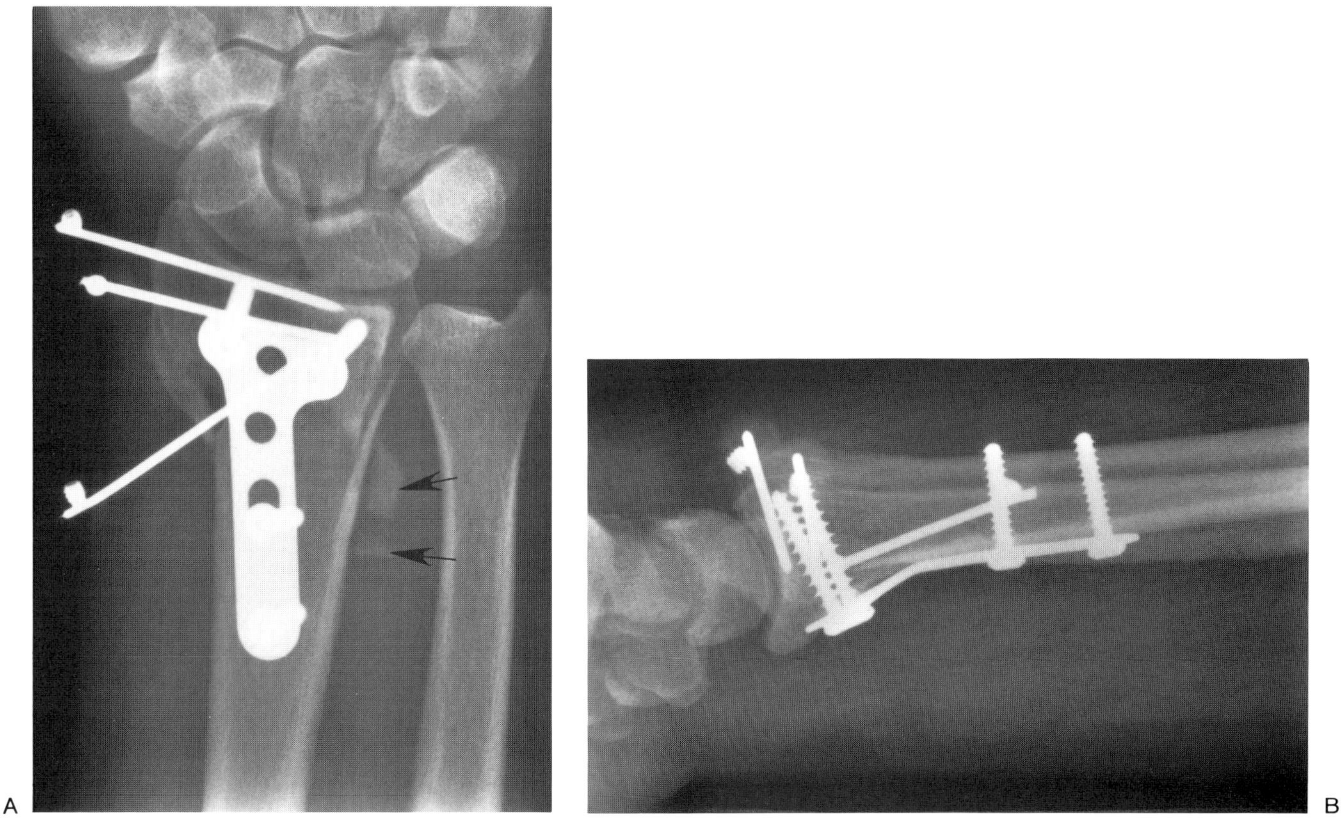

FIG. 13-28. The PA **(A)** and lateral **(B)** radiographs of an unstable intraarticular distal radial (Smith) fracture (note bone fragments, *arrows*) with an oblique T buttress plate volarly and three K-wires for fixation. The articular surface is reduced.

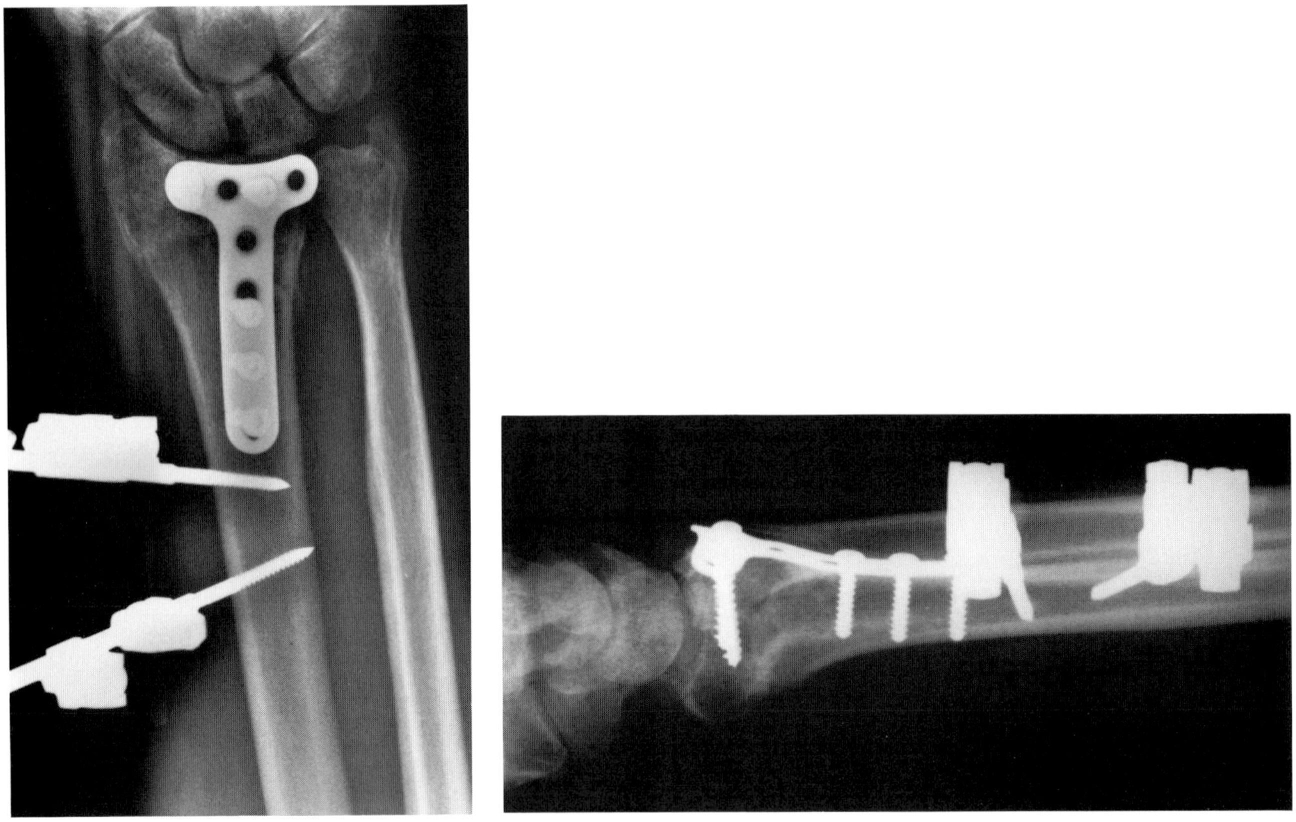

A B

FIG. 13-29. The PA **(A)** and lateral **(B)** radiographs showed internal fixation with a T buttress plate and five screws. The external fixator is still in place.

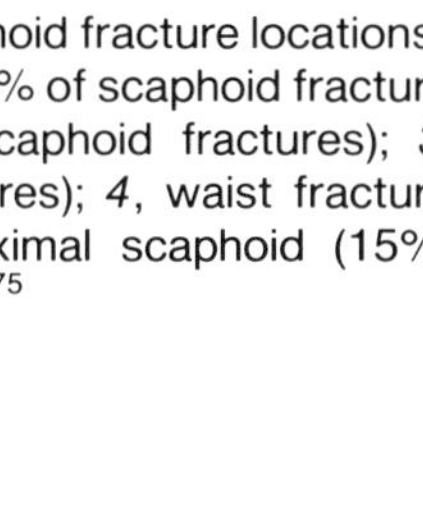

FIG. 13-30. Scaphoid fracture locations. *1*, Capsular attachment or tubercle (8% of scaphoid fractures); *2*, distal articular surface (2% of scaphoid fractures); *3*, distal third (10% of scaphoid fractures); *4*, waist fracture (65% of scaphoid fractures); *5*, proximal scaphoid (15% of scaphoid fractures).[72,82,85,93,102,175]

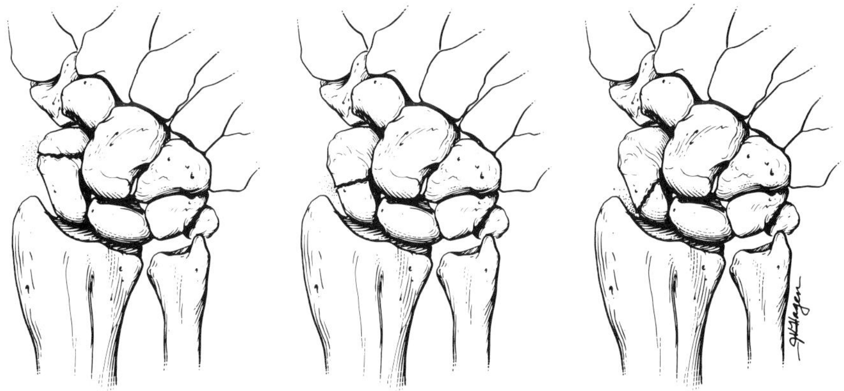

A,B C

FIG. 13-31. Russe[147] classification of scaphoid fractures. Type I **(A)**, type II **(B)**, and type III **(C)**. (From Berquist TH. *Imaging of orthopedic trauma,* 2nd ed. New York: Raven Press, 1992.)

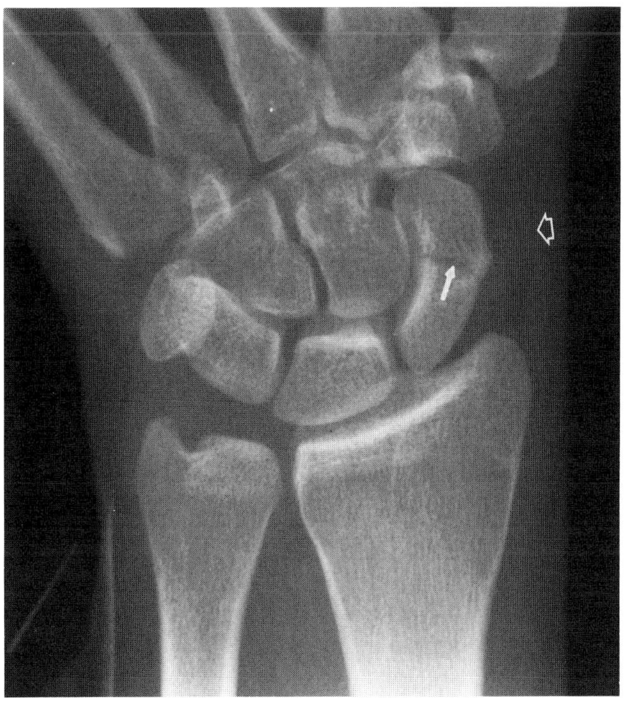

FIG. 13-32. Scaphoid view demonstrating an undisplaced fracture of the midscaphoid (*arrow*) with obliteration of the fat stripe (*open arrow*).[13–33]

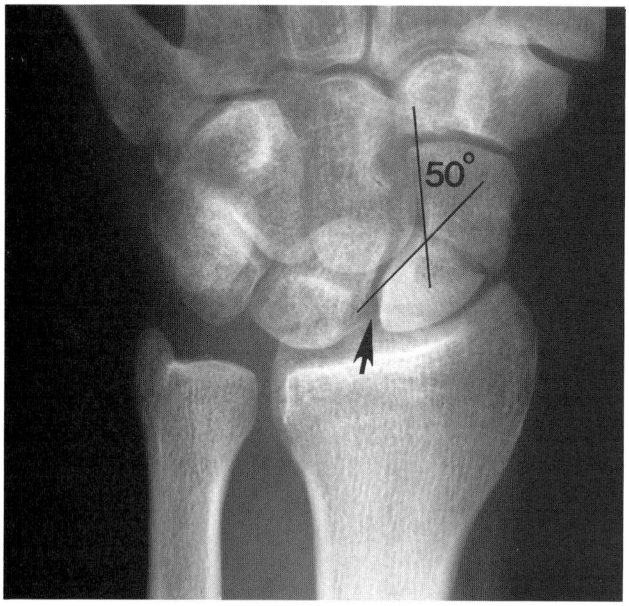

A

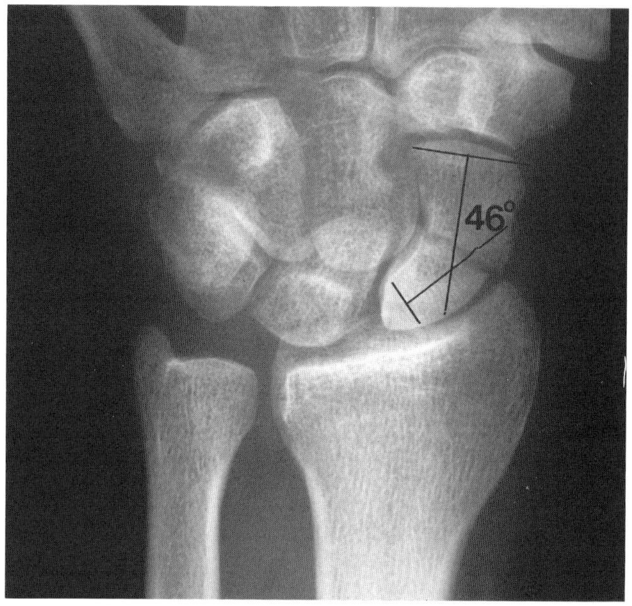

B

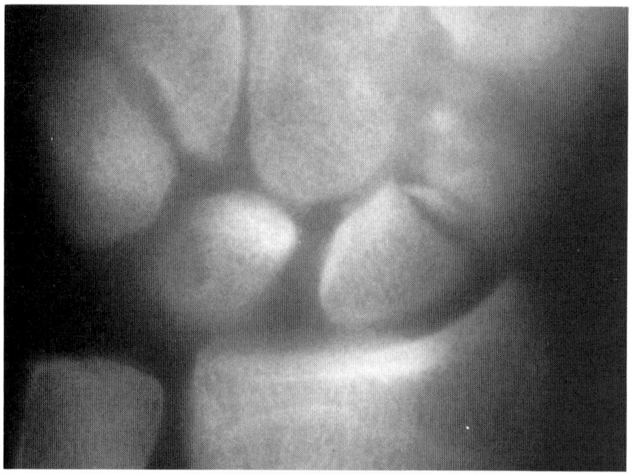

C

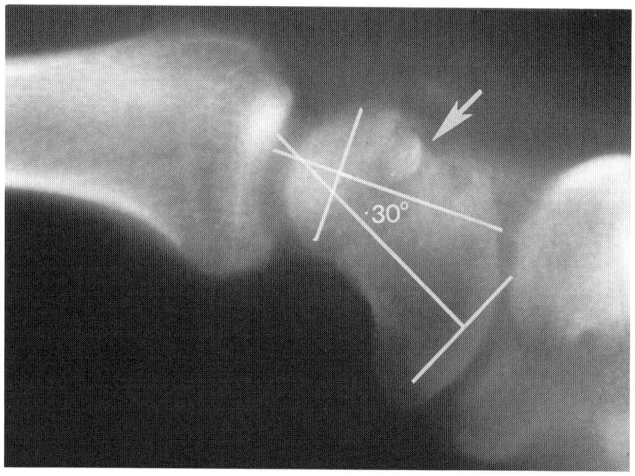

D

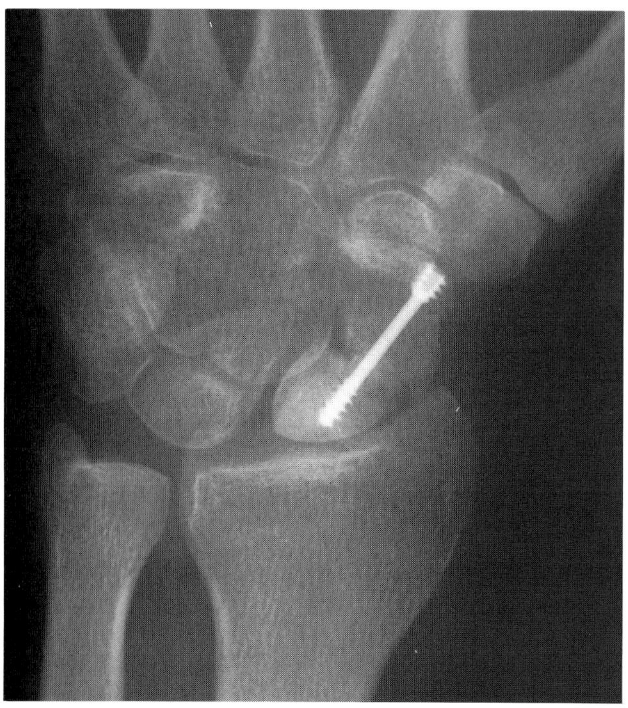

E

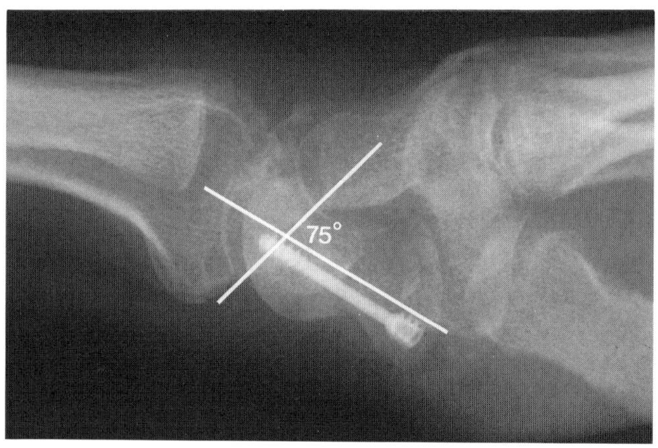

F

FIG. 13-33. Displaced fracture of the scaphoid **(A)**; PA radiograph demonstrates a fracture through the scaphoid waist with articular step off. The scaphoid angle is 50° using the cortical technique. This technique uses lines along the distal and proximal articular surface as shown (normal, 40° ± 3°; abnormal, < 35° or > 46°). This technique is more easily reproduced than the articular technique demonstrated in B.[153] Note also the widened scapholunate space caused by a ligament injury (*arrow*).

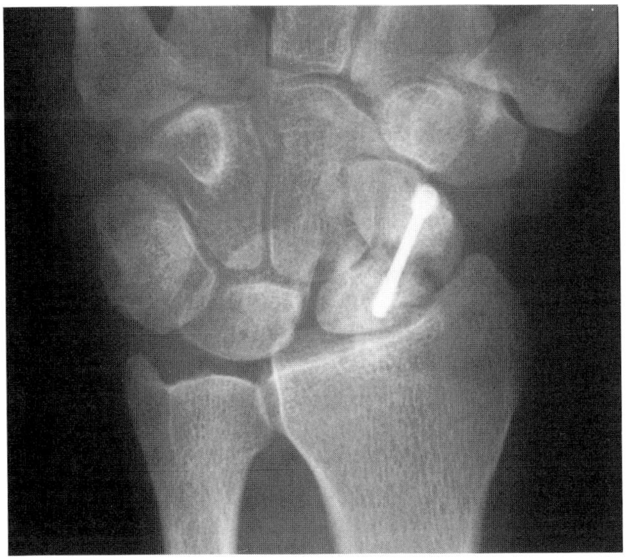

G

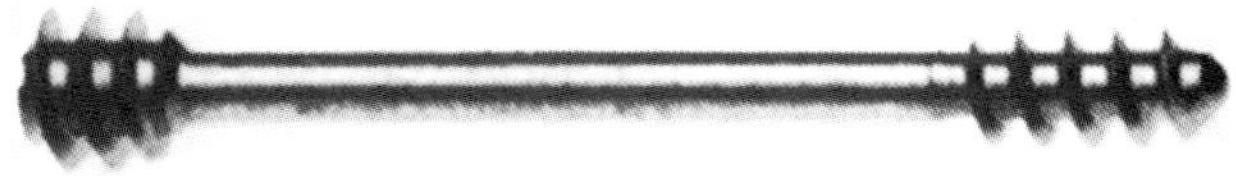

H

FIG. 13-33. (*Continued.*) **B:** A PA radiograph of the same patient demonstrating the articular technique. This technique uses the orientation of the proximal and distal pole articular surfaces. Lines are drawn perpendicular to the articular surface to measure the angle. This technique is more difficult to reproduce. The angle in this case is 46° (normal, 40° ± 4°; abnormal, < 32° or > 49°).[153] **C:** A PA tomogram demonstrating the fracture with fragmentation along the fracture line. **D:** Lateral tomogram showing dorsal comminution (*arrow*). The lateral angle can be measured using the cortical or articular techniques. The articular technique shown here reveals an angle of 30° (normal with cortical technique, 32° ± 5°; normal with this articular technique, 24° ± 5°). Angles of > 42° with the former or 33° with the latter have a 95% confidence of predicting malunion.[153] **E:** A PA radiograph after reduction with a Herbert screw. **F:** Lateral radiograph with Herbert screw. Note the DISI deformity with a scapholunate angle of 75°. **G:** A PA radiograph at 9 months shows widening and irregularity of the fracture line and lucency around the proximal screw indicating motion and nonunion. **H:** A Herbert screw. (Courtesy of Zimmer, Warsaw, IN.)

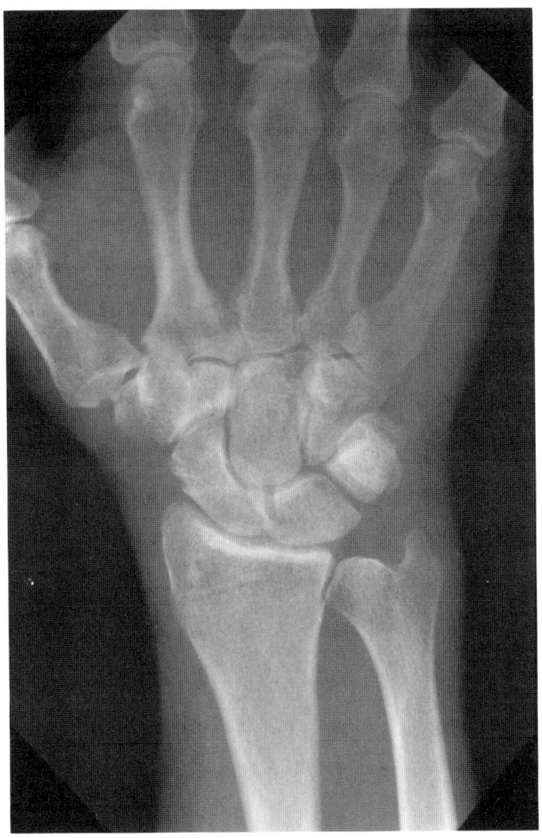

A

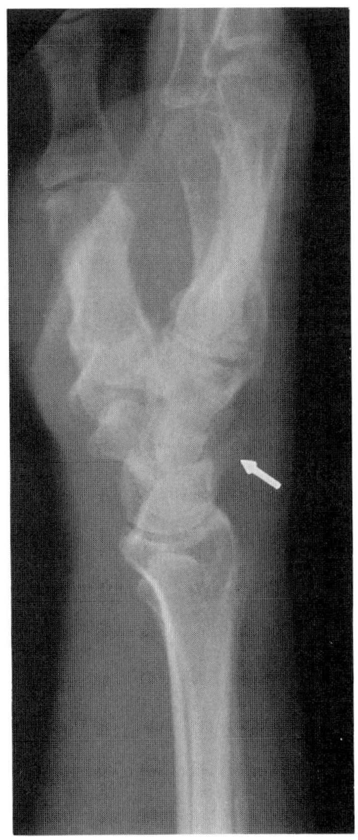

B

FIG. 13-34. The PA **(A)** and lateral views **(B)** of the wrist demonstrating a dorsal triquetral fracture (*arrow*). This is only clearly demonstrated on the lateral view.

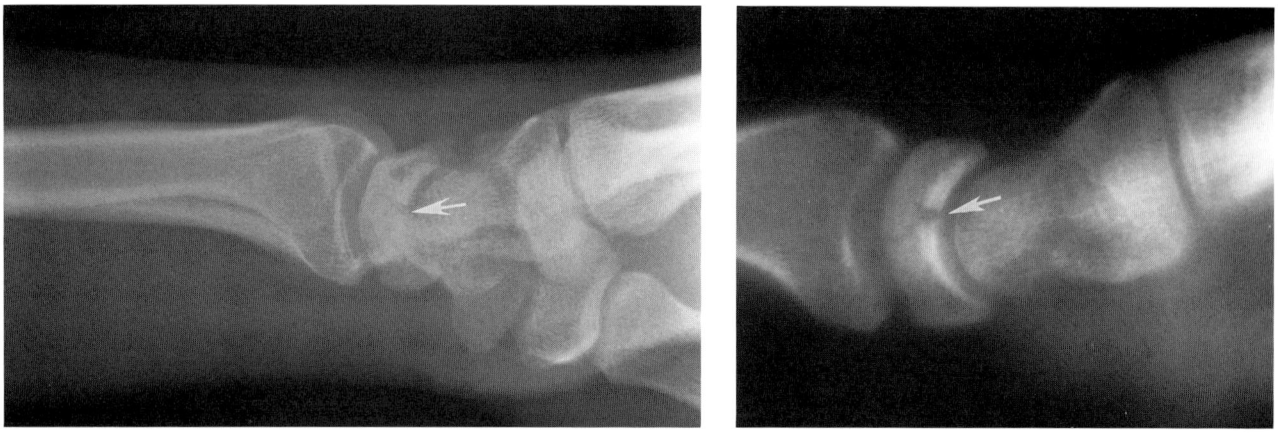

A B

FIG. 13-35. A: Lateral radiograph of the wrist shows a questionable fracture (*arrow*) and apparent compression of the lunate. **B:** Lateral tomogram clearly demonstrates the fracture (*arrow*).

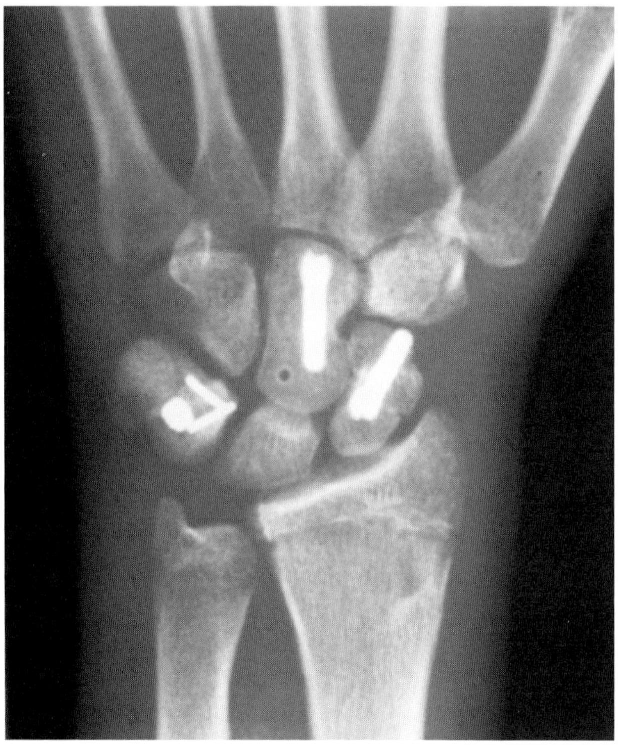

A

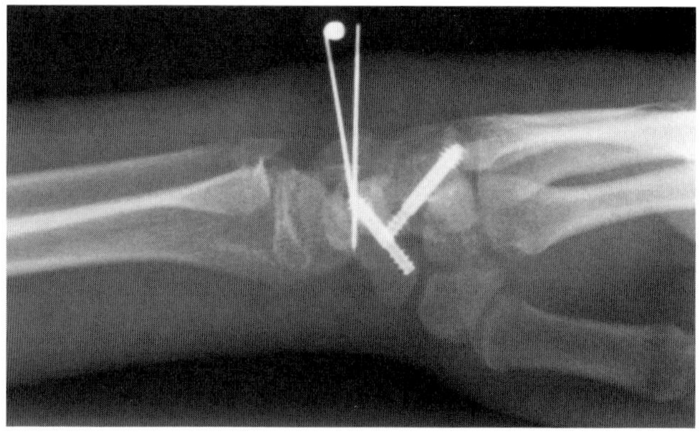

B

FIG. 13-36. Complex wrist injury with multiple carpal fractures involving the scaphoid, capitate, and triquetrum. The PA **(A)** and lateral **(B)** radiographs demonstrate compression screw fixation of the scaphoid and capitate and K-wire fixation of the dorsal lunate fragment.

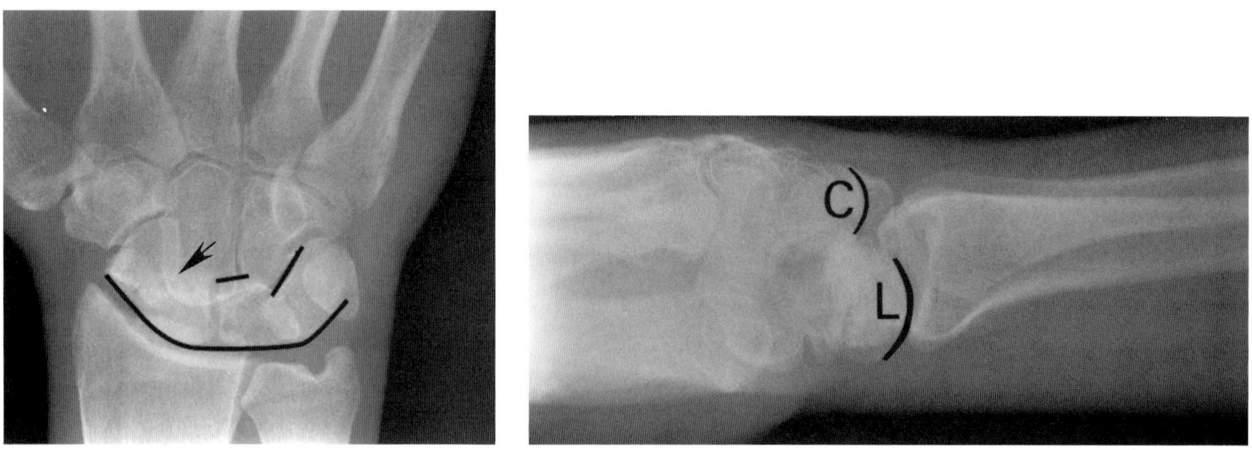

A B

FIG. 13-37. The PA **(A)** and lateral **(B)** radiographs demonstrating a transscaphoid (*arrow* to fracture) perilunate dislocation. The lunate and proximal scaphoid are in a relatively normal position on the PA view. The second arc is clearly interrupted. The position of the lunate (*L*) and capitate (*C*) are marked on the lateral radiographs.

maintained using conservative measures. Fractures of the hook of the hamate often require internal fixation or resection because conservative treatment is usually unsuccessful.[136,140,157,158,165]

Carpal and Carpometacarpal Dislocations

Dislocations of the carpus are most often associated with perilunate injury.[85,131,173] The transscaphoid perilunate dislocation is the most common. In this setting, the lunate and proximal scaphoid may maintain their normal relationships to the distal radius (Fig. 13-37). The remainder of the carpus and distal scaphoid are displaced dorsally.[72,93,111,115]

Dorsal perilunate dislocations are similar, but there is no associated scaphoid fracture. Isolated dorsal or volar dislocations of the lunate also occur. However, as we expand beyond perilunate dislocations to dislocation of the other carpal bones, the injuries become increasingly uncommon.[85,111,149]

Carpometacarpal dislocations are most frequently associated with distal carpal row or metacarpal base fractures (Fig. 13-38).[70,72,101,116,124,128,141,148] These injuries may be subtle or difficult to define clearly because of their complexity without CT or conventional tomography.[72] Multiple articulations are generally involved, although isolated dislocation of the fifth metacarpal has been reported.[138] These injuries are usually unstable, particularly when the first or fifth metacarpal is involved. In this setting, open reduction with internal fixation is advisable.[72,85,128] Unless a perfect and stable closed reduction can be achieved with carpal dislocations, many authors also recommend open reduction and internal fixation for these injuries (Fig. 13-39).[72,85,111]

Metacarpal Fractures

Metacarpal fractures are common. The fourth and fifth metacarpals are the most frequently involved. For purposes of discussion and because of the variations in treatment, it is best to discuss three categories of injury. The fourth and fifth metacarpals have more mobility than the second and third. Therefore, we discuss the thumb, mobile rays (fourth and fifth), and stable rays (second and third) separately (Fig. 4-40).[72]

Thumb

The thumb is highly mobile, resulting in more tolerance of angulation and rotation after fracture.[72,112] However, pinch strength is critical so there is less room for error in fractures involving the carpometacarpal articular surface.[72,156,159]

Fractures of the thumb (Fig. 13-41) can be divided anatomically as listed in order of decreasing frequency.

1. Intraarticular basilar fractures, most common.
2. Proximal metaphyseal fractures, common.
3. Transverse or spiral diaphyseal fractures, uncommon.
4. First metacarpal neck fractures, uncommon.

The PA, lateral, and oblique images are required to identify and characterize the fracture (oblique, spiral, transverse, rotation, shortening, angulation, and articular involvement).[72] Most neck and diaphyseal fractures are treated conservatively. Up to 20° of angulation is acceptable because of the mobility of the thumb.[112,127] Spiral fractures tend to be unstable. These injuries or fractures that cannot be adequately reduced are treated with open reduction and K-wire, tension-band wire, or plate and screw fixation.[72,112,119,127,156]

Basilar intraarticular fractures are the most common and most difficult to treat. Anatomic reduction is essential.[112,154] Two common fracture patterns are the Bennett and Rolando fractures. The Bennett fracture (Fig. 13-42) is actually a fracture subluxation of the first carpometacarpal joint. The fracture is usually oblique, with the volar (ulnar) fragment remaining behind attached to the ulnar oblique ligament (Fig. 13-42). The main fragment is displaced proximally because of the abductor pollicis longus and flexor pollicis longus tendons, which pull on this unattached fragment.[72,112] The second fracture pattern is the Rolando fracture (Fig. 13-43), which is a Y- or T-shaped intraarticular fracture.[72,156]

Intraarticular basilar fractures can be reduced using traction. However, reduction is difficult to maintain without internal fixation. With their external ends curved to allow easy removal and prevent migration, K-wires (percutaneous or with open reduction) are used to attach the main metacarpal fragment to the trapezium (Fig. 13-44). It is not essential to cross the fracture line and include the small ulnar (volar) fragment (1 in Fig. 13-42).[72,112,127,156]

Second and Third Metacarpals (Stable Rays)

The second and third metacarpals are considered stable because of the lack of motion at the carpometacarpal joint (Fig. 13-40). This reduces the latitude for angulation and rotational deformity that is acceptable after fracture compared with that of the thumb and fourth and fifth metacarpals.[72,112]

Fractures of the second and third metacarpals occur most commonly in the neck of the bone. The injury usually is the result of an axial loading force, and muscle forces tend to angulate the distal fragment in a palmar direction (Fig. 13-45).

Transverse or spiral fractures of the diaphysis occur less frequently. Spiral fractures have more tendency to shorten and rotate.

(*text continues on page 862*)

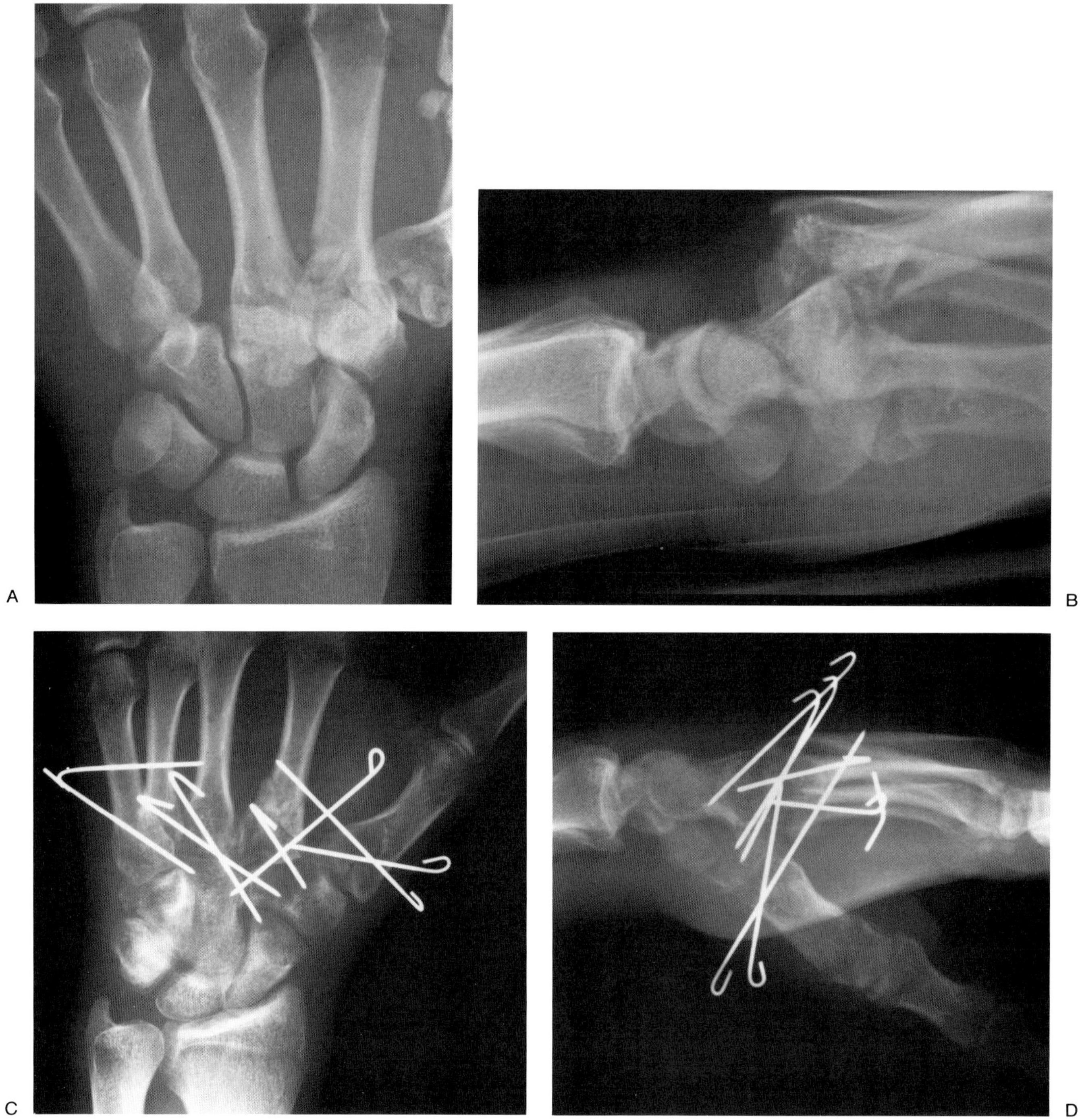

FIG. 13-38. The PA (A) and lateral (B) radiographs of a carpometacarpal fracture dislocation with comminuted fractures of the first to third metacarpal bases. The fourth metacarpal is dislocated to the ulnar side. Postreduction PA (C) and lateral (D) radiographs after reduction and K-wire fixation.

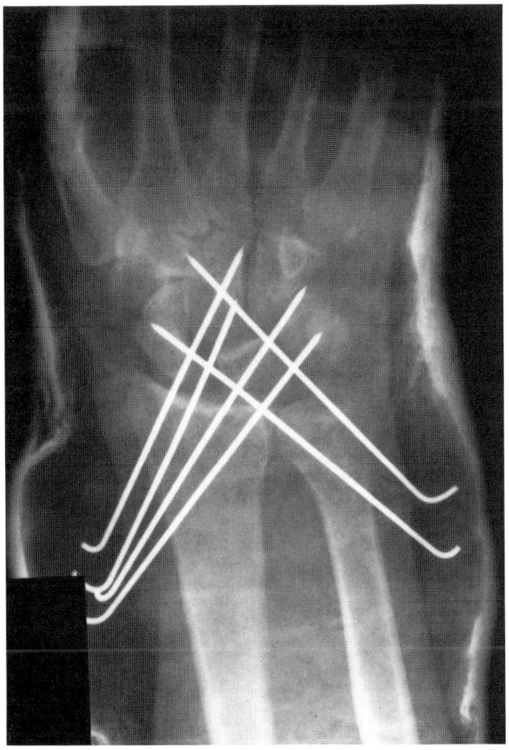

A

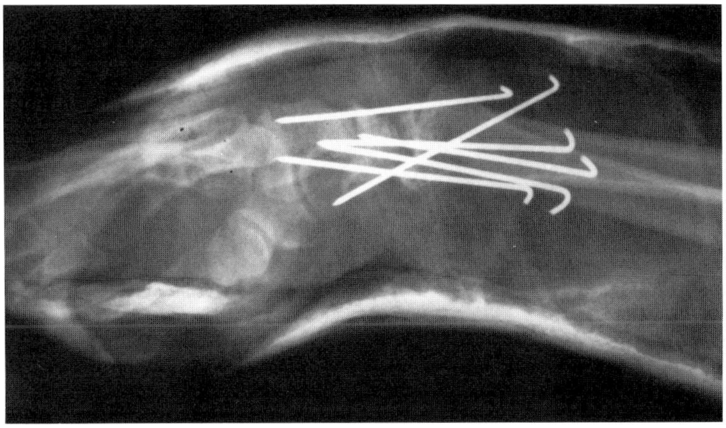

B

FIG. 13-39. The PA **(A)** and lateral **(B)** radiographs of the wrist demonstrating internal fixation of a perilunate dislocation with K-wires and cast immobilization.

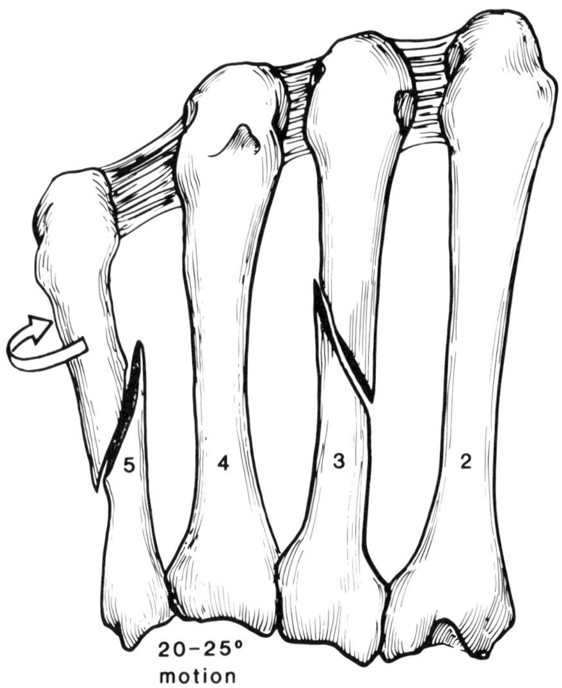

FIG. 13-40. The second through fifth metacarpals and transverse metacarpal ligament distally. There is 20° to 25° of motion at the bases of the fourth and fifth metacarpal, and the ligament laxity is also more apparent. Therefore, fractures of these rays, especially oblique or spiral, tend to shorten and rotate. (From Berquist TH. *Imaging of sports injuries.* Gaithersburg, MD: Aspen Press, 1992.)

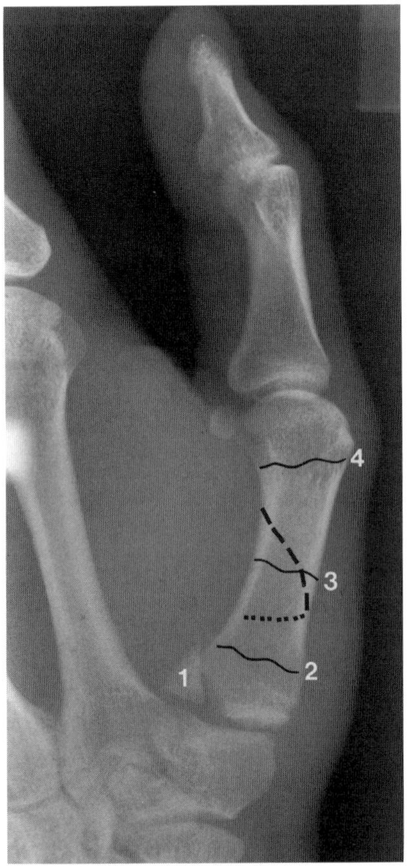

FIG. 13-41. Fractures of the first metacarpal in order of decreasing frequency. Lateral view of the thumb demonstrating a basilar intraarticular fracture (*1*), which is the most common. *1*, Intraarticular basilar fracture; *2*, metaphyseal fracture; *3*, transverse or spiral diaphyseal fracture; *4*, neck fracture.

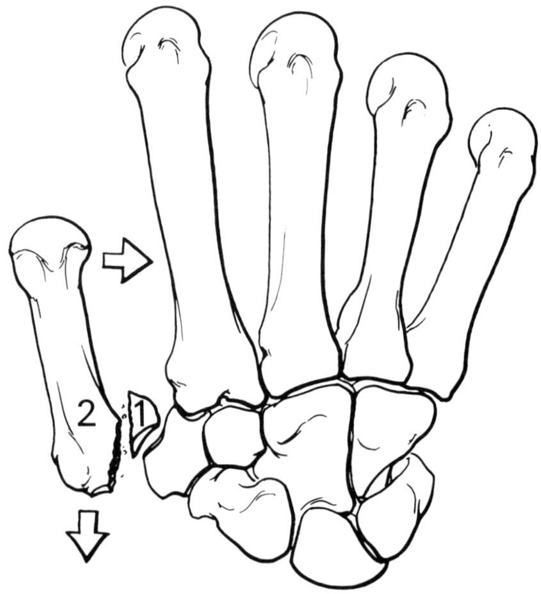

FIG. 13-42. Bennett fracture of the thumb. The small ulnar (volar) fragment (*1*) remains in place because of the strong ulnar oblique ligament. The remainder of the metacarpal (*2*) is pulled proximally and flexed by the abductor pollicis longus and flexor pollicis longus tendons.

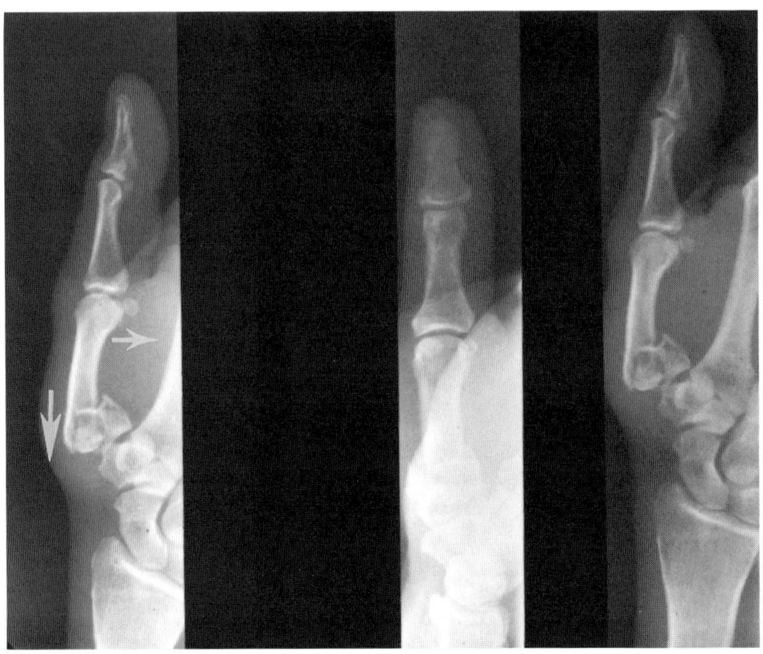

FIG. 13-43. Radiographs of a T-shaped Rolando fracture. The first metacarpal is pulled proximally and flexed (*arrows*), which is similar to the Bennett fracture.

A

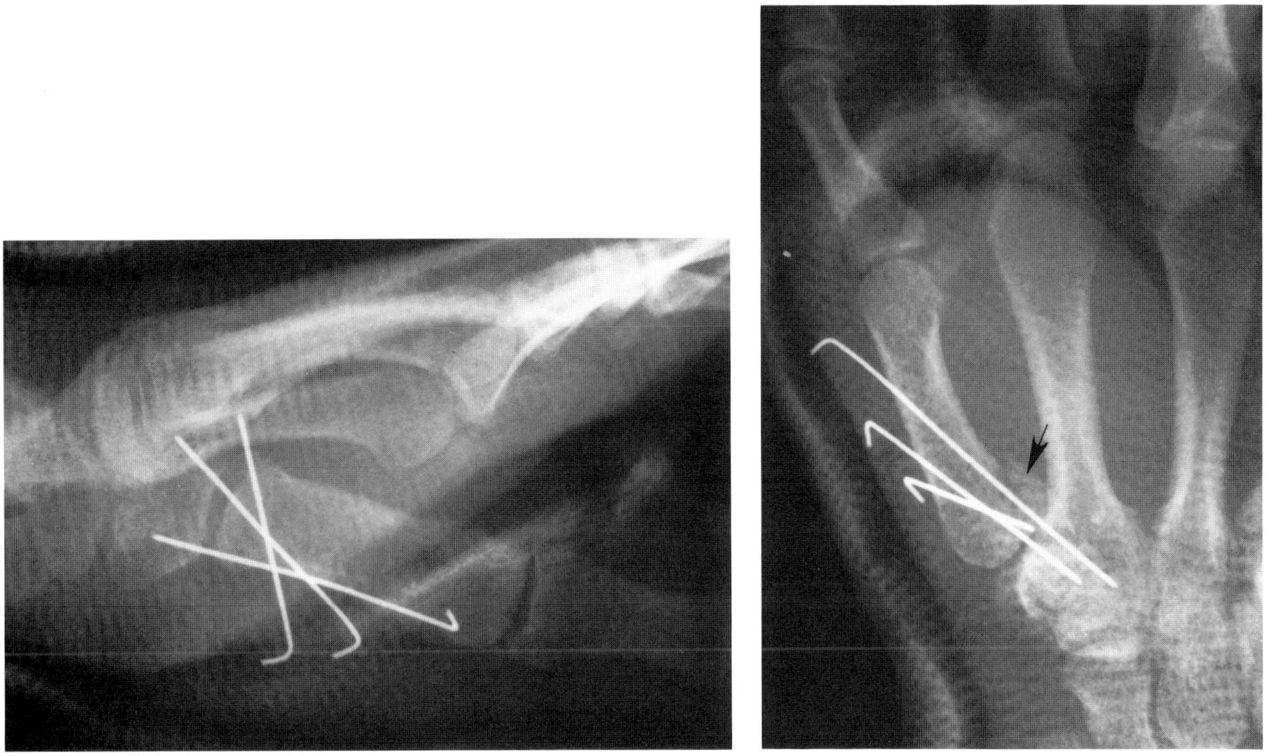

B

FIG. 13-44. The AP **(A)** and lateral **(B)** radiographs of the thumb with three K-wires for fixation of the first metacarpal after a Bennett fracture. The small ulnar fragment (*arrow*) is pinned by the lower wire (*3*). The upper two wires (*1, 2*) attach the main fragment to the trapezium.

A

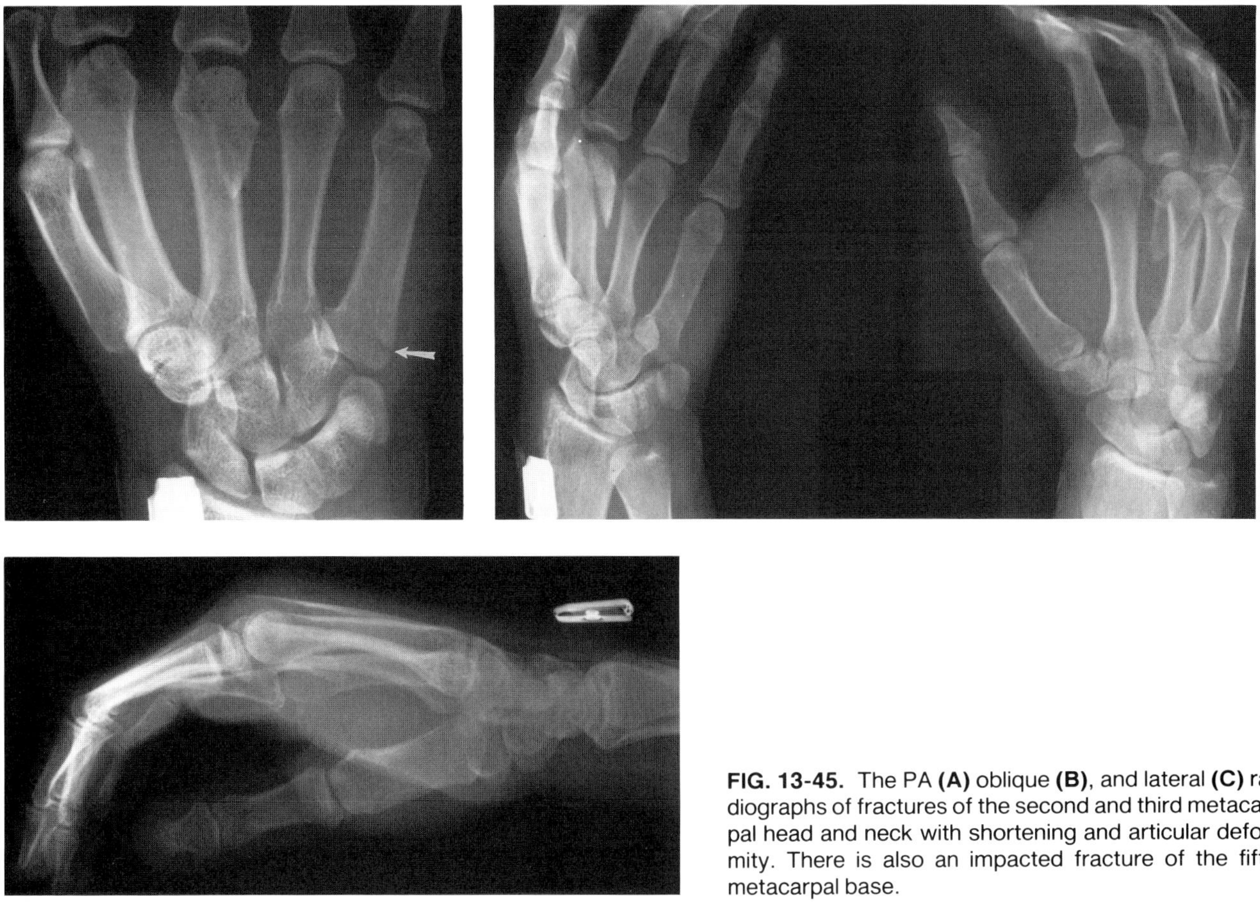

B

C

FIG. 13-45. The PA **(A)** oblique **(B)**, and lateral **(C)** radiographs of fractures of the second and third metacarpal head and neck with shortening and articular deformity. There is also an impacted fracture of the fifth metacarpal base.

Proximal fractures of the second and third metacarpal are usually stable. Fortunately intraarticular basilar fractures are uncommon.[112]

Fractures of the second and third metacarpals can usually be reduced by using longitudinal traction. However, maintaining reduction may be difficult. Plate and screw fixation or transverse K-wires through the adjacent metacarpal may be necessary to maintain the length and prevent rotation or angulation.[72,112,125] Basilar intraarticular fractures may also require internal fixation or primary arthrodesis.[72]

Fourth and Fifth Metacarpals (Mobile Rays)

Mobility at the fourth and fifth carpometacarpal joints allows more latitude for fracture angulation in these metacarpals. However, excessive malrotation, shortening, or angulation is not acceptable.[72] Fractures of the neck and metacarpal bases, especially the fifth, are common. Transverse and spiral shaft fractures occur less frequently.

Fracture of the fifth metacarpal neck (boxer's fracture) is common. The distal fragment is typically angulated in a palmar direction (Fig. 13-46). The functional limitation is minimal with up to 40° of angulation of the fifth and 25° for the fourth metacarpal neck. The lateral view is essential to measure the degree of angulation properly (Fig. 13-45).[72]

Reduction, when required, is usually easily accomplished with dorsal pressure at the fracture site or longitudinal traction. Stable fractures are managed with an ulnar gritter splint. Unstable fractures can be managed with percutaneous K-wires placed across the fracture (Fig. 13-46) or transversely into the adjacent metacarpal.[72,112]

Transverse or spiral diaphyseal fractures are not common. However, displacement and instability are more common. Spine fractures are particularly prone to shortening and rotation. Therefore, percutaneous K-wire fixation or internal fixation are more often required to maintain stable fixation (Figs. 13-47 and 13-48).[72,112,166]

Intraarticular fractures of the metacarpal base most often involve the fifth metacarpal. The extensor carpi ulnaris tendon can displace the metacarpal proximally, which is similar to the Bennett fracture. This injury is frequently unstable. Reduction and stabilization with percutaneous K-wires is frequently required.[72,112]

Phalangeal Fractures and Fracture-Dislocations

Phalangeal fractures are the most common fractures in the hand.[68,78,110,146,156,160] Treatment depends on which phalanx (proximal, middle, or distal) is fractured, the fracture type and location, and the presence of associated articular or soft tissue injury.[72,112,132,156]

Fractures of the proximal phalanx occur most frequently. Problems with malunion, shortening, rotation, or tendon dysfunction caused by adherence at the fracture site are more common with proximal phalangeal fractures.[66,71,75,112,146,156]

Fractures of the proximal phalanx may be due to direct blows, trauma from falls, or athletic injuries.[66,71,146] Fracture management depends on the fracture plane and location. Unicondylar or bicondylar fracture of the distal articular surface are frequently unstable, even though they may appear minimally displaced radiographically.[78,119,156] Bicondylar fractures (Fig. 13-49) tend to displace outwardly because of axial forces. Undisplaced fractures can be treated with cast or splint immobilization and careful radiographic monitoring to be certain the fragment does not displace.[72] If the fracture is displaced or displaces, K-wire or wire loop internal fixation is usually required (Fig. 13-50).[72,109,126,174]

Phalangeal shaft fractures are also common. When the fracture is undisplaced, it can be managed conservatively. However, there is a tendency for these fractures to angulate in a palmar direction (Fig. 13-51).[71,72,112] Angulation occurs as a result of the intrinsic muscles of the hand flexing the proximal fragment.[71,72]

When angulation exceeds 20° in adults or 30° in children, it should be corrected. This is usually accomplished by using longitudinal traction for reduction followed by K-wire or tension-band wire for fixation (Fig. 13-52). Rotation and shortening are not usually a problem with transverse fracture. However, maintaining the reduction of these fractures without K-wire or internal fixation of some type (K-wire, plate and screw, or intramedullary fixation) may be difficult.[71,72,78,88,89,112,113,122,166]

Basilar phalangeal fractures are particularly common in the fifth finger in children. Closed reduction is almost always possible in this setting. Intraarticular fractures at the phalangeal base are often impacted and stable. In this setting, buddy taping to the adjacent finger may be adequate. When displacement is identified, especially when greater than one third of the articular surface is involved, K-wires, sutures, or a single bone screw may be required to reestablish the articular surface (Fig. 13-53).[72,97,110,112,171]

Fracture patterns for the middle phalanx are similar to those described in the proximal phalanx. The treatment options are also similar. The most common middle phalangeal fracture is the volar plate hyperextension injury, which avulses a fragment of bone from the volar base of the middle phalanx. This injury can be subtle radiographically. Oblique or lateral radiographs of the isolated finger are essential for the diagnosis (Fig. 13-54).[72] Small fragments are treated in a splint with the proximal interphalangeal (PIP) joint flexed 20° to 30°.[72,112] Even larger fragments involving up to one third of the articular surface can be treated conservatively if they are undisplaced. When displaced, K-wire reduction is usually required. Dorsal subluxation should be watched for radiographically because the long-term results are poor if it is left unattended.[66]

Fractures of the distal phalanx are rarely treated aggressively. An exception is the dorsal lip or mallet fracture involving greater than one third of the articular surface (Fig. 13-55) and when there is associated volar displacement of the distal fragment. When reduction cannot be maintained or there is associated subluxation, internal fixation is recommended.[112] Volar segment fractures also occur, and associated instability is fairly common (Fig. 13-56).[112,135,171]

Dislocations of the phalangeal joints usually occur dorsally and may be associated with articular fractures (Fig. 13-56).[66,71,174] The PIP joint is involved most frequently. If there is no fracture, closed reduction is adequate. When a fracture is also present, the injury is treated as described previously.

TABLE 13-2. *Fractures of the distal radius and ulna: complications*[72,81,83,85,86,100,105,114,117,118,120,123,137,151,172]

Early
Loss of reduction
Dislocation or subluxation in distal radioulnar joint
Median nerve injury (contusion, entrapment, compression, or disruption)
Carpal tunnel syndrome
Forearm compartment syndrome
Tendon entrapment, adhesive tendinitis, or rupture
Carpal fracture or ligament injury
Pin tract infection (external fixators)
Pressure sores (cast immobilization)
Delayed
Loss of reduction or malunion
Shoulder-hand syndrome
Median nerve compression
Tendinitis or stenosing tendinitis
Contractures
Reflex sympathetic dystrophy
Nonunion

Complications

An evaluation of complications and chronic pain or dysfunction following hand or wrist trauma can be difficult. A thorough knowledge of the clinical history and physical examination findings is essential when determining how to workup the patient from an imaging standpoint. Conventional radiographs, fluoroscopic examination, radionuclide scans, CT, MRI, arthrotenography, and diagnostic injections must all be considered. For our purposes, we discuss the imaging of postoperative complications anatomically.

Distal Radius and Ulna

The complications of fractures or fracture-dislocations of the distal radius, ulna, and radioulnar joint are fairly similar with all the varieties of injury (e.g., Colles's, Smith, or Barton's fractures).[85,86,155,161,168] They may be related to the injury or the fixation technique used to treat the injury.[72,85,86,92,98,123] Table 13-2 summarizes early and late complications.

Most early and delayed osseous complications can be detected with routine radiographs or fluoroscopically positioned spot views. On occasion, CT or radionuclide scans are required. It is essential to understand what the orthopedic surgeon is looking for when evaluating postreduction radiographs or later follow-up studies.[72,129] Mann et al.[129] described important measurements and relationships that we should all be familiar with when evaluating posttraumatic or other wrist disorders. Figures 13-57 to 13-61 summarize these features and demonstrate certain complications of distal radioulnar injuries. The carpal height and carpal ulnar ratio were demonstrated in Figs. 13-4 and 13-5. The abnormal features demonstrated in Figs. 13-57 to 13-61 result in reduced function and a guarded prognosis.[72,85,129]

Serial radiographs are the most useful to evaluate the loss of reduction and fracture healing. Nonunion is unsual except for the ulnar styloid. Differentiating fibrous union from nonunion can be most easily accomplished by using MRI. This should be reserved for patients treated with external fixators because local image distortion may be too significant with plate and screw fixation. In this setting, reformatted CT images may be the most effective.[72]

Soft tissue complications are frequently not detected until fracture healing has occurred and the patient complains of persistent symptoms. Exceptions or early complications might include compartment syndrome and tendon or nerve entrapment.[123] Delayed soft tissue or DRUJ disorders are studied with MRI and arthrography (CT or arthrography for the DRUJ, Fig. 13-62).[72] Tenography with an anesthetic injection may be most useful in patients with suspected tendon adhesions or stenosing tenosynovitis. The latter is most common in the first dorsal compartment.[72,123]

Carpal Fracture-Dislocations

Most significant complications of fracture-dislocations of the carpal bones relate to osteoarthritis and persistent discomfort with or without associated functional loss. These problems may develop long term, even when the fractures have healed.[94]

Scaphoid fractures occur most frequently and present particular problems with imaging in the immediate postreduction phase and later, even if healing has occurred.

(*text continues on page 873*)

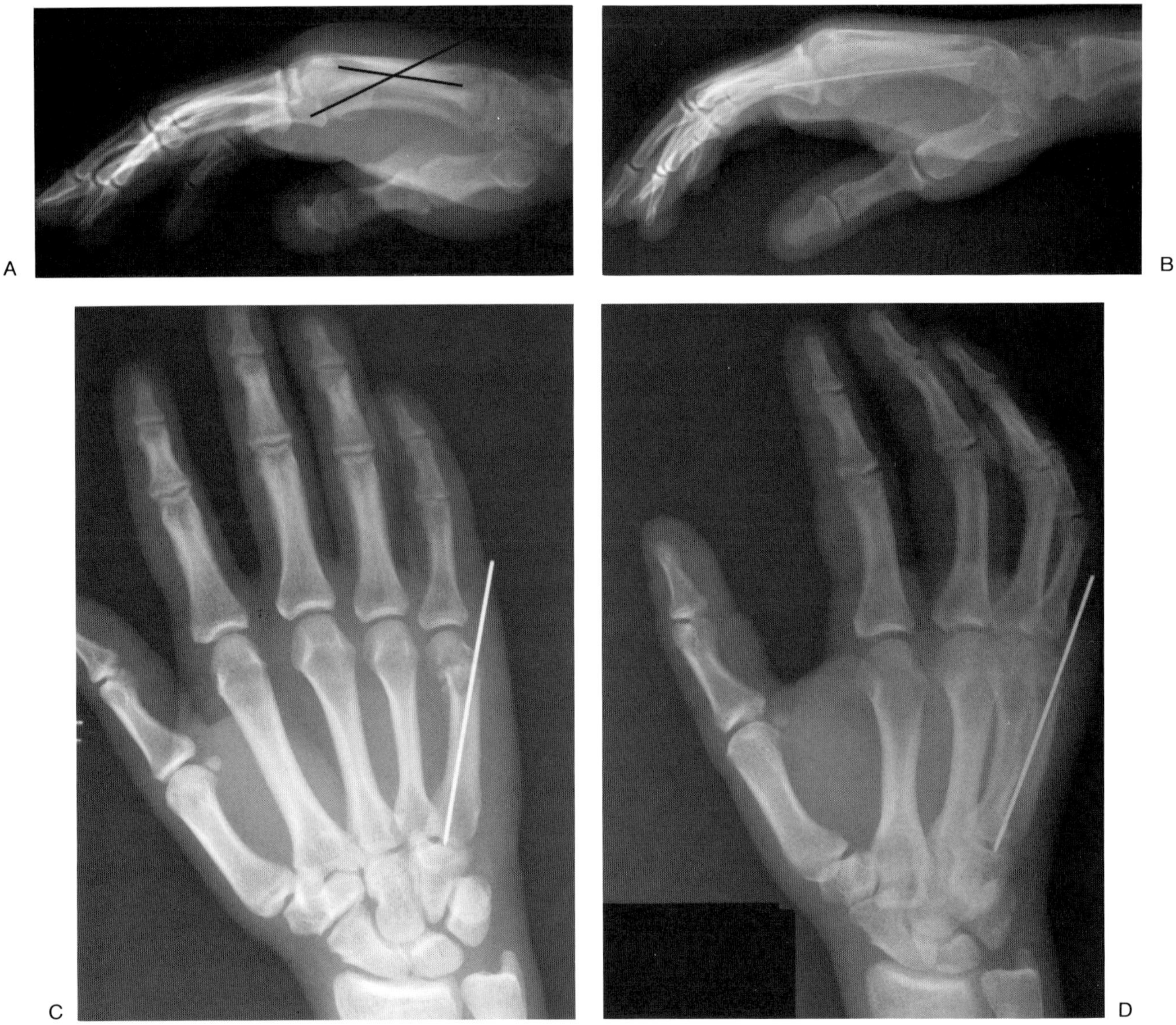

FIG. 13-46. **A:** Boxer's fracture of the fifth metacarpal seen on the lateral radiograph. The lateral view is best for determining the degree of angulation. In this case, there is 35° of angulation. **B:** The fracture was reduced and fixed with a percutaneous K-wire. The PA **(C)** and oblique **(D)** postreduction radiographs show the K-wire through the distal fragment but avoiding the articular surface.

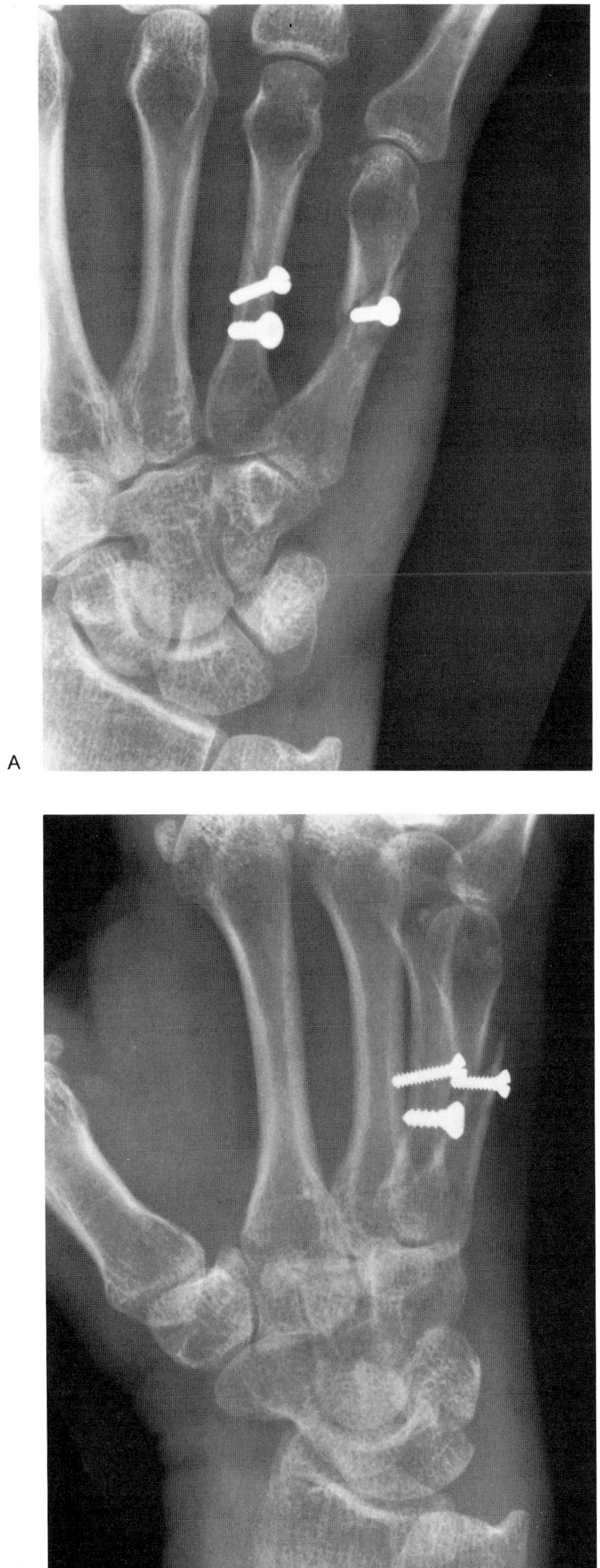

FIG. 13-47. The PA **(A)** and oblique **(B)** radiographs of spiral fractures of the fourth and fifth metacarpals internally fixed with bone screws. The screw in the fifth metacarpal has pulled out, and the fracture has displaced and shortened.

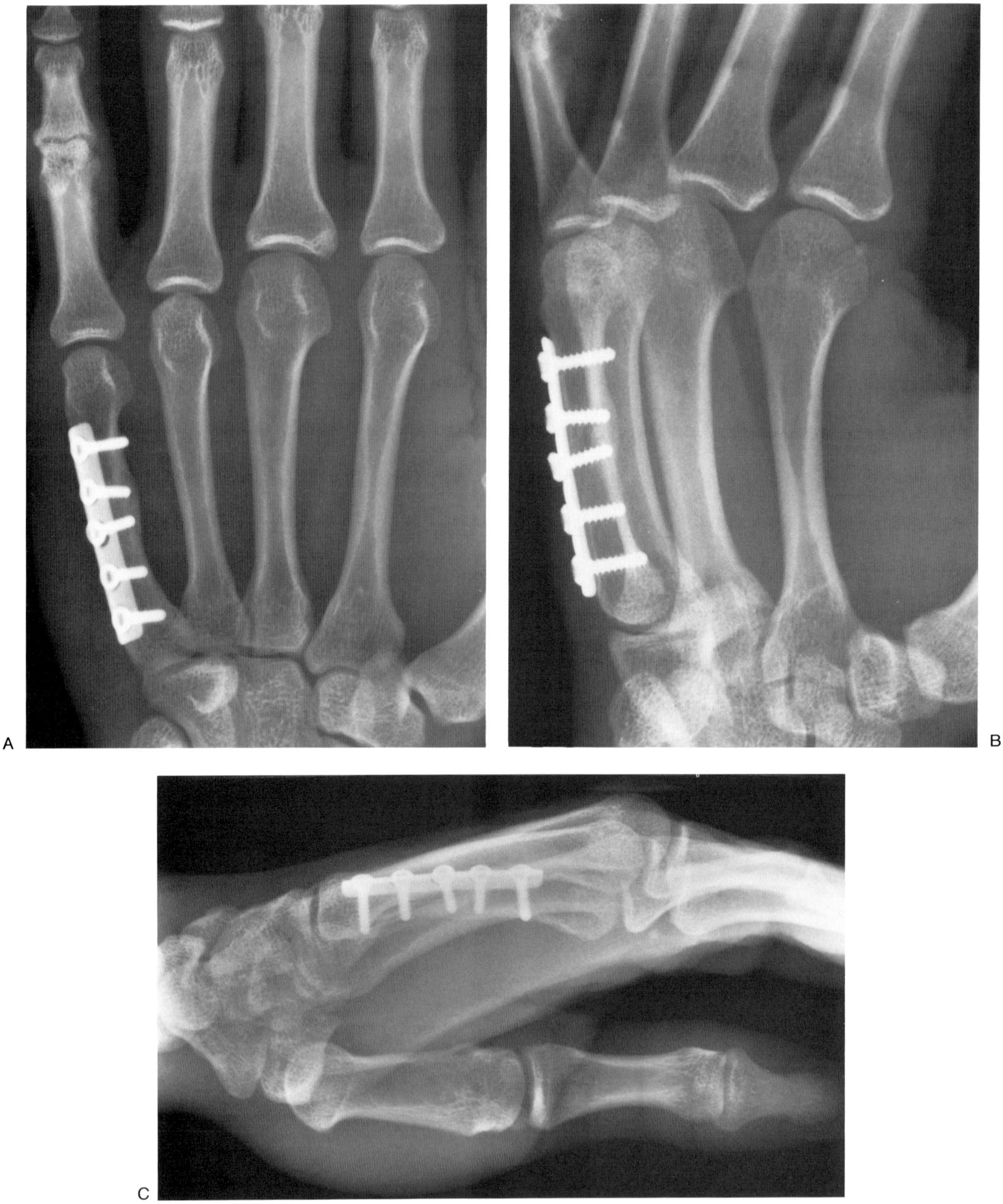

FIG. 13-48. The PA (A), oblique (B), and lateral (C) radiographs of a healing oblique fracture of the fifth metacarpal diaphysis treated with a one-third tubular plate and five cortical screws.

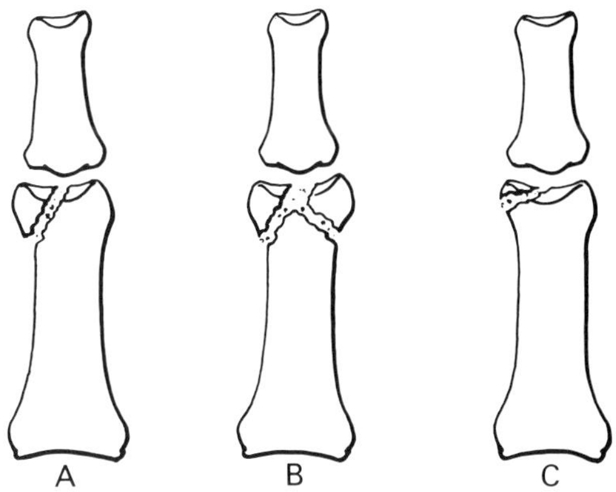

FIG. 13-49. Intraarticular fractures of the proximal phalanx. Unicondylar **(A)**, bicondylar **(B)**, and osteochondral shear fracture **(C)**. (From Berquist TH. *Imaging of sports injuries.* Gaithersburg, MD: Aspen Press, 1992.)

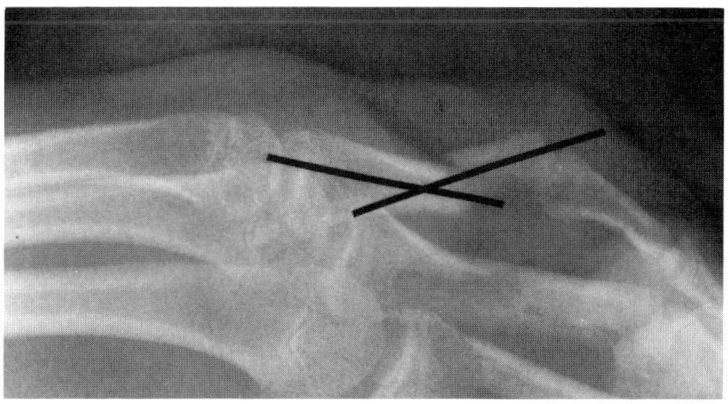

FIG. 13-51. Fracture of the left fifth proximal phalanx with palmar angulation. This is most easily detected and measured on the lateral view.

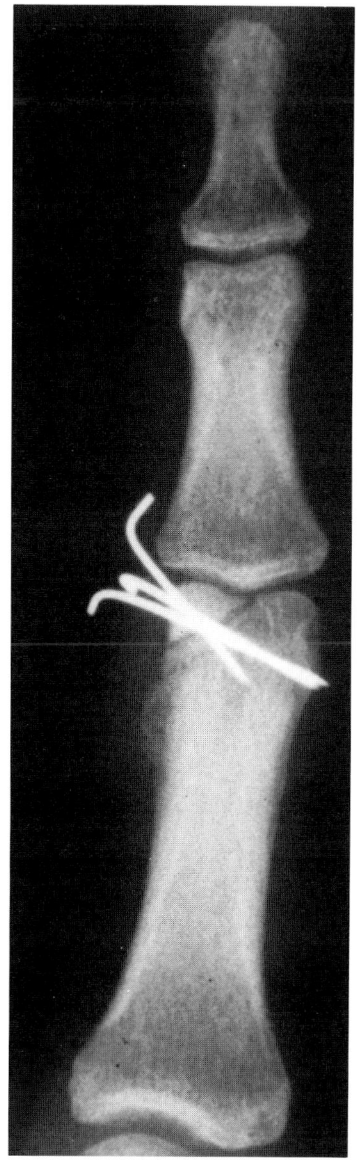

FIG. 13-50. A PA radiograph of the second proximal phalanx with an intraarticular unicondylar fracture that is reduced and fixed with three percutaneous K-wires.

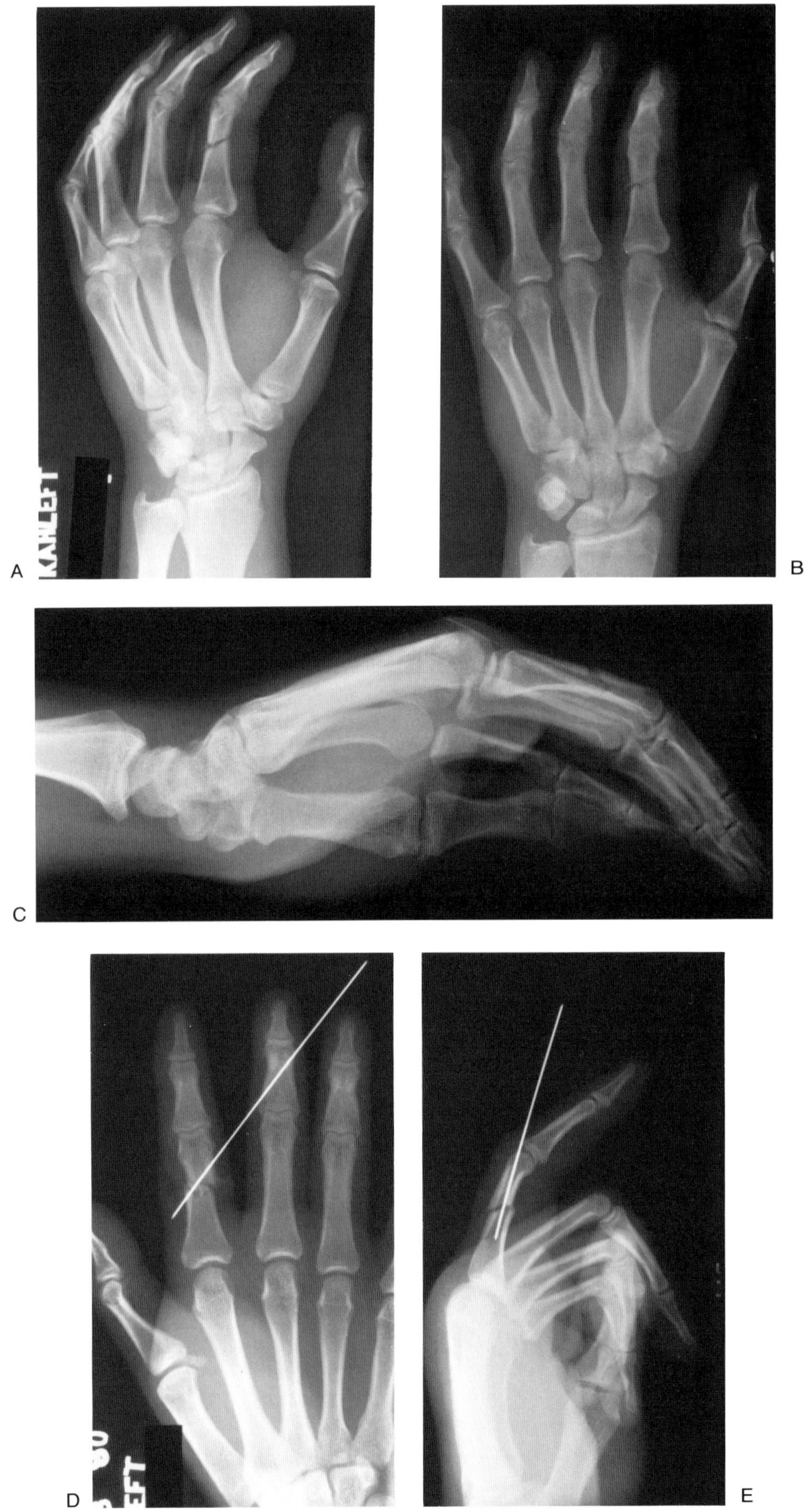

FIG. 13-52. Oblique **(A)**, PA **(B)**, and lateral **(C)** radiographs of the left hand demonstrating an oblique fracture of the left second proximal phalanx. There is no rotation or shortening. Reduction was maintained by using a single K-wire, which is obliquely positioned across the fracture line. The PA **(D)** and lateral **(E)** radiographs demonstrate slight displacement of the distal fragment during pinning.

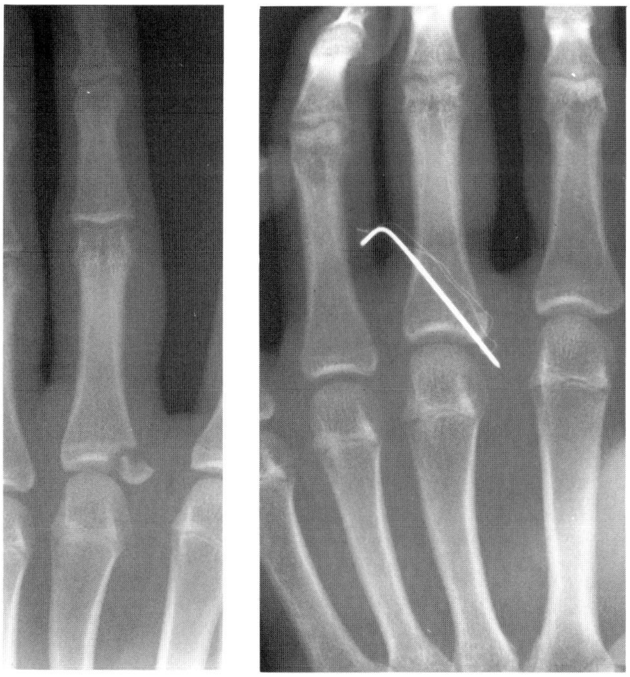

A B

FIG. 13-53. **A:** The PA view of the left hand demonstrating a displaced intraarticular fracture of the proximal phalanx. **B:** The fracture was reduced with a single K-wire, and the articular surface was reestablished.

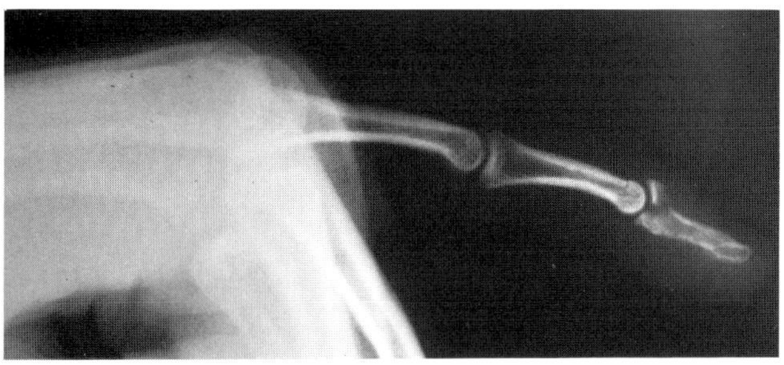

FIG. 13-55. Lateral views of the index finger demonstrating a displaced dorsal intraarticular fracture involving greater than 50% of the articular surface.

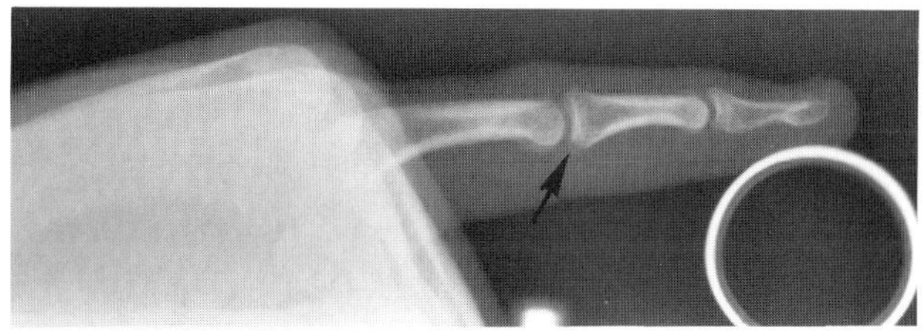

FIG. 13-54. Isolated lateral view of the index finger demonstrating a small volar plate fracture (*arrow*) of the middle phalanx.

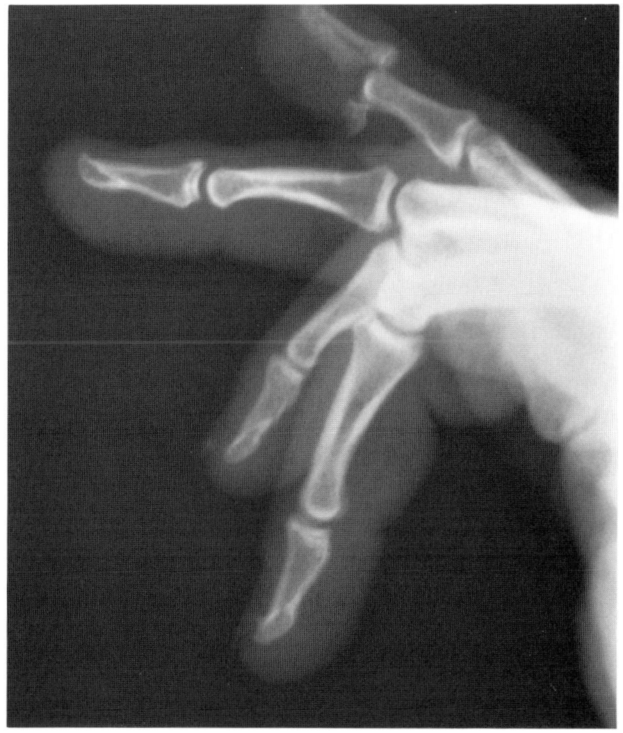

FIG. 13-56. Lateral radiographs of the fingers demonstrating a volar plate fracture of the fifth distal phalanx with dorsal dislocation of the main fragment and proximal rotation and displacement of the volar fragment.

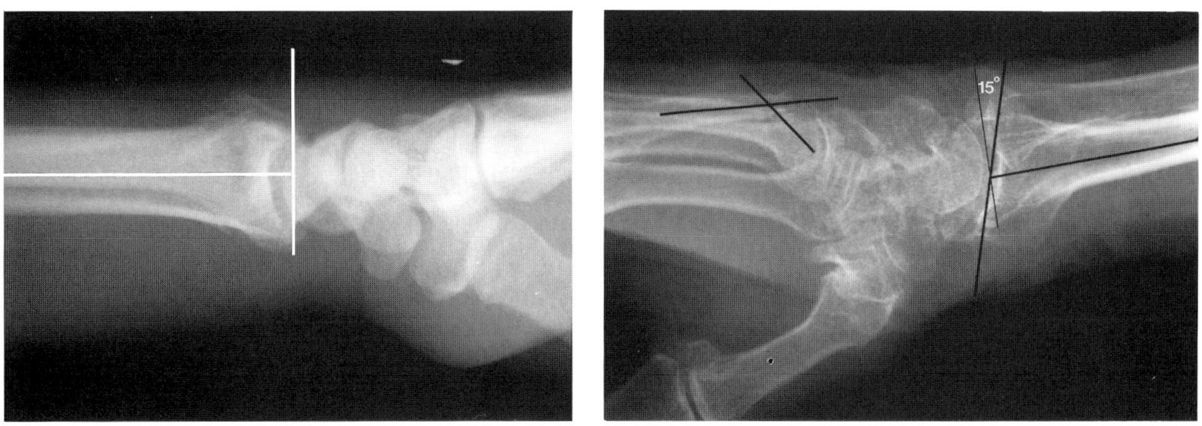

A B

FIG. 13-57. Palmar (volar tilt). This is the angle of palmar inclination of the distal radius measured on the lateral radiograph. The normal angle is 14.5° ± 4.3° in males and 12.4° (range, 11.3° to 13.5°) in females. Dorsal tilt can result in reduced grip and function. The carpus repositions dorsally with dorsal tilt, especially when the angle exceeds 20°. A line is drawn longitudinally through the axis of the radius, and a perpendicular line is constructed to it. The angle is measured along the dorsal to volar articular surface of the radius. **A:** Impacted distal radial fracture. The impaction dorsally creates a neutral angle with no palmar tilt. **B:** Poorly positioned lateral demonstrating a dorsal distal radial tilt of 15°. There is also an angulated fifth metacarpal fracture.

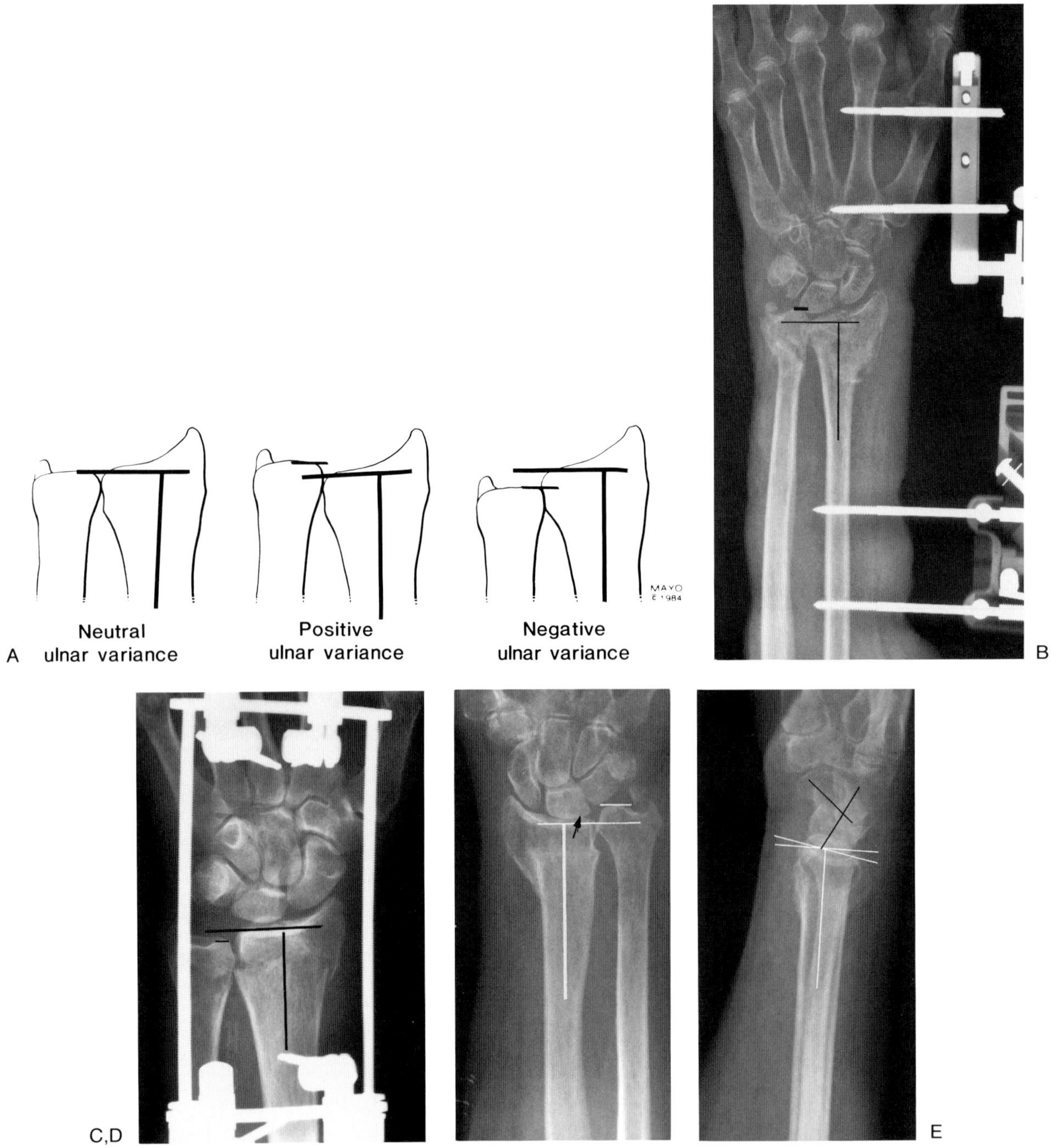

FIG. 13-58. Ulnar variance. This is described as neutral, positive, or negative compared with the radial length at the margin of the lunate fossa. This is evaluated on a neutral PA radiograph. **A:** The perpendicular method is the most useful because no aids are required. A line longitudinal to the radius is connected to a perpendicular line through the radial margin on the ulnar side. The length of the ulnar is neutral (i.e., the same), positive (i.e., a number of millimeters longer), or negative (i.e., a number of millimeters shorter).[72,129] **B:** A PA radiograph of the left wrist taken in external fixation with an Agee wrist jack. There is 3 mm of ulnar positive variance. **C:** Fractures of the distal radius and ulnar taken in an external fixator demonstrating 3 mm of ulnar minus variance. **D,E:** Old healed Colles's fracture with radial shortening and ulnar styloid nonunion. The PA radiograph (D) demonstrates ulnar positive variance of 5 mm with a lucent area in the lunate (*arrow*) caused by ulnar lunate abutment (compression) syndrome. There is slight dorsal radial tilt (*white lines*) and DISI deformity (*black lines*) on the lateral view (E). Posttraumatic ulnar positive variance is associated with ulnar lunate abutment syndrome, and patients with $\geq$ 5 mm of ulnar positive variance after distal radial fracture have a more guarded prognosis.[129]

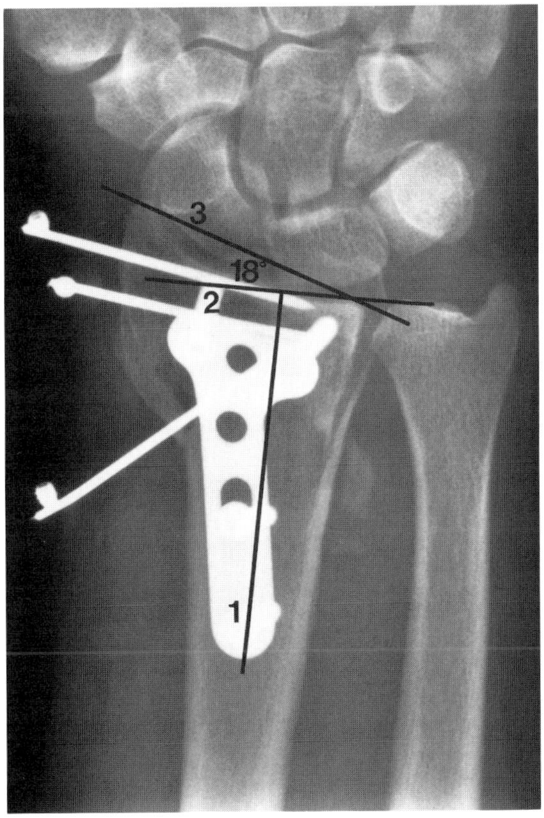

A

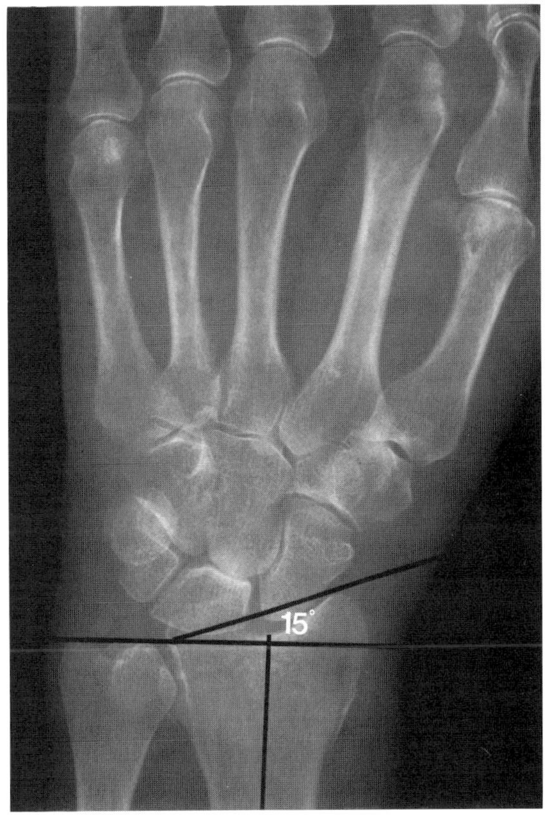

B

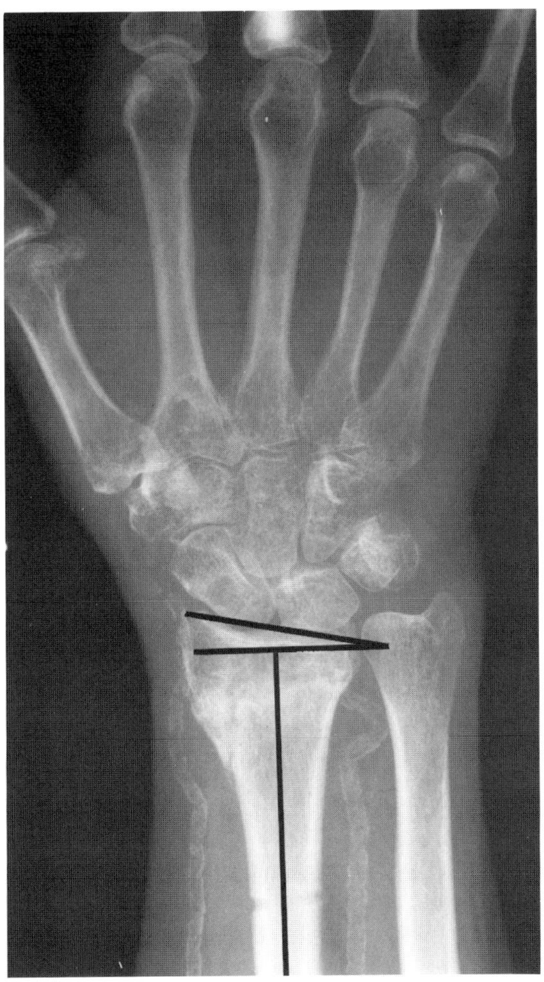

C

FIG. 13-59. Radial inclination is evaluated on the PA radiograph (normal, 16° to 28°); < 5° indicates a poor prognosis.[129] A line is drawn along the longitudinal axis of the radius, and a perpendicular line is constructed to this. A third line is drawn from the radial styloid to the ulnar margin of the radius. The radial inclination angle is the angle formed by the second and third lines (A). **A:** Comminuted distal right radial fracture with oblique T plate and K-wires for fixation. The line perpendicular (*2*) to the radial axis (*1*) and the third line (*3*) from the radial styloid to the ulnar margin demonstrate a radial inclination angle of 18°. **B:** Colles's type of fracture of the left wrist with slight ulnar minus variance and a radial inclination angle of 15°. **C:** Old distal radial fracture with radial shortening and ulnar positive variance of 4 mm. The radial inclination angle is 6°.

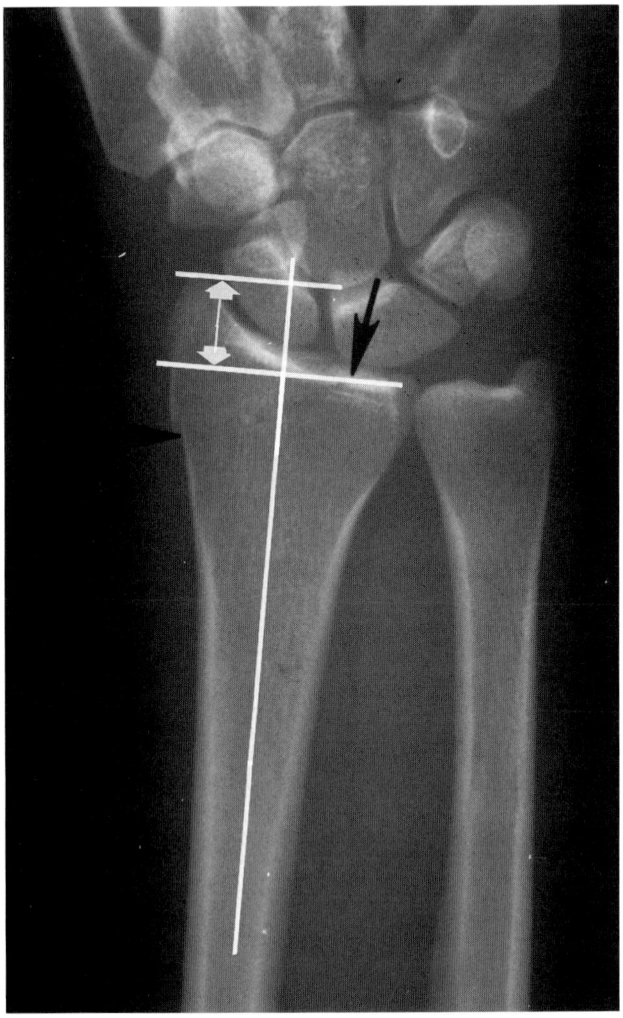

FIG. 13-60. Radial height measures the distance between the tip of the radial styloid and the ulnar margin. This distance along with the other measurements is also a predictor of the prognosis (normal, 13.5 ± 3.8 mm).[129] Frykman type III fracture (*arrows*) with lines perpendicular to the radial axis line to measure the radial height (*white arrows*).

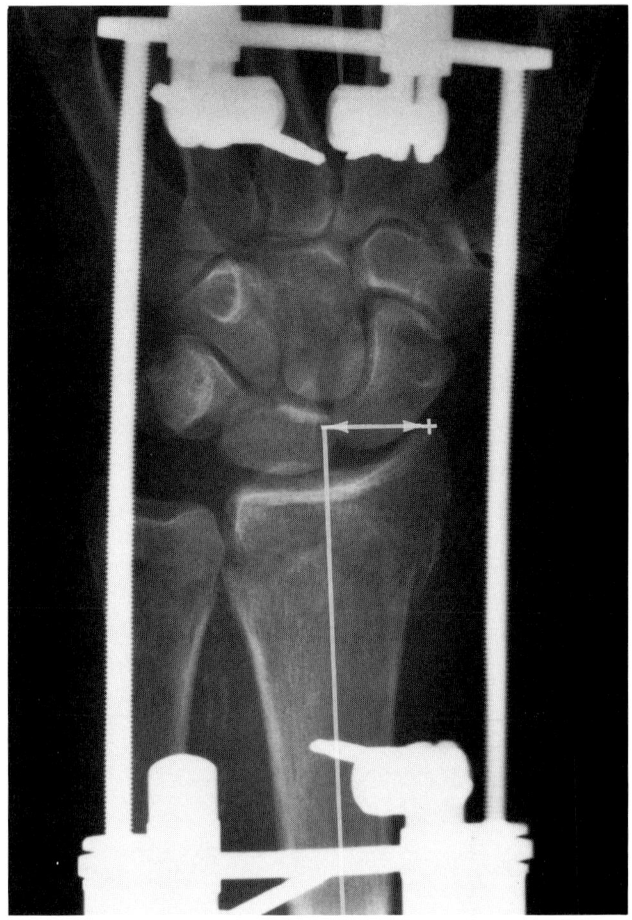

FIG. 13-61. Radial shift demonstrates the offset of the radial fragments with respect to the radial axis. Both wrists are required for comparison. Measurement differences of greater than 1 mm are abnormal.[129] Fractures of the distal radius and ulna (Frykman type VI) with slight radial shift measured from the axis of the radius to the styloid tip. External fixator in place.

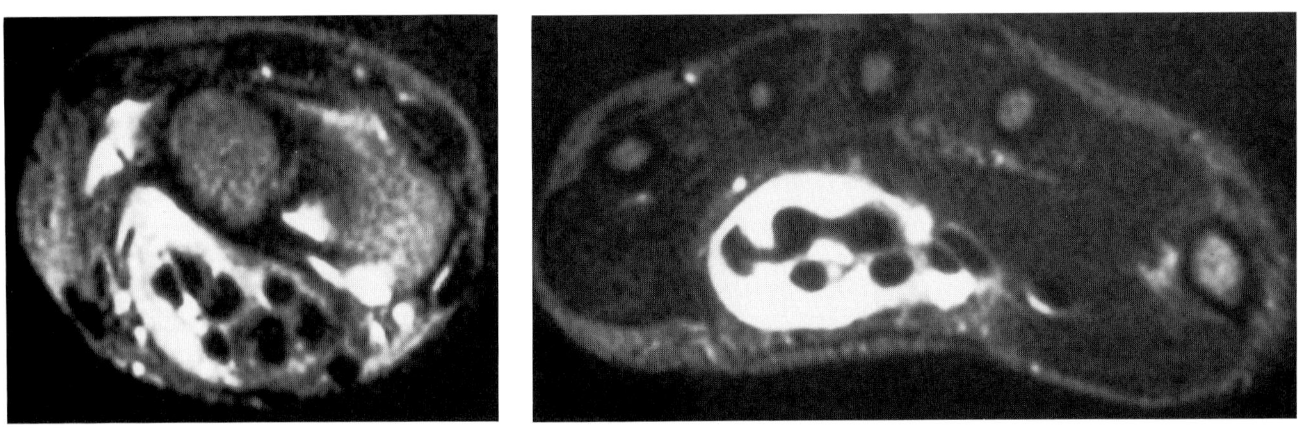

A B

FIG. 13-62. Axial SE 2,000/80 images of the wrist in a patient with chronic posttraumatic pain. There is high signal intensity around the flexor tendons at the level of the DRUJ **(A)** and into the hand **(B)** caused by tendonitis.

Although the incidence of nonunion (Fig. 13-63) is 10%, delayed union (failure to heal in 3 months) is a more common problem.[72,85,147,167] These problems are especially common with proximal and Russe III type injuries (Fig. 13-31).[147,167] Tomography or reformatted CT to demonstrate coronal and sagittal planes is essential for the early detection of a "humpback" deformity or palmar displacement of the distal scaphoid fragment (Fig. 13-64).[152,153] Treatment complications can also occur (Fig. 13-65), which require reformatted CT or tomograms for diagnoses.[72,152,153]

In addition, MRI is valuable for the detection of soft tissue abnormalities (Figs. 13-62 and 13-66), nonunion, and avascular necrosis (Fig. 13-9).[72,73] Therefore, chronic posttraumatic conditions are a common indication for MRI. Arthrography or tenography with anesthetic agent injections are also useful in sorting out the cause and site of posttraumatic wrist pain.[72,119]

Arthrosis and recurrent instability are the most common complications after carpal dislocations (Fig. 13-67).[72,85] Routine radiographs, motion studies, and arthrography are the most useful for evaluating these disorders in our practice.[72]

Fracture-Dislocations of the Hand

Arthrosis and malunion are the most significant osseous problems following fractures and dislocations of the metacarpals and phalanges.[72] Improper reduction or loss of reduction can result in functional loss and may require revision surgery (Fig. 13-68).[72,112] Reconstruction using bone graft or arthrodeses may be indicated in some situations (Fig. 13-69).[72,112]

ARTHROPLASTY

Joint-replacement arthroplasty for the hand, thumb, and wrist evolved as an alternative to arthrodesis or synovectomy for patients with pain and joint deformity.[178] For the purposes of the review in this atlas, the wrist (including carpal bones), hand, and thumb are discussed separately.

Wrist

Arthroplasty of the wrist began to evolve soon after the early successes with hip-replacement surgery.[181] Much of the early research and development is credited to Meuli, Volz, and Lodi.[208] Meuli designed his implant system in 1972 (Figs. 13-70 and 13-71).[178,184] Using this implant, the radial styloid and distal ulna were resected along with the scaphoid, lunate, triquetrum, and proximal capitate (Fig. 13-72).[207]

The Volz prosthesis (Arizona Health Science Center) was developed in 1973. The original implants were configured of cobalt-chromium alloy with an ultrahigh molecular weight polyethylene interface (Fig. 13-73).[226] This system allowed 90° of flexion and extension and 50° of radioulnar deviation. The original system was modified in 1977 so that there was only one distal stem and small fixation pegs (Fig. 13-74).[206,226,227]

Swanson developed the Silastic™ wrist prosthesis in the early 1970s (Fig. 13-75).[190] This implant was used with resection arthroplasty primarily for rheumatoid arthritis. The original design had a Dacron™ core to increase its strength and reduce rotary torque.[216,217] The newer modified component has a shorter distal stem and wider hub with a protective metal grommet (Fig. 13-76).[181] Silastic™ prostheses tend to reduce forces across the component, lessening the likelihood of loosening compared with that of rigid metal-polyethylene arthroplasties. In addition, revision or additional procedures are more easily performed. Silicone-induced synovitis has not been a significant problem with radiocarpal arthroplasty.[181,216,218]

The trispheric wrist arthroplasty (Fig. 13-77) is a more constrained device that reduces the likelihood of ulnar drift, and there are fewer problems with dislocation. However, because of its limited motion, loosening is more common. Figgie et al.[191] reported excellent or good results using the trispheric system in 86% of patients with rheumatoid arthritis.

Newer designs are also available that have attempted to reduce cement requirements and provide more normal anatomic function. The biaxial type (Biax™, Depuy, Warsaw, IN) simulates the biaxial motion of the wrist. This system (Fig. 13-78) has a short porous-coated trapezoid fixation stem (see arrow in figure) with a porous-coated distal base and long partially coated stem for insertion into the third metacarpal. The radial stem is also partially porous coated with a polyethylene bearing. Flexion, extension, and radioulnar deviation are possible with this articulation.[179]

Indications

Most wrist arthroplasties are performed for rheumatoid disease because upper extremity involvement frequently drives the need for improved wrist function. In other arthritides, the other joints (shoulder and elbow) are often uninvolved, reducing the need for wrist arthroplasty.[178,180] Poor bone stock and previous fusion make arthroplasty difficult, but they do not exclude the technique.[178,218]

The contraindications include infection, paralysis, or a loss of muscle function or heavy activity. After wrist arthroplasty, patients are not suited for athletic activities or lifting more than 10 pounds.[178,208,218]

(text continues on page 882)

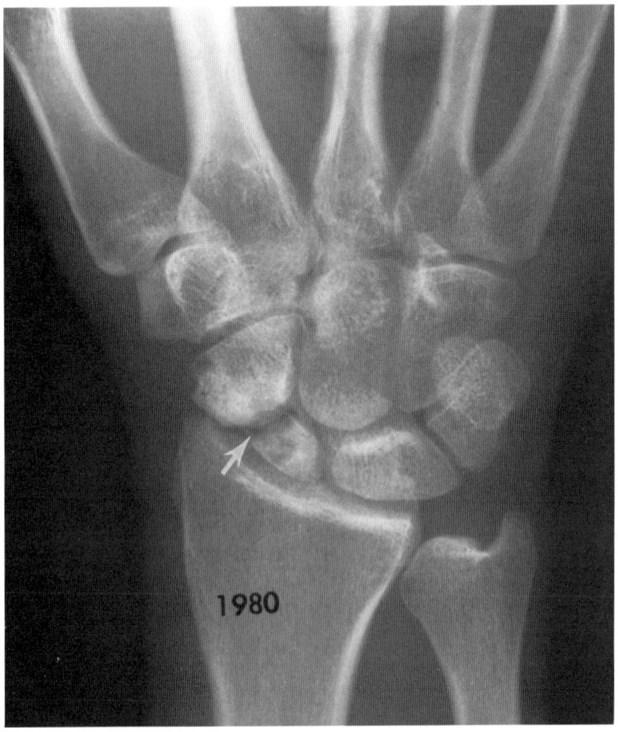

FIG. 13-63. A PA radiograph of the wrist demonstrating an obvious scaphoid nonunion (*arrow*).

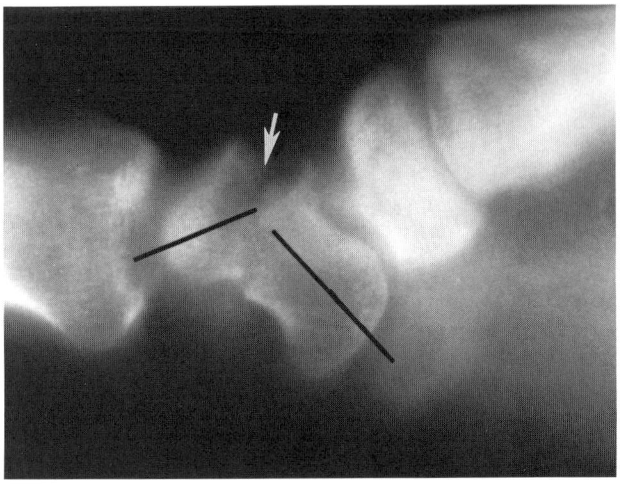

FIG. 13-64. Lateral tomogram demonstrating displacement of the distal fragment with opening of the fracture dorsally (*arrow*).

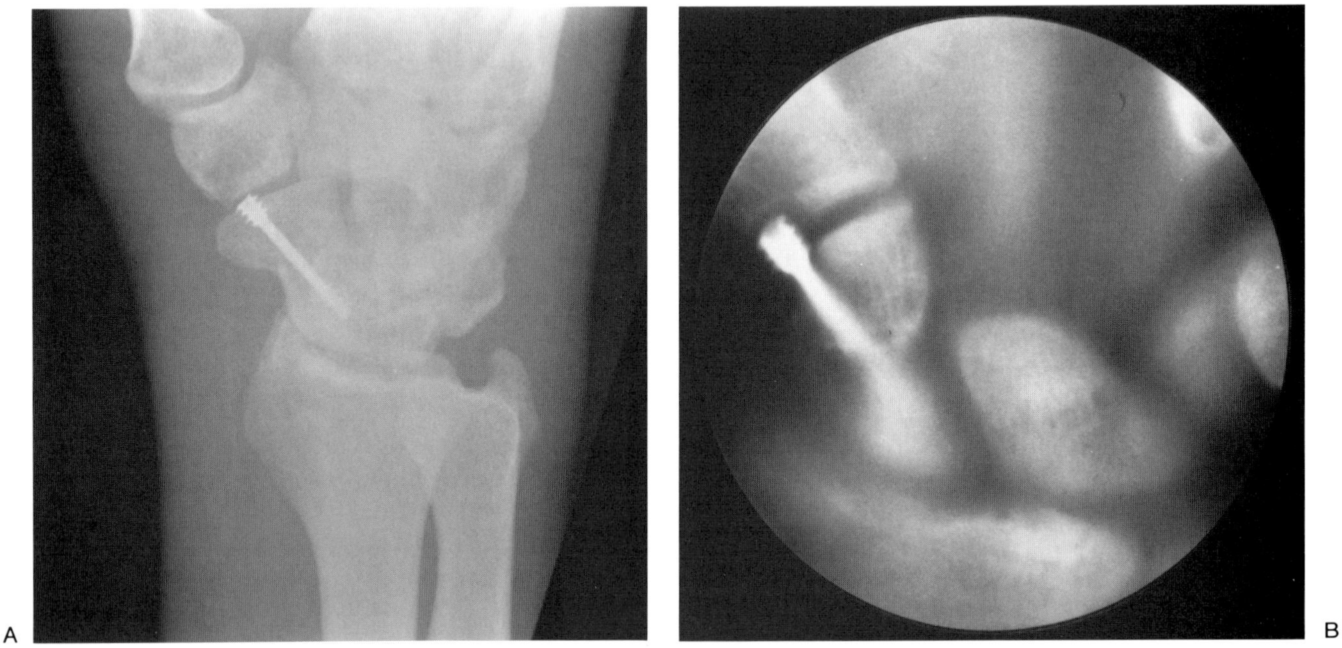

FIG. 13-65. A: Scaphoid view of the wrist with Herbert screw for fixation. There was pain at the base of the thumb. B: Tomogram demonstrating a protruding Herbert screw with erosion into the trapezium.

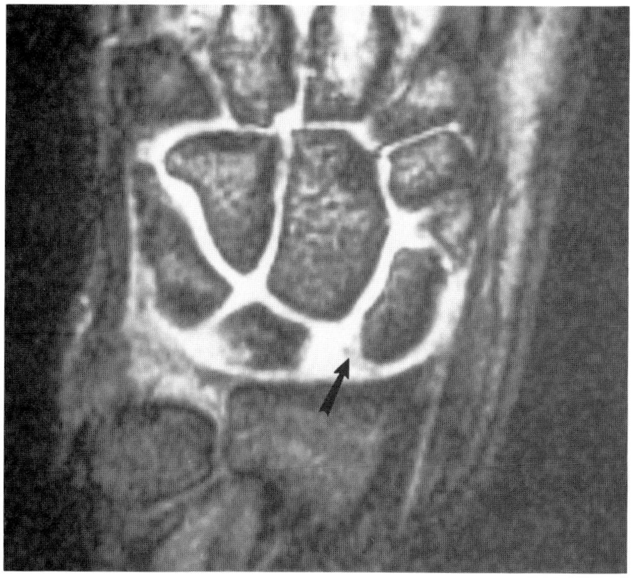

FIG. 13-66. Coronal gradient-echo T2* image demonstrating a scapholunate ligament tear (*arrow*).

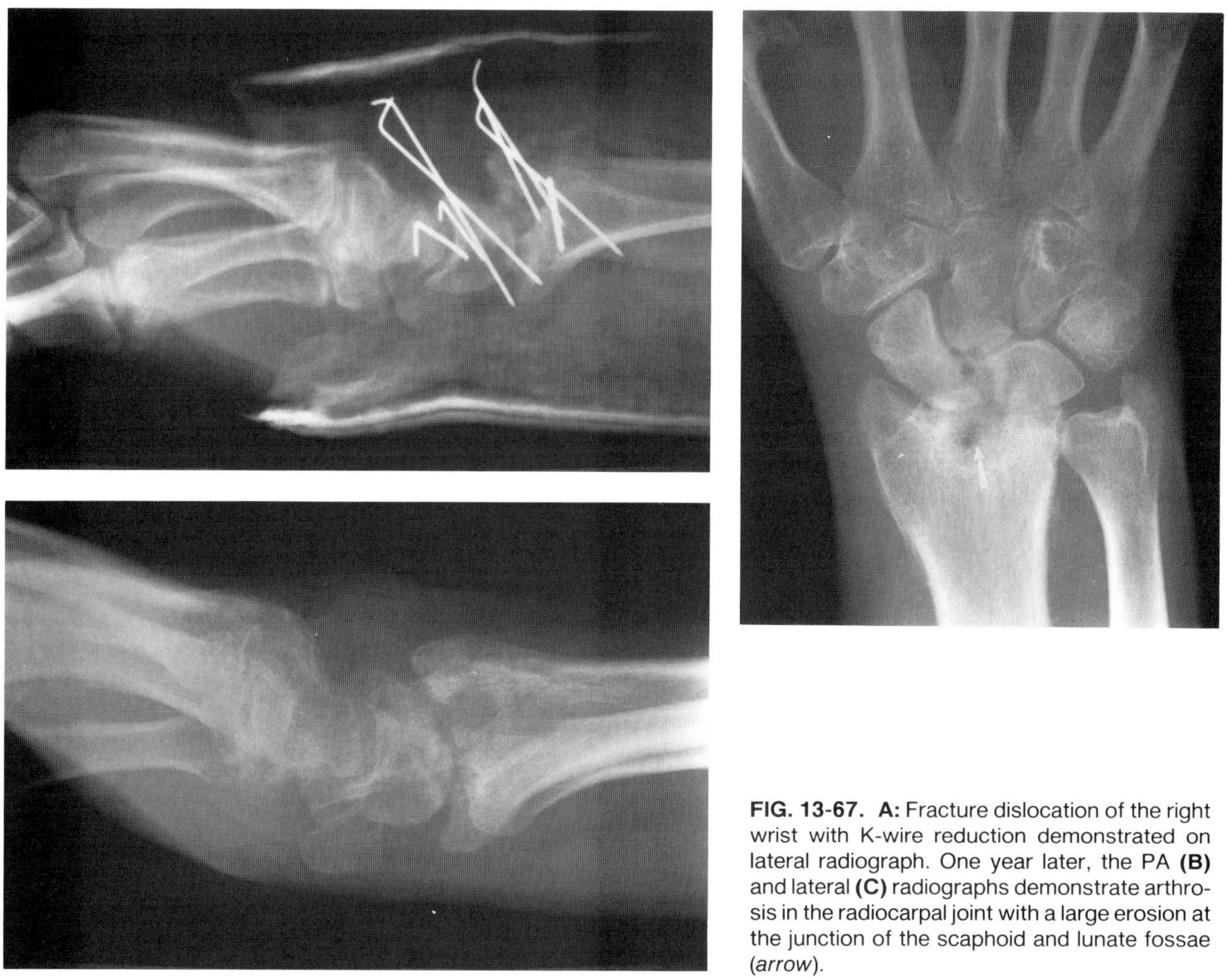

A

B

C

FIG. 13-67. A: Fracture dislocation of the right wrist with K-wire reduction demonstrated on lateral radiograph. One year later, the PA **(B)** and lateral **(C)** radiographs demonstrate arthrosis in the radiocarpal joint with a large erosion at the junction of the scaphoid and lunate fossae (*arrow*).

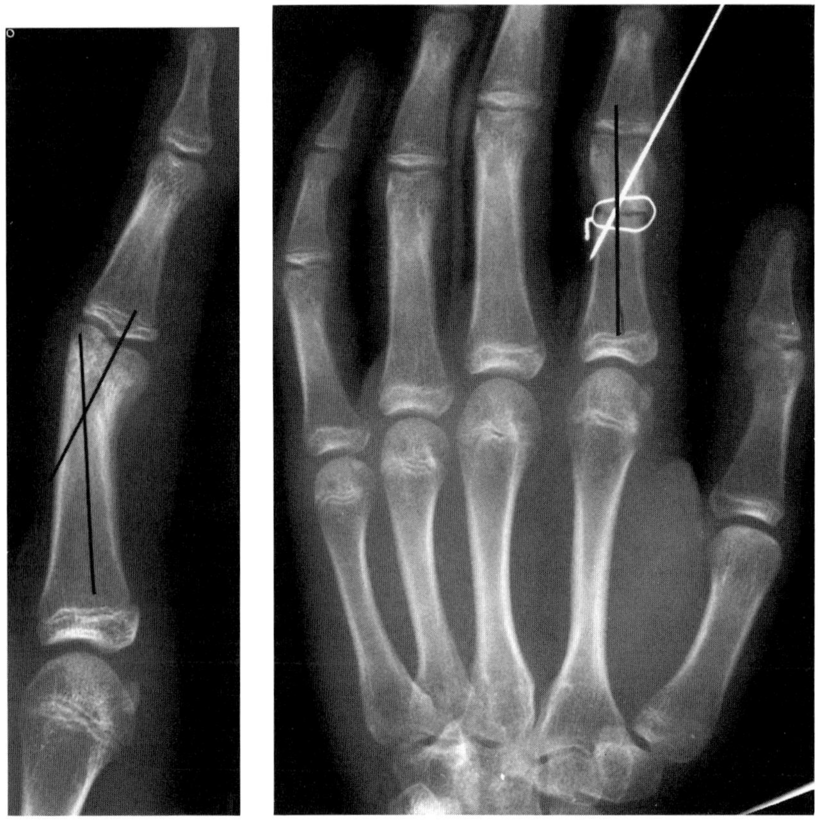

A B

FIG. 13-68. A: Old oblique fracture of the proximal phalanx with rotation and angulation distally. **B:** Osteotomy was performed, and the fragments were fixed with a wire loop and K-wire.

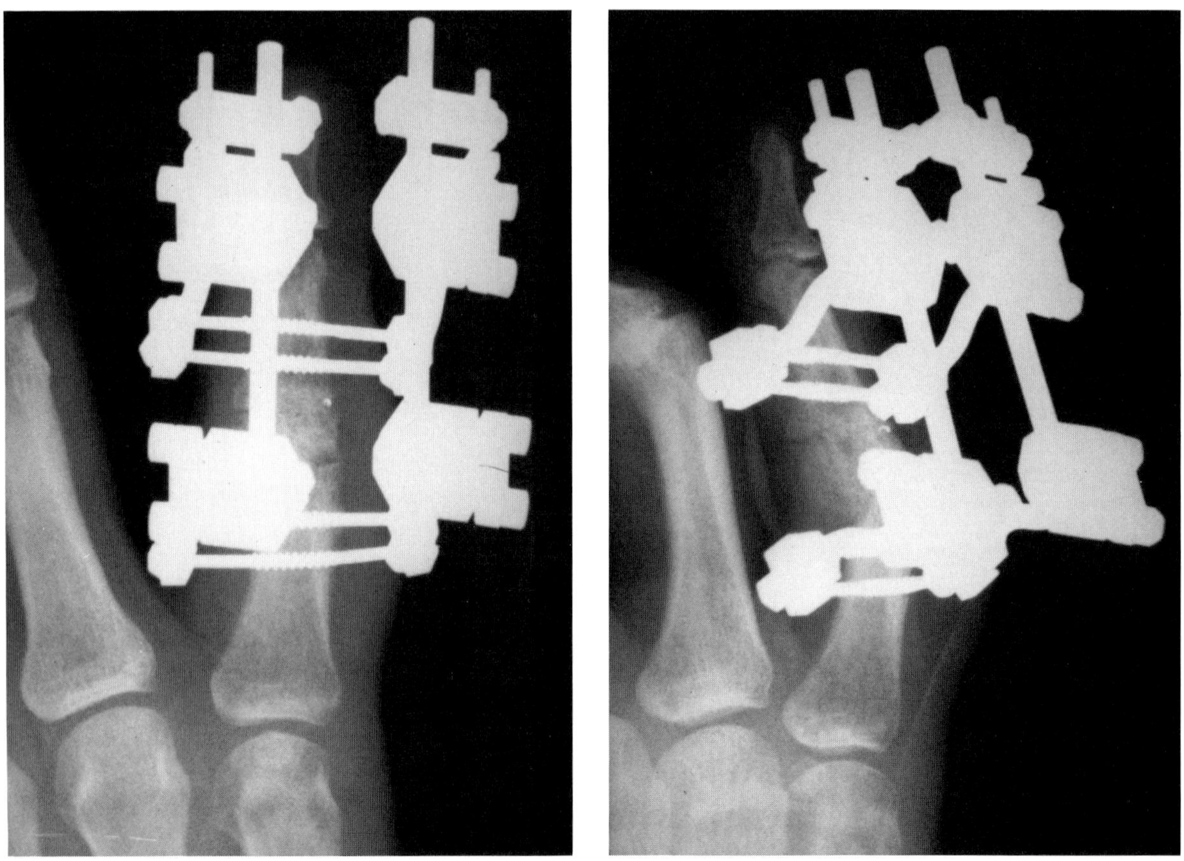

A B

FIG. 13-69. Old fracture with deformity and function loss in the right fifth PIP joint. Resection of a portion of the middle phalanx with bone graft and external fixation for arthrodesis was performed. The PA **(A)**, oblique **(B)**, and lateral **(C)** radiographs show the finger with arthrodesis in flexion (*black lines*) with a miniexternal fixator in place.

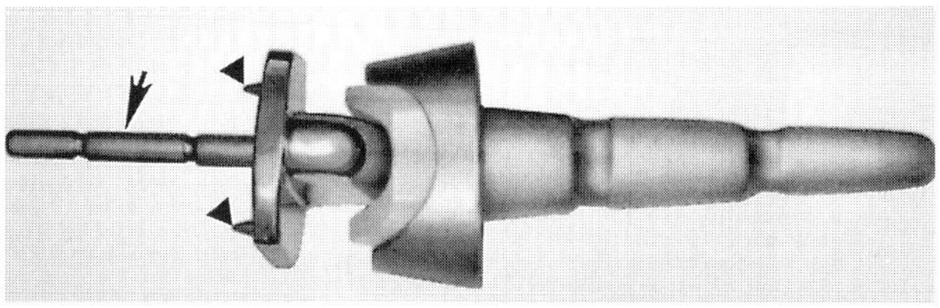

A

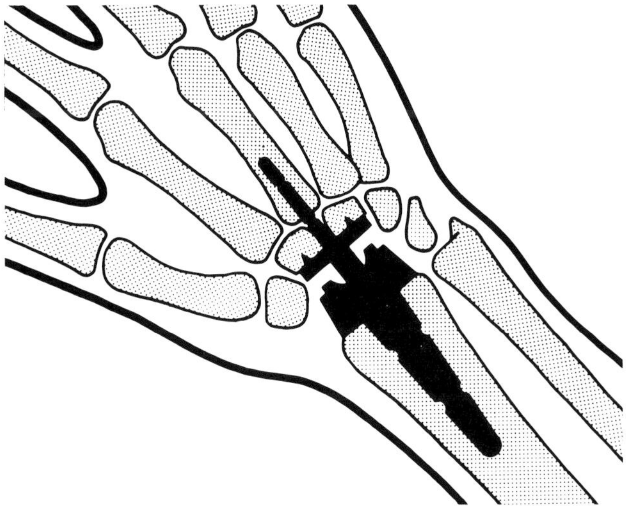

B

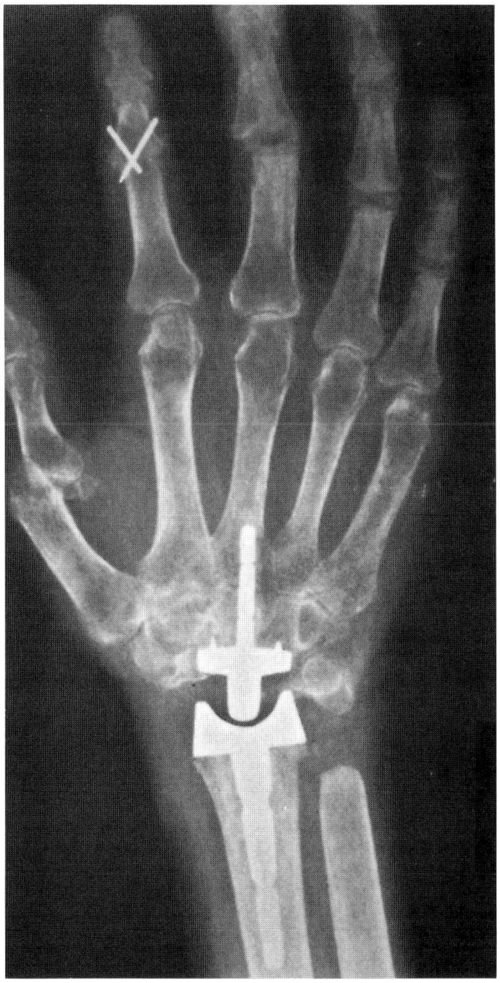

C

FIG. 13-74. A: Modified Volz prosthesis with single distal stem (*arrow*) and two short pegs (*arrowheads*). **B:** The modified Volz prosthesis in place after a resection of the scaphoid, lunate, triquetrum, and proximal capitate and hamate. (A,B: Courtesy of Howmedica, Rutherford, NJ.) **C:** A PA radiograph demonstrating the modified Volz prosthesis in a patient with rheumatoid arthritis. The distal ulna has been resected along with the scaphoid, lunate, and proximal capitate. Note the subluxation of the thumb and PIP joint arthrodesis with K-wire fixation. (From Menon J. Total wrist replacement using the modified Volz prosthesis. *J Bone Joint Surg* [*Am*] 1987;69A:998–1006.)

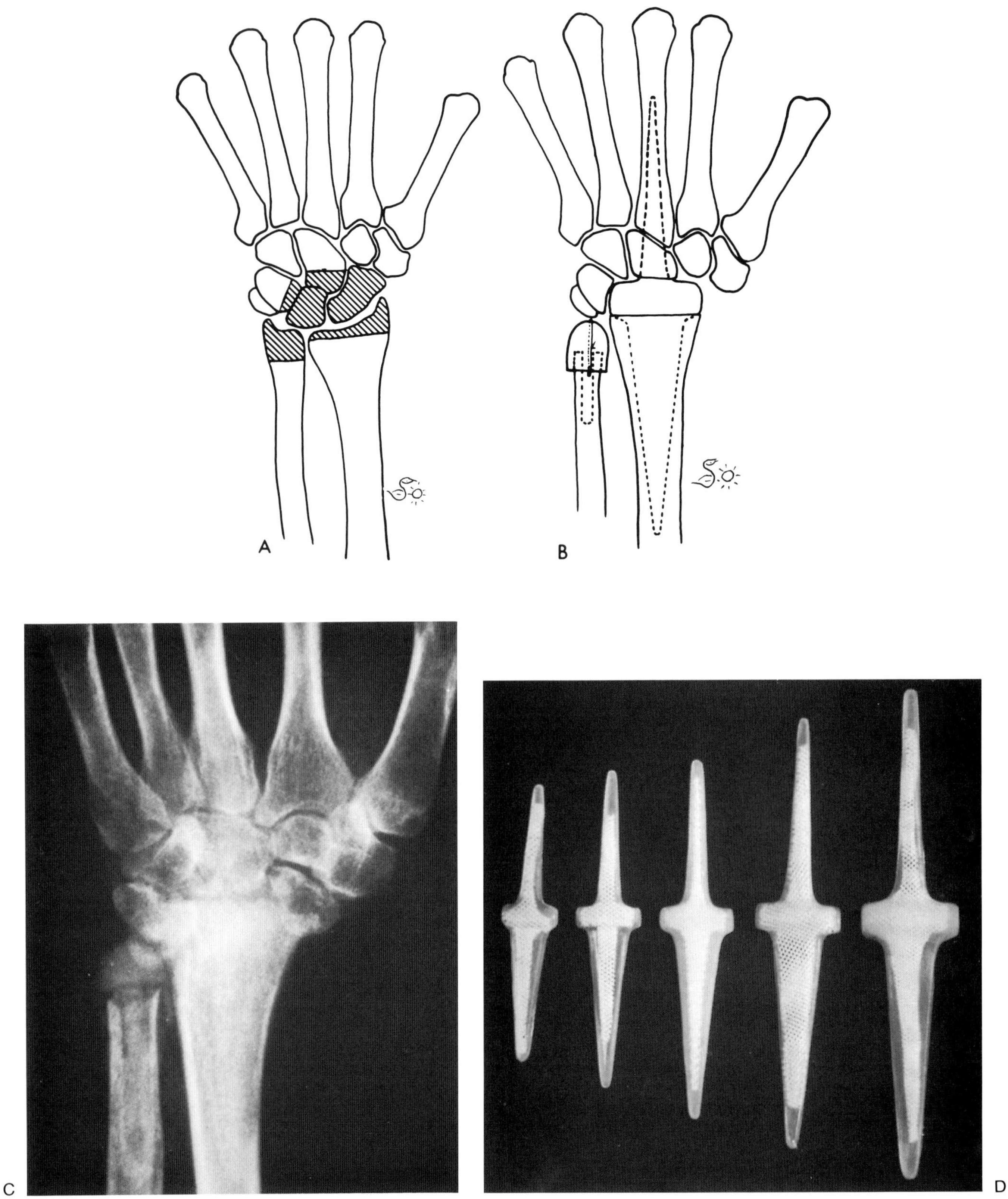

FIG. 13-75. **A:** The usual resection of the ulna, radius, and carpal bones prior to Silastic™ wrist implant insertion. **B:** The proximal stem fits into the radius and the smaller distal stem, into the capitate and third metacarpal (*dotted lines*). Ulnar head implant in place. **C:** A PA radiograph with an uncemented Silastic™ radiocarpal and ulnar head implant. **D:** Intramedullary stems with Dacron™ core to provide greater stability and reduce rotary stress. Flexible implants used with resection arthroplasty. (From Swanson AB, de Groot Swanson G. Flexible implant arthroplasty of the radiocarpal joint: surgical technique and long-term results. In: Inglis AE, ed. *AAOS symposium on total joint replacement of the upper extremity.* St. Louis: CV Mosby, 1982;301–315.)

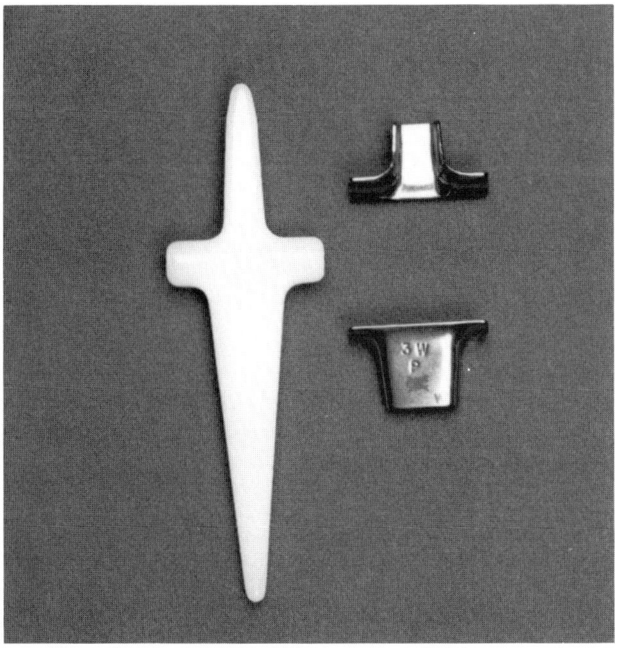

FIG. 13-76. The newer Swanson Silastic™ implant and metal grommets. The distal stem is shorter. See Fig. 13-75D for comparison. (Courtesy of Sutter, San Diego, CA.)

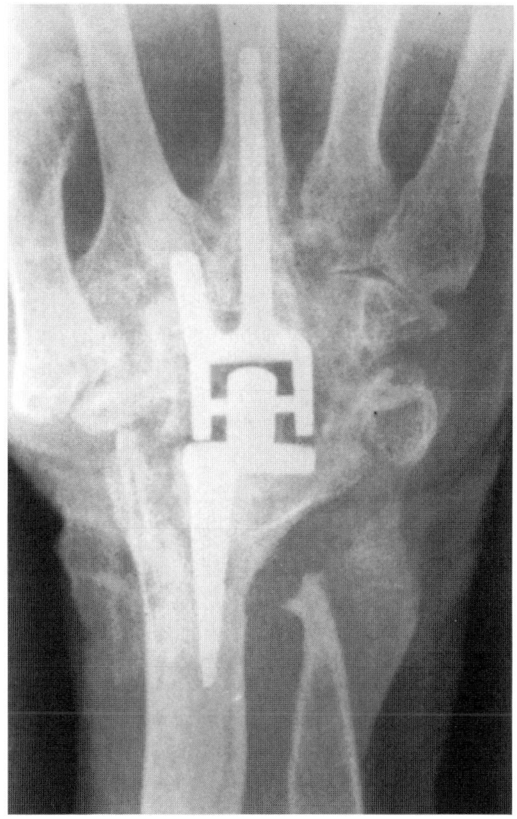

FIG. 13-77. A PA radiograph demonstrating wrist arthroplasty with a trispheric system. The long distal stem is inserted into the third metacarpal. The distal component is fixed to the proximal with an axis pin. (From Figgie HE III et al. Preliminary results of total wrist arthroplasty in patients with rheumatoid arthritis using a trispherical total wrist arthroplasty. *J Arthroplasty* 1988;3:9.)

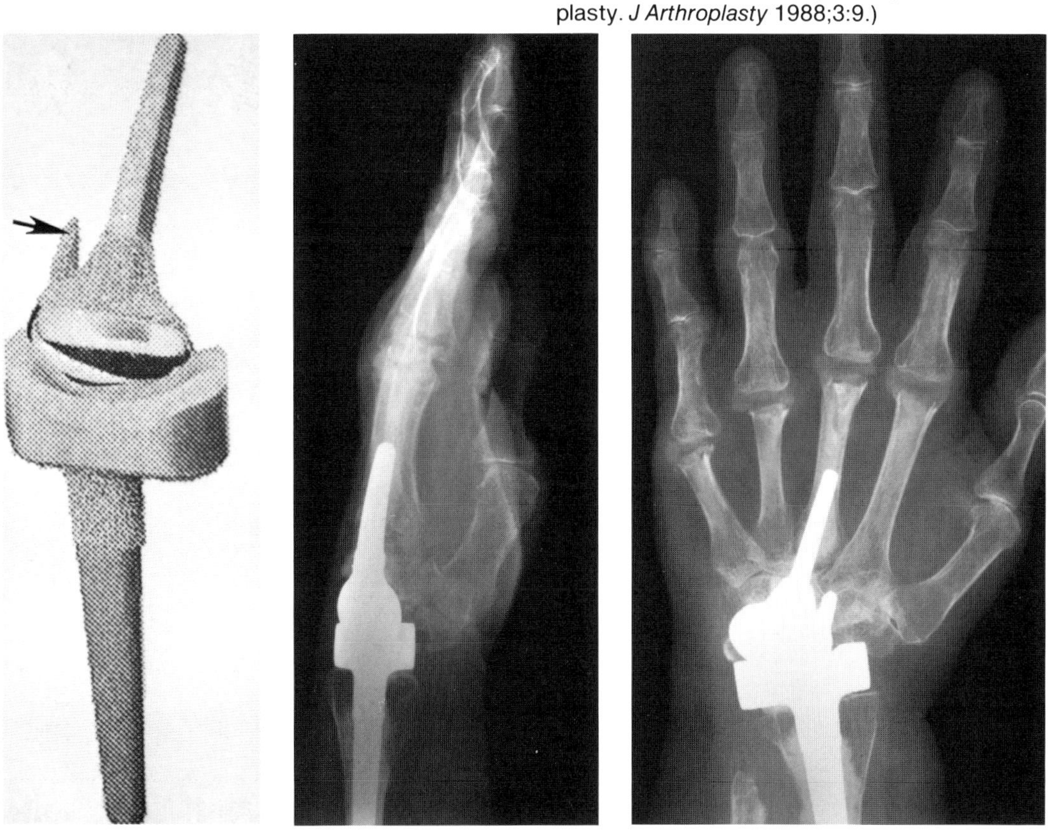

A B,C

FIG. 13-78. A: The Biax™ total wrist. (Courtesy of DePuy, Warsaw, IN.) Lateral **(B)** and PA radiograph in radial deviation **(C)** demonstrate the radiographic appearance. There are metacarpophalangeal joint silicone implants in the second to the fifth metacarpophalangeal joints. The distal ulna is resected.

Preoperative Evaluation

The goals of wrist arthroplasty are to improve motion, relieve pain, and increase stability.[226,227]

Normal wrist motion includes flexion (85° to 90°), extension (80° to 85°), and radial and ulnar deviation. The degree of motion, pain level, and function are used to evaluate patients prior to surgery. The same criteria can be used following arthroplasty to judge the results.[206,218,223] A 100-point scoring system, which was developed by Lamberta et al.,[197] evaluates balance, motion, and pain relief. This system is summarized in Table 13-3. These measurements are made clinically, but radiographs can also be used to assess the degree of motion with flexion, extension, and radial and ulnar deviation. Patients with instability or dislocation or who are receiving corticosteroids tend to do more poorly after wrist arthroplasty.[223]

The preoperative imaging should include routine PA, lateral, and oblique radiographs. Motion studies are also useful to assess preoperative motion restriction, to serve as a baseline, and to detect preoperative instability or subluxation; CT is used in some cases to assess bone stock preoperatively.

Postoperative Evaluation

The postoperative clinical evaluation includes the relief of pain and wrist function. Pre- and postoperative wrist scores are compared to assist in the quantitation of results.[197,206]

Routine radiographs are obtained at 3, 6, and 12 months and then yearly unless otherwise indicated by changes in clinical status.[218]

Fewer wrist procedures are performed than hip or knee arthroplasties; therefore, the data are more limited. The results and complications vary with the extent of disease preoperatively, the type of system used, and patient compliance.[178,180,201,206,225,226]

TABLE 13-3. *Wrist arthroplasty scoring*[197,206]

Category	Points
Balance	Maximum, 30 points
Flexion-extension	15
Radioulnar deviation	15
Motion (flexion and extension)	Maximum, 25 points
70–90° Excellent	25
50–69° Good	20
15–49° Fair	15
< 15° Poor	0
Pain relief	Maximum, 35 points
No pain	35
Mild pain	30
Moderate pain	7
Severe pain	0
Grip strength	Maximum, 10 points

TABLE 13-4. *Wrist arthroplasty: complications*[178,179,182,190,201,207,224–226]

Complication	Incidence rate[a] (%)
Soft tissue imbalance (drift)	20–35
Soft tissue contracture	12
Cement failure or loosening	4–30
Dislocation	4–10
Tendon rupture	6
Wound healing	5
Component fracture	8–20 +
Loosening	2–5
Nerve compression	2–3
Deep infection	1
Silicone-induced synovitis	—[b]

[a] Varies due to multiple series and experience with multiple component systems.
[b] Unusual with radiocarpal arthroplasty compared with carpal bone implants.

As with other joint-replacement arthroplasties, loosening is more common with the more constrained or hinged devices.[179,184,201,206,207] The complications related to wrist arthroplasty were divided into three major categories by Cooney et al.[184] Implant failures were most often related to component centering, fixation, or soft tissue imbalance. Centering of the implant is often difficult in the deformed rheumatoid wrist. Fixation, except for the silicone hinged implant, is achieved with cement and fraught with the same problems described in arthroplasty of the knee and hip. Soft tissue imbalance is the major cause of implant failure. This is largely due to muscle deficiency, tendon imbalance, or tendon subluxation.[182,184,190,225]

Table 13-4 summarizes the complications described with wrist arthroplasty.[182,184,190,225]

Serial radiographs using PA, lateral, PA (radial and ulnar deviation), lateral (flexion and extension), and PA compression-distraction views are useful for evaluating most postoperative complications and the range of motion.[198,201] Fluoroscopic positioning provides optimal positioning and component alignment, and it should be performed on at least the initial postoperative study so that a baseline is available to evaluate subtle changes later. As can be seen from the images that are used to demonstrate complications, this technique is all too often forgotten.

Imbalance, contractures, subluxation, or dislocation can be detected with routine radiographs (Figs. 13-79 to 13-82).[184,201,224–226] Serial radiographs (Figs. 13-82 and 13-83) provide the simplest method of evaluating changes in lucent lines, which may indicate component loosening. Lucent lines greater than 1 mm at the bone-cement interface should be carefully followed (Fig. 13-82).[179,184]

The fracture of components occurs with Silastic™ hinge components. The incidence is about 8% during the first few years and increases to more than 20% after 5

(*text continues on page 887*)

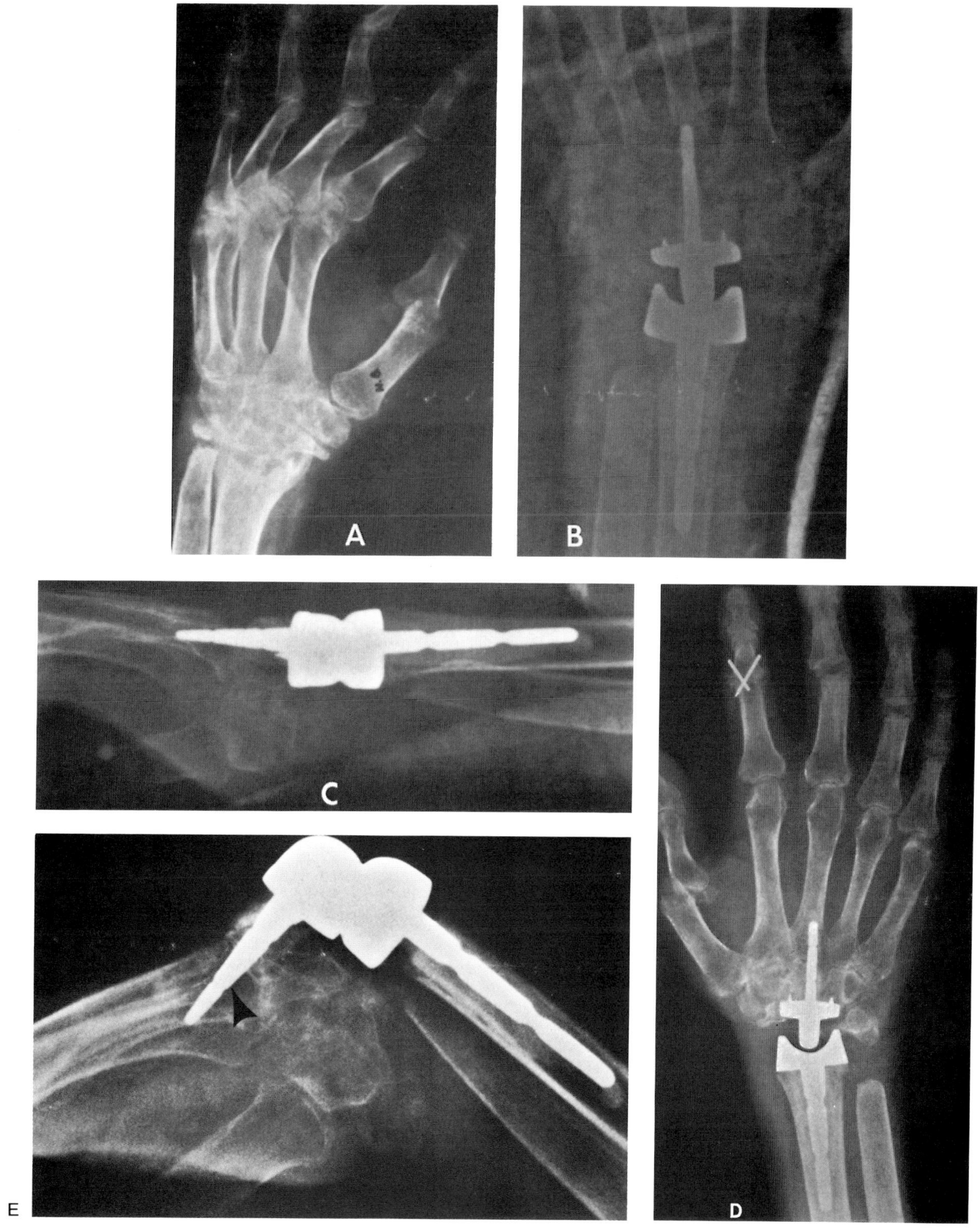

FIG. 13-79. A: Preoperative radiograph demonstrating advanced rheumatoid arthritis with carpal collapse and metacarpophalangeal subluxations. The PA **(B)** and lateral **(C)** radiographs with a modified Volz prosthesis postoperatively. The PA **(D)** and lateral **(E)** radiographs on later follow-up demonstrate an apparent good position with no lucency to suggest loosening on the PA view (D). The lateral view demonstrates a fixed flexion contracture with fracture of the distal stem (*arrow*) out of the third metacarpal. (From Menon J. Total wrist replacement using the modified Volz prosthesis. *J Bone Joint Surg* [*Am*] 1987;69A:998–1006.)

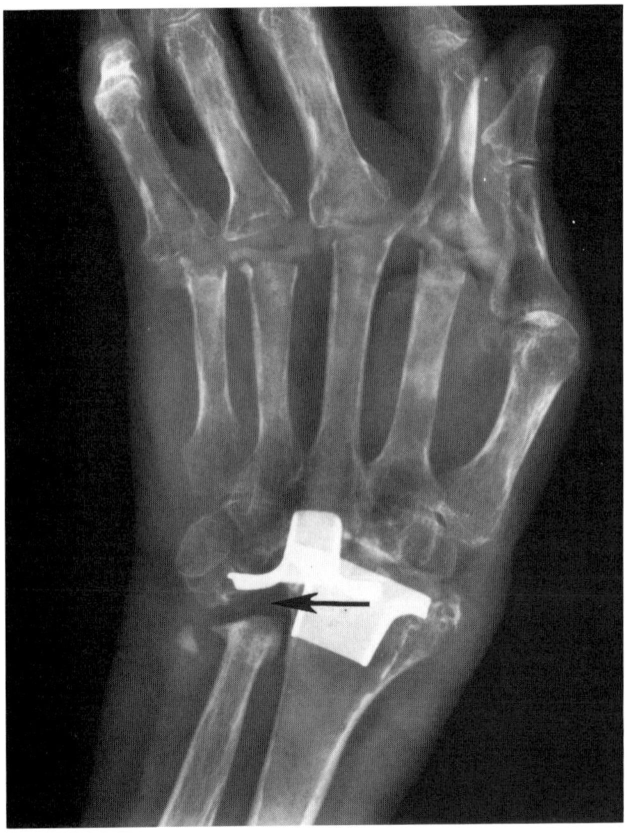

FIG. 13-80. A PA radiograph of the wrist with a silicone implant with metal grommets in place. The implant has fractured and displaced (ulnar translocation) to the ulnar side (*arrow*). There are silicone implants in the second through fifth metacarpophalangeal joints and ulnar drift.

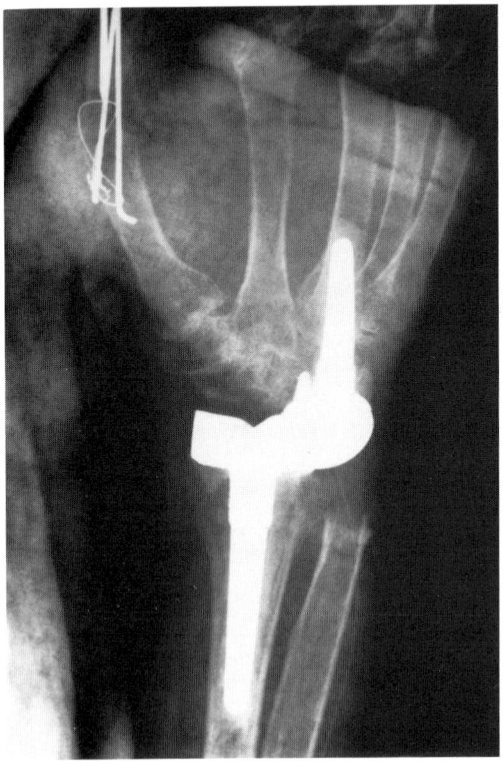

A

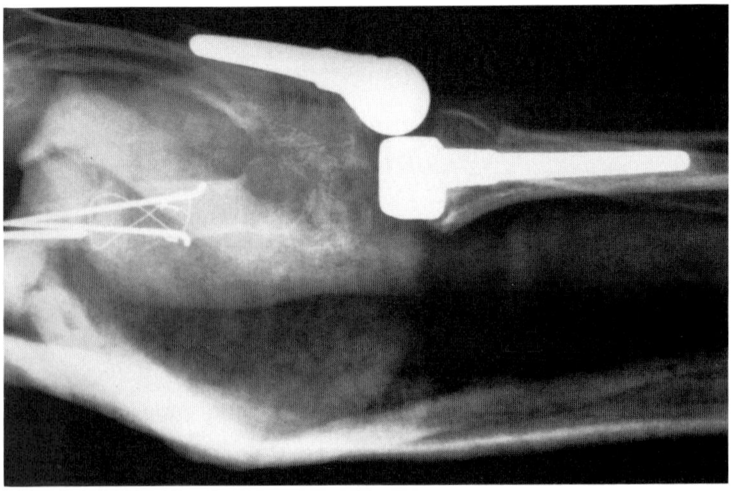

B

FIG. 13-81. The PA **(A)** and lateral **(B)** radiographs of a biaxial wrist arthroplasty with dorsal dislocation of the distal component dorsally. There is also ulnar rotation of the hand and distal stem. Arthrodesis of the right thumb with K-wire and figure-eight tension-band wiring.

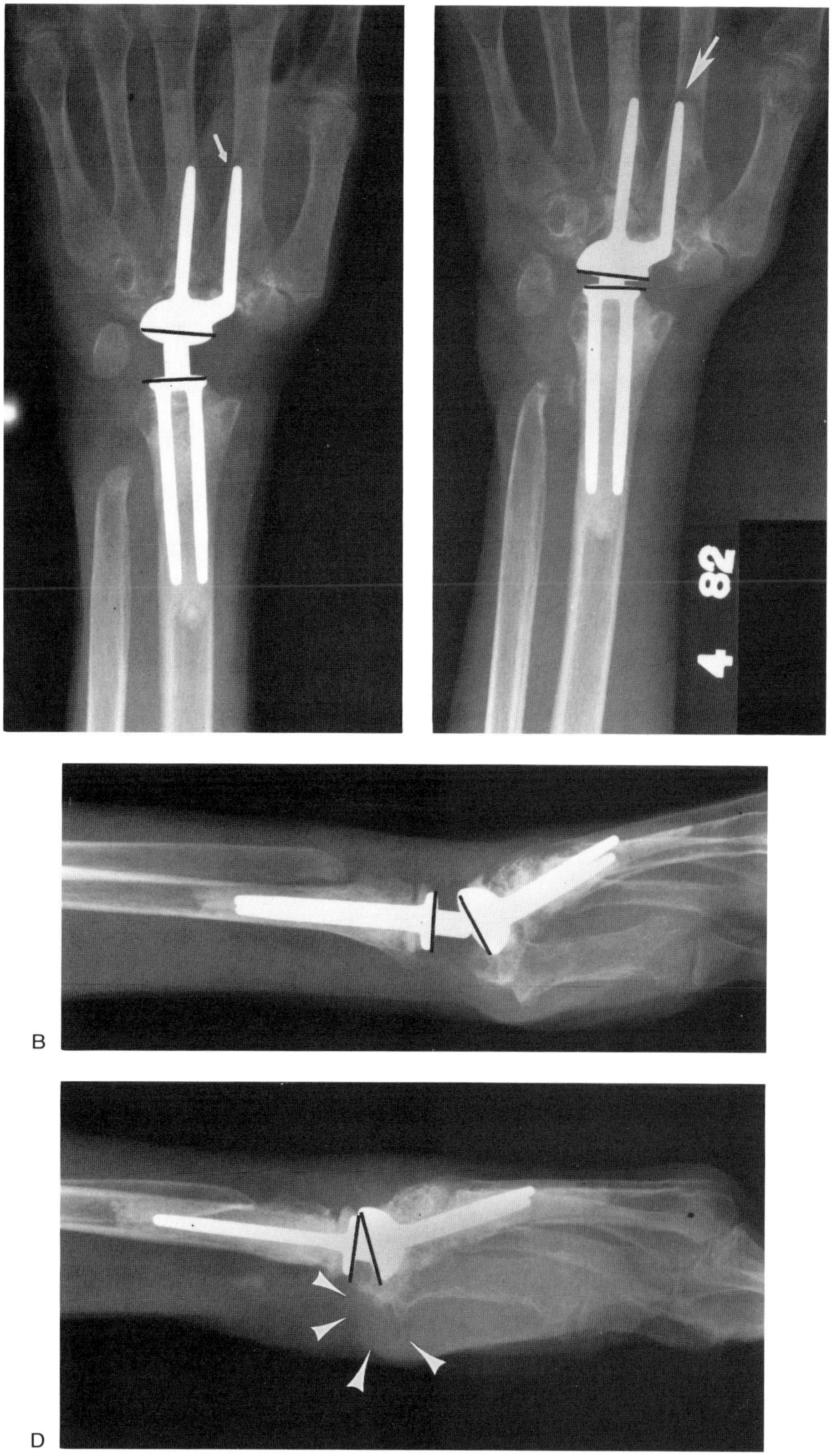

A C B D

FIG. 13-82. The PA **(A)** and lateral **(B)** radiographs of a Meuli modified wrist arthroplasty. There is loosening of the stem in the second metacarpal with cortical thinning on the PA and dorsal breakthrough seen on the lateral view (*arrow*). Eighteen months later, the patient complained of increasing pain and palpable mass in the palm. The PA **(C)** and lateral **(D)** radiographs demonstrate decreased distance (*lines*) between the distal and proximal components (compare with the distance in A and B). The polyethylene bearing (*arrowheads* in D) had dislocated from the component. There is further cortical thinning and loosening of the component in the second metacarpal (*arrow* in C).

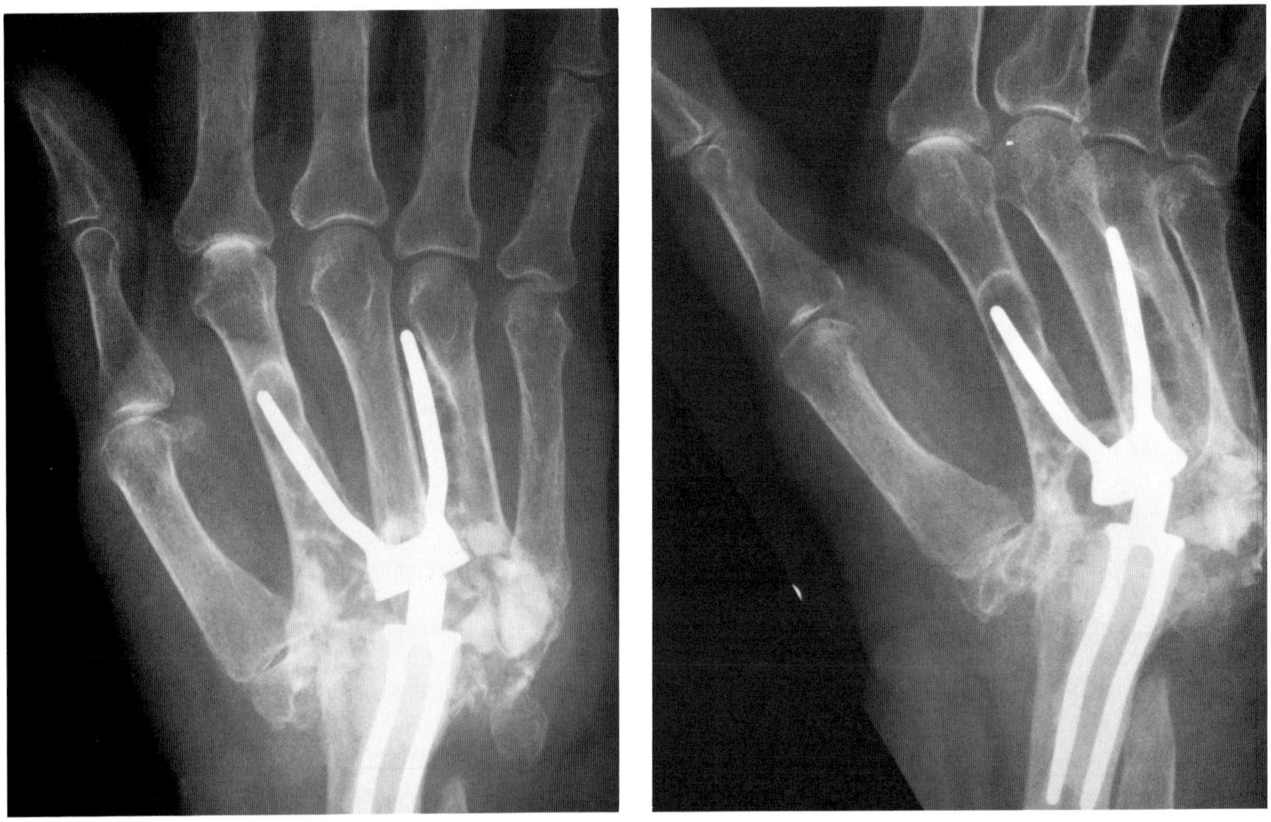

A

B

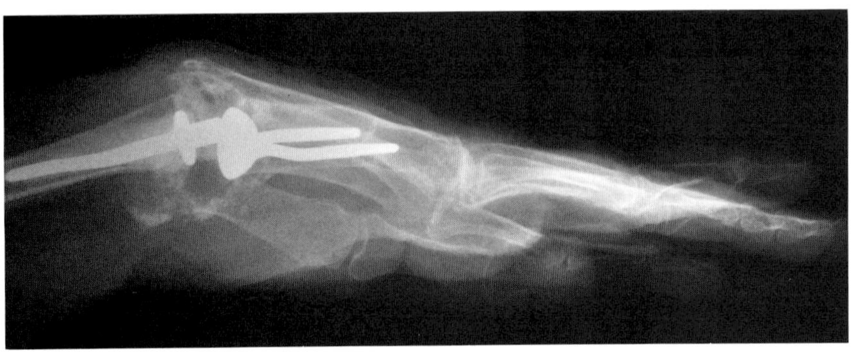

C

FIG. 13-83. The PA **(A)**, oblique **(B)**, and lateral **(C)** radiographs of a Meuli prosthesis with the two distal stems prebent to improve the metacarpal alignment. There is gross loosening of the stem in the second metacarpal, and the stem has pulled out of the fourth metacarpal.

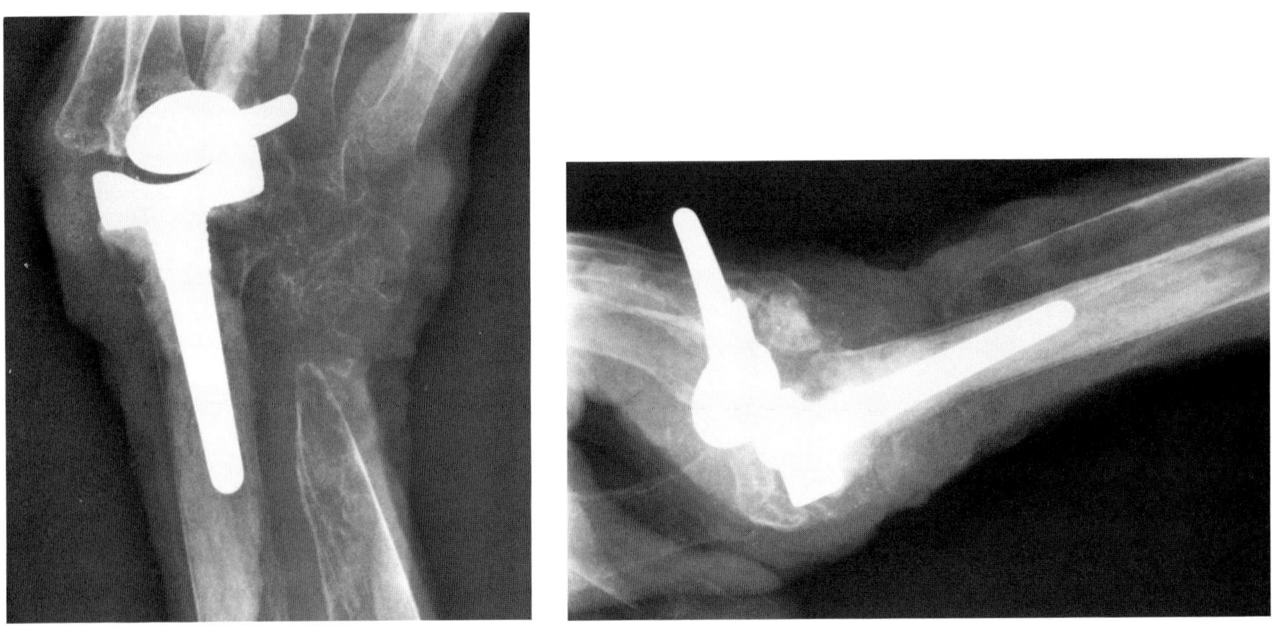

A

B

FIG. 13-84. The PA **(A)** and lateral **(B)** radiographs of a biaxial component. The distal component has fractured dorsally through the third metacarpal.

years.[182,224–226] Failure or fracture of the silicone implant does not necessarily correlate with a deterioration of clinical results or function. Metal implants rarely fracture, but cortical breakthrough (Fig. 13-84) is fairly common.[179,184]

The imaging of infection and soft tissue complications requires additional procedures. Radionuclide imaging is most useful for infection. Combined technetium-99m and indium-111 studies are preferred. Usually, MRI is best for soft tissue pathologic conditions. However, the metal artifact may degrade the images, resulting in suboptimal studies. Tenography or alternative techniques may be used instead.

Carpal-Replacement Arthroplasty

The replacement of individual carpal bones, most commonly the scaphoid and lunate, has been successful using Silastic™ implants.[210,221,224] The indications include posttraumatic arthritis, osteoarthritis, avascular necrosis, and inflammatory conditions.[210] Although silicone implants are typically used, Vitallium and other metal alloys have also been attempted for scaphoid replacement.[219]

The results with silicone implants have been successful in most cases. However, with time, the components can fibrillate, resulting in silicone-induced synovitis and osteolysis (Figs. 13-85 and 13-86). Therefore, patients should be followed clinically and radiographically for up to 8 years.[210,224] Synovitis causes pain, swelling, osteolysis, and decreased range of motion. Arthrography may be indicated in these patients to confirm the diagnosis (Fig. 13-85).[210]

Thumb-Replacement Arthroplasty

The first carpometacarpal joint is one of the most frequent sites of osteoarthritis in the hand.[177] Women older than age 40 years are most commonly affected.[199,213] The pain from this condition can be disabling, reducing pinch and hand use. Some type of surgical repair is required in up to 20% of patients.

Rheumatoid arthritis also affects the trapezium and first metacarpal. Generally, other joints are also involved, which may require multiarticular replacement procedures.[211,226]

Preoperative Assessment

Clinical findings (e.g., age, activity, and pain) and radiographic features are used to select candidates for surgical repair. There are several procedures that can be selected, depending on the clinical and radiographic features.

Eaton et al.[185,186] classified or staged patients based on stability and radiographic features. Stage I disease is degenerative arthritis confined to the trapeziometacarpal joint without clinical evidence of instability. The radiographs are normal in stage I so the findings are purely clinical (local pain and reduced pinch strength). Stage II disease demonstrates a loss of joint space radiographically with lateral or dorsal subluxation but no definite clinical instability. Stage III disease has similar or slightly more advanced radiographic features with the addition of instability of the joint. Stage IV disease extends beyond the thumb to involve the scaphoid, trapezoid, and trapezium (STT) arthrosis (Table 13-5).[185,186]

Arthroplasty Options

The goals of joint-replacement procedures for the thumb are to relieve pain, improve function, and correct instability.[195]

Silicone replacement arthroplasty, with resurfacing of the thumb base and shaving or partial trapezium resection or complete replacement of the trapezium, has been successful but is less commonly used today.[183,195] Complete resection of the trapezium is usually reserved for stage III or IV disease.[183,185,186] The common options for silicone arthroplasty are demonstrated in Figs. 13-87 to 13-91.[195]

Total joint-replacement procedures can also be used. This technique is usually reserved for patients with stage II or III degenerative disease (Table 13-5).[183] The Braun implant system consists of a titanium metacarpal component designed to be cemented in the metacarpal. The trapezial implant is a short-stemmed polyethylene cup, which is also cemented. This results in a ball and socket design (Fig. 13-91).[185] Other ball and socket designs include the de la Caffiniére and Lewis systems (Fig. 13-92).[185] The implants were configured to improve the

TABLE 13-5. *Trapeziometacarpal joint: staging and treatment*[183–188]

Stage	Treatment options
I Normal or mild Joint space narrowing with no subluxation	Splints Nonsteroidal antiinflammatory drugs
II Joint space narrowing with lateral (radial) subluxation	1. Ligament repair with osteophyte resection 2. Interposition arthroplasty 3. Osteotomy
III Loss of joint space (Fig. 13-94A), subluxation 750% of articular surface	1. Silastic arthroplasty 2. Soft tissue interposition arthroplasty
IV Advanced osteophytes with pantrapezial disease, including STT joints	1. Complete trapezial excision 2. Silicone spacer

(*text continues on page 897*)

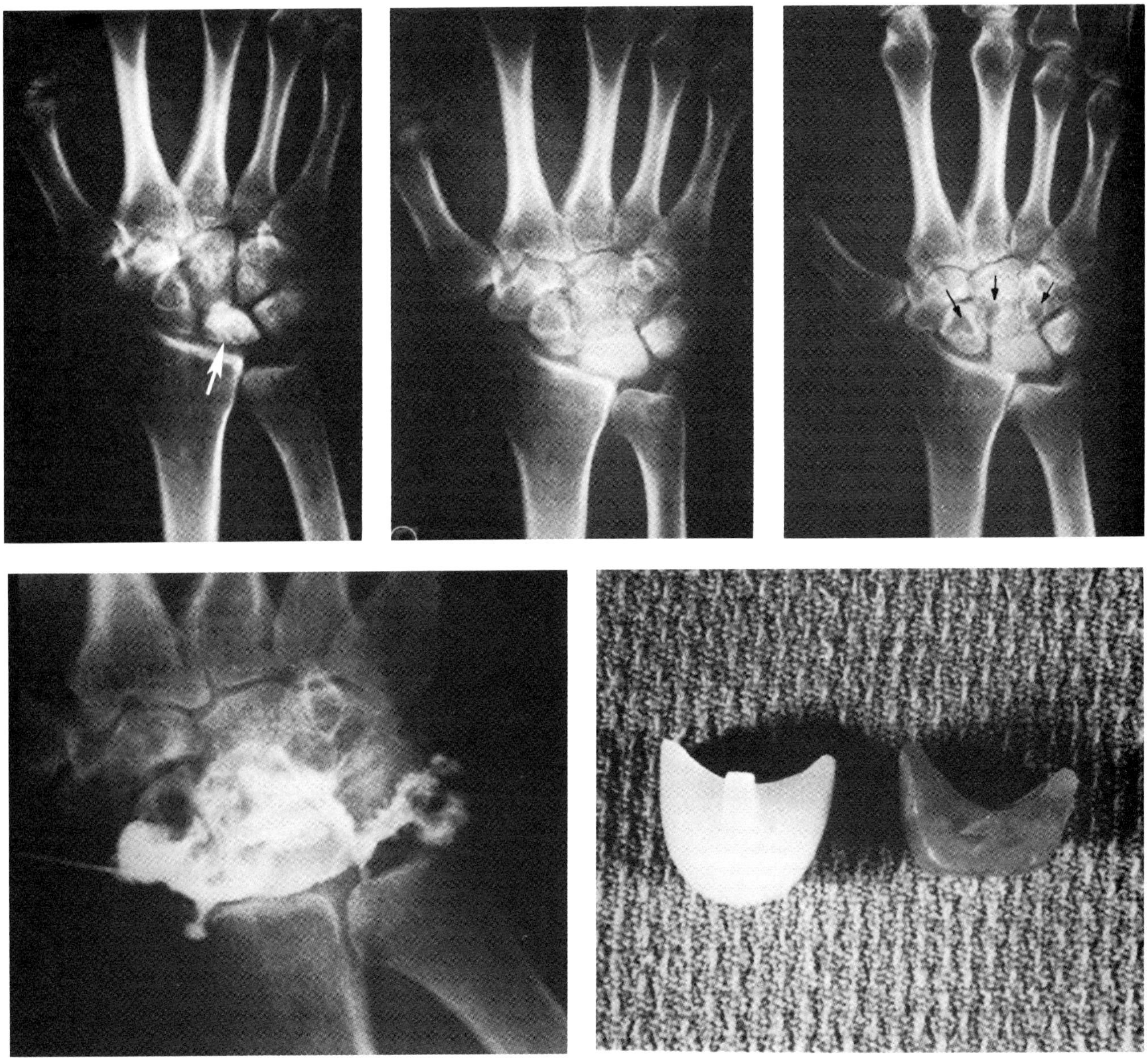

A B,C D E

FIG. 13-85. A: A 29-year-old woman with avascular necrosis of the lunate (*arrow*). **B:** A PA radiograph after replacement with a silicone lunate implant. **C:** Seven years later, the lunate is slightly flattened, and the scaphoid is rotated with erosions in the scaphoid, hamate, and capitate (*arrows*). **D:** Arthrogram demonstrates synovitis with multiple irregular filling defects. **E:** New normal implant (*left*) compared with the implant in B (*right*) removed after 7 years.

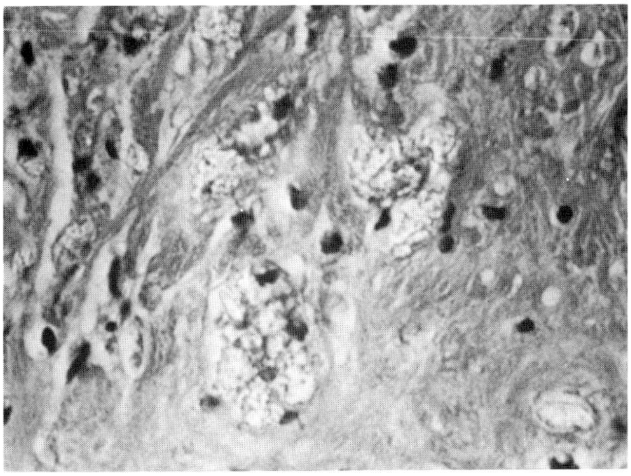

F

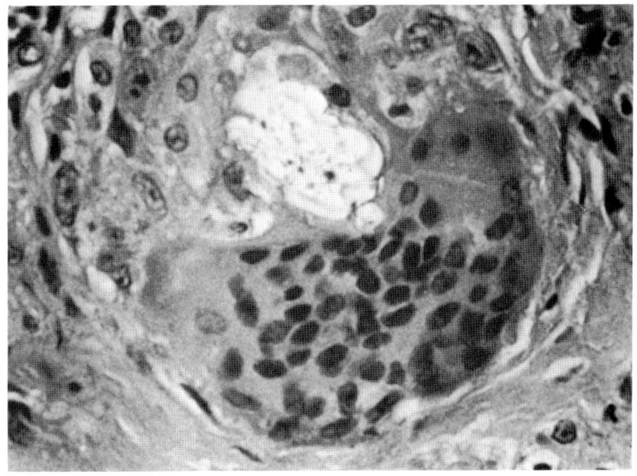

G

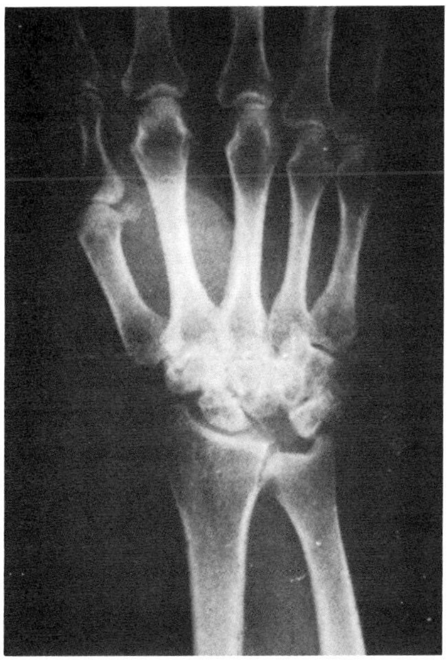

H

FIG. 13-85. (*Continued.*) **F,G:** Histologic specimens demonstrating multinucleated grant cells and foreign bodies. **H:** A PA radiograph after synovectomy implant removal and trapezoid capitate-hamate arthrodesis. (From Smith R, Atkinson R, Jupiter B. Silicone synovitis of the wrist. *J Hand Surg* [*Am*] 1985;10A:47–60.)

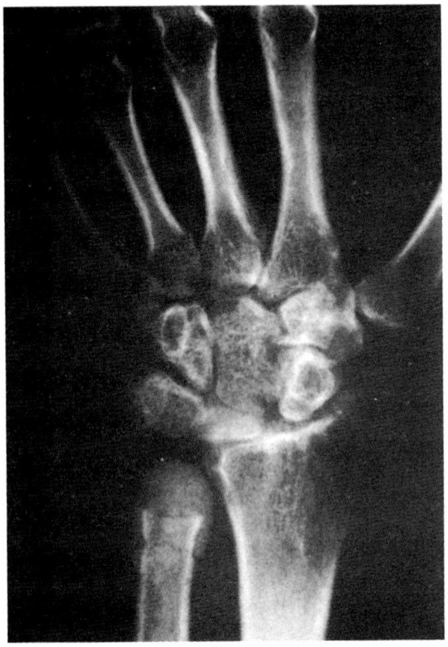

A

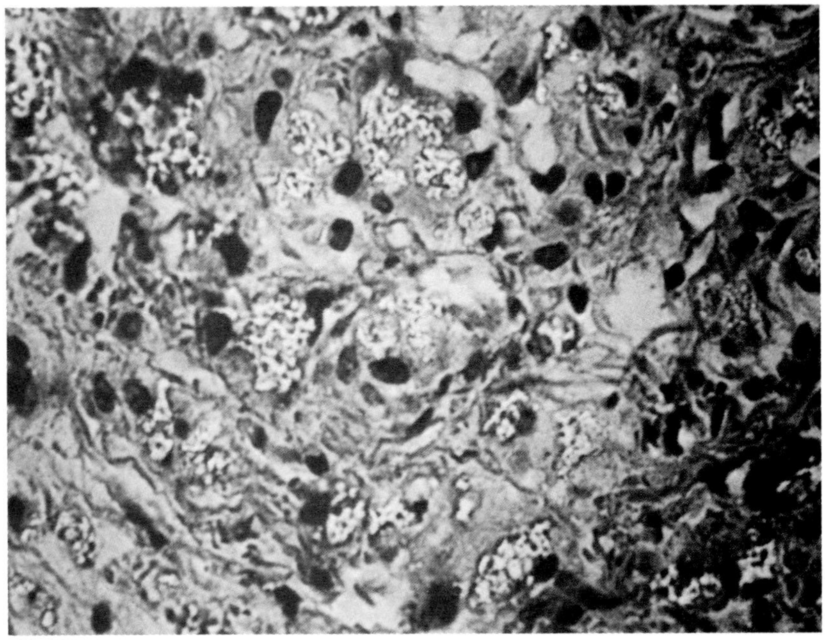

B

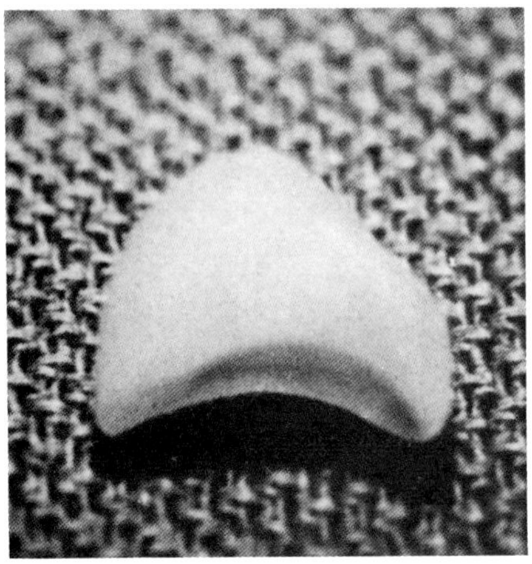

C

FIG. 13-86. A: The PA radiographs 6 years after lunate and distal ulnar replacement with silicone implants. **B:** Histologic specimen of proliferative synovial tissue resected with implant removal. **C:** Deformed resected lunate implant. (From Smith R, Atkinson R, Jupiter B. Silicone synovitis of the wrist. *J Hand Surg* [*Am*] 1985;10A:47–60.)

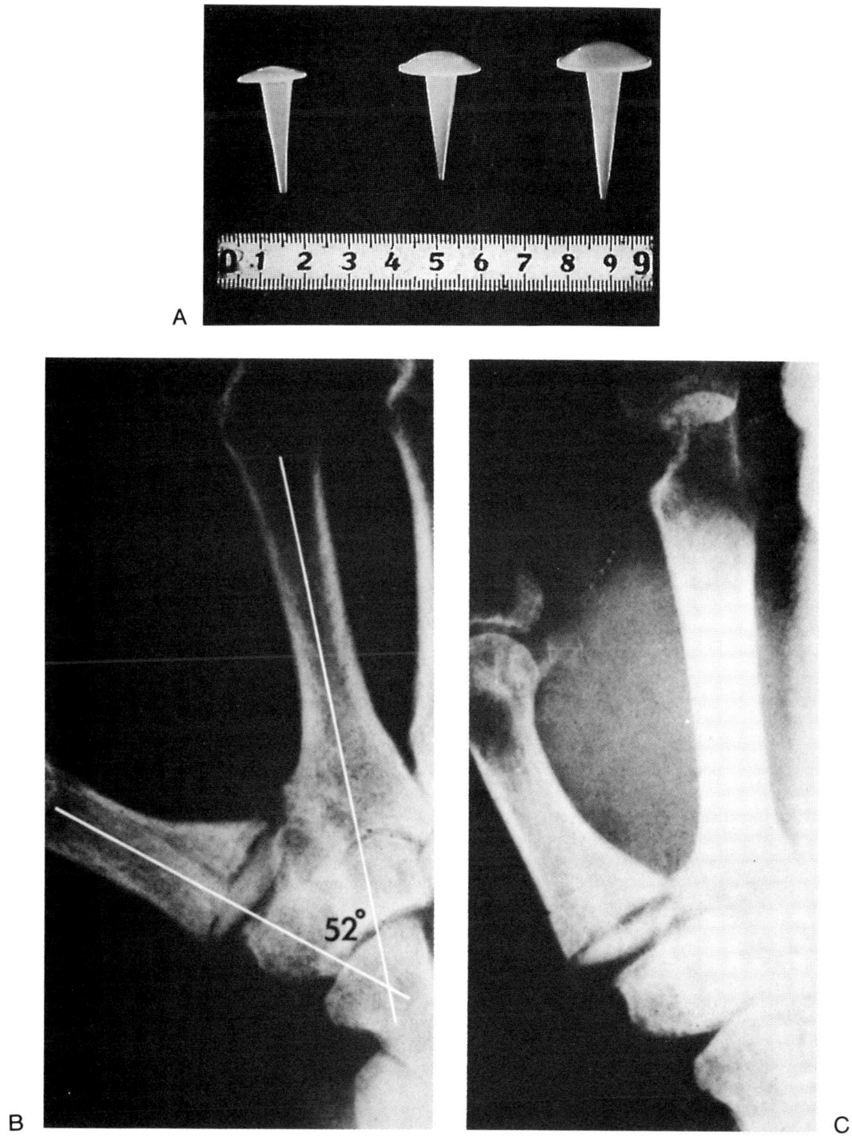

FIG. 13-87. **A:** Three different sizes of metacarpal silicone implants for resurfacing the base of the first metacarpal. Abducted **(B)** and **(C)** neutral positions of the thumb after implant placement demonstrate a metacarpal angle of 52°. These measurements can be made pre- and postoperatively to assist in judging a response to the procedure. (From Kessler I. Silicone arthroplasty of the trapeziometacarpal joint. *J Bone Joint Surg* [*Br*] 1973;55B:285–291.)

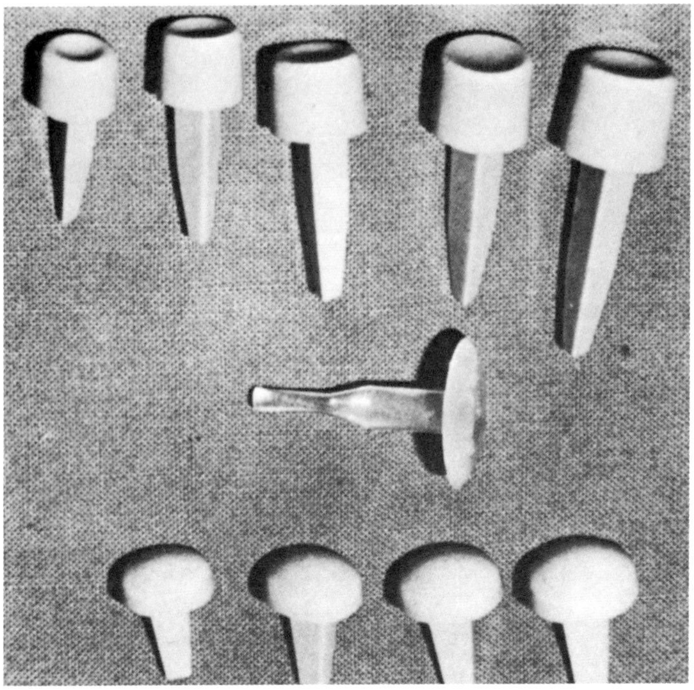

A

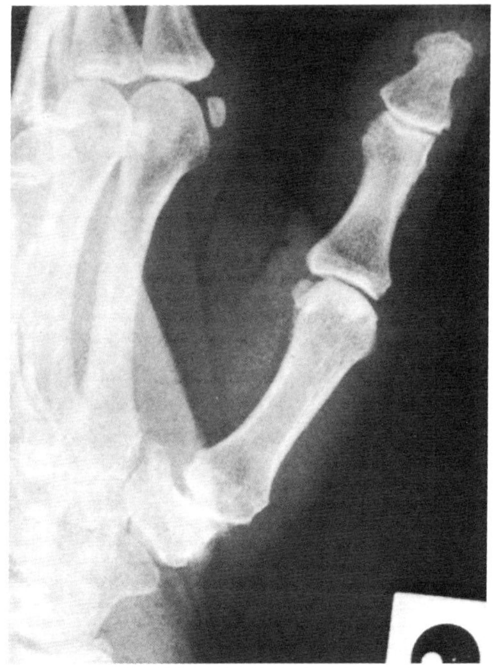

B

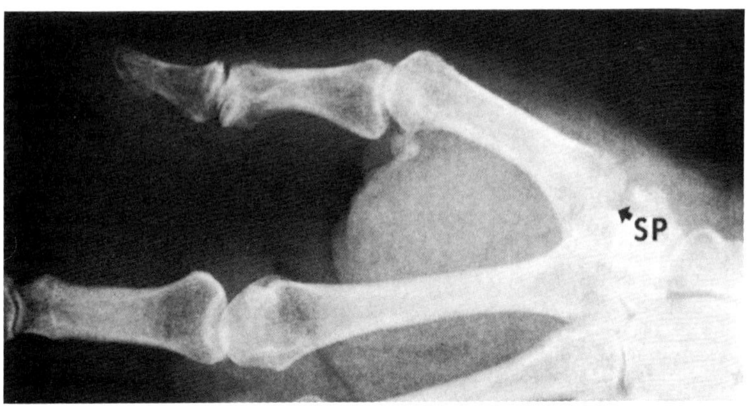

C

FIG. 13-88. A: Thumb base implants. *Top,* trapezium implant with stem for first metacarpal; *middle,* silicone burr hole implant for resurfacing first metacarpal; *below,* condylar thumb base implants. Preoperative **(B)** and postoperative **(C)** radiographs with spacer (*SP*) in place. (From Howard FM, Simpson LA, Belsole RJ. Silastic condylar arthroplasty. *Clin Orthop* 1985;195:144–150.)

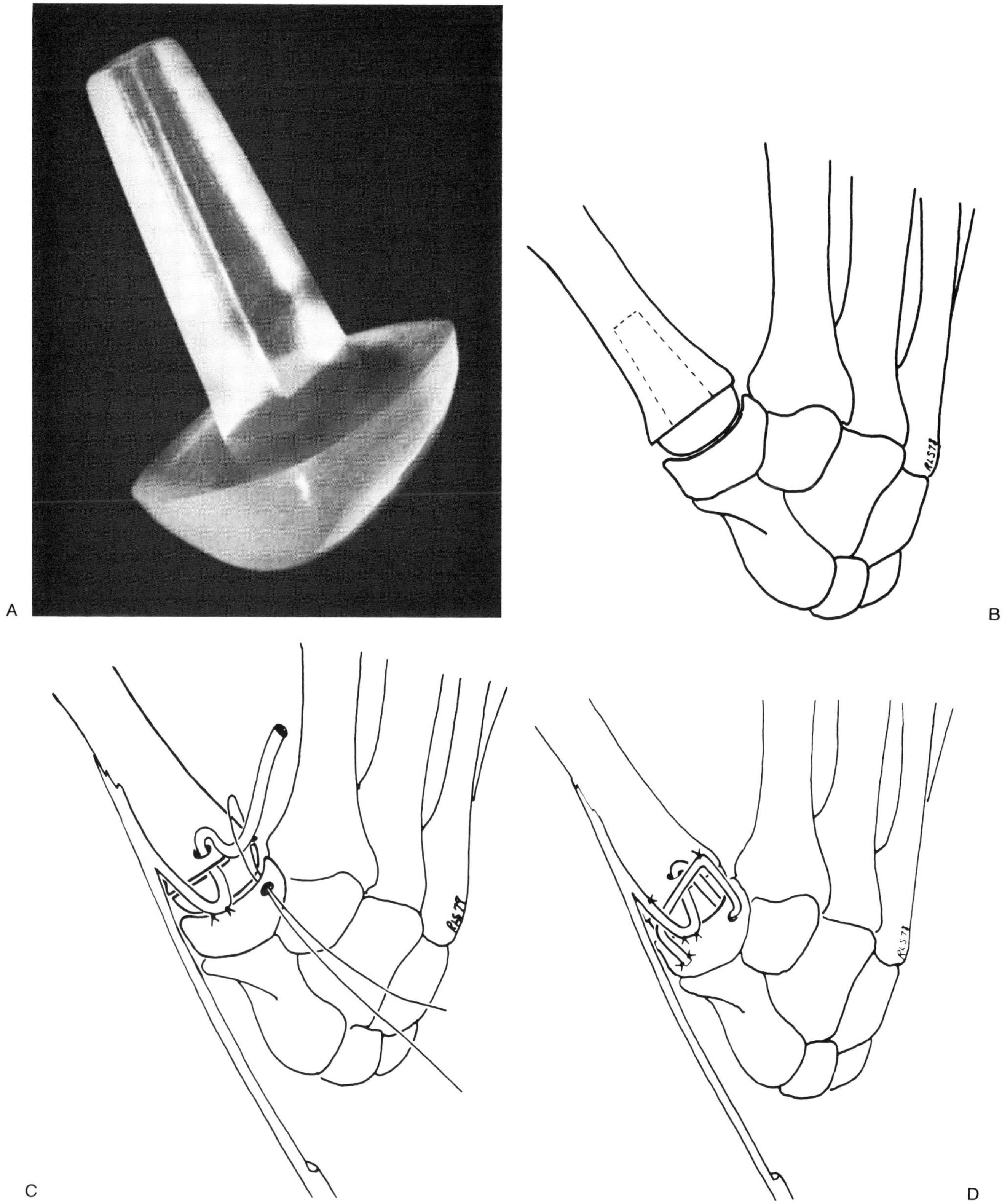

FIG. 13-89. A: Silicone condylar implant. **B:** Condylar implant in place with resection of the distal surface of the trapezium. An 8-cm segment of the abductor pollicis longus is prepared **(C)** and interwoven with the two osseous segments **(D)** for reinforcement. (From Swanson AB, de Groot Swanson G, Watermeir JJ. Trapezium implant arthroplasty: long-term evaluation of 150 cases. *J Hand Surg* 1981;6:125–141.)

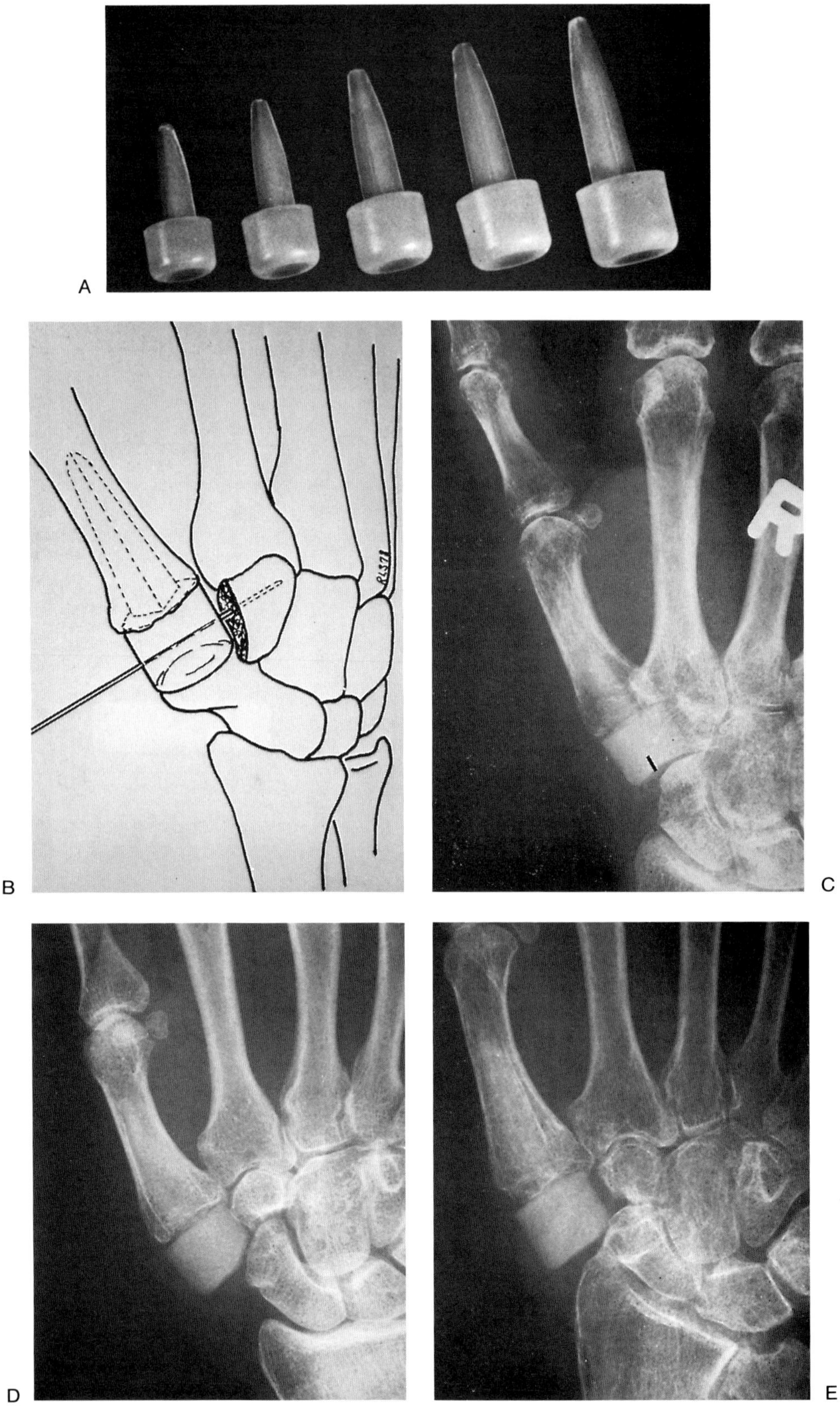

FIG. 13-90. A: Intramedullary stemmed trapezial silicone implants. **B:** Implant in place with temporary K-wire. Implants in place are shown next. **C:** Implant with mild displacement of implant on scaphoid. One third of the implant (*line*) is not articulating with the scaphoid. The results were good in spite of the radiographic appearance. **D:** Moderate displacement. Only a portion of the implant articulates with the scaphoid. The results were still good with no instability. **E:** Implant articulating with the radial styloid. Cosmetic deformity but no instability. (From Swanson AB, de Groot Swanson G, Watermeir JJ. Trapezium implant arthroplasty: long-term evaluation of 150 cases. *J Hand Surg* 1981;6:125–141.)

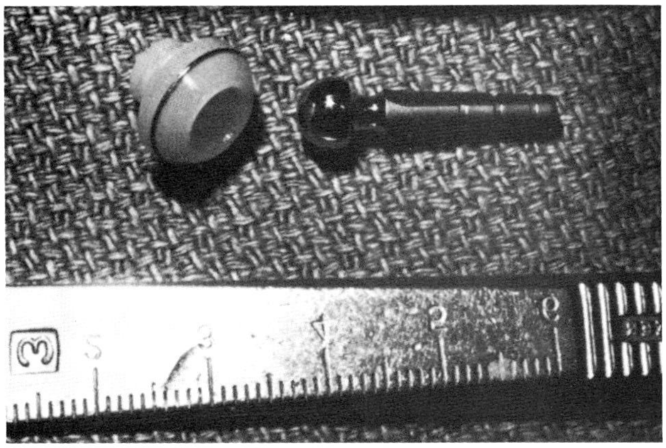

A

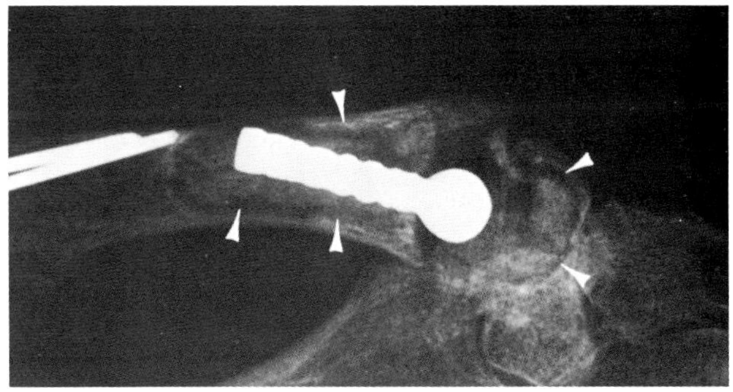

B

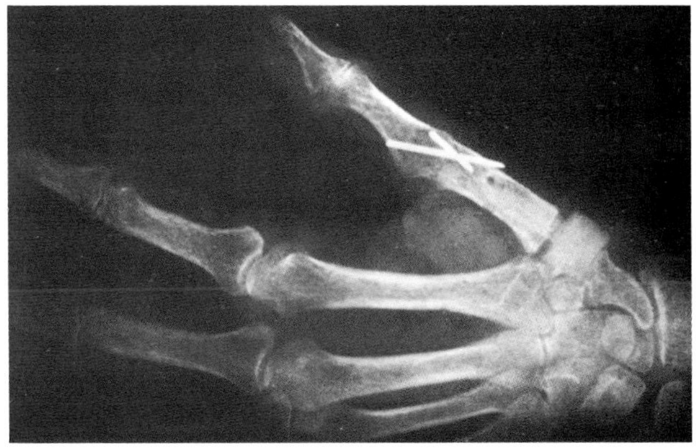

C

FIG. 13-91. **A:** The titanium metacarpal and polyethylene trapezial components of the Braun system. **B:** Braun total joint system with lucency (*white arrows*) at the bone-cement interface caused by loosening after a fall. **C:** Revision accomplished using a Swanson Silastic™ spacer. K-wire arthrodesis of the metacarpophalangeal joint.

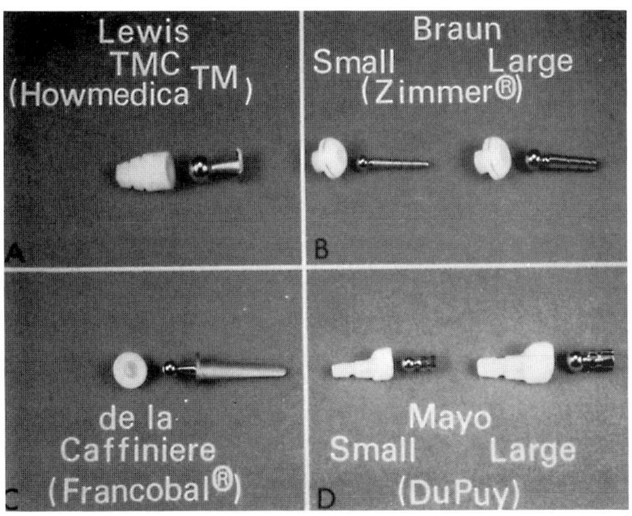

FIG. 13-92. Thumb trapeziometacarpal total joint-replacement systems. **A:** Lewis system is of the ball and socket type with a polyethylene metacarpal component with a ball and a pedestal metal trapezium component (Howmedica, Rutherford, NJ). **B:** Braun system has a metal metacarpal stem with a ball and a trapezial polyethylene cup (Zimmer, Warsaw, IN). **C:** The de la Caffiniére system is a cobalt-chromium metacarpal component with a cupped polyethylene trapezial component (distributed by Howmedica, Rutherford, NJ). **D:** The large and small Mayo implants each have a symmetric polyethylene metacarpal component and metal ball trapezial component (DePuy, Warsaw, IN). (From Cooney WP III, Linscheid RL, Askew L. Total arthroplasty of the thumb trapeziometacarpal joint. *Clin Orthop* 1987;220:35–45.)

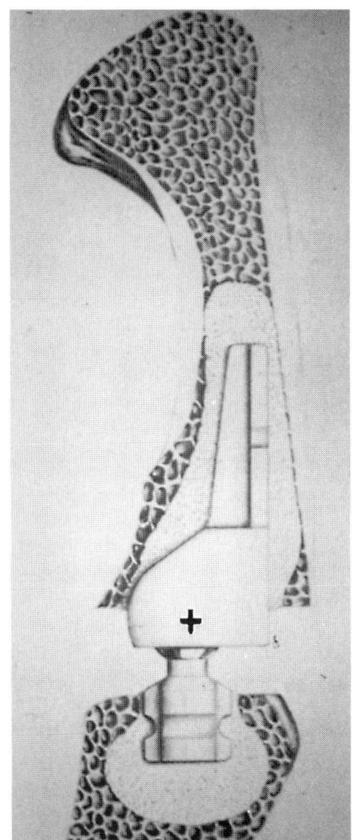

FIG. 13-93. The Mayo total joint trapeziometacarpal arthroplasty. The center of rotation (+) is at the base of the first metacarpal instead of the trapezium. (From Cooney WP III, Linscheid RL, Askew L. Total arthroplasty of the thumb trapeziometacarpal joint. *Clin Orthop* 1987;220:35–45.)

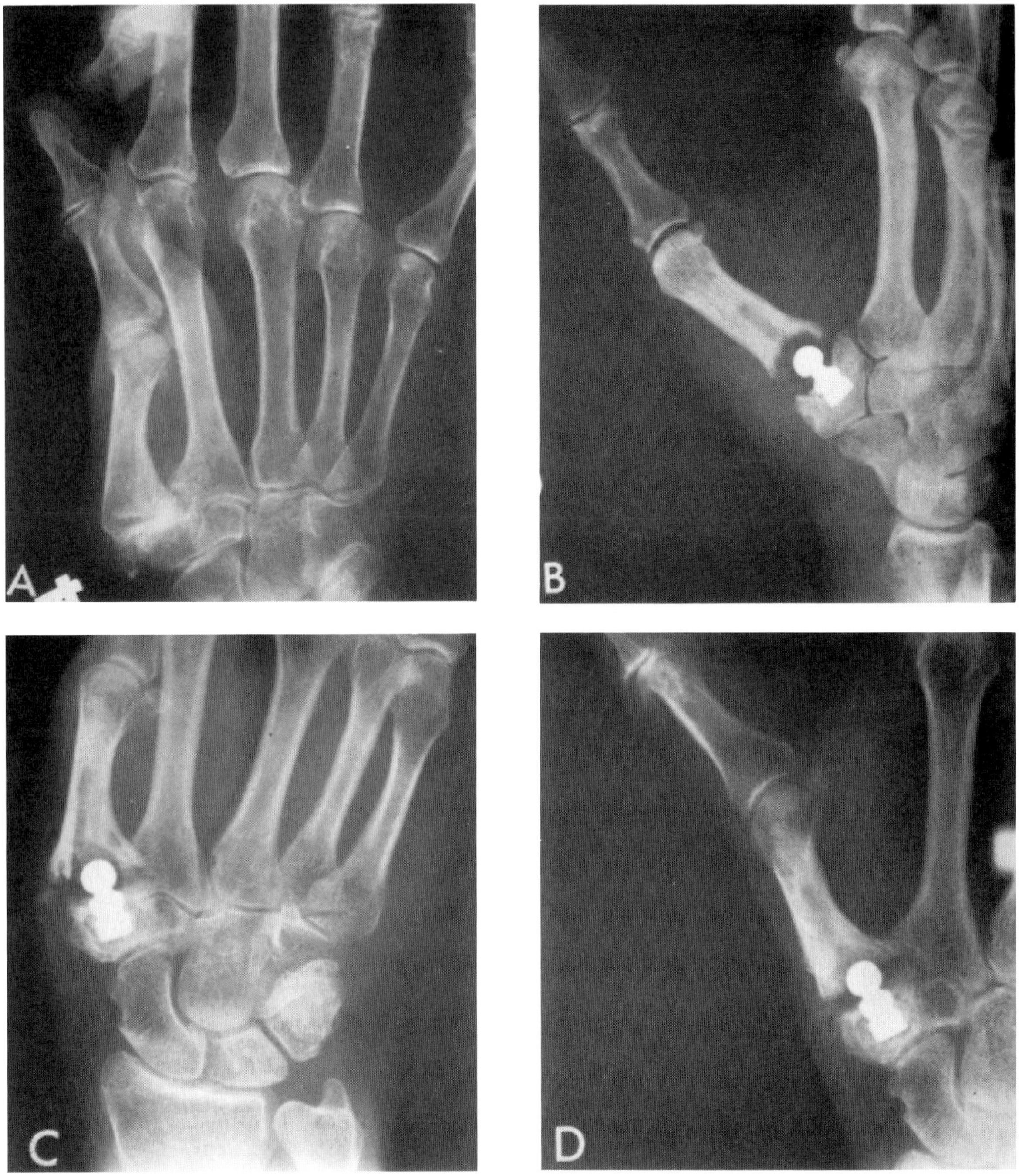

FIG. 13-94. **A:** A PA preoperative radiograph with stage III arthritis at the trapeziometacarpal joint. **B:** Mayo total joint system in place. **C:** Pinch or flexion 4 years postoperatively. **D:** Extension 4 years postoperatively.

pinch and grasp strength, which creates significant compression and shearing forces at the trapeziometacarpal joint. Total joint replacement should, in theory, improve function compared with that after silicone spacers and alleviate the problems of implant fracture and silicone-induced synovitis.[185] The ball and socket designs (Figs. 13-91 and 13-92) serve this purpose. The Mayo asymmetric design (Figs. 13-93 and 13-94) was based on a fixed fulcrum prosthesis centered in the trapezium with an extended ball and socket joint articulating with the first metacarpal. This places the center of rotation at the base of the first metacarpal instead of the trapezium, which should improve the biomechanical parameters.[183,228]

Postoperative Evaluation and Complications

Improved motion and significant decrease in pain can be achieved with most trapeziometacarpal arthroplasty techniques.[177,180,189,192,193] Cooney[183] reviewed interposition and silicone implant arthroplasty and found decreased pain in 90% to 95% of patients and improved range of motion in 42% to 46% with both techniques. The large number of procedures and variations in implant design suggest that none of the techniques is perfect; the surgeon's selection depends on the cause and extent of the disease and the patient's age, activity, and compliance. For example, total trapeziometacarpal joint replacement is only possible in patients with good bone stock and suitable functional demands.[181,183,185]

A radiographic evaluation is important to determine function and detect complications. Baseline studies should include PA and lateral views. In addition, abduction-adduction (pinch) views should be obtained with the hand in the prone position. Measuring the motion of the first metacarpal compared with that of the second and the arc of motion (abduction to adduction) can be used to judge the treatment response (Figs. 13-87B,C and 13-94C,D). Lateral views with the thumb palmoflexed and dorsiflexed measure this arc of motion.[195,203]

The complications are similar to those described with wrist arthroplasty (Table 13-4). Implant failures vary with individual circumstances, but the rates of failure are reported to be as high as 15%.[195] This figure was reported for metacarpal condylar implants at 4.5 years by Jennings and Livingstone.[195]

Instability, loosening (Fig. 13-91B), and infection (Fig. 13-95) can occur, although the last is uncommon.[183,195,220] Silicone-induced synovitis (Fig. 13-96) is a fairly common complication.

Metacarpophalangeal and Interphalangeal Arthroplasty

The treatment of disorders of the metacarpophalangeal and interphalangeal joints consists of several options. Soft tissue imbalance and maintaining or improving function of the involved and adjacent articulations is a significant challenge.[200,202,215] The surgical options include synovectomy, resection arthroplasty, interposition arthroplasty, and replacement arthroplasty.[209,213,214,217] Arthroplasty techniques and implant categories are summarized in Figure 13-97.[217]

Metacarpophalangeal Joint

A number of techniques and implants have been designed to meet the challenges of metacarpophalangeal joint arthroplasty. When discussing this procedure or designing implants, we must consider the function of the interphalangeal joints of the involved finger, matching the implant's position to the other metacarpophalangeal joints, and soft tissue balance.[177,200,202]

Metacarpophalangeal arthroplasty is primarily considered for rheumatoid arthritis with progressive deformity. The procedure is contraindicated in patients with infection, poor bone stock, or soft tissue and cutaneous abnormalities.[200,202]

The implant designs have varied since the late 1950s.[213,217] Brannon developed a hinged metal implant in 1956. This was later modified by Flatt in 1961. Steffee developed a metal-polyethylene system in 1964, and Swanson and Niebauer originated the flexible silicone implants in 1962.[204,212,213,217] Figures 13-98 to 13-105 demonstrate metacarpophalangeal arthroplasty systems.

PIP Joint

The PIP joint has the greatest arc of motion of any of the finger articulations.[176] Surgical reconstruction is most often considered to correct inflammatory, degenerative, or posttraumatic arthropathies. Impairment results in decreased motion and deformities (e.g., boutonniere and swan neck). In most cases, the options are arthrodesis *versus* arthroplasty. Arthrodesis may be preferred for the index finger.

The preoperative evaluation includes variables, such as the patient's occupation, hobbies, handedness, age, and compliance. Routine radiographs (PA, lateral, and oblique) and, on occasion, stress views are helpful in surgical decision making.

Most implants are either metal-plastic hinge or flexible silicone designs. Figures 13-106 to 13-109 summarize phalangeal implants. The Silastic™ Swanson implant (Fig. 13-105) has a similar appearance to the slightly larger implant used for the metacarpophalangeal joint.[219]

Postoperative Evaluation

Patients are evaluated for stability, pain relief, and function after arthroplasty. A radiographic evaluation is

(*text continues on page 908*)

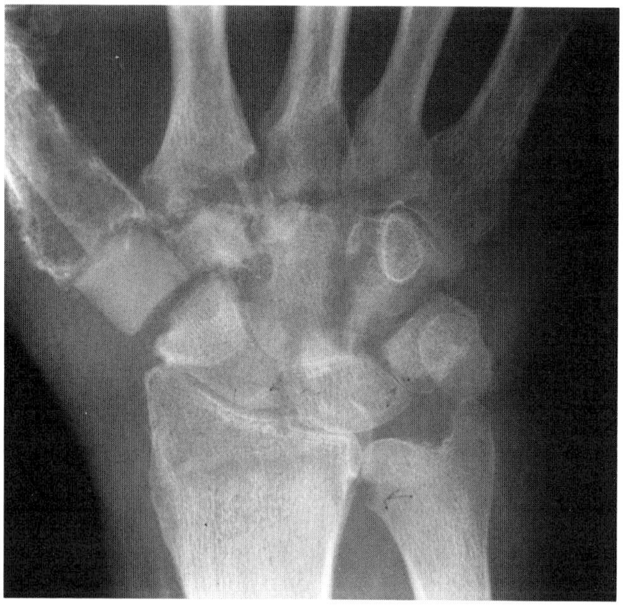

FIG. 13-95. The PA radiographs of the wrist after silicone trapezial implant. The first metacarpal is eroded, and there are multiple carpal erosions caused by infection.

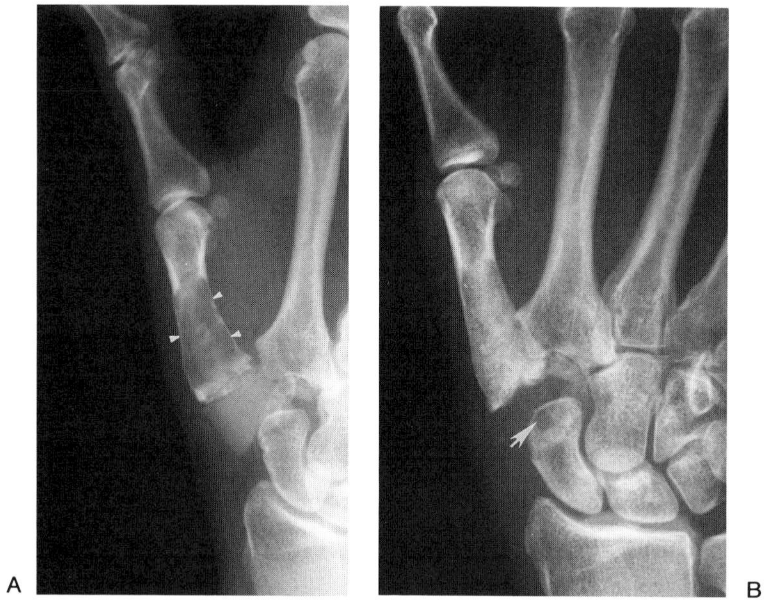

FIG. 13-96. A: Radiograph of the thumb after trapezial spacer placement with resorption of bone (*arrows*) around the implant stem. **B:** The implant was removed because of silicone-induced synovitis. The defect was filled with bone graft. There is a lucent area in the scaphoid as a result of synovitis or osteolysis (*arrow*).

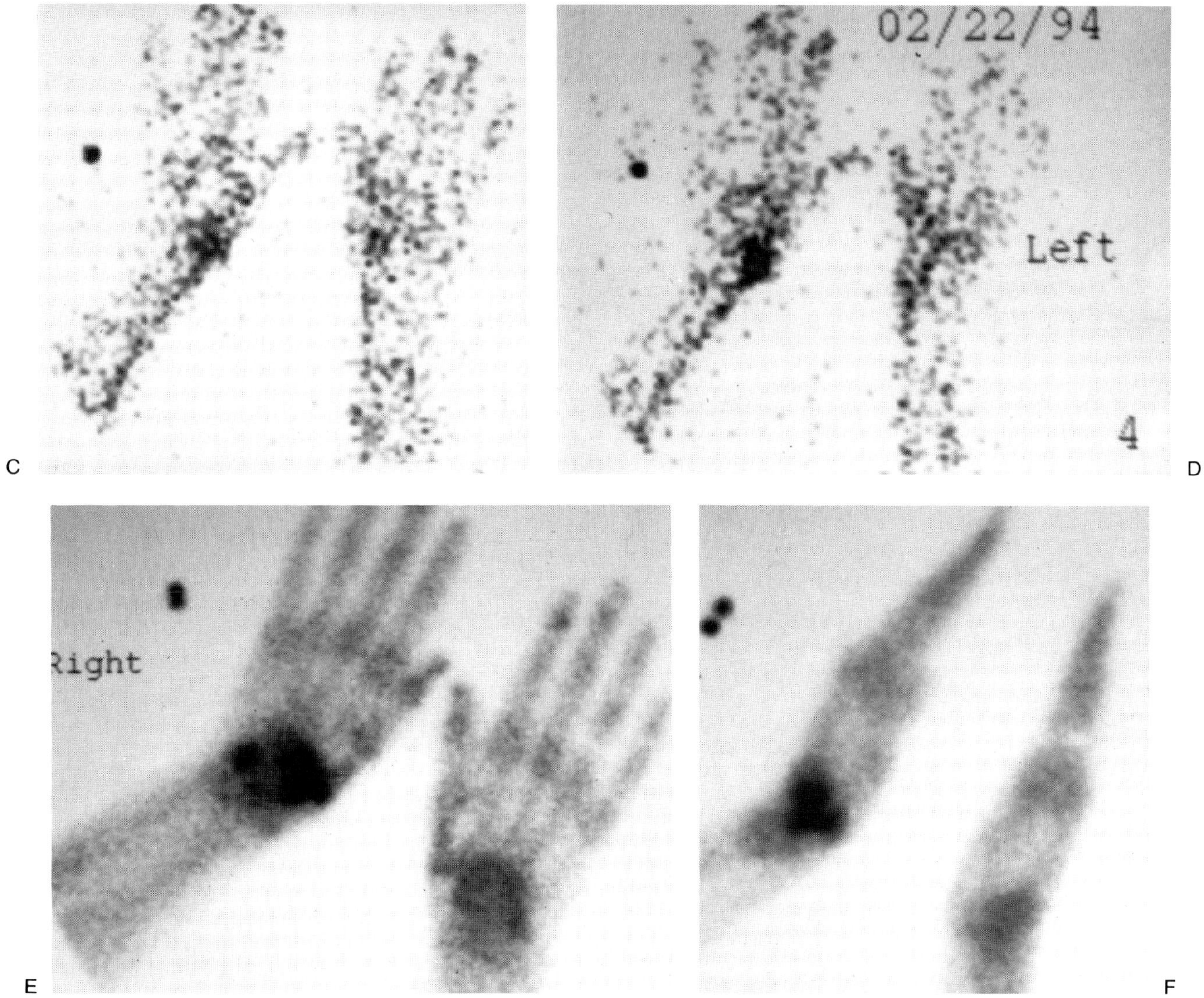

FIG. 13-96. (*Continued.*) Three-phase bone scan later demonstrates increased flow **(C,D)** and diffuse increased tracer on delayed images **(E,F)** caused by synovitis.

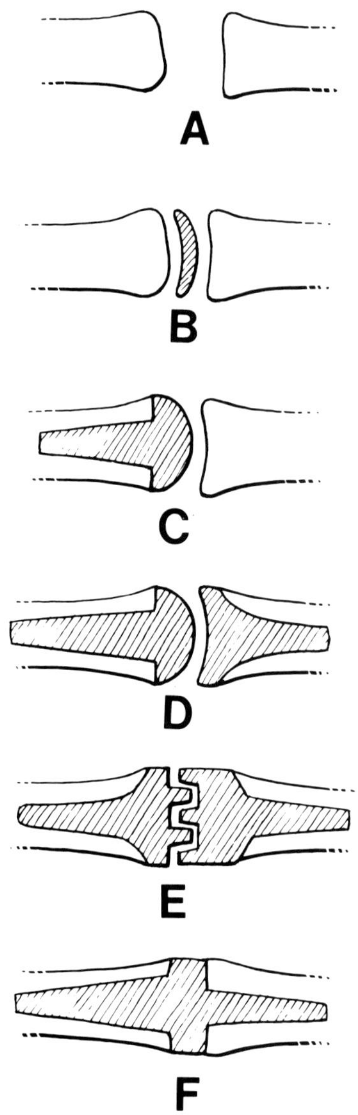

FIG. 13-97. Categories of arthroplasty used in the hand. **A:** resection arthroplasty. **B:** Interposition arthroplasty. **C:** Condylar replacement. **D:** Ball and socket configuration. **E:** Interlocking hinges. **F:** Flexible Silastic™ implant.

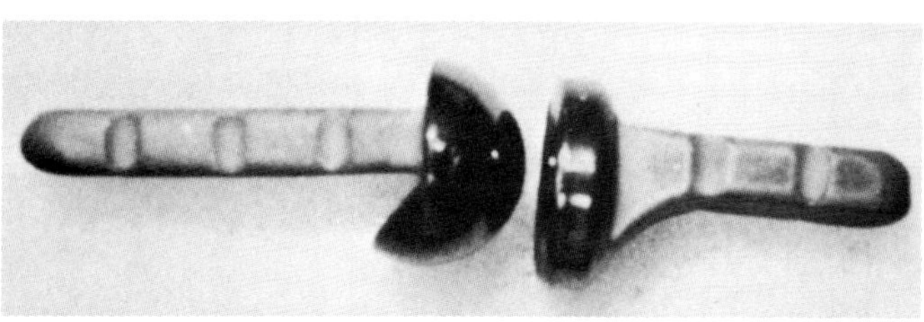

FIG. 13-98. Pyrolytic carbon implant with nonhinged components that are used without cement. Good soft tissue support is required because of the unconstrained configuration. Therefore, this system is limited to patients with minimal deformity. (From Beckenbaugh RD. Implant arthroplasty in the rheumatoid hand and wrist: current state of the art in the United States. *J Hand Surg* 1983;8:675–678.)

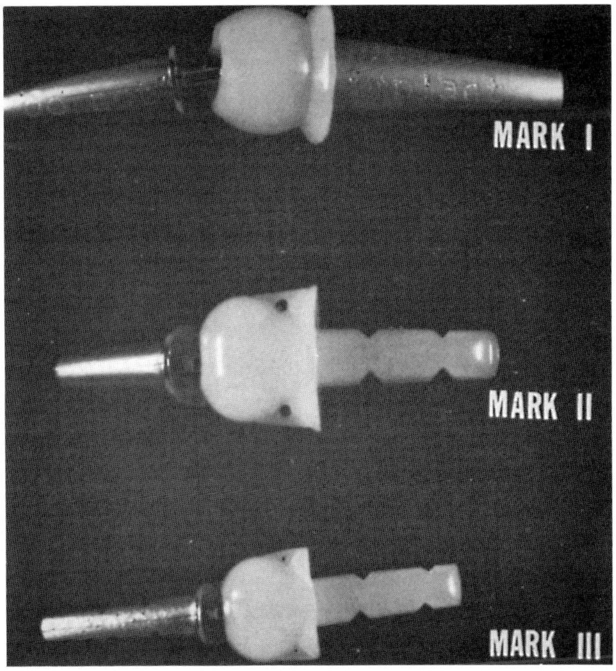

FIG. 13-99. Steffee implants.[204,212,213] Snap-fit T-shaped distal stem with hollow proximal polyethylene component. The Mark I has cemented components. Flexion contractures are common on follow-up. The Mark II has dorsally offset proximal and distal stems. Stems are shorter than in the Mark I. The Mark III has lengthened stems. Side flanges are for alignment and suspension of the volar plate. (From Linscheid RL, Dobyns JH. Total joint arthroplasty: the hand. *Mayo Clin Proc* 1979;54:516–526.)

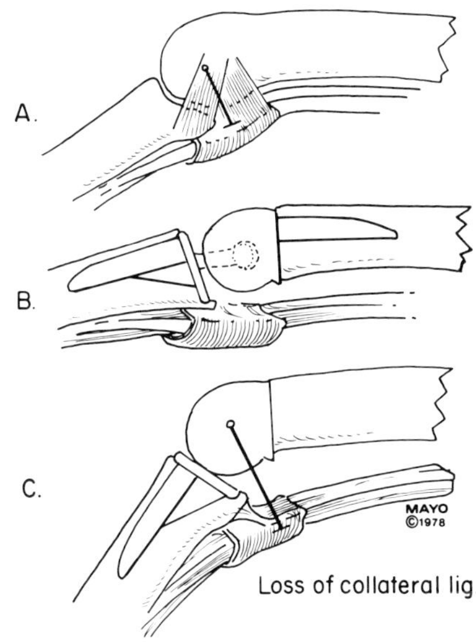

FIG. 13-100. A: The normal moment arm of flexor tendons as they cross the metacarpophalangeal joint, which is determined by the attachment of the accessory collateral and collateral ligaments to the volar plate. B: When the metacarpal head is removed (Steffee implant demonstrated), the fixation is lost. C: The flexor tendons and volar plate may sublux volarly, increasing the moment arm of the tendons and leading to flexor contraction. (From Linscheid RL, Dobyns JH. Total joint arthroplasty: the hand. *Mayo Clin Proc* 1979;54:516–526.)

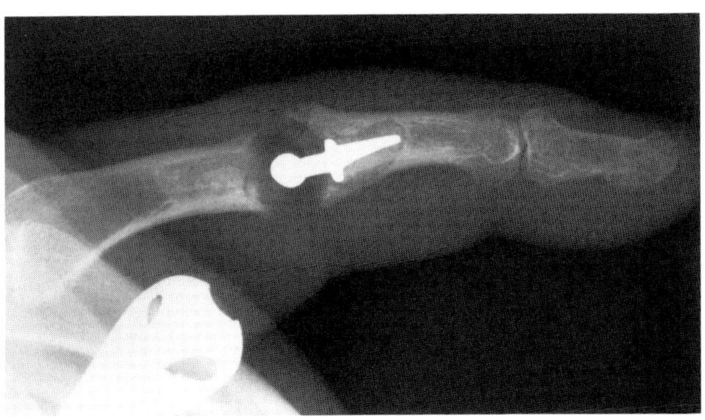

FIG. 13-101. Lateral radiograph of the finger demonstrating a cemented Steffee Mark II implant.

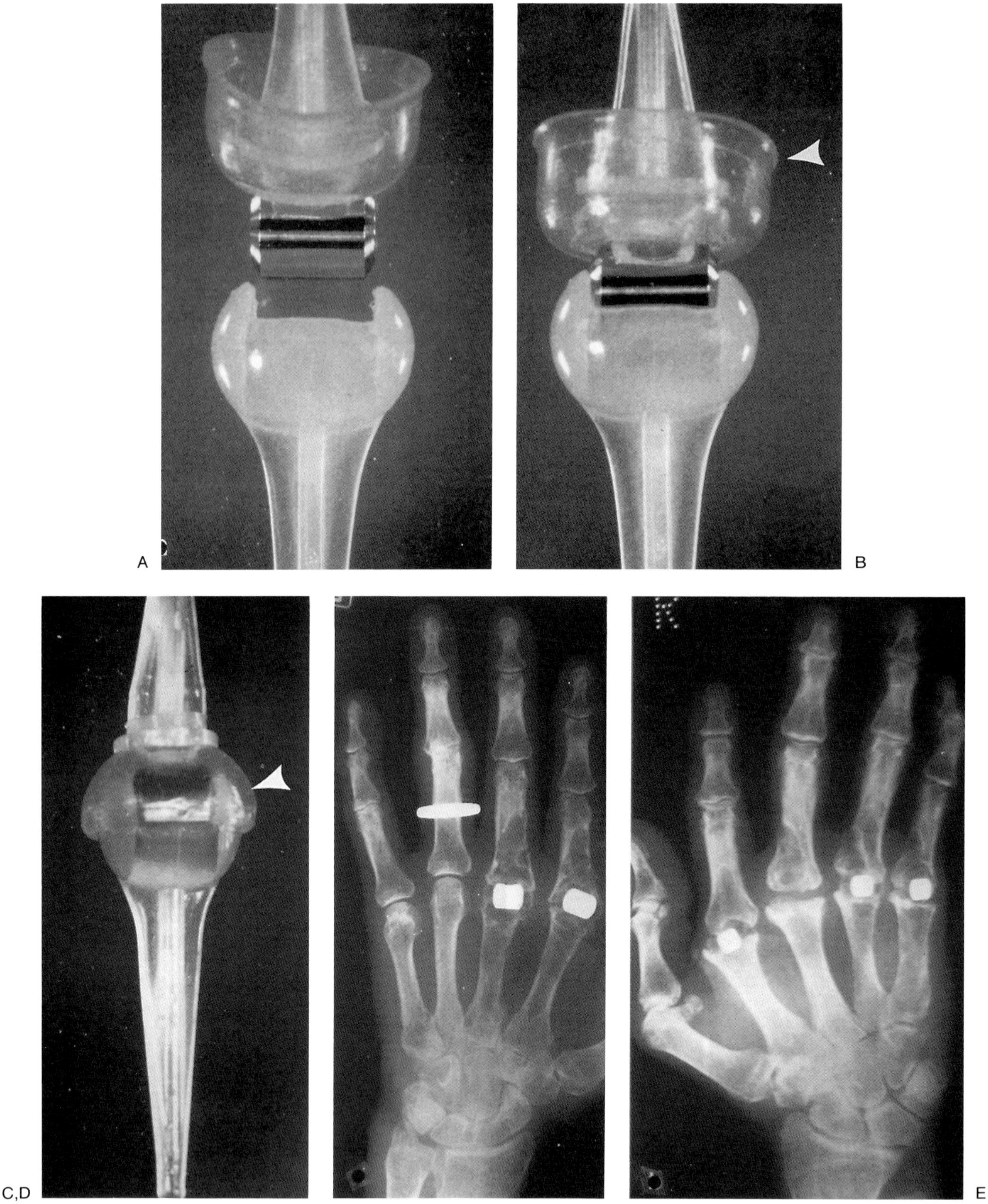

FIG. 13-102. Nicolle prosthesis, which was introduced in 1973.[222] The prosthesis is an articulated hinge with polypropylene stems and a stainless steel bearing. **A:** Disarticulated components. **B:** Prosthesis articulated with cuff (*arrow*) retracted. **C:** Components assembled with cuff covering joint (*arrow*). **D:** A PA radiograph of the left hand with Nicolle prosthesis in the second and third metacarpophalangeal joints; the components are not cemented. Cystic bone changes seen in 5%. **E:** A PA radiograph of the right hand with implants at the second to the fifth metacarpophalangeal joints. There are erosions with ulnar deviation. (From Varma SK, Milward TM. The Nicolle finger joint prosthesis: a reappraisal. *Br J Hand Surg* 1991;16B:187–190.)

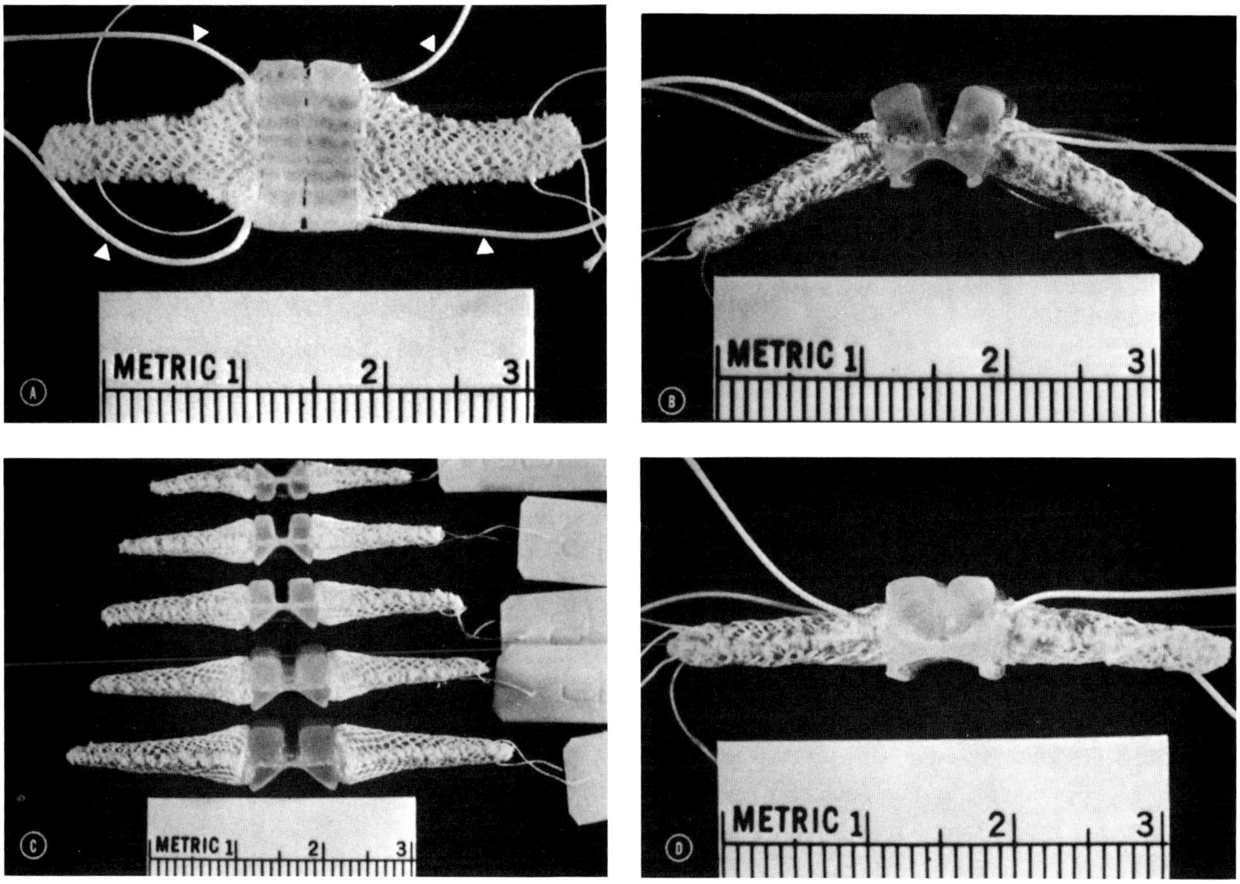

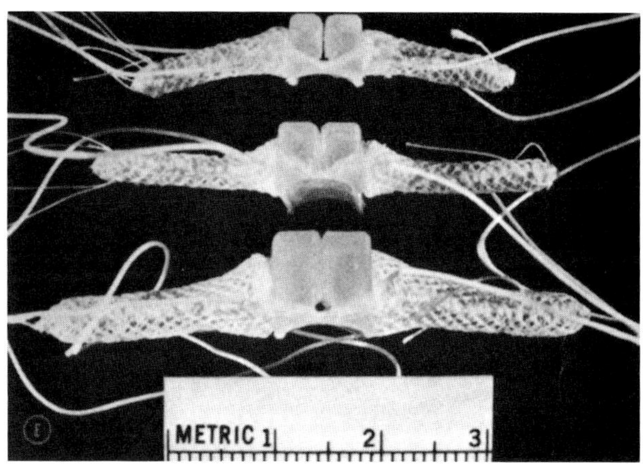

FIG. 13-103. Silicone-Dacron™ Niebauer prostheses.[209] **A:** Silicone-Dacron™ metacarpophalangeal prosthesis. Silicone is molded over a Dacron™ mesh with proximal and distal stem. There is a Dacron™ mesh sleeve to enhance ingrowth of fibrous tissue. Dacron™ ties (*arrows*) are used to assist with immediate bone fixation. **B:** Metacarpophalangeal prosthesis seen from the side with biconcave hinge, which allows 15° of extension and 90° of flexion. **C:** Original silicone-Dacron™ prosthesis with lighter hinge and no ties at the articular surface. **D:** Modified heavier hinge prosthesis with ties. **E:** New model heavier hinge in three available sizes. (From Goldner JL, Gould JS, Urbaniak JR, McCollum DE. Metacarpophalangeal joint arthroplasty with silicone-Dacron prosthesis (Niebauer type): six and a half years experience. *J Hand Surg* 1977;2: 200–211.)

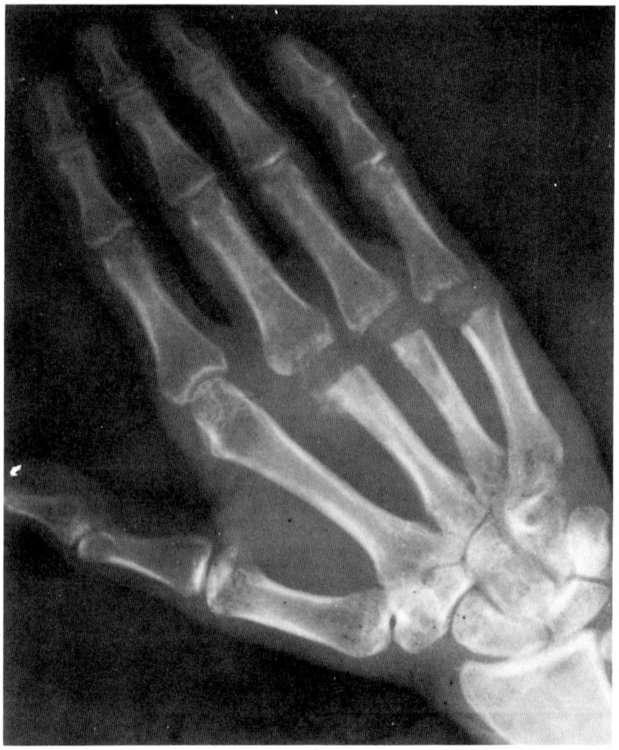

A

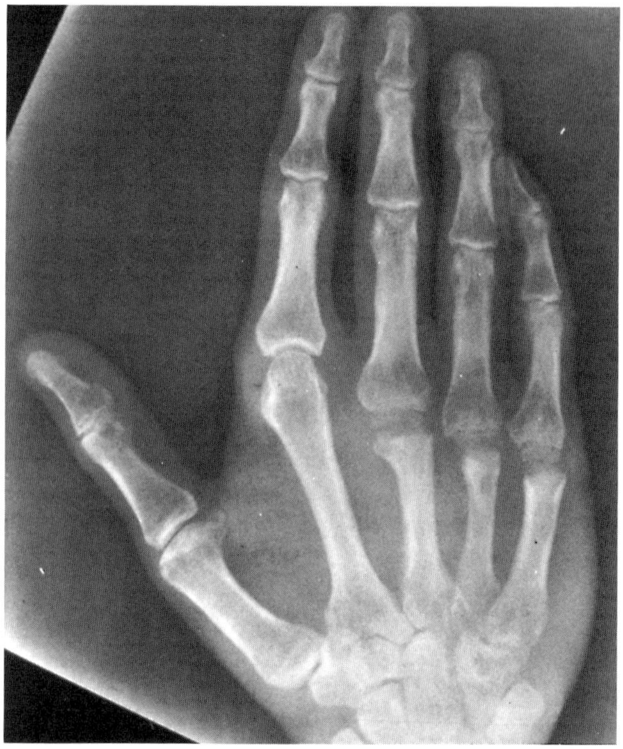

B

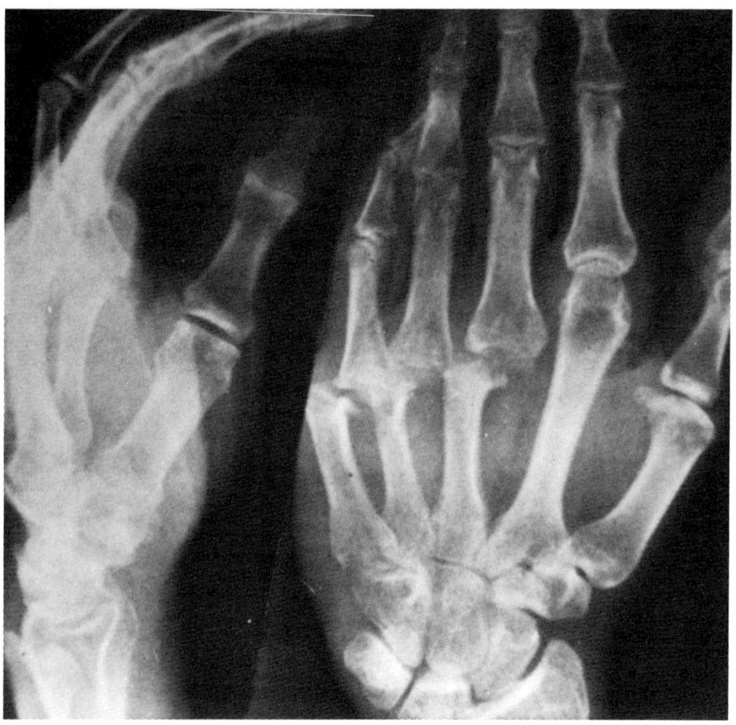

C

FIG. 13-104. A: Niebauer prostheses in the third to fifth metacarpophalangeal joints. **B:** Patient was doing heavy work 1 year later with the prosthesis intact. **C:** Lateral and PA radiographs 5 years after insertion. All prostheses have fractured, and there is volar subluxation. The patient continued to work and was unaware of the changes in function. (From Goldner JL, Gould JS, Urbaniak JR, McCollum DE. Metacarpophalangeal joint arthroplasty with silicone-Dacron prosthesis (Niebauer type): six and a half years experience. *J Hand Surg* 1977;2:200–211.)

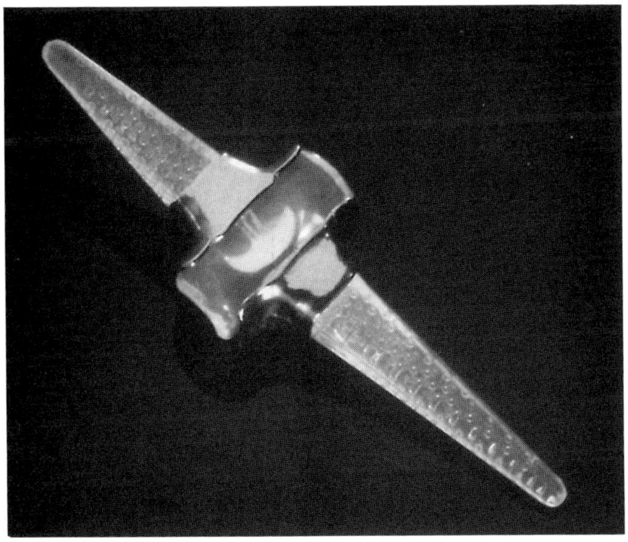
A

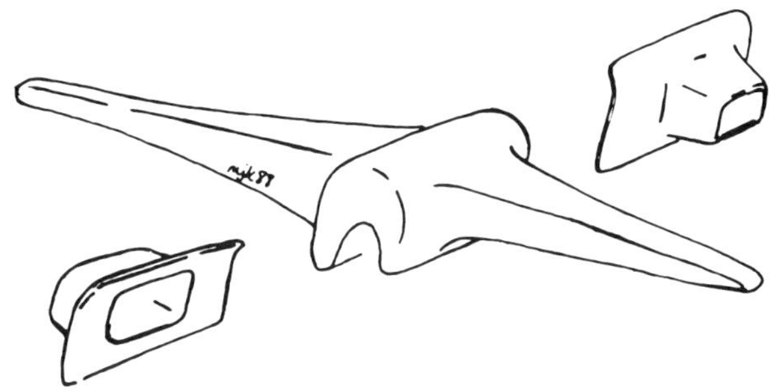
B

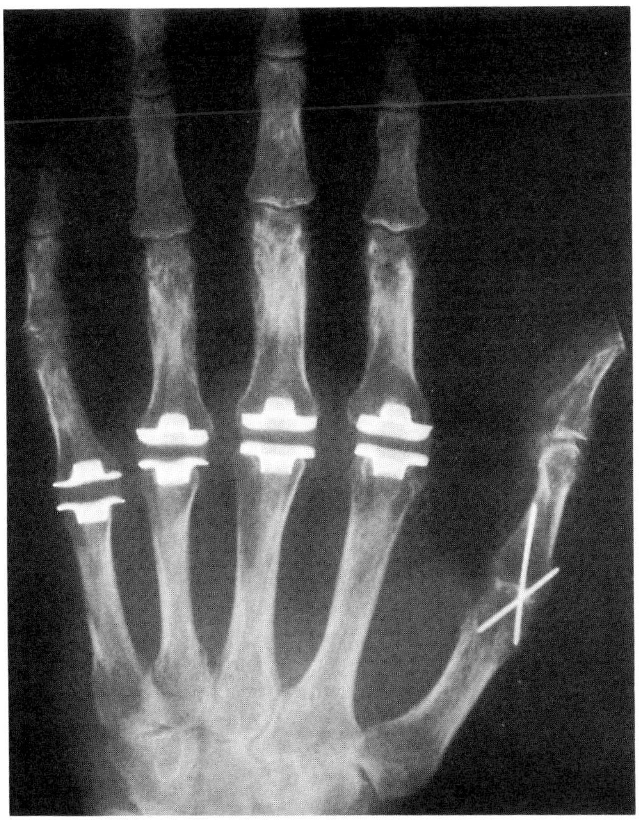
C

FIG. 13-105. Swanson finger implant for the metacarpophalangeal joint and interphalangeal joint. **A:** Silastic™ implant with metal grommets in place. **B:** Implant and metal (titanium) grommets separated. The grommets reduce wear and protect the Silastic™ implant from bone, providing more even load distribution. **C:** Postoperative radiograph of Swanson implants with metal grommets at the second to fifth metacarpophalangeal joints. K-wire arthrodesis of the first metacarpophalangeal joints. (Courtesy of Wright Medical Technology, Arlington, TN.)

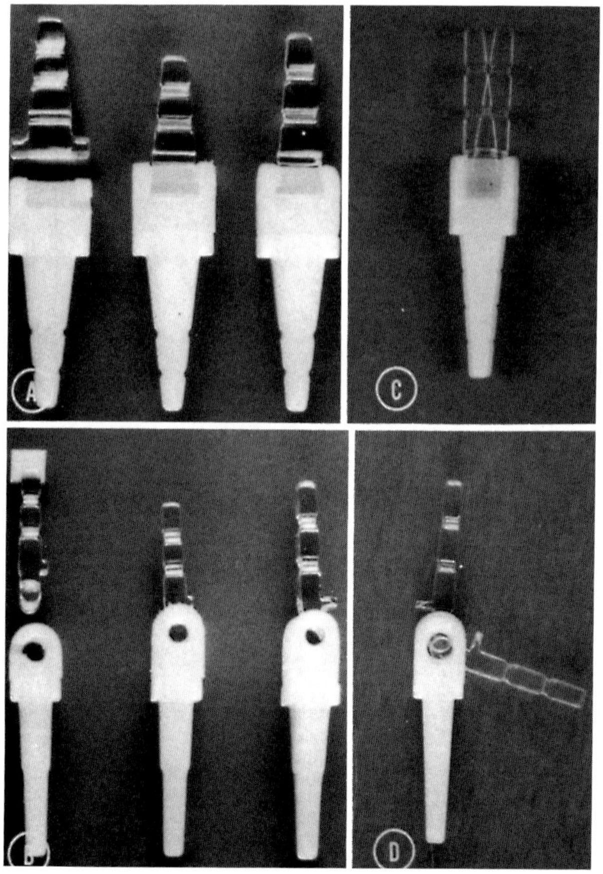

FIG. 13-106. Alumina ceramic finger implants composed of alumina ceramic and high-density polyethylene hinged components.[186] **A:** Initial designs seen from the front (first, *left;* second, *middle;* third, *right*). **B:** Initial design seen from the side (first, *left;* second, *middle;* third, *right*). **C:** Fourth design seen from the front. **D:** Fourth design seen from the side. The initial three designs had a monoaxial hinge. The fourth design (C,D) allowed 120° of flexion-extension and 20° of abduction-adduction. (From Doi K, Kuwata N, Kavai S. Alumina ceramic finger implants: a preliminary biomaterial and clinical evaluation. *J Hand Surg* [*Am*] 1984;9A:740–749.)

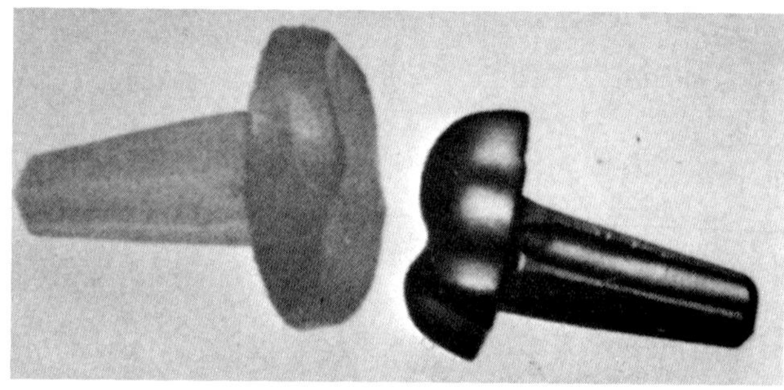

FIG. 13-108. Unconstrained polyethylene interphalangeal joint replacement. This requires intact soft tissue support. (From Linscheid RL, Dobyns JH. Total joint arthroplasty: the hand. *Mayo Clin Proc* 1979;54:516–526.)

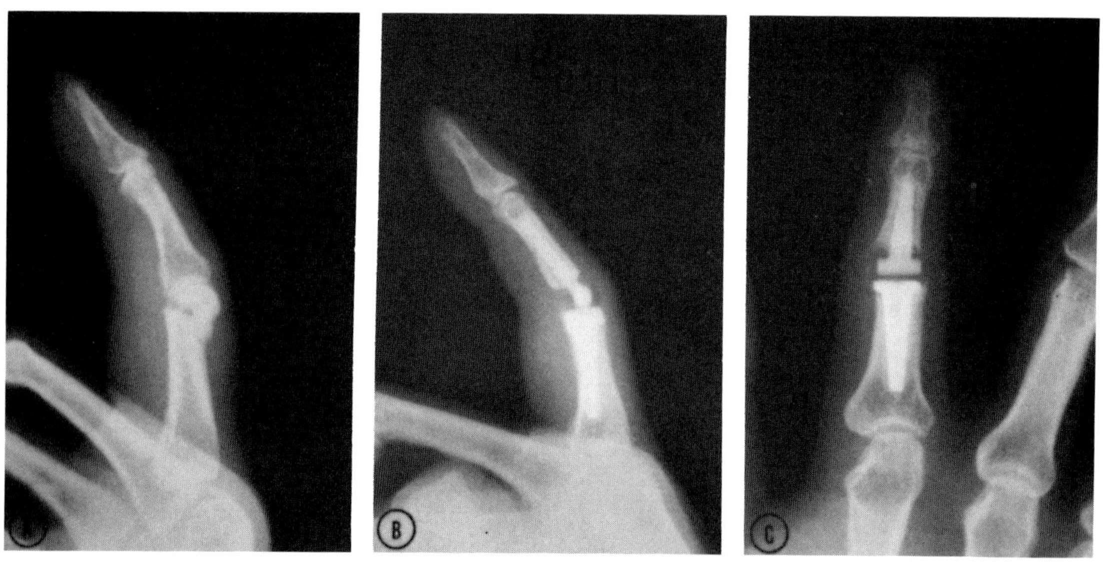

FIG. 13-107. **A:** A 50-year-old man with traumatic ankylosis of the left index PIP joint. Lateral **(B)** and PA **(C)** views after alumina ceramic implant placement. (From Doi K, Kuwata N, Kavai S. Alumina ceramic finger implants: a preliminary biomaterial and clinical evaluation. *J Hand Surg* [*Am*] 1984;9A:740–749.)

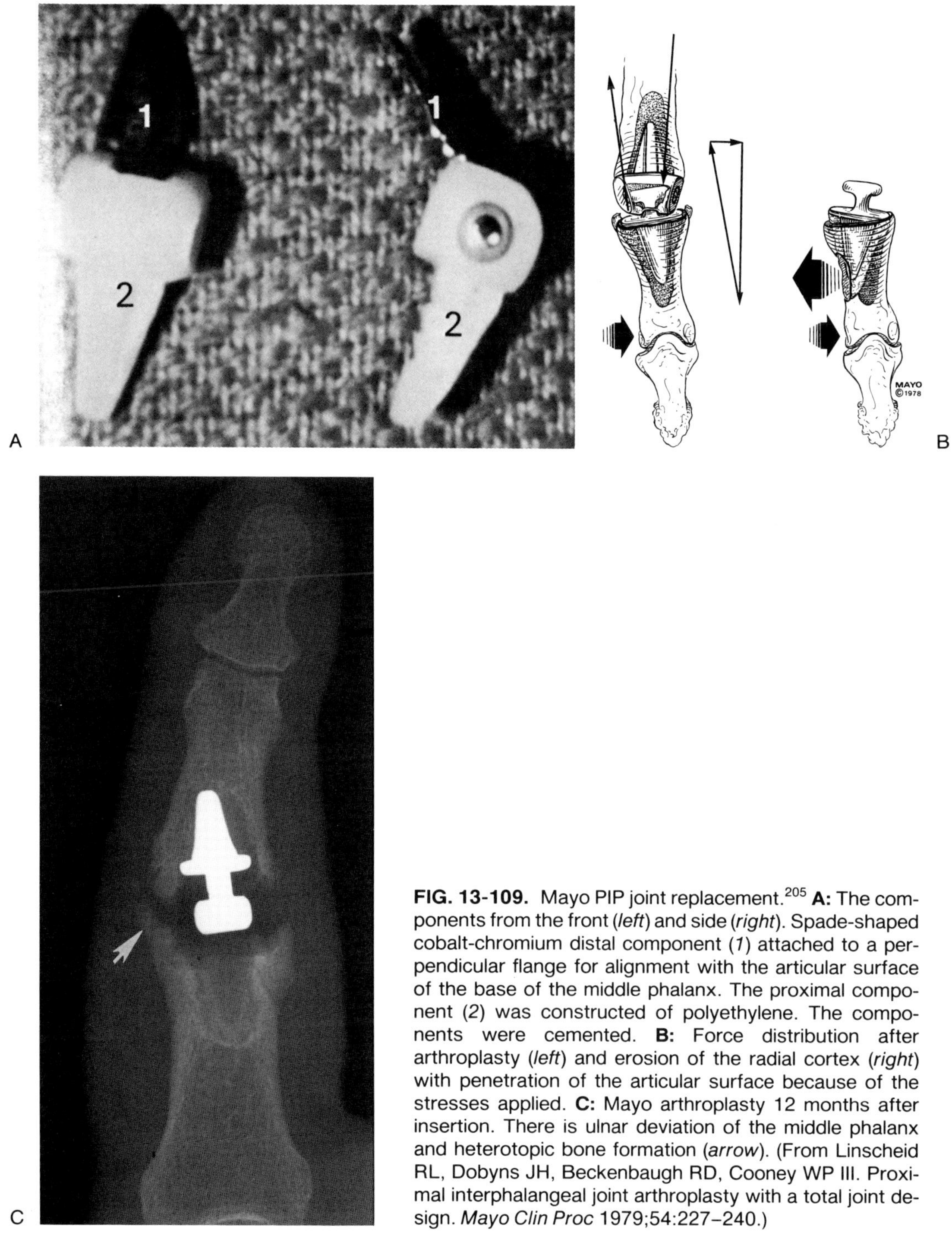

FIG. 13-109. Mayo PIP joint replacement.[205] **A:** The components from the front (*left*) and side (*right*). Spade-shaped cobalt-chromium distal component (*1*) attached to a perpendicular flange for alignment with the articular surface of the base of the middle phalanx. The proximal component (*2*) was constructed of polyethylene. The components were cemented. **B:** Force distribution after arthroplasty (*left*) and erosion of the radial cortex (*right*) with penetration of the articular surface because of the stresses applied. **C:** Mayo arthroplasty 12 months after insertion. There is ulnar deviation of the middle phalanx and heterotopic bone formation (*arrow*). (From Linscheid RL, Dobyns JH, Beckenbaugh RD, Cooney WP III. Proximal interphalangeal joint arthroplasty with a total joint design. *Mayo Clin Proc* 1979;54:227–240.)

also important to confirm motion measurements and evaluate component position. Serial radiographs are most useful to detect changes about the component, such as loosening, heterotopic bone formation, and component fracture.[176,190,194,200,202]

Most large series have evaluated the silicone flexible hinge implants.[194] The results are predictably satisfactory, and revision is facilitated compared with that of cemented components.[176] The results with Swanson PIP implants demonstrated 38° to 60° of motion. The incidence of fracture was 5%, and 11% required revision. Infection is rare, occurring in less than 1% of patients.[176,194] Similar results have been obtained with metacarpophalangeal arthroplasty. However, component fracture is reported more frequently with both Swanson and Niebauer implants: 26% and 38%, respectively.[180,196,198] Routine radiographs (Figs. 13-104 and 13-110) are usually adequate for evaluating silicone implants. Although silicone-induced synovitis is not as significant as that reported with carpal implants, Varma and Milward[222] reported cystic and erosive changes around the stems of the Nicolle implant (Fig. 13-102D,E), presumably caused by reactive changes.

The results with most metal-metal or metal-polyethylene hinged devices have been less satisfactory. As with hinged components in other regions, the failure rates are usually higher and, in some cases, unacceptable.[213] Linscheid et al.[205] reported satisfactory results in only 20% of patients. The complications included loosening (10%), heterotopic bone formation (27%), infection (4.5%), tendon erosion, bone erosion, and stem fractures.[201] Steffee et al.[213] abandoned the type I design (Fig. 13-99) for the type II in 1974. The results with this implant system were also disappointing. Although pain was initially improved, problems with ulnar drift (> 20°) and loosening were also reported. Figures 13-111 to 13-114 demonstrate problems with metal-polyethylene hinge implants.

ARTHRODESIS

There are several options for the reconstruction or salvage of the articulations of the hand and wrist in addition to arthroplasty. Resection arthroplasty, with or without soft tissue interposition, is an effective alternative to joint replacement for joints requiring motion with reduced mechanical load demands.[238] Joint débridement with cheilectomy, partial or complete arthrodesis, and denervation are additional options.[230,237,238] Because this atlas is primarily concerned with orthopedic devices, this section concentrates on arthrodesis.

Arthrodesis can be used to treat pain and instability in any of the joints of the hand and wrist. This technique, first performed in 1910, is still useful because of the limited application and varied success of joint-replacement arthroplasty.[232,238]

Arthrodesis of the distal interphalangeal joint is not performed commonly. Although arthritic deformity is common, pain is not a typical complaint. Procedures are more often performed for cosmetic deformity or instability. K-wires (Fig. 13-112), with or without a tension-band wire, or a single cancellous screw can be used in this setting.[231,233,238]

Pain is a more frequent problem in the PIP joint. In most cases, function and pain relief are important. Therefore, arthroplasty may be preferred.[233,234] Arthrodesis is an effective salvage procedure, especially for pain or failed arthroplasty (Fig. 13-110). The technique is most useful for the index and fifth fingers. As a rule, the PIP joint should be fused in slight to moderate flexion.[233,234] In general, the index finger is fused in 15° of flexion and the third through the fifth PIP joints, in 25°, 35°, and 45° of flexion, respectively.[238]

Fusion of the metacarpophalangeal joints is more difficult and usually reserved for isolated joint involvement.[234] K-wires (Fig. 13-105C), with or without tension-band wire, or staples (Fig. 13-115) can be used.[238]

Arthrodesis of the wrist is still an excellent technique to provide pain relief and a stable wrist. This technique is primarily used for salvage of arthroplasty, instability, paralytic imbalance, and after septic arthritis.[238] Total or partial fusions can be used. Total arthrodesis usually includes the radius, scaphoid, lunate, capitate, trapezoid, and third metacarpal. Occasionally, the second metacarpal is also included.[229,237,238] Partial arthrodesis is also performed for more localized arthrosis. The STT fusion is most frequently involved.[229,238] The DRUJ is excluded from the fusion when possible.

Multiple techniques have been described for wrist arthrodesis, with and without the use of bone grafts.[229,235–238] Figure-eight wire and bone graft, medullary pins or rods, compression plates and screws, and external fixators can all be used alone or in combination. The wrist is often fused in 10° to 30° of extension and slight ulnar deviation to improve grip and function.[236] Figures 13-116 to 13-119 demonstrate fusion techniques.

The complications of arthroplasty include pseudarthrosis, carpal tunnel syndrome, and implant failure or irritation, which may necessitate removal. Vicar and Burton[235] reported 18% complications but 97% good results. Most complications were minor, and there were no pseudarthroses.

Radiographic evaluation of complications can usually be accomplished with serial radiographs. The angles, position of the wrist, and bone fusion should be evaluated (Fig. 13-116). Pseudarthrosis can be evaluated with conventional tomography, but CT in the coronal and axial planes is more useful. Reformatted images in multiple planes are useful and reduce artifacts (Fig. 13-120). Radionuclide scans or diagnostic injections can be used in difficult cases. Soft tissue complications, such as carpal tunnel syndrome, are best evaluated with electromyog-

(*text continues on page 917*)

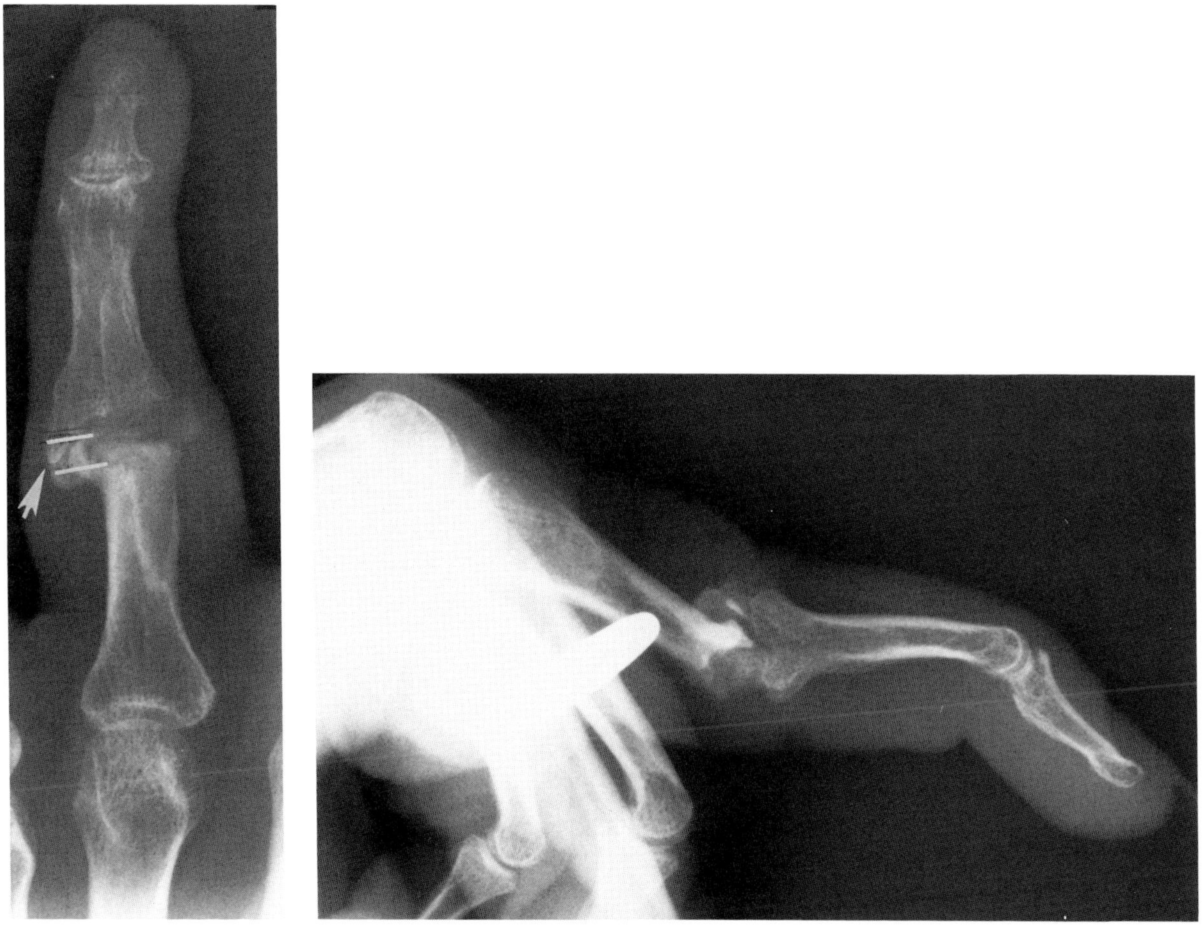

A B

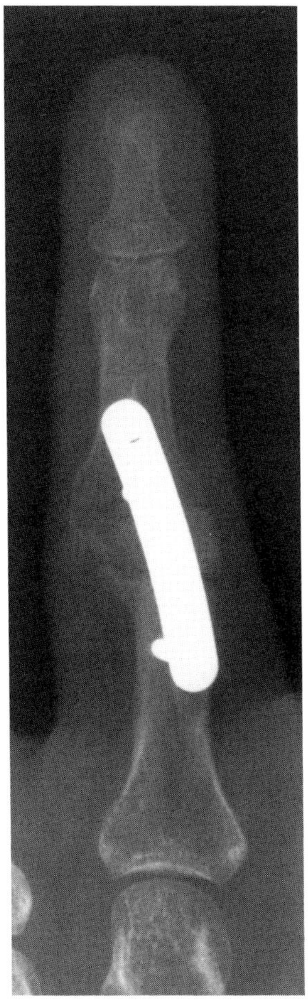

C

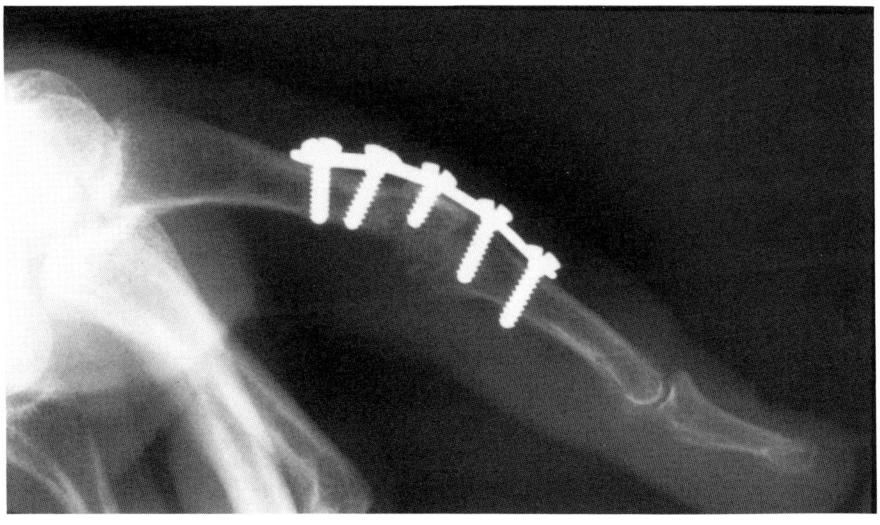

D

FIG. 13-110. The PA **(A)** and lateral **(B)** radiographs of a failed silicone implant with a swan-neck deformity. There is heterotopic bone bridging the ulnar side of the PIP joint (*arrow, lines*). The PA **(C)** and lateral **(D)** radiographs after removal of the implant and arthrodesis with iliac bone graft and a dorsal miniplate with five cortical screws for fixation.

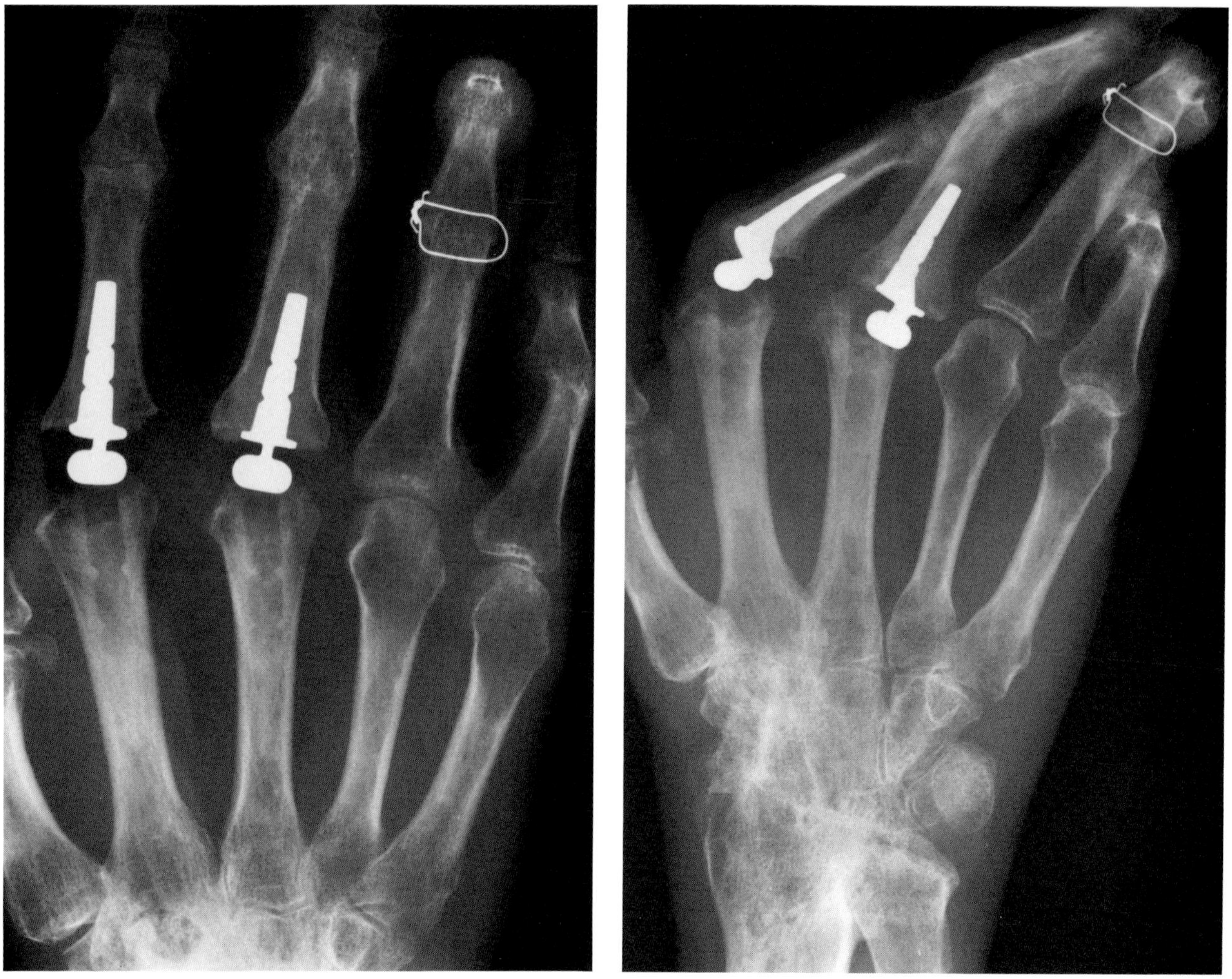

A B

FIG. 13-111. A: A PA radiograph after insertion of Steffee Mark III implants in the second and third metacarpophalangeal joints. Healed arthrodesis of the third to fifth PIP joints. **B:** Twenty months later, there is significant ulnar deviation and deformity.

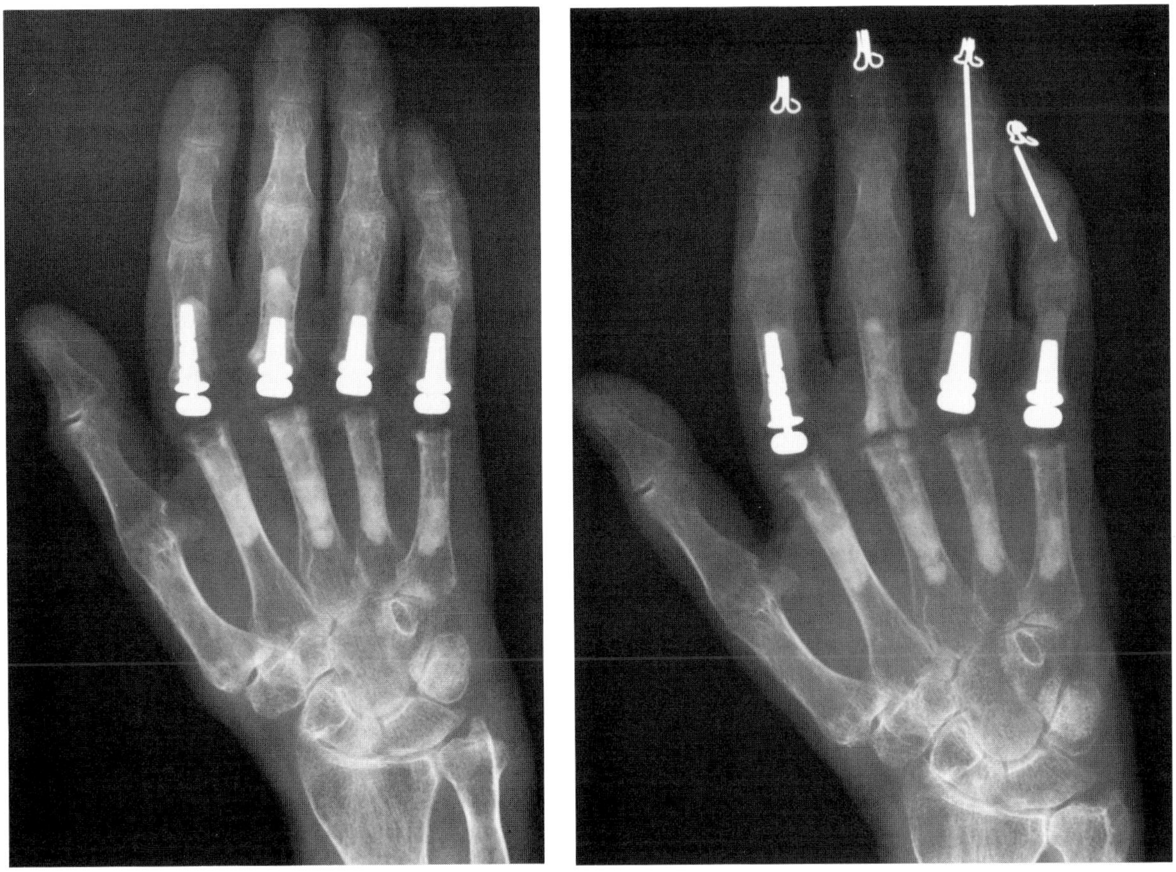

A B

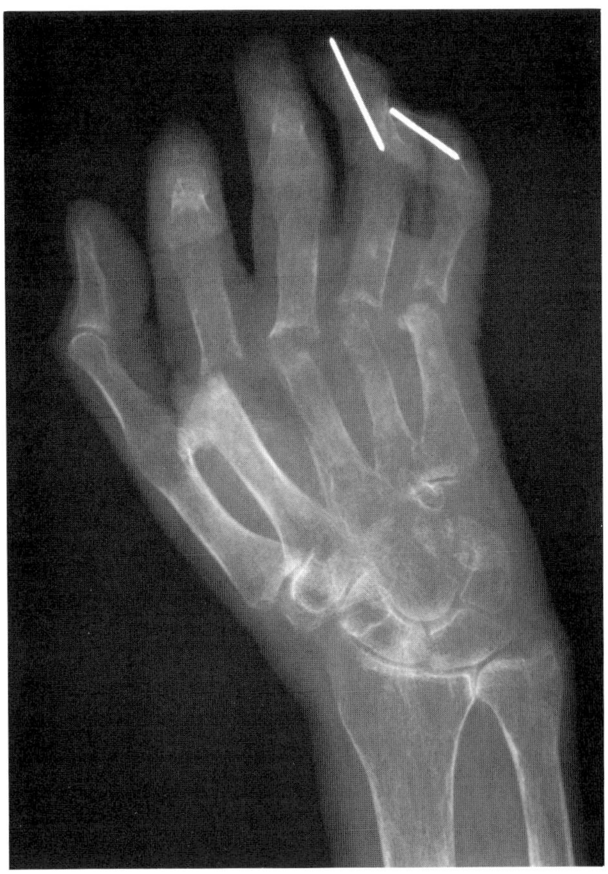

C

FIG. 13-112. **A:** Advanced rheumatoid arthritis with arthrodesis of the thumb. There are Steffee Mark II implants in the third to fifth metacarpophalangeal joints and a Mark III (Fig. 13-98) in the second. The components appear well positioned. There are no lucent lines around the cement. **B:** Fourteen months later, the implant in the third finger was removed. Arthrodesis of the fourth and fifth distal interphalangeal joints. **C:** Two months later, all implants were removed.

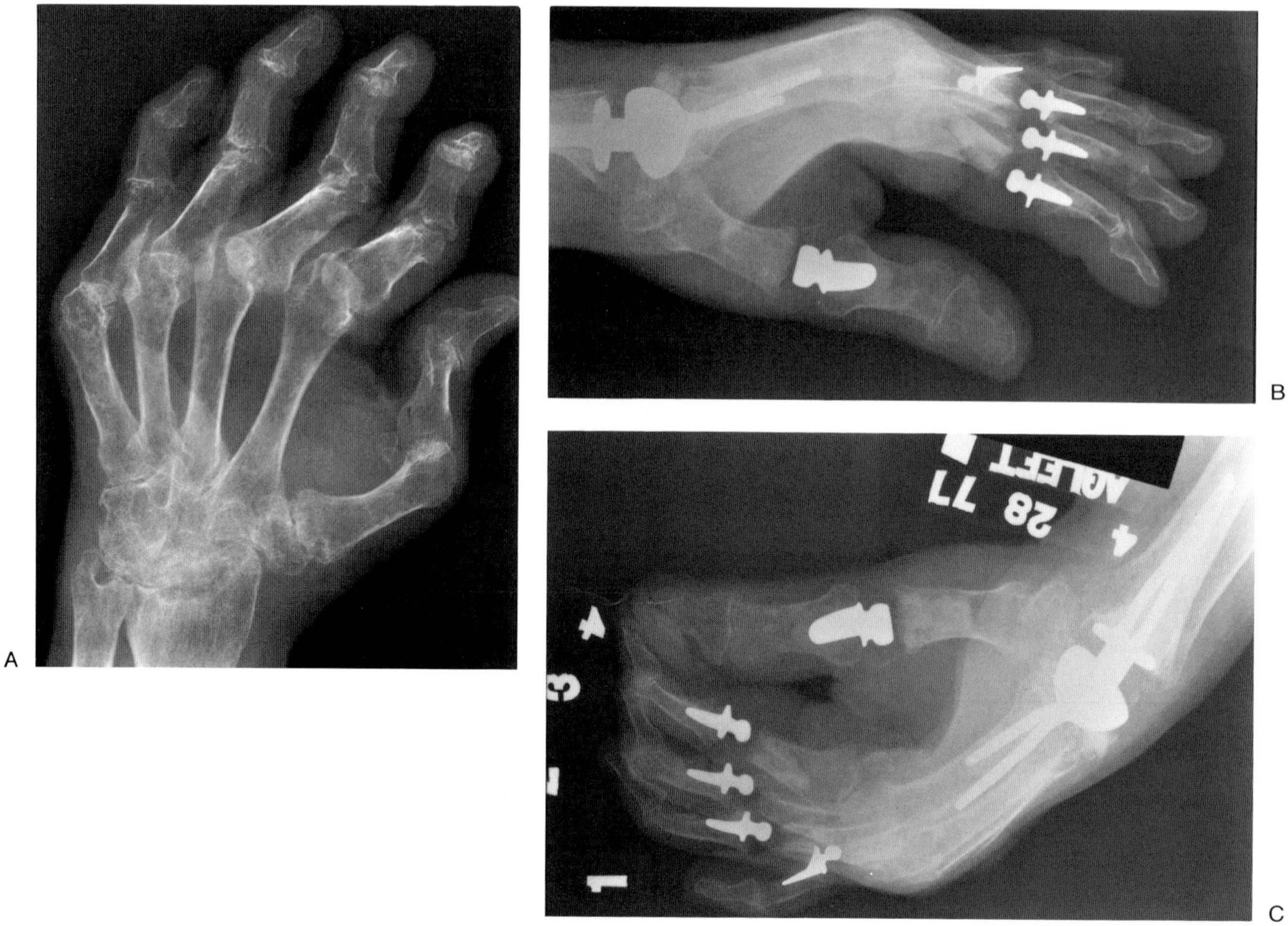

FIG. 13-113. A: Advanced changes of rheumatoid arthritis in the left hand and wrist. Lateral **(B)** and pinch **(C)** views after arthroplasties of the second to the fourth PIP and the first metacarpophalangeal joints with Mayo prostheses. A Meuli wrist prosthesis was used. The range of motion was improved, but the overall results were disappointing. (From Linscheid RL, Dobyns JH. Total joint arthroplasty: the hand. *Mayo Clin Proc* 1979;54:516–526.)

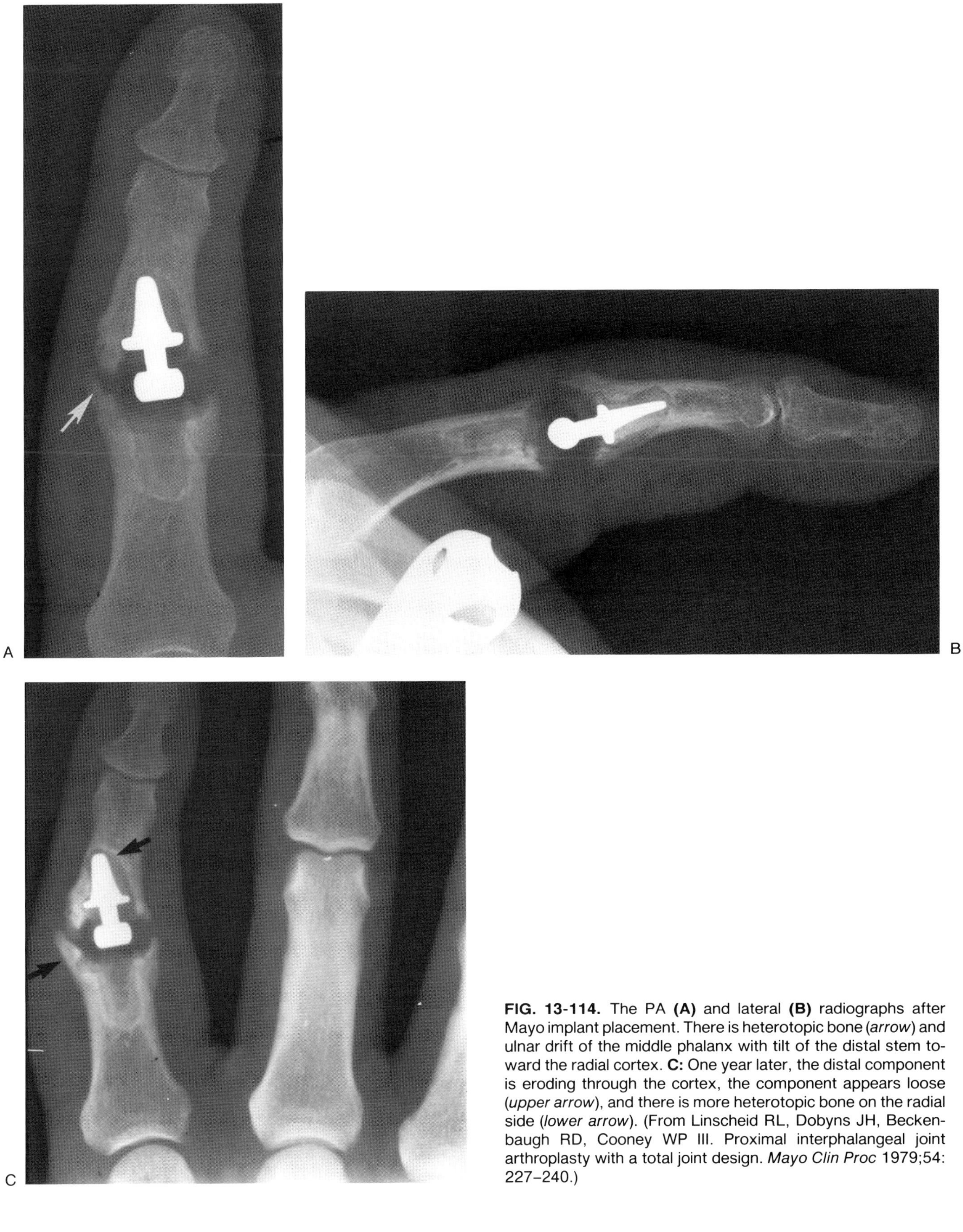

FIG. 13-114. The PA **(A)** and lateral **(B)** radiographs after Mayo implant placement. There is heterotopic bone (*arrow*) and ulnar drift of the middle phalanx with tilt of the distal stem toward the radial cortex. **C:** One year later, the distal component is eroding through the cortex, the component appears loose (*upper arrow*), and there is more heterotopic bone on the radial side (*lower arrow*). (From Linscheid RL, Dobyns JH, Beckenbaugh RD, Cooney WP III. Proximal interphalangeal joint arthroplasty with a total joint design. *Mayo Clin Proc* 1979;54:227–240.)

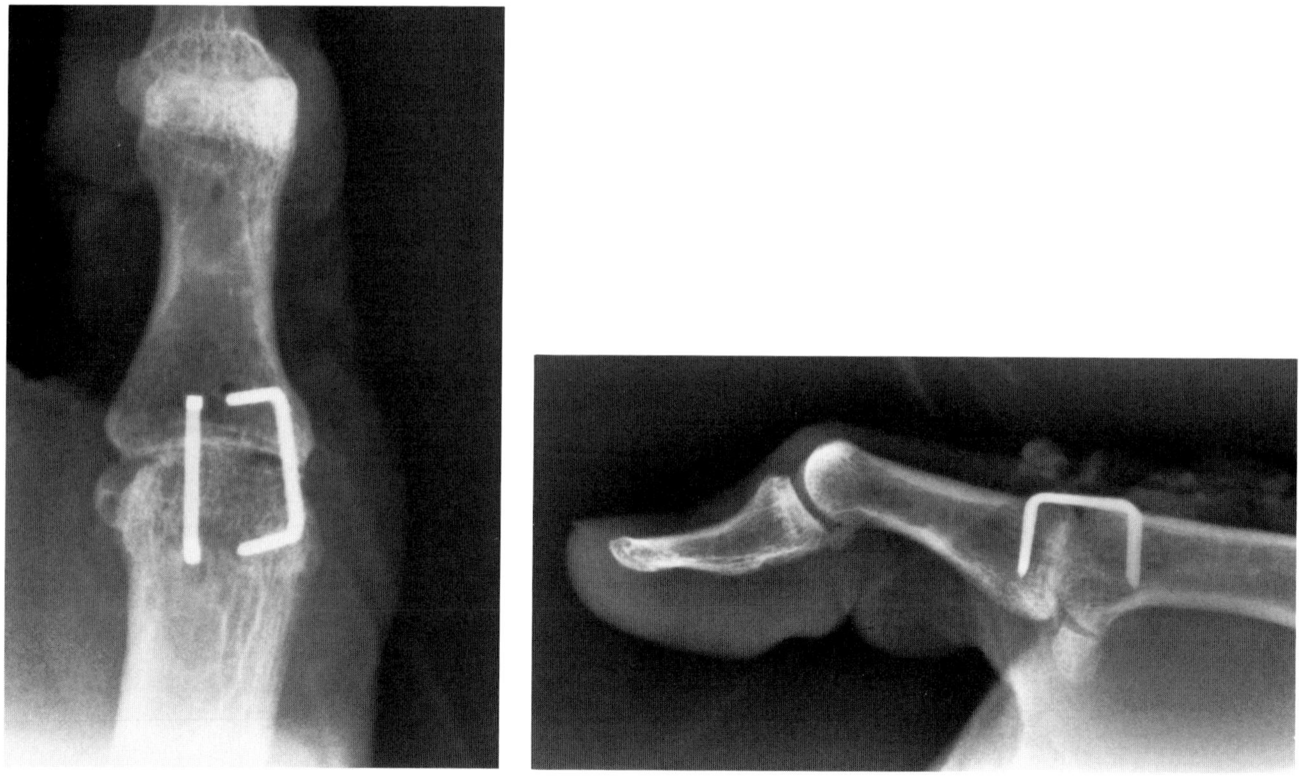

A B

FIG. 13-115. The PA **(A)** and lateral **(B)** radiographs after staple arthrodesis of the first metacarpophalangeal joint.

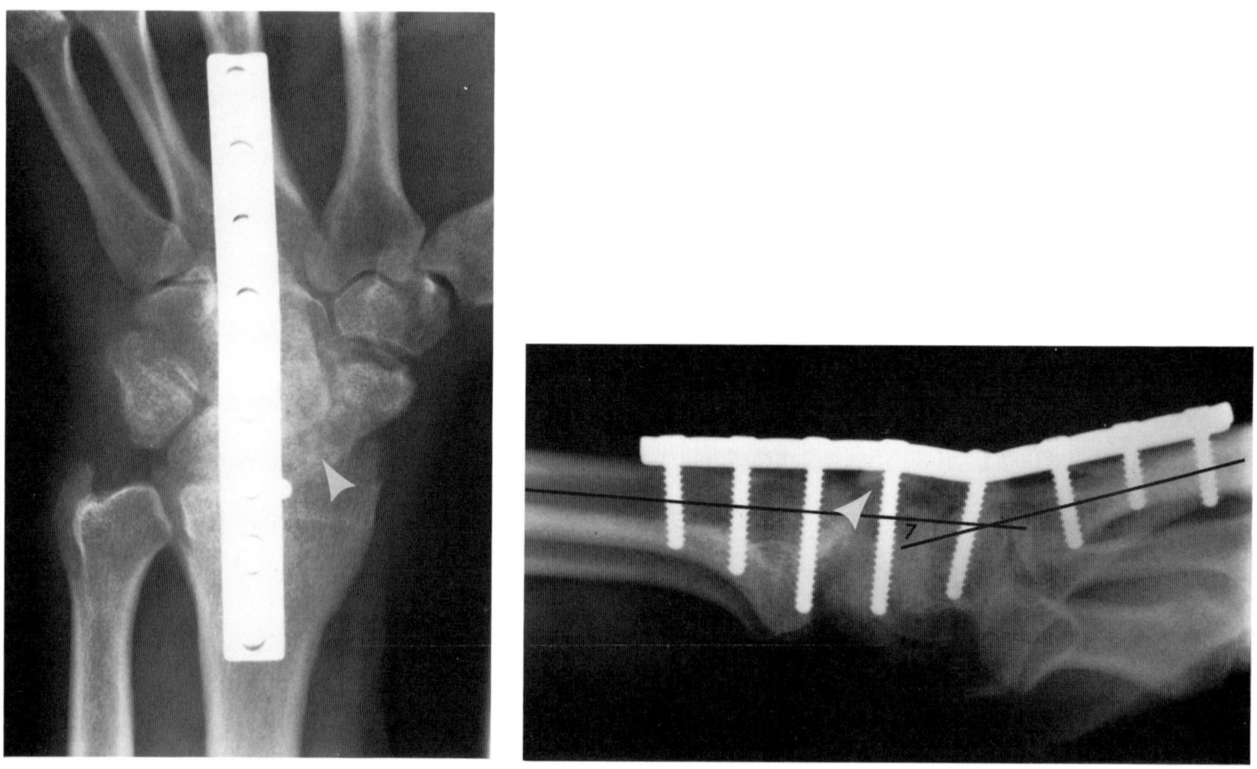

A B

FIG. 13-116. The PA **(A)** and lateral **(B)** radiographs after wrist arthrodesis with an eight-hole DC plate and cortical screws for fixation. The wrist is extended 17°. There is bone graft (*arrows*), and the lunotriquetral, distal radioulnar, and STT articulations are excluded.

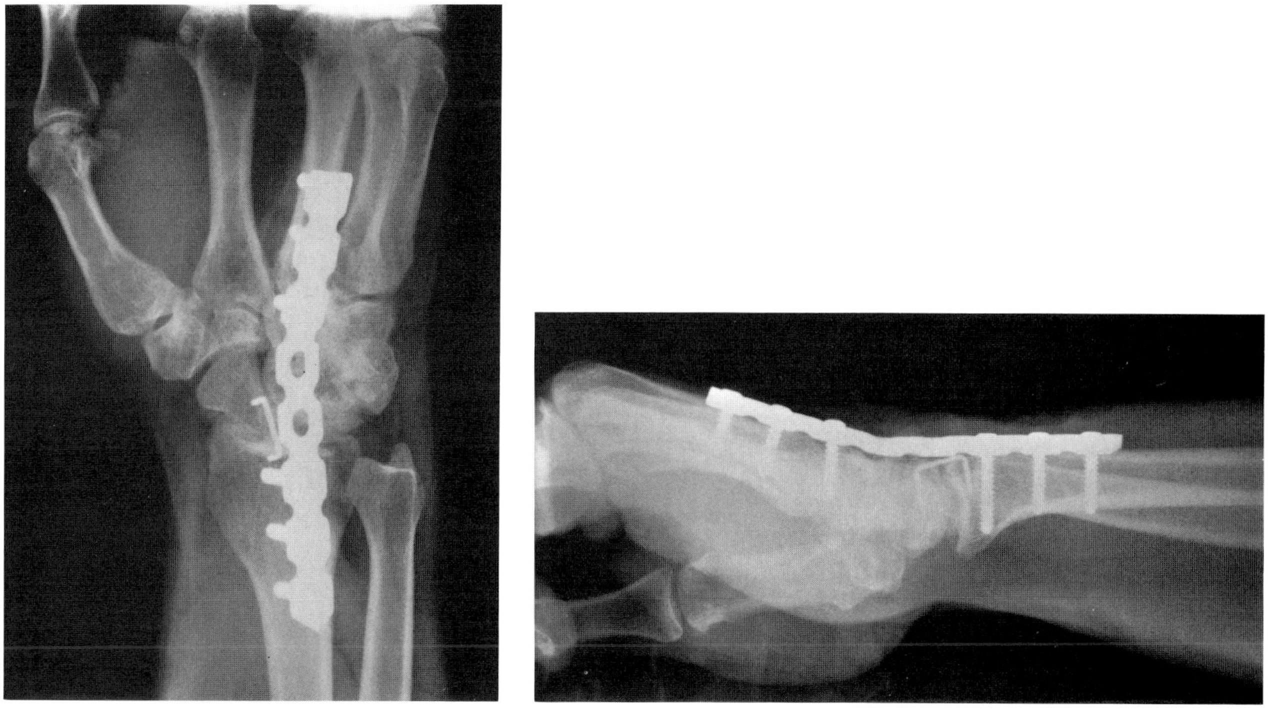

FIG. 13-117. The PA **(A)** and lateral **(B)** radiographs after wrist arthrodesis with an eight-hole reconstruction plate (notched edges) and six cortical screws. A single dorsal radioscaphoid staple is also used.

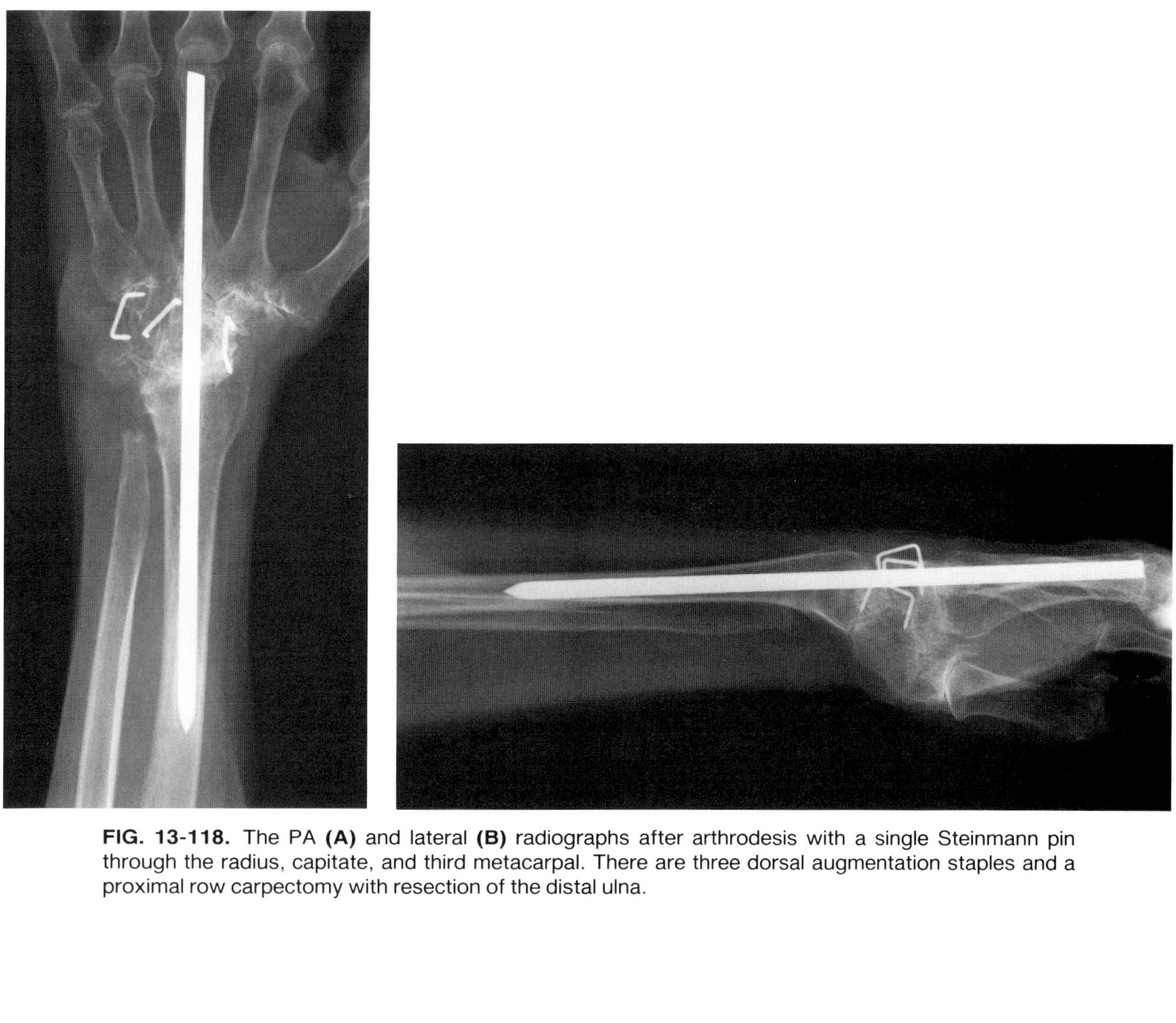

FIG. 13-118. The PA **(A)** and lateral **(B)** radiographs after arthrodesis with a single Steinmann pin through the radius, capitate, and third metacarpal. There are three dorsal augmentation staples and a proximal row carpectomy with resection of the distal ulna.

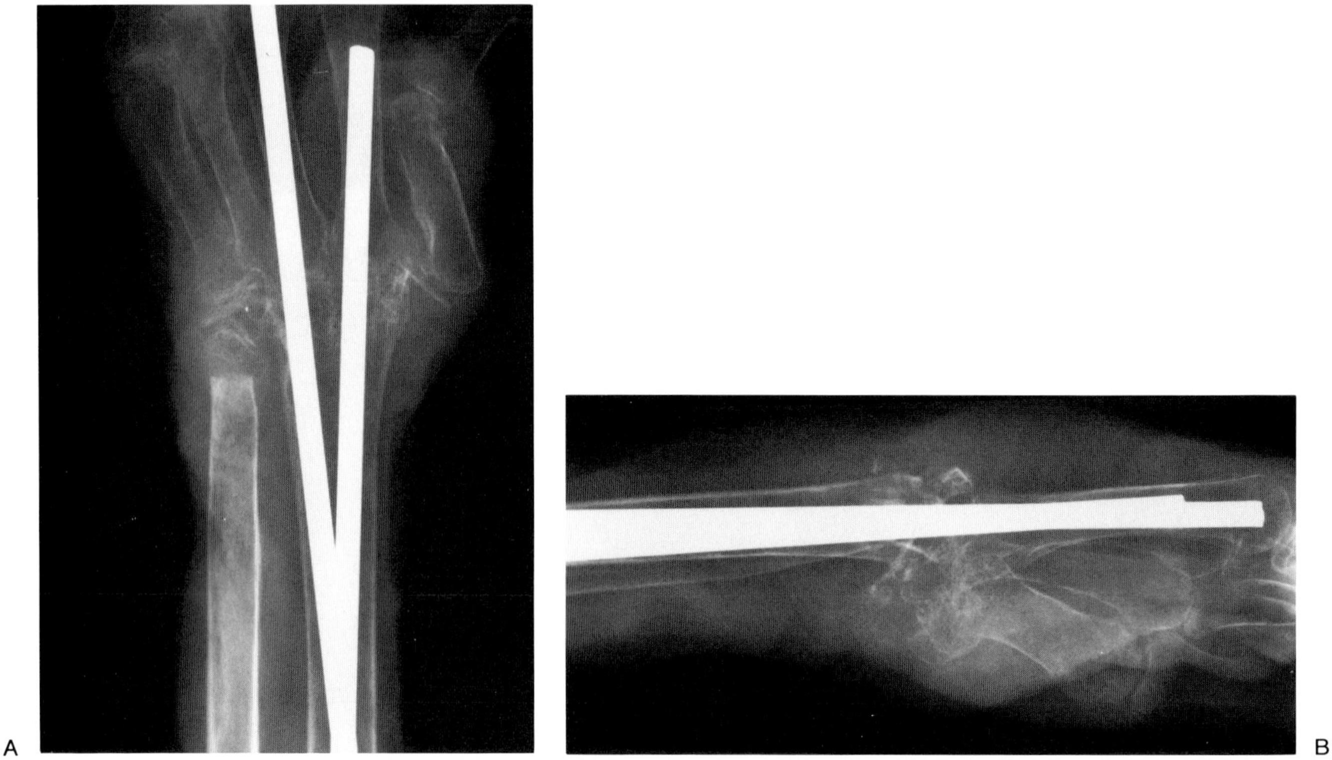

FIG. 13-119. Advanced rheumatoid arthritis with removal of arthroplasty components and fusion using two Steinmann pins in the radius and second and third metacarpals.

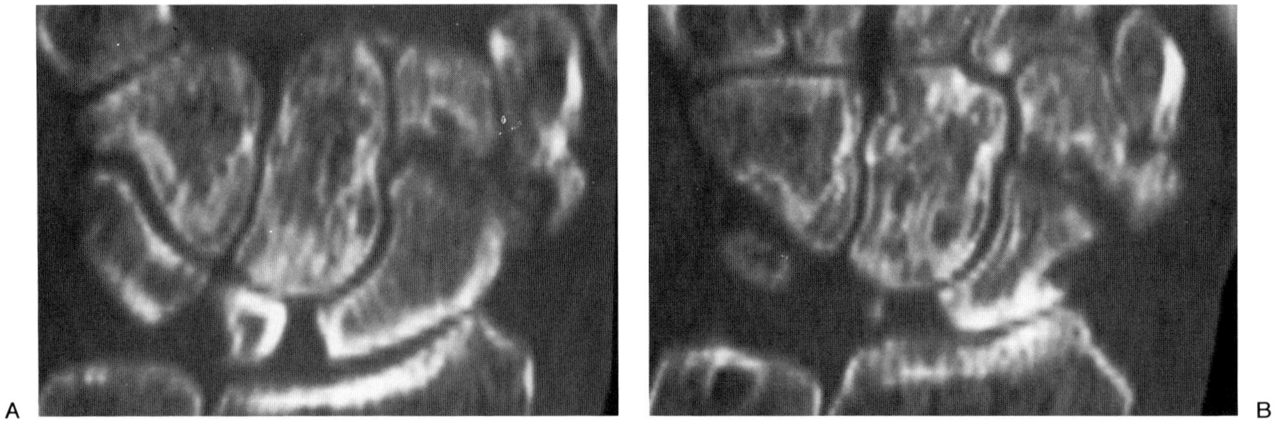

FIG. 13-120. The CT images after STT fusion. A,B: Reformatted coronal images demonstrate marked irregularity and no bone fusion because of pseudarthrosis.

raphy and clinical findings because MRI scans are often degraded by the metal artifact.

REFERENCES

1. Abbitt PL, Riddervold HO. The carpal tunnel view: helpful adjuvant for unrecognized fractures of the carpus. *Skeletal Radiol* 1987;16:45–47.
2. Ballinger PW. *Merrill's atlas of roentgenographic positions and standard radiologic procedures.* 5th ed. St. Louis: CV Mosby; 1982.
3. Berger RA, Blair WF, EL-Koury GY. Arthrotomography of the wrist. The palmar radiocarpal ligaments. *Clin Orthop* 1984;186: 224–229.
4. Bernau A, Berquist TH. *Orthopedic positioning in diagnostic radiology.* Baltimore: Ulrban and Schwarzenberg; 1983.
5. Berquist TH. *MRI of the musculoskeletal system.* 2nd ed. New York: Raven Press; 1990.
6. Berquist TH. The elbow and wrist. *Top Magn Reson Imaging* 1989;1:15–27.
7. Berquist TH. *Imaging of orthopedic trauma.* 2nd ed. New York: Raven Press; 1992.
8. Berquist TH. Diagnostic and therapeutic injections as an aid to musculoskeletal diagnosis. *Semin Intervent Radiol* 1993;10:326–343.
9. Bond JR, Berquist TH. Radiologic evaluation of hand and wrist motion. *Hand Clin* 1991;7:113–123.
10. Bowers WH, Hurst LC. Gamekeeper's thumb. Evaluation by arthrography and stress roentgenography. *J Bone Joint Surg [Am]* 1977;59A:519–524.
11. Braunstein EM, Louis DS, Greene TL, Hankin FM. Fluoroscopic and arthrographic evaluation of carpal instability. *AJR Am J Roentgenol* 1985;144:1259–1262.
12. Brewerton DA. A tangential radiographic projection for demonstrating involvement of the metacarpal head in rheumatoid arthritis. *Br J Radiol* 1967;40:233–234.
13. Bridgman CF. Radiography of the carpal navicular bone. *Med Radiogr Photogr* 1949;25;104.
14. Burman M. Anteroposterior projection of the carpometacarpal joint of the thumb by the radial shift of the carpal tunnel view. *J Bone Joint Surg [Am]* 1958;40A:1156–1157.
15. Bush CH, Gillespy T, Dell PC. High-resolution CT of the wrist: initial experience with scaphoid disorders and surgical fusions. *AJR Am J Roentgenol* 1987;149:757–760.
16. Cone RO, Szabo R, Resnick D, Gelberman R, Taleisnick J, Gilula LA. Computed tomography of the normal soft tissues of the wrist. *Invest Radiol* 1983;18:541–545.
17. Cooney WP III, Linscheid RL, Dobyns JH. Fractures and dislocations of the wrist. In: Rockwood CA, Green DP, Bucholz RW, eds. *Rockwood and Green's fractures in adults.* 3rd ed. Vol. 1. Philadelphia: JB Lippincott; 1991:563–678.
18. Crittenden JJ, Jones DM, Santarelli AG. Bilateral rotational dislocation of the carpal navicular. *Radiology* 1970;94:629–630.
19. Curtis DJ, Downey EF Jr. A simple first metacarpophalangeal stress test. *Radiology* 1983;148:855.
20. Downey EF, Curtis DJ. Patient induced stress test of the first metacarpophalangeal joint: a radiographic assessment of collateral ligament injuries. *Radiology* 1986;158:679–683.
21. Epner RA, Bowers WH, Guifford WB. Ulnar variance—the effect of wrist positioning and roentgen filming technique. *J Hand Surg* 1982;7:298–305.
22. Fodor J III, Malett JC, Moulton J. Carpal tunnel ring artifact. *AJR Am J Roentgenol* 1985;144:765–766.
23. Ganel A, Engel J, Oster Z, Farene I. Bone scanning in the assessment of fractures of the scaphoid. *J Hand Surg* 1979;4:540–543.
24. Gilula LA. Carpal injuries: analytic approach and case exercises. *AJR Am J Roentgenol* 1979;133:513–517.
25. Gilula LA. Mid carpal wrist arthrography. *AJR Am J Roentgenol* 1986;146:645–646.
26. Gilula LA, Distouet JM, Weeks PM, Young LV, Wray RC. Roentgen diagnosis of the painful wrist. *Clin Orthop* 1984;187:52–64.
27. Gilula LA, Totty GW, Weeks PM. Wrist arthrography: the value of fluoroscopic spot filming. *Radiology* 1983;146:555–556.
28. Gilula LA, Weeks PM. Post-traumatic ligamentous instability of the wrist. *Radiology* 1978;129:641–651.
29. Greyson ND, Tepperman PS. Three-phase bone studies in hemiplegia with reflex sympathetic dystrophy and the effect of disuse. *J Nucl Med* 1984;25:423–429.
30. Gundry CR, Kursimoglu-Brahme S, Schwaighofer B, Kang HS, Sartoiris DJ, Resnick D. Is MR better than arthrography for evaluating the ligaments of the wrist? In vitro study. *AJR Am J Roentgenol* 1990;154:337–341.
31. Ham SJ, Konings JG, Wolf RFE, Mooyuart EL. Functional anatomy of the soft tissues of the hand and wrist: in vivo excussion measurement of the flexor pollicis longus tendon using MRI. *Magn Reson Imaging* 1993;11:163–167.
32. Holder LE, Mackinnon SE. Reflex sympathetic dystrophy in the hands: clinical and scintigraphic criteria. *Radiology* 1984;152: 517–522.
33. Howard FM, Fahey T, Wojcik E. Rotary subluxation of the navicular. *Clin Orthop* 1974;104:134–139.
34. Hudson TM, Caragal WJ, Kaye JJ. Isolated rotary subluxation of the carpal navicular. *AJR Am J Roentgenol* 1976;126:601.
35. Kindynis P, Resnick D, Kang HS, Haller J, Satoris DJ. Demonstration of the scapholunate space with radiography. *Radiology* 1990;175:278–290.
36. Lane CG. Detecting occult fracture of the metacarpal head: the Brewerton view. *J Hand Surg* 1977;2:131–133.
37. Levinsohn EM, Palmer AK. Arthrography of the traumatized wrist. Correlation of radiography and the carpal instability series. *Radiology* 1983;146:647–651.
38. Levinsohn ME, Palmer AK, Coren AB, Zinberg E. Wrist arthrography: the value of the three compartment injection technique. *Skeletal Radiol* 1987;16:539–544.
39. Levinsohn ME, Rosen DI, Palmer AK. Wrist arthrography: value of the three-compartment injection method. *Radiology* 1991; 179:231–239.
40. Magid D, Thompson JS, Fishman EK. Computed tomography of the hand and wrist. *Hand Clin* 1991;7:219–234.
41. Maloney MD, Sauser DD, Hanson EC, Wood VE, Theil AE. Adhesive capsulitis of the wrist. Arthrographic diagnosis. *Radiology* 1988;167:187–190.
42. Manaster BJ. Digital wrist arthrography: precision in determining the site of radiocarpal-mid carpal communication. *AJR Am J Roentgenol* 1986;147:563–566.
43. Manaster BJ. The clinical efficacy of the triple-injection wrist arthrography. *Radiology* 1991;178:267–270.
44. Mauer AH. Nuclear medicine in evaluation of the hand and wrist. *Hand Clin* 1991;7:183–200.
45. Metz VM, Mann FA, Gilula LA. Lack of correlation between site of wrist pain and location of noncommunicating defects shown by three-compartment wrist arthrography. *AJR Am J Roentgenol* 1993;160:1239–1243.
46. Metz VM, Mann FA, Gilula LA. Three compartment wrist arthrography: correlation of pain site with uni or bidirectional communication. *AJR Am J Roentgenol* 1993;160:819–822.
47. Nattrass GR, King JW, McMurtry RY, Brant RF. An alternative method for determination of carpal height ratio. *J Bone Joint Surg [Am]* 1994;76A:88–94.
48. Poznanski AK. Useful measurements in the evaluation of hand radiographs. *Hand Clin* 1991;7:21–36.
49. Protas JM, Jackson WR. Evaluating carpal instability with fluoroscopy. *AJR Am J Roentgenol* 1980;135:140–147.
50. Quinn SJ, Belsole RS, Green TL, Rayhack JM. Post-arthrography computed tomography of the wrist: evaluation of the triangular fibrocartilage complex. *Skeletal Radiol* 1989;17:565–569.
51. Quinn SF, Murray W, Watkins T, Kloss J. CT for determining results of treatment of fractures of the wrist. *AJR Am J Roentgenol* 1987;149:109–111.
52. Resnick D. Roentgenographic anatomy of the tendon sheaths of the hand wrist: tenography. *AJR Am J Roentgenol* 1975;124;44.
53. Resnick D, Dalinka MK. Arthrography and tenography of the wrist. In: Dalinka MK, ed. *Arthrography.* New York: Springer-Verlag; 1980.
54. Rosenthal DI, Murray WT, Smith RJ. Finger arthrography. *Radiology* 1980;137:647.

55. Smith DK. Volar carpal ligaments of the wrist: normal appearance on multiplanar reconstruction of three-dimensional Fourier transform MR imaging. *AJR Am J Roentgenol* 1993;161:353–357.
56. Smith DK, Linscheid RL, Amadio PC, Berquist TH, Cooney WP. Scaphoid anatomy: evaluation with complex motion tomography. *Radiology* 1989;173:177–180.
57. Tehranzadeh J, Davenport J, Pas MJ. Scaphoid fracture; evaluation with flexion-extension tomography. *Radiology* 1990;176: 167–170.
58. Terry DW, Ramin JE. The navicular fat stripe. A useful roentgen feature for evaluating wrist trauma. *AJR Am J Roentgenol* 1975;124:25.
59. Viegas SF, Hillman GR, Elder K, Stoner D, Patterson RM. Measurement of carpal bone geometry by computer analysis of three-dimensional CT images. *J Hand Surg [Am]* 1991;18a:341–349.
60. Wechsler RJ, Wehbe MA, Rifkin MD, Edeiken J, Branch HM. Computed tomography diagnosis of distal radioulnar subluxation. *Skeletal Radiol* 1987;16:1–5.
61. Weeks PM, Vanner MW, Steven WG, Gayon D, Gilula LA. Three-dimensional imaging of the wrist. *J Hand Surg [Am]* 1985;10A:32–39.
62. White SJ, Lous DS, Braumstein EM, Hankin FM, Greene TL. Capitate-lunate instability. Recognition by manipulation under fluoroscopy. *AJR Am J Roentgenol* 1984;143:361–364.
63. Yeager BA, Dalinka MK. Radiology of trauma to the wrist: dislocations, fracture dislocations, and instability patterns. *Skeletal Radiol* 1985;13:120–130.
64. Zlatkin MB, Chis PC, Osterman AL, Schmoll MD, Dalinka MK, Kressel HY. Chronic wrist pain: evaluation with high-resolution MR imaging. *Radiology* 1989;173:723–729.

Trauma

65. Adler JB, Shaftan GW. Fractures of the capitate. *J Bone Joint Surg [Am]* 1962;44A:1537–1547.
66. Agee J. Unstable fracture-dislocations of the proximal interphalangeal joint of the fingers: a preliminary report of a new treatment technique. *J Hand Surg* 1978;3:386–389.
67. Albert SM, Wohl MD, Reachtman AM. Treatment of the disrupted radio-ulnar joint. *J Bone Joint Surg [Am]* 1963;45A: 1373–1381.
68. Baldwin LW, Miller DL, Lockhart LD, Evans EB. Metacarpophalangeal-joint dislocations of the fingers. *J Bone Joint Surg [Am]* 1967;49A:1587–1590.
69. Bartone NF, Grieco RV. Fractures of the triquetrum. *J Bone Joint Surg [Am]* 1956;38A:353–356.
70. Bellinghausen H, Gilula LA, Young LV, Weeks PM. Post-traumatic palmar carpal subluxation. *J Bone Joint Surg [Am]* 1983;65A:998–1006.
71. Belsole R. Physiologic fixation of displaced and unstable fractures of the hand. *Orthop Clin North Am* 1980;11:393–404.
72. Berquist TH. *Imaging of orthopedic trauma.* 2nd ed. New York: Raven Press; 1992.
72a. Berquist TH. *Imaging of sports injuries.* Gaithersburg, MD: Aspen Press; 1992.
73. Berquist TH. *MRI of the musculoskeletal system.* 2nd ed. New York: Raven Press; 1990.
74. Bowen TL. Injuries of the hamate bone. *Hand* 1973;5:235–238.
75. Bowers WH. Management of small joint injuries in the hand. *Clin Orthop* 1983;14:798.
76. Bradway JK, Amadio PC, Cooney WP. Open reduction and internal fixation of displaced, comminuted intra-articular fractures of the distal end of the radius. *J Bone Joint Surg [Am]* 1989;71A: 839–847.
77. Bryan RS, Dobyns JH. Fractures of the carpal bones other than lunate and navicular. *Clin Orthop* 1980;149:107–111.
78. Burton RJ. Fractures of the proximal phalanx of the finger. *Contemp Surg* 1977;11:32–37.
79. Carter PR, Eaton RG, Littler JW. Ununited fracture of the hook of the hamate. A case report. *J Bone Joint Surg [Am]* 1975;57A: 276–277.
80. Clyburn TA. Dynamic external fixation for comminuted intra-articular fractures of the distal end of the radius. *J Bone Joint Surg [Am]* 1987;69A:248–254.
81. Cooney WP III, Beckenbaugh RD, Bryan RS, Dobyns JH. External minifixators: clinical applications and techniques. In: Johnston M, ed. *Advances in external fixation.* Chicago: Year Book Medical; 1980.
82. Cooney WP III, Dobyns JH, Linscheid RL. Fractures of the scaphoid: a rational approach to management. *Clin Orthop* 1980;149:90–97.
83. Cooney WP III, Dobyns JH, Linscheid RL. Complications of Colles' fractures. *J Bone Joint Surg [Am]* 1980;62A:613–619.
84. Cooney WP III, Linscheid RL, Dobyns JH. External pin fixation for unstable Colles' fractures. *J Bone Joint Surg [Am]* 1979;61A: 840–845.
85. Cooney WP III, Linscheid RL, Dobyns JH. Fractures and dislocations of the wrist. In: Rockwood CA, Green DP, Bucholz, eds. *Fractures in adults.* 3rd ed. Vol. 1. Philadelphia: JB Lippincott; 1991:563–678.
86. Cooney WP III, Smith DK. External fixation of the upper extremity. In: Griffin BP, ed. *Inst course lectures AAOS.* CV Mosby, 1987;36:455–496.
87. Cordrey LJ, Ferrer-Torells M. Management of fractures of the greater multangular. *J Bone Joint Surg [Am]* 1960;42A:1111–1118.
88. Crawford GP. Screw fixation for certain fractures of the phalanges and metacarpals. *J Bone Joint Surg [Am]* 1976;58A:439–451.
89. Cziffer E. The use of the Manuflex disposable mini external fixator. *Orthopedics* 1989;12:163–166.
90. Desser TS, McCarthy S, Trumble T. Scaphoid fractures and Kienböck's disease of the lunate: MR imaging with histopathologic correlation. *Magn Reson Imaging* 1990;8:357–361.
91. De Oliveira JC. Barton's fractures. *J Bone Joint Surg [Am]* 1973;55A.
92. Dingman PVC. Resection of the distal end of the ulna (Darrach operation). End-result study of 24 cases. *J Bone Joint Surg [Am]* 1952;34A:893–900.
93. Dunn AW. Fractures and dislocations of the carpus. *Surg Clin North Am* 1972;52:1513.
94. Düppe H, Joknell O, Lundbarg G, Karlsson M, Redlund-Johnell I. Long-term results of fracture of the scaphoid. *J Bone Joint Surg [Am]* 1994;76A:249–252.
95. Edwards HC. Mechanism and treatment of backfire fracture. *J Bone Joint Surg [Br]* 1965;47B:724–727.
96. Ellis J. Smith's and Barton's fracture—a method of treatment. *J Bone Joint Surg [Am]* 1956;38A:681–684.
97. Fahmy NRM. The stockport serpentine spring system for the treatment of displaced intra-articular phalangeal fractures. *J Hand Surg [Br]* 1990;15B:303–311.
98. Fenton RL. The naviculo-capitate fracture syndrome. *J Bone Joint Surg [Am]* 1956;38A:681–684.
99. Fernandez DL. Radial osteotomy and Bowers arthroplasty for malunited fractures of the distal end of the radius. *J Bone Joint Surg [Am]* 1988;70A:1538–1550.
100. Fernandez DL. Irreducible radiocarpal fracture-dislocation and radioulnar dissociation with entrapment of the ulnar nerve, artery, and flexor profundus II-V—case report. *J Hand Surg* 1981;6:456–461.
101. Fisher MR, Rogers LF, Hendrix RW, Gilula LA. Carpometacarpal dislocation. *Crit Rev Diagn Imaging* 1984;22:95–126.
102. Fisk GR. An overview of injuries of the wrist. *Clin Orthop* 1980;149:137–144.
103. Frykman G. Fractures of the distal radius including sequelae—shoulder-hand-finger syndrome, disturbance in the distal radioulnar joint, and impairment of nerve function. *Acta Orthop Scand Suppl* 1967;108:1–55.
104. Frykman GK, Tooma GS, Bayko K, Henderson R. Comparison of eleven external fixators for treatment of unstable wrist fractures. *J Hand Surg [Am]* 1989;14A:247–254.
105. Funk DA, Wood MB. Concurrent fractures of the ipsilateral scaphoid and radial head. *J Bone Joint Surg [Am]* 1988;70A:134–136.
106. Garland JJ Jr, Wesley CW. Evaluation of Ledel Colles' fractures. *J Bone Joint Surg [Am]* 1951;33A:895–907.
107. Gelberman RH, Welock BS, Siegel DB. Fractures and nonunions

of the carpal scaphoid. *J Bone Joint Surg [Am]* 1989;71A:1560–1565.
108. Gilula LA, Destouet JM, Weeks PM, Young LV, Wray RC. Roentgen diagnosis of the painful wrist. *Clin Orthop* 1984;187:52–64.
109. Gingrass RP, Fehring B, Matloub H. Intraosseous wiring of complex hand fractures. *Plast Reconstr Surg* 1980;66:383–394.
110. Green DP, Anderson JR. Closed reduction and percutaneous fixation of fractured phalanges. *J Bone Joint Surg [Am]* 1973;55A:1651–1653.
111. Green DP, O'Brien ET. Classification and management of carpal dislocations. *Clin Orthop* 1980;149:55–72.
112. Green DP, Rowland SA. Fractures and dislocations of the hand. In: Rockwood GA, Green DP, Bucholz RW, eds. *Rockwood and Green's fractures in adults*. 3rd ed. Vol. 1. Philadelphia: JB Lippincott; 1991:441–561.
113. Grundberg AB. Intramedullary fixation for fractures of the hand. *J Hand Surg* 1981;6:568–573.
114. Hamlin C. Traumatic disruption of the distal radioulnar joint. *Am J Sports Med* 1977;5:93–96.
115. Hill NA. Fractures and dislocations of the carpus. *Orthop Clin North Am* 1970;1:275–284.
116. Hsu JD, Curtis RM. Carpometacarpal dislocations of the ulnar side of the hand. *J Bone Joint Surg [Am]* 1970;52A:927–930.
117. Hughston JC. Fracture of the distal radial shaft—mistakes in management. *J Bone Joint Surg [Am]* 1957;39A:249–264.
118. Hui FC, Linscheid RL. Ulnotriquetral augmentation tenodesis: a reconstructive procedure for dorsal subluxation of the distal radioulnar joint. *J Hand Joint Surg* 1982;7:230–236.
119. Hung LK, So WS, Leing PC. Combined extramedullary K-wire and inter-osseous wire loop for fixation of finger fractures. *J Hand Surg [Br]* 1989;14B:171–176.
120. Johnson RP. The acutely injured wrist and its residuals. *Clin Orthop* 1980;149:33–44.
121. Jupiter JB. Fractures of the distal end of the radius. *J Bone Joint Surg [Am]* 1991;73A:461–469.
122. Jupiter JB, Sheppard JE. Tension wire fixation of avulsion fractures of the hand. *Clin Orthop* 1987;214:113–120.
123. Kozin SH, Wood MB. Early soft tissue complications after fractures of the distal part of the radius. *J Bone Joint Surg [Am]* 1993;75A:144–153.
124. Lawlis JF, Gunther SF. Carpometacarpal dislocations. *J Bone Joint Surg [Am]* 1991;73A:52–58.
125. Lewis RC, Nordeyke M, Duncan K. Expandable intramedullary device for treatment of fractures of the hand. *Clin Orthop* 1987;214:85–92.
126. Lister GD. Intraosseous wiring of the digital skeleton. *J Hand Surg* 1978;3:427–435.
127. Lucas GL. Internal fixation in the hand: a review of indications and methods. *Orthopedics* 1980;3:1083–1092.
128. MacLaughlin HL. Complex "locked" dislocations of the metacarpophalangeal joints. *J Trauma* 1965;5:683–688.
129. Mann FA, Wilson AJ, Gilula LA. Radiographic evaluation of the wrist: what does the hand surgeon want to know? *Radiology* 1992;184:15–24.
130. Maudsley RH, Chen SC. Screw fixation in the management of the fractured carpal scaphoid. *J Bone Joint Surg [Br]* 1972;54B:432–441.
131. Mayfield JK, Johnson RP, Kilcoyne RK. Carpal dislocations: pathomechanics and progressive perilunar instability. *J Hand Surg* 1980;5:226–241.
132. McElfresh EC, Dobyns JH, O'Brien ET. Management of fracture-dislocation of the proximal interphalangeal joint by extension-block splinting. *J Bone Joint Surg [Am]* 1972;54A:1705–1711.
133. Meyers MH, Wells R, Harvey JP Jr. Naviculocapitate fracture syndrome. *J Bone Joint Surg [Am]* 1971;53A:1383–1390.
134. Mikic ZD. Galeazzi fracture-dislocations. *J Bone Joint Surg [Am]* 1975;57A:1071–1080.
135. Mikio T, Uamamuro T, Kotoura Y, Tsuji T, Shimizu K, Itakura H. Rupture of the extensor tendons of the fingers. *J Bone Joint Surg [Am]* 1986;68A:610–614.
136. Milch H. Fracture of the hamate bone. *J Bone Joint Surg* 1934;16:459–462.
137. Morrissy RT, Nalebuff EA. Dislocation of the distal radioulnar joint: anatomy and clues to prompt diagnosis. *Clin Orthop* 1979;144:154–158.
138. Nalebuff EA. Isolated anterior carpometacarpal dislocation of the fifth finger. Classification and case report. *J Trauma* 1968;8:1119–1123.
139. Nielsen PT, Hederboe J, Thommesen P. Bone scintigraphy in the evaluation of fracture of the carpal scaphoid bone. *Acta Orthop Scand* 1983;54:303–306.
140. Normal A, Nelson J, Green S. Fracture of the hamate: radiographic signs. *Radiology* 1985;154:49–53.
141. North ER, Eaton RG. Volar dislocation of the fifth metacarpal. *J Bone Joint Surg [Am]* 1980;62A:657–659.
142. Olsen N, Schousen P, Dirksen H, Christoffersen JK. Regional scintimetry in scaphoid fractures. *Acta Orthop Scand* 1983;54:380–382.
143. Peltier LF. Eponymic fractures: John Rhea Barton and Barton's fractures. *Surgery* 1953;34:960–970.
144. Peltier LF. Eponymic fractures: Robert William Smith and Smith's fracture. *Surgery* 1959;45:1035–1042.
144a. Prince H, Worlock P. The small AO external fixator in treatment of distal forearm fractures. *J Hand Surg* 1988;13B:294–297.
145. Radford JP, Matthewson MH, Meggilt BF. The Herbert screw for delayed and nonunion of scaphoid fractures: a review of 50 cases. *J Hand Surg [Br]* 1990;15B:455–459.
146. Ruby LK. Common hand injuries in the athlete. *Orthop Clin North Am* 1980;11:819–839.
147. Russe O. Fracture of the carpal navicular. *J Bone Joint Surg [Am]* 1960;42A:759–768.
148. Russell TB. Intercarpal dislocations and fracture-dislocations. A review of 59 cases. *J Bone Joint Surg [Br]* 1949;31B:524–531.
149. Sebald JR, Dobyns JH, Linscheid RL. The natural history of collapse deformities of the wrist. *Clin Orthop* 1974;104:140–148.
150. Seitz WH, Froimson AI, Brooks DB, Postak PD, Parker RD, LaPorte JM, Greenwald AS, Phil D. Biomechanical analysis of pin placement and pin size for external fixation of distal radius fractures. *Clin Orthop* 1990;251:207–212.
151. Shall J, Cohn BT, Froimson AI. Acute compartment syndrome of the forearm in association with fracture of the distal end of the radius. *J Bone Joint Surg [Am]* 1986;68A:1451–1454.
152. Smith DK, Gilula LA, Amadio PC. Dorsal lunate tilt (DISI configuration): sign of scaphoid fracture displacement. *Radiology* 1990;176:497–499.
153. Smith DK, Linscheid RL, Amadio PC, Berquist TH, Cooney WP. Scaphoid anatomy: evaluation with complex motion tomography. *Radiology* 1989;173:177–180.
154. Smith RJ. Post-traumatic instability of the metacarpophalangeal joint of the thumb. *J Bone Joint Surg [Am]* 1977;59A:14–21.
155. Stahelin A, Pfeiffer K, Sennwald G, Segmuller G. Determining carpal collapse. *J Bone Joint Surg [Am]* 1989;71A:1400–1405.
156. Stark HH. Troublesome fractures and dislocations of the hand. *Instr Course Lect* 1970;19:130–149.
157. Stark HH, Chao E, Zemel NP, Rickard TA, Ashworth CR. Fracture of the hook of the hamate. *J Bone Joint Surg [Am]* 1989;71A:1202–1207.
158. Stark HH, Jobe FW, Boyes JH, Ashworth CR. Fracture of the hook of the hamate in athletes. *J Bone Joint Surg [Am]* 1977;59A:575–582.
159. Stener B. Displacement of the ruptured ulnar collateral ligament of the metacarpophalangeal joint of the thumb. *J Bone Joint Surg [Br]* 1962;44B:869–879.
160. Swanson AB. Fractures involving the digits of the hand. *Orthop Clin North Am* 1970;01:261–274.
161. Talersnik J. Carpal instability. *J Bone Joint Surg [Am]* 1988;70A:1262–1268.
162. Tehranzadeh J, Davenport J, Pais MJ. Scaphoid fracture: evaluation with flexion-extension tomography. *Radiology* 1990;176:167–170.
163. Thomas FB. Reduction of Smith's fractures. *J Bone Joint Surg [Br]* 1957;39B:463–470.
164. Thompson GH, Grant TT. Barton's fracture-reverse Barton's fracture: confusing eponyms. *Clin Orthop* 1977;122:210–220.
165. Torisu T. Fracture of the hook of the hamate by golf-swing. *Clin Orthop* 1972;83:91–94.
166. Varela CD, Carr JB. Closed intramedullary nailing of metacarpal and phalanx fractures. *Orthopedics* 1990;13:213–215.

167. Verdan C, Narakas A. Fracture and pseudoarthrosis of the scaphoid. *Surg Clin North Am* 1968;48:1083–1095.
168. Vesley DG. The distal radioulnar joint. *Clin Orthop* 1967;51:75–91.
169. Viegas SF, Ferren EL, Self J, Tencer AF. Comparative mechanical properties of various Kirschner wire configurations are transverse and oblique phalangeal fractures. *J Hand Surg [Am]* 1988;13A:246–253.
170. Weber ER, Chao EYS. An experimental approach to the mechanism of scaphoid waist fracture. *J Hand Surg* 1978;3:142–148.
171. Wehbe MA, Schneider LA. Mallet fractures. *J Bone Joint Surg [Am]* 1984;66A:658–669.
172. Weiss A, Weiland AJ, Moore R, Welges EFS. Radial shortening for Kienböchs disease. *J Bone Joint Surg [Am]* 1991;73A:384–391.
173. Wesely MS, Barenfield PA. Trans-scaphoid, transcapitate, transtriquetral, perilunate fracture-dislocation of the wrist. *J Bone Joint Surg [Am]* 1972;54A:1073–1078.
174. Wilson JN, Rowland SA. Fracture-dislocation of the proximal interphalangeal joint of the finger. Treatment by open reduction and internal fixation. *J Bone Joint Surg [Am]* 1966;48A:493–505.
175. Yeager BA, Dalinka MK. Radiology of trauma of the wrist: dislocations, fracture dislocations, and instability patterns. *Skeletal Radiol* 1985;13:120–130.

Arthroplasty

176. Amadio PC. Arthroplasty of the proximal interphalangeal joint. In: Morrey BF, ed. *Joint replacement arthroplasty.* New York: Churchill Livingstone; 1991:147–157.
177. Beckenbaugh RD. Implant arthroplasty in the rheumatoid hand and wrist: current state of the art in the United States. *J Hand Surg* 1983;8:675–678.
178. Beckenbaugh RD. Total joint arthroplasty: the wrist. *Mayo Clin Proc* 1979;54:513–515.
179. Beckenbaugh RD. Arthroplasty of the wrist. In: Morrey BF. *Joint replacement arthroplasty.* New York: Churchill Livingstone; 1991:195–215.
180. Beckenbaugh RD, Dobyns JH, Linscheid RL, Bryan RS. Review and analysis of silicone-rubber metacarpophalangeal implants. *J Bone Joint Surg [Am]* 1972;58A:483–487.
181. Braun RM. Total joint replacement at the thumb—preliminary report. *J Hand Surg* 1982;7:245–251.
182. Comstock CP, Louis DS, Eckenrode JF. Silicone wrist implant: long-term follow-up study. *J Hand Surg [Am]* 1988;13A:205–210.
183. Cooney WP III. Arthroplasty of the thumb axis. In: Morrey BF, ed. *Joint replacement arthroplasty.* New York: Churchill Livingstone; 1991:173–194.
184. Cooney WP III, Beckenbaugh RD, Linscheid RL. Total wrist arthroplasty: problems with implant failure. *Clin Orthop* 1984;187:121–128.
185. Cooney WP III, Linscheid RL, Askew L. Total arthroplasty of the thumb trapeziometacarpal joint. *Clin Orthop* 1987;220:35–45.
186. Doi K, Kuwata N, Kavai S. Alumina ceramic finger implants: a preliminary biomaterial and clinical evaluation. *J Hand Surg [Am]* 1984;9A:740–749.
187. Eaton R. Replacement of the trapezium for arthritis of the basal articulations: a new technique with stabilization by fusion. *J Bone Joint Surg [Am]* 1979;61A:76.
188. Eaton R, Lane L, Littler JW, et al. Ligament reconstruction for the painful thumb metacarpal joint: a long term assessment. *J Hand Surg [Am]* 1984;9A:692.
189. Eaton RG, Malerech MM. Volar plate arthroplasty of the proximal interphalangeal joint: a review of 10 years experience. *J Hand Surg* 1980;5:260–268.
190. Fatti JF, Palmer AF, Greenky S, Mosher JF. Long-term results of Swanson interpositional wrist arthroplasty: part II. *J Hand Surg [Am]* 1991;16A:432–437.
191. Figgie HE III, Ranawut CS, Ingles AE, Straub LM, Mow C. Preliminary results of total wrist arthroplasty in patients with rheumatoid arthritis using a trispherical total wrist arthroplasty. *J Arthroplasty* 1988;3:9.
192. Goldner JL, Gould JS, Urbaniak JR, McCollum DE. Metacarpophalangeal joint arthroplasty with silicone-Dacron prosthesis (Niebauer type): six and a half years experience. *J Hand Surg* 1977;2:200–211.
193. Howard FM, Simpson LA, Belsole RJ. Silastic condylar arthroplasty. *Clin Orthop* 1985;195:144–150.
194. Iselin F, Pradat G. Resection arthroplasty with Swanson's implant for post-traumatic stiffness of the proximal interphalangeal joints. *Bull Hosp Jt Dis Orthop Inst* 1984;44:233–247.
195. Jennings CD, Livingstone DF. Convex condylar arthroplasty of the basal joint of the thumb: failure under load. *J Hand Surg [Am]* 1990;15A:573–581.
195a. Kessler I. Silicone arthroplasty of the trapeziometacarpal joint. *J Bone Joint Surg [Br]* 1973;55B:285–291.
196. Kirschenbaum D, Schneider LH, Adams DC, Cody RP. Arthroplasty of the metacarpophalangeal in patients who have rheumatoid arthritis. *J Bone Joint Surg [Am]* 1993;75A:3–12.
197. Lamberta FJ, Ferlic DC, Clayton ML. Volz total wrist arthroplasty in rheumatoid arthritis. A preliminary report. *J Hand Surg* 1980;5:245–252.
198. Lane CS. Les implants in Dacron-silicone are niveau des articulations interphalangiennes. *Ann Chir* 1975;29:1011–1014.
199. Leslie BM, O'Malley M, Thilodeau AA. A forty-three year follow-up of a Vitallium scaphoid arthroplasty. *J Hand Surg [Am]* 1991;16A:465–468.
200. Linscheid RL, Beckenbaugh RD. Arthroplasty of the metacarpophalangeal joint. In: Morrey BF, ed. *Joint replacement arthroplasty.* New York: Churchill Livingstone; 1991:159–172.
201. Linscheid RL, Beckenbaugh RD, Dobyns JH. Total wrist arthroplasty. In: Inglis AE, ed. *AAOS symposium on total joint replacement of the upper extremity.* St. Louis: CV Mosby; 1982: 255–264.
202. Linscheid RL, Beckenbaugh RD, Dobyns JH, Cooney WP III. Metacarpophalangeal arthroplasty with Steffee prosthesis. In: Inglis AE, ed. *AAOS symposium on total joint replacement of the upper extremity.* St. Louis: CV Mosby; 1982:187–198.
203. Linscheid RL, Cooney WP III, Dobyns JH. Metacarpophalangeal arthroplasty. In: Inglis AE, ed. *AAOS symposium on total joint replacement of the upper extremity.* St. Louis: CV Mosby; 1982: 289–299.
204. Linscheid RL, Dobyns JH. Total joint arthroplasty: the hand. *Mayo Clin Proc* 1979;54:516–526.
205. Linscheid RL, Dobyns JH, Beckenbaugh RD, Cooney WP III. Proximal interphalangeal joint arthroplasty with a total joint design. *Mayo Clin Proc* 1979;54:227–240.
206. Menon J. Total wrist replacement using the modified Volz prosthesis. *J Bone Joint Surg [Am]* 1987;69A:998–1006.
207. Meuli HC. Arthroplasty of the wrist. *Clin Orthop* 1980;149:118–125.
208. Ranawat CS, Green NA, Inglis AE, Straub LR. Spherical-tri-axial total wrist replacement. In: Inglis AE, ed. *AAOS symposium on total joint replacement of the upper extremity.* St. Louis: CV Mosby; 1982:265–272.
209. Schultz RJ. Total metacarpophalangeal joint arthroplasty with limited metacarpal head resection. In: Inglis AE, ed. *AAOS symposium on total joint replacement of the upper extremity.* St. Louis: CV Mosby; 1982:199–215.
210. Smith R, Atkinson R, Jupiter B. Silicone synovitis of the wrist. *J Hand Surg [Am]* 1985;10A:47–60.
211. Sondergaard L, Konradsen L, Rechnagel K. Long-term follow-up of the cemented Caffiniere prosthesis for trapezio-metacarpal arthroplasty. *J Hand Surg [Br]* 1991;16B:428–430.
212. Steffee A. History, design and development of Stiffee metacarpophalangeal prosthesis. In: Inglis AE, ed. *AAOS symposium on total joint replacement of the upper extremity.* St. Louis: CV Mosby; 1982:179–186.
213. Steffee A, Beckenbaugh RD, Linscheid RL, Dobyns JH. The development, technique and early clinical results of total joint replacement for the metacarpophalangeal joint of the fingers. *Orthopedics* 1981;4:175–180.
214. Stothard J, Thompson AE, Sherris D. Correction of ulnar drift during Silastic metacarpophalangeal joint arthroplasty. *J Hand Surg [Br]* 1991;16B:61–65.
215. Straub LR. Anatomy of the metacarpophalangeal joint in rheumatoid arthritis: etiology of ulnar drift. In: Inglis AE, ed. *AAOS*

symposium on total joint replacement of the upper extremity. St. Louis: CV Mosby; 1982:171–178.

216. Swanson AB. Flexible implant arthroplasty for arthritic disabilities of the radiocarpal joint. *Orthop Clin North Am* 1973;4:383–394.
217. Swanson AB, de Groot Swanson G. Joint replacement in the rheumatoid metacarpophalangeal joint. In: Inglis AE, ed. *AAOS symposium on total joint replacement of the upper extremity.* St. Louis: CV Mosby; 1982:217–235.
218. Swanson AB, de Groot Swanson G. Flexible implant arthroplasty of the radiocarpal joint: surgical technique and long-term results. In: Inglis AE, ed. *AAOS symposium on total joint replacement of the upper extremity.* St. Louis: CV Mosby; 1982:301–315.
219. Swanson AB, de Groot Swanson G, Leonard J. Post-operative rehabilitation program for flexible implant arthroplasty of the finger. In: Inglis AE, ed. *AAOS symposium on total joint replacement of the upper extremity.* St. Louis: CV Mosby; 1982:238–253.
220. Swanson AB, de Groot Swanson G, Watermeir JJ. Trapezium implant arthroplasty: long-term evaluation of 150 cases. *J Hand Surg* 1981;6:125–141.
221. Toby EB, Glisson RR, Seaber AV, Urbaniak JR. Prosthetic silicone scaphoid strains: effects of intercarpal fusion. *J Hand Surg [Am]* 1991;16A:469–473.
222. Varma SK, Milward TM. The Nicolle finger joint prosthesis: a reappraisal. *Br J Hand Surg* 1991;16B:187–190.
223. Vicar AJ, Burton RI. Surgical management of the rheumatoid wrist-fusion or arthroplasty. *J Hand Surg [Am]* 1986;11A:790–797.
224. Viegas SF, Patterson RM, Peterson PD, Crassley M, Foster R. The silicone scaphoid: a biomechanical study. *J Hand Surg [Am]* 1991;16A:91–97.
225. Volz RG. Total wrist arthroplasty. *Clin Orthop* 1984;187:112–120.
226. Volz RG. Total wrist arthroplasty: a clinical and biomechanical analysis. In: Inglis AE, ed. *AAOS symposium on total joint replacement of the upper extremity.* St. Louis: CV Mosby; 1982: 273–287.
227. Volz RD. The development of a total wrist arthroplasty. *Clin Orthop* 1976;116;209–214.
228. Zancolli EA, Ziadenberg C, Zancolli E. Biomechanics of the trapeziometacarpal joint. *Clin Orthop* 1987;220:14–26.

Arthrodesis

229. Campbell CJ, Keokarn T. Total and subtotal arthrodesis of the wrist. *J Bone Joint Surg [Am]* 1964;46A:1520–1523.
230. Carroll R, Dick H. Arthrodesis of the wrist for rheumatoid arthritis. *J Bone Joint Surg [Am]* 1971;53A:1365–1369.
231. Culver JE, Fleegler EJ. Osteoarthritis of the distal interphalangeal joint. *Hand Clin* 1987;3:385.
232. Ely LW. Study of joint tuberculosis. *Surg Gynecol Obstet* 1910;10:561–572.
233. Hill NA. Small joint arthrodesis. In: Green DP, ed. *Operative hand surgery.* 2nd ed. Vol. 1. New York: Churchill Livingstone; 1988:121.
234. Moberg E. Arthrodesis of finger joints. *Surg Clin North Am* 1960;40:465.
235. Vicar AJ, Burton RI. Surgical management of the rheumatoid wrist-fusion or arthroplasty. *J Hand Surg [Am]* 1986;11A:790–797.
236. Viegas SF, Rimoldi R, Patterson R. Modified technique of intramedullary fixation of the wrist. *J Hand Surg [Am]* 1989;14A: 618–623.
237. Wood MB. Wrist arthrodesis using dorsal radial bone graft. *J Hand Surg [Am]* 1987;12A:208–212.
238. Wood MB. Alternative reconstruction procedures. In: Morrey BF, ed. *Joint replacement arthroplasty.* New York: Churchill Livingstone; 1991:217–235.

Imaging Atlas of Orthopedic Appliances and Prostheses,
edited by T.H. Berquist.
Mayo Clinic Foundation © 1995.
Published by Raven Press, Ltd., New York.

CHAPTER 14

Musculoskeletal Neoplasms

Thomas H. Berquist and Mary I. O'Connor

Musculoskeletal neoplasms are treated with surgical excision, radiation therapy, chemotherapy, and combination therapeutic approaches. This chapter concentrates on orthopedic procedures used to treat neoplasms. Techniques and implants not already presented in previous chapters are emphasized.

PREOPERATIVE EVALUATION

Decisions regarding the approach to musculoskeletal neoplasms may be relatively simple (i.e., localized benign lesion) or complex, depending on the histologic type; location; bone and soft tissue involvement; and patient-related factors, such as age, activity, and the prognosis of the lesion. Limb-salvage procedures, defined as surgical techniques to restore skeletal continuity after en bloc excision of musculoskeletal neoplasms, have become more feasible and performed more frequently in recent years.[17,21,24,29,30] Decisions as to the type of procedure depend on clinical and imaging staging of lesions preoperatively.[1–3,17,29,30] Limb-salvage procedures, often with extensive reconstruction, are usually considered when the lesion is located in a region that allows complete resection with a wide surgical margin. Preoperative chemotherapy is often used in conjunction with these procedures. Limb-salvage procedures are generally contraindicated in patients with neurovascular encasement, which would result in reduced function of the extremity after resection, and in patients with significant pathologic fractures, which might result in the dissemination of tumor cells.[17,29,30] Lower-extremity procedures that may compromise growth in an immature skeleton can also be a problem. However, new prosthetic designs and other surgical options do not definitely exclude limb-salvage procedures in children in whom the growth plate is at risk.[17,45,54] When considering limb-salvage procedures, the clinician must consider the risk of local recurrence, long-term survival rate, functional outcome compared with amputation, psychological benefit, and the immediate and delayed morbidities of the surgical procedure.[17]

Functional analysis can be used pre- and postoperatively to evaluate patients. Enneking[12] and Enneking et al.[14] developed a 35-point system (category range, 0 to 5) with seven categories for evaluation or scoring. The criteria include (1) motion, (2) pain, (3) stability, (4) deformity, (5) strength, (6) functional activity, and (7) emotional acceptance.

Imaging plays a significant role in detection, staging, and operative planning for the treatment of musculoskeletal neoplasms. Routine radiographs, computed tomography (CT), magnetic resonance imaging (MRI), radionuclide scans, and angiography may be used for diagnosing, characterizing, and staging the lesions.[1–4,13,18,24,35] The extent of bone, soft tissue, neurovascular, and distant (i.e., ship lesions or metastases) tumor involvement should be clearly defined prior to treatment plan preparation.[1–4,13]

When selecting the imaging techniques to define the type and extent of the lesion appropriately, it is important for the radiologist to understand the staging systems used. The Musculoskeletal Tumor Society (MSTS) staging system is commonly used for musculoskeletal neoplasms.[11,13,15] This system is based on the tumor grade (G), the tumor site (T), and the presence of local or distant metastasis (M). Histologically low-grade lesions (Table 14-1) are classified as G1 and high-grade lesions, as

T. H. Berquist: Mayo Medical School and Department of Diagnostic Radiology, Mayo Clinic Jacksonville, Jacksonville, Florida 32224.

M. I. O'Connor: Department of Orthopedics, Mayo Medical School and Mayo Clinic Jacksonville, Jacksonville, Florida 32224.

TABLE 14-1. *Staging of malignant musculoskeletal neoplasms*[11,12,15]

Stage	Grade	Site	Metastasis
I			
IA	G1	T1	No metastasis
IB	G1	T2	No metastasis
II			
IIA	G2	T1	No metastasis
IIB	G2	T2	No metastasis
III	G1 or G2	T1 or T2	Metastasis

G1, low grade histologically; G2, high grade histologically; T1, intracompartmental (i.e., confined to bone); T2, extracompartmental (i.e., extends beyond bone).

G2. Tumors that are confined to their compartment (i.e., intraosseous with no extraosseous extension) are classified as T1 and tumors that extend beyond bone or their compartment, as T2. On the basis of these categories and the presence or absence of metastasis, the MSTS system divides tumors into three stages (Table 14-1).[11,13,15] Stage I lesions are low grade (G1) without metastases. Subcategories are included, depending on whether the lesion is intracompartmental (stage IA) or there is extracompartmental extension (stage IB). Stage II lesions are high grade (G2) but there are no metastases. Again, the lesions may be intracompartmental (stage IIA) or extracompartmental (stage IIB). Stage III lesions have metastatic disease and may be high or low grade with intra- or extracompartmental disease locally (Table 14-1).[11,13,15]

The imaging of primary skeletal tumors, soft tissue neoplasms, and potential metastases requires several imaging techniques to optimize their detection and staging. Significant improvement in these capabilities has been achieved with CT and MRI. The ability to predict the histologic type of lesions is still imperfect.[1-4]

Primary Skeletal Lesions

Routine radiographs are still useful for the detection of benign and malignant skeletal neoplasms. The appearance of benign and malignant lesions is well documented, and the ability to characterize lesions on routine radiographs is well established.[1-4] In addition, CT is useful in patients with subtle bone or soft tissue calcification or when there is thin cortical bone and little marrow (e.g., scapula, ilium, and fibula; Fig. 14-1).[2] Radionuclide imaging can be used for lesion detection and to determine the extent of osseous involvement. However, MRI has become the most commonly used staging technique for local disease because of its superior soft tissue contrast and ability to evaluate marrow and soft tissue involvement (Fig. 14-2).

The entire osseous structure should be included on MRI scans. This may require the body coil or a license plate coil. T2-weighted sequences (spin-echo [SE] TR 2,000/TE 80/20) are most often used for cortical, periosteal, and soft tissue involvement. A STIR sequence can be used for subtle changes as a result of its increased contrast and improved lesion conspicuousness. Gradient-echo sequences or vascular protocols may be used to evaluate vascular involvement. T1-weighted (SE 500/20) or fat-suppressed T2-weighted or STIR sequences can be used for marrow involvement. The images should be obtained in at least two planes. An oblique or off-axis plane may be required to depict entire the osseous structure within the image plane so the extent of signal abnormality can be more accurately measured (Fig. 14-3).[1-4]

Angiography may be necessary in some cases for a classification of the anatomy, definition of vascular involvement (encasement or displacement), and evaluation of neovascularity and the status of run-off vessels (Fig. 14-4). Angiography can also be used preoperatively to embolize tumor vessels or to administer chemotherapy infusions prior to surgery.[34] Figure 14-5 demonstrates the utility of various imaging techniques in a young patient with a chondrosarcoma with extensive extraosseous involvement.

Soft Tissue Neoplasms

Routine radiographs are useful to evaluate bone and soft tissue calcification or other soft tissue changes that may be useful in selecting the most definitive radiographic studies. In most cases, MRI is the technique of choice for characterizing and staging soft tissue tumors. Features such as signal inhomogeneity, irregular margins, and neurovascular involvement are more commonly seen with malignant tumors.[1,3] At least two image planes and two pulse sequences are required to characterize and evaluate the extent of soft tissue tumors (Fig. 14-6). Generally, SE T1- and T2-weighted sequences are sufficient. Occasionally, STIR and angiographic sequences are required. Dynamic gadolinium studies are still being investigated.[1,3,16] Angiography may be useful in selected cases.[34]

Metastasis

For the staging of new primary neoplasms, bone scintigraphy provides a good skeletal screening technique for most neoplasms.[1,18] Multiple myeloma, osteosclerotic myeloma, and some metastases are not as clearly defined with bone scintigraphy. In addition, MRI can be useful because the image features are more specific and the technique is also sensitive.[1,3] Screening techniques using phased-array spine coils with sagittal T1-weighted sequences and coronal T1-weighted sequences of the pelvis and upper femurs can be performed quickly. When necessary, fat-suppressed T2-weighted or STIR sequences can be used to define more subtle changes (Fig. 14-7). In

(text continues on page 932)

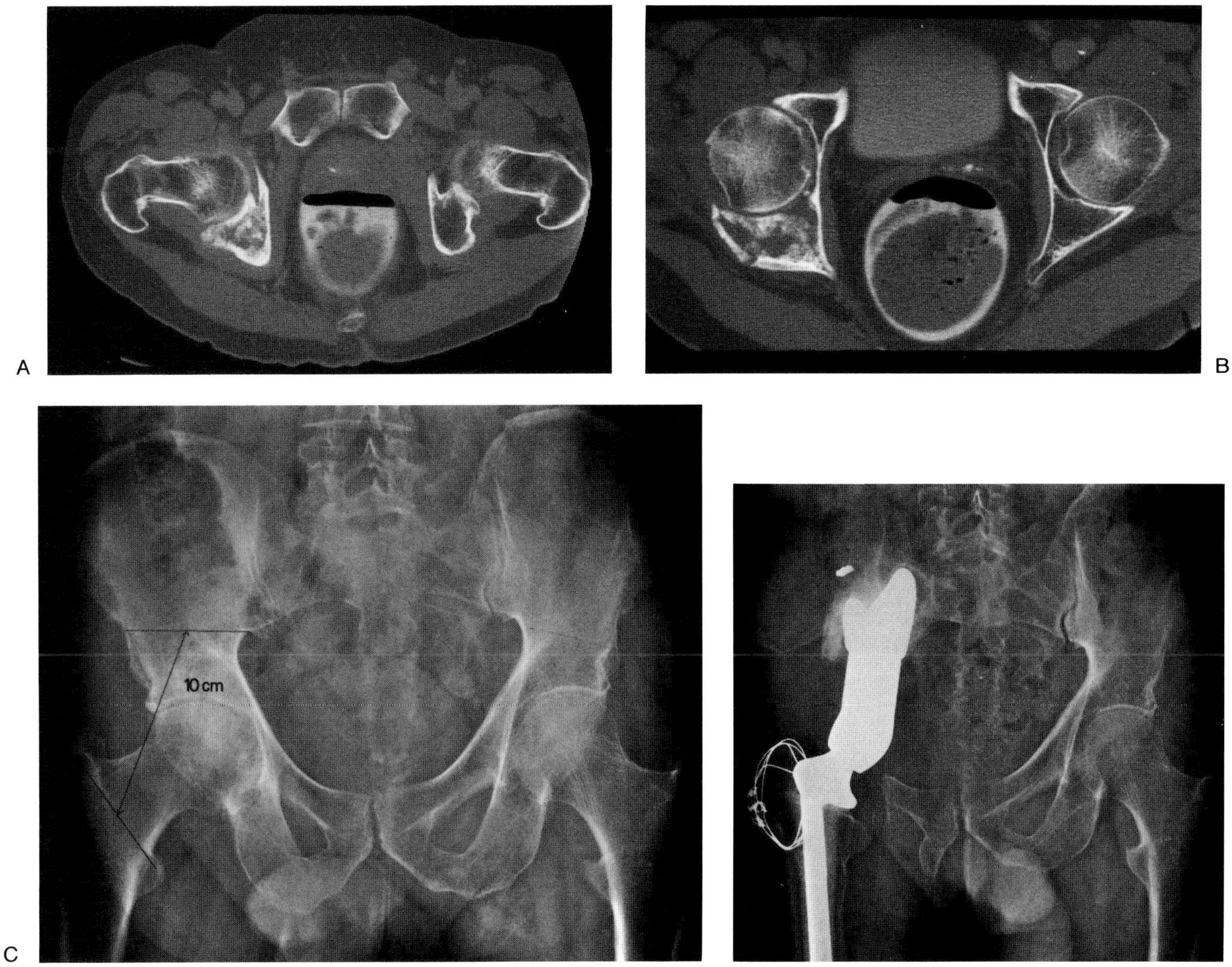

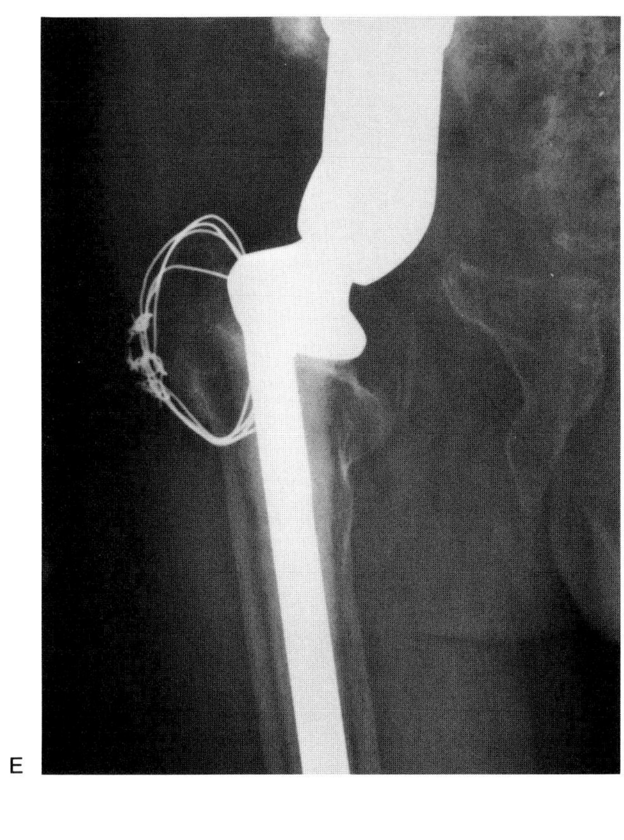

FIG. 14-1. A,B: CT images of the pelvis and hips demonstrating a destructive lesion in the right acetabulum with calcification characteristic of a chondrosarcoma. There is a pathologic fracture. **C:** Preoperative anteroposterior (AP) view of the pelvis marking the area to be resected. Postoperative AP views of the pelvis **(D)** and femur **(E)** after wide excision and reconstruction with a saddle prosthesis with a long-stem cemented femoral component.

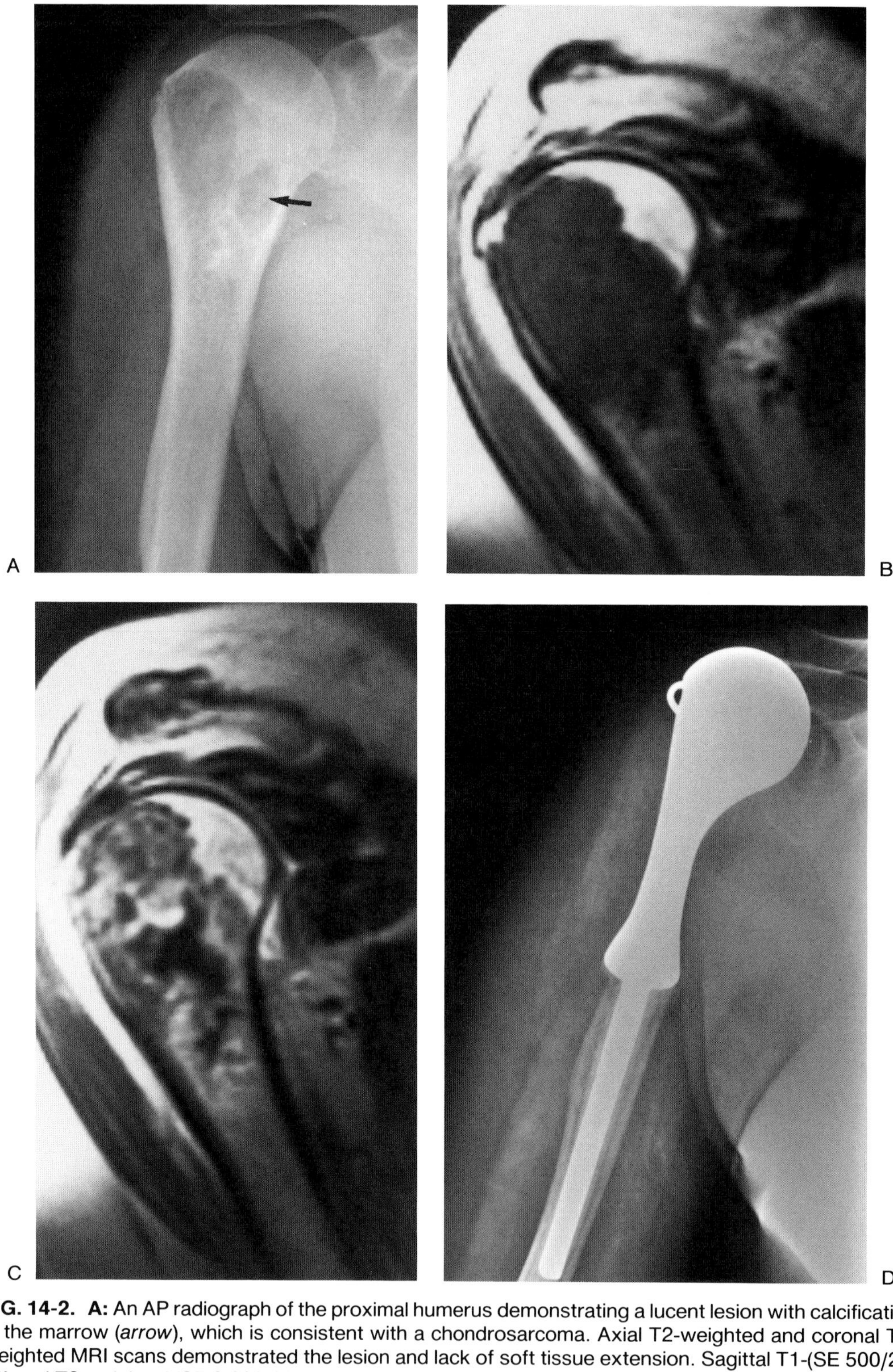

FIG. 14-2. A: An AP radiograph of the proximal humerus demonstrating a lucent lesion with calcification in the marrow (*arrow*), which is consistent with a chondrosarcoma. Axial T2-weighted and coronal T1-weighted MRI scans demonstrated the lesion and lack of soft tissue extension. Sagittal T1-(SE 500/20) **(B)** and T2-weighted (SE 2,000/80) **(C)** images more clearly demonstrate the extent of marrow involvement to allow proper resection and selection of the appropriate customized shoulder prosthesis **(D)**.

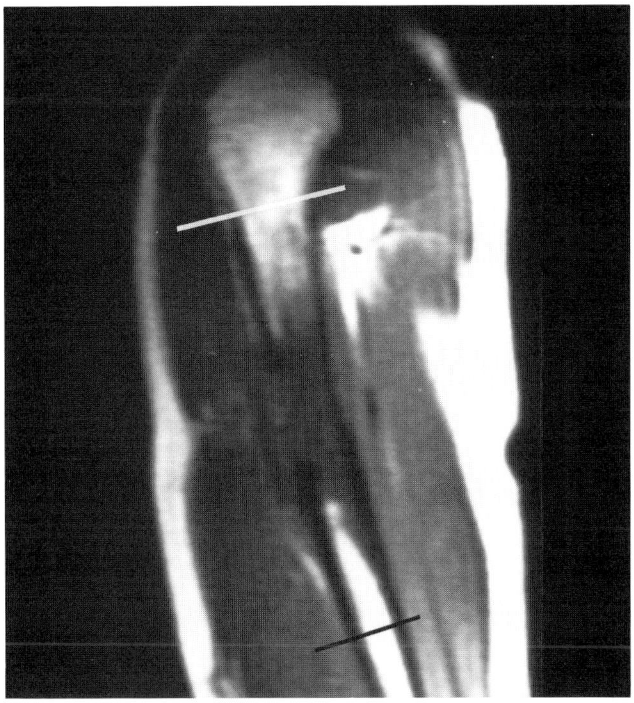

FIG. 14-3. Sagittal T1-weighted (SE 500/20) image of the humerus clearly demonstrates the extent of abnormal signal so the extent of resection can be evaluated (*lines*) when considering limb-salvage procedures. Generally, 5 to 7 cm of normal margin is included with the resection when possible.

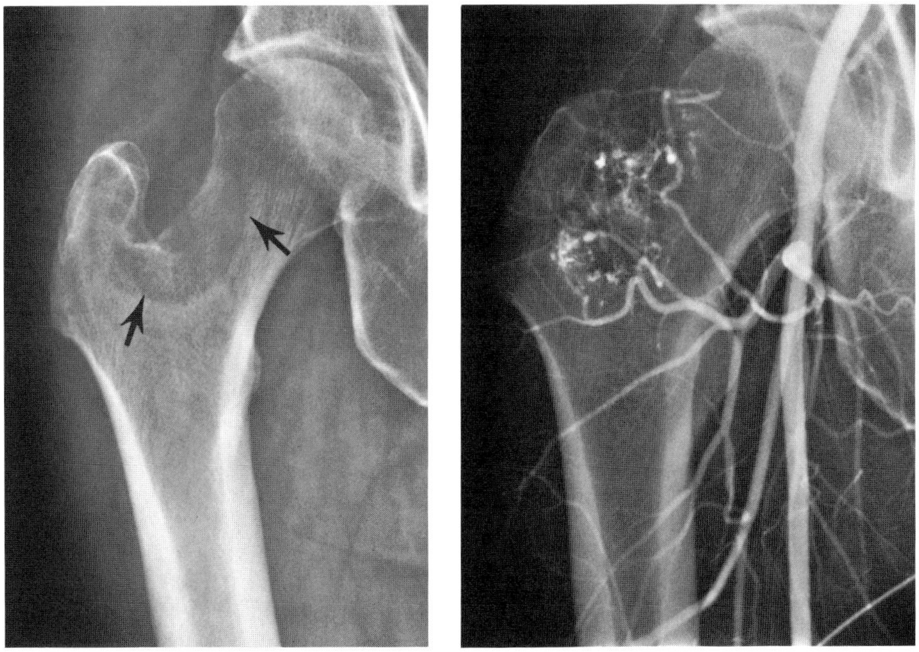

A B

FIG. 14-4. Solitary renal cell metastasis. **A:** An AP view of the femur demonstrating a lytic lesion in the femoral neck (*arrows*). **B:** Angiogram demonstrates a vascular lesion with multiple small tumor vessels; preoperative embolization was performed. (See **C** on next page.)

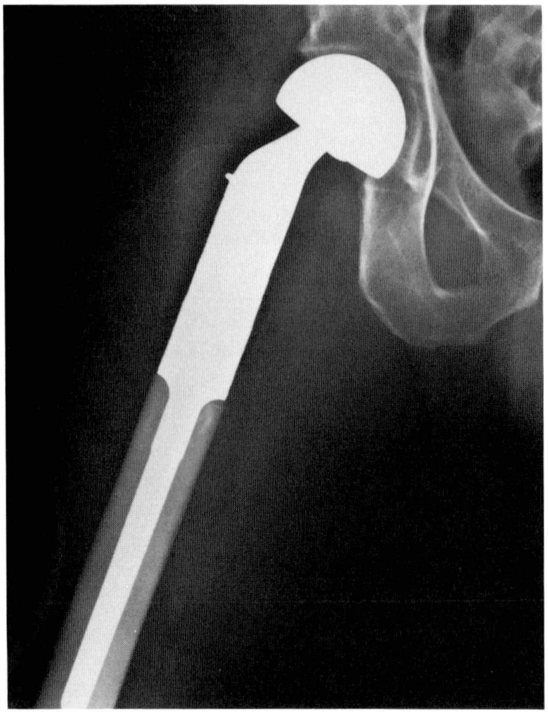

C

FIG. 14-4. (*Continued.*) **C:** The upper femur was resected, and a bipolar femoral custom-designed prosthesis was inserted.

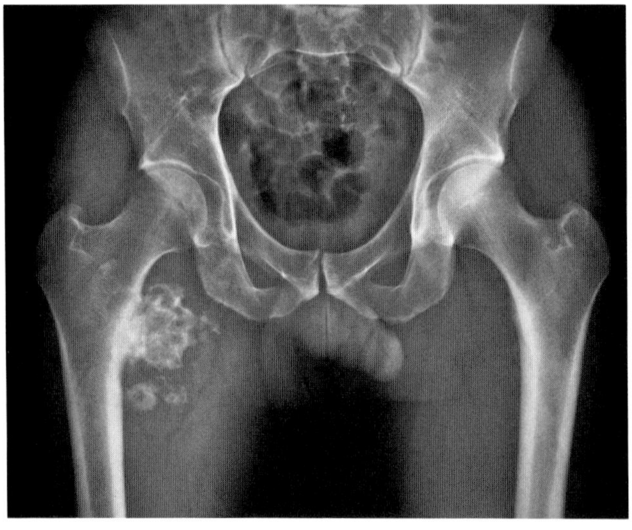

A

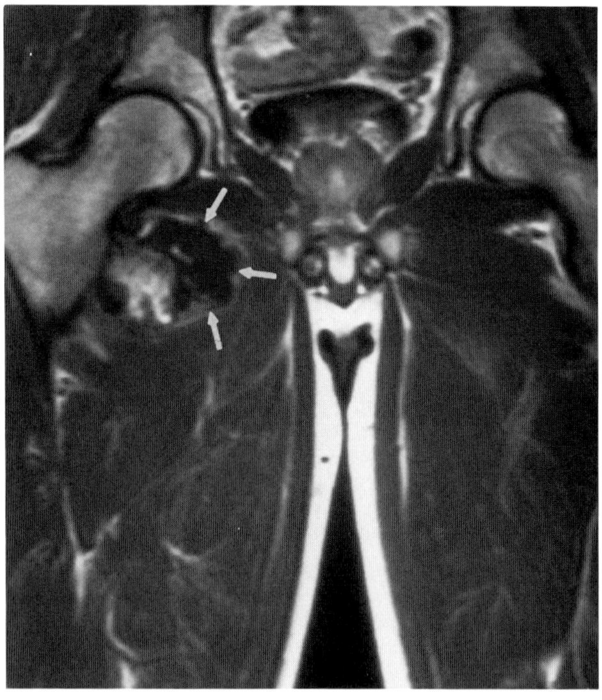

B

FIG. 14-5. Chondrosarcoma with a soft tissue extension. **A:** An AP radiograph demonstrating a chondrosarcoma with extensive soft tissue calcification and ossification arising from the upper right femur. **B:** Coronal SE 500/20 MRI scan demonstrates a large area of low intensity (*arrows*) extending medially from the margin of the osseous portion of the tumor.

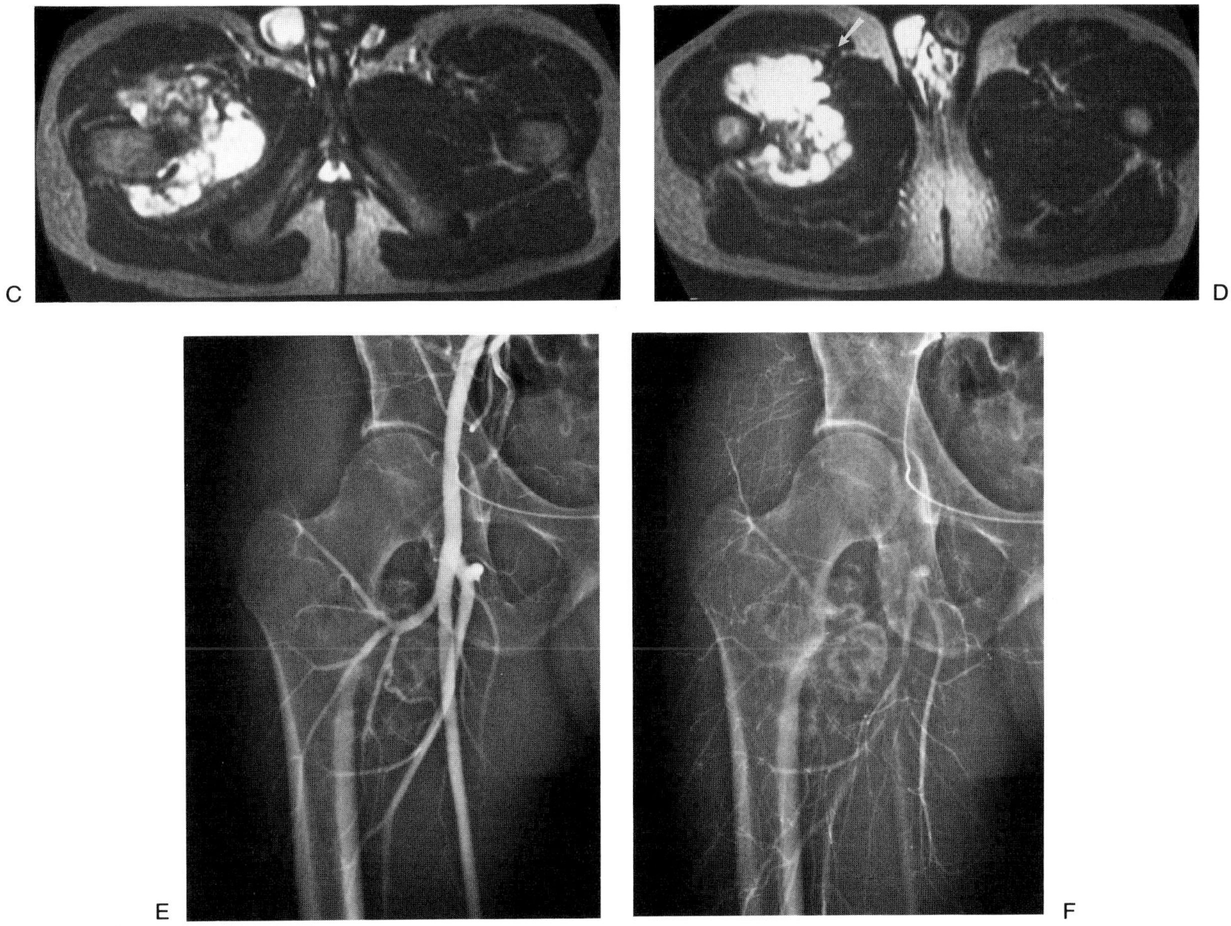

FIG. 14-5. (*Continued.*) **C,D:** Axial SE 2,000/80 images show a high signal intensity in the periphery of the lesion. The vascular structures appear displaced (*arrow*) inferiorly (D) but are not clearly defined at the level of the femoral neck (C). Angiograms during early **(E)** and late phases **(F)**. The superficial femoral artery was easily dissected free from the tumor. The medial and posterior branches were involved. The profunda was displaced but not encased. (See **G–I** on next page.)

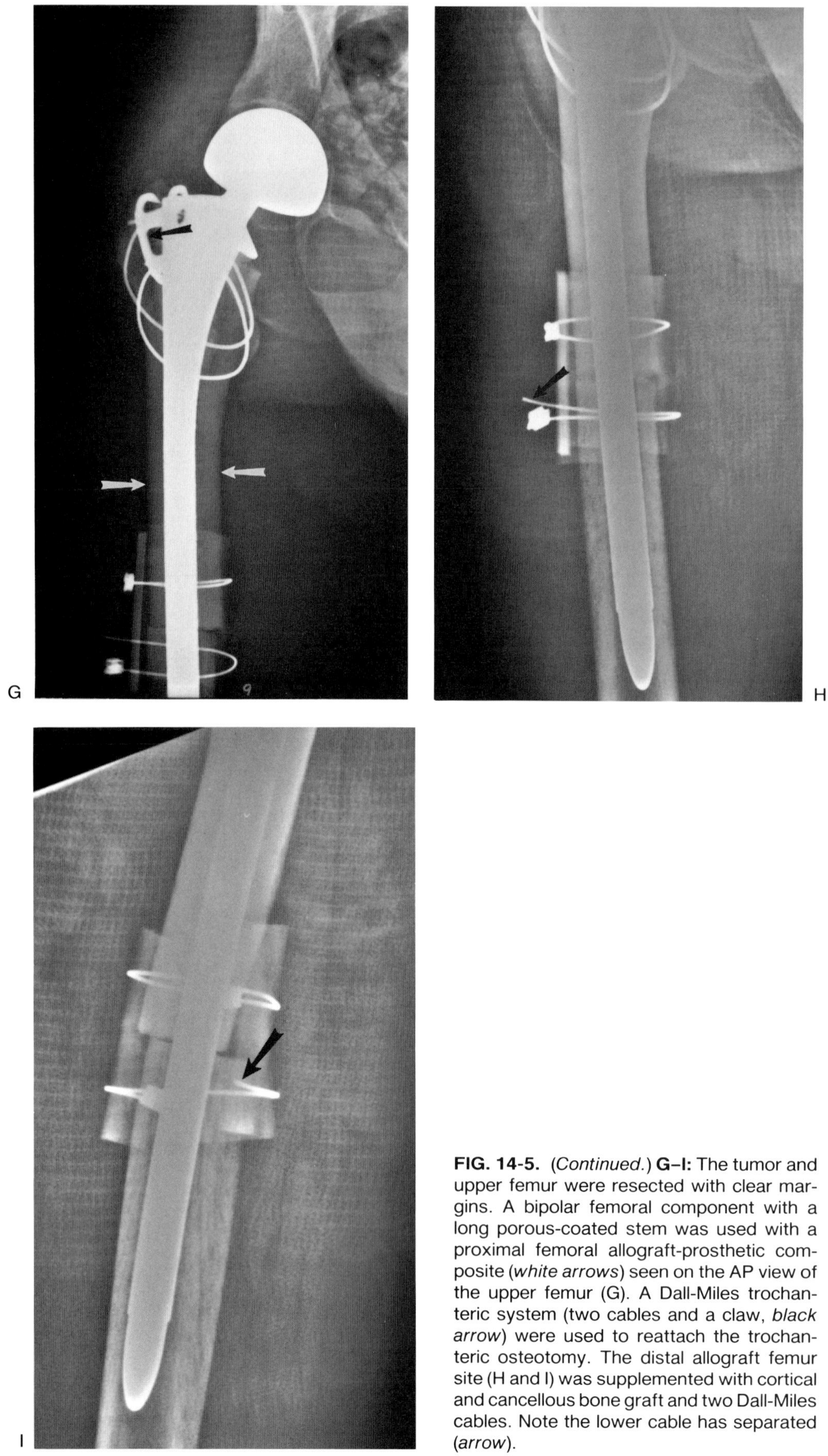

FIG. 14-5. (*Continued.*) **G–I:** The tumor and upper femur were resected with clear margins. A bipolar femoral component with a long porous-coated stem was used with a proximal femoral allograft-prosthetic composite (*white arrows*) seen on the AP view of the upper femur (G). A Dall-Miles trochanteric system (two cables and a claw, *black arrow*) were used to reattach the trochanteric osteotomy. The distal allograft femur site (H and I) was supplemented with cortical and cancellous bone graft and two Dall-Miles cables. Note the lower cable has separated (*arrow*).

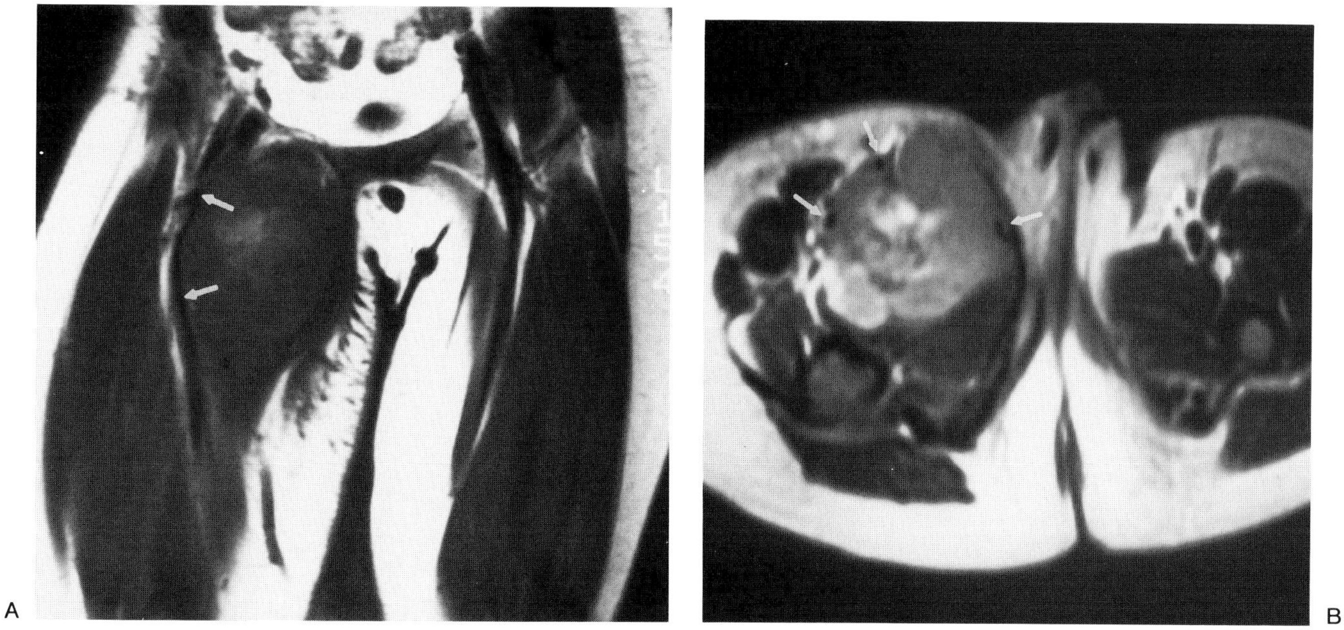

FIG. 14-6. High-grade liposarcoma. A: Coronal SE 500/20 sequence demonstrates a large isointense mass compared with muscle with lateral displacement and compression of the femoral vessels (*arrows*). B: Axial SE 2,000/30 sequence demonstrates a high-signal-intensity inhomogeneous mass. The vessels (*arrows*) are at least partially encased.

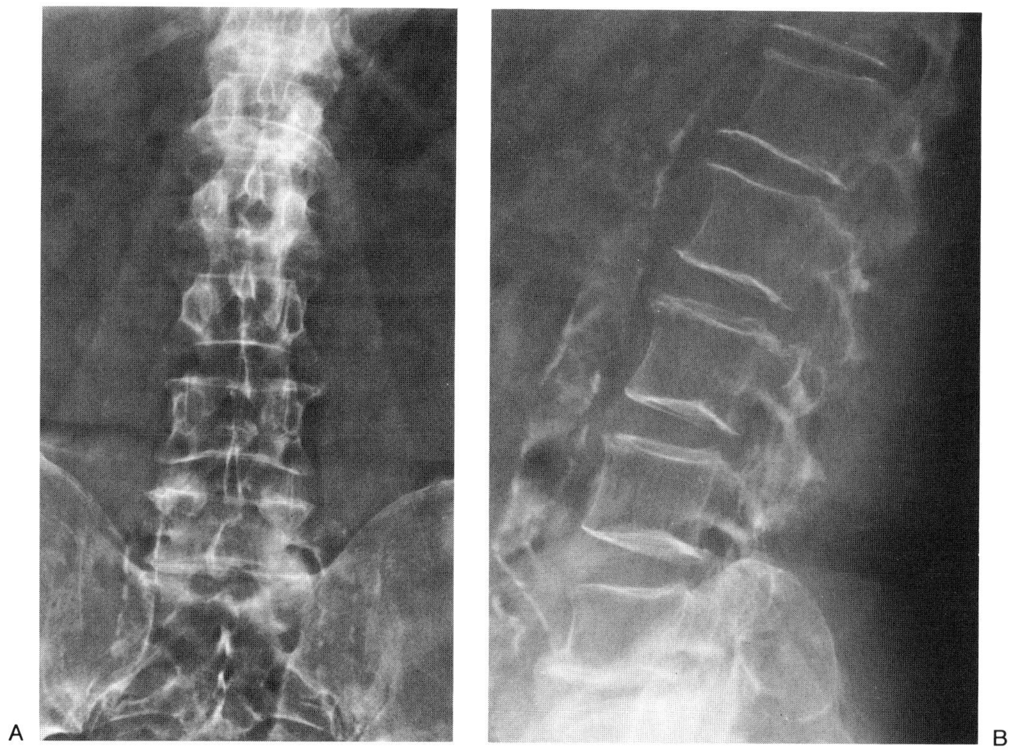

FIG. 14-7. In a 76-year-old man with a suspected metastasis, AP (A) and lateral (B) radiographs of the lumbar spine do not show metastases. (See C–F on next page.)

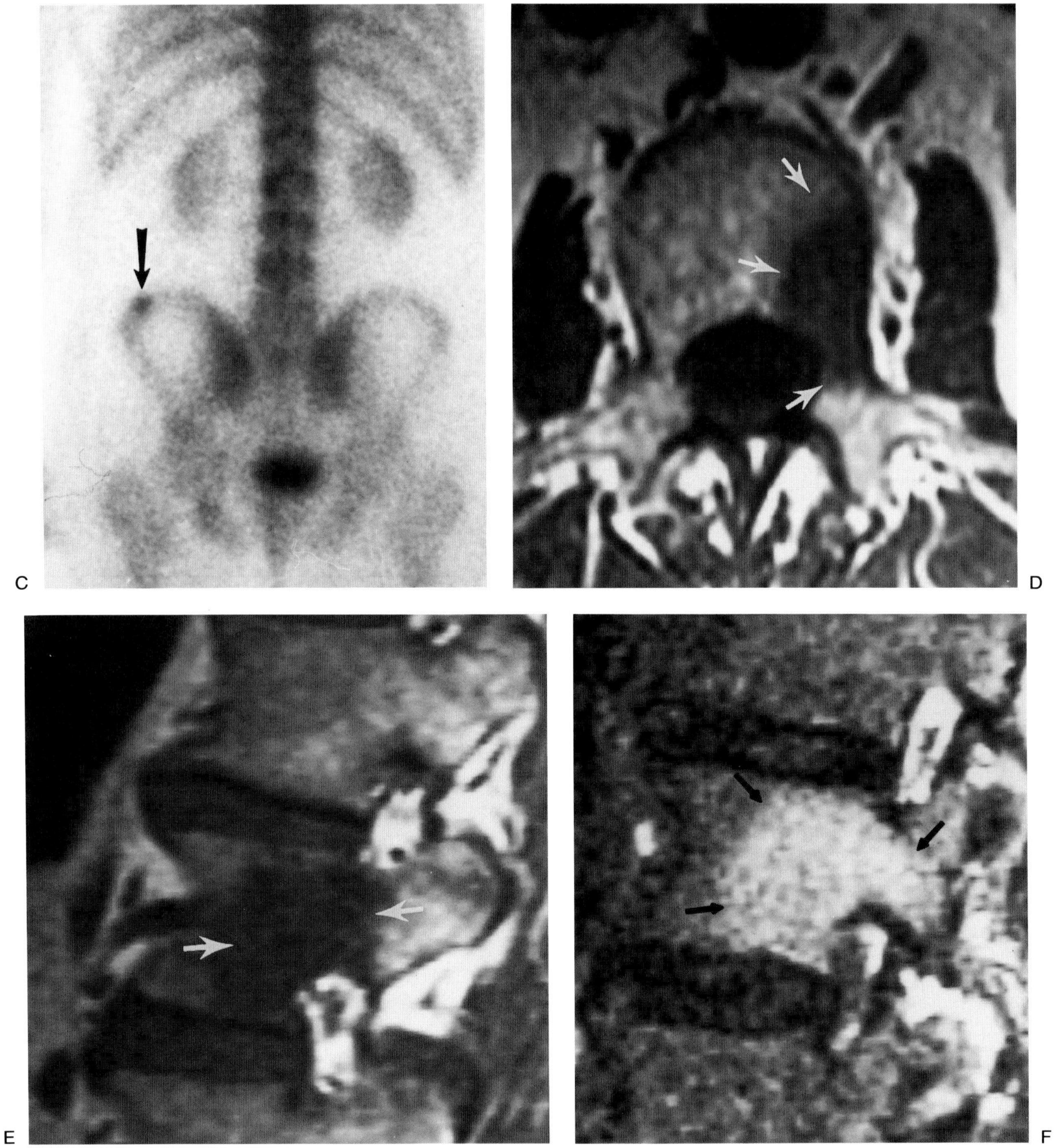

FIG. 14-7. (*Continued.*) **C:** Technetium-99m bone scan demonstrates a focal abnormality in the right ilium (*arrow*) and no definite spinal abnormalities. Axial **(D)** and sagittal **(E)** SE 500/20 and sagittal SE 2,000/80 **(F)** images demonstrate a definite abnormality in L-2 (*arrows*) caused by metastases.

general, CT is used for the screening of pulmonary and abdominal metastases.[1–4]

TREATMENT OPTIONS

The treatment options vary, depending on the site and extent of tumor involvement. In certain cases, implants used for trauma or conventional arthroplasty can be used. In other situations, more customized implants are required (Figs. 14-1 and 14-2).

Bone Grafts

Bone grafts are used for many situations in orthopedic practice. Cancellous or cortical grafts can be used for fracture treatment or filling bone deficits created by other conditions. Autografts (autogenous grafting) are taken from one site and positioned where they are needed in the same patient. These grafts may be vascularized or nonvascularized. Frozen allografts (graft taken from another individual) are more commonly used for neoplasms or other reconstructive procedures in which large segments of bone must be replaced (Fig. 14-5).[25,56]

Autogenous grafts have the advantages of more rapid and reliable incorporation, and the vascularized grafts can hypertrophy, providing long-term stability. Vascularized fibular grafts are used commonly. These grafts are commonly attached using screws or plate and screw fixation (Figs. 14-8 and 14-9).[43,56] Surgery is technically demanding and long (can require > 12 hours). Fibular grafts typically heal in 3 to 8 months. As expected, healing occurs more readily in children, as is the case with ordinary fracture healing, compared with the rate in more elderly patients.[56]

Allografts may be used to fill in segments of long bone, as osteoarticular replacements (Figs. 14-5 and 14-10 to 14-12). The most common problems with allografts are nonunion, fracture, and infection.[24,36,52,56] Collapse of the subchondral region of osteoarticular allografts has prompted the use of such allografts in conjunction with a prosthesis (i.e., an allograft-prosthetic composite; Fig. 14-5). The use of an allograft-prosthetic composite allows the attachment of the soft tissues to the remaining tendon of the allografted bone, improving the functional result.[24] Allografts may also be used in an intercalary fashion to achieve an arthrodesis (Figs. 14-10 and 14-12).

Nonarticular Implants and Methyl Methacrylate

The treatment of benign lesions can be accomplished with curettage by using a bone graft or methyl methacrylate to fill the bone defect. The technique can be used with benign lesions, such as most giant cell tumors (Fig. 14-13).[19]

Methyl methacrylate is also used in conjunction with other orthopedic implants for the treatment of diaphyseal lesions. Methyl methacrylate provides immediate stability when placed in the marrow defect created by the tumor.[22,25,53] Fixation is most often achieved with intramedullary nails (see Chapters 5, 7, and 10). In the past, implants, such as Ender nails or Rush rods, were typically used. Currently, interlocking intramedullary nails are favored.[6,22,53] Spacers and revision arthroplasty components can also be used for diaphyseal lesions (Figs. 14-14 and 14-15).[6,8,53] Miller et al.[33] configured a fluted intramedullary nail so that methyl methacrylate could be injected into the nail and distributed around the entire implant.

Plate and screw fixation can also be used, but most authors prefer the intramedullary nail-methyl methacrylate technique (Fig. 14-16).[22,25,53]

Customized Joint Prostheses

Most neoplasms occur in the metaphyseal or epiphyseal regions of the long bones. Therefore, some type of joint prosthesis is commonly used for limb-salvage procedures. Osteoarticular allografts were discussed earlier. Metal or ceramic prostheses that are custom designed or designed for revision arthroplasty may be selected based on the extent of tumor involvement.[24,40,43,44,54] The entire long bone can also be replaced.[40,51] An allograft-prosthetic composite (Fig. 14-5G,I), as previously discussed, can also be used. This section focuses on prosthetic types of reconstruction following tumor resection. Nonprosthetic options are not reviewed.

Expandable components are available for use in the skeletally immature patient to allow periodic leg lengthening. Although initial results are encouraging, there are no long-term follow-up studies at this time.[17,24] Figure 14-17 demonstrates various custom-designed prostheses.

Upper Femur and Hip

Limb-salvage procedures for the upper femur and hip vary with the lesion; tumor extent; and the patient's age, activity level, and expected longevity.[24] Lesions of the proximal femur may be treated with endoprostheses (Figs. 14-17A, 14-18, and 14-19) or an allograft-prosthetic composite. Lesions involving the acetabulum or hip may be reconstructed with an allograft-prosthetic composite or a saddle prosthesis with variable femoral stems (Figs. 14-20 and 14-21).[37,38] Total femoral replacement is usually performed for limited indications. These include repeated treatment failure with more conventional components, major femoral bone loss, and infection.[40,51]

(text continues on page 947)

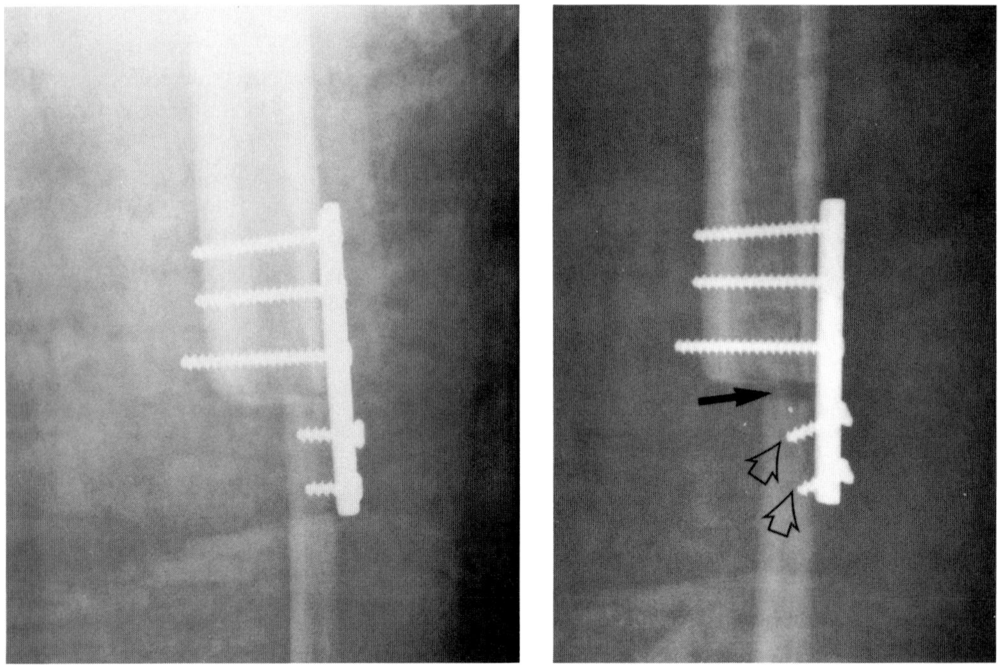

A B

FIG. 14-8. Vascularized fibular graft. **A:** Postoperative radiograph demonstrating the fibular graft with a five-hole DC plate and screws for fixation. The lower two screws (fibular graft) do not have purchase in the opposite cortex. **B:** One week later, the graft separated (*black arrow*), and the screws (*open arrows*) pulled out.

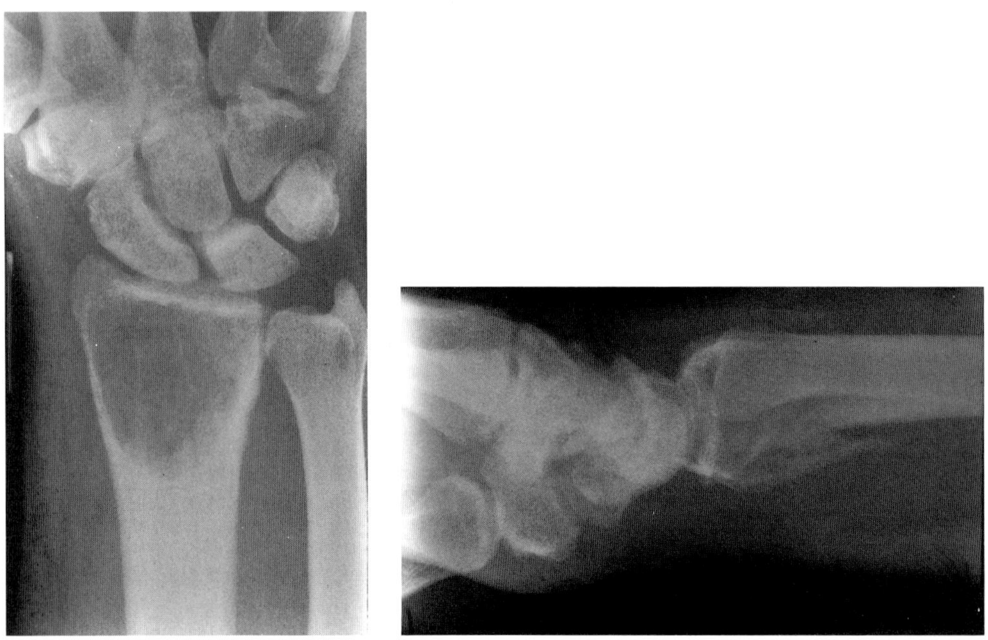

A B

FIG. 14-9. Aggressive giant cell tumor of the distal radius. The AP **(A)** and lateral **(B)** radiographs demonstrate the typical lytic appearance of a giant cell tumor with pathologic fracture seen on the lateral view.

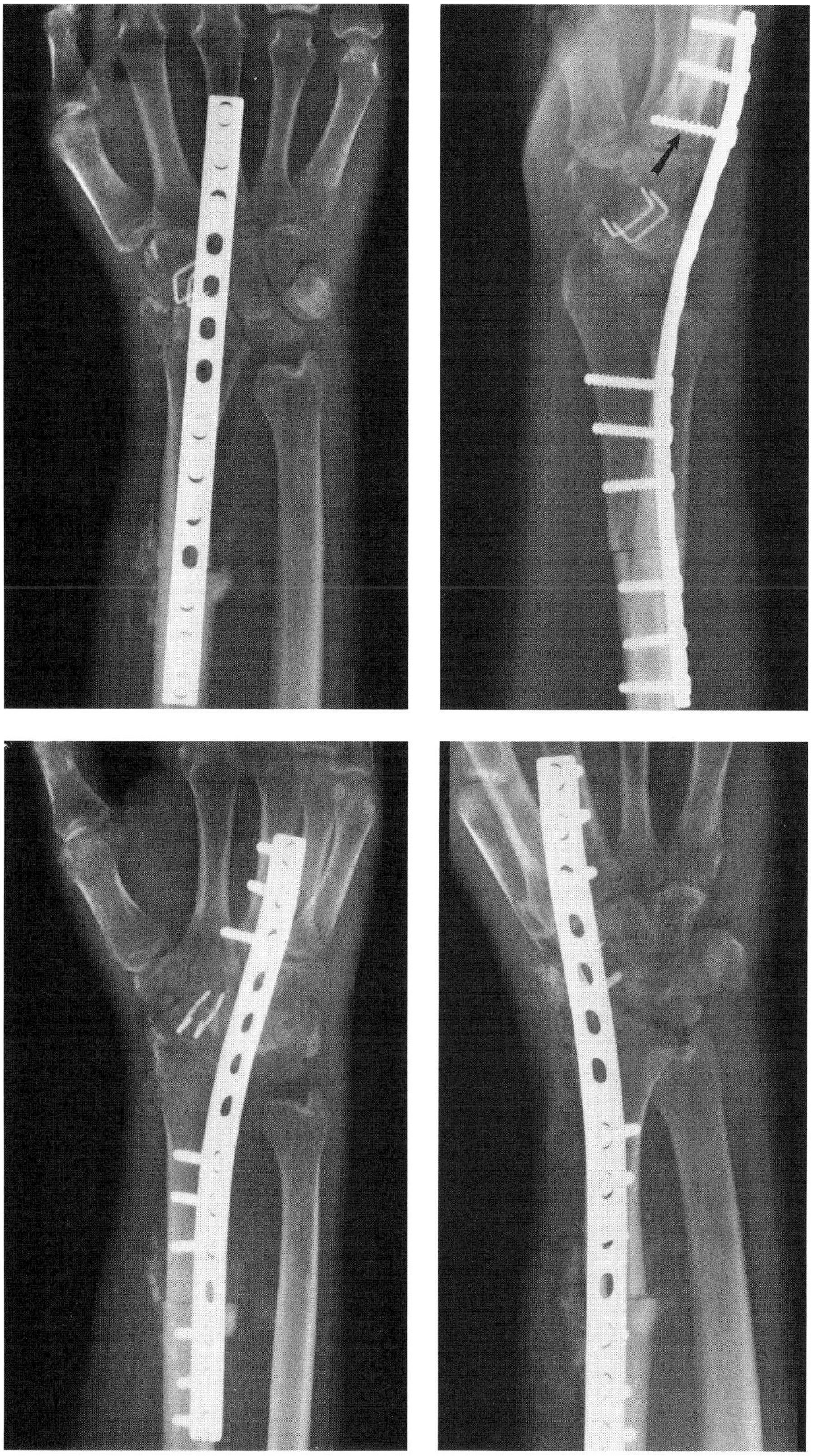

FIG. 14-9. (*Continued.*) The AP **(C)**, lateral **(D)**, and oblique **(E,F)** radiographs obtained after tumor resection and reconstruction with autograft proximal fibula and morcellized allograft in the carpal and radiofibular junction. The scaphoid and lunate were denuded, and graft fixation to the radius and third metacarpal was fixed using a DC plate with 14 holes and cortical screws. One cancellous screw was used distally (*arrow*). There are two dorsal carpal staples.

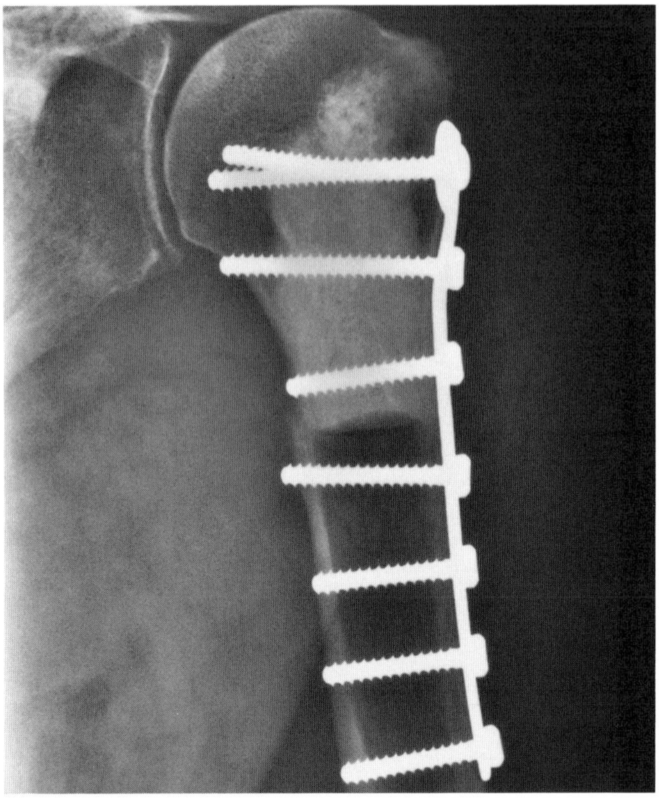

A

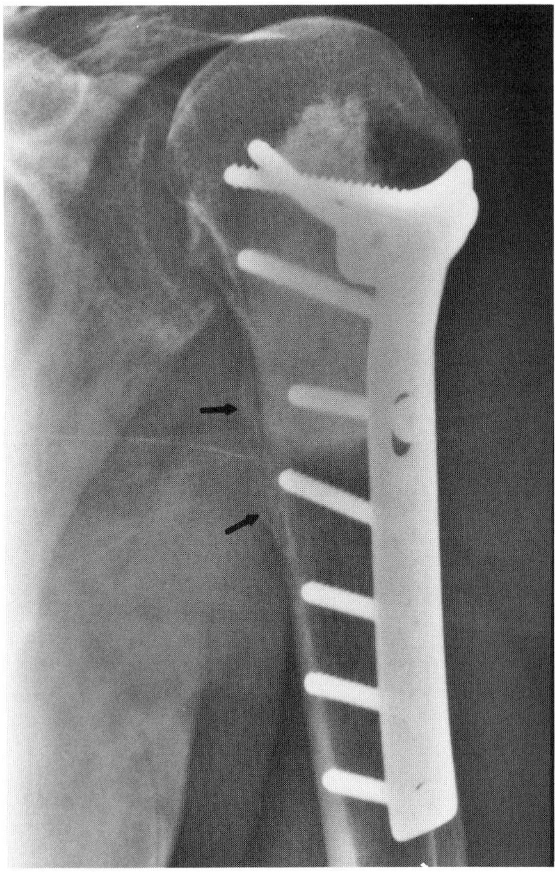

B

FIG. 14-10. Healing osteoarticular allograft in the proximal humerus. The allograft has antibiotic-impregnated methyl methacrylate to improve screw purchase and potentially decrease the risk of infection. It is internally fixed with a long T buttress plate with six cortical screws distally (note both cortices are properly engaged) and two cortical screws in the proximal plate. The patient's rotator cuff tendons were repaired to the corresponding tendon on the allograft. **A:** The positions of the screws are clearly seen on the AP external rotation view. **B:** Callus (*arrows*) can be appreciated on the internal rotation view. Allografts can take up to 77 weeks to heal radiographically.[23]

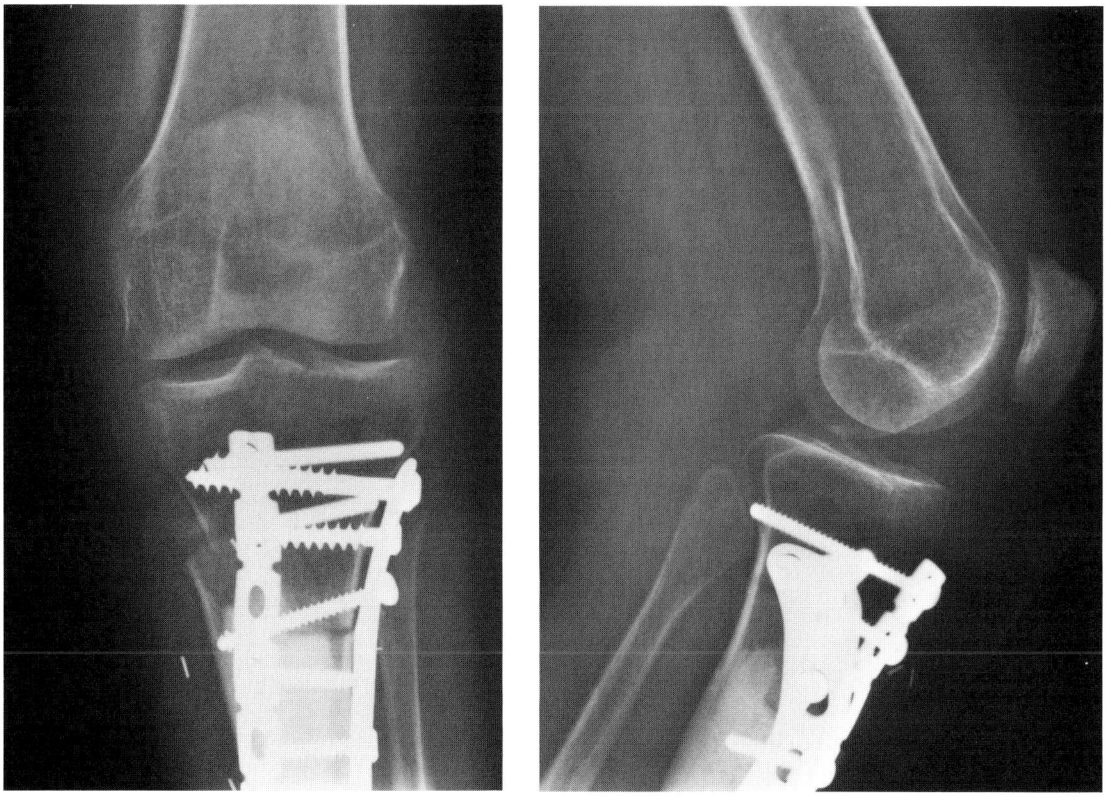

A B

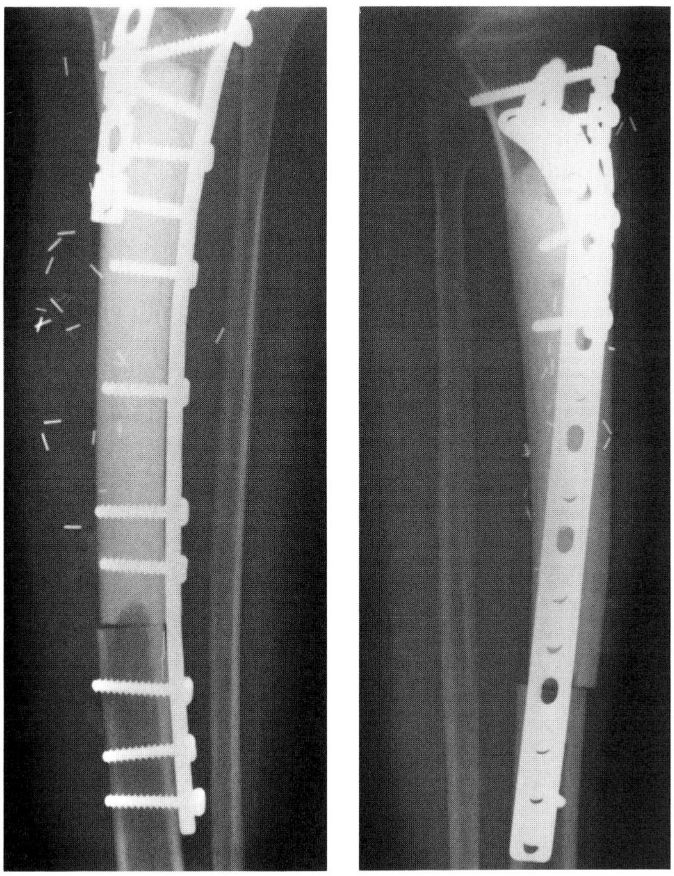

C,D

FIG. 14-11. Resection of the upper tibial diaphyses for neoplasm. An allograft has been inserted between the upper articular portion of the native tibia, which is best seen on the AP **(A)** and lateral **(B)** radiographs of the knee. The distal contact is demonstrated on the AP **(C)** and lateral **(D)** radiographs of the leg. The allograft has been fixed with a long 15-hole lateral condylar plate and ten cortical screws distally with cancellous screws in the expanded upper plate. There is a second reconstruction plate with screws medially.

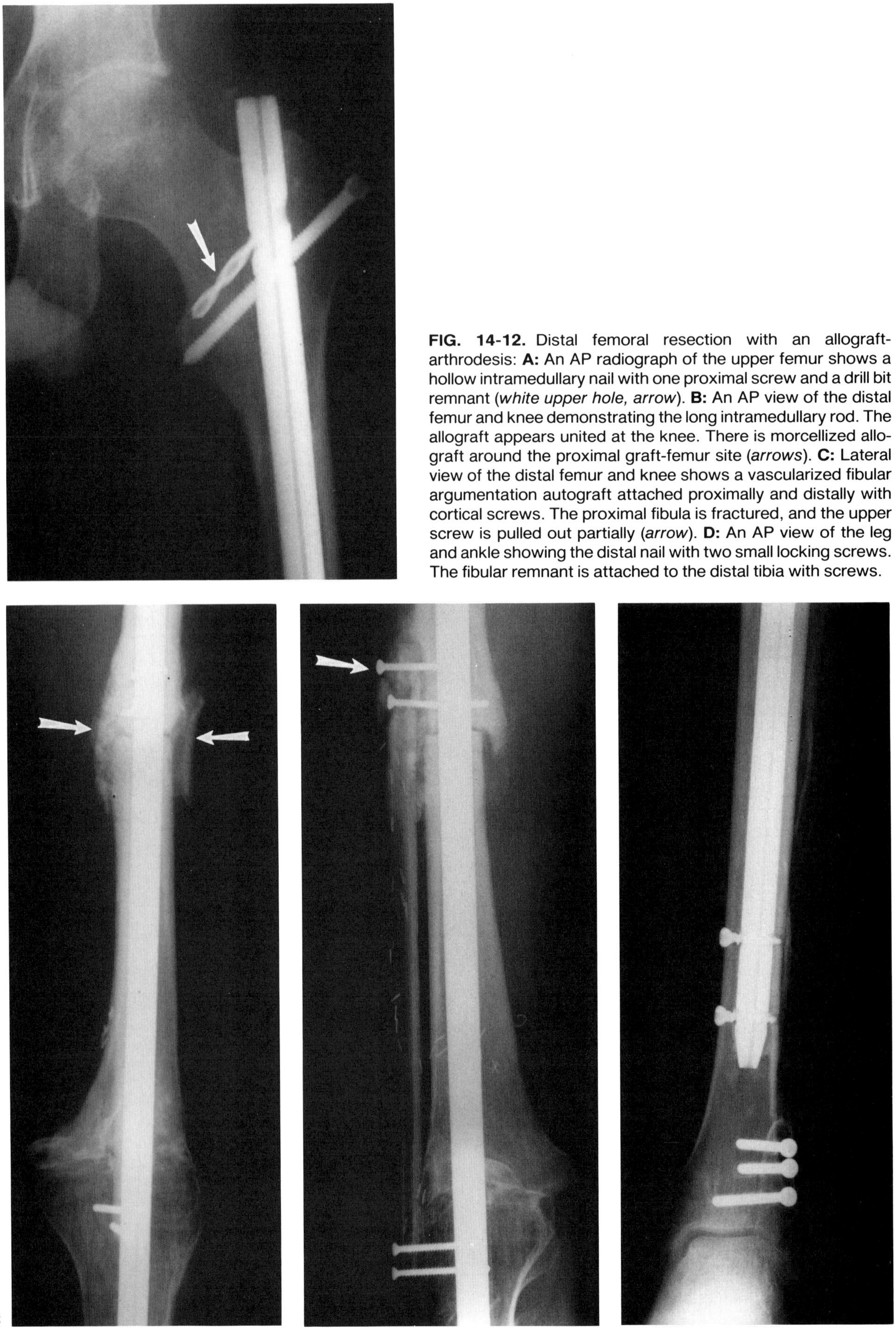

A

B,C

D

FIG. 14-12. Distal femoral resection with an allograft-arthrodesis: **A:** An AP radiograph of the upper femur shows a hollow intramedullary nail with one proximal screw and a drill bit remnant (*white upper hole, arrow*). **B:** An AP view of the distal femur and knee demonstrating the long intramedullary rod. The allograft appears united at the knee. There is morcellized allograft around the proximal graft-femur site (*arrows*). **C:** Lateral view of the distal femur and knee shows a vascularized fibular argumentation autograft attached proximally and distally with cortical screws. The proximal fibula is fractured, and the upper screw is pulled out partially (*arrow*). **D:** An AP view of the leg and ankle showing the distal nail with two small locking screws. The fibular remnant is attached to the distal tibia with screws.

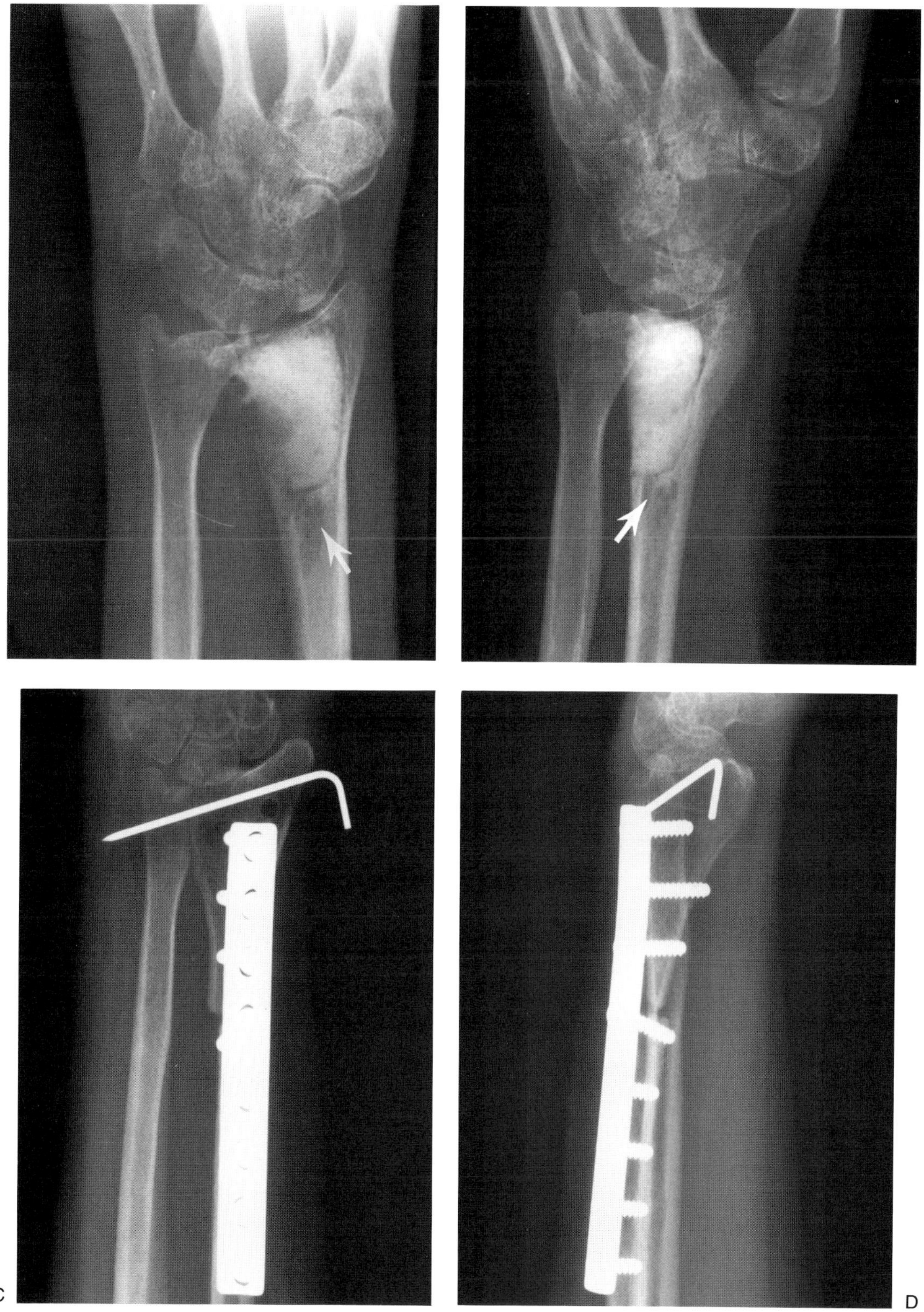

A B C D

FIG. 14-13. Giant cell tumor of the distal left radius. Posteroanterior **(A)** and oblique **(B)** radiographs after curettage and filling of the bone defect with methyl methacrylate. The patient had symptoms, and recurrence was suspected. The radiograph shows irregular lucent areas (*arrows*) near the operative site, which suggested a recurrence. The AP **(C)** and lateral **(D)** radiographs after resection of the distal radius. A fibular autograft was positioned using an eight-hole DC plate and a temporary K-wire to stabilize the distal radioulnar joint.

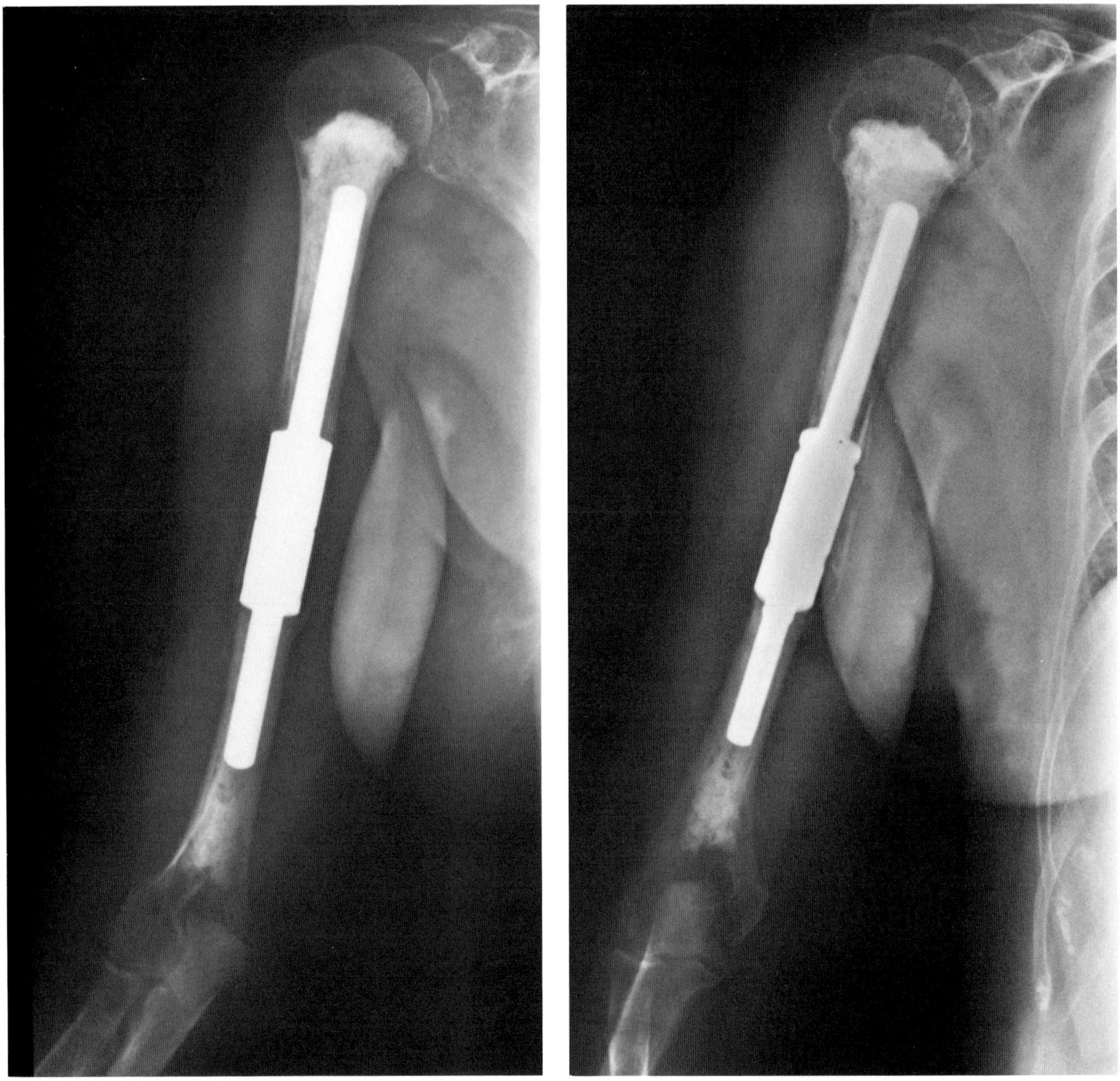

A B

FIG. 14-14. Plasmacytoma of the right midhumerus with a pathologic fracture. The midhumeral region was resected *en bloc* and a 50-mm spacer inserted. The AP external **(A)** and internal **(B)** rotation views of the humerus demonstrate the spacer and cement in place.

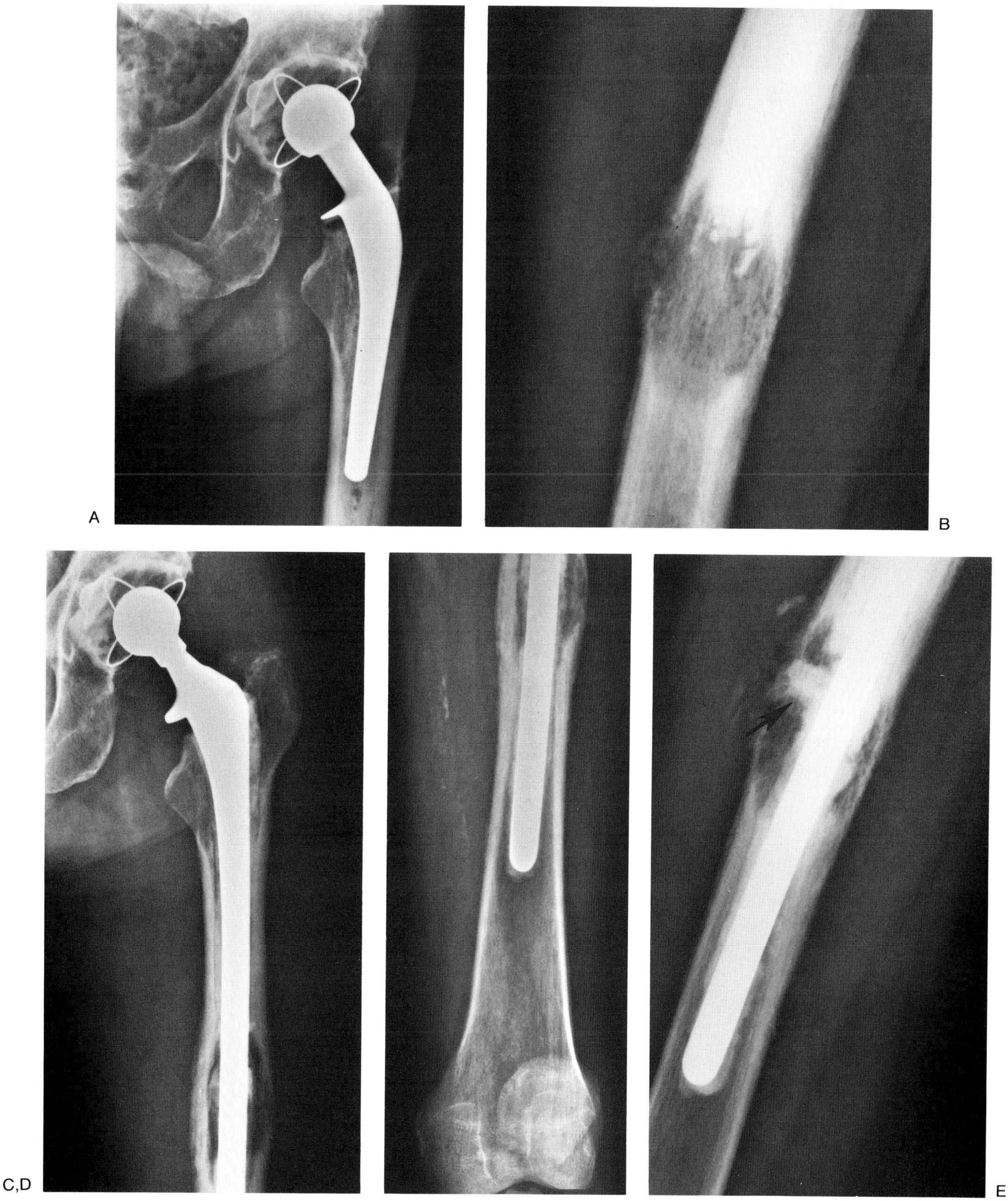

FIG. 14-15. Metastatic lung cancer to the left midfemur below a conventional hip arthroplasty. The AP **(A)** and lateral **(B)** radiographs of the hip and tumor site show a lytic destructive lesion with anterior cortical disruption. The femoral component was replaced with a long-stem prosthesis that extended well below the destructive lesion. The AP (**C,** upper; **D,** lower) radiographs of the hip and femur demonstrate the cemented component crossing the tumor site. Cement does not fill the tumor site. **E:** Lateral view of the tumor site shows cement in the anterior region of cortical disruption (*arrow*).

A,B 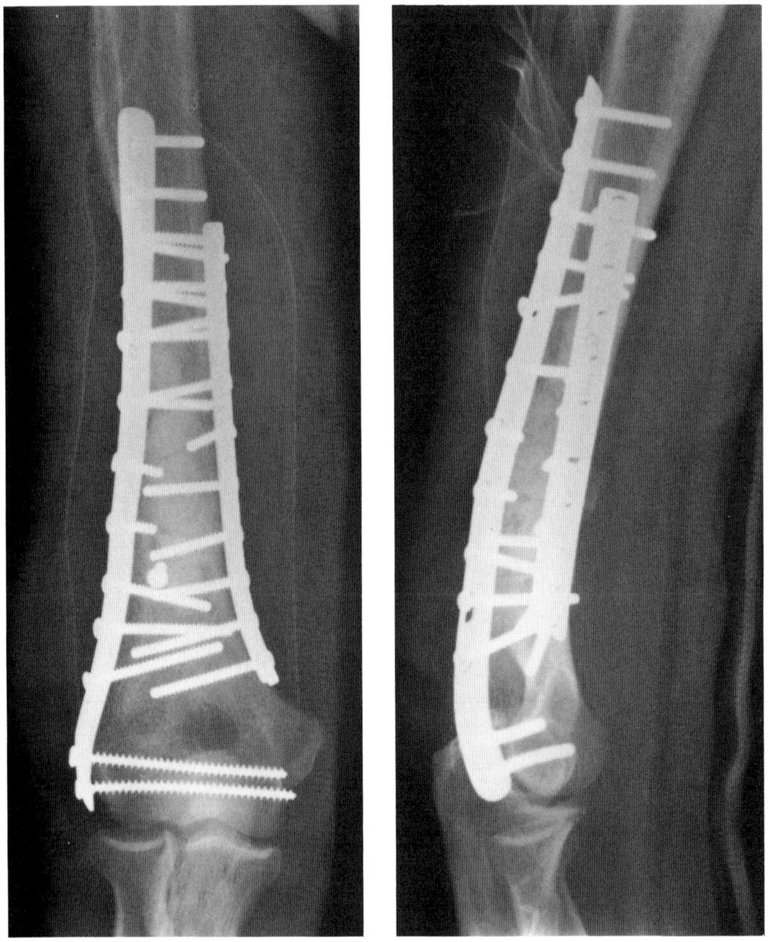

FIG. 14-16. The AP **(A)** and lateral **(B)** radiographs of a distal humeral destructive lesion treated with methyl methacrylate and dual plates and screws.

A 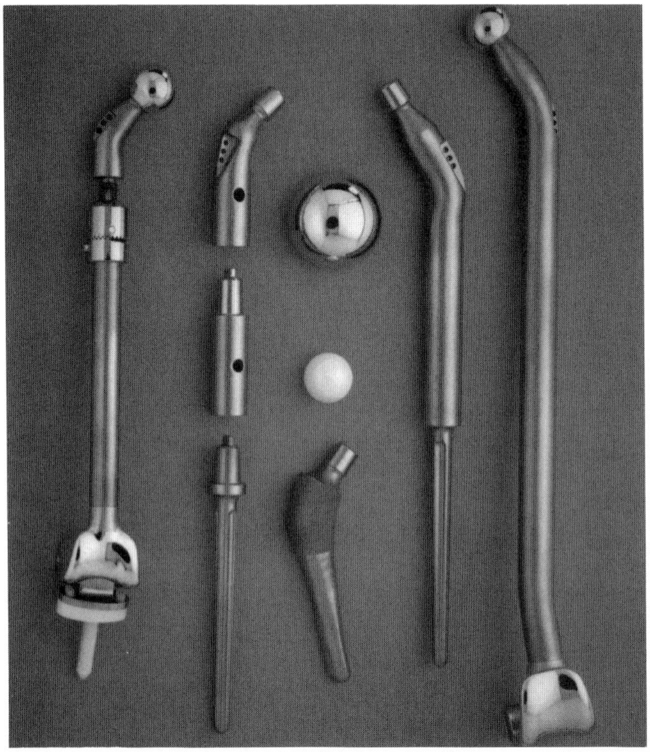

FIG. 14-17. A: Hip, femur, and femoral-knee components. *Right,* Total femoral component with expandable upper shaft and knee articulation; *center,* modular femoral components; *left,* total femoral component.

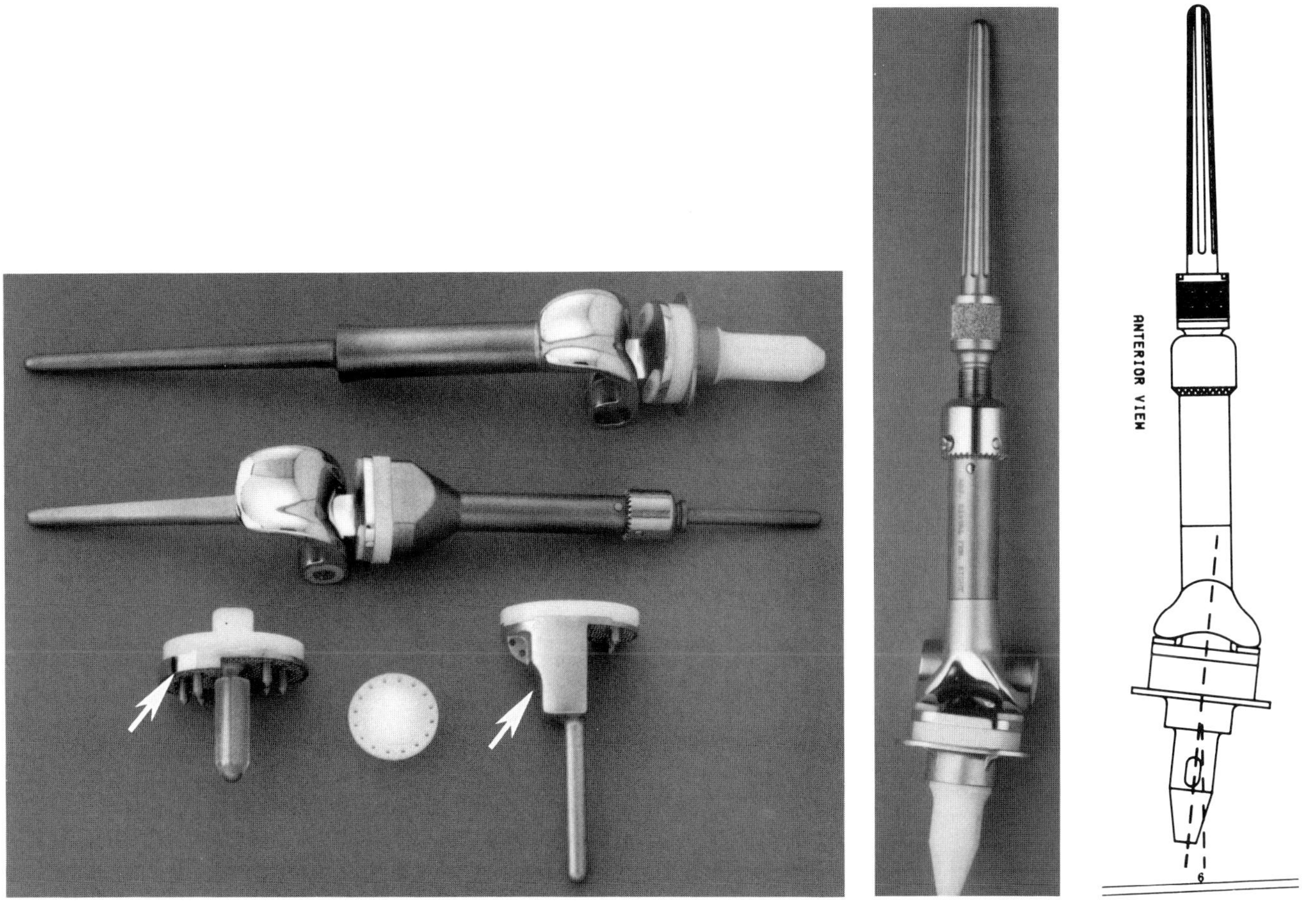

B,C

D

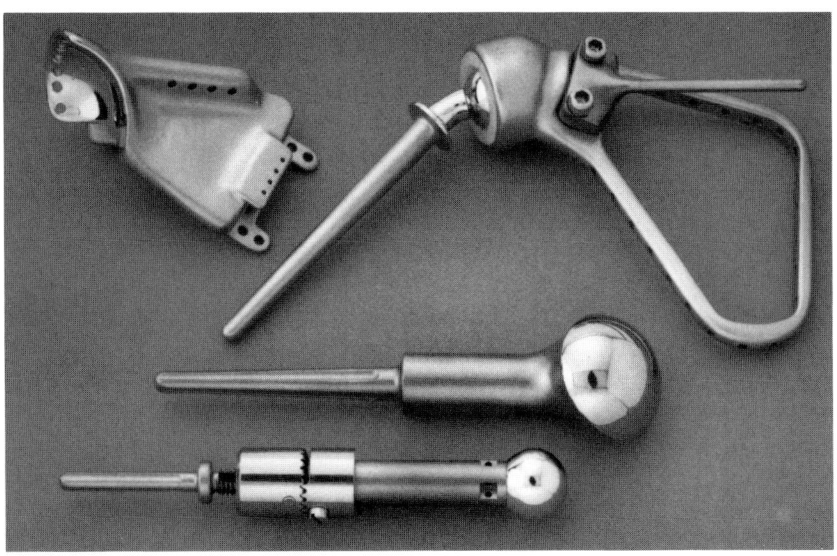

E

FIG. 14-17. (*Continued.*) **B:** Customized distal femoral-knee components. *Top,* long-stem femoral component; *center,* long-stem expandable tibial design; *below,* revision knee systems with tibial augmentation (*arrows*) for bone loss and polyethylene patellar component (*center*). Custom-designed distal femoral component **(C)** with expansion capability and illustration showing normal valgus angle of the knee **(D)**. **E:** Customized scapular (*upper left*), total shoulder (*upper right*), and humeral endoprostheses (*below*). The lower humeral endoprosthesis is expandable. (Courtesy of Wright Medical Technology, Arlington, TN.)

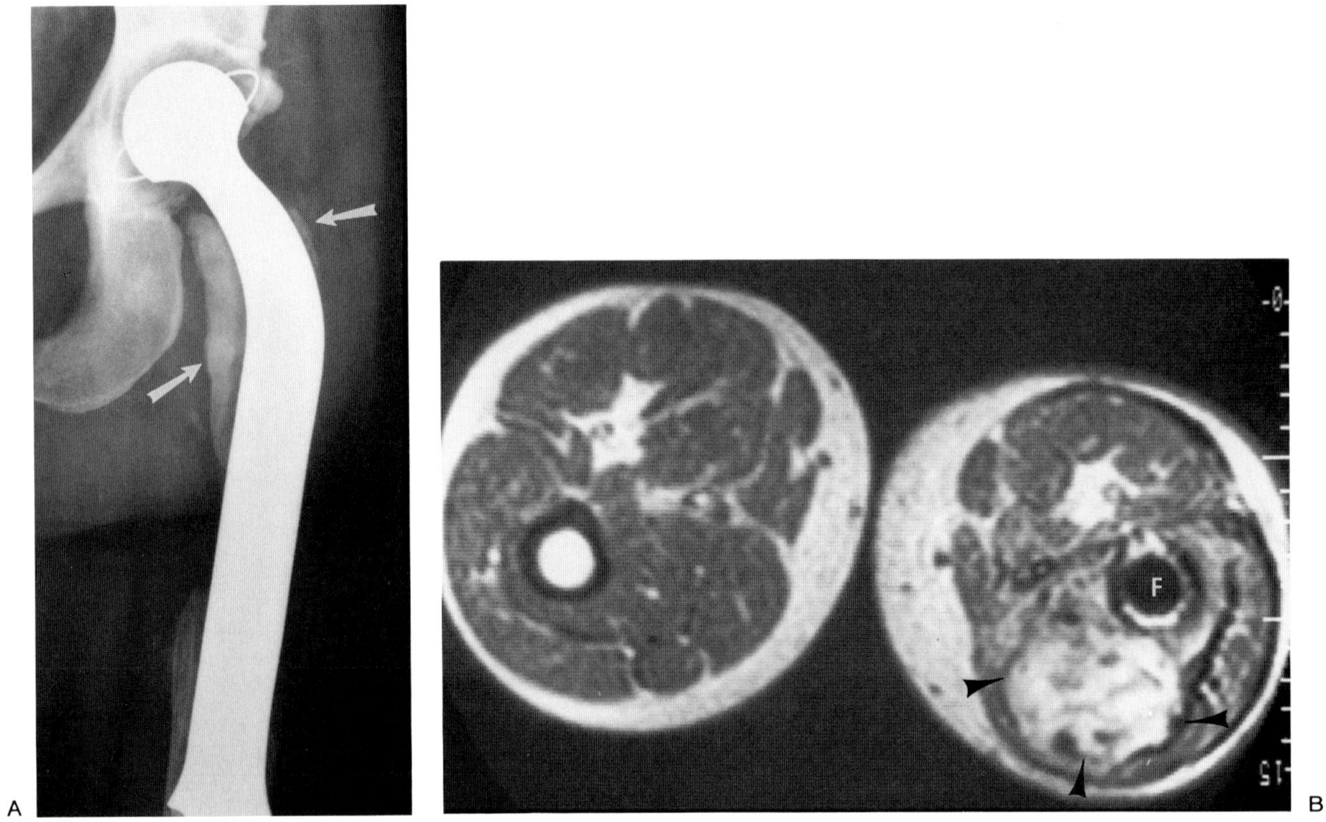

FIG. 14-18. Chondrosarcoma of the proximal femur. **A:** An AP view of the hip and upper femur demonstrating a left hip arthroplasty with a custom-designed femoral component. There is new bone formation (*arrows*) along the component. **B:** Axial SE 2,000/30 MRI scan shows recurrence in the soft tissues (*arrows*). Note the minimal artifact from the femoral component (*F*).

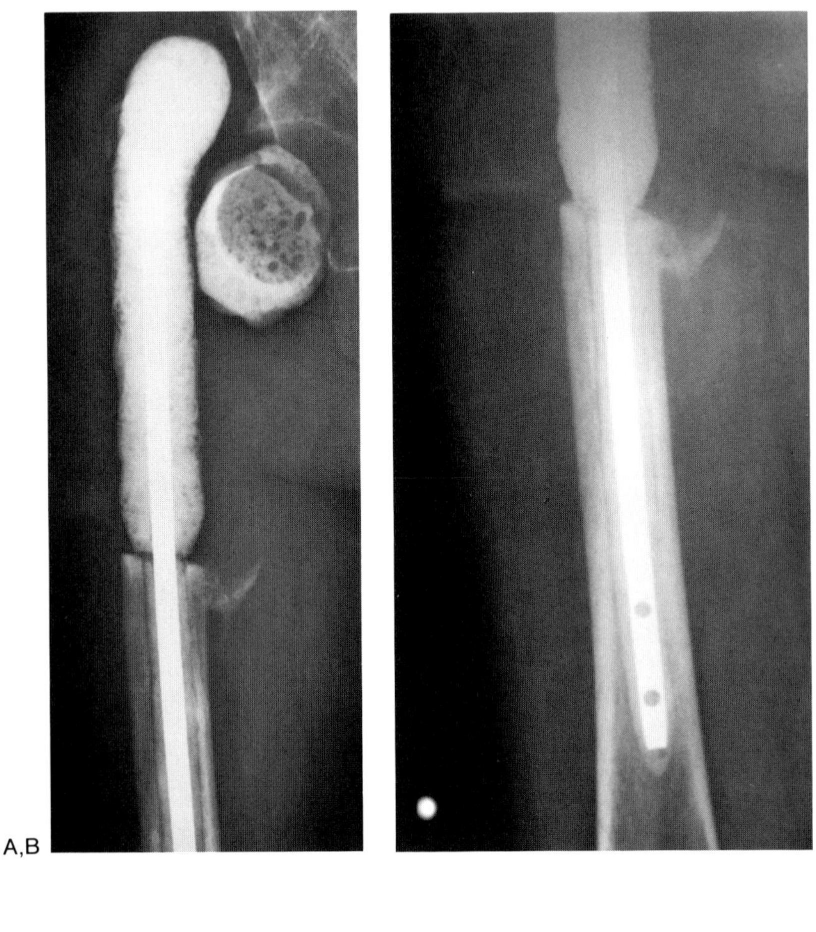

FIG. 14-19. Chondrosarcoma of the right femur with extensive osseous extension. The upper femur was resected and reconstructed using an allograft-prosthesis composite with a bipolar configuration, which subsequently became infected. The implant was removed, and an antibiotic-impregnated spacer (over an intramedullary rod) was inserted during antibiotic therapy. The rod-methyl methacrylate construct dislocated from the methyl methacrylate acetabular spacer. The patient had no discomfort related to this and could ambulate with crutches. The patient subsequently had these spacers removed and reconstructed with a (revision) allograft-prosthesis composite and fixed acetabular component. Long femoral allograft structure held with Dall-Miles cables. The AP radiographs of the upper femur **(A)** and distal femur **(B)** demonstrate the cemented intramedullary nail distally. The composite looks like methyl methacrylate. The cup is dislocated, and the femur is subluxed superiorly.

A,B

C

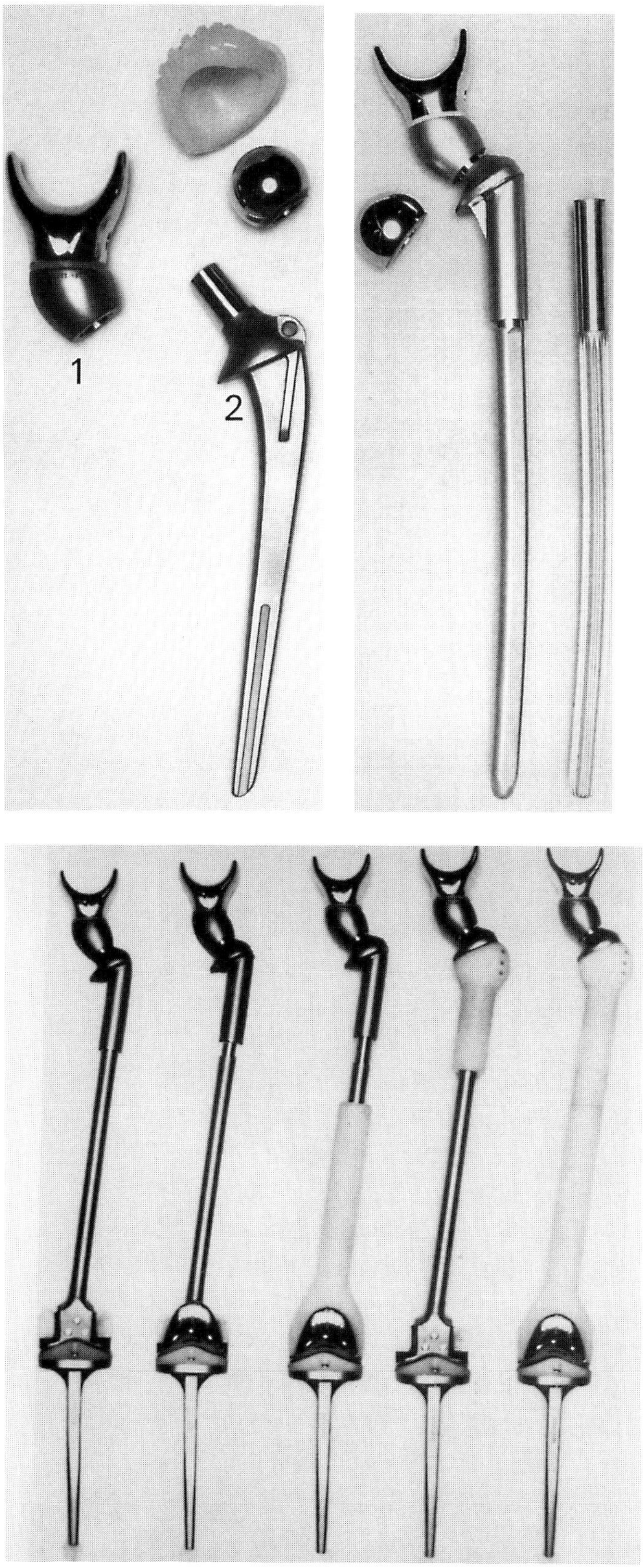

FIG. 14-20. Photographs of the Mark II saddle prosthesis. **A,***1***:** Iliac component. *2*: Standard anatomic stem with modular heads. **B:** Long femoral stem for major proximal bone loss. **C:** Various femoral replacement stems. (From Neider E, Elson RA, Engelbrecht E, Kasselt MR, Keller A, Steinbsink K. The saddle prosthesis for salvage of the destroyed acetabulum. *J Bone Joint Surg* [*Br*] 1990;72B:1014–1022.)

A

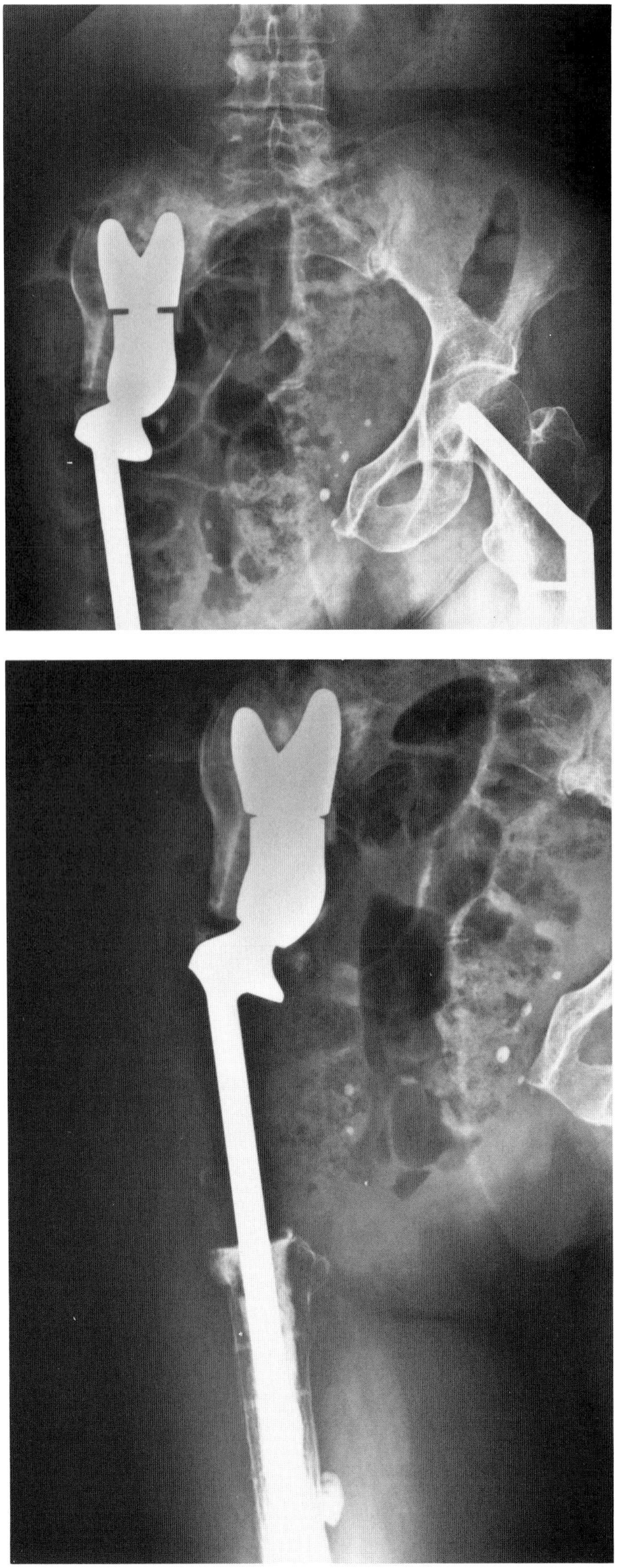

B

FIG. 14-21. Resection of the right acetabulum and upper femur with a saddle prosthesis and long-stem femoral component. The AP radiographs of the pelvis **(A)** and upper femur **(B)**. The entire femoral component should be included on the film.

Distal Femur, Knee, and Proximal Tibia

Neoplasms of the distal femur and upper tibia can be treated with various revision or customized prostheses.[23,41,44] Hinged or rotating-hinge components are commonly used (Fig. 14-22). Roberts et al.[44] reported 72% success rates at 5 years and 64% at 7 years by using a customized Stanmore prosthesis (Fig. 14-23). The incidence of infection was 68%, and loosening was reported in 6% of patients. Shih et al.[47] reported on the Mayo Clinic experience with 61 patients treated from 1972 to 1990. Early in this series, the Walldius type of hinged arthroplasty was used in 13 of 45 patients (34%) who underwent subsequent revision at 5 years. The Kinematic rotating hinge prosthesis, the design currently used, has not failed to date in 16 patients with an average follow-up of 2 to 3 years. Figure 14-24 demonstrates treatment of a giant cell tumor with a kinematic rotating hinge prosthesis with a customized femoral component.

Shoulder

Shoulder-salvage procedures may require significant resection with the replacement of the scapula and upper humerus (Fig. 14-17E). More often, tumors of the upper humerus are treated with various custom-designed humeral endoprostheses.[26,27,43] Humeral endoprostheses are configured of various materials, including metallic alloys (Fig. 14-25) and, in the past, ceramic (Fig. 14-26) components.[7,46]

Spine

Spinal procedures for neoplasms are most often performed for metastatic disease with vertebral destruction and correctable neurocompromise or spinal instability.[28,48,50] The goals of these procedures are to reduce pain, improve neurologic function, provide stability, and allow more normal patient activity.[21,28,39]

Spinal implants have been described in Chapter 3. As in other spinal disorders, anterior, posterior, and combined approaches can be used.[5,10,20,21,26,31,39,42,49,50] The technique used is determined by the spinal level or levels, the tumor's location (vertebral body or posterior elements) the patient's status, and surgical preferences. Anterior decompression with vertebrectomy is well accepted.[21] However, combined and posterior procedures are also used.[9,31,39,42]

Figures 14-27 to 14-31 demonstrate radiographic examples of different techniques. The reader should also refer to the instrumentation described in Chapter 3.

POSTOPERATIVE IMAGING AND COMPLICATIONS

Imaging after limb-salvage or other stabilization or reconstructive procedures is required to evaluate fixation and stability and to detect tumor recurrences.[1-3] The type of complication varies with the location (e.g., upper *versus* lower extremity or spine), the extent of the procedure, and the type of implant used (e.g., allograft or metal implant).[27,34,50] The evaluation can be difficult because of the presence of the implants, which can create significant artifacts on CT or MRI scans.[1]

Recurrence after the resection of primary neoplasms is a common problem, even with "nonmalignant" tumors. Giant cell tumors are a particular problem.[19] The detection of skeletal recurrence begins with routine radiographs (Fig. 14-13). A comparison with the immediate postoperative radiographs is essential. Significant destruction must occur before the radiographic findings are positive. Therefore, MRI or CT are generally performed to evaluate patients with suspected recurrences.[1-3]

Artifact and image distortion is created by metal implants. However, the degree of artifact can be reduced by using short SE sequences or intermediate echo time (TE)/repetition time (TR) sequences (TE, 30; TR, 1000 to 1500; Fig. 14-18). This may be the ideal situation for gadolinium with a short TE/TR T1-weighted SE sequence. Recurrent tumors enhance to a greater extent than do normal tissue. However, granulation tissue also enhances.[1-3,16] Scar tissue, once organized, has a low signal intensity on T1- and T2-weighted sequences. However, the scar may require 6 months or longer to organize to this degree. Methyl methacrylate does not cause an artifact (Fig. 14-22) and does not hinder MRI examinations.

When using MRI for following patients with limb-salvage procedures, it is best to obtain a baseline 4 to 6 weeks after surgery to allow the operative changes to subside. This study can serve as a baseline for future comparison. Dynamic gadolinium studies and spectroscopy have been suggested as methods of improving the detection of recurrence, but insufficient data exist to confirm this presently.[1-4,16,55]

Allograft, autogenous, and vascularized grafts present a different set of problems. Nonunion, fracture (12% to 40%), graft resorption (10%, Fig. 14-18), and deep infection (5%) are the most frequent problems with allografts.[36,52] Most allograft fractures occur in about 26 months. There is usually no history of trauma. These fractures are probably due to stress rises (including defects created at the time of implantation) or to soft tissue or vascular ingrowth.[52] Nonunion of grafts also occurs (Figs. 14-8 and 14-32).[36,52]

Joint-replacement procedures should be evaluated for recurrence and typical problems noted with arthroplasty

(text continues on page 961)

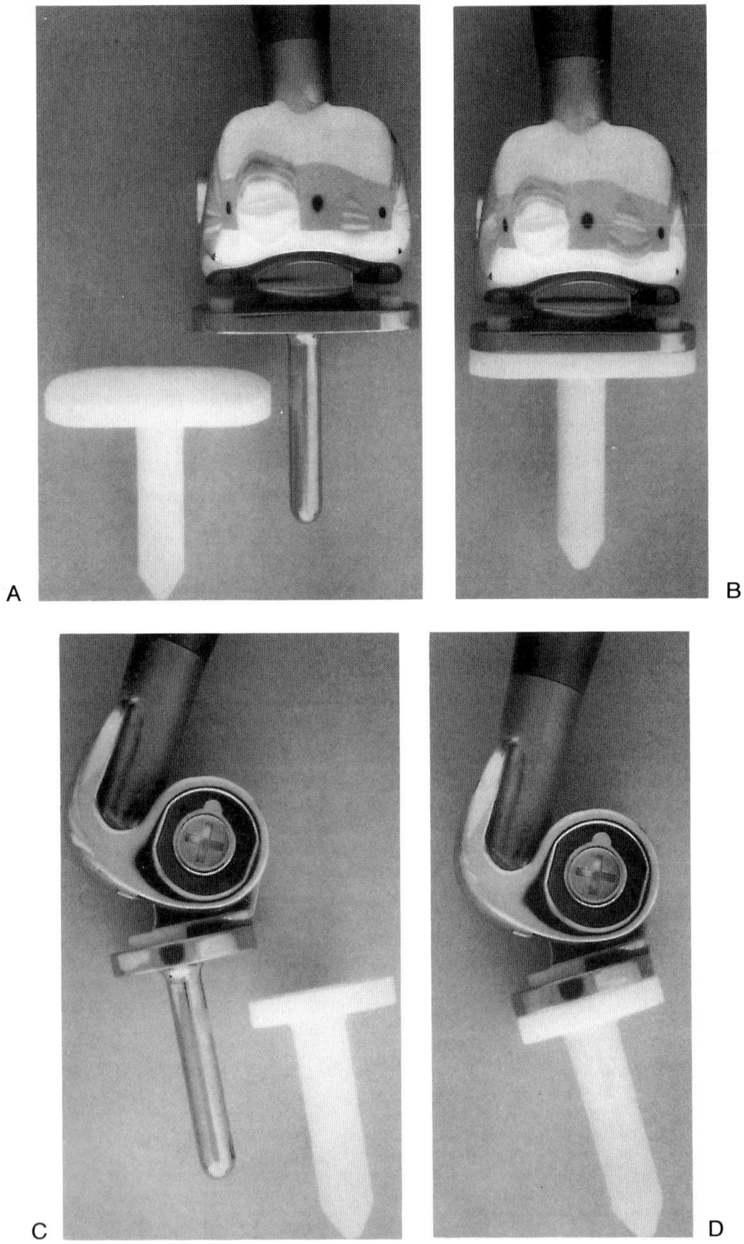

FIG. 14-22. Lewis expandable adjusting prosthesis (LEAP) incorporates Lacey rotating hinge (Wright Medical Technology, Arlington, TN). **A:** Frontal photograph with tibial component out of the sleeve. **B:** Frontal photograph with tibial component in the sleeve. **C:** Lateral photograph with the tibial component out of the sleeve. **D:** Lateral photograph with the tibial component in the sleeve.

E

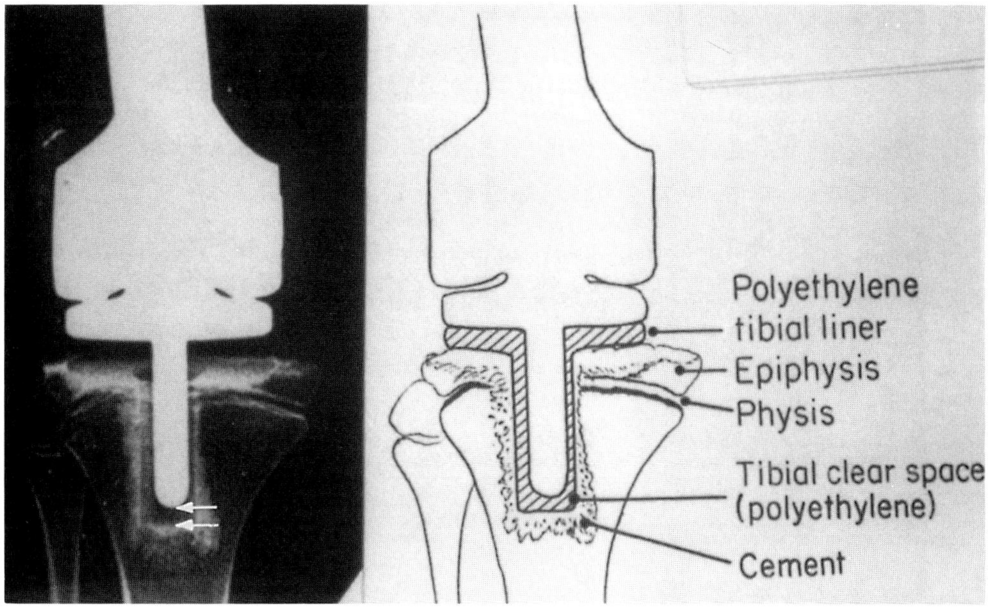

F

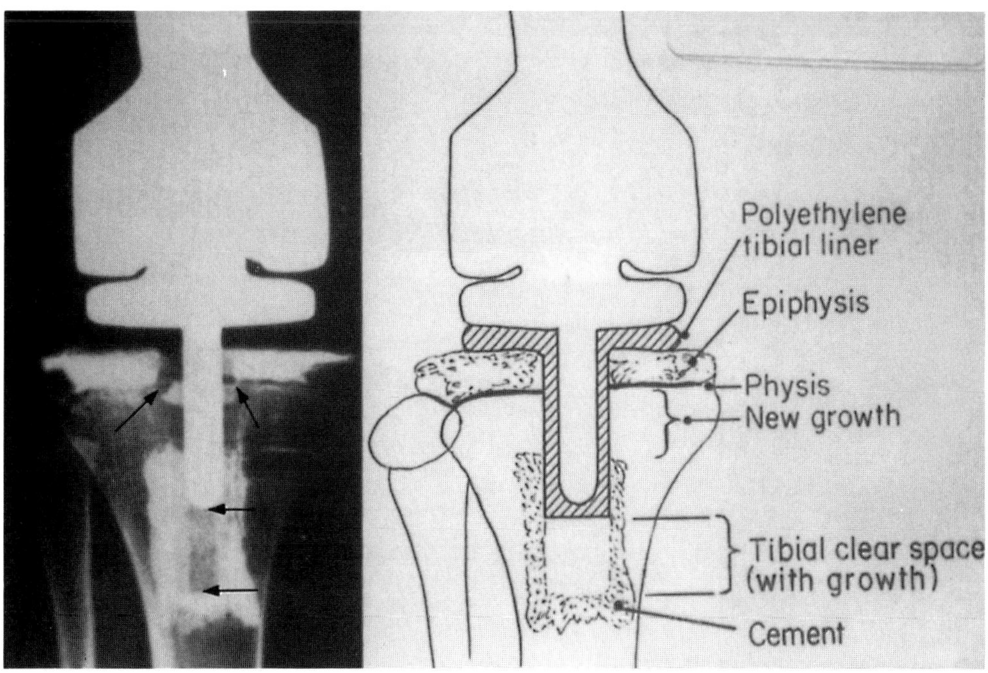

FIG. 14-22. (*Continued.*) **E:** Radiograph with corresponding line drawing demonstrating the components immediately after surgery. Note the distance of the tibial insert from the cement (*arrows*). **F:** Twenty-six months postoperatively, the tibial cement mantle has fractured (*upper black arrows*), and growth has occurred. Note the distance from the tibial insert to the cement at this time (*arrow*).

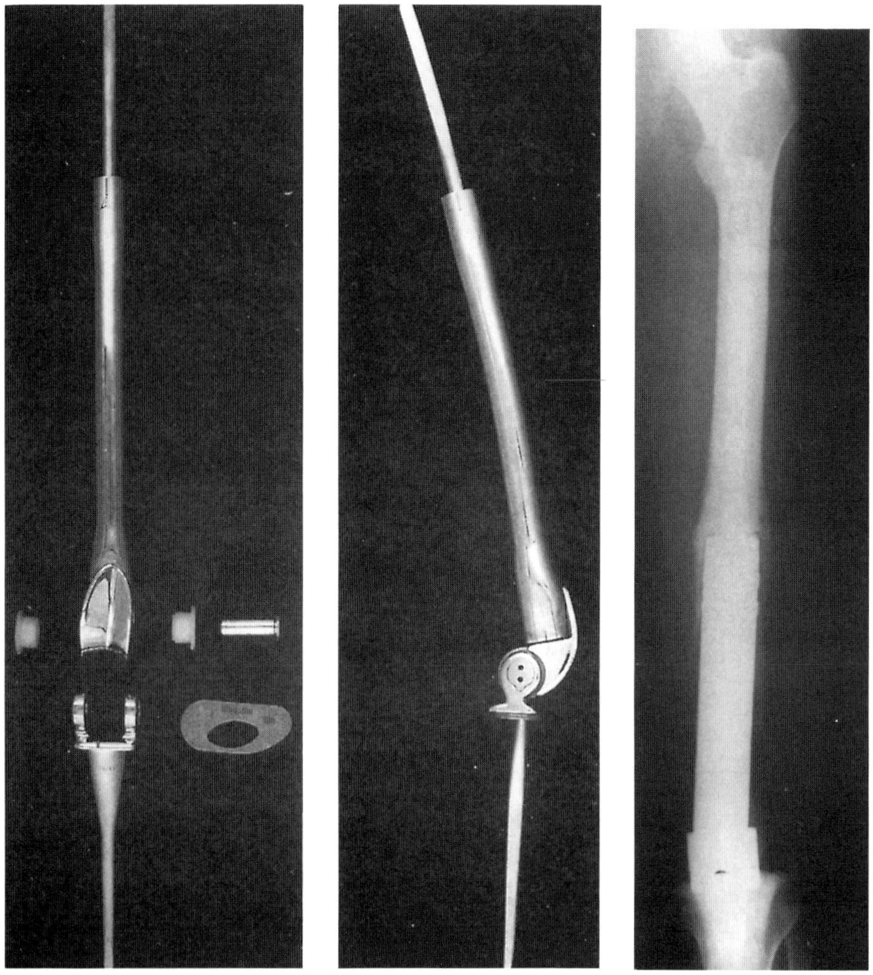

A,B C

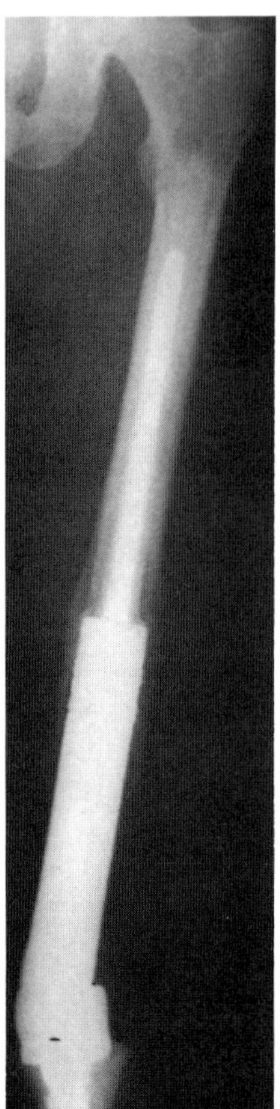

D

FIG. 14-23. Frontal **(A)** and side **(B)** views of a Stanmore-type prosthesis with a custom-designed femoral component. **C:** The AP radiographs at 1 year show a lucent line at the bone-cement interface. **D:** There was no progression at ten years. (From Roberts P, Chan D, Grimer RJ, Sneath RS, Scales JT. Prosthetic replacement of the distal femur for primary bone tumors. *J Bone Joint Surg* [*Br*] 1991;73B:762–769.)

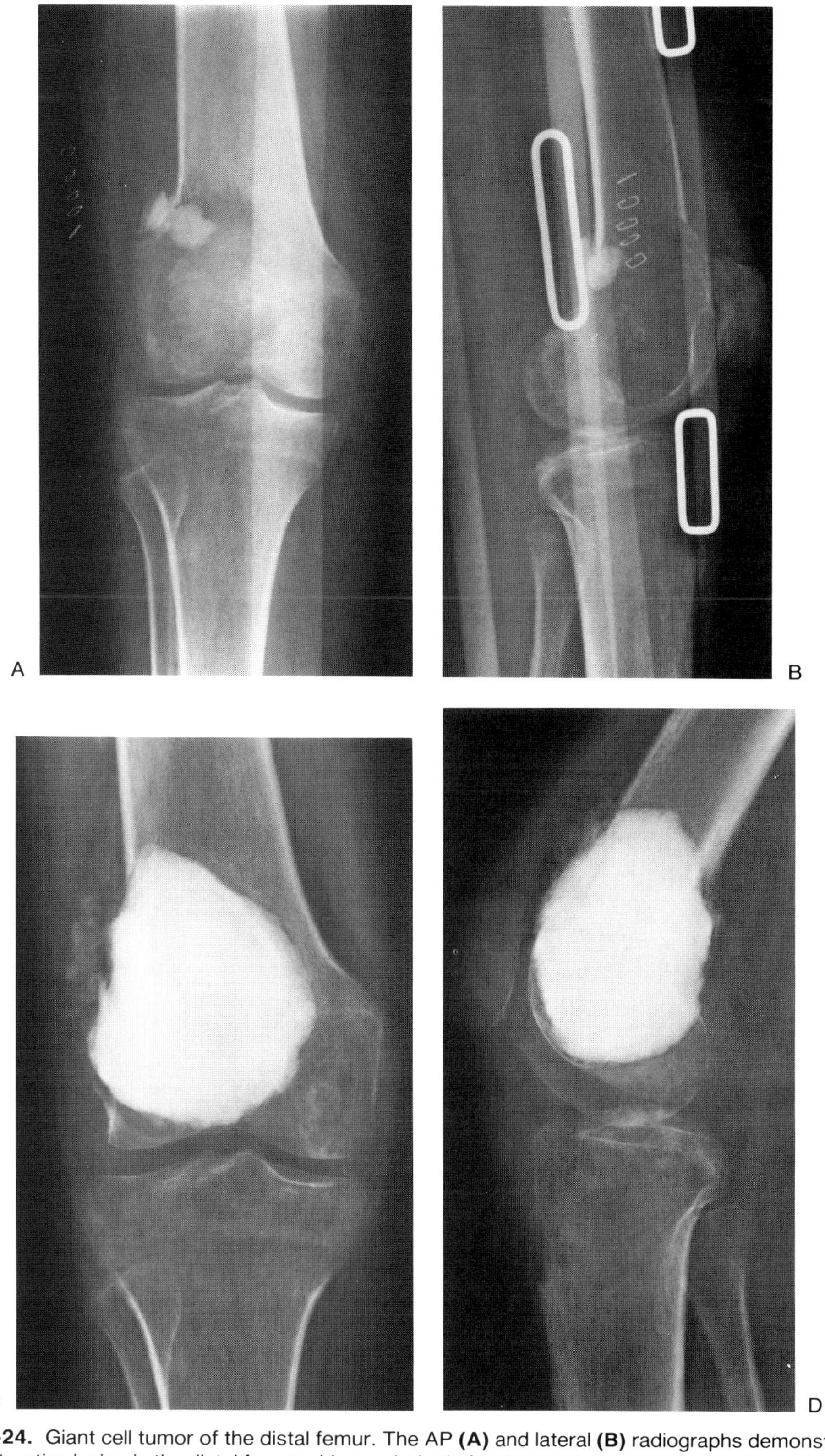

FIG. 14-24. Giant cell tumor of the distal femur. The AP **(A)** and lateral **(B)** radiographs demonstrate a lytic destructive lesion in the distal femur with a pathologic fracture and a small methyl methacrylate plug in the biopsy site. The AP **(C)** and lateral **(D)** radiographs after curettage and methyl methacrylate packing. Bone graft was placed along the subchondral bone prior to cement use. (See **E–I** on next page.)

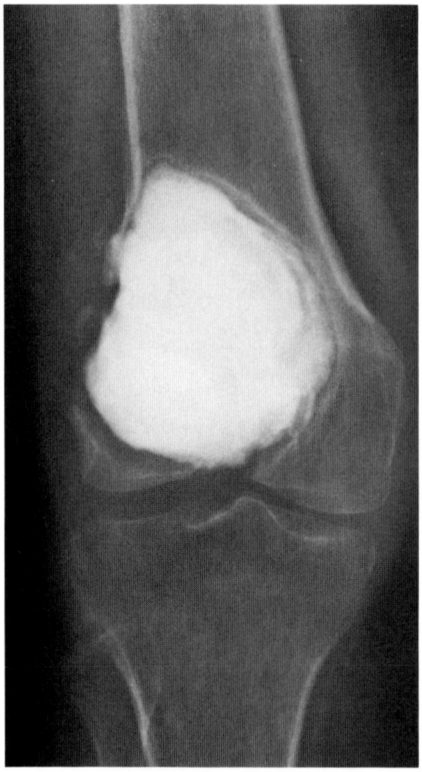
E

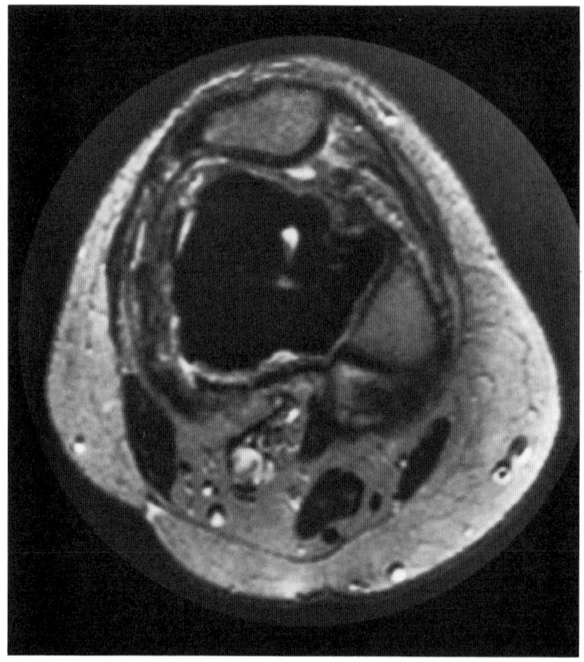
F

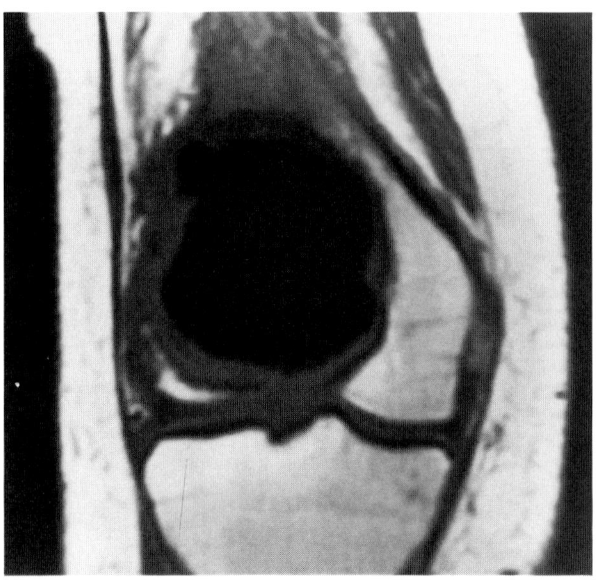
G,H

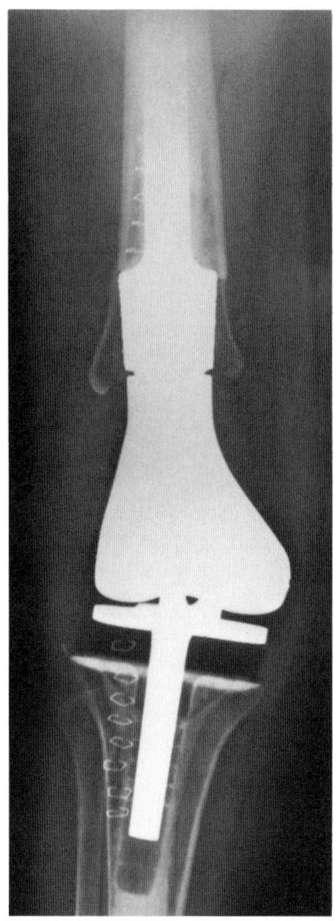

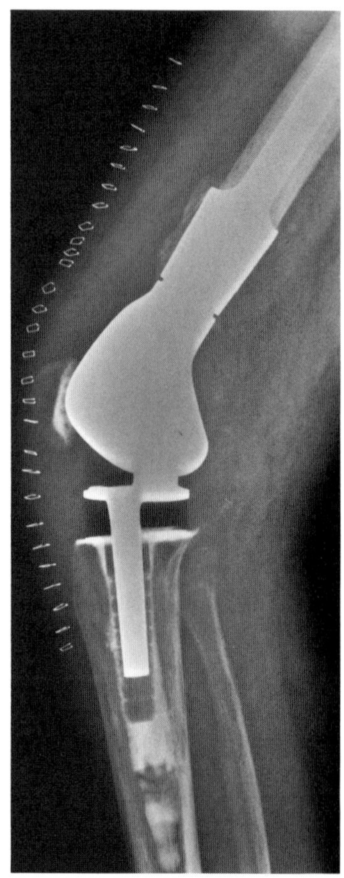
I

FIG. 14-24. (*Continued.*) **E:** Five months later, the intraarticular fracture has not healed and has now displaced. Axial T2-weighted (SE 2,000/80) **(F)** and coronal T1-weighted (SE 500/20) **(G)** images show no recurrence around the methyl methacrylate. There is no signal in the cement and no artifact. The distal femur was resected, and the knee was replaced using a Kinematic rotating hinge arthroplasty (see Chapter 6) with a customized femoral component. The AP **(H)** and lateral **(I)** views postoperatively and at 1 year **(J,K)**. Note the extracortical bone bridging along the porous shoulder (*arrows*). The thin lucent zone around the superior and medial aspect of the cement typically occurs.

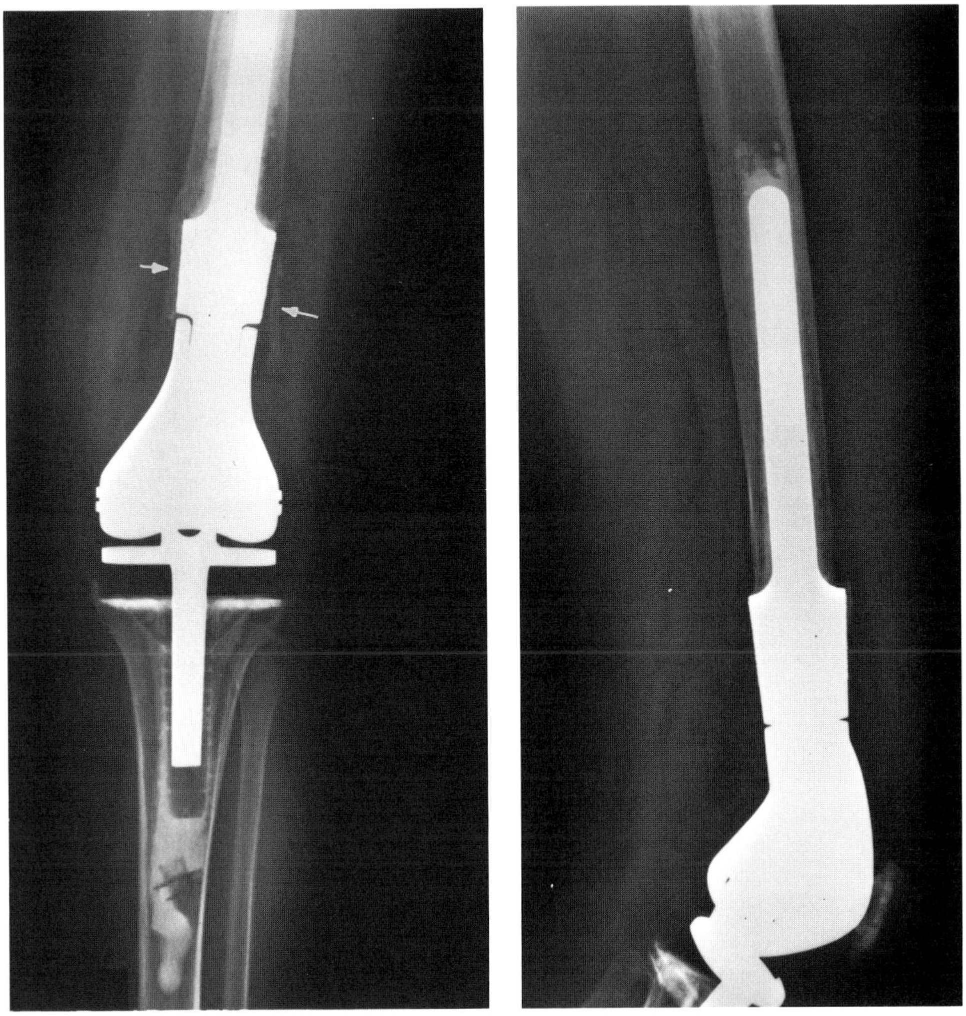

J K

FIG. 14-24. *Continued.*

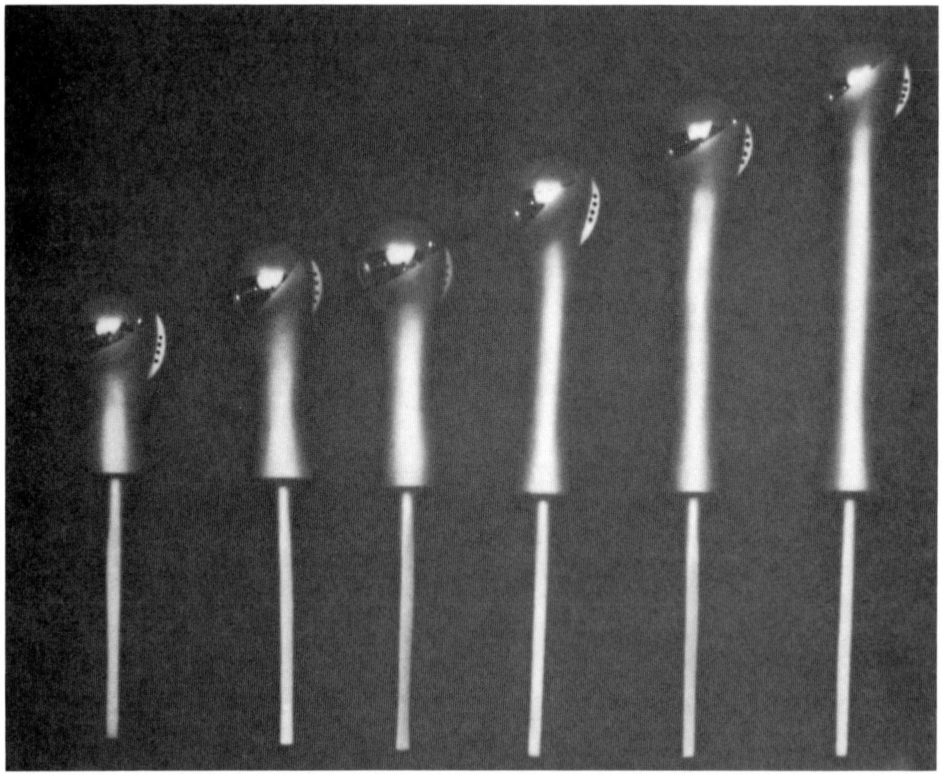

A

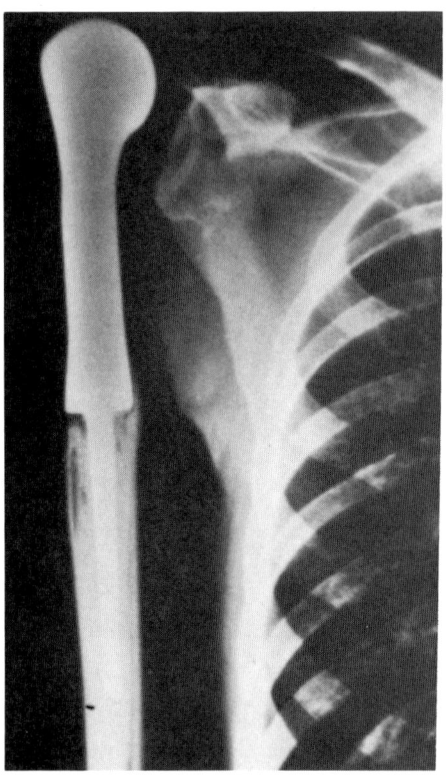

B

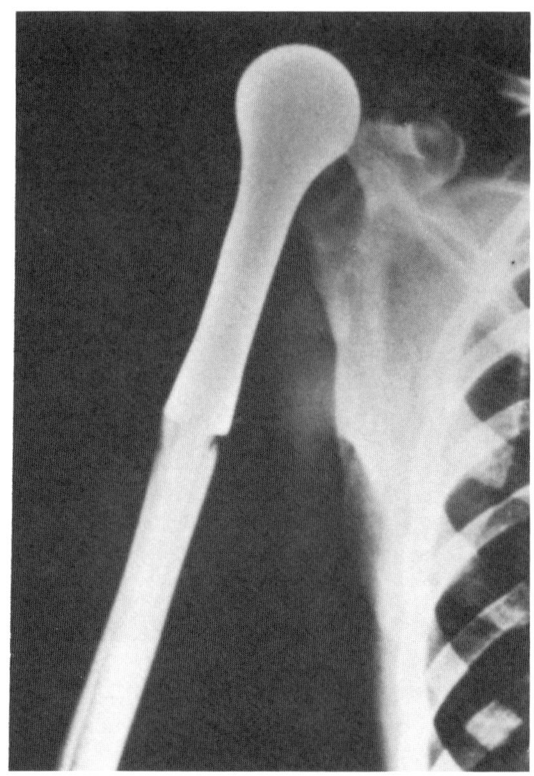

C

FIG. 14-25. A: Metal humeral endoprosthesis with incremental length variation (Howmedica, Rutherford, NJ). The AP external **(B)** and internal rotation **(C)** radiographs show the component is well seated. The humerus is subluxed superolaterally. Despite this, function was satisfactory. (From Bos G, Sim FH, Pritchard D, et al. Prosthetic replacement of the proximal humerus. *Clin Orthop* 1987;224:178–191.) Today, modular endoprotheses (see Chapter 9) are often used in this setting.

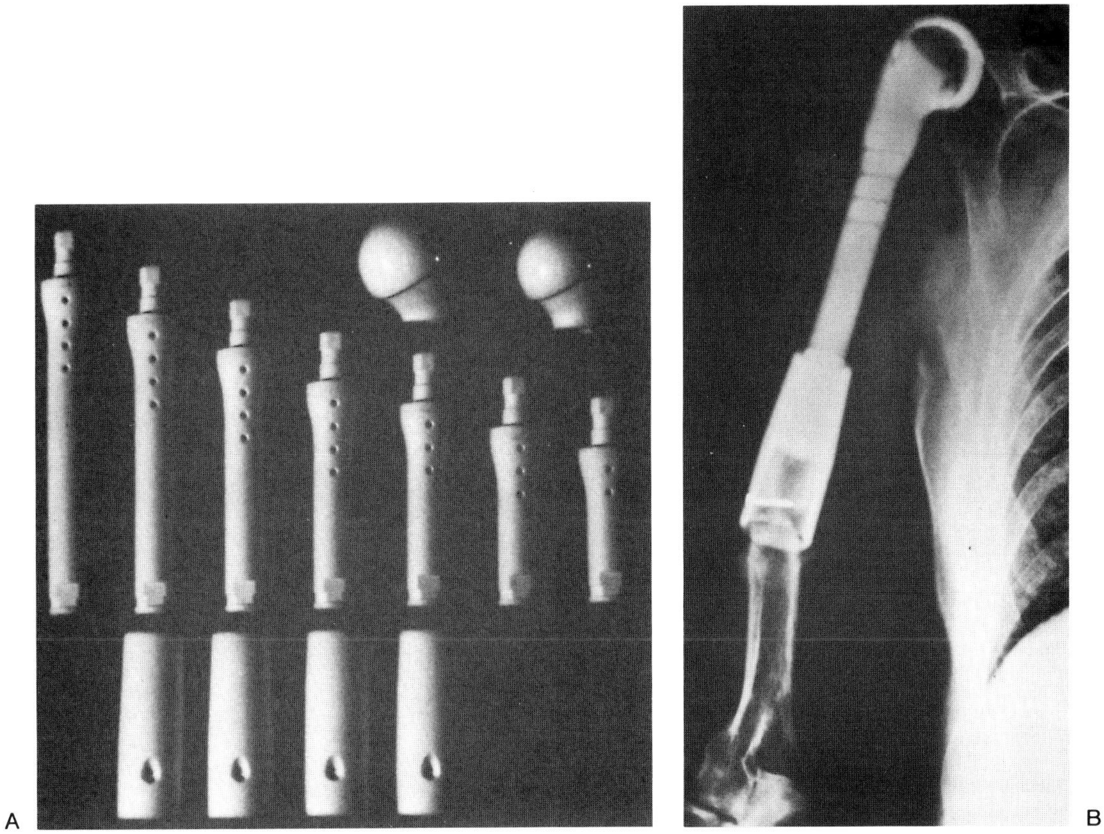

FIG. 14-26. A: Modular ceramic humeral endoprosthesis. B: The AP radiographs with a ceramic implant. There is a fracture at the humeral-implant junction with callus formation, (From Bos et al.,[7] with permission.)

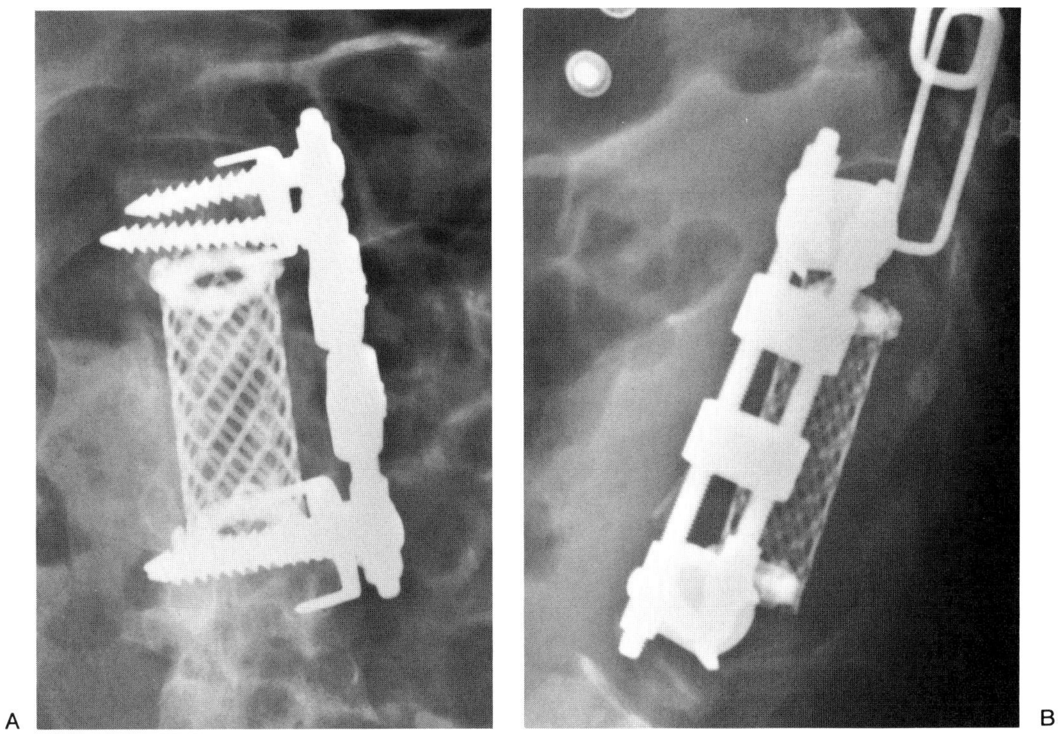

FIG. 14-27. Large destructive lesion in the upper lumbar spine. Anterior decompression and instrumentation was used. The AP (A) and lateral (B) demonstrate a Kaneda device from T-12 to L-3 with a metal cage and bone graft to replace the resected L-1 and L-2 vertebra.

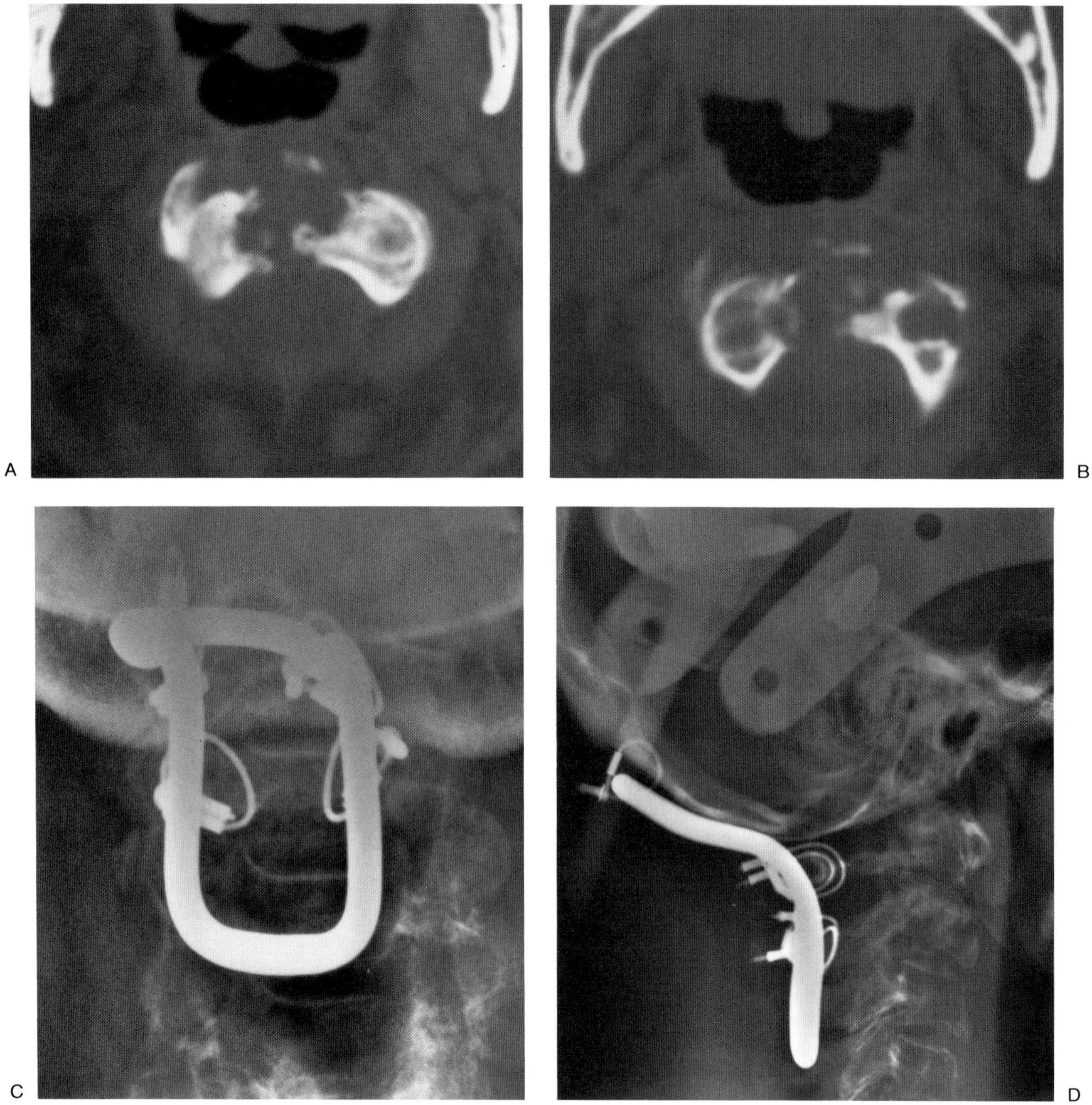

FIG. 14-28. A,B: Destructive C-2 metastases demonstrated on axial CT images. The AP **(C)** and lateral **(D)** radiographs after fusion with posterior bone graft, Songer cables, and a Luque rectangle.

A,B

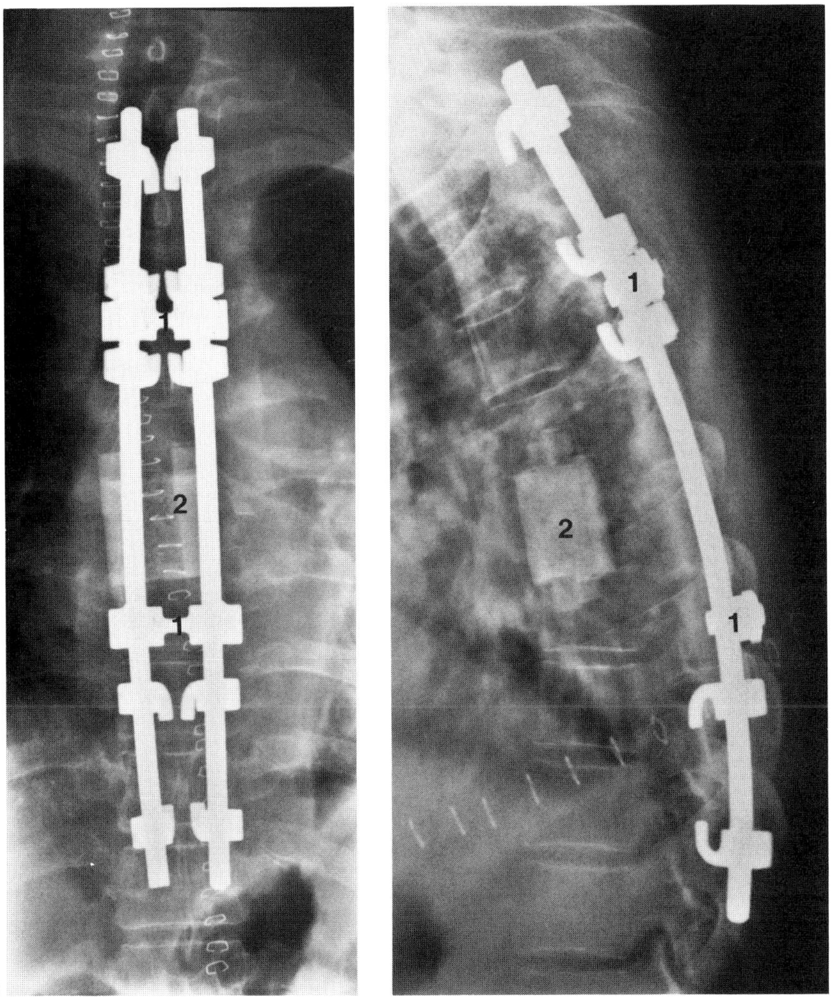

FIG. 14-29. T-6 chondrosarcoma with previous T-6 and T-7 laminectomies. The AP **(A)** and lateral **(B)** radiographs demonstrate posterior instrumentation with ISOLA rods and hooks and Danek cross-links (*1*). Iliac bone graft at the T-6 level (*2*).

A

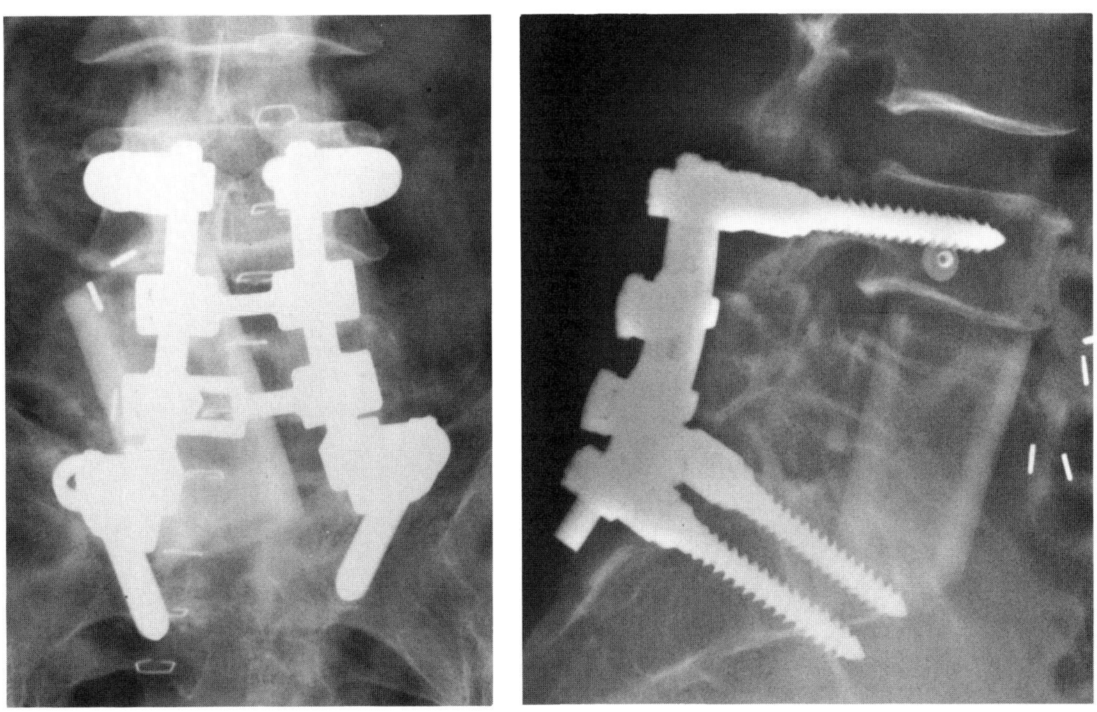

B

FIG. 14-30. Partial vertebrectomy at L-5. The AP **(A)** and lateral **(B)** radiographs demonstrate iliac bone graft bridging L-4 to the sacrum, with ISOLA rod and pedicle screw instrumentation posteriorly. The sacral screw on the left enters the prevertebral soft tissues.

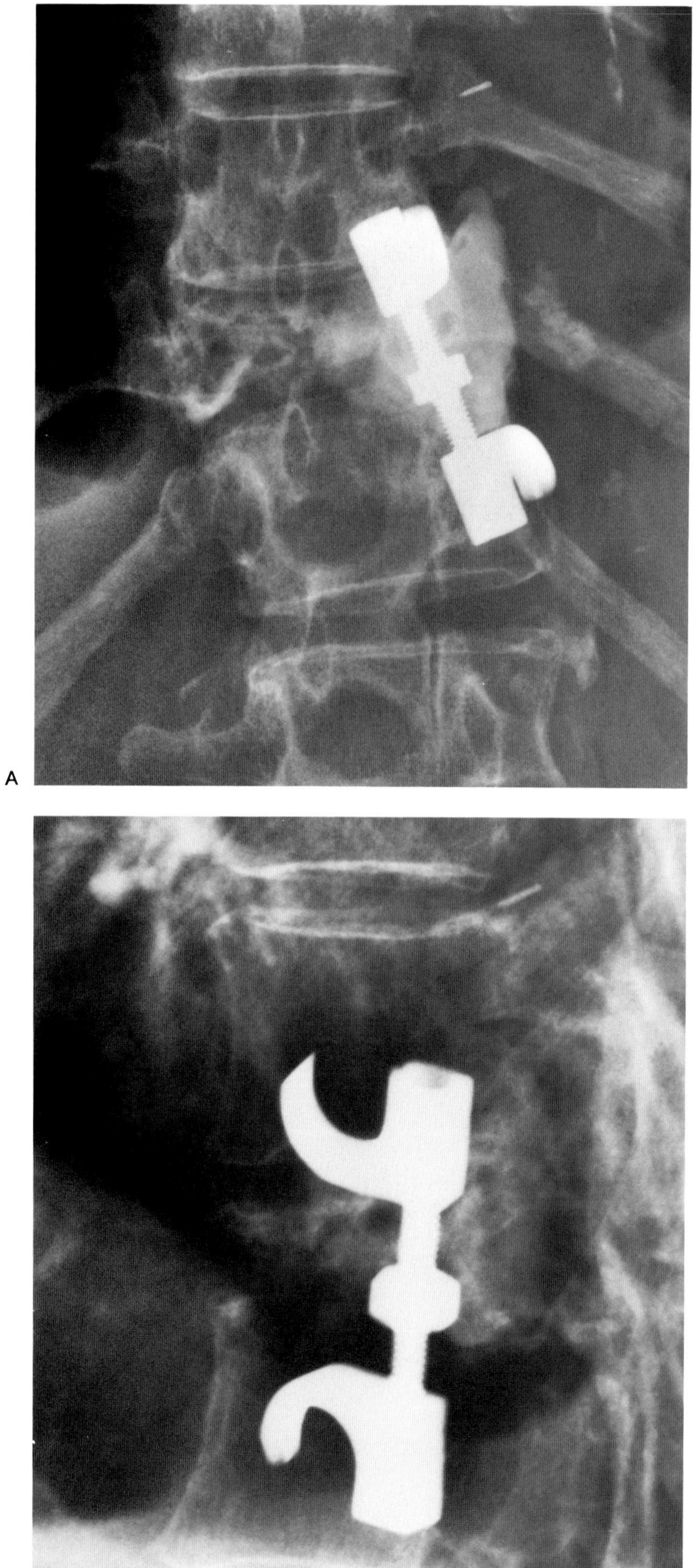

FIG. 14-31. T-11 compression fracture with epidural mass. Partial vertebrectomy at T-11. The AP **(A)** and lateral **(B)** radiographs demonstrate stabilization with methyl methacrylate and a Knodt distraction rod on the left.

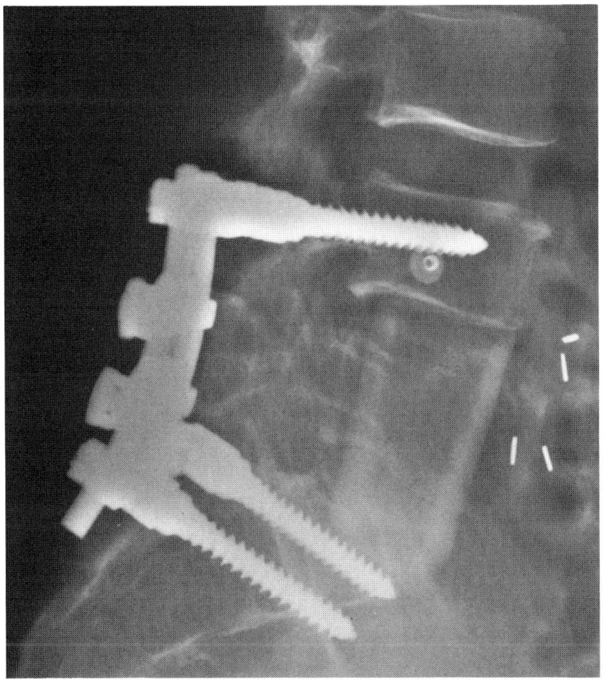

A

FIG. 14-32. **A:** Lateral radiograft after partial L-5 vertebrectomy with iliac bone graft and ISOLA posterior rod-pedicle screw fixation. **B,C:** Lateral tomograms show bone resorption (*arrows*) and failure of the upper graft to incorporate with L-4.

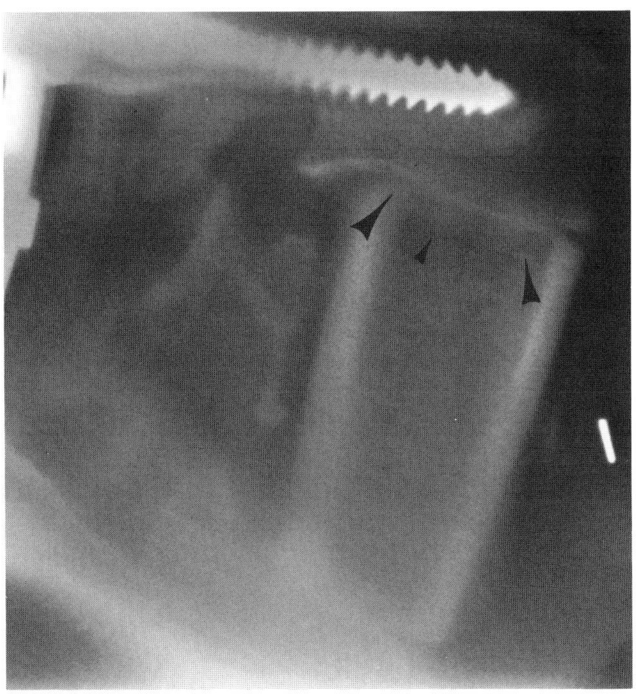

B

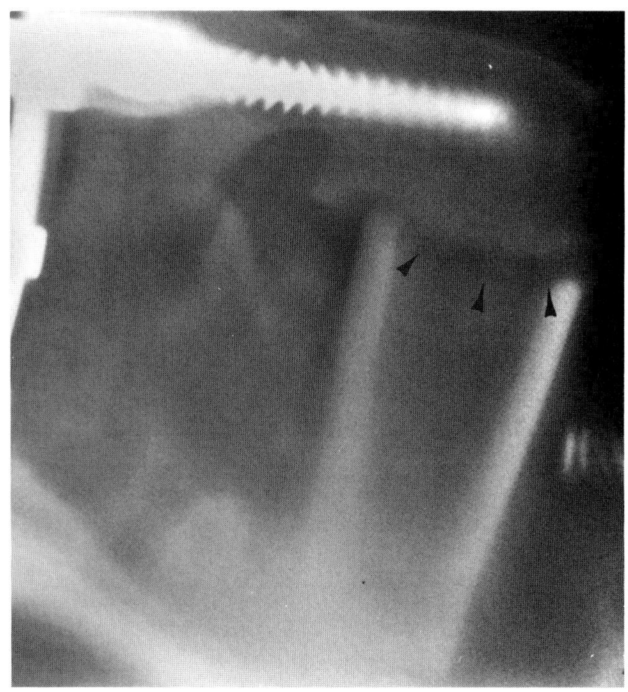

C

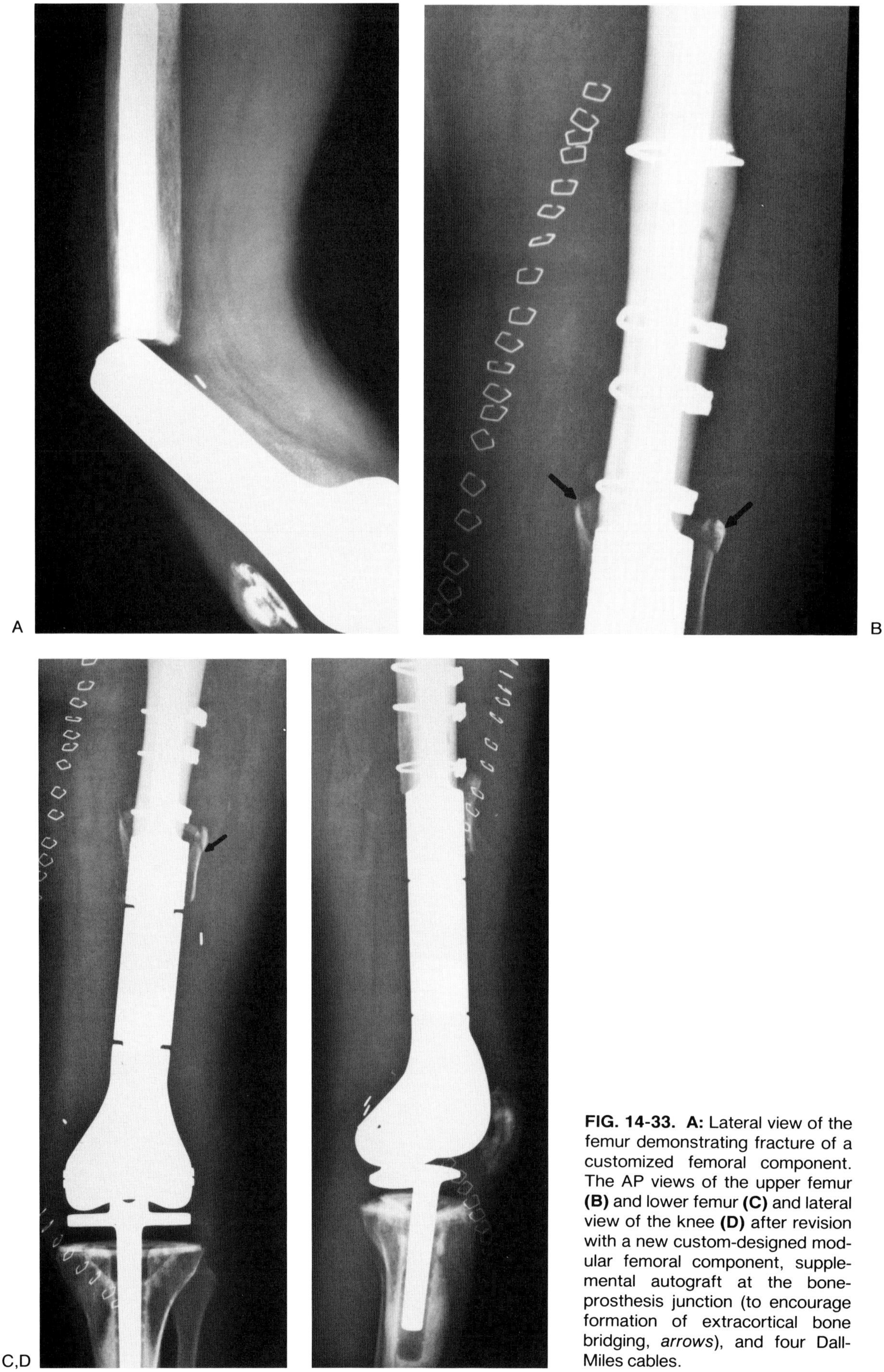

FIG. 14-33. A: Lateral view of the femur demonstrating fracture of a customized femoral component. The AP views of the upper femur **(B)** and lower femur **(C)** and lateral view of the knee **(D)** after revision with a new custom-designed modular femoral component, supplemental autograft at the bone-prosthesis junction (to encourage formation of extracortical bone bridging, *arrows*), and four Dall-Miles cables.

procedures. Loosening and deep infection can be evaluated with serial radiographs (Fig. 14-23). Short patient life expectancies, which depend on the neoplasm, may artificially reduce the incidence of loosening. The incidence rates of loosening with the constrained types of prostheses are high when used in nonneoplastic joint replacement. Fractures of the adjacent bone (Fig. 14-26) or the components themselves also occur (Fig. 14-33).[23]

Other orthopedic complications, such as leg-length discrepancy, can be evaluated with scanograms or CT. Nonorthopedic complications include urinary tract infection, pneumonia, deep venous thrombosis, and pulmonary emboli. These complications are more common in patients with cancer and in elderly patients who have long hospital recoveries.[21,26,31]

REFERENCES

1. Berquist TH. *Magnetic resonance imaging of the musculoskeletal system.* 2nd ed. New York: Raven Press; 1990.
2. Berquist TH. Magnetic resonance imaging of the primary skeletal neoplasms. *Radiol Clin North Am* 1993;31:411--424.
3. Berquist TH. Magnetic resonance imaging of musculoskeletal neoplasms. *Clin Orthop* 1989;244:101–118.
4. Berquist TH. Magnetic resonance techniques in musculoskeletal diseases. *Rheum Dis Clin North Am* 1991;17:599–615.
5. Black RG, Eng P, Gardner V, Armstrong G, O'Neil J, St. George M. A contoured anterior spinal fixation plate. *Clin Orthop* 1988;227:135–142.
6. Bocchi H, Lazzeroni L, Maggi M. The surgical treatment of metastasis in long bones. *Ital J Orthop Traumatol* 1988;14:167–173.
7. Bos G, Sim FH, Pritchard D, Shives T, Rock M, Askew L, Chao E. Prosthetic replacement of the proximal humerus. *Clin Orthop* 1987;224:178–191.
8. Capanna R, Mapelli S, Ruggieri P, Biqiui R, Ferruzzi A, Zucchi V, Giuntic A. Resection of the proximal humerus and I.O.R. medullar prosthesis in the treatment of metastatic lesions. *Ital J Orthop Traumatol* 1988;14:143–148.
9. Dombrowski ET. The Rezaian fixator in the anterior stabilization of unstable spine. *Orthop Rev* 1986;15:65–69.
10. Dunn HK. Anterior stabilization of the thoracolumbar injuries. *Clin Orthop* 1984;189:116–124.
11. Enneking WE. *Musculoskeletal tumor surgery.* Vol. 1. New York: Churchill Livingston; 1983:69–122.
12. Enneking WF. Modification of the system for functional evaluation of surgical management of musculoskeletal tumors. In: Ennecking WF, ed. *Limb salvage in oncology.* New York: Churchill Livingston; 1987:626–639.
13. Enneking WF. Staging of musculoskeletal neoplasms. *Skeletal Radiol* 1985;13:183–194.
14. Enneking WF, Durham W, Gebhardt MC, Malavar M, Pritchhard DJ. A system for the functional evaluation of reconstruction procedures after surgical treatment of tumors of the musculoskeletal system. *Clin Orthop* 1993;286:241–246.
15. Enneking WF, Spamer SS, Goodman MA. A system for surgical staging of musculoskeletal sarcomas. *Clin Orthop* 1980;153:106–120.
16. Erlemann R, Reisor MF, Peters OE, et al. Musculoskeletal neoplasms: static and dynamic Gd-DTPA-enhanced MR imaging. *Radiology* 1989;171:767–773.
17. Finn HA, Simon MA. Limb-salvage surgery in treatment of osteosarcoma in skeletally immature individuals. *Clin Orthop* 1991;262:108–118.
18. Frank JA, Liurg A, Patronas NJ, et al. Detection of malignant bone tumors. MR imaging, US, scintigraphy. *AJR Am J Roentgenol* 1990;155:1043.
19. Gitelis S, Mallin BA, Piasechi P, Turner F. Intra-lesional excision compared with en bloc resection for giant cell tumors of bone. *J Bone Joint Surg* [*Am*] 1993;75A:1648–1655.
20. Guyen DW, Wiltse L, Peek RD. The Wiltse pedicle screw fixation system. *Orthopedics* 1988;11:1455–1460.
21. Hall DJ, Webb JK. Anterior plate fixation in spinal tumor surgery. Indication, techniques and results. *Spine* 1991;16:580–583.
22. Healey JH, Lane JM. Treatment of pathologic fractures of the distal femur with a Zickel supracondylar nail. *Clin Orthop* 1990;250: 216–220.
23. Horowitz SM, Lane JM, Otis JC, Healey JH. Prosthetic arthroplasty of the knee after resection of a sarcoma in the proximal end of the tibia. *J Bone Joint Surg* [*Am*] 1991;73A:286–293.
24. Johnson ME, Mankin HJ. Reconstruction after resections of tumors involving the proximal femurs. *Orthop Clin North Am* 1991;22:87–103.
25. Karkala OL, Karaharju EO. Metastatic fractures in long bones. *Int Orthop* 1991;15:105–109.
26. Kostuik JP. Anterior Kostuik-Harrington distraction systems. *Orthopedics* 1988;11:1379–1391.
27. Malawer MM. Tumors of the shoulder girdle. Techniques of resection and description of surgical classification. *Orthop Clin North Am* 1991;22:7–35.
28. Malawski SK. The results of surgical treatment of primary spinal tumors. *Clin Orthop* 1991;272:50–57.
29. Mankin HJ, Gebhardt MC. Advances in the management of bone tumors. *Clin Orthop* 1985;200:73–84.
30. Mankin HJ, Gebhardt MC, Tomford WW. The use of frozen cadaveric allografts and management of patients with bone tumors of the extremities. *Orthop Clin North Am* 1987;18:275–289.
31. Marchesi DG, Thalgott JS, Aebi M. Application and results of the AO internal fixator system in non-traumatic indications. *Spine* 1991;16:162–169.
32. Mathys R. Isoelastic prosthesis for shoulder joint: materials, instruments, types of prosthetic devices. In: *Endoprostheses and internative for the arm-shoulder joint.* Bern: Hans Huber; 1977.
33. Miller GJ, VanderGriend RA, Blake SP, Springfield DS. Performance evaluation of a cement-augmented intramedullary fixation system for pathologic lesions of the femoral shaft. *Clin Orthop* 1987;221:246–254.
34. Mitty HA. Musculoskeletal neoplasms. Role of angiography in diagnoses and intervention. *Semin Intervent Radiol* 1993;10:277–283.
35. Mjoberg B, Pettersson H, Rosenquist R. Bone cement thermal injury and the radiolucent zone. *Acta Orthop Scand* 1984;55:597–600.
36. Muscolo DL, Azerza MA, Calabrese ME, Gruenberg M. The use of a bone allograft for reconstruction after resection of giant-cell tumor close to the knee. *J Bone Joint Surg* [*Am*] 1993;75A:1656–1662.

36a. Neider E, Elson RA, Engelbrecht E, Kasselt MR, Keller A, Steinbsink K. The saddle prosthesis for salvage of the destroyed acetabulum. *J Bone Joint Surg* [*Br*] 1990;72B:1014–1022.

37. Nieder E, Englebrecht E, Steinbrink K. The saddle prosthesis for salvage of the destroyed acetabulum. *J Bone Joint Surg* [*Br*] 1990;72B:1014–1022.
38. Nieder E, Keller A. The saddle prosthesis Mark II Endo-Modell™. Yamamuro T, ed. In: *New developments for limb salvage in musculoskeletal tumors.* Tokyo: Springer-Verlag; 1989:481–490.
39. O'Neil J, Gardner V, Armstrong G. Treatment of tumors of the thoracic and lumbar spinal column. *Clin Orthop* 1988;227:103–112.
40. Present DA, Kuschner SH. Total femur replacement: a case report with 35 years follow-up study. *Clin Orthop* 1990;251:166–167.
41. Raneda K, Abwni K, Fujiya M. Burst fractures with neurologic deficits of the thoracolumbar spine. Results of anterior decompression and stabilization with anterior instrumentation. *Spine* 1984;9: 288–298.
42. Rezaian SM. The Rezaian spinal fixator for management of fractures of the thoracolumbar spine. *J Neurol Orthop Med Surg* 1991;12:1307–1313.
43. Riebel G, Webster DA. Proximal humeral replacement for tumor. A preliminary report. *Orthopedics* 1989;12:833–836.
44. Roberts P, Chan D, Grimer RJ, Sneath RS, Scales JT. Prosthetic

replacement of the distal femur for primary bone tumors. *J Bone Joint Surg* [*Br*] 1991;73B:762–769.

45. Safran MR, Echardt JJ, Kabo JM, Orpenheim WL. Continued growth of the proximal part of the tibia after prosthetic reconstruction of the skeletally immature knee. *J Bone Joint Surg* [*Am*] 1992;74A:1172–1179.
46. Salzer M, Knahr K, Locke H, Stark N, Matejovski Z, Plenk H, Punzet G, Swey Muller K. A bioceramic endoprostheses for replacement of the proximal humerus. *Arch Orthop Trauma Surg* 1979;93:169–184.
47. Shih H-Y, Sim FH, Prithcard DJ, Rock MG, Chao EYS. Segmental total knee arthroplasty after distal femur resection for tumor. In: Brown KLB, ed. *Complications of limb salvage. Proceedings of the Sixth International Symposium on Limb Salvage, Montreal, Canada.* 1993:403–408.
48. Siegal T. Vertebral body resection for epidural compression by malignant tumors. *J Bone Joint Surg* [*Am*] 1985;67A:375–382.
49. Steffee AD, Biscup DO, Sitkowski DJ. Segmental spine plates with pedicle screw fixation. *Clin Orthop* 1986;203:45–53.
50. Steffee AD, Sitowski DJ, Topliam LE. Total vertebral body and pedicle arthroplasty. *Clin Orthop* 1986;203:203–208.
51. Steimbrunk K, Engelbrecht E, Fenelon GCC. The total femoral prosthesis. *J Bone Joint Surg* [*Br*] 1982;64B:305–312.
52. Thompson RC, Pickvance EA, Garry D. Fractures in large segment allografts. *J Bone Joint Surg* 1993;:1663–1673.
53. Vail TP, Harrelson JM. Treatment of pathologic fracture of the humerus. *Clin Orthop* 1991;268:197–202.
54. Ward WG, Johnston KS, Dorey FJ, Eckardt JJ. Extramedullary porous coating to prevent diaphyseal osteolysis and radiolucent lines around proximal tibial replacements. *J Bone Joint Surg* [*Am*] 1993;75A:976–987.
55. Zlatkur MB, Lenkinski RE, Shunkwin M, et al. Combined MR imaging and spectroscopy of bone and soft tissue tumors. *J Comput Assist Tomogr* 1990;14:1–10.
56. Zwierzchowski H, Zwierzchowski D, Snyder M. The value of fibular autografts in block resection of bone tumors and tumor like conditions. *Int Orthop* 1989;13:113–117.

Subject Index

Page numbers followed by *f* refer to figures; page numbers followed by *t* refer to tables.

G

L

N

O